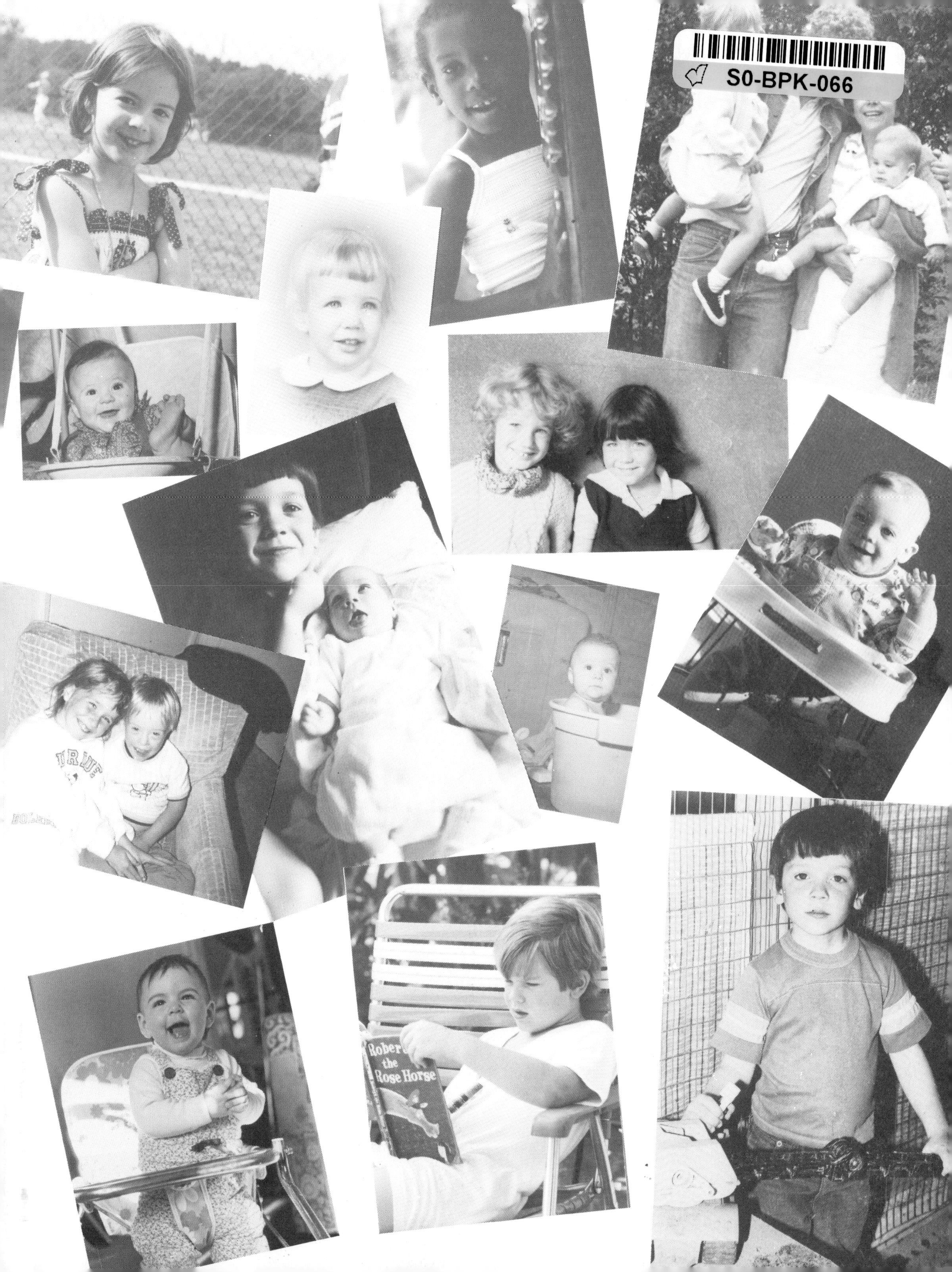
Rober
the
Rose Horse

Child
Health Nursing

Essential Care of Children and Families

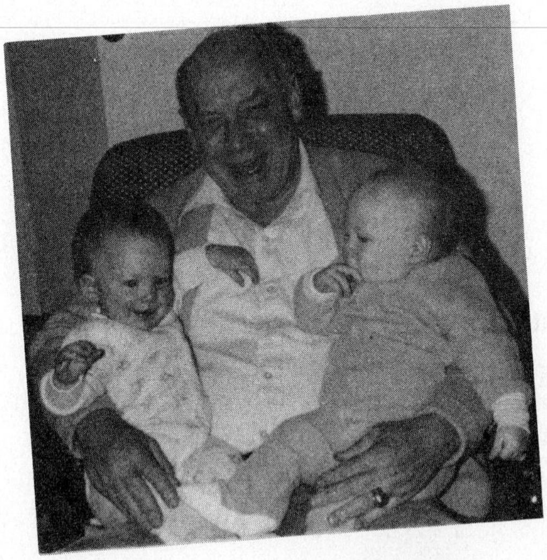

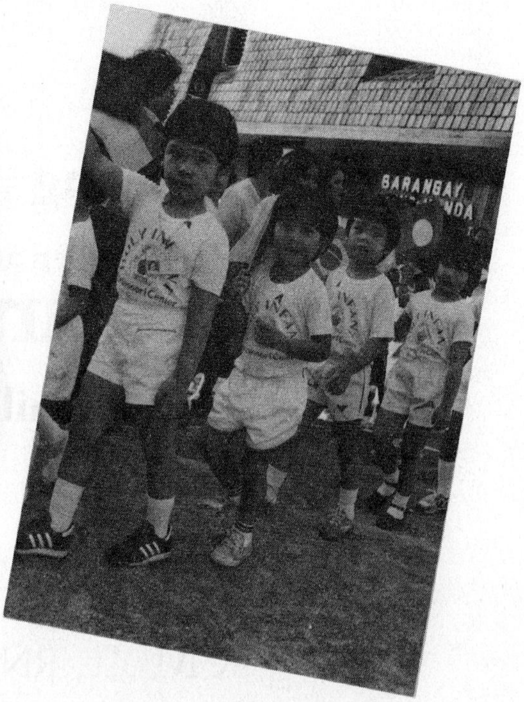
BARANGAY

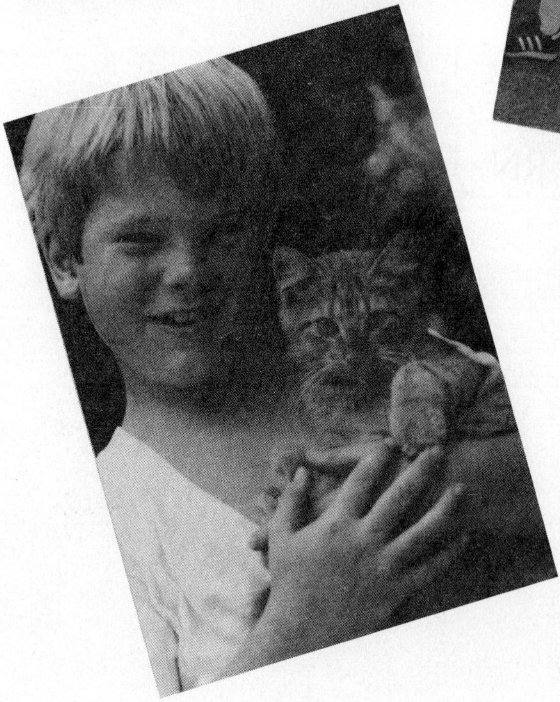

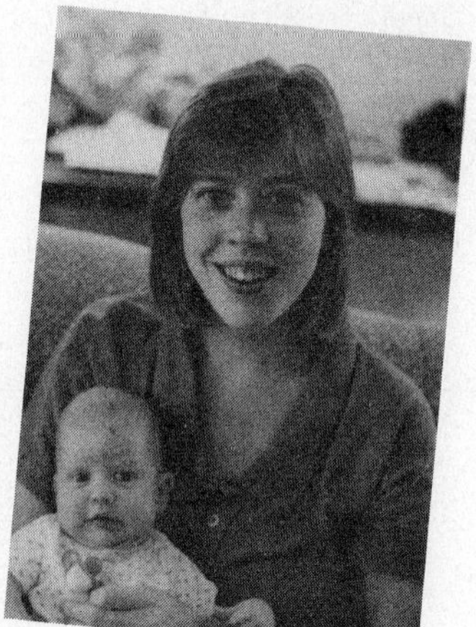

Child Health Nursing

Essential Care of Children and Families

Susan Rowen James, RN, MSN

Sandra R Mott, RN, MSN

Addison-Wesley Publishing Company

Reading, Massachusetts · Menlo Park, California · New York
Don Mills, Ontario · Wokingham, England · Amsterdam
Sydney · Singapore · Tokyo · Madrid · Bogotá
Santiago · San Juan

To Bob, whose love, patience, and support enriches my life and to Richard, Elena, and Carolyn who have taught me the most about the wonders of childhood.

Susan James

To my husband, Stephen, and children, Adam, Rachel, and Sarah for their love, cooperation, patience and support.

Sandy Mott

Sponsoring Editor: Debra Hunter
Production Supervisor: Anne Friedman
Interior Designer: Wendy Calmenson
Cover Designer: Rudy Zehntner
Copyeditor: Melissa Andrews
Proofreaders: Jenny Pulsipher, Judith Hibbard, Toni Murray, Elliot Simon
Indexer: Elinor Lindheimer
Typesetter: G&S, Austin, Texas
Illustrators: Susan Strawn, Irene Imfeld, Nori Tolson
Photographers: George Fry III, William Thompson, Joseph Greco, Judy Koenig, Frank Keillor
Endsheets: Designed by Detta Penna. Photographs supplied by the families of Addison-Wesley employees.

Library of Congress Cataloging-in-Publication Data

James, Susan Rowen, 1946–
Child health nursing : essential care of children and families / Susan Rowen James, Sandra R. Mott.
p. cm.
Includes bibliographies and index.
ISBN 0-201-14178-7
1. Pediatric nursing. 2. Children—Care. 3. Family—psychology. 4. Nursing Process. 5. Pediatric Nursing. I. Mott, Sandra R., 1942– . II. Title.
[DNLM: 1. Child Health Services—nurses' instruction. WY 159 J29c]
RJ245.J36 1988
610.73'62—dc19
ISBN 201-14178-7
ABCDEFGHIJ-RN-891098

The authors and publisher thank the following institutions and agencies for their kind permission to photograph many of the children and families who appear in this book:

Children's Hospital at Stanford, Stanford, California
Community Association for Retarded, Inc., Palo Alto, California
Peninsula Center for the Blind, Palo Alto, California
Peninsula School, Menlo Park, California
University of Massachusetts Medical Center
Valley Medical Center, San Jose, California

The authors and publishers have exerted every effort to ensure that drug selection and dosage set forth in this text are in accord with current recommendations and practice at the time of publication. However, in view of ongoing research, changes in government regulations and the constant flow of information relating to drug therapy and drug reactions, the reader is urged to check the package insert for each drug for any change in indications of dosage and for added warnings and precautions. This is particularly important where the recommended agent is a new and/or infrequently employed drug.

Addison-Wesley Publishing Company
Health Sciences Division
2725 Sand Hill Road
Menlo Park, California 94025

Contents

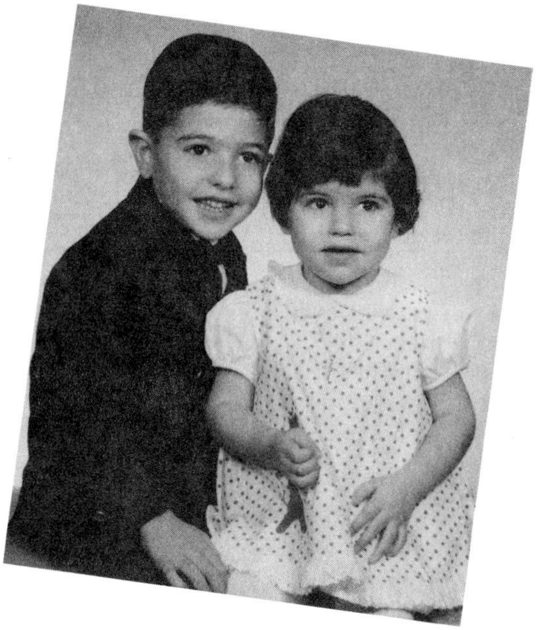

UNIT II: Growth and Development: The Child and Family 53

Preface

In 1985 we published a new text *Nursing Care of Children and Families* that came to be widely accepted throughout the nursing community. We'd like to thank the many nurses who wrote to us and to our publisher to tell us what you liked about the book. You praised the emphasis on family and on health promotion, the nursing care plans and many other aspects of the book. Many of you from many different kinds of nursing programs also sent us one very strong request—for a book with the same forward-looking emphasis, but one shorter and more manageable for students. The book you now hold answers those many requests.

Child Health Nursing: Essential Care of Children and Families covers both the ill child and the well child, including health maintenance and prevention of illness and disability. Like its parent text, *Child Health Nursing* consistently addresses the emotional, social, cultural, and psychologic needs of children and families. All the information included is based on nursing research and theories. Home care, patient and family teaching, and discharge planning are emphasized throughout the text.

Child Health Nursing improves on its parent text in many ways. We present straightforward explanations of difficult topics. The clarity and consistency of presentation are enhanced. We have improved the tables and pedagogic devices that emphasize nursing care. We updated information throughout, including, for example, the most recent developments in AIDS, blood transfusions in children, and dietary treatment of children with PKU. We use the latest NANDA-approved nursing diagnoses. The pedagogy is streamlined and refined. A second color has been added to highlight key information, to add to the overall visual appearance of the book, and to help students absorb the information.

Our goals in presenting this text to you are: (1) to provide the student with a basic ability to assess the factors affecting the child's and family's responses to preserving wellness, preventing illness or injury and hospitalization, and dealing with long term or chronic illness or disability; (2) to use this knowledge in formulating and implementing nursing care to meet the physical, cognitive, and psychosocial needs for both the immediate situation and the future; and (3) to accomplish these objectives in a text that is the right size for students in both abbreviated and conventional courses in child health nursing.

To create a shorter, manageable text we concentrate on providing essential principles of nursing care of children and families, with an emphasis on ongoing care and situations that are seen most frequently in nursing practice. Unlike other short texts, we did not eliminate information we consider essential for holistic nursing care, for example, normal structure and function of body systems, patient and family teaching and specific discharge planning, and preparation for and interpretation of validating diagnostic studies.

Conceptual Framework

The text builds three major components into its conceptual framework:

Nursing process
Wellness to illness and general to specific format
Integration of growth and development

Nursing Process

The five-step nursing process (assessment, nursing diagnosis, planning, implementation, and evaluation) is applied in a consistent manner throughout the text. The nursing process as it applies to children is introduced in Chapter 1 with a step-by-step illustration of how to construct a nursing care plan for a child (pages 12–25). Diagnoses accepted by the North American Nursing Diagnosis Association (NANDA) are used whenever possible.

Assessment is addressed in Chapter 9, *Principles of Assessment,* which provides a description of assessment tools frequently used with children and families. Successful approaches to conducting a health interview, the initial assessment tool, are discussed. Chapter 10 continues with an in-depth presentation of physical assessment including a step-by-step physical examination. Assessment Guides appear in most of the chapters in Unit VI.

Nursing diagnoses are highlighted for emphasis and woven throughout the text. Nursing diagnoses serve as organized heads for material on nursing care. An example is on pages 639–642, where nursing care for a child with an imbalance of fluid regulatory mechanisms is explained by using nursing diagnoses as a framework. The logo ❀ identifies these headings as nursing diagnoses. The diagnoses are derived from assessment data clearly presented in each chapter. Planning, implementation, and evaluation are illustrated in accompanying nursing care elements. Throughout, the text demonstrates how a comprehensive assessment leads to individualized nursing diagnoses and interventions for a child and family.

Wellness to Illness/General to Specific

Accepting the teaching principle of presenting simple information before presenting that which is complex, this text is organized around progression of wellness to illness and general to specific. The first chapters present general data about nursing care of children, followed by an overview of the well child, including growth and development, and principles of maintaining wellness and preventing illness and injury.

The subsequent chapters begin to cover the more complex aspects of the acutely or chronically ill child, each following the principle of general to specific. Illness chapters begin with general assessment data, nursing diagnoses, and interventions directed toward children with dysfunctions affecting body structures. These general principles of nursing care are then applied to the care of children with specific dysfunctions.

Integration of Growth and Development

We have elected to discuss a given health problem in a single place, as much as possible, and to incorporate the variations of and reactions to this health problem as it affects children and adolescents, rather than discussing deviations for each age group. This approach allows us to highlight such general themes as assessment, prevention, acute and chronic care needs, and principles of nursing care, in a consistent manner. More importantly, this approach also permits easier access to information about a specific problem than does the sometimes arbitrary and misleading assignment of a disease to a specific age category.

Nursing Care Features

We believe in presenting nursing care as specific principles and in presenting a role model of creative and individualized use of the nursing process in child health. Throughout this text, features present nursing care resources and references for the student. They are:

1. Essentials of Structure and Function
2. Assessment Guides
3. Standards of Nursing Care
4. Nursing Care Plans
5. Procedures

All nursing care elements are specially highlighted by the ❀ symbol so they can be easily located.

The *Essentials of Structure and Function* is a brief visual review of pertinent anatomy and physiology. We feel that in order to understand dysfunction, the student needs a brief review of normal function. This feature is distinguished by a glossary of terms essential to the comprehension of structure and function by various body systems and by clear figures illustrating the norm. Examples are found on pages 659–660 (The Respiratory Tract) and page 767 (The Skin).

Assessment Guides pull together the significant assessment questions and supporting data for physiologic alterations in each body system. Nursing diagnoses based on the assessment data are highlighted throughout each chapter in the general principles sections. Examples of Assessment Guides are found on page 718 (The Child with a Cardiovascular Problem) and page 877 (The Child with a Gastrointestinal Problem).

Standards of Nursing Care tables offer guidelines for nursing management of general dysfunctions that can result from disease or other threats to health. They address such topics as the child following abdominal surgery (pages 886–889), or the care of the child with a major burn (pages 793–796). At the suggestion of our colleague Marjory Gordon, these tables are divided into two parts to distinguish those nursing actions that reflect colleagiality between nursing and medicine from those that are specifically part of independent nursing practice. "Risks" covers nursing action related to complications such as postoperative bleeding, adverse effects of medications, and increased intracranial pressure. "Guide for Nursing Management" presents nursing diagnoses, interventions, rationale, and outcomes (evaluation).

Nursing Care Plans present individual cases of children and families with specific health problems or concerns. They demonstrate the progression of gathering assessment data to identifying nursing diagnoses, outcomes, and interventions. Rationales are included for every intervention. Nursing care plans, such as the Child with Juvenile Rheumatoid Arthritis (pages 823–825) and the Child with Classic Hemophilia A (pages 865–868), give the student a perspective that encourages holistic and individualized approaches.

Procedures give step-by-step technical information and patient education guidelines for clinical nursing procedures such as Bone Marrow Aspiration (page 845) and Cardiac Catheterization (page 724).

Organization and Content

The text is organized around six units that progress from wellness to illness. Each unit addresses a particular aspect of child health nursing.

Unit I "Overview of Child Health Nursing" sets contemporary child health nursing in its historic context, explains legal and ethical responsibilities, and delineates the various roles and functions of nurses as they relate to children and their families. The role of the family and its culture is explained.

Unit II "Growth and Development: The Child and Family" presents a comprehensive look at the growth and development of the child and family and current theories. Included in this unit are assessment techniques to obtain data about the physical, social, environmental, and developmental aspects of the child at various developmental levels. Included also is nursing management of frequently seen health problems of well children.

Unit III "Preventive Child Health Nursing: Strategies for Health Promotion" presents preventive measures for illness, injury, and poisoning. Each chapter is organized around the primary and secondary levels of prevention and identifies factors at each level that predispose the child of various developmental stages to health risks. Emphasis is on health teaching and parent counseling that will promote wellness behaviors for both child and family.

Unit IV "The Child and Family at Psychosocial Risk" deals with risks and conditions that upset the psychosocial functioning of the child and family. Chapters examine such issues as dysfunctional parenting, stressors associated with the physically or developmentally disabled child, maladaptive coping strategies, and dysfunctional behaviors leading to psychiatric illness. The psychosocial factors discussed in this unit are presented from the perspectives of both the community and the acute care setting, with an emphasis on prevention through detection of early cues to potential problems, and on the expanding role of the nurse in health promotion.

Unit V "The Impact of Illness on the Child and Family" applies general principles of nursing care to the ill child in home and hospital settings. Special consideration is given to adaptations of play as part of nursing care. We stress attention to the viewpoints of the child, parent, and siblings in assessing the effects of hospitalization on the ill child and family. Teaching and discharge preparation are covered in depth.

Unit VI "Nursing Care of the Ill Child" is the largest unit in the book. It concerns the nursing care of children with specific health problems and is organized by physiologic alteration. The unit begins with a chapter on fluid and electrolyte balance, because the theories and applications of this important concept are relevant to pathology in almost all body systems.

Emphasizing the nursing process, each remaining chapter in this final unit reflects the holistic perspective of the book's conceptual framework. The chapters reinforce the nurse's synthesis and application of nursing process to the care of children and families. Since dysfunctions in one area of the child's functioning affect other areas, explanations and cross references are given.

Organization of content in each of these final chapters is consistent. Each begins with a review of essential facts necessary to grasp an understanding of the structure and function of the body system being discussed. Nursing assessment including history, physical examination, and validating laboratory data follows, summarized and supported by *Assessment Guides.*

Nursing management for procedures and treatments are then discussed. Many procedures are illustrated by *Procedure boxes,* each of which describes the procedure and the child's reaction to it, illustrating how the nurse can explain the procedure in terms the child will understand. General principles of nursing care follow. These principles are organized around diagnoses that have been developed from assessment data. The commonalities and the general pathophysiology of each physiologic alteration are thus learned before the specific details of each disease entity are presented. The remainder of each chapter considers the essential and significant physiologic deviations, explaining specific treatment and nursing interventions for each condition.

Pedagogic Features

In addition to a wide variety of tables and boxes that summarize essential information or topics of related interest, the standard pedagogic features of each chapter include a chapter outline, list of objectives, a summary of the essential concepts covered, references, and additional readings. To help students find the content they need, a *Cross Reference Box* appears at the beginning of many chapters to indicate where discussions of related topics can be found. Examples are on pages 632 and 872.

Supplements

To assist instructors in taking full advantage of this text, we have the following ancillary materials available:

- *Nursing Care of Children and Families: A Workbook,* by Barbara Michaels, offers a balanced review of theoretic, psychosocial, and physiologic aspects of child health nursing care. A variety of learning activities emphasize the application of the nursing process and development of important assessment skills. Self-assessment guides help reinforce the student's grasp of principles, facts, and rationales for nursing actions in the child health nursing setting. The workbook is designed to accompany any child health nursing text.
- *Test Bank* provides approximately 700 questions for faculty use, written by respected educators in the field of child health nursing. All questions are presented in NCLEX format and classified according to content area, subclassification, cognitive level, and nursing process step. A computerized version is available for IBM-PC *or* APPLE-II users.
- *Slide Package* provides 60 color and black-and-white slides selected from the outstanding art program in *Child Health Nursing* and the parent text.

Acknowledgements

We would like to acknowledge the enthusiastic interest and efforts of the following people who have contributed their talents and time throughout the project:

Debra Hunter, whose assistance and support have been invaluable, even though she was not part of the project from its inception. Her rapid comprehension and enthusiastic support of the goals of the project and her ability to cooperatively set a reasonable and realistic schedule was immensely appreciated.

Debi Osnowitz, developmental editor and friend, who not only contributed her immense talent but also her empathy and caring when it was most needed.

Tom Eoyang, whose vision and efforts initiated this book and whose creativity has greatly enhanced the finished product.

Anne Friedman, production supervisor, Brian Jones, assistant, and the entire production and design staff at Addison-Wesley who kept production moving in a patient manner and used their talents to create from manuscript a book that is entirely consistent with our vision and goals.

The employees of Addison-Wesley and Benjamin Cummings who contributed photographs of their families to the endpapers of this book.

Judy Koenig for her ability to photograph children in a manner that enhances the creative and educational value of the book, and for her patience during many a hectic photographic session.

Evelyn Anderson, the public relations personnel, nursing staff, and children at the University of Massachusetts Medical Center for their cooperation in our search for additional photographs, and to the Town of Sandwich Nursing Agency personnel for their assistance with this endeavor.

Marjory Gordon for her generous guidance in assisting us to clarify nursing diagnoses and apply them consistently to the nursing care of children.

To the many reviewers whose helpful suggestions and comments allowed us to improve the clarity of the text, and who helped us to decide which vital information to include.

To the original contributors to *Nursing Care of Children and Families* whose literary efforts provided the core of this text:

Carole C Arenge, RN
The Children's Hospital, Boston

Michelle Burns, RN, MS, CPNP
Sandwich, Massachusetts

Carolyn Clayton Cahn, RN, MSN
Kaweah Delta District Hospital, Visalia, CA

Annette Calvi, RN, MSN
University of Colorado Health Science Center

John Conley, RN, BSN
Medical College of Georgia

Diane Holditch Davis, RN, MS, PhD
University of North Carolina

Cynthia E Degazon, RN, MA, EdD
New York University

Maureen De Maio, MS
Rutgers, The State University of New Jersey

Margaret Marusek Dozois, RN, MSN
National Jewish Center for Respiratory and Immunology Research

David J Driscoll, MD
Mayo Medical School, Mayo Clinic, Rochester, MN

Deanna Edwards
Provo, Utah

Mary Jo Eoff, RN, MSN
Indiana University

Wendy J Fibison, RN, PhD, FAAN
formerly, Doctoral Candidate
University of Pennsylvania

Juanita Fleming, RN, PhD, FAAN
University of Kentucky

Beverly Piper Giordano, RN, MS
The Children's Hospital, Denver

Cathryn L Glanville, BSN, MA, MEd
Medical College of Georgia

Janet A Grossman, MSN, CS
Rush-Presbyterian-St. Luke's Medical Center

Christine Hermann, RN, MS
Milwaukee Children's Hospital

June Andrews Horowitz, RN, PhD
Boston College and Lamaze Childbirth Education, Inc

Nancy Houlder, RN, BSN
formerly, Rocky Mountain Poison Control Center, Denver, CO

Cynthia B Hughes, RNC, PNP, EdD
Seton Hall University

Mary Virginia Jacobs, RN, MSN, CFNP
Yoakum Catholic Hospital, Yoakum, TX

Lorna N Kaufman, MEd
formerly, Doctoral Candidate
Boston College

Gretchen L Kelly, RN, MA
University of Virginia

Elizabeth Laliberte, MSN
University of Connecticut

Barbara J Leonard, RN, PhD
University of Minnesota

Betty M Lovelace, MS
Retired from Stanford University Medical Center

Noreen Mahon, MS, PhD
Rutgers, The State University of New Jersey

Lyn Marshall, RN, MSN
Langley Porter Hospital, San Francisco, CA

Bonnie McMillin, RN, MSN
Rochester Methodist Hospital, Rochester, MN

Karen Mitchell, MSN, PhD
Editor, Pediatric Nursing

Judith Surveyor Mitiguy, RN, MS
The Children's Hospital, Boston, MA

Kathleen Hardin Mooney, RN, PhD
University of Utah

Gayle Doerner Olsen, RN, MS, PNP
Winona State University, Rochester, MN

Jean A O'Neil, MS, EdD
Boston College

J Craig Peery, PhD
Brigham Young University

Joy Hinson Penticuff, RN, MSN, PhD
University of Texas

Bobbie Jean Perdue, MSN
Rutgers, The State University of New Jersey

Joan Orchardo Pernice, MS, CPNP
Doctoral Candidate
Boston College

Margo Pinney, MSN
University Hospital, Denver CO

Marva Mizell Price, RNC, MPH, CFNP
North Carolina Department of Human Resources

Virginia Caponetti Prout, RN, MS
Boston College

Frances Ward Quinless, RN, PhD
University of Medicine and Dentistry of New Jersey

Robert G Riedel, PhD
Southwest State University, Marshall, MN

Gwendolyn C Robinson, RN, MA, CPNP
formerly, Director, Child Development Associates, Tolland, CT

Jean Marie Rockenhaus, RN, MSN
Montana State University

Mary Ann Scoloveno, RN, EdD, PNP
Rutgers, The State University of New Jersey

Ellen Shuzman, MS
Rutgers, The State University of New Jersey

Rosemary A Simkins, RN, BSN, MN
National Jewish Center for Immunology & Respiratory Medicine, Denver, CO

Margaret P Smith, RN, MS
Kennedy Memorial Hospital for Children, Brighton, MA

Charlotte M Spicher, RN, PhD
University of Cincinnati

Sandra K Spiller, RN, BSN
Rocky Mountain Poison Control Center, Denver, CO

Mary E Walker, RN, PhD, FAAN
Consultant, Austin, TX

Patricia A Woodbury, RN, MSN, CPNA
Child & Family Services
Children's Hospital of St Paul, MN

Kathleen M Wruk, RN, BSN
Certified Poison Information Specialist
Rocky Mountain Poison Center, Denver, CO

Susan Rowen James, RN, MSN
formerly, Instructor, School of Nursing, Boston College, Chestnut Hill, Massachusetts

Sandra R Mott, RN, MSN
Associate Professor, School of Nursing, Boston College, Chestnut Hill, Massachusetts

Contributors

Susan Miller, RN, MSN
Director of Education and Development
Cape Cod Hospital
Hyannis, Massachusetts
formerly, Associate Professor of Nursing
Cape Cod Community College
West Barnstable, Massachusetts

Barbara Michaels, RN, MSN
Instructor and Level Coordinator
Health Occupations Division
El Centro College
Plano, Texas

Nancy Fiero Fazekas, RN, MN
formerly, Assistant Professor
School of Nursing
Doctoral Student
Boston College
Chestnut Hill, Massachusetts

Reviewers

Anne Batchelder, BSN, MSN
New Hampshire Vocational School, Manchester, New Hampshire

Carolyn Belz
St Francis College, Pittsburg, Pennsylvania

Pamela Cassirer, BSN, MSN
Brookdale Community College, Lincroft, New Jersey

Jeannette Chambers
Riverside Methodist Hospital, Delaware, Ohio

Mary Dillon, BSN, MN
Trocaire College, Buffalo, New York

Nancy Eppich, BSN, MSN
Rainbow Babies & Children's Hospital, Cleveland, Ohio

Pamela K Evans, BSN, MN
Butler County Community College, El Dorado, Kansas

Carol Holsonback, BSN, MSN
St Petersburg Junior College, Pinellas Park, Florida

Mary P Khoury, BSN, MSN
Cape Cod Community College, West Barnstable, Massachusetts

Joyce Kliesen
St. Francis College, Pittsburg, Pennsylvania

Katherine Kniest
St Francis Hospital, Evanston, Illinois

Karen Kristensen, BSN, MS
North Dakota State University, Fargo, North Dakota

Judith McDonald, BSN, MSN
Thornton Community College, South Holland, Illinois

Bette Michel, BSN, MSN
El Paso Community College, El Paso, Texas

Susan Miller, BSN, MSN
Cape Cod Community College, West Barnstable, Massachusetts

Pat Murray, CCRN, RN
Amarillo College, Amarillo, Texas

Linda Olivet, MSN, DSN
University of Alabama, Tuscaloosa, Alabama

Sharon Pontious
University of Texas, El Paso, Texas

Nancy Potts, BSN, MSN
St Petersburg Junior College, Pinellas Park, Florida

Constance Powell, BSN, MS
Hartnell College, Salinas, California

Janice Selekman, RN, DNSc
Thomas Jefferson University, Philadelphia, Pennsylvania

Bobbie Siler
Macon Junior College, Macon, Georgia

Marilyn Stamp, BSN, GN
Clinton Community College, Clinton, Iowa

Judy White, BSN, MSN
Rockland County Community College, Suffern, New York

I

Overview of Major Influences on Child Health Care

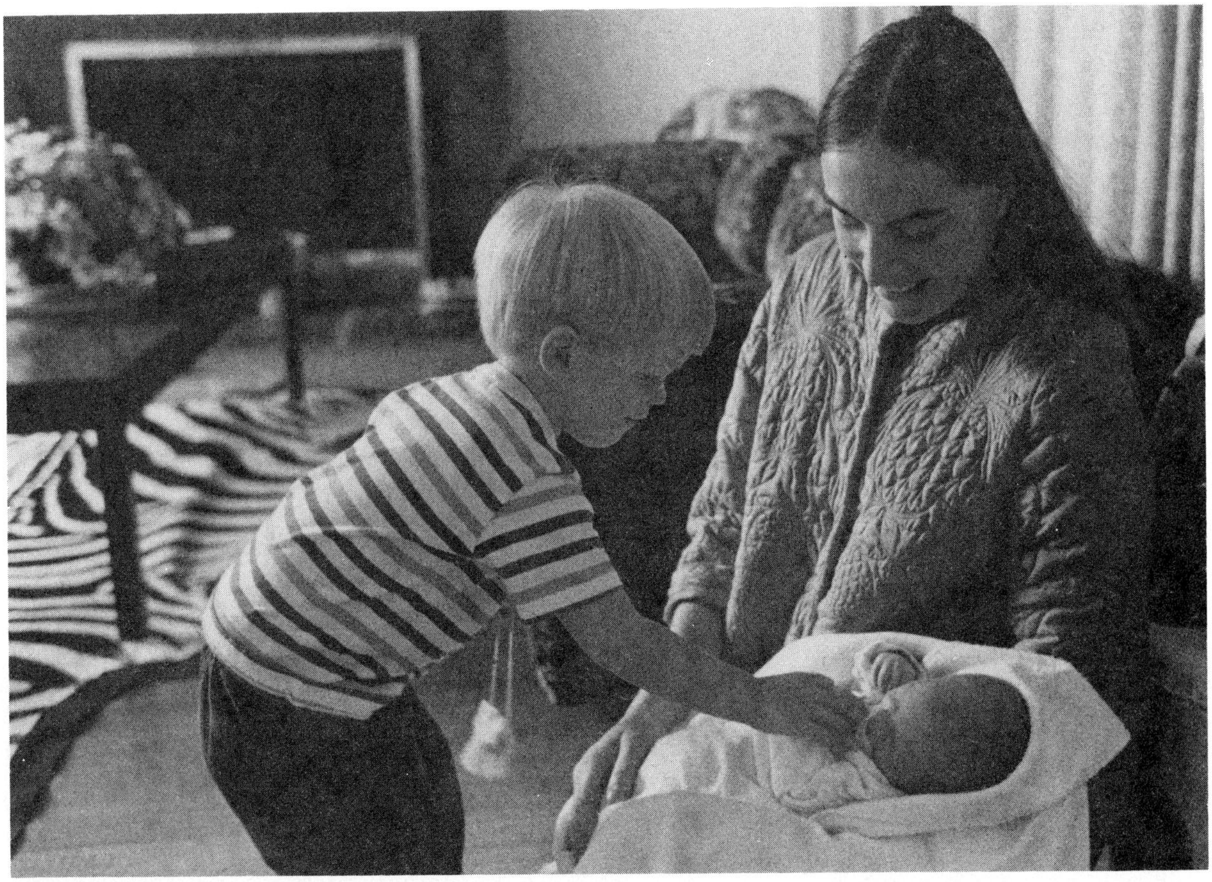

Chapter 1

Perspectives in Child Health Care

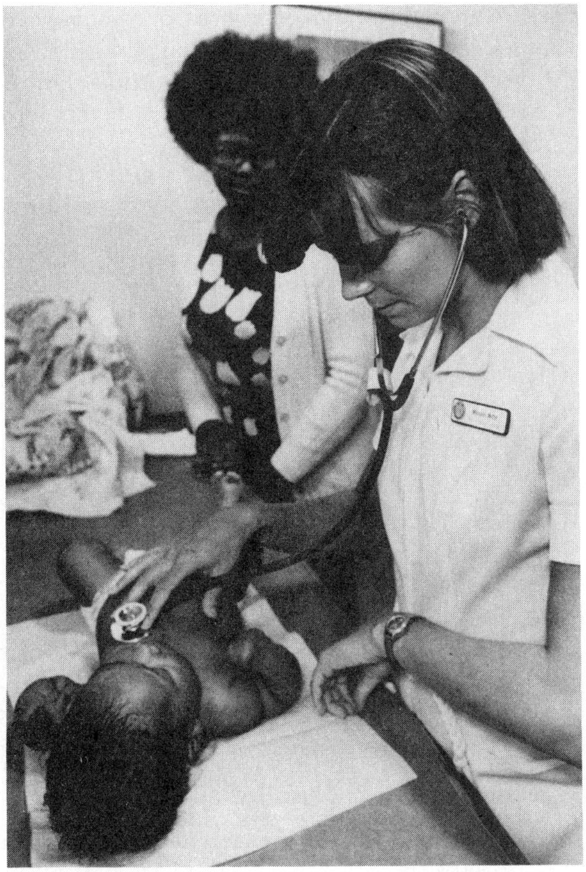

Chapter Contents

(Continues)

Informed Consent
Legal Accountability of the Child Health Nurse

Future Directions in Child Health Nursing Care

Computer Applications in Health Care
Advances in Nursing Research
DRGs: Impact on the Health Care System

Objectives

- Describe the origins of child health nursing and its subsequent evolution.
- Explain how social and economic changes and advances in medical science helped determine the role of child health nurse.
- Describe the roles of the child health nurse.
- Discuss the relationship between the child and the child's internal and external environments.
- Discuss the relationship between the child's basic developmental needs and health deviation needs, together with the nurse's ability to facilitate self-care.
- Define the phases of the nursing process—assessment, nursing diagnosis, planning, intervention, and evaluation.
- Describe how nursing theory relates to the nursing process.
- Describe the legal and ethical factors that affect child health nursing.

In the past 150 years a remarkable shift of emphasis has occurred in health care, particularly in the care of the child. Historically, although both children and adults needed medical assistance, children were considered to be the property of their parents, and their value was essentially economic. That view contrasts significantly with the current feeling that children are the future of the world and therefore are entitled to health care that meets their special needs.

This evolving attitude is apparent in child health care over the last two centuries. Child health care has changed from a strictly curative approach to a holistic approach that encompasses every aspect of health—physical, emotional, social, and environmental—and not just the absence of disease. Nowhere is this approach more noticeable than in the emerging role of the nurse, who has become a child advocate rather than simply a child caretaker.

Development of Child Health Nursing

Child Health: Some Background

Changes in child health nursing are reflected in statistical data from the turn of the twentieth century to the present. Statistics help to analyze trends and are useful tools for observing changes occurring over an extended period of time. For child health care, important statistical data include birth rates and mortality rates.

Birth rates are particularly helpful to agencies planning for quality health care. Public funding then can be channeled to areas that are most in need of assistance. As a statistical measure, the *birth rate* is the number of live births compared to the population being analyzed. The birth rate usually is expressed in figures that reflect the number of live

Nursing textbook, 1855. (Courtesy of the Children's Hospital of Philadelphia.)

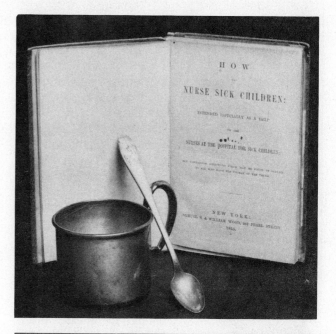

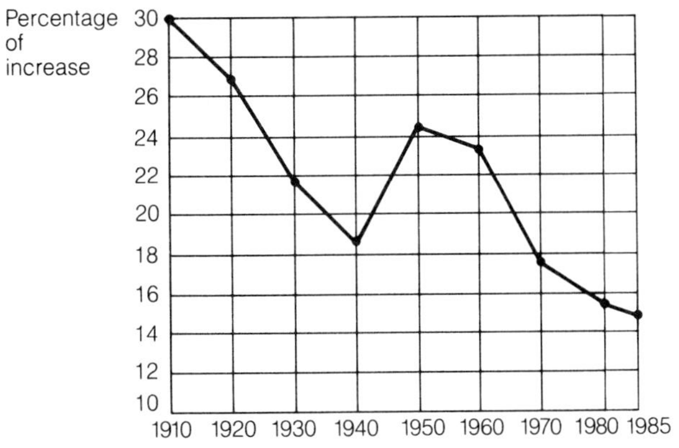

FIGURE 1-1

Birth rates 1910–present. The birth rate is the number of live births per total population, or the rate at which the population increases.

TABLE 1-1 Differences by Sex—Male to Female Ratio of Birth

Year	Male	Female
1940	1055	1000
1950	1054	1000
1960	1049	1000
1970	1066	1000
1980	1053	1000

births per 1000 people. Figure 1-1 shows that the birth rate for the United States in the twentieth century has fluctuated greatly. Throughout this time, birth rates have ranged from a high in 1910 to an unprecedented low in 1980. The graph illustrates this change and also shows some commonly recognized trends—wartime lows and the post-World War II "baby boom." One current prediction is that birth rates in the near future might accelerate slightly as a greater number of postwar "baby boomers" reach childbearing age. Table 1-1 shows that although birth rates have been inconsistent, the ratio of male to female births has remained steady.

Mortality rates reflect the number of deaths per 1000 people in a geographical area being studied. Mortality rates focus attention on areas of health care delivery that might need intervention, either through additional funding or widespread education. For example, an increased infant mortality rate in a certain area might indicate the need for greater funding of prenatal services or for better availability of neonatal intensive care services. Mortality rates also reflect improvements in health care delivery over a specified period of time.

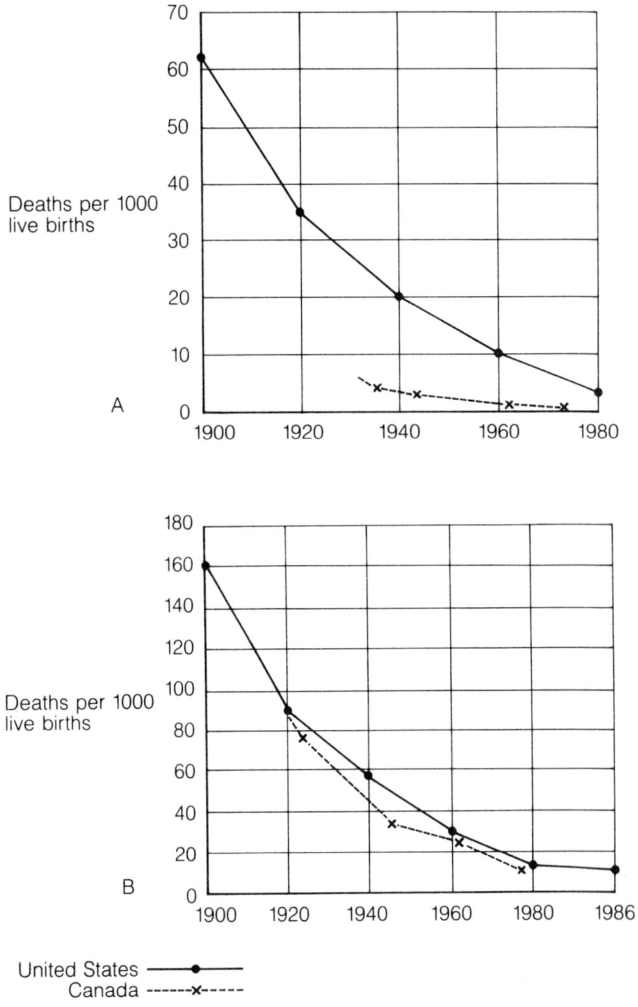

FIGURE 1-2

Infant and child mortality rates in the United States and Canada, 1910–present. **A.** *Childhood mortality (for children under 14 years).* **B.** *Infant mortality.*

Mortality rates in the United States and in other countries have declined consistently. The circumstances that made life precarious for children in 1900 (62 deaths per 1000 children in the United States versus 3.9 deaths per 1000 children in 1985) have changed, along with improvements in medical and nursing care. Figure 1-2 shows these changes.

Changes in mortality rates also reflect improved public health practices and scientific discoveries. For example, in 1900 the leading cause of death in children was gastroenteritis, followed closely by pneumonia (Table 1-2). After the mandatory pasteurization of milk and the discovery and

TABLE 1-2 Leading Causes of Childhood Deaths—United States *

1900	1920	1940	1960
Gastroenteritis	Pneumonia	Pneumonia	Congenital malformations
Pneumonia†	Gastroenteritis	Congenital malformations	Pneumonia
Tuberculosis	Tuberculosis	Gastroenteritis	Accidents‡
Cardiovascular disorders	Syphilis	Accidents	Gastroenteritis
Cancer	Cancer	Syphilis	Cancer

* Includes causes of infant death.
† Pneumonia includes influenza and other respiratory problems.
‡ Accidents includes motor vehicle accidents.

SOURCE: Information from US Department of Health and Human Services. *1900–1980 Vital Statistics Rates in the United States*, 1983.

TABLE 1-3 Leading Causes of Childhood Death—1985

Age	Cause of death
0–1	Birth associated and perinatal
	Congenital anomalies
	Other causes
	Sudden infant death syndrome
	Respiratory distress syndrome
1–14	Accidents
	Congenital anomalies
	Leukemia
	Cancer
	Homicide
15–24	Motor vehicle accidents
	All other accidents
	Homicide
	Suicide
	Cancer

SOURCE: US Department of Health and Human Services. *Monthly Vital Statistics Reports*, 1986. September 19, 1986.

use of antibiotics, the significance of both problems decreased. The most common cause of childhood deaths today (aside from neonatal deaths due to congenital or mechanical problems) is accidents. Apparently, as children are raised in a more complex world, the potential increases for household and environmental hazards to be the instruments of death. Prevention is the only cure for this type of epidemic (Table 1-3).

Infant mortality rates also have declined dramatically, although both the United States and Canada have lagged behind many of the European countries. In 1978, at 13.8 deaths per 1000 infants in the United States and 12.4 deaths per 1000 infants in Canada, these two nations followed Sweden, Norway, Switzerland, and Denmark, among others (WHO, 1982). More current statistics show that the United States has an infant mortality rate of 10.5 deaths per 1000 infants.

Better prenatal care and parent education programs have contributed to these improved rates, as have improved neonatal intensive care facilities. Medical care for mothers and children has become more available. Nursing care, particularly health supervision, has improved as the roles and functions of nurses have expanded. These factors will continue to have positive effects on mortality rates. Other contemporary factors, however, threaten positive trends. Local and national cutbacks in funding for programs assisting women and infants have the potential to affect the infant mortality rate adversely. Child health nurses thus need to understand how these trends affect the health care system so that nurses can be advocates for improved services.

Historical Development of Child Health Nursing

The evolution of child health nursing in many ways has paralleled the improvement in children's health. Child health care in the western hemisphere took root in the mid-seventeenth century with the establishment of an orphan-

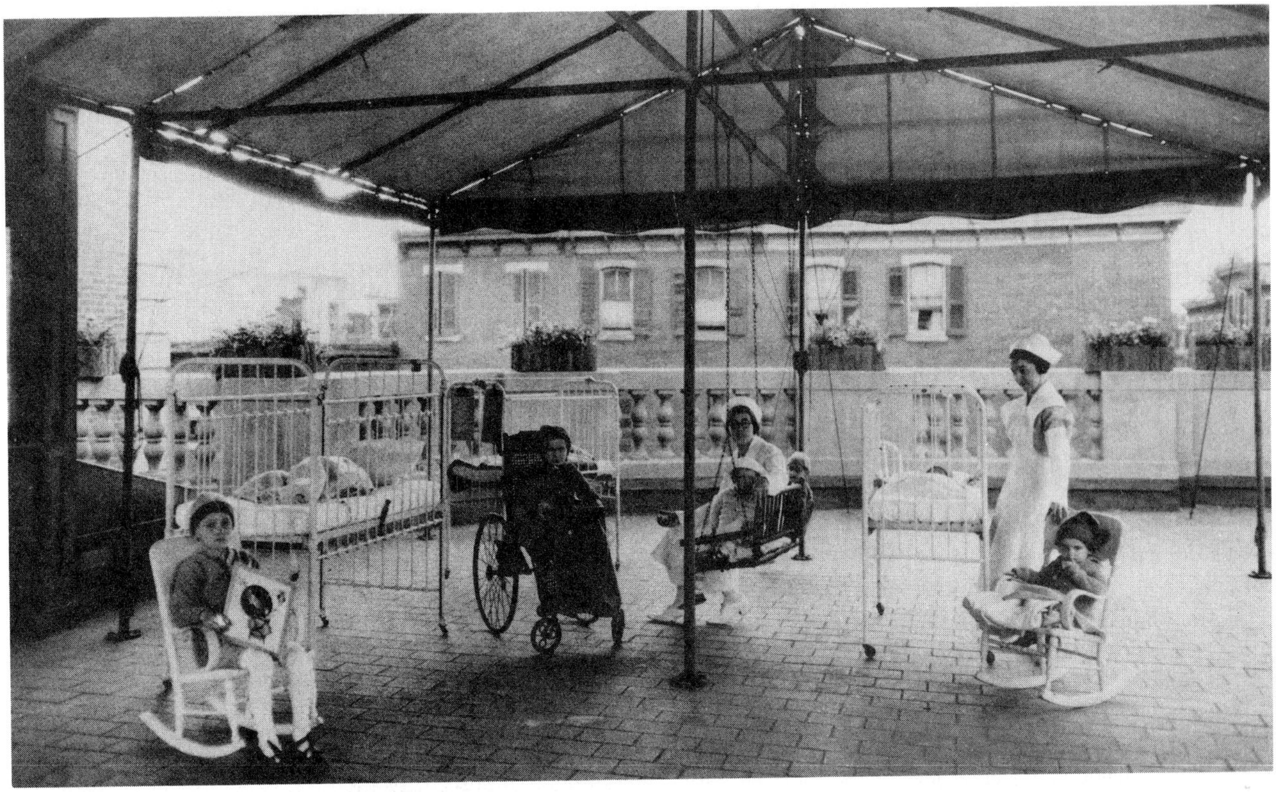

Roof garden, 1921. (Courtesy of the Children's Hospital of Philadelphia.)

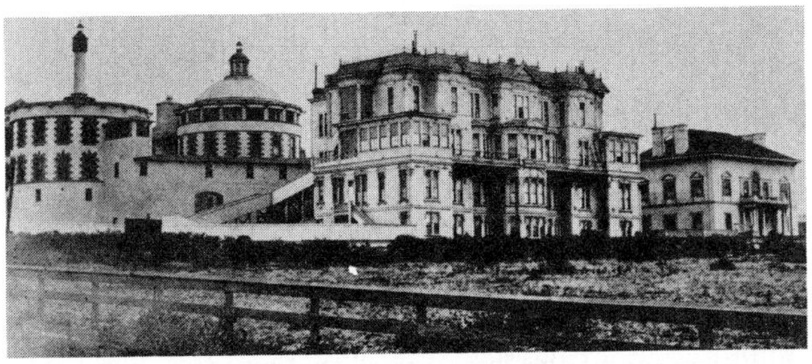

Children's hospital in San Francisco.

age and school for the children of the settlers in Quebec. Through subsequent centuries, *child health nursing,* once entirely dependent on the pediatric medical speciality, has become an autonomous nursing specialty.

Today's child health nurses are nursing specialists, the colleagues of pediatricians and other child health care professionals. The evolution of child health nursing has come through advances, not only in the nursing profession but also in medicine and the social sciences. Changes in nursing thus reflect changes in society as a whole.

The Science and Art of Child Health Nursing

Science and art often are seen as opposites, but in the best nursing care, they are combined creatively. As a science, nursing requires the theoretic knowledge and skill to manage all aspects of a child's health and response to a health problem. The theoretic base of nursing practice includes an understanding of normal physiologic processes that occur during the child's maturation and of the impact of pathologic processes on specific body systems. The nurse also needs to know how normal developmental crises, illnesses, and injuries affect children of different ages and how to identify resources that can help the child respond in the most effective way to a given health problem.

The art of nursing lies in the skill with which each nurse applies the necessary knowledge anew to each individual child. Just as no two children are alike, no two children will respond in the same way to a health problem. Like adults, children respond to events and people in ways that reflect their own personalities, past experiences, growth and developmental levels, cultural heritages, coping patterns, and current states of health. The nurse needs to take these factors into account when adapting the principles and details of nursing care to the unique requirements of each child. The more the nurse knows about each of these factors, the more sensitive, appropriate, and complete the nursing care will be.

Understanding the Individual Child

Being attentive to the values, beliefs, customs, and rituals of clients is important regardless of age, but for children this attention can present special challenges to the nurse. The nurse needs to be sensitive to the child's stage of development. A child is not a "little adult" but is living through a period of rapid development in all respects: biophysical, emotional, cognitive, and social. Although nurses often can rely on certain shared assumptions and understanding with other adults, a child is in the process of discovering those shared assumptions and of achieving an adult understanding.

This process takes place through the child's interaction with the surrounding environment—sending messages or presenting behavior to significant others and obtaining feedback about the appropriateness, expectedness, or adequacy of the behavior or message. The child then interprets this information and either maintains the behavior or communication pattern or adjusts it accordingly. This constant dynamic feedback process begins in childhood and continues throughout life, although the environment and the people in it change over time. A child seems to develop simultaneously in many directions with a rapid and undiscriminating abandon that can be wondrous to the observer.

Nurses need to be particularly alert to a child's unique characteristics when assessing needs and establishing a therapeutic relationship. For instance, the level of cognitive understanding is a critical factor in the child's response to care. One nurse described the case of a 4-year-old girl who seemed to be unreasonably terrified of vomiting and became upset when it happened. Later, the nurse discovered that the girl equated this experience with the stuffing that fell out of her torn rag doll. Reassurance and a simple explanation dispelled the girl's fears. The nurse explained to the girl that her body was not made like her rag doll's and that vomiting did not mean that her insides were falling out (Pontious, 1982).

A child's inner abilities and developmental status are part of the resources available to that child. The nurse also will identify additional resources, such as education, prior health care, religion, relatives, friends, socioeconomic status, and community services, that might contribute to the child's response to illness and nursing care. All of these factors influence the child's interpretation of and response to the events of daily life. For most children, however, none of these external factors will be as significant as the support, love, and caring found with the child's own parents and siblings.

Including the Family

Nursing a child always involves that child's family. From birth, a child is continually influenced by the beliefs, values, rituals, traditions, attitudes, and practices of the family. The family not only endows the child biologically but also fosters moral development and provides psychologic support. The nurse can thus look to the family for much of the information needed to understand the child accurately.

The family is a primary resource for the child. The nurturing and support a family provides can be crucial factors in determining how well a child responds to a health problem and to the nursing care provided. Each member of the family may contribute something to the child's abilities to cope with the health problem. The strong, supportive interactions of the family as a whole can provide the child with a foundation of security and love, which is an extremely important resource.

On the other hand, the child's health problem and inability to function in the usual or expected manner have definite effects on the other family members, both individually and collectively. Latent problems with family members or family functioning might be brought to the fore by a crisis in the child's health. Such problems, if neglected, might not only impair the family's ability to provide the needed support for the child but also could have long-term implications for the family's continued healthy development.

Including the family in the various aspects of nursing management is therefore extremely important. The family is involved directly in decisions and activities related to the child's care, and the family itself is treated as a client in potential need of nursing care. Nurses in child health settings are therefore responsible for goals that address the needs of families. These goals include:

1. Focusing on all family members while providing direct nursing care to a specific member
2. Assessing the impact of the child's health problem on individual family members
3. Assessing the relationships among individual family members
4. Appreciating and incorporating the cultural heritage and values of the family
5. Promoting the health and growth of the family, both during the child's illness and after recovery

The Nurse's Role in Child Health Care

Primary Health Care

Essential to an understanding of how a child health nurse functions is an understanding of primary health care. In an age of increasing medical specialization, the role played by the general medical practitioner came to be sadly neglected. As a result, clients no longer had a primary contact person in the health care system. Their health concerns became scattered among specialists, none of whom viewed clients as whole persons. *Primary health care,* which provided clients with a single physician who approached their needs in a more comprehensive and humanistic manner, became a rarity.

Standards of Maternal—Child Health Nursing Practice

Standard I—The nurse helps children and parents attain and maintain optimum health.

Standard II—The nurse assists families to achieve and maintain a balance between the personal growth needs of individual family members and optimum family functioning.

Standard III—The nurse intervenes with vulnerable clients and families at risk to prevent potential developmental and health problems.

Standard IV—The nurse promotes an environment free of hazards to reproduction, growth and development, wellness, and recovery from illness.

Standard V—The nurse detects changes in health status and deviations from optimum development.

Standard VI—The nurse carries out appropriate interventions and treatment to facilitate survival and recovery from illness.

Standard VII—The nurse assists clients and families to understand and cope with developmental and traumatic situations during illness, childbearing, childrearing, and childhood.

Standard VIII—The nurse actively pursues strategies to enhance access to and utilization of adequate health care services.

Standard IX—The nurse improves maternal and child health nursing practice through evaluation of practice, education, and research.

SOURCE: American Nurses' Association, Division on Maternal & Child Health Nursing Practice.

As consumers became more vocal about the lack of a primary contact person in the system, medical schools developed family practice specialties that prepared physicians for the role of family doctor. Meanwhile, child health nurses expanded their roles, adding health promotion to acute care as standard parts of nursing practice. Child health nurses came to fill the need for primary health care in a number of ways. As part of the nursing process, they obtained health histories, assessed client needs, performed health screening procedures, and developed comprehensive plans of care. They were able to handle common health concerns and make referrals. Community nurses met the health needs of the well client in addition to the sick client. The community nurse ultimately came to be viewed as the ideal person to administer primary health care to clients.

The nurse is essentially a contact person who provides primary health care for child and family in various health care settings. All nurses perform similar functions. These functions include:

1. *Facilitating therapeutic care by applying the nursing process.* Nurses obtain histories and assess child growth and development, family interactions, parenting, and general lifestyle. Part of this assessment is observing the family's and child's response to stress. Nurses identify problems and intervene to correct them before further complications occur.
2. *Health education.* Child health nurses counsel and educate children and families as well as society as a whole. Education is specific to a child's medical problem and includes anticipatory guidance to prevent the development of disease. Child health nurses play an important educational role in facilitating positive changes in attitudes toward health in individuals and groups.
3. *Referral.* Child health nurses refer children and families to appropriate community resources.
4. *Accountability.* Nurses are autonomous in their nursing practice within the states' Nurse Practice Acts and are accountable for their actions.
5. *Child advocates.* In their roles as child advocates, nurses initiate changes for better-quality health care.

Many practicing nurses might find these role definitions somewhat idealistic. Nurses striving for excellence in care, however, function well within this framework.

In practicing the art and science of nursing, nurses function in many ways that fit within the primary health care framework. They teach simple and complex facts about the human body, how it works, and how to protect it from injury and disease. They answer questions about the principles of growth and development and how they apply to the problems of a specific child. They provide care during times of illness, injury, or recovery. Nurses also are instrumental in motivating children and their families to take personal charge of and make responsible decisions about their own health.

Settings and Roles for Child Health Nurses

Nurses have traditionally functioned in a variety of settings, each with specific roles and expectations for the nurse. Today, the expanding roles of the child health nurse also have influenced the development of autonomous nursing practice. Nurses now may be educated as nurse practitioners and clinical specialists, so that they are further qualified to provide specialized care for children and families.

Primary nursing in the hospital Because a child's contact with the health care system is often through hospitalization, the child health nurse working in an acute-care setting might become the primary contact person.

Primary nursing, not to be confused with primary health care, is a staffing pattern that facilitates the execution of primary health care in the hospital setting. In essence, primary nursing is a system whereby the health needs of clients are met on a 24-hour basis. Children and parents seem to respond more rapidly if they can depend on one nurse. Primary nurses obtain nursing histories and construct care plans for their clients. They are accountable for the care they give and for seeing that the plans are followed and evaluated.

In the hospital, the role of the child health nurse encompasses the holistic assessment of the child's needs and the development of a care plan to facilitate recovery. Nurses assist the child and family in adjusting to a threatening situation. In addition to following a medical regimen designed to correct an existing medical problem, the nurse treats each child as an individual and attempts to incorporate as much of the child's normal routine as possible in the care plan. Child health nurses include parents in the care of their children. They provide information about the disease, hospital procedures, and general health. Nurses also coordinate the efforts of other members of the health care team to promote an optimal environment for recovery. Discharge preparation is an important function of the child health nurse, easing the transition from the hospital to the home environment.

The nurse's role in a chronic or rehabilitative hospital is similar to that in an acute setting. Greater emphasis is placed on the maintenance or improvement of the child's ability to function at maximum potential. Here, too, nurses use anticipatory guidance for health promotion. Child health nurses are concerned with the needs of the disabled child, and they collaborate with members of the community to ease the child's adjustments to daily living. Most important is the skill with which the nurse can assist the child and family to adjust emotionally to a chronic illness.

The pediatric nurse practitioner The 1960s brought an awareness that quality health care must become more available to children in rural areas. In response to this, Henry K. Silver, MD and Loretta C. Ford, RN, PhD established a program at the University of Colorado that was designed to educate a new category of health worker, the pediatric nurse practitioner. The nurse practitioner's role filled a gap caused by the physician's increasing attention to the complex curative aspects of pediatric care.

Pediatric nurse practitioners collaborate with physicians to provide better health care for children and families and serve as primary contact persons for children in the health care system. They conduct health screenings, give well-child care, manage simple medical problems, and provide support during medical emergencies. Nurse practitioners learn to perform a physical assessment using some of the tools (eg, otoscope, ophthalmoscope) that formerly were used only by physicians (Ford, 1976).

In addition to screening and health supervision activities, the nurse practitioner can order laboratory tests, prescribe selected medications, and diagnose and treat minor illnesses and emergencies using established protocol. The nurse practitioner often will answer health questions posed by parents during "call-in time" (scheduled time when parents may call to discuss problems their children are experiencing).

Initially, the role of the nurse practitioner appeared to combine traditional roles of medicine and nursing because the activities of health screening and health promotion were superseded by an emphasis on assessment tools—the otoscope, ophthalmoscope, palpation, and auscultation. As pediatric nurse practitioners continue to define their roles, however, a wide range of nursing services will be offered to children and families that are unique and separate from medicine.

As originally envisioned, the pediatric nurse practitioner would provide care in rural areas, where physician accessibility was limited. As the specialty developed, however, nurse practitioners came to practice in both urban and rural areas (Silver, 1971).

The program at the University of Colorado was followed closely by programs in other areas of the country. These programs prepare practitioners to function not only in rural areas but also in urban health centers and physicians' offices.

The pediatric nurse practitioner was the prototype for other expanded nursing roles in a variety of specialties. Equally important, this role continues the movement to change the focus of nursing from curative to preventive. In

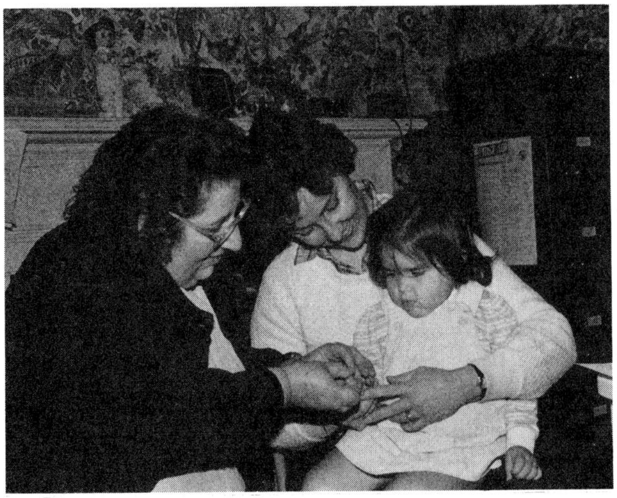

Community nurses meet the health needs of well clients in addition to the sick.

recent years, the education of nurse practitioners generally has been incorporated into nursing programs at the graduate level to prepare better primary care nurses.

The community health nurse *Community health nurses* follow children from infancy throughout the life cycle. Working in a given community, these nurses have a unique opportunity to observe children and families in their normal environment. Community health nurses assess children within their family structures and intervene to assist children and families to develop positive health habits. At well-baby clinics, they perform simple screening tests, administer immunizations, observe and record developmental progress, and provide anticipatory guidance for normal developmental problems.

Community health nurses receive referrals from hospitals and other sources, and, as health care becomes more home centered, they care for acutely ill children in the home. They are particularly knowledgeable about specialized community resources. Like all nurses, community health nurses communicate information about medical progress to the other members of the health team and are accountable for nursing actions.

The school nurse and school nurse practitioner The *school nurse* is gaining increasing recognition as a primary provider of health care. In the past the school nurse's role was more or less restricted to the administration of minor first-aid and emergency care. Because children do need more comprehensive health care during the school years and because greater numbers of children with special needs are being "mainstreamed" in the school environment, the role of the school nurse has gained new dimensions.

The responsibilities of school nurses include the following:

1. Maintaining a health record for all schoolchildren, including an assessment and identification of special health problems
2. Following up communicable diseases, including the maintenance of immunization records
3. Counseling children and families with physical, emotional, or social difficulties
4. Managing accidents and illnesses occurring in school
5. Recognizing and counseling pregnant adolescents, substance abusers, and victims of domestic violence
6. Collaborating with the school physician in conducting routine physical examinations of schoolchildren, including screening for visual or hearing impairments, scoliosis, and other health problems
7. Identifying potential health and safety hazards in the school environment

School nurses also play an active role in health promotion. They become involved with the school health education program by teaching about stress reduction, diet, exercise, and other principles for healthful living. They provide information related to problems of substance abuse, pregnancy, sexuality, and domestic violence. School nurses confer with teachers about health problems occurring in the classroom and assist teachers in the management of children with special needs (Igoe, 1980).

Programs for school nurse practitioners emphasize the problems of well-child care and health and developmental screening. They vary in length from several months to 2 years, depending on the educational goal. A certificate is awarded on completion of the program. School nurse practitioners also assist teachers in identifying and treating children with learning or perceptual disorders. They are actively involved with community planning for disabled children and for those with other special needs.

The camp nurse Nurses in camp settings function autonomously within a medical framework authorized by an attending physician. The *camp nurse* is responsible for maintaining the health of campers and staff, administering ordered prescriptions, and managing acute illness and emergencies under the medical director's standing orders. While assessing campers upon their arrival, camp nurses identify health problems and needs for health education. Because children in new settings often exhibit maladaptive behaviors, communication among parents, staff, and nurse is essential for a unified approach to problems. Camp nurses communicate directly with the camp administration about unsafe conditions, especially regarding high-risk areas such as the waterfront and archery and riflery ranges.

The office nurse *Office nurses,* although capable of skilled nursing care, traditionally have been assigned routine tasks, such as obtaining measurements, immunization administration, routine specimen collection, and office paperwork. In the past, pediatricians have been reluctant to allow nurses to assume more responsibility for health promotion. As nurses have become better educated and more prepared to be autonomous practitioners, however, they have assumed greater responsibility for child health care. Office nurses perform preliminary assessments, counsel parents by phone, and assist parents in coping with normal developmental difficulties.

The clinical nurse specialist Clinical specialties originated at a time when nursing was functional and fragmented. Nursing leaders envisioned a nurse who not only would function as a coordinator of care but who also would demonstrate expertise in a specialized area of nursing (Kinsella, 1973). This clinical nurse specialist would act as a role model and a change agent, improving the quality of care.

Initially, the role was ill-defined. At present, a *clinical nurse specialist* is defined as a nurse with a master's degree in a specialty, who is prepared to function with an increased depth of knowledge and capacity to make high-level nursing judgments. In child health care, specialists concentrate on the general care of children or on the nursing care problems stemming from alterations in specific body systems. Both concentrations include the responsibility for consultation, application of change theory, research design, role modeling, and expertise in the specialty field.

Those specializing in general child health care usually practice in community hospitals, where patients are fewer and the disease entities are less acute. Specialists act as liaisons between the hospital and community, planning care for clients as they move through the health care system. Their major focus is the quality and continuity of care. They handle referrals from other nurses and from physicians, and they find cases and initiate appropriate health care.

Specialists maintain continuous, updated records on their clients and communicate essential information to other members of the health care team. Participation in staff educational development and in research to improve nursing care is implicit in the role. As Nurse Practice Acts change and third-party insurers recognize the value and cost-effectiveness of the clinical specialists, more of these nurses will establish independent nursing practices as primary caregivers.

Specialists who focus on a narrower aspect of child health care usually practice in the larger teaching hospitals. They are experts in a single aspect of care, such as oncologic nursing. They, too, are physicians' colleagues, often working closely with physicians in research and publication. In addition to providing expert nursing care, these specialists assist the nursing staff by conducting care conferences and by coordinating care for individual clients.

The Nursing Process: Role Enhancement for the Child Health Nurse

A goal for the child health nurse is to administer systematic, holistic, and comprehensive nursing care to children and families. A primary way of achieving this goal is through consistent use of the nursing process. The nursing process has been defined as a

> . . . problem-identification and problem-solving approach to client care. It is the basis for a helping relationship characterized by knowledge, reason, and caring. Structurally, the nursing process is adapted from the scientific approach to solving problems. (Gordon, 1982)

The nursing process has five phases: assessment, nursing diagnosis, planning, intervention, and evaluation. The nursing process is dynamic. It is an ongoing process for each child and family. It enables the nurse to respond quickly as the needs of the child or family change. Although the word "phase" implies a time span with a well-defined beginning and an end, the "phases" in the nursing process very often are carried out simultaneously (Fig. 1-3). For example, when performing a specific *intervention,* such as teaching the parent the skills to treat a child's illness at home, the nurse also might be *evaluating* the parent's understanding of the disease process itself and *assessing* the potential problems that might affect the ability of the parent to care for the child at home.

A Framework for Applying the Nursing Process

Effectively applying the nursing process depends on organizing a system for obtaining information. Such a framework is essential in facilitating holistic nursing care for each child and family. For example, two children might have similar infections but require very different plans for nursing care. Such differences might be due to a parent's avail-

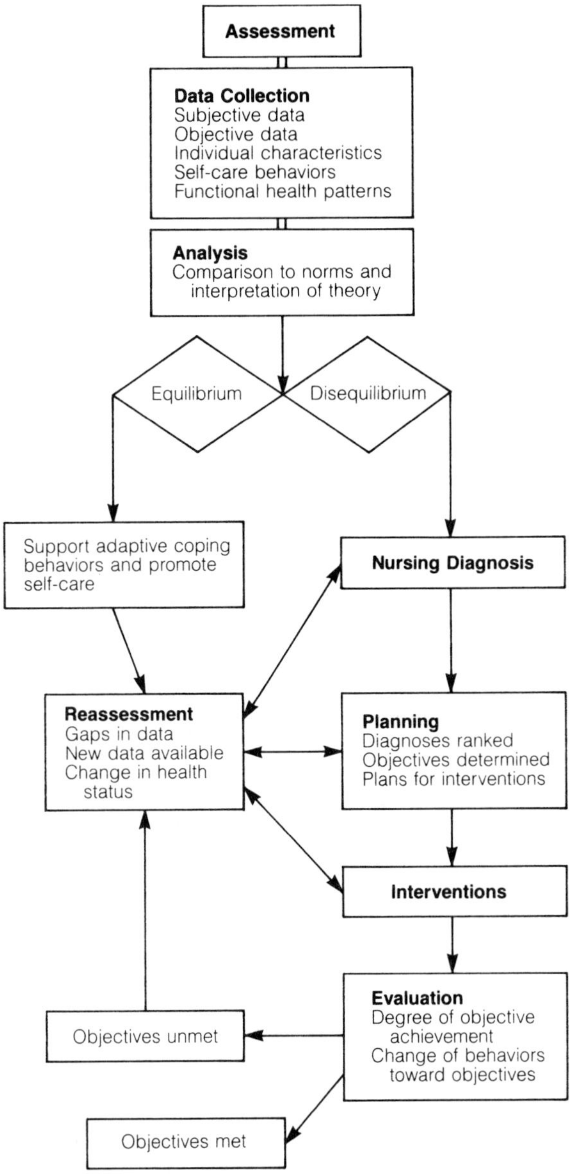

FIGURE 1-3

The interrelated phases of the nursing process.

ability to provide care at home, to the children's ages, or to other existing health problems. To provide nursing care, the nurse needs an organized system for all the information obtained in assessing a child and family. An effective way of doing this is to examine children in relation to themselves and in relation to their external environments.

Children interact with both their external and internal environments to maintain a state of balance, or *equilibrium*. Because factors in a given child's life are constantly changing, the child's relationship to external and internal environments change correspondingly. More simply stated, any

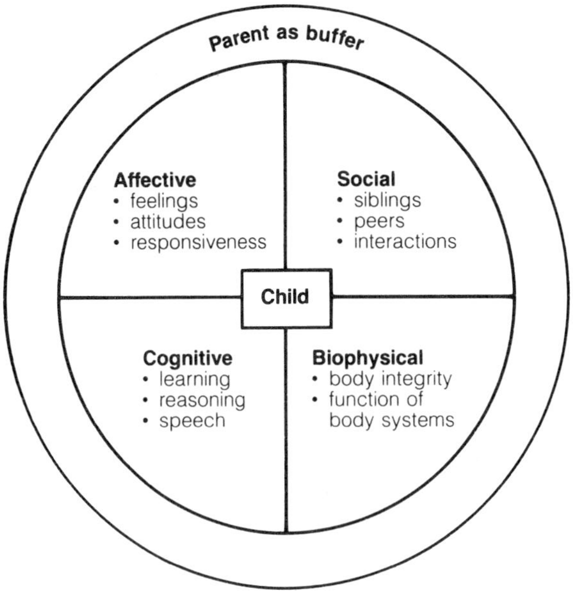

FIGURE 1-4

The child's four areas of development define each child's internal functioning.

alteration in one facet of a child can alter the others. For example, the state of emotional balance that exists between child and parents clearly will be redefined if those parents divorce. The divorce would put *stress* on the parents' emotional relationship with the child and might adversely affect the child physically and socially. Illness also places stress on a particular body system, thus altering the body's internal equilibrium. Other body systems and the other aspects of the child's internal and external environments are affected also.

Children in relation to themselves Like adults, children maintain intimate interaction with their physical and psychologic selves. Each child's unique characteristics can be grouped into four internal realms: biophysical, affective, cognitive, and social (Fig. 1-4). These areas are useful for categorizing, defining, and describing the main aspects of individual growth and development. Growth and development in each area is a continual process. The ongoing interaction among these areas helps distinguish children from each other. It also helps to determine each child's response to illness through such mechanisms as coping behaviors.

The *biophysical* component refers to the child's body integrity, including development and function of body systems. The *affective* component includes the child's feelings, attitudes, responsiveness, and other factors that help determine the development of ego and self-concept (see Chapter 3). Children who participate in activities to the best of their abilities, and who know their strengths and limitations

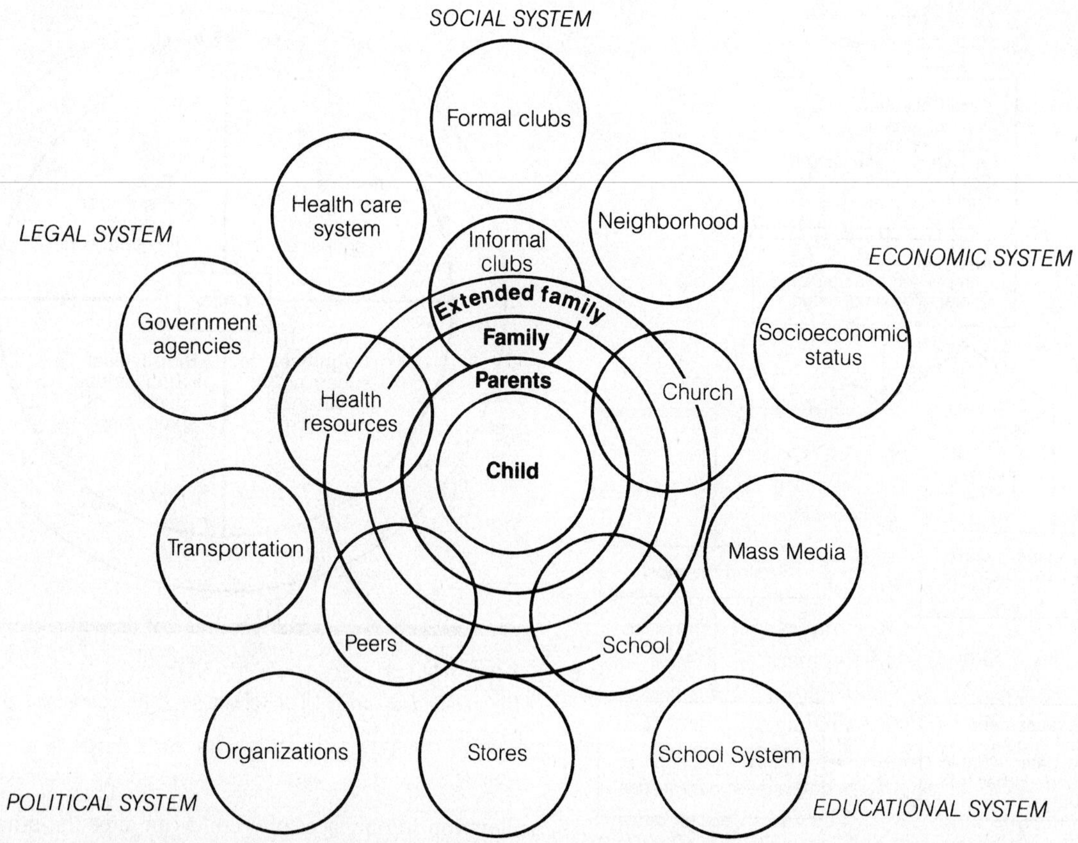

FIGURE 1-5
Throughout the process of growth and development, the child interacts with a variety of resources in the external environment.

have achieved a realistic sense of self. The child's affective development is related to opportunities to interact with the environment.

Learning, reasoning, and communication comprise the *cognitive* realm. *Social* factors include those that help the child interact with others in ways that are considered appropriate by the society or culture in which the child lives. Learning to express one's feelings responsibly is part of social development, as is learning to respect the rights and feelings of others.

Children in relation to the external environment Children are not isolated entities. Each child maintains a relationship with the surrounding environment. The child contributes to the environment, and environmental influences help shape the child's life and character. The child interacts with important resources in the environment, and the specific nature of this interaction helps to distinguish one child from another. These resources include the family, the extended family, school, friends, the community, religious and ethnic groups, government agencies, and the nation. These environmental resources interact not only with the child but also with each other (Fig. 1-5).

In the early years of development, the child often does not interact directly with some resources within the environment but relates to them through the mediation of parents. Thus, the parent acts as a buffer between the young child and the environment (Fig. 1-6). As the child grows, other spheres of influence, such as school and peer relationships, become more important.

Self-care Looking at children simply as the sum of their internal and external environments gives a flat, rather than a multidimensional, view of each child. The interaction with these internal and external resources, however, adds the missing dimension to a holistic perspective of nursing care. The child does not merely exist in an environment but actively uses the environment to enhance growth. If nurses expect to provide holistic nursing care to children and families, they need to examine how children and families ac-

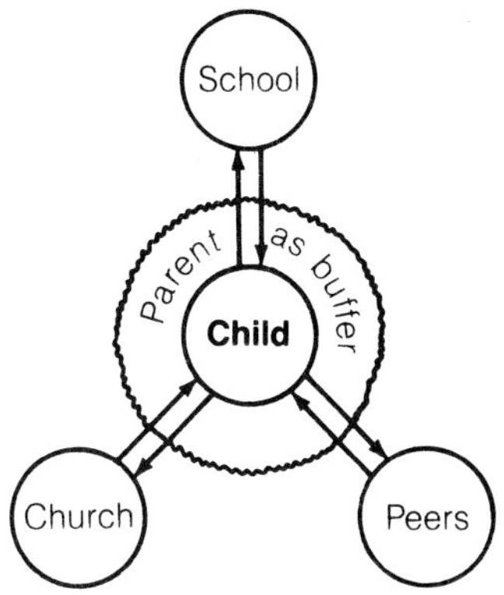

FIGURE 1-6

During the early years of a child's development, the parent acts as a buffer between the child and the external environment.

tively use their environmental resources to maintain health and to promote growth and development.

Self-care is a response by the child or parent to a need presented by the external or internal environment (Orem, 1980). For example, the sensation of hunger alerts the child to the body's need for nutrients and results in activities directed toward obtaining food. Likewise, the sensation of cold prompts a child to dress warmly.

An individual's means of satisfying these environmental needs also can be termed *activities of daily living* (ADL). These are behaviors basic to human existence, functioning, and development. Activities of daily living also define an area of special interest to nursing because nursing emphasizes health maintenance, health promotion, and disease prevention. In performing routine ADL, the child—or adult if the child is incapable—initiates self-care activity. Activities of daily living are learned behaviors and learning differs from child to child.

Activities of daily living are those activities directed toward responding to the basic human needs. (Table 1-4 summarizes these needs and some corresponding self-care activities.) These needs and activities apply to both children and adults.

Other self-care behaviors of children and parents specifically promote a child's development and so are important to the child health nurse. *Developmental self-care behaviors* are actions used by the child or parent to support the normal process of growth and development. These behaviors are particularly important to children, whose growth, development, and maturation are continually progressing to higher levels of achievement. As the child's perspective and abilities change, the child and parent's self-care activities for health maintenance and the prevention of illness change as well.

Nurses need to know the child's developmental status in order to teach, and encourage parents to teach, self-care skills appropriate for the child's development. For example, a developmental self-care behavior to promote biophysical development might be providing the child with supplies (eg, crayons, pencils, and blunt scissors) that help to develop fine motor skills. Self-initiated exploration of the environment is a developmental self-care behavior that promotes cognitive growth. In their exploration, children apply concepts by using them in systematic thinking and problem solving.

Self-care is an area in which nurses have the opportunity to teach the principles of health and to assist children and families to identify and use their resources in achieving health. The nurse, however, needs to be cautious before introducing changes in self-care activities, to be certain that these changes will not upset the balance between the environmental resources. For example, before encouraging a teenager to seek routine gynecologic care on her own, the nurse would want to assess the adolescent's relationship with the parent and determine whether the relationship is stable and whether this self-care activity would adversely affect that relationship.

For a child health nurse to give holistic nursing care to children and families, an assessment of developmental self-care activities is necessary. Guidelines for assessing children and families and assisting them with developmental self-care behaviors are presented in Chapters 4–8.

Decision making The philosophy of self-care suggests that the child or parent takes an active role in the decision-making process and then follows through with behaviors that are directed toward achieving the desired goal. Children imitate actions more than words. They look to parents and other family members, friends, and significant people as role models—as demonstrators of self-care behaviors. The actions and responses children observe tend to be the ones they choose when the decision-making responsibility is theirs.

Decision making is a learning experience that begins during childhood and continues throughout adulthood. This experience helps the child grow from dependence on parents for care to independence in self-care. The child becomes aware of the meaning, significance, and/or insignificance of events from experiences, from observing role models, and from education. "Children learn responsible self-care when they are allowed to choose from alternatives, take action and evaluate consequences" (Eichelberger et al., 1980). Although the child's decision might not always be the best one, the opportunity to make choices concerning self-care and to evaluate the results is an important part of the child's learning.

Individuals have their own definitions of health and make their own decisions about seeking health information

TABLE 1-4 Self-Care Activities

Basic need	Self-care activity	Implications
Air, Water, Food		
Air—includes exchange of gases in the lungs and within the cells as well as the body's ability to metabolize hemoglobin and utilize oxygen	Avoid air pollutants. Decrease high altitude activity. Rest after running. Perform regular aerobic exercise.	Basic needs are initially met by parents responding to neonate's cry. As child develops, self-care is assumed by the child. Adequate provision for these needs depends on knowledge and acceptance of their importance. Methods of self-care are related to cultural influences.
Water—demands vary according to activity, fluid loss, and dietary intake	Take in fluid.	
Food—essential for growth and repair of body tissue	Take in a nutritious, well-balanced diet.	
Elimination—includes urine, feces, perspiration, menstrual flow, and seminal fluid	Practice personal hygiene and take responsibility for care of the environment. Properly dispose of excrements. Attend to sanitation principles to prevent disease spread.	
Activity and Rest—activity expends energy; rest is a change from one activity to another that provides restoration of energy	Select stimulating activities that balance physical movement, affective response, intellectual effort, and social interactions. Attend to and respond to needs for rest and activity.	Infants might become irritable with overstimulation and might require parental intervention to provide rest. Children often have conflicts between the body's need for rest and their interest in the stimulating activity. Parental intervention might be necessary, even though the child is old enough to seek appropriate rest.
Solitude and Social Interaction—balance of being alone and being with others	Make choices that balance need for social contact and solitude.	Social interactions with adults and peers are important, but children need time periods for regrouping.
Safety—includes all aspects of preventing hazards such as acute disease and accidents	Use strategies that protect the self and promote normal function and development. Avoid known hazards.	Good health habits and safety principles are accepted more readily if demonstrated and practiced by parents.
Being Normal—includes being physically and mentally healthy relative to cultural norms	Select health maintenance activities, such as physical and dental examinations, immunizations, and good personal hygiene.	

SOURCE: Orem DE: *Nursing Concepts of Practice*. McGraw-Hill, 1980.

or assistance. Nursing plays an important role in preparing children and families to make these decisions. Nurses influence decision making by sharing information and by their ability to discuss different options and their potential results.

Health deviation Sometimes the child's self-care activities or the parental caretaking activities need to change in response to disease or injury. The extent of this alteration is related to the severity or complexity of the health deviation or its management. Some situations are relatively minor, such as a head cold, and the child and/or parent have the knowledge and experience to cope. When this is the case, adjustments are made in self-care activities until the disease or injury is healed and health is restored. At other times, the health deviation might exceed the parent and/or child's knowledge, experience, or ability, and the child might need to become a receiver of health care.

Health deviation results in subtle or obvious changes in the child's appearance, functioning ability, and/or feelings of well-being. Recovery from a health deviation may happen quickly, with few, if any, lasting effects, or after a prolonged healing period with many episodes of pain and disability. The specific course over time will determine the kinds of care demands the child and family will experience.

When an illness or injury is beyond their ability to manage, parents seek assistance from health care professionals. They exercise self-care in assuming responsibility and in deciding whose advice to seek. Treatments often require a change in lifestyle or living habits. For instance, medical diagnostic tests and treatments may necessitate changes in behavior and limit freedom of choice, with such requirements as having to take medication, modify normal activities, or change dietary habits. Surgical procedures usually result in pain, limitation of mobility, an intentional wound, a temporary or permanent change in appearance, and some modifications in self-concept.

The nature of the treatment determines, in part, the role of the child or parent. Some treatments exceed a parent's abilities and require the skill and knowledge of professionals. Such treatments include surgical interventions and intensive medical and nursing management. Many other treatments or procedures can benefit from the child's and/or parent's participation, either as active participants or as informants about preferences and dislikes.

Health deviation and its treatment thus require adjustments by the child and family. These adjustments will range from minimal to major depending on the individual situation. They are related to the ability and support the child and parent have (1) to adapt to new ways of meeting universal and developmental self-care needs, (2) to establish new techniques of self-care, (3) to modify expectations and self-image, (4) to revise the routines of daily living, (5) to develop a new lifestyle compatible with the health deviation, and (6) to cope with the effects of the health deviation or its medical management.

Assessment

The assessment phase of the nursing process consists of two parts—data collection and analysis. During assessment, the nurse applies the framework for organizing information about the child and family. Keeping in mind the child's interactions with the environment and the child's basic self-care needs and activities, the nurse gathers data both formally and informally.

Data collection The nurse uses all available methods in collecting data, including observation, communication, inspection, palpation, auscultation, percussion, and laboratory results. The sources of these data include the child, family, friends, environment, health records, and other members of the health care team. Whatever the source or method, the cooperation and trust of the child or family is important, because to be valuable, the information must be accurate.

The nurse also is careful to gather both subjective and objective data. *Subjective data* are derived from the child's or parent's perceptions. These data usually describe what the child is thinking or feeling and often take the form of a complaint. For example, the child might describe shortness of breath, nausea, or itching.

Objective data, on the other hand, are what the nurse observes. Objective data might include diminished breath sounds, vomiting, or a skin rash. The nurse needs to take into account the child's own perception of the data, as determined by personal values, cognitive abilities, or cultural background.

To give the data collection activity a systematic order, an organizing framework is a useful nursing tool. Gordon (1987) describes 11 functional health patterns that not only provide an organized framework for assessment but also assist with grouping nursing diagnoses—the next phase of the nursing process. The following list provides an ordered, structured method for collecting data about the child according to self-care behaviors and Gordon's functional health patterns.

- Introduction
- Brief health history
- Internal environment—growth and development
  - Biophysical (physical examination)
  - Cognitive
  - Affective
  - Social
- Functional health patterns
  - Health perception—health management
    - Hygiene
    - Physical checkups
    - Immunizations
    - Dental health
    - Safety
  - Nutritional-metabolic (food and fluids)
  - Elimination
  - Activity-exercise
  - Sleep-rest
  - Cognitive-perceptual (sensory, memory)
  - Self-perception—self-concept (body image, emotions)
  - Sexuality-reproductive
  - Role relationship

Family (immediate and extended)

Culture (language and traditions)

Peers

Clubs, hobbies, organizations

Socioeconomic status

Community resources

Housing

Play space

School

Coping-stress tolerance (coping mechanisms, soli tude, and social interaction)

Value-belief (religion)

Health deviation

Response to alteration in function

Response to treatment

Other nurse theorists have proposed alternate methods of organizing assessment data. As the nursing profession continues to evolve, the theoretic basis for nursing care will be more clearly defined.

Assessing internal factors Using a structured approach, the nurse assesses the child's self-care activities with reference to internal and external environmental factors. For example, the nurse would assess the biophysical component by observing the child's ability to perform appropriate gross and fine motor skills. Other parameters, such as height, weight, anatomic proportions and functions, physiologic functioning and intactness, and general health status, also would be assessed.

Cognitive functions to be assessed include acquisition of knowledge, logical thinking, and ability to learn related to the developmental level. The child's adaptability to change, ability to cope with stress, or any dysfunction or delays in cognitive development are noted. (Chapters 4–8 describe age-appropriate developmental norms.)

Data from the affective realm indicate whether the child's personality development has been steady, resulting in a positive self-image. The nurse notes any expressed or implied feelings of anger and dissatisfaction with self, which can indicate a negative self-concept.

Finally, the nurse assesses such characteristics as the child's ability to interact with others, preferences for peers or adults as companions, and the contribution of social interaction on the child's growth and development. Whichever area is being assessed, both assets and deficits are identified.

Assessing external factors Equally important to a complete assessment is information gathered about external environmental resources, especially the parents, and about activities of daily living. This assessment would include parental roles, parenting style, and the parents' own styles of interacting with each other.

Additional information also can be valuable. Such data might include religion—type, use, and importance to the child and family; culture, including nationality; language spoken at home; traditions; rituals; beliefs; folklores; and definition of health.

Also valuable is information regarding the influence of extended family members as well as the family's socioeconomic status, living conditions, and financial concerns. Important to note is the hierarchy of values for both child and family and especially the place of health in that hierarchy.

The knowledge base the nurse needs to make an assessment of the external environment includes several elements. It is essential, for instance, that the nurse have a working knowledge of, or an available resource that describes, the important beliefs and traditions of the various religions, cultures, and socioeconomic groups. The nurse also needs a theoretic knowledge of family roles and dynamics that can be applied to specific families.

One way of observing the child's use of internal and external resources is to assess behavior related to the activities of daily living. The individual's performance of these basic functions of living will reveal characteristic choices and behaviors.

The nurse learns from the child or significant others how facts are perceived and what they mean to those involved. The following questions are a useful guide:

1. What are the child's or family's attitudes, perceptions, values, or beliefs about health?
2. What are the significant influences from culture, socioeconomic status, education, or past experience?
3. Does this particular encounter with the health care professional represent a crisis for the child or family?
4. What are the child's and family's typical coping behaviors and available resources?

Analysis *Analysis* is the thought process that leads from assessment to the nursing diagnosis. It combines inductive and deductive reasoning. In the art of analysis, the nurse takes the assessment data, sorts them according to a conceptual framework, compares them with accepted norms, identifies areas of potential or actual deficit and areas of strength, and, finally, identifies the diagnostic description that best fits the data.

A nurse's analytic and diagnostic skills develop as experience accumulates. These skills are based on the theoretic and factual knowledge acquired in the biologic, behavioral, and social sciences. This knowledge provides the norms against which the nurse can assess variations and their significance. A broad base of knowledge allows for a holistic view of the child and family, of their environment, and of their abilities to adapt to life's stressors. Recognizing these areas for assessment forms the basis for the nurse's analytic interaction with the child (Brodish, 1982).

In performing the task of analysis, the nurse necessarily is influenced to some extent by personal perceptions, values, attitudes, and expectations. For this reason, the nurse needs to be as conscious as possible about personal values and biases to ensure they are not substituted for those of the child and family. If the nurse obtains insufficient data during assessment, the likelihood is greater that gaps will exist and that some of the information will be interpreted from a personal perspective rather than from the child's or parent's viewpoint. The perspectives may or may not coincide, but the nurse is always alert to the possibility of a difference.

Nursing Diagnosis

The product of data collection and analysis is the nursing diagnosis. The *nursing diagnosis* is a comprehensive summary statement of actual or potential alterations in the child's health status. The diagnostic statement is the result of the nurse's analysis of the data.

The nursing diagnostic statement is composed of two parts: The first part is the response—the category label derived from the assessment data; the second part defines the contributing factor as it relates to the response. The following examples illustrate both parts:

Impaired mobility (response) related to bilateral corrective leg casts (contributing factor)

Potential for poisoning (response) related to developmental stages and presence of lead paint (contributing factors)

Parental anxiety (response) related to anticipation of child's surgery (contributing factor)

Knowledge deficit (response) related to nutritional needs of infant (contributing factor)

Those problems that are potential do not necessarily require definition of the contributing factor. Often the contributing factor is not identifiable until the problem becomes actual. However, potential problems require interventions to prevent them from becoming actual. Therefore, they are identified.

The summary statement, or diagnosis, is chosen by referring to the list of categories for accepting nursing diagnoses. The current diagnostic categories are not complete and generally are oriented to adult situations. Sometimes the diagnostic category is too general and needs a modifying statement to make it appropriate for the child. Occasionally, the nurse needs to construct a new diagnosis because of the unique characteristics of the child's health situation. Child health nurses can contribute to the development and formulation of nursing diagnoses by defining those that are specific for the health status of the developing child and family.

One diagnosis that is encountered frequently, for instance, is altered growth and development. This general category needs to be individualized by stating the nature of the delay, such as cognitive, biophysical, or a combination of several areas, and by providing relevant assessment criteria. Another example is parental anxiety or parental fatigue caused by the child's health deviation or its treatment and the resulting change or increased demands placed on the parent.

Although the current taxonomy is incomplete, it still provides a valuable source of categories that have a common meaning and implication for subsequent nursing actions. "No diagnostic classification scheme is ever complete, owing to increasing knowledge and precision in differentiating various syndromes" (Mallick, 1983).

Each of the established diagnoses has assessment data that support it. These are cues that help the nurse arrive at the diagnosis. Thus, if the assessment of the child reveals data specific for a particular diagnosis, the nurse can more easily see which diagnoses apply to the child. For instance, Daniel is an 18-month-old boy seen by the nurse for a routine health checkup. The nurse notes the following:

> *Objective data:* Eight white teeth—four upper and four lower incisors visible; mouth appears in a healthy state.
>
> *Subjective data:* Parents state they give Daniel a bottle of juice or milk when putting him to bed for the night; parents report that they do not brush Daniel's teeth and ask questions about how to proceed with this; parents state they have fluoridated water.

Looking at the data, the nurse might arrive at the following nursing diagnosis: alteration in health maintenance related to knowledge deficit about dental health.

Nursing diagnoses are distinct from medical diagnoses. Medical diagnoses focus on pathologic processes and the means of cure, whereas nursing diagnoses focus on the child's and/or parent's response to the physical, psychosocial, or cognitive effects of the health deviation or its treatment. (See Table 1-5 for a comparison of other characteristics of the two models.)

Nursing diagnoses are holistic and can include responses

List of Approved Nursing Diagnoses (North American Nursing Diagnosis Association)

Activity intolerance
Activity intolerance, Potential
Adjustment, Impaired
Airway clearance, Ineffective
Anxiety
Body temperature, Alteration in: Potential
Bowel elimination, Alteration in: Constipation
Bowel elimination, Alteration in: Diarrhea
Bowel elimination, Alteration in: Incontinence
Breathing pattern, Ineffective
Cardiac output, Alterations in: Decreased
Comfort, Alteration in: Chronic pain
Comfort, Alteration in: Pain
Communication, Impaired: Verbal
Coping, Family: Potential for growth
Coping, Ineffective family: Compromised
Coping, Ineffective family: Disabling
Coping, Ineffective individual
Diversional activity deficit
Family processes, Alteration in
Fear
Fluid volume, Alteration in: Excess
Fluid volume deficit, Actual
Fluid volume deficit, Potential
Gas exchange, Impaired
Grieving, Anticipatory
Grieving, Dysfunctional
Growth and Development, Altered
Health maintenance alteration
Home maintenance management, Impaired
Hopelessness
Hyperthermia
Hypothermia
Incontinence, Functional
Incontinence, Reflex
Incontinence, Stress
Incontinence, Total
Incontinence, Urge
Infection, Potential for
Injury, Potential
Knowledge deficit
Mobility, Impaired physical
Neglect, Unilateral
Noncompliance
Nutrition, Alterations in: Less than body requirements
Nutrition, Alterations in: More than body requirements
Nutrition, Alterations in: Potential for more than body requirements
Oral mucous membranes, Alterations in
Parenting, Alterations in
Parenting, Alteration in: Potential
Poisoning, Potential for
Posttrauma response
Powerlessness
Rape trauma syndrome
Self-care deficit: Feeding, bathing/hygiene, dressing/grooming, toileting, total
Self-concept, Disturbance in: Body image, self-esteem, role performance, personal identity
Sensory-perceptual alteration: Input deficit
Sensory-perceptual alteration: Input excess
Sexual dysfunction
Sexuality patterns, altered
Skin integrity, Impaired
Skin integrity, Impaired, potential for
Sleep pattern disturbance
Social interaction, Impaired
Social isolation
Spiritual distress
Suffocation, potential for
Swallowing, Impaired
Thermoregulation, Ineffective
Thought processes, Alteration
Tissue integrity, Impaired
Tissue perfusion, Alteration in: Cerebral, cardiopulmonary, renal, gastrointestinal, peripheral
Urinary elimination patterns, Altered
Urinary retention
Violence, Potential for: Self-directed or directed at others

SOURCE: Lederer JR et al: *Care Planning Pocket Guide*. Addison-Wesley, 1986, Proceedings from the NANDA conference, 8/1/86, and Gordon M: *Manual of Nursing Diagnosis*. McGraw-Hill, 1987.

TABLE 1-5 Characteristics of Medical and Nursing Diagnoses

Medical diagnosis	Nursing diagnosis
Describes a specific disease process	Describes an individual's response to a disease process, condition, or situation
Is oriented to pathology	Is oriented to the individual
Remains constant throughout the duration of illness	Changes as the patient's responses change
Guides medical management, some of which may be carried out by the nurse	Guides independent nursing care, that is, nursing orders (therapies) and evaluation
Is complementary to the nursing diagnosis	Is complementary to the medical diagnosis
Has a well-developed classification system accepted by the medical profession	Has no universally accepted classification system; such systems are in the process of development

SOURCE: Kozier B, Erb G: *Fundamentals of Nursing*. 3rd ed. Addison-Wesley, 1987.

resulting from the child's interaction with various adverse aspects of the environment. Air pollution created by industrial wastes, for example, may result in an ineffective breathing pattern for the child with asthma.

Lack of knowledge can be a contributing factor to nursing diagnoses that describe an inability to meet self-care needs. This area has particular importance for the child health nurse, whose role often includes teaching, role modeling, and supporting learning behaviors.

Nursing diagnoses are an integral part of the nursing process and are the means by which nurses communicate with each other concerning the identified health alterations for which nurses assume responsibility and therapeutic decision making. By arriving at a commonly agreed on standard and a complete list of nursing diagnoses, the nursing profession can achieve greater consistency in communication with the public about exactly what nurses do.

Price (1980) suggested the following five questions the nurse could ask to validate the nursing diagnosis formulated:

1. Are the data sufficient, factual, accurate, and conceptually based?
2. Is there a pattern to the data as analyzed?
3. Are the child's or parent's data consistent with that of the nursing diagnosis?
4. Does the nursing diagnosis correspond to scientific nursing knowledge and clinical experience?
5. Would most other nurses concur with the diagnosis?

Nursing diagnoses facilitate outcome-directed nursing care. The data that enable the nurse to diagnose actual or potential health alterations or deficits in self-care also indicate the type of assistance the child or family requires. Nursing activities can then focus on stated goals, or outcomes. Achievable outcomes over long and short periods of time are the basis for a plan of care. Once nursing diagnoses are formulated, the nurse can develop a nursing care plan that is appropriate, individualized, and promotes health.

Planning

A nursing care plan that will help the child and family maintain or regain health is developed in the *planning* phase of the nursing process. Planning is a dynamic, goal-oriented process. The plan needs to be specific, needs to relate to the stated diagnosis, and needs to reflect the child's and/or parent's participation.

The nurse and child and/or parent discuss and agree about assessment data, analysis, and nursing diagnoses. Together they define and set mutual goals. Listing expected outcomes gives direction to the actions of the nurse, the child, and the parent, thus ensuring cooperation and collaboration.

Expected outcomes Expected outcomes are specified for each nursing diagnosis. Goals need to be realistic and attainable, and they need to be agreed on by child and parent. In addition, they need to be compatible with the desired result. Statements of outcomes provide the nurse with a standard by which to evaluate nursing actions, that is, to determine whether nursing actions are indeed helping to reach the goal.

Some expected outcomes might take a long period of time to achieve. They might pertain to rehabilitation, to prevention of complications from a health deviation, or to the adaptations needed for self-care. Statements of these outcomes are general and relate to an overall goal.

Other outcomes are specific behaviors or changes in behavior that are steps toward achieving an overall goal. Regardless of the time period for attaining an outcome, outcomes are stated as observable and measurable actions or responses that are clearly defined and understood by all. Outcomes change as some are attained and new ones are identified according to the child's new status.

The active participation by the child and parent in helping to define goals, to determine priorities, to request additional information, or to be involved in decisions about treatment is an important component of planning. When plans take into account the parent's values, ideas, and beliefs, communication is improved, and the nurse's perspective will be more holistic.

Nursing care plan The second aspect of planning is the identification of appropriate nursing actions that will assist the child or parent to reach the goals and thus will resolve the problems identified by diagnoses. These nursing actions are the *nursing interventions.*

The planning phase enables the nurse to organize the interventions so that they are purposeful, thorough, and based on scientific principles. The plan provides direction, so that nurses can use their time and energy efficiently and effectively. Together the nurse and child or parent discuss each nursing diagnosis and decide whether (1) no intervention is required at this time; (2) another resource or health team member is more appropriate (for example, social worker for financial concern, minister for spiritual problem); or (3) nursing intervention (assistance, support, teaching) is indicated.

Usually, several nursing interventions are required for each diagnosis. Armed with knowledge, previous experience, and scientific principles, the nurse formulates interventions and writes them down in an accessible location. Each intervention describes a specific action and its frequency.

Interventions (Implementing the Plan)

Interventions may be thought of as the doing, or action, part of nursing. This action is not routine but is "intellectual, interpersonal, and technical in nature" (Stanton, Paul, & Reeves, 1980). Orem (1980) divided the extent of nursing interventions into three general categories: wholly compensatory, partly compensatory, and supportive-educative. These categories reflect the balance of active participation in the intervention by child, family, and nurse.

While performing interventions, the nurse continually evaluates their appropriateness in relation to the individual's abilities and health status. This ongoing evaluation guides the nurse in the selection and extent of interventions required by the individual (Table 1-6).

Wholly compensatory interventions The individual who is totally dependent because of age or health status requires assistance to meet needs. For example, the infant requires total care, as does someone who is unconscious or severely ill. In most cases the situation is temporary because as the infant grows and the ill recover, the nurse uses other interventions that begin to involve the individual in self-care. At other times, the ill person does not regain the ability for self-care and requires total care until death. Because the nurse wholly compensates for a child or family's needs, these interventions are termed "wholly compensatory."

Partly compensatory interventions In some situations the nurse and child-parent unit work together to meet needs. For example, the child and/or parent might provide self-care except for the technical maneuvers necessary to treat an illness or injury.

The nurse's role varies and is related to (1) the patient's degree of mobility, (2) the nursing knowledge and skills required, and (3) the patient's psychologic readiness to participate in self-care activities. In the event of illness or injury, the parent and child usually continue as much as possible to maintain the same caregiving and receiving relationship while the nurse performs and/or teaches the parents about the technical aspects of care. Partly compensatory interventions might include the nurse's assessing breath sounds, monitoring or adjusting equipment that provides increased humidity, and evaluating the hydration status and adequacy of gas exchange for an infant with a respiratory infection, while the parent feeds, changes, comforts, and plays with the infant.

Some nursing interventions are directed to the parents as caregivers instead of to the child. This would especially be true for parents of children who have chronic congenital conditions or acquired illnesses or injuries. In these situations the nurse initially performs and demonstrates the prescribed care and procedures as they are adapted to the particular situation. Support and assistance are then provided until the parents are psychologically and technically ready to perform the care.

Supportive-developmental (educative) interventions Supportive-developmental nursing actions are primarily teaching-learning activities. The participants are capable of providing for their self-care needs but require additional information, guidance, or direction to do so. As nurses interact with parents and children, they continually assess self-care activities, provide direction when change is required, and offer support and anticipatory guidance regarding developmental and safety issues.

By providing support and information, nurses assist individuals in decision making. The nurse's focus frequently is health promotion, with all areas of human functioning considered. When a health-related question arises, parents can seek the advice and counsel of the nurse, whose knowledge, experience, and judgment they respect.

The nurse continues to teach and to provide support as the child's condition or ability changes but adapts the extent

TABLE 1-6 Extent of Nursing Assistance Required*

	Wholly compensatory	Partly compensatory	Supportive–developmental
Individual	Passive—unable to provide self-care or health-related care, may or may not be able to verbalize preferences	Able to meet all or most self-care needs but not health-related or technical care needs; learning new or better ways to meet basic needs	Meets self-care and health-related needs
Nurse	Active—takes care of individual so basic, developmental and health-related needs are met—supports individual in independent role (decision-making control resides with the nurse)	Supports and guides individual learning, provides technical care; assists in decision making about health-related concerns; performs care for unmet self-care needs (decision-making control shared)	Teaches, supports, guides individual in decision making related to health (decision-making control resides with client)
Examples	Infant or young child when parent is absent—unconscious individual; total paralysis; severe, acute, or degenerative illness; major trauma	Mild to moderate acute or chronic illness or injury; growing, developing child learning self-care activities; adaptive behaviors being learned	Primary level care consultation

*The respective assistance in terms of nursing actions according to individual limitations, alterations, or deficits in providing self-care.

SOURCE: Adapted from Orem DE: *Nursing: Concepts of Practice*. McGraw-Hill, 1980.

of interventions to meet changing needs. The ideal is for children and parents to be self-sufficient, well-informed, and able to provide their own care or care of their dependent children. Child health nurses in some respects are like wise parents, who not only take care of their infants and provide basic necessities during the dependent years but also teach the children how to provide for their own needs and become independent. Knowledgeable and capable, the parents step aside yet remain available for consultation and additional help if and when needed and requested by the children. So too, nursing adjusts its involvement according to individual need (as illustrated in Table 1-6).

Evaluation

Evaluation is a continual part of the nursing process. In *evaluating*, the nurse determines whether the outcomes are being met or whether a new approach is indicated. If the results are those desired and change is in the planned direction, the interventions continue as planned. If the results are not those desired, the process is restarted, beginning with a reassessment and concluding with new interventions and further evaluation.

Evaluation includes both objective and subjective measurements. The child and parent provide an important means of evaluation as the nurse scrutinizes the care plan and determines whether the child and parent were assisted most effectively in regaining or improving health status or in resuming self-care activities.

Interacting with the child and parent to provide care, the nurse continuously evaluates their responses. These responses are compared with the stated outcomes to ascertain whether the nursing actions selected are assisting the child and parent to resolve the nursing diagnosis. The feedback gathered from their responses directs further nursing action.

Evaluation is central to the nursing process because it informs the nurse whether behavioral changes are occurring and whether they are occurring in the desired direction. (Table 1-7 summarizes the phases and activities of the nursing process.)

Implications of the Nursing Process

The use of nursing process requires gathering and integrating a considerable amount of assessment data because the environmental resources, the functioning of the child, and the characteristics of the parent-child interactions are all considered significant. The nursing process is an ongoing, dynamic process that works with child and family even when the setting for nursing action changes (eg, goes from

TABLE 1-7 Definitions and Activities Associated with the Nursing Process

Term	Definition	Activities
Nursing process	A series of planned steps or phases directed toward assisting patients and their support persons; the underlying scheme or methodology of nursing practice.	
Assessment	Obtaining and organizing essential information about a client	Data collecting History Nursing examination Reviewing records Interviewing Data analysis Comparing with standard Relating data collected Identifying gaps in information
Nursing diagnosis	A statement about the patient's response to actual or potential health problems and the etiologic and contributing factors	Sorting data Grouping data into patterns Identifying alterations in function or deficits in meeting self-care needs Comparing patterns to taxonomy of diagnostic categories Identifying response
Plan	A written guide for nursing intervention assisting the client to meet health needs and coordinating the care of nursing staff	Priority setting Goal setting Developing nursing orders Forming a nursing care plan Determining evaluation criteria
Intervention	Putting the nursing care plan into action (wholly compensatory, partly compensatory, or supportive-educative care)	Updating the data base Reviewing the plan with the patient Adjusting the plan as necessary Identifying and providing for safety precautions Determining needs for assistance Intervening as per the plan Analyzing feedback Communicating findings
Evaluation	Assessing the patient's response against predetermined standards	Identifying the appropriate standard Collecting and organizing the data Comparing the data with the criteria Establishing conclusions

SOURCE: Adapted from Kozier B, Erb G: *Fundamentals of Nursing*. 3rd ed. Addison-Wesley, 1987.

hospital to home). Nursing diagnoses that are the result of a thorough assessment of the interaction between child, parent, and the environment can delineate which self-care activities require nursing intervention. The written plan serves as a means of communication, so that nursing interventions are consistent, individualized, and outcome-directed. Ongoing evaluation ensures that the plan is current and effective. Once the nursing care plan is developed, the task of achieving health becomes a manageable and collaborative project for the nurse, child, and parent.

NURSING CARE PLAN *Sample*

Phase 1 (Assessment)

Assessment Data: Daniel — Age: 18 months

Objective Data: Eight white teeth—four upper, four lower; mouth appears in a healthy state.

Subjective Data: Parents give juice or milk in bottle to take to bed; parents report they do not brush the child's teeth and ask for assistance with the method of proceeding; drinking water is fluoridated.

Phase 2 (Diagnosis) Nursing diagnosis	Phases 3 and 4 (Planning and Interventions) Interventions	Rationale
Alteration in health maintenance related to knowledge deficit about dental health	Discuss what happens when food or sugar is held in the mouth overnight. Explain that saliva decreases during sleep so that substances remain on the teeth initiating excessive acid formation and erosion of tooth enamel	Foods, especially carbohydrates and sugar, are damaging to dental enamel if allowed to remain on teeth. The enzyme that breaks these substances down also destroys tooth enamel and causes dental caries. During sleep the process is faster because of decreased saliva
	Suggest switching Daniel to water at night. Begin by diluting the juice with water and increase the amount of water by 1 oz a night until by the end of a week the bottle contains only water	Diluting juice rather than going directly to water will allow the child to gradually adjust to the new taste and will avoid upset from an abrupt change in routine
	Have Daniel drink water after each meal to rinse the food from his mouth. This can be followed by brushing by the parent if the child will allow it	Rinsing the mouth after eating removes any leftover pieces of food. Brushing should be gentle at this age
	Begin to introduce the toothbrush by allowing Daniel to "brush" his teeth so that he can learn with time to play and practice	Brushing that is introduced as fun should be a positive experience. Time to play and experiment allows the child to learn by imitation. Parents will need to brush the child's teeth until the child is able to assume the task independently

Phase 5 (Evaluation)

Outcome: As a result of good dental hygiene, Daniel will be prevented from experiencing dental caries. Daniel's parents will describe the process of tooth decay and will discuss the relationship between putting Daniel to bed with a bottle and the occurrence of dental caries. His parents will demonstrate how to care for Daniel's teeth. Daniel will begin to brush his own teeth

Legal and Ethical Considerations

Rights of the Child and Family

Child health care has been affected by some important legislative landmarks facilitating improvements in the health and welfare of children. Some of the basic rights of the child and family have undergone much change and scrutiny in this century.

The creation of the Children's Bureau in 1912 was a major step in the improvement of health care for children. The functions of the Children's Bureau were as follows:

1. To recognize the rights of children for a safe birth and optimal healthy development to adulthood

2. To remove obstacles impeding the achievement of this goal
3. To prevent harmful conditions (Dolan, 1978, pp. 255–256)

Subsequent White House Conferences on children and youth (held approximately every 10 years) created state divisions on maternal-child health, modified child labor laws, accepted federal responsibility to assist in the development of healthy children, made it mandatory to report certain health problems such as phenylketonuria (PKU) and child abuse, and directed attention to minorities and the disabled (Dolan, 1978).

The United Nations declared the year 1979 as the International Year of the Child, stating, "The main objective of the year—to encourage raising significantly the level of services benefiting children on a permanent basis—ultimately implies an increase in financial resources dedicated to this end" (International Year of the Child 1979, p. 244).

In preparation for the International Year of the Child, the United Nations reaffirmed the *Declaration of the Rights of the Child,* which calls for freedom, equality of opportunities, the social and emotional benefits of love and security, and the enhancement of maximum potential for all children. Nurses have been working toward these goals as long as nursing of children has been recognized as a specialty. Nurses care for children in developing countries. As child advocates, nurses have vastly improved health services to the poor and underprivileged.

When applying the principles set forth in the *Declaration of the Rights of the Child,* it is evident that specific health rights can be applied to both children and families. These rights include provisions for adequate medical and dental care, including preventive and prophylactic treatment, regardless of the family's ability to pay. Access to adequate nutrition, whether at school or at home, also is of primary importance for good health (Parks, 1982).

The United States has enacted legislation to attain the goals listed in the *Declaration of the Rights of the Child.* The improvement in maternal and child health service (MCH) was guaranteed when written into the Social Security Act of 1935. Since then, the federal government has supported improved accessibility of services for women and children through additional legislation (Table 1-8). At present, many of these programs have been taken over by state and local governments under the block grant services. Block grants are awarded by the Office of Human Development Services, Administration for Children, Youth and Families, United States Department of Health and Human Services.

In addition to basic human rights, children and families

United Nations Declaration of the Rights of the Child

Principle 1

All children without exception shall enjoy the rights expressed in the Declaration, and they shall not be subject to discrimination for any reason.

Principle 2

Children have the legal right of access to opportunities and facilities, which promote optimal, holistic, development under conditions of freedom and dignity.

Principle 3

The child shall be entitled from birth to a name and nationality.

Principle 4

Children and mothers shall have access to adequate protection and security; this includes pre- and postnatal care, and adequate medical, nutritional, housing, and recreational services.

Principle 5

The disabled child has the right to receive special treatment, education, and care.

Principle 6

Children shall have access to services that enable them to stay with their parents and to grow in an atmosphere of affection and security.

Principle 7

Children have the right to receive a free and compulsory elementary education that will help them develop to their full potential as useful members of society.

Principle 8

The child under all circumstances shall be among the first to receive protection and relief.

Principle 9

The child shall be protected against all forms of neglect, cruelty, and exploitation. Provides for employment restrictions for children.

Principle 10

All children have the right to be brought up in an atmosphere of peace and universal brotherhood free from discrimination and intolerance.

TABLE 1-8 Health Care Legislation Affecting Children

Title	Year	Function
Social Security Act	1935	Provides matching state and federal funds to encourage quality care for mothers and children as well as crippled children. Supports health promotion (screening, immunizations, and so on)
Maternal Child Health Maternal Infant Care Project	1963	Reduces infant handicaps and complications due to inadequate care of childbearing women. Decreases infant and maternal mortality. Provides diagnostic services and treatment for women for whom care is inaccessible
Children and Youth Project	1965	Meets health needs of children from targeted low-income areas or those for whom care is inaccessible
Medicaid	1965	Provides reimbursement for medical care to low-income families through state aid
Crippled Children's Services	1965	Locates, diagnoses, and treats disabled children under 21 years of age
National School Lunch Act and Child Nutrition Act	1966	Provides meals to children from low-income families for free or a reduced price according to income guidelines
Public Law 94–142—Education for All Handicapped Children Act	1975	Guarantees free public education with support services to all children regardless of handicap. Requires an updated educational plan specific to each child and encourages children to be placed as much as possible in an educational environment similar to peers of their age.

NOTE: Most of these programs formerly under the US Department of Health, Education, and Welfare are now administered by Block Grants to the states under the supervision of the US Department of Health and Human Services.

also possess legal rights that are particularly relevant for health personnel. While children contend with societal problems, such as sexually transmitted disease, drug addiction, birth control, and abortion, the courts have been interpreting the laws to ensure the child's access to adequate health care. Although children previously were regarded as possessions of their parents and therefore under total parental control concerning decisions regarding health care, the courts recently have reinterpreted this assumption to give some children more freedom to seek treatment or counseling.

Informed Consent

Children and parents have the right to know and understand the implications of any treatment or surgical procedure, including its possible adverse effects on health. Often, the parent needs to sign a consent form prior to any procedure that carries inherent danger to the child. It is a nursing responsibility to find out from child and parent their understanding of the procedure and its possible complications before any written consent is given.

Problems often occur in ill-defined areas, particularly those subject to interpretation of the laws. Two of these areas are particularly important to caregivers: (1) minors' consent for treatment, and (2) children's participation in research.

All children are minors, but some fall into one or both of the following categories:

Emancipated minor—a child who for various reasons is making responsible life decisions without parental supervision. This might include the minor who is pregnant or married, who is self-supporting and living away from home, or whose parents have abdicated responsibility for them willingly or unwillingly.

Mature minor—a child who by statutory regulations (age differs by state, but usually over 15 years) is of an age to make informed decisions and to understand the risks of medical interventions.

Emancipated minors may give consent for treatment. Depending on their financial status, college students may or may not be emancipated minors. Mature minors may give consent for treatment under some circumstances, particularly in emergency situations when parents are unavailable.

If minors give their own consent for treatment, they become financially responsible for the treatment given (Eldridge, 1979).

Certain issues are sensitive, and children often are unwilling to discuss them with parents. States differ concerning when treatment can be given without parental consent. Most states allow minors to obtain treatment for sexually transmitted disease and drug abuse and allow access to birth control without parental consent. Abortion is a more difficult issue, and laws concerning abortion vary by state.

Generally, strict adherence to confidentiality is the rule when children seek treatment for any of these reasons. Recently at issue, however, is whether parents should be informed after the treatment has taken place. Sources differ concerning the appropriateness of breaches of confidentiality but generally accepted practice dictates that if the physician feels duty-bound to inform parents about treatment, the child needs to be told before treatment begins.

Young children in the care of their parents cannot legally seek medical treatment on their own. Also, if the child is in the care of parents, other adults—such as relatives or school personnel—cannot initiate treatment without parental consent, except in emergency situations. Even in emergency situations, every effort is made to contact parents prior to treatments.

Children have rights when decisions are made to include them in research projects. Even very young children can understand explanations about treatments, and common practice is to enlist their cooperation in their care. When considering whether to include a child in research, decisions need to be made about whether the research will directly benefit the child and whether the research procedure is painful. Generally speaking, parents can give consent for the child to be a research subject in a project that will benefit the child directly, even if that research is invasive. In almost all cases, however, it is preferable to enlist the cooperation of the child. If the research is to benefit society or another individual, the child's right to refuse participation assumes greater importance. This becomes a difficult issue, particularly in organ transplants where the child's refusal to donate could result in later feelings of guilt. Options need to be presented carefully, so that the best decision for all can be made (Fromer, 1981).

In cases where the research is nontherapeutic, such as screening procedures, young children have the right to refuse participation after receiving adequate information (Fromer, 1981). If the children or parents refuse to participate or choose to withdraw from a research study, their decision cannot affect the quality of care they receive.

Legal Accountability of the Child Health Nurse

All nurses are responsible for maintaining high-quality standards of care regardless of the age of the client. Child health nurses are in a special position because of children's integral relationships with their families. The child health nurse is accountable for care given to the child within the family unit because rarely is a child seen as separate from family. Nurses giving less than high-quality care to the child-family unit are accountable for their actions to all members of the unit.

In addition to practicing high standards of health care, child health nurses are also responsible for considering rights of clients in the health care system, most specifically those of confidentiality, privacy, and self-determination. Nurses are responsible for maintaining accurate and descriptive records and for respecting the confidentiality of communications with their clients.

In a child health-care setting, respecting privacy and maintaining confidentiality can be difficult. Health professionals differ in their attitudes toward children. Some do not really accept the premise that children have the right to privacy. Behaviors such as talking freely about the child's problem with others or examining the child in front of others can become commonplace. Nurses need to be advocates for children's rights under these circumstances and can be held accountable if they are not.

Another problem with maintaining confidentiality often occurs in crowded settings. Well-meaning parents will ask questions about other children they see, placing nurses in the position of finding an acceptable method for tactfully avoiding answers that would compromise other patients' privacy.

Because children have certain rights of self-determination, and because some children will refuse treatments or medications, nurses need to use acceptable choices creatively in their care. Children should be allowed, as much as possible, to maintain control while still accepting necessary care. To force a child to accept a treatment can be construed as assault or battery, and the nurse can be liable for consequences (Cazalas, 1978). The overuse of restraints also is included in this category. The child health nurse therefore needs to be certain that restraints are necessary for the protection of the child and others and that the minimum amount of restraint is used.

Nurses also are accountable for reporting certain problems peculiar to children. For example, some communicable diseases (such as sexually transmitted disease and salmonella) must be reported to state public health departments. A positive test for phenylketonuria (PKU) also should be reported.

Most states make it mandatory to report suspected child abuse or neglect (see Chapter 13). Here the emphasis is on the word *suspected*. Nursing personnel must report any case of suspected child abuse to the appropriate agency. In their child abuse laws, most states also protect the informant from prosecution if the report is made with a sincere interest in protecting the child from harm.

Nurses have a responsibility to teach parent and child what they need to know about caring for the child after discharge from the hospital. Instructions need to be written, so that the parent can refer to them should there be any questions. Instructions include how to care for the child, a description of any necessary treatments or procedures, how to recognize complications, and whom to contact if complications should occur.

The final legal issue unique to child health nurses concerns the accountability of nurses who assume expanded roles. The increasing numbers of certified nurse practitioners have forced states to reexamine their Nurse Practice Acts to accommodate these expanded roles. There is still an ill-defined overlap in some states between medical duties and the duties of the nurse practitioner. This overlap has caused different interpretations of legal accountability. All nurses, however, are accountable for their actions and are autonomous regarding nursing decisions. As nurse practitioners establish practice as colleagues of physicians, Nurse Practice Acts will adjust accordingly. Meanwhile, it is the mandate of all nurses, regardless of their roles, to be familiar with the provisions of the Nurse Practice Acts in their states.

Future Directions in Child Health Nursing Care

The future directions of child health nursing are rooted in its past. Child health nursing as a specialty has affected the entire health care system. Large children's hospitals provide care for critically ill children, whereas the community hospitals manage children with less life-threatening medical conditions. Nursing, regardless of the setting, is becoming increasingly challenging and complex. When caring for children, nurses need to view themselves as primary client contacts and need to demand greater continuity of care. Many facilities still linger in the past, refusing to relax visiting hours and ignoring the fact that primary nursing facilitates the recovery and improved health care of the child-family unit. In their role as child advocates, nurses need to initiate changes and to accept the responsibility and accountability for the future directions of child health care.

Children growing and developing in a fast-paced world must be able to cope with the stresses of everyday living. Child health nurses will assume a more active teaching role in the hospital and community in their contacts with children of all ages. They will teach a variety of concepts designed to assist children and families in developing and using effective coping mechanisms. These concepts will include the following:

1. The importance of self-care activities in becoming responsible for one's own health
2. The interrelationship between mind and body—emotional and physical health
3. The effects of proper diet and exercise
4. The avoidance of health hazards and harmful substances
5. Stress reduction techniques

The emphasis is, and will be, on disease prevention. Nurses will be more creative, structuring health teaching to the child's age. They will more actively secure clients, both in a structured setting and as independent practitioners. Nurses will effect changes in health care through consumer education in the same way they have demonstrated the value and cost-effectiveness of health promotion.

In addition to health promotional activities, nurses will expand their role in the early identification of and intervention with high-risk families, particularly those with the potential for child abuse. Early prenatal and postpartum management of teenage mothers and their children will be essential because the rate of teenage pregnancies is rising dramatically. The greater number of single parents is a consequence of the increasing divorce rate and the number of unwed mothers. Additional concern is needed for the special needs of single-parent households, both within the community and when a child from this type of family is hospitalized.

Greater attention to the additional needs of children and youth is an important nursing goal. These "unmet needs" were described by an American Nurses' Association special committee in 1979 and included exploration into the problems of child abuse, substance abuse, adolescent sexual behavior, including adolescent pregnancy and sexually transmitted disease, mental health and suicide, and other more common health problems (Durand, 1979).

Computer Applications in Health Care

Hospitals are entering the computer age, heralding great changes in the delivery of health care. Nurses in large children's medical centers will need to be experienced in handling computers. Computerized medical information facilitates communication among members of the health care team and may lead to greater mobility and effectiveness of nurses. Children's health records retained in computer data banks facilitate a continuous monitoring of children's health status. Much more information is available to the child health nurse, enabling better care planning. Researchers will have access to lifelong health information, which they will use to identify the positive and negative influences contributing to health and disease.

This stored information can vastly improve the continuity of care. Consequently, however, a greater number of ethical questions will need to be addressed. Nurses need to be aware that the dangers of the computer age are similar to those of the mechanized age: that the uniqueness and humanness of clients will be lost without careful attention to their personal needs.

Advances in Nursing Research

To ensure a future of improved health care for children, advances need to take place in the area of nursing research. Nursing research has been conducted for years, but its focus has changed as its quality has improved. Historically, researchers investigated specific nursing procedures, curriculum theory, nurse-client relationships, and hospital management effectiveness (Gortner, 1980). Future research needs to be more comprehensive, examining the holistic approach to health care and consumer involvement in the health care system. Research will contribute to nursing theory.

Studies need to be conducted to evaluate the effectiveness of therapeutic intervention. Nursing's theory base needs to be defined further by the scientific replication of research (Gortner, 1980). Nurse researchers need to examine children's reactions to stress and the appropriate interventions to set patterns for good health practices and disease prevention. New techniques of nursing practice in nurses' relationships with children and families need to be evaluated and their practicality and cost-effectiveness tested.

Faced with an imminent nursing shortage, researchers can discover innovative approaches to increasing job satisfaction and generating new interest in nursing. Perhaps one of the major goals of nursing research should be "nurse advocacy." A definite, methodologic approach is needed to create and retain interest in nursing. If the profession is to survive, concerted efforts need to be directed toward this end.

DRGs: Impact on the Health Care System

In the spring of 1983, President Reagan signed into law House Bill 1900 (P.L. 98-21), the Social Security Amendment of 1983. This bill would begin to reform the health care industry by restricting the high escalation in medical costs. All of the implications of this bill for the health care system are not yet known, but, in the first few years since the passage of the bill many changes have occurred in health care delivery. These changes have had tremendous impact on the roles and functions of nurses.

Historically, hospitals were reimbursed by Medicare, Medicaid, and other third-party insurances according to the actual costs of caring for patients. As a result, medical costs have risen dramatically as new, expensive, technologic developments have come into more widespread use. Hospitals charged patients a per diem rate that calculated in the costs of equipment, supplies, nursing care, and other ancillary personnel, among other costs. Because Medicare and Medicaid payments to hospitals are government funded, the rising cost of medical care placed a greater burden on the taxpayer.

H.B. 1900 established a *prospective* payment plan to hospitals for Medicare and Medicaid patients. Under this new plan, the hospital would know ahead of time how much money it would be reimbursed for any particular patient. To assess standard payment rates, a classification system known as *diagnosis related groups (DRGs)* was developed.

A DRG is a combination of a medical diagnosis, the age of the patient at the time of admission, surgical procedures needed, and complications. There are 23 major diagnostic categories (MDCs) from which DRGs are derived and 467 DRGs, each with a code number as a subcategory of a major diagnostic category. Each code number prescribes the length of hospital stay and the prospective payment the hospital will receive. If the hospital discharges the patient earlier than prescribed and has kept the patient costs down, the hospital may keep the amount saved. If, however, the patient uses more of the hospital resources of time and money, the hospital loses money by having to absorb the extra cost.

For example, Bobby, age 2 years, is admitted to the hospital with the medical diagnosis of pneumonia. Pneumonia is in MDC 4, *Diseases and Disorders of the Respiratory System.* Because Bobby is under 17 years old and without complications, his projected length of stay would be 4.6 days—DRG 91. (DRG 91 and other DRGs associated with pneumonia are illustrated in Fig. 1-7.) If at some point during his admission he should develop complications from the disease, the DRG might be changed, or "upcoded," to a DRG that reflects a longer hospital stay with greater reimbursement for the hospital.

Implications for nurses Although DRGs were signed into law for hospitals serving Medicare patients, many third-party insurance companies are following suit by establishing prospective payment systems of their own. Thus, the child-health nurse needs to be aware of the effects of this system on nursing care of the child and family.

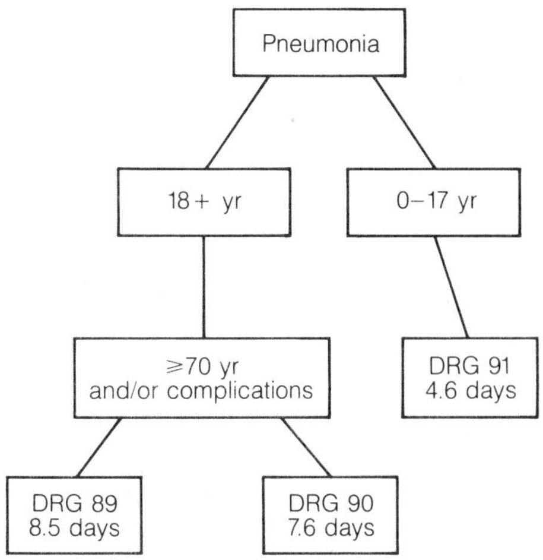

FIGURE 1-7
Major diagnostic category 4—diseases and disorders of the respiratory system—and associated diagnosis related groups (DRGs).

There are several immediate implications for nurses: (1) Nurses are required to know how the DRGs are assigned and to know the DRG status of their patients; (2) nurses need to become more conscious of keeping hospital costs down while still providing high-quality nursing care; (3) the nursing process will become even more important to quality patient care, particularly in evaluating the effectiveness of nursing actions; (4) discharge planning will begin at the time of admission and might have to be accelerated to prepare a family for discharge properly; and (5) to maximize the delivery of high-quality nursing care, nurses will have to decrease the time spent on nonnursing activities (Henderson and Sullivan, 1985).

Implications for the health care system The health care system will see increased emphasis on health promotion and disease prevention in an attempt to keep children out of the hospital setting. Children will be discharged earlier, requiring more complicated care at home. Hospitals might try to cut back on personnel or supplies, requiring careful monitoring by nurse advocates to preserve the standard of health care. Nurses might begin to reassume some of the functions of ancillary personnel, such as respiratory therapists and play therapists.

Other implications to the health care delivery system include the following: (1) the expense of primary nursing might indicate a return to the team nursing concept of care; (2) community health nurses will be required to care for children with more complex health care needs in the home; (3) nursing care will be closely studied to determine cost effectiveness; (4) a greater number of nurses will become independent practitioners moving from hospital to home to give care, with their fees charged to the patient or to insurers (Smith, 1985).

Nurses are at a crossroads. The future of nursing depends on how well nurses can demonstrate their value and cost effectiveness to the health care system. In their roles as consumer advocates and with their use of the nursing process as a vehicle for communication, nurses will be crucial to providing high-quality, holistic health care to children and families. As nurses practice the science and art of nursing, they play a pivotal role in focusing on the clients, the human rather than the mechanical aspects of health care.

Essential Concepts

- In the past 150 years child health care has altered its focus from a strictly curative approach to a holistic approach that encompasses every aspect of health.
- Child health nursing has evolved as a specialty keeping pace with the changes in child health care, society's view of women, quality control, and development of nursing standards.
- Over the years statistical data relative to child care have demonstrated a variable birth rate along with a steadily declining infant and child mortality rate.
- The most common cause of childhood death in the United States today is accidents.
- The child health nurse of the present may function autonomously in a variety of roles in both the community and the hospital, including the expanded roles of clinical specialist and nurse practitioner.
- The best nursing care creatively combines science and art: science as the knowledge of human biology, pathophysiology, and psychology and art as the creative and specific application of this knowledge to the health care needs of each individual child and family.
- The nurse involves the family in the decisions and activities of the child's care and considers the family itself as a client in potential need of care.
- Effective, holistic nursing care depends on an organized system for obtaining information that examines children in relation to their inner selves and to their external environments.

- The attributes of the child are the result of the combined functioning of four internal realms: the biophysical, cognitive, affective, and social domains of growth and development.
- Important resources in the child's environment interact with the child and help distinguish one child from another. The family, perhaps the most influential environmental resource, mediates the young child's interactions with the environment, thus creating a "buffer" while the child matures.
- The child and family do not merely exist in an environment but actually use the environmental resources to maintain health and promote growth and development. The activities used by the child and family are referred to as self-care activities.
- Nursing has an important role in preparing children and families to make choices with regard to health. These choices can be related to the resolution of eight basic needs.
- For the child, whose rapid rate of maturation is one of the most important characteristics, the nurse's assessment of the growth and development status with respect to physical, cognitive, affective, and social development is crucial.
- Health deviations affect the child and family's capacity for self-care and may require new adaptations and techniques to meet basic and developmental needs.
- Self-care is the result of making decisions to meet needs, and of taking appropriate actions based on the decisions.
- Assessment, or data collection and analysis, addresses the child in relation to the internal and external environments, identifying both assets and deficits. In assessment, the nurse uses a variety of methods, such as observing the child's own activities of daily living, physical assessment techniques, and assessment of family functioning.
- Nursing diagnoses are comprehensive summary statements of actual or potential alterations of health status, and are the means by which nurses communicate with each other about the identified health deviations or self-care deficits for which they assume responsibility and make decisions.
- Planning for the child's health care involves cooperation and agreement by the child and/or parent in setting mutual goals, identifying appropriate nursing actions to help the child or parent to reach these goals, and synthesizing these into a systematic and prioritized nursing care plan.
- Intervention, or implementing the plan, can fall into one of three categories, as described by Orem: wholly compensatory, as for an infant who requires total care; partly compensatory, as for the child or parent who can participate in some aspects of self-care; and supportive-developmental (educative), which consists of teaching and learning activities.
- Evaluation, a continual part of the nursing process, is the means by which the nurse determines whether the interventions were adequate or appropriate to meet the stated outcomes.
- Children in this society hold certain basic and legal rights, which child health nurses are responsible to protect.
- Child health nurses are accountable for their actions and have a responsibility to maintain high-quality standards of care regardless of the age of the child.
- Future directions in child health nursing include expanding such activities as promoting self-care within a holistic framework, advocating a clean and healthy environment for children, reducing child and family stress, effecting changes in health care delivery through consumer education, and intervening with high-risk families.

References

Brodish MS: Nursing practice conceptualized: An interaction model. *Image* (Feb/March) 1982; 14:5–7.

Cazalas MW: *Nursing and the Law.* Aspen, 1978.

Dolan J: *Nursing in Society.* Saunders, 1978.

Durand B: The ANA hearings on the unmet needs of children and youth. *Am J Matern-Child Nurs* (Nov/Dec) 1979; 6–8.

Eichelberger KM et al: Self-care nursing plan: Helping children to help themselves. *Pediatr Nurs* (May/June) 1980; 6:9–13.

Eldridge T: Adolescent health care—the legal and ethical implications. *Pediatr Nurs* 1979; 51–52.

Ford LC: U.S. circa 1976: Change and challenges in nursing education and practice. *Aust Nurses' J* 1976; 5:26–30.

Fromer MJ: *Ethical Issues in Health Care.* CV Mosby, 1981.

Gordon M: *Nursing Diagnosis Process and Application.* McGraw-Hill, 1982.

Gordon M: *Manual of Nursing Diagnosis.* McGraw-Hill, 1987.

Gortner S: Nursing research: Out of the past and into the present. *Nurs Res* 1980; 29:204–207.

Henderson D and Sullivan T: Diagnosis related groups: Effects on nursing. *JEN* (1985):117–118.

Holder A: *Legal Issues in Pediatrics and Adolescent Medicine.* Wiley, 1977.

Igoe J: Changing patterns in school health and school nursing. *Nurs Outlook* 1980; 28:487–488.

International Year of the Child 1979. *Nurs J India* 1978; LXIX:244.

Kinsella C: Who is the clinical nurse specialist? *Hospitals* 1973; 47:72.

Mallick MJ: Patient assessment—Based on data, not intuition. *Nurs Outlook* (Oct) 1983; 29:600–605.

Orem DE: *Nursing: Concepts of Practice.* McGraw-Hill, 1980.

Parks P: Student nurses' attitudes toward children's health rights: Implications for advocacy. *Child Health Care* (Summer) 1982; 11:25–29.

Pontious SL: Practical Piaget: Helping children understand. *Am J Nurs* (Jan) 1982; 82(1):114–17.

Price MR: Nursing diagnosis: Making a concept come alive. *Am J Nurs* 1980; 80(4):668–671.

Silver HD: The school nurse practitioner program. *JAMA* 1971; 216:1332–1334.

Smith C: DRGs—making them work for you. *Nurs '85* (January) 1985; 15(1):34–41.

Stanton M, Paul C, Reeves JF: An overview of the nursing process. In: *Nursing Theory: The Base for Professional Nursing Practice.* Nursing Theory Conference Group. Prentice-Hall, 1980.

Van Eys J (editor): *Research on Children.* University Park Press, 1978. *World Health Statistics Annual—1982.* World Health Organization, 1982.

Additional Readings

Avant KC, Walker LO: The practicing nurse and conceptual frameworks. *Matern-Child Nurs J* 1984; 9(2):87–90.

Bilitski JS: Nursing science and the laws of health: The test of substance as a step in the process of theory development. *Adv Nurs Sci* (Oct) 1981; 4:15–29.

Chance S: Nursing models: A requisite for professional accountability. *Adv Nurs Sci* (Jan) 1982; 5:57–65.

Chang BL: Evaluation of health care professionals in facilitating self-care: Review of the literature and a conceptual model. *Adv Nurs Sci* (Oct) 1981; 3:43–58.

Curtin L, Flaherty MJ: *Nursing Ethics: Theories and Pragmatics.* Brady, 1982.

Cushing M: Legal lessons on patient teaching. *Am J Nurs* 1984; 84(6):721–722.

Czupryna L: Primary prevention in a camp setting. *MCN* (May/June) 1984; 9:197–199.

DeStefano LK, Thomson H: *Manual of School Health.* Addison-Wesley, 1986.

Felton G: Harnessing today's trends to guide nursing's future. *Nursing and Health Care* (April) 1986; 211–213.

Fulginiti V: Pediatrics. *JAMA* (October 25) 1985; 254(16): 2293–2295.

Hauck MR, Roth D: Application of nursing diagnosis in a pediatric clinic. *Pediatr Nurs* 1984; 10(1):49–52.

Hemelt MD, Mackert ME: *Dynamics of Law in Nursing and Health Care.* 2nd ed. Reston, 1982.

Hollen P: A holistic model of individual and family health based on a continuum of choice. *Adv Nurs Sci* (July) 1981; 4:27–42.

Jameton A: *Nursing Practice: The Ethical Issues.* Prentice-Hall, 1984.

Justus M, Montgomery J: Current status of nursing process in ADN programs. *J Nurs Educ* (March) 1986; 25(3):118–120.

Kim MJ, McFarland GK, McLane AM: *Classification of Nursing Diagnoses: Proceedings of the Fifth National Conference.* Mosby, 1984.

King C: The self-help/self-care concept. *Nurs Pract* (June) 1984; 5(6):34.

Lederer JR et al: *Case Planning Pocket Guide.* Addison-Wesley, 1986.

McKibbin R et al: Nursing costs and DRG payments. *Am J Nurs* (December) 1985; 85(12):1353–1356.

Murchison I, Nichols T, and Hanson R: *Legal Accountability in the Nursing Process.* Mosby, 1982.

Nichols A: Physician extenders, the law, and the future. *J Fam Pract* 1980; 11:101–108.

O'Leary J: What employers will expect from tomorrow's nurses. *Nursing and Health Care* (April) 1986; 7(4):207–209.

Piper L: 10 ways to win the DRG game. *RN* (March) 1985; 48(3):18–20.

Romano C, McCormick KA, McNeely LD: Nursing documentation: A model for a computerized data base. *Adv Nurs Sci* 1982; 4(2):43–56.

US Department of Health and Human Services: *Monthly Vital Statistics Reports,* August 11 and October 18, 1983.

Walker LO, Avant KC: *Strategies for Theory Construction in Nursing.* Appleton-Century-Crofts, 1983.

Wajdowicz E: The Americanization of Florence: A look at associate degree nurses. *Nurs Health Care* (Feb) 1986; 7(2):97–99.

Waters S, Arbeiter J: Nurse practitioners: How are they doing now? *RN* (Oct) 1985; 48(10):38–43.

Woolley A: Defining the product of baccalaureate education. *Nurs Health Care* (April) 1986; 7(4):199–201.

Chapter 2

Environmental, Cultural, and Family Influences on the Child

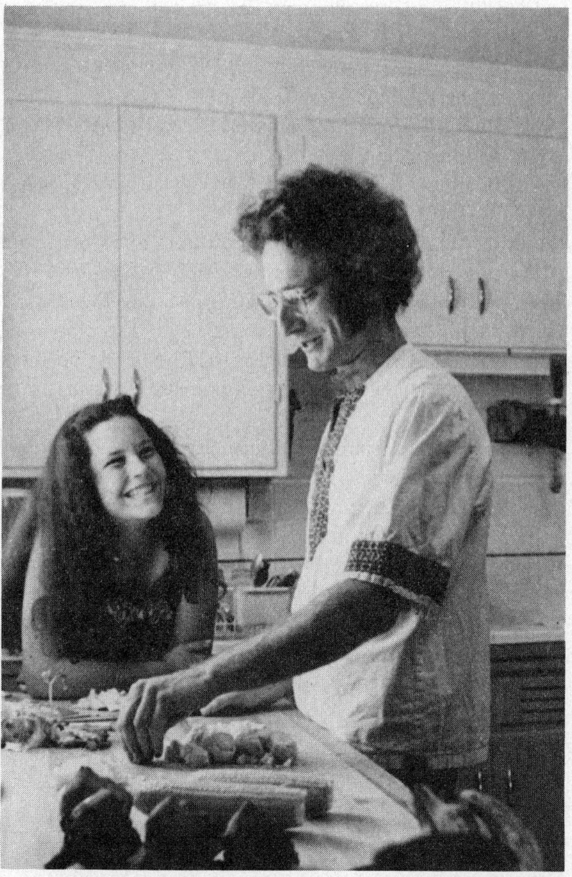

Chapter Contents

Objectives

- Define race, culture, ethnicity, community, and family.
- Discuss how the external environment of community, peers, school, and family influences the social development of children.
- Define current types of families and the needs they commonly present to the nurse.

- Define authoritative, authoritarian, and permissive parenting.
- Define the responsibility of the nurse in relation to awareness, communication, and accommodation in providing health care and teaching.

The acts and events that occur in the lives of children and their families take place in a broad social and cultural context. The more completely the nurse understands that context, the more realistic and accurate will be the view of the developing child. Understanding the society and culture in which the child lives allows the management of that child's health problems to be more humanistic and holistic.

The External Environment

The external environment includes both a social sphere and a cultural atmosphere. The social sphere includes people, such as the child's family, peers, and members of the larger community, and it includes influences from school, media, health care, government, and economy. The cultural atmosphere encompasses more intangible entities, such as norms, values, beliefs, morals, customs, knowledge, and attitudes. American society is extremely diverse ethnically, and it would be difficult to specify a single, uniform culture. Instead, the immigration of various groups, from colonial settlers to the more recent political refugees, has created a complex fabric in which some elements of culture are shared among most or all of the various ethnic or racial groups. Other elements of culture remain unique to a specific group. Effective nursing care of children and their families includes an understanding of and sensitivity to the complexity of cultures in American society.

American communities encompass the environmental, social, and economic conditions that typify local areas, whether these areas are small towns or identified sections of a large city. Housed within each community are services, such as the neighborhood schools, churches, shops, clubs, and health care centers. As the child grows older, the community takes a greater role in influencing attitudes and behavior. The family, however, is the basic social unit for the child. The composition of the family varies greatly from child to child, but the primary function—socialization of its members—remains the same. The family transmits values, knowledge, skills, and culture from one generation to the next.

The Community's Influence on the Child

The community defines for the child and family many of the educational, health care, recreational, social, protective, and support services available to them. To a certain extent, the community also interprets the goals and realities of day-to-day living. Whether or not the community is able to respond to the individual needs of its children and families is closely linked to its economic health and the awareness of its leaders.

Nurses are in a key position to observe the issues, deficits, and strengths of the community as they affect the health of the child and family. Helping local health care programs and agencies identify and meet children's health care needs—whether the need is for preventive well-child visits or for special programs—is a contribution nurses are well equipped to make. The programs available within a community are often a reflection of the social and economic status of its inhabitants. The family's status is closely related to assumptions and values concerning health and health care.

The health care system as a whole, however, reflects dominant middle-class values. Nurses therefore need to learn and understand the conditions and needs of children and families whatever their position in society. For instance, the realities of an affluent lifestyle and the forces that affect the child of an affluent family are different from those of the child in a middle-class family. Likewise, the expectations and concerns of the middle-class child differ from the pressures and stressors affecting the child who lives in poverty. Stereotyped beliefs and prejudices affect each one of these seemingly diverse groups, an irony that transcends social class.

Poverty One definition of social class is the unequal distribution of material goods, power, and prestige that cuts across society. Because of this inequality, a sense of powerlessness often accompanies poverty. Feelings of powerlessness can be a major obstacle to the nurse-client relationship and to the self-care abilities of the poor family. For example, families that can afford to seek medical care only in emergencies may be unable to maintain schedules of immunizations for their children. Parents in such families may lack the necessary information and the means to learn what they need to know about health care.

Growing up in impoverished conditions thus has a direct effect on health maintenance, and poverty can have further implications for persons seeking to restore or improve health. For various reasons, the poor may not use the health care system to the same extent or in the same ways as people from other economic strata use it. Poor families may feel that the quality of care available to them is not as good as that available to families able to pay more. They may not seek treatment for health problems for several reasons: lack of funds, inaccessibility of services, fear of lost time from work, unawareness of services, or the need to maintain pride in self-sufficiency.

Some poor families are excluded from the health care delivery system because it is too expensive. Access to quality health care also may be problematic.

> Many rural and urban poor lack qualified professionals to attend to them. Even in the cities, health care facilities are not always located where the poor can reach them. At present there has been significant improvement in health care services for the poor, but we still have a significant way to go, both in delivering effective health care and in getting the poor to effectively utilize what is available. (Bullough and Bullough, 1982, p. 154)

For the child growing up in poverty, a consistent lack of material advantage can lead to a continuing sense of powerlessness, a narrowly confined world of experience, and a constant sense of frustration. Conditions of substandard and insufficient housing and sanitation, poor nutrition, and inadequate or inappropriate stimuli can all seriously impair a child's health and general well-being. Even when a poor family is able to obtain health care, the contrast between the health care facility and the family's home environment may cause culture shock or may lower self-esteem. A sterile, quiet, orderly hospital may bewilder a child and family from a dirty, noisy, chaotic neighborhood.

The nurse can help both child and family to adjust to a new environment and to participate in their own health care. This process requires alert, sensitive, and individually planned care. The key lies in finding the strengths of the family and using this knowledge to help empower family members to use the resources available to them. The goal is to promote optimal health.

Affluence Although a wealthy family would seem to have the resources needed to take advantage of the health care system, affluence creates other potential risks of which the nurse should be aware. Although few studies have described the very rich, the nurse can expect wealth to create some differences between affluent families and those in the larger middle class.

For instance, the child from a wealthy home may be subject to inconsistent or apathetic care given by a succession of nannies or governesses. Large, isolating homes may limit the social contacts and attachments available to the child. The result can be poor communication skills and dispersed attachments. A strong sense of family heritage and explicit codes of behavior are often strengths for these families, but these standards may also impair the development of close, continuous parent-child relationships. The work and social demands of affluent parents may also encroach on their time and availability for nurturing their children.

The nurse cannot assume, however, that wealth and poverty by themselves necessarily impair the development of children or create problematic family relationships. Obviously, many children have achieved and prospered regardless of their initial economic position. How the family perceives and copes with its economic situation is more important than the actual dollars available to that family. The relative stability of family life has been found to be significant. Stability of family life helps in predicting the chances of a child's growing up either to have problems that might be classified as dysfunctional or to have adequate coping strategies to deal with daily stressors.

The School's Influence on the Child

Schools are major forces of social development in Western countries. Most children spend 12 or more years in formal schooling. School affects the lives of children in many ways, including role transition (from son or daughter to pupil), change in setting (from home to classroom), and adaptation to a different authority figure (from parent to teacher). Each child perceives school differently and builds on both positive and negative experiences as they contribute to personal development.

Decisions concerning curriculum, textbooks, and teaching methods often reflect the beliefs and perceived ideology of the dominant culture. The textbooks selected frequently portray happy, intact, two-parent, white families working or playing together. The actual diversity of family life and its numerous forms is often overlooked. The frustration, loneliness, fear, sadness, or anger, which are realities for many children, might be ignored.

Children usually attempt to meet adult expectations. Children who have high aspirations most likely have parents and teachers reaffirming them. Teachers have different expectations and goals for students and their parents. Their expectations for students may be reflected in the attitude, the time, and the energy that teachers are willing to spend on the students' learning. Teachers' expectations for parents are reflected in their efforts to communicate with parents.

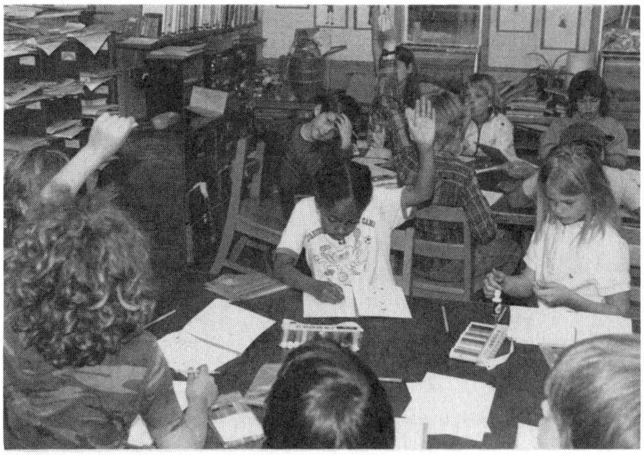

A

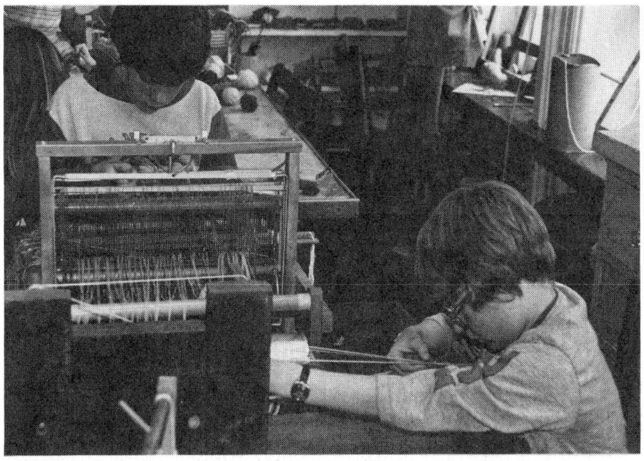

B

Schools are a major force for social development, although teaching methods differ. **A.** *Traditional classroom.* **B.** *Nontraditional classroom.*

School promotes the child's cognitive development (learning), but it also contributes in a significant way to the child's social and affective development. The interaction that occurs between teacher and student and among classmates communicates approval or disapproval for the student's behavior and class participation. When the child experiences approval, that child is motivated to excel; when the child experiences disapproval, that child may become discouraged or disruptive. The classroom conditions and atmosphere influence children's attitudes toward learning and toward their feelings about themselves.

The Peer Group's Influence on the Child

The child's social horizons broaden as the child interacts with people outside the family. The larger group outside the family grows as the child grows older and forms new relationships with peers. The child's developing language skills, cognition, and motor skills provide the vehicles for this social exchange and entry into a world outside the family. This expanded environment provides the child with a wide range of experiences in which to learn to adapt to different situations.

For most children, their peer group is a significant socializing force in which social roles are practiced and perfected. The reinforcement that children receive from one another either supports or negates their actions. New skills are shared, and children learn new behavior by imitating each other's actions and responses.

Children's play is not only activity for fun and enjoyment but also is an arena for testing and exploring the environment, for developing a sensitivity to the feelings of others, and for refining skills and interactive abilities.

The Family's Influence on the Child

The family is the earliest environment, and the primary one, in which social development takes place. It is in the family that the child first experiences human interaction.

Beginning at birth and continuing throughout childhood and into adolescence, the family transmits to the child what it means to be a member of society. Although other factors determine the child's development, the family is the primary socializing agent. The family mediates the forces and conditions that affect the child and acts as a screening device for cultural influences and experiences. Through the family, the child first learns what it means to be male or female, what constitutes acceptable social behavior, and what roles and achievements society values.

Each child comes from and belongs to a family. Identifying the family, in personal terms, is relatively easy for most people. Devising a single definition that includes the multiple conditions and commonalities that exist in families today, however, is no easy task. The previously accepted biologic definition of the family—a couple and their offspring—does not adequately describe today's changing family relationships. Current definitions should therefore include persons who are not biologically related but view themselves and are viewed by others as a social unit. Such a comprehensive definition includes persons who are adopted, who are "significant others," who are stepparents, or who are distantly related.

The form that a family takes and the style that it adopts are distinct characteristics for each family. Even so, the family remains a primary environment for a child's social development. The bonds that hold family members together persist, and the strength of family life may be its ability to endure change without being destroyed. The resilience of families has allowed them to restructure, adapt, and survive throughout history to the variety of forms that exist today. The assets and strengths of families do not rest on the particular structure or form they take, the culture in which they exist, or the values they hold. Rather, their strength is their ability to nurture their members; to meet their physical, emotional, and social needs; to develop group norms; and to adapt to stress and change.

Types of families Many types of families make up today's society. This variation in American families has come about through significant changes in the structure of the traditional family, the roles of its members, and its patterns of childrearing. Historically, mothers shared childrearing responsibilities with nearby members of the extended family, especially grandparents. As society became more mobile, the distance between parents and grandparents made shared childrearing impossible for some families. Today, the nuclear famly and its variations have emerged as the predominant form of family life, and an increasingly mobile and urban society continues to limit opportunities for extended family interactions.

Nuclear families The *nuclear family* commonly is defined as a small, functional group composed of a mother, a father, and their children. The primary social development of the child in a nuclear family is the shared responsibility of two parents. Although the nuclear family generally is considered traditional, and is sometimes considered preferable, it is also somewhat restrictive and deficient in the range of possible role models it provides for the child. In the nuclear family, parent-child relationships tend to be intense. Parents are concerned about and feel responsible for their child's future and for the recognition of special abilities or needs. This peculiar combination in which the parent is both the authority figure and the provider of emotional comfort creates tension in the parental role, especially in families with few community ties. The absence of community assistance and support, or even sociability, however, is considered to be the norm in most of American society. Thus, parents and children become dependent on each other for fulfilling their needs.

Dual-career families Although the nuclear family persists as a family form, it has undergone significant alterations. The most notable change is the increasing number of women who, either by choice or by economic necessity, are employed outside the home. The economic changes that have occurred since the 1950s have caused many more families to need two incomes. This trend toward *dual-career families,* in which both parents are employed, has created a need for child-care alternatives, which have in turn exposed the children to a wide range of people and experiences.

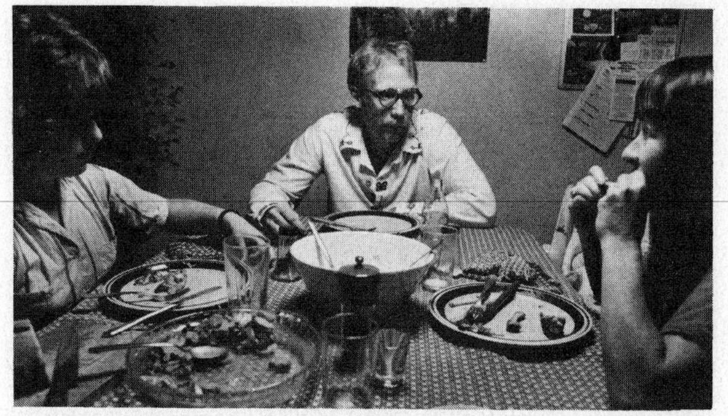

In nuclear families, a mother and father are traditionally responsible for the social development of their children.

The demands of dual careers have caused other changes in the roles of family members. Since the 1960s, the long-accepted norm in which men are socialized away from child-care responsibilities has been changing. Some fathers are making a conscious choice to participate in the daily household chores and child-care activities. Fathers are learning to nurture their children in ways similar to those traditionally associated with mothers. Fathers are spending more time with their children. Some parents alternate working hours, with one parent working days and the other one working evenings, thus making it possible for one parent to be home with the children. When this working arrangement is not possible and both parents have similar working hours, limited time is available to care for the children and also to complete routine household chores.

Dual-career families need to work out their own arrangements to create a balance between the strains and benefits of their chosen lifestyle. In essence, they must carve out a new niche for themselves that differs from the prevailing social assumptions about families but that better fits their personalities and goals.

Reconstituted families In recent years, the relative stability of the nuclear family has been rocked by an increasing number of marital separations and divorces, which has created a variation on the nuclear family known as the *reconstituted family.* Reconstituted, or blended, families are established through remarriage and in many instances result in larger kinship systems for the children involved.

The occurrence of reconstituted families is more frequent now than at any other time. One of the problems is a limitation imposed by language. By what term do children address their mother's new husband or father's new wife, other than by their first names? Mothers and fathers often comment that their children refuse to allow the new spouse's children to call them "mom" or "dad." The enforced distinction makes it difficult for them to enact the parental role equally toward both sets of children.

Symbols are used to define roles, but the language has yet to describe the roles in a reconstituted family. For example, the term *stepparent* originally was reserved for the parent who replaced a deceased parent, but in situations of divorce and remarriage, the child has an additional parent or even two additional parents. Relationships in these families are complex, and few guidelines are available to help with the problems that arise. Clearly, there are more questions than answers, and each family has to work out its own solutions.

Extended families The *extended family* consists of two or more nuclear families arranged either across generations to include grandparents or among siblings to include aunts, uncles, and cousins. Today, few children grow up in extended families in which related adults other than two parents comprise the household and provide for the daily care of the household and children on a regular basis. The current emphasis on mobility necessitated by school or occupation often separates related adults by hundreds of miles or more. In spite of physical separation, emotional attachment and loyalty can remain high, and a special relationship exists between grandparents and grandchildren and among cousins, aunts, and uncles. For example, 4-year-old Mark was hesitant to talk with adults or to play with children that he did not know. When some relatives visited whom he had never seen, he immediately interacted with them as if they were best friends. His mother commented that Mark placed relatives in a different category and that if people were family, they were special and were automatically friends.

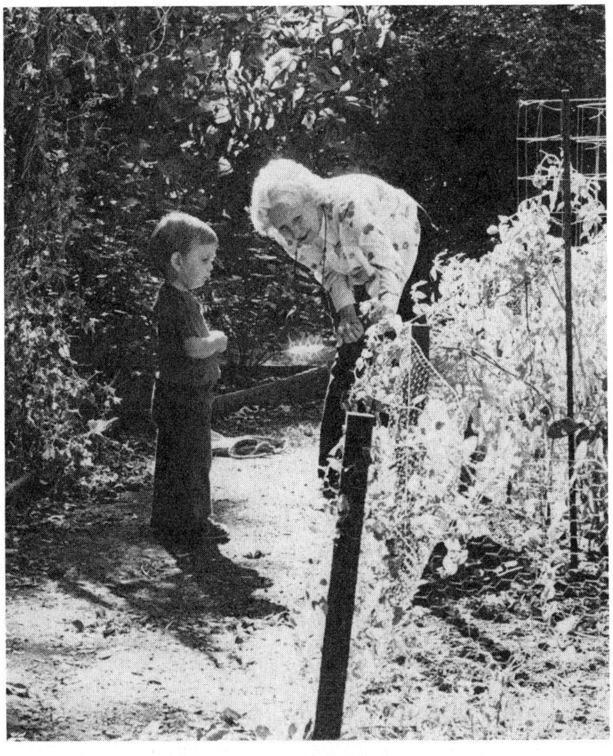

In extended families, grandparents and children develop special relationships.

Today, kinship ties are important more for friendship and emotional support than for economic cooperation. Of all types of visiting and socializing activities, the most common is visiting with relatives. The intensity and extent of kinship ties vary with each family. For some families, the trend for mothers to return to work has revived the practice of depending on relatives, albeit those living in separate households, to care for children while the parents are working. In fact, over 30% of child care in the United States is provided by relatives (Fantini and Rossi, 1980).

Communal families For some families, the attributes of an extended family lifestyle have been sought by establishing communal living arrangements. The result is a communal family and shared childrearing, which is neither a new nor an exclusively American phenomenon. The number of communal families and children reared in them rose significantly during the 1960s and 1970s. Many of these arrangements have since dissolved; some, however, continue to exist, and new ones still emerge.

Communal families exist in a variety of settings and forms but generally are defined as groups of unrelated adults who come together to form a committed unit. The structure of these families and the functions they share vary considerably from formal and defined patterns of roles and relationships to informal groupings with diffuse roles and relationships. The Israeli kibbutzim exemplify the structured and functionally defined approach to communal childrearing. A less structured and less defined pattern of role relationships is the "hippie" commune popular in the late 1960s.

In general, communal families are established as alternatives to the family forms that these family members reject. Particular ideologies and a search for belonging and for kindred relationships often are impetus for establishing communal arrangements. Most communal families regard themselves as an extended family that contains nuclear family units. Usually, the tie between infant and mother is fostered, but as the child grows, the family stresses the importance of the child's relationships with other adults in the group. These relationships may cause ambiguity in the parent-child relationship as may conflicts that arise among adults over the consistency of child discipline and guidance.

Because of the wide variation that can exist in these arrangements, no definition encompasses their characteristics and their respective influences on child development. In

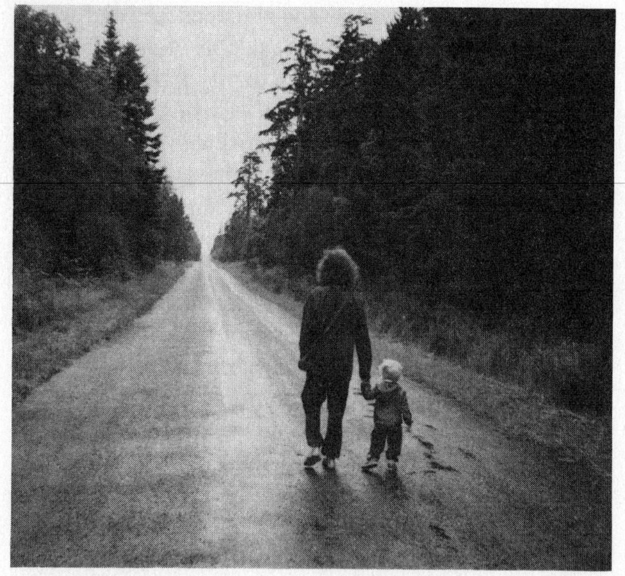

When single parents have the necessary supports, single-parent families can be effective and reliable in the social development of young children.

the health care setting, the nurse therefore assesses the characteristics of each child and family to determine how the variables are influencing that child.

Single-parent families *Single-parent families,* in which children have day-to-day contact with only one parent, usually result from the death of one parent, marital separation, divorce, or birth of a child to an unmarried woman. A recent trend in which an unmarried individual adopts a child also creates a single-parent family. In most instances, single-parent families are headed by a female parent. For many of these families, issues of companionship and support for the available parent, financial solvency, and role modeling of adult interactions in a family setting are sources of concern for future child development. For some cultural groups, however, single-parent households have been traditionally and effectively structured as the dominant family form with relatively satisfactory child development. What seems to be significant for the health professional is the coping ability of the parent during times of stress and the overall functional stability of the family.

Because of the number of marriages that end in divorce, many children must cope with the disruptive and separating effects that divorce brings. The actual crisis of the divorce is often preceded by a long period of conflict and discord within the family, and at times, the child may be torn between conflicting allegiances. For some children, the divorce actually brings a sense of relief as tempers calm and battles end.

In all instances, the children of the divorcing parents find themselves in a situation that significantly affects them but over which they feel they have no control. This sense of powerlessness is for many children translated into self-doubt and guilt. They cannot comprehend that they did not somehow contribute to the problem. For these families, the divorcing partners and their children need support to cope with the difficulties inherent to loss, separation, and a sense of failure. New patterns of relationships must be defined as channels of communication and interaction change.

Gay families The *gay family,* in which the adult partners are the same sex, is a relatively recent family type, and it is one that often has special problems. The dilemma of the gay family is the prejudice and discrimination with which the larger society has traditionally treated homosexuals. This complex issue takes many forms. For instance, children and parents living in gay families must cope with such issues as society or family disapproval and conflicts in adopting and enacting sexual roles.

Homosexuality is still condemned by many people. For the health care professional, sensitivity and acceptance are necessary prerequisites to helping these families cope with the day-to-day issues of childrearing and health maintenance. In some communities, several organizations and support groups can assist the gay family in achieving its goals and carrying on its everyday activities with dignity and self-acceptance. The nurse needs to be informed of these resources so that necessary referrals can be made and current literature can be used when working with these families.

Foster-care families Over 250,000 children currently are living in foster-care families in the United States. A *foster-care family* is a family in which children, whose natural parents are unable or unwilling to care for them, are cared for by adults who might or might not be related to them. Foster-care placement has almost entirely replaced the institutional housing of children who would otherwise be without homes.

Because a child's family is the base from which the child ventures to explore the world and initially develops an awareness of affectionate bonds to others, a foster-care experience can have considerable impact on a child's life. Understanding this impact is especially important for the nurse who is working with a child in foster care either to maintain or to restore health. In addition, several dilemmas characterize the foster-care family. Some of these include:

1. The lack of formal parental rights for foster parents
2. The ambiguity of the foster parent's role
3. The constant possibility of removal of the child from the foster-care home, which often prevents the foster parents and/or foster child from becoming too attached

Family tasks Families exist as a vital force in the social and emotional fabric of life. Many reasons may account for this vitality, not the least of which are the unique roles that families play in the social and intimate needs of people. In addition, families are charged with the responsibility of meeting the physical needs of their members, such as food, shelter, clothing, and health care. The specific needs of family members, especially those of the children, change with the advancement or decline in self-care skills.

A parent's knowledge of child care is especially important during times of transition in the family's development. The birth of a child, for example, regardless of whether it is the first child, presents new challenges and stressors for all family members. New parents might be unaware of the changes a child will bring to the family. Parents expecting an additional child might not anticipate the needs of siblings and the difficulties of meeting the needs of an infant plus one or more older children. Gathering information about a parent's knowledge of normal growth and development, about expectations of the child's needs, and about available child-care resources enables the nurse to construct a plan for providing the parent with the necessary information. The nurse's knowledge of typical family stressors and family development is therefore important in identifying and alerting parents of potential needs during times of additional stress.

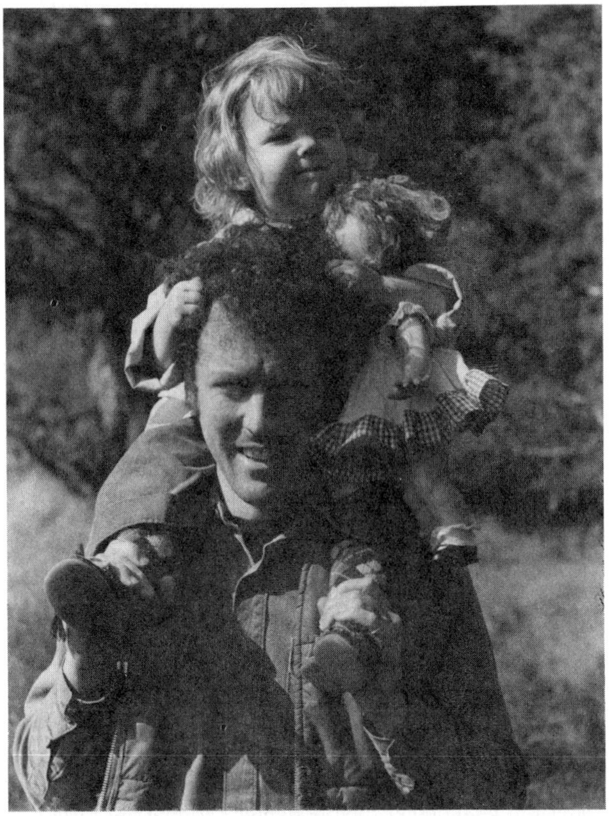

Building time into family schedules for pleasurable moments together is important for developing the relationship between parent and child.

Styles of parenting *Parenting* is the process by which a child within a family is supported in learning about the norms, rituals, and requirements of becoming a contributing member of a social group. Whether or not they are acting consciously, parents adopt various models of behavior for raising their children. The model selected often reflects the parent's experience as a child, perceived societal expectations, and awareness of the parent and child's personalities.

Brink (1982) found, in her research with parents and children, that the most important ingredient for good parenting was giving the child a sense of belonging to a particular family group. Children need love, but even more they need to know that they are securely attached to someone. Good parenting can be accomplished in different ways, depending on the model of parenting behavior adopted, but good parenting is always healthy and growth-producing. Specific parenting behaviors are therefore not as important as the degree of fit between parental actions and parental beliefs and abilities.

Childrearing is a complex socialization process that is expressed uniquely by every family. Many factors determine how a specific family will carry out its childrearing responsibilities. The expectations of the society in which the family lives define the acceptable limits of behavior, whereas the cultural, religious, and emotional characteristics of the family shape its approach to this goal. The essential factor is not the style of parenting but the recognition that someone is institutionally sanctioned and supported to provide child care. Even so, the experiences and outcomes vary for each child, even for children within the same family.

Each child brings to a family a particular set of characteristics that affect both that child's behavior and the behaviors evoked in others. The personality traits, birth order, and gender of the child are a few of the child's characteristics. The parent's response to these attributes, the way in which the parent interacts with the child, and the parent's methods of discipline are the characteristics of that individual's style of parenting.

The parental behaviors and childrearing practices that make up a parenting style generally can be broadly categorized as authoritative, authoritarian, or permissive (sometimes termed *laissez-faire*). In practice, however, most parents mix parenting styles. Some parents actually vary their responses so often that children receive both authoritarian and permissive messages at the same time. Nurses therefore need to know the working definitions of parenting styles to recognize them in both their pure and mixed forms. Parents sometimes need nurses to explain that any style of parenting can be effective as long as the expectations for children's behavior are consistent and age-appropriate.

Authoritative parenting According to Baumrind (1979), the most effective parenting style is authoritative. *Authoritative parenting* involves guiding the child's behavior in a rational, issue-oriented manner. Parents who interact with their children in this way set standards and establish limits that are clearly conveyed. In addition to valuing disciplined behavior, parents encourage self-assertion and independence by respecting their children's actual abilities and capacities. Authoritative parents try to be open and receptive to children's thoughts and feelings. They respect children's opinions and right to disagree, but they retain ultimate control when a particular behavior is deemed unacceptable. Authoritative parents temper rules with reasonable flexibility and an understanding of the child's developmental stage and abilities. Explanations appropriate to the child's age and level of understanding are offered when disagreements arise so that parental empathy, sensitivity, and responsibility are balanced. For example, if a 16-year-old girl asked her parents for permission to attend a weekend party, the parents might respond authoritatively by asking whether there would be adult supervision or by determining whether their daughter had met her responsibilities at home and at school during the week. An authoritative response to an adolescent would therefore involve consistent behavioral norms and clear explanations for parental limits.

Authoritarian parenting In contrast to the authoritative parents, those with *authoritarian parenting* styles value obedience over independent development and rely on many inflexible rules and regulations to govern behavior. Authoritarian parents seek to shape the child according to a series of rigid, clearly defined rules and limits. The parent retains strict control over definitions of acceptable behavior. Discipline often is achieved by punishing the child rather than by explanation or positive example. Deference and respect for parental authority are expected, and little room is left for questioning or choice.

An authoritarian response to the same 16-year-old girl's request might therefore be based on a predetermined rule. For instance, the parents might arbitrarily choose to limit their daughter's social activities to two parties a month and would base their decision on the number of parties she had attended so far that month.

Permissive parenting *Permissive parenting* takes many forms, but in the extreme it refers to the absence of restraints and the allowance of maximum freedom for the child, with little or no parental input. Permissive parents provide little direction to their children's behavior. Limits usually are not clearly defined, if they are defined at all. Punishments also are rare because the child is encouraged to develop personal standards of behavior. For example, a permissive response to this same adolescent girl's request is likely to be a question asking the child whether she wants to attend the party.

Some permissive parents emphasize happy homes and assume that their children will develop according to behavioral norms. Permissive parenting can provide older children with experience in making their own decisions, but some children do not always welcome such freedom or are not yet mature enough to accept complete responsibility for their actions. Conflicts also might arise for young children who are suddenly confronted by teachers, peers, and others who have clear expectations for their behavior. Children who are unused to acting within prescribed limits often find socialization at school particularly difficult.

Families as clients: The nurse's role When parents enter the health care system through the hospital, community health clinic, or physician's office, they arrive with some preconceived notions about those problems or issues that nurses are equipped to handle. They often assume that nurses are interested solely in illness or physical complaints because traditionally these have been considered the concerns of health care providers. Therefore, the parent who may have an array of psychosocial concerns frequently presents only those physical problems perceived as appropriate to the situation.

Nurses therefore need to convey to parents that they are interested in learning about and assisting with all concerns parents may have about their children, whether these are physical or psychologic, major or minor. The first step in analyzing a parenting concern is identifying the major issues of concern. The nurse assists the parent to clarify key concerns regarding the child, so that, from a parent's diffused, nonspecific feeling of concern, specific target behaviors for intervention can be defined.

When focusing on the family as the client, the nurse needs to be aware that the child's behavior problems may be symptomatic of larger difficulties within the family. If the parent is under stress, normal childhood behaviors may be perceived as abnormal and disruptive. Children may be reacting to unrealistic parental expectations or stressful events within the home or community. Therefore, the nurse needs to understand the complete context of the child's family, school, and community environment to assess the possible reasons for a child's problematic behavior. Recognizing that within the family each family member influences the other members, nurses focus on those behaviors that need to be altered to achieve smooth family functioning.

Race, Culture, and Ethnicity

Race, culture, and *ethnicity* are terms that are often confused with each other, but important distinctions must be made among their actual meanings. *Race* refers to the classification of human beings into groups based on particular physical characteristics, such as skin pigmentation, head form, and stature. Caucasoid, Mongoloid, and Negroid are the three racial types generally recognized. *Culture,* on the other hand, is the learned patterns of behavior and thinking shared by a particular group and transmitted over time by group members to other group members. These patterns provide tested and acceptable solutions to the problems of living. *Ethnicity* is the condition of belonging to a group whose members share a unique cultural, social, and linguistic heritage.

Each child, as a member of an ethnic group, shares to some degree a common background and culture with other members of the group. This common background frequently emerges from a sense of shared beginnings in a particular geographic area of the world and from a common language, religion, and history. Depending on the group, one or another of the common elements will have more significance; for example, religious characteristics are the main features that distinguish the Amish and Mennonites from the larger culture.

The ways in which significant behavioral and personality characteristics evolve depend to a large measure on these ethnic traditions. The sex-role development of the child, attitudes toward competition, and willingness to accept or reject the attitudes, practices, and values of the dominant culture are just a few of the ways in which the child's development is influenced by ethnic background.

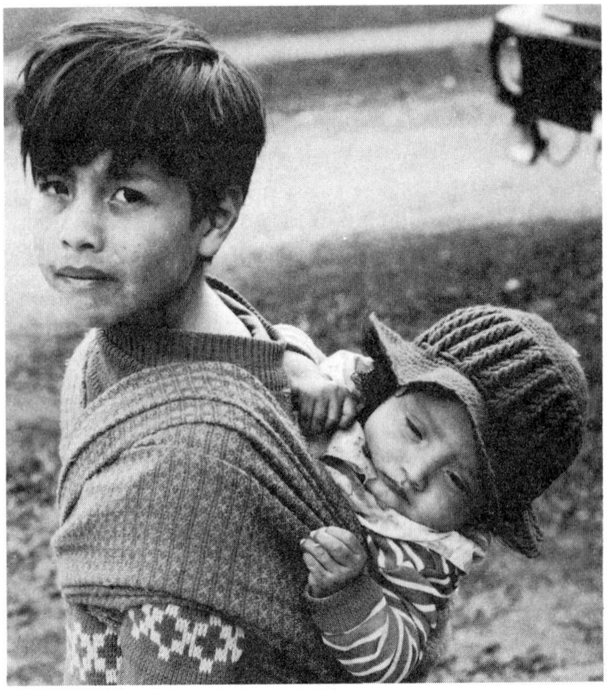

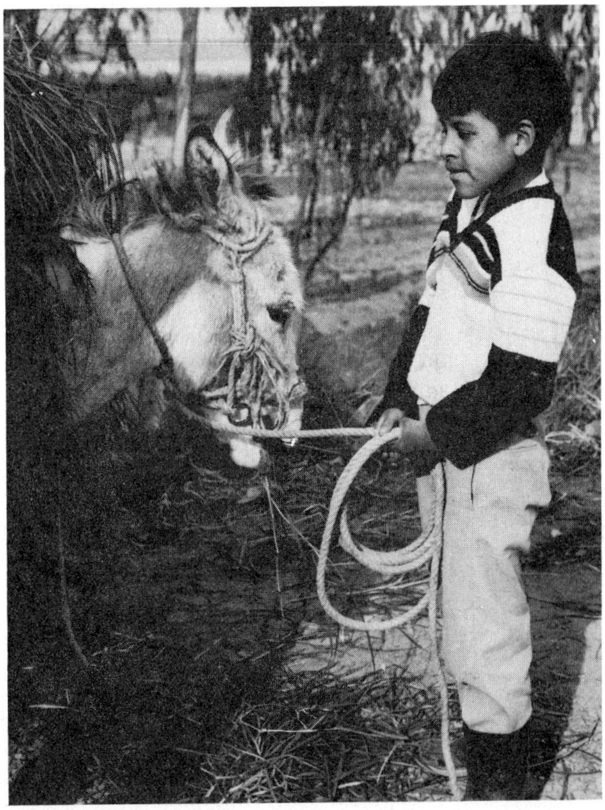

In some cultures, older children are responsible for assuming some adult responsibilities. Caring for younger siblings may be the responsibility of the older child, and children may help to support the family economically.

Impact of Ethnicity on Health Care

Nurses who care for children have many reasons for learning more about ethnic characteristics among people. Among these reasons are the variations in physical and behavioral norms that define wellness for a particular group, the different views concerning the value of children among different cultures, the impact of folk beliefs and practices on a client's health behaviors, and the perception of the health care industry and its delivery of care. (Table 2-1 summarizes a variety of health-related factors that may affect nursing care.)

There is a range of physical variation among people of different races with regard to growth rate, dentition, body structure, blood group, and susceptibility to certain diseases, and a great many other variables. Although a thorough and detailed knowledge of every physical variation

TABLE 2-1 Comparison of Health-related Factors and Subcultures

	Definition of health	Cause of illness—is prevention possible; if so, how?	Name of healer, healing practices	Problems of entry to health care system	Communication patterns	Sexuality and family life	Beliefs about death
Navajo Indian	Harmony between individual, earth, and supernatural, as well as the ability to survive difficult circumstances[1,2]	Disease is disharmony and can be caused by violating taboo or attack by witch; illness prevented through elaborate religious rituals; do not believe in germ theory[1,2]	Medicine man, who is more than average human being, is therefore influential figure; medicine man diagnoses and treats problem; treatments include yucca root, massage, herbs, and chanting; his chant states person will get well, and person believes him[1,2]	Language; will first visit medicine man; general beliefs are not compatible with health care system and structure; problems also include money and past experiences of disrespect; fear of spirits of dead may influence decision to leave hospital early[1,2]	Time of silence after each speaker to show respect and reflection on what they said; little eye contact; time orientation not very strict; recording of conversation invasion of privacy[1,2]	Family, extended family, and tribal ties strong; cooperation emphasized; consider children as individuals as soon as they can talk, therefore can make own decisions[1,2]	Fear of spirits of dead; children and family should be with dying person[1]
Hispanic-American	Gift from God; also good luck; can tell healthy person by robust appearance and report of feeling well[1,3,4]	Illness is punishment from God for wrongdoing, to be suffered; it can be prevented by eating well, praying, being good, and working; wearing medals may help; physically, illness is an imbalance between "hot" and "cold" properties of body[1,3,4]	Healer called *curandero;* cures hot illness with cold medicine and reverse; classification of hot and cold diseases varies; penicillin is hot medicine; massages and cleanings are common[4]	Language; will first go to woman for advice, then if needed, to "señora," then to curandero, then to physician; many migrant workers are Hispanic, and frequent moves may make access to medical care difficult; belief that hospital is place to go to die causes underuse of system; modesty may result in woman bringing friend to physician with her[1,3,4]	Confidentiality and modesty important; too many questions are insulting; it is more acceptable to make tentative statement to which they can respond; time orientation not strict; politeness essential[1,3-5]	High degree of modesty, may prefer home births for this reason; men are breadwinners, women homemakers; women are healers, men make all decisions[1,3-5]	Afterlife of heaven and hell exists

TABLE 2-1 ***(Continued)***

	Definition of health	Cause of illness—is prevention possible; if so, how?	Name of healer, healing practices	Problems of entry to health care system	Communication patterns	Sexuality and family life	Beliefs about death
Traditional black	Harmony with nature, no separation of mind and body[4]	Disease is disharmony caused by spirits and demons; it can be prevented through good diet, rest, cleanliness, and laxatives to clean out system; some use of copper and silver bracelets for prevention	Some belief in voodoo still prevalent; religious healing practiced; geophagia (eating of clay) and pica (eating of starch) practiced[4,6]	May seek folk or religious healer first; money and type of service affect decision; emergency room frequent entry point; black women have high "noncompliance" rate[4,6]	Racism toward blacks still prevalent; common names for symptoms should be known by health worker; time orientation not strict	Matriarchy prevalent; almost 30% of black families have woman head of household; therefore women make decisions[4,6]	Death is passage from evils of this world to another state; blacks have shorter life expectancy than national average[6]
Chinese-American	Balance of yin and yang (negative and positive energy forces); healthy body is gift from parents and ancestors[4,7,8]	Illness caused by imbalance of yin and yang, which may be due to overexertion or prolonged sitting; disease is prevented through better adaptation to nature[4,7]	Acupuncture and moxibustion (which is a therapeutic application of heat to skin) restore balance of yin and yang; herbal remedies such as ginseng used for many illnesses; healer is called physician[4,7]	Language; traditional Chinese physicians were paid to keep their patients well and cared for sick without fees because illness indicated they had failed in their job; Chinese physicians are available in community and may encourage patients to use Western physician; family spokesman may accompany patient to Western physician[4,7]	Open expression of emotions not acceptable; therefore might not complain about pain or symptoms; may smile when does not understand[4,7]	Women subservient to men; patriarchal family; ancestor worship and respect for parents observed; divorce considered disgrace[1,4,5]	Reincarnation[7]

(Continues)

TABLE 2-1 Comparison of Health-related Factors and Subcultures *(Continued)*

	Definition of health	Cause of illness—is prevention possible; if so, how?	Name of healer, healing practices	Problems of entry to health care system	Communication patterns	Sexuality and family life	Beliefs about death
Low income	Functional definition; if you can work, you are healthy[5,9]	Belief that illness is not preventable; fatalism common; future orientation minimal because present problems are too great[1,5,9]	Will often rely on folk healers and remedies because of belief and problems gaining access to health care system[5]	Use of public funding may limit access and type of care; present time orientation and beliefs about prevention may cause delay in obtaining care; inability to afford health insurance; may lose day's pay to go to physician[5,9]	May use slang and language of subculture; may view providers as authoritarian; time orientation not strict[5]	Many single-parent families with woman head of household[9]	Depends on culture and religion
High income	No data available	General belief in prevention of illness through diet, exercise, and good health habits; motivators such as previous experience or family tradition are influential in actual practice of prevention[5]	Combination of traditional practices of religion and culture, frequent use of health care system and self-help information[5]	Access not too difficult, usually through private physician; most have health insurance through employer[5]	Most like health care culture; cannot be expected to understand jargon	Women more likely to have career by choice than financial necessity	Depends on culture and religion

among racial groups is beyond the abilities of any one nurse, all nurses need to know that biologic variations exist.

In assessing a child, the nurse not only collects data but also compares the data to the established norms. If the norms chosen are not appropriate for the individual—if, for example, an Asian child's growth is assessed on the basis of norms for Caucasian children—the comparison information will not be accurate.

Like physical norms, standards of behavior can differ from one ethnic group to another. For instance, individuals brought up in a traditional Asian culture may be much more formal than is usual in American society. A nurse caring for the child of Asian heritage may never succeed in getting to a first-name basis with family members and will need to understand that the more formal address is a sign of mutual respect and appropriate personal distance.

Psychologic characteristics, such as self-concept, also can differ along ethnic lines. These characteristics can be the result of centuries of cultural development, or they may be the products of specific, more recent historical events, such as the adjustments forced on Vietnamese immigrants by years of violent upheaval.

TABLE 2-1 (Continued)

	Definition of health	Cause of illness—is prevention possible; if so, how?	Name of healer, healing practices	Problems of entry to health care system	Communication patterns	Sexuality and family life	Beliefs about death
Health care culture	Optimal level of functioning; more than absence of disease; physical, emotional, social, and mental health included[5]	Scientific approach to cause of illness; prevention involves periodic physical examinations, laboratory studies, inoculations, as well as avoiding smoking and overeating, etc.[4]	Healing done by physician, usually takes place in office or hospital; treatments based on scientific knowledge and are frequently embarrassing or uncomfortable; often emotional component of disease is ignored[4]	Physician is main access to system; focus is basically curing illness rather than prevention; encouragement given to population to seek care as soon as symptoms appear; consider health care system as only provider	Widespread use of jargon and specialized language; large percentage of workers from middle class; often expect gratitude for care given; time orientation strict; written records kept[4]	Hierarchy, with physicians making decisions	Death usually means workers have failed to do their job; elaborate means are used to keep people alive; ethical and legal questions are being discussed and tested

[1]Data from Brownlee AT: *Community, Culture, and Care: a Cross-cultural Guide for Health Workers.* Mosby 1978.
[2]Data from Wood R: The American Indian and health. In: *Ethnicity and Health Care.* NLN publ. no. 14–1625, 1976, pp. 29–35.
[3]Data from Gonzales H: Health care needs of the Mexican-American family. In: *Ethnicity and Health Care.* NLN publ. no. 14–1625, 1976, pp. 21–28.
[4]Data from Spector R: *Cultural Diversity in Health and Illness.* Appleton-Century-Crofts, 1979.
[5]Data from Murray R, Zentner J: *Nursing Assessment and Health Promotion through the Life Span.* Prentice-Hall, 1975.
[6]Data from Martin B: Ethnicity and health care: Afro-Americans. In: *Ethnicity and Health Care.* NLN publ. no. 14–1625, 1976, pp. 47–55.
[7]Data from Wang R: Chinese Americans and health care. In: *Ethnicity and Health Care.* NLN publ. no. 14–1625, 1976, pp. 9–18.
[8]Data from Channing G: What is a Christian Scientist? In Rosten L (editor): *A Guide to Religions of America.* Simon & Schuster, 1955.
[9]Data from Fromer M: *Community Health Care and the Nursing Process.* The Mosby 1979.

SOURCE: Gingrich-Crass J: Structural variables: Factors affecting adaptation. In: *School Nursing: A Framework for Practice.* Wold S.J. Mosby, 1981, pp. 136–141. Copyright 1981. Reprinted with permission of the C. V. Mosby Co.

Views of children Ethnicity also will affect the value placed on children, the child's role within the family structure, and the choice of adult family members who are most likely to assume child-care responsibilities. Economic necessity also has a major influence on these matters. The nurse caring for children of varying ethnic backgrounds would benefit by knowing, for example, that the childrearing attitude that stresses obedience to parents stems from the Confucian value system of some Asian families. The nurse might also expect a more active role to be played by extended family members (grandmothers, aunts, cousins, and older siblings) in the social development of black children. This type of childrearing is seen especially in families requiring more than one income to meet basic needs. Extended family members often provide child care while parents are working.

One of the cultural beliefs to which many nurses subscribe is the Western scientific concept of health and disease. This belief suggests that today's technologically advanced medical system is the most effective model for health restoration, but this view is not necessarily shared by people from other cultures. Some cultural groups have developed their own comprehensive methods of health care that have little in common with the Western model. Herbs, folk remedies, the evil eye, spiritualism, and the Yin/Yang dualism are some of the particular beliefs or practices rooted in the cultures of various ethnic groups.

Although these beliefs and practices may not have been scientifically validated, they can nevertheless have a powerful influence on what a client believes to be an accurate description of an illness or an effective method of cure. For some clients, the rituals and traditions of a familiar culture are a source of comfort during the stress of illness. "Although folk medicine may be defined as primitive by outsiders, it is functional for the persons within a culture" (Henderson and Primeaux, 1981, p. 175). Therefore the more nurses learn about the ethnically derived health beliefs and practices of the children and families in their care, the better able they will be to create a relationship of mutual respect and trust, which is necessary for effective health care.

Effect on participation Behaviors and attitudes that relate to family customs, rituals, priorities, and ideals are values that endure over time because they provide a sense of identity, belonging, and continuity. No one is born with these values. Rather, they are learned through verbal and nonverbal exchanges with society as its members represent the cultural and ethnic traditions. Value acquisition is a dynamic process that begins at birth and continues throughout life. A family's customs seem perfectly natural to the family members, and customs and beliefs of children and families from various cultural and ethnic traditions are a valued, natural, and important part of their lives.

In the United States today, the growing recognition and pride in ethnic diversity point to the value of cultural variation in society as a whole. The total assimilation once promoted by those who saw the United States as a "melting pot" is increasingly seen as unrealistic and undesirable. This increased ethnic awareness has significance for nurses. Unless nurses adapt their teaching and other interventions to the family's ethnic characteristics, they risk giving inappropriate and ineffective care. Sometimes, for example, the dietary preferences of a family can influence the family's participation in health promotion. A case in point is a young mother who continued to feed her 15-month-old child strained, prepared baby food rather than table food, as she had been advised. The nurse was concerned about the child's nutritional status and about opportunities for independent feeding experiences. It occurred to the nurse that the ethnicity of this family might offer some clues. This possibility was validated when the nurse learned that the family was of West Indian heritage and that their dietary preference was for food that was highly spiced with curry and pepper. The mother had remembered an earlier admonition by the nurse to restrict salt and spices for the child and therefore felt she was complying with the nurse's advice. The nurse then worked with the mother to identify ways to serve the child table foods prepared without adding strong spices. The mother was encouraged to participate in finding methods to meet the child's dietary needs, and she was happy to comply with the eventual plan.

Every ethnic group and subgroup has its own historical and contemporary details that are fascinating and that influence health care beliefs. When the nurse is knowledgeable about these specific values and beliefs, health-related information can be adapted to achieve congruence between nursing interventions and the family's values. When congruence occurs, cooperation and understanding usually follow.

Implications for the Nurse

The social and cultural influences on children and their families also have a major impact on the role nurses play in their health care. Nursing care requires not only manual skill or applied knowledge but also the nurse's complete participation.

Personal preparation Everyone is the product of a long process of socialization that lasts a lifetime—a process by which individuals learn how those around them expect them to behave and what behaviors they expect and value in others (Goode, 1964). The nurse, therefore, needs not only to define and enact many nursing roles but also to acknowledge, modify, and use as best as possible the strengths and attributes, weaknesses, and human frailties that each individual brings to an encounter. In their personal and professional lives, nurses' beliefs, values, and attitudes are enmeshed in their behavior and actions, views of health and illness, and decisions about themselves and others. How well nurses understand themselves has a direct effect on their abilities to understand and care for others.

Considerations for nursing care

Clarifying values Providing optimal and humanistic health care requires that nurses first understand the values that they bring to a situation. Clearly, a multicultural society, such as the United States, consists of several dominant cultures and subcultures that specify the desirable behaviors and attitudes of their members. Each person belongs and ascribes to a unique set of norms and values on which assessments, decisions, and actions are based. The key is to recognize and accept the uniqueness, freedom, and autonomy of oneself and others in a given situation.

Values clarification is a process by which the individual explores the many attitudes and beliefs that govern personal behavior. The goal of this process is to discover those concepts and misconceptions that color actions and attitudes, thereby freeing the professional to enter a nurse-client relationship with greater objectivity and sensitivity.

Several frameworks have been developed to clarify one's values and to produce greater self-awareness and objectivity. The philosopher Martin Buber (1958) defined one approach as the "I-Thou" relationship. The focus of the nurse-client relationship, based on the "I-Thou" framework, requires sensitivity and acceptance of the cultural differences that each person brings to an encounter.

Numerous other frameworks for values clarification also have been developed. Although each identifies a different series of steps or strategies, the ultimate goal of each method is a clearer understanding and appreciation of the values and attitudes of oneself and others. This kind of awareness can free the nurse to empathize with the client and, in so doing, act as a true advocate and effective health care provider. This process can assist in distinguishing assessments that are value-laden and based on cultural biases from assessments that are based on objective, scientifically supported rationales.

Interacting with clients If nurses continue to work toward improving their cultural and ethnic sensitivity, three beneficial effects will enhance their interactions with children and families: (1) an informed awareness on the part of the nurse, (2) more effective nurse-client communication, and (3) greater flexibility in making appropriate accommodations. (Table 2-2 illustrates some questions that the nurse might use in a cultural assessment.)

Awareness of cultural variation Many of the assessments and interventions that nurses employ in caring for clients are imbued with the values of the health care system, which may differ sharply from the values of clients. How often have nurses provided nutritional guidelines to clients based on their own dietary practices or those of the dominant culture? Nutritional guidance would be more effective if it were provided in the context of the family's customs and food preferences. The nurse could then discuss meals and methods of preparation with appropriate terms and familiar ingredients.

Childrearing practices also are heavily laden with cultural values and norms. Nurses need to remember that practices that conflict with the values of the health care provider and the dominant culture are not necessarily wrong; rather, they are different. Discussions about such common issues as toilet training, discipline, and sleeping arrangements should reflect an awareness of the cultural beliefs and values of the child and family. The nurse and family then plan interventions with these factors in mind. Whenever possible, the nurse designs and presents alternatives and modifications in the context of cultural awareness and empathy for the conditions that the child and family share. The direct involvement of the parents in developing the plan can help to ensure its relevance and appropriateness.

TABLE 2-2 Questions for Cultural Assessment of Hospitalized Children

Family characteristic	Possible questions
Religion	What is your family's religion?
	Do you have any religious beliefs or practices that the staff needs to be aware of?
Diet	What foods do you suggest for your child's meal and snack times?
	Are there any foods that your family does not eat? If yes, what are they? Why?
Language	What language(s) do you speak in your home?
	What is your family's communication style (for example, talkative, quiet, tactile)?
Healing beliefs and practices	What do you think caused your child's illness?
	Has the child been treated for this illness at home?
	Is there anyone else involved in the health care of your child besides your physician?
	How do you think your child should be cared for?
Parenting practices and family values	Who takes care of the child most of the time?
	Who disciplines the child? How?
	How will the family be involved in the child's care during this hospitalization?
	Who makes the final decision about family matters?

SOURCE: Adapted from Maheady DC: Cultural assessment of children. *MCN* 1986; 11 : 128.

Patterns of communication Culture and ethnicity can affect a great range of nurse-client communication. For example, in some ethnic and cultural groups, members are free to vocalize their pain and to convey clearly their feelings of physical discomfort. People from Oriental cultures, however, respond to pain much more subtly, and stoicism in response to physical discomfort is a cultural expectation. When working with such clients, the nurse needs to recognize nonverbal signs of pain and discomfort and cannot expect the client to report these feelings.

Perhaps the most significant barrier to effective nurse-client interactions is the confusion and misunderstanding that can result from the process of communication. Communication is affected by culture in a variety of ways. The appropriateness of terms, the nuances of meaning, and the contextual aspects of the interaction are vital aspects to any relationship. For most people, the concept of space and the distance between individuals as they speak is a culturally determined behavior. The use of voice tones, hand and arm movements, and other nonverbal cues illustrates carefully prescribed differences from one culture to another. The dominant culture of North America deemphasizes the personal and physical contact that is integral to the communication process of several other groups. When admiring Mexican-American infants, for instance, it is essential to include touch. Otherwise, the mother is convinced that the infant will develop symptoms of "mal ojo," which consists of fitful crying, fever, diarrhea, and vomiting. Mexican-Americans tend to believe that nurses who do not touch an infant cannot be trusted.

For each family, methods of communicating, loving, disagreeing, and sharing develop. The ways in which they convey information, support, a sense of urgency, or calm understanding messages are vital to each family's integrity. These very basic behaviors, which are essential to daily living, can be at odds with the expectations of individuals outside the family unit. It is helpful, for example, for the nurse to ascertain who has the authority for decision making, how disagreement with this authority is expressed, and what the acceptable methods are of expressing feelings of respect and love between family members. In traditional Italian families, for example, the father is viewed as the central authority, but true power regarding major household and childrearing decisions lies with the mother. This distinction has clear implications for the parental roles that each parent adopts.

Accommodation to cultural differences The nurse working with children and families needs to accommodate the family's expressions of culture and ethnicity with identified health care needs. Nurses who are sensitive and evaluate all forms of communication objectively are an important link between the family and the health care establishment. They are in the unique position of being informed about both the health care system and the family traditions and values and are able to interpret the one to the other.

Direct and indirect observation of family interaction, knowledge of cultural values, and familiarity with a variety of subcultural practices all enhance the nurse's assessment and interventions. The nurse is then able to include the child-family unit in formulating the plan of care. In this way, the nurse can incorporate specific health care beliefs, taboos, and rituals and can accommodate cultural differences. Many folk traditions are an integral part of the cultural response to a health need; some are basic childrearing practices, and some have religious significance. Whenever possible (and this is most of the time), these traditions should be included in the nursing care plan.

For example, a Laotian infant was hospitalized because of diarrhea and dehydration. The infant's mother roomed-in and was therefore available to participate in the infant's care. The nursing staff initially viewed the mother as uncooperative because every night she would take the infant out of the crib and into her cot to sleep with her. The staff feared for the infant's safety, and the sleeping arrangement created a slight inconvenience when monitoring the infant's treatment during the night. Some of the staff even questioned whether this mother might be resistant in other aspects of her infant's health care regimen because she had several herbal combinations at the bedside and performed various rituals "to appease the errant spirit." Fortunately, a part-time nurse who knew the cultural traditions was available. She explained the Laotian customs and beliefs to the staff members, who then were able to understand and incorporate them into the plan of care. The nurse discovered that the herbs were for the mother's back pain and were not being used to treat the infant's condition; the rituals were related to a belief that illness is disharmony with the universe. The part-time nurse explained that parents in this culture always sleep with their young children. That nurse was then designated to interpret the medical regimens and goals to the mother. With improved communication, the mother and nursing staff respected and trusted each other, and the mother gained self-confidence in caring for the infant.

Accommodations to cultural differences might create minor changes in nursing routine. This is inconsequential however, because the nurse's goal is to provide holistic health care.

Essential Concepts

- Social development for children includes interactions with the family, community, peers, and school, together with the influences of culture, race, and ethnicity.
- A family's socioeconomic status influences childrearing and health-related attitudes and behaviors in specific ways, including preventive health care practices.
- The family is the earliest environment, and the primary one, in which social development of the child takes place.
- Types of families common today include nuclear and reconstituted families, extended families, communal families, single-parent families, gay families, and foster-care families.
- The family assumes the task of providing for the specific developmental needs of the children. The nurse assesses the family's knowledge of child care and provides teaching or support as needed.
- Parenting generally takes on one of three unique styles: authoritative, authoritarian, or permissive.
- Childrearing practices are intimately related to the cultural beliefs and traditions of the family.
- Nurses cannot generalize their interventions but must be sensitive to the unique characteristics of each family.
- The response to health needs often involves a combination of traditional fólk treatments and modern scientific health care practices.
- Nurses play a vital role in interpreting the family's cultural traditions and the scientific health care system to each other with the goal of enhancing mutual understanding and decreasing mutual fear and mistrust.
- Accommodating nursing interventions to include the family's beliefs and values benefits the client and enhances participation.
- Nurses need to discover their own values and to explore the relationships among their values, perceptions, actions, and methods of processing information.

References

Baumrind D: Parents as leaders: The role of control and discipline. In: *Families Today.* DHEW Publication No. 79–815. US Department of Health, Education, and Welfare, 1979.

Brink PJ: An anthropological perspective on parenting. In: *Parenting Reassessed: A Nursing Perspective.* Horowitz JA, Hughes CB, Perdue BJ (editors). Prentice-Hall, 1982, pp. 66–84.

Buber M: *I and Thou.* Smith RG (translator). Scribner, 1958.

Bullough VL, Bullough B: *Health Care for the Other Americans.* Appleton-Century-Crofts, 1982.

Fantini MD, Rossi A: Parenting in a pluralistic society: Toward a policy of options and choices. In: *Parenting in a Multicultural Society.* Fantini MD, Cardenas R (editors). Longman, 1980.

Goode W: *The Family.* Prentice-Hall, 1964.

Henderson G, Primeaux M: *Transcultural Health Care.* Addison-Wesley, 1981.

Additional Readings

Carpio B: The adolescent immigrant. *Can Nurse* (March) 1981; 77(3):27–29.

Clark A (editor): *Culture and Childrearing.* Davis, 1981.

D'Antonio WV, Aldous J: *Families and Religions: Conflict and Change in Modern Society.* Sage, 1983.

Davies M, Yashida M: A model for cultural assessment. *Can Nurse* (March) 1981; 77(3).

Drakulic L, Tanaka W: The East Indian family in Canada. *Can Nurse* (March) 1981; 77(3).

Ehling MB: The Mexican-American (El Chicano). In: *Culture and Childrearing.* Clark A (editor). Davis, 1981.

Farris LS, Farris CE: The Native American. In: *Culture and Childrearing.* Clark A (editor). Davis, 1981.

Fox MF, Hesse-Biber S: *Women at Work.* Mayfield, 1984.

Garbino J: *Children and Families in the Social Environment.* Aldine, 1982.

Friedman MM: *Family Nursing: Theory and Assessment.* Appleton-Century-Crofts, 1981.

Goode WJ: Why men resist. In: *Rethinking the Family: Some Feminist Questions.* Thorne B, Yalom M (editors). Longman, 1982.

Gough K: The origin of the family. Reprinted In: *Family in Transition.* Skolnick AS, Skolnick JH (editors). Little, Brown, 1983.

Greathouse B, Miller V: The black American. In: *Culture and Childrearing.* Clark A (editor). Davis, 1981.

Hall E, Whyte WF: Intercultural communication: A guide to men of action. In: *Transcultural Nursing: A Book of Readings.* Brink P (editor). Prentice-Hall, 1976.

Hareven TK: *American Families in Transition: Historical Perspectives on Change in Normal Family Processes.* Walsh F (editor). Guilford Press, 1982.

Joe V: A new lifestyle in a new land. *Can Nurse* (March) 1981; 77(3).

Kodama K: Nursing in Japan. *Can Nurse* (March) 1981; 77(3).

Lacay G: The Puerto Rican in mainland America. In: *Culture and Childrearing.* Clark A (editor). Davis, 1981.

Lamb M: What can research experts tell parents about effective socialization? In: *Parenting in a Multicultural Society.* Fantini MD, Cardenas R (editors). Longman, 1980.

Lein L, Blchar MC: Working couples as parents. In: *Family in Transition.* Skolnick AS, Skolnick JH (editors). Little, Brown, 1983.

LeMasters EE, DeFrain J: *Parents in Contemporary America.* Dorsey Press, 1983.

Leyn RB: The challenge of caring for child refugees from Southeast Asia. *Ethnic Nursing Care: A Multicultural Approach.* Orque MS, Bloch B, Monrroy LSA (editors). Mosby, 1983.

Lewis M: The social network systems model. In: *Review of Human Development.* Field TM et al (editors). Wiley, 1982.

Maheady DC: Cultural assessment of children. *MCN* 1986; 11(2): 128.

Meleis AJ, Sorrel L: Arab American women and their birth experiences. *MCN* (May/June) 1981; 6: 171–176.

Miller JR, Janosik EH: *Family Focused Care.* McGraw-Hill, 1980.

Orque MS, Bloch B, Monrroy LSA: *Ethnic Nursing Care: A Multicultural Approach.* Mosby, 1983.

Olson DH, McCubbin HI: *Families: What Makes Them Work.* Sage, 1983.

Prout V: Emotional deprivation and the privileged child. In: *A Call for Action on Behalf of Children.* American Nurses' Association, Publication No. MCN 11: 11–12, March, 1980.

Rapoport R, Rapoport RN: Three generations of dual-career family research. In: *Dual-Career Couples.* Pepitone-Rockwell F (editor). Sage, 1982.

Report of the Select Panel for the Promotion of Child Health: *Better Health for our Children: A National Strategy.* Vol. 1. Public Health Service Publication No. 79-55071. US Department of Health and Human Services, 1980.

Ritzer G: *Contemporary Sociological Theory.* Knopf, 1983.

Skolnick AS, Skolnick JH (editors). *Family in Transition.* Little, Brown, 1983.

Sodetani-Shibata AE: The Japanese-American. In: *Culture and Childrearing.* Clark A (editor). Davis, 1981.

Staples R, Mirandi, A: Racial and cultural variations among American families: A decennial review of the literature on minority families. In: *Family in Transition.* Skolnick AS, Skolnick JH (editors). Little, Brown, 1983.

Strengfellow-Liem N, Liem L: The Vietnamese in America. In: *Culture and Childrearing.* Clark A (editor). Davis, 1981.

Suzuki R: The Asian-American Family. In: *Parenting in a Multicultured Society.* Fantini MD, Cardenas R (editors). Longman, 1980.

Swanson AR, Hurley PM: Family systems: Values and value conflicts. *J Psychosoc Nurs Ment Health Serv* 1983; 21(7): 24–30.

Tripp-Reimer T, Brink PJ, Saunders JM: Cultural assessment: Content and process. *Nurs Outlook* (March/April) 1984; 32(2): 7882.

Yussen SR, Santrock JW: *Child Development: An Introduction.* Brown, 1982.

II

Growth and Development: The Child and Family

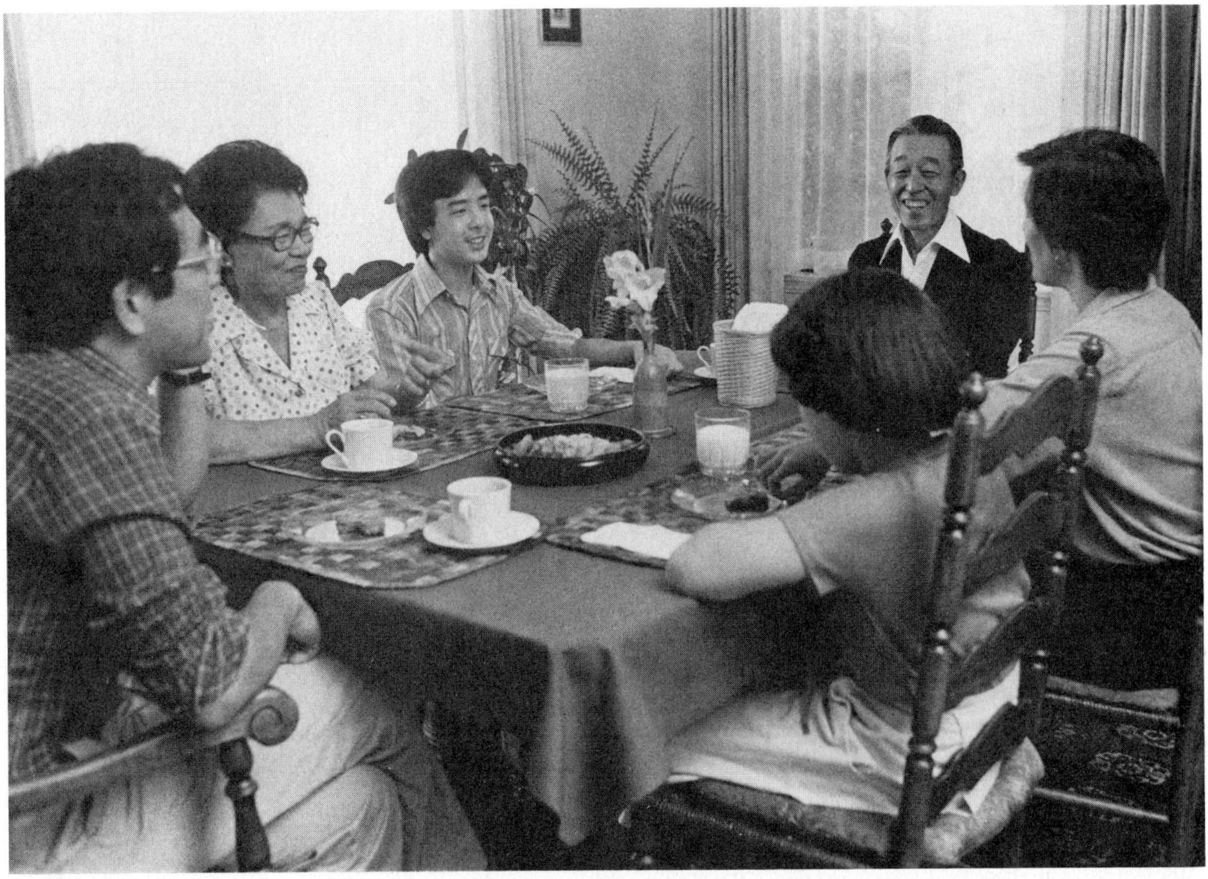

Chapter 3

Developmental Theories: How the Child Grows

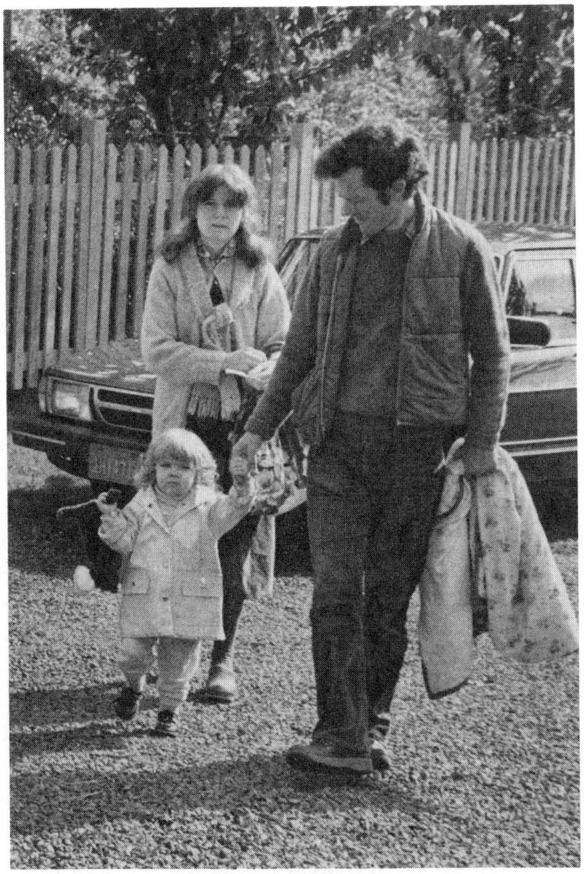

Chapter Contents

Objectives

- Define the concepts that underlie growth and development theories.
- Relate the principles of growth and development theory to the child's personality, behavior, and skill levels.

(Continues)

- Explain the importance of growth and development theories to child health nursing.
- Identify the principal growth and development theorists.
- For each of the principal theorists, explain the assumptions, terms, areas of interest, research methods, and findings that support the theory.
- Identify general patterns and expectations of physical, cognitive, affective, and social development of the child from birth through adolescence.

Human growth and development—the unfolding of the child's personality, characteristics, and potential—are processes that are unique to each child. Growth and development occur, however, in an orderly sequence of stages. This sequential process is guided and infuenced by both genetic endowment and the external environment, especially the child's family, culture, and community. To understand these processes, the nurse looks not only at the child but also beyond the child.

The child does not and cannot develop in a vacuum. Various external environmental factors play a significant role in the child's development. The community, school, peers, and family members interact with each child and thereby affect children directly. In addition to these external factors, a number of internal regulators moderate the way the child perceives and interprets, organizes, and responds to stimuli.

Theories provide *guidelines* or possible explanations for behavior, responses to events, or adult-child interactions. A theory is the way in which data are organized and presented for use by others.

Developmental theorists have proposed a variety of hypotheses to explain the phenomenon of growth and development. Some have contributed new theories, whereas others have discussed new interpretations or applications of an existing theory or combinations of theories. Most theorists have studied one aspect of development, such as ego development, cognitive development, moral development, or psychosocial development in great detail. Each of these aspects of development helps to explain the behaviors and characteristics of children. The nurse often needs to consider several explanations together, however, before fully understanding a child's behavior. The nurse also needs to remember that *the child does not develop in isolated segments. Rather, development occurs as a whole, and that whole is greater than the sum of its individual parts.*

Applying Theories to Nursing Practice

Developmental theorists basically seek to describe the ways in which the human organism grows and changes, asking why certain characteristics tend to appear at certain ages or in similar situations. In an attempt to answer these questions, theorists select certain facts and discard others, and in so doing they identify the facts they consider important to the phenomenon of development. The facts they select relate in part to the theorists' education and experience and in part to the method used to collect data. This is one reason why there are so many theories and why it is necessary to know both the limitations and the contributions of each theory.

Theories can be useful to nurses in providing insight into the child's thinking, capabilities, and probable responses. As such, the nurse uses the theory as a resource for planning client interactions, such as selecting the method to teach one child about a procedure or to prepare another child for elective surgery. The nurse uses theory to provide a rationale for behavior and to assist others, primarily parents, in understanding the child's thought processes, verbal expressions, and actions.

At the same time, theories can be limiting, usually not so much for what is said but for what is left unsaid. Growth and development are complex processes, and seldom can a situation be explained by a single theory. Rather, human communication, whether expressed by acts or words, can be better understood as a synthesis of biophysical, cognitive, affective, and social processes. At any time, one or another process might be more dominant, but all have an influence on the growing child. These influences, although similar in some respects, are different for each child. Thus, as nurses apply the theories that explain growth and development, they always take into account individual differences.

Some nurses assess development by surveying the child's achievement of major milestones. *Milestones* are standards of reference based on the assumption that a child should undertake certain tasks or display certain behaviors by a given age. If the child's behavior matches the age-appropriate milestones, all is assumed to be well. Comparing the child's behavior with well-known developmental milestones is a useful technique, although it is only part of the nurse's assessment.

Nurses use the understanding of growth and developmental sequences to assess the child's health status: "Growth and development has been termed, appropriately, the basic science of child health" (Haggerty, 1977). Variations in a child's growth pattern or plateaus in development may be cues to underlying problems. For example, a child's failure to gain weight as anticipated may be related to a nutritional deficit, hormonal deficiency, or parental neglect. Additional information and diagnostic tests would be needed to identify the cause of the variation, but an altered growth pattern often is a clue that something is amiss and that further investigation is needed.

Knowledge of usual growth and development patterns provides the basis for the nurse's explanations to parents. When parents are informed about what to expect next from their chlidren—a nursing role called *anticipatory guidance*—they are better prepared to take measures to support their children's progress. Parenting is a learned role; nurses can aid parents in this endeavor by providing them with appropriate information and advice. For example, children who are able to pull themselves to a standing position will soon be walking, first by holding onto objects and eventually on their own. A parent who is aware of this sequence and of the child's needs will prepare for the child's safety, will provide encouragement and practice for the child to master this skill, and will remain sensitive to the child's readiness and learning pace. A knowledgeable parent is better able to participate in and enjoy a child's accomplishments and learning.

Nurses need to help parents interpret the great quantity of information that is available to them. The collection of "how to" literature is vast, and parents, especially first-time parents, often seek answers and guidance from a variety of resources. This variety might cause confusion and even more uncertainty, as the advice of one source often contradicts that of another. Sometimes, the guidelines given are so minimal that they cannot be implemented without further direction. Nurses who understand developmental theories can convey this information to parents, thereby helping parents to understand themselves and their children better. In this way the nurse can be instrumental in helping both parent and child grow together in a way that accommodates and enhances the development of each.

Growth and Development: Dynamic Processes

Growth and development are lifelong dynamic processes. Changes that occur during each phase of development are critical to this ongoing process. Some changes, such as those that occur during infancy and adolescence, are dramatic and obvious. At other times, such as middle childhood, the changes are slower and subtler. Nevertheless, change is continuous, and each child is affected by both the internal and external environments and in turn interacts with and affects the environment in a reciprocal process (Fig. 3-1).

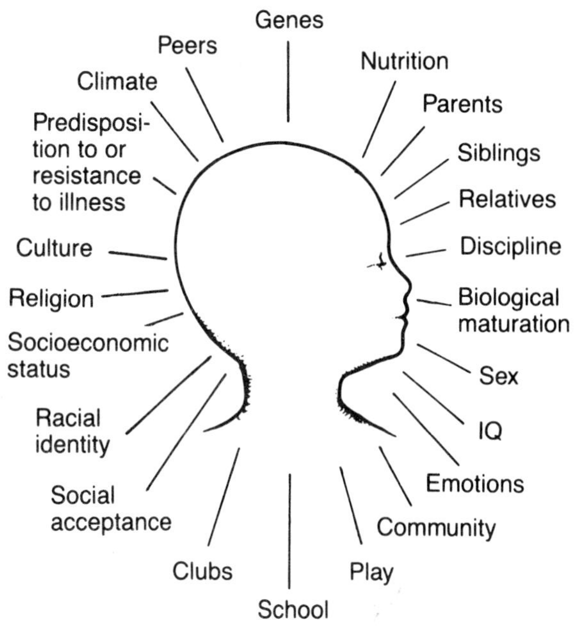

FIGURE 3-1

Interplay of heredity and environment in the development process. Many different influences shape the child's personality.

Definitions and Principles

Growth and development are terms that are often used together because they are not synonymous and interchangeable. The terms identify independent processes, but they are interrelated and refer to complex phenomena occurring in the human body (Table 3-1).

Nine specific principles are helpful in providing a framework for interpreting the changes that occur in the child from birth through adolescence. The extent to which these principles evolve is the result of the interaction between genetic potential and environment.

Principle 1: growth and development are orderly and sequential A child's maturation is predictable and follows a generally universal timetable. Certain characteristics common to the human species include rapid growth during the first year, slow growth during middle and late childhood, the loosening of primary teeth during middle childhood, and the appearance of secondary sex characteristics during early adolescence. The onset, length, and effects of each phase vary with each child, but the basic developmental sequence is the same for all chldren.

TABLE 3-1 Key Terms Describing Growth and Development

Term	Definition
Growth	An increase in size of either the whole organism, as evidenced by an increase in height and weight, or any of its parts, such as bones or organs. Growth can be measured quantitatively
Development	An increase in complexity of function and progression of skills. These are qualitative changes, such as the older infant's ability to digest and metabolize meats and vegetables, the acquisition of eye-hand coordination to master self-feeding, the building of block towers during early childhood, or the perfection of fine motor control during middle childhood. In essence, development is the fine tuning and perfecting of functions
Maturation	The sequence of physical changes that are related to genetic factors. These changes occur in healthy children. They are independent of the external environment, but their timing may be influenced by environmental factors. For example, children are able to walk once nerve myelination is complete, but the stimulated child will accomplish this task earlier than the deprived or malnourished child
Adaptation	The body's adjustment and accommodation to environmental factors. These may be momentary, such as widening of the eye's iris upon entering a dark room, or they may be permanent, such as the enlargement of the remaining kidney following a nephrectomy

Principle 2: growth and development are related to environment Family, peers, and community are among the important factors creating the social and emotional climate for the child. Family and community settings vary considerably and, as a result, so do their rules and regulations, institutions, economics, values, expectations, and resources. As the children grow and interact with others, they are socialized as members of their environmental groups. Because environments differ, learned behaviors also differ. What is true and correct behavior for one group may not be so for another. For example, in most Western cultures competitiveness is recognized as a positive virtue, but the same competitive behavior is viewed negatively in some Eastern societies.

Principle 3: the pace of growth and development is specific for each child Although growth and development are essentially continuous, they are not synchronous. Each body system has a timetable for increments in size, weight, and maturity of function. For instance, the nervous and cardiovascular systems mature before the immune or reproductive systems. Likewise, changes in appearance, behavior, and skill acquisition vary within each child. Frequently, a child appears to be developing in only one area while the other areas show little, if any, change. A child who is learning to walk, for example, devotes so much energy and time to this task, that development of fine motor skills and language skills seems to stop. Each child's timetable for these aspects of growth and development, however, is unique. Nurses therefore need to consider the child's overall behavior and not focus on specific skills or only one aspect of development. The same rationale explains the wide range of ages for developmental norms on most assessment guides. The combination of development in the various areas—biophysical, cognitive, affective, and social—determines a child's uniqueness.

Principle 4: growth and development occur in a cephalocaudal direction This means that the areas closest to the brain or head develop first and that development proceeds in a downward direction to the trunk and then to the legs and feet. The direction of growth is evident at birth as the head is disproportionately large, comprising one quarter of the infant's length. During the embryonic state, the brain and central nervous system also develop first and most rapidly, thus accounting for the infant's appearance. Further developmental progress follows myelination of nerves and maturation of muscles, thus explaining the advances in motor ability that progress from head control to sitting to crawling to standing and finally to walking (Fig. 3-2).

Principle 5: growth and development occur in a proximodistal direction Controlled movements closest to the center of the body occur before controlled movements that are distant to the body axis. The infant rolls over before skillfully using a pincer grasp (thumb and forefinger) to pick up a raisin (Fig. 3-2).

Principle 6: growth and development become increasingly differentiated In all aspects of development, general responses progress to skilled, specific, responses. The infant's early responses to stimuli involve total body activity. The newborn cries with the whole body: legs kick, arms thrash, shoulders twist, and the face becomes red and contorted. The older child cries only with the eyes and face. The young child responds in general when unhappy, de-

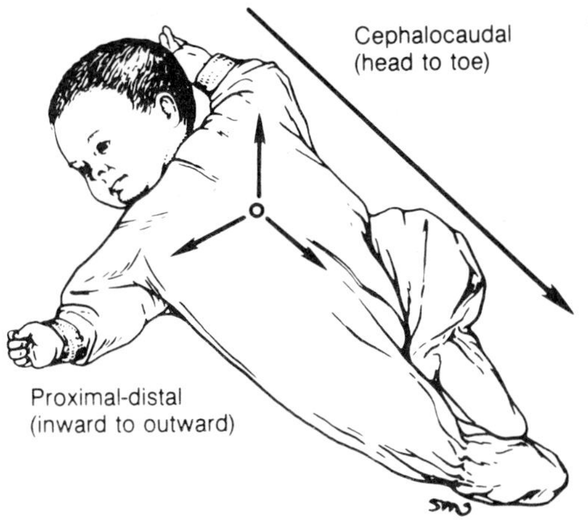

FIGURE 3-2

Principles of development: cephalocaudal (head to toe) and proximo-distal (inward to outward).

lighted, excited, afraid, or in pain. With maturation and experience, these emotions and feelings become better defined, and the chlid's responses become more specific.

Principle 7: growth and development become increasingly integrated Behavior and function progress from simple to complex as the child gains new skills and combines previously learned skills to accomplish more difficult tasks. For instance, the young child learning to drink from a cup first combines eye-hand, grasping, and hand-mouth coordination. Then, once the cup reaches the mouth, the child adds controlled tipping and mouth, lip, and tongue movements to drink and swallow the liquid. What seems so natural to the adult is, for the child, the result of considerable prior effort in connecting previously learned single behaviors to attain new skills. Childhood is a foundation, a period during which basic learning and skills are acquired, combined, and perfected in preparation for the increasingly complex functions and skills required by the growing organism.

Principle 8: certain periods are critical during growth and development This principle is often not well understood, but it has a variety of applications. For instance, during times of rapid cell division and growth, the organism is most vulnerable to insults from abnormal conditions. The increased incidence of congenital anomalies in children of mothers exposed to certain viruses, chemicals, or drugs during the first 10–12 weeks after conception is evidence of this. Early malnutrition is more likely to result in cognitive deficits, whereas later nutritional deprivation does not have the same adverse effects.

Whether critical periods exist for other learning and skill development is a question requiring additional investigation before a definitive answer can be given. Educators have noted that the notion of sensitive periods for learning new skills and tasks seems to have some validity. Although learning is not precluded beyond this sensitive time, it occurs with greater difficulty (Nelms and Mullins, 1982). Human resiliency, which compensates for less-than-ideal conditions for children's common patterns of development, also needs further investigation.

Principle 9: growth and development are continuous and are influenced by many factors Although both environment and genetic factors influence growth and development, this last principle emphasizes the total picture of a complex, multidimensional, ongoing process. To understand the growth and development of the human organism, it is necessary to identify the way in which a multitude of factors combine and contribute to the whole. The growth and development process is integrated. Heredity and environment work together in important ways. Genetic factors provide the potential and set in motion the process that is stimulated and nurtured by the environment, which affects the degree to which the individual's potential is fulfilled.

Concepts Integral to Growth and Development Theories

Developmental theories offer explanations of the various facets of growth and development, but no one theory answers all the questions about the nature of being human, the how and why individuals are both similar and dissimilar, and the relative roles of biology and environment. Each theory describes a segment of the growth and development process and is helpful in understanding the process as a whole. One might think of the individual as a house with the window shades pulled and the doors closed. As information and insight are gained from each theory, a door opens or a shade is raised, thus shedding light on the human condition and the human capability of interacting with others.

Studying and then synthesizing the many growth and development theories provides the nurse with a framework within which to comprehend the dynamic organization of internal and external stimuli. Individuals relate to their environments in ways that are both common to all human beings and also unique to each person. Such a synthesis, therefore, requires an examination of each theory and a clarification of what it does and does not reveal about human growth and development.

Theories of Growth and Development

Maturation Theories

Maturation theorists emphasize the role of genetics as the determiner of how and in what order developmental changes occur. Dating back to Jean Jacques Rousseau, the French philosopher of the late seventeenth century, this theoretic view was proposed as one that coincided with the natural growth of children.

Heredity and environment The maturationists further explain development as *autogenetic*, suggesting that the child plays the active role, and the environment plays the supportive role. In other words, the environment provides the stage for the expression of genetically endowed physical, cognitive, and psychosocial abilities that become evident in the mannerisms, interactions, and skills of the child. Mastery of one skill provides the impetus toward learning another, more complicated skill; the process then repeats itself and thus becomes self-generative.

Theory of Gesell Arnold Gesell (1880–1961) is the theorist credited with adopting the term *maturation* to refer to the developmental changes that result from the genes. His initial fascination with the orderly, sequential patterns of embryonic development motivated him to study human development over time in an effort to verify that the same processes continued after birth. Gesell dedicated his life to observing and gathering detailed, descriptive, longitudinal data of characteristic behavior and skills of children from birth through 16 years of age. He noted that behavior becomes progressively organized as the child grows. He attributed this organization to the unfolding of the child's genetic inheritance. He observed that similar skills and behaviors seem to appear at about the same time in all children. This finding provided him with evidence of the progressive maturation of the neuromuscular system, a process that enables the child to perform and organize motor skills and other behaviors. Through extensive studies with identical twins, Gesell ultimately concluded that certain universal skills are preprogrammed and that prior practice or teaching makes little, if any, difference in the time of their appearance.

Gesell and his assistants did not limit their observations to one aspect of development. They used observations, films, and interviews with parents to collect data that presented a composite picture of each child studied. This multitude of data was then categorized into ten major areas for which gradations of maturity were correlated with specific traits. (These areas and their subheadings are outlined in Table 3-2; taken together, they form a data base for a personality profile.)

TABLE 3-2 Areas of Behavior Observed for Personality Profiles

Type of behavior	Observable traits
Motor characteristics	Body activity; eye and hand movements
Personal hygiene	Eating, sleeping, elimination; bathing and dressing; health and somatic complaints; outlets for tension
Emotional expression	Affective attitudes; crying and related behaviors; assertion and anger
Fears and dreams	—
Self and sex	—
Interpersonal relations	Maternal-child interactions; child-child interactions; groups in play
Play and pastimes	General interests; reading; music; radio; cinema
School life	Adjustment to school; classroom demeanor; reading; writing; arithmetic
Ethical sense	Blaming and telling alibis; responses to directions, punishment, praise, or reason; sensing good from bad; understanding truth and property
Philosophic outlook	Attitudes toward time, space, language, thought, war, death, deity

SOURCE: Gesell A, Ilg FL: *Child Development: An Introduction to the Study of Human Growth.* Harper & Row, 1949, p. 69.

Gesell described cycles of behavioral trends that tend to coincide with chronologic ages. With each cycle, a characteristic pattern alternating between equilibrium and disequilibrium occurs. Times of *equilibrium* are defined as years in which the child is in good balance, "having relatively little difficulty within himself or with the world about him" (Ilg and Ames, 1960, p. 20). Times of equilibrium are followed by periods of *disequilibrium* when behavior becomes disorganized and the child appears to be "at odds with his environment and with himself" (Ilg and Ames, 1960, p. 21). As a result of their analysis, Gesell and his group outlined ages and stages, each lasting from 6 months to 1 year, in a sequence in which better and worse times

TABLE 3-3 Gesell's Cycles of Behavior

Age in years			Description
Cycle 1	Cycle 2	Cycle 3	
2	5	10	Smooth, consolidated
2½	5½–6	11	Breaking up
3	6½	12	Rounded, balanced
3½	7	13	Inwardness
4	8	14	Vigorous, expansive
4½	9	15	Inwardness-outwardness troubled, "neurotic"
5	10	16	Smooth, consolidated

SOURCE: Adapted from Ilg FL, Ames LB: *The Gesell Institute's Child Behavior.* Dell, 1960, p. 22.

follow each other repetitively. Each stage and corresponding age was described as though it brought its own personality, clearly definable and resulting from maturational changes. Thus the phrases "terrible twos," "trusting threes," "frustrating fours," and "fascinating fives" were used to typify children at those ages. Because the theory predicted that better years would follow worse years, the phrase, "It's just a stage," became popular, and parents were admonished to be patient and tolerant of difficult times because these times were only temporary (Table 3-3).

Although still assuming the predominant importance of heredity, some of Gesell's followers later accepted the idea that the environment has some influence on development. As one team of researchers explained (Ilg and Ames, 1960)

> All of this does not mean that human behavior is *entirely* determined by hereditary factors. What it does mean is that the body structure provides the raw material out of which personality is formed: that is the instrument upon which the life forces, both internal and external, play.

Their painstakingly constructed atlas of chronologic growth and development according to motor, affect, language, and social domains (Table 3-4) serves as a guide for parents to assess the current status of their children and to anticipate a child's next stage. Although Gesell's behavioral profiles are subject to criticism because of his small sample size and the similar socioeconomic backgrounds of his subjects, the idea of cataloging the expected appearance of skills and their order laid the foundation for the various developmental assessment guides currently in use.

Cognitive-Structural Theories

The focus of cognitive-structural theories is *cognition,* or the manner in which children learn to think, reason, and use language. Cognitive-structural theorists are interested primarily in defining the developmental patterns of intelligence, that is, the orderly progression of mental thought and problem solving as it advances from simple to complex.

Cognitive theorists study qualitative changes in children's thinking from illogical to logical thought and finally to the ability to handle abstract concepts. They describe and analyze *how* children learn rather than *what* they learn, an analysis that includes the child's experiences and processing of information. Unfortunately, the study of these processes is limited to inferences made from observable behaviors; there is no other way for the theorist to "see" what is transpiring in the child's mind.

Cognitive theorists propose that development in cognition is the result of the child's active interaction with the environment together with maturation, especially maturation of the central nervous system. The rate and potential for change is assumed to be determined genetically, an assumption that partly accounts for individual differences. These theorists thus assume that the continuous, repetitive interaction between one's genetic endowments and environment results in growth.

Theory of Jean Piaget The most widely read and well known of the cognitive theorists is Jean Piaget (1896–1980). His cognitive development theory has provided the basis for other theories such as Kohlberg's theory of moral development. Piaget was primarily interested in how knowledge is acquired and how learning takes place. Piaget systematically explained the growth and development of intellectual knowledge.

Piaget's theory initially resulted from field studies of children, first his own and neighborhood children and later those of other cultures and countries. He viewed development as an inherent, unalterable, evolutionary process. In successive studies Piaget explored the growth of intelligence, attainment of moral perspective, and concept of physical reality as they develop during childhood. He concluded that a child's knowledge is neither inborn nor passively constructed by society; rather, children construct their own intelligence through actions performed on objects, thus creating or recreating logical principles.

Piaget's hypotheses about learning Piaget proposed that development preceeds learning. He suggested also that learning, or the development of logical and rational thinking, occurs as a result of the active manipulation of objects

TABLE 3-4 An Example of Gesell's Developmental Schedules

54 months	Key age 60 months	72 months
Motor development		
Hops on one foot Articulation not infantile Drawing: traces cross	Skips using feet alternately Stands on one foot for more than 8 seconds Walking backwards: 6 cm board, no step off Pellets: 10 into bottle in 20 seconds	Jumps from height of 12 in.; lands on toes Ball: advanced throwing Stands on each foot alternately with eyes closed Walking backwards: length 4 cm board Drawing: copies diamond
Adaptive development		
Manipulates cubes: makes gate from model Drawing: copies square Drawing: three bubbles correct Geometric forms: points to nine Counts four objects and answers "how many?" Aesthetic comparison: correct Missing parts: two correct Digits: repeats four (one of three trials)	Manipulates cubes: builds two steps Drawing: Unmistakable man with body and so forth Drawing: copies triangle Drawing: copies rectangle with diagonal at 66 mo Drawing: adds seven parts to incomplete man Drawing: four bubbles correct Counts: 10 objects correctly Counts: 12 objects correctly at 66 mo Weights: only one error in five block test (at 72 mo) Fingers: correct no. on each hand	Manipulates cubes: builds three steps Drawing: man with neck, hands, clothes Drawing: man's legs are two-dimensional Drawing: copies diamond Drawing: adds nine parts to incomplete man Weights: five weights, no error, best trial Missing parts: all correct Digits: four correct (two of three trials) Fingers: correct no. 1 hand; on both hands Adds and subtracts within 5
Personal-Social		
Communication: calls attention to own performance (at 60 mo) Communication: relates fanciful tales (at 60 mo) Communication: bosses and criticizes (at 60 mo) Play: shows off dramatically (at 60 mo)	Dressing: dresses and undresses with no assistance Communication: asks meaning of words Play: dresses up in adult clothes Play: prints a few letters at 60–66 mo	Dressing: ties shoelaces Communication: differentiates A.M. and P.M. Communication: knows right and left (three of three) or complete reversal (six of six) Communication: recites numbers to 30s

NOTE: Four different areas of development are examined: motor, adaptive (fine motor), language, and personal-social.

SOURCE: Bigner JJ: *Human Development*. Macmillan, 1983, p. 16. Reproduced from various copyrighted books by Arnold Gesell and associates, all rights reserved. The Psychological Corporation, 304 East 45th St, New York, NY 10017.

followed by internal mental structuring of the event. This continuing process of manipulation and internal structuring enables the child to perform increasingly complex mental activities. Intellectual growth occurs as the child becomes capable of higher levels of problem solving.

The possession of operations, of special mental processing, is the heart of intellectual growth. According to Piaget, *operations* are generalized mental activities or actions that develop from internalization of the child's behavior. Operations are organized, follow logical rules, and are reversible. Learning is an internal action that enables the child to interpret reality by knowing, modifying, and transforming objects and by understanding the process of the transformation and thus the construction of the object (Piaget and Inhelder, 1969). Intellectual growth is therefore more than an accumulation of facts. It is an active processing of objects and information.

As the child interacts with the external environment, new objects are discovered and new problems are uncovered. As these activities occur, the child is creating mental *schemes,* Piaget's term for patterns of related thought with which the child comes to understand the environment. A child's developing intelligence is the result of two continual processes, assimilation and accommodation, both of which help the child to relate information to existing schemes, or develop new schemes. *Assimilation* is the continuous process by which the child integrates new experiences into already-existing schemes. The process of *accommodation* is used when a child is confronted with a new stimulus and is unable to assimilate it into an existing scheme, necessitating modification of the scheme or creation of a new scheme (Fig. 3-3).

According to Piaget, the quality of a child's thinking changes with progressive development. This is not an abrupt change. It is gradual and signifies the process of adaptation to the environment and new organization of structures of thought. Children of similar ages respond to intellectual tasks in a similar manner, and their responses are reflections of their levels of reasoning. Piaget therefore postulated the following principles of development:

1. All development proceeds through the same sequence of stages.
2. All development progresses from simple to complex.
3. Development begins from experience with concrete objects and situations and proceeds to abstraction only after mastery of the concrete.
4. Personality development includes experience with the physical world, then the social world, and finally the world of ideas.
5. Personality development begins with an egocentric (self) orientation and progresses to objective assessment and finally to an internal sense of reality.
6. Intellectual behavior begins with activity and progresses to activity and thought and then to thought with minimal activity.

Piaget's stages of cognitive development Piaget defined four stages and related substages that mark this sequence of development and maturation of intellectual thought. Between each stage is a period of transition in which a combination of behaviors exists. At the end of each stage is a brief time of *equilibrium,* or balance, characterized by distinct, sequential changes in the way that thinking is organized. Imbalance quickly resumes as the child finds new ways of problem solving and is dissatisfied with the old answers to questions or old methods of structuring thought.

The sensorimotor stage According to Piaget, the *sensorimotor stage,* which comprises the first 2 years of life, is the time during which the foundation for future cognitive functioning is laid down. This stage is a time for relating and organizing sensations and motor movements. Piaget defined this stage as a series of discrete and qualitatively different substages (see Chapter 4) in which the child responds to the environment in increasingly complex ways, leading to early problem-solving ability. The infant's innate reflexive responses become more purposeful. Behaviors that initially center on the infant's own body become outwardly focused during the sensorimotor stage. This reveals development in understanding of the concepts of space, object permanence (the idea that an object exists even when it has been moved out of sight), and causality, as well as development in the ability to use memory for early problem solving.

The preoperational stage Piaget suggested that in early childhood children learn to think and understand by characterizing new experiences according to past experiences. A child might, for example, try to bounce a new ball because an old ball bounced when it was dropped. This is the preoperational stage, a time of trial-and-error learning, which Piaget divided into two substages:

1. The *preconceptual substage,* from about 2 to 4 years of age, which is characterized by the increased use of symbols, especially language, and by representational thought, egocentrism, assimilation, and symbolic play.
2. The *intuitive substage,* from about 4 to 7 years of age, during which the child demonstrates increased symbolic functioning, with a more sophisticated use of language, decreasing egocentricity, more exact imitation of reality through symbolic play, better balance between assimilation and accommodation, and incessant questioning. Piaget further defined and illustrated a

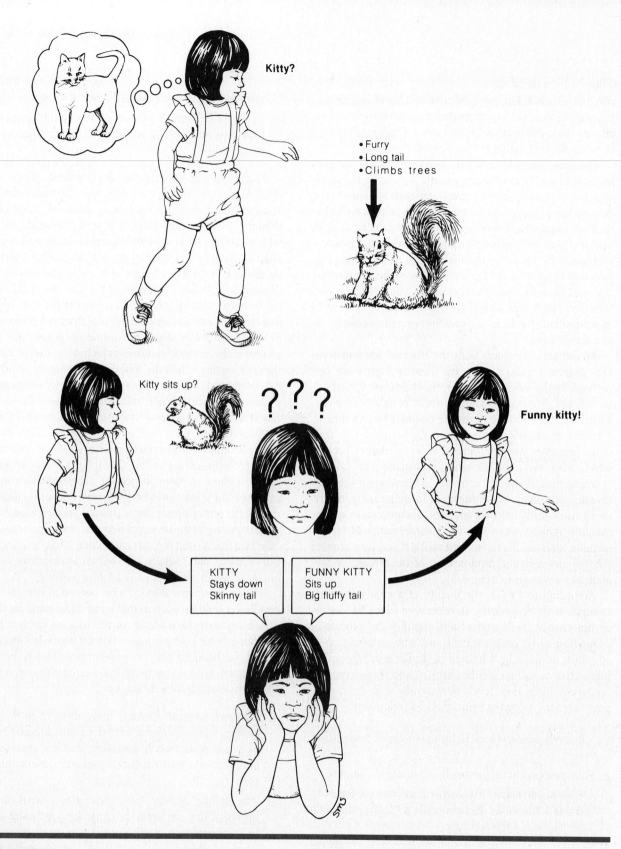

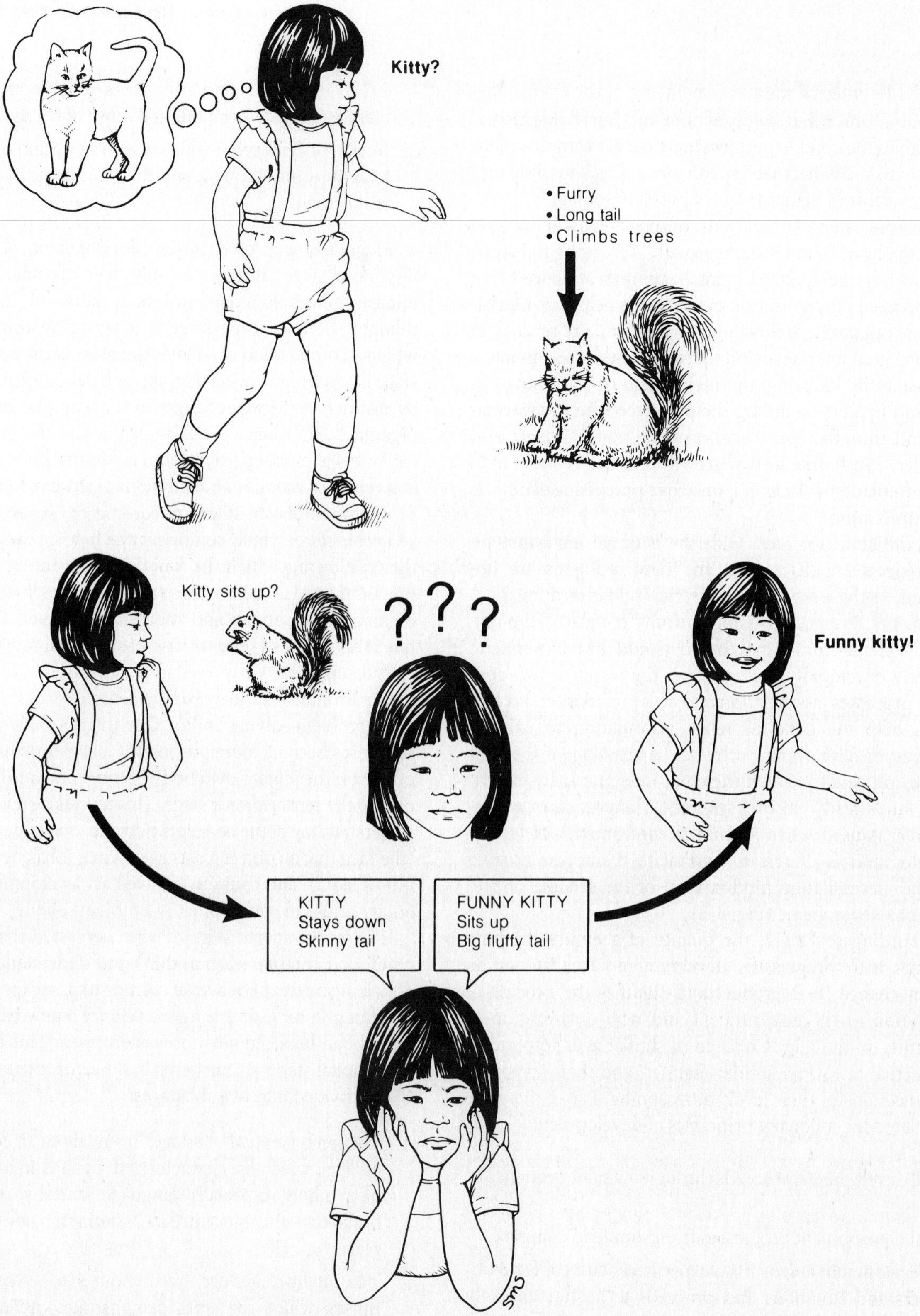

FIGURE 3-3

Process of accommodation, by which the child alters cognitive structures to comprehend new data from the environment.

TABLE 3-5 Characteristics of the Piagetian Stage of Preoperational Thought

Term	Definition
Egocentrism	Inability to take role or perspective of another; viewing the self as the center of reality
Centration	Focus on one aspect of situation; inability to manipulate two dimensions at the same time; child easily deluded by appearance
Animism	Belief that inanimate objects have human feelings and are capable of human actions
Artificialism	Belief that everything that exists in the world has been created either by human beings or by a supernatural force specifically for humans and in the same manner as humans build things
Finalism	Belief that every question has a simple and direct answer, every event a direct cause, and that nothing happens spontaneously or by chance
Imminent justice	Sense that world is equipped with built-in system of law and order so that things, as well as humans, can punish
Transductive thinking	Specific to specific thinking. Difficulty understanding comparisons or relational terms; the child concentrates on either the parts or the whole but is unable to relate the two
Monologue	Talking to oneself out loud for a prolonged period of time without regard for the presence of a listener
Collective monologue	Talking "at" instead of "with" another person; two or more conversations occurring simultaneously, each at an egocentric level, neither child taking account of the other's words
Irreversibility	Inability to reverse an action, situation, or physical properties of an object. Associating a change in appearance with a qualitative or quantitative change in the identity of the object or event. Focusing on the end result
Nonconservation	Inability to retain identity of two dimensions at the same time. Influenced by perceptual changes; difficulty understanding compensation (eg, when one dimension changes, a corresponding offsetting change occurs in another dimension)
Symbolic play	Pretend or imaginary play; use of one object or self to represent that of another (eg, block can be a boat, car, or building). Play-acting events experienced in everyday living, often with role change or extension. Blending of fantasy with reality

number of characteristics that are specific to this stage of cognitive development (Table 3-5).

The concrete operational stage Children in Piaget's concrete operational stage learn by manipulating concrete objects but are still unable to perform mental operations requiring abstraction. They may, for example, understand the principles of addition but will recognize that $8 + 7 = 15$ only after previous manipulation of the numbers represented by tangible objects. Logical thinking is therefore limited to tangible, known, or directly perceived information.

Children learning at the concrete operational stage do understand the concept of relation. They are able to classify objects according to two or more characteristics. They also understand the concept of seriation, or the ordering of a series of objects according to a given principle. Children in this stage understand the principle of conservation—that is, that certain properties of objects, like volume or mass, remain constant (are conserved), even though the shape or appearance of an object may change.

The following are further characteristics of concrete operational thought:

1. Ability to understand the rules of reversibility
2. Ability to understand the concept of number through improved spatial operations and object identification
3. Ability to focus on several dimensions of a situation simultaneously, a principle that Piaget called *decentration*
4. Ability to see another's perspective—decreased egocentricity
5. Ability to imitate details, often manifested through intricate rules for collective games
6. Ability to understand equality and justice in which wrongdoing is punished and the wrongdoer must compensate for damage done

TABLE 3-6 Stages of Moral Development According to Kohlberg

Stage	Definition
Preconventional level	Behavior abides by cultural rules because of punishment or reward consequences
Stage 1—punishment and obedience orientation	Good and bad and right and wrong are thought of in terms of consequences of an action; avoidance of punishment
Stage 2—instrumental realistic orientation	Right action is whatever satisfies one's own needs and occasionally the needs of others; exchange of favors; "do for me and I do for you"
Conventional level	Behavior is self-controlled due to expectations of others and desire to conform to and accept social expectations
Stage 3—interpersonal acceptance of "good boy," "nice girl" social concept	Good behavior is what pleases and is approved by others; response to stereotype; social units are loose and flexible
Stage 4—the "law and order" orientation	Right behavior accepts and shows respect for authority; doing one's duty for the good of the social order; laws are permanent and not likely to change
Postconventional, autonomous, or principles level	Effort to define moral values and principles that are valid beyond the authority of the group and even beyond the self
Stage 5—social contract, utilitarian orientation	Adherence to legal rights commonly agreed on by society but with laws subject to interpretation and change in terms of rational consideration for the rights of the individual while maintaining respect of self and others
Stage 6—universal ethical principle orientation	Right behavior is defined in terms of ethical principles based on logical comprehensiveness, universality, and consistency and respects the inherent dignity of human beings as individuals

SOURCE: Data from Kohlberg L: Stage and sequence: The cognitive-development approach to socialization. In: *Handbook of Socialization: Theory and Research.* Gaslin D (editor). Houghton Mifflin, 1969.

The formal operational stage Piaget's formal operational stage, which begins at about 11 years of age, corresponds with the beginnings of adolescence. This is the phase in which children learn to evaluate the environment without relying on concrete phenomena. Adolescents develop logical thinking, the ability to work with abstract ideas and the ability to speculate. Their mental capacities now allow them to follow a train of thought to a logical conclusion and to test hypotheses with deductive reasoning. Adolescents' reasoning abilities are increasingly multidimensional, and they are able to synthesize and integrate concepts into larger schemes. By this stage, they can manipulate facts, ideas, and consequences.

Other characteristics of the formal operational stage are as follows:

1. Understanding mathematics and scientific principles, such as concepts of variables and proportion
2. Showing evidence of reflective, futuristic thinking
3. Establishing personal rules and values based on a more developed sense of equality

Theory of Lawrence Kohlberg Lawrence Kohlberg (1927–1987) studied one aspect of development: the changes that occur in the child's thinking about moral judgments or the process by which the child learns to reason about what is right or wrong. Unlike Piaget, who based his study of moral development on the concept of rules and respect for rules, Kohlberg identified morality with justice. He stressed that the orientation to justice is defined as "relations of liberty, equality, reciprocity, and contract between persons" (Kohlberg, 1976, p. 40). Moral behavior is culturally related, however, and reflects the extent to which a person internalizes societal rules and expected behaviors. Kohlberg's studies therefore reflect some specific cultural characteristics.

On the basis of responses given by research volunteers to a series of stories containing different moral dilemmas, Kohlberg isolated three levels of thinking reflected in the criteria that respondents used for making judgments. Within each of the three levels, he then defined two further stages (Table 3-6).

The *preconventional level* of moral development is characterized by egocentricity or self-interest arising first out of fear of punishment and then as a means of serving one's own desires. Decisions are made according to their consequences and effects on the decision maker. The second level of moral development, the *conventional level,* recognizes group values. Decisions at this level demonstrate respect and allegiance to these ideals, regardless of the consequences. The third level of moral development is the principled thinking, or *postconventional level.* He proposed three conditions that must be met for a person to achieve autonomous or principled thinking: (1) skepticism, or the tendency to be intellectually disillusioned by the supposed benefits of society's laws; (2) egocentricity, or a sense of deciding in one's own mind what is right and wrong; and (3) relativism, or the ability to see how certain rules are relative to the beliefs and needs of a particular society (Duska and Whelan, 1975, p. 70). The consequences of an action for Kohlberg are not as important as the reasoning or motivations behind the action. For example, does one give to charities because of the tax incentive or because it is not right for any human to be deprived of basic needs for food, shelter, clothes, or medical care? The results are the same, but Kohlberg's scheme indicates that the moral reasoning providing the rationale for the action is very different.

The child's capacity to make moral decisions is related to the whole complex process of social development. This process includes learning rules, observing models, and taking different roles, first vicariously in play and later during life events. Although the external environment and social interactions are important, Kohlberg viewed the child's overall cognitive development as the primary determiner of moral development.

Within Kohlberg's sequential stages, each successive stage builds on the previous stage and adds one or two new dimensions. The stages do not correspond to any chronologic age. Rather, they describe an orientation to morality that is based on "normative order, utility consequences, justice or fairness and ideal-self" (Kohlberg, 1976, p. 40).

Kohlberg's theory is interesting but not problem-free. Because it is difficult to assess and to eliminate the role of culture, his analysis of moral development seems to be more characteristic of Western civilizations than of other civilizations. This limitation presents problems for any claim of universality in moral behaviors. Furthermore, the theoretic emphasis on reasoning as the sole determiner for developmental stage excludes the importance of human behavior and feelings. Other theorists have noted a considerable variance between what one thinks is the right decision and what one actually does.

The dilemmas Kohlberg suggested also are not relevant for children who are concerned with friendships, peer relations, or parent and family relations that involve them. Posing more common dilemmas could help in assessing the moral decision-making processes in children's lives. Finally, Kohlberg's theory was formulated according to the responses of a group of males. Carol Gilligan (1982) has noted that females' thoughts and actions involve significantly different dimensions with different objectives and goals. For example, relationships and cooperation are more highly valued by women, and these values are reflected in the rationales women use in confronting moral dilemmas.

Psychodynamic Theories

Psychodynamic theorists are interested in the emotional forces reflected in the individual's personality. Early psychodynamic theorists sought to define and describe the motivations and inner workings of the mind as they were manifested and developed during the individual's lifetime.

Personality is an extremely complex term to define, probably with as many definitions as persons attempting to formulate them. A very basic definition is that personality is the outward expression of the inner self. Personality encompasses the traits related to temperament and style of interaction. Personality development as described by psychodynamic theories also includes the related notions of self-esteem and self-concept. The way a person feels, personally looks, and acts is *self-esteem.* The way a person thinks others perceive his or her looks and actions is *self-concept.*

Theory of Sigmund Freud One of the earliest developmental theories and the one that has influenced thinking and theory formation since its inception is that of the Viennese neurologist-psychoanalyst Sigmund Freud (1856–1939). In an effort to identify the etiology of the puzzling physical symptoms that were without known medical cause in some of his patients, Freud became interested in the seemingly powerful but consciously unknown infuences of early experiences on behavior and physical health. Essentially, he sought to find a connection between the mind and the body. Freud hypothesized that this connection was related to the unconscious. The unconscious, which is present at birth, was to Freud the source of instinctual drives. He defined the *unconscious* as a deep depository for ideas, emotions, problems, fears, and pains within the mind. According to Freud, the individual was not cognizant of these feelings, yet they influenced and often determined behavior and personality characteristics (Freud, 1923).

Freud's component's of personality The newborn's behavior is one example of the response to instinctual needs. Whenever hungry, wet, or uncomfortable, the newborn

TABLE 3-7 Freud's Stages of Psychosexual Development

Stage	Age Range	Erogenous zone	Sexual activity
Oral	0–18 months	Mouth, lips, tongue, teeth	Sucking, swallowing, chewing, biting
Anal	8 months–4 years	Anus, buttocks	Expulsion and retention of waste products
Phallic (Oedipus complex)	3–7 years	Genitals	Masturbation
Latent	5–12 years	—	—
Genital (Oedipus complex)	12–20 years	Genitals	Masturbation, sexual intercourse, feelings for others

SOURCE: Fong C, Resnick R: *The Child.* Benjamin/Cummings, 1980, p. 352.

cries until the need is met. The instinctual drives that cause this self-serving behavior are what Freud termed the *id.* Freud noted, however, that with time, repetition of familiar patterns, and social interaction, the demand for immediate gratification is modified. This is related to the development of the ego and to the recognition of other ways to fulfill needs.

Freud described the *ego* as a mediator, or "reality principle." The ego takes the demands of the unconscious, rechannels them, and makes them compatible with other people and events. Functioning on the conscious level, the ego helps the child cope with reality. The other component of personality is the superego. The *superego* is roughly equivalent to the conscience and is the result of internalizing society's rules and values. The child's experiences of praise for obeying and punishment for disobeying teach the foundation for the superego. It serves as disciplinarian by creating feelings of guilt and remorse for transgressing rules and pride and self-praise for adhering to rules.

Freud described the process of socialization and personality development as a lifelong struggle among the instinctual pleasure drives of the id, expectations of reality and demands for acceptable behavior as expressed by the ego, and the moral standards, beliefs, values, and rules internalized by the superego.

Freud's stages of psychosexual development Freud elaborated on the steps of personality development by identifying five stages of pleasure-seeking, or psychosexual, growth. Each stage related to the body part, called an *erogenous zone,* which brought primary pleasure during that phase of growth and development. The stages are identified as oral, anal, phallic, latent, and genital. (Table 3-7 summarizes these five stages.)

Freud viewed the reduction of tension during the *oral stage* as both pleasurable and critical for infant survival. Freud also saw sucking and mouthing of objects as important for early learning about the environment. The *anal stage* was seen as a major hurdle in the child's life because this was the first time that delay of gratification became required and expected through toilet training. Knowledge of gender differences, identification with one's own gender, conflict, and then identification with the parent of the same sex constituted the *phallic stage.* During this stage, Freud posited the famous *Oedipus complex* (derived from the Greek tragedy, *Oedipus Rex*), which appears when sons have an intense love for their mothers. The *Electra complex* is the corresponding phenomenon in girls, in which they have intense love for their fathers. *Latency* followed and was a period of transition. The sexual conflict was resolved, and the child developed other interests with peers. A rekindling of earlier sexual (Oedipal and Electra) conflicts marked the *genital stage.* During this time, Freud theorized that the individual vacillated between dependence and independence, eventually establishing personal autonomy and adult relationships. Freud built this theory on the retrospective memories of his maladjusted patients, and this has created difficulties for others trying to reproduce his results. Freud's theories have established for nurses and others, however, the importance of childhood and its role in developing adult personality characteristics.

Theory of Erik Erikson The developmental theory of Erik Erikson was based on and expanded from Freudian analysis. Erikson acknowledged the contribution of biologic factors to the developmental process but also gave equal emphasis to the cultural and social aspects of environment. He proposed a theory of psychosocial development of

TABLE 3-8 Erikson's Timetable of Developmental Stages

Stage	Psychosocial crisis	Radius of significant others	Theme
I	Trust vs. mistrust	"Maternal" person	To get; to give in return
II	Autonomy vs. shame/doubt	"Paternal" person	To hold on; to let go
III	Initiative vs. guilt	Family	To make; to make like—play
IV	Industry vs. inferiority	"Neighborhood," school, instructive adult	To make things; to make together—complete
V	Identity vs. role confusion	Peer groups (in and out groups)	To be oneself; to share being oneself or not being oneself
VI	Intimacy vs. isolation	Partners in friendship, sex, competition	To lose and find oneself in another
VII	Generativity vs. self-absorption	Partner	To make be; to take care of
VIII	Integrity vs. despair	Humanity	To be, through having been; to face not being

SOURCE: Adapted from Erikson, E: Identity and the life cycle: A review. By permission of WW Norton and Company Inc. © 1980 by WW Norton and Company Inc. © 1959 by International University Press Inc.

the healthy individual from birth to death that focused on the interrelationships between physical and emotional variables during the individual's lifetime.

The psychosocial development of the ego was for Erikson an interactive process whereby the individual reconciles current internal polar struggles and establishes a new orientation to self and society. This process is continuous. Each mastery of opposing "pulls" sets the stage for a different set of polarities. Erikson suggested that all new development is rooted in prior accomplishments, experiences, and behaviors. These provide the impetus for the additional acquisition of skills and the opportunity for correcting or improving earlier skills.

Erikson believed that although development is a continuous process, it also has distinct stages characterized by the achievement of developmental goals. Each stage presents a developmental crisis to be mastered. These crises are represented in the eight stages of life that describe the development of the self in relation to the demands and expectations of society (Table 3-8). The stages form the life span, beginning with birth and concluding with old age and death. Erikson was one of the first theorists to acknowledge that development continues during adulthood and is not completed with adolescence.

Childhood for Erikson was the beginning of a growing process that culminated in the achievement of ego identity. He saw the process as a series of steps with gradually increased differentiation. Ego identity consists of two aspects: an inner-focused aspect that involves personal knowledge and acceptance of oneself and an outer-focused aspect that includes the sharing of group values and ideals or "some kind of essential character with others" (Erikson, 1968).

Erikson's theory was based on Freud's psychosexual concepts but expanded to include adult development and the role of the environment, especially the interplay between the self and significant others. Erikson created a grid to illustrate the process of ego development. Each step represented the psychosocial crisis or conflicting personality traits that characterized that stage (Fig. 3-4).

The resolution of each crisis could result either in positive growth and preparation for future crises or in frustration and difficulty in coping with the crisis in subsequent stages. Failure to succeed at any one of the developmental stages does not doom the child to failure for life. There is always the hope that mastery will be attained, even though at a delayed rate. Difficulty at any one stage may slow progress through the other stages, but Erikson's theory is essentially optimistic, and he believed that the child eventually would develop the necessary competencies for healthy functioning in society.

The approximate ages of the first five stages of Erikson's theory corresond to those of Freud's. Erikson integrates biologic instincts with the process of self-development in relation to significant others and society in general.

Stage	1	2	3	4	5	6	7	8
Maturity								Ego Integrity vs. despair
Adulthood							Generativity vs. stagnation	
Young adulthood						Intimacy vs. isolation		
Puberty and adolescence					Identity vs. diffusion			
Latency				Industry vs. inferiority				
Locomotor Genital			Initiative vs. guilt					
Muscular Anal		Autonomy vs. shame						
Oral Sensory	Trust vs. mistrust							

FIGURE 3-4
Erikson's phases of psychosocial crisis in ego development.

Erikson's last three stages deal with adult development and are therefore not applicable to child health nursing. An important aspect of Erikson's theory is that development is not concluded with adolescence.

Trust versus mistrust Trust versus mistrust is Erikson's first stage and involves the period of infancy. The focus of the infant's activities is to establish mutual giving and getting between the self and the caregivers. The infant learns to trust both self and environment because of the consistency with which the basic needs of food, comfort, and warmth are met. "The general state of trust, furthermore, implies not only that one has learned to rely on the sameness and continuity of the outer providers, but also that one may trust oneself and the capacity of one's own organs to cope with urges . . ." (Erikson, 1963).

Mistrust may result if needs are met unpredictably or inadequately. When caregivers are inconsistent or convey a sense of confusion and chaos, the infant is unable to feel that the world is a safe and reliable place but rather feels that the environment must be regarded with wariness and mistrust.

Autonomy versus shame and doubt Erikson's second stage, autonomy versus shame and doubt, spans the initial years of early childhood and involves the child's newly developing physical and mental skills. The child begins to discover the many things that can be accomplished with motor skills and language. Self-assertiveness and an intense desire to practice and perfect these new skills characterize this stage. As parents support the child and allow for gradually increasing independence in such tasks as eating, dressing, toileting, and bathing, they enhance the child's sense that muscles, impulses, self, and the environment can be controlled for mutual cooperation and benefit.

Shame and doubt are the result of the parent's always doing for the child the things that are being learned. The child treated in this way is thus made to feel inadequate or incapable. A parent who overly criticizes a child and expects perfection rather than making allowance for learning and mistakes also conveys a sense of shame and doubt about the child's ability to control the self and the world.

Initiative versus guilt Erikson's third stage of development is initiative versus guilt. The later years of early childhood involve the crisis of initiative, the instigating of activity rather than imitating or responding to the actions of others. The skills perfected previously and the sense of self-confidence gained now motivate the child to initiate activities and ask questions. The child spends time inventing new ways to use known skills, trying out new combinations and imagining how it would feel to be someone or something else. This is also a time of learning to take responsibility for one's behavior.

Guilt is the negative side of this stage and is the result of frequent reprimands for using initiative. Children who are severely restricted in their activities and whose questions are belittled and unanswered will develop a sense of guilt about their thoughts and actions. Guilt developed during this stage may be manifested as passivity and reluctance or even a refusal to initiate any action requiring motor or language skills.

Industry versus inferiority The fourth stage of development is industry versus inferiority. During the middle and later childhood years, the challenge is sufficient mastery of the skills needed to create and complete projects. Whereas doing was of utmost importance in the previous stage, the satisfactory completion of the project is now all important. Peers often are included to help plan and produce the result. Children become increasingly competitive both in school and in play because the sense of industry is benefited by being first, best, smartest, or fastest.

Children who can never measure up to adult expectations or who are ridiculed by their peers are likely to develop a sense of inferiority. Their status within their group and their self-evaluation becomes endangered once they believe that whatever they do or however much they try is not good enough.

Erikson noted that at this time the child spends as much time outside the home as in it. This allows for negative feedback given by those at one place to be countered with support and sensitivity at the other place. By this time, parents, teachers, and peers all contribute to the development of industry or inferiority.

Identity versus identity diffusion The task of the adolescent is to achieve a stable sense of who the self really is. This is accomplished in Erikson's fifth stage of development, identity versus identity diffusion, by integrating the past knowledge of using tools and social interaction with the present development of physical and sexual maturity.

> The growing and developing youths, faced with this physiological revolution within them, are now primarily concerned with what they appear to be in the eyes of others as compared with what they feel they are, and with the question of how to connect the roles and skills cultivated earlier with the occupational prototypes of the day. (Erikson, 1963)

Adolescence is a time of trying on different roles to evaluate how they "fit"—how one feels playing the role and how others, especially peers, respond to the role. Identity formation is a crucial point in an adolescent's life because it affects the quality of decisions and commitments that one will make as an adult.

Although identity occurs eventually in most cases, identity diffusion may be the result if the adolescent is unable to acquire a sense of self, direction, or place in the world. Erikson stated that in the contemporary world, "We are witnessing a situation where youths sport identity confusion very openly and almost mockingly, for they prefer to find their own way to new ethical commitments" (Maier, 1978, p. 86). This attitude is related to the rapid social and technologic changes that make it more difficult for one to find continuity from the past to the present to the future. Such times involve a longer adolescence because of the increased difficulty experienced in integrating ideals and reality, past events and future possibilities.

Development throughout the life span Erikson's stages are distinct, however he made allowances for development to move in either direction at any time during the individual's lifetime. Although his theory lacks scientific measures and statistics, that does not diminish its value to nurses for understanding the process of personality development. His theory is a tribute to his perceptive observations and descriptions of human development. The sensitivity with which he conveys the individual's relation to self, others, and society as a whole, together with his commonsense approach, is to be applauded.

Recognition of the complexity and diversity of the human personality is the reason he emphasized that life is constant change. That is why crises confronted at one stage of life may reappear at another, why crises not completely resolved may return for new and better resolutions, and why failure to achieve a positive balance between the two traits the first time does not mean that the individual will not have a second chance to do so.

Behaviorism

Behaviorism is a general theoretic explanation for human actions and interactions. Behaviorists assume that human behavior is the result of learned responses to environmental stimuli. The behaviorist does not research individual personality development but rather seeks to identify general laws of human behavior that can be applied to everyone. Behavioral research largely is conducted in a laboratory, where variables can be controlled. Behaviorists are skeptical about the vague concepts of mind and mental functions because these cannot be seen or measured.

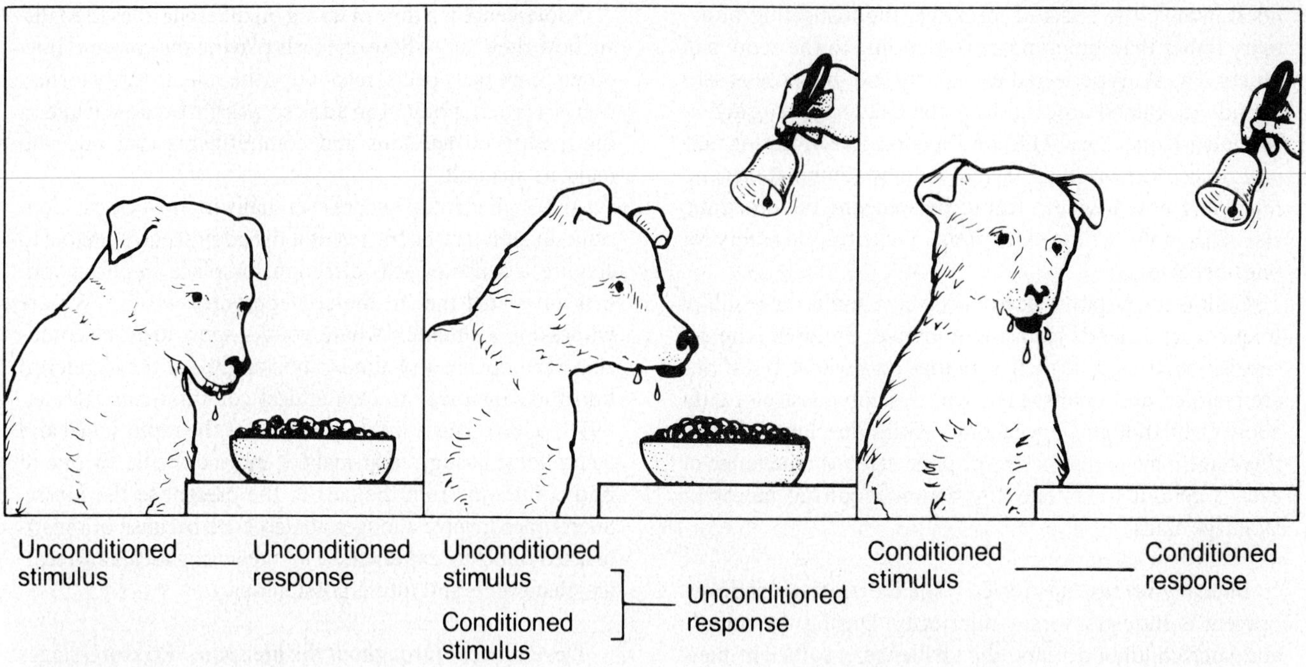

FIGURE 3-5

Pavlov's classical conditioning paradigm. Pairing of unconditioned stimulus (food) and unconditioned response (salivation) with conditioned stimulus (bell) causes a conditioned response when food is eliminated and the only stimulus is the ringing bell.

Behaviorists concentrate on the present and the means by which the environment influences human behavior. The past is not considered the root of all behavior, as it is for the psychodynamic theorist. Maturation is not as central to learning as it is for the cognitive-structuralists. The environment and the way a person modifies and controls it are the variables that determine human action.

Theory of B. F. Skinner B. F. Skinner (1904–) assumed that the child is a passive recipient of environmental influences and therefore is malleable. Skinner believed that learning could be controlled by proper structuring and response to the child's action. For him learning was the result of responses received from the environment. The child is considered to be a miniature adult, therefore all learning is cumulative. Adults are responsible for creating optimal conditions so that the desired learning can be achieved.

Skinner postulated that there are two types of *conditioning,* or behavioral responses to a *stimulus,* that cause the response. The first type of conditioning is termed *classical conditioning* and is illustrated by Pavlov's well-known experiments with dogs. Pavlov caused his dogs to salivate by ringing a bell when they received food. He thus linked an unconditioned response (salivating with food) with a second stimulus (the ringing bell). After several times with both stimuli, the original stimulus (food) was eliminated, and only the second stimulus (bell) was used. The dogs, however, still salivated at the sound of the bell (Fig. 3-5). Classical conditioning is thus a procedure in which conditioned responses are established by the association of a new stimulus with a stimulus that is known to cause an unconditioned response. The resulting response is the conditioned response to the unrelated (new) stimulus.

The second type of response is what Skinner referred to as *operant conditioning,* a procedure by which the frequency of a response can be increased or decreased, depending on when, how, and to what extent it is reinforced. Convinced that humans, like animals, will always repeat an action that brings pleasure, Skinner noted that the consequences of action, what he termed *reinforcement,* are all important. Positive consequences will foster repetition of the action. The absence of consequences will cause the action to stop.

To demonstrate his theory, Skinner designed cages with electronic levers that delivered food when they were pressed. The animal learned that these two events were related through the repeated consequence of a primary reinforcer (food) that rewarded its pushing the lever (the conditioned response). Thus, whenever it desired food, attention, or relief from boredom, the animal would push the lever, fully expecting some food to appear.

Skinner and his associates later discovered that learning was more permanent if reinforcers were provided intermittently rather than continuously. They also concluded that time, patience, and steps that were carefully graded from simple to complex were needed when teaching complicated behaviors.

Nurses can use the principles of behaviorism to change certain actions in some children. This approach is called *behavior modification.* The focus of behavior modification is changing behavior by manipulating the response, or reinforcement, evoked by the behavior. For example, if a group of participants repeatedly arrives late for appointments or for a health education class, the nurse first speaks to them about this and then commends them for attempts to arrive on time. The first few times, this praise may be for being 7 minutes late instead of 10. The reinforcer is then given only for being even more punctual until punctuality finally becomes the norm. The principle is that positive, cooperative behavior is praised and rewarded rather than disobedience punished.

A negative behavior may, however, become inadvertently rewarded and thus conditioned. For example, the small child who cries for candy at the store may be given some candy to stop the crying and to decrease parental embarrassment. The next time the parent and child go to the store the child will cry for candy again because last time that behavior (crying) was successful in obtaining the desired object. The parent may once again comply with the child's wishes or anticipate the wish and provide the candy even before the behavior begins. Denying the request and ignoring any outbursts would start the process of *extinction,* in which the behavior is "unlearned" because the reinforcement has been removed. Extinction does, however, take longer; greater effort is required to extinguish a behavior than to condition it.

To use behavior modification effectively, it is important to be accurate in identifying what will be a positive reinforcer and what will be a negative reinforcer from the child's perspective. It is also important to be attentive to what behavior is being reinforced, whether positively or negatively. For example, a child stands under her mother in the kitchen and whines until the mother surrenders and gives her a cookie before supper. The child then stops whining. Although the mother may feel that she stopped the whining behavior, she is in fact positively reinforcing the behavior of whining to obtain a desired end. The child learns that whining does obtain the cookie after all and will use this strategy again. In another case, the child may not perceive a punishment such as spanking as a negative reinforcer if, in fact, the child's desired goal was to obtain the parent's attention.

Theory of Albert Bandura Although he agreed with the concepts of conditioned learning, Albert Bandura (1925–) was not convinced that all learning had to occur in such a trial-and-error fashion. He proposed that many behaviors were the result of imitation. His *social learning theory* emphasizes the social variables and the ways in which they are responsible for the child's behavior.

An important variable in social learning is whether observed actions are rewarded or punished. Two other variables are the similarity of the imitated model to the self and the degree of prestige accorded the model. The two concepts that are central to Bandura's research are (1) *imitation,* the process by which an individual copies or reproduces what has been observed; and (2) *modeling,* the process by which an individual learns by observing the behavior of others.

In a study designed to assess delayed imitation of aggressive models in the absence of the models, Bandura assigned nursery school children to one of the following groups: aggressive adult models, nonaggressive adult models, human aggression on film, aggression on filmed cartoons, or a control group. For the groups assigned to aggressive models and filmed human aggression, the model demonstrated various acts of physical and verbal aggression toward a large, inflated plastic doll. The model in the cartoon film was a cartoon character participating in pranks and fights aimed at overpowering another character. The nonaggressive model sat quietly in the room and ignored both the doll and the instruments of aggression that were present. After viewing the model's behavior according to their assigned groups, the children were mildly frustrated. The researchers then counted the number of imitative and nonimitative aggressive behaviors each child performed in a setting identical to the one previously viewed but without the model present.

The children who observed the aggressive models performed many aggressive behaviors, many of which imitated precisely those they viewed. The children in the nonaggressive and control groups demonstrated few aggressive acts. Furthermore, those in the nonaggressive group displayed inhibited behavior characteristic of their model to a greater extent than did the control children. The children not only demonstrated that modeling occurs in the later absence of the model but also showed that film-mediated models are as effective as real-life models in transmitting social attitudes, values, actions, beliefs, and behaviors that may be appropriate or deviant (Bandura and Walters, 1963).

In another study, Bandura assigned nursery school children randomly to one of four groups: (1) a group in which the aggressive model was rewarded, (2) a group in which the aggressive model was punished, (3) a control group without models, or (4) a control group with expressive nonaggressive models.

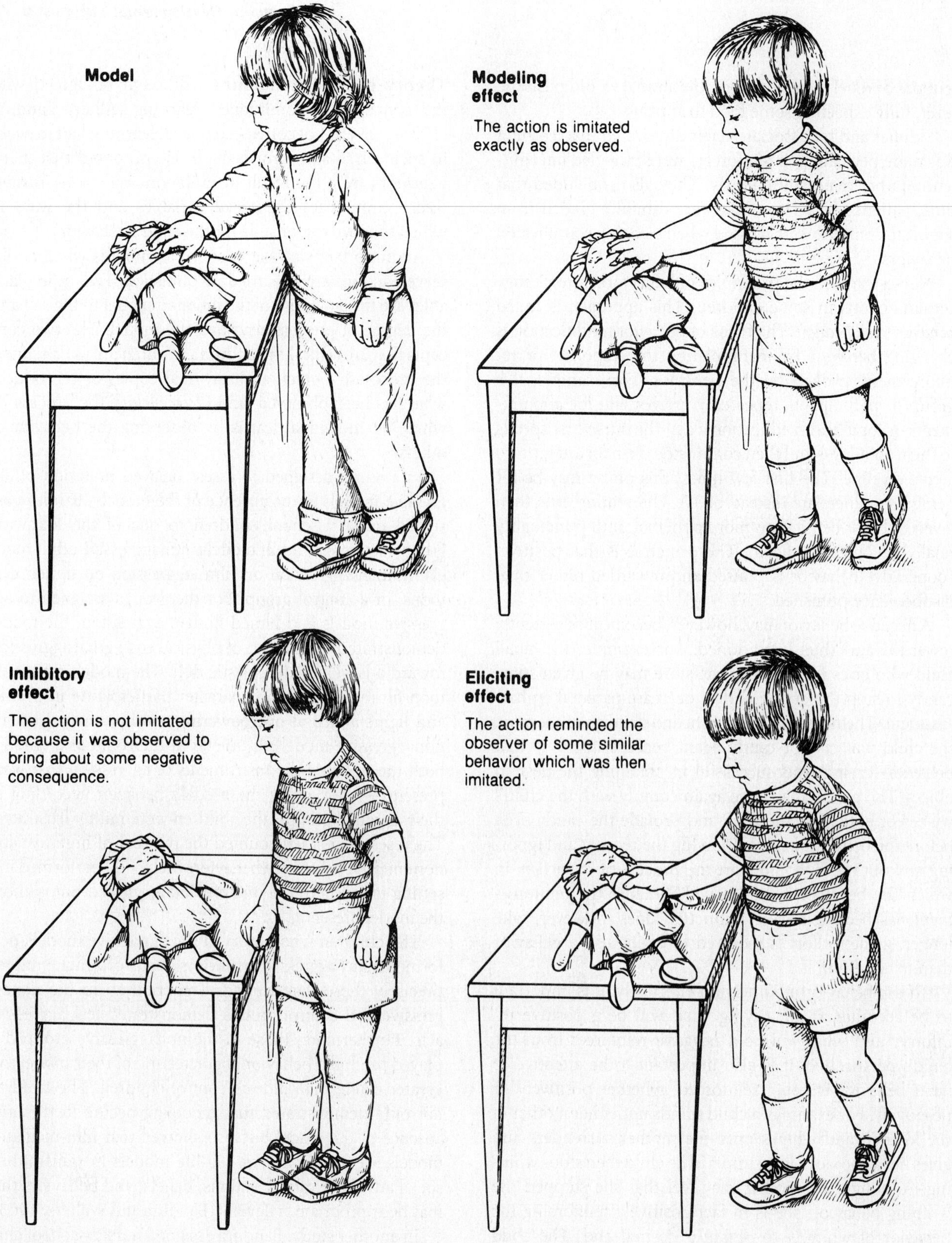

Model
Modeling effect
The action is imitated exactly as observed.
Inhibitory effect
The action is not imitated because it was observed to bring about some negative consequence.
Eliciting effect
The action reminded the observer of some similar behavior which was then imitated.

FIGURE 3-6

Bandura's modeling effects on social learning.

Children who observed the aggressive model rewarded imitated many more verbal and physical aggressive acts than did those who saw the model punished. The latter group did not differ significantly from the control groups, thus demonstrating the inhibitory effect of exposure to punishment. On the basis of the children's responses to seeing behavior rewarded and punished, Bandura predicted that if the behavior of an aggressive model is rewarded, the child will be more likely to imitate it than if the behavior is punished.

To a greater or lesser extent, imitative behaviors occur throughout the life span, but not all learning or acquisition of new behaviors can be explained by imitation. Social learning theorists have difficulty accounting for creativity and changes in thinking about moral dilemmas. Nevertheless, Bandura distinguished between the acquisition of a response set and the actual performance of the behavior. The child may acquire a new way of thinking or responding to a situation but may save it for a more appropriate time (Fig. 3-6). That the child does not immediately imitate a performance does not mean that imitation has not occurred. Imitation is therefore more than mere mimicking; it is learning a whole behavior pattern from observing and evaluating another's behavior.

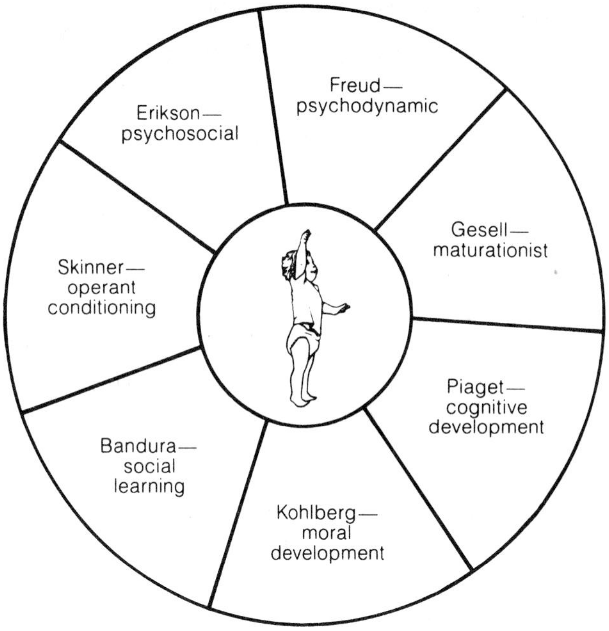

FIGURE 3-7

Human development as a composite of various theories. Each sheds light on the process and helps explain human behavior and personality.

Framework for Developmental Stages

Child development theories provide an analysis of the various components of the child's growth and development (Table 3-9). Each theory contributes to a better understanding of the child and the process of development (Fig. 3-7). (Chapters 4 through 8 focus on the application of these theories to children in the various stages of development.)

Infancy, the first phase, is the period of birth and early beginnings in the life of the child. An infant is essentially a preverbal child, generally from 0 to 18 months of age. During this time, the child experiences rapid growth in all areas, the most noticeable of which is physical growth. The infant's initial social interactions are formed, and the sense of trust in self and others is developed; learning about the external environment is closely related to motor and sensory experiences.

Early childhood is the time from 18 months through 4 years of age. Physical skills and gross motor activities become well learned, and fine motor activities are being learned. For the child in this phase, language has opened new horizons in thought and interaction, but understanding is still limited, and the world is perceived from an egocentric perspective. Social interactions continue to develop, and the child, no longer dependent on others, becomes increasingly independent. The child now wants to do things without help and to decide when and how to do them.

Early childhood encompasses the phase of toddlerhood, with its beginning assertions for self-recognition and independent mobility. The continuation and refinement of these is sometimes called the preschool phase. Children in Western cultures increasingly have early social and peer group experiences away from home and are exposed to early learning of language and mathematical concepts. This progressive learning effectively compresses this early period into one more homogenous period rather than two separate phases.

Middle childhood is the time of the early school years. The first four years of school, from kindergarten through third grade, are times of new discoveries. New learning and ways of thinking develop as the child becomes less tied to fantasy and more realistic. New fine motor skills are learned and others perfected. Social relations expand as the child becomes increasingly peer-oriented. The child's sense of self is gained from satisfaction in tasks performed and recognition from others.

Late childhood is the time in which the child becomes increasingly sophisticated in thinking, behavior, and interactions. The ability to think logically and solve problems

TABLE 3-9 Comparison of Major Developmental Theories

Developmental stage	Erikson (psychosocial development)	Piaget (logical and cognitive development)
Infancy	Trust vs. mistrust	Sensorimotor period Substage 1—pure reflex adaptations Substage 2—primary circular reactions Substage 3—secondary circular reactions Substage 4—coordination of secondary schemes Substage 5—tertiary circular reactions
Early childhood toddler	Autonomy vs. shame and doubt	Substage 6—invention of new solutions through mental combinations Transition—early preconceptual
Preschool	Initiative vs. guilt	Preoperational stage Preconceptual—uses representational thought to recall past, represent present, and anticipate future Intuitive—Increased symbolic functioning; able to see simple relationships
Middle childhood	Industry vs. inferiority	Concrete operations—categoric classification; reversible concrete thought
Later childhood	Industry vs. inferiority (continued)	Formal operations Substage 1—relations involving the inverse of the reciprocal (ability to form negative classes and to see relations as simultaneously reciprocal)
Adolescence	Identity vs. role diffusion	Substage 2—capacity to order triads of propositions or relations
Mid	Identity vs. role diffusion (continued)	Substage 3—true formal thought; construction of all possible combinations of relations; deductive hypothesis testing
Late	Identity vs. role diffusion (continued)	(Note: all relations between Piaget and Kohlberg are that attainment of the logical stages is necessary, but not sufficient, for attainment of the moral stage)

is, for this later school-age child, both fun and challenging. Competition with others is a motivating force. Instead of thinking only about the self, the child can now take the perspective of others and respond accordingly. This phase includes children from about 9 years of age, or fourth grade, until about 12 years of age, or the beginning of preadolescence.

Adolescence is the time from prepubescence through high school. The key characteristics of this phase are the physical changes associated with hormonal maturation and

Kohlberg (development of moral reasoning)	Freud (psychosexual development)	Integration of theories
	Oral stage	Phase 1—establishing primary independence from parent; focus on motor and sensory experiences
Stage 0—the good is what I want and like	Anal stage	Phase 2—establishing self as independent decision maker concerning use of acquired skills; focus on increased mobility and use of language for communication; doing for the sake of doing; increased learning about the environment and relation of self to it
Stage 1—punishment—obedience orientation; obey rules to avoid punishment	Phallic stage (Oedipus complex; Electra complex)	
Stage 2—instrumental; hedonism and concrete reciprocity; conform to obtain rewards, favors	Latent stage	Phase 3—establishing self in new relations with peers and goals for project construction; focus on the satisfactory completion of the project; use of fine motor skills
Stage 3—seeking good relations and approval of family group; oriented to interpersonal relations of mutuality	Latent stage (continued)	Phase 4—establishing self as a logical thinker and problem solver with the ability to expand one's perspective to others, focus on concrete problems and their solutions; sophisticated motor and social skills involving group cooperation and organization
Stage 4—obedience to law and order in society; maintenance of social order—show respect for authority	Genital stage	Phase 5—establishing new ways of relating to parents and peers; increased attraction to opposite sex; new ways of thinking and ability to solve hypothetic problems and think about the future; focus on resolution of dependence vs. independence in all modes of behavior
Stage 5A—concern with individual rights and legal contract; social contract; utilitarian lawmaking perspective	Genital stage (continued)	
Stage 5B—higher law and conscience orientation; orientation to internal decisions of conscience but without clear rationale or universal principles	Genital stage (continued)	

development of secondary sex characteristics. Changes in thinking and reasoning become evident, and the child is now able to solve abstract and hypothetic problems.

The growth and development of the child from a helpless newborn to an independent, self-functioning adolescent are marvelous, yet complex, phenomena that are only partially understood. The more nurses know about these ongoing processes, however, the more effectively they can be involved in planning interventions, whether in teaching healthy behavior, preventing illness, or providing care.

Essential Concepts

- Developmental theorists seek to discover how human beings grow and develop and why identifiable characteristics appear at certain ages or in similar environments.
- Developmental theories can direct nursing actions and explain a child's behavior or thought processes as long as the nurse considers chlidren's individual differences.
- Each theory describes a segment of the development process and provides part of the nurse's understanding of the process as a whole.
- Growth and development occur as orderly, sequential processes, although their pace varies from child to child.
- Growth and development are continuous processes influenced by a variety of internal and external factors.
- Maturation theorists, such as Arnold Gesell, emphasize the role of genetics as the determiner of the way and the order in which developmental stages occur.
- Cognitive-structural theorists study the qualitative changes in children's thinking, reasoning, and language skills by observing behaviors and making inferences.
- Jean Piaget, a cognitive-structural theorist, defined learning as an active process in which the child develops intelligence and logic skills by manipulating the environment.
- Lawrence Kohlberg, a cognitive-structural theorist, studied moral development and identified stages of moral judgment as represented in decision making about moral dilemmas.
- Psychodynamic theorists examine the emotional forces reflected in personality.
- Sigmund Freud, an early psychodynamic theorist, studied unconscious motivation and defined the stages of personality development that were related to psychosexual growth.
- Erik Erikson expanded on Freud's work by analyzing the role of the external environment and significant persons in influencing personality development.
- Behaviorists, such as B. F. Skinner and Albert Bandura, explained development as the result of learned responses to environmental stimuli.
- B. F. Skinner defined learning as a process of conditioning, or response to a stimulus, and thereby suggested principles that nurses can use in influencing behaviors of some children in some situations.
- Albert Bandura explained behavior as a result of social learning, which functions through imitation and role modeling of others in the environment.
- The variety of developmental theories, taken together, suggest a series of developmental stages; at each stage, the child makes critical progress in one or more areas of development.

References

Bandura A, Walters R: *Social Learning and Personal Development.* Holt, Rinehart & Winston, 1963.

Duska R, Whelan M: *Moral Development, A Guide to Piaget and Kohlberg.* Paulist Press, 1975.

Erikson E: *Childhood and Society.* Norton, 1963.

Erikson E: *Identity: Youth and Crisis.* Norton, 1968.

Freud S: *The Ego and the Id.* Hogarth, 1974. (Translation of 1923 work.)

Gilligan C: *In a Different Voice: Psychological Theory and Women's Development.* Harvard University Press, 1982.

Haggerty R: Foreword. In: *Physical Growth and Development.* Valadian I, Porter D (editors). Little, Brown, 1977.

Ilg FL, Ames LB: *The Gesell Institute's Child Behavior.* Dell, 1960.

Kohlberg L: Moral stages and moralization: The cognitive-developmental approach. In: *Moral Development and Behavior.* Likona T (editor). Holt, Rinehart & Winston, 1976.

Maier HW: *Three Theories of Child Development: The Contributions of Erik H. Erikson, Jean Piaget, and Robert R. Sears and Their Applications.* Revised ed. Harper & Row, 1978.

Nelms BC, Mullins RG: *Growth and Development—A Primary Health Care Approach.* Prentice-Hall, 1982.

Piaget J, Inhelder B: *The Psychology of the Child.* Basic Books, 1969.

Additional Readings

Baldwin AL: *Theories of Child Development.* Wiley, 1968.

Berkenfield J, Schwartz JB: Nutrition intervention in the community—the "WIC" program. *N Engl J Med* 1980; (10): 579–580.

Bigner JJ: *Human Development—A Life-Span Approach.* Macmillan, 1983.

Brainerd CJ: *Piaget's Theory of Intelligence.* Prentice-Hall, 1978.

Field TM et al: *Review of Human Development.* Wiley, 1982.

Fong BC, Resnick MR: *The Child: Development Through Adolescence.* Benjamin/Cummings, 1980.

Fowler JW: *Stages of Faith: The Psychology of Human Development and the Quest for Meaning.* Harper & Row, 1981.

Frieberg KL: *Human Development: A Life-Span Approach.* Jones and Bartlett, 1987.

Freud S: Beyond the pleasure principles. In: *The Standard Edition of the Complete Psychological Works of Sigmund Freud.* Vol 18. Strachey J (editor). Hogarth, 1957.

Gesell A, Ilg FL: *Child Development: An Introduction to the Study of Human Growth.* Harper & Row, 1949.

Hess EH: Ethology and developmental psychology. In: *Carmichael's Manual of Child Psychology.* Vol 1. Mussen H (editor). Wiley, 1970.

Kohlberg L: Moral development. In: *International Encyclopedia of the Social Sciences.* Macmillan, 1968.

Kohlberg L: Stage and sequence: The cognitive-development approach to socialization. In: *Handbook of Socialization: Theory and Research.* Goslin D (editor). Rand McNally, 1969.

LaBarba RC: *Foundations of Developmental Psychology.* Academic Press, 1981.

Labinowicz E: *The Piaget Primer.* Addison-Wesley, 1980.

Lazar I: The persistence of preschool effects. Education Commission of the States. US Department of Health, Education, and Welfare (DHEW Publication No. (OHDS) 78-30130), September, 1977.

Lazar I, Darlington R: Lasting effects after preschool. Final Report, HEW Grant 90C-1311. US Department of Health, Education, and Welfare (DHEW Publication No. (OHDS) 79-30179), 1979.

Lewis M: *Clinical Aspects of Child Development.* Lea & Febiger, 1982.

Lickona T (editor): *Moral Development and Behavior: Theory, Research, and Social Issues.* Holt, Rinehart & Winston, 1976.

Lowrey GH: *Growth and Development of Children.* Year Book, 1978.

Maier HW: *Three Theories of Child Development.* Harper & Row, 1965.

Omery A: Moral development: A differential evaluation of dominant models. *ANS* 1983; 6(1): 1–17.

Piaget J: *The Development of Thought.* Viking Press, 1977.

Ramey CT, Campbell FA, Finkelstein NW: Course and structure of intellectual development in children at high risk for developmental retardation. In: *Learning and Cognition in Mental Retardation.* Brooks P, Baumeister A (editors). University Park Press, 1983.

Schell RE, Hall E: *Developmental Psychology Today.* Random House, 1983.

Schuster CS, Ashburn SS: *The Process of Human Development: A Holistic Approach.* Little, Brown, 1986.

Sheldon WH: *Varieties of Physique.* Harper & Row, 1940.

Sheldon WH: *Varieties of Temperament.* Harper & Row, 1942.

Siegler RS, Liebert DE, Liebert RM: Inhelder and Piaget's pendulum problem. *Dev Psychol* 1973; 9:97–101.

Skinner BF: *Beyond Freedom and Dignity.* Knopf, 1971.

Skinner BF: *Walden Two.* Macmillan, 1948.

Tanner JM: *Education and Physical Growth.* University of London Press, 1966.

Tanner JM: Growing up. *Sci Am* 1973; 229(3): 34–43.

Thomas RM: *Comparing Theories of Child Development.* Wadsworth, 1979.

Tulman, LJ: Theories of maternal attachment. *ANS* 1981; 4(3): 7–14.

Vurpillot E: The development of scanning strategies and their relation to visual differentiation. *J Exp Child Psychol* 1968; 6:632–650.

Wadsworth B: *Piaget's Theory of Cognitive Development.* Longman, 1979.

Watson R, Lindgren HC: *Psychology of the Child and the Adolescent.* Macmillan, 1979.

Yussen SR, Santrock JW: *Child Development: An Introduction.* Brown, 1982.

Zeskind PS, Ramey CT: Fetal malnutrition: An experimental study of its consequences on infant development in two caregiving environments. *Child Dev* 1978; 49:1155–1162.

Zeskind PS, Ramey CT: Preventing intellectual and interactional sequelae of fetal malnutrition: A longitudinal, transactional, and synergistic approach to development. *Child Dev* 1981; 52:213–218.

Chapter 4

Infancy

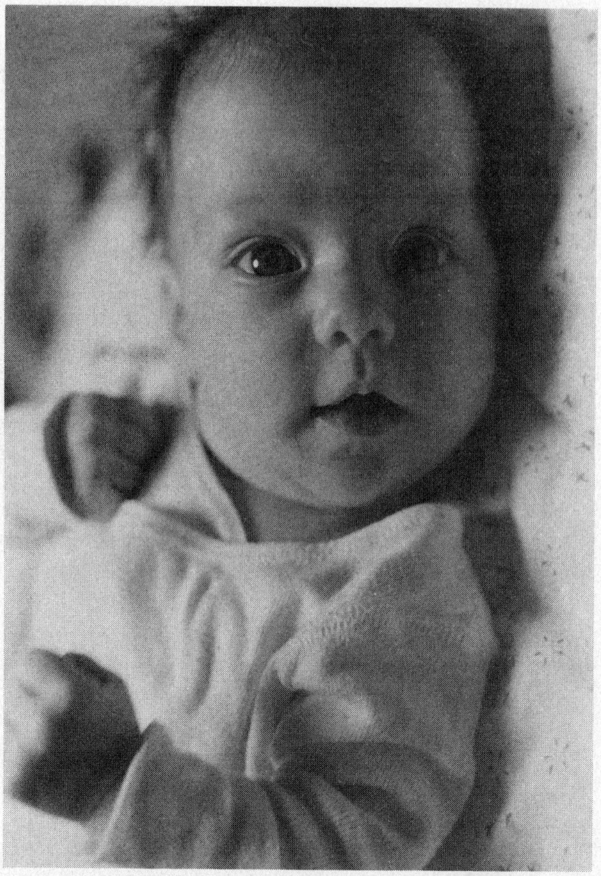

Chapter Contents

Objectives

- Explain the influences of the external and internal environments on infant development.
- Define the major criteria for neonatal assessment.
- Explain the essential biophysical changes that occur in infancy.
- Describe the principal theoretic explanations for cognitive, affective, and social development in infancy.
- Identify the basic health care needs for infants.

The word *infant* is derived from Greek and Latin and means literally "one who does not speak." Infancy is defined as the time from birth to approximately 18 months of age, when children begin to speak in sentences consisting of two words. During infancy, rapid physical growth and maturation are primarily important.

Shortly after birth, the infant appears to be relatively helpless. A number of reflexes are present, as well as some rudimentary control over eye and head movements, but that is the extent of physical skills. During the first few months, the infant progresses from this relatively helpless state to a level of substantial skill in motor coordination and mobility. By the end of infancy, the child can sit up, crawl, walk, and even run. Infants can reach out and grasp objects to examine them, pass them from hand to hand, and manipulate them with increasing skill. The combination of neuromuscular maturation and practice leads to improved coordination, which the infant quickly puts to practical use. By the end of infancy, children can feed themselves with utensils and can manipulate and play with toys in ways that were entirely impossible a few short months before.

Language development and communication skills progress from the ability to cry to the ability to babble in a broad range of sounds and then to the ability to imitate sounds common to the language spoken in the environment. When the child begins to put words together into two- and three-word sentences, this preverbal phase concludes, and the infant progresses to early childhood.

During the first 18 months of life, the infant develops a number of social skills and abilities. A warm and deep relationship with the parent is soon translated and expanded into relationships with relatives, caregivers, or siblings. Infants show an ability to enjoy socializing with peers at a very simple level. In the beginning, the infant's personality is evident predominantly in satisfying immediate needs: eating when hungry, being changed when wet, sleeping when tired. This natural egocentricity begins to broaden during the first few months, and the infant comes to recognize and respond to the emotional communication received from others. This is preparation for an emerging sense of self and for the struggle for autonomy and independence during early childhood.

The infant experiences transitions from the intrauterine environment to the outside world and then from a neonate to a walking, talking person at 18 months of age. These changes can demonstrate a wide variation of developmental rates and personality styles, but the development of motor skills and personality characteristics proceeds in a relatively ordered and sequential fashion. First infants roll over, then they crawl and sit, and then they walk (Figure 4-1). A neonate will respond to all caregivers but prefers the parent after a few days. By 9 months of age, the same child may have a substantial aversion to strangers. Within this normal sequence, each child forges a unique path across the developmental landscape. A precocious infant may start walking at 8 months, whereas next door, the infant born fifth into a busy family may not begin to walk until 13 months of age. These two individuals, however, eventually may play side by side on their high school basketball team. The infant born as the fifth child in a family of active older siblings may never exhibit stranger anxiety because a wide range of family, friends, neighbors, and extended family is always available in the environment. Next door, the baby born first in the family might exhibit substantial stranger anxiety at 9 months. Once again, however, both may be perfectly well-adjusted children when they enter preschool together.

For all the changes and developments that take place in infancy, the development of most infants proceeds remarkably well. The nurse's role is first to understand the sequences of development and then to discuss them with the parent, to help the parent appreciate and facilitate developmental changes. Helping parents to anticipate children's needs is an important nursing intervention. Likewise, analysis of developmental progress is critical because delays in development can indicate biophysical or pyschosocial difficulties. Astute observations compared with the child's developmental history provide important cues to the infant's overall development, as well as to the accomplishment of specific tasks.

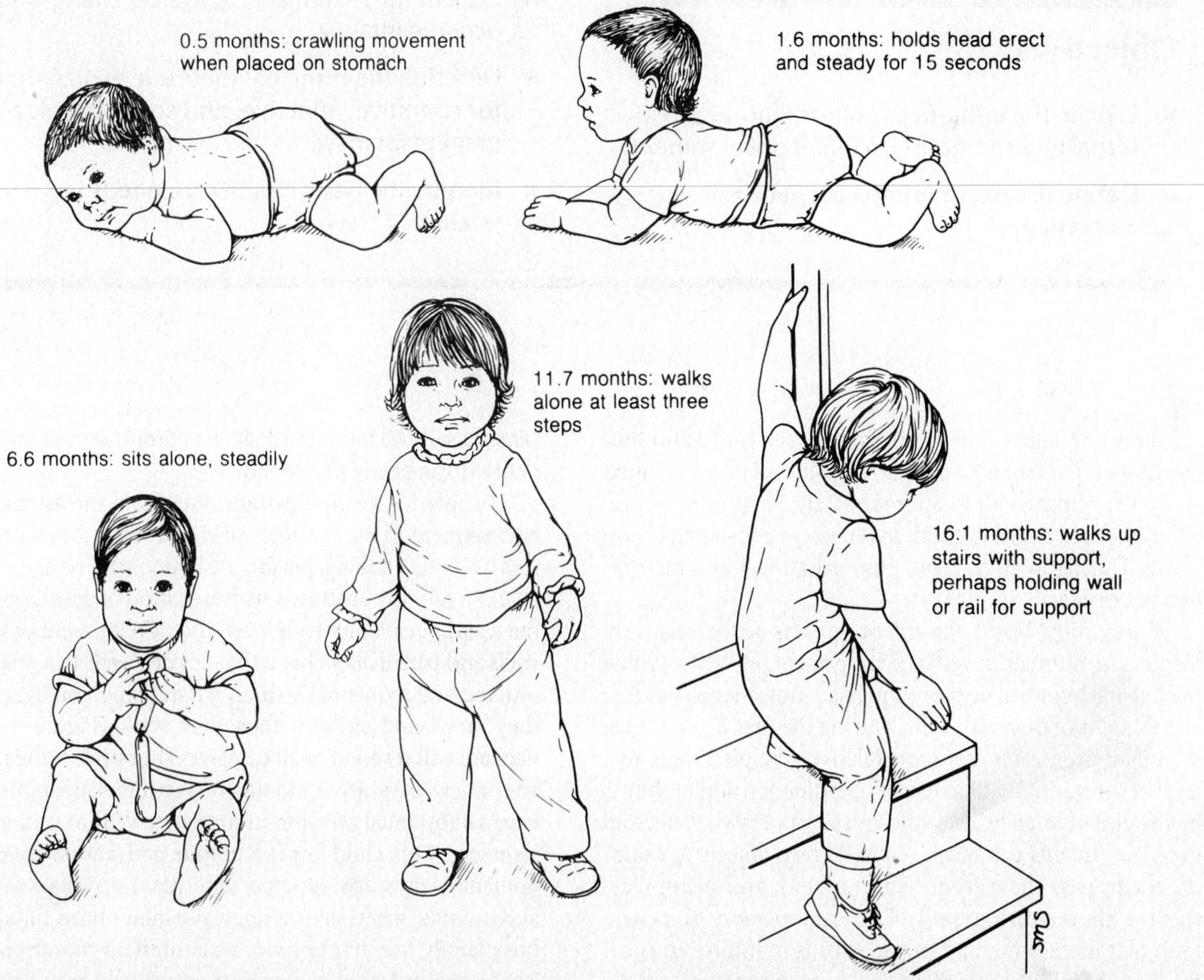
0.5 months: crawling movement
when placed on stomach
1.6 months: holds head erect
and steady for 15 seconds
11.7 months: walks
alone at least three
steps
6.6 months: sits alone, steadily
16.1 months: walks up
stairs with support,
perhaps holding wall
or rail for support

FIGURE 4-1

Sequence of motor development with average ages at which the infant achieves coordination.

The External Environment's Influence on the Infant

Influence of the Family

Infants are innately attractive to adults, and parents tend to lavish them with attention and care without any encouragement. A firstborn can be a source of delight and wonder for parents, but firstborn chldren also are subjected to first-time parental errors, occasional overconcern, and sometimes unrealistic expectations. With subsequent infants, the parents' skills are more developed, but the time available to spend with the child is decreased. Older siblings and extended family members often come to play a significant role in the social interaction and socialization process of subsequent infants.

Parental preparation Parents perceive their infants in substantially different ways. Most parents eagerly await the arrival of their infants and anticipate this event as a positive, life-enhancing experience. A relatively high proportion of infants, however, are "unplanned" in that their parents were not trying actively to conceive when the pregnancy occurred. Sometimes, these infants interrupt career plans, come in the middle of schooling, or add an undesired burden on family finances and resources. Parents' reactions to their infants can also vary with the infant's temperament. An infant who makes few demands and is easy to manage might be more enjoyable initially than one who is active, vocal, and intrusive. The infant with the difficult temperament is likely to establish a place within the family structure more quickly because of this demand for attention.

Social and economic differences also affect parents' motivations for having an infant. For some parents, having a baby fulfills the primary purpose of marriage. For others, especially unmarried teens, the value of an infant is the increase in status and attention from society that the mother enjoys for a time. For some families, the increased demands on parental resources (both time and money) are easily accommodated. For others, these demands are sources of stress.

For example, the unplanned pregnancy for a couple who thought that they had completed their family and were starting to prepare for college tuitions and long-delayed travel plans resulted in a crisis. Rather than obtain a part-time job as planned, the mother stayed home to care for this new infant. The father took a second job to supplement the family's income, which necessitated weekend and evening work. The family was seldom together; the older children resented the infant, whom they blamed for changing all their plans; the mother was tired and felt "tied down" all over again; and the father did not have the energy to play games or the time to attend the numerous events in which the older children participated. The parents finally realized that changes had to be made if the family was to survive. Family life had deteriorated to the point where each member was living and acting as if no one else mattered. Fortunately, this family was able to identify the problem and were willing to work together to solve it and restore family equilibrium.

Family resources The economic position of the family determines to a large extent how infant care needs are met. Whether the infant is the firstborn or the fourth, the impact on the family is considerable. Plans and roles must consider the needs of this dependent member. It has been estimated that a child costs at least $2000 a year without any extras such as day care or private school. One mother figured that she spent as much on day care per year as she would spend in sending the child to a mid-priced private college.

When the mother has a career, attends school, or needs to be employed for financial reasons, infant care must be provided by someone else during her absence. Sometimes, relatives live nearby and can be of assistance. Many parents, however, do not have the convenience of a family member who is capable and willing to be a caregiver and must find other resources. Such sources may be a friend, on-site child care, traditional day care, a child-care co-op, or even a nanny.

Some families adapt easily and consider the infant a planned extension of their lives and an experience to share. Other families find the infant's arrival to be a stressor that creates anxiety and turmoil and severely taxes their ability to cope. Nurses need to recognize the behaviors, questions, and comments that indicate stress. Assessment, planning, and intervention to assist and support the family then can follow.

Influence of the Community

The birth of an infant represents different norms and expectations for various cultural and ethnic groups. For some groups, it is a time of religious celebration, and the entire family gathers around while the infant is baptized or given a blessing by the father in a formal religious service. In some cultures, taking care of the infant is strictly "women's work," and fathers keep their distance. In some American subcultures taking care of an infant becomes largely an extended family activity.

Each of these variations provides the infant with a different experience in family dynamics and socialization, which can influence personality and social development. Infants are remarkably robust and flexible, and each adapts to variations in care and social environment. Infants thrive in the snowbound wilderness environment of the Eskimo family and on the tropical islands of Fiji. There is more than one way to raise a child successfully. A great many social and emotional environments are all healthy and wholesome for an infant. Even in less-than-ideal circumstances, infants adjust remarkably well. Nurses assessing infants and their families therefore need to distinguish between unusual or less-than-optimal family environments and families that are genuinely at risk, such as those cases of abuse or neglect so severe that the infant will fail to thrive and damage may result. (Families at risk are discussed in Chapter 13.)

Developmental Changes in Infancy

Transition at Birth

During the first few days of life, the neonate makes the transition from the warm, secure, fluid-filled intrauterine environment to the outside world, which is filled with sounds, sights, and a variety of new experiences. This transition is not without substantial adjustment; it is both abrupt and traumatic. During labor and delivery, the neonate is literally forced through the pubic opening in the pelvis and through the birth canal by the muscular contractions of the uterus. The pressure on the head is frequently so great that it is elongated and stretched at the leathery fontanels (see Fig. 10-2).

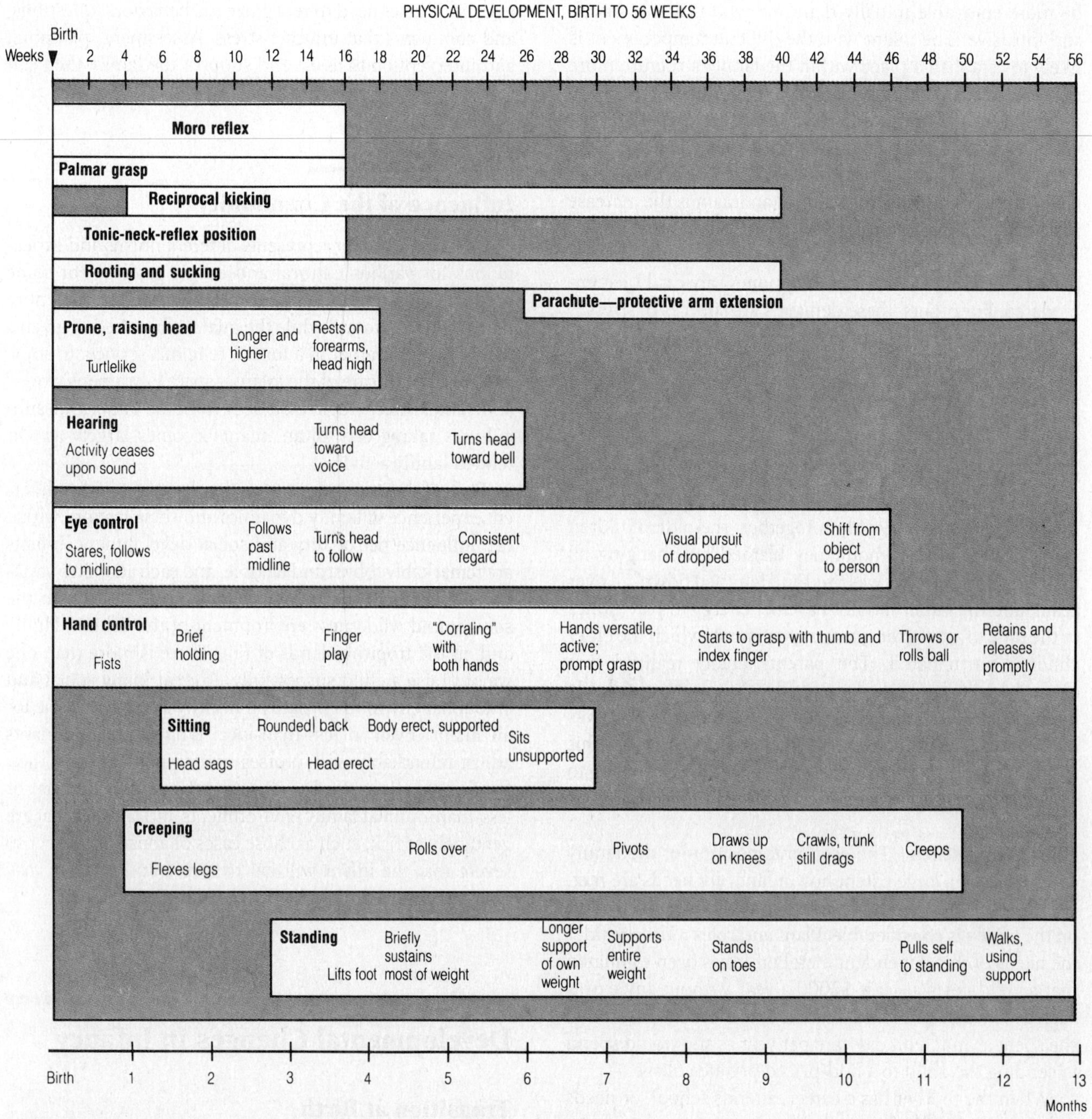

FIGURE 4-2
Developmental changes from birth to 56 weeks of age.

In addition to the abrupt environmental change at birth, the neonate experiences abrupt physiologic changes. For the first time, the heart takes on the full responsibility for pumping blood through the circulatory system; for the first time, the bronchioles and air sacs in the lungs fill with air, and the lungs begin to supply oxygen to the blood. With the first few breaths comes the possibility of making a sound with the vocal cords and of hearing the sound of one's own voice.

An hour or so after birth, the neonate frequently drifts off into a deep sleep that can last for many hours. Like the mother, the neonate seems to welcome the opportunity to rest after the stressful and difficult experience of birth. Far from looking like the "Gerber baby," the neonate's skin is

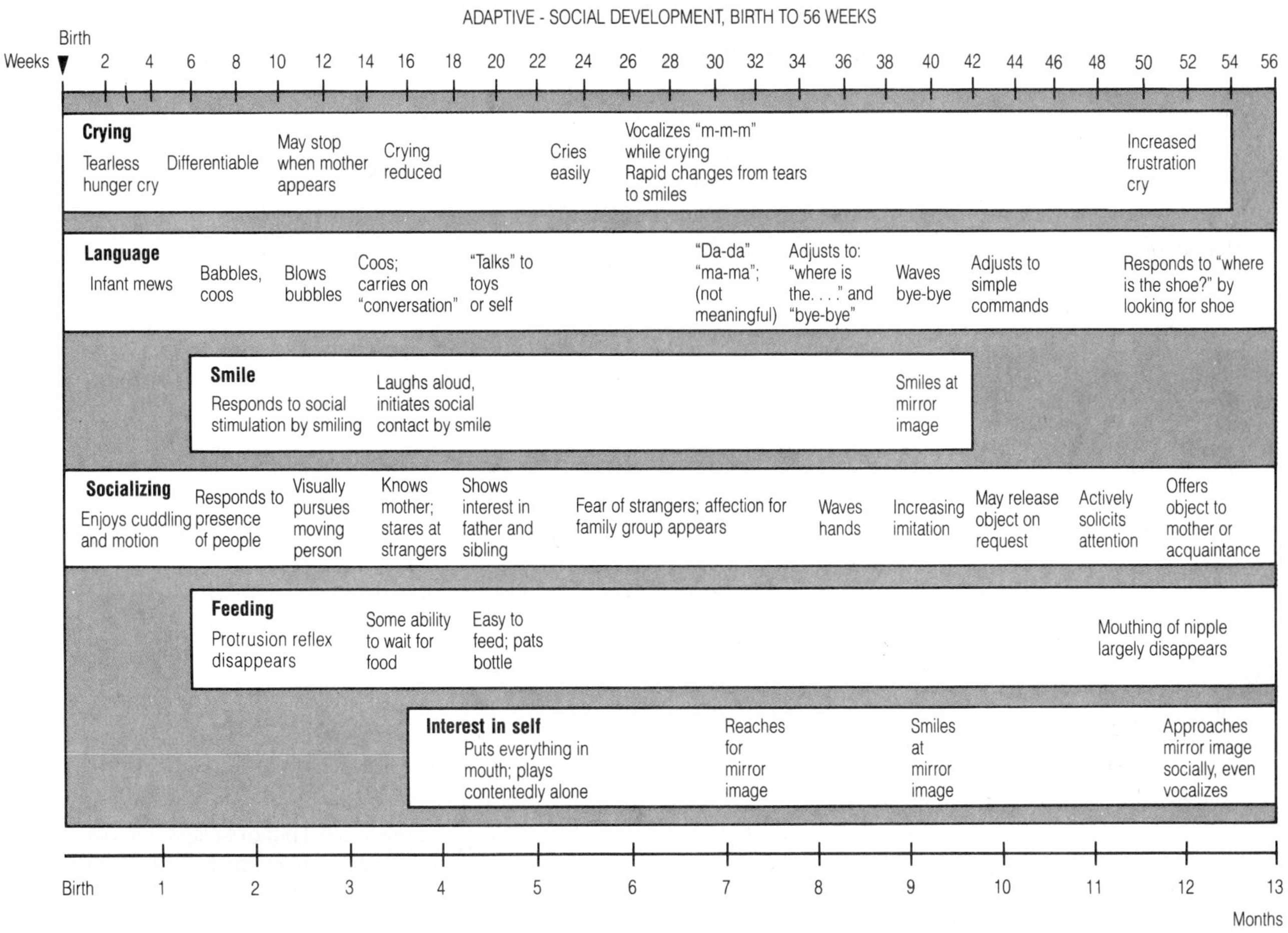

FIGURE 4-2 ***(Continued)***

red, wrinkled, and covered with fine, light hair and a white, cheesy coating. An infant's skin often looks one or two sizes too large. Some neonates have heads full of hair (which sometimes falls out during the first few months), whereas others are completely bald. During the next year or so, this dependent neonate makes tremendous strides toward becoming a more independent being. (Figure 4-2 indicates the variety of developmental changes that occur from birth to about 56 weeks of age.)

Neonatal assessment A number of measurements and comparisons to standardized norms are employed to evaluate the neonate: the Apgar evaluation (Apgar, 1953); birthweight and length; physical assessment, including a neurologic examination; and the Brazelton Neonatal Behavioral Assessment Scale (Brazelton, 1973).

Assessment guides The *Apgar evaluation* was developed by Virginia Apgar (1953) and is particularly helpful in identifying oxygen deprivation, which may have occurred during labor and delivery or is evident in infants with neurologic or respiratory disorders. The Apgar evaluation is administered at 1 minute and again at 5 minutes after birth to evaluate the neonate's ability to support vital functions. Five variables—heart rate, respiratory effort, muscle tone, reflex irritability, and body color—are given a score of 0, 1, or 2 (Table 4-1). A high score, from 8 to 10 at 5 minutes, indicates that the neonate is in good condition in that the blood is oxygenated. A score of 3 or lower indicates that immediate emergency steps are necessary to help the infant survive.

Although the standard physical assessment parallels the physical examination (Chapter 10), the neurologic examination evaluates the gestational age and neuromuscular response of the neonate. These are critical concerns at birth. The *Brazelton Neonatal Behavioral Assessment Scale* (BNBAS) (1973) includes some elements of the neurologic examination and some fundamental social interaction behaviors. It

TABLE 4-1 Apgar Scoring Chart for Evaluating the Status of the Newborn

Sign	0 points	1 point	2 points
Heart rate	Absent	Slow (less than 100)	Greater than 100
Respiratory effort	Absent	Slow, irregular	Good strong cry
Muscle tone	Limp	Some flexion of extremities	Extremities well flexed, active motion
Reflex—irritability (response to catheter in nostril)	No response	Grimace	Cough, sneeze, or cry
Color	Blue, pale	Body pink, extremities blue	Completely pink

SOURCE: Apgar VA: The newborn (Apgar) scoring system. *Pediatr Clin North Am* 1966; 13:645.

TABLE 4-2 Common Reflexes of the Neonate

Reflex name	Evoking stimulus	Response
Blinking reflex	Light flash	Closing eyelids
Pupillary reflex	Light flash	Constriction of the pupil to brighter light
Rooting reflex	Light touch of finger on cheek close to mouth	Head rotation toward the stimulation; mouth opening and attempting to suck finger. Disappears by about 4 months of age
Sucking reflex	Finger (or nipple) inserted into mouth	Rhythmic sucking
Moro reflex	Infant lying on back with head slightly raised; head is suddenly released. Or infant is held horizontally, then lowered quickly about 6 in. and stopped abruptly	Arms extended out, head thrown back, fingers spread wide; arms then brought back to center convulsively with hands clenched; extension of spine and lower extremities. Disappears by about 6 months of age
Startle reflex	Loud noise	Similar to Moro reflex flexion in arms; fists clenched
Grasping reflex	Finger placed in palm of hand	Infant's fingers closed around and grasped
Babkin reflex	Infant lying on back, pressure applied on both palms	Head turned to midline, mouth open, eyes closed. Disappears by about 4 months of age
Tonic neck reflex	Head turned to one side while infant lies on back	Arm and leg extended on the side the infant faces. Opposite arm and leg are flexed
Abdominal reflex	Tactile stimulation or tickling	Contraction of the abdominal muscles
Withdrawal reflex	Slight pinprick to the sole of the infant's foot	Leg flexes
Walking reflex	Infant supported in an upright position with feet lightly touching a flat surface	Rhythmic stepping movement. Disappears by about 4 months of age
Babinski reflex	Gentle stroking on the sole of the foot	Fanning and extension of the toes (adults respond with flexion of toes to this stimulation)
Plantar, or toe-grasping, reflex	Pressure applied with the finger against the balls of the infant's feet	A plantar flexion of all toes. Disappears by the end of the first year of life
Swimming reflex	Infant placed prone in 2 in. of water (avoid water in nose and mouth)	Arm and leg swimming-like movement

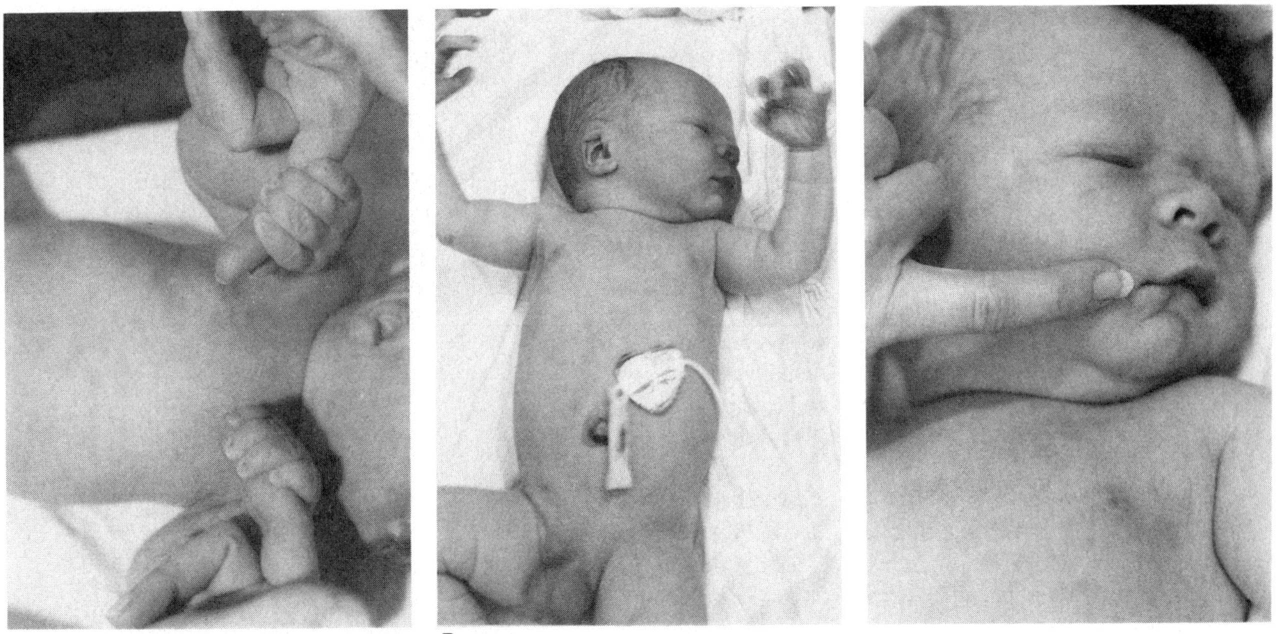

A B C

Neonatal reflexes. ***A.*** *Grasping reflex.* ***B.*** *Moro reflex.* ***C.*** *Rooting reflex. (From Swearingen PL:* The Addison-Wesley Photo-Atlas of Nursing Procedures. *Addison-Wesley, 1984).*

has been found to predict potential problems in development reasonably well, and it is used increasingly in a number of professional settings.

Birthweight and length The birthweight for neonates is between 2500 and 4300 g (5.5 and 9.5 lb). Birth length is between 46 and 56 cm (18 and 22 in.), with the average being 50 cm (20 in.). Birthweights above 4550 g (10 lb) may be an indication of problems with developmental physiology or problems associated with the mother's physiology during the last weeks of pregnancy. A low birthweight is considered to be less than 2500 grams (5.5 lb). A low birthweight frequently indicates some kind of developmental problem during gestation and is associated with multiple risks. The frequency of low birthweight is higher for minority women, those with lower socioeconomic status, and those who have experienced complications during pregnancy.

Reflexes Although neonates appear to be fragile and perhaps slightly alien, their behaviors are very well directed. Behaviors that initially seem to have little to do with mature human functioning are closely related and even predictive of later-developing perceptual and motor skills. Among the best evidences of the sophistication of the neonatal nervous system are the neonate's reflexes. Reflexes are specific patterns of behavioral response to directly focused stimulation. (Table 4-2 indicates some of the most common reflexes.)

Alterations in these reflexes resulting in consistent weakness, absence, or asymmetry may indicate defects or neurologic damage in the areas tested. Reflex testing is, consequently, included in the standard neurologic and behavioral examinations. Some reflexes have obvious adaptive purposes, and some are directly related to later-developing competencies. The pupillary and blinking reflexes, for example, are lifelong and serve an obvious protective function for the visual system. Grasping and walking reflexes, although initially strong, fade, and these tasks have to be relearned later. Rooting and sucking reflexes have great survival value. Some reflexes, such as the Babinski, abdominal, and tonic neck reflexes, are not obviously tied to later-developing behaviors. They are, nevertheless, helpful in assessing the functioning and maturation of the neonate's central nervous system.

As the infant makes the transition from the prenatal environment through birth, these reflexes facilitate emerging from one kind of world into another. At birth, the cerebral cortex is not fully capable of controlling the infant's body and directing the infant's behavior. Reflexes provide some necessary involuntary responses and give the brain and central nervous system time to mature and begin to take over the controlled coordinated behaviors. During the neonatal transition phase, many of these reflexes are prominent enough to have predictive value for later levels of functioning. Early assessment is important because neonatal reflexes are often more valuable in predicting neurologic problems than similar examinations conducted later in infancy. Some abnormal functioning that can be detected using reflexive evaluations may not appear for several months or even years. Although these abnormalities can be detected in the neonate, they may disappear during a "silent" period until they emerge as problems in later development (Prechtl and Beintema, 1964).

The Moro reflex serves as a barometer of central nervous system functioning. Its presence, absence, and hyper- or hyporesponsiveness at various ages is often a clue that some other problem exists. Because the Moro reflex is strongest for a full-term normal infant during the first 8 weeks of life, the nurse should be suspicious if the infant demonstrates obvious diminished response during these weeks. Reasons for a diminished reflex might indicate a birth injury, postbirth injury, or a congenital anomaly that has caused cerebral pressure. Sometimes, the cerebral pressure is related to cerebral edema or other factors present at birth. In these situations the Moro reflex may be absent initially and gradually appear as the edema decreases or other factors, such as hemorrhage, are treated.

The characteristics of the Moro reflex show a normal transition. From the vigorous, total-body, easily elicited response, the reflex becomes more controlled, deliberate, and refined. By 6 months of age, the Moro reflex should no longer be present. When the reflex persists after 6 months, it could have developmental or neurologic significance.

More important than any one indicator or single abnormal reflex pattern is the presence of a cluster of warning signs. Primitive reflexes present at birth should give way to righting reflexes (neck, head, and body righting), which are followed by protective reactions (parachute reflex) and finally by equilibrium or balance reactions (sitting, standing). Reflexes should disappear or appear at standard ages (see Fig. 4-2). The infant's pattern can be compared with the standard to assess neuromotor development. Progressive development is complex and involves more than neuromotor behaviors.

Social interactions The infant actively learns about the environment and its properties while assimilating experiences into innate schemes or modifying the schemes to accommodate the events and objects that are different. In addition, the infant's subjective experience and perception of events further contributes to behavior organization. Early parent-child interactions are important to confirm or disconfirm the child's sense of being able to influence the environment.

Development is never one-dimensional; rather, it is the combination of the infant's characteristics, original tenden-

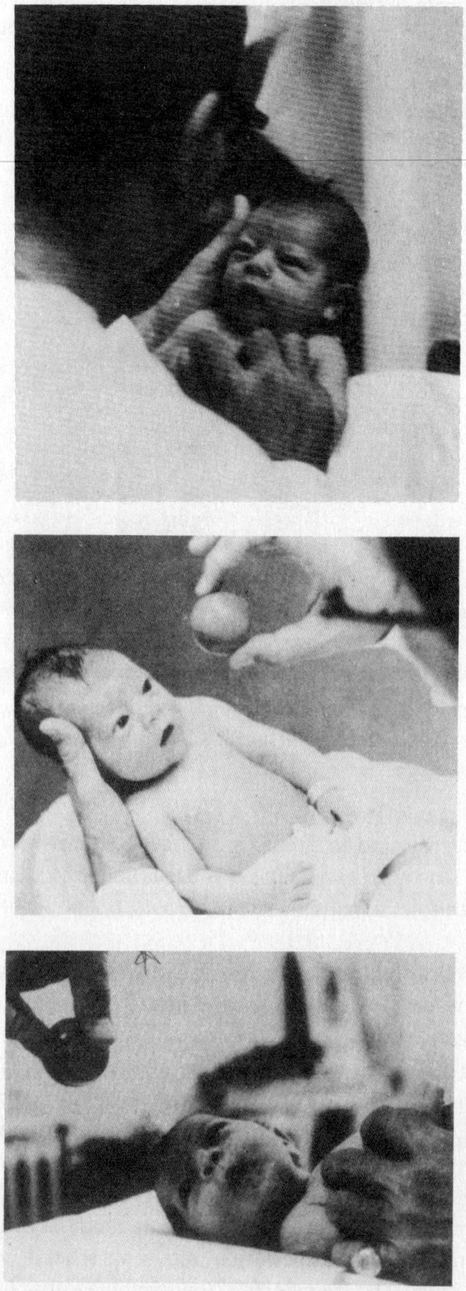

A B C

A. Neonate shows intense interest in the human face. B. Infant follows a red ball. C. Infant turns head to follow a human face. (From Avery ME, Talusch, HW: Diseases of the Newborn. *5th ed. Saunders, 1984. Reprinted by permission.)*

cies, and responses to intricate environmental influences. (Guidelines for assessing neonatal development are presented in Table 4-3). A lag in physical development, for example, may be the result of an unresponsive or chaotic social environment. Gesell (1954) commented that an

TABLE 4-3 Guidelines for the Assessment of the Neonate

Developmental area	Expected characteristics
Perinatal behaviors—assessment of gestational age	
State control	Attains and maintains the quiet alert state; changes state gradually rather than abruptly
Habituation to offending stimuli	Response decrement to shining of light in eyes during light sleep, noise of rattle and bell during light sleep
Consolability	Consoles self or accepts consolation from adult
Visual orientation	Fixates on object and/or face; follows object or face with eyes; attains eye contact with adult
Auditory orientation	Attends to rattle and/or voice; turns toward source of sound
Motor skills	Predominantly positioned with arms and legs flexed; moves symmetrically; moves smoothly; moves purposefully; responds normally to elicitation of reflexes
Biophysical development	
Body proportion	Head ¼ of total length; legs ⅓ of total length
Weight	3.23 kg (7 lb) girls
	3.27 kg (7¼ lb) boys
	Neonates lose 5%–10% of birthweight following birth before stabilizing and beginning to gain
Length	49.9 cm (19¾ in) girls
	50.5 cm (20 in) boys
Head circumference	34.3 cm (13½ in) girls
	34.8 cm (13¾ in) boys
Neuromuscular	Development of motor skills occurs in conjunction with myelination and increase in number and size of nerves in the central and peripheral nervous systems (see Chapter 31)
Gross motor skills (major combination of muscles)	Substantial control over eye, head, and mouth movements; random kicking of legs and arms; Moro, tonic neck, and walking reflexes
Fine motor skills	Undeveloped; random movements of extremities; grasp reflex

Developmental area	Expected characteristics
Cardiovascular	Overall change from an essentially singular, or mixed circulatory pattern to a well-defined, two-sided circulation (see Chapter 23)
Heart	Horizontal position
Heart rate	120–140 beats/min
Blood pressure	78 systolic
Temperature	Stabilizes after several weeks
Blood values	Elevated hemoglobin and red blood cells
Respiratory rate	30–80 breaths/min; trachea is 4 cm long and diameter ¼ that of the adult; epiglottis and bifurcation of the trachea are high, making the infant vulnerable to respiratory distress; infants younger than 3–4 months of age are obligatory nose breathers
Gastrointestinal	
Stomach capacity	90 ml (3 oz); requires feeding every 2 ½–4 hours; rooting, sucking, and swallowing reflexes aid ingestion; tongue thrust reflex facilitates expressing milk from the nipple; first stools are meconium (greenish, sticky substance)
Genitourinary	
Bladder capacity	15 ml
Urine specific gravity	1.008 Voids 20 or more times per day; unable to concentrate urine effectively; kidney reabsorption and filtration not well developed
Integumentary	Thin and sensitive skin; susceptible to blistering, chafing, and rashes; milia (sebaceous retentive cysts) appear around nose and chin as tiny white spots; might lose original hair to be replaced by hair of different color and texture; long nails need to be cut while infant is sleeping to prevent injury
Immune	Receives passive immunity from mother for protection against major childhood diseases; additional immunities against influenza, mumps, chickenpox provided by breast milk

(Continues)

TABLE 4-3 Guidelines for the Assessment of the Neonate *(Continued)*

Developmental area	Expected characteristics
Sensory-perceptual	
Vision	20/600–20/800; can discriminate both brightness and color; limited visual accommodation (see Chapter 32); can see objects held 8–12 in. from face with reasonable clarity
Hearing	Short, wide eustachian tube facilitates passage of organisms into the middle ear (see Chapter 32); can discriminate sounds, particularly mother's voice
Taste and smell	Prefers sweet tastes; will refuse salty; turns to avoid noxious odors; can smell and turn toward breast milk
Tactile	Very sensitive to tactile stimuli, particularly when hungry or awake
Social development	
Infant	Gives clear cues; responds with eye contact; attends to adult face and/or voice; accepts feeding readily; displays satisfaction; cuddles close to adult when held
Parent	Perceives infant positively; might feel some ambivalence toward infant; displays sensitivity to needs and cues of infant by recognizing and responding to infant's signals; recognizes infant's alert periods and attempts interaction; uses en face position and attempts eye contact; holds infant close to trunk; speaks positively about or to infant; shows awareness of infant's capabilities

infant cannot learn to smile in response to a smiling person if a smiling person seldom is present.

Each infant has a unique pattern, including intensity of reaction, ability to delay gratification, self-comforting behaviors, ability to elicit assistance from others, and skills or resources for diversion. This combined interplay becomes evident in what has been described as the quiet, average, and active infant (Brazelton, 1974).

Some infants move rapidly from one new skill to another. The child attacks each challenge vigorously, seeking instant success, and then moves on to confront the next challenge. These infants may walk at 9 or 10 months of age. Other infants tend to practice and delight in each skill attained and have no desire to hurry on to the next one. They may not walk until they are 15 or 16 months old. The third group, or average infants, progress from skill to skill at a rate somewhere between the two extremes. Although enjoying each new skill, they are eager for a new challenge and are usually walking around 12-13 months of age. All three groups are developmentally normal expressions of general response patterns. (Tables 4-4 through 4-8 describe developmental characteristics of infants of various ages in five major areas—temperament, biophysical, language, cognitive, and social/affective.)

Affective Development

Sigmund Freud provided the first theoretic model for understanding affective development in infancy. Since he first introduced his theory, his ideas have been criticized, modified, and expanded by others in an attempt to better understand the process of affective development.

Egocentricity According to Freud's psychodynamic model, the neonate is driven primarily by the id. The ego functions emerge only gradually during the first year (Freud's oral stage of development), and the infant has no superego at this time. The neonate's primary concern is having instinctual needs for food and comfort met. The infant's primary mode of interacting with the environment is *incorporation,* the process by which needs are met through the mouth (hence the oral stage). If the infant's needs for care, food, cuddling, warmth, and comfort are met, movement through the oral stage is relatively smooth.

After the first few months of life, an emerging ego begins to develop that distinguishes between "self" and "not self." The infant begins to understand that the performance of certain behaviors leads to the gratification of desires. A parent becomes a primary source of "goods and services," and thus infants develop a primary dependency on their parents.

Erik Erikson (1977) believed that the child is preprogrammed to develop certain psychologic capacities at different ages (a concept that Erikson termed the *epigenetic principle*). Whether the outcome of these stages is successful or frustrated depends on the support of significant people and on the social environment the infant experiences.

Erikson's first stage, trust versus mistrust (described in Chapter 3) lasts through the first year or so. Like Freud, Erikson saw the infant as fundamentally dependent and egocentric, demanding the satisfaction of basic biologic needs without understanding how those needs are met. According to Erikson, if an infant is fed, caressed, and cared for when uncomfortable, hungry, cold, or wet, the world is seen as a fundamentally friendly place that can be trusted and relied on to satisfy one's needs. A basic sense of trust then develops. If, by contrast, the infant experiences frustration, punishment, confusion, and deprivation when attempting to have needs met, the world is seen as a harsh, capricious, and unreliable place, and a basic sense of mistrust develops.

Erikson also believed that experiences in each stage have a major, long-lasting influence on personality. If an infant develops a basic sense of mistrust, that sense can be diminished by later positive experiences but never thoroughly eliminated, and vestiges of that mistrust will be seen in the individual's adult personality.

The psychodynamic models of both Freud and Erikson note the importance of an environment that is warm, supportive, and capable of meeting the infant's egocentric demands and biologic needs. Both theorists also agree that it is unrealistic to make demands requiring cognitive skills of infants when the necessary personality characteristics are not yet available. In this they agree with Piaget.

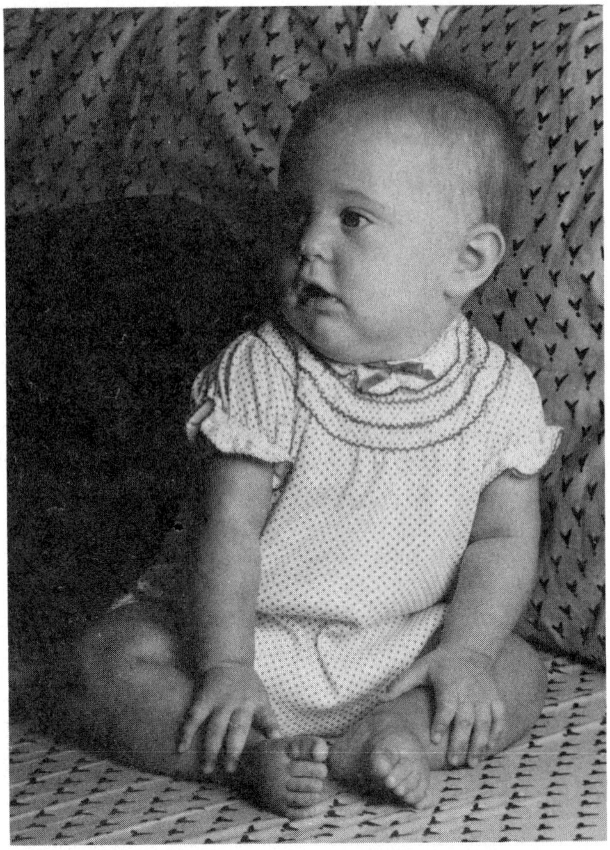

Infants show temperamental characteristics that indicate developing personality differences.

Temperament *Temperament* is the child's basic behavioral style, which affects that child's interactions. Infants have individual characteristics even as neonates, and these characteristics differentiate infants from one another. Temperamental characteristics frequently appear in clusters that define the characteristics of a child. These characteristics have been grouped into three classes: (1) the easy child, (2) the difficult child, and (3) the slow-to-warm-up child (Table 4-9). The easy child has a positive mood, rhythmic behaviors, ready adaptability, and a positive reaction to new toys. This child makes little fuss when a family schedule is changed and is as adaptable to traveling on vacation as to staying at home with the baby-sitter.

The difficult child is irregular, does not adapt to new routines, has a high intensity of reaction and negative moods, and frequently responds negatively to new stimuli. The difficult child spits out new food, cries when left with the baby-sitter, and fusses during a first car trip and during subsequent trips as well.

The slow-to-warm-up child also reacts negatively to novel stimuli but has a low intensity of reaction and tends to have irregular habits. This child may respond in an initially negative way to changes in life patterns or circumstances but will eventually adjust and adapt positively.

Many parents with more than one child are convinced that differences between children are not solely related to differences in parenting. "They are as different as night and day" is an expression commonly used by parents when describing their children. Subtle differences related to the vigor of the infant's suck, ease of consolability, and preferred position are noted at birth and provide clues to this infant's temperament. Children seem to have their own personalities and their own approaches to dealing with the world, and these characteristics do seem to persist over time. However, instruments used to measure temperament do not have the ability to satisfy the scientific requirements of validity and reliability. Although temperament remains an

(Text continues on page 102)

TABLE 4-4 Guidelines for Assessment of the 1- to 3-Month-Old Infant

Developmental area	Expected characteristics	Assessment techniques
Temperament	Parent perceives the infant's temperamental characteristics	Ask the parent about the infant's temperament
Biophysical development		
Weight	Weight gain of approximately 0.9 kg (2 lb) per month	Weigh unclothed on infant scale (see Appendix A)
Length	Length gain of approximately 2.54 cm (1 in.) per month	Mark length at crown of head and heel of feet
Head circumference	Increases at a steady rate along normal growth curve (see Appendix A); head circumference larger than chest circumference	Measure with metal or paper tape three times for accuracy; palpate fontanels
Neuromuscular		
Gross motor skills	Minimal head lag when pulled to a sitting position; head bobs when supported in sitting position	Observe and provide performance opportunity
1 month	Lifts head and turns from side to side when prone	Ask the parent about the infant's daily opportunity for development of motor skills
2 months	Lifts head 45° when prone	
3 months	Lifts head 90° when prone	
Fine motor skills	Palmar grasp present but fading; hand-to-mouth tendency; hands open (not clenched) most of time; follows object 180° with eyes by 3 months; swipes at objects suspended above eyes; becomes excited by object but is unable to grasp unless put in hand	Observe the infant's visual response to objects and whether followed by reaching, touching, and grasping attempts Ask parent about infant's opportunity for development of fine motor skills (eg, presence of cradle gym, mobile, or reachable hanging toys)
Cardiovascular		
Heart rate	130 beats/min	Take apical pulse for a full minute
Blood pressure	86 systolic	
Respiratory rate	30–60 breaths/min	Count respirations for a full minute with the infant's clothing removed
Gastrointestinal	Between feeding time increases; stools are soft yellow (breast-fed) or brown (formula-fed)	

TABLE 4-4 *(Continued)*

Developmental area	Expected characteristics	Assessment techniques
Genitourinary	Bladder capacity gradually increases	
Immune system	Immunity provided by immunizations (see Chapter 25); passive immunity from mother begins to decrease	
Sensory-perceptual		
Vision	Acuity 20/300; fixates and follows objects in horizontal and vertical direction	Observe infant's ability to follow a light or brightly colored toy
Hearing	Turns head toward sound, particularly high-pitched voices	Elicit startle reflex with a bell; see if older infant turns toward a high-pitched voice at each ear
Language development	Attends to noises and voices; responds differentially to voice of primary caregiver; pattern, pitch and intensity of cry varies; begins prelanguage vocalization (small throaty noises and early cooing); vocalizes more to primary caregiver	Listen to the infant's vocalizations in response to the parent or toy Ask whether the parent can differentiate pain and hunger Assess the quality and quantity of language stimulation
Cognitive development	Begins to replace reflex activity with more deliberate behavior; begins to repeat pleasurable chance movement (eg, thumb sucking, swiping at musical toy)	Observe difference in response between pacifier and thumb Observe ability to locate sound Ask the parent about quality and quantity of environmental stimulation
Social and affective development		
Infant	Watches faces intently and engages in eye contact; shows preferential behavior toward primary caregiver; occasionally smiles (birth to 6 weeks); shows consistent social smile (6 to 8 weeks); follows caregiver around room with eyes; shows increasingly predictable behavior and routines; cues increasingly clear; cries for increased periods; begins reciprocity in interaction with parents	Observe parent-infant interaction, the infant's attempts to initiate attention Ask the parent if infant is awake and alert for increasing periods
Parent	Holds the infant closely and securely; shows sensitivity to the infant's cues and responds appropriately; interacts reciprocally with the infant; maintains eye contact with the infant; takes pleasure from interacting with the infant; continues to feel fatigued because of night feedings; reports frustration caused by increased crying	Observe parent's response to the infant's movements and vocalizations Ask the parent about adjustments to infant care

TABLE 4-5 Guidelines for Assessment of the 3- to 6-Month-Old Infant

Developmental area	Expected characteristics	Assessment techniques
Temperament	Parent perceives the infant's temperamental characteristics	Ask the parent about the infant's temperament
Biophysical development		
Weight	Birthweight doubles by 5 months; weight gain slows to 0.45 kg (1 lb) a month	
Length	Growth rate decreasing	
Neuromuscular		
Gross motor skills		
3 months	Minimal head lag; back rounded when supported in sitting position	Observe the infant's movements when prone, supine, and pulled to a sitting or standing position
4 months	Decrease in reflexes, increase in controlled movements; head steady when supported in sitting position; back less rounded when sitting; raises head and chest when prone, supporting weight on arms	Ask the parent about the infant's opportunities to develop gross motor skills
5 months	Rolls over intentionally; back straight when in a sitting position; bears most of weight when held in a standing position; no head lag when pulled to a sitting position	
Fine motor skills		
3 months	Regards hand; grasp reflex disappears; begins to hit at objects, missing often; begins to reach for objects but does not usually obtain them	Ask the parent about the infant's opportunities to develop fine motor skills—types of toys preferred and available
4 months	Brings hands together to midline; holds objects intentionally but is unable to let go; plays with object in hands; puts objects in month; begins to pick up objects, often misses; uses both hands when attempting to pick up object	Observe the infant's ability to manipulate rattle, blocks, toys of different sizes
5 months	Picks up objects voluntarily, misses less frequently; alters hand position to accommodate size of object; if holding one block, drops it to pick up another; plays with toes; regards hand less; begins thumb opposition in picking up object, but skill is not refined	
Cardiovascular		
Heart rate	130 beats/min	
Blood pressure	90 systolic by 6 months	
Blood values	Iron stores depleted; might need supplementation	
Respiratory rate	30–50 breaths/min	

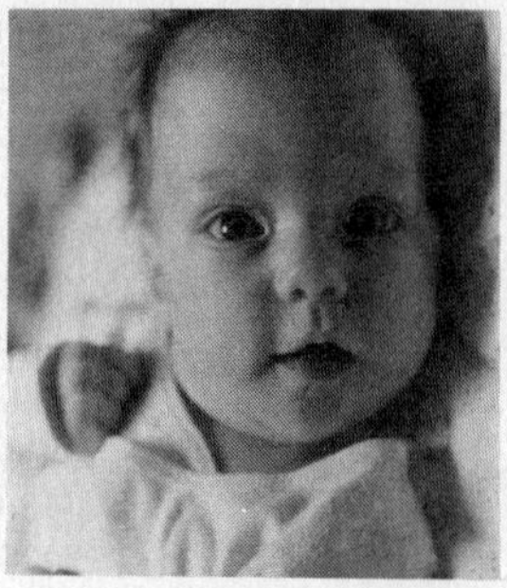

TABLE 4-5 (Continued)

Developmental area	Expected characteristics	Assessment techniques
Gastrointestinal	Between feeding time increases; begins solid foods at 6 months; stools are soft yellow (breast-fed) or brown (formula-fed)	Look for disappearance of the tongue-thrust reflex and coordinated jaw movements
Genitourinary	Bladder capacity gradually increases; reabsorption and filtration become better developed	
Immune system	Immunity provided by immunizations (see Chapter 25); active immunity develops by exposure to infectious agents	
Sensory-perceptual	Visual acuity 20/300; tearing begins at 3 months; ability to perceive colors	
Language development		
3 months	Squeals, coos; "talks" when spoken to; searches for sound in room; localizes sound by turning head to side	Listen to the infant's verbalizations while playing with a toy or interacting with parent
4 months	Laughs aloud; begins to use consonant sounds (h, n, k, g, p, b); varies tone and intensity of vocalizations; varies quality of vocalizations with mood	Ask the parent if the infant imitates sounds and differentiates human sounds
5 months	Localizes sound made below level of ear; uses simple vowel sounds such as "ah-goo"	Ask the parent about the quality and quantity of verbal interaction with the infant
Cognitive development		
3 months	Repeats behaviors found to be interesting; engages in activity more for the pleasure of the activity than the result; recognizes familiar faces and objects (such as a bottle or toy); discovers parts of own body; does not search for objects dropped from sight	Observe the infant's use of objects, imitation of gesture Observe the infant's response to a hidden object
4–5 months	Directs interest toward result of action; attempts to maintain interesting events discovered by chance; becomes more skilled at grasping, mouthing; shows interest in novelty	Ask the parent to describe the infant's environmental stimulation, for example, how and where the infant spends the day, toys and individuals available for interaction
Social and affective development		
Infant	Reciprocal interaction in parent-infant relationship (turn taking, infant's expecting response from parent, parental sensitivity to infant's cues); preferential response to family members and especially primary caregiver; discriminates familiar persons from strangers; might show early stranger wariness	Observe parental response to infant distress and the infant's response to parental comforting

TABLE 4-6 Guidelines for Assessment of the 6- to 9-Month-Old Infant

Developmental area	Expected characteristics	Assessment techniques
Temperament	Parental perceptions of the infant's temperamental characteristics	Ask the parent about the infant's temperament
Biophysical development		
Weight	Gains weight at approximately 0.45 kg (1 lb) per month	
Length	Steady increase (see Appendix A)	
Neuromuscular	Disappearance of the Moro reflex	
Gross motor skills	Bears weight on legs when held; no head lag when pulled to a sitting position; sits alone without support; stands holding on (75% of infants are able to do this by 9 months); moves around by hitching, rolling, crawling, and creeping	Observe the infant sitting; ask the parent to estimate the length of time the child is able to sit before falling over
Fine motor skills	Reaches and grasps well; picks up two blocks; transfers object from hand to hand; obtains small object using raking motion of fingers; improves finger-thumb opposition; turns wrists to better examine objects	Observe the infant's activity when prone; ask the parent about the infant's skill performance Observe the infant's hand positions when reaching, grasping objects of different sizes Ask parent about the environment and opportunities to learn and practice new behaviors
Cardiovascular		
Heart rate	115 beats/min	
Blood pressure	90 systolic	
Blood values	Hemoglobin usually greater than 11g/dL; might need iron supplementation if hemoglobin values are low	
Respiratory rate	25–45 breaths/min	
Gastrointestinal	Taking solid foods; appearance of deciduous teeth; begins to feed self with hands and hold the bottle; shows food preferences; stools are soft yellow (breast-fed) or brown (formula-fed); stools become fewer in number and more regular	Observe for presence of teeth, signs of teething such as irritability, excessive drooling, increased mouthing activity Ask parent whether infant holds own bottle or feeds self

TABLE 4-6 *(Continued)*

Developmental area	Expected characteristics	Assessment techniques
Genitourinary	Bladder capacity increases; number of voids decreases	
Immune system	Immunity provided by immunizations (see Chapter 25); active immunity increases	
Sensory-perceptual		
Vision	Can recognize fine differences in facial characteristics; responds more positively to familiar people than to strangers; depth perception is developed	Ask the parent if the infant appears cautious when faced with a visual drop such as the edge of a bed
Hearing	Becomes more precise about locating sounds	Observe the infant for vocalizations, imitation of sounds
Language development	Laughs and squeals; enjoys listening to own voice; combines vowels and consonants ("ga," "ba"); "talks" to toys; imitates sounds; combines syllables ("mama," "dada"); recognizes familiar words—own name; vocalizes emotions	Listen to the infant's vocalizations; access the infant's ability to imitate sounds Observe the parent-infant verbal interaction Ask the parent how much time is spent "talking" to the infant
Cognitive development	Uses well-developed behaviors for mouthing, shaking, banging, and dropping when examining objects; looks for object that is dropped from sight; wary of strangers; imitates simple sounds and gestures; develops awareness of means-ends relationships; obtains object by pulling on string	Observe the infant's response to a hidden object Observe the infant's ability to repeat actions purposefully Ask the parent about the infant's play opportunities and the introduction of new toys or objects
Social and affective development		
Infant	Reciprocity evident in parent-child relationship; displays more initiative in interactions and explorations; increasingly interested in objects; begins finger feeding of simple foods such as crackers; plays peek-a-boo; enjoys looking at self in mirror; demonstrates clear emotional states; communicates likes and dislikes; displays joy and anger; shows displeasure if activity is interrupted; aware of strangers	Observe parental response to the infant's initiative and infant's interest in objects Ask the parent how time is spent with infant, nature of activities, interaction

TABLE 4-7 Guidelines for Assessment of the 9- to 12-Month-Old Infant

Developmental area		Expected characteristics	Assessment techniques
Temperament			Assess the infant's temperamental characteristics; discuss parental perceptions
Biophysical development			
Neuromuscular			
	Gross motor skills	Sits steadily; twists around without falling; rights self if falls	Place the infant in a sitting position; place an interesting object on side and toward back of the infant; observe whether the infant obtains the object
		Gets to a sitting position from a lying position	Observe; ask the parent whether the infant does each behavior
		Pulls to a standing position; sits down with a bump; stands alone either momentarily or longer; creeps with abdomen off the floor; "walks" holding onto furniture; walks with help; might take first step	Hold the infant's hands and observe walking; assess parental responses to increased motor activity
	Fine motor skills	Bangs two objects together	Give the infant two blocks and observe activity; may demonstrate activity first
		Thumb-finger grasp	Place a small object such as a raisin on the table and observe how the infant picks up the object
		Puts objects into a container	Provide small objects and a container and see whether the infant puts objects into the container
Language development		Might say "mama" and "dada" specifically; uses expressive sounds	Observe; ask the parent about the infant's vocabulary
		Continues to imitate speech sounds	Have the parent present simple speech sounds and see whether the child repeats the sounds
		Understands simple words (5 words by 12 months of age)	Ask the parent whether the infant consistently responds to specific words
			Assess the quality of communication between the parent and infant
Cognitive development		Continues to be interested in environment	Observe exploratory behavior and assess parental response to the infant's exploratory efforts
		Displays intentional behavior	See whether the infant purposefully seeks an interesting experience

TABLE 4-7 *(Continued)*

Developmental area	Expected characteristics	Assessment techniques
	Imitates novel behavior	Ask the parent to perform simple activity (something the infant does not ordinarily do) and to get the infant to imitate
	Associates symbols with events	Ask the parent whether the infant understands simple expressions like "pat-a-cake" and "bye-bye"
	Differentiates means and ends	Place a toy out of reach of the infant with a string attached to the toy and near the infant; see whether the infant obtains the toy
	Searches for a hidden object	Show an interesting toy to the infant, then cover it with a cloth; see whether the infant uncovers the object
		Assess opportunities for cognitive growth
		Assess parental awareness of the infant's developmental interests
Social and affective development		
Infant	Many infants show a heightened attachment to mother	Assess parent-child interaction; assess the infant's use of the parent (especially the mother) as a resource; assess parental response to the infant's focus on primary caregiver
	Shows separation anxiety	Discuss the infant's behavior at separation with the mother; discuss parental responses to separations
	Protests at bedtime or awakens during night	Assess sleep patterns; discuss how the parent manages protest at bedtime or night waking (if these are concerns)
	Shows sensitivity to approval or disapproval	Assess the infant's response when the parent says "no"; assess parental perceptions of and response to infant "misbehavior"
	Affection; enjoys simple games	Observe interaction

TABLE 4-8 Guidelines for Assessment of the 12- to 18-Month-Old Infant

Developmental area	Expected characteristics	Assessment techniques
Temperament		Assess the infant's temperamental characteristics; discuss parental perceptions
Biophysical development		
Weight	Birthweight triples by 1 year	
Length	Increases 50% of birth length by 1 year	
Head circumference	Equals chest circumference at 1 year; 46 cm–47 cm (18 in.–18.5 in.)	
Neuromuscular	Anterior fontanel closed by 18 months	Gently palpate fontanel
Gross motor skills	Stands alone	Observe the infant in a standing position
	Walks well	Observe the infant's gait
	Creeps up stairs	Ask the parent whether the infant creeps up stairs or climbs on furniture
	Stoops to recover an object on the floor; throws objects but might fall in the process	While the infant is standing, drop a toy on the floor near the feet and observe how the infant obtains toy
	Has difficulty walking around corners or stopping suddenly	Discuss with the parents the infant's opportunities to develop gross motor skills
Fine motor skills	Builds tower of two blocks	Present two blocks and demonstrate how to stack; observe the infant's ability
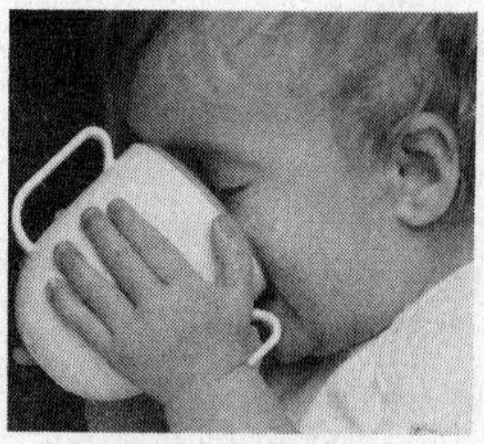	Drinks from cup	Observe or ask the parent how well the infant drinks unaided
	Uses spoon without rotating the wrist; spills when bringing utensils to mouth	Observe or ask the parent whether the infant uses a spoon and the amount of spillage
	Scribbles spontaneously; removes shoes and socks	Offer paper and crayon or pencil
	Turns pages in heavy cardboard book	Offer infant cardboard book and observe
Cardiovascular		
Heart rate	110 beats/min	
Blood pressure	96/65 mm Hg	
Respiratory rate	20–40 breaths/min	
Gastrointestinal	Intestinal length increases by 50% over birth; adult proportions of digestive enzymes; bowel pattern regular; feeds self with spoon and cup	Inquire about infant's bowel pattern. Assess parental knowledge about toilet training. Ask parent whether the infant is feeding self
Genitourinary	Voiding becomes more regular	
Sensory-perceptual		
Vision	20/100; permanent color of the iris	
Language development	Uses expressive sounds	Listen to the quality of verbalization
	Uses gestures to ask for objects	Ask the parent how the infant indicates wishes and observe the infant's gestures
	Shakes head "no"	Observe or ask the parent
	Says several intelligible words	Observe for the use of words; ask the parent whether the infant uses words; observe parental response to verbalization and the quality of parent-infant verbal interactions

TABLE 4-8 *(Continued)*

Developmental area	Expected characteristics	Assessment techniques
Cognitive development	Continues curiosity and exploration	Ask the parent about the infant's exploratory efforts; assess how parent feels about the infant's explorations and the amount of freedom the infant is given to explore; assess parental awareness of infant's development
	Interest in books	Offer infant simple, colorful book and observe response
	Finds hidden object with successive visible displacements	Place an interesting, visible toy under cover; then move under another cover and drop while infant watches and with toy visible; see whether the infant locates the toy; allow several trys if necessary
	Inserts circle into formboard or puzzle	Present foamboard without circle and see whether the infant can insert the circle into the foamboard
	Imitates behavior of parent (such as housework)	Ask the parent for examples of imitations; assess opportunity for cognitive growth; assess parental response to exploratory behavior
Social and affective development		
Infant	Increasing autonomy	Assess parental feelings regarding the infant's increasing autonomy
	Ventures away from parent to explore but returns frequently for reassurance	Observe the infant's exploratory behavior in the assessment setting
	Tolerates separations better than before	Discuss with the parent how the infant reacts to separations, how parents feel about separations, and how frequently separations occur; observe separation directly, noting the behavior of both the parent and infant during leave taking, behavior of both during separation, and infant's ability to play, interact, and be comforted in the absence of the parent; note their behavior when reunited
	Temper tantrums might occur	Assess frequency and intensity of tantrums; assess parental response
	Feeds self, usually refuses attempts of others to feed	Discuss mealtime behavior; assess parental attitudes regarding infant's self-feeding
	Protests at bedtime	Assess sleep behavior, noting especially protest or night waking and parental reactions
	Notices strangers but is less wary than before	Observe infant's reaction to nurse
	Affectionate and loving; might kiss and hug parent	Observe interaction, noting affectionate interchanges, who initiates them, and how the infant and parent respond
	Changes moods quickly and frequently (emotional lability)	Assess parental reaction to the infant's mood changes
	Begins to be provocative; purposely does things that are forbidden and watches for parental response	Assess parental reactions to "misbehavior"; discuss parental discipline and the infant's response; observe parental limit setting and reactions to the infant's breaking the limit.

TABLE 4-9 Personality Types and Temperament

Aspect of personality	Type of Child		
	Easy	Slow to warm up	Difficult
Activity level (proportion of active periods to inactive ones)	Low to moderate	Varies	Varies
Rhythmic (regularity of hunger, excretion, sleep, and wakefulness)	Very regular	Varies	Varies
Distractibility (degree to which extraneous stimuli alter behavior)	Varies	Varies	Varies
Approach-withdrawal (response to a new object or person)	Positive approach	Initial withdrawal	Slowly adaptable
Adaptability (ease with which a child adapts to changes in environment)	Very adaptable	Slowly adaptable	Slowly adaptable
Attention span and persistence (amount of time devoted to an activity and the effect of distraction on the activity)	High or low	High or low	High or low
Intensity of reaction (energy of response, regardless of its quality or direction)	Low or mild	Mild	Intense
Threshold of responsiveness (intensity of stimulation to evoke a discernible response)	High or low	High or low	High or low
Quality of mood (amount of friendly, pleasant, joyful behavior as contrasted with unpleasant, unfriendly behavior)	Positive	Slightly negative	Negative

intriguing approach to understanding individual differences, it is not understood exactly how temperamental factors can be identified and how they influence a child's behavior.

Cognitive Development

Behavioristic principles suggest that young infants learn through operant conditioning (see Chapter 3). Infants respond to a number of reinforcers, including colored lights and novel sounds, a smiling parent, or a pleasing taste. For example, three-day-old neonates will control the rate of their sucking to have an opportunity to hear their parents' voices (DeCasper and Fifer, 1980).

Very young infants are difficult subjects for conditioning experiments because neonates have a limited behavioral repertoire and because the amount of energy required for a given response may be more than the infant is willing to expend. Certain situations are, however, conducive to infant learning. Infants who receive attention, are talked to, tickled, played with, and generally stimulated by a normal home environment learn faster and learn a wider variety of things than infants in institutional settings (Clarke-Stewart and Apfel, 1979).

According to Piaget (1952, 1969), on the other hand, an infant's thinking does not advance much beyond rudimentary reflexive behaviors during early infancy. Gradually, the infant develops a repertoire of behaviors and learns to accommodate existing schemes to new situations, thereby developing memory and recognizing representations of objects. During infancy, the tie between the infant's behavior and understanding of the world is very direct. This tie between behavior and thought distinguishes Piaget's study of infant thinking and is the source of many of his insights about learning in the first months of life.

Cognitive development during the sensorimotor stage Piaget divided cognitive development into several stages (see Chapter 3). The first of these stages, the sensorimotor stage, is in turn divided into six substages of developing cognitive ability (Table 4-10).

Substage 1 During the first month of life, or the *reflexive substage,* the infant learns little but exercises innate reflexive behaviors (schemes). In this way, the infant begins to develop some fundamental control over body activity.

Substage 2 The *primary circular reactions substage* (1–4 months of age) is the time during which behaviors occur at random but give rise to pleasant sensations and so are repeated. Wiggling the legs or sucking the thumb, for

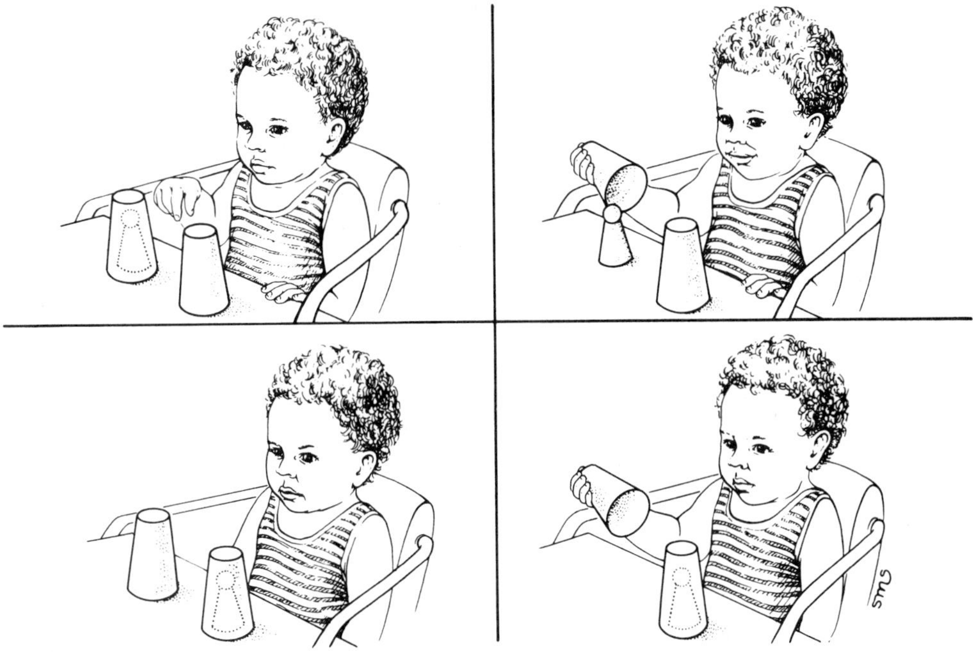

FIGURE 4-3

The search for a hidden object. The infant looks for an object where it is first hidden and does not look further. Piaget suggested that the infant is not yet able to differentiate between the object and the act of reaching for it. This is an example of the A-not-B phenomenon.

example, occurs initially in a random way but then is repeated because the activity brings intrinsic enjoyment. These activities are centered on the body, therefore are "primary," and they are circular because they repeat patterns of behavior that initially have no specific meaning.

Substage 3 *Secondary circular reactions* (occurring at approximately 4–8 months of age) change the focus of the infant's attention from centering on the body to centering on items of interest in the environment. Such reactions are termed secondary because they are centered outside the body. For the first time, the infant understands that behavior can have an effect on the environment. For example, the infant might be wiggling one foot and might accidentally tap the side of the crib, producing an interesting sound. The behavior is repeated to reproduce the sound.

Substage 4 The next substage is the *coordination of secondary schemes,* or, purposeful coordination of means and ends (at approximately 8–12 months of age). Now the infant begins to coordinate more than one scheme to reach a goal. For example, looking, reaching, and grasping become coordinated to facilitate reaching out and grasping a desired object. Also, during this substage, infants demonstrate what is called the A-not-B phenomenon. This is manifested experimentally by placing a ball in a cup to the infant's right side and letting the infant reach in and take the ball out. After several trials, the ball is placed in a cup on the left side. Even though the infant can see the ball being placed in the cup on the left and can see the ball, the infant still will attempt to find the ball in the cup on the right side (Fig. 4-3). This kind of behavior lends credence to Piaget's hypothesis that thinking and cognition have their roots in motor behavior. According to Piaget, an infant at this substage does not differentiate between the concept of the ball and the concept of reaching for the ball in the cup on the right side. The ball and reaching for the ball are one, so the infant is not able to displace the ball mentally into the cup on the left.

Substage 5 During the first four substages, the infant's primary means of adapting to the environment is assimilation. With the development of *tertiary circular reactions* (at approximately 12–18 months of age), the infant begins to develop accommodation. No longer are behaviors repeated identically for their own sake; rather, the repetition includes modification of the behavior to reproduce new results or sounds. For example, the infant may say "dada" and then practice the new sounds "daddy," "dad," and so on. These modifications are called tertiary because they are modifications in the behaviors themselves to produce novel ends. The infant is coming to understand that an important factor

TABLE 4-10 Sensorimotor Stage: Multidimensional Development at Each of Six Substages

Substage	Object permanence	Means-ends relations	Schemes
1. Reflective, ready-made schemes Characterized by predictable, innate, survival reflexes (0–1 mo)	No expectations; out of sight, out of mind, egocentric	No intentionality; unable to distinguish between need and action; adapts to world through reflexes that change as a function of experience	Looking; hearing; sucking; rooting; grasping
2. Primary circular reactions Characterized by stereotyped repetition; own body center of interest (1–4 mo)	Visual pursuit; no motor pursuit but visual following of object to point of disappearance, expecting it to reappear	Different responses to objects; visually directed grasping; acquisition of elementary habits without distinguishing means from ends; rudimentary distinction of need and action	Mouthing; attentive; looking; grasping-letting go; hand-mouth coordination; beginning distinction of assimilation and accommodation
3. Secondary circular reactions Characterized by environment and objects as center of attention; acquired adaptations (4–8 mo)	Recognizes partially visible object and will search briefly for partly hidden ones at location of disappearance	No intentional goal-directed behavior; functional differentiation between need and act; repeats behaviors found novel or interesting	Hand-eye coordination; multiple schemes capable of producing interesting results: hitting; kicking; shaking; pulling; patting; grabbing
4. Coordination of secondary schemes Characterized by intentionality—goal in mind prior to any action; consolidation and coordination of schemes (8–12 mo)	Begins to internalize conceptions of objects; systematic search for object hidden under single barrier in same place; unable to sustain search through multiple barriers or displacements	Differentiation of means and ends; behaviors repeated with intended goal in mind at onset; distinguishes objects from related activity; active problem solving; beginning of intelligence	Addition of breadth to previously acquired schemes to increase adaptation and intentionality: dropping; throwing; examining
5. Tertiary circular reactions Characterized by interest in novelty, creativity; discovery of new means by active experimentation (12–18 mo)	Follows series of visible displacements in search for hidden object; retains image of visible moving object	Trial-and-error learning; discovery of new means through experimentation; use of objects in systematic ways to discover new possibilities; modifies means (discovers new ways) of reaching same end (goal); accommodation	Social schemes showing systematic creation of new schemes for specific situations; coordinates schemes; generalizes existing schemes to fit variety of situations
6. Inventions of new means through mental combinations Beginning of thought; mental problem solving ends dependence on overt trial and error (18–24 mo)	Awareness of permanency of objects; follows series of invisible displacements; retains mental image of absent object	Discovery of new means by internalized combinations resulting in insight; uses objects for their innate qualities; foresight in problem solving—mentally manipulates event prior to acting	Invents new schemes through mental representations of symbols and their combinations; increased capacity for and use of mental symbols; naming

→

Causality	Objects in space	Imitation	Play
No real signs of understanding causal relationships	Alternate glancing; no appreciation of relationships; objects do not have definite boundaries	Immediate reflexive imitations; no true imitation	Practice or exercise of basic reflexes
Magical-phenomenalist; believes that self is cause of all action; exact repetition of accidental or random self-initiated event that brought pleasure—diffuse connection between action and result	Localization of sound begins; heterogeneous, unrelated, centered spaces on infant's body (perceptual systems); no distinction between internal and external stimuli	Pseudoimitation; reproductive assimilation—self-imitation of behaviors already possessed (i.e., sounds and gestures)	Repetitive practice of new results of behavior for pleasure; apparent voluntary repetition of actions
Observes actions and consequences and repeats those that bring pleasure; separates actions from internal feelings; formation of action patterns with external world	Increasing awareness of own behavior acting on different objects—separates objects spatially according to actions; separates self from environment; differentiates internal and external stimuli; follows trajectories of objects dropped anticipating landing spot	Imitation (true) of familiar sounds and gestures already a part of infant's repertoire	Repetition of interesting actions applied to familiar objects
Conceives of end results, then acts to achieve result; aware that objects other than self cause results; anticipates events and actions of others	Improved space concept; able to assign objects spatial locations independent of own actions; object constancy—object exists outside of perception	Use of generalized schemes to express unfamiliar sounds and gestures	Beginning of ritualization in actions; means become enjoyable and prolonged as ends in themselves
Recognizes independent causality—outside of infant's wishes; able to view cause-and-effect relations more objectively; solicits adult help to cause desired action; other people seen as autonomous actors	Understands relationships between objects and their use; spatial relations further refined and objectified; combines and relates objects in different spatial configurations, reversals, and rotations	Quicker, more precise, true imitation based on ability to discern differences between objects; confined to action phase of model; unable to internalize familiar words, invisible gestures	Expressive function; repetition of learned behavior for self-satisfaction; repetition of action phase—activity to amuse; predominance of assimilation
Searches for independent causality; infers cause when observes effect—predicts effect when observes causes	Symbolic representation of spatial features of objects; able to locate objects in familiar space—solves detour problems; relates objects to each other through internal system of representation	Capable of delaying the imitation for several days; imitation of complex, inanimate, and/or absent models, unfamiliar words, invisible gestures	Increased possibilities of play activities through mental representation; symbolically reenacts event with objects at hand to represent reality; ritualized symbolic play begins

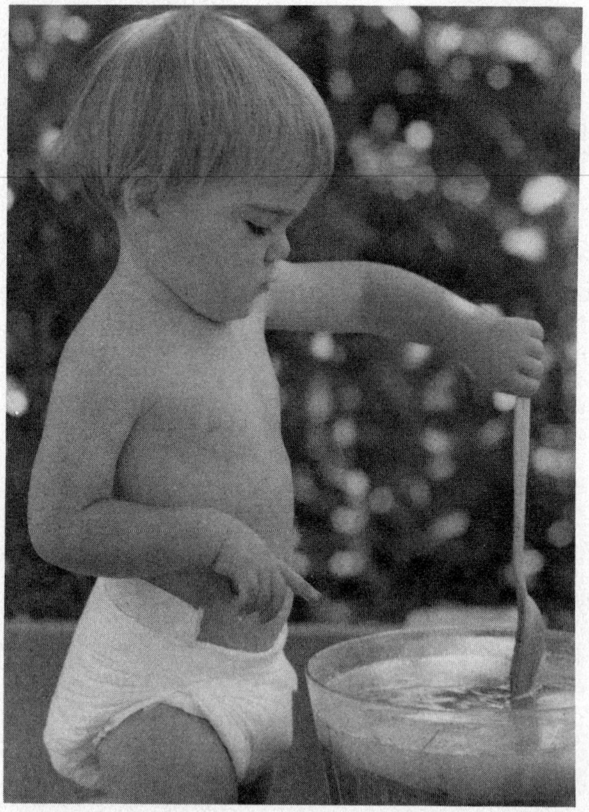

From 12 to 18 months, the infant develops accommodation and learns to repeat behaviors to produce desired results.

in bringing about change in the environment is personal action and interaction. Insights arising from experimenting with new behaviors become incorporated into the ability to deal more effectively with the world. Infants are now capable of responding to simple requests, such as obtaining a toy from another room.

Substage 6 Mental representation, (or, the *mental combinations substage* at approximately 18–24 months of age), is the sixth and final substage of the sensorimotor period. It is really a transition from sensorimotor intelligence to a cognitive intelligence that relies less directly on repeated behaviors and is more of an internal cognition. Rather than going through the process of trial and error in solving the A-not-B problem, for example, the older infant can anticipate that the ball will be found in the left cup after seeing it put there. The emerging abilities of mental representation are necessary for the second stage of congitive development, or preoperational thought (see Chapter 5).

Object permanence One of the major difficulties in studying cognitive development in infants is understanding what it is that an infant is "thinking."

A great deal of attention has been given to the skills and abilities that enable the infant to perceive the environment using the senses. Piaget believed that the infant actively integrates perceptual experiences with developing motor behaviors to develop concepts about how the world operates.

The rudimentary concept studied most intensively is *object permanence,* the fact that an object exists even when it is not seen. According to Piaget, an infant in the secondary circular reaction substage (substage 3) lacks an understanding of object permanence. Thus, a toy hidden under a blanket may "cease to exist" for an infant under 8 months of age.

Piaget proposed that the infant's understanding of object permanence begins during the coordination of secondary schemes substage (substage 4). Aspects of it are completed in substage 5, and by the time the infant is in the sixth substage, the concept of object permanence is well developed.

Evidence actually shows that object permanence occurs somewhat before Piaget originally thought. The development of object permanence seems to occur at some point between the third and ninth month of life. For example, a 3-month-old infant who is simultaneously presented with three mothers (with the use of mirrors) is quite delighted, but a 5-month-old infant presented with three mothers simultaneously shows signs of distress. Bower (1974) concluded that this kind of distress indicates that a child is beginning to understand that there is only one mother for any given place and time.

Although some psychologists have questioned Piaget's theory, Piaget's original observations about infants and the concepts he derived from those observations have been remarkably resilient to empiric demonstration.

Communication and language

Nonverbal communication Among the most important milestones in infancy is the development of the ability to communicate with others. During most of infancy, communication is nonverbal, and young infants develop considerable skill in communicating without the use of language. During the second year of life, these nonverbal communication skills become matched with verbal communication skills. By the end of infancy, the infant's capacity for communication is well developed for many of the practical social encounters that occur daily, even though the infant's actual vocabulary is limited. Communication takes place through movement, mutual gazes, touch, facial expression, and various forms of vocalization (Figure 4-4).

Because vision is controlled voluntarily from birth, gazing is an important part of an infant's nonverbal communication. Eye contact is important social communication and early eye contact makes a significant difference in a parent's feelings toward a child. Eye contact is thought to be one of the cardinal factors in developing parent-infant attach-

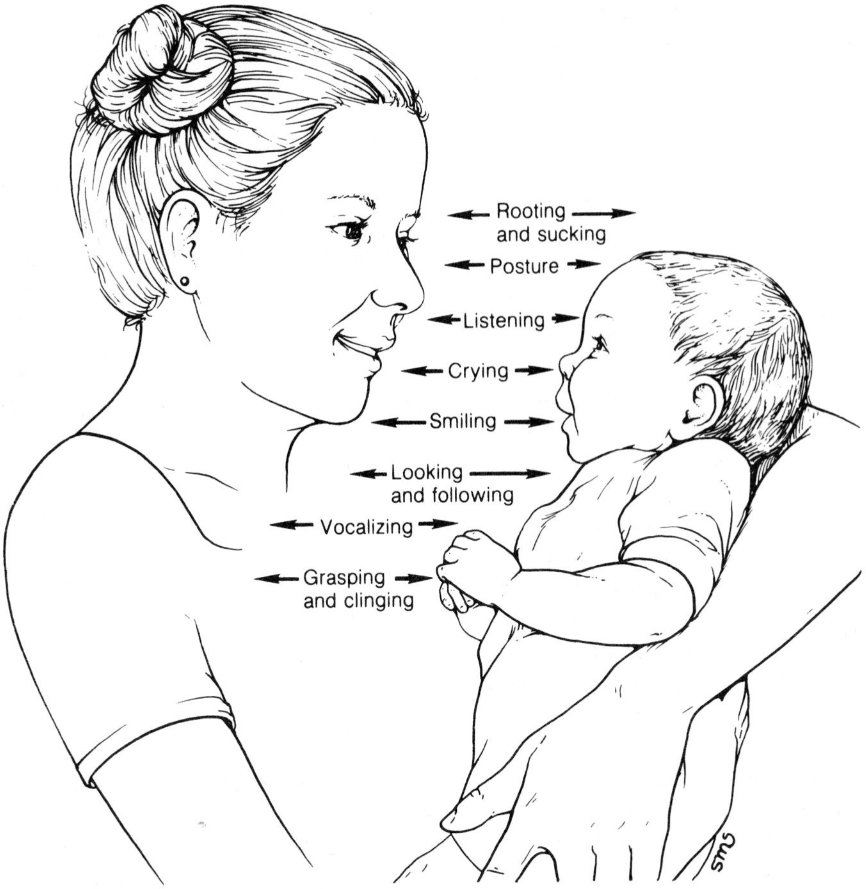

FIGURE 4-4

Behaviors that enhance parent-infant communication.

ments. By 3 months of age, the coordination of adult-infant gazing shows some remarkable similarities to the interactional synchrony of adult dialogue. Neurologic mechanisms that control gazing and dialogue might therefore be similar, and the gaze and vocal communication might share some fundamental properties of human communication that are evident in the infant's gaze long before language develops.

Parents and infants engage in long mutual gazes during play and feeding activities. Gazing then becomes integrated with touching and vocalizing behaviors, and both parent and infant participate in the mutual regulation of social behavior during the early months. As the infant becomes able to turn toward adults and engage them visually and then turn away and avert the gaze, the infant develops fundamental control over the intensity of social involvement. Head turning therefore might be the child's first expression of "no" or "yes."

Touching also is a form of communication. Adults communicate warmth and affection to their children by touching, stroking, patting, and kissing. Infants respond positively to gentle touch and attention. Just as 4-month-old infants first reach to touch inanimate objects when developing fine motor control, so they will reach out and touch an adult's face or put their fingers in an adult's mouth when they are being held. This expression of interest may be an early form of communication. Later an infant's touch or a pat on the parent's leg can be a way of seeking adult attention.

Adults usually are interested in an infant's facial expressions, especially smiling. The 6-week-old infant's smile clearly results from human stimulation. Infants first smile when presented with parts of human faces, and they particularly enjoy smiling human faces. Infants might smile for many reasons and with great variation in the degree of emotional involvement. Behaviors associated with smiling range from bright-eyed attention to laughing and giggling at 9 or 10 months of age. They also learn that smiling and laughing prolong adult attention and play.

Infants also might present very sad and distressed faces when crying. An infant's crying face combined with the compelling sound of a cry is a very powerful mechanism for communicating displeasure and is virtually impossible for adults to ignore. Crying is therefore the infant's first form of communication.

Verbal communication During the first 8 or 9 months of life, infants develop substantial ability at nonverbal communication. They can express happiness, laughter, sadness, or frustration. They can obtain attention from adults and can participate with adults in closely regulated social interaction without every saying a word. Before infants are able to speak, they are apparently able to understand communication and language. An infant's first words usually are spoken around 10–12 months of age. A few months later, the infant begins to use rudimentary phrases.

Before actually using language, however, infants progress through universal stages of prespeech development. Babbling, cooing, and gurgling accompany the infant's smiling at 1 month of age. Infants soon begin to produce the sounds of their native language in a sequence that is believed to be invariant from culture to culture. By 6 months of age, infants engage in verbal dialogue that is somewhat similar to adult speech. These fundamental speech sounds are transformed into words at about 8–10 months of age.

Early language is *holophrastic speech,* in which the infant uses a single noun to convey the entire meaning of the sentence. For example, a child will use "car" to mean "I want to go in the car" or "There is a car." The infant then progresses to *telegraphic speech,* which is produced by focusing on the content words. A child of 18 months will say "more cookie" to communicate meanings that are more specific and better understood than the earlier single words. This is the stage of language development that marks the end of infancy and the beginning of early childhood.

Social Development

Parental attachment Attachment is an affectionate tie between the infant and a primary caregiver. Freud and Erikson theorized that neonates, who can do little to provide for their survival instincts, need to become attached to another person for survival. Infants therefore manifest wants by crying and demonstrate satisfaction by sleeping and by rudimentary playing. Because parents are the primary sources for meeting the infant's needs, the infant comes to associate parents with need fulfillment. Thus, the infant becomes dependent, both physically and emotionally, on the parents for meeting needs, and need fulfillment becomes the foundation for building a basic sense of trust.

Harry Harlow and colleagues (1959, 1966) discovered that attachment is more than supplying food to the infant. Harlow's classic studies involved using two kinds of "surrogate mothers" in raising infant monkeys. The surrogate mothers had wire bodies, one covered with terry cloth and one with a wire mesh. Harlow discovered that infants preferred clinging to and associating with the "terry cloth mother" even though they might be fed exclusively by a bottle in the "wire mother." The infant monkeys would cling to the terry cloth mother when frightened and would use the terry cloth mother as a secure base of operations. This finding emphasized the importance of tactile stimulation and bodily contact.

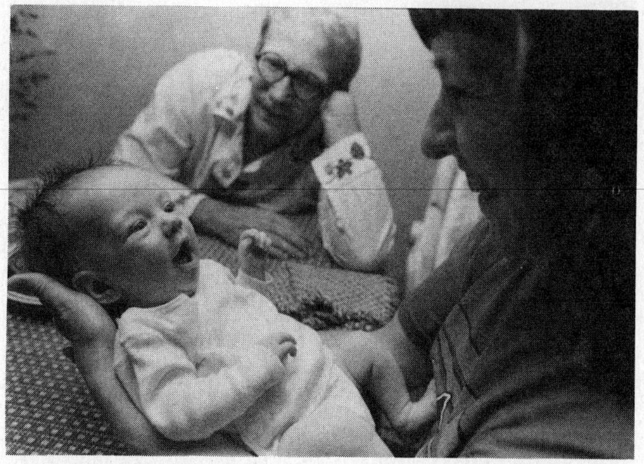

Eye contact between infants and parents is important in the process of attachment.

Seven-month-old infants begin to develop specific attachments to parents, and by 10 months of age, most seem to be attached to their parents. These infants become distressed when left alone, particularly in a strange situation. Studies of the parent-infant attachment show that between 9 and 24 months of age, the strength of attachment can be measured by the infant's attempt to seek proximity when left alone in a room by the parent. Contact-seeking and proximity-maintaining behavior peak at around 18 months of age and then decrease.

At around 8–9 months of age, many infants develop stranger anxiety and negative reactions to strangers, usually at the same time that parental attachment first develops. Infants recognize familiar faces as different from strangers, and they become centered on primary caregivers. They feel distress when these primary attachment figures are not present or are replaced with unfamiliar figures. These behaviors also are related to their increasing awareness of their dependence on their parents and, likewise, their vulnerability when their parents are not present.

Although stranger anxiety is not manifested by all infants, it is thought to be related to the infant's emerging

TABLE 4-11 Behaviors and Interactions with Others That Influence the Process of Socialization

Behavioral system	Social behaviors
Attachment	Staying near, asking to be held, crying. The presence of a caring adult to whom the infant is strongly attached provides a sense of protection
Fear, wariness	Avoiding objects, persons, and situations that might be harmful. Most infants older than 7 or 8 months are cautious of or distressed by strangers. Wariness declines as the infant grows older (over 2 years) and begins to interact with strangers
Affiliative	Smiling, vocalizing, and showing toys to persons other than those to whom infants are strongly attached
Exploratory	Presence of attachment figures lends security to infants' first "voyages" of exploration. Based on initial strong attachment to a caregiver, as infants grow older they gain more confidence in "going it alone"

SOURCE: Adapted from Lamb ME: Social interactions in infancy and the development of personality. In: *Social and Personality Development.* Lamb ME (editor). Holt, Rinehart, Winston, 1978.

understanding that parents have a permanent relationship with them. Infants who have been surrounded by many people, such as extended family members or friends of older siblings, tend to manifest less distress when parents leave. Although they prefer their parents, these infants have learned that other familiar, and even not so familiar, persons can meet their needs. For example, one young mother was concerned that her 10-month-old infant seldom complained when she left. She also was both pleased and puzzled that he readily interacted with strangers. This infant had several health problems that were being treated and monitored by physical therapists, nutritionists, and visiting nurses. He had become accustomed to positive experiences from a variety of people and thus did not have that sense of vulnerability experienced by infants who have received all their care from their parents.

Infants engage in a variety of complex interactions, not only with their parents but also with other family members, strangers, and friends. The emotional bond between the parent and child is only one of the important variables in infant social development (Table 4-11).

Siblings and peers Birth order is an influencing factor in family dynamics because parents often have more time to spend with the firstborn infant than they do with subsequent infants. Parents also tend to "practice" with their firstborn child and frequently make changes in their parenting with later infants.

Siblings sometimes are assigned to infant caregiving, especially in large families where the older siblings are considerably older than the new infants. Little is known about sibling interaction during infancy, but research on social interaction between peers during infancy has yielded interesting results. Early in the first year, infants will begin to respond to social advances made by other infants. Infants who have older brothers and sisters seem to have more social skill and seem to be more responsive to these social advances by their peers.

Although less formal research has been done with infants, infants do learn substantially from watching the social interactions in their families. Although they do not understand language, infants are clearly sensitive and responsive to nonverbal communication and learn from the behavior exhibited in their social environment.

Integrating Development Through Play

Play during infancy is an important way of becoming acquainted with the environment. Playing first with the parents and family and then with toys and peers, the infant learns about cause and effect, interactions and expectations, and personal skills and abilities. Initially, infant play seems to be object-centered, and infants pay more attention to toys than to each other. During the second year, this gradually decreases, and actual social interaction increases. Play, moreover, is fun. It is repetitious activity that is done for the sole enjoyment of practicing a known or comfortable pattern of behaviors.

Piaget (1962) noted that play during infancy involved the pure assimilation of sensorimotor actions because they are enjoyed. The infant will pick up the rattle and shake it; will watch the movement and listen to the sound; and then will drop the toy, look around, and repeat the action. Why? Because play brings pleasure and is fun. The schemes of reaching, grasping, lifting, and shaking are so well mastered that they are done without effort. The activity is no longer work but pleasure. It is the means to the end; it is the activity itself that is satisfying.

Play begins as soon as the sensations are enjoyed. Play is the link that enables the infant to become a social being. From the early smile in response to parental coaxing to total involvement in a world of toys and their manipulations, the infant learns and practices becoming like others in the environment.

Themes of Play

Many different theories describe the process of play and its value. Psychodynamic theorists tend to describe play around its theme.

Body-centered behavior Early play focuses on the infant's own body. The fascination of moving, touching, and intertwining one's own fingers or hands or of bringing them into sight singly or together and then watching them will occupy an infant for long periods of time. This activity might be accompanied by babbling or cooing sounds that express additional pleasure. These positive experiences are repeated over and over again for the satisfaction of the movement and sensation. This type of play allows infants to increase their awareness and control of desired actions involving their own bodies.

As the infant becomes aware that the parent is not an extension of the self, the theme of play shifts. Now the infant extends play to the parent, with face patting or poking and, unfortunately, hair pulling. Play is enhanced by the parent's participation and willingness to be the "object." The infant vocalizes and masters the production of various sounds and their combinations. The infant creates utterances and squeals of various pitch and intensity and practices these sounds solely because of their intrinsic enjoyment.

Objects Toward the end of the first year, the infant extends play to the objects, which serve as an extension or substitute for the parent when the parent is not present. In addition, the infant learns little games, such as pat-a-cake and peek-a-boo. Infants will play these games endlessly and often beg for them to be continued long after the adult has tired of the activity.

Toys gain importance as objects to manipulate and to work out themes at the beginning of the second year. Erikson defined this play as the microsphere stage. The infant uses small objects and toys to work out or manage larger events experienced in the real world. The world is put in order and better understood as the older infant controls these small toys and thus achieves a sense of mastery. While playing with a dollhouse, a toy gas station, cars, trucks, dolls, stuffed animals, or puppets, the older infant becomes engrossed in creating and controlling events. This type of play becomes more elaborate during early childhood. Erikson viewed this fantasy type of play as preparatory for interaction with peers.

Toys increasingly become a medium for play and skill perfection. The push-pull and dump-fill activities popular with infants at this age provide practice of fine and gross motor skills, manipulation of objects at will, and trial-and-error experiences with objects of different sizes and shapes. Thus, doing things with and to objects becomes the theme of the play. Play also is used to overcome the fear of parental loss when object permanence is acquired. The peek-a-boo game, retrieval of rolled or tossed objects, and doll play are means of playing out this fear.

Using toys as a medium, older infants increasingly enjoy play with the parent. Rolling a ball back and forth, mutual stacking of shapes or blocks, shape-sorter toys involving searching and finding the right hole for the shape, top spinning, and looking at picture books are but a few activities that encourage parent-infant play.

Content of Play

Theorists who focus on the content of play note the exploratory nature of infants' first play (Hurlock, 1978). Initial exploration is visual, and the 1- to 3-month-old infant spends long periods of time staring at objects and people, especially faces. Parents and infants often spend several minutes locked into each other's gaze as if trying to absorb all the details of each other's appearance.

As neuromuscular maturation progresses, infants gain control over arms, hands, and upper body and use them to explore both their own bodies and other objects. The manipulation of objects thus is influenced by biophysical maturation and coordination. First, the infant pats or swipes at things. The young infant finds hours of enjoyment hitting the mobile or cradle gym and watching the result, which usually includes both sound and movement. Improved coordination permits better eye-hand-mouth control, and objects soon are grasped, maneuvered, and brought to the mouth for further exploration. The infant delights in the increased voluntary control over self and objects. Time is passed happily surrounded by toys, which are picked up, mouthed, banged, shaken, and dropped, and the same or similar actions are repeated on another toy. As mobility improves, the object world and its combinations becomes even greater.

Gross motor play encourages the exploration of the physical self in relation to the environment. The older infant walks back and forth because the skill that had once been work is now mastered, and the infant takes pure delight in this accomplishment. Once the infant masters a skill, the attraction to practicing it again and again is irresistible. Many parents express frustration that once climbing is perfected, nothing is safe. The infant climbs up stairs but can-

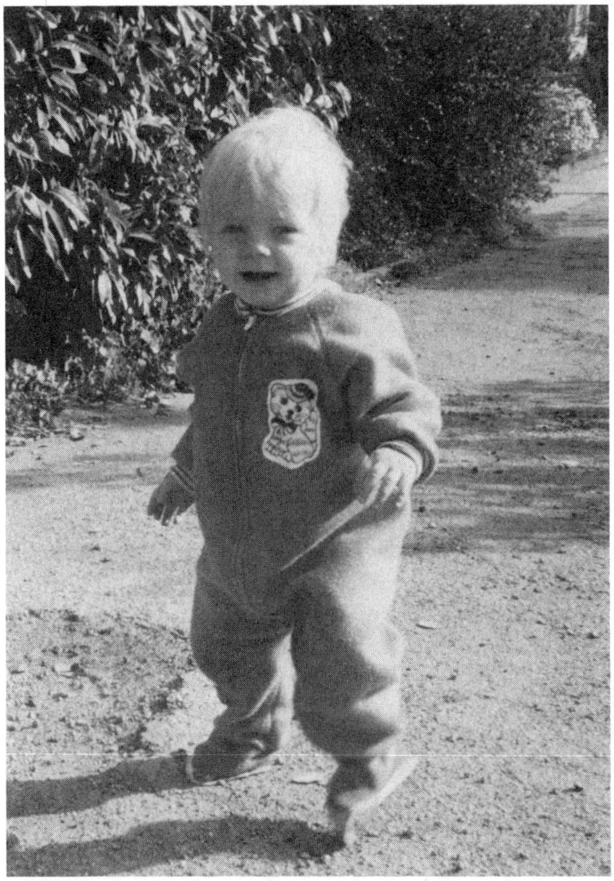

Developing motor skills allows the infant to explore the environment and practice new skills.

not get down or climbs up onto a chair or couch and from there to the windowsill or lamp table, but once there is both proud and helpless.

Fine motor skills are activities that generate coordination and the control of more precise movements. The infant manipulates toys and other external objects. The repetitive building and knocking down of the block tower facilitates the use of a mastered skill involving the precision of motor-perceptual movement.

Near the end of infancy, play becomes constructive. The skill acquired in the manipulation of objects and in understanding their function is now put to use in creating structures. This encourages the expression of feelings and the use of self as the creator of the event. Play construction helps children to create a world through their own eyes and according to their own styles.

Exploratory play is an extension of exploratory activities that are directed toward learning and therefore requires effort and concentration. Exploratory play is doing or practicing what has already been learned, purely for the pleasure the activity brings. Initially, matching shapes is a learning process, and finding the right spot for a circle, square, or triangle is difficult. A few weeks later, this same infant quickly matches all objects and shapes and is ready to repeat the performance. The early exploratory activity has now become exploratory play. When the parent is paying attention, this infant may tease and purposefully place a circle over the square hole, mischievously look up at the parent for a response, laugh, find the correct hole, and repeat the game just created.

Interest in specific toys peaks and wanes in relation to the infant's own interest, sense of achievement, and desire to practice new skills. A toy that has multiple uses will return to a favored spot as the infant discovers each new use to which it can be put.

Structure of Play

Play can also be defined by its structure, which reflects its degree of complexity. The complexity of the infant's play is related to the complexity of the available materials and to the infant's cognitive development. Piaget noted that stages of cognitive functioning often can be marked by an understanding of the structures of objects. An infant must first learn properties of an object, such as roundness. Then, putting a round form into a circular hole can be repeated endlessly for the sheer joy of it.

According to Piaget, such practice games occupy all of infancy, an explanation related to the importance he placed on the process of learning about the environment by actively interacting with it. (Table 4-12 shows the progressive sequence the infant employs in learning about an object and its properties.) Practice games are demonstrated by infants shaking, grasping, throwing, clapping, winding up the jack-in-the-box or the music box, running, or climbing for the pleasure of the activity itself. Play in this sense is the process of reexperiencing, reexploring, and reinvestigating the familiar because it is there to be done. (Table 4-13 provides a list of suggested toys and activities appropriate for the 12–18-month-old.)

Symbolic play appears near the end of infancy. Symbolic play contains the element of make-believe and pretending and provides opportunities for imaginary games and reenactment of fantasies. Symbolic play has no limits; anything can become what is desired. A block is a car, a plane, a house, or a bed because of the power of magical assignment. One knows what the object is because of the sounds or functions associated with it rather than because of its appearance.

TABLE 4-12 Progression in Schemes Used by Infants to Explore Objects in Their Environment

Behavior observed in most infants	Age in months
Mouthing	2
Holding	2
Visual inspection	3
Hitting	4
Shaking	5
Examining	6
Pulling, tearing, rubbing	6
Squeezing, sliding	6
Pushing	7
Dropping	8
Throwing	9
Socially instigated behaviors	10
Showing	14
Naming	18

SOURCE: Uzgiris IC: Ordinality in the development of schemas for relating to objects. In: *Exceptional Infant. The Normal Infant.* Vol 1. Helmuth J (editor). Bruner/Mazel, 1967.

TABLE 4-13 Toys and Activities for Infants 12–18 Months of Age

Types of toys or activities	Developmental benefits
Pull toys	Stimulates gross motor development and awareness of object even when not seen
Picture books	Teaches page manipulation, stimulates guided language development, teaches remembered properties of objects (for example, form and color), provides social experience when assisted
Books of rhymes	Provides fine distinctions in hearing, social experience, and humor, and stimulates language development
Toys as symbols of adult activities	Symbols represent actions (eg, lunch pail equals going to work)
Scribbling on paper	Stimulates creativity and fine motor development
Medium-sized push-and-pull toys (cars, trucks)	Stimulates gross motor development and walking; provides active experimentation with toys, objects, and movements; develops gross motor skills and self-expression
Large crawl-into boxes	Teaches gross motor skills, creates own environment
Large cardboard blocks	Stimulates two-handed movement, lifting, placing, and stacking; stimulates self-expression
Stuffed animals (without glass or button eyes) or blanket or blanket surrogate	Comforts and provides security through familiarity, stimulates social interaction
Filling-and-emptying toys (stack and dump truck)	Provides self-satisfaction with repetition
Puzzles with squares and pegs	Provides awareness of simple shapes

Parental Actions to Facilitate Play

Parents provide a supportive role in the infant's play and need to monitor the infant's environment to provide opportunities for play. Some of the dimensions of play are determined by the physical nature of the materials available. If the infant never has anything to see or to reach, or if the object grasped is not interesting in its color, noise, or movement, the infant has little incentive to play.

Parents can make desirable objects available. Objects or toys do not have to be expensive; some of the best toys are those created by the parent. Universally favorite toys seem to be boxes, pots and pans with lids, wooden spoons, and other kitchen-related containers. For several months, a 1-year-old will spend hours playing with a large plastic dishpan, a bag of potatoes, a wooden spoon, and a dishtowel. Some actions are ritualistically performed, and others are newly created, but the infant engages in the playing process of pretending, exploring, manipulating, and fantasizing and obviously enjoys the activities.

Another important supportive role of the parent during this stage is interactive playing with the infant. The first games involve visual gazing and responding to facial interactions. The parent who enjoys an activity with the infant encourages the infant to be perceptive and responsive. The complex interactional process that is established between the parent and child around play is usually positive. Parent and child enjoy each other mutually. They orient each other

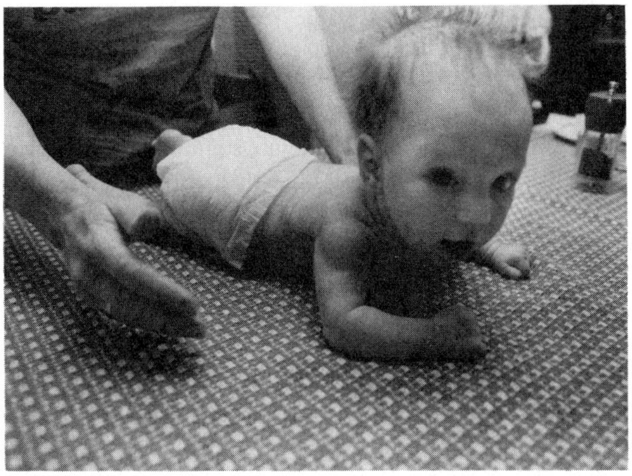

As infants develop motor skills, parents need to develop safety-related behaviors to protect the child.

to the environment. Specific stimuli, causal relations, and social conventions all become standard aspects of their play together.

Health Care Needs of Infancy

Hygiene

The infant depends on the parent for skin care and cleanliness. During early infancy, sponge baths are appropriate because the infant does not need to be immersed daily in a tub. For both infants and parents, bath time is usually a time for playful interaction. The frequency of baths depends on the condition of the infant's skin (whether dry, moist, or oily), the temperature of the environment, and the infant's schedule. Few infants require a daily bath, and applying lotion or petroleum is preferred for infants with dry skin. For all infants, the diaper area should be cleansed carefully with each diaper change. After feeding, hands and faces may need to be cleaned, depending on the infant's age and neatness in eating.

Miliaria—Prickly heat During hot, humid summer days, infants are prone to a rash that is technically termed *miliaria* but is commonly called prickly heat. It appears suddenly and can disappear just as quickly once the skin is cooled. The rash is caused by inflamed or blocked sweat glands and consists of tiny, pinhead-sized erythematous, papular lesions with vesicles in the center. Because infants do not perspire until after the first month of life, neonates are particularly susceptible. Miliaria also occurs throughout the life span and is harmless. It develops whenever body warmth is excessive because of the weather, indoor overheating, or overdressing. Removing excess clothing; leaving an overheated room; finding a cool, shady spot outdoors; or giving the infant a tepid sponge bath will decrease body warmth and reverse the appearance of prickly heat. Powder, if used, should be applied in a thin layer. Cornstarch, creams, and ointments should not be used. Gently patting the infant's skin to keep it dry and changing damp clothing and bed linen also help to prevent and treat miliaria.

Seborrheic dermatitis—Cradle cap Although the infant is clean and the head and hair are washed frequently, *seborrheic dermatitis,* or cradle cap, may occur. Its cause is unknown but appears to be related to activity of the sebaceous glands. The scalp is the most frequent site, but seborrheic dermatitis also might be found on the eyebrows and eyelids, behind the eyelids, behind and in the ears, on the sides of the nose, and in the inguinal region. Cervical lymph node enlargement may also be associated with the condition.

Cradle cap appears as thick, yellowish, oily, scaly, nonpruritic patches. Often, the area of greatest involvement is the anterior fontanel. Parents need to be reassured that this "soft spot" is not fragile but similar to skin and will not be harmed by routine washing. A simple method of removing the scaly patches is to use a cotton ball to apply baby oil on each site, allow the oil to penetrate the crusts, and then thoroughly wash the scalp with a dandruff-control shampoo. Fine-tooth combing or brushing with an old toothbrush then removes the flakes from the hair. Daily shampooing should follow. This same procedure can be used for other sites except the eyes. Parents need to be cautioned not to pick at the crusts to remove them but first to soak them and then wash the site thoroughly.

In most instances, the condition is temporary. It appears sometime between 2 and 12 weeks of age and usually disappears by 8–12 months of age. If the sites become infected, the physician should be consulted because additional treatment is necessary.

Diaper dermatitis—Diaper rash Experienced parents know that it is easier to prevent *diaper dermatitis,* or diaper rash, than to treat it. The nurse is responsible for emphasizing to all parents the importance of thoroughly cleansing the perineal area with each diaper change as the best way to prevent diaper rash. Sponging the area with warm water or mild soap and water followed by gentle drying is recommended. Other measures that help to promote dryness and adequate aeration of the area include frequently changing wet or soiled diapers, limiting use of plastic or rubber pants because they retain moisture (making the perineal area wet and warm—a perfect medium for bacteria growth), and exposing the perineal area to the air for 5–10 minutes, three or four times a day. This often can be accomplished around diaper-changing times. In addition, applying a thin film of medicated powder helps to promote dryness. Powder must be used carefully. It should not be shaken vigorously because inhaling the powder dust can cause respiratory problems (Chow et al., 1979). Excess powder is a hazard because the powder will cake in the body creases, particularly the groin, and will result in skin excoriation. Rather, a small amount of powder should be put in the parent's hand and then lightly rubbed onto the infant's skin so that a thin film covers the entire diaper area. Medicated powder is preferred over powder containing talc because talc does not absorb water and has no antifungal or antibacterial properties.

Cornstarch, creams, and petroleum jelly generally are contraindicated. Any ointment or powder containing boric acid must never be used because of the associated risk of systemic poisoning. Petroleum jelly, once a favorite, is no longer used because it is too occlusive and does not allow adequate aeration. Furthermore, its use causes excessive softening and thinning of the protective layers of the skin, predisposing that area to yeast infections. Cornstarch tends to cake once wet, which irritates the skin and promotes skin breakdown. With any loss of skin integrity in a wet, warm, dark environment, bacteria and fungi thrive. Preventing this combination is the goal of providing for the infant's hygiene needs.

Diaper rash has numerous causes, including contact with external irritants, bacterial or fungal infections, ammonia irritation, and reaction to certain foods ingested. To a large extent, the management of a diaper rash resembles the measures recommended for its prevention. Identifying the causative agent is especially helpful in preventing a recurrence of the rash. Parents are usually good detectives and can identify what has been changed or is new and different in the infant's routine and care. Known irritants are soaps, fabric softeners, disposable diapers, acid from urine and feces, certain breakdown products from foods (such as orange juice and tomatoes), and the use of plastic pants, cornstarch, excess powder, or ointments.

Some infants are more prone to diaper rash than others. Infants with fair complexions tend to have more sensitive skin and tend to be less tolerant of wet diapers and irritants in general. Many times, an infant who has a diaper rash is uncomfortable. The addition of a wet diaper can be painful, resulting to increasing restlessness and irritability.

The nurse can advise the parents that preventive measures instituted from the beginning quickly become routine. The advantage is a happy infant with few, if any, diaper rashes.

Sleep and Rest

Sleep patterns during infancy vary greatly. The neonate averages 16 hours of sleep a day, with some neonates requiring as little as 10 hours and others as much as 22 hours. Sleep patterns vary from infant to infant, and sleep-wake routines vary from month to month for individual infants. The neonate sleeps in a series of naps. Some naps last 30 minutes, whereas other naps last 3–4 hours. Approximately half of the neonate's sleep time is spent in light sleep. During this stage of sleep, involuntary muscle movements and dreaming occur, which account for the many coughs, gurgles, sighs, squirms, and squiggles the young infant makes while sleeping. When the nurse shares this information with parents, they can better understand that the sounds their infant makes are not necessarily waking-up sounds. Therefore, it is best to wait until the infant is obviously awake before picking him or her up to be changed or fed.

During infancy, the organization of sleep and wakefulness changes significantly, whereas the total amount of sleep decreases only by 2–3 hours. The average sustained sleep of the neonate seldom exceeds 4 hours; it increases to 7 hours for the 5-month-old and 11–12 hours for the 18-month-old. With longer sleep periods come longer times of wakefulness. Instead of the six naps a day needed by the neonate, the older infant does well with only one or two naps. The sleep-wake patterns tend to be a stable characteristic for the individual infant. The 18-month-old who required less than an average amount of sleep as a neonate continues to thrive on less sleep, whereas the infant who required more than an average amount of sleep as a neonate still requires more.

One indicator of maturation appreciated by parents is sleeping through the night. Having an infant begin to sleep through the night, however, does not mean an end to night wakings. Infants commonly wake up during the night between 5 and 9 months of age and again during their second year of life, even after months of having slept through the night.

Whether night wakings are considered to be problematic depends on the parent's perception. Some parents find themselves so tired from being awakened at night that they are irritable during the day, whereas other parents are able to tolerate the sleep interruptions better. Parents vary in their sleep-wake needs, just as infants do. Some parents become very discouraged when an infant who has been sleeping through the night starts to awaken again during the night. Therefore, when assessing an infant's total sleep time, the nurse compares these sleep-wake patterns to those of the family and the ways in which each member is affected when the patterns do not coincide.

Parents often need reassurance that night wakings are common and that they appear to be related to maturational, temperamental, and environmental factors. Each situation needs to be assessed and changes planned to fit with the needs and lifestyles of the family. Like so many aspects of parent-child interactions, there is no one "right way" but rather as many variations as there are parents and children. The goal is to establish a good fit between the parent and infant so that the relationship can thrive.

Crying and fussiness One of the disturbances in infant rest is the inevitable crying periods that occur during infancy. The infant's crying often is misinterpreted by the parent, who might feel rejected by the infant or might view the crying as a signal of failure to meet the infant's needs. The nurse therefore reassures the parent while providing possible explanations for the infant's behavior.

To assist parents, the nurse can first assure the parent that crying is extremely common in infancy and then can assess the nature and pattern of the crying. Specific information should include the following:

1. The time of day that the crying occurs
2. The duration of each crying episode
3. The onset of the crying: When did the parents begin to consider the crying a problem?
4. Situational factors: What is going on when the crying occurs; how is feeding related to these crying episodes?
5. Feeding techniques: Is the infant bottle- or breast-fed; are solid foods or cereals included; how is the infant held or not held during feedings; how frequently is the infant burped?
6. Pattern of elimination: Does the infant experience diarrhea, constipation, flatus, or abdominal pain?
7. Parent's reaction to the crying (level of anxiety, fatigue, depression): What is the primary emotional response that the parent has to the infant's crying episodes?
8. Handling of the crying by parents and others: What has been tried; what worked; and what did not work?
9. The infant's behavior pattern when not crying: Is the infant's behavior easy and predictable or difficult and unpredictable?

In addition to questioning the parent, the nurse also observes the parent's interaction with the infant. Observing a feeding might provide some cues. Perhaps all that is needed is to suggest ways of decreasing the infant's ingestion of air. Also helpful are compliments about positive parental responses to the infant in feeding and holding.

A crying period for the infant between 3 and 10 weeks of age is extremely common at the end of each day and is a possible precursor to the social period of infancy. The nurse can reassure the parent that a 1- to 2-hour period of fussiness or crying a day during the early weeks can be expected and will resolve with time. Infants seem to need this crying period to release energies and will stop this behavior when they are able to participate in interesting activities.

If feeding or other physical problems can be ruled out as reasons for the crying, parents can be reassured that the crying is a normal, although frustrating, part of the infant's development.

Colic *Colic* is unexplained periods of crying within the first 3 months of infancy and is associated with abdominal distention, spasms, and/or the passage of flatus. The symptoms usually occur late in the day. The infant cries loudly, clenching fists, extending legs, and acting as if searching for food. Feeding, however, does not quiet the infant. From a usual 2–3 hours of daily crying, colicky infants can cry 8–12 hours per day. With crying, the infant's entire body becomes tense and hyperactive. Crying then causes the further intake of air, and the vicious cycle of abdominal distention and pain results. There is little agreement on the specific causes of colic. Possible explanations include feeding problems, parental tension, milk allergy, physiologic immaturity of the gastrointestinal system, and hyperactivity and overresponsiveness of the infants themselves. Colic usually disappears when the infant is 3–4 months old.

Colic is nerve-wracking, frustrating, and terribly stressful to parents. The nurse again observes parent-infant interactions and feeding procedures. Sometimes changes in the feeding procedure bring some relief. Possible changes include feeding the infant in an upright position, burping more frequently, changing the formula, changing the type of nipple, and holding or positioning the infant upright after the feeding. In addition, other comfort measures, such as wrapping the infant warmly and providing rhythmic activities, might be tried.

Parents of colicky infants need reassurance and support. They should understand that their infants are not ill and will stop this behavior usually when 3–4 months of age. Guilt feelings should be acknowledged and parents should be encouraged to designate free time for their enjoyment to decrease their anxiety and frustration.

Nutrition

Infant nutrition is a subject that combines a great quantity of current information with cultural attitudes and traditions about food and feeding routines, together with socioeconomic factors that influence food choices. The child health nurse not only needs to be well-informed about traditional or middle-class ways of meeting nutritional requirements but also needs to be knowledgeable about cultural and ethnic preferences and individual variations. Good nutritional habits begin in infancy and are one of the best preventive health care practices available. Nutrition education therefore needs to be directed to parents during the prenatal period. Often, a first step is examining the belief that fat babies are healthy babies or the stereotype that good parents have fat babies. Infantile obesity has become a major concern, especially as obesity can jeopardize optimal development.

Milk The food of choice for infants under 6 months of age is milk, either human milk or prepared formula. Adequate intake of either one provides all known nutritional requirements, with the possible exception of vitamin D and fluoride for breast-fed infants, and provides an optimal balance of carbohydrate, protein, and fat in readily digested forms. The addition of solid foods prior to 6 months of age only adds excess calories and imposes a heavy renal solute load while increasing water demands. A variety of prepared formulas is available, including some formulas to accommodate infants who are allergic to milk or who have specific nutritional needs (Table 4-14). Human milk has the additional advantage of providing protection against disease in the form of immune factors and resistance to antigen absorption from the small intestine. Infants, furthermore, are rarely allergic or unable to digest and metabolize their mothers' milk.

The American Academy of Pediatrics (1976) has recommended that infants receive either human milk or prepared formula during their first year of life. The use of homogenized cow's milk during the first year places the infant at risk for iron-deficiency anemia. The iron in cow's milk is poorly absorbed, and intake in excess of a quart per day may cause intestinal bleeding and occult blood loss.

Solid foods Around 6 months of age the infant is physiologically and developmentally ready to have solid foods added to the diet. An indicator on which to base an infant's nutritional care is the development of motor functions (Table 4-15). For example, the normal neonate initially is capable of rooting, sucking, and swallowing fluids; at first, the sucking is an up-and-down tongue movement that matures to a back-and-forward tongue movement. Nutritional care plans depend on an understanding of these developmental changes, so that the nurse can help the parent to recognize specific behaviors. For instance, the strong tongue thrust reflex during the first 6 months of life inhibits an infant from accepting spoon-feeding but assists in the intake of breast milk or formula. Infants can better learn solid-food-feeding once they can sit up, reach, grasp, and exercise lateral tongue movements and good hand-to-mouth coordination. Waiting until 6 months of age to introduce solids allows not only neuromuscular maturity but also development of the digestive system's ability to handle foreign proteins with the enzymes necessary for the absorption and use of specific nutrients.

By 6 months of age, most infants need an external source of iron because prenatal stores have been depleted. Iron-fortified cereals are recommended at this time and are continued daily at least until the child is 18 months old. Three level tablespoons of dry cereal diluted with milk or formula make a serving of about 60 g, providing 7 mg of iron. The RDA for iron for infants 6–12 months of age is 15 mg. Therefore, if the infant takes two feedings of cereal per day, these would adequately meet the daily requirement. The infant who has been on an iron-fortified formula need not start with cereal but may choose to take fruits or vegetables.

Traditionally, the sequence in which foods are introduced is (1) cereals, particularly rice for its nonallergenic properties; (2) fruits, such as peaches, pears, or applesauce; (3) vegetables, with yellow vegetables, such as squash, sweet potatoes, or carrots (being careful to avoid a buildup of carotene) given before green vegetables, such as peas or beans; and (4) strained meats, such as nonallergenic lamb or veal. High-protein foods, such as meats, are not given before 6 months of age because of the increased chance of an allergic reaction. In families with histories of allergies, the nurse advises parents to read all baby food jar labels carefully. Many strained fruits are preserved with orange juice, and many of the meat and vegetable dinners contain tomato, both of which are allergenic. The potentially allergic infant should not be given orange juice until after the first birthday.

By 7–9 months of age, teething allows the infant to chew, and the infant has a mature swallowing ability that makes it possible to experience foods with different textures. By 9–12 months, the infant indicates a readiness to self-feed appropriate finger food. Finger foods might include sliced and peeled apple, sliced peach, a piece of cheese, or few pieces of dry cereal. These foods are readily softened by saliva, thereby preventing choking. Peanuts, popcorn, or hard candy, which can be inhaled or choked on, should be avoided at this age.

It is most important that the parent be advised to introduce one new food at a time and no faster than once every 5 days, so that any symptoms of intolerance can be traced. The more simple the choice of foods, the less is the chance of providing excess calories. The infant can tolerate the simplicity and limited choices better than the parent. Parents should know that prepared dinners provide more starch fillers than meat and vegetables provide, and that desserts, although attractive, offer no more than empty calories. Strained fruits offer mostly carbohydrate and some vitamin C. Vegetables are a good source of vitamin A.

Strained meats contain protein and minerals. Orange juice and other juices are good sources of vitamin C. Juices are best offered from the cup and initially diluted with water to assist in eventual weaning. Egg yolks are a poor source of iron and need not be offered until the infant reaches 1 year of age.

Manufacturers of commercially prepared infant foods recently have reduced or eliminated the sugar and salt from their products because of concern about the development of hypertension and obesity in later life. Home-prepared infant foods, which some parents prefer, usually have a higher caloric density because of lower water content and may have significant amounts of added salt if parents are not guided in the preparation of these foods.

Infants respond differently to the introduction of solid food. Some infants adapt quickly to the new tastes and textures, whereas others initially resist and only gradually make the adjustment to eating solids. When the infant refuses a food, it is best to stop and try again in a few days. Force-feeding at this stage paves the way for mutual frustration and future power plays involving food. When solids are introduced at 6 months of age, most infants progress rapidly to table foods. Soft foods, such as mashed potatoes, cooked carrots, squash, beans, canned fruits, yogurt, toast, cereals, soups, and cottage cheese, are managed well. Foods that splinter, such as raw carrots and celery sticks, should be avoided because of the danger of aspiration. Commercially prepared strained or junior meats or home-pureed meats need to be continued until the infant has an adequate chewing ability because meat is such an important source of iron.

By 9 months of age, the infant should be eating three meals a day and drinking about 24 oz of formula. If breast-feeding continues, the number of feedings should decrease to around four per day. At 1 year of age, the infant can be completely fed on table food and the daily milk intake can be decreased to 18–24 oz.

Feeding difficulties The hallmark of good parenting is the contented, thriving infant. When the infant appears to be hungry all the time or refuses to eat, parents, particularly the breast-feeding mother, are under stress. Parental anxiety transmitted to the infant sets up a cycle that creates a real dilemma for the family. In assessing this situation the nurse should first ascertain whether the infant gained 4–7 oz/week for the first 6 months of life. Next, the adequacy of fluid intake and output should be determined. The infant should have at least six wet diapers per day, and, if adequately nourished, the infant should fall quietly asleep for several hours after a feeding.

Breast-feeding mothers who are having difficulty feeding their infants are concerned immediately about the adequacy of their milk production. Supporting the nursing mother requires that the nurse transmit knowledge and confidence. The signs of successful lactation include milk dripping from the breast before feeding and at the sight or sound of the baby, milk dripping from the opposite breast during the feeding, uterine cramps during the feeding, cessation of any nipple discomfort during the feeding, milk dripping during sexual arousal, and a tingling sensation of the nipple seconds after the feeding starts. These signs all indicate the presence of a good "let-down reflex," which is essential for successful lactation. The initiation of the let-down reflex requires a strong suck from the infant.

Regurgitation Regurgitation, or spitting up, of predigested milk frequently occurs in the early months but can continue for most of the first year. One advantage of breast-feeding is that the regurgitation is odorless, whereas regurgitated formula smells sour. Although regurgitation can be most disconcerting to parents, it is not necessarily indicative of a nutritional problem. Evidence of a satisfactory growth pattern often reassures the family.

The amount, force, and character of the contents of regurgitation should be investigated, however, to rule out any significant gastric problem. Observing a feeding is helpful in determining any changes to suggest. The nurse might, for example, encourage adequate burping during the feeding to eliminate air bubbles. The neonate should be burped after every ounce of formula or every 5 minutes of breast-feeding. The infant should be held in a relaxed, comfortable position with the bottle tipped so that milk fills the nipple to prevent swallowing air. If regurgitation is caused by an immature gastric sphincter, placing the infant in a semi-upright position, as in an infant seat, following the feeding allows the milk or food to settle.

Gastrointestinal changes Constipation can be a concern for parents, particularly if they do not understand the normal bowel patterns of infants. Breast-fed and formula-fed infants are rarely constipated. Parents first need to know that it is the consistency and not the frequency of the stool that characterizes constipation. A hard, formed, marble-sized, dry, hard-to-pass stool is descriptive of a constipated condition. Most infants have stools at least once a day. Some infants may have stools as infrequently as once every 2–3 days and still have a normal stool pattern if the stool is of a normal, soft consistency. If the infant does have an occasional hard stool, the nurse might recommend an increase in fluid intake or, if the infant is on solid foods, an increase in fruits and fruit juices.

A very watery stool occurring more than five times in a day is diarrhea. Parents sometimes confuse diarrhea with the frequent, loose, yellowish, seedy stool of the breast-fed infant or with the stool of the infant using certain types of formula (Table 4-14). Because diarrhea is unusual in the breast-fed infant, it suggests an infection, and the parent

TABLE 4-14 Pediatric Formulas

Formula (Company)	Carbohydrate	Protein	Fat	Stool characteristics	Explanation
Enfamil (Mead Johnson)	Lactose	Nonfat milk	Soy, coconut oils	Formed, greenish-brown with very little free water around stool	Can be used with infants with fat intolerance. Appropriate formula for normal infants who have no special nutritional requirements
Similac (Ross)	Lactose	Nonfat milk	Soy, coconut, corn oils	Formed, greenish-brown with very little free water around stool	Iron may be added to any of these formulas to supply a dependable daily intake; for premature infants; for off-spring of anemic mothers; for infants of multiple births; for infants with low birthweights and those who grew rapidly; for infants who have lost weight
SMA (Wyeth)	Lactose	Electrolyzed whey, nonfat milk	Coconut, safflower, soybean oils	Similar to breast-milk stools: small volume, pasty yellow, some free water	
Isomil (Ross)	Sucrose, cornstarch, corn syrup solids	Soy protein isolates	Soy, coconut, corn oils	Mushy, yellow-green with more free water than cow's milk stools	Used for children with milk allergies
Neomulsoy (Syntex)	Sucrose	Soy protein isolates	Soy oil		
Nursoy (Wyeth)	Sucrose, corn syrup	Soy protein isolates	Coconut, oleic, safflower, soybean oils, and soy oil		
Prosobee (Mead Johnson)	Sucrose, corn syrup	Soy protein isolates	Soy oil		Metabolic defects (eg, galactosemia)
Lofenalac (Mead Johnson)	Corn syrup solids, tapioca starch	Hydrolyzed casein (most of phenylalanine removed)	Corn oil	Similar to cow's milk formula: formed, greenish-brown with very little free water around stool	Used in children with phenylketonuria in whom a low phenylalanine diet is needed
Lanala (Mead Johnson)	Lactose	Casein	Coconut oil	Similar to cow's milk formula stool	Sodium-free. Used in infants with severe renal/cardiac disease. Not recommended for long-term use without a sodium supplement
Similac PM 60/40 (Ross)	Lactose	Demineralized whey and nonfat milk	Coconut and corn oil	Similar to cow's milk formula stool	Cow's milk base. Low renal solute base. Low-sodium but supplies daily sodium requirements. Used in long-term renal/heart disease patients

TABLE 4-14 *(Continued)*

Formula (Company)	Carbohydrate	Protein	Fat	Stool characteristics	Explanation
Portagen (Mead Johnson)	Sucrose, corn syrup solids	Sodium caseinate	Fractionated coconut oil, corn oil	Similar to cow's milk formula	Indicated in a child with liver or pancreatic disease because the medium-chain triglycerides are absorbed into the portal system and do not require bile and pancreatic enzymes for digestion (eg, cystic fibrosis)
Nutramigen (Mead Johnson)	Sucrose, tapioca starch	Enzymically hydrolyzed 8 casein	Corn oil	Low-volume, green stools with some mucus	Used in protein hypersensitive disorders where intact proteins are not tolerated; this formula's proteins are broken into amino acids and polypeptides (eg, congenital galactosemia). Also used in cases of multiple food allergies
Pregestimil (Mead Johnson)	Dextrose, tapioca starch	Enzymically hydrolyzed 8 casein	Fractionated coconut oil, corn oil	Low-volume, green stools with mucus	Used in some cases of fat or carbohydrate malabsorption because formula is composed of simple structures that are easily absorbed (eg, cystic fibrosis). High intestinal osmolarity; therefore may result in diarrhea. Must be started at half-strength and gradually increased to full-strength. Can be used for protein supplementation
Cho-Free (Syntex)	None	Soy protein isolate	Soy oil	Similar to soy formula stools	Carbohydrate-free formula. Provides 12 calories/oz. Used in short-term carbohydrate intolerance
Lytren (Mead Johnson) Pedialyte (Ross)	—	—	—	—	Used for dehydration, loss of electrolytes, and the replacement and prevention of electrolytes. Indicated in diarrhea and vomiting. Postoperative fluid for oral electrolyte replacement. Contraindicated in infants with impaired renal function

TABLE 4-15 Infant Feeding Behaviors

Age	Hunger behavior	Feeding behavior	Satiety behavior
Birth to 13 weeks (0–3 months)	Cries; hands fisted; body tense	Rooting reflex; medial lip closure; strong suck reflex; suck-swallow pattern; tongue thrust and retraction; palmomental reflex; gags easily; needs burping	Withdraws head from nipple; falls asleep; hands relaxed; relief of body tension
14–24 weeks (4–6 months)	Eagerly anticipates; grasps and draws bottle to mouth; reaches with open mouth	Aware of hands; generalized reaching; intentional hand-to-mouth; tongue elevation; lips purse at corners—pucker, shifts food in mouth—prechewing; tongue protrudes in anticipation of nipple; tongue holds nipple firm; tongue projection strong; suck strength increases; coughs and chokes easily; preference for tastes	Tosses head back; fusses or cries; covers mouth with hands; ejects food; distracted by surroundings
28–36 weeks (7–9 months)	Reacts to food preparation sounds; vocalized hunger; reaches out	Biting (first teeth); turns palm toward face; draws lower lip with food; thumb-finger grasp and palmar grasp; increased dexterity of hands; lateral tongue movement; mature swallow; chewing begins—vertical jaw protrusion; sucking decreases; holds bottle; handles cup awkwardly	Changes posture; closes mouth; shakes head "no"; plays with and throws utensils
40–52 weeks (10–12 months)	Vocalizes; grasps utensils	Tongue licks food from lower lip; holds and transfers to mouth; drinks from cup with spillage; lateral chewing movements; sticks out tongue; demands to feed self	Shakes head "no"; sputters

should be referred for medical diagnosis. For the bottle-fed infant, the nurse first might want to investigate the formula preparation, source of water supply, and possibility of contamination. If the infant is on solids, the diarrhea may reflect the introduction of a new food, fruit juice, or excess fruit intake. For mild diarrhea, which lasts only a day or two, the cessation of solid food may be indicated along with diluting the formula with water, either half-and-half water or one-quarter of formula to three-quarters of water. Diarrhea in infants, particularly those under 6 months of age, is considered serious because it may lead to dehydration. The nurse therefore should seek medical supervision for the parent and child.

Weaning Weaning historically refers to the infant's loss of the mother's milk, although the term can refer to a change from breast milk to cow's milk formula, a change from bottle to cup, or the introduction of solid food in the diet. Weaning should be a mutually satisfying experience for both parent and child. Infants feel strong emotional attachments related to the security surrounding the original source of nourishment. The transition to other sources and means of food intake must therefore be easy and comfortable. The nurse guides and encourages the parent to recognize the infant's cues of readiness for weaning.

Weaning usually occurs sometime during the last half of the first year, but it is also determined by parental preference. Prepared formula is best continued throughout the first year. Once cow's milk is the infant's main source of milk, it should be limited to 1 qt/day, although if the infant is already receiving a significant amount of calories from solid food, milk intake will have decreased. Cup feeding can be introduced at about 5 months of age. Many infants who are breast-fed until at least 7 or 8 months of age are weaned directly to a cup with no intervening bottle-feeding.

Another option during weaning is to use the cup at mealtimes and allow a bottle before naps and bedtime, taking care to prevent "bottle-mouth syndrome." Some children initially want the security of going to bed with their bottle. Many parents find that diluting the formula or milk with gradually increasing amounts of water is a convenient method of weaning. They begin with a dilution of three parts formula to one part water and gradually add a greater percentage of water to formula until the infant is drinking plain water. Few infants enjoy drinking water and willingly substitute a stuffed toy or blanket for the bottle.

TABLE 4-16 Sequence of Tooth Eruption

Location of tooth	Approximate age	Range
Lower central incisors	6 mo	5–11 mo
Lower lateral incisors	7 mo	6–15 mo
Upper central incisors	8 mo	6–12 mo
Upper lateral incisors	9 mo	7–18 mo
Lower first molar	12 mo	10–30 mo
Upper first molar	14 mo	10–20 mo
Lower cuspid	16 mo	11–24 mo
Upper cuspid	18 mo	11–24 mo
Lower second molar	24 mo	13–31 mo
Upper second molar	26 mo	13–31 mo

Dentition

The first tooth appears at about 6 months of age. The timing of tooth eruption is hereditary. Some infants get their first tooth for their first birthday. Additional studies should be done if the infant is born with a tooth. It may be either a normal or supernumerary lower deciduous tooth. Supernumerary teeth are loose, have no roots, and need to be removed because of their defective structure and chance of being aspirated.

The teething experience is different for each infant. Some parents are surprised to discover that the first tooth has erupted because there was no noticeable change in their infant's behavior. Other parents have anxiously awaited the tooth's eruption because their infant has been irritable, uncomfortable, awake at night, and eating fussily for several weeks. After the first tooth erupts, a new one follows at intervals of approximately 1–2 months (Table 4-16). Dental development coincides with the general pattern of skeletal development.

When teething occurs, the infant's gums are red, swollen, and sensitive. Having the gums rubbed with a clean, wet cloth or gauze or chewing on hard objects seems to relieve the tension and discomfort. Hard rubber teething rings, beads, ridged toys, or teething pretzels seem to be favorites for chewing. One infant kept a hard rubber bead necklace in his mouth for hours at a time while cutting his lateral incisors. He would secure the toy behind his present teeth and then massage his sore gums by constantly biting down on the beads.

Sometimes infants find comfort in toys that have been cooled in the refrigerator. One parent provided relief by freezing water in popsicle containers and then rubbing the infant's gums with it. The plastic, liquid-filled teething toys are not recommended because the infant may puncture the plastic with a sharp tooth and ingest the liquid, which is often contaminated.

Primary teeth are important for speech development, maintaining space for permanent teeth, and the proper development of the facial muscles and ligaments that support upper and lower jaw development. It is essential to provide good care of the primary teeth. Loss of primary teeth may cause overcrowding when the permanent teeth erupt. Early dental care consists of following meals and the intake of sweetened liquids with a drink of water. In addition, several times a day the parent should gently rub the teeth with gauze wrapped around a finger. Good nutrition is also important for healthy teeth and gums. Teeth require calcium, phosphorus, vitamins C and D, and fluoride for the growth and formation of enamel. Chewing helps to develop strong teeth. The inclusion of crackers, cereals, raw fruits, and hard rolls provides the infant with opportunities for strenuous chewing.

Coincidental to teething is the lowered resistance to infections that results from the depletion of maternal antibody reserves. Teething does not cause illness. Fevers, diarrhea, or other signs of illness need to be assessed separately and medical care sought.

Exercise

The kicking, stretching, crying infant is an exercising infant. Crying has both physiologic and psychosocial benefits. It is a normal discharge of tension and way of maintaining homeostasis. Infants enjoy movement and exercising the large body muscles. Some infants are very active and seem to be in perpetual motion. One concerned young mother needed to be reassured by the visiting nurse that she was a good mother because she thought her daughter, although healthy, was too thin. The nurse spent a few hours observing mother and daughter at their home and assessing the infant's growth history and food intake. The nurse noted that the infant was thin only in relation to a neighbor's infant but was gaining weight and following her own growth curve. This girl was very active, always kicking, reaching, rolling over, waving her arms, and squealing, in contrast to the more passive activity engaged in by the neighbor's infant. The nurse demonstrated the infant's firm extremity muscles and strong neck and abdomen muscles by pulling her up to a sitting position, having her resist a toy's being pulled away, and other similar games. Together, the nurse and mother concluded that this infant was never going to be "fat" but was healthier for all of her spontaneous exercising.

Young infants who do most of their exploring visually benefit from parent-guided exercises. These can be done at bath time, and some communities have special postnatal exercise programs for the infant and mother. For the infant, the program begins with passive range-of-motion exercises, frequently done to music or nursery rhymes. Other activities then are added to enhance muscle development and flexibility, such as pull-ups, roll-ups, playing airplane, and later, wheelbarrow walking.

Infant movement, activity, and play have the added advantage of fostering social interaction and learning about the environment. Young infants can exercise better when placed on a firm surface. Older infants who have started to crawl need safe spaces in which to practice and further develop the associated muscles. Playpens are actually more appropriate for the young infant because they provide a safe, firm surface and nearby toys for stretching and reaching exercises than for the older infant, who needs a larger area for optimal development.

Transition to Early Childhood

The first 18 months of a child's life are marked by rapid development in all areas. The horizontal neonate is now an active, vertical child. Secure with the gross motor skills of walking, climbing, and running, the infant is now ready to practice coordination and fine motor skills. The once-dependent neonate has become secure in the immediate environment and is ready to exert some control over it. Through exploration and play, objects have acquired meaning and relationships to other objects or events. The infant has become increasingly aware of the self as an individual, as an actor, and as a creator of action. In addition, the infant is beginning to acquire language and the ability to use symbols.

Language opens up a whole new world to the child. It brings "an all-pervasive transformation of perceiving, feeling, thinking and general intelligence" (Stone and Church, 1975). The ability to communicate through language marks the end of infancy and the beginning of early childhood.

Essential Concepts

- Developmental progress during infancy involves major changes in the infant's biophysical, affective, cognitive, and social development.
- Infancy encompasses the developmental phase from birth until the beginnings of language (around 18 months of age).
- The family plays a major role in the infant's life, while acting according to family beliefs, values, and traditions of culture.
- As a result of growth, development, and maturation, the infant progresses from reflexive behaviors to independent mobility.
- The infant initially communicates by crying but rapidly adds cooing, babbling, and then words.
- The neonate views the self and environment as one, then gradually differentiates between the two and develops a sense of self.
- The infant learns to trust the self, the environment, and the caregivers through the consistent response to and satisfaction of needs.
- Exploration and active experimentation with objects in the environment enable the infant to begin to learn the properties of objects.
- The concept of object permanence is learned during the fifth substage of Piaget's sensorimotor phase of development and completed during substage 6. The infant now searches for the hidden object in more than one place.
- The neonate's body's systems all function but are immature. Most systems (except the reproductive system) achieve near mature levels of functioning by the end of infancy.
- Play is an important part of infancy; the infant develops gross and fine motor skills through practice play.
- The content of play includes the infant's own body, toys, exploratory play, repetitive play, and early symbolic play.
- Developmental theorists characterize infancy as a time of the rapid acquisition of developmental skills and growth. Piaget emphasized the infant's use of reflexes, emerging motor capacities, and sensory abilities to learn actively about the environment. Erikson noted the foundation of trust established between parent and infant and its relation to the gratification of oral needs.
- Dependence also characterizes the infant. For example, the parent needs to provide for hygiene and skin care needs, especially preventing diaper rash.

- Sleep patterns mature and consolidate so that longer sleep periods occur at night. This coincides with longer wakeful periods during the day.
- Good nutrition is essential for optimal development. Human milk or formula is sufficient for the first 6 months of life, after which solids are added to the infant's diet.
- The first tooth erupts around 6 months of age, and teething continues until 20 deciduous teeth are present.

References

American Academy of Pediatrics, Committee on Nutrition: Commentary of breast-feeding and infant formulas, including proposed standards for formulas. *Pediatrics* 1976a; 57: 278–285.

Apgar VA: A proposal for a new method of evaluation of the newborn infant. *Curr Res Anesthes Analg* 1953; 32: 260, 267.

Ball W, Tronick E: Infants' response to impeding collision: Optical and real. *Science* 1971; 171: 818–820.

Bower TGR: *Development in Infancy.* Freeman, 1974.

Bower TGR, Broughton JM, Moore MK: Infant responses to approaching objects: An indicator of response to distal variables. *Percept Psychophysics* 1970; 9: 193–196.

Brazelton TB: *Infants and Mothers.* Delacorte Press/Seymour Lawrence, 1974.

Brazelton TB: *Neonatal Behavioral Assessment Scale.* Clinics in Developmental Medicine. No. 50. Spastics International Medical Publications and Lippincott, 1973.

Brazelton TB: Behavioral competence of the newborn infant. *Sem Perinatol* 1979; 3(1): 35–44.

Chow MP et al: *1979 Handbook of Pediatric Primary Care.* Wiley, 1979.

Clarke-Stewart KA, Apfel N: Evaluating parental effects on child development. In: *Review of Research in Education,* vol. 6. Shulman LS (editor). Peacock, 1979.

DeCasper A, Fifer W: Of human bonding: Newborns prefer their mothers' voices. *Science* 1980; 208: 1174–1176.

Erikson E: *Toys and Reason.* Norton, 1977.

Gesell A: The ontogenesis of infant behavior. In: *Manual of Child Psychology.* Carmichael L (editor). Wiley, 1954.

Harlow HF, Zimmerman RR: Affectional responses in the infant monkey. *Science* 1959; 130: 420–431.

Harlow HF, Harlow MH: Learning to love. *Am Sci* 1966; 54: 244–272.

Hurlock EB: *Child Development.* McGraw-Hill, 1978.

Kessen W, Haith MM, Salapatek PH: Human infancy: A bibliography and guide. In: Carmichael's *Manual of Child Psychology.* Mussen PH (editor). Wiley, 1970.

Lowrey GH: *Growth and Development of Children.* Year Book, 1978.

Peery JC: Neonate-adult head movement: No and yes revisited. *Dev Psychol* 1980; 6: 245–250.

Piaget J: *The Origins of Intelligence in Children.* International Universities Press, 1952.

Piaget J: *Play, Dreams and Imitation in Childhood.* Gattengo C, Hodgson FM (translators). Norton, 1962.

Piaget J, Inhelder B: *The Psychology of the Child.* Basic Books, 1969.

Prechtl H, Beintema D: The neurological examination of the full-term newborn infant. *Clinics in Developmental Medicine,* no. 12. Spastics Society and Heinemann, 1964.

Stone T, Church J: *Childhood and Adolescence.* Random House, 1975.

Additional Readings

Ainsworth MDS, et al: *The Strange Situation: Observing Patterns of Attachment.* Erlbaum, 1979.

American Academy of Pediatrics, Committee on Nutrition: Iron supplementation for infants. *Pediatrics* 1976b; 58(5): 765.

American Academy of Pediatrics, Committee on Nutrition: On the feeding of supplemental foods to infants. *Pediatrics* 1980; 65: 1178–1180.

Bernal J: Night waking in infants during the first 14 months. *Dev Med Child Neurol* 1973; 15: 760–769.

Bloom L: *Language Development: Form and Function in Emerging Grammars.* MIT Press, 1970.

Bornstein MH: Infants are trichromats. *J Exp Child Psychol* 1978; 21: 425–445.

Bowlby J: *Attachment and Loss,* vol 1. Hogarth Press and Institute for Psychoanalysis, 1969.

Brown R, Belugi V: Three processes in the child's acquisition of language. In: *New Directions in the Study of Child Language.* Lennenberg EL (editor). MIT Press, 1964.

Carey WB: Clinical appraisal of temperament. In: *Developmental Disabilities: Theory Assessment and Intervention.* Lewis M, Taft L (editors). SP Medical, 1982.

Condon WS, Sauder LW: Neonate movement is synchronized with adult speech. *Science* 1979; 183: 99–101.

Erikson EH: *Childhood and Society.* Norton, 1963.

Fagan JF: Origins of facial pattern recognition. In: *Psychological Development from Infancy.* Bornstein MH, Kessen W (editors). Erlbaum, 1979.

Fantz RL: A method for studying depth perception in infants under 6 months of age. *Psychol Record* 1961; 11: 27–32.

Field T: The adjustment of reaching behavior to object distance in early infancy. *Child Dev* 1976; 47: 304–308.

Fomon SJ et al: Recommendations for feeding normal infants. *Pediatrics* 1979; 63:52–59.
Gordon FR, Yonas A: Sensitivity to binocular depth information in infants. *J Exp Child Psychol* 1976; 22:413–422.
Gulick EE: Infant health and breast-feeding. *Pediatr Nurs* 1983; 9(5):359–362.
Jacklin C et al: Sleep pattern development from 6 through 33 months. *Pediatr Psychol* 1980; 5:295–303.
Kessen W, Levine J, Wendich KA: The imitation of pitch in infants. *Infant Behav Dev* 1979; 2:93–100.
Korner AF: Conceptual issues in infancy research. In: *Handbook of Infant Development*. Osofsky JD (editor). Wiley, 1979.
Lamb ME, Campos JJ: *Development in Infancy*. Random House, 1982.
Lawton JT: *Introduction to Child Development*. Brown, 1982.
Levine MD et al: *Developmental-Behavioral Pediatrics*. Saunders, 1983.
Ludington-Hoe SM: What can newborns really see? *Am J Nurs* 1980; 83(9):1286–1289.
MacFarlane A: Olfaction in the development of social preferences in the human neonate. In: *Parent-Infant Interaction*. CIBA Foundation Symposium, 33, 1975.
Maddi B: *Personality Theories: A Comparative Analysis,* 4th ed. Dorsey, 1980.
Osterholm P, Lindeke LL, Amidon D: Sleep disturbance in infants aged 6 to 12 months. *Pediatr Nurs* 1983; 9(4):269–271.
Peery JC, Aoki E: Leave-taking behavior between preschool children and their parents. *J Genet Psychol* 1982; 140:71–81.
Peery JC, Crane PM: Personal space regulation: Approach-withdrawal-approach proxemic behavior during adult-preschooler interaction at close range. *J Psychol* 1980; 106:63–75.
Richards JE, Rader N: Crawling-onset age predicts visual cliff avoidance in infants. *J Exp Psychol* 1981; 7:382–387.
Schiamberg LB, Smith KU: *Human Development*. Macmillan, 1982.
Schuster CS, Ashburn SS: *The Process of Human Development*. Little, Brown, 1986.
Smilansky S: *The Effects of Sociodramatic Play on Disadvantaged Preschool Children*. Wiley, 1968.
Spitz RA: Hospitalism: An inquiry into the genesis of psychiatric conditions in early childhood. In: *The Psychoanalytic Study of the Child*, vol 1. Eissler RS et al. (editors). International Universities Press, 1945.
Spitz RA: Hospitalism: A follow-up report. In: *The Psychoanalytic Study of the Child,* vol 2. Eissler RS et al. (editors). International Universities Press, 1946.
Wagner TJ, Hindi-Alexander M: Hazards of baby powder? *Pediatr Nurs* 1984; 10(2):124–125.
Weir L: Auditory frequency sensitivity in the neonate: A signal detection analysis. *J Exp Child Psychol* 1976; 21:219–225.
Yussen SR, Santrock JW: *Child Development: An Introduction*. Brown, 1982.

Chapter 5

Early Childhood

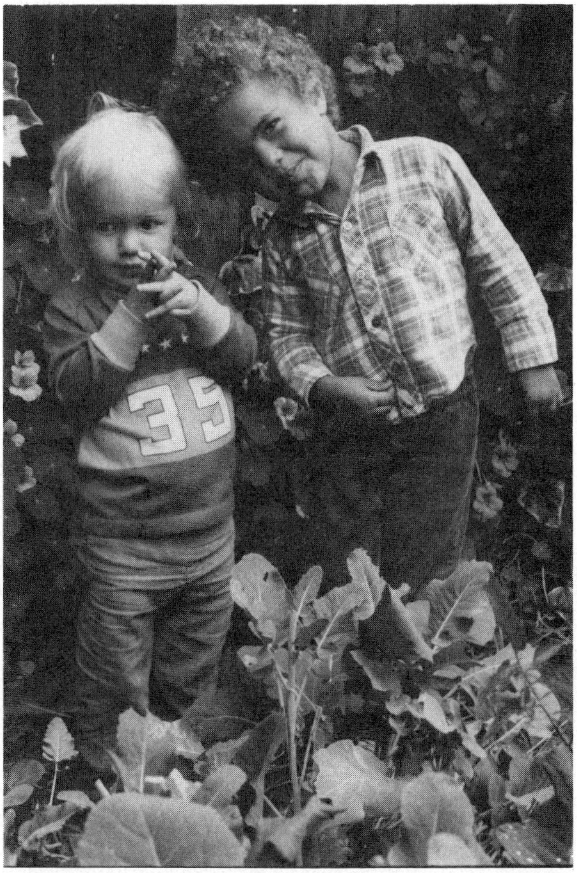

Chapter Contents

(Continues)

Objectives

- Discuss the ways that the family and community contribute to the socialization process of the child.
- Define the major parameters of development in early childhood.
- Explain the essential biophysical changes that occur in early childhood.
- Describe the principal personality and cognitive developments in early childhood.
- Explain the purpose of play in early childhood.
- Identify the basic health care needs of preschool children.

Early childhood is the time from about 18 months to 4 1/2 years of age. Locomotion and language distinguish this stage from infancy. Early childhood is the time for learning skills that enable the young child to begin the move toward independence. Being able to walk and talk are the important, self-enhancing skills that support the child's interaction with others, allowing the child freedom to explore the environment and further develop a unique personality.

The child at this stage acquires the ability to use symbols or words to describe experiences and thoughts. This ability to describe events and thoughts gives the child a powerful tool in exploring and manipulating the environment. The ability to communicate serves as a catalyst for the child's cognitive and social development.

The child also shows an increased awareness of the self, of "me." This awareness is accompanied by tensions that pull the child's emotions and behavior in opposite directions. These tensions are demonstrated in many of the behaviors that characterize this age. Independence-seeking behaviors, such as running from the parent, saying "no" to all requests, and having temper tantrums are contrasted by increasing demands for parental attention, needing assistance with previously mastered tasks, and/or showing hesitancy with strangers.

Thus transition from infancy into early childhood is marked by disequilibrium as the child first tries to control the environment while not being controlled by it. Such efforts reflect the child's dilemma—the need to hold on and yet to let go—since the desire for independence still is not matched by an ability to be independent.

Fortunately for parents, a calmer, more delightful period follows. Although the 3- to 4 1/2-year-old does have periods of disequilibrium, these are tempered by the acquisition of important self-care skills, greater problem-solving skills, and more emotional and social maturity. The child at this age bursts into a time of creativity, imagination, and fantasy, all of which make the child an amusing, delightful companion. In addition, the child at age 3 is learning from experience and from parental admonitions to recognize and set personal limits.

The increased mobility and feeling of independence characteristic of this period culminate in such behaviors as the child's ability to walk to school. A child about to enter school has achieved a relative degree of independence in communication, locomotion, and self-care.

The External Environment's Influence on the Child

Influence of the Family

The child interacts with objects and people in the environment, which in turn contributes to the child's unique course of development. During early childhood, the child's environment is primarily the immediate family, and young children therefore experience and interpret events, activities, and decisions as their families perceive them. As observed by Erik Erikson, the child's world of significant others is first the immediate family, then the extended family, and last the neighborhood friends. Therefore, during early childhood the intense infant-parent bonds are transformed into broader relationships, but the safety, trust, and stability provided by the family remain critical. Not until middle childhood does the child step beyond the family and develop truly independent relationships.

Parents Through the family, the child is introduced to society and to the rituals and traditions that become associated with holidays, annual events, or celebrations. Although today's children often are introduced to society through day care or nursery school at younger ages than children of earlier generations, families still are the primary socializers.

The family plays the predominant teaching role and provides the necessary continuity in the child's development. During early childhood, children observe, then imitate through play, and eventually claim as their own the behaviors, values, and expectations demonstrated by family members. The adults' approval or disapproval of these actions determines whether the child continues the same patterns of behavior. In this way, the family provides the child with feedback to help guide a developing sense of self.

As the child is exposed to ideas and demands of others, the availability of parental support is critical. Children who have learned about trust from the nurturing, consistent responses of parents are able to trust others. Those who have acquired basic knowledge and information from parental teaching are better able to learn from others, such as teachers. Secure children can adapt to different standards or demands of others because they have learned self-control and have a sense of who they are. They also can begin to learn goal-directed and appropriate self-initiated activity.

The family sets the stage for reciprocal interactions. A firstborn child might, at this time, need to adapt to a younger brother or sister, or a second or third child might be part of a family that is expanding and adjusting to incorporate a new member. Children with siblings learn about sharing, compromise, and the social power of age. The firstborn who enters this phase as an only child might have learned to interact primarily with adults and might experience initial difficulty interacting with peers (Bigner, 1979).

The first experiences of having to share toys or adults' attention can be rather traumatic. For example, 4-year-old David was an only child in a nuclear family and experienced a rude initiation when he attempted to join his neighborhood peer group. At first, these children were curious about David and his toys, yard, house, and family. They asked many questions while exploring the area. They then took over and told David what he could do, what toys he could use, and that he had to be the baby when they played "house." David made some initial attempts to comply, but soon he could be heard to say, "But my daddy always lets me be the boss," and "Mommy bought that truck for me, it's mine, and I want it now. I'll tell my mommy." Frustrated, he ran into the house and informed his mother that he did not like these children and wanted to play with only her or with daddy because they were nicer.

Extended family In extended families more family members might be psychologically, socially, and physically present for the developing child. A network of close relationships expands the complexity of interactions, diffuses intense parent-child ties, and broadens social support systems. In extended families the child has more role models and a greater diversity of occupations and personalities to imitate through play.

A child growing up in an extended family has grandparents, aunts, uncles, and cousins available either within the same house or nearby, such as next door, around the corner, or on the next farm. If a parent is busy, another adult can be found to help or to listen as needed.

For example, 4-year-old Susie likes her big family because she never has to be alone. If her parents are busy, she goes downstairs to her grandparents, and one of them usually has time to play a game or talk. Although she is the youngest in her family, she thinks she knows all about caring for and playing with infants because she spends a lot of time with her 6-month-old cousin, who lives next door. She talks to another aunt about being a schoolteacher and visits her uncle while he is working at the bank. She knows all about tools and carpentry because her grandfather is a carpenter, and together they built her dollhouse. When her siblings and cousins play ball, she is right there, learning what to do and how to do it. The extended family provides a great variety of resources, role models, and teachers for the child.

Patterned family behaviors are passed on from previous generations and encompass the developing child. A "family script" that expresses expectations for this child is influenced by cultural, social, or ethical values. The young child growing up in an extended family that is both psychologically and physically close will have experiences that are different from those of the child in a more isolated family.

Comparing the experiences of Susie and David helps to illustrate the difference in orientation experienced by children from extended families and those from small nuclear families. David's play activities and approval-seeking were oriented toward his parents. Susie's sphere of orientation involved a variety of adults and children of different ages. David was exposed to one set of standards and expectations from his parents, who also were responsible for fulfilling all of the other numerous roles related to family maintenance. Susie related intimately with several families and observed different interpretations of the same standards and different ways of performing similar roles. She had a larger radius of people from whom to receive recognition or approval. In Susie's situation the extended family was a supportive and positive experience; unfortunately, this is not always the case. Sometimes extended families have more negative, competitive experiences than positive ones.

The child's role in the family Clinical work and research done by Stanley Greenspan and his group noted the importance of the emotional tone of the family environment on the child's adaptive functioning. "By age three or four, children . . . are learning to regulate behavior and emotion, or they are learning to be impulsive and destructive . . . are learning positive self-esteem or they are learning to be sad and have negative self images" (Kagan and Greenspan,

1986). Early patterns of interaction relate to later patterns and set the stage for more complex patterns. Providing the child with an early foundation in the pattern of supportive, loving interaction among family members is essential. Positive interactions provide the opportunity to learn about more complex human relationships and about causes and effects of behavior.

To varying degrees the child's social experience within the family might be influenced by birth order and gender. Attitudes toward the gender of the child are derived partly from family values and sex stereotyping that prevail in society. Evidence of this can be seen in chores assigned to children or in intimacy allowed between children and parents, particularly between young boys and their fathers. Parental expectations and acceptance of independent or dependent behaviors might vary according to the child's birth order. The youngest child is allowed to remain dependent longer than the older children, especially if the youngest is female.

Influence of the Community

Adult family members take on roles such as the breadwinner, caregiver, teacher, and disciplinarian. Family breadwinners, and in turn other family members, are assigned status or position in society based on income, education, and occupation.

Community resources Income and prestige determine the section of town in which the family lives; the child's opportunities to participate in various activities, such as music lessons, swimming, or art; the presence of a second or third vacation home; and the type, amount, and quality of toys available. Some indicators of the family's status are subtler. These might include the manner in which the town bankers, merchants, or officials respond to the family (especially the father), the particular school the child attends, or the amount of attention, level of expectation, and degree of responsiveness from school teachers. All these indicators provide cues to the child about the family's status in the community (Coles, 1977).

Other indicators are related to the community's economy and ideology. School facilities, the living and play environment, the purity of the air and water, the educational and technical resources, and the availability of quality support services are evidence of the community's position in society as a whole. The community's resources for young children relate to its potential to provide quality early childhood experiences. These resources might include nursery schools, a Head Start program, child care for working parents, or YWCA-YMCA programs, all of which have the potential to affect the child positively. A community that chooses to provide such resources enriches the lives of its young children by providing positive interaction with the surrounding environment.

Health care system The accessibility of health care also influences the character of community life. The quality and diversity of screening, counseling, and intervention programs available for children and their families enhance or inhibit healthy development. Many communities provide tax-supported health services through federal, state, or local monies. Communities differ, however, in their ability to provide and in their philosophy about providing screening programs as one of the health services.

Early childhood is the ideal time to detect the precursors of some diseases and identify certain correctable disorders. For screening programs to be of value, however, they must be convenient, free or of minimal cost, well advertised, and connected to follow-up programs when problems are detected. Providing screening programs requires a commitment to health education, prevention, and early intervention rather than the traditional practice of crisis intervention. This progressive philosophy conveys the community's concern for the quality of life of its residents and a willingness to spend the resources of time, money, and energy to achieve a better-quality life.

In the past, immunization programs were the most widely known and accepted means of preventing illnesses. These are still important today, but other equally important programs have been added. Newer approaches to improve and maintain health during the early childhood years include blood tests to screen for anemia, lead levels, sickle cell trait or disease; vision screening to detect strabismus, amblyopia, and color blindness; auditory and speech screening to identify hearing loss or articulation problems; and developmental screening to assess gross and fine motor skills, including coordination and balance.

The extent to which these programs are accessible before the child enters school also is significant. Vision, hearing, speech, or other physical disorders can adversely affect the child's ability to learn. In addition, the child's achievement of a positive self-concept is thwarted if others tease, mock, or make fun of an existing deficiency.

Developmental Changes in Early Childhood

Both the genetic endowment and the child's interaction with the external environment contribute to making each child's growth pattern unique. A child's internal environment matures according to key genetic and phylogenetic phases.

The direction and sequences of growth are, however, predictable. Normal children reach developmental milestones, such as walking, language acquisition, and bladder and bowel control, within a certain time frame. The patterns of the separate behaviors that lead to these milestones might differ, but the results are stable and consistent for all children. If the child reaches developmental milestones within the standard time frame, development is likely to be normal. The ages at which children normally reach their milestones do, however, vary widely. Children progress at paces that are optimum for them.

The child continuously learns new skills, which in turn help the child interact with the environment and influence growth in other areas of development. Social growth during early childhood is facilitated by language acquisition, cognitive growth, and fine and gross motor skills. Similarly, motor skills, such as bicycling and ballplaying, may be facilitated by social interactions. Emotional growth, evidenced by learning to tolerate separation from parents, is made easier by the mental achievement of what Piaget termed object permanence, or the ability to retain a mental image. The child who cried at 9 months when a parent or caregiver was out of sight can now understand that objects that have disappeared from view are not gone forever. (Developmental norms and assessment techniques for 18- to 24-month-olds are summarized in Table 5-1; those for 2- and 3-year-olds are summarized in Table 5-2; and those for 4-year-olds are summarized in Table 5-3.)

Affective Development

Characteristics of the child's personality take form during the early childhood period. During infancy, temperamental differences, coupled with environmental and genetic influences, account for individuality, but around 18 months of age, the child exhibits more complex and unique personality traits.

Self-control and limit setting The first phase of early childhood (also known as toddlerhood) corresponds to Sigmund Freud's second stage of development, the anal phase (see Chapter 3). Freud thought that the maturation occurring at this time was responsible for the child's shift in focus from oral to anal interests. Additional factors contributing to this shift, as observed by Freud, were society's expectations and parental demands regarding toilet training and cleanliness.

Parents of toddlers know that children use their newly learned toileting behaviors to dominate others in their search for increased independence. The child is able to control powerful others, usually parents, by withholding and expelling during toilet training. One 2-year-old girl, for example, discovered that she could refuse to "go potty" before a family outing and then create great turmoil by demanding to make a bathroom stop once the trip had begun.

Related to this withholding characteristic is the tendency to say "no." Young children constantly hear prohibitions against their actions during this time of increased locomotion and exploration. They become aware of the power that the word *no* has to govern behavior, and they mimic their parents with automatic recitals of "no" in response to every request or demand. This is one of the ways in which they test limits and identify areas of acceptable independence. Parents need tremendous patience and an understanding of the interplay of developmental tasks as their children attempt to discover and define their place. This process is facilitated by giving the young child some measure of control and then clearly and consistently presenting the consequences of the actions.

Other researchers also have defined this stage of affective development. The second stage of Erik Erikson's theory (autonomy vs. shame and doubt) suggests that these interactions with the environment will either support the child's sense of autonomy or engender feelings of shame and doubt. Parental attitudes and behaviors, which are a significant part of this environment, therefore influence the child's sense of self. If socializing experiences, such as toilet training, eating correctly, and self-dressing, are fraught with anxiety and become a battle of wills, the child is likely to feel shame and doubt. If, however, the child is encouraged and supported in these developmental tasks, a realistic and positive sense of autonomy is likely to result.

The child's need for autonomy leads to other characteristic behaviors. One of the more frequently heard demands is "Me do it." One 2 1/2-year-old astonished her proud grandmother in front of a group of friends at church. This young girl loudly insisted that she was going to put on and button her new coat, and offers of help were refused defiantly. The wise grandmother stepped aside and covertly watched as the child struggled for 20 minutes until she got the coat on and partly buttoned. Proudly she showed her grandmother, who praised her accomplishment. Parents often find that they need to allow extra time before an outing so that young children can express their autonomy in dressing. Otherwise, a battle of wills is likely to ensue, and the child is chastised for making everyone late.

Another major issue for the young child is the development of self-control. Toilet training, limits on behavior, and peer interactions all require the child to curb impulses and control actions. Some youngsters engage in a battle of wills and resist parental guidance, so temper tantrums are fairly common during this period. Children become enraged when their wishes are not gratified. These outbursts of screaming, thrashing, and kicking are triggered even more

(Text continues on page 140)

TABLE 5-1 Guidelines for the Assessment of the 18- to 24-Month-Old Child

Developmental area	Expected characteristics	Assessment techniques
Temperament		Discuss temperamental characteristics of the child and parental perceptions
Biophysical development		
Weight	Average (50th percentile) 11.4 kg (25 lb)	The child can be weighed and measured on a stand-up scale if the child can cooperate; all clothing is removed except underpants
Length—averages 2 to 3 inches growth/year	Average 76.8 cm (32 in.)	
Neuromuscular	90% of adult brain size achieved by 2 years of age. Anterior fontanel closed	
Gross motor skills	Runs clumsily	Observe the child's running or ask parent to describe
	Pushes and pulls toys	Provide push toy for the child
	Seats self on small chair	Provide small object for the child to sit on or ask parent whether child does this
	Walks backward	Observe the child walking backward
	Kicks ball forward	Demonstrate kicking a ball and tell the child to do this
	Walks up steps with one hand held	Ask the parent how the child manages stairs; discuss with the parent the child's opportunities to develop gross motor skills
Fine motor skills	Builds tower of three to four blocks	Provide blocks and demonstrate stacking
	Grasp and release are well controlled	Observe the child picking up a small object and the release of blocks when stacking
	Attempts to imitate drawing straight line	Provide paper and crayon, demonstrate a line, and ask the child to draw
	Uses spoon with little spilling	Ask the parent to describe the child's skill at eating
	Turns pages in book, may turn two to three at a time	Provide book and observe how the child handles it
Cardiovascular		
Heart rate	110 beats/min	
Respiratory rate	20–40 breaths/min—abdominal breathing	
Sensory-perceptual		
Vision	Convergence; accommodation to both near and far	
Hearing	At adult levels	Assess through observing language development and response to speech or environmental noise
Language development	Uses several single words	Listen to the child's verbalizations and ask the parent what words the child uses
	Combines two words in a phrase	Ask the parent whether the child combines two or more words
	Points to body part	Ask the child (or have the parent ask the child) to point to eyes or nose
	Names an object	Show the child a picture of a common, interesting object and ask the child to name it
	Follows simple directions	Tell the child to "take the ball (or other object) to mother"; "give it to me," or "put the ball on the table"; observe the quantity and character of the verbal interchanges between the parent and child

TABLE 5-1 ***(Continued)***

Developmental area	Expected characteristics	Assessment techniques
Cognitive development	Dumps a raisin from a bottle spontaneously or with demonstration	Place a raisin in a bottle and tell the child to get it out; may demonstrate
	Locates hidden object with invisible displacements	Place a small screen in front of the child, put a toy in a small cup, put the cup behind a screen and dump the toy, show the child the empty cup and observe the child's reaction; the child should locate the toy behind the screen; ask the parent whether the child goes through cupboards to get objects
	Obtains an object by using a tool	Place an interesting toy on a table just out of reach, place a toy rake or stick near the child and observe whether the child uses a rake to obtain the toy; may demonstrate; ask the parent whether the child drags a chair across the room to climb and obtain an object that is out of reach
	Deferred imitation	Ask the parent whether the child imitates non-present behaviors
	Begins to "pretend"	Ask the parent whether the child does any simple "pretending" behaviors
	Infers a cause while only seeing an effect	Watch for behavior during assessment; assess the child's learning environment (parental encouragement, appropriate toys, books); assess parental response to exploratory behavior
Social and affective development		
Child	Increasing autonomy but continues marked dependence on parent	Assess parental feelings about child's increasing independence
	Insists on self-feeding	Assess feeding situation, noting particularly whether the child feeds self independently and how the parent handles food refusal
	Beginning negativism, temper tantrums	Ask the parent whether the child is becoming more negative, assess the frequency and intensity of temper tantrums, assess parental response
	Separation anxiety but the child is learning to cope better	Discuss the child's behavior during separation, ask the parent to compare the child's current behavior with behavior at an earlier age to identify evidence of more adaptive coping, assess the parental reaction to separation
	Uses "transitional objects" for comfort	Ask whether child has a "security" object and the situations in which it is used, assess the parents' perception of a transitional object
	Might begin to be ritualistic	Ask the parent about family routines and how the child responds if routines are altered
	Changes moods rapidly and frequently (emotional lability)	Discuss the child's mood changes with the parent, assess parental perceptions and reactions
	Understands most limits but does not have self-control	Discuss with the parent the limit set, how the child responds, and what happens if the child disobeys and assess the parent's perception of the child's "misbehavior"
	Begins to be possessive	Ask the parent whether the child demonstrates possessiveness, ask the child to give the nurse an object (shoe or toy) and see how the child responds
	Might indicate readiness for toilet training	Discuss parental views concerning toilet training techniques and how to handle accidents; assess the child for signs of readiness

TABLE 5-2 Guidelines for Assessment of the 2- and 3-Year-Old Child

Developmental area	Expected characteristics: 2-year-old	Expected characteristics: 3-year-old	Assessment techniques: 2-year-old	Assessment techniques: 3-year-old
Temperament			Assess temperamental characteristics of the child and parental perceptions of the child's temperament	Assess tempermental characteristics and parental perceptions
Biophysical development				
Weight	Average (50th percentile) 12.3 kg (27 lb)	14.5 kg (32 lb)		
Length	Average (50th percentile) 86.4 cm (34 in)	94 cm (37 in)		
Neuromuscular				
Gross motor skills	Jumps in place	Alternates feet going up stairs	Tell the child to jump; demonstrate if necessary	Observe or ask the parent to describe
	Broad jumps 8 in.	Rides a tricycle	Place sheet of paper on the floor and tell the child to jump over it	Ask the parent whether the child pedals a tricycle
	Tip-toes		Tell the child to walk on tiptoes; demonstrate if necessary	
	Goes up and down stairs alone; places both feet on each step		Ask the parent to describe how the child manages stairs; observe if possible	
	Balances on one foot for 1 second	Balances on one foot for 2 seconds	Tell the child to stand on one foot for as long as possible; demonstrate if necessary	Tell the child to stand on one foot as long as possible; demonstrate if necessary
Fine motor skills	Might copy a circle	Copies circle Copies cross	Show the child a circle but do not let the child observe the circle being drawn and do not name the circle; ask the child to "draw one just like this" and see whether the child draws an enclosed shape that is not necessarily perfectly round	Show the child a circle but do not let the child observe the circle being drawn and do not name the circle; ask the child to "draw one just like this"; use the same technique as with the circle but with a cross
	Imitates a circle		Allow the child to watch the circle being drawn and tell the child to "draw one just like this"	
	Imitates a vertical line		Allow the child to watch a line being drawn and tell the child to "draw one just like this"	

TABLE 5-2 *(Continued)*

Developmental area	Expected characteristics		Assessment techniques	
	2-year-old	3-year-old	2-year-old	3-year-old
	Builds tower of seven to eight blocks	Builds "bridge" from blocks	Provide 1-in. cubes and tell the child to build a tower; demonstrate if necessary	Assemble a bridge and tell the child to build one
	Hold pencil with fingers rather than fist	Puts pellets into a narrow-necked bottle	Observe how the child uses pencil or crayon	Provide a narrow-necked bottle and pellets and tell the child to put the pellets into the bottle; demonstrate if necessary
	Turns doorknobs		Observe the child opening a door or ask the parent whether the child does this	
			Assess the opportunities for the development of fine motor skills	
Cardiovascular				
Heart rate	90–110 beats/min	90–110 beats/min	Apical or carotid pulse	
Blood pressure	90–95 mm Hg systolic 65 mm Hg diastolic	90–95 mm Hg systolic 65 mm Hg diastolic	Use blood pressure cuff 1.5 times the diameter of the extremity part being used; no less than ½ or more than ⅔ of the extremity part to be covered	
Respiratory rate	20–30 breaths/min	20–30 breaths/min		
Sensory-perceptual				
Vision	20/70 acuity	20/50		Use Allen cards to test vision if the child can identify the pictures (see Chapter 10)
Language development	Combines two and three words	Speaks in sentences using adverbs and adjectives	Listen to the child's spontaneous speech; ask the parent for examples of the child's word combinations	Listen to the child's speech and sentence structure
	Names pictures of common objects		Present realistic pictures of common objects, such as a dog, cat, and ball, and ask the child to name them	

(Continues)

TABLE 5-2 Guidelines for Assessment of the 2- and 3-Year-Old Child *(Continued)*

Developmental area	Expected characteristics		Assessment techniques	
	2-year-old	3-year-old	2-year-old	3-year-old
	Follows simple directions; uses plurals; uses "I," "me," and "you"; knows one color	Understands "up" and "down"; understands "loud" and "soft"; gives first and last name; understands "tired," "cold," and "hungry"; asks many questions, very talkative; knows two colors; improved articulation	Tell the child to "Give the ball to mommy," "Put the ball on the table," and "Put the ball on the floor," and see whether the child can do two of three tasks Listen to the child's spontaneous speech for the use of plurals; place several blocks on the table and ask the child, "What are these?" and listen for "s" at the end of blocks; ask the parent whether the child uses plurals Listen to the child's speech; ask the parent whether the child uses these words at home Place blocks of different colors on the table and ask child to give the nurse the red block (or another color) Assess the quality of verbal interaction between the parent and child	Tell the child to put hands "up" and then "down" Tap an object softly or loudly on the desk and ask the child to describe Ask the child to say his or her whole name Ask the child, "What do you do when you are tired?" "Cold?" "Hungry?" and expect two of three appropriate answers Assess the quality of the interaction between the parent and child; assess parental responses to the child's questions Place blocks of different colors on the table and ask the child for the red (blue, yellow, or green) block Should be able to understand half of the child's speech
Cognitive development	Dumps a raisin from a bottle spontaneously Places circle, square, and triangle in formboard Unscrews lid Infers cause from observing effect Characteristics of thought: egocentricity, animism, transductive thinking, perception-bound thinking, and magical thinking	Imaginative play Repeats three digits States own sex Classifies according to one characteristic Characteristics of thought include egocentricity, transductive thinking, animism, perception-bound thinking	Place a raisin in a bottle and tell the child to get it out; the child should be able to do so readily Present formboard with three forms and tell the child to place the forms in the right places Provide a small jar with a screw top, place a toy inside and tell the child to obtain the toy Allow the child to see a wind-up toy in action but do not allow the child to observe the toy being wound up; give the toy to the child and see whether the child can wind the toy up Listen to the child's spontaneous speech and observe spontaneous activities; engage the child in conversation and attempt to elicit the child's perceptions	Discuss with the parent the child's evidence of imagination Ask the child to repeat three single numbers (should do so in two of three trials) Ask whether the child is a boy or a girl Present 12 forms: four triangles (two red, two blue), four squares (two red, two blue), and four circles (two red, two blue); ask the child to put like forms together Observe the child's speech and activity; engage the child in conversation and attempt to elicit perceptions

TABLE 5-2 *(Continued)*

Developmental area	Expected characteristics		Assessment techniques	
	2-year-old	**3-year-old**	**2-year-old**	**3-year-old**
Social and affective development				
Child	Increased independence from parents but still needs "refueling"	Depends less on parents but needs reassurance and support	Observe parent-child interaction, noting the child's ability to function alone and to use the parent as a resource; discuss parental reactions to the child's increasing independence	Assess parent-child interactions, noting how independently the child functions, how the child approaches tasks, and whether the parent allows the child to perform a task without interference
	Undresses self and attempts to dress self Independent, refuses certain foods Protests at bedtime, awakens during night Separation anxiety, but child is better able to tolerate separations Might continue use of transitional objects Achieves bowel and bladder control during day Remains dry at night	Actively initiates many projects and explorations but does not necessarily complete them Performs simple tasks around the house Tolerates separations from parent for short periods Demonstrates an awareness of sex role behavior and family roles	Observe the child's dressing and undressing directly; ask the parent to describe who dresses and undresses the child, who selects the clothes, and how willing the child is to accept help Assess feeding behaviors and parental response to food refusal Assess sleep behaviors and parental response Discuss the child's behavior before, during, and after separation; discuss parental feelings about separation; might ask parent to leave room and observe behavior directly Discuss with the parent whether and how toilet training has been established Assess the frequency of "accidents" and how these are managed; assess the child's reactions to training procedures and accidents	Assess the child's behavior in exploration and interaction; note how the child approaches tasks; assess parental feedback to the child Discuss with the parent what tasks the child does; assess parental satisfaction with the child's performance Discuss the child's behavior before, during, and after separation; assess parental reactions; discuss the extent of these with the parent Ask the child such questions as, "What do mommies do?" and "What do daddies do?"
	Negativism continues but begins to decrease as child becomes more secure about autonomy	Negativism and ritualism are significantly decreased	Observe the child for instances of negativism, discuss parental perceptions of the child's negative behavior and note whether the parent sees change; assess parental response to negative behavior	

(Continues)

TABLE 5-2 Guidelines for Assessment of the 2- and 3-Year-Old Child *(Continued)*

Developmental area	Expected characteristics		Assessment techniques	
	2-year-old	3-year-old	2-year-old	3-year-old
	Temper tantrums begin to diminish as the child develops more mature strategies to cope with conflict and frustration		Discuss the occurrence of tantrums with the parent and note precipitating factors, the child's behavior, and parental responses	
	Ritualism (begins to diminish)		Discuss the child's special routines and reaction to disruption of routine	
	Dawdling		Observe for dawdling in assessment setting and observe parental response	
	Indicates an understanding of unacceptable behavior but has limited self-control	Shows a willingness to conform to parental expectations Exerts more self-control but is not reliable; continues to need supervision	Observe limit setting by the parent and the child's response to the limit; discuss parental responses to "misbehavior"; ask the parent to describe the limits set at home, how these are enforced, and the responses when the child breaks a limit	Observe limit setting by the parent and observe the child's response to limits Discuss with the parent any concerns about misbehavior, type of discipline usually used, and child's response
	Demonstrates specific fears	Evidences specific fears	Discuss with the parent whether the child has special fears and how the parents respond	Ask whether the child is especially fearful of anything and how the parent responds
	Parallel play with other children	Associative play; begins to share; plays interactive games with other children but with little regard for rules	Observe the child's play; discuss with the parent how the child interacts with other children; assess opportunities for peer relationships	Ask the parent to describe the child's interaction with peers and siblings

TABLE 5-3 Guidelines for Assessment of the 4-Year-Old Child

Developmental area	Expected characteristics	Assessment techniques
Temperament		Assess temperamental characteristics and parental perceptions
Biophysical development		
Weight	Average (50th percentile) 16.4 kg (36 lb)	
Length	101.6 cm (40 in)	
Neuromuscular	One-sided functioning is fully established	
Gross motor skills	Balances on one foot for 5 seconds; might balance on one foot for 10 seconds	Tell child, "Do this as long as you can," while demonstrating; time the number of seconds the child can balance and expect the child to balance for 5 seconds on two of three trials
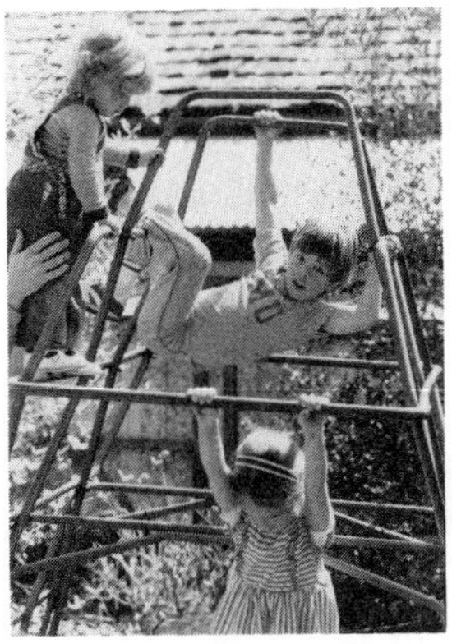	Hops twice on one foot	Tell the child to hop on one foot; demonstrate if necessary
	Forward heel-to-toe walk, heel within 1 in. of toe, for at least four steps; runs with good leg-arm coordination	Tell the child to do heel-to-toe walk; demonstrate if necessary; helpful to have line on floor for the child to follow
	Goes up and down stairs using alternate feet; begins climbing jungle gyms and other playground equipment	Observe the child or ask the parent to describe how the child manages stairs and playground equipment
	Catches bounced and tossed ball with arms; might trap ball against body	From a distance of 3 ft, have the child catch a bounced ball and a tossed ball; note if catching or trapping ball with arms and body; expect the child to either catch with arms or trap ball on two out of three attempts
Fine motor skills	Might imitate square after demonstration	First see whether the child can copy a square from a picture without being shown; if not, demonstrate how to draw a square by drawing two opposite sides first and then the other two sides; corners should be about 90°
	Copies cross	Show the child a cross but do not let the child see it being drawn and do not name it; tell the child to draw one like the picture; lines need not be straight to pass
	Draws a person with three identifiable parts; draws house crudely	Tell the child to draw a person but do not tell the child which parts to draw; the child's picture should include three identifiable body parts, but if one part of a pair (eyes, arms) is not drawn, that part does not count
	Uses scissors	Provide the child with scissors and paper with the outline of a simple shape and tell the child to cut out the shape; ability to use scissors effectively is more important than precision in cutting; assess the child's opportunities to practice fine motor skills
Cardiovascular		
Heart rate	105 beats/min	
Blood pressure	99/65 mm Hg	
Respiratory rate	20–30 breaths/min	

(Continues)

TABLE 5-3 Guidelines for Assessment of the 4-Year-Old Child *(Continued)*

Developmental area	Expected characteristics	Assessment techniques
Sensory-perceptual		
Vision	20/40 acuity	Use Allen cards; or Snellen Alphabet Cards if the child can identify letters (see Chapter 10)
Hearing		May begin audiometric testing if the child can cooperate (see Chapter 10)
Language development—expression and comprehension	Uses sentences of four to five words	Listen to the child's spontaneous speech
	Understands prepositions such as "under," "on top of," "behind," "in front of"	Ask the child to place an object in various positions (eg, "Place the block on top of the table"); the child should perform three of four trials correctly
	Understands analogies	Ask the child the following: "If fire is hot, ice is _____?" "Mother is a woman, Daddy is a _____?" "A house is big, a mouse is _____?"; the child should perform two of three trials correctly
	Recognizes three colors	Place four colored blocks on a table, ask the child to give the nurse the red (blue, green, or yellow) one; replace the block on the table and repeat using another color; ask for four colors; the child should perform three correctly
Cognitive development	Understands concepts of "long" and "short	Present two lines, one of which is longer; ask the child to point to the longer line; change the position of the lines; the child should consistently choose the longer line
	Understands "heavy" and "light"	Present two objects, one of which is noticeably heavier; ask the child to hold the objects and say which is heavier
	Repeats four digits	Tell the child to listen carefully, then say four single digits and ask the child to repeat; the child should succeed in one of three trials
	Counts three objects	Present ten blocks and tell the child to "take two blocks and put them here," indicating a place on the table; put the blocks back into the group and tell the child to "take three blocks" and so on
	Continues to classify objects according to one characteristic	Present 12 forms: four triangles (two red, two blue), four squares (two red, two blue), and four circles (two red, two blue); ask the child to put like forms together
	Does not perceive conservation of matter	Present two identical glasses with the same amount of water in each; as the child watches, pour the water from one glass into a tall, narrow glass; ask the child which glass has more water; present two balls of clay the same size; roll one ball into a long, narrow shape; ask the child which shape has more clay
	Continues to be imaginative; tells stories mixing fantasy and reality but with little regard for accuracy	Discuss the child's imaginative play with the parent; ask whether the child exaggerates or "tells tales"
	Considers other's perspectives (less egocentric)	Observe for spontaneous examples of the ability to consider another's point of view during the assessment

TABLE 5-3 (Continued)

Developmental area	Expected characteristics	Assessment techniques
Social and affective development		
Child	Demonstrates independence in daily activities; dresses and undresses without supervision; buttons clothes (except in back); knows front from back	Observe how child dresses and undresses self in assessment; discuss with the parent and child who selects clothes and dresses child and how much help the child needs
	Washes own face and hands	Discuss with the parent how the child handles hygiene
	Manages toileting without help, remains dry at night with an occasional "accident"	Inquire about toileting habits and assess frequency and responses to accidents
	Generally separates easily from parents	Discuss with the parent how the child reacts to separation and how the parent feels about separation; ask the parent to leave the room and observe how the child and parent react to separation
	Verbalizes feelings	Observe how the child handles feelings during the assessment; observe parental responses; ask the child such questions as, "What is the happiest (saddest, scariest) thing you can think of?" and discuss with the parent how the child acts when sad, angry, or frightened
	Fears about body integrity emerge; other fears might remain or diminish	Discuss with the parent any concerns about the child's fears and how the parent responds
	Judges acts according to consequences but does not take intention into account	Present a moral dilemma to child and observe the child's behavior in the assessment setting; note parental limit setting and the child's response
	Defines acceptable and unacceptable behavior but might not always accept limits; controls behavior in assessment setting	Discuss with the parent how the child responds to limits; what happens if the child breaks a limit, what type of discipline the parent uses, and how the child responds; explore the child's perceptions of discipline
	Regularly performs household tasks but might need reminders	Discuss with the parent and child what jobs the child does around the house
	Displays sexual curiosity and interest in bodily differences between girls and boys; might have own private theories to explain sexual differences and reproduction	Ask child such questions as, "How can you tell if someone is a girl or a boy?" "Why are girls and boys different?" "Where do babies come from?" and ask the parent whether the child has engaged in sexual exploration of self or others; discuss parental response
	Shows strong attachment to parent of opposite sex	Discuss the parent-child relationship, including how the child gets along with each parent, whether the child prefers one parent or the other in certain situations, how much time each parent spends with the child, and the types of activities parents and child do together
	Might exhibit jealousy of siblings	Discuss the relationship between the child and siblings, noting how the child gets along with each sibling, the incidence of conflicts, and how conflicts are resolved; might ask the child directly, "What do you like best about your brother (sister)?" "Is there anything you don't like about _____?" "Do you ever fight with _____?" "What happens then?"

(Continues)

TABLE 5-3 Guidelines for Assessment of the 4-Year-Old Child *(Continued)*

Developmental area	Expected characteristics	Assessment techniques
	Engages in cooperative play with peers; shares but frequently reminds others of ownership of objects	Discuss with the parent how the child interacts with other children, what types of play the child engages in, and the child's ability to share; assess opportunities for the child to interact with peers
	Looks for parental support and encouragement	Note parental response to the child's performance, whether the parent allows child to proceed independently or intervenes; note whether the parent makes encouraging or discouraging remarks
	Displays confidence in approaching tasks	Observe how the child approaches tasks during the assessment; note any hesitancy, carelessness, expectation of success or failure, use of parent as a resource, and reaction to successful or unsuccessful performance

quickly if children are tired or hungry. When parental limits are consistent and reasonable, most children will learn to cope with frustrations, and temper tantrums will cease. (Methods of discipline are covered in Chapter 13.)

To achieve the upcoming tasks of the school years, the child begins to learn how to interact appropriately with others in various situations. This necessitates self-control over the undisciplined expression of self-centered feelings.

Self-concept and self-esteem The early childhood period is crucial in the development of a healthy self-concept. In early childhood, self-concept develops as attitudes about the self are formed by social interactions. A child's *self-concept* develops from perceiving others' views of the child during social learning situations. *Self-esteem*, the evaluative component of self-concept, is a measure of how competent, pleased, worthy, and loved the child feels within. Children require support to gain a realistic sense of their abilities and limitations. The healthy development of self-esteem forms the basis for self-confidence in trying out new things and new relationships in early childhood and in later developmental stages. Children with a high degree of self-esteem are more active and demonstrate more leadership than those with low self-esteem.

Children assume that what adults tell them about themselves is true. A child who fears water is not helped to develop a positive self-concept if significant others make comments such as, "See, Amy is your age, and she is not afraid of the water, so why are you?" Or "Last year you went in up to your chin, and now you are afraid to get your feet wet; what is wrong with you?" Thus, parents, siblings, teachers, peers, and community leaders play a role in the way a child organizes temperament, personal attributes, and feelings to achieve positive feedback. If the child is unable to please the significant others or if the effort to do so is judged too costly, a sense of failure and feelings of "bad me" result. Adults who are insensitive to the young child's perspective and who belittle childhood fears might contribute to the development of a negative self-concept. If, on the other hand, the child receives approval, love, and support from significant others, a positive self-concept is engendered.

Gender identification Freud's theory postulates that successful mastery of the tasks of toilet training gradually shifts the child's attention to the genital zone. The ensuing Oedipal phase is the period in which children discover anatomic differences between the sexes. Libidinal investment is then focused on the boy's penis or girl's clitoris, and, according to Freud, this discovery and interest is related to concerns over threats or fears of harm and castration among boys and envy and sadness over the absence of visible male genitalia among girls. Freud's theory of the Oedipus complex further claimed that the healthy outcome of this conflict is that the young boy represses his unacceptable wishes for his mother and identifies with his father. Although Freud failed to develop a completely satisfactory description of this process for the young girl, he theorized that girls follow a similar course. Initially they desire their fathers, thus viewing mother as a rival, but eventually they identify with mother for fear of retaliation (Freud, 1969).

When parents are comfortable with their own sexuality and recognize that behavior associated with the Oedipal period is normal, problems need not result. For example, one 4-year-old boy told his mother that he hoped Daddy would never come home from his business trip and that he would be the "new Daddy." The mother understood the child's message and let him know that she was glad to have him care for her but that it would be wonderful for the entire family to be together again. When the father returned, the mother encouraged the son to tell his father what they had done during his absence so that he would not feel threatened by his father's renewed presence.

The development of the superego, which Freud equated with conscience, coincides with the Oedipal phase. Freud described the superego as the "heir" to the Oedipus complex, meaning that the superego can only emerge after the resolution of the Oedipal complex. As he grows older, the 4-year-old who wanted to replace Daddy will therefore want to identify with his father and take on similar behaviors.

Independence and separation During early childhood, the child begins a gradual shift from complete dependence to the beginning of independence. This initial sense of independence is, however, a fragile thing. Young children experience acute *separation anxiety,* the fear and frustration that come with parental absences. Parents remain central figures in their children's lives, and protection, nurturance, and the provision of basic needs are still parental responsibilities. Experience with separation helps the child cope with parental absences. Two-year-olds act out their frustrations with loud protest and tantrums. The 2-year-old might excitedly examine a new object or corner of the house only to break into tears when suddenly noticing that a parent is no longer nearby. At the same age, the child might have difficulty accepting a babysitter or day care provider.

To help establish feelings of security, young children often carry familiar objects with them. Blankets and stuffed toys are characteristic objects of security at this age. These objects help the child make the transition to independent behavior and tolerate unfamiliar people and situations. From 3 to 4 1/2 years of age, the child is faced with increasing challenges that help develop independence. As more mothers work outside the home, independence may be learned at an even earlier age. During this time, the child's social world begins to expand beyond the family boundaries to the playground, neighborhood, and nursery school. The external environment then requires that the child tolerate separation from parents and learn to play with other children.

Erikson's theory defines the psychosocial issue of this stage of early childhood as "initiative versus guilt." As in the development of autonomy, protective and supportive limits encourage the child to initiate interactions and foster self-esteem. Overly restrictive controls and global prohibitions tend to create a sense of guilt, dampen the child's initiative, and lower self-esteem. A child who has learned appropriate limits is developing a healthy self-concept.

The child's ability to take pride in new accomplishments and to have that pride validated by parental approval provides the basis for a sense of initiative. The mother who praises her daughter's early attempts at selecting her clothes and dressing herself encourages autonomy and supports initiative, whereas the mother who criticizes the daughter's combination of colors or uneven buttoning of her blouse paves the way for a sense of guilt and fear of failure in meeting expectations. "From a sense of self-control without loss of self-esteem comes a lasting sense of good will and pride; from a sense of loss of self-control and of foreign overcontrol comes a lasting propensity for doubt and shame" (Erikson, 1973). The young child's learning to function without the constant support of an adult is crucial in making a successful transition to school and middle childhood.

Related to the child's tolerance of separation is the development of personal boundaries. The young child moves from the normal mother-child symbiosis of infancy to a separate identity. Although emotional connections remain, the child begins to feel like an individual with feelings, reactions, and abilities attributed to no other person. For example, the child no longer bursts into tears when a peer is distressed but can differentiate between personal distress and that of someone else.

The healthy process of separation prepares the young child to enter the world of peer interactions. The child learns that initiative and exploration are rewarding and, at the same time, learns that the secure parent-child relationship need not be sacrificed when the network of relationships is expanded.

Cognitive Development

Reasoning and logic The child's ability to learn about the consequences of actions and to manipulate the environment is fundamental to development. Cognitive development is not an isolated phenomenon. It results from the contributions of the child's genetically inherited characteristics, life experiences, and social interactions. For example, the 3-year-old child who manipulates pebbles is learning by experience. By feeling, dropping, and tossing the pebbles, the child learns about some of their properties. By counting and ordering the pebbles in a row, the child learns about ordering objects and thus develops skills involving logic and mathematics.

During early childhood, a major change in cognition takes place: the child begins to use symbols to represent the outside world, a phase that Piaget labeled the *preoperational stage* of thought (Piaget and Inhelder, 1969) (see Chapter 3). For the first time, the child can learn about the course of an event without actually experiencing it.

Early in this stage, the child experiences severe limitations in internalizing events, and because the child still is unable to form abstractions or generalizations, cognition is restricted to concrete actions. In addition, children learn sequences and routines, so that once the sequence of steps begins, the child's mental review proceeds systematically, step-by-step, with little variation. For example, the child cannot state what number follows eight without counting from one to eight first and then responding with the answer nine.

The child also has a limited ability to classify objects. The tendency at this stage is to focus on the dominant characteristic of an object and to exclude the other characteristics. For example, when 2- or 3-year-olds place all blue blocks in a pile, they are not necessarily demonstrating their ability to categorize. Rather, they are responding to the dominant characteristic—the blue color. This ability to classify objects is limited because the child's inductive reasoning tends to deal with a limited range of available information. Lindsay and Norman (1977) provided an apt description of the preoperational child's system of categorization:

> A child is likely to group a bat with a ball (because you play with them), then a tomato with a ball (because they are round), and then put a rose with the tomato (because they are red). An adult does not do this. The adult will attempt to find a logical connection or one single rule that applies to all objects.

During this stage, children are described as *egocentric,* that is, viewing everything in relation to themselves. They are intolerant when told, "I don't understand you," because they think that everyone else has the same thoughts as they do. The young child cannot imagine how an object would look from another direction nor can the child recognize that other people have experiences or feelings that are different from one's own. For example, when told not to take the truck from his friend, Johnny replied, "But it's mine, and I need it." When told, "But Lee is sad and crying," Johnny replied, "He knows I need it; he should give it to me." At this age, Johnny is unable to be objective. The egocentric behavior of early childhood means that he is unable to consider that Lee also might want the truck.

Another characteristic of preoperational thought is *irreversibility,* that is, the inability to reverse a process and return it to its original state. In the child's thinking, once an action is completed, it cannot be mentally reversed.

Piaget's familiar water glass problem illustrates the concept of irreversibility. Three glasses are set side by side. One glass is tall and narrow, and the other two glasses are low and wide. The two wide glasses are filled with equal amounts of water. Next, the water is poured from one wide glass to the narrow glass; the level of the water rises to a higher point. When the child is asked whether the narrow glass has the same amount of water as the other wide glass the answer is likely to be "no." Most children will explain that the level is higher, meaning that there is more water in the narrow glass. Height is the most obvious, so their reasoning is based solely on that one characteristic. In preoperational thought the concept of conservation of volume does not yet have meaning (Piaget, 1952).

Imagination and fantasy Preoperational thought also is characterized by *symbolic play.* It is during symbolic play that the child pretends and reenacts events. Part of the delight of children at this stage is their ability to pretend and fantasize. A broomstick becomes a motorcycle, a stack of pillows a fort, a doll, a crying baby to comfort. Although thought is symbolic, the symbols are not necessarily organized into a cohesive set of concepts and rules. Organizational ability occurs during the following stage of development, concrete operations. Not until then do children become aware of the difference between pretending and reality and require more realistic props and/or toys for play.

The young child's understanding of dreams also blends the real world and fantasy. In dreams, real events seem to be happening in a real place. After a frightening dream, the child might be reluctant to return to his or her room because "the bad dream is still in there." For example, for weeks after being scared by a birthday party clown and then having a bad dream about it, one 3-year-old girl made her mother chase all of the clowns out of her room every night before turning off the light. A 4-year-old boy had a recurring dream about a vicious dog. He would escape to his parents' room and refuse to return to his own room until both parents joined him in inspecting his room to make certain that the dog was not there.

Imaginary playmates also are created from the young child's active imagination and serve as examples of the child's cognitive processes. Estimates indicate that 20%–50% of children 4 and 5 years of age have imaginary companions (Stone and Church, 1975). The invisible playmates may serve a specific need by expressing feelings, such as resentment or hostility, that the child is unable to verbalize safely. Imaginary playmates often serve as the scapegoat for a child's lapses in behavior, as in "Susie spilled the milk," or paradoxically, as the developing conscience or superego that guides the child's behavior. The playmate embodies the child's conscience by reminding what should or should not be done and by gently scolding when infractions are committed.

Frequently, children who have imaginary playmates are characterized as imaginative and bright, but this phenomenon occurs at all intellectual and socioeconomic levels. One researcher suggested that these playmates are introduced during times of stress or developmental tension and represent a healthy way of coping with this stress (Nagera, 1969). For example, to cope with the realities of learning right from wrong, one boy created an imaginary adult friend. "Mrs. Legger" told his mother when she could go downstairs or outside and where she could walk in his room. He also used her when he wanted something, such as, "Mrs. Legger wants Robert to have a drink of juice and a cracker now."

Imaginary playmates also serve to reduce loneliness and provide the child with an opportunity to try out interactions during play. Many parents tell about having to dress, set the table, or hold the hand of some imaginary friend. The child often becomes very upset if the parent does not cooperate. For example, 3-year-old Sarah would not get in the car because her mother had left Amy (her imaginary friend) in the shopping cart in the store. They had to go back and get Amy, who (according to Sarah) was crying because she had been left and thought no one loved her. Once Amy was retrieved, Sarah was her happy self once again.

Self-awareness During early childhood, children are able to separate their own action from events in the environment. They also sense, and sometimes exaggerate because of their active imaginations, their own vulnerability to danger or harm. Parents of 4- and 5-year-olds frequently report a sudden explosion of fears. A minor illness or medical procedure sometimes leads to the expression of panic and fear of body mutilation or dying. Support by parents, caregivers, and health professionals can assist the young child during times of stress or illness. For example, the child's imagination can be guided through play to master the frightening situation. Using a doll and a syringe, the child can be helped to play out the sequences of receiving an injection. By taking the roles of the giver and receiver of the injection, the child can be helped to work through the fear of receiving an injection (see Chapter 20).

Language

Changes in children's speech One of the most dramatic developments in childhood—the beginning of language—occurs during the second year of life. Names of objects and a few simple verbs are learned first. The average 2-year-old has a vocabulary of about 200–300 words. From this basic language, the young child begins to construct sentences.

A 2-year-old puts two to three words together using primarily nouns and verbs. The 4 1/2-year old already has learned to speak in complicated sentences, using and understanding all structures of grammar. The child's early sentences are telegraphic, shortened versions of adult sentences, composed of nouns and verbs with an occasional adjective. These short sentences can express a range of meanings and have been found in the speech of young children from various cultures speaking different languages.

After the child learns to use sentences, vocabulary appears to increase suddenly. By about 30 months of age, the child no longer uses "baby talk" or babbling, and all verbal output has communicative intent. The young child will show frustration if adult listeners cannot interpret his or her meaning. Sentences become more complicated and are characterized by some prepositions, particularly "in" and "on"; occasional articles, such as "an"; forms of the verb "to be," including "is" and "are"; nouns with plural and possessive endings; and some verb tense inflections, such as the past (ed) and the progressive (ing). These additions are developed gradually over a period of 2–3 years (Mussen, Conger, & Kagan, 1979). A 22-month old asks, "Mommy, change Carolyn?" Ten months later the same question is asked as, "Mommy, did you just change Carolyn?"

By about 3 years of age, the young child has a vocabulary of some 1000 words and approximately 80% of communication is understandable, even to strangers. Although grammatical mistakes occur, the child's speech takes on the quality of colloquial adult speech. Nurses assessing children's language development therefore need to know that young children will learn basic grammar from the colloquial language they hear and not according to textbook guidelines. Thus, their language competence should be assessed in light of the language forms and communication styles to which they have been exposed.

Although many formal grammatical rules are not learned until the school-age years, the child's language is well established by about 4 1/2 years of age. Deviations from the spoken adult language appear more in word selection and variety than in grammar. Some errors still occur in questions that involve inserting the question word (why, who, what, where) and inverting the subject and part of the verb, but the child has nearly mastered the proper use of negation, so that these errors do not interfere with the child's meaning.

Adults may be able to assist children in learning language by simplifying their own speech when engaging young children in conversation. It is important for the nurse to talk with the child at the child's level of comprehension and to use terms with which the child is familiar, rather than more formal or medically correct terms. The young boy who knows the meaning of the term "throw-up" but has never heard the word "vomit" cannot answer the nurse's question correctly when asked if he feels he has to vomit.

In general, adults can help the child's conversation to

progress by using both informal and formal words and, as the child gets older, by using only the more complex word. Active encouragement and placing value on verbal communication are additional parental factors that can enhance the child's language development.

Moral thinking During early childhood, children begin to learn rudimentary standards of behavior and a sense of right and wrong. Freud and his followers explain moral development as the emergence of the conscience or superego. Kohlberg (1969) and his followers offer another explanation of moral development (see Chapter 3).

According to Kohlberg, the premoral 2-year-old is just starting to learn that some actions are forbidden and others rewarded. This is the time when the child gains a simple understanding that actions have consequences and that some limits must be learned. Three- and 4-year-olds are also in Kohlberg's premoral, or pre-conventional, stage of moral development, but they have developed a larger repertoire of moral judgments. They can judge behavior as good or bad according to the rewarding or punitive response it will elicit. They learn not to repeat a behavior, such as throwing sand in the sandbox, because it causes parental disapproval, which is expressed in punishments, such as having to spend time in the house or losing a privilege.

At 4 1/2 years of age, children are just starting to evaluate actions according to inherent labels of good and bad, and they are beginning to understand moral concepts beyond reward and punishment. Transition to Kohlberg's conventional moral stage is gradual, and the consistent conformity to rules that characterizes this stage does not appear until middle childhood.

Simple religious beliefs often are taught to children during the early childhood years. These in turn foster the development of faith. Part of moral development in many families also includes learning about the moral teachings of a religion. For some children, moral development is fostered by the parents' faith and by participating in major religious practices or holidays.

Social Development

Social development involves learning the customs of society and adopting culturally defined behaviors. The tasks of social development are interwoven with those of biophysical, affective, and cognitive development. The following tasks need to be accomplished during early childhood: (1) to form simple concepts of social and physical reality; (2) to learn to relate oneself emotionally to parents, siblings, and other people; (3) to learn to distinguish right and wrong; and (4) to develop a conscience (Havighurst, 1972).

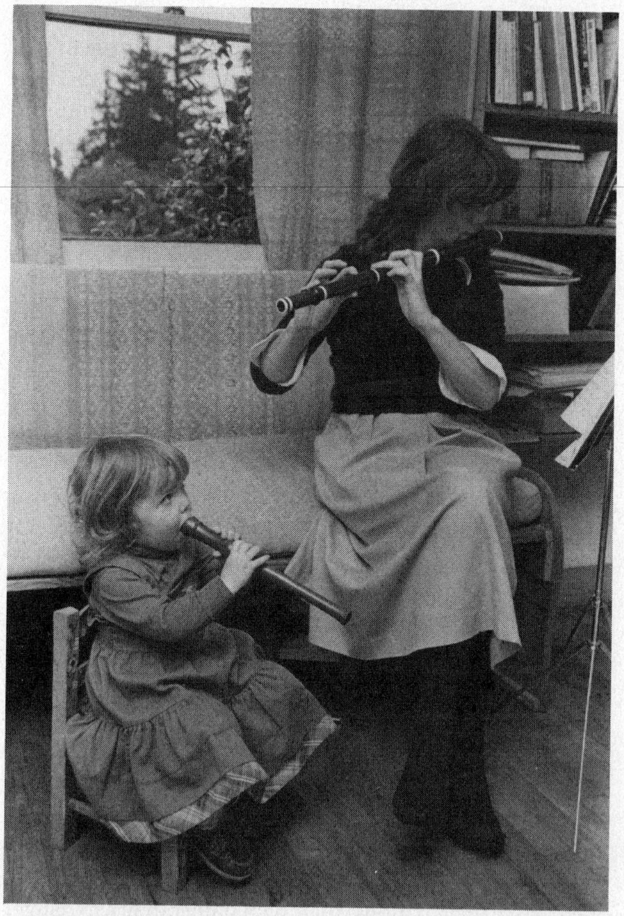

Imitation is an essential part of social development in early childhood.

By this stage, the child's interactions with other children, both siblings and friends, are important. The nurse therefore explores with the parent the child's opportunities to interact with other children and ability to get along with them. In addition the nurse discusses how siblings interact and how conflicts between siblings are managed.

Imitation Imitating others, whether peers or adults, is a major component of social development in early childhood. Gewirtz and Stingle (1972) suggested that the first imitative behaviors occur by chance, through assistance, or through direct training. When the child reproduces these responses, they are strengthened by positive reinforcement from socializing agents, particularly the parents. Gradually, the child adopts a set of varied but "functionally equivalent" behaviors that are maintained by intermittent reinforcement. Over time, the behaviors take on intrinsic value and need only occasional reinforcement from the social environment to be continued.

The child first learns to say "thank you" by responding to parental direction to do so. After being rewarded verbally or with a show of affection for saying "thank you," the behavior is extended to a variety of situations. Soon the child is heard to say "thank you" whenever given something.

One outcome of identification during the early childhood years is the child's adoption of gender-related traits, attitudes, and behavior. Young children imitate behaviors of both sexes, although behaviors of their own sex usually predominate. Sometime after 2 years of age, the young child gains a sense of gender identity; that is, "I am a girl" or "I am a boy." From 3- to 4 1/2 years of age, the child learns to adopt characteristics, views, and behaviors that are consistent with culturally prescribed roles of males and females. Through identification with the parent of the same sex and reinforcement by parents and others, children gradually develop male or female identities.

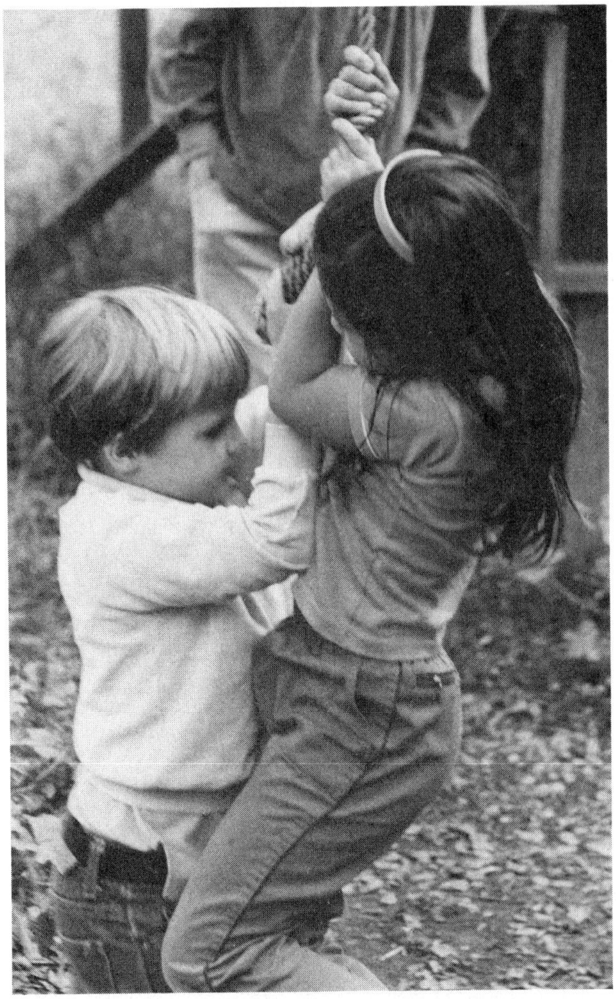

Sibling rivalry occurs in most families. First-born siblings appear more dominant in all situations, especially when they are female.

Sibling rivalry Competition among siblings and an intense need to receive equal and fair treatment from the parent are the most pervasive characteristics of sibling relationships. Sibling rivalry occurs in almost every family with more than one child. It is most common in families where the age range between children is small, with brothers close in age having the least harmonious relationship of sibling pairs (Yussen and Santrock, 1982). Firstborn siblings appear more dominant in all situations, especially when the firstborn is also female.

For most families, sibling rivalry is typified by behavior problems among children who are close in age. Parents who want to count on their older children to stop or limit inappropriate behavior are then faced with a dilemma. Should they expect the same standards of behavior in both the older and the younger child? In most situations the solution is to reinforce age-appropriate behavior in both children without blaming either child for the behavior problem.

Younger children are more likely to fight with each other over toys than to challenge differences in parental standards. In minimizing the unacceptable behavior, parents need first to define what is acceptable and age appropriate. If, for instance, the older of two young children has been taught to share, this behavior might be rewarded when the child is observed sharing a toy. At times when willingness to share does not exist, it might be necessary to modify the environment by separating the children and removing the toy.

Dawdling Dawdling is a common behavior in young children and seems to be related to children's ambivalence about complying with parental wishes. The nurse needs to note whether a child uses dawdling as a strategy for dealing with parental pressure and how the parents manage this behavior. Some children simply become so involved in whatever activity they are doing that they find it very difficult to heed their parents' requests to stop and do something else.

Temper tantrums Temper tantrums often cause extreme parental responses. Tantrums are characterized by earsplitting noise, flailing of arms, and kicking. These performances seem to occur spontaneously whenever the parent denies the child's request. Parents feel embarrassed when tantrums occur in such public places as supermarkets or stores. Tantrums are most common in children 18 months to 3 years of age and signal the child's negativism and struggle for autonomy. Regardless of the motives, this behavior is socially unacceptable and intolerable to the nerves of most parents.

Temper tantrums in early childhood are most common when the child must cope with frustration (see Chapter 16). The frequency, intensity, and duration of tantrums are influenced by events, temperamental characteristics, and parental response.

Most parents with a shouting child feel the urge to punish the child physically. A light tap on the bottom might relieve the parents' frustration but might also be ineffective in preventing recurrent outbursts. The parents might need reassurance that the child's behavior is attention seeking and evidence of immature and inadequate coping strategies.

Many children calm down if taken to their rooms until they have settled down. A more difficult technique for parents is ignoring the behavior when the tantrum is being performed as an attention-seeking mechanism. The nurse can also advise the parents that children who are tired or hungry are more likely to have a tantrum because their ability to cope with fatigue or hunger is limited. In these situations, it is best to modify plans and provide for the child's basic needs and thereby avoid the unpleasant experience of dealing with a temper tantrum.

Integrating Development Through Play

The various components of a child's development—biophysical, affective, cognitive, and social—all interact to produce a unique child. Growth in one sphere influences growth in another.

Play is an important mechanism through which such integration occurs, although play was not always considered the meaningful part of childhood that it is now. In the past, play was considered devilish, frivolous, or worthless. Today, however, play is understood to be a valuable tool that enhances growth and aids in the development of fine motor skills, as well as sensory and perceptual capabilities. Play enhances coping strategies and releases tension. Play allows the child to reenact and reconstruct events and interactions that occur in daily life. Through play the child practices physical and perceptive skills and also develops the social skills of cooperation, sharing, and assertiveness. The child learns and assimilates cultural norms and adult occupational, family, and sex roles. The child safely experiments with and evaluates moral and ethical questions of right and wrong through play.

Types of Play

Ideas for play vary. Samples include "Let's play house. I'll be the mommy, you be the big sister," "Let's pretend our mother is dead, and we're lost in the woods," "Let's play school and do homework" (this after a day at nursery school or kindergarten), "Let's play war," "Let's pretend we're turkeys," "Let's be birds or airplanes" (this when jumping off the living room couch), and "I'm making presents for Holly and Andrea." From this potpourri of play ideas, work and family roles are assumed, separation and aggression issues are played out, and fine and gross motor skills are practiced. Fun, high spirits, and silliness are a part of some, but not all, play scenes.

A traditionally accepted categorization of play is the one developed by Parten and Newhall (1943), who described play according to the relationship between the players. *Unoccupied behavior* is at one end of a continuum. Here, the child is not involved in any activity that teaches or promotes development, and the child's attention drifts. Two-year-olds normally spend 10%–12% of their time this way, and normally developing 3-year-olds spend 7%–8% of their time doing this.

In *onlooker play,* the child observes others' activities. Included in this category is time spent watching television as well as watching other children play. Television watching often increases during early childhood, and its effect on children is of interest to researchers and parents. Although the findings are inconclusive, some of the evidence certainly points to an alarming proportion of time spent in this form of play, which diminishes the time spent in more active types of play.

Solitary play, in which children are engrossed in their own independent play with toys or projects, is apparent at all levels of development. The younger child, who is limited in the social, affective, and cognitive skills necessary for more advanced and prolonged interaction, spends a greater proportion of time in this type of play. Nevertheless, it is equally important for the 4 1/2-year-old to spend some time in this form of play because having privacy and personal space has been linked to creativity in children (White, 1975).

Parallel play is characteristic of the 2-year-old, who plays alongside others without interaction or cooperation. Although 2-year-olds frequently engage in this type of play, they are not limited to it. Similarly, 4-year-olds, who are better able to engage in cooperative play, also enjoy activities like coloring, which is a form of parallel play.

Associative play involves interaction and a common activity within a loosely structured environment. Several 2- and 3-year-olds might enjoy a simple ball game or play

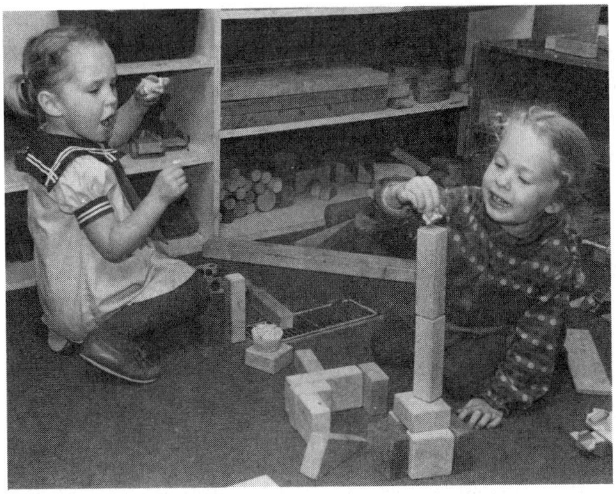

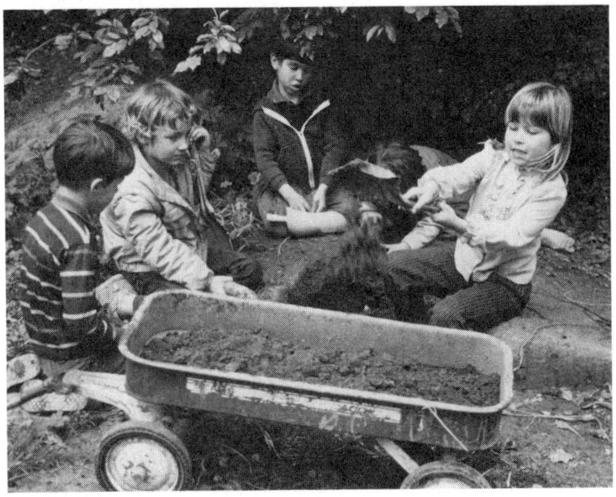

Play in early childhood takes various forms. Parallel play does not involve cooperation between children, whereas cooperative play involves more interaction, with clearly defined roles.

together with a truck. The time and tolerance for this kind of play increases with age.

Cooperative play, often considered the most complex form of play because it involves a common interactive activity, is characterized by a variety of roles assigned through interaction among children. In cooperative play, tasks are all allocated, and the plot is delineated; children clearly belong or do not belong to the play. The 4-year-old will begin to get involved in the casting and directing of this type of play and the 5-year-old will start to add new ideas and drama to the plot. Parts usually are assigned according to age, ability, or popularity within the group.

Play also might be described according to the type of activity (Piers, 1972). *Functional play,* or physical play, is action play and may be social, boisterous, and competitive or it may be manipulative and include doing jigsaw puzzles. *Symbolic play*—pretending, make-believe, or fantasy—is a type of play in which reality is transformed through language, action, or physical objects. Symbolic play can occur as early as 18 months of age but certainly is evident by 3 years of age and increases steadily thereafter.

Games that mutually involve the participants and include taking turns and repeating behaviors are a final way of characterizing play. Although recent evidence and opinion suggest that gamelike interaction occurs during infancy, actual game-playing is certainly evident in the 3- to 4-year-old. Hide-and-seek, tag, and some simple board games (such as Candyland® and Winnie the Pooh®) exemplify this kind of play. Play for children can be characterized further as fun and as an end in itself. Play is a safe medium for learning and practicing; it should therefore provide a reasonable challenge for the child and take place in a relaxed setting.

Parental Actions to Facilitate Play

How can parents facilitate or enhance their children's play? Experts agree that the freedom allowed in a child's environment is a chief ingredient in successful play. This freedom implies reasonable physical freedom (that is, some reasonable space without excessive rules regarding the use of the space). The child also should have the freedom to make mistakes, to be imperfect, to be silly, and to regress—in short, to be socially and emotionally free of parental evaluation.

How adults play with children is also important. Both increased imagination and complexity of play result from parents who play with their children.

Parents can also enhance play by providing toys appropriate for children during early childhood. Toys or household articles that accomplish more than one kind of play can serve the child well. Building blocks can enhance fine motor skills and creativity while the child engages in solitary or associative play. Swings, slides, or balls encourage gross motor activity and associative kinds of play. Crayons, scissors, and paper encourage fine motor skills and creative activities. Props that allow for creative and dramatic play include dress-up clothes, toy stoves, dishes, refrigerators, stores, puppets, and doctor and nurse kits. To facilitate all aspects of development, play should involve large muscle groups, fine motor skills, imagination, and creativity, and it

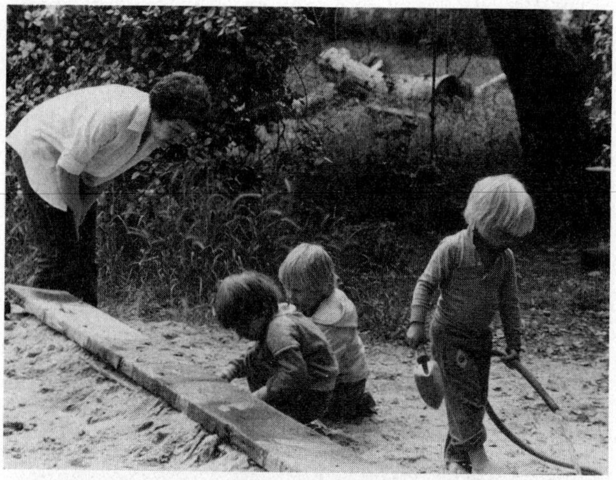

In early childhood, children learn from adults facilitating play.

should be at different times active, quiet, associative, and solitary.

Imaginary companions are also certainly a normal part of early childhood. Although a parent should not rearrange the family for this new member, parents can certainly play along and accommodate these temporary visitors.

Health Care Needs of Early Childhood

The change from dependence to independence occurs dramatically in a relatively short time. The 18-month-old who can pull off socks and diapers learns in the next few years to dress, button, zip, select clothes, and even tie shoelaces. The young child who splashes instead of washes hands in the sink (with some supervision) becomes one who can brush teeth, take care of toileting, practice basic hygiene, and even help wash hair. The spoon- and finger-feeder is replaced by a knife and fork user and even part-time assistant kitchen helper in setting the table, buttering bread, or baking. The 2-year-old who absolutely refuses to go to bed or take a nap is replaced by a fairly logical, reasonable participant in limit-setting decisions, although this child is still occasionally illogical and unreasonable.

Hygiene

One of the important and stressful milestones of self-care in early childhood is control of the bowel and bladder. Readiness for toilet training is a composite of neurophysiologic, personal-social, adaptive, and cultural characteristics of the child. Because of the enormous amount of folk wisdom passed down from generation to generation about when and how to toilet train, nurses need to anticipate this milestone much earlier than readiness criteria might indicate.

Readiness for toilet training Brazelton (1962) reported in his survey of toilet training among 672 boys and 491 girls that the average age of completion of both bladder and bowel training was 33.3 months. Daytime training was achieved somewhat earlier, at 28.5 months. Girls were trained on an average of 2.46 months earlier than boys. Most 4- and 5-year-olds remain dry both day and night. About 10%–15% of them experience nocturnal enuresis (bedwetting) of varying frequency. Although most children with nocturnal enuresis do not have underlying problems, further assessment is recommended.

Some parents begin toilet training at a much earlier date than these figures would indicate. The nurse can introduce the concept of readiness and encourage the parent to look for the following adaptive and psychomotor readiness signs: the ability to walk well, the balance and ability to climb and sit on a potty chair, and the ability to undress oneself. Standing and walking indicate myelination of the spinal tract to the level needed for bowel and bladder sphincter control. Behavioral readiness is reflected in the child's awareness of the need to urinate or defecate. These signs include a word, increased fussiness, clinginess, silence, or actual movement toward the bathroom. The child's ability to imitate people and maintain an attention span of at least 5 minutes as well as letting go of a toy when requested are also readiness signs.

Parents must be "ready" too. Toilet training requires time, consistency, patience, and understanding. Optimally, there is congruence between the child's readiness and that of the parents. Before discussing methods for toilet training, the nurse assesses the readiness of the entire family. Overly high expectations about toilet training from family members might result in overly rigid or harsh toilet-training methods. A new sibling in the family might significantly alter a child's readiness. A family with two working parents might have to involve the child's other caregiver(s) in toilet-training methods.

Methods of toilet training Although frequently a source of great parental anxiety, toilet training may be viewed as an educational process. As children learn increased control over bodily function, they can progress toward becoming socially acceptable members of society.

The first premise of toilet training is that the process occurs according to the child's own speed and level of readiness. Once readiness is determined, the parent can begin toilet training in a manner that the family finds comfortable.

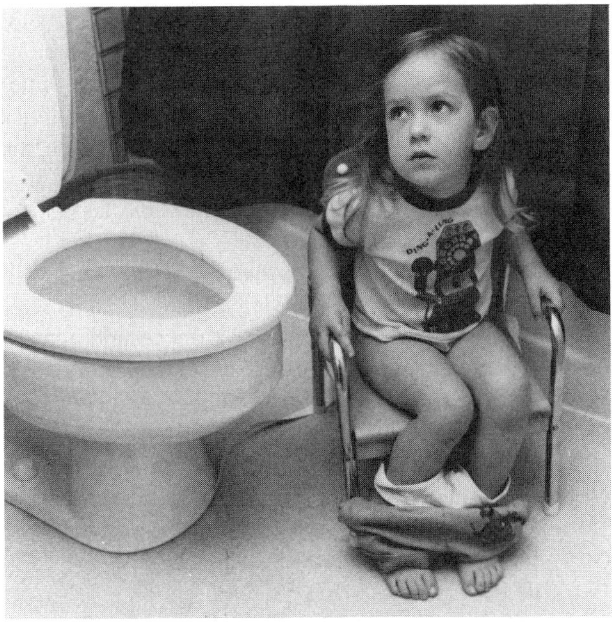

Emphasis on the child's independence and self-care, together with attentiveness to the child's physiologic and psychologic readiness, can make toilet training a nonstressful experience.

One method uses the following steps. First, a potty chair is placed in the bathroom, and the child is informed that this chair is the child's. The deflector provided for male potty chairs should be removed because it can hurt the child getting up and down. Once daily, with all clothes on, the child is taken to sit on the chair for a few minutes and allowed to get up whenever desired. The parent tells the child what is supposed to happen in the chair (for example, "This is where you go dudu").

Second, once accustomed to the chair, the child can be taken to sit on it without clothes or diapers. This should be done at a time when a bowel movement might be expected. When the child does have a bowel movement in the diaper, the parent undoes the diaper and places it in the chair, saying something like, "One day you will be able to dudu in the chair."

Third, if the child begins to become interested, the parent takes the child to the chair several times a day to see whether the child can urinate or have a bowel movement. The parent can praise the child for positive results. Fourth, once the child seems ready to monitor his or her own actions, the parent can allow the child to remain undressed from the waist down as much as possible with the potty chair handy in the room. The child is reminded that this is the child's business but that the parent will help remind the child to go. Eventually, training pants, which are easy for the child to pull up and down, can be worn.

This method is only one of many options available to families. An important concept in evaluating methods of toilet training is its appropriateness for the individual child and family. Regardless of the particular method chosen, parents need to remember that children should be rewarded for successful efforts but not punished for unsuccessful attempts.

Sleep and Rest

Normal needs Sleep needs during the early childhood period slowly decrease. The 2-year-old needs 12–14 hours of sleep per day (including naps), but unlike the infant, most of this sleep is at night, although one afternoon nap of 1–2 hours is still common. The percentage of rapid-eye-movement, or REM, sleep has decreased to 25% (Powell, 1981). The sleep needs of the 3- to 4-year-old decrease to 10–12 hours per day. This is a time when a nap frequently is eliminated and all sleep takes place at night.

Bedtime difficulties Behavioral problems related to rest and sleep needs frequently occur, and resistance to going to bed might reach an all-time high. Equilibrium is assisted by adhering to repetitive or patterned behavior in the form of rituals. Consistent rituals around bedtime help make the transition from awake to asleep easier, although attempts to prolong these indefinitely warrant parental limit-setting.

In contrast to the infant's normal awakening during the night and parents' social and cultural willingness to tend to infants at night, the young child who awakens at night is considered a problem. Developmentally, sleep is a form of separation from parents, and separation at this stage is sanctioned culturally by most families in the United States. Because one of the developmental themes of this stage is separation, nurses can assist parents in looking at their child's sleep habits from this perspective.

Although REM sleep decreases to 20%, vivid dreams and nightmares may result in night terrors or awakening during this period (Powell, 1981). Many young children also are afraid of the dark. Parents should respect these fears and attempt to assist the child by providing a nightlight or flashlight for the child to hold. When awakened by a nightmare, the child should calmly be told by a parent that it was only a dream and that everything is fine. The parent may remind the child that a parent is always nearby.

Children generally love to sleep with their parents if they are allowed to do so, and such habits as having a parent present while falling asleep frequently become problematic for this age group. The young child who is acquiring a more sophisticated repertoire of coping and cognitive abilities can participate in a routine nighttime plan. Generally, parents can plan and explain a bedtime ritual with the children (for example, brush teeth, hear a story, hug goodnight, then lights out). The parent also can reassure the child that someone will comfort him or her if need be in the middle of the night. "Daddy will come to pat you on the back and see if you're ok, but you must stay in your bed and sleep in your own bed all night, then Daddy will go back to bed." Crucial to any communication with the child are consistent and appropriate behaviors that reinforce the spoken message. Parents can promote good sleep habits by creating a consistent and nurturing environment in which firm expectations about good sleep habits for the whole family are upheld.

Nutrition

During early childhood, there are few nutritional problems. In general, the child's diet resembles that of the parents, except that the quantity is less. Early childhood appetites are erratic, and a parent might worry that the child is not eating enough food. The child's metabolic needs, however, have decreased, and growth has slowed so the child's bodily needs are not as great. Calorie requirements decrease to an average of about 100 kcal/kg (45 kcal/lb). Because caloric needs are reduced, these must be quality calories. The recommended intake of protein is 1.5–1.8 g/kg of bodily mass, which can be obtained by two 8-oz glasses of milk and 2 oz of meat (Enders and Rockwell, 1980). The most common dietary insufficiency in this age group is iron, followed by ascorbic acid, calcium, and vitamin A (Hussey and Kanoff, 1979).

With the development of bones and teeth, calcium intake becomes important. Two to three glasses of milk per day will meet the daily requirement of 800 mg of calcium. Other sources of calcium, such as cheese, yogurt, and ice cream, can be used as substitutes for milk. To maintain 15 mg of iron per day during this frequently iron-deficient period, children should be encouraged to eat foods high in iron. Such food sources include meats (especially liver), legumes, green vegetables, and enriched whole-grain products. In addition, a daily source of vitamin C is important because it facilitates iron absorption and might be helpful in preventing infections. (Table 5-4 translates the recommended daily nutrient requirements into the number of required servings in the basic four food groups for this age.)

During early childhood, children are more selective about their food and the way it is served, and some of the tensions of this developmental era are manifested during meals. Children tend to have definite food preferences. *Food jags,* as they are commonly called, might result in the child's requesting some chosen food three times a day. The child's need for rituals also can be a cause of food jags. The child's ability to say "no" is frequently practiced at mealtime by refusing food. One child had a peanut butter and jelly sandwich and a glass of milk or juice three times a day for 6 months. Whenever any other food was offered, the answer usually was "no," but the sandwich was always happily eaten. Usually, these strong food likes or dislikes will disappear if they are ignored.

The intrusiveness and talkativeness of the 3-year-old may manifest itself by not allowing anyone else to control dinner conversation. The physically active and intense 4-year-old might have to leave the table for bathroom expeditions and might fidget frequently. Table manners at this age are only minimally acceptable.

Despite these immaturities, the nutritional habits of the young child reflect the independence and skill observed in other areas. Hussey and Kanoff (1979) summarized the developmental skills of feeding as follows:

Fifteen to eighteen months—child holds own spoon, although spilling occurs because of lack of wrist and hand coordination; child holds a cup and drinks well from it

Twenty-four months—wrist-hand coordination is established; child eats well with spoon and drinks from glass

Two and one-half years—rotary chewing skills are established; corn and meats are therefore acceptable

Three to four years—child can begin to use a fork

Four years—child uses a fork well; can begin to cut soft foods

Five to six years—child uses a knife to cut soft foods

Because of the often-dramatic change in quantity and variety of food eaten during early childhood, parents frequently worry about their children's nutritional intake. Some health professionals recommend assessing the child's diet for a week to determine the number of servings eaten in the basic four food groups. This can reassure parents and encourage them not to focus unduly on individual mealtimes. Parents can be reassured that the refusal to eat all food at all meals is normal. As long as frequent high-carbohydrate snacks are not responsible for a diminished appetite parents can avoid power struggles by not insisting that the child eat everything.

Pipes (1981) suggested that most well-developing children seem to get all their required nutrients at mealtimes and do not need many snacks. Others recommend smaller, more frequent feedings for young children, emphasizing that meals and snacks should contain high-quality protein, fiber, and vitamin-rich foods. For snacks, protein and fiber

TABLE 5-4 Recommended Daily Food Groups

Food group	Daily servings: 1 to 3 years	Daily servings: 4 to 6 years	Portion size
I. Milk and cheese group (1.5 oz cheese = 1 cup of milk)	3 to 6	4	4 oz of milk or milk substitute; 1 oz hard cheese
II. Meat, eggs, poultry, fish, peanut-butter group (protein high here)	2 or more	2 or more	Meat, fish, and poultry = 2 to 3 tbsp baby meat; 2 to 3 oz Eggs = 1 Peanut butter = 1 to 2 tbsp; 2 to 3 for older child Legumes = ¼ to ½ cup cooked
III. Fruit and vegetable group	4 to 5 Include one green leafy vegetable or yellow vegetable; one citrus fruit or other vegetable or fruit rich in ascorbic acid	4 to 5	Cooked vegetables = 2 to 4 tbsp; ¼ cup for older child Raw vegetables = few pieces Canned fruit = 4 to 8 tbsp; ½ cup for older child Fruit juice = 3 to 4 oz Raw fruit = ½ to 1 small
IV. Cereal and bread group	4 or more	4 or more	Bread = ½ to 1 slice Cooked cereal = ¼ to ½ cup Dry cereal = ½ to 1 cup Pasta = ¼ to ½ cup Crackers = 2 to 3
Fats—bacon, butter, or vitamin A fortified margarine	3	3 to 4	Bacon = 1 slice (not to be substituted for meat) Butter or margarine = 1 tsp
Desserts	As needed to meet calorie demands		¼ to ½ cup

SOURCE: Adapted from Baker S and Henry R: *Parent's Guide to Nutrition*. Addison-Wesley, 1986.

might be provided by cheese squares, peanut butter on celery, apples, or milk; vitamins might be obtained from fresh fruits, fruit juices, or raw vegetables, such as carrot, celery, or green pepper sticks.

Children in early childhood enjoy simple foods that are colorful and attractively served. Giving the child small portions sets reasonable expectations that the child will be able to finish the meal. Children often refuse casseroles and mixed foods but enjoy raw vegetables and finger foods. Meats are often not a favorite food, and parents must substitute other high-protein foods.

Attitudes toward food and mealtime are formed in these early years. Food can easily take on secondary meanings that do not foster healthy nutrition. Food can become a bribe or a pacifier for tired, irritable, or bored children. Parents are heard to coax compliance by saying, "If you are good, I will buy you an ice cream cone" or "Finish your vegetables and you can have an extra cookie." Treats come to be expected and used as a weapon against well-meaning parents. Food given for love can lead to obesity and overall poor nutrition because of the over-representation of certain food groups.

Parents can achieve sound nutritional habits by following some simple rules (Hussey and Kanoff, 1979):

1. Avoid confrontations over disliked foods and table manners.
2. Give nutritious, appropriate-sized, well-timed, between-meal snacks.

3. Avoid tensions at the table.
4. Avoid the inappropriate use of food.
5. Include the child in dinnertime conversations.
6. Offer a well-balanced variety of nutritious food types that are colorful and attractively served.
7. Avoid introducing sugared desserts as a necessary part of the meal.
8. Develop reasonable expectations about eating (for example, the child cannot have a dessert if other foods are not touched).

Dentition

All 20 deciduous, or primary teeth, normally have erupted by 30 months of age. The cuspids and the bicuspids (first and second molars) are usually the teeth erupting during the second year. The care of primary teeth is important because of their role in the development of good speech habits, their need for proper eating habits, their importance for cosmetic purposes related to body image, and their relation to the health of the permanent teeth. Diseased primary teeth can seriously affect the structure of permanent teeth. Brushing of teeth should begin in infancy, and children should increasingly assume partial responsibility for brushing their teeth. Children need supervision by parents because they lack the fine motor skills and persistence to brush their teeth well. Nevertheless, young children should be allowed to initiate and participate in toothbrushing.

One of the crucial variables contributing to dental health is the child's diet. Poor nutritional habits have been linked to dental diseases. Some studies have shown that (1) carbohydrate consumption (mostly sugar) increases tooth decay, (2) the risk of caries is greater if the sugar is in a form that will be retained (for example, caramel or candy), and (3) the risk of caries is related to the frequency of between-meal snacks containing sugar (Wei, 1981).

Optimal fluoride intake improves dental health. The consumption of fluoridated water is a preventive dentistry regimen; a fluoridated dentifrice is another source of fluoride in the growing child (Wei, 1981). If the water in a community does not meet the minimum standards for fluoridation, a system of fluoride supplementation might be needed.

Suggestions to parents vary about the optimal age for a routine check-up by the dentist. Three-year-olds or certainly 4-year-olds should have the maturity to cooperate with the dental examination and teeth cleaning. Good preparation for the visit can come from role-playing, doll-playing, stories, or a visit to the dentist with an older sibling.

Exercise

Physical activity is important for muscular development, gross motor skills, and social skills and is an outlet for tension. Exercise also benefits the circulatory system.

During early childhood, there is no difference in muscle size between the sexes. Children of both sexes show wide differences in muscle tone and the amount of adipose tissue, which is directly related to exercise. Obesity might begin to develop in these early years, as lifelong patterns and attitudes toward exercise are being formed.

Children of this age enjoy the vigorous exercises of running, jumping, going down slides, or swinging. Older children refine their exercise skills by adding skipping, hopping, tumbling, bicycling, and swimming. Engaging in these exercises helps develop muscle strength, balance, coordination, and social skills.

Exercise helps consume the child's seemingly endless energy and is particularly important for very active children. After vigorous exercise, children are emotionally and mentally better able to deal with challenging cognitive tasks, to practice fine motor skills, or to engage in solitary play.

Wise parents also alternate vigorous exercise periods with quiet periods. For the 2-year-old, this quiet time might be a nap or solitary play; for the 4-year-old, quiet time might be spent coloring or looking at a book. Parents need to be alert to the clues in their children's behavior that signal overfatigue. Children of this age frequently have difficulty making transitions from one type of activity to the next, from active, boisterous play to quiet play. Parents play an important role in helping their children to make this transition.

Transition to Middle Childhood

The theme of early childhood is the child's progress toward independence, self-care, responsibility, and accountability. Although the 4 1/2-year-old emerging from this stage is by no means an adult, important social, cognitive, cultural, and psychomotor skills have been acquired. At the end of the early childhood period, a distinct personality has been formed, and the 4 1/2-year-old is ready to venture out into the world of school.

Essential Concepts

- Early childhood encompasses the developmental phase from about 18 months to 4 1/2 years of age. This phase is characterized by increased independence as the child develops communication, locomotion, and self-care skills.
- The process of maturation and experiences with objects and obstacles in the environment result in the learning and mastery of many gross motor skills and fine motor skills.
- Parents can minimize common behavior problems in early childhood—such as temper tantrums, sibling rivalry, and dawdling—by enforcing consistent, clearly defined limits.
- Developmental issues of early childhood include toilet training, learning to share, and learning to control impulses.
- Gender identity is related to cultural definitions and the imitations of significant role models.
- The ability to tolerate separation from parents and other familiar caregivers is an essential part of affective development in early childhood.
- The acquisition of self-concept and self-esteem is an important aspect of development; adults who are supportive of children's questions, needs for increased reassurance, and expression of initiative communicate to the child a positive self-concept.
- Early childhood is characterized by incessant questioning as the child learns about the organization and functioning of the environment.
- The ability to use information is limited by the lack of concrete experiences, and the child accepts any answer, whether it is logical or not.
- The child fuses fantasy and reality in searching to understand the world but increasingly learns to distinguish between them.
- The learning of language and its use to express needs, requests, ideas, or plans develops rapidly and includes all speech parts and the ability to construct complicated sentences by the end of early childhood.
- Moral development begins as children learn right from wrong in response to punishment and reward.
- Rituals help children gain some control over events and put their lives in order.
- Developmental theorists have characterized early childhood. Piaget defines this stage as a time of egocentricity, limited logical thinking, and active and creative imagination. Erikson describes it as a time of developing autonomy and initiative leading to either a positive sense of self or a negative sense of self. Freud emphasized gender and role identification with the parent of the same sex, following resolution of love for the parent of the opposite sex.
- Play enhances all types of learning and enhances all aspects of development through the use and practice of motor, mental, and social skills.
- The child engages in various types of play—solitary, onlooker, parallel—and, by the end of early childhood, engages in associative and cooperative play.
- These are important years for learning about basic self-care activities and participating in screening programs to detect any potential problems, especially those that are correctable with early intervention.
- The parent's role in protecting and educating the child changes as the child gains independence and spends time away from home.

References

Bigner JJ: *Parent-Child Relations*. Macmillan, 1979.

Brazelton TB: A child-oriented approach to toilet training. *Pediatrics* 1962; 29:121–128.

Coles R: *The Privileged Ones*. Little, Brown, 1977.

Enders JB, Rockwell RE: *Food, Nutrition and the Young*. Mosby, 1980.

Erikson EH: *Childhood and Society*. Norton, 1973.

Freud S: An outline of psychoanalysis. In: *The Complete Psychoanalytic Works of Sigmund Freud*. Norton, 1969.

Gewirtz JL, Stingle KG: Learning of generalized imitation as the basis for identification. In: *Readings in Child Behavior and Development*. Lavatelli CS, Stendler F (editors). Harcourt Brace Jovanovich, 1972.

Havighurst RJ: *Developmental Tasks and Education*. McKay, 1972.

Hussey C, Kanoff N: Toddler and preschool nutrition. In: *Maternal and Child Nutrition Assessment and Counseling*. Slatterly J, Pearson G, Torre C (editors). Appleton-Century-Crofts, 1979.

Kagan J, Greenspan SI: Milestones of development: A dialogue. *Zero to Three* 1986; 6(5):1–9.

Kohlberg L: Stage and sequence: The cognitive-development approach to socialization. In: *Handbook of Socialization: Theory and Research*. Goslin D (editor). Rand McNally, 1969.

Lindsay PH, Norman DA: *Human Information Processing: An Introduction to Psychology*. Academic Press, 1977.

Mussen PH, Conger JJ, Kagan J: *Child Development and Personality*. Harper & Row, 1979.

Nagera H: The imaginary companion. *Psychoanal Study Child* 1969; 24:165–196.

Parten MB, Newhall S: Social behavior of preschool children. In: *Child Behavior and Development*. Baker BG (editor). McGraw-Hill, 1943.

Piaget J: *The Origins of Intelligence*. International Universities Press, 1952.

Piaget J, Inhelder B: *The Psychology of the Child*. Basic Books, 1969.

Piers MW (editor): *Play and Development*. Norton, 1972.

Pipes PL: *Nutrition in Infancy and Childhood*. Mosby, 1981.

Powell ML: *Assessment and Management of Developmental Changes in Children*. Mosby, 1981.

Stone LJ, Church J: *Childhood and Adolescence*. Random House, 1975.

Wei S: Nutrition, diet, flouride and dental health. *Pediatr Basics* 1981; 30:5.

White B: *The First Three Years of Life*. Prentice-Hall, 1975.

Yussen SR, Santrock JW. *Child Development: An Introduction*. William C. Brown, 1982.

Additional Readings

Brill E, Kilts D: *Foundations for Nursing*. Appleton-Century-Crofts, 1980.

Brink P: An anthropological perspective on parenting. In: *Parenting Reassessed: A Nursing Perspective*. Horowitz J, Hughes C, Perdue B (editors). Prentice-Hall, 1982.

Chance P: *Learning Through Play*. Gardner Press, 1979.

Chess S, Hassibi M: *Principles and Practice of Child Psychiatry*. Plenum, 1978.

Chomsky C: Language development before age six. In: *Readings in Child Behavior and Development*. Lavatelli CS, Stendler F (editors). Harcourt Brace Jovanovich, 1972.

Chow M et al: *Handbook of Pediatric Primary Care*. Wiley, 1979.

Duvall EM: *Marriage and Family Development*. Lippincott, 1980.

Epstein S: The self-concept revisited: Or a theory of a theory. *Am Psychologist* 1973; 28:407.

Fowler J, Keen S: *Life Maps: Conversations in the Journey of Faith*. Word Books, 1978.

Horner M, McClellan M: Toilet training: Ready or not? *Pediatr Nurs* 1981; 7:12–18.

Horowitz JA: *The Relationship of Father Absence/Presence and Daughter's Perception of Mother's Gender-Related Traits to the Daughter's Views of her own Gender-Related Traits and Women's Roles*. (Doctoral Dissertation.) New York University, 1981.

Hughes CB: *Stressors, Roles, Strain, and Coping Mechanisms in the Continuously Employed Nurse-Mother*. (Doctoral Dissertation.) Columbia University, 1980.

Illingsworth RS: Sleep problems of children. *Clin Pediatr* 1966; 5:45–58.

Keniston K and the Carnegie Council on Children: *All Our Children: The American Family Under Pressure*. Harcourt Brace Jovanovich and the Carnegie Corporation, 1977.

Kohlberg L: The development of children's orientations toward a moral order: Sequence in development of moral thought. *Vita Humana* 1963; 6:311–333.

Kohlberg L: Development of moral character and moral ideology. In: *Review of Child Development Research*. Vol 1. Hoffman ML, Hoffman LW (editors). Russell Sage Foundation, 1964.

Labov W et al.: A study of non-standard English of Negro and Puerto Rican speakers. In: *Cooperative Research Reports*, vol 1. US Regional Survey, 1971.

Lichtenberg P, Norton DG: *Cognitive and Mental Development in the First Five Years of Life*. National Institute of Mental Health, 1970.

Liss M: *Sex Roles and Children's Play*. Academic Press, 1983.

Mitchell S: Imaginary companions—friend or foe? *Pediatr Nurs* 1980; 6:30.

Nelms BC, Mullins RG: *Growth and Development—A Primary Health Care Approach*. Prentice-Hall, 1982.

Pelton LH (editor): *The Social Context of Child Abuse and Neglect*. Human Sciences Press, 1981.

Piaget J: Development and learning. In: *Readings in Child Behavior and Development*. Lavatelli CS, Stendler F (editors). Harcourt Brace Jovanovich, 1972.

Piaget J: *The Grasp of Consciousness: Action and Concept in the Young Child*. Harvard University Press, 1976.

Rubin LB: *Worlds of Pain*. Basic Books, 1976.

Schuster CS, Ashburn SS: *The Process of Human Development*. Little, Brown, 1980.

Slobin DL: Seven questions about language development. In: *New Horizons in Psychology*, no 2. Dodwell PC (editor). Penguin Books, 1972.

Slobin DL, Welsh CA: Elicited imitation as a research tool in developmental psycholinguistics. In: *Language Training in Early Childhood Education*. Lavatelli CS (editor). University of Illinois Press, 1971.

US Department of Health and Human Services: *Monthly Vital Statistics Reports*, Aug. 11, 1983.

Chapter 6

Middle Childhood

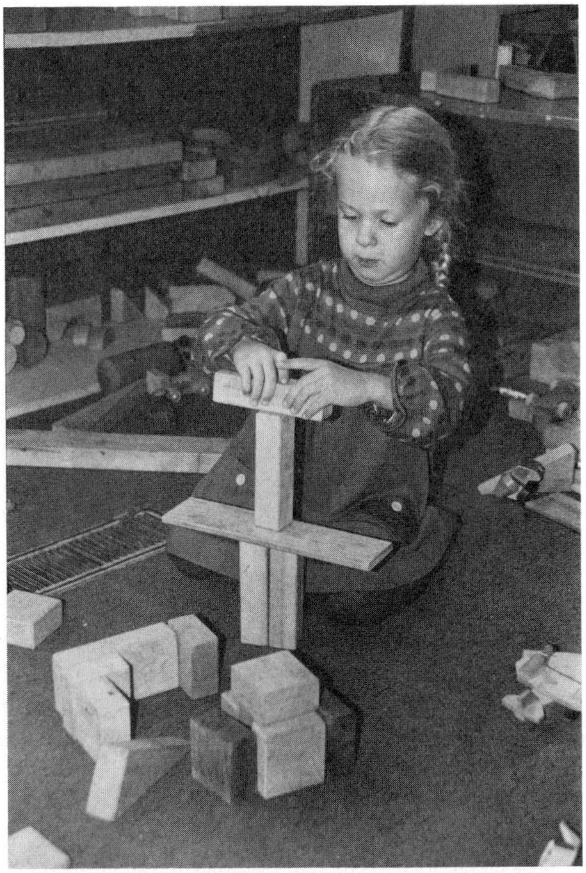

Chapter Contents

(Continues)

Objectives

- Explain the influence of external environment on middle childhood development.
- Define the major developmental changes that occur in middle childhood.
- Explain the essential biophysical changes that occur in middle childhood.
- Describe the principal explanations for affective, cognitive, language, moral, and social developments in middle childhood.
- Explain the purpose of play in middle childhood.
- Identify the basic health care needs of children in middle childhood.

Middle childhood is the period of time encompassing the early elementary school years, roughly kindergarten through third grade. The physical and cognitive changes that occur between the ages of 4 1/2 and 8 years correspond to the new social roles adopted during this developmental period. Middle childhood is a time of transition, during which the child is challenged to learn new skills and adapt to new environments. Relationships with authority figures change as the child is expected to respond to the expectations of teachers and school rules. In the school environment the child is exposed to new peer groups and learns to interact with a wide variety of people outside the family.

The transition from early to middle childhood is a more difficult change than many people realize. Although children enter middle childhood with many skills and significant advances occur in language, thought, feeling, yet to be gained are symbolic thoughts, moral consciousness, independence, and self-awareness. In some ways, these areas of new learning are equal in significance to those that occur during puberty.

Among the challenges of middle childhood are (1) the search for independence, (2) the need to become part of a group, and (3) the need to succeed in school. Children might be particularly uncertain of others' expectations of them during this time of change and stage of social development. The structures that children enter at this time force them to include peers and teachers in their social system and therefore to confront their limitations in social skills.

To meet these challenges, children become resourceful in using their energies and their developing assets to complete the goals they set for themselves. In addition to the child's intrinsic strengths, many other factors influence the successful completion of these goals. Family characteristics, socioeconomic conditions, ethnic and cultural heritage, and the values shared by family, school, and community all play vital roles in a child's ability to master the immediate environment.

The External Environment's Influence on the Child

In contrast to early childhood, middle childhood socialization is characterized by greater contact with adults and children who reside outside the home (Fig. 6-1). During this developmental period, children expand their contacts to include new social relationships. Interactions with adults and children in each of the new settings provide information for the development of the child's emerging self-concept and sense of competence.

Influence of the Family

The socializing functions of the family continue to be important during middle childhood. These functions do, however, change in relation to the child's overall social development as the child spends increasingly larger blocks of time away from home. Although the socializing responsibility now is shared, the family's contribution still is critical in such areas as the development of the child's self-concept, self-esteem, sex-role identification, interpersonal skills, social role as a family member, and social norms.

During middle childhood, the family's support is invaluable as the child embarks on new experiences. The family provides stability and security in a world where everything else seems to be changing. Within the family context, the child needs to feel free to express the tensions, fears, and anger that would be unacceptable in front of peers or teachers. One 5-year-old, for example, eagerly left for kindergarten every morning accompanied by her sibling and friends. When she returned home at noon, however, she needed some special "love time." It was safe for her to "be

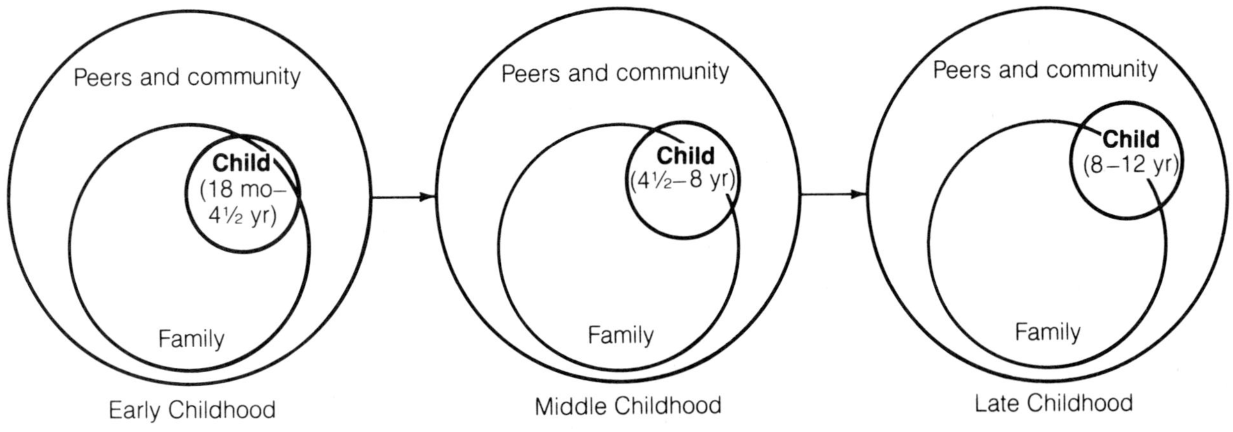

FIGURE 6-1

With age and maturity, the child gradually progresses through the boundary of the family to immediate interaction with the environment.

little" and to sit on her parent's lap recounting the morning's experiences.

Children who feel secure with their families know that someone who understands them will be there to help them in times of difficulty. Knowing this enables them to cope with new experiences, problems, or demands when away from home. Once they return to the secure confines of home and family, however, they become free to express their feelings of anger, disappointment, or self-doubt. They no longer have to work at meeting someone else's expectations but rather know that they can reveal their true emotions and still be loved and accepted. Parents sometimes need to be reassured that this "Dr. Jekyll and Mr. Hyde" phase of affective development is a characteristic expression of the struggle during middle childhood in which the child must integrate new behaviors and attitudes with those previously known. Thus, the child begins a process of self-evaluation and self-acceptance in a world now composed of a multiplicity of rules and values.

Children in this age group tend to hold their families in high regard. When children are exposed to alternative ways of doing things or different attitudes, they reduce their tension by reaffirming to others that "My mom or dad said to do it this way." Parents are idealized, and their manner of performing their roles is accepted as the best way. This loyalty may range from basic skills, such as how to throw or catch a ball, to lifestyle decisions.

Parents Parents who have given their children freedom within consistent guidelines and explanations for their expectations and values have prepared their children for new experiences and the judgments of others. For example, siblings who have difficulty getting along with each other at home help and defend one another in unfamiliar or troublesome situations because of family love and loyalty. These children know how their parents expect them to behave when they are at school, a friend's house, or a community activity. Commonly, however, these children misbehave and become demanding or whiny when they return home. At home it is safe to relieve the tension that was generated by consciously performing within parental guidelines. Explaining this tendency to parents helps them to understand why their children behave the way they do and the importance of the family. The angel at school who becomes a hellion at home does so because of the trust and security already established within the family. The child also anticipates that the family will limit "out-of-bounds" behavior and help sort out and put into perspective confusing ideas and feelings.

Middle childhood often is the time when children are given increased responsibilities. In rural areas these responsibilities might include doing farm-related chores, either alone or with a parent. In urban areas the child might have to sweep the stairs, take out the trash, or walk the dog. The child at this stage also might be expected to care for younger siblings. Participation in family chores increases the child's sense of responsibility for each family member's well-being.

A correlation is evident between family experiences and the development of high self-esteem during middle childhood (Coopersmith, 1967). Parents who are self-reliant, comfortable in their parental role, and confident of their abilities convey to their children the importance and benefits of showing respect to others. Children who receive positive feedback from significant adults also develop high self-esteem. Parents with definite values and standards of behavior who take the time to communicate them to their

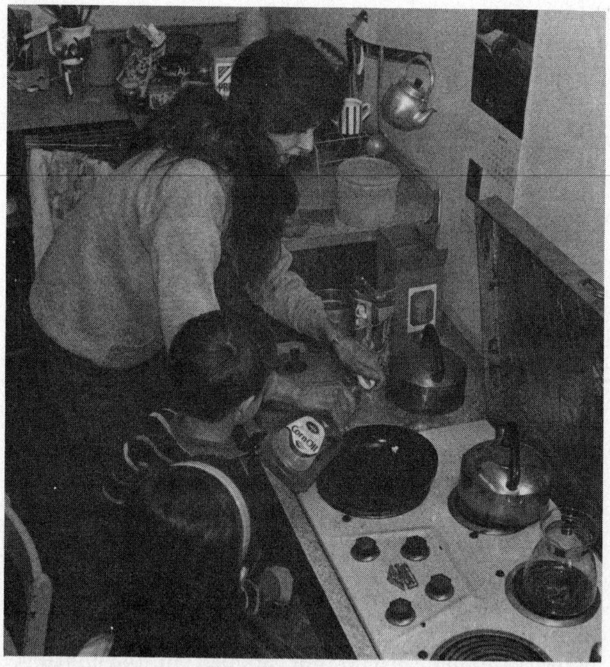

Parents continue to be important agents to socialization as children in middle childhood learn new skills and participate in family functioning.

offspring tend to have children capable of making good judgments and feeling good about themselves.

The parental role during this time of middle childhood is essential. Parenting demands considerable time and effort because parents must have confidence in presenting and enforcing their beliefs, as well as acting as role models. Parents who show sensitivity to their children's needs and abilities are more likely to have close, loving relationships with their children. Although children in this age group are increasingly influenced by others, they still look to their parents for guidance.

Parenting styles do make a difference. Parents who are restrictive and authoritarian require strict adherence to rules but take little time to explain the rules and their importance. This lack of communication also does not allow a parent to discover a child's unique needs and abilities. Children of authoritarian parents tend to be passive, shy, socially inept, immature, and dependent. On the other hand, authoritative parents exert firm control but take time to explain the reasoning behind their rules and encourage discussion about the rules. The children of authoritative parents appear to feel secure in their knowledge of parental expectations and tend to demonstrate behaviors that reflect self-reliance, self-control, self-assertiveness, curiosity, and competence. Although these trends are true when studying large groups, it generally is impossible to predict how parental characteristics and practices will affect the individual child.

Siblings Siblings also exert some influence on the child's behavior. During middle childhood, the number of siblings present and the number of years between their ages are important components of the home setting in which the child is socialized. The social learning environment is different for the firstborn child, the middle child, and the last child born. The most obvious difference is the number of members and the variety of personalities and ages comprising the family unit.

Researchers have made some generalizations concerning parental interactions with children of different birth order. Parents tend to be more involved, participate in more play activities, and have higher expectations for their firstborn child (Dunn and Kendrick, 1982; Sutton-Smith and Rosenberg, 1970). Parents appear to be more casual and less demanding of their successive children. Later-born children also have the advantage of older siblings with whom to identify. This identification sometimes takes the form of competition, as when each strives to excel in the same activity and to receive parental recognition for being the best.

Influence of the Community

By middle childhood, cultural rituals, values, beliefs, language, and customs begin to have a greater impact than biologic maturation on the child's growth and development. At this time the child is exposed to other children in school and to clubs and informal activities where lifestyles and living conditions are different. To a certain extent the family's social class influences the access to power, community influence, and economic resources. Children become aware of these differences, whether obvious or subtle, as they compare toys, vacations, and family routines. In addition, children are exposed to different religious practices and belief systems as they make new friends. This introduction to a greater collection of beliefs, values, norms, rituals, rules, and expectations opens the door to new learning experiences.

The nurse needs to note the roles of these factors in orienting the child to the environment outside the home. The nurse plans teaching or guidance to include the child's and family's values. For example, one of the cultural characteristics of Western civilizations in general and the United States in particular is competition. The overarching, unspoken, motivating factor is to learn a skill as quickly and completely as possible because those who are best are rewarded. Thus the child becomes oriented toward achievement as the ultimate goal. In school this phenomenon is manifested by the awarding of stickers, spending time at special-interest tables, or having extra quiet-reading time. The child quickly concludes and the teacher confirms that those who are most skilled and the first to finish assigned work are rewarded. The child works for the reward rather than for the joy of learning. Such a child, for example, might read books at home only when the school holds a reading contest because reading is perceived as a worthwhile activity only if rewarded by teachers and peers rather than as a stimulating activity in itself.

Television Television has become an integral part of the American culture and, as such, influences the child's growth and development. When used appropriately, television can enrich the child's world, introducing new ideas and concepts. Television can, however, have a negative impact. Often children watch developmentally inappropriate programs that portray violence, explicit sexuality, and racial and cultural stereotypes. Studies have shown that heavy television viewing by children in the early elementary grades may lead to increased aggressive behavior and distorted perceptions of the world (Rubinstein, 1983).

Another detrimental aspect of television is the behavior it prevents. Bronfenbrenner (1972) noted that television is one of a host of factors that conspire to isolate children from parents, peers, and society in general. Hours spent being entertained limit children's contact and interaction with others, their participation in the give-and-take of relationships, and the use of imagination in creative play experiences.

Television is a powerful socializing force on children, and the child's social attitudes and behavior are affected by it. Whether the influence is more positive than negative or vice versa remains a question for social scientists.

School As the child prepares to enter elementary school, certain temperamental characteristics might help or hinder the transition to formal education. Some of these characteristics are the child's activity level, adaptability to change, reaction to new situations, persistence, and distractibility. Children who might need special help in making the transition to school are those who are particularly active or passive, who have typically been slow to adjust to change, or who tend to withdraw or be distractible. Such temperamental characteristics are not necessarily "problems," but information about the child's responses might be helpful in planning interventions to ease the transition.

Despite the continuing importance of the family, much social development is transferred from home to the playground and classroom. The function of education is twofold: (1) to perpetuate the culture, and (2) to stimulate thinking, learning, and creativity. The beginning of formal schooling is a rite of passage for children in modern industrial countries. Entry into school also coincides with the phase in cognitive development in which children begin to think more logically. Formal schooling provides the child with a landmark in the growing-up process. Interests and energy become shared among family, school, and peers. The educational community now actively participates in the transfer of information and skills, such as reading, writing, problem solving, and interpersonal relations.

Teachers are important people in the child's life. Some are chosen as role models, while others are viewed as directors or motivators toward achievement. The kind of teachers that children have will influence whether the school experience will be positive or negative. Success in school confirms feelings of self-confidence and contributes to a sense of industry.

The transition from home to school is a significant milestone in the young child's life. It involves learning new skills considered basic to life, namely, reading and writing. It also entails becoming familiar with a new environment, schedule of activities, peers, and authority figures. How successful the child is in making these initial adjustments will influence future school-related experiences. Children's attitudes toward school and toward adult authority figures in general are correlated with their level of school achievement and with their teachers' expectations.

Peer groups In the peer group, children learn to interact with age-mates and to participate in both competitive activities and cooperative projects. In a peer group the 4 1/2- to 8-year-old child's friends are playmates. This group tends to be informal and transient, consisting of small groups of children who usually are of the same sex. The peer group provides a supportive environment for the child's move from family to school and community. Initially, the peer group consists of those children who are in close physical proximity to each other. Children play together because they live near each other, or are in the same swimming, ballet, or gymnastics class. Later, these children become more selective and seek friends with common interests and abilities.

The peer relationship is dynamic and necessitates mutual give-and-take. Friendships are earned; they are not acquired automatically. Children quickly learn that peers have different opinions about how a game is played, how a skill is performed, or how a task is completed. Children who insist on doing everything their way soon find themselves left out of games and activities. They learn that they must adapt, share ideas, and then follow mutually agreed-on rules if they want to be included. For example, while investigating the rising crescendo of an argument, one parent discovered that five girls who wanted to play "neighbors" could not agree on the location of their houses. It seemed that one girl was threatening the harmony of the group by insisting on locating her house in someone else's "pretend" driveway. This violated their rule that the houses had to be far apart so that no one could spy on another's "dress up" plans. Sometimes, such disagreements can be resolved if the other children allow an exception or reach a compromise. Often, the children go their separate ways, complaining that a friend does not play fairly, always has to be the boss, or is selfish and spoiled. During middle childhood, children tend to be very expressive and fairly uninhibited when justifying their behavior with their friends.

During this stage, peer relations are sociable, aggressive, experimental, and somewhat calculated. The child has to concentrate on prosocial behaviors with peers, and adults need to encourage and support these actions. Children meet each other as equals, and their understanding of each other differs from the views of adults. Children who have minimal peer contact are limited in their abilities to understand others' points of view (Fischer and Lazerson, 1984). Children now find it becomes very important to maintain status with peers, and their behavior increasingly reflects the norms and values of their peer group. The middle childhood peer group begins to foster conformity to social norms and expectations. In this respect the peer group is a powerful agent for cultural continuity. Within the context of the peer group, children learn what to expect from each other and subsequently how to maintain harmony in a variety of situations.

Peers also help to organize and refine the child's self-concept. What the adult might view as "silly" the peer might view as "terrific." A child's humor or antics might not be appreciated by serious-minded adults, but peers will applaud such behavior and view the child as special. In this way, peers help a child to categorize certain behaviors as appropriate for adults and other behaviors as appropriate for peers. Peers help one another to become less egocentric and to think about situations from another person's perspective. Social interaction with age-mates is necessary for the development of this skill.

Developmental Changes in Middle Childhood

The developmental tasks of middle childhood push the child outward into more concentrated interactions with the environment. Physically, the child begins engaging in games and other activities requiring practice and coordination. Socially, the child moves from home and family to the world of school, peers, and playground, learning social skills and how to get along with age-mates. Cognitively, the child learns how to communicate symbolically and to question the "how's" and "why's" of life. (Table 6-1 summarizes the biophysical development and other developmental changes associated with middle childhood and notes guidelines for assessment.)

Affective Development

Affective development in childhood correlates highly with development in other areas. As in infancy and early childhood, the personality attributes of 4 1/2- to 8-year-old children influence their thought processes. As the child develops, personality traits remain a factor in decision making, even though cognition and social awareness take on additional meaning.

The affective qualities demonstrated by a child in middle childhood stem from an emerging self-identity based on values learned at home. Friendship, kindness, caring, and sharing are positive emotional expressions that contribute to feelings of psychologic well-being among children of this age. Fear, anger, and anxiety are expressions of negative emotion.

Gender identification Middle childhood is a time when gender and social identity become solidified. Lamb (1978) explained that gender identity is not secure until the child is satisfied and feels comfortable being male or female. Once this occurs, the child identifies first with the same-sex parent and then with other role models, imitating their behaviors and usually taking on stereotypic sex-role attitudes and actions.

This explanation of the process of identification is a refinement of Freud's concept (1969). He presented identification as the resolution of the Oedipal complex (or Electra complex in girls) and claimed that it was the major task the child accomplished during the phallic stage of development (see Chapter 3). Freud assumed that by the time the child reaches 6 years of age, the Oedipus complex is usually resolved and the child enters the latency period. During latency, the development of intellectual skills becomes paramount.

Cognitive theorists, as represented by Kohlberg (1966), have noted that gender identity is a two-step process. The child first acquires a basic sense of identity. This usually occurs in early childhood, when, for example, Mark will identify himself as a boy and his sister, Lisa, as a girl. The second step occurs during middle childhood and entails the concept of gender constancy. Now, Mark affirms that boys will always become men and girls will always become

(Text continues on page 168)

TABLE 6-1 Guidelines for Assessment of the 4½- to 8-Year-Old Child

	Expected characteristics		
Developmental area	**4½- to 5-year-old**	**6- to 8-year-old**	**Assessment techniques**
Temperament			Assess temperamental characteristics of child and parental perceptions Ask how easily the child becomes upset and how the child responds to disappointments, being teased, and new experiences
Biophysical development			
Weight–average annual increase of 2.3 kg (5 lb)	Weight at age 5 years is 2 times that at age 1 Average (50th percentile) 18.1 kg (40 lb)	Weight at age 7 is 7 times birth weight 19.5 kg (43 lb)–24.5 kg (54 lb)	
Length	109.2 cm (43 in.)	114.3 cm (45 in.)–127 cm (50 in.)	
Neuromuscular	Definite hand preference by 4½ years of age		
Gross motor skills	Balance on one foot for 10 seconds	Runs, skips, hops, jumps, climbs with increased speed and improved accuracy (can walk a 2-in. wide balance beam, jump and hop into small squares); learns to climb trees and an interval-knotted rope; learns to roller skate	Tell child, "Do this as long as you can," while demonstrating; time the number of seconds the child can balance and expect the child to balance for 10 seconds on two of three trials
	Jumps rope	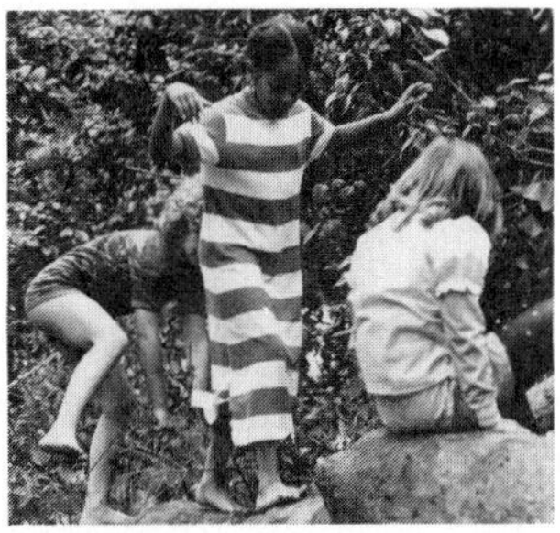	Ask the child to jump rope; demonstrate if necessary
	Performs heel-to-toe walk, toe within 1 in. of heel, for at least four steps backward		Tell the child to do backward heel-to-toe walk; demonstrate if necessary; helpful to have line on floor for the child to follow
	Runs on toes; skips by alternating feet; becomes proficient at climbing playground equipment		Observe the child or ask the parent about the child's running, skipping, and playing on playground equipment
	Catches bounced ball; catches small tossed ball with hands	Can throw small ball about 40 ft fairly accurately	Tell the child to stand 3 ft away and catch a bounced ball with hands (not with arms or by trapping against body); do again except tossing instead of bouncing ball Ask what the child can do best when playing ball and what aspect (throwing or catching) needs work
	Rides bicycle with training wheels	Rides bike without training wheels	Ask the child and parent about bicycle-riding abilities
		Learns to swim; improved coordination allows activities to be more purposeful, such as dance lessons, gymnastics, relay races, and kickball	Ask questions to elicit child's interest and participation in sports, dance lessons, and physical activity

TABLE 6-1 Guidelines for Assessment of the 4½- to 8-Year-Old Child *(Continued)*

	Expected characteristics		
Developmental area	**4½- to 5-year-old**	**6- to 8-year-old**	**Assessment techniques**
Fine motor skills	Copies square and triangle	Prints numbers, letters, and words; printing becomes smaller and more accurate; learns cursive writing	Show the child a square and a triangle but do not let the child see the shapes being drawn and do not name the forms; tell the child to draw one like each of the pictures
	Might print a few letters or even simple words (such as own name)		Ask child about writing skills; may have child print or write name
	Draws a person with at least six parts; improved drawing of house	More precise in artwork, including drawing, coloring, painting, and cutting; chosen designs and projects are reproduced more accurately 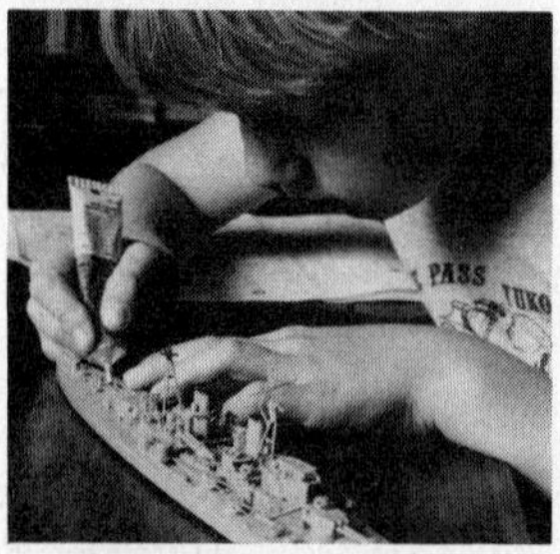	Tell the child to draw a person but do not tell the child which parts to draw; the child's picture should contain six identifiable parts; if one part of a pair (eyes, arms) is not drawn, that part does not count; ask the child and parent about crafts, artwork, and other projects that might be hobbies or special interests
	Cuts along a straight line for 6 inches		Give the child a piece of paper 6 inches wide with a line drawn straight across and tell the child to cut along the line
	Begins to tie shoelaces	Most children can tie a bowknot by the time they are 8 years old	Tell the child to tie shoelaces—either own or on doll
		Improved hand-eye coordination for board games, puzzles, and playing musical instruments	Assess hand-eye coordination by the child's performance on the neurologic examination
Cardiovascular		Heart becomes more vertical; by age 7, the left ventrical is adult thickness	
Heart rate	95±30 beats/min	95±30 beats/min	Assess by taking radial pulse
Blood pressure	105–95/65–60 mm Hg	105–95/65–60 mm Hg	
Blood values	Hemoglobin and hematocrit increase while the white blood cell count decreases		
Respiratory	Alveolar multiplication probably complete by age 8 years		
Respiratory rate	20–24 breaths/min	20–24 breaths/min	
Gastrointestinal	The stomach enlarges, reducing frequency of eating; stools one to two times a day; elimination controlled		
Genitourinary		Output 1000 ml/day; urine values similar to adult	
Immune	Increase in antibody production with increased exposure to antigen; enlargement of lymphatic system, especially tonsillar tissue		
Sensory-perceptual			
Vision	Changes from hyperopic to normal 20/30	20/20	Use Snellen alphabet test
Hearing	Episodes of otitis media decrease		Use audiometric testing and tympanogram

TABLE 6-1 *(Continued)*

Developmental area	Expected characteristics: 4½- to 5-year-old	Expected characteristics: 6- to 8-year-old	Assessment techniques
Language development—expression and comprehension	Uses complete sentences with nouns, pronouns, verbs, adverbs, adjectives, prepositions, and articles		Listen to the child's spontaneous speech and use of grammar and syntax, noting the child's ability to listen and to comprehend verbal messages throughout the assessment
	Defines words according to shape, composition, or general category	Oral vocabulary of 2500 words by 6 years of age; sentence length approximately five words in length	Ask the child to define words, one at a time, with such questions as "What is a ______?" and words such as ball, lake, house, shoe, desk, banana, ceiling; expect the child to define most words (six of nine) appropriately
	Decodes verbal messages	Makes use of all the various parts of speech Asks questions that indicate a quest for information about the purpose of objects Able to arrange stories of events objectively and begins to write "pretend" stories	Say to the child, "Guess what I have. It is long and hard and you write with it," "It is made of paper, it has pictures and stories and pages in it," or use other examples
	Identifies the composition of objects	Defines words according to their related action (eg, apple = something to eat)	Ask the child what a spoon (shoe, door, etc) is made of
	Follows three commands		Note the child's ability to listen and follow directions Ask the child to relate some event in school or at an after-school activity; note sentence structure, objectivity, and whether the story is told logically Ask the child to define several words, such as orange and snow
Cognitive development	Identifies four colors	Increased attention span allows for improved visual discrimination and processing of information from the environment	Place colored blocks on the table, point to the blocks, and tell the child to identify the color or to give the red (blue, yellow, etc) block to the nurse Ask the child and parent about the types of books the child enjoys reading
	Identifies basic geometric shapes		Show the child a circle, triangle, and square and ask the child to name each shape
	Repeats ten-word sentence	Memory improves; remembers best the material that is meaningful to them; begins to use imagery as a memory aid	Tell the child to "listen carefully to what I say and then say what I say. We are going to the store to buy some bread" or use another simple sentence
	Reproduces a pattern of four objects in the correct order		Place a block, pencil, ball, and book on the table; ask the child to name each object, then scramble the objects and tell the child to put them back the way they were

(Continues)

TABLE 6-1 Guidelines for Assessment of the 4½- to 8-Year-Old Child *(Continued)*

Developmental area	Expected characteristics: 4½- to 5-year-old	Expected characteristics: 6- to 8-year-old	Assessment techniques
			Ask the child to recite the Pledge of Allegiance; show a box with ten objects, then cover the box and ask the child to name as many objects as possible; ask the child to explain the method used for remembering
	Classifies objects according to similarities in relationship	Knows number combinations up to ten; can count by 1, 2, 5, or 10; has basic idea of addition and subtraction; can tell time	Ask the child, "How are bread and milk alike?" "How are a jacket and a hat alike?" and expect the child to identify similarities between the objects
	Might be able to classify objects according to more than one characteristic		Present 12 forms: four triangles (two red, two blue), four squares (two red, two blue), and four circles (two red, two blue); ask the child to put like forms together, first according to color and then according to shape
		Knows comparative value of coins	Have the child identify various coins and then ask child to provide change for word problem about buying milk or something else that costs less than the money given to the salesperson
		Takes an interest in learning facts and solving problems	Ask the child to solve problems; include both written and oral problems
		Is learning to read	
		Developing a sense of humor; tells a joke repeatedly	Ask the child to repeat a riddle or joke and assess the type of humor
		Preoperational to concrete operational thinking; able to perform mental operations of conversation of liquid amount and solid amount	Use the Piagetian task for conservation; may use two clay balls—roll one into a sausage shape and ask the child if the amount of clay has changed; ask the older child if the weight of the clay balls has changed
		Has acquired operations of reversibility, basic class inclusion, class hierarchy of visible objects, seriation of visible objects	Have the younger child place a series of blocks in order according to descending size; observe for frequency of size and comparison; ask the older child a representation question, "If Karl's red shirt is darker than Mathew's, and Karl's shirt is lighter than Adam's, who has the darkest shirt?"

TABLE 6-1 *(Continued)*

Developmental area	Expected characteristics: 4½- to 5-year-old	Expected characteristics: 6- to 8-year-old	Assessment techniques
		Does not understand relationships among time, speed, and distance; solves problems by trial and error; has difficulty verbalizing rationale for solution; considers two factors simultaneously but not more	Provide the child with a small balance and series of weights; request the child to position the weights so that the sides balance, then ask the child why it balanced and how things are related
		Less egocentric, able to take another's viewpoint; can consider someone else's feelings or needs; internalizes sense of conscience; follows rules to avoid punishment	Tell the child about someone who cheated by going out of turn while playing a game because of wanting to win so badly and someone else who won by forgetting a penalty and ask what should be done; assess how the child solves the problem and the use of rules
	Shows imagination but accurately describes events		Discuss the child's imaginative play with the parent; ask how often the child exaggerates or "tells tales"
		Able to differentiate fantasy and reality but still thinks that radio and television characters are real	Ask the child if events that happen on a favorite program are real and why
	Precausal ideas about reasons for illness	Shows more realistic sense of causality	Ask the child why someone gets sick and note the child's response and understanding of realistic, logical, or scientific cause-and-effect relationships
Affective and social development			
Child	Independently dresses, washes, and performs toileting		Discuss the child's daily habits with both the parent and child, assess how the child performs these tasks during the assessment exam and whether the parent interferes
		Awareness of individual attributes; further development of sense of self-esteem	Have the child describe self; note the statements that indicate positive or negative attitudes about self
	Displays sexual curiosity; might have own private theories to explain sexual differences and reproduction	Understanding of sexuality more realistic	Ask the child questions such as, "How can you tell if someone is a boy or a girl?" "Why are boys and girls different?" "Where do babies come from?" and ask the parent whether the child has engaged in sexual exploration of self or others; discuss parental response
			Ask the child about reproduction and differences between sexes, and note the child's understanding of facts

(Continues)

TABLE 6-1 Guidelines for Assessment of the 4½- to 8-Year-Old Child *(Continued)*

Developmental area	Expected characteristics: 4½- to 5-year-old	Expected characteristics: 6- to 8-year-old	Assessment techniques
	Looks for parental support and encouragement		Note parental response to child's performance, whether the parent allows the child to proceed independently or intervenes; note whether parent makes encouraging or discouraging comments
		Becoming self-critical—wants to do things well; completes projects; becomes upset if performance not up to personal expectations	Have the child draw a picture and explain what is good, what needs improvement, and why; assess the child's demand on self to do well
	Might exhibit jealousy of siblings		Discuss the relationship between the child and siblings, noting how the child gets along with each sibling, the incidence of conflicts, and how conflicts are resolved; might ask the child directly, "What do you like best about your brother/sister?" "Is there anything you don't like about ______?" "Do you ever fight with ______?" "What happens then?"
	Separates easily from parents		Discuss with the parent how the child handles separation and how parents react to separation (school entry may temporarily cause renewed separation anxiety)
	Verbalizes feelings		Observe how the child handles feelings during assessment; observe parental responses; ask the child such questions as "What is the happiest (saddest, scariest) thing you can think of?" and discuss with the parent how the child acts when sad, angry, or frightened
	Judges acts according to consequences but does not take intention into account		Present a moral dilemma to the child; observe the child's behavior, noting parental limit setting and the child's response
	Controls behavior in assessment setting, defines acceptable and unacceptable behavior		Discuss with the parent how the child responds to limits, what happens if the child breaks a limit, what type of discipline the parent uses, and how the child responds; explore the child's perceptions of discipline

TABLE 6-1 *(Continued)*

Developmental area	Expected characteristics: 4½- to 5-year-old	Expected characteristics: 6- to 8-year-old	Assessment techniques
		Delay of gratification possible; can control emotions and assume responsibility for own behavior but has difficulty if tired or hungry	Ask the child about own behavior if someone teases, picks an argument or fights, or does not complete their work and the child has to do it; have the child compare what ideal and actual responses are and note the child's ability to accept responsibility
	Habitually performs certain household tasks		Discuss with the parent and child what jobs the child does around the house
		Able to complete chores with reminding at times; might bargain to get paid for work around the house	Ask the parent about the child's cooperation in completing tasks, need for reminders, and response when reminded
	Displays confidence in approaching tasks		Observe how the child approaches tasks during the assessment; note any hesitancy, expectation of success or failure, use of parent as resource, and reaction to successful or unsuccessful performance
		Begins collections and hobbies	Ask the child to describe any hobbies or collecting; assess interest and use for self-concept
		Learns and begins to use social manners of greeting	Ask the parent to evaluate the child's manners
		Fears decreasing but might be stimulated by reading, television, or movies; might fear shadows or strange noises; worries about being late for school, not being liked, and not having someone to play with at recess	Ask whether the child is afraid of certain objects, animals, the dark, injury, or pain and note the child's response
	Engages in cooperative play Relates appropriately to adults outside family	Expands social environment because of school and peer-group activities; peer group gains importance; usually same age and boys and girls play together	Discuss with the parent how the child interacts with other children, what types of play the child engages in, and the child's ability to share; assess opportunities for the child to interact with peers
		Learns to relate to new authority figure; notices differences in cultural, ethnic, and religious traditions; friends often reside in neighborhood; beginning to be more selective in choosing friends	Note the child's response to the examiner Ask the child to name and describe friends and their favorite activities; ask the child and parent about the child's adjustment to school, new expectations from teacher, and ability to relate to children of different backgrounds

women and that this fact can never change. Even if a boy grew his hair long and wore dresses and makeup, he would still be a boy. Thus, the child has an intellectual grasp of the concept and meaning of gender.

Once children learn to identify with their parents, they judge actions as right or wrong according to their parents' evaluations of these actions. This developing conscience in turn influences how children act in situations involving moral judgment.

Although they have more freedom to choose friends, games, and activities, children during middle childhood tend to prefer to be with others of the same sex. They play games, establish rules, and assign roles that often are exclusive and reflect their perceptions about their future roles. Boys will participate in such play activities as football, police, or space rangers and temporarily take the names of their heroes. Girls will play house, school, or television studio, assigning names and roles accordingly. The two groups often stake out their own territory and post "No Girls Allowed" or "Entrance Limited to Girls Only" signs. Each group regards its sex as superior, more intelligent, and more talented.

In their peer groups, characterized by the separation of interests and activities, boys and girls develop their skills, values, and roles with others most like themselves. This division according to gender facilitates the socialization process, aids in the attainment of competence, and reduces the risk of failure. Children gain a better sense of who they are by establishing who they are not. Likeness is rooted in gender identity and the internalization of behaviors, roles, attributes, and mannerisms of the same-sex role models.

Masturbation Masturbation is a normal exploration of the body, particularly the genital area. Almost all children engage in touching or exploring themselves. Masturbation is pleasurable and might be used for the sensation itself or to release anxiety or tension.

Parents' values concerning modesty and sexuality are crucial to handling this behavior. Parents might need to understand that children's touching of themselves in private might best be ignored to prevent unnecessary attention or anxiety. Nurses can reassure parents that this is a normal process that often increases around 4 1/2 years of age and disappears if ignored. The parent should, however, differentiate between masturbation in private and in public. Without causing fear or guilt in the child, the parent can simply let a child know that touching oneself is not appropriate in front of other people. The child, already incorporating the concepts of pride and modesty, usually will accept this advice without difficulty.

Sense of self The contributions of others to the child's development is a consistent theme in the theory of Erik Erikson (see Chapter 3). During middle childhood, developmental tasks focus on interacting appropriately and creatively with the environment. According to Erikson (1963), the 3- to 6-year-old child must resolve the dilemma of initiative versus guilt by learning to explore beyond the self. Children's initiative can be seen in the increasing number of questions they ask and in the world they create.

The ways that parents and other adults react to the child's inquisitive posture is important because these people influence the child's leaning toward initiative or guilt. Children need families to assist them in striving to master initiative. The family should (1) teach the child where play ends and responsibility and purpose begin, (2) clearly define the dos and don'ts with reference to words and actions, and (3) develop a mutually loving relationship between father and son or mother and daughter based on worth and acceptance, thereby fostering behaviors that are similar to those of the same-sex parent.

Feelings of satisfaction stimulate the child first in the development of initiative and second in the production of work, or industry. Constructing new behaviors is satisfying. Children derive pleasure from building, discovering new knowledge, and learning. Initially, the child is rewarded for beginning a task. The child's attempt to replicate a mental image of a city by building a block city or drawing many buildings demonstrates initiative. The quality or exactness of the final product is not as important as the attempt to replicate reality or to transcribe a creative idea accurately.

Erikson saw the child's conflict after 6 years of age as one of industry versus inferiority. As children apply their recently learned skills, they focus more on the product than on the process. They gain a sense of satisfaction when the product does, in fact, replicate reality and they have successfully transcribed an image or idea accurately. This accomplishment allows them to attain a sense of industry, but if they fail to meet the tasks at hand, children acquire a sense of inferiority. Parent, teacher, and peer evaluation of a child's "work" are influential in establishing self-worth. Encouragement from others assists and encourages the child in the work of mastering school tasks.

As children interact with others and accomplish the tasks of middle childhood, they refine their sense of self. They increasingly understand how they are seen by others. Their self-concept reflects how others respond to them, what others appear to think of them, and how others evaluate their skills. The acquisition of self-concept is a complex process that is influenced by the expectations of many others and therefore does not follow a smooth continuum.

The child with a positive self-concept feels capable, worthy, important, and likable, all feelings that translate into self-respect and self-confidence. Children with a negative self-concept feel unacceptable, doubt their ability to do well or to have friends, and develop a sense of inferiority.

Educators have observed that improvement of a negative self-concept is best achieved by the child's learning basic skills and thus becoming capable of changing behavior. This is important for nurses to remember, especially when caring for children with chronic illnesses or disabling conditions. It is more beneficial for nurses to teach such children the skills that will help them to function optimally than to give them falsely inflated views of themselves.

Fears Middle childhood is the time when early childhood fears wane, to be replaced by new fears. As the child matures, imagination and fantasy are replaced by more realistic thinking. Between the ages of 4 1/2 and 6 years, fears related to physical injury increase. The child, who now is very aware of the body and its functioning parts, is fearful that injury will result in body mutilation. They might overreact to a minor injury because they fear for the intactness of their body. The fear of body mutilation might be related to the appearance of masturbation during middle childhood. Children fear injuries from animals (especially dogs) and activities such as swimming that relate to drowning. Their active imaginations might recreate or invent threatening creatures and harmful situations. The child naturally is fearful of things that are different, unexpected, or not understood.

Nurses especially need to be cognizant of the child's fears, to respect the fears as real, and to be patient and understanding of their influence on the child's behavior. The nurse must never belittle the child or ignore the fear. The child might need frequent reassurances or actual checkings under the bandage to be certain that their body is intact and not changing shape or disappearing while they cannot see it. In addition, it is common for children to be very fearful of the strangeness of the personnel and environment in health care facilities.

Around 7 or 8 years of age, these fears for personal well-being become replaced by anxieties and fears about school and social relationships. Seven-year-old children tend to be anxious about (1) school performance, (2) peer acceptance, (3) teacher acceptance, and (4) school conduct.

Cognitive Development

According to Piaget, children 4–7 years of age are in the *intuitive substage* of the preoperational stage. During this substage the child seems to understand intuitively the rules that govern the social environment. In reality, the child is more able to cope with the physical world than to understand how it is governed. The child's thinking processes are still limited to the appearance of things, egocentricity, and illogical reasoning. Even so, children at this stage are less egocentric than in the preconceptual substage and can distinguish between their own perception of the real world and the reality of the physical and social environment (Piaget, 1973).

Intuitive thought processes are characteristic of *transductive thinking*. A precursor of inductive reasoning, transductive thinking involves drawing conclusions from one specific, current event to another equally specific and immediate event. For example, the child who sees the wind blowing leaves away might conclude that it is possible for children to be blown away by a strong wind. Until the child is able to classify or discern similar from dissimilar objects, conclusions about their operations might be illogical.

Imitation and learning Social learning theories have integrated some aspects of both behaviorism and psychosocial stage theories. Whereas Freud and Erikson focused on dependence and identification as the antecedents for learning, social learning theorists stress imitation and reinforcement. To social learning theorists, a child 4–7 years old learns when behavior is reinforced. Other social learning theorists go further and suggest that observing another person might be sufficient to lead to a learned response.

Bandura (1963) argued that when placed in social situations, children often learn much more rapidly by observing the behavior of others (see Chapter 3). Observational learning is a cognitive process that teaches the child the outcomes of the behavior without the child's having experienced the outcomes firsthand. The child's experience with a model reflects an experience that may be direct or indirect, real or symbolic, but the child interprets the model's behavior and selects the information to retain. Learning in middle childhood might therefore be a vicarious process in which the child need not directly experience the reinforcer to learn.

Bandura postulated that cognition is influenced by the child's own motivation. Hence, learning through modeling varies from child to child. Children particularly observe models who are rewarded, who have personal characteristics that are favorable, and who are somewhat similar to them. The 6-year-old taking gymnastic lessons might watch Olympic or national competition on television and then try to perform similar tricks. A young boy who met a professional basketball star decided to pursue a career in basketball. He spent hours practicing, trying to imitate everything this player did. As a result, he was the best player on his midget basketball team.

Egocentricity Egocentric children believe that everyone perceives and interprets the world in exactly the same way that they do. In middle childhood egocentricity is not an intentional act of disregarding but rather the inability to see another person's point of view. Four-year-old children have difficulty comprehending such concepts as "share," "fair," "right," or "wrong." Not until they reach 6 years of age and begin to recognize that other people have personal reasons for their behavior can they fully understand socially prescribed rules.

Before 4 years of age, there is no evidence that children can understand another's point of view. Four-year-olds, however, can show empathy toward others who are placed in unfortunate situations. Significant changes occur in the child's ability to take another's perspective as the child advances toward concrete operational thinking. The 6-year-old child can begin to understand whether another person's actions are accidental or intended and can recognize that other people might act on the basis of their own personal feelings.

As the child gradually learns about others through interaction with peers, teachers, and neighbors, egocentric thinking decreases. For example, while playing with blocks in school, 4 1/2-year-old Jack decided he needed another large yellow block. He looked around for one, but none was in sight. Then he saw a long row of blocks where Carolyn was playing. Quickly he went over to Carolyn's area and took two of the blocks. As she attempted to reclaim them, an argument ensued. Jack shouted that he needed them to complete his building, and Carolyn protested that he had taken her yellow brick road. Neither child could understand the other's point of view, and both children were outraged that someone was interfering with their projects.

Self-knowledge, or the development of conscious awareness of self, progresses during the early phase of middle childhood, when the child's emphasis is on images of physical events, to the latter phase of middle childhood, which is the beginning of Piaget's concrete operational stage (see Chapter 3). Eventually, children learn to organize and interpret stories, dreams, and images. Initially, when children tell stories or relate dreams, they omit large portions because they assume that the listener shares their perspective. In fact, they have little tolerance if the listener requests additional information. By 6 or 7 years of age, they realize that the listener only knows what they relate and thus provide detailed accounts of the events.

Conservation, centration, and irreversibility The notion that objects can be transformed from one state to another and still preserve their integrity is foreign to the 4- and 5-year-old. At this stage, children simply cannot comprehend that two equal quantities remain equal as long as nothing is added or subtracted. The child has not grasped the principle of *conservation,* that certain properties of objects remain the same despite transformations.

Lack of conservation is best demonstrated with 4- and 5-year-olds when two equal-size balls of clay are put before them. Children of this age correctly respond that the balls have the same amount of clay. When the perceptual properties are changed by rolling one into a sausage shape in front of the children, they will change their minds, select the longer of the two pieces, and state that it has more clay. Piaget (1969) said that children in the intuitive phase think that if things look different, they must be different.

At approximately 6 or 7 years of age, children begin to comprehend conservation of substance. To gain an understanding of this concept, children first focus on only one aspect or dimension of the object without recognizing relationships among such dimensions as height, weight, length, and width. This lack of multidimensional perception is termed *centration.*

Because children cannot recognize reversibility, they also are easily deceived by appearance. They do not mentally reverse the process, that is, change the sausage shape back into the ball shape. Eventually, children vacillate in comprehending this concept and might be able to focus on more than one dimension simultaneously but without understanding the relationships among the dimensions observed. At this point, the child will be able to recognize that the mound of clay is the same but can do so only by concrete experimentation. Logical explanations for such phenomena usually are not given until the child is 10–12 years old and can reason abstractly.

Until abstraction is possible, the child can understand events in the present but is limited by irreversibility and is unable to retrace the process. Another example of irreversibility is the reasoning of a 5-year-old child who is able to tell his teacher that he has a brother but replies "no" when asked whether his brother has a brother.

Most 6- and 7-year-olds are in transition. They can reverse familiar, concrete events when they have direct experience or when they have the objects to manipulate back and forth. One child moved childlike characters back and forth between a toy vehicle and doll house while verbally problem solving: "In the car you are crowded, in the house you have lots of room, but there are the seven in the car and seven in the house, so there must be more room in the house and less room in the car."

The child's ability to conserve begins with the conservation of number. The 4-year-old preconserver focuses on a single dimension. If 20 coins are arranged in two rows of ten so that the rows are of equal length, the child will identify them as equivalent. If one row is then pushed together, the child will center only on the length of the rows and claim that the longer (original) row has more coins than does the pushed-together row. The 5-year-old generally is at the transitional phase, which is characterized by inconsistency of response. By 7 years of age, most children have the mental ability to count and a basic understanding of addition and subtraction. Instead of focusing on the length of the rows, they count the number of coins. If the number is the same, they know the rows are equivalent even though the rows are of different lengths. In addition to number, conservation tasks that are mastered during middle childhood include length, liquid amount, solid amount, and sometimes area. The final conservation task involves displaced volume and is not gained until the end of late childhood.

Time, space, seriation, and classification Like all learning during middle childhood, children's experiences with time are perceptual. By 4 years of age, children are able to remember time sequences and the repetition of events in particular places. They have also mastered such concepts as next summer, last summer, daily events, and months. Concepts such as the time of day and clock time are developed around 5 or 6 years of age.

Piaget (1973) maintained that spatial knowledge develops so that the child eventually can locate an object in reference to other objects and without self-reference. Before this is possible, however, the child must first represent space by formulating a "cognitive map" and placing objects in relation to the self. When 4-year-olds are shown a community scene and then asked to place the doll figures in their model scene in the positions that they had observed them, they will place the figures in the same general proximity. They will not be concerned, however, with replicating left-right or before-behind distances. Five- and 6-year-olds demonstrate a heightened awareness of spatial relations and will place the dolls more exactly. If the model is turned 180 degrees, these children will place the dolls in relation to themselves as if the rotation had not occurred. Until the child's egocentricity diminishes, objects are assumed to be positioned in relation to the child. Seven-year-olds have a better understanding of relationships in space and are able to account for the rotation and replicate the model when positioning their dolls (Labinowicz, 1980).

During middle childhood, children master such quantitative terms as *more, less, all, some, none,* and *another.* The ability to arrange objects according to increasing or decreasing size is *seriation.* The 4 1/2-year-old can identify which of two sticks, labeled A and B, is longer. If A, the longer stick, is replaced by a very short stick, C, the child then will identify B as longer than C. If asked whether A or C is longer, this child would have to guess at the answer because the ability to order events mentally that occur sequentially has not been attained. The child also has not mastered the concept of greater or lesser and thus lacks a principle with which to solve the problem. The 7-year-old has no difficulty answering the question. This child can reason that if A is longer than B and B is longer than C, then A is longer than C.

During middle childhood, children learn to classify objects according to their properties. Among 4- and 5-year-olds, objects are grouped perceptually rather than according to a category. Many studies demonstrate that these children are more likely to group objects on the basis of color rather than form. If given blocks in various shapes, sizes, and colors, the child is likely to put a yellow cube next to a yellow block and a green triangle next to a green block. This kind of classification, in which each object is related to the one beside it but without an overall relationship tying them together, is called *chaining.* The shift from color preference to form preference occurs at about 5 years of age. Most 6-year-olds, after having grouped objects on the basis of color, will further subgroup them on the basis of shape and then size.

The 5-year-old has difficulty understanding that something might be included in more than one class. The child focuses on one property of the object and is unable mentally to abstract and compare two of its properties. For example, if there are five oranges and two apples in the bowl, the child will state that apples are a fruit and oranges are a fruit. When asked whether there is more fruit or more oranges, the child confidently answers more oranges. By 8 years of age, the child usually is able mentally to retain and compare several properties of an object and will answer that apples and oranges are both fruits, so there is more fruit.

Memory and attention By the time children are 5 years old, they have excellent recognition memory and can readily identify objects they have seen before. Both quantitative and qualitative memory have improved. Children at this age can recall and repeat an increasing amount of information, and the repeated information is increasingly accurate. With their developing cognitive abilities, they begin to create strategies for remembering, such as repeating the list, grouping objects, and relating an event to the situation.

Major advances in memory occur during middle childhood. The child learns to use relations to recall the sequence of observations and some social interactions. Fantasy and imitative play might help children to remember how to behave or perform certain skills. This freedom to practice remembering during play fosters better retention and practice in monitoring their memories. For example, when Sam is sent to the store for milk, butter, and bread, he memorizes the list by repeating the items several times, holding up three fingers, each one representing a different item, or by mentally visualizing the items. When he gets to the store, he repeats the list as he obtains the items. If he were to forget an item, he would attempt to remember it by repeating his original method for memorizing the list.

Although children's attention spans are short, they are able to concentrate on activities for longer periods of time. They are not as easily distracted by other children, toys, and noise. Improved attention enables them to organize the input of information better, that is, more systematically. This in turn facilitates memory retention.

Creativity The creativity evident throughout early childhood prepares children for concrete operations. As children creatively fashion their own world, they constantly modify and change the external environment to correspond to their internal world. Young children are always seeking new experiences to exercise old skills and develop new ones; they use creativity to achieve this task. Children who experience success and have high self-esteem are more adventuresome and creative. They do not relate conformity to approval to

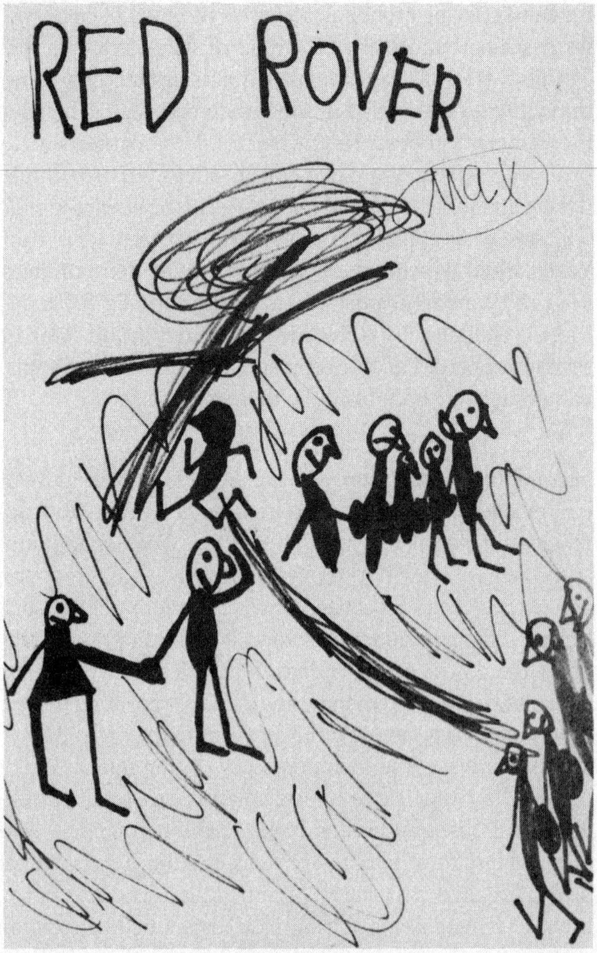

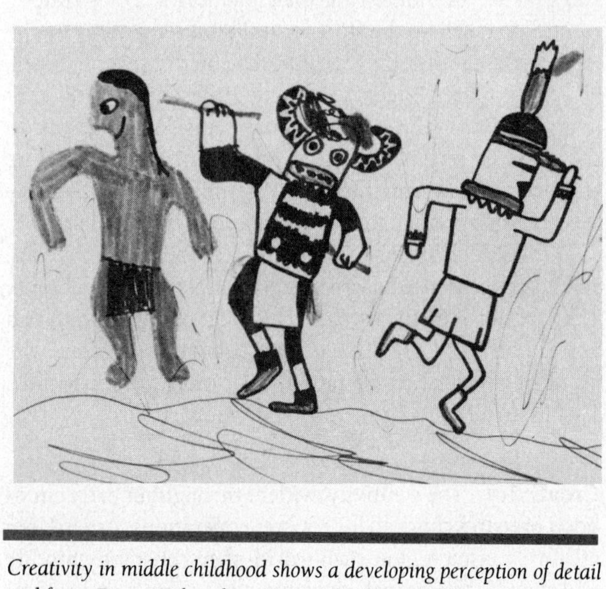

Creativity in middle childhood shows a developing perception of detail and form. Drawing done by a 6-year-old shows an elementary sense of human form, whereas drawing done by the same child two years later reflects awareness of detail in dress and position.

the same extent as do children with low self-esteem (Coopersmith, 1967).

The creative child derives pleasure from inventing a tune on the piano, such as expressing joy by lightly playing a series of high notes or expressing sadness by playing the low notes slowly and methodically. A less creative child will attempt to play a known tune rather than experiment with something new. Art is another area where the creative child expresses mood, feeling, and ideas or experiments with color and design. The more self-confidence and self-esteem children have, the freer they feel to invent, experiment, and create.

Creativity and intelligence, however, cannot be equated. Both are concepts composed of multiple parts and are difficult to define, but their focus is different. The key to fostering creativity in children is for adults to encourage flexibility, the exploration of ideas, and imagination.

A commonly held stereotype is that creativity declines with age because of social pressures to conform. As middle childhood moves toward late childhood, the manner of expressing creativity changes. Feeling and imagery do not disappear from the child's work but are complemented by realistic perceptions of the world. Spontaneity takes on more complexity in its revelation but is not decreased as the child's thinking becomes more concrete.

Language At 5 years of age, the child's language is well developed and bears a striking resemblance to what is spoken in the immediate environment. Grammatic structure and voice control of the 4 1/2-year-old match the meaning of what is said. These children have the ability to put together sentences indicating future and past tense. They can also blend sounds together, a prerequisite for learning to read. All children's speech, however, assumes the characteristics of what is spoken by their parents and other familiar adults and reflects such variables as socioeconomic class and geographic region.

By 5 years of age, the child's vocabulary increases to 2500 words and is understandable to all adults. By 6 years of age, when the child enters first grade, the child's vocabulary approaches 3000 words. Children in kindergarten and first grade use words as tools to explore the social environment of school. Additional improvements in the child's speech patterns develop as a result of the linguistic stimuli produced by television and other informal teaching media.

The increase in vocabulary is significant because words aid the child in moving away from egocentricity. Three- and 4-year-old children in particular use the names of objects to make inferences about the world. Their inferences can result in their making connections between objects and actions.

Not only parents but also other significant adults and peers influence the type of words the children use. Researchers have observed that in families where parent-child

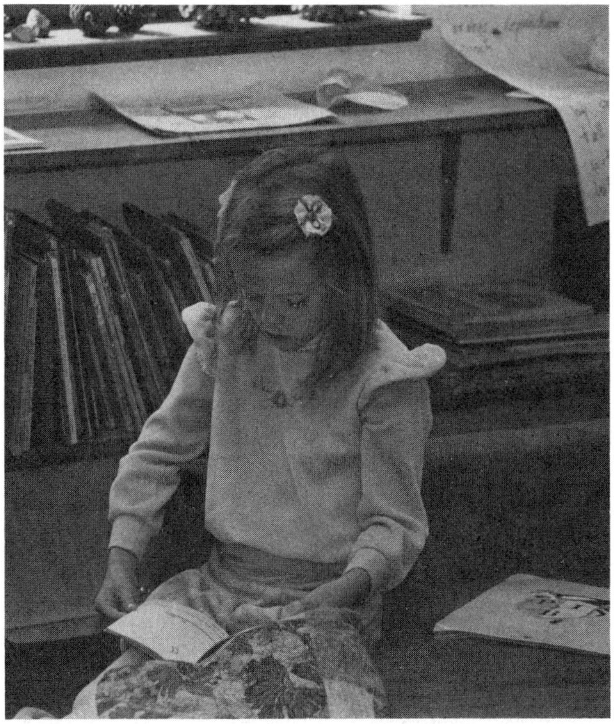

In middle childhood, the environment affects the child's developing use of language.

interactions were characterized by the parents' talking about objects rather than feelings or relationships, the child's language also reflected the parents' emphasis. Moreover, parents adjust their speech to their children's speech in their choice of topics and length of utterances (Moerck, 1976), and they adapt their use of language to their children's performance and achievement levels.

The educational level and socioeconomic status of the parents is reflected in speech. Children from better-educated and advantaged families are more likely to have larger vocabularies and be more fluent in expressing themselves. The speech patterns and words chosen when speaking to adults often are less casual and quite different from those used when conversing with peers.

Children who live in a bilingual environment usually speak one language at home and English at school. In some European countries, two or more languages are learned by everyone. Some educators debate whether the child is confused by having to learn two words and grammatic forms for everything or whether the child benefits from the intellectual stimulation such learning provides. Research with bilingual children in Geneva, Switzerland indicated that language confusion is minimal when children only speak the second language with specific people and at specific places (Dale, 1976).

Moral thinking As children progress through middle childhood, they learn, organize, and internalize the values of significant adults as a basis for decision making. Moral development is a process that involves stimulation from the social environment and transformation of cognitive thought patterns. It is more than the imprinting of rules and virtues from adults to child.

Piaget and Inhelder (1969) observed a rigid obedience to rules by children from 4 to 7 years old, as if the rules were sacred and therefore unalterable. Although these children would express an obligation to the rules of a game, they were unable to practice these rules consistently while playing the game. Their egocentricity and limited ability to think abstractly prevented them from applying the rules except by imitation.

For example, while playing a board game, Chris recited the rules exactly. When she noticed that she was behind, however, she changed some of the rules to her advantage. When confronted by her father, she claimed that she and her brother always played the game as she had redefined it. She did not perceive that she was altering the rules.

During middle childhood, the child is primarily self-centered and can consider other people's welfare only if such consideration is personally beneficial. Children in this stage behave in morally acceptable ways in the presence of enforcement agents, but they lack the internal controls necessary to act responsibly when left on their own.

Gradually, as the result of cooperative play and of the maturation of thought processes, children view rules as a code for social behavior rather than as laws handed down by some authority during middle childhood. As children gradually learn about others' perspectives, they become aware that self-perspective is different. They thus begin the process of acquiring an awareness of the thoughts, ideas, feelings, and intentions of others.

As children become able to take another's perspective, they judge the concept of wrong according to intention rather than to degree of material damage. They begin to understand that the important difference is whether someone intended to do wrong (cheat, steal, lie) rather than the extent of damage resulting from the act. Prior to 8 years of age, guilt is assigned regardless of motive. As children become able to identify with others, they start to compare intentions. Gradually, their attitudes change, and guilt is defined by intention.

With maturation, the child transfers authority from the caregiver to the peer group. At this stage, the child conforms to all the rules of the group and assumes an absolute stance when interpreting the rules of the game. The child has a less egocentric understanding of morality and experiences guilt and shame when violating the group norm.

The 7- to 10-year-old recognizes that rules are necessary to regulate the game and facilitate fair competition. Rules are no longer viewed as absolute but as flexible according to the situation. Once the rules are agreed on, however, everyone must adhere to them. Children of this age have a very strong sense of justice.

According to Kohlberg (1969), most children during middle childhood operate at the second stage of the preconventional level (see Chapter 3). "Taking care of number one" is the objective of the child at this stage. A wrong act is defined as one that elicits punishment, whereas a correct act is rewarded. The criteria used to determine right or wrong are related to cultural rules, adult responses, and the desire to satisfy the child's own needs. Children do what is expected or requested of them if it is in their own interests. For example, Tommy told his friend on the way to school that the only reason he was going to school that day was because he wanted to play outside after school. Earlier that morning his mother had warned him, when he started complaining about vague aches and pains, that if he did not go to school, he could not play outside after school. Once he heard that ultimatum, Tommy decided it was more advantageous to go to school, even though he did not feel like going that particular day.

Kohlberg's second stage of the preconventional level is also characterized by the exchange of favors, that is, "Do for me and I will do for you." Children bargain and trade with others to obtain a desired object. For example, during recess, one boy who forgot his snack was overheard making a deal to satisfy his hunger. In exchange for a cookie, he offered his friend two baseball cards. Children's motivations for doing right, sharing, and being kind are based on the positive response they receive from others.

Social Development

One of the most important aspects of development during middle childhood is learning to get along with age-mates. The child with a wholesome self-attitude feels secure enough to establish good relations with peers. Acceptance by peers is crucial to the child's development, because at this time the child's dependence begins to shift from parents to peers and community. The child's social environment expands as more contacts make possible increased involvement in activities away from the home. Not only does the child learn to get along with a greater variety of children, but the increased experiences also enable the child to begin to select as friends children who have similar interests. Moreover, social habits developed during middle childhood provide the basis for future interactions.

Learning appropriate masculine or feminine social roles is a task that begins during middle childhood after the child has a sense of gender identity. Even though anatomic differences between boys and girls are not evident until after middle childhood, expectations for sex roles begin to form the basis for social behavior. Children imitate sex roles that are expected by others for them.

Achieving personal independence by becoming less dependent on parents is another task in the area of social development. The child begins to learn that adults (parents and teachers) are not infallible and can be wrong at times. Although this process continues throughout all stages of development, children in middle childhood begin to think of themselves as future adults, making decisions about activities to perform around the home, books to read, games to play, and those with whom to play. They gradually spend longer periods away from home and might, for example, spend a night with a friend. At a relatively early stage, American children are encouraged to develop personal independence. Parents with high expectations for achievement tend to expect their children to grow up fast, get ahead, be alert, and take the initiative.

In middle childhood the child also develops attitudes toward social groups and institutions. Children learn attitudes by imitating people whom they believe to have prestige and by associating simple, deeply emotional, pleasant or unpleasant experiences with given objects or situations. Attitudes toward religious, social, political, and economic groups are formed after the child starts interacting with the world outside the family. Such attitudes are an outgrowth of experiences with the family, teachers, and peers and of knowledge gained from movies, radio, television, books, and the larger community.

Younger children (4–6 years of age) have a global, undifferentiated concept of their religious identity. They group people as either religious or not religious, basing the classification on whether or not they go to religious services. Children seem to believe that God makes people of different denominations as well as of different skin colors. The child's knowledge of religion is a combination of what significant others have said and personally formulated descriptions. These descriptions often relate to a concrete object. For example, when asked to describe or draw a picture of God, children frequently will equate God with their grandfather or an elderly friend.

The 7- and 8-year-old is able to distinguish religious fact from fantasy. Ideas about religion in this age group are based on concrete, objective experiences. They take on characteristic beliefs and observances that symbolize their religion, such as baptism, communion, attendance at church or synagogue, and observance of feast or holy days. Fowler and Keen (1978) noted, however, that although children expressed a more orderly, concrete view of the world, they also had private, speculative fantasies. They drew on this fantasy world to explain abstract concepts such as evil and events such as death. Events beyond their understanding were rationalized by assigning them to "God's power," creating a mythic and powerful character, or by expanding on an idea about space or UFOs seen on television or at the movie theater. The child is able increasingly to make sense out of the world but must rely on concrete experiences to do so.

Aggressive behavior As children progress in their social development, they might engage in certain behaviors or adopt certain tendencies that are distressing for parents. One such tendency is the use of aggression when frustrated. Many children commonly engage in aggressive behavior, such as fighting, hitting, biting, and scratching. Naturally, these activities are antisocial and not productive in building healthy relationships.

The nurse should help parents to identify what behavior is acceptable and what behavior is not acceptable. The parent then needs to make these limits clear to the child. Parents need to explore the motives for their children's behavior and attempt to deal with the underlying stresses and anxieties. During an aggressive episode, the parent might remove the child to another place to "cool off." After calm is restored, the parent helps the child to talk about the frustrations and angry feelings. The child might be reminded that angry thoughts and feelings are normal and acceptable but that acting out this anger in uncontrolled behaviors that hurt others is unacceptable. The child and parent might explore alternative coping methods when anger occurs. These might include walking away to cool off or hitting a punching bag or pillow.

Parents might be well advised to stay out of a situation unless it is obviously dangerous. By doing this, the parent eliminates parental attention as a motivation for this behavior. Children then have to resolve their conflicts within their peer group. When tempers are hot and children become irrational, however, external measures, such as removing the "out of control" child, might be the better choice.

Sibling rivalry Some children control their aggressive tendencies when with peers but are very aggressive with siblings. This sibling rivalry might be caused by daily proximity of interactions and constant competition for the attention from the same household members.

Older siblings who have been on their "best behavior" all day, perhaps even being the peace-maker or problem listener within a peer group, might be easily frustrated and react negatively to the demands for attention from younger siblings.

Parents need to be sensitive to the personal needs of their children. Parents who find time for each of their children help to minimize sibling rivalry. Children often fight to compete for parental attention but are less likely to do so if they feel individually loved and appreciated. Finding time to give each child singular attention is difficult, especially in single-parent families in which one parent must divide what time is available among the children. Time spent actively listening to the child and communicating about expectations, however, minimizes the occurrence and the severity of behavior problems.

Noncompliance Noncompliance is a child's seemingly constant refusal to cooperate. Commonly known as "not minding," this behavior can be extremely frustrating and aggravating for parents. The parents' frustration stems from their seemingly endless repetition of the same request before the child even responds. Noncompliance often begins as the child seeks independence from adults and tests limits. The behavior is an outward manifestation of the search for answers to questions about decisions the child is allowed to make, about decisions the parents make, and about the expectations and choices allowed.

Key guidelines for parents who are concerned about noncompliant behavior are setting consistent limits and avoiding power struggles whenever possible. Parents need to agree about expectations for their children's behavior and to respond consistently. Limits are provided and children are encouraged to exercise as much self-care and responsibility as appropriate. By encouraging children's responsibility for their own behavior, parents may eliminate the potential for many power struggles. When conflict does occur, parents should employ the "no-lose" method of conflict resolution, which involves mutual discussion and compromise.

Integrating Development Through Play

Middle childhood is a transitional time in which the child has gained basic gross and fine motor skills and is now in the process of perfecting these skills. Language is now used as a tool, and although language is initially limited to speech, the child at the end of this phase has learned the significance of written words.

During this time, children participate in cooperative play as they exlore their environments and learn about their cultures. Their play becomes more realistic and complex. They enact roles with greater detail and accuracy through sociodramatic play, which in turn allows the child to resolve conflicts, fill in gaps of understanding, change roles or power structures, change outcomes, or invent new problems to solve. This is a time of increased peer interaction and the challenge of learning to get along with others both in pairs and in groups. Cognitive skills are developing, and the child is entering a transitional phase of thinking. Gradually, the limitations of preoperational thought are giving way to

TABLE 6-2 Toys and Activities for Children 4–7 Years Old

Type of toy or activity	Developmental benefits
Clay	Enhances fine motor skills; teaches representations of reality
Housekeeping toys	Facilitates role play and imitation; stimulates social interaction
Tool bench	Provides outlet for aggression
Scissors and paste	Stimulates creativity and fine motor skills
Dolls	Provides vehicles for fantasy
Old adult clothes and costume box for "dress-up'	Provides opportunity for role play; stimulates interaction with others
Chalk and blackboard	Stimulates creativity, concept of erasability, writing
Storytelling by child	Stimulates self expression; stimulates imagination and fantasy
Puppets	Stimulates imagination; provides outlet for emotional expression
Punching bag	Provides outlet for anger, tension, and energy; teaches realization related to infliction of pain
Guessing games and simple races (task or physical)	Teaches coordination, organized thinking, and playing with others
Building a city of blocks	Stimulates creativity and reality representation; fosters higher levels of thinking and social interaction
Sandcastles	Stimulates creativity
Transport toys (trucks, wagons)	Teaches rules of driving and walking on busy streets; provides social interaction
Simple jigsaw puzzles	Stimulates problem solving; causes preoccupation with parts, not the whole; teaches fine motor coordination
Seesaw	Stimulates sharing, cooperation, and participation in group activities
Group outdoor trips	Stimulates social interaction and participation in group activities; play is increasingly a social activity; helps build self-confidence
Jungle gym	Enhances active play, coordination, and balance
Color books and coloring sets	Stimulates creativity; teaches colors and how to color between the lines; teaches fine motor coordination
Small pet	Encourages responsibility and social interaction with an animal
Construction toys	Teaches hand-eye coordination; stimulates creativity, invention, and use of tools (instruments and functions, specialization of functions); teaches role imitation
Jump rope	Teaches timing, rhythm, and social interaction; stimulates motor skills and balance
Bicycle with training wheels	Stimulates coordination, balance and locomotion
Simpler electronic games	Stimulates problem solving and teaches a variety of physical skills or memory skills depending on the game; a wide range of games are available
Hide-and-seek	Teaches motor skills through movement; teaches problem-solving group interaction and cooperation through collective rules; objects need not be present to be known to exist; teaches play, work, and fantasy as coequal activities

an increased awareness of objects, their transformations, and their reversibility. Numbers and letters become meaningful as they also become useful. Games with rules are increasingly important because they lend order and structure to play and provide a neutral means of settling arguments. (Tables 6-2 and 6-3 provide some examples of appropriate toys or activities and the corresponding aspects of development they promote.)

Play in middle childhood is both associative and cooperative. Children learn to share, borrow, and lend toys, and they eventually learn to cooperate with three or four people in a highly organized way. Play also contributes to the refinement of gross and fine motor skills and sensory and spatial perception, the release of emotional tension, the positive imitation of powerful others, and the development of leader and follower skills. Favorite games include tag; hide-and-seek; jump rope; rhythmic games, such as ring-around-the-rosy; farmer-in-the-dell; follow-the-leader; red-rover; and fruit-basket upset. Children's improved fine motor coordination enables them to manipulate objects

TABLE 6-3 Toys and Activities for School-Aged Children 6–8 Years Old

Type of toy or activity	Developmental benefits
Simple collection (eg, leaves, flowers, or other nature specimens)	Stimulates exploration of the environment, categorization and fine distinctions; objects may have multiple properties; child knows simple relationships between objects rather than complex relationships
Other collections	Stimulates observation, categorization, and distinctions, facilitates abstract thinking—examples include rocks, shells, insects, stamps
Magic tricks	Stimulates imagination; teaches illusion versus reality
Word games	Stimulates social communication and language skills
Books	Stimulates the development of new concepts and self-expression
Bicycle	Teaches locomotion and balance
Books and storytelling	Develops vocabulary and logic; demonstrates reversibility through storytelling; provides outlet for emotional development; fosters language skills, creativity, and social relationships
Comics	Teaches about the supernatural and quasi-real fantasy; stimulates imagination
Drama	Encourages imagination and new experiences; stimulates social planning as a group
Art	Stimulates creativity and self-expression
Group games	Stimulates competitiveness, self control, and social conformity; develops relationship to rules; teaches cooperation and prosocial behavior

such as clay, models, paints, small construction blocks, and needle and thread. From initially exploring the possibilities with these objects, they advance to the satisfactory completion of their project. At first, the clay might be pounded and rolled into a simple ball or snake, but eventually the child learns to make a bowl, basket, seal, or dog with the clay. Likewise, the threaded needle is first pulled in and out of the cloth haphazardly. Then a design is made on the cloth, and the child carefully follows the outline, creating a picture with the stitching.

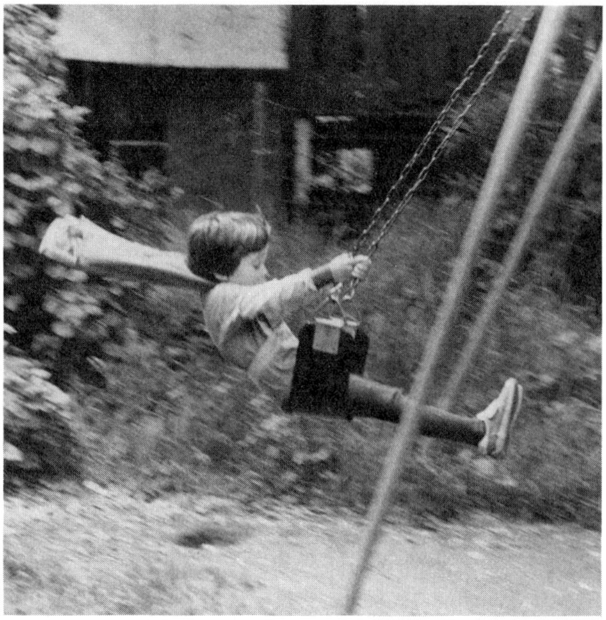

Play in middle childhood contributes to the development of motor skills while providing the child with an outlet for fantasy.

Symbolic play, in which symbolic thought is used to simulate reality, is a significant part of middle childhood. Ideas, rather than features of objects, govern the child's thinking about a particular toy. Aided by fantasy and imaginary playmates, 4- and 5-year-old children are capable of creating realms of play from a single object just by pretending. The discarded appliance box becomes a fort, clubhouse, or spaceship according to the group's desire. Once the game is decided, roles are assigned, and children imitate and create actions to correspond to their role's expected performance.

Although a few games with rules are mastered by 4 1/2 years of age, the ability to master games with complex rules rarely occurs before 7 years of age. Parents who foster inner controls in their children provide a supportive environment for their children's play activities. Children want to win, and they experience intense emotions in game situations. Parents who help their children put into perspective the short-term consequences of a game versus long-term friendships and lessons learned from being a good loser help prepare them for life experiences. Play facilitates the important developmental tasks of learning to cope with defeat, controlling one's emotions, and praising another's skills.

With adequate reinforcement for independent mastery during middle childhood, the child learns to internalize two crucial ideas: (1) the idea of self-reward and (2) the notion of standards. Self-reward allows children to praise and reinforce themselves for successes. Children also internalize the standards of the socializing agents who have rewarded or punished them. As the internalization process occurs, the need for and dependence on external social reinforcement decreases.

Health Care Needs of Middle Childhood

Hygiene

The 4 1/2-year-old child shows beginning competence in self-care, which is continually refined during middle childhood. By the time children reach 6 years of age, they are toilet trained and perform the activities associated with toileting, that is, manipulating their clothing, wiping themselves, flushing the toilet, and washing their hands. The female child should be taught to wipe from front to back (toward the rectum) after urination and defecation to decrease the possibility of introducing bacteria into the vagina or urethra.

At this age, children may be too busy with play to perform self-care activities, and parental monitoring is therefore essential. Parents must ensure that children caring for themselves properly wash their hands, face, ears, and body when taking baths. Children should not, however, be expected to give themselves complete baths until they are 7 years old. Children can dress and undress themselves when their clothing is simple and at 7 years of age can graduate to combing their hair.

Parental guidance aids children in self-care activities. Left alone, the child will wear the same clothing repeatedly. Therefore, the selection of clothing appropriate for activity and weather requires parental assistance. A child of this age can change clothes at will, but if unsupervised, the child will leave clothes wherever they were removed. This requires frequent reminders from the parent to return clothes to their correct location.

Sleep and Rest

Children in middle childhood require about 12 hours of sleep per night, particularly during the school year. Failure to obtain adequate sleep can contribute to daytime irritability, fatigue, poor attention span, and poor learning. The 4 1/2- to 6-year-old might still require a daytime nap or quiet period to restore their energy levels.

Most children in this age range dislike bedtime. They might be immersed in play or television, or they might use stalling tactics to keep from going to bed. The parent can help the child prepare for bed by setting a time limit for the child and assisting the child to meet it by issuing reminders as the time approaches for bed, enabling the child to conclude activities gradually. Incorporating relaxing activities, such as stories, religious readings, prayers, and hugs and kisses, is helpful in preparing for bed. Sharing affectionate confidences, selecting appropriate television programs that do not introduce excessive stressors, and restricting games that may be too stimulating are other measures that parents can use to encourage cooperation.

Just as children need time to prepare for bed, they also need time to prepare for the start of the day's activities. On wakening, children usually are still very sleepy and stumble around before they are fully awake. Therefore, children should be awakened early and given adequate time to get ready for the day without being rushed.

Nutrition

As children grow, their nutritional requirements change. Requirements per unit of body weight decrease while total intake increases. The 5-year-old requires about 90 calories/kg of body weight, whereas the 8-year-old needs about 80 calories/kg of body weight. (Table 6-4 lists the recommended daily food intake for children during the middle childhood period.)

Growth in this age group is slow and steady. Children need a nutritional intake that will facilitate growth and development to meet the basal metabolic needs and keep the body functioning at an optimal level. Nutrients must meet the body's growth needs, allow for cellular growth, meet cellular replacement needs, and meet cellular repair needs.

The child generally has a good appetite, likes variety, and is usually not fussy but might maintain food preferences and aversions characteristic of early childhood. A child's eating habits change with increasing maturity as table manners are learned and practiced.

The child's nutritional patterns and habits also are strongly associated with cultural and socioeconomic identification. For example, in Puerto Rican families, red beans are a common source of protein, whereas rice and fish provide protein for Vietnamese children. Several studies have shown positive correlations between the child's socioeconomic status and height and weight. Children from families with fewer economic resources or less education tend to be shorter and leaner.

Because the focus for children in middle childhood is play, they are little interested in spending time at the table eating. They frequently use their fingers to pick food up off

TABLE 6-4 Daily Food Guide for Middle Childhood

Types of food	Recommended amounts	Average servings 5–8 years	Foods included	Contribution to diet
Milk and cheese (1.5 oz cheese = 1 cup of milk; 1 cup = 8 oz or 240 g)	4 servings per day	¾–1 cup	Milk—fluid, whole, skim, evaporated; cheeses (natural or processed); ice cream	Calcium, magnesium, riboflavin, protein, phosphorus, vitamins A and B_{12}, and vitamin D, if milk is fortified
Meat group (protein foods)	2 or more servings per day	2 oz	Beef; veal; lamb; pork; variety meats such as liver and sausages; poultry; fish; shellfish; eggs. Alternates include dry beans, dry peas, lentils, nuts, peanut butter	Protein, iron, thiamine, riboflavin, vitamins B_6 and B_{12}, phosphorus, and niacin
Egg				
Lean meat, fish, poultry (liver once a week)				
Peanut butter				
Dried beans				
Fruits and vegetables	At least 4 servings, including:			Vitamins C, A, riboflavin, folic acid, iron, and magnesium
Vitamin C source	1 or more (twice as much tomato as citrus)	1 medium orange; ½–1 cup juice	Citrus fruits, berries, tomato, cantaloupe, mango	
Vitamin A source	1 or more	¼ cup	Green or yellow fruits and vegetables	
Other vegetables	2 or more	½ cup	Potatoes, legumes	
or				
Other fruits		1 medium	Apple, banana	
Bread and cereals (whole grain or enriched)	At least 4			Protein, iron, thiamine, riboflavin, niacin, vitamin E, and food energy
Bread		1–2 slices		
Ready-to-eat cereals		1 oz		
Cooked cereal		½ cup	Includes macaroni, spaghetti, rice, grits, noodles	
Fats and carbohydrates	To meet caloric needs			
Butter or margarine (1 tbsp = 100 calories)		2 tbsp	Mayonnaise, oils	Vitamins A and E
Desserts and sweets		3 portions	100 calorie portion = ⅓ cup of pudding or ice cream, 2 cookies, 1 oz of cake, 1⅓ oz of pie, 2 tbsp of jelly, jam, honey, or sugar	

SOURCE: Adapted from US Department of Health, Education and Welfare. Four food groups of the daily food guide. USDA Institute of Home Economics and Publication No. 30, Children's Bureau, 1977 and Baker S, Henry R: *Parent's Guide to Nutrition*. Addison-Wesley, 1986.

their plates, stuff food in their mouths, and swallow without thoroughly chewing. They talk with their mouths full of food and at times cause accidents. At breakfast, they eat in a hurry and sometimes rush off without completing the meal. Breakfast, however, is an important meal for this age group because the child needs a high-protein, nutritious meal in the morning to provide the energy needed to perform academically. Many children prefer fortified, ready-to-eat cereals but also should have orange juice and a protein, such as a hard-boiled egg or peanut butter or cheese on toast. These foods prevent low blood sugar, which lowers efficiency. Active children need snacks, particularly after school, and usually accept cheese, fruit, yogurt, raw vegetables with cream cheese dip, or peanut butter. Instead of soda pop, children should be encouraged to drink fruit juices, milk, or ice cream drinks, which provide quality calories and a better source of nutrients.

Once the child enters school, both peers and teachers influence the child's food consumption and provide new ideas about nutrition. Peers encourage the child to taste new foods and to assume new food preferences. Lunch might be served in school or brought from home, but the child frequently is free to select what to eat. The 6- and 7-year-old enjoys selecting food from vending machines but needs to be reminded about the nutritional value of the foods selected.

Recognizing that the child in this age group is extremely active, parents should refrain from imposing too rigid an environment at mealtime. It is important to balance teaching the child table manners with promoting a healthy atmosphere conducive to eating. The child also should be taught to select nutritious snacks, including fresh and dried fruits, vegetables, cheese, peanut butter, nuts, and granola. Snacks high in refined sugar such as candy, cookies, and cake should be avoided. Between 4 1/4 and 8 years of age, close parental monitoring of nutrition is crucial. Children need continuous nutritional supervision to obtain the right nutrients and in the proper amounts so that excess weight does not become a problem.

Dentition

Oral hygiene is part of the child's daily needs. Toothbrushing helps to remove bacteria, carbohydrates, and other leftover food materials from the teeth. If these residues are not removed, plaque forms in the child's mouth. The two methods of oral hygiene for this age period are brushing and flossing the teeth.

Using a medium-bristle toothbrush, the child should brush the teeth immediately after eating both meals and snacks. When this is not practical, the child should be taught to "swish and swallow" as an alternative to brushing after eating. The technique consists of taking mouthfuls of water and swishing it around and through the teeth to remove excess food particles from the mouth. Not until they reach approximately 9 years of age can children fully master the technique of flossing, so flossing during middle childhood should be performed by parents. Dental floss should be placed between the teeth in areas where the toothbrush cannot reach. Flossing should be done at least once per day (usually at bedtime).

Self-care activities must be promoted if children are to develop proper dental health, but until they are able to manipulate a toothbrush adequately, parents need to brush their teeth for them. The selection of a toothbrush and dentifrices is an important aspect of oral hygiene and should not be underplayed. When teaching oral hygiene, the parent should emphasize the frequency of brushing and the role carbohydrates play in the development of dental caries. Appointments with the dentist should be made every 6 months to ensure that dentition is following a normal course and to assess any need for corrective work.

Children are somewhat anxious and fearful about dentists. Parents can promote a positive attitude about a trip to the dentist so that children will be more relaxed. Parents also can monitor their children's diets to ensure adequate intakes of calcium and vitamin D, which are necessary for the calcification of teeth.

One of the most striking biophysical changes occurring during middle childhood is the process of replacing deciduous (baby) teeth with permanent teeth. This process begins at about 5 or 6 years of age. At this time, the child begins to lose primary teeth, which are replaced by larger secondary (permanent) teeth. The central incisors are the first teeth to be lost and account for the "toothless gap" appearance of many first-graders and the introduction of the myth about the tooth fairy. One first-grader felt very left out because he had not yet lost a tooth, an event regarded as a status symbol by his classmates. His greater concern, however, was that the tooth fairy might run out of money before he had a chance to collect.

Unless children are prepared, losing teeth can be very frightening. Once prepared, children view the experience very positively because they associate it with receiving gifts from the "tooth fairy" and because it indicates that they are finally beginning to enter the adult world.

The age at which children lose teeth is variable and related to genetic factors. Girls tend to lose teeth earlier than do boys. Prolonged undernutrition might delay eruption of secondary teeth. Cultural factors also play a crucial role in determining when children cut their first permanent teeth. For example, American children get their first incisors at about 6.5 years of age, children from Ghana at 5.3 years of age, and children in Hong Kong at 6.2 years of age.

The new central incisors usually appear much too large for the child's mouth and face, but as nasomaxillary and mandibular growth continue, the child assumes a more adult face to accommodate the permanent teeth. Malocclusion in middle childhood occurs when the upper and lower teeth do not meet properly in the horizontal or vertical position. As a result, the child's normal chewing and biting are impaired. A National Health Examination Survey of children between 6 and 11 years of age reported that about two-thirds of children have normal occlusion. Fourteen percent of the remaining one-third of children had problems related to appearance, chewing, or speech (Kilman and Helpin, 1983).

For the child in this age group, malocclusion develops from three major sources: oral habits, tooth crowding, and trauma. Oral habits are mainly thumb- and finger-sucking that continue after the eruption of permanent teeth. Crowding, which starts when the child is between 5 and 6 years of age, occurs when the new permanent teeth crowd out the remaining primary teeth. This situation should be monitored closely by a dentist. It might be temporary and disappear with growth and elongation of the maxilla and mandible. If crowding persists, braces might be necessary. Another dental concern during middle childhood is crossbite, that is, the lower teeth crossing over the upper teeth when the mouth is closed. This condition usually necessitates braces early, before the bones of the maxilla are fused. The braces stretch the upper jaw until the bite is corrected. Good oral hygiene is essential with braces, and gum, toffee, and caramels are forbidden.

Exercise

Children in middle childhood are constantly on the move. Exercise influences normal growth and increases the size of bones and the degree of mineralization. The child's cardiovascular, skeletal, and neuromuscular systems benefit from maximum physical activity. The child needs space to run, jump, and skip and needs freedom from parental restriction to exercise.

Even so, the play activities of children in middle childhood must be monitored. Because these children are so energetic and always willing to play, they do not always recognize their own capacities and will play continually unless asked to take breaks. The child who fails to take breaks and allow the body to reenergize can become overtired and exhausted. The 6-year-old is goal-oriented and will use energy to complete specific tasks. The 8-year-old is conservative and will plan games that permit periods of sitting and resting. Unless children are assigned rest periods, they will not normally rest on their own. Parents should learn to recognize cues of fatigue or irritability before overexertion occurs.

Transition to Late Childhood

The theme of middle childhood is the child's movement from the family to peers and community, along with growth toward independence and responsibility for self-care and decision making. New skills, maturing cognitive structures, and orientation toward others mark the child's emergence from egocentricity toward taking another's perspective. The child now is less imaginative and is able to separate reality from fantasy. Answers to questions that were illogical but satisfactory no longer make sense. Advances in cognitive thought motivate the child to find more logical, rational answers to questions about everyday reality.

The child's venture into the world of school results in meeting new friends, learning new concepts, and exploring new surroundings. The child learns to communicate through the written as well as the spoken word. Stories are created and written, and adventures and fantasies are read and then shared with others.

Physical skills and coordination improve during this stage and prepare the child for more serious competition. The social and emotional skills that are learned also prepare the child for smooth interaction with others.

For each child a unique set of genetic and environmental factors combine to foster development. During middle childhood, children learn more about their culture, religion, values, and socioeconomic status, as well as those of other groups. Supportive adults who take the time to answer children's many questions will encourage open, honest curiosity and an eagerness and pleasure in learning throughout life.

Essential Concepts

- Middle childhood is characterized by the child's movement from the home and family as a primary resource to that of school, peers, and community.
- The family remains a critical influence, although its role has changed to one of behind-the-scenes support.
- Children gain new insights and understanding about their own culture, ethnicity, and values as well as those of others with whom they play and attend school.
- The peer group becomes an increasingly important

influence, and friends are chosen on the basis of similar interests rather than physical proximity.

- Physical growth slows during middle childhood. The long bones continue to grow, which gives the child a more adultlike appearance.
- Primary teeth are lost and replaced by permanent teeth.
- The child perfects gross motor skills and uses them in combination for games, advanced skills, and competition.
- The child refines fine motor skills and uses these skills in writing, model-building, crafts, and projects.
- Characteristics of affective development are fairly well established during this developmental phase. Self-concept continues to be developed as a result of social interaction with a wider spectrum of people.
- Fears relate more to performance at school and play than to personal safety.
- At the beginning of middle childhood, the child is egocentric and possesses limited cognitive structures. By the end of this stage, the child's developed thinking allows the child to take another's perspective.
- The advance in cognitive skills is related to increased attention and improved memory.
- The child internalizes roles, values, expectations of behavior, and an understanding of right and wrong and good and evil from the words and actions of significant adults.
- Initially, the child does right (follows rules) for fear of punishment or for desire of reward; with increased understanding and experience, the child views rules as social organizers to ensure justice.
- Development of moral and religious thinking continues to be linked to concrete experience and the imitation of others.
- Aggression, sibling rivalry, and noncompliance are best handled with parental consistency, clear limit setting, and avoidance of power struggles with the child.
- Play takes on more organization, and games involve groups and early competition between teams. Gross and fine motor skills and social interaction behaviors of sharing, coping with disappointment, and controlling emotions are developed through play.
- Games that mix fantasy and reality remain popular, but now the children know where one leaves off and the other begins.
- Self-care activities related to hygiene, dress, nutrition, rest, and exercise increase as the child becomes more independent and spends more time away from home.

References

Bandura A, Walters R: *Social Learning and Personality Development.* Holt, Rinehart & Winston, 1963.

Bronfenbrenner U: *Influence on Human Development.* Dryden Press, 1972.

Coopersmith S: *The Antecedents of Self-Esteem.* Freeman, 1967.

Corbin CB: *A Textbook of Motor Development.* 2nd ed. Brown, 1980.

Dale P: *Language Development: Structure and Function.* Holt, Rinehart & Winston, 1976.

Dunn J, Kendrick C: *Siblings: Love, Envy and Understanding.* Harvard University Press, 1982.

Erikson E: *Childhood and Society.* Norton, 1963.

Fischer KW, Lazerson A: *Human Development.* Freeman, 1984.

Fowler J, Keen S: *Life Maps.* World Books, 1978.

Freud S: *The Complete Psychoanalytic Works of Sigmund Freud.* Norton, 1969.

Holm VA: Childhood. In: *The Biologic Ages of Man.* Smith DW, Bierman EL, Robinson NM (editors). Saunders, 1978.

Kilman C, Helpin ML: Recognizing dental malocclusion in children. *Pediatr Nurs* 1983; May/June: 204–208.

Kohlberg L: A cognitive-developmental analysis of children's sex-role concepts and attitudes. In: *The Development of Sex Differences.* Maccoby EE (editor). Stanford University Press, 1966.

Kohlberg L: Stage and sequence: The cognitive-developmental approach to socialization. In: *Handbook of Socialization: Theory and Research.* Goslin D (editor). Rand McNally, 1969.

Labinowicz E: *The Piaget Primer.* Addison-Wesley, 1980.

Lamb ME: *Social and Personality Development.* Holt, Rinehart & Winston, 1978.

Londe S et al.: Blood pressure and hypertension in children: Studies, problems, and perspectives. In: *Juvenile Hypertension.* Neal MI, Lechvine LS (editors). Raven, 1977.

Lowrey GH: *Growth and Development of Children.* Year Book, 1978.

Moerck EL: Process of language teaching and training in the interactions of mother-child dyads. *Child Develop* 1976; 47: 1064–1078.

Piaget J: *Child and Reality.* Grossman, 1973.

Piaget J, Inhelder B: *The Psychology of the Child.* Basic Books, 1969.

Rubinstein EA: Television and behavior. *Am Psychol* 1983; 38: 820–825.

Sutton-Smith B, Rosenberg BG: *The Sibling.* Holt, Rinehart & Winston, 1970.

Additional Readings

Birren JE, et al.: *Developmental Psychology.* Houghton Mifflin, 1981.

Bordzinsky D: Sex differences in children's expression and control of fantasy and overt aggression. *Child Develop* 1979; 50(2): 372–379.

Bullock M, Gelmen R: Preschool children's assumptions about cause and effect: Temporal ordering. *Child Develop* 1979; 50(1):89–96.

Comstock GA: The impact of television on American institutions. *J Communication* (Spring) 1978; 28:12–18.

Crain W: *Theories of Development.* Prentice-Hall, 1980.

Dudek S: Creating in young children—attitude or ability. *J Creative Behav* 1974; 8(4):282–292.

Durio HF: Mental imagery and creativity. *J Creative Behav* 1975; 9(4):233–244.

Harter S: Developmental perspectives on the self-system. In: *Carmichael's Manual of Child Psychology.* Vol IV. Hetherington EM (editor). Wiley, 1982.

Harter S: A model of mastery motivation in children: Individual differences and developmental change. In *Minnesota Symposium on Child Psychology.* Vol 14. Collins, WA (editor). Erlbaum, 1981.

Johnson TR, Moore WM, Jeffries JE (editors). *Children Are Different: Developmental Physiology.* Ross Laboratories, 1978.

Kagan S, Madsen MC: Experimental analysis of cooperation and competition of Anglo-American and Mexican children. *Dev Psychol* 1972; 6:49–59.

Kay P: The imaginary companion. Review of the literature. *Matern Child Nurs J* (Spring) 1980; 9:8–11.

Kenny SL: Developmental discontinuities in childhood and adolescence. In: *Levels and Transitions in Children's Development* (New Directions for Child Development, No 21). Jossey-Bass, 1983.

Mitchell C, Ault R: Reflection, impulsivity and the evaluation process. *Child Develop* 1979; 50(4):1043–1049.

Mitchell S: Imaginary companions: Friend or foe. *Pediatr Nurs* 1980; 6(6):29–30.

Moore K: Childhood enuresis. *Can Nurse* (March) 1984; 80: 38–42.

Piaget J: *The Child's Conception of Physical Causality.* Harcourt Brace Jovanovich, 1930.

Piaget J: *Play, Dreams, and Imitation in Childhood.* Norton, 1962.

Rapp R: Family and class in contemporary America. In: *Rethinking the Family.* Thorne B, Yalom M (editors). Longman, 1982.

Rubin Z: *Children's Friendships.* Harvard University Press, 1980.

Santrock JW: *Life-Span Development.* Brown, 1983.

Schell RE, Hall E: *Developmental Psychology Today.* Random House, 1983.

Schiamberg LB, Smith KU: *Human Development.* Macmillan, 1982.

Schuster CS, Ashburn SS: *The Process of Human Development.* Little, Brown, 1986.

Selman RL, Selman AP: Children's ideas about friendship: A new theory. *Psychol Today* (October) 1979; 9:71–80.

Chapter 7

Late Childhood

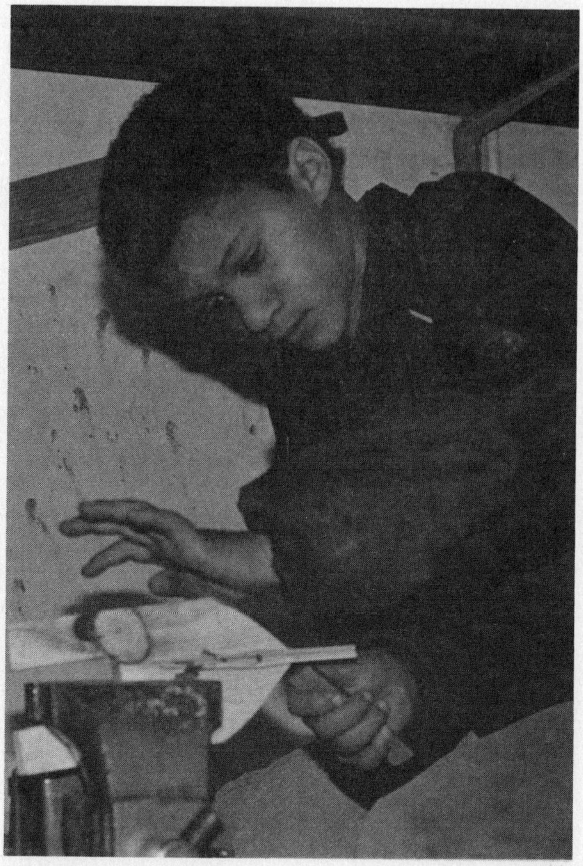

Chapter Contents

Objectives

- Explain the influences of both external environment and developmental changes on late childhood development.
- Explain the essential biophysical changes that occur in late childhood.
- Describe the principal components of affective, cognitive, language, moral, and social development in late childhood.
- Explain the purpose of play in late childhood.
- Identify the basic health care needs of children in late childhood.

In late childhood the child lives in a world of ups and downs, and transitions occur frequently and dramatically. From about 8 to 12 years of age, the child's development is a continuous, complex process. This is a dynamic period in which the child learns social skills and independence. The child moves away from dependence on the home and family and toward the growing influence of school and peer groups.

During late childhood, the child's life is accentuated by newfound independence and the ability to solve problems and plan strategies. The child's world is characterized by friendships, activities, and new experiences. This developmental stage is one of mastery, integration, and refinement of gross and fine motor skills, coupled with increased cognitive powers involving seriation, conservation, logical thinking, and space-time concepts. Children in this phase are more oriented to the world outside the home. These children consolidate their earlier psychosocial development with their present world—a world that becomes increasingly diverse and complex as they encounter new situations and people with differing opinions, attitudes, and values. Parents, teachers, and peers take on new dimensions for children during this time. Parents lose their omnipotence; peers become more important; and other adults assume greater influence.

The External Environment's Influence on the Child

Influence of the Family

The family continues to be an important source of influence, comfort, and support for the child in late childhood. The reciprocal relationship that has been developed between the parent and child remains fairly stable. Although the basic relationships continue, the child's need for attention decreases, and parents find themselves moved to the background. Now they primarily are giving guidance and support, monitoring activities, and providing assistance when requested. Parents are accepted as participants in family activities but not in peer group activities.

By 8 years of age, children no longer think of their parents as omnipotent. These children have been exposed to other perspectives, are more independent, and view their parents more realistically. They will ask their parents for advice or help with homework problems or a project, but they do not appreciate it if parents try to help without being asked or if their parents try to do the work for them. Relations between parent and child become delicate and complicated. Parents often comment that they never know when to help or how much assistance to give. The 8-year-old is torn between wanting parental advice but being unable to tolerate criticism or suggestions. Parenting takes patience and tact to gain the child's confidence during this struggle to develop a sense of industry and accomplishment. The 10-year-old is able to tolerate constructive criticism and may be self-critical. At this age, children are more independent and responsible for themselves and for completing their projects. They are also more respectful of their parents' knowledge and abilities.

As children demonstrate increased maturity and independence, their parents' expectations usually increase. Most children are given chores, which might be limited to responsibility for their bedroom and belongings or might include responsibilities for other aspects of the household. Some children need to earn money by mowing grass, shoveling snow, delivering papers, or babysitting. Whether they are expected to share that money, save it, or spend it as they desire depends on family needs and values.

Family responsibilities and peer activities may conflict, necessitating difficult decisions. For example, a 12-year-old boy was given the job of splitting and stacking some wood for the wood-burning stove used to heat the house. His friends were going sledding and urged him to join them. Although the snow was perfect for sledding and he had the fastest sled in the neighborhood, this boy knew that if the

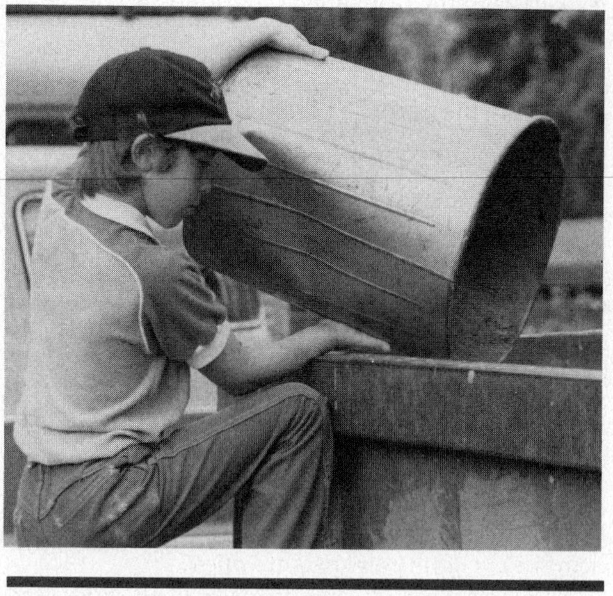

In late childhood, children are able to assume some responsibility for family chores.

wood was not split, his house would not be warm. Difficult decisions such as this become more frequent during late childhood.

Family composition can change during this period. A new sibling might be born; an elderly grandparent might move in; the parents might separate or divorce; or one parent might die. Family roles sometimes change if the mother begins working outside the home or if a parent goes to school or changes jobs. How well children adapt to these changes depends on how well they are prepared, whether they are included in family discussions, and whether they are able to understand the reasons for the change.

Once children are able to consider alternative points of view, they can perceive and respond to the needs and attitudes of others. For example, in one family the father decided to change careers, which meant that he had to return to school. Family discussions were held during the decision-making period, and the children were encouraged to voice their opinions, questions, and concerns. Although initially angry about the plan because it necessitated moving and a change in lifestyle, the 9-year-old and 11-year-old children were able to understand their father's reasoning and future goals, to place the decision within a realistic time perspective, and to look for the positive aspects of the plan.

Children whose parents separate or divorce during this developmental period seem to cope better with the experience than do younger or older children. Conflict, hurt, and confusion exist, especially during the first painful year or two following the separation. Children in this age group do not experience the strong sense of guilt that younger children feel or the sense of loss and betrayal that older children feel. The level of cognitive functioning and prior experiences enable the 8- to 12-year-old child to view the process fairly realistically, to resolve feelings of loyalty, and to assign responsibility more objectively (Wallerstein and Kelly, 1980). The end of conflict between the parents and the provision of adequate support systems, both financial and emotional, appear to be key factors in how well children cope with divorce.

Studies of the relationship between patterns of parenting and the child's self-concept have produced fairly consistent findings (Baumrind, 1965; Coopersmith, 1967). Self-confident and independent children usually have parents who are warm, supportive, directive, trusting, minimally punitive, and who provide opportunities for autonomy and responsibility. Dependent children with low self-confidence frequently have parents who are restrictive, punitive, fearful, aloof, and who provide few opportunities for autonomy or experimentation. The experiences and support that parents provide for their children are key factors in the child's ongoing social development.

Influence of the Community

To a large extent, the child's social environment is determined by the community in which the family lives, whether urban, suburban, rural, affluent, or disadvantaged. The child's schooling and leisure-time activities are likewise influenced by the environment. The values, beliefs, rituals, and goals transmitted to children from their parents reflect the family's lifestyle and experiences. Affluent children might be sent to boarding or private schools to obtain the best education available and to prepare for entry into prestigious prep schools and colleges. Children from disadvantaged communities might be struggling to mesh conflicting values between home and school.

The child's leisure activities also reflect environmental resources. Whereas certain sports, such as basketball and baseball, are more egalitarian and include children from all social strata, other sports, such as tennis and golf, necessitate expensive lessons and generally exclude those from lower socioeconomic strata. Some communities have recreational organizations that are partially supported by public funds and provide group activities and lessons. Parents from suburban communities tend to encourage their children to join clubs, take music or dance lessons, and participate in sports programs. Some children have little free time for spontaneous neighborhood play.

School By late childhood, children have developed fundamental skills in spelling, reading, handwriting, phonics, arithmetic, and arts and crafts. They have some familiarity with the natural sciences and geography (for example, students plan nutritional meals, talk about the earth and solar system, and make maps of their rooms). By 8 and 9 years of age, children's education broadens as history, social studies, and current events become part of the school curriculum. Children at this age learn to use maps, discuss distant countries and their cultures, and debate current issues.

Initially, these subjects are difficult for most students to learn. Children's personal experiences provide few examples that are similar to those of the ancient Greeks or Romans or to those of the people and governments that characterized medieval times. In addition, children who have done little traveling might know their own towns or cities but only vaguely understand the size of their states, the locations of state capitals, the names of neighboring states, and the names and locations of other countries. In late childhood, children still have difficulty relating events that happened in the past or in other locations to their present or future lives. The child therefore still needs concrete examples, often supplied by visual aids and other creative means. For example, when studying about the Far East, one fourth grade class rearranged the classroom to resemble an Oriental home. The children then invited their families to join them for a program to demonstrate what they had learned, including a typical meal prepared in advance by the children.

By 11 years of age, most children can deal with abstract concepts beyond actual experiences and can work with new problems. They therefore are able to learn about other parts of the world without the aid of models and simulated experiences.

Mathematics and geometry deal with patterns and relationships. Children learn to recognize the patterns and relationships between addition and subtraction and multiplication and division. Later, they can deal with spatial arrangements and find the areas of triangles, squares, and rectangles. Learning mathematic concepts is evident as the child begins to note these patterns and relationships outside the classroom. A child in this stage can manage an allowance, monitor game scores and players' averages, and know which glass really does contain more lemonade.

Early in this developmental period, language is a major focus. Children learn to describe events and work with numbers in both oral and written form. The acquisition of language is a vital component of more complex learning, such as problem solving and interpreting the natural and social sciences. Children need language for writing, reading and following directions, communication of ideas, and overall social development.

Children need little extrinsic prompting to learn about the natural sciences. They are inquisitive and readily ask questions about causes and effects. Among other questions, children ask about trees, insects, rain, water, rocks, life, birth, death, and sexuality. The child learns about the natural sciences through experimentation and by rediscovering what others before have discovered. Children collect insects, play with rocks, and build model cars; they explain phenomena and point out items of interest to peers and siblings.

Although children can have difficulty learning about geography, history, and current events, they demonstrate an awareness of societal problems, politics, and values. Children might not fully understand poverty or a congenital disease, but they will collect money for charities or donate a part of their allowance, demonstrating that they have learned social rules and values. They observe game rules, classroom rules, and parental rules. They detest cheating among peers. By the end of late childhood, they have developed more sophisticated notions of morality.

In some school systems, sixth grade is part of middle school, whereas in other systems, sixth graders remain in elementary school and enter junior high school in seventh grade. The transition from elementary school to either middle school or junior high school usually includes being exposed to new teaching styles, meeting new classmates and teachers, becoming familiar with a new setting, and adapting to new expectations. These schools often are considerably larger than the smaller, more familiar elementary schools, and this is a major adjustment for many children. The experiences of a sixth grader in elementary school are quite different from those of a sixth grader in middle school. One study noted that middle school sixth-grade girls were more interested in boys and had a higher level of self-esteem than elementary school sixth-grade girls (Yussen and Santrock, 1982). Conversely, elementary school boys had a higher level of self-esteem, but there was little or no difference in their interest in girls. This finding corresponds to the difference in the onset of puberty between the sexes. The more adolescent-like atmosphere of middle school promotes the girls' earlier developmental changes. In fact, sixth-grade girls might begin telephoning boys and arranging for mixed-group activities. Boys, especially those who are late developers or who are shy or immature, might find this transition difficult. Status among boys frequently is measured by physical strength or athletic ability. As they compare themselves to the older boys in middle school, feelings of inferiority might increase in sixth-grade boys, whereas in elementary school they are the oldest and usually the strongest and most competent in sports.

Peer groups Peer groups are an important aspect of development during late childhood. Children spend more and more time with their peers. The 8- to 10-year-olds spend most of their time with peers of the same sex. The 11- and 12-year-olds begin to venture into activities and organizations in which both sexes participate. Most children find that doing things with another person, especially a best friend, is far more fun than doing things alone. Two boys found that mowing grass changed from a weekly chore to a fun activity when they did it together. Some children prefer to have one or two close friends, whereas other children are happiest in a crowd.

Children acquire much information about themselves from peer interactions. They also learn that to have friends, they have to be a friend, that is, be trustworthy, empathetic, happy, and modest. For example, one 9-year-old girl was feeling lonely and sorry for herself because her best friend was away at camp for the summer. One day while riding her bike around the neighborhood, she stopped to help a girl who had fallen. Although she initially did not know this girl, she soon discovered that they were the same age and both lonely (the injured girl was new in town). The summer brightened for both as they discovered mutual interests and learned from each other. When the other girl returned from camp, they became a happy trio.

The peer group is also a strongly influential group that controls its members by promoting conformity to group norms, style of dress, and activities. As 8- to 12-year-olds assume responsibility for hygiene practices, they become interested in their appearance. Interest in current fads and fashions becomes a favorite pastime and is fostered by the mass media, which beckons children in this age group to buy and wear designer jeans, shoes, and other status symbols. The urge to conform, which is so much a part of socialization in late childhood, makes the children a ready target for such marketing efforts.

Developmental Changes in Late Childhood

Late childhood is a time to learn to interact with others within the greater society. Most adults in the United States view childhood as a time to learn and have fun before being required to take on many responsibilities. Although parents and children do have differences during this time, adult expectations and peer norms coincide more frequently than they conflict. An adult who expects a child to do well and who provides honest encouragement and support helps the child to develop a positive self-concept and self-esteem. Children also need to relate achievement to their own efforts. Social experiences during late childhood are of critical significance to the adolescent's and adult's orientation toward achievement. (Table 7-1 summarizes biophysical development and developmental characteristics of late childhood and provides some guidelines for assessment.)

Affective Development

Self-concept Self-concept, the mental picture of oneself formed in the process of growing and developing, is composed of psychologic, sociologic, and physiologic experiences. Children learn about themselves through self-exploration, comparison to others, and response from others.

As the child's environment broadens to include both home and school, the child might be subject to feelings of inadequacy and inferiority. For instance, a child might note that other children speak better, run faster, and perform more effectively. Children might ostracize peers who are exceptionally slow or exceptionally bright. Children who have actual or imagined limitations can develop negative self-concepts because they do not meet the expectations of themselves or others. Even wearing corrective glasses can lead to a disturbance in the body image.

Children who fail to develop positive self-concepts require a greater degree of physical stimulation (Blaesing and Bruckhaus, 1972). These children often meet this need independently through rocking, clapping hands, and initiating other stimulating actions. A positive self-concept emerges for those children who develop friendships and are able to perform physical and cognitive tasks at levels relatively equal to their peers. Self-concept in late childhood is closely related to gender, and gender-role identification develops from an increasing awareness of self-concept. Sexual self-exploration and comparison of one's genitals with another's helps to sharpen self-concept as well as sexual identity. As multiple body changes begin to occur at the end of late childhood, the emerging adolescent focuses much attention on the body.

Sexuality Human sexuality denotes not only physical actions but also includes the concept of self-identity. Freud (1962) believed that late childhood is a period of continued sexual latency. Latency is characterized by the suppression of sexual impulses and channeling of energies into the acquisition of new skills, learning new roles, mastering educational tasks, and developing moral and ethical standards.

Freud did not equate latency with complete cessation or lack of sexual activity but noted that sexual impulses are present throughout late childhood. Although the child learns to deny the direct sexual or instinctual gratification, masturbation, thumb-sucking, and other sensual activities can persist. Tension and frustration might induce sexual impulses. Tackling a difficult task or studying for an examination might stimulate the child sexually, but the child might react with disgust, shame, and guilt when these impulses are overt.

TABLE 7-1 Guidelines for Assessment of the 8- to 12-Year-Old Child

Developmental area	Expected characteristics	Assessment techniques
Temperament		Assess the child's temperamental characteristics and parental perceptions Ask how easily the child becomes upset and how the child responds to disappointments, being teased, and new experiences
Biophysical development		
Body proportion	Begins to exhibit adult body proportion	
Weight—average gain is 3–3.5 kg (5–7 lbs) per year	Average (50th percentile) *Girls:* 24.5 kg (54 lb)–41.8 kg (92 lb) *Boys:* 25.4 kg (56 lb)–40 kg (88 lb)	
Length—5–6.4 cm (2–2.5 in.) per year	*Girls:* 127 cm (50 in.)–152.4 cm (60 in.) *Boys:* 127 cm (50 in.)–149.8 cm (59 in.)	
Neuromuscular	Head reaches 95% of adult size	
Gross motor skills	Does tricks on bikes; has races; begins to use bike for transportation	Ask questions to elicit child's interest and participation in sports; dance lessons, and physical activity
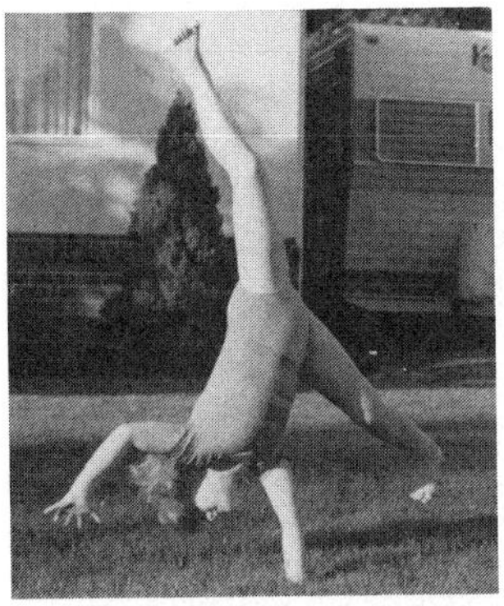	Increased skill fluidity, and control of skipping, running, hopping and jumping actions; running spead increases to 5 m/sec, broad jump distance reaches 4–5 ft, and vertical jump height measures 8–10 in.; adept at tree climbing; learns to shinny up a rope Improves swimming and adds new strokes Continued improvement in coordination and ability to participate in organized competition, either individually or as a team member Increased stamina, identification and practice of individual skills	Observe or inquire about the child's coordination in running, skipping, jumping, climbing, or hopping Question the child's perception of ability and performance in physical activities Ask the parents about their expectations in relationship to the child's performance and participation in activities
Fine motor skills	Fluent printing of numbers and letters in correct alignment; cursive writing improves Uses tools increasingly well; more advanced art, carpentry, and crafts projects	Ask child about writing skills; may have child print or write name Ask the child and parent about crafts, artwork, and other projects that might be hobbies or special interests
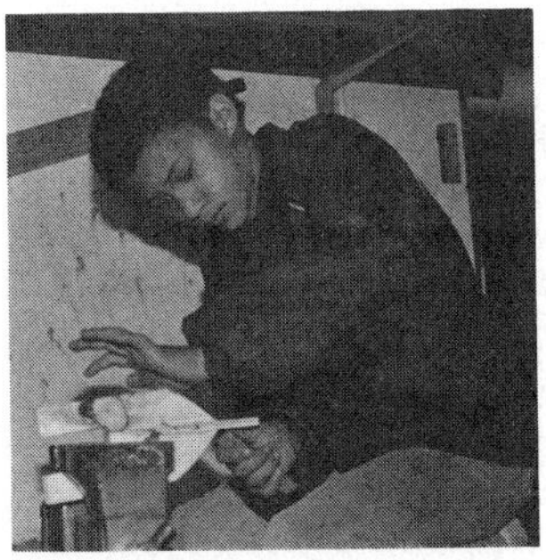	Increased precision and speed in manipulating small objects into place, such as stamps in an album; improved skill and finger dexterity in playing musical instruments Can catch and/or intercept pathways of small balls when thrown from a distance; throws ball overhand and underhand	Ask what the child can do best when playing ball and what aspect (throwing or catching) needs work
Cardiovascular		
Heart rate	Approaches adult norms	
Blood pressure	110–115/60 mm Hg	
Respiratory	Lung tissue matures and tidal volume doubles	
Respiratory rate	17–22 breaths/min	
Gastrointestinal	Achieves adult functional maturity	
Genitourinary	Bladder capacity increases; girls might begin development of secondary sex characteristics (rare in boys of this age)	

TABLE 7-1 Guidelines for Assessment of the 8- to 12-Year-Old Child *(Continued)*

Developmental area	Expected characteristics	Assessment techniques
Immune	Lymphoid tissue decreases; allergies are frequently seen and might be severe	Allergy testing (see Chapter 25)
Sensory-perceptual		
Vision	20/20; possible growth spurt of the eye might result in myopia (nearsightedness); ocular muscle movements, peripheral vision, and color discrimination fully developed	
Language development—expression and comprehension	Increased expansion of oral vocabulary to 7200 words; greater use of language for socialization; reading vocabulary of 50,000 words; speech is entirely understandable; improved grammar and correct use of parts of speech; uses language to solve problems; talks through options before making a decision	Listen to the child's speech and use of grammar and syntax
	Oral and written stories become more logical; characters and events are described in detail; able to create suspense; uses metaphors and personifications; gives precise, dictionary-type definition to words	Ask the child to relate some event in school or at an after-school activity; note sentence structure, objectivity, and whether the story is told logically
Cognitive development	Major advancement in ability to do more complex intellectual tasks; improved attention fosters focusing on details	Ask the child about school and ability to listen and follow directions; might use drawing of four objects, each slightly different, and ask the child to identify the differences
	Wants to acquire large store of facts because they're useful and interesting; enjoys reading the Guinness World Record books; may focus on a special interest; multiplication and division concepts fairly well mastered; uses numbers beyond 100 with understanding; uses and understands simple fractions	
	Gathers factual information for reports from a variety of sources; is interested in learning about foreign places	Ask the child and parent about the types of books the child enjoys reading
	Makes change for small amounts of money	
	Develops strategies and uses a greater variety of memory aids, including rehearsal and organization	Ask the child to recite the Pledge of Allegiance; show a box with ten objects, then cover the box and ask the child to name as many objects as possible; ask the child to explain the method used for remembering
	Skeptical of "realness" of television and radio programs	Ask the child if events that happen on a favorite program are real and why
	More sophisticated sense of humor; uses double meanings and metaphors; enjoys riddles; begins to read comics in newspaper	Ask the child to repeat a riddle or joke and assess the type of humor
	Concrete operational to beginning of formal operational thinking; able to perform additional mental operations of conservation of area, weight, and solid volume	Use the Piagetian task for conservation; might use two clay balls—roll one into a sausage shape and ask the child if the amount of clay has changed; ask the child if the weight of the clay balls has changed
	Has acquired additional operations of class inclusion, hierarchy of representation; seriation tasks presented verbally are accomplished by 12 years of age	Ask the older child a representation question, "If Karl's red shirt is darker than Matthew's, and Karl's shirt is lighter than Adam's, who has the darkest shirt?"

TABLE 7-1 *(Continued)*

Developmental area	Expected characteristics	Assessment techniques
	Understands relationships among time, speed, and distance; still uses trial-and-error approach to problem solving but is more logical in approach; has difficulty verbalizing answer; considers two and maybe three factors by 12 years of age but may omit the fourth factor	Provide the child with a small balance and series of weights; request the child to position the weights so that the sides balance, then ask the child why it balanced and how things are related
Affective and social development		
Child	Better able to take another's perspective; focuses on the intention of a behavior rather than on the act itself; follows conscience in decision making; obeys rules because they are instrumental; expects favor in return, views rules as instruments for own or other's satisfaction of needs	Tell the child about someone who cheated by going out of turn while playing a game because of wanting to win so badly and someone else who won by forgetting a penalty and ask what should be done; assess how the child solves the problem and the use of rules
	Social environment expands with activity; involvements, friends outside of immediate neighborhood; peer group influences become stronger; usually same-age, same-sex peers	Ask the child to name and describe friends and their favorite activities
	Increase in new authority figures with organized club and team membership; increased interest in sociocultural differences; tends to categorize peers according to skills; more selective in friends—chooses friends who have similar interests and skills; friendships usually loosely knit for boys and more tightly knit for girls	Ask the child and parent about the child's adjustment to school, new expectations from teacher, ability to relate to children of different backgrounds
	Self-critical; proud of accomplishments; refuses to accept recognition perceived as undeserved	Assess the child's demand on self to do well
	More invested in hobby or collection	Ask the child to describe any hobbies or collecting; assess interest and use for self-concept
	Gradual improvement of social manners but might use selectively	
	Able to assume more responsibilities but tends to argue about what parents expect done; constant comparison with peers	Assess the verbal interaction of the parent and child
	Self-concept redefined in relation to peer's and new authority figures' perspectives; self-esteem related to self-perception of skill mastery; able to delay gratification; controls and expresses emotions more appropriately and takes responsibility for own behavior; fears more appropriate and reasonable, such as exams, school or sport performance, or personal failure; fears body injury or pain	Have the child describe self; note the statements that indicate positive or negative attitudes about self
	Understands human reproduction	Ask the child about reproduction and differences between the sexes, and note the child's understanding of facts
	Understands health concepts	Ask the child why someone gets sick and note the child's response and understanding of realistic, logical, or scientific cause-and-effect relationships

At 8 or 9 years of age, children are no longer satisfied with simple answers about sexuality and reproduction. They want to know about respective male and female roles and often will wait for an appropriate time and then ask a barrage of questions about birth and procreation. Because late childhood is characterized by a concern for body image and integrity, it is also a time when children become concerned about how birth occurs. They might have been told that the baby leaves the mother through an opening, but even until 9 years of age, some children believe that babies are born through the mother's abdomen. The older child wants explicit information and will ask peers if unable to obtain this information from parents.

Sexual awareness and curiosity increase for both sexes. Children are more exposed to nudity, sexual innuendos, and behavior from television, music, radio, and movies than their parents were. The implications of increased exposure and decreased restraint concerning topics related to sex are open to speculation. In some families, children feel freer to ask questions and discuss with their parents what they have heard or seen. Parents can then clarify or correct any misconceptions. In other families, children feel embarrassed to mention sexual issues, especially if they think their parents might disapprove. Among peers, children share information, giggle, whisper, or create codes for words dealing with elimination and sex.

The age at which pubertal changes begin varies considerably. Eleven-year-old girls might or might not evidence signs of breast development. The early-maturing girl might attempt to hide her breasts by wearing large sweatshirts or loose blouses, whereas the late-maturing girl observes her with envy, dreaming of the day when she will be able to wear a brassiere. Boys experience few pubertal changes during late childhood, although some boys experience initial growth in their genital organs.

As they begin to experience changes in their bodily appearance, personality traits, feelings, and moods, children become more interested in the relationship of these changes to puberty. Sometime before puberty and usually around 10 years of age, children need to be given the basic information about menstruation, intercourse, and reproduction. Although it is best that they get this information from their parents or responsible adults, most youth acquire their knowledge about sex from peers.

Self-esteem Self-esteem becomes increasingly important to children as their growing cognitive powers permit them to gain and master new skills. A child's feelings of self-worth can be encouraged by (1) a high degree of acceptance by family and others, (2) clearly defined and consistent limits, and (3) flexibility within those limits to permit individual activity. Depending on their self-esteem, children will differ in their reactions to new situations, praise, or criticism. Children with high self-esteem can accept criticism, feel more confident, and usually think they will be successful. Children with low self-esteem will demonstrate opposite behaviors.

During late childhood, the child's feelings of self-esteem are influenced by many factors. Parents and teachers are influential persons during this time. They help children learn acceptable behavior by directing children's energies into constructive activities. Although children need encouragement and praise from significant persons, even more important is their own evaluation and sense of satisfaction in their personal development.

Erik Erikson (1963) called this phase of development "industry versus inferiority" and viewed it as the "entrance into life." This developmental stage is marked by the child's determination to master particular tasks and experiences that enable more competent, more accomplished, and less dependent behavior. The concept of industry is delineated by self-control, cooperation, and compromise, which go beyond playful expressions.

Children are proud of their accomplishments and want to be recognized for them. Erikson suggested that the child forms basic attitudes toward work during this period in response to systematic instruction provided by society. Such instruction often includes the skills, such as reading and writing, needed to become a useful, productive member of society. Children are eager to learn at this stage, and successful learning increases their self-esteem.

Children are motivated by peer approval and by such extrinsic stimuli as grades, material rewards, and privileges. It is not only important to be able to manipulate the environment but is also essential to do so successfully. If children do not succeed in accomplishing these tasks, they develop a sense of inadequacy or inferiority, often losing status among their peers. This experience might discourage them from identifying with peers and others in society.

Erikson proposed that unsuccessful or delayed resolution of this psychosocial crisis results in the child acquiring a sense of inferiority. Difficulty achieving a sense of industry might reflect incomplete resolution of previous psychosocial crises or limited parental support and encouragement for independent behaviors.

For example, the only recognition that satisfied one 10-year-old girl was the occasional praise she received from her mother. To her, it seemed that everything her mother did was perfect and that everything she herself did, whether it was making her bed, baking a cake, running a race, or writing a story, made her susceptible to criticism. She labored over simple projects for hours to earn a rare positive comment from her mother. She therefore had little time, energy, or interest in exerting similar efforts to obtain recognition from others. She also discounted praise received from others if her effort had not been affirmed by her mother.

A sense of inferiority also might occur if children feel defeated. Children with a sense of inferiority might never finish a task for fear of failing or will sometimes be afraid to try mastering a new task for fear of being shamed. How children perceive their success or failure at mastering certain tasks depends on the reinforcements provided by significant persons. As children begin to master any task, they need both constructive criticism and positive reinforcement from parents, teachers, and peers. In this way, they acquire a sense of accomplishment and self-esteem during this period.

Lack of self-esteem, Erikson pointed out, also might be caused by the child's constricting the world and focusing entirely on mastering one particular skill, such as playing a musical instrument, and thereby neglecting relationships with other people. Ideally, the environment provides a balance between mastering developmental tasks or skills and strengthening interpersonal skills. Without this balance, the child might develop a poor self-concept and a sense of inferiority, which will lead to difficulty in mastering the tasks of adolescence.

Independence Late childhood is a period during which the child makes great strides toward becoming independent. Increased cognitive power, coupled with refined gross and fine motor skills, provides the necessary tools for becoming self-reliant. During their struggle for independence, however, children are extremely dependent on their families for encouragement and support.

During late childhood, a child can assume more responsibilities that are relatively complex. A gradual increase of responsibilities helps children learn new skills and gain confidence—both vital to developing self-reliance and becoming independent. In addition, learning to be responsible for completing chores and assignments creates a sense of being a contributing member of the family. This sense of belonging provides a prelude for becoming a cooperative, reliable, and productive member of society.

At times, attempts to be independent and self-reliant meet with frustration and failure. These episodes should be viewed as potential growth experiences rather than as lost opportunities. For example, one 11-year-old boy worked hard one summer mowing grass. By the end of the summer, he had earned over $100. His parents told him that he could decide what he wanted to do with his money. Initially indecisive, this boy spent a considerable portion of his savings on a spur-of-the-moment trip to an amusement park with some of his friends. He had a wonderful time and considered the money well spent until a month later when he wanted to buy a new bike. He wished that he had not spent his money so freely at the amusement park when he discovered that he did not have enough money left to purchase the bike he wanted, and he realized the consequences of spending his money without first considering the options carefully. The experience provided a good lesson in making decisions as he learned to take responsibility for his actions. Because the decision had been his, he could not blame someone else, and although frustrated, he accepted the outcome.

Cognitive Development

Concrete operations During late childhood, a transition in thinking and problem solving occurs. The child begins to develop what Piaget called *concrete operations.* This transition appears after the child has demonstrated the ability to represent mentally what has been perceived and to view the self and actions objectively (Piaget and Inhelder, 1969). Concrete operations, which relate directly to objects and not to ideas or hypotheses, concern the child's grouping of actions, objects, and events according to general coordinating structures and relationships. The attainment of concrete operations, along with the decrease in egocentricity and increase in language skills, allows the child to think, act, and interact at a more sophisticated level.

The child's ability to group falls into the following categories (Piaget and Inhelder, 1969):

1. *Closure or composition grouping*—two or more classes can be combined to produce a general inclusive class. For example, children might combine cats and dogs into the class of animals and apples and oranges into the class of fruit.
2. *Tautology grouping*—a class can be added to itself to yield the same class (for example, apples plus apples equals apples). This type of action, however, does not hold true for numbers (for example, 2 plus 2 equals 4, not 2).
3. *Inverse relationship or reversibility grouping*—once formed, a class is reversible (that is, can be transformed back into their original, less-inclusive classes). The child who has mastered this concept is able to subtract when addition was previously performed or divide when multiplication was carried out (for example, fruit minus apples equals oranges). Reversibility, a factor in effective problem solving, enables the child to anticipate the results of actions.
4. *Identity grouping*—a class united with its opposite is obliterated. This type of grouping is apparent in sub-

traction (for example, ten apples minus ten apples equals zero apples). Grouping by identity operates in the concept of conservation. The child learns that 10 oz of water is 10 oz of water whether the water is in a short, wide glass or a long, thin glass.

5. *Association grouping*—three or more elements can be combined in any manner to produce the same result. For example, $(2 + 1) + 3 = 2 + (1 + 3)$. The child thus understands the properties of addition but at 8 years of age might not yet know that this grouping does not hold true for all actions, for example, $3(3) - 2 = 7$, but $3(3 - 2) = 3$.

Classification Children in late childhood learn to classify items according to shared characteristics. The child can easily divide classes into subclasses and thus can form a hierarchy. For example, when presented with groups of animals, children can construct the following hierarchy:

- Animals
  - Dogs
    - Beagles
    - German shepherds
  - Cats
  - Rabbits

They also can respond correctly to questions such as: "Are there more beagles or more dogs?" "If all the dogs ran away, would there be any animals left?" "Are rabbits and cats both animals?" and "If all the animals died, would there be any rabbits?" Eight- and nine-year-olds are able to construct hierarchies only when they can visualize the actual objects, whereas 10- to 12-year-olds can construct hierarchies when given verbal representations of the objects.

The ability to classify and sort items indicates that the child can identify a concept and mentally represent the concept prior to taking action. When children under 7 or 8 years of age are asked to sort items according to shape or size, they approach the task by comparing one item with another and rarely look at the whole. Children who have mastered concrete operations, however, examine the whole and consider more than one concept at a time to arrive at a decision. As the child's operational skills increase, double classifications become common (that is, classifications that are based on more than one shared characteristic, such as size and shape or function and color).

Classification is manifested in many of the activities of children. Most common is the proliferation of collections in late childhood: stamps, baseball cards, stickers, posters, seashells, records, T-shirts, postcards, coins, and magazines. In school, children learn to classify countries according to geographic location, population, type of government, economics, and natural resources.

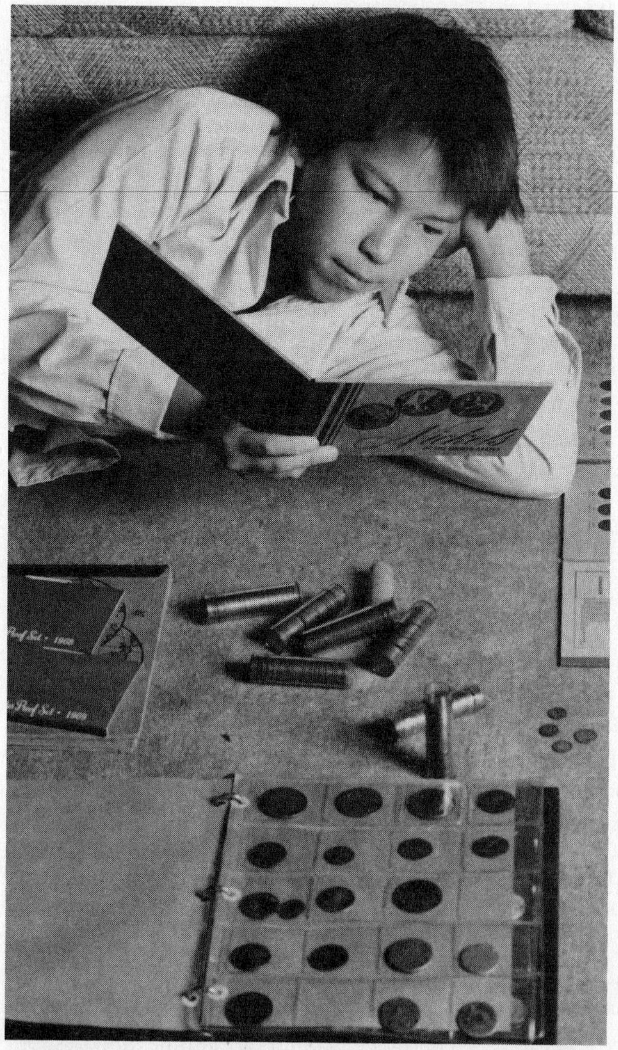

Coins are just one of the many things collected in late childhood.

Seriation Prior to 7 or 8 years of age, children learn to build a limited sequence of objects in successive, related pairs. In late childhood this process develops into seriation, in which objects and events are arranged and related according to distinguishing characteristics (Piaget and Inhelder, 1969).

For instance, children often rank members of their peer group according to toughness or degree of success in a given sport. They select members of a baseball team on the basis of seriation and often line up in school in an order based on height. In school children learn to read maps, interpret graphs, and compare gradations in color intensity, all of which require viewing the whole, comparing the items, and arriving at a conclusion. With increasing skill, the child begins to seriate in more than one dimension or with more than one set of characteristics.

Conservation The concept of conservation is one of the complex operations that is progressively mastered during late childhood. By 8 years of age, children understand the concept of conservation of liquid. Experiments using the conservation of weight, however, demonstrate that this operation is not learned until 9 or 10 years of age (Labinowicz, 1980). At 11 or 12 years of age, children recognize that volume is conserved regardless of the size or shape of the container, and the 12-year-old does not merely know that volume has been conserved but also can explain the concept of conservation.

Understanding the concept of conservation is essential if the child is to perform mathematic skills, solve problems, and comprehend other operations involving space, time, movement, and speed. In problem solving, children need to recognize how different combinations or equivalents can be used. One child who collected coins, for example, learned the concept of conservation by determining how many and which types of coins were equal amounts of money.

Numbers At 7 or 8 years of age, the child learns to use numbers to measure quantity, weight, time, and space through classification and seriation. After the child perceives that each number has a meaning, regardless of the various characteristics of the elements, the child is prepared to examine relationships that are expressed numerically. The child can tell time, manipulate numbers for solving mathematic problems, and understand monetary figures, making it possible to go to the store and purchase an item independently or manage an allowance.

Space, time, movement, and speed With the ability to classify, seriate, conserve, and comprehend the meaning of numbers, the child begins to examine the concept of space, an understanding that remains limited during most of late childhood. Not until 12 or so years of age does the child usually come to appreciate space as an abstraction.

Children first learn to make spatial measurements by dividing a line into segments and measuring the distances between them. Children in late childhood comprehend geometric space (that is, the measurements of length and angles) but cannot incorporate space successfully into their activities. A child might, for example, understand that a given triangle consists of two smaller triangles, but when attempting to replicate the triangles precisely, the child fails because applying concepts still requires a concrete object for reference.

Children learn to appreciate proximities, distances, openness, closedness, and the coordination of positions. They learn to read and draw maps. They deal with geography and astronomy in school and, by 9 years of age, can appreciate projections (Piaget, 1962). The child can imagine or draw shadows, the projections for simple objects, sticks, disks, and rectangles and by 11 and 12 years of age can draw more complex objects.

In late childhood, time is initially sequential and purposeful. The child at 7 years of age is time conscious and likes to wear a watch, and within a year is acutely aware of time. Up until 9 years of age, the child uses time to plan the day, and with maturation, time becomes a conceptual measurement for planning not only activities of daily living but also future events.

As soon as time becomes a functioning operation, the child can comprehend the concept of speed (Piaget, 1970). First, the child merely assumes that a moving object is in motion longer than another if it has traveled a longer distance. Using the concept of time, however, the child can view motion temporally. The child then understands speed as a function of time and distance.

Intelligence and creativity The increased capacity for logical thinking enables children at this age to respond to a situation as a whole rather than to the part affecting them. In describing a science experiment such as a pendulum problem, they accurately describe the results of each trial regardless of who did it. They vary the length of string, the weight, and occasionally the point of release to determine which variables make the pendulum swing the fastest. Although they are precise observers and no longer view the impetus of the swinging action as the contributing factor, they have difficulty systematically eliminating variables to arrive at a conclusion.

The child's conclusions are the result of multiple trial-and-error attempts to find by chance which variable makes the difference. Gradually, the child learns to deal with multiple stimuli of varying complexity. Initially, the child can deal only with abstractions that resemble actual experiences, but eventually, the child understands representative concepts removed from actual experiences.

The 8-year-old develops an appreciation for logical reasoning and the implications of events and actions. At 9 years of age, the child is intrigued with details and at 11 years of age is inquisitive. Eight- and nine-year-olds can understand the physical sciences, but these children do not grasp more complex concepts, such as morality, social relationships, and death, until 10 or 11 years of age. As children grow older, they manifest the intellectual ability to deal with abstractions—an intellectual ability that is developed further in adolescence and adulthood.

Intelligence has numerous different facets. Piaget defined intelligence as the qualitative changes that occur in the child's thinking as a result of maturation and experience. Psychometricians measure intelligence quantitatively by means of various tests. Definitions of intelligence therefore vary depending on the aspect being studied. Wechsler (1958) defined intelligence as "the global capacity of the individual to act purposefully, to think rationally, and to deal effectively with the environment."

Intelligence seems easier to define than to measure because it is strongly influenced by the environment, home, culture, and school. During late childhood, various group tests are given in school to assess the child's ability to perform at grade level and the appropriateness of advanced placement. A major problem in intelligence testing is cultural bias. In general, the tests reflect the vocabulary and culture of the educated, middle-class, white society. Children from minority and low-income groups score lower even with nonverbal tests because subtle cultural biases influence the child's performance. Although widespread testing continues, psychologists and educators are quick to point out the limitations of standard intelligence tests. The narrow range of cognitive functioning that is tapped by such tests relates primarily to the content taught at school. Many other facets of intelligence, such as social adaptability, everyday problem solving, and general work performance, are not tested. If administered and interpreted carefully, intelligence tests are useful measurements of one aspect of the child's mental capacity. They are abused, however, when they are used to label children.

Some children who demonstrate intellectual superiority and academic achievement in school participate in special programs. These programs usually take one of three forms: enrichment, grouping, or acceleration. Enrichment programs seek to broaden the child's academic experience to include advanced courses, independent study, and exposure to the fine arts. Grouping is the same concept as "tracking," a plan that groups children of similar abilities together. Although this might benefit the better students, it deprives the others, often minority and disadvantaged children, from the classroom stimulation provided by the questions and discussions of these more academically adept students. Acceleration occurs when the student skips a grade or compresses a grade into a semester.

Another component of intelligence and one not measured by the standard tests is creativity. Creativity is illusive; historically, some of the world's most creative individuals were thought to be unable to learn. Perhaps this mistaken judgment was made because their inquisitive minds took them beyond the basic, simpler answers requested by their teachers. Today, educators often try to foster creativity, and exercises in creative thinking are part of many classroom activities. Brainstorming and playing with improbabilities are two techniques frequently used to foster creative thinking. Both of these techniques encourage the free flow of ideas, release from conventional answers, and freedom to fantasize.

Creativity can be stifled if not allowed expression. Children need to be permitted, and even encouraged, to follow through with their ideas. Teachers and parents who provide opportunities for creative expression sustain an atmosphere that supports curiosity and investigative problem solving, skills beneficial for learning during adolescence. Putting words and sentences together to form poems, rhymes, and stories is a manifestation of creativity. The following was written by a 9-year-old.

> Snowfights
> fun, exciting
> turning faces red
> ducking, dodging, and throwing
> Exciting.

Memory During late childhood, the child uses short-term memory frequently in school. For example, the child looks at a word and repeats the spelling. If short-term memory were the only way to remember, however, the child would lose the ability to spell the specific word. Long-term memory therefore allows the child to learn and store information. Long-term memory requires organizing information into a purposeful form, a process called *encoding*. Encoded information may be retrieved when external or internal stimuli are matched appropriately.

By late childhood, information can be organized as concepts, visual representations, and verbal complexes. Thus, the 10- to 12-year-old is able to retrieve information to apply to new situations. Long-term memory is crucial for the child to succeed in school and at play. Words, numbers, concepts, and rules must therefore be encoded so that they can be retrieved when needed.

Cognitive conceit *Cognitive conceit,* a feeling of great pride in intellectual achievements, is a manifestation of the child's new cognitive powers (Elkind, 1974). In early and middle childhood, prior to concrete operational thought, children perceive adults as powerful, omnipotent beings. During late childhood, that aura of power begins to dissipate. Children are delighted when they discover that their parents or teachers can make mistakes, and they take this discovery a step further with the notion that all adults are stupid or foolish. For example, a teacher who makes a little mistake in the class might cause the children to roar with almost uncontrollable laughter.

Cognitive conceit is also evident in children's stories that

TABLE 7-2 Jokes and Riddles of Late Childhood, Classified by Type of Language Ambiguity

Type of ambiguity	Joke	Riddle
Lexical (word formation)	"Order! Order in the court!" "Ham and cheese on rye, please, Your Honor."	"Why did the farmer name his hog 'Ink'?" "Because he kept running out of the pen."
Phonologic (speech sound)	"Waiter, what's this?" "That's bean soup, ma'am." "I'm not interested in what it's been, I'm asking what it is now."	"Why did the cookie cry?" "Because its mother had been a wafer so long."
Surface structure (regrouping of words to give two meanings)	"I saw a man-eating shark in the aquarium." "That's nothing. I saw a man eating herring in the restaurant."	"Tell me how long cows should be milked." "They should be milked the same as short ones, of course."
Deep structure (two different relations between noun and verb possible)	"Call me a cab." "You're a cab."	"What animal can jump as high as a tree?" "All animals; trees cannot jump."

SOURCE: Adapted from Gibson J: *Living: Human Development Through the Lifespan*. Addison-Wesley, 1983.

are made up, read in comics or books, or seen on television and in movies. Adults play inconsequential roles in stories in which superheroes are featured. Children perceive themselves as having all the answers and skills necessary in life, whereas adults, those bungling fools, lack those talents.

Language A child's language at the beginning of late childhood differs from an adult's because of dissimilar patterns of thought, a less sophisticated vocabulary, and fewer experiences to draw on.

By 8 years of age, children begin to depend more on speech and use fewer gestures to communicate. Using the telephone becomes a social activity. Children might play with language, and they sometimes make up words or speak pig latin. At 8 years of age, children begin to put order into their storytelling, and at later ages they narrate events in order and use appropriate pronouns.

During late childhood, children encounter and learn new words and concepts. They master complicated sentence structure, and they make fewer grammatical errors. Vocabulary increases rapidly, partly because of the more advanced reading level and exposure to new words within the context of familiar ones. Children 9–12 years old are more adept at spoken language than younger children because older children are more prone to ask questions about what is unfamiliar. Older children also have developed the ability to use concrete operations and can analyze and interpret language. At the end of late childhood, spoken language resembles that of adults.

Schooling facilitates the child's use of language, especially as a means of exchanging and processing information. The child uses language to give meaning to the properties of objects. Language enables the child to explain the rationale for a decision, the rules of a game, or the steps for conducting a science experiment.

During late childhood, the child comes to understand many of the inconsistencies in vocabulary and sentence structure of the English language. Mastering these ambiguities of language and sentence structure sets the stage for jokes and riddles. (Table 7-2 shows how these ambiguities are used to create humor.) This improved comprehension of word usage enables children to manipulate meaning and structure to their advantage. They delight in creating riddles and repeating traditional ones.

Moral thinking During late childhood, the child's cognitive and moral development evolve simultaneously. Prior to late childhood, children are confined by external sanctions, where rewards or punishments govern their behavior. Adults are assumed to be right, and there is little understanding of the reasoning behind certain judgments. The older child now is able to judge an act with some reasoning. For the first time, a child can see beyond the result of an action.

Piaget (1965, 1969) observed that the child's concept of justice progresses from a rather rigid idea of right and wrong to the notion of equity in moral judgments. A progressive idea of egalitarianism evolves from 8 to 11 years of age. In making a judgment, the older child takes into account the interpretations and viewpoints of others. Still governed by rules, these children now have more insight into the rationale for rules.

Children begin to demonstrate their understanding of right and wrong in all aspects of their lives. For the 8-year-old, lying is a natural means by which to protect one's self-interest. The 8-year-old definitely knows that certain acts result in punishment. The child therefore avoids punishment by lying, but the lie is not an intentional, planned deception. For example, two sisters were describing their afternoon of neighborhood play experiences. The older sister described in detail how her younger sister had not shared her ball and had teased one of their friends. The younger sister, aware that punishment follows when rules of conduct are broken, explained the incident quite differently and blamed the afternoon quarrel on their young friend. At 10 years of age, the older sister had a better understanding of the importance of the need to tell the truth. The 8-year-old viewed truth-bending, or lying, as a way of stating her perspective and thereby avoiding punishment.

The older child also relinquishes egocentric thought processes and learns how to relate to others. Through experience in cooperative activity, the child develops an understanding of the rationale for rules. Prior to playing a game, these children will spend considerable time reviewing the rules to establish mutual consent. They no longer consider themselves submissive to rules but create and use rules to organize the game and ensure fair play. During this period, children tend to be more forgiving as rules of conduct focus on cooperation or mutuality.

Continuing with Piaget's work, Lawrence Kohlberg studied cross-cultural moral development and noted that children from 8 to 12 years of age tended to demonstrate characteristics of his third stage, "interpersonal acceptance of 'good boy, nice girl' social concept," and fourth stage, "the 'law and order' orientation." These two stages, part of Kohlberg's defined "conventional level of morality," suggest that up to about 10 or 11 years of age, children seem to interpret right and wrong according to physical consequences or the power of authorities (Kohlberg, 1969). From 8 to 10 years of age, moral development consists of seeking and gaining approval.

Children during this time also seek to establish and maintain good relationships with their peers, teachers, and families. From 10 to 12 years of age, children's moral reasoning is characterized by concern for showing respect for authority and for maintaining rules and social order. They view rules more objectively and genuinely understand their implications.

When questioned why they have to go to school, the responses of children who reason at Kohlberg's third stage demonstrate their concern for doing what others expect of them. For example, one boy stated simply that he went to school because everyone expected him to—his friends, parents, and teachers. Being good is important and that means being kind, showing respect, helping others, obeying, and being trustworthy. A child thinking at Kohlberg's fourth stage will add that school attendance is part of obeying the law. As one boy commented, "whether you like it or not, you have to attend school until 16; that is the law." Doing right is related to observing laws. Upholding the law is viewed as a social duty and one way of contributing to the good of society.

Because laws are made by adult authorities, these people are highly respected. During late childhood, children often claim that they want to be like a teacher, minister, coach, or club leader. They daydream of what they would do with such power if they were in a similar leadership position or if they were parents.

Religion Eight-year-olds might still subordinate the religious attitudes of peers to those of their family (Fowler, 1974). They conceptualize God or the Supreme Being as having human characteristics—sometimes as a kindly, benevolent being who grants their requests when they are good and at other times as a judge who doles out punishment for wrongdoing. The 11- and 12-year-olds are exposed more to different religious beliefs and tend to question the rightness or wrongness of beliefs that differ from theirs. They usually seek advice from some authority figure, whether their minister, Sunday school teacher, or youth group leader.

These children often find it difficult to resolve conflict in belief systems because they are striving for acceptance and conformity in other parts of their lives. They resolve this conflict either by dismissing all other beliefs as wrong and being convinced that theirs is the only true religion or by excluding religion as a basis for their friendships.

Social Development

During late childhood, children want to be accepted by their peers, and they feel that friendships are important. By 8 years of age, children have best friends, most often of the same sex. As the child approaches adolescence, friendships with the opposite sex reappear, and gangs of friends begin to form.

Competition and compromise Competition appears among all children, regardless of culture, at approximately 6 years of age. Competition is highly valued and vigorously encouraged in Western technologic society—so much so that a child who cannot compete because of physical or mental limitations is labeled nonfunctional. During late childhood, children must learn to deal with the forms of competition that are accepted within their society. These range from such competitive situations as the spelling bee in school to team sports. Children like to set up situations where they either win or at least meet their self-prescribed goals. When children play together, the child who expects to win usually sets up the challenge. In the game of "hide and seek," for example, the child who volunteers to be "it" usually expects to find everyone.

The alternative to competition is compromise, which means give and take. Through compromise, children learn the rules of the game and understand that they will sometimes win and sometimes lose. Children often make their own rules and require strict adherence to those rules within either the game or the relationship. Reciprocity is typical in late childhood, and "If you do this for me, I'll do this for you" is a common comment. In this way both parties define themselves as winners and therefore maintain self-esteem. Children's rules involve strict adherence; those who break the rules are "cheaters," and fights between cheaters and noncheaters are common.

With compromise also comes cooperation, which is essential for a child's developing sense of industry. Compromise and competition should be balanced so that neither becomes a troublesome trait. The person who is only competitive and feels a vital need to be ahead of everyone else will have problems with social functioning, as would the person who is always willing to defer to almost anyone.

The very competitive child frequently is intense and self-demanding in all that is undertaken, whether the undertaking is a game, schoolwork, or home project. Highly competitive individuals appear to be engaged in a constant struggle to obtain an unlimited number of poorly defined rewards from their environment in the shortest period of time. Highly competitive persons are often willing to work, if necessary, against the opposing efforts of others.

Siegal and Matthews (1983) hypothesized that there are four general ways that parents, teachers, and health care personnel can help children alter some of these highly competitive behaviors, especially excessive anger and overachievement. First, children should be advised to exercise, to eat a balanced, low-cholesterol diet, and not to smoke. During late childhood, children begin to eat more meals away from home and experience peer pressure. Knowing what foods and activities are good for them and having adult support and role models as guides will help them in the decision-making process. Second, these children should be guided to identify appropriate times and settings to be competitive. They might need to learn to have fun. For example, one boy who was an excellent swimmer and on a youth swim team had to learn to have fun swimming. Whenever he went swimming, he wanted either to race or to challenge someone in long-distance swimming. With guidance, he realized that it was healthier to limit competition to the practices and swim meets and to enjoy water games and relaxed swimming with his friends.

Third, these children need assistance in formulating well-defined goals. Characteristically, they tend to push themselves beyond their abilities, strength, and endurance because the activity has no defined goal or identifiable end. For example, a sixth grader who stayed up later and later each evening to complete her homework was tired and grouchy during the day. On investigation, her parent discovered that she was doing not only her homework but also some extra-credit work. She and her parent discussed family expectations and academic achievement concretely and together set well-defined, reachable goals. Fourth, these children need help in identifying and dealing with anger in constructive ways. When challenged, they tend to respond aggressively and impatiently in an attempt to control the situation. They benefit from learning relaxation techniques (see Chapter 16).

Two other factors contributing to social development during this period are social subordination and social accommodation (Sullivan, 1953). *Social subordination* is a redefinition of the authorities to whom the child must answer. At this stage, the family is no longer the only authority, and other authorities, such as teachers, counselors, or crossing guards, have become a part of the child's environment. These people have limitations on their authority, however, and children must understand their power and how this differs from family authority at home. *Social accommodation* is the process by which children learn that the environment consists of people different from each other and from themselves. Children first label such differences as right or wrong but begin to learn to approach a person or situation with some degree of flexibility.

During this time, however, children's social accommodation is incompletely developed, and they are often cruel to other children who are considered different. Children with eyeglasses or dental braces, those who are poor students or clumsy athletes, or those whose skin color, name, religion, or style of dress varies from that of the majority are common targets for ridicule.

Through social accommodation, children form peer subgroups, such as clubs or gangs. These may facilitate socialization, or they might generate rebellion against parental figures or other authorities. Children at this time often discover what other children can or cannot do, what they can get away with, and what they get punished for. They see differences in their peers' parents' expectations that they never imagined could exist. Children now integrate competition, compromise, social accommodation,

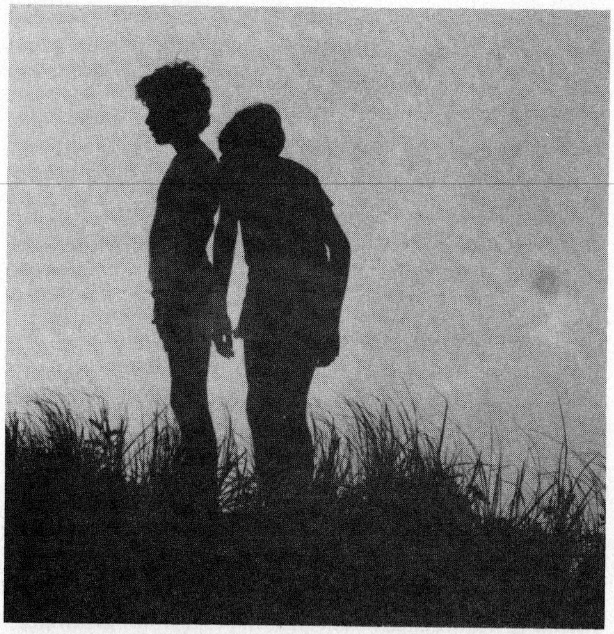

Late childhood is a time of close same-sex friendships, which are part of the process of social accommodation.

and social subordination into their personal development, and they gain a more accurate and realistic self-concept.

Solitude and social interactions At times during late childhood, the child needs solitude and respite from a complex and changing world. At other times, social interactions are crucial to development and survival within the growing number of groups that involve the child. Most children seek moments of solitude through such activities as reading, playing in their own rooms, or fantasizing in private. Social interactions vary depending on the child's environment and companions; interactions take place at home, on the playground, or in school. Social interactions are a testing ground for children's newly acquired skills, and each child handles interactions in a characteristic way. Whether timid or aggressive, each child incorporates both solitude and interaction into social development.

Developmental tasks Developmental tasks define what behaviors and skills the child is attempting to accomplish while growing up in society. A *developmental task* is something that the child must learn during a specified time of growth and development to have happiness and success in the future. The principal developmental tasks of late childhood are gaining mastery over one's own body and developing intrapersonal and interpersonal skills (Havighurst, 1972). The specific developmental tasks that define this stage are as follows:

1. Learning the physical skills necessary for ordinary games
2. Building wholesome attitudes toward oneself as a growing person
3. Learning to get along with age-mates
4. Learning an appropriate masculine or feminine role
5. Developing fundamental skills in reading, writing, and calculating
6. Developing the concepts necessary for everyday living
7. Developing conscience, morality, and a scale of values
8. Achieving personal independence
9. Developing attitudes toward social groups and institutions

Mastering one's body is important to the child's self-image. Children concentrate on developing the dexterity and control needed to master new tasks or skills. Late childhood is a time when children ally themselves with those most like themselves. Same-sex peers become increasingly important as children develop their feminine and masculine roles. Now that the once-rigid differentiation in gender-related roles has been replaced, children of both sexes are encouraged to participate in activities according to their interests and abilities. For example, many Little League and soccer teams are composed of both boys and girls. In school and organized clubs, everyone is required to learn sewing, cooking, and carpentry.

Integrating Development Through Play

During late childhood, play strengthens the child's self-concept, self-esteem, and emerging sexuality. Play, alone or with peers, provides an environment in which a sense of industry can develop. The child takes pride in new tasks mastered in play; for example, riding a bicycle as well as or better than peers promotes self-concept, self-esteem, and a sense of industry.

Organized play can promote or diminish a child's self-esteem. There is little more humiliating than always being the last one selected to play a team sport, and such a child usually is categorized as having little talent or few friends. This child learns to dread organized sports and might develop a sense of inferiority. On the contrary, being the first child selected or being the team captain who does the selecting provides the child with a sense of accomplishment and affirmation.

TABLE 7-3 Toys and Activities for Children 8–10 Years Old

Type of toy or activity	Developmental benefits
Table games	Teaches ability to apply rules; stimulates competition; promotes higher level of thinking
Construction sets	Stimulates creativity and problem solving
Complex collections	Stimulates ability to classify objects systematically; enhances movement of thinking from myths to science and logic; teaches that the world has order
Sports activities (team play)	Teaches ability to apply rules; provides outlet for energy and reduction of tension; encourages fair play and teaches importance of team effort; stimulates large muscle development; teaches cooperation and prosocial behavior
Magnifying glasses	Teaches that objects known to be one size can seem to be larger
Puzzles and mental games	Helps child move from inductive to deductive reasoning
Reading	Teaches new concepts and stimulates logical and sequential thinking
Bicycle riding	Enhances large muscle development and balance
Electronic games	Stimulates curiosity and problem solving

Fantasy during this stage becomes a vehicle with which the child considers new roles. Daydreams and make-believe play allow children to be heroes or heroines and superstars. Goals and wishes are attained through fantasy.

Play also maintains and promotes cognitive, social, and physical skills (Tables 7-3 and 7-4). During late childhood, the social component of play takes on a new dimension. Interest develops in group play as children join baseball and soccer teams, Boy or Girl Scouts, Boys Club, Girls Club, 4-H clubs, as well as nonstructured group play. Team sports help to develop the sense of competition and compromise as children learn to work together to accomplish a goal. If the team wins, each child feels responsible, and self-esteem is enhanced; if the team loses, self-esteem need not be hampered because team members can commiserate over the loss together.

Toys and Activities for School-Aged Children 10–12 Years Old and Older

Type of toy or activity	Developmental benefits
10–12-year-old children	
Collections	Teaches classification of objects and similarities and distinctions
Books	Increases reading and language ability; teaches implications of sentence structure versus individual words
Construction sets	Enhances creativity; stimulates problem solving and imagination
Board games (cards, chess)	Teaches fair play and competitiveness; play becomes more intellectual and experimental
Team games	Teaches rules, fair play, and team effort; teaches how to be fair and adhere to established standards; rules become more variable and complex and play becomes more intellectual
Parties	Provides interaction with others, including those of the opposite sex; develops notion of social position and roles; sometimes reduces tension but can be very difficult for shy children
Swimming	Enhances large muscle development
Cooking	Teaches creativity and self-expression
Sewing	Teaches creativity, imagination, and self-expression
Carpentry	Enhances self-expression, creativity, accomplishment and imagination; enhances fine motor skills
Electronic games	Enhances problem-solving and decision-making skills
Movies	Enhances ability to concentrate; peer activity
12-year-old and older children	
At these ages, most, but not all, children reach the level of formal operations. In many instances, children will, after reaching this, participate in board games, sports, hobbies, and other activities shared by adults	

Health Care Needs of Late Childhood

Hygiene

Children 8 years of age and older are capable of carrying out personal hygiene practices daily. They can be held responsible, in varying degrees, for bathing, grooming, and dressing. Because brushing teeth, cutting nails, and cleaning under nails require manual dexterity, however, children up to 9 years of age still might need assistance.

At 8 years of age, children are busy with play and other activities and might need to be reminded to carry out hygienic practices. Some children choose to assert their independence with noncompliant behavior involving personal hygiene. They might refuse to brush their teeth, take showers, or change their clothes from one day to the next. Parents who are concerned about the cleanliness and attractiveness of their children might find that they need to discuss these issues with the children and clarify decision-making responsibilities. Most often this apparent disdain for cleanliness is the outward evidence of the child's search for independence in decisions of a personal nature. Parents might find solace in learning that this behavior is epidemic in this age group.

By 9 and 10 years of age, many children can assume full responsibility for personal hygiene. They can select their own clothes and place soiled clothing in the proper receptacle. Many children by 11 and 12 years of age, and especially girls, become conscious of fashionable clothes and hair grooming.

Sleep and Rest

Despite their abundance of energy, children in late childhood do tire and need to restore and repair their bodies. The 8-year-old needs about 10–11 hours of sleep each night. Bedtime is usually at 8 or 9 PM, although children seldom fall asleep immediately. Some children read, daydream, or talk privately before drifting off to sleep. Others might want a parent to read a story or tuck them into bed. In the morning they awaken spontaneously.

As they grow, children deny or are unaware of the need for sleep. The child might resist bedtime to finish an activity or go to bed later than a younger sibling. Bedtime is progressively delayed, so that although the 8-year-old might go to bed at 8 PM, the 9- or 10-year-old might not go to bed until 9 PM. By 10 years of age, less sleep is required, and in some households 10-, 11-, and 12-year-olds have the same bedtimes as the adults. By 12 years of age, the child also resists going to bed less and enjoys quiet, private moments. From 8 or 9 years of age on, listening to the radio or reading a book becomes a common presleep activity. Although sleep time is delayed, children might waken purposefully early so that they can play alone, watch television, or read before going to school. By late childhood, the child's awakening time depends on bedtime and on personal preference.

In general, sleep is peaceful during late childhood. Occasional nightmares are often the result of a scary television program or event. Children often independently choose not to watch a scary television program to avoid nightmares.

Nutrition

Nutrition during late childhood is no longer closely monitored by the parents. The child, whose world has expanded and who spends more time outside the home, is influenced by others' eating habits and dietary intake. Children in this age group begin to determine their own nutrition.

Mealtime is a social event. The child still enjoys eating with the family and, by 10 or 11 years of age, might help prepare part of the meal. Children particularly enjoy preparing recipes learned at school or taken from cookbooks written especially for children. The child gradually learns table manners and might criticize the manners of others, especially those of younger siblings.

At school, friends are also meal partners, and children frequently share or swap parts of their lunches with their friends. Because conformity is the social norm, a child usually wants to buy lunch at school if friends do.

Children have definite food likes and dislikes, but by 8 years of age, they will try new foods or foods previously not liked. In general, children prefer plain foods to gourmet foods, but as they mature, their food likes resemble those of adults.

By 8 years of age, children have greater appetites, and by 10 years of age, their appetites are similar to those of adults. Despite their increasing appetites, children seldom voluntarily interrupt play and other activities for meals. If unsupervised, they might either neglect to eat a meal or simply grab high-carbohydrate, high-fat snacks until the next meal, which diminishes their appetite for it. Sometimes they are so eager to return to their game or to meet a friend that they hurry through their meal, not taking time to eat a well-balanced diet or satisfy their bodily needs. When hunger and fatigue return, they might become irritable and disagreeable, or they might resort to snacks, usually of the high-carbohydrate, high-fat variety. Poor eating habits might result in obesity, a fairly common problem during late childhood that is often related to replacing balanced meals with frequent empty-calorie snacks.

To promote growth and development, children need at least four servings of milk and cheese, three servings of meat and eggs, four servings of fruits and vegetables, and four servings of breads and cereal. Boys and girls between 8 and 10 years of age require approximately 2400 calories per day. Boys over 11 years of age require an additional 400 calories per day. (Table 7-5 compares the physical indicators of a well-nourished child with those of a malnourished child and notes the deficient nutrient.) The nurse can use this information when teaching the child and family about meal planning and the components of good nutrition.

Dentition

During late childhood, the permanent teeth erupt, and therefore, dietary and hygienic habits in this period will have a lasting effect on the teeth in later years.

Dental caries (cavities) are common in late childhood. Plaque, a film composed of bacteria and waste products, forms and hardens on tooth enamel. The accumulation of plaque attracts fermentative carbohydrates and provides bacteria with a nutritive environment in which to grow. The interaction of plaque, carbohydrates, and bacteria promotes tooth decay. Plaque is removable. If the plaque has been allowed to harden, a dentist or dental hygienist needs to remove it, but because plaque does not harden immediately, frequent toothbrushing might remove a large portion of it.

Children should be taught to brush their teeth after meals and snacks and to use dental floss between their teeth once a day. Frequent brushing is rarely practiced either by children or by their adult role models, so that children up to 9 or 10 years of age need to be reminded to brush and floss their teeth and taught how to do both properly. Children under 10 years of age often lack the manual dexterity to brush the posterior teeth correctly; therefore, parents should assist.

Fluoride in toothpaste and fluoridated water impede tooth decay. Children should be taught to use an appropriate toothpaste and encouraged to drink fluoridated water. Children's diet and eating patterns also should be carefully monitored. Snacks should not be overloaded with soda pop, dark chocolate, cakes, and cookies. Snacks composed of carbohydrates and sugars should be followed by toothbrushing. Frequent dental screening and early treatment of problems will help keep the child's teeth healthy.

Exercise

Most children engage in sufficient physical activity to support normal structure growth. Many children walk to and from school, participate in various sports, or play games that involve running, climbing, jumping, or bike riding. In addition, some schools have a daily exercise program in which all students perform progressive sets of exercises. Physical activity increases mineralization and bone width, which are important for both muscle and skeletal strength.

Attitude, interests, and habits regarding exercise are developed during childhood. Active children often become active adults, whereas inactive children become sedentary adults. The types of activities children choose are related to the social systems in which they participate. Peer pressure, adult expectations, and role models influence values and behavior. A child with a talent for a particular motor skill will not develop it if the peer group spends its free time playing video games at the neighborhood arcade. Parents still need to supervise their children's activity to ensure a balance between active exercise and quiet pursuits. Children benefit when parents support them in their activities. They usually want to have family members watch them participate in races or ball games. If parents are unable to attend, the child is eager to tell them about the race or game afterward.

The child experiences physical, cognitive, and social maturation between 8 and 12 years of age, which contribute to improved coordination, speed, understanding of events, and ability to plan strategies. Activities and expectations must coincide with development. Children often place unrealistic demands on themselves to perform beyond their abilities. They need to be recognized for the skills they demonstrate, not criticized for something that is beyond their ability to perform. Parents, too, must have realistic expectations of their children's abilities, making sure that the child does not become discouraged and feel inferior. This pressure for excellence might be as strong for video or computer games as for competitive play or organized sports.

Transition to Adolescence

The theme of late childhood is the child's growing independence and responsibilities for self-care, decision making, and perfecting motor skills. Late childhood is also a time for learning new combinations of physical skills and mental powers and for understanding the successes and failures of human life. It is a time when adults outside the home exert an increasing influence on children, and peers take on increased value.

During late childhood, children attempt to master the roles and responsibilities needed for socialization in their culture, with the comfort of knowing they can still enjoy

TABLE 7-5 Physical Indications of Nutritional Stress in Late Childhood

Physical aspect	Well-nourished child	Malnourished child	Deficiency
Height and weight	Within growth norms—steady gain and increase from year to year	Above or below growth norms—failure to gain or excessive weight gain each year	Protein, calorie, other essential nutrients
Skin	Clear, smooth, elastic, and firm	Rough, dry, scaly, xerosis	Vitamin A
	Reddish-pink mucous membranes	Petechiae, ecchymoses, poor wound healing	Vitamin C
		Depigmentation of skin	Protein, calorie
		Lesions	Riboflavin
		Dermatitis, sensitivity of skin to sunlight	Niacin
		Pallor	Vitamin B_{12}, iron, folacin
Musculoskeletal	Well-developed, erect posture Shoulder blades flat Arms and legs straight	Head sags, winged scapula, bowed legs, costochondral beading, cranial bossing	Calcium, vitamin D
	Skull and jaw well developed	Epiphyseal enlargement of wrists	Vitamins D, C
	Firm muscles with good tonus	Small, flabby muscles, muscle weakness	Phosphorus, protein
	Moderate amount of fat	Faulty epiphyseal bone formation	Vitamin A
		Pretibial edema bilateral	Protein, calorie, thiamine
Head	*Hair*—smooth, good amount, lustrous	Dull, dry, depigmented, abnormal texture, easily pluckable, thin	Protein, calorie
	Eyes—clear and bright	Dull with dark circles and hollows. Bitot's spots, conjunctivitis, xerosis, night blindness (nyctalopia), light sensitivity (photophobia)	Vitamin A, riboflavin
	Mouth—pink, moist lips; pink, firm gums; full set of teeth	Cracking and scaling lips, cheilosis, fissuring of mouth corners	Riboflavin
		Spongy, swollen gums, bleed easily (gingiva)	Vitamin C
		Irregular or missing teeth with cavities; defective tooth enamel	Vitamin D, A
		Glossitis	Folacin, B_{12}, niacin, iron
		Tongue fissuring	Niacin
Neck	Normal size	Enlarged thyroid	Iodine
		Enlarged parotids	Protein, calorie
Neurologic		Listlessness	Protein, calorie
		Loss of ankle- and knee-jerk reflexes, motor weakness, sensory loss	Thiamine
		Headache	Niacin, thiamine
		Polyneuritis, motor weakness	Thiamine
Abdomen	Flat	Distended, protrudes, hepatomegaly	Protein, calorie
Cardiac	Normal heart size and sounds	Cardiac enlargement and tachycardia	Thiamine, potassium

SOURCE: Pearson GA: Nutrition in the middle years of childhood. Copyright © 1977 American Journal of Nursing Company. Reproduced with permission from *Matern Child Nurs* (Nov/Dec), Vol 2:6.

being children at the same time. Through school, play, and interpersonal relationships within the home environment and the outside world, children perfect the first steps they took as younger children to walk into adolescence with a sense of accomplishment, self-esteem, independence, industry, and affiliation.

Essential Concepts

- Late childhood is a time of coordinating, perfecting, and using the skills gained through earlier experiences and a time of learning and increased independence as the child spends more time away from home at school, clubs, lessons, and play.
- Peers become constant companions, selected on the basis of similar interests, compatible personalities, and traits such as honesty and trustworthiness.
- The child interacts increasingly with the community, learning in the process that the beliefs, rituals, and values other subscribe to might differ from the child's.
- The family remains a significant influence in the child's life, but it moves to the background as peers and other adults assume greater importance.
- Biophysical growth continues at a steady, although slower, pace. Most organs have reached maturity in structure and function. Motor skills are expanded and refined, enabling the child to perform more complex tasks.
- Major changes occur in the child's cognitive thought processes. Piaget refers to this stage as the concrete operational phase.
- Late childhood is characterized by a general decentering of cognitive thought processes. The child can take the perspective of another and can reverse or reconstruct the events or problem to reach a solution.
- Children use language to express thought, explain the logic they used to solve the problem, and communicate new knowledge.
- During late childhood, operations of seriation, class inclusion, reversibility, and conservation of length, weight, and volume are mastered.
- Long-term memory improves during late childhood, allowing children to use and apply previously learned material more efficiently.
- Moral and religious thinking advances to include the social implications of behavior.
- The child in this phase spends much energy completing projects and accomplishing goals. Success is judged by the recognition received from others.
- Self-esteem grows when the child is successful in some endeavor; feelings of inferiority grow if success and recognition are not attained.
- Children with high self-esteem are more autonomous and creative and less likely to conform.
- Sexual awareness increases, as does the need for accurate information about pubescent changes and reproduction.
- Responsibilities increase as children participate in household chores.
- Health care maintenance becomes the child's responsibility. Children in late childhood make more decisions about nutrition, and they eat more and more meals away from home.
- Late childhood is an active and generally healthy phase. Basic exercise habits and endurance, as well as attitudes toward exercise, are formulated.
- During late childhood, children learn more about themselves, their interests, and abilities and begin to prepare for adolescence.

References

Baumrind D: Parental control and parental love. *Children* 1965; 12:230–234.

Blaesing S, Bruckhaus J: The development of body image in the child. *Nurs Clin North Am* (Dec) 1972; 7:560–592.

Coopersmith S: *The Antecedents of Self-Esteem.* Freeman, 1967.

Elkind D: *Children and Adolescents: Interpretative Essays on Jean Piaget.* 2nd ed. Oxford University Press, 1974.

Erikson EH: *Childhood and Society.* 2nd ed. Norton, 1963.

Fowler JW: Toward a developmental perspective on faith. *Relig Educ* 1974; 69:207–219.

Freud S: *Three Essays on the Theory of Sexuality.* Basic Books, 1962.

Havighurst RJ: *Developmental Tasks and Education.* 3rd ed. McKay, 1972.

Kohlberg L: Stage and sequence: The cognitive-development ap-

proach to socialization. In: *Handbook of Socialization: Theory and Research.* Goslin D (editor). Rand McNally, 1969.
Labinowicz E: *The Piaget Primer.* Addison-Wesley, 1980.
Piaget J: *The Child's Conception of Movement and Speed.* Ballantine Books, 1970.
Piaget J: *The Child's Conception of Space.* Basic Books, 1962.
Piaget J: *The Moral Judgment of the Child.* The Free Press, 1965.
Piaget J, Inhelder B: *The Psychology of the Child.* Basic Books, 1969.
Siegal JM, Matthews KA: Type A behavior, achievement striving and their childhood origins. In: *Advances in School Psychology.* Vol 3. Krachtochwill TR (editor). Erlbaum, 1983.
Sullivan HS: *The Interpersonal Theory of Psychiatry.* Norton, 1953.
Wallerstein JS, Kelly JB: *Surviving the Breakup: How Children Actually Cope with Divorce.* Basic Books, 1980.
Wechsler D: *The Measurement and Appraisal of Adult Intelligence.* Williams & Wilkins, 1958.
Yussen SR, Santrock JW: *Child Development.* Brown, 1982.

Additional Readings

Albinson JG, Andrews GM: *The Child in Sport and Physical Activity.* University Park Press, 1976.
Allen MT: An overview of the Type A behavior pattern in children and adolescents. *Pediatr Nurs* (Nov/Dec) 1983; 9(6):407–412.
Betz CL: Faith development in children. *Pediatr Nurs* (March/April) 1981; 7:22–25.
Boettcher J, Boettcher K: Sex education for fifth and sixth graders and their parents. *Am J Matern Child Nurs* (July/Aug) 1978; 3(4):218–220.
Bridgewater SC, Voignier RR, Smith, CS: Allergies in children: recognization. *Am J Nurs* (April) 1978; 78(4):613–621.
Chinn PL: *Child Health Maintenance: Concepts in Family Centered Care,* 2d ed. Mosby, 1979.
Fischer KW, Lazerson A: *Human Development.* Freeman, 1984.
Hetherington EM, Cox M, Cox R: The aftermath of divorce. In: *Mother-Child/Father-Child Relations.* Stevens JH, Matthews M (editors). National Association for the Education of Young Children, 1978.
Inhelder B: Memory and intelligence in the child. In: *Studies in Cognitive Development: Essays in Honor of Jean Piaget.* Elkind D, Flavell J (editors). Oxford, 1979.
Kaluger G, Kaluger MF: *Human Development.* Mosby, 1984.
Magnusson D, Allen VL: *Human Development.* Academic Press, 1983.
McCown DE: Moral development in children. *Pediatr Nurs* (Jan/Feb) 1984; 10:42–45.
Oda DS: Community nursing in schools: Developing a specialized role. In: *Community Health Nursing.* Archer S, Fleshman R (editors). Duxbury Press, 1979.
Pearson G: Nutrition during the middle years of childhood. In: *Maternal and Child Nutrition: Assessment and Counseling.* Slattery J, Pearson G, Torre C (editors). Appleton-Century-Crofts, 1979.
Santrock JW: *Life-Span Development.* Brown, 1983.
Sarnoff C: Normal and pathological psychological development during the latency age period. In: *Development in Normality and Psychopathology.* Bemporad J (editor). Brunner/Mazel, 1980.
Schuster CS, Ashburn SS: *The Process of Human Development.* Little, Brown, 1980.
Sieman M: Mental health in school age children. *Am Matern Child Nurs* (July/Aug) 1978; 3(4):215.
Slattery J: Dental health in children. *Am J Nurs* (Feb) 1976; 76(2):1159–1161.
Strickland D: Friendship patterns and altruistic behavior in preadolescent males and females. *Nurs Res* (July/Aug) 1980; 30(4):222, 228, 235.
Tuan Y: *Landscapes of Fear.* Pantheon Books, 1979.

Chapter 8

Adolescence

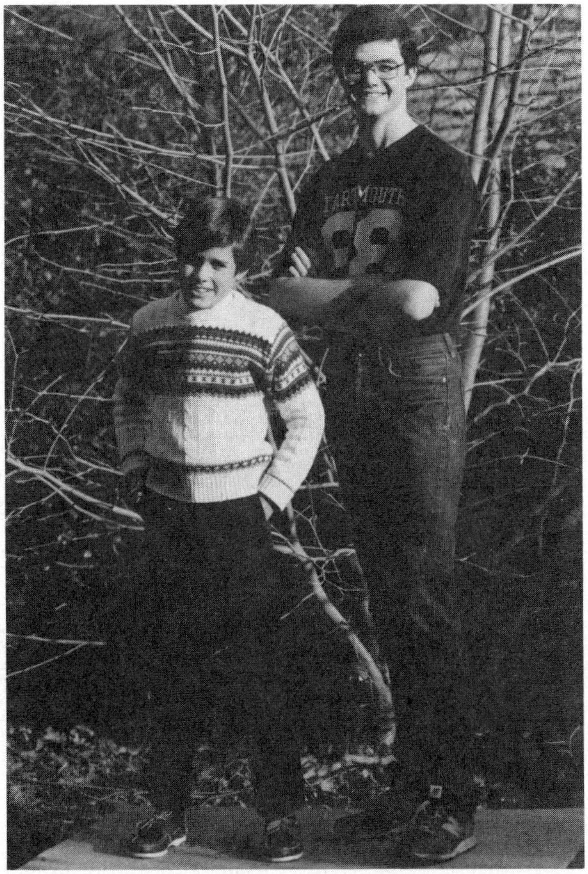

Chapter Contents

(Continues)

Objectives

- Explain the influences of both the external environment and developmental changes on the adolescent's development.
- Define the major areas of development in adolescents.
- Explain the essential biophysical changes that occur in adolescence.
- Describe the principal explanations for affective, cognitive, and social development in adolescence.
- Identify the basic health care needs of adolescents.

Adolescence is the longest developmental stage and the most difficult to define. Some authorities define it chronologically as the teenage years or the years when the reproductive system matures, a process that might begin as early as age 8 1/2 and extend into the 20s. Others define adolescence as a time of emerging legal and economic independence and place it in a social framework. If that social framework is the school system, adolescence in the United States may begin in the sixth or seventh grade, or middle school or junior high school, and may end after graduation or withdrawal from senior high school or college, depending on the person's legal age, maturity, or occupational status. Psychologically, adolescence is an optimistic time of rapid growth in physical, intellectual, and social achievement, but it is also a period of moodiness, rebellion, or even a sad loss of childhood innocence and ease.

The universally recognized biologic changes that mark the transition from childhood to adulthood tend to focus on size, strength, and reproductive system changes. In adolescence metabolic and hormonal changes affect almost every body system, and psychosocial development is further affected by the interaction among biophysical, cognitive, and affective capacities. Physical growth and development are hallmarks of adolescence, but physical development does not occur in isolation from psychosocial development.

Many words used to describe this phase of life are biologically based. The most general term, *maturation,* applies to the physical changes that occur as a result of internal body processes or internal regulation. For example, rapid height increments are evidence of a growth spurt and signify maturation. An adolescent's decision to use weights to build muscles will not succeed unless these coincide with maturation of the hormonal system. Social environment and internal developmental processes are also factors affecting the physical changes that occur at this stage.

The term *puberty* is less well defined. Puberty sometimes describes a process involving numerous changes and considerable time, but it may also refer to a specific event. For example, puberty as an event is definitely signaled in the female by menarche, or the first menstrual period. In the male, puberty is signaled to some by the presence of pigmented pubic hair and to others by the first ejaculation. As a general concept, puberty involves the relationship between physiologic and psychologic changes that occur during adolescence.

Although the sequence of maturation is universal, the rate is highly variable between sexes and among individuals of the same sex. The average age of onset of puberty is 2 years earlier in females than in males, but factors other than sex differences can affect pace. For example, differences in body type often are correlated with the tempo of maturation (Tanner, 1962).

The first body type to complete maturation is the *mesomorph,* a body type characterized by rectangular shape, hardness, apparent bone and muscle development, and strength. Individuals with this body type tend to be taller and fatter before puberty but may be the same height or even shorter than age and sex peers at reproductive maturity. At the opposite extreme is the linear, fragile, flat-chested, thin, lightly muscled, large-brained *ectomorph.* While late-maturing, the ectomorphic individual may reach the greatest height. In the middle is the *endomorph,* who is soft, spheric, low in muscle and bone development, but high in digestive system development. The endomorphic individual might begin puberty before the mesomorphic person and end it after the ectomorphic individual, taking the longest time in puberty. Even with standard differences between the sexes, a female ectomorph, or late-maturing girl, might begin maturation later than a male mesomorph, or early-maturing boy.

The External Environment's Influence on the Adolescent

Influence of the Family

The adolescent searches for explanations of culture, ethnicity, socioeconomic factors, and family structure. Understanding these aspects of family life ultimately leads to a recognition of the values held by parents. These values then affect the adolescent's choices in education and career. Family structure, parenting styles, and parental aspirations are consistently believed to be more influential factors than schooling in a child's achievement motivation. For adolescents, communication patterns, educational attainments of parents and siblings, and parental aspirations are repeatedly noted to correlate with achievement in education.

In a given family one or more children often follow in the careers of the parents, provided that the parents are satisfied with their own career choices. Years ago, when opportunities for women were limited, this tendency was more evident. If the mother were a housewife, nurse, or teacher, the daughter often would choose the same occupation. With expanding opportunities for women, adolescent girls, while using the mother as a role model, might also consider the father's occupation as a valid career choice.

Size of the family also is significantly related to achievement, with more success demonstrated by children from small families or older children from larger families. Adolescents from families where parents and/or siblings have demonstrated high achievement levels often tend to follow the same course. Small families often can more easily promote intellectual growth and achievement because more attention generally is given to each individual. This is more difficult in larger families. The oldest child initially receives a greater deal of attention and stimulation. As the others arrive, time constraints usually make it impossible to do the same for successive children. Oldest children therefore might be more motivated than their siblings to pursue advanced education.

Another important factor is the role modeling of adult behavior, a form of imitation common to adolescents. Role models for behavior are diverse and important at this stage. Other relatives or esteemed adults such as teachers, Scout leaders, coaches, religious leaders, or political leaders serve as role models for occupational choices that the adolescent may choose to pursue. If the adult is positive about the career and the rewards are obvious, the likelihood of the adolescent's following an early interest in a similar career are increased.

Differences in parenting styles often are reflected in the emphases placed on future-oriented goals and standards. Authoritative parenting, aimed at aiding the young to achieve self-control, autonomy, and concern for others, focuses on the intent of a person's actions. The adolescent who experiences authoritative parenting learns that the give-and-take of communication is necessary to evaluate a person's intent. In contrast, authoritarian parenting focuses on achieving respectability, as demonstrated by obedience to situational rules. The adolescent from an authoritarian environment faces preset guidelines, thus diminishing the capacity for decision making. This adolescent might demonstrate behavior extremes of conformity or rebellion.

For example, in making judgments about whether to use alcohol, the adolescent from the authoritarian family will decide whether or not to abide by the rules. The adolescent from the authoritative family is more apt to examine the options and discuss the advantages and disadvantages of the situation with family members. Thus, the final decision ultimately is made by the adolescent, with the understanding that the adolescent accepts the consequences of the decision.

Influence of the Community

The community's recognition of the change from child to adult status is specific in the rites of passage, or initiation ceremonies marking the start of adulthood, that are common to many societies worldwide. Vestiges of transitional rituals remain in certain religious practices and in the significance attached to certain social events, school progressions, and laws. For example, Christian confirmation and Jewish Bar and Bat Mitzvah reflect the need and ability of an adolescent to affirm through personal decision a belief in the religious doctrines he or she has been taught. The laws governing the assumption of adult rights and responsibilities, such as the legal age for marriage, consent for health care, compulsory education, employment, driving, military service, criminal procedures, and drinking alcoholic beverages, vary but are also forms of recognition of adult status.

Social class, particularly income level and the interaction patterns associated with it, seems to be more influential than race or ethnicity in determining the social involvement and achievement of adolescents. Adolescents in the lower socioeconomic classes are often needed to help support the family financially. This necessitates after-school employment or increased school absenteeism. School work suffers, leading to failure and/or withdrawal from school. The adolescent might be unable to participate in enriching extracurricular activities. Opportunities for peer activities and involvement in school clubs or projects are limited. The lower-class adolescent is influenced by family expectations that encourage early adulthood. As a result of this, the adolescent might perceive school as drudgery and leave at the first available opportunity.

Expectations of adolescents at the middle- to upper-income level emphasize that the child not embarrass the family. Adolescents who are intellectually motivated benefit from the educational advantages and parental support for their goal achievement. Goal achievement often entails many years of schooling, all or most of which are provided by their parents.

Prolonged schooling in postindustrial societies, which creates the social framework for some adolescents, is a pattern of deferred gratification that is not available to those who lack basic necessities. Because basic necessities are of

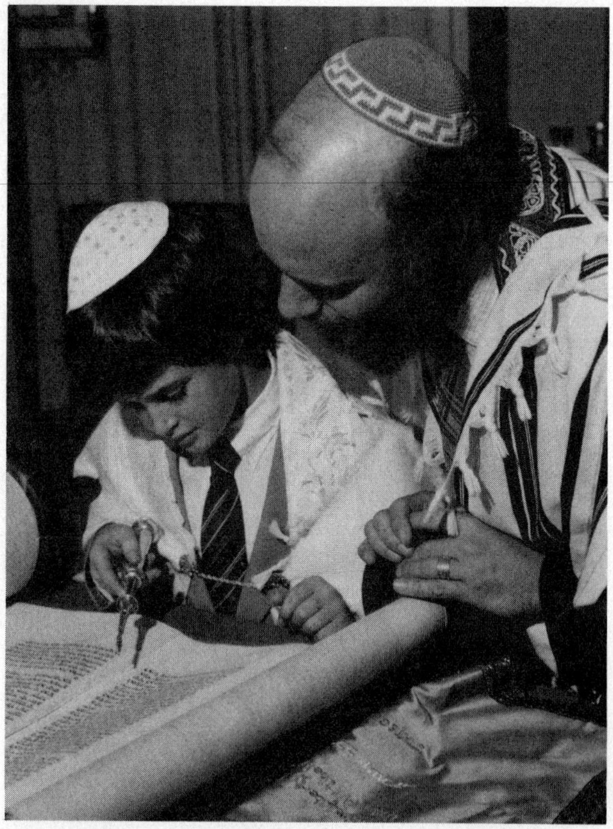

Rites of passage, such as the Jewish Bar Mitzvah, traditionally mark the transition to adulthood and are common to many cultures.

paramount importance, they, in turn, intrinsically affect the quality of the adolescent's life. The needs, goals, and actions of adolescents involved in a daily struggle for economic survival are therefore very different from those for adolescents with family resources.

Social class lines tend to be rigidly drawn in school social groups and activities. Social class is often influenced by the amount of money available for dress and membership dues. The early tracking of students into vocational paths also might accentuate differences in potential development.

School School has a multifaceted effect on the adolescent because it provides an environment for promoting completion of tasks. From the learning tasks of late childhood, the child gains confidence in personal achievement and the ability to initiate and achieve projects and to compete or cooperate with peers. In addition to encouraging cognitive development, schools establish a climate of social interaction. Adolescents, in contacts with their peers and teachers in the school setting, validate thoughts and test new ideas in the process of developing unique identities. During the high school years, adolescents assume responsibility for learning (one hopes). These years are a time for finding and developing the self and for being accountable for personal behavior.

The learning climate in school allows the adolescent to explore avenues of future goals and directions while being guided by significant others outside the family structure. During the high school years, many adolescents make preliminary decisions about vocations or careers and take definite steps toward achieving their goals, such as applying for college admission, obtaining job experience, or receiving vocational training.

Extracurricular activities offered by most school systems allow the adolescent opportunities to engage in team participation or the in-depth pursuit of a hobby or other constructive activity. Some schools offer a variety of sports as well as theater groups, bands, newspapers, television and radio stations, ski clubs, and more. These activities not only promote special interests but also provide structured opportunities for contacts with members of the opposite sex in nonthreatening situations. These opportunities promote the development of a sense of confidence in future heterosexual relationships.

Peer group The school years expand the child's peer interactions. During late childhood and early adolescence, a progression occurs from same-sex, informal play groups to more structured, competitive, and cooperative group activities and then to exclusive, same-sex partnerships or "chumships." All of these interactions precede apparent interest in the opposite sex. Expressed interest in the opposite sex and in marriage as a goal frequently occurs with the onset of puberty.

Perhaps at no other stage in development do one's peers have as major an influence as during adolescence. As children mature and begin to separate from the family, the peer group becomes important as a judge of ideas, morality, mode of dress, and activity participation. Being "one of the group" becomes extremely important for the adolescent. Popularity seems to be an important goal. In any setting, however, the groups vary according to informal standards established by the members. For instance, the most popular adolescents in one group may be those who wear designer clothing and are judged to be the most physically attractive. Other groups may have an activity, such as sports, auto mechanics, or computer programming in common, or they all may be particularly talented in music, art, dance, or science. Even those who are considered unpopular by their peers might be members of a group whose basis is their unpopularity. The sense of belonging is a basic need.

Peer groups do, however, provide a dilemma for many adolescents. Attempts to live up to the standards of the group or to become more popular might force them to depart from the family standards. Decisions about whether to engage in substance abuse or to participate in sexual relations, for example, are major decisions with far-reaching consequences. The ability to resist peer pressure at the risk of losing popularity requires a constantly supportive attitude from parents and teachers. Adolescents eventually learn to internalize standards, but often as a result of trial and error. Unfortunately, in some cases experimentation as a result of peer pressure has undesirable and even tragic consequences, such as teenage pregnancy and death from drunk driving. A successful beginning in developing standards eases the transition into adulthood, where peers more often are judged by their unique qualities than by a common appearance or actions.

Developmental Changes in Adolescence

Adolescence is marked by clearly evident secular trends in development. A secular trend is a phenomenon manifested through many years or generations; it has no connotations of or opposition to religion. Secular trends related to adolescence are (1) increasingly earlier ages of onset of puberty and (2) attainment of greater height and weight during puberty. For example, since 1900, research in Western countries has demonstrated that average menarche occurs 4 months earlier, height has increased 1.0–2.5 cm, and weight has increased 0.5 kg (Tanner, 1972). The trend toward the earlier onset of puberty does, however, seem to be leveling off. Physiologically, developmental age is calculated by skeletal age, not chronologic age. Although trunk growth eventually accounts for 60% of the adolescent's increase in height, the sequence of growth begins in the extremities, with closure of the epiphyseal plates in the long bones under the influence of sex-specific hormones. During this sequence, members of either sex might appear and feel awkward and uncoordinated; both sexes might worry about sex-inappropriate changes. For example, girls might worry about disproportionately large hands and feet, a problem that is usually temporary. Young people need reassuring information about expected growth patterns during this period of asynchrony, in which maturation of different body parts occurs at different rates.

The nurse's knowledge of earlier developmental progress is useful in assessing the impact of puberty. Children may experience relatively short or long periods of slow growth, during which they may direct energy into motor skill coordination, competence, and satisfaction in peer relationships and both formal and informal pursuit of knowledge. All these areas of human development are challenged in adolescence. Specific, definite expectations of self and others are more uncertain in adolescence. Even social opportunities are influenced by variations in the pace of puberty, a phenomenon over which the adolescent has no control.

During late childhood, the child becomes more graceful and coordinated as body proportions slim, legs lengthen, and posture straightens. Longer legs and arms and a lower center of gravity aid gross motor skills of running, reaching, climbing, and bike riding. Continued myelination of the nervous system enhances achievement in writing and other fine motor skills. Then, certain features of the adolescent growth spurt disrupt steady progress in gross and fine motor skills. First, a disproportionate phase occurs during the growth spurt, and, second, the outward manifestations of change increase self-awareness. (Table 8-1 describes normal biophysical development and other development in the adolescent and notes assessment guidelines.)

Restlessness, moodiness, and fluctuations between independence and dependence are signals of transition that reflect lability, or lack of stability, in emotions and behavior. Lability is often made evident by spoken desires unmatched by preparation and by behavior that seems extreme for a given situation. For example, one 15-year-old who was still unable to drive legally asked to borrow the car to accompany some older friends on an overnight trip. When turned down by his parents, he reacted violently and put his hand through a window.

Adolescents show lability of impulse control, which might relate to loss of body control. In puberty, both sexes must deal with body functions over which they initially have no control: menstruation in the female and penile erection in the male. Feeling out of control might interfere with an adolescent's need for increasing independence. Young people need information to explain and validate what is "normal."

Affective Development

Several leaders in psychodynamic thinking have made important contributions to understanding adolescent affective development. Theorists suggest that both unconscious and conscious elements from past and present experiences contribute to affective development. The following aspects of development are important.

1. *Sexuality* To integrate gender, affection, and genital function, the adolescent reviews earlier identifications and attractions to parents, expands and intensifies friendships with same-sex peers, and experiments with opposite-sex relationships.
2. *Leader/follower role* Adolescents use peer group activities to test their interpersonal influence and their needs for others to achieve goals.

TABLE 8-1 Guidelines for Assessment of the Adolescent

Developmental area	Expected characteristics	Assessment techniques
Temperament		Ask adolescent and parent, if present, to describe adolescent's temperamental characteristics, discipline, and response
Biophysical development		
Weight—see Appendix A. Major weight gain in girls is from subcutaneous fat; major weight gain in boys is from muscle	Growth spurts occur with weight gain and eventual closure of the epiphyseal (growth) plate	
Length—see Appendix A; 60% of increase in length is increase in trunk	*Girls:* growth corresponds with breast development and preceeds menarche (10–18 years of age) *Boys:* growth follows testicular enlargement and corresponds with penile elongation (12–20 years of age)	
Neuromuscular		
Gross motor skills	Progressing from awkward, clumsy stage to adultlike motor skills; activity level varies—may become involved in organized and/or competitive sports; choice of activities is influenced by personal preferences	Ask the adolescent about participation in physical activities; have adolescent state activity preferences and why they are favored; have the adolescent assess own perception of performance; ask about parental perceptions of child's skills, use of talents, choice of activities
Fine motor skills	Refined fine motor skills; eye-hand coordination adultlike Precise movements when building models and doing fine sewing or other crafts; speed and individuality in handwriting; capable of small printing or writing; art skills perfected if interested; improved dexterity in fingers for playing musical instruments	Assess the adolescent's performance during a neurologic examination Ask about any hobbies, interests, crafts; have the adolescent describe and evaluate abilities
Cardiovascular		
Heart rate	Approaches adult norms 70–80 beats/min	
Blood pressure	112/55–70 mm Hg	
Blood values	Red blood cells and hemoglobin increase (greater in boys)	
Respiratory rate	15–20 breaths/min	
Genitourinary	Puberty begins with hypothalamus induced pituitary output of sex hormones (see Chapter 29) causing growth of the gonads and production of sex-specific hormones *Girls:* growth of pubic hair, development of the clitoris, growth of the ovaries, uterus, and vagina *Boys:* growth of pubic hair, elongation of the penis, testicular enlargement and enlargement of the scrotum	

TABLE 8-1 *(Continued)*

Developmental area	Expected characteristics	Assessment techniques
	Girls: hormones produced by the anterior pituitary (see Chapter 29) stimulate ovulation and formation of the corpus luteum; ovarian follicles secrete *estrogen,* which stimulates development of secondary sex characteristics (axillary and pubic hair, breast enlargement, darkening of the nipples, and female contours) and *progesterone,* which thickens the uterine lining that sheds during menstruation	
	Boys: testosterone (an androgen) produced by the testes influences development of secondary sex characteristics (voice changes, pubic, facial, and axillary hair) and growth of the sex organs including maturation of sperm; influences sexual drive and potency	
Integumentary	Increased sweat gland activity; development of acne	
Immune	Lymphoid tissue produces immunoglobulins at a steady rate (see Chapter 25); the thymus decreases in size as other lymphoid tissue assumes its function	
Sensory-perceptual		
Vision	Ability to fixate and focus on objects with fixation and focusing becoming fused; might experience visual fatigue	Test vision at age 14 years
Language development	Speech and writing totally understandable; expands oral and reading vocabulary; reads and writes complex sentences; follows abstract ideas; enjoys fantasy and scientific literature; peer dialect commonly used	Ask about favorite or current book being read
Cognitive development	Concrete to formal thinking; works with decimals; increased ability to reason abstractly; understands abstract ideas—"justice," "honesty"; aware of moral codes; able to generate hypothesis—to consider "possible" and follow idea through to a logical conclusion	Ask the adolescent about school, academic performance, and favorite subject; ask the adolescent to define justice and relate the concept to a recent event
	Systematically solves verbal and mental problems using the scientific method	Present the pendulum problem and observe the process used to solve it; note the adolescent's ability to consider and systematically eliminate variables
	Plans ahead—oriented toward personal future, such as college, career; tends to be idealistic	Discuss future goals—assess adolescent's perception of options
	Capable of imaginative, creative, inventive thinking; of mentally testing the hypothesis and critically evaluating it	Ask the adolescent, "If you could change the world in only one way, what would that change be and why?"
Social and affective development		
Adolescent	Establishing sense of self-identity; may try out different roles in the process	Ask such questions as, "Do you like yourself?" "Do you fear being rejected?"
	Introspective; demands privacy and spends time daydreaming	Discuss importance of time alone to daydream

(Continues)

TABLE 8-1 Guidelines for Assessment of the Adolescent *(Continued)*

Developmental area	Expected characteristics	Assessment techniques
	Emotionally labile	Might ask if moody, tense, easily angered, or anxious
	Establishes sexual identity; knowledgeable of bodily changes and implications for relationships	
	Adopting lifestyle that fits with sense of self and goals for future; concentrates on special interests	Ask the adolescent to provide a word picture of personal characteristics; favorite and disliked traits and behaviors; goals and aspirations
	Predominant orientation is the peer group; becomes increasingly involved with peers and "excuses" self from family activities; chooses own friends of both sexes; contacts widen with increased mobility	Ask the adolescent about friends, favorite activities, and frequency of group activities; might ask if it is easy or difficult to make friends
	Vacillates between independent and dependent behavior; family stress might be present; might opt to follow rules and values of peers over those of society; generally decides right and wrong according to the majority	Discuss the adolescent's relationship with the family, especially the parents; ask, "What is the best thing about your parents, what 'bugs' you the most?"; note the adolescent's responses
	Formulates personal beliefs and values; might or might not explain them to others, especially parents	Present moral dilemma such as, "Your brother tells you a secret. He was going to a rock concert but was telling the parents he was going to a friend's house. Later, there is a need to contact your brother. Should you tell your parents where he is? Why?"
	Establishing own identity within family; moving to more adult relationship of love and respect but independence; process of establishing identity one of storm and stress	Discuss with the parent the adolescent's behavior and attitude at home, relationships with siblings and adults in family

3. *Response to authority* An appearance of rebellion against authority might mask an unconscious desire for control. The adolescent might challenge limits and appreciate them at the same time. The adolescent seeks guidelines but must experience decision making and its consequences.
4. *Values* Experiments in role playing, from the superficial level of appearance to more essential human behaviors, are used to test both self-image and the response of others to self. Such role playing represents an effort to resolve confusion about values in practice. Adolescents carefully observe adults for the consistency of stated values and action behavior.
5. *Emotional control* Appropriate outlets for the release of tension, as well as physical maturation, resolve the problems of emotional lability that are most pronounced in early adolescence.
6. *Self-esteem* Self-definition and self-evaluation, the essential components of self-esteem, require involvement in interpersonal relations in which the self can be seen in interactions with others.
7. *Belonging* The adolescent turns from family acceptance, which may be taken for granted, to choice and a new level of mutual closeness in relationships outside the family. This may involve a search for belonging, for being accepted by chosen others.
8. *Self-assertion* The adolescent learns to share thoughts and feelings, first to validate them and later to contribute to human interactions.
9. *Daydreams* The reverie of daydreams for anticipation, review, and tension release can facilitate development but needs to be controlled. An excessive daydreamer might withdraw from human relations. Fantasy life might interfere with the use and evaluation of real inter-

personal relations or might create ideals that human interactions cannot achieve.

Physical and emotional changes in adolescence have a profound impact on personality development in the adolescent. In addition, familial and societal attitudes impinge on the teenager and might exacerbate the inner turmoil the young person is experiencing.

Freud's final stage of psychosexual development, the genital stage, occurs at puberty. At the beginning of this stage, the initial focus of libido (energy) is on one's own genital activity. Freud believed that to successfully complete this stage, the sexual drive must be turned to a person of the opposite sex outside one's family. The second major drive, the aggressive drive, must be channeled into productive work to benefit society and into hobbies to sublimate energies.

Derek Miller (1974) offered a three-stage description of adolescence. This description is roughly age-related and encompasses five factors: (1) physiologic basis, (2) emotional control, (3) self-esteem, (4) activities, and (5) relationships. Miller's conception of early adolescence, corresponding to ages 11–15, is characterized by turmoil. This turmoil has a physiologic basis in body changes, loss of body control, and hormonal influence on the emotions. According to Miller, adolescents are consciously aware of restlessness and tension and unconsciously look for control. Therefore, they show overt defiance of parents and other authorities. Miller described boys as experiencing physical discomfort that they release in jokes, physical play, and masturbation. At this stage, the boy denies his father as a model. Miller cautioned the mother to avoid sexually stimulating action on her part. Girls demonstrate shy embarrassment and defensive behavior, such as hostile giggling. The girl may seek solitude but can use both diaries and friends to draw herself out. Miller stressed the importance of the father's reaction to the girl's development, encouraging him to express verbally his appreciation of her attractiveness.

Extremes in hairstyles or modes of dress are obvious examples of the adolescent's urge to achieve autonomy. Adolescents themselves might not even like the look but feel compelled to try it. If parents understand the directive force that prompts the adolescent behavior, they can be supportive rather than authoritarian until the phase passes, which it eventually does.

Middle adolescence, at approximately 14–18 years of age, features, according to Miller (1974), identification of "what I am" and self-realization. Although physical changes are stabilizing, two problems reach their peak: (1) acne affects appearance, and (2) adolescents face the possibility of pregnancy. The middle adolescent's sense of sexual power might be overwhelming, and the young person might be made anxious by overpermissive parents. Sexual activity at this time is more apt to be a test of oneself and response to peer pressures than a loving relationship. Miller designated this period the peak of the need for adult models other than parents because middle adolescents tend and need to test the quality of people in their environment. Middle adolescents need to bounce ideas, values, and feelings about morality and sexual desires against significant adults other than family members. In this way adolescents determine ways to be similar as well as different, thus further developing autonomy and clarifying identity.

In late adolescence, the years from 17 to 20 (or later for those in college), the characteristic described by Miller (1974) is coping. The late adolescent needs the opportunity to try out the personality confirmed in middle adolescence. Here, the adolescent might forgive parents for parental failures and omissions or might rebel, depending on how the young person's first steps into adulthood were confirmed by the parents.

Interpersonal relationships Interpersonal relationships in early adolescence are characterized by "chumships." A *chumship* is a special relationship with one same-sex friend, which marks the transition from juvenile indifference to peers, except as competitors or task helpers, to adolescent interpersonal intimacy. Through chumships, adolescents learn to be close to others before developing relationships with the opposite sex. Two major benefits are gained from chumship: (1) one gets a look at oneself through the chum's eyes, and (2) one learns about another because it is of great interest to observe and analyze one's experiences with the other. Sullivan (1953) deemed chumship a prerequisite for eventual heterosexual intimacy and mature sexuality.

Accordingly, only later in adolescence should the need for intimacy be directed to a person of the opposite sex. Fondness for a special friend can manifest itself in common interests and activities, as well as modes of dress, hairstyles, and makeup. Close friends often are inseparable. Through their friends, adolescents have an opportunity to see themselves reflected honestly and can practice communication techniques that can be used later in a heterosexual relationship. Girls in early adolescence might support one another and exchange confidences. They often can be seen dancing together at junior high school dances while prompting one another to be the first to ask a boy to dance. Very often, close friends will have parents with similar expectations of behavior, and the friends can insulate each other from social ostracism if their social mores do not match those of their peers.

Older adolescents must integrate feelings of lust and a

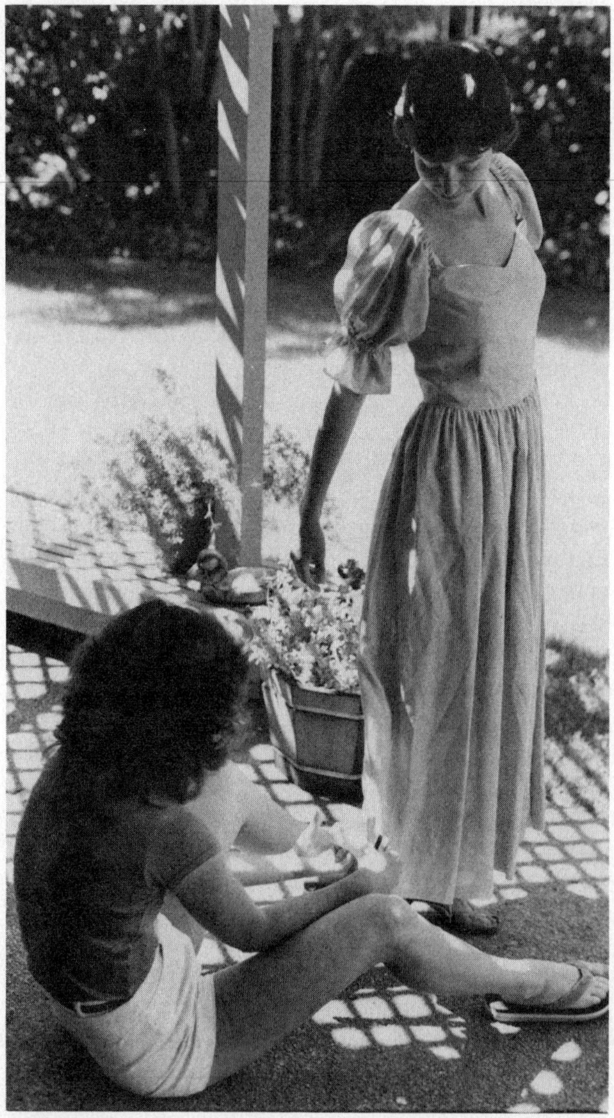

"Chumship" in adolescence is a special relationship with a same-sex friend and marks the transition to interpersonal intimacy.

need for intimacy into their affective development (Sullivan, 1953). These are interwoven but not identical drives. Integrating feelings of lust into personal identity involves (1) acknowledging genital-based urges for heterosexual unity, (2) organizing the individual system of motives that makes a person become involved with others or avoid others, and (3) organizing an appropriate heterosexual interpersonal situation of choice.

Identity crisis The identification that Miller suggested characterizes midadolescence is similar to the psychosocial crisis of adolescence that Erikson (1968) described as "identity versus role diffusion." According to Erikson's view of human development, adolescent identity achievement depends on a favorable resolution in each prior psychosocial crisis. The adolescent therefore can use ego strengths achieved in resolving the crises of infancy and early, middle, and late childhood.

Erikson's concept of identity has several components of self-definition and self-evaluation: (1) a temporal perspective that enables a person to realize continuity of identity, that is, being the same person in the past, present, and future; (2) a value orientation based on personal decision and commitment; (3) vocational orientation with active preparation for a work goal; and (4) specific gender sexuality of being male or female. To resolve the identity crisis, the adolescent may experiment with several roles. Erikson cautioned parents and other authorities not to react too strongly to such experimentation because some adolescents are so fragile that they will accept a label and persist in a role that gains attention. Successful progress in resolving the adolescent identity crisis fosters the ego strength of fidelity. The person then finds someone and something to be true to.

Whether evidence of resolution of the adolescent identity crisis can be found in young adults is the question posed by James Marcia (1966, 1980). He used two criteria: (1) crisis, in the sense of dealing with questions and doubt, and (2) commitment, meaning a personal decision. Marcia applied two of Erikson's components of identity, the vocational and the value orientation, in his studies. His initial work with male college students included questioning each subject about how certain he was about the appropriateness of his chosen major and whether he had ever doubted his religious beliefs. Marcia found the following four types of identity crisis outcomes:

1. *Identity achievement*—subject experienced crisis (questions) and reached commitment (personal decision)
2. *Moratorium*—subject is experiencing crisis and has not yet reached but expects to reach a commitment
3. *Foreclosure*—subject has never experienced crisis but is strongly committed to a goal or value fostered by family or other external influence
4. *Diffusion*—subject might have experienced a crisis but is not interested in commitment

For example, the high school student considers many different roles when attempting to decide on a career. Some entering college may choose a liberal arts program to postpone making any commitment to a specific academic area. Even those who make a commitment because the program requires it, as nursing does, often experience a period of disequilibrium as specialty courses begin. The final out-

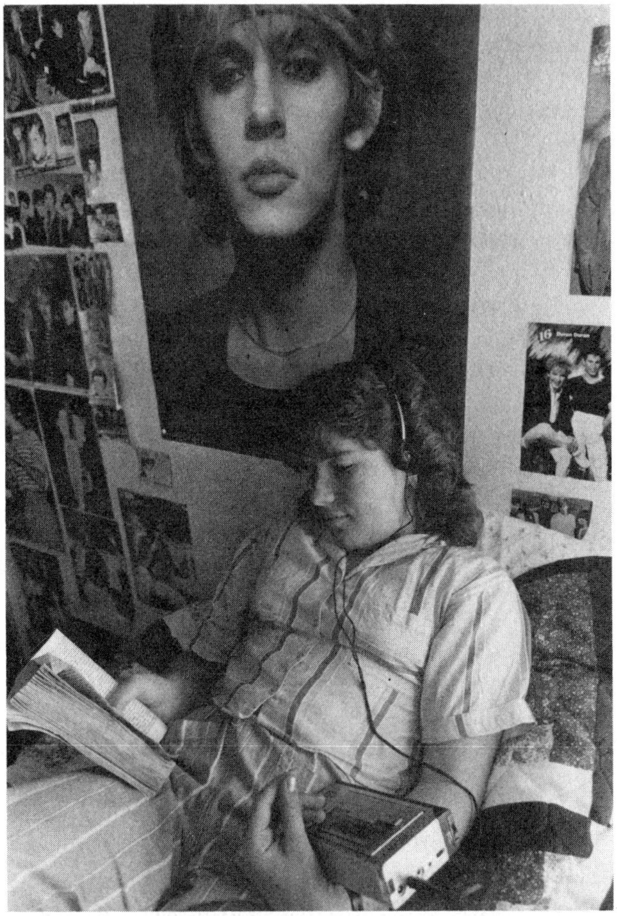

Adolescence is a time of questioned identity. Adolescents need time to consider and reflect in the process of self-definition.

comes of this crisis may be a commitment to the chosen profession, change in the subject area, or a continuing search.

Cognitive Development

Formal operations Cognitive theorists relate important advances in thinking to the physical and social maturation of the adolescent. Piaget's theory of cognition describes operations of cognition as activities through which the individual attempts to transform reality by applying procedures to various data (Piaget, 1952). According to Piaget, maturation of the nervous system, combined with material and social experience and personal activity, enables the adolescent to achieve formal operations. Piaget's stage of *formal operations* is defined as the ability to reason from the possible to the actual.

Formal operational thought possesses several characteristics. First, the individual learns to hypothesize, or to use propositional thinking, which is free from the evidence of experience essential to earlier concrete operations. At this stage, the adolescent is able to imagine several alternatives to the same phenomenon. A person using formal operational thinking can imagine a view from various spatial positions and can think about an abstract concept from another person's point of view.

Formal operations and the ability to hypothesize facilitate scientific problem solving. The adolescent can envision multiple relations of cause and effect, can control variables mentally, and can plan a systematic combination of possibilities prior to actual experimentation. This abstract thinking requires some caution because of the danger of losing touch with reality. This problem, known as cognitive slippage, might occur in adolescents who push thinking to its limits in mentally constructing an ideal world. The problem with this fantasy is that adolescents might then experience major difficulties adjusting to the futility of attaining their imagined utopia.

Second, formal operations are exemplified by what Piaget called the INRC group of transformations (identity, negation, reciprocity, correlation). These processes enable the person to call on many available operations and therefore to be flexible when considering possible solutions to problems (Piaget, 1954). Through formal operational, or abstract, thinking, the individual also can order relations, such as big, bigger, biggest, without tangible evidence.

Piaget's transition from concrete to formal operations usually is assumed to occur in early adolescence but is not age specific. In fact, some people never achieve formal operations, and most people achieve formal operations only with limited types of data.

Motivation and learning In North America, organizing and understanding information is emphasized more than the acquisition and memorization of facts, especially in the high school grades. Basic academic subjects, however, also include formulas and rules for processing information. Piaget's theory describes the process of learning to organize and understand information. Behavioral theories describe the acquisition of information by identifying the external controls in an individual's learning (see Chapter 3). Current thinking incorporates both processes, suggesting that for optimal learning to occur, the learner must have various opportunities for learning. The learner needs to be an active participant, both in the decisions about which learning tasks to undertake and in the evaluation of his or her success.

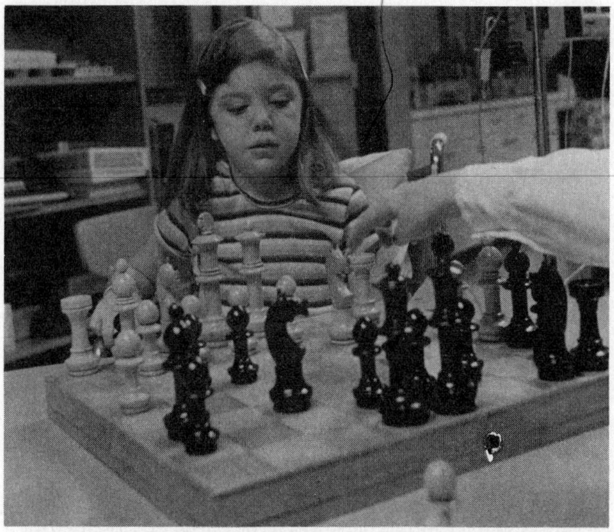

Games using abstract thinking are ways of assessing formal operations.

Personal responsibility for learning requires motivation, which is linked with enjoyment of school and/or with perceived rewards for the effort expended. For most adolescents, family-derived motivating factors are a predominant influence in school achievement. In the school setting the relevance of school studies to occupational goals provides an effective motivation. For example, the process of vocational choice during adolescence demonstrates a gradual transition from fantasy about potential occupational goals to a realistic appraisal of one's own abilities and interests in comparison with the demands of different occupations. Planning for the future in this way is part of the experience of most high school students.

Social learning theorist Albert Bandura (1977), whose experiments concentrated on the response to the role modeling of behavior, believed that motivation could be affected by external factors. His research showed that children learned from observing other people's behavior and its consequences. According to Bandura, creating an environment that is conducive to learning is the responsibility of adults. Adolescent learners then observe, remember, judge, decide, and create a response according to their own values. For example, an adolescent often will use a teacher as both a role model and a motivational influence.

Adolescents are more highly motivated to learn in an atmosphere that fosters excitement about the subject area. Students motivated in this way become self-motivated in other areas and expand their interests.

Memory Some personal capabilities important to school learning peak in adolescence. Memory, which is certainly important to knowledge acquisition, becomes a more active process during adolescence. The adolescent's efficient use of mnemonic schemes or memory aids is an indication of the active nature of memory.

For example, one 14-year-old girl used mnemonic devices to aid her memory in various school subjects. She remembered the sons of Leah for her theology class with the phrase "Reuben saw lice (or lines) just in zebras." This gave her the first letters of the names Reuben, Simeon, Levi, Judea, Issachar, and Zebulun.

Creativity The adolescent who achieves abstract thinking differs from the child intent on collecting facts and finding the one right answer. Formal operations therefore promote creative thinking, which produces many possible anwers to a problem. The adolescent who achieves formal operations can switch readily from realistic thinking to fantasy. Fantasy, in turn, is part of the adolescent's process of setting long-term goals. Literature popular with adolescents also indicates their enjoyment of fantasy as a leisure-time pursuit.

Large, long-term studies of people considered to be creative in adolescence show good health and social adjustment as well as academic and career productivity. Creativity is clearly more than a way to compensate for a physical or social handicap. Some of the inhibitors to creativity are an extremely peer-oriented culture, sanctions against questioning and exploring, and overemphasis on stereotypic sex roles. Facilitators of creativity include a social setting in which a variety of talents and achievements are rewarded, assistance with social skills so that creative individuals interact with peers and are less isolated, attention to the development of values, and aid in coping with fears. Overall, an environment that respects unusual questions and unusual ideas and provides opportunities for self-initiated and unevaluated learning promotes creative thinking.

Recently, high school students are being encouraged more and more to demonstrate creative thinking. Creative problem-solving courses are available through some school systems, which result in such competitions as "Olympics of the Mind." These competitions confer status on the creative child and enhance acceptance by peers. To nourish their creativity, adolescents need time for reflection and planning. Reflection leads to better self-awareness and personal insight in many adolescents.

Nurses can assist parents to encourage artistically, athletically, or intellectually creative adolescents. Nurses need to be aware of the adolescent's creative interests. For instance, fantasy games involving unstructured play and the use of imagination as well as strategy are popular with adolescents. In an acute-care setting nurses can encourage group contacts to promote creative interaction among adolescents. Incorporating specific interests into the therapeutic regimen encourages participation in self-care.

Language As cognitive abilities develop in adolescence, so does the learning of new words, structures, and purposes of language. For example, reading, writing, and speaking depend on the coordination of visual skills, maturation, and experience. Adolescents develop skills in written language involving both the style of writing and the expression of personality characteristics.

Writing in adolescence may be used to put thoughts about oneself on paper for evaluation in a diary or journal. For many adolescents, the evaluation process is a private one. In the hospital setting the nurse therefore must respect the limits that adolescents set.

Health problems require communication, and language barriers must be surmounted. The adolescent's special vocabulary words and variations of language often are used in conversing with peers. The vocabulary that the nurse uses must permit the comfortable discussion of body changes between the adolescent and the nurse. Adolescents vary greatly in their knowledge and use of language. Some know anatomic terms, whereas others know only lay or even crude terms to refer to body parts and functions. Inquiring about a student's school progress may reveal the level of language skills to the nurse who is selecting health teaching methods and materials for the adolescent.

Moral thinking Piaget's (1952) theory of cognition involves a component of moral development. Piaget described a progression from a rigid morality, in which the young child believes rules are made by authority and cannot be broken, to an autonomous morality based on social experiences with peers. This progression helps the child to realize that people make and change rules and that rules are important for their organizing and unifying function. In the process the child learns that there is nothing sacred or untouchable in the rule itself.

In Kohlberg's theory (Kohlberg, 1963, 1976), the common achievement of moral reasoning in adolescence is the second, or conventional, level. The two stages at this level are stage 3, an orientation to interpersonal relations of mutuality, sometimes called a "good boy, good girl" conception, and stage 4, in which the theme is the maintenance of social order, fixed rules, and authority. This is often called the "law and order" stage. Both stages of moral reasoning at this level require a formal operational level of cognition to adopt alternative frames of reference or to understand the viewpoints of others.

Kohlberg's stage 3 is the stage in which the adolescent focuses on the approval of others and often looks to the peer group to determine norms for approval. This is the time in which moral dilemmas are solved by appealing to a group standard. The adolescent who cheats on a test might justify cheating in this way: "Everybody does it; besides, I wouldn't have been allowed to stay on the team if I hadn't passed and that would have let the team and the coach down." Adolescents at Kohlberg's stage 4 are inclined to do what the law or their own sense of duty requires. Some might, for example, register for the draft "because that's the law," regardless of their personal views or group expectations.

Kohlberg's educational experiments also were intended to stimulate the development of moral reasoning. His experiments with high school students included discussions of moral issues in groups where members could be exposed to the next higher level of reasoning from their own. Findings suggest that education can foster moral reasoning in adolescents. Kohlberg and Turiel's (1971) studies have demonstrated that individuals understand reasoning at or below their own dominant levels and are interested in and attracted to the next higher level. For instance, the student who would register for the draft "because that's the law" can discuss the consequences of being drafted with a veteran. A veteran of a war such as Vietnam, which evoked many conflicting moral issues, can provide an alternate viewpoint for the adolescent's consideration.

Religion James Fowler (1976) likened early adolescence to stages, in his description of faith development. Faith progresses so that the adolescent first respects authorities as the providers of meaning, the ones who answer the hard questions about life in general. This view is congruent with much of the schooling in early adolescence, which at this time focuses on the learning of facts about history, grammar, and rules for setting up and solving math problems.

A transition of faith occurs when the individual begins to assume responsibility for his or her own commitments, lifestyle, beliefs, and attitudes. This transition begins during late adolescence. The person at this stage faces the tensions between individuality and belonging to community, between subjectivity and objectivity, between self-fulfillment and service to others, and between the relative and the absolute (Fowler, 1976). The crisis of faith common in late adolescence illustrates these tensions. Being exposed to values and beliefs that may differ from those held by the family often precipitates questioning and exploring in an attempt to apply these beliefs to one's own life. This exploration causes tension, as conflicts with family and long-held traditions arise. The outcome is the ability to extrapolate and use what most closely fits the lifestyle the individual has chosen.

Social Development

Developmental tasks The adolescent faces a series of developmental tasks that are derived from the pressures of physical maturation and the development of individual values and goals in the context of cultural expectations. Havighurst (1972) described eight tasks of adolescence, as follows:

1. Achieving new and more mature relations with agemates of both sexes
2. Achieving a masculine or feminine social role
3. Accepting one's physique and using one's body effectively
4. Achieving emotional independence from parents and other adults
5. Preparing for marriage and family life
6. Preparing for an economic career
7. Developing an ideology—a set of values and an ethical system as a guide to behavior
8. Achieving socially responsible behavior

Albert Bandura (1977) emphasized the continuity of adolescence rather than its disruptions. His views are based on studies that demonstrated harmonious, if not completely communicative, parent-child relations. He criticized the mass media for sensational depictions of troubled individuals as role models for adolescents. Bandura, like Erikson, cautioned against overinterpretation of superficial signs of nonconformity such as following fads. He deplored the tendency to focus attention on negative role models of adolescent behavior, noting the hazard of self-fulfilling prophecies, a phenomenon in which people behave in the way they believe others expect them to behave.

Maturation and social interaction Differences in psychologic and social adjustments between early and late maturers are a factor in the social development of adolescents. Early maturers of both sexes usually demonstrate more positive self-concepts; late maturers demonstrate more anxiety. The expanded social opportunities available to girls seem to be limited to early adolescence but continue for early-maturing boys. Parents and peers accept maturity and readily provide opportunities to assume responsibility and leadership to early-maturing males. Although dating opportunities are available earlier to early-maturing girls, parents might be anxious about premature sexual activity and its possible consequences. Late maturers appear more childlike and are treated as children longer, so that early dating is not an issue.

The early maturers are rated by peers to be more attractive and popular as dates. Thus, development-stimulating opportunities are rewarded on the basis of physical characteristics. By late adolescence, physical differences are less apparent, but late maturers report more negative feelings about themselves and seek more attention and affection.

Early developers continue to be socially successful in adulthood but tend to be conforming and somewhat overcontrolled. Late maturers appear to benefit from adaptive compensation by being insightful, exploring, independent, and spontaneous. One hypothesis suggests that late maturers have happier marriages because of their greater psychologic insight (Jones, 1965).

Integrating Development Through Play

Adolescence is the period when the child's conceptions of play develop into those of the adult. Erikson (1963) aptly described this difference when he defined play as "the work for a child," rather than the escape from work pressures that defines play for the adult. Many forms of play, however, continue to promote growth and preservation of function in all ages. Speed of reaction, strength, endurance, and coordination are all aspects of physical fitness that are enhanced by physical play in the form of gross motor skills. Bone growth, muscle size and strength, and the blood's oxygen-carrying capabilities are a few body functions that need to be stimulated by regular exercise. Both adults and children can enhance fine motor precision and dexterity with arts and crafts. Both children and adults can relieve physical and psychic anxiety or tension by a balance between work and play. Physiologically, such a balance supports the interaction of the complementary branches of the autonomic nervous system—the stress-stimulated sympathetic responses and the restorative-maintenance parasympathetic functions.

Three types of play predominate in adolescence. Cooperative play in adolescence is exemplified in games, clubs, and dating; team play in organized sports; and construction and creativity in hobbies. The content of play includes fantasy through daydreaming, art, reading, and dramatics; role playing in dramatics and some games, club activities, and dating; and both cognitive and motor skills in hobbies, sports, and arts and crafts.

In team sports girls are less apt to participate in games requiring motor skills of organized teamwork after the onset of puberty. Many girls thus miss opportunities for learning to respond to criticism, to settle disputes, to organize activities, and to compete in a structured environment. They also miss the chance for improved physical fitness that exercise provides. Male concentration on organization and competition in team sports might, however, deny boys the opportunities to develop a sense of intimacy or commitment. The traditional expectations, interest, and assistance of parents in the play activities (as well as in the education of both boys and girls) might need to be evaluated critically in light of the life challenges to be faced by both sexes.

As adolescents begin dating, sex-role experimentation and appraisal of self in male-female interaction become more important. Developing relationships is usually the stated purpose of dating among older adolescents. Younger adolescents tend to describe dating simply as participation in socially desirable activities.

Because parents of adolescents tend to stress the importance of preparing for future goals, such as getting good grades in high school to get into college, nurses might need to remind them of the adolescent's need for real play and relaxation. Any tendency for parents to overidentify or compete with their children also might impinge on certain activities, such as sports or dating, and might interfere with the adolescent's emerging sense of identity.

Health Care Needs in Adolescence

Basic physical and health care activities during adolescence require some modifications because of maturational changes and because parents need to foster independent decision making by the adolescent.

Hygiene

Complete self-direction in the area of hygiene is achieved by midadolescence.

Skin care Increased sweat gland activity requires careful cleansing of the body and airing and cleaning of clothes. Deodorants and body powders become necessary because of the interaction of bacteria with the secretion of the newly active apocrine sweat glands, resulting in a pungent odor. The choice of appropriate deodorants or antiperspirants is based on effectiveness, cost, and any existing allergies. A deodorant or antiperspirant that causes a skin irritation should be discontinued, and a girl who shaves axillary hair should not apply a deodorizing agent immediately after shaving. Skin care concerns are intensified first because of the increased activity of the sebaceous glands. This factor, over which the adolescent has no control, contributes to acne. These glands produce *sebum,* a mixture of fatty acids, lipids, and sterols, which helps to keep the skin moist by inhibiting the evaporation of water. The environment influences the amount of secretion; more sebum is produced in hot, humid climates. Androgens also stimulate glandular activity, so that more secretion occurs in males.

Acne can produce skin lesions, including varying numbers and combinations of comedones (blackheads), papules (inflamed tissue), pustules (pus-containing lesions), and cysts (fluid-filled sacs). These lesions are caused by a plug of sebum blocking the hair follicles and by the inflammatory response of surrounding tissue. The areas affected are the face, upper chest, back, shoulders, and forehead. The earlier the onset, the more severe will be the manifestations. The average ages of the onset of acne are 14–17 years in girls and 16–19 years in boys.

Nurses might find that adolescents must be told to avoid handling or squeezing the lesions to prevent further infection and scarring. Cleanliness and attention to dietary elements that aggravate the condition might help, but medical care often is needed. Parents sometimes blame adolescents' diets or hygienic practices for the occurrence or severity of acne; nurses might need to explain that acne cannot be blamed solely on diet or hygiene.

Menstrual hygiene For girls, menstrual hygiene requires special attention because the irregularity of girls' early menstrual cycles often leads to embarrassment caused by soiled clothes. Exposure of this body secretion to air and/or stasis of the secretion on unchanged absorbent materials also causes odor. Menstrual flow can convey a sense of the unknown and lack of control because it is secreted from the vagina, which is located in a less visible body area and surrounded by the hair-covered labia. Girls can achieve some control by learning the signs that forecast the menstrual period, such as skin eruptions, tender breasts, weight gain, and unusual hunger.

A variety of comfortable, unobtrusive, absorbent materials are available for use during menstrual periods, for anticipated periods, or for midcycle discharges. External absorbent materials are usually called sanitary pads but may be referred to as napkins, towels, or cloths. These are constructed with a waterproof backing and hydrostatic packing to draw fluid away from the vulva. Some are biodegradable, easing disposal problems. They are available in various sizes, thicknesses, and shapes to accommodate varying ages, amounts of flow, and body configurations. They may be secured by belts or, more recently, by adhesive attachment to close-fitting panties.

Internal absorption may be achieved by inserting a plug of absorbent material, called a tampon, into the vagina, but the recently demonstrated incidence of a serious, sometimes fatal, systemic illness called toxic shock syndrome (TSS) has drawn attention to factors affecting tampon use in women of all ages. Estimates indicate that 95% of documented cases of TSS occur during menses, and a significant relationship has been found between tampon use and the development of TSS.

Tampon users of all ages are advised to be cautious in

tampon use. Women may alternate tampon use with external sanitary pads; current advice is to use an external pad at night or during sleep. Pad use during the lighter first and last days of menses decreases the trauma potential on these days, when tampon insertion is more difficult because of less lubrication. Thorough handwashing before insertion, perineal cleansing, frequent changing of tampons, and careful and complete removal of tampons can decrease local infection with *Staphylococcus aureus,* a possible antecedent to TSS. Baths, showers, and soap and water cleansing of the genital area, with separate wiping from front to back, offer sufficient cleaning of the vulva so that douching is not needed.

Parents need to understand the involuntary and often confusing nature of these hygienic concerns. Ridicule and blame are destructive to the self-esteem of the young person, who is trying to gain control over a changing body and, at the same time, trying to be accepted in peer social interactions. Parents may seek resources or refer young people to health professionals for current, accurate information. The best assistance is offered by alertness to signs of the onset of puberty and anticipatory guidance.

Sleep and Rest

During adolescence, the range of bedtimes becomes more variable. As adolescents become more aware of body needs, they go to bed because they think they need sleep, and they dawdle less. Some adolescents spend the entire evening in their bedrooms. Adolescents find more pleasure in sleeping and will sleep late when possible. They often have problems getting up.

Parents can encourage the greater awareness of body needs occasioned by fatigue. Parents also can use bedtime and awakening time as opportunities for adolescents to exercise control and recognize the consequences of their decisions. Alarm clocks usually decrease family tension and increase individual responsibility if arousal is a problem.

The major complaint of parents of teenagers probably is that teens sleep too much.

Nutrition

Especially during the growth spurt, adolescents show a markedly increased need for calories. The observation that teens, especially males, seem to be hungry and eating all the time might relate to an imbalance between the size of the stomach and the amount of calories needed. Nutrient intake is important for growth, energy, emotional control, appearance, and the health of the next generation. Problems in this area might be mild and easily solved or complex and controlled only with professional help.

Adolescence is a nutritionally vulnerable time because of the increase in physical growth and the changes in lifestyle and food habits. Because of the adolescent's process of development, nutrition education seldom affects eating practices. Eating and food choices are reactions to a variety of physical, emotional, and psychosocial motivations or impulses.

Nutritional requirements are closely related to the rate and timing of the adolescent growth spurt, which begins in males about 12 years of age, peaking at around 14 years of age, and begins in females at approximately 10 years of age, peaking at around 12 years of age. During the growth spurt, males increase their lean body tissue and skeletal mass while concurrently decreasing total body fat. Females gain proportionately more fat, so that by 20 years of age, they have about twice as much body fat as males. Males have a later, larger, and more prolonged growth period.

Because of their larger and longer growth period, the nutrient requirements of adolescent males are greater than those for adolescent females. These requirements vary not only with sex but also with age, body build, activity, and physiologic state. Males generally increase their caloric intake with greater physical maturity, whereas females decrease their caloric intake because their growth precedes sexual maturity. The 1980 recommended daily allowances (RDAs) for average caloric intakes based on chronologic age are as follows:

Females 11–14 years—2200 calories
Males 11–14 years—2700 calories
Females 15–18 years—2100 calories
Males 15–18 years—2800 calories

After 10 years of age, energy allowances decline to 45 calories/kg for adolescent males and 38 calories/kg for adolescent females (Committee on Dietary Allowances, 1980). After 11 years of age, the allowances for most of the nutrients are increased as follows:

Protein—56 g for males and 46 g for females
Vitamin A—1000 μg for males and 800 μg for females
Vitamin C—60 mg
Calcium—1200 mg
Iron—18 mg
Zinc—15 mg

These significant increases come at a period in life in which the eating habits may be poorest. Calcium and iron are most important because of the increase in skeletal mass, the expansion of blood volume and muscle mass in the male, and iron loss in the female menstrual flow. Adolescents should be advised to increase their milk intake to four servings a day and to select high iron-containing foods, such as animal proteins, to meet these increased nutrient needs. Males usually are better able to meet their nutrient requirements because of larger food intake. Most females are calorie conscious and are not willing to consume a larger amount of food.

Despite claims that adolescents have the poorest dietary intake of the general population, the findings of past national surveys show no evidence of extensive nutrient deprivation for adolescents (National Dairy Council, 1981). Nutrients most often consumed in inadequate amounts are iron, calcium, riboflavin, and vitamin A. Calcium and riboflavin are generally associated with a decrease of dairy food in the diet and the drinking of soft drinks rather than milk. It is difficult to consume 18 mg of iron each day when caloric intake is low, as is particularly common with adolescent females.

Three problems of insufficient nutritional quality may occur. The first is the problem of empty calories, evidenced by the popularity of snacks, soft drinks, chips, and candy in North American culture. Such an intake leads to a sufficient calorie intake but a deficiency of nutrients. The problem is intensified if it is derived from a lifelong pattern of poor eating habits and is lessened if it is a temporary adaptation to peer culture. Second, some adolescents select vegetarian diets, which can be adequate with careful planning but are more frequently inadequate in protein. The third dietary concern is weight control, where excessive or inadequate intake might be caused from or might itself cause both psychologic and physical problems.

Nurses can help parents to focus on the adolescent's need to make individual decisions in many areas of life and to prevent food intake from becoming the center of an independence-dependence struggle. For example, parents may refer to nutritionists for information in planning a nutrient-adequate diet and to consumer groups to influence the quality of snacks available in schools. Severe problems such as anorexia nervosa or bulimia require both psychiatric and medical treatment (see Chapter 16). Milder problems, such as obesity, may be resolved within community support groups.

Dentition

If malocclusion exists, correcting it during adolescence is usually advisable. Later correction is possible, but physical, psychologic, and social factors make it more difficult. The eruption of third molars ("wisdom teeth") during this period may intensify the degree of malocclusion.

Self-direction in the care of teeth usually has been established by midadolescence, but the adolescent might need to be reminded to obtain regular professional care. An increased incidence of dental caries between the ages 14 and 17 years is thought to be due to maturational changes (Valadian and Porter, 1977). Parents are urged to provide regular dental checkups and treatment of problems but to avoid blaming dietary or self-care practices of teens for the seemingly involuntary increase in caries in this age group.

Exercise

Research demonstrates that physical activity is necessary to support normal growth, especially of bones and muscles; to prevent adult health problems, especially arteriosclerotic vascular disease; to motivate lifelong activity involvement; and to enhance learning in the classroom. Therefore, regular habits of exercise through individual or group activities yield short- and long-term physical and psychologic benefits.

Parents can set examples that benefit themselves as well as their offspring. Current reports of participation indicate that parents might need to encourage girls and academically oriented adolescents to increase the balance between sedentary and active pursuits in favor of more exercise. Parents also might need to urge a greater range of activity for girls.

Sexual Maturation and Activity

Female growth sequence Breast growth is the first visible sign of female sexual maturation and usually coincides with the beginning of the growth spurt (Fig. 8-1). A mild asymmetry in this growth is normal. There are five stages of breast growth: (1) elevation of the nipple; (2) enlargement of the areola, the darkened area around the nipple; (3) enlargement of the breast; (4) projection of the areola and nipple; and (5) recession of the areola, leaving only the nipple projecting. (The 2-year transient breast growth that occurs in males reaches only the second stage.)

The second sign, pubic hair growth, sometimes precedes breast development (Fig. 8-2). Again, five stages have been distinguished: (1) no true pubic hair during puberty; (2) pale, fine hair, mainly at the sides of the labia in the female; (3) darker, coarser, curled hair; (4) hair of adult character; and (5) hair of adult quantity with an inverted triangle at the mons pubis. In the final stage, hair covers the sides of the labia and the perianal area. Stages 2 to 4 take 2 years; stages 4 to 5 may take 4–5 years. The rate of axillary hair growth corresponds to the growth of pubic hair.

The external female organs collectively are called the vulva, or pudendum. They include the mons pubis, the labia majora and labia minora, the clitoris, and the vaginal opening, which is usually partly covered by the hymen

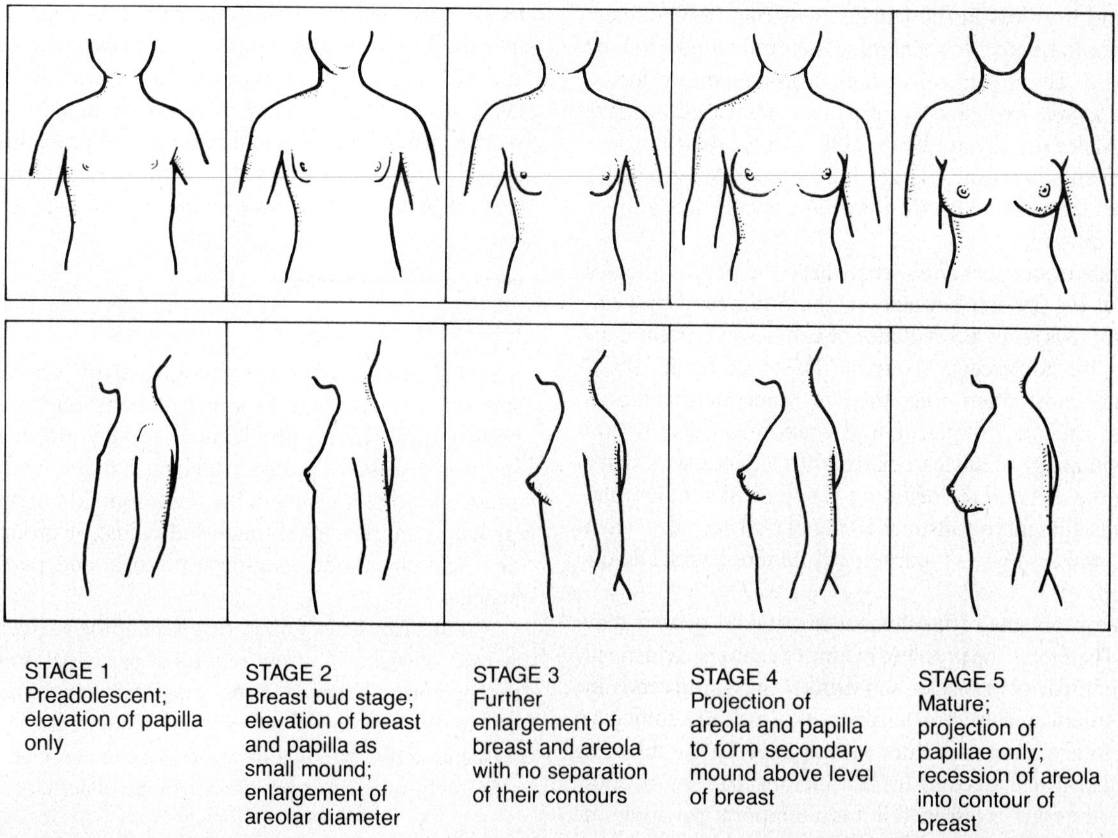

STAGE 1
Preadolescent; elevation of papilla only
STAGE 2
Sparse growth of long, downy, straight, slightly dark hair, chiefly along labia
Breast bud stage; elevation of breast and papilla as small mound; enlargement of areolar diameter
STAGE 3
Darker, coarse, curly hair, spreading slightly
Further enlargement of breast and areola with no separation of their contours
STAGE 4
Hair adult in type, but area covered smaller than in adult
Projection of areola and papilla to form secondary mound above level of breast
STAGE 5
Hair adult in quantity and area
Mature; projection of papillae only; recession of areola into contour of breast

FIGURE 8-1

Maturational stages of female breast development.

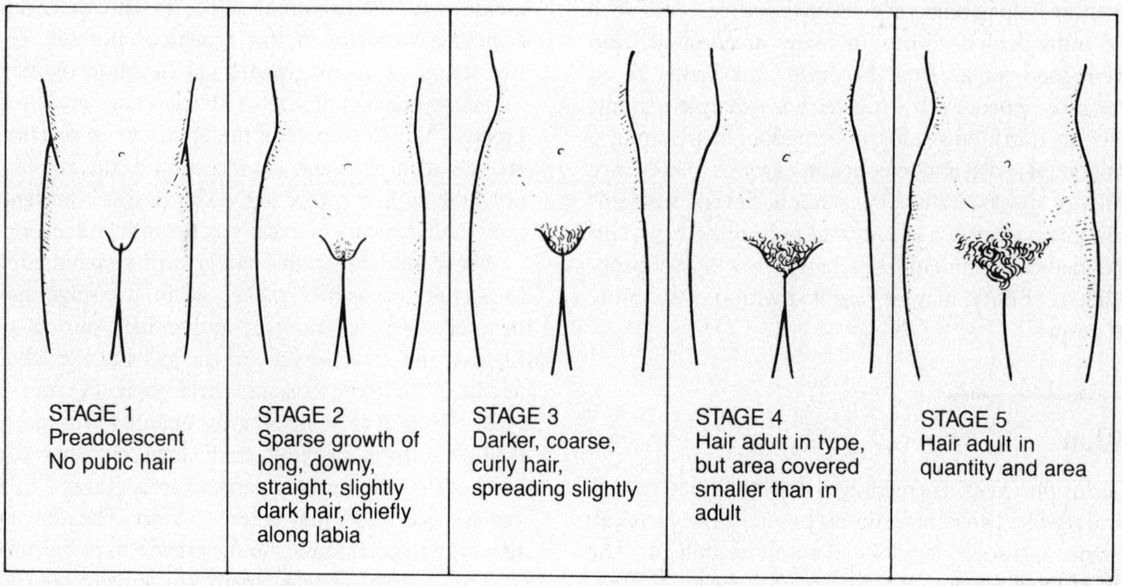

FIGURE 8-2

Maturational stages of female pubic hair development.

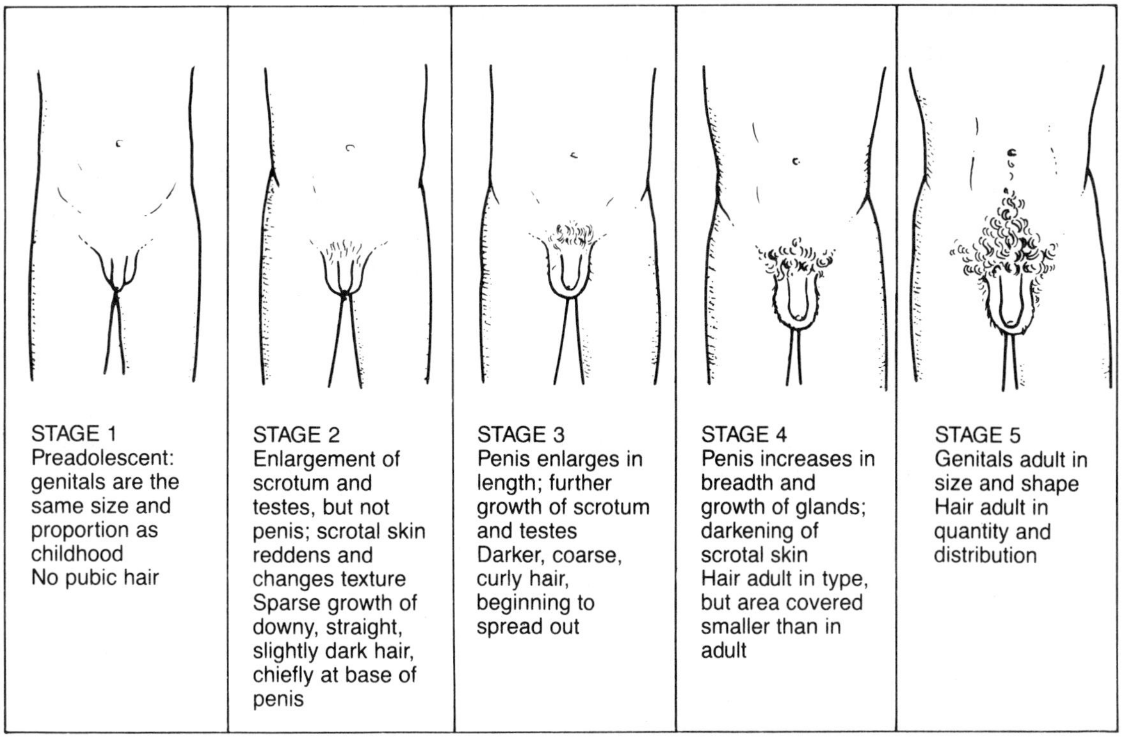

FIGURE 8-3

Maturational stages of male genital development.

in virgins. During puberty, these organs, especially the clitoris, become enlarged and increase in erotic sensitivity. The internal organs—the paired ovaries, the fallopian tubes, the uterus, and the vagina—increase in weight and musculature at this time. The cellular changes of the vagina, which cause its lining to thicken and the organ to enlarge, are the first internal changes of puberty. The vaginal contents also become acidic.

Finally, the onset of menstruation and the establishment of menstrual cycles provide a definite observable sign of reproductive maturation, although the first cycles may be anovulatory. For menstruation to occur, both the uterus and the ovaries undergo changes. The inner lining of the endometrium expands, with longer, thicker muscles, to become functional.

Male growth sequence The male's first visible sign of sexual maturation is testicular enlargement, which begins between 10 and 13 years of age and is completed between 14 and 18 years of age (Fig. 8-3). Two associated events follow testicular growth, but their timing is highly variable. The first is postpubertal orgasm, a neuromuscular event that is usually accompanied by the second event, ejaculation, the discharge of semen. Ejaculation is necessary for fertilization. Adolescent ejaculation most often is elicited by masturbation and less frequently occurs as nocturnal emission.

The male external genitalia are the penis and scrotum. A four-stage sequence of growth progresses from (1) prepubertal consistency in the size of both organs; (2) scrotal sac enlargement and a coarsening, wrinkling, and reddening (darkening) of the scrotal skin, which indicates enlargement of the enclosed testes; (3) penis lengthening; and (4) further enlargement of the penis and darkening of the scrotal sac. It is common for one side of the scrotum to grow faster than the other side. Penile growth occurs later than testicular and scrotal growth.

The growth of male pubic hair follows stages similar to those of the female, but the hair initially is distributed at the base of the scrotum, then the base of the penis, and eventually spreads over the pubic area. Approximately 40% of males also experience enlargement of the nipple area of the breast as a transient, 2- to 3-year phenomenon.

Sexual activity Major potential dangers in adolescence are unplanned pregnancy and sexually transmitted disease. The incidence of both is increasing as 55% of adolescents 13–19 years of age are sexually active (Zelnik and Kantner, 1980). Improved methods of contraception and the increased provision of sex education in public schools reach

TABLE 8-2 Advantages, Disadvantages, and Effectiveness of Different Forms of Contraception

Method	Major advantage	Major disadvantage
Oral contraceptive (0.3)*	Highly effective, does not interrupt sexual activity	Must be taken daily on a prescribed schedule; might produce side effects such as break-through bleeding, thrombus formation, nausea, headaches, depression; contraindicated for heavy smokers and those with any hypertensive disorder
Diaphragm with spermicide (15)	No major side effects, protects against sexually transmitted disease	May cause minor irritation and discomfort, must be fitted correctly and checked frequently for tears, may interfere with spontaneity
Condom (5)	No major side effects, protects against sexually transmitted disease, nonprescription	May cause vaginal irritation, possible dulled sensation, may interfere with spontaneity, must be checked for breaks or tears, must be removed properly to avoid spillage of semen
Spermicide (foams, jellies) (20)	Protects against sexually transmitted disease, nonprescription, most effective when used in conjunction with diaphragm or condom	Generally ineffective when used alone
Contraceptive sponge	Easier to use but slightly less effective than the diaphragm, does not require fitting, can be used for multiple coitus up to 48 hours	Can be difficult to remove, expensive
Fertility awareness (combined calendar rhythm, basal body temperature, cervical mucus observation)	Requires nothing artificial, inexpensive, no major side effects	Requires meticulous attention to body changes, abstinence during fertile periods, partner cooperation needed, effectiveness depends on conscientiousness
Douche (35–40)	Nonprescription, inexpensive, no major side-effects	Generally ineffective method, may cause irritation
Withdrawal (15–23)	Nonprescription, inexpensive, no major side effects	Semen may be deposited during pre-ejaculation, generally ineffective

*Numbers in parentheses represent pregnancies per 100 woman-years of use.

SOURCE: Adapted from material in Ladewig PA, London ML, Olds SB: *Essentials of Maternal-Newborn Nursing*, Addison-Wesley, 1986.

only a small percentage of the adolescents. Cognitive and affective development for the adolescent involves integration of sexuality into a continuous personal and social identity and the need for social support and responsible decision making.

Parents and professionals need to recognize cognitive, affective, social, and physical development in planning sex education. Many of the typical adolescent's perceptions of sexual intercourse are myths and stereotypes about how to be popular with peers, to achieve adult status, and to prove one's identity. During routine examinations, the nurse therefore assesses the young adolescent's knowledge about sex, intercourse, contraception, and reproduction. Being well-informed and understanding the personal and physiologic dynamics of a heterosexual relationship are the first steps in preventing unwanted pregnancy. The knowledgeable adolescent is less likely to take risks thinking that "it (pregnancy) can't happen to me" or that "my partner would use some protection."

Adolescents must know the facts but also must be aware of the personal responsibility each has regarding sexual activity. Education in the use of contraceptives is secondary, for example, to efforts to enhance the adolescent's self-concept and the ability to refuse unwanted sexual intercourse. Similarly, a responsible decision to be sexually active when one is socioeconomically unable to care for a child requires that contraception be considered. The nurse needs to explain the advantages, disadvantages, and effectiveness of each contraceptive method and then needs to support the adolescent in the proper use of the method chosen. (Table 8-2 provides a perspective of the various contraceptive methods available.)

Transition to Adulthood

The prime objective of adolescence is achieving a sense of self or personal identity. The definite and obvious changes of puberty, the cognitive development of an increasing ability to think about one's own thinking, and the highly variable rate of development among individuals of the same age challenge the teenager's sense of self. The adolescent's physical, and especially reproductive, maturation occurs in a context of economic dependence, creating an individual who is neither wholly child nor adult and causing both grief and anticipation at some level of consciousness.

The social setting, and especially the responses of significant people in this setting, influence the adolescent's ability to achieve a positive self-concept. Nurses might interact with adolescents or the significant people, such as parents and teachers, to provide information and clarify misconceptions about many issues of human growth and development. Nurses also have to consider how health problems affect the adolescent's ongoing efforts to confirm personal identity.

Essential Concepts

- Adolescence involves definite changes that affect the person's interactions with the family, community, school, and peers.
- Some physical and psychologic signs of the onset of puberty are evident, and some are less obvious.
- Physical signs include maturation of the sweat glands and sexual organs, as well as changes in body configurations. Psychologic changes are evident in behavior.
- The onset of puberty is a major transition and is often associated with disequilibrium.
- Male and female reproductive systems follow specific patterns of maturation that are related to the interaction of neurologic and hormonal controls.
- Affective development involves sexuality, leader-follower roles, response to authority, values, emotional control, self-esteem, belonging, self-assertion, and daydreaming.
- The components of self-esteem and self-concept are challenged in the psychosocial crisis of adolescence described by Erik Erikson as a conflict resolution between identity and identity diffusion or confusion.
- Adolescents need to experiment with several roles to achieve identity. James Marcia developed a method for evaluating identity achievements by applying the components of vocation choice and value orientation.
- Adolescence is a time of developing formal operations, described by Jean Piaget as the ability to manipulate ideas as well as objects. Schooling of adolescents, especially tasks requiring motivation and memory, is best designed so that the adolescent is an active participant in an environment conducive to learning.
- Language development is linked to cognitive development, school tasks, and self-concept.
- Moral reasoning for most adolescents involves consideration of group norms and fixed rules. Development of religious faith involves exploring the differing values and beliefs of the adolescent's experience.
- Social development in adolescence is a process of developmental tasks through which the adolescent acquires independence, a sense of self in relation to others, and the skills to assume adult roles.
- The varied purposes and forms of play, including dating, in adolescence are exemplified by cooperative play, team play, and construction and creativity.
- Hygienic concerns in adolescents include special attention to skin care, sweat gland activity, and menstrual hygiene. Development concerns relate to sleep and rest, nutrition, dental care, exercise, and sexual activity.

References

Bandura A: *Social Learning Theory.* Prentice-Hall, 1977.

Committee on Dietary Allowances, Food and Nutrition Board, National Research Council: Page 28 in: *Recommended Dietary Allowances.* 9th ed. National Academy of Sciences, 1980.

Erikson EH: *Childhood and Society.* Norton, 1963.

Erikson EH: *Identity: Youth and Crisis.* Wiley, 1968.

Fowler J: Stages in faith: the structural-developmental approach. In: *Values and Moral Development*. Hennessy T (editor). Paulist Press, 1976.

Gesell A, Ilg F, Ames LD: *The Years From Ten to Sixteen*. Harper & Row, 1956.

Havighurst RJ: *Developmental Tasks and Education*. 3rd ed. McKay, 1972.

Jones MC: Psychological correlates of somatic development. *Child Dev* 1965; 36:899–911.

Katchadourian H, Lunde D: *Fundamentals of Human Sexuality*. Holt, Rinehart & Winston, 1975.

Kohlberg L: Moral development and identification. In: *Child Psychology*. Stevenson H (editor). University of Chicago Press, 1963.

Kohlberg L: Moral stages and moralization: The cognitive-developmental approach. Pages 31–53 in: *Moral Development and Behavior: Theory, Research and Social Issues*. Lickona T (editor). Holt, Rinehart & Winston, 1976.

Kohlberg L, Turiel E: Moral development and moral education. In: *Psychology and Educational Practice*. Lesser GS (editor). Scott Foresman, 1971.

Marcia J: Development and validation of ego-identity status. *J Pers Soc Psychol* 1966; 3:551–558.

Marcia J: Identity in adolescence. In: *Handbook of Adolescent Psychology*. Adelson J (editor). Wiley, 1980.

Miller D: *Adolescence: Psychology, Psychopathology and Psychotherapy*. Jason Aronson, 1974.

National Dairy Council: Nutritional concerns during adolescence. *Dairy Council Dig* (March/April) 1981; 52:7–11.

Piaget J: *The Construction of Reality in the Child*. Cook M (translator). Ballantine Books, 1954.

Piaget J: *The Origins of Intelligence in Children*. Cook M (translator). International Universities Press, 1952.

Sullivan HS: *The Interpersonal Theory of Psychiatry*. Perry HS, Gavel ML (editors). Norton, 1953.

Tanner JM: *Growth of Adolescence, With a General Consideration of the Effects of Hereditary and Environmental Factors Upon Growth and Maturation from Birth to Maturity*. 2nd ed. Blackwell, 1962.

Tanner JM: Sequence, tempo, and individual variation in growth and development of boys and girls aged twelve to sixteen. In: *Twelve to Sixteen: Early Adolescence*. Kagan J, Coles R (editors). Norton, 1972.

Valadian I, Porter D: *Physical Growth and Development From Conception to Maturity*. Little, Brown, 1977.

Zelnick M, Kantner JK: Sexual and contraceptive experience of young unmarried women in the United States, 1976 and 1971. In: *Adolescent Pregnancy and Childbearing*. Chilman CS (editor). US Department of Health and Human Services. Publication No. (NIH) 81–2077, Dec 1980.

Additional Readings

Bailey DA: The growing child and the need for physical activity. In: *School-Age Children: Development and Relationships*. Smart MI, Smart RC (editors). Macmillan, 1978.

Bell R: *Changing Bodies, Changing Lives: A Book for Teens on Sex and Relationships*. Random House, 1981.

Borow H: Career development. In: *Understanding Adolescence*, 3rd ed. Adams JF (editor). Allyn and Bacon, 1976.

The Boston Women's Health Book Collective: *Our Bodies Ourselves: A Book By and For Women*. Simon & Schuster, 1976.

The Boston Women's Health Book Collective: *Ourselves and Our Children: A Book By and For Parents*. Random House, 1978.

Brown LK: Toxic shock syndrome. *Matern-Child Nurs J* 1981; 4:57–59.

Coles R: *Privileged Ones: The Well-Off and the Rich in America*. Little, Brown, 1977.

Comer JP, Poussaint AF: *Black Child Care: How to Bring Up a Healthy Black Child in America: A Guide to Emotional and Psychological Development*. Simon & Schuster, 1975.

Comfort A, Comfort J: *The Facts of Love: Living, Loving and Growing Up*. Crown, 1979.

Douvan E, Adelson J: American dating patterns. In: *Issues in Adolescent Psychology*. Rogers D (editor). Appleton-Century-Crofts, 1969.

Erikson EH: *Youth: Change and Challenge*. Basic Books, 1963.

Flavell J: *The Developmental Psychology of Jean Piaget*. Van Nostrand, 1963.

Freud A: *The Ego and the Mechanisms of Defense*. International Universities Press, 1967.

Frisch RE: Weight at menarche: similarity for well-nourished and under-nourished girls at differing ages and evidence for historical constancy. *Pediatrics* 1972; 50:445–501.

Ginsburg HJ, Opper S: *Piaget's Theory of Intellectual Development*. Prentice-Hall, 1979.

Gruen W: Adult personality: an empirical study of Erikson's theory of ego development. In: *Personality in Middle and Late Life*. Neugarten B (editor). Atherton Press, 1964.

Guttmacher A: *Teen Pregnancy: The Problem that Hasn't Gone Away*. The Alan Guttmacher Institute, 1980.

Jones IH: The history of sanitary protection. *Nurs Times* (March 6) 1980; 76:407–408.

Kagan J, Coles R (editors): *Twelve to Sixteen: Early Adolescence*. Norton, 1972.

Katchadourian H: *The Biology of Adolescence*. Freeman, 1977.

Kohlberg L, Gilligan C: The adolescent as a philosopher: The discovery of self in a post-conventional world. *Daedalus* (Fall) 1971; 100:1051–1086.

Neimark ED: Adolescent thought: transition to formal operations. In: *Handbook of Developmental Psychology*. Prentice-Hall, 1982.

Neimark ED: Intellectual development during adolescence. In: *Review of Developmental Research*, vol 4. Horowitz FD (editor). University of Chicago Press, 1975.

Nelms BC: What is a normal adolescent? *Am J Matern-Child Nurs* (Nov/Dec) 1981; 6(6):402–406.

O'Hara R, Tiedeman D: Vocational self-concept in adolescence. In: *Issues in Adolescent Psychology*. Rogers D (editor). Appleton-Century-Crofts, 1969.

Olds SB, London ML, Ladewig PA: *Maternal-Newborn Nursing.* Addison-Wesley, 1984.

Peterson AC: Can puberty come any faster? *Psychol Today* (Feb) 1979; 12:45–46.

Piaget J: *The Moral Judgment of the Child.* Gabain M (translator). Free Press, 1965.

Rivers C, Barnett R, Baruch G: *Beyond Sugar and Spice: How Women Grow, Learn and Thrive.* Putnam, 1979.

Schestowsky B: Helping your adolescent client become more physically fit. *Can Nurse* (April) 1983; 79:24–25.

Schowalter JE, Anyan R: *The Family Handbook of Adolescence.* Knopf, 1979.

Schuster CS, Ashburn SS: *The Process of Human Development: A Holistic Approach.* Little, Brown, 1986.

Sheldon WH, Stevens SS, Tucker WB: *The Varieties of Human Physique.* Harper & Row, 1940.

Sommer BB: *Puberty and Adolescence.* Oxford University Press, 1978.

Stone LJ, Church J: *Childhood and Adolescence: A Psychology of the Growing Person.* Random House, 1973.

Torrance EP: Fostering creative thinking during the high school years. In: *Issues in Adolescent Psychology.* Rogers D (editor). Appleton-Century-Crofts, 1969.

Vick RL: *Contemporary Medical Physiology.* Addison-Wesley, 1984.

White JE: Initiating contraceptive use: how do young women decide? *Pediatr Nurs* 1984; 10:347–352.

Yeaworth RC et al.: The development of an adolescent life change event scale. *Adolescence* 1980; 15(57):91–97.

Chapter 9

Principles of Assessment

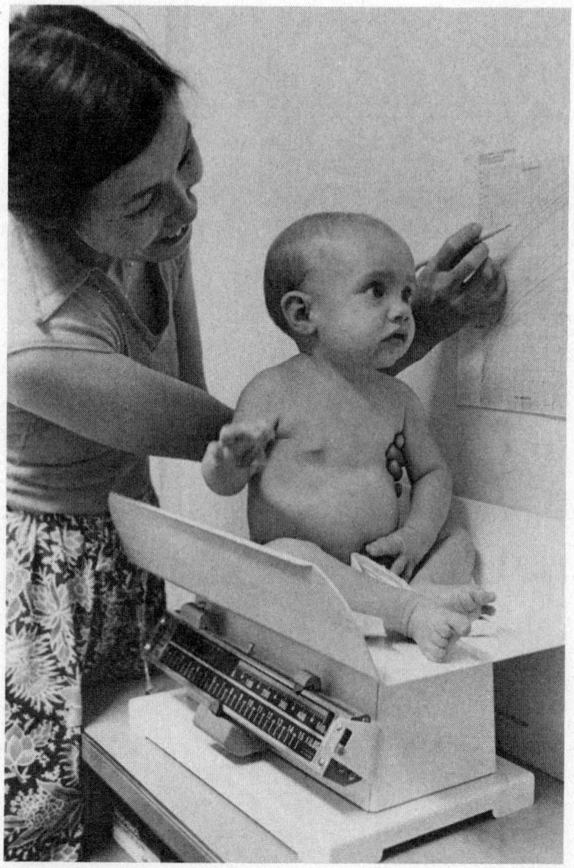

Chapter Contents

Objectives

- State the goals of a child health history.
- Discuss the nurse's role in child health assessment.
- Describe communication techniques used to interview the child and family.

- Explain the purpose of observations and screening tests in the assessment process.
- Define the nurse's role in identifying developmental delays.
- List the component parts of the child health history.
- Explain the purpose of including the family health history.

Nurses are often the first contacts that children and families have with the health care system. During well-child visits, the nurse frequently is responsible for conducting the health history and initiating the assessment process. When the child is ill, the nurse first asks questions, makes observations, and interprets the information concerning the child's state of health before referring the child and family to the physician. The nurse is responsible for collecting health-related information and for interpreting the information for early identification, intervention, or referral to other members of the health team. Assessment therefore is a vital part of the child health nursing process.

A comprehensive health assessment begins with the health history interview. The health history includes data concerning the past and current physical and developmental status of the client. While gathering this information, the nurse interprets it and uses it to direct further data collection and to plan nursing interventions. In the absence of specific medical problems, nursing responsibilities focus on providing teaching and reassurance to parents.

Techniques for Interviewing the Child and Family

The verbal and nonverbal exchange of information between the nurse and the client (or in the case of young children, the parent) is essential to the nursing process. The client interview requires good communication skills, as the nurse needs to set the tone and establish trust with both the child and parent. The success of the client-nurse relationship often depends on this initial contact.

The ability to communicate purposefully and skillfully, however, is seldom a natural gift. Communication skills must be learned and practiced. Good communication between the nurse and client consists of a mutual understanding of each other's questions and answers. This understanding is accomplished by amplifying, elaborating, giving examples, setting a respectful tone, and conveying a willingness to be of assistance. During the interview, the nurse uses both learned techniques and personal characteristics that seek to put the client at ease and to establish a trusting relationship.

The goals of the health interview are to (1) gain information concerning the health status of the client, (2) understand the client as a unique person, (3) establish rapport and a trusting relationship, and (4) provide support by answering questions and preparing for treatments and procedures. To accomplish these goals, the nurse employs basic interviewing skills that allow a purposeful and flexible exchange of information. The interview is not only a process of obtaining information but also an opportunity for health teaching and anticipatory guidance. Parents often need basic information about normal growth and development and about preventing injury and illness (see Chapters 11 and 12). The interview provides a setting in which the nurse can address the parent's needs and concerns.

While it is important to attend to the concerns and questions of the client, the nurse also guides the interview process so the client does not digress at length from pertinent material. The nurse who knows what information is needed and has a plan for obtaining the information is better able to refocus the interview and guide the client back to the topics of concern. By asking questions that show respect for what the client has said, the nurse can develop rapport with the client and, at the same time, emphasize data that are most pertinent to the health history.

Communicating Nonverbally

Central to the interviewing process is being alert and responding to nonverbal cues provided by the client. These nonverbal cues include the child's and parent's posture and use of gestures. Voice quality, sentence structure, and choice of words often provide more information than what is actually said. Facial expression, eye contact, physical distance, and touch also are valuable cues to the quality of interaction, both between client and nurse and between parent and child. Body hygiene, skin color, dress, and grooming are additional cues that may be helpful in understanding the client's socioeconomic situation and potential needs for assistance.

Nonverbal communication places verbal communication in better perspective. The nurse's response to nonverbal cues also sets the tone of the interview. Responding to these cues indicates concern for the client as a person and shows the nurse's desire to be of assistance. By being sensitive and exploring the meaning of nonverbal cues, the nurse conveys to the client a sense of individual importance and indicates that the client is not "just a number."

Standard communication techniques of reflection, validation, and clarification are useful in the interview. The nurse reflects the client's message by repeating and summarizing what the client has said, validates the message by affirming its importance, and clarifies the information by asking further questions. By using these techniques, the nurse lets the client know that feelings, fears, and concerns—whatever they are—can be discussed and will be accepted as genuine and worthy of attention. Effective communication, identification of areas of concern, verification of client strengths, and a relationship of trust occur more quickly when attention is given to nonverbal cues.

Communicating Verbally

The health history interview is likely to be more complete if clients are provided with privacy and receive the nurse's undivided attention. The client who feels important and worthy of the nurse's time and energy throughout the interview is more likely to cooperate and provide the requested information. While conducting the interview, it is essential for the nurse to maintain professonal composure. Common traps in the interviewing process are social conversation, hasty reassurance, use of medical jargon, and questions that create defensiveness in the client. Rather than fall into these traps, the nurse needs to demonstrate supportive and empathic behavior that facilitates the development of a therapeutic relationship. The nurse therefore chooses vocabulary that the client can understand, repeats information or rephrases questions as necessary, and gives clear definitions of all technical terms, thus treating the client with dignity and respect.

What the nurse says to the client, in addition to the nurse's tone and action, greatly determines what the client says and how completely the client answers the question. The kinds of questions asked or statements made by the nurse influence the kinds of responses made by the client. Phrasing a question in an open-ended manner, for example, allows the client to answer in descriptive statements rather than with "yes" or "no" statements. Making statements that call for descriptive responses also helps clients fully describe their present and past experiences. Statements such as "Go on," "Tell me more," "Oh?" "When?" "What?" "Start at the beginning and tell me," "Then what happened?" "And?" or "Describe . . ." call for descriptive elaboration of an experience. The client who is given the opportunity to respond in this way is more likely to feel comfortable asking questions and voicing concerns.

Open-ended questions thus are broad questions that leave the client free to describe a situation or problem from a personal perspective. The response can then assist the client in recalling further aspects of the experience or in clarifying concerns. In contrast, closed, direct questions do not encourage the client to talk freely but ask instead for specific responses to specific questions. The information gained from closed questioning usually is biased according to the questions asked and often suggests a judgment. For example, asking "Does the child behave during mealtimes?" requires the parent to evaluate the child's behavior and answer "yes" or "no." Asking instead, "How does the child behave during mealtimes?" allows the parent to elaborate and gives the nurse clues about family functioning.

Some closed questions are appropriate during the health history, but these need to be used selectively. For example, "How old is the baby?" or "What medication did you take?" are closed, direct questions. This format elicits information that can be used in formulating additional open-ended questions and directing the interview. The wording of questions is thus a component of nursing care and involves the nurse in initial planning and evaluation of the client's response. Throughout the interview, the nurse notes the way in which the client describes problems, why the client is concerned, and whether stated problems are related to specific life events.

Clients also can learn during the health interview, through the interpersonal process between the client and the nurse. The nurse is often able to identify and study a parent's degree of skill in struggling with the responsibilities of parenting and can help parents meet problems that involve their child's health and parent-child relations. These difficulties often are identified during the health interview. By using communication skills, the nurse develops effective methods for helping parents learn more constructive behavior and provides parents and other family members with opportunities to increase their knowledge and develop the skills necessary to improve. (Table 9-1 reviews child development and relates it to family responsibilities and suggests relevant questions for the nurse to gain insight into the parent-child interaction.)

Addressing Parental Concerns

If a parent has a particular concern about a child's development, it is helpful to discover this early in the assessment process by clarifying with the parent the exact nature of the problem. To discover whether the problem is old or new, the nurse asks when the parent first became concerned. Next, the nurse determines whether the problem has seemed to

(text continues on p. 237)

TABLE 9-1 Areas of Child and Family Assessment

Child development	Family responsibilities	Relevant child-care questions
Infancy		
Biophysical development Normal fine and gross motor milestones	Provide safe, comfortable environment with proper nutrition and health care Maintain a nurturing relationship with infant by parent through mutual regular feeding and sleeping patterns Learn to care competently for infant	Is the environment safe, with adequate food and clothing? Does the family have a regular source of medical care and an adequate income? Does family provide muscle activity, toys, or equipment to enhance motor development? Does parent restrict infant's physical movement? Is child at an appropriate weight?
Cognitive development Sensorimotor stage	Provide environment with appropriate level of interaction and stimulation for sensorimotor development (auditory, visual, and tactile stimulation) Spend time with infant to enhance language and sensorimotor development	Does parent consciously encourage language development through labeling and verbal interchanges with the infant? Does parent invest time and interest in enhancing developmental milestones? Does parent provide appropriate toys to foster sensorimotor development (books and toys that require eye-hand coordination)?
Affective development Oral stage Trust vs. mistrust	Develop attachment between infant and caregivers Provide an environment that consistently satisfies infant's needs	Does parent have appropriate perceptions and expectations of the infant? In what ways does parent spend time on a regular basis interacting with infant? Is there a continuity and consistency in caregivers? Is the home free of conflict?
Social development	Maintain relationship with relatives and community Have sources of emotional and tangible support	Does the family see or communicate with relatives at least once a month? Is family involved in community organizations (church, leisure activities, etc)? Is the parent pleased with the role of parent?
Early childhood		
Biophysical development Development of gross and fine motor control; use of utensils to feed self; beginning self-dressing; scribbling; copying simple geometric designs; toilet training accomplished during this period; eating habits might become idiosyncratic	Provide safe environment to allow child an opportunity for motor development Encourage gross and fine motor activity through appropriate toys, permitting required space to experiment with walking and other movements Facilitate beginning skills in self-care (feeding, dressing, and toileting) Encourage gradual independence in self-care activities (dressing, bathing) Provide opportunities for successful toilet training	Has the home been childproofed? Is parental supervision adequate for activity levels of this age? Is the child allowed to move around the home? How much time is spent in crib, playpen, or highchair? Does the family provide appropriate toys or equipment to enhance both fine and gross motor development? Does child receive regular medical care?

(Continues)

TABLE 9-1 Areas of Child and Family Assessment *(Continued)*

Child development	Family responsibilities	Relevant child-care questions
Early childhood (*Continued*)	Adjust family meal and sleep patterns to include child	Does the family respect the child's food likes and dislikes? Is there respect and consideration for changing sleep needs? What are the family's accident prevention behaviors?
Cognitive development Ability to solve new problems through representation; object permanence with invisible displacement; prediction of cause-and-effect relationships; development of spoken language (egocentric speech) with eventual mastery of speech; preoperational stage of development of such conceptual modes of thought as transformation, concentration, reversibility, and conservation; thought becomes representational	Encourage language development through continual verbal interaction with child by labeling objects and reading Encourage sensorimotor development through appropriate toys Take the child into areas of the community that provide variety and stimulation	Do family members spend time talking to the child? Do parents have any structured play time with the child? Do parents read to the child? What do parents do to consciously encourage cognitive development? How much time is spent on this? Is the child included in family activities and outings? Does the child get out of the house regularly? Do parents provide appropriate toys? How do the parents support/encourage the child in beginning decision making and responsibility for actions and behavior? To what extent is the family involved with a preschool experience, nursery school, organized day care, or a play group?
Affective development Autonomy vs. shame and doubt Initiative; ability to use physical and emotional energy for self-direction, self-exploration, and experience with a multitude of new adventures; development of the superego through resolution of the Oedipus or Electra conflict; continued emergence of the child's ego structures; development of gender identity	Provide ratio of control to freedom in toilet training, mobility, and satisfaction of needs Be available to help child deal with conflicts between mental images and reality Provide appropriate ratio between restrictions and permissiveness Reinforce child's appropriate sense of body image	Are parents either overly restrictive or overly permissive in toilet training, allowing mobility, and "messy" play activities? How does the family handle the child's fears? What role does the "imaginary playmate" have in the family? What are the discipline practices? How are fathering and mothering roles delineated in the family? How do these roles support and affect the child's identification process?
Social development Development of autonomy through self-control	Provide child with opportunities to interact with other children Provide opportunities to visit with relatives Help child in learning how to share and interact with others Set appropriate limits on child's behavior Plan for family-oriented extracurricular activities	If child is in day care, is amount of time acceptable? Is it quality day care? Is the child in a play group? What are the size, frequency, and supervision? How is time spent with siblings? Does the child have regular visits with relatives? How do parents assist the child with social interactions? What is the family's mode of discipline? How frequently do parents punish?

TABLE 9-1 *(Continued)*

Child development	Family responsibilities	Relevant child-care questions
Early childhood (*Continued*)	Support interactions with larger social environment and interactions to validate the child's emerging perceptions of the larger social world	What are the specific opportunities available to the child for engaging with a wider social environment? How do the family members relate to the child's larger world?
Middle and late childhood		
Biophysical development Lower growth rate but increased self-awareness of bodily changes and increased efficiency in motor skills	Continue to meet child's nutritional and physical needs Be sensitive to changes in eating and sleeping patterns of the child	Does the parent allow the child a choice in foods occasionally? Is there negotiation on bedtime when appropriate? Does the family provide an environment that supports expanding motor skills (ie, amount of play space available, use of public playgrounds, involvement in cooperative sports)?
Cognitive development Period of concrete operations; cognitive ability to use logic; use of symbols, classification of information; social communication; preconventional stage of moral development	Foster child's emerging cognitive style (the way the child organizes information and finds solutions to problems)	Does the family reinforce and support the learning that is taking place in school? Is attention paid to the child's homework? Is the parent involved in the child's school activities and communicating with teachers regarding the child's progress?
Affective development Industry vs. inferiority	Provide for and support the child's entrance into larger society and into school, social organization (community, sports, clubs, etc.), and peer groups	Does the home/school environment provide a wide array of opportunities and materials for creative and productive work?
Social development Development of self-concept, self-esteem	Be sensitive to child's developmental abilities and limitations Foster child's developing ego through unconditional acceptance, continued love, and affective nurturance	Are family members honest with the child? Does the family guide the child into setting limits to behavior (eg, taking turns with others or caring for own room and personal belongings)? Does the family provide age-appropriate play materials? Do play materials differ for sons and daughters? In what ways does the family allow the child to test out new ideas and concepts? What are the family's attitudes toward and practice of television viewing, video games, and other media? How do the family members perceive the child's developing sense of right and wrong? What is their style of discipline toward the child? Do they allow the child limited responsibility for actions?

(Continues)

TABLE 9-1 Areas of Child and Family Assessment *(Continued)*

Child development	Family responsibilities	Relevant child-care questions
Middle and late childhood (*Continued*)		How does the family foster the child's strivings for personal accomplishments? Do family members encourage and support involvement in extracurricular activities, membership in organizations, or self-expression through individual interests? How do family members convey acceptance to the child? Do they set clear and consistent limits to behavior? Is there flexibility with these limits to permit individual changes? Are the family members sensitive to the importance of the child's peer group? How accepting are they of the child's peer group?
Adolescence		
Biophysical development Growth spurt with development of primary and secondary sexual characteristics	Provide health education to adolescent regarding physical bodily changes Provide sex education and/or seek out health care providers to assist in this task	Is there an open, honest approach toward sexuality? How do family members feel about sexual identity? How is love and affection expressed?
Cognitive development Period of formal operations (ie, abstract mental functioning) Conventional stage of moral development		How does family encourage and/or support adolescent in vocational or professional pursuits? In what ways does the family help prepare the adolescent for adult work life? How does the family give the adolescent an opportunity to act on own problem-solving strategies?
Affective development Identity (ie, clarifying and becoming aware of one's personal self) vs. diffusion	Appropriately adjust family roles to move from parental protectiveness and sole responsibility to guided and increased adolescent individuality, independence, and autonomy	What are methods of parental control (ie, authoritative, permissive, or bureaucratic parenting styles)?
Social development Self-definition, personal uniqueness, and independence	Continue stability in family acceptance and affection within atmosphere of mutual trust	How does the family exhibit an atmosphere of mutual trust? How do family members handle the issue of privileges (ie, use of family car, dating, and choice of social activities)? How has family handled issues of sexuality, drinking, and drugs? How does the parent handle the adolescent's swings in behavior from childlike to adultlike? How does the parent react to the adolescent's increasing dependence on the peer group and decreasing dependence on the family?

improve or worsen, noting any factors that appear to make the problem better or worse. In addition, the nurse questions whether or not the child thinks that this concern of the parent's is a problem. Also important is whether this is the only problem or one of several.

Finding out whether the child has developed any symptoms attributable to the problem will help to direct the rest of the interview and later the physical exam. The nurse explores any recent changes in the child's family life (such as moving, separation, death, divorce, illness), the family members' response to the change, and whether the change might be related to the problem. Finally, the nurse discusses the impact of the problem on the family and child, what measures the family has taken to deal with the problem, and whether any of these measures have been effective. Parents often need to hear the nurse validate and encourage positive aspects of their parenting styles.

For example, 4-year-old Mark appeared to be a normally developing child but showed some inability to tolerate separation from his mother. By questioning the mother, the nurse learned that the family had recently moved to the area and that the mother was concerned about Mark's loss of neighborhood playmates. She also expressed feelings of loneliness herself and reported some recent attempts to make friends. Recognizing the needs of both Mark and his mother, the nurse was able to encourage the family to make contacts in the community and could refer the mother to a neighborhood nursery school for Mark.

Involving the Child in the Interview

Early childhood By 2 years of age, the child should start to be included in the interview process. The nurse approaches the young child gradually, at eye level, respecting the child and yet showing interest. The child can better relate to the nurse if the nurse sits on the floor or bends down to the child's level. The nurse who stands up is viewed by most children as an imposing authority figure.

Using puppets or toys is an excellent way to involve very young children in communication. Although children at this stage can respond to simple questions and can follow simple commands, they will do so more readily if these are seen as a game. Involving the child and praising the child's responses also help to gain the child's cooperation. The child is also more likely to cooperate when the nurse is viewed as a trusted and "safe" person by the parents.

As the young child matures, the nurse includes the child in the history taking to the extent that is developmentally appropriate. During early childhood, the child has little perception of time and is oriented in the present. The nurse therefore focuses on the present. The nurse might ask the child about a favorite toy or book or the toy with which the child was just playing. If the child has been using crayons or markers, the nurse might comment on the drawing and ask the child to tell about it. The nurse can establish rapport by asking the child to do some easily performed and fun-producing behaviors. The child who experiences success with initial skills is more likely to attempt more difficult skills than the child who met failure with the initial behaviors. The communication process also helps the child to cooperate during the physical examination (see Chapter 10).

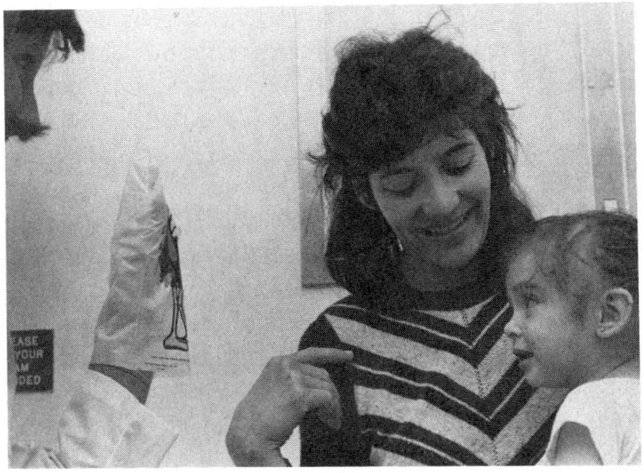

Puppets and dolls can help the nurse communicate with young children. Developing trust in this way can also help the nurse gain the child's cooperation during the physical examination.

Middle and late childhood During middle and late childhood, children generally like to participate in answering questions. They like to tell the nurse what their favorite foods are, what game they like the best, and who their best friends are. Integrating the child into the interview in this way gives the child a sense of control over the situation, acclimates the child to the environment, and helps the child begin to trust the nurse. Conversing with the child also gives the nurse important information about the child's speech patterns, developmental level, and ability to relate with an adult.

When conversing with the child, the nurse will be more effective in obtaining information if the questions are well formulated. Questions should be clearly stated in language and terms that the child can understand. Children at these stages do not appreciate being asked too many questions. The child who feels bombarded with questions will view the nurse as a source of irritation instead of a source of help. Also irritating are questions that have obvious or readily apparent answers. Children do not like to answer questions that they consider obvious or "dumb"; they either might not respond or might purposefully give incorrect answers.

Because new knowledge and problem-solving skills are learned through concrete objects during this time, the nurse uses charts, diagrams, and models when explaining health-related concepts. These children are curious about their bodies and how they function. With the use of actual objects or illustrations, they can begin to understand the body's internal functioning and the relationship between infection and preventive measures such as rest, diet, and exercise. It is important to give these children appropriate choices and to allow them to assist in procedures so that they gain some sense of control.

Adolescence Adolescents, especially older adolescents, might come to the health center by themselves. The nurse then focuses the interview and history taking on the adolescent's concerns, asking questions about information that the adolescent is likely to know. When an adolescent is accompanied by a parent or other adult, the nurse needs to determine whether the two should be seen together or separately. If seen separately, each should know that confidentiality is assured. If an issue arises that the nurse feels ought to be shared, the nurse suggests that the adolescent and adult meet together but does not violate confidentiality.

The concerns that either parent or adolescent chooses to discuss when the other is absent can be revealing. Some families communicate openly and discuss problems directly, so that family members are not likely to discuss different concerns during separate interviews. Other families do not discuss concerns openly with each other, and during separate interviews, these family members might bring up topics they are hesitant to discuss in front of each other.

For example, an adolescent girl who was comparatively healthy and doing well in school mentioned to the nurse that she wished her parents would give her more freedom. She knew they loved her and wanted her to be happy, but at the same time she thought their fears for her safety and their resulting restrictions were extreme. She cooperated with them because she did not want to hurt them but admitted to feeling increasingly resentful. After further discussion of her concerns, the nurse suggested that she talk to her parents about this matter. The nurse and girl identified some areas in which additional responsibility for making decisions would be appropriate for her. When interviewing the parents, the nurse discussed normal adolescent growth and development and asked the parents to give their impressions of their daughter's developmental status. This discussion provided an opportunity for the nurse to suggest ways in which they could comfortably foster their daughter's independence and sense of identity. The nurse also encouraged the parents to discuss this idea with their daughter. In this way the nurse was able to help the family members gain new insights into their own and each other's concerns and, more important, to suggest ways to enhance individual and family development.

Because adolescents have learned to think in hypothetical or abstract terms and can use analogies, the nurse can ask them about their ideas of why illness occurs and ways to stay healthy. The adolescent who is encouraged to suggest ways to recover from a present illness or to prevent future occurrences tends to cooperate more fully with planned interventions. Furthermore, the adolescent can identify future implications of illness or injury and can relate behaviors to prevention or susceptibility. For adolescents, however, a common problem is the gap between knowing healthful behaviors and actually practicing them. It therefore is best to concentrate on the present concern and its current effects. Directing the adolescent's attention and energies to a single focus tends to be more successful than encouraging the adolescent to change too many behaviors at the same time.

Components of the Health Interview

As a result of questions and observations, the nurse should be able to do the following:

1. Determine that the child is developing normally or detect problems early
2. Provide guidance and counseling for both the child and the parent
3. Help the parent understand the child's behavior
4. Identify the child's concerns
5. Foster optimal development

The parent who has an opportunity to discuss concerns with the nurse and participate in the child's developmental assessment is better able to recognize normal development. This recognition reassures the parent not only that the child is doing well but also that the parent is doing a good job as a parent.

Developmental History

Until adolescence, children usually are accompanied to the health center by a parent, guardian, or other relative, so that assessment involves both the child and the family. With the nonverbal infant, the nurse gathers information concerning the infant's health and development from the adult, most often the parent who usually is the primary caregiver. If more than one adult is present, the nurse identifies the primary caregiver and addresses most of the questions to that person. (Components of the developmental history are listed in Table 9-2.)

TABLE 9-2 Components of the Developmental History

Developmental factor	Specific criteria
Parental view of the child's development	
Concern of some aspect of the child's development	Definition of the concern
	Chronology (when the parent first became concerned, whether the problem has improved or worsened)
	Aggravating or alleviating factors
	Associated symptoms
	Associated changes in the child's life
	Impact of the problem on the child and family
	Actions taken to deal with the problem
Prenatal factors*	Duration of pregnancy
	Exposure to chemicals
	Exposure to infectious agents or radiation
	Complications (bleeding, hypertension, toxemia, excessive or inadequate weight gain, diabetes, malnutrition)
	Emotional adjustment to pregnancy
Intrapartum factors*	Length of labor
	Rupture of membrane
	Presentation and type of delivery
	Complications (precipitous or prolonged labor, bleeding, fever, fetal distress)
	Condition of infant (Apgar evaluations, need for resuscitation)
	Parental reactions and perceptions regarding labor and delivery
Neonatal factors*	Birthweight, height, and occipitofrontal circumference
	Birth defects or injuries
	Complications (respiratory problems, jaundice, cyanosis, apnea, sepsis, poor suck, meningitis, lethargy)
	Behavioral characteristics of the infant (alertness, state changes, consolability)
	Parental responses and perceptions of the infant
Family history*	Mental retardation, genetic disorders, learning disabilities, "slow" development, birth defects in blood relatives (including grandparents, aunts, uncles, and cousins)
Past development	Parental perceptions of past development
	Problems in infancy (excessive crying, colic, poor feeding, poor weight gain)
	Parental reaction to infant and feelings about parenthood
	Ages of major milestones (smiling, rolling over, sitting alone, crawling, walking, first word, first sentences, prehension, toilet training)
Temperament	Activity level
	Regularity of body functions
	Ease of adaptability
	Approach and withdrawal reactions to new situations
	Responsiveness to stimuli
	Quality of mood (usually positive or usually negative)
	Intensity of mood
	Distractibility
	Persistence
	Parental response to child's temperament
Gross motor skills	Survey of child's gross motor abilities (sitting, walking, climbing, sports)
Fine motor skills	Survey of child's fine motor skills (reaching for objects, grasping, copying, coloring, writing)
Opportunities for child to develop fine motor skills	
Language development	Receptive language (ability to comprehend the spoken word)
	Expressive language (ability to communicate through symbols, vocabulary, grammar)
	Speech (articulation, fluency)
	Opportunities to develop language skills

(Continues)

TABLE 9-2 Components of the Developmental History ***(Continued)***

Developmental factor	Specific criteria	Developmental factor	Specific criteria
Cognitive development	Characteristics of the thought process Problem-solving ability Interest in learning Academic performance Type of school experience Parental awareness of child's interests Opportunities for development of cognitive skills	Social development	Relationships (parent-child, sibling, peer, teacher, grandparent) Self-concept (child's view of self, perceptions of strengths and weaknesses) Level of responsibility Independence (eating, sleeping, decision making, time management, reaction to separation) Self-control (management of emotions and impulses) Discipline (method used, child's responses)

NOTE: The specific data for each component depend on the age of the child.
*Often obtained elsewhere in the health history.

Observations of development The interview includes aspects of the child's developmental progress. Near the beginning of the interview it is helpful to ask for the parent's perception of the child's development. Questions that can be asked to elicit this information include (1) What questions would you like to ask me about your child's development? (2) How would you describe your child's development? and (3) How does this child's development compare with that of any brothers and sisters or other children of similar age?

While conducting the interview, the nurse also observes the interactions between the parent and child. For infants, noting infant temperament and parental responsiveness to the infant's signals is important. Direct observations of both the child and the parent are an extremely important part of data collection. Virtually all behavior of both children and parents provides data; therefore, nurses need to attend even to seemingly minor incidents. Not all behavior is significant, but the nurse will not be able to make that judgment if the behavior was not first observed and noted.

There are two types of observation: (1) structured and (2) unstructured. *Unstructured observations* of the child's behavior occur throughout the entire visit. Unstructured observations are more frequently used in data collection because the child and family are generally more relaxed and performing in a more natural manner. *Structured observations* occur when the child is asked to perform certain tests or demonstrate certain behaviors or skills. Because the child's behavior in an unfamiliar setting might not be representative of usual behavior, structured observations require the nurse to validate the data with the parent.

Sometimes, the nurse might note discrepancies between observed data and information given by the parent. For example, the parent might tell the nurse that the child is doing fine and has no problems, but the nurse might observe behavior such as unequal extremity movement, squinting, or resistance to being consoled. Whenever a discrepancy exists, the nurse points out the difference to the parent and discusses the issue. In this way, the quality of the relationship between the nurse and the parent is enhanced, which in turn will affect the accuracy and the completeness of future data.

Sometimes, the nurse perceives a problem that the parent does not express. This difference in perception might exist because the parent does not interpret the child's behavior as unusual or indicative of a problem, because the parent has become so accustomed to the behavior that it is no longer noticed, or because the parent is not sufficiently comfortable with the nurse to mention the behavior as a problem.

The information obtained from the interview guides the nurse in adapting approaches to the expressed concerns of the child and family as well as in identifying any concerns that are not expressed. By integrating the developmental assessment into the health history, the nurse gains valuable data to plan individualized, comprehensive care for the child and family.

Parents (and older children) need to feel that the nurse is

a caring, capable, and trustworthy person before they will share their thoughts, feelings, and experiences. The nurse therefore needs to communicate warmth, concern, competence, and acceptance. A nurse who cares always addresses and talks about the child by name; remembers little idiosyncrasies such as a preferred position, food, or toy; and takes the time to provide comfort when the child is distressed or stimulation when the child is bored.

Screening tools A few standardized screening tools that many nurses find helpful can be part of a developmental assessment. Screening tools help organize observations and provide a guide for discussing the child's development with the parents. Screening tools are not predictive of future development or performance but are indicative of the child's present performance level. Serial measurements of some tools are more useful than a one-time screening because serial measurements allow development to be observed over time.

The Denver Prescreening Developmental Questionnaire (PDQ) is valuable because of its brevity and the information it provides about the parent's awareness of the child's behavior (Fig. 9-1). The PDQ consists of 97 questions, grouped according to age. Only the ten questions that correspond to the child's age are answered by the parent. When compared with other more elaborate tools and methods, the PDQ has a good record for reliability in identifying children whose development needs further evaluation.

Probably the most popular screening test is the Denver Developmental Screening Test-Revised (DDST-R) (see Appendix C). It is a widely used standard developmental screening tool for children from birth to 6 years of age. The DDST-R is used to screen children for possible deviations from anticipated developmental behaviors. A child with a questionable or failing score should be referred for further testing.

The four broad areas of development assessed in the DDST-R are (1) personal-social, (2) fine motor-adaptive, (3) gross motor, and (4) language. For each behavior a given age range indicates when 25%, 50%, 75%, and 90% of the children perform the behavior. The test usually is administered by asking the child to perform behaviors of increasing difficulty according to standard instructions. A few items are scored according to the parent's report. Because scoring and instructions are connected, nurses who uses this tool must study the instruction manual carefully and review the material periodically for their results to be valid.

The DDST-R is a valuable test to use whenever some aspect of a child's development seems inappropriate or the parent expresses concern about the child's progress. The form quickly compares the child's abilities and behavior with the norm for that age. The nurse can then either offer reassurance or suggest the need for referral.

Developmental delays A developmental assessment also should detect developmental problems as early as possible. In many cases, although not all, identifying developmental problems early can lead to interventions that significantly improve outcomes and minimize future or more severe problems. A *developmental delay* is an aspect of development that lags behind the normal range for a given age. The diagnosis of developmental delay is usually a complex process that involves a multidisciplinary team and extensive assessment of both the child and family. The nurse's suspicion, however, might be the first step in this process.

Some developmental delays are caused by a lack of parental knowledge or by misinformation. Guidance and information that is obtained during a careful health and developmental history interview often can address these concerns. When a knowledge deficit is the problem, the nurse can devise and implement a teaching plan for the family. For example, one nurse identified that a child's motor skills were delayed. The parent did not perceive the child as delayed and thought that a 3-month-old was too young to do anything except sleep and eat. The nurse then planned with the parent to include a "play time" in the infant's day and suggested toys and exercises that could be used to enhance the child's motor skills.

Throughout the interview, the nurse needs to be alert to any information that could be related to developmental problems. These factors may occur any time during the child's life. Some factors are reversible, whereas others are not, but a child should never be labeled as developmentally delayed too quickly. What appears to be delayed development might be only a delay in experience.

Health History

Child health history The purpose of the health history is to identify potential nursing diagnoses that will then assist the nurse in planning nursing interventions. The content of a child health history varies depending on the reason for the visit and the severity of any present illness. The prior knowledge of the child and family also directs the depth of information sought. The basic format remains the same, but the amount of information collected on certain topics will increase or decrease according to the nurse's judgment about the information needed to plan for the current problem or overall health needs.

Identifying data The initial phase of the health history involves a limited amount of information recorded concisely. Much of the data already might be included on the child's chart and therefore needs only verification. The informant (mother, father, grandparent, neighbor) is noted,

(*text continues on p. 245*)

DENVER PRESCREENING DEVELOPMENTAL QUESTIONNAIRE

Child's Name

Date

Birthdate

Please read each question carefully before you answer. Circle the best answer for each question. YOUR CHILD IS NOT EXPECTED TO BE ABLE TO DO EVERYTHING THE QUESTIONS ASK.

4 year

YES—CHILD CAN DO NOW or HAS DONE IN THE PAST
NO —CHILD CANNOT DO NOW, HAS NOT DONE IN THE PAST or YOU ARE NOT SURE THAT YOUR CHILD CAN DO IT

R —CHILD REFUSES TO TRY
NO-OPP—CHILD HAS NOT HAD THE CHANCE TO TRY

4 year check — Answer 71 through 80

71. Can your child pedal a tricycle at least ten feet? If your child has never had a chance to ride a tricycle his size, circle NO-OPP. YES NO R NO-OPP

72. After eating, does your child wash and dry his hands well enough so you don't have to do them over? Circle NO-OPP if you do not allow him to wash and dry his hands by himself. YES NO R NO-OPP

4 year, 3 month check — Answer 73 through 82

73. Does your child put an "s" at the end of his words when he is talking about more than one thing such as block<u>s</u>, shoe<u>s</u>, or toy<u>s</u>? YES NO R NO-OPP

74. Without letting your child hold onto anything, have him balance on one foot for as long as he can. Encourage him by showing him how, if necessary. GIVE HIM THREE CHANCES. Estimate seconds by counting slowly. Did your child balance 2 seconds or more? YES NO R NO-OPP

75. Without letting your child take a running jump, ask him to jump lengthwise over this paper. Did he do this without landing on the paper? YES NO R NO-OPP

76. Have your child draw this figure in the space below. DO NOT SAY "CIRCLE." *Do not help or correct your child.* Say to your child, "Draw a picture just like this one," and point to the picture on the right.

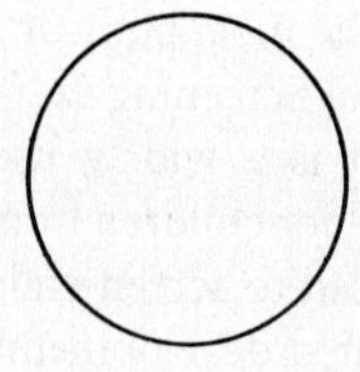

Look at these examples when scoring your child's drawing.

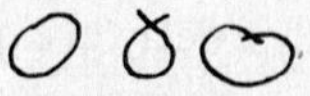

Answer YES

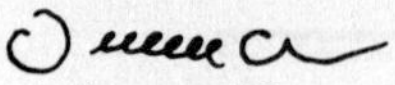

Answer NO

Did your child draw a circle? YES NO R NO-OPP

4 year, 6 month check — Answer 77 through 86

77. Can your child put *eight* blocks on top of one another without the blocks falling? This applies to *small* blocks about 1 inch in size and not blocks more than 2 inches in size. YES NO R NO-OPP

4 year, 9 month check — Answer 78 through 87

78. Does your child play hide-and-seek, cops-and-robbers or other games where he takes turns and follows rules? YES NO R NO-OPP

79. Can your child put jeans, shirt, dress or socks on without help except snapping, buttoning and belts? YES NO R NO-OPP

80. *Without your coaching or saying his name so he can repeat it,* does your child say both his first and last name? Nicknames may be used in place of first name. Circle NO if he only gives his first name or is not easily understood. YES NO R NO-OPP

FIGURE 9-1

Denver Prescreening Developmental Questionnaire. (Reprinted with permission of William K. Frankenburg, MD, University of Colorado Medical Center.)

Child Health History

Date and Initial Data

Identifying Information

1. Name (nickname or preferred name)
2. Age, birthdate
3. Sex
4. Primary care and other health resources

Source of Information (Referral Source)

1. Parent, child, or other (medical records)
2. Reliability of source

Chief Concern (CC)

1. Any concern of child, family, or other person working with family
2. Usually described in a brief statement, using the patient's words

Definition of CC or History of Present Illness (HPI)

1. Onset—sudden or gradual, previous episodes
2. Location of complaint—anatomically precise
3. Quality—dull, sharp, aching, burning, itching, etc.
4. Quantity—intensity and degree of discomfort
5. Chronology—previous health, onset of problem, duration, frequency, change over time
6. Setting (home, school)
7. Alleviating or aggravating factors
8. Associated symptoms
9. Associated changes in child or family's life
10. Actions taken to relieve problem
11. Epidemiologic information—exposure, contacts, travel

History

Birth History

Pregnancy—gravida, para, abortions, miscarriages, onset and place of prenatal care

1. Duration—EDC, number of weeks
2. Complications and time of occurrence
   a. Drugs—self-prescribed, prescribed by doctor, street drugs, alcohol, tobacco
   b. Exposure to infectious disease—STD (sexually transmitted disease), rubella, other
   c. X-ray exposure
   d. Kidney infection
   e. Vaginal bleeding
   f. Hypertension
   g. Swelling of extremities
   h. Excessive or inadequate weight
   i. Diet during pregnancy
   j. Trauma, surgery
   k. Ultrasound
   l. Amniocentesis
3. Was pregnancy planned?
4. Emotional adjustment to pregnancy
5. Problems with previous or subsequent pregnancies

Labor and Delivery—Hospital

1. Length of labor
2. Rupture of membranes
3. Medications
4. Presentation of infant
5. Type of delivery
6. Forceps
7. Complications—bleeding, fever, etc.
8. Did infant breathe spontaneously?
9. Apgars, if available

Neonatal History

1. Birthweight, height, and OFC (occipital frontal circumference)
2. Complications: jaundice, cyanosis, apnea, incubation, seizures, skin eruptions, vomiting, refusal tc eat, weight loss or gains during hospital stay, other
3. Temperament of infant
4. Any abnormalities

Infancy

1. Temperament of infant
2. Feeding pattern—type, frequency, addition of new foods and reaction
3. Problems in infancy—illnesses, excessive crying, vomiting, etc.
4. Parental response

Development

1. Motor: sat alone, crawled, walked, tricycled, prehension, weaned, self-feeding, toilet training
2. Language: babbled, single words, sentences (one word, two words, or more), easy or difficult to understand

(Continues)

Child Health History *(Continued)*

3. Psychosocial behavior: smiles, fears, tantrums, detachment, transitional object, toleration of separations

Illnesses—age when each occurred and treatment received; pneumonia, croup, asthma, high fevers; childhood diseases; meningitis, nephritis, etc.; any complications or sequelae

Hospitalization—date, cause, child's reaction

Surgery—date, hospital, doctor, reason for surgery, any complications

Accidents or Injuries

Allergies—drugs, foods, other items; type of reaction; skin, respiratory, behavioral, neurologic, other

Medications—over the counter, prescribed, or home remedies; taken in past; taking presently

Immunization—dates, reactions

Family History

Family Members—age and state of health (parents, siblings, grandparents, maternal and paternal aunts and uncles)

1. EENT—deafness, blindness, glaucoma, cataracts, myopia, strabismus, nosebleeds, sinus problems
2. Cardiovascular and respiratory—TB, asthma, hay fever, emphysema, hypertension, heart disease, strokes, rheumatic fever, anemia, leukemia
3. GI—ulcers, colitis, other problems
4. GU—kidney infections, kidney stones, bladder problems
5. Musculoskeletal—arthritis, multiple sclerosis, muscular dystrophy, congenital hip or foot problems, other problems
6. Neurologic—seizures, epilepsy, nervous disorder, mental retardation, learning disorders or problems
7. Chronic—diabetes, cancer, tumors, serious allergies, thyroid problems, birth defects, substance abuse
8. Miscellaneous—any other medical problem not mentioned

Psychosocial Family History

1. Education of parents
2. Occupation of parents
3. Living arrangements—type of housing, number of rooms, persons in household, sleeping arrangements, water supply tested?, proximity to playground, schools, transportation
4. Religious affiliation and/or philosophical outlook
5. Racial or ethnic background
6. Financial status, particularly method of payment for medical expense
7. Family crises or stress—recent death, divorce, separation, hospitalization, accidents, natural disasters
8. Family profile—how family members relate to each other, family activities, social outlet for members, support system, philosophy of parenting
9. Family's use of health care resources, attitudes and participation in preventive health
10. School and community involvement

Review of Body Systems

Pertinent Negatives Related to CC

1. General—overall state of health, ability to perform normal daily functions
2. Head—trauma, headaches, size, fontanelles
3. Eyes—redness, drainage, unusual movements, visual acuity, strabismus, cataracts, tearing, infections, photophobia
4. Ears—infections, drainage, hearing, care habits, ringing
5. Nose—drainage, congestion, bleeding, smelling ability, sinus pain
6. Mouth—condition of teeth, lesions on mouth or tongue, palate, condition of gums, pattern of dental care, odor
7. Speech and voice—hoarse, stridor, voice changes, articulation problems, fluency problems
8. Throat—frequent sore throats, tonsillitis
9. Neck—stiffness, masses, tenderness, goiter
10. Lymph—swollen nodes, tenderness, inflammation, pain
11. Breasts—discharge, masses, pain, self-examination pattern
12. Respiratory—cough, sputum, wheezing, dyspnea, pain, smoking, hemoptysis, stridor, pain, shortness of breath, pneumonia, other infections, cyanosis
13. Cardiac—exercise intolerance, pain, murmurs, cyanosis, syncopal episodes, hypertension
14. GI—appetite, swallowing difficulty, constipation, diarrhea, abdominal hernia, thirst, pain, jaundice,

Child Health History (Continued)

changes in bowel habits, food intolerances, nausea, vomiting, hemorrhoids

15. GU—urgency, frequency, dysuria, polyuria, nocturia, dribbling, enuresis, hematuria, STD, vaginal or penile drainage, menarche, menstrual history, pruritis, OB history
16. Musculoskeletal—pain, redness, swelling of joints, limitation of movement, fractures, edema
17. Skin—texture, lesions, bruising, petechiae, hair loss, dryness, itching, care habits
18. Neurologic—seizures, ataxia, unconsciousness, loss of sensation, unusual movements as twitches or tremors, slow learning, clumsiness, memory loss

Current Health

Habits

1. Nutrition
   a. Diet—frequency of meals, amount and types of food
   b. Eating habits—likes and dislikes
   c. Vitamins—kind, how often, how much, iron, fluoride
2. Elimination
   a. Urine—frequency, color, odor, character of stream
   b. Bowel—frequency, character, and color of stools
   c. Toilet training—age, accidents, day or night
3. Sleep
   a. Difficulty putting to bed
   b. Hours
   c. Disturbances—nightmares, night terrors (if so, what does the parent do?)
   d. Daytime naps

Development

1. Client's view of development—how does child compare to siblings and peers? What can child do now?
2. Gross motor—timing of achieved major milestones (rolling over, walking, biking)
3. Fine motor—feeding self, writing, copying, coloring, using scissors, tying shoes
4. Language—words, vocabulary, articulation, fluency
5. Cognitive—general understanding level, curiosity, major interest in learning (not necessarily in school), academic performance, grades in school, concepts of sex and death
6. Social
   a. Emotions
   b. Temperament
   c. Trust and attachment to parents
   d. Independence in activities—feeding, toileting, hygiene; ability to entertain self; ability to go around neighborhood; ability to separate from parents; self-concept; self-control (management of impulses and feelings such as love, anger, aggression, fear, jealousy); social relationships with parents, siblings, peers; reaction to new situations; response to discipline, type of discipline; responsibilities; general interests and activities (indoors, outdoors); annoying or deviant behaviors (tantrums, lying, stealing, meanness, thumbsucking)

Sexual Understanding of Adolescents—birth control methods if appropriate

Environmental Factors

1. Pollutants—noise, air, chemical
2. Safety risks

along with an assessment of the informant's reliability in providing accurate data.

In the health history, the identifying data always include the child's age, date of birth, and sex. Frequently, the child's race is included. This information is useful when the child might be at risk for diseases that occur more frequently in a particular racial group.

If the child's and family's primary language is not English, the nurse notes the extent to which the family does understand and speak English to assess the need for an interpreter.

Chief complaint The chief complaint is the client's perception of the primary reason for the visit. The chief complaint should be recorded as a concise statement or statements in the client's own words. For example, if the opening question is "Tell me why you came here to the clinic" and the client responds with "We are here for a checkup," the nurse records "well-child care" or "health maintenance." If the client is seen for assessment and care of an illness, the chief complaint then includes the symptoms and their duration as described by the client. The nurse might need to guide the client to describe the most relevant and pertinent symptoms. Asking which one problem or symptom brought the client to the clinic or office often helps.

The duration of the chief complaint indicates whether the problem is acute or chronic. Duration also is useful in assessing severity. For instance, if a client describes having "headaches for 3 years" and the symptoms are not described as very severe, the client might have different underlying reasons for the visit. The nurse then asks further exploratory questions to uncover the real problem.

History of present illness The history of the present illness (HPI) is the detailed narrative of the client's chief complaint. This portion of the health history might not be needed in a health maintenance visit, unless the client presents a specific physical or psychosocial problem. In collecting information about symptoms, the nurse asks about the total duration, date of onset, characteristics at onset, aggravating or relieving factors, treatments tried and their results, and course since onset.

Total duration refers to the client's recall of the day the problems began and is recorded as the date of onset. The nurse asks, "How did the problem start?" and "Was it gradual or sudden?" Depending on the nature of the chief complaint, the nurse also might assess any precipitating and/or predisposing factors related to onset. These might include emotional disturbances, infections (for example, exposure and incubation period), allergies, physical exertion, fatigue, and environmental factors.

Characteristics at onset (or at any other time) refers to a description of pain or discomfort because this usually denotes a physical problem. The nurse might, for example, ask, "Is the pain sharp, dull, or aching?" Having the child point to, or having the parent describe, the location and radiation of the pain also is useful. Children should attempt to describe the intensity of the pain and its temporal character in their own words. To facilitate the child's description, the nurse asks whether the pain is continuous, intermittent, sharp, throbbing, aching, or stabbing. Finding out how the pain has affected the child's normal eating, playing, and sleeping behaviors is a good method of assessing the severity of the problem.

Aggravating factors or relieving factors cause a change in the type, location, severity, or duration of the pain. (Aggravating factors worsen and relieving factors lessen the client's perception of pain.) They need to be documented in the client's words, usually by asking what made the client feel worse or better. The course since onset includes the circumstances related to the problem: whether it is a single, acute attack; recurrent acute attacks; or daily, periodic, or continuous occurrences. The nurse notes whether the child or parent reports that at the time of the visit the problem is better, worse, or unchanged and records data about the medical attention provided, if any, and its effects.

Past health history and birth history The nurse asks whether anything unusual or any problems occurred during the client's neonatal history or the mother's maternity history. Because events during pregnancy and in the perinatal period can have long-range organic and psychologic effects, the details of the birth history are important in planning health maintenance and problem management.

Pregnancy, labor, and delivery histories begin with open-ended questions such as, "How was your pregnancy?" Often, beginning the history taking with the mother's own health enlists her cooperation and assistance with the remainder of the history and examination. Direct questions then can be used to obtain the relevant information regarding any problems of prenatal health and events of labor and delivery. An assessment of the parent-child relationship is best begun by assessing parental feelings toward the pregnancy.

The child or adult is asked to list any illnesses, hospitalizations, surgery, and accidents, with details of the events. Equally important is the child's reaction to these events. Most parents recall only serious medical problems and need to be asked directly about common childhood diseases, such as chickenpox, strep throat, and tonsillitis. Also important is historical information about childhood injuries, such as falls, cuts, or burns, which parents might not consider serious accidents. A large number of such incidents might suggest a need for parental guidance and education regarding childhood safety (see Chapter 12).

Allergies are recorded with details about symptoms, etiology (if known), treatment, and results. The nurse also asks about any unusual reactions to food, drugs, or environmental agents, even if the reaction was an isolated incident. A single reaction might indicate an early allergic predisposition, or a seasonal cycle might suggest an allergy (for example, "Every spring she gets sick"). Current medications are documented by listing all prescribed or nonprescribed drugs taken and the reason for their use. Immunizations are documented on the child's immunization schedule. Most parents have a separate record that can be copied into the chart. If the parent is a reliable informant and states that the child's schedule is complete, this is noted as such in the chart.

Review of body systems The review of body systems is a thorough checklist of any and all possible medical problems the child has experienced or is experiencing. If the review uncovers a problem, the nurse documents the duration, frequency, intensity, course, associated factors, and results of treatment. It is extremely important to go through each body system thoroughly with the child or adult to discover any past or current health deviation or concern. Any significant positive response needs to be recorded. Further questions may be asked during the examination of the affected body part.

Because most parents and children are not familiar with medical terminology, the nurse phrases questions in appropriate ways. For example, "Has Johnny had any ear infec-

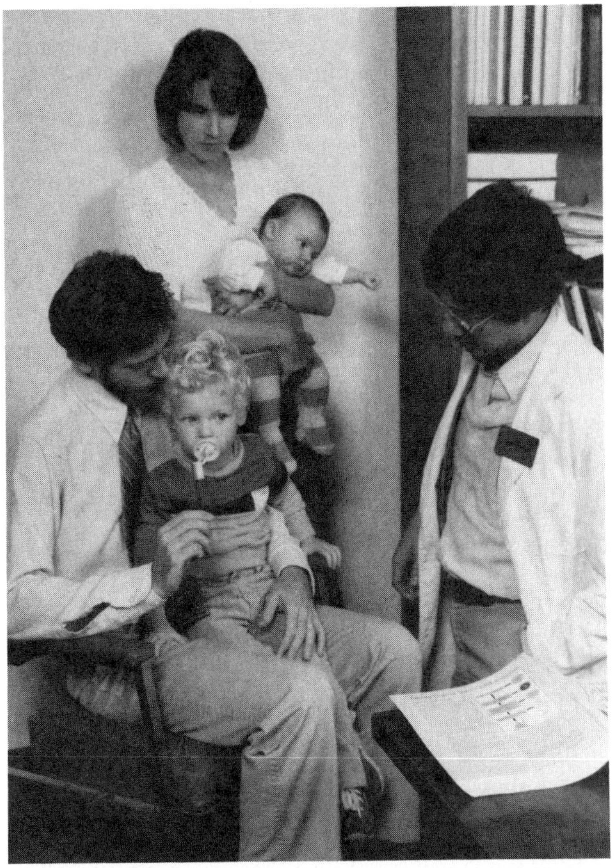

During family assessment the nurse focuses on the family's characteristics, concerns, roles, and relationships.

tions?" might be understood but "Has Johnny had any otitis media?" might not.

Current health The nurse asks about current health by including data on the child's habits of eating, eliminating, sleeping, and current developmental profile. With an older child or adolescent, this component includes questions about use or experimentation with alcohol, drugs, and cigarettes. Given a supportive, trusting relationship, the nurse can discuss openly with the child the reasons for this behavior and its potential consequence.

Family health history The family health history is best introduced to the parent by stating its purpose for inclusion. Most parents understand that the child's health might be affected by family health, especially congenital or familial health problems. A simple statement such as, "I would like to ask you some questions about the health of family members" is appropriate. Significant features of the medical histories of all immediate family members are then documented; for any serious problems, details about the diagnosis, cause, treatment, and management are included. A family history of medical problems also might have psychologic ramifications for the family due to stress, financial burdens, or turmoil.

A narrative format commonly is used to describe the family and its environment. The purpose is to begin assessment of the family in which the child is a member. The nurse focuses the assessment on the family's characteristics, concerns, roles, and relationships. Some of the factors that should be included in a family assessment are the family composition (names, genders, and ages of immediate family), the occupations of the parents, the resources for child care, and the involvement of others (relatives, friends, or babysitters) in providing child care. The socioeconomic status, cultural and ethnic identity, and religious affiliation also assist the nurse in understanding family dynamics and adapting teaching and health care management plans accordingly.

Depending on the data collected, a further, in-depth family assessment might be needed, especially if preliminary data reveal problematic family relationships or social, psychologic, or financial concerns. (Risk factors related to family dysfunction are discussed in Chapter 13.)

Essential Concepts

- A health history requires effective interviewing skills and a systematic method for documentation.
- A developmental history is an integral part of the health history.
- Open-ended questions addressed to both the parent and the child assist the nurse in identifying developmental concerns early in the interview.
- Observations of development might be structured or unstructured.
- A developmental assessment should foster optimal development by validating that the child is developing normally or by detecting problems early so that necessary interventions can be planned.
- To assist the child in cooperating and performing well in the assessment setting, the nurse proceeds slowly and involves the child in the interview.
- Young children can participate through puppet or doll play; those in middle and late childhood can under-

stand models and illustrations and can answer straightforward questions; adolescents are often interviewed separately from their parents and might be chief informants about their health.

- Common tests for developmental screening include the Denver Prescreening Developmental Questionnaire (PDQ) and Denver Developmental Screening Test-Revised (DDST-R).
- A health history includes identifying the purpose of the visit; the history of the present illness (if any); the past, birth, and family health history; and the child's current state of health.
- The overall goal of a family health history and assessment is to gather data about a family and its members to promote family growth by identifying needs for teaching and referral.

Additional Readings

Bernstein L, Bernstein R: *Interviewing: A Guide for Health Professionals.* Appleton-Century-Crofts, 1980.

Cadman D et al: The usefulness of the Denver Developmental Screening Test to predict kindergarten problems in a general community population. *Am J Public Health* (Oct) 1984; 74 (10): 1093–1097.

Casey P, Bradley R: Developmental screening for the pre-school-child: Practical recommendations. *J Arkansas Med Soc* 1980; 77: 175–179.

Casey P, Bradley R: The impact of the home environment on children's development. *J Dev Behav Pediatr* 1982; 3: 146–152.

Castiglia PT et al: Selecting a developmental screening tool. *Pediatr Nurs* (Jan-Feb) 1985; 11(1): 8–17.

Chinn P: *Child Health Maintenance.* Mosby, 1974.

Chow M et al: *Handbook of Pediatric Primary Care.* Wiley, 1979.

Cohn DH, Stern V: *Observing and Recording the Behavior of Young Children.* Teachers College Press, 1978.

Edison C: Family assessment guidelines. In: *Family Health Care—General Perspectives,* 2nd ed. vol. 1, 1979.

Eichel E: Assessment with a family focus. *J Psychiatr Nurs* (Jan) 1978; 11–14.

Ferholdt JD: *Clinical Assessment of Children: A Comprehensive Approach to Primary Pediatric Care.* Lippincott, 1980.

Frankenburg WK: *The Denver Prescreening Development Questionnaire.* LADOCA Project and Publishing Foundation, Inc. 1975.

Frankenberg WK, Goldstein AD, Camp B: The revised Denver Developmental Screening Test: Its accuracy as a screening instrument. *J Pediatr* 1971; 79: 988–995.

Frankenburg WK, Sciarillo W, Burgess D: The newly abbreviated and revised Denver Developmental Screening Test. *J Pediatr* 1981; 99(6): 995–999.

Greenspan SI: *The Clinical Interview of the Child.* McGraw-Hill, 1981.

Greenspan SI, Lieberman AF: Infants, mothers and their interaction: A quantitative clinical approach to developmental assessment. In: *The Course of Life: Psychoanalytic Contributions Toward Understanding Personality Development,* Vol 1. Infancy and Early Childhood, 1980.

Korsch A: *Pediatric interviewing techniques. Curr Prob Pediatr* (May) 1973; 3(7).

Lewis M, Rosenblum LA: *The Effect of the Infant on its Caregiver.* Wiley, 1974.

Lewis M, Taft LT: *Developmental Disabilities: Theory, Assessment and Intervention.* SP Medical and Scientific Books, 1982.

Lichtenstein R, Ireton H: *Preschool Screening.* Grune & Stratton, 1984.

McCall R. A hard look at stimulating and predicting development: The cases of bonding and screening. *Pediatr Rev* 1982; 3: 205–212.

Mendell F, Yogman M: Developmental aspects of well child visits. *J Dev Behav Pediatr* 1982; 3: 118–121.

Mickalide AD: Children's understanding of health and illness: Implications for health promotion. *Health Values* (May-June) 1986; 10(3): 5–21.

Murphy-Alexander M, Brown M: *Pediatric History Taking and Physical Diagnosis for Nurses.* McGraw-Hill, 1979.

Nilms C, Mullins G: *Growth and Development. A Primary Health Care Approach.* Prentice-Hall, 1982.

Parish L. Communicating with hospitalized children. *Can Nurse* (Jan) 1986; 82(1): 21–24.

Powell M: *Assessment and Management of Developmental Changes and Problems in Children.* 2nd ed. Mosby, 1981.

Robischon P, Smith JA: *Family Assessment: Current Practice in Family Centered Community Nursing.* Vol 1. Mosby, 1977.

Siegel BS: Counseling and health screening for children entering sports and physical exercise. *Nurs Pract* (May) 1985; 10(5): 11–12, 17–18, 20–21.

Speer JJ: Selecting the appropriate family assessment tool. *Pediatr Nurs* (Sept-Oct) 1985; 11(5): 349–355.

Strangler S, Huber C, Routh D: *Screening Growth and Development of Preschool Children—A Guide for Test Selection.* McGraw-Hill, 1980.

Szumowski E, Chamberlin R: Typical behaviors of one-year-old children and their mothers. *J Dev Behav Pediatr* 1980; 1: 122–127.

Vaughn B, Deinard A, Egeland B: Measuring temperament in pediatric practice. *J Pediatr* 1980; 96: 510–514.

Ventura JN: Parent coping behaviors, parent functioning and infant temperament characteristics. *Nurs Res* (Sept-Oct) 1982; 31(5): 269–273.

Yoos L: A developmental approach to physical assessment. *Am J Matern-Child Nurs* 1981; 6(3): 168–170.

Chapter 10

Physical Assessment

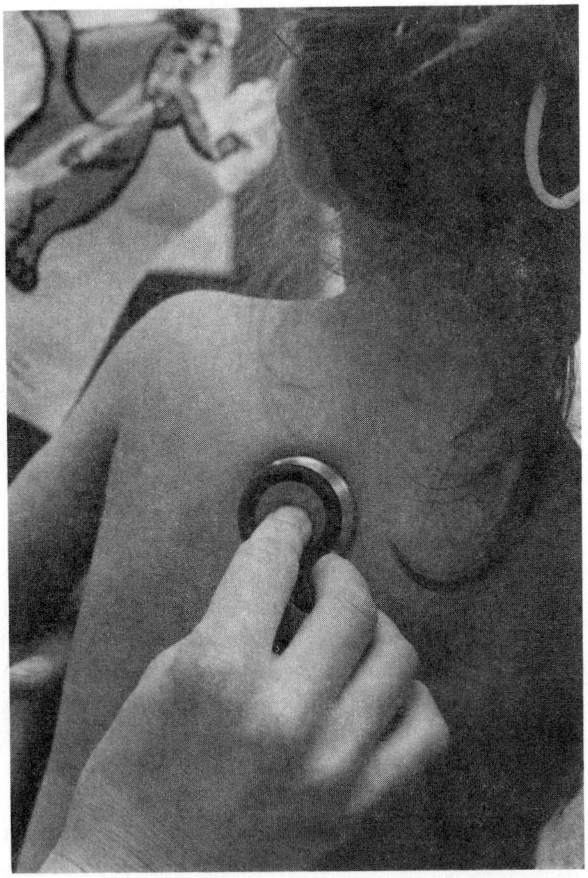

Chapter Contents

(Continues)

Objectives

- Identify the factors that determine the nurse's approach to the physical examination.
- Explain the methods used to reduce the child's anxiety in the physical assessment setting.
- Identify the body systems assessed by the physical examination.
- Identify the assessment criteria associated with each body system.
- Describe the four basic physical examination techniques.

The physical assessment, a component of both well-child and sick-child health care, includes both a health history and a physical examination in conjunction with physical screening tests. The emphasis and methods used vary, depending on the purpose of the visit and the age and developmental level of the child. The nurse therefore plans the assessment according to the needs of both child and family.

The physical assessment process is continuous and actually begins with the nurse's initial contact with the child and parent. During the health interview, the nurse observes the child's developmental level, the quality and effectiveness of the parent-child relationship, and the child's overall growth pattern and health status (see Chapter 9). The physical examination usually follows the health interview.

A systematic method for organizing the physical assessment ensures thoroughness and consistency in performing and recording physical findings. Whereas the actual written document may be in a format used by physicians, the nurse collects data and analyzes information to formulate nursing diagnoses. As in all aspects of the nursing process, these are followed by planning and intervention.

Health Screening

In the physical assessment process, screening and laboratory tests are useful in augmenting the health history and physical examination findings. They provide quick, inexpensive measures for detecting those children most likely to have a specific problem. Screening and laboratory tests often provide information about the accuracy of the entire health assessment and have become common and accepted practice.

Measurements

Because children grow rapidly, screening measurements of height, weight, and head circumference are important. Failure or delay in any one of these areas of growth might be an early indicator of a serious problem, especially because failure in one area eventually affects the others.

Measurements of height, weight, and head circumference document the child's rate of growth and changes from previous examinations. Therefore, they need to be taken periodically and plotted on a graph.

Height Height usually is measured at every well-child visit; the method used varies with the age of the child. Measuring the length of a young infant usually requires two people. One person secures the child's head as the child lies flat, and the other extends the child's legs and marks the length between the head and heel. The distance is then measured using a metal or paper tape and recorded. Cloth tapes should not be used because they stretch. An infantometer, which is a sliding ruler that is positioned at the infant's head and heel, allows a single person to measure an infant.

For older children who can stand, height measurement is easier and more accurate because these children can be positioned on a standard scale. The child is instructed to stand straight and quiet in stocking or bare feet as the attached tape measure is placed on the top of the head. As a safety measure, the base of the scale should be against the wall, and the nurse should steady the scale as the child stands on it.

Height is generally a familial trait; therefore, a child who has tall parents and grandparents and is healthy and well nourished is likely to be tall. Abnormally short stature can be due to family growth patterns or chronic illness.

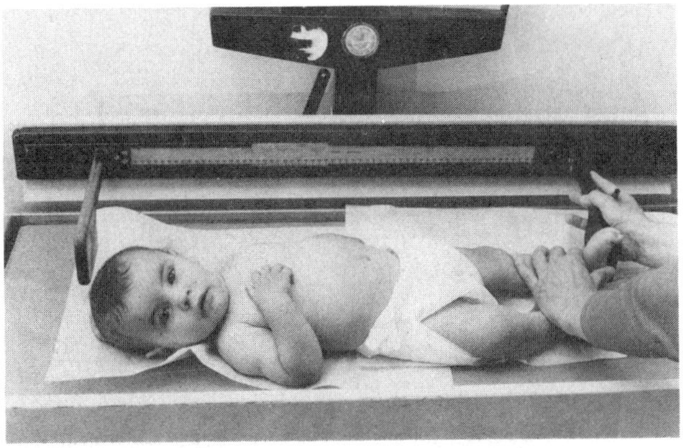

A

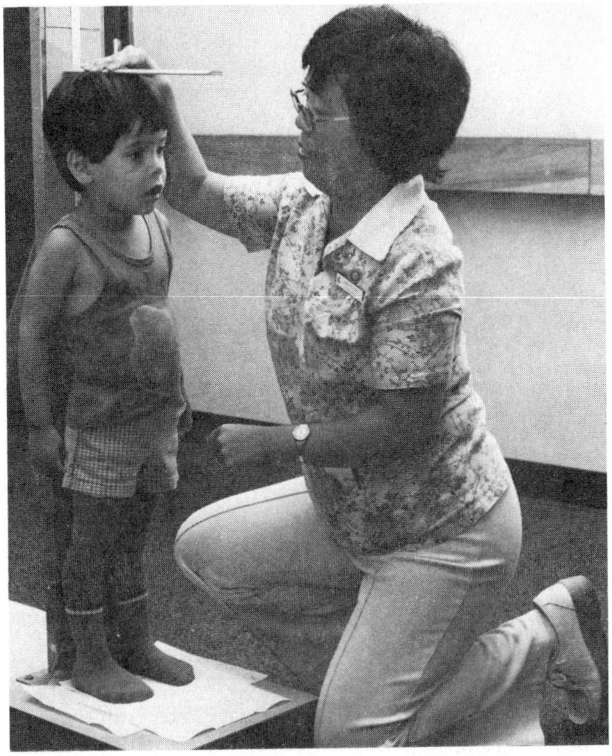

B

Measuring height. **A.** *An infant's length is measured from the crown of the head to the heels of the feet, with the legs fully extended.* **B.** *A child's height is measured by having the child stand straight, without shoes, and by placing the measuring marker on top of the child's head. (From Kozier B, Erb G:* Techniques in Clinical Nursing, *2nd ed. Addison-Wesley, 1987.)*

Weight Weight is another important index of the child's general growth and nutritional status and therefore is measured at every well-child visit. Because sudden and often drastic fluctuations can occur, weight also should be checked at every sick-child visit.

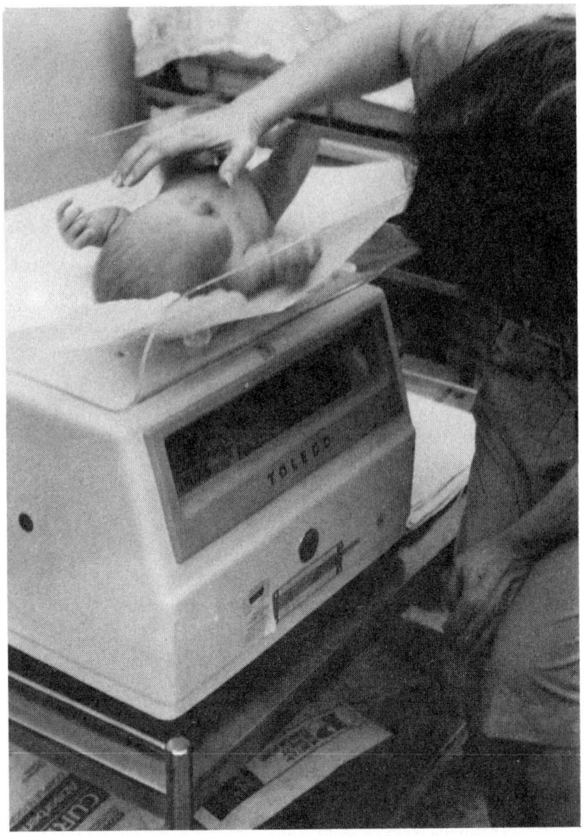

Infants are weighed on a draped balanced scale and are protected from falls at all times. (From Swearingen PL: The Addison-Wesley Photo-Atlas of Nursing Procedures. *Addison-Wesley, 1983.)*

Infants are weighed without any clothing, including diapers, on a balanced infant scale. The infant should be protected from direct contact with the scale by cloth or paper. Infants should be protected from falls and should not extend beyond the length of the scale. Young children who are walking usually can be weighed on the adult standing scale and should be weighed with all clothing removed except underpants. Older children can remain clothed but without shoes and be weighed on the standing scale.

As with height, the weight measurement is plotted on a growth chart (Appendix A). Weight generally remains on or near the same percentile curve from one visit to the next, and any sudden decrease or increase should therefore be evaluated. The most common cause of a significant weight increase is obesity. Weight decrease usually is caused by chronic disease, acute infections, or emotional problems.

Head circumference Most health practitioners include head circumference measurements in every well-child visit from birth to 2 or 3 years of age. Head circumference is

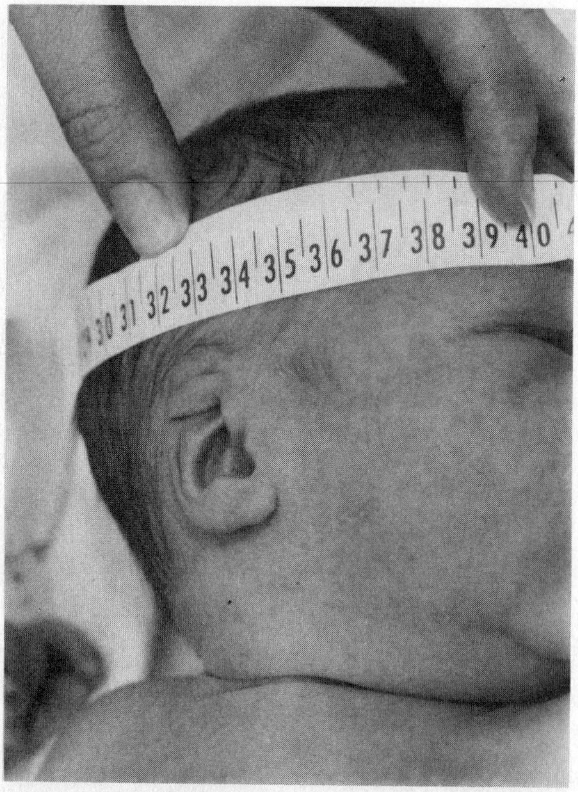

Head circumference is measured with a paper or metal tape held securely over the child's forehead and occipital protuberance. (From Swearingen PL: The Addison-Wesley Photo-Atlas of Nursing Procedures. *Addison-Wesley, 1983.)*

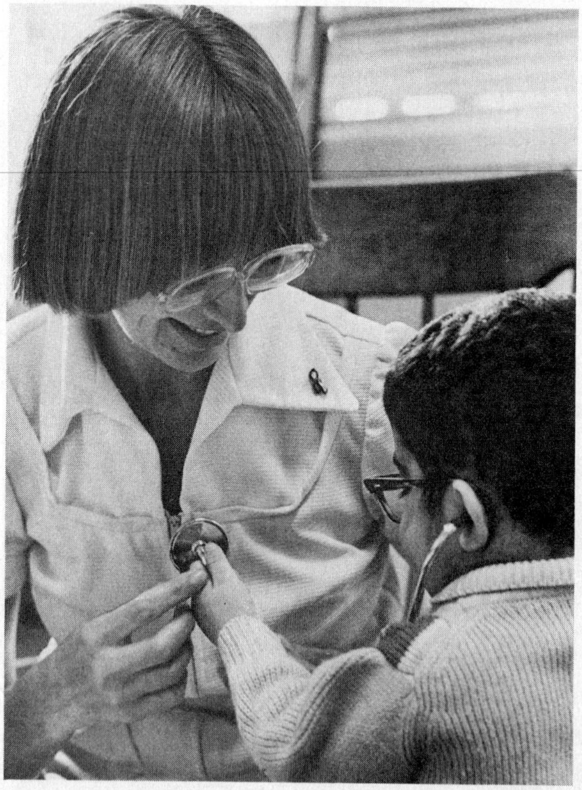

Children are less fearful if they are allowed to manipulate equipment before the nurse takes vital signs.

documented in centimeters and often is recorded as "OFC" (occipital frontal circumference) or "HC" (head circumference) in children's health records.

The most reliable method for obtaining the head circumference is to measure with a metal or paper tape three times and record the largest measurement on a head circumference graph (Appendix A). The tape should be held securely on the child's head over the forehead and the occipital protuberance. The tape should not cover the ears. Although it is often not possible, having the same practitioner measure the head circumference at every well-child visit further ensures accuracy.

In general, the neonate's head circumference is slightly larger than chest circumference. This ratio is fairly constant until the child is 2 years old, when the chest circumference becomes greater than head circumference. If head measurement deviates from the norm or from the infant's established percentile, the additional measurement of the infant's anterior and posterior fontanelles becomes crucial.

At birth, both fontanelles and all sutures are palpable, and the anterior fontanelle is easily measured in centimeters on vertical and horizontal planes. The anterior fontanelle is 1–2 in. across and closes at some time between 9 and 18 months of age. The posterior fontanelle may be closed at birth or closes by 3 months of age; it is one-fourth to one-half inch across. Premature or delayed closing can cause or indicate serious neurologic problems.

Vital signs The frequency with which vital signs are assessed on well children varies from clinic to clinic, but most nurses follow general guidelines. Temperature might not necessarily be taken at every well-child visit during infancy but should be taken during the older child's annual physical examination. The choice of taking an oral, axillary, or rectal temperature depends on the child's age, cooperation, and general health.

Pulse and respiration should be measured at every well-child visit because these measurements directly indicate functioning of the cardiac and respiratory system. The pulse should be taken for a full minute. The pulse should be auscultated in the apical area of the heart, palpated in the radial and femoral areas, and assessed for rate and rhythm.

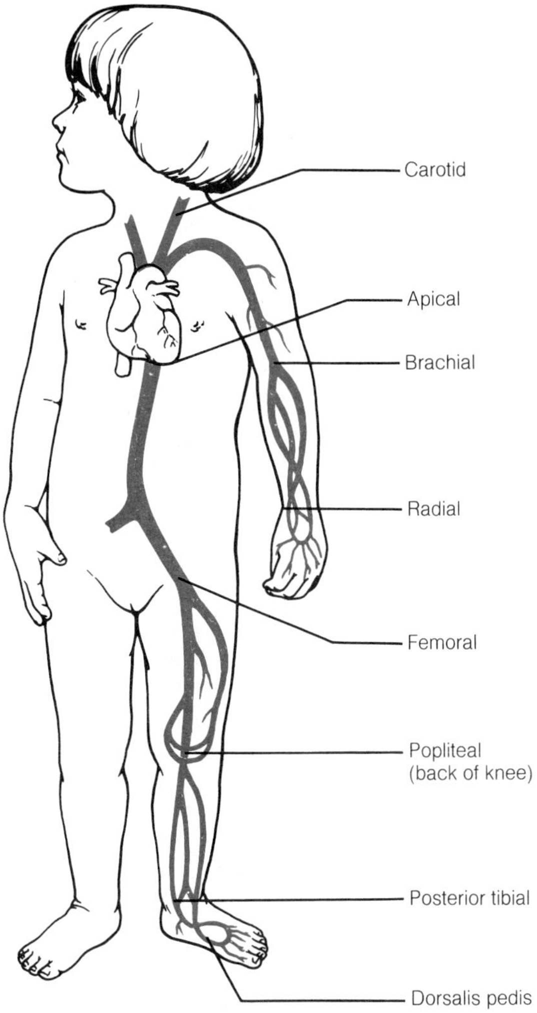

FIGURE 10-1
Location of pulses.

(Locations of pulses are indicated in Fig. 10-1.) Heart rate that is more rapid than normal for the child's age is *tachycardia;* abnormally slow heart rate is called *bradycardia.* The rhythm is described as regular or irregular. If the rhythm is irregular, the nurse describes it in detail.

The rate, rhythm, and depth of a child's respiratory pattern should be observed at every well-child visit and especially at sick-child visits. Infants and children should be observed and their respirations counted for a full minute with their upper clothing removed. Older, more cooperative children can be observed as they sit quietly on the examining table during examination of the chest and lungs. Abnormally rapid respirations are called *tachypnea;* slow breathing is *bradypnea.*

Blood pressure also should be measured at every well-child visit. Hypertension may be detected early in life if blood pressure is consistently assessed in children. The blood pressure cuff must be the correct size for the child. It should be 1.5 times the diameter of the part of the extremity to be measured or no less than one-half and no more than two-thirds of the part of the extremity to be measured (Table 10-1).

TABLE 10-1 Guidelines for Blood Pressure Cuff Selection

Age	Size
Neonate	2.5–3 cm
Infant	4–5 cm
1- to 4-year-old	6–7 cm
5- to 10-year-old	8–10 cm
10-year-old and older	10–12 cm

Laboratory Tests

Although the nurse's role in screening blood and urine tests varies from one setting to another, all nurses should be familiar with how these tests are performed, how specimens are obtained and tested, and how results are interpreted.

In ambulatory settings, protocols for well-child visits usually involve hematocrit, hemoglobin, lead screening, urinalysis, and urine tests for culture and sensitivity. Children who are at risk for sickle cell trait or disease, thalassemia, glucose-6-phosphate-dehydrogenase deficiency (G-6-PD), or galactosemia are screened at the appropriate time, as determined by the characteristics of the potential disease and the reliability and validity of the screening test. (Disorders of the blood are described in Chapter 26.)

As screening tests, the blood and urine tests determine whether a child is within a normal range or whether intervention is required. For example, anemia in childhood might first be detected through a routine hematocrit and hemoglobin check or a complete blood count. An asymptomatic urinary tract infection in a 4-year-old-girl might be detected through a routinely scheduled clean-catch urinalysis or urine test for culture and sensitivity and treated before more serious upper urinary tract disease could occur. (Disorders of the urinary tract are described in Chapter 28.) When obtained in conjunction with subjective and objective findings, laboratory tests used as screening aids or diagnostic tools provide comprehensive data.

TABLE 10-2 Techniques Used in Physical Assessment

Technique	Purpose	Comments
Inspection	Evaluation of visible characteristics	First step in assessment Adequate exposure of area inspected and good direct lighting necessary Nurse uses eyes to examine thoroughly and unhurriedly the area inspected, may also use senses of smell and hearing Most valuable but most difficult to learn; requires sensitivity and keen observations Each body part inspected for color, tone, texture, firmness, masses, hair distribution, movement, and symmetry
Palpation	Hands used to touch or feel area being assessed for temperature, texture, vibration, size, or position Light palpation is gentle pressure applied with the fingertips or palms Deep palpation is firm pressure applied with the fingertips to evaluate organs within the abdomen; deeper palpation is achieved by placing the fingers of one hand over the fingers of the hand that is palpating Ballottement is application of pressure by tapping or bouncing of several fingers to note pressure within an organ (for example, ocular pressure) or rebound tenderness (for example, of the abdomen or specific organ)	Temperature (for example, of the skin) assessed best with the dorsum of the fingers Texture, size, or position (for example, texture of the hair, size or position of an organ or mass) best assessed with palmar surface of the fingertips; also assessed are moisture, consistency, pressure (for example, pulses), form, and movement Vibration or pulsation (for example, air or sound moving through the lungs or cardiac thrills) assessed best with the palms Validates visual impression used to assess organs, glands, bones, muscles, hair, skin, and mucosa The child must be relaxed to assess internal organs adequately. Tight, tense muscles act as a barrier
Percussion	Rapping motion used to determine the density of an area assessed or the borders of a specific organ Blunt or direct percussion done by striking the surface assessed with a partially flexed finger (usually the middle finger) Bimanual or indirect percussion accomplished by placing the middle finger of one hand on the surface to be percussed (other fingers should not rest on the surface to be percussed as this will diminish the sound created by percussion); the middle finger or index and middle fingers of the other hand strike the middle finger resting on the body surface on the upper phalange; only the very tip(s) of the striking finger(s) used	Direct percussion used most often to percuss the nasal sinuses or tendons or inflamed organs; indirect percussion used to percuss any area of the body Percussion sounds include resonance, hyperresonance, tympany, dullness, flatness (see Table 10-6)
Auscultation	Listening to or studying sounds arising from organs through the direct contact of the ear on the body surface over the organ or, more commonly, with the aid of a stethoscope The diaphragm (flat side) of the stethoscope picks up high-frequency sounds and is used for auscultation of most organs Bell (curved or cupped side) of the stethoscope when applied lightly picks up low-frequency sounds such as heart murmurs	Done over the lungs, heart, and abdomen to determine the functional status of these organs; the skull, thyroid gland, and carotid arteries are auscultated for bruits (swishing sounds) Requires concentration, listening to only one sound at a time, disregarding all others; then systematically proceeding from one area to another

Physical Examination

Physical examination uses four assessment skills: (1) inspection, (2) palpation, (3) percussion, and (4) auscultation. (Details of these techniques are presented in Table 10-2).

Adaptations for Children

The "systems approach," the head-to-toe physical assessment technique recommended for adults, is often not feasible with children, although the head-to-toe format is generally used to document assessment findings. The nurse's approach to assessment of the child depends on the developmental and chronologic age of the child; the amount of stress and anxiety the child associates with the examination; the trust developed among the nurse, child, and parent; and the child's state of health or illness.

The nurse first considers these factors and then adjusts the approach to fit the needs of the child and parent. Performing a physical assessment in a supportive, nonthreatening, and educative environment is an art that is part of comprehensive nursing care. (A guide for approaching the pediatric client during physical assessment is provided in Table 10-3. Such a guide, however, is only a starting point for assessing the child's and parent's physical needs, cognitive understanding, and emotional functioning.)

Those parts of the examination that require a quiet child, such as auscultation of the heart and lungs, should be done first with infants and young children, who are initially cooperative. The nurse then proceeds from the least traumatic procedures, engaging the child in the examination as much as possible. Adequate preparation increases the child's sense of security. For example, providing time for the child to relax and feel comfortable, to manipulate stethoscopes, and to switch the "flashlight" of the otoscope on and off can ensure a quick and efficient examination later on.

Combining knowledge, skill, and sensitivity to the child's and parent's physical and emotional needs, the nurse can execute a complete physical appraisal. Enlisting the help of the parent is of utmost importance, but respecting the parent's needs is also crucial. Therefore, although it is often possible to have the parent help to gently restrain the child's head for an ear examination, the child's unhappiness might make the parent anxious, and the nurse might instead enlist the help of a colleague. For children up to 2 years old, the entire examination often is best performed with the child on the parent's lap.

When a child is ill or in pain, the nurse quickly assesses the healthy body systems first and then proceeds to the areas associated with the health problem. For example, a child whose history reveals a potential ear infection should have chest and lungs evaluated first to rule out respiratory involvement before the more stressful and possibly painful otoscopic exam.

Whenever the nurse's assessment findings deviate from the normal or expected findings, referral is made to the appropriate professional for further evaluation.

General Appearance

The physical examination should begin with an overall impression of the child. This is a cumulative, subjective impression of the child's physical appearance, nutritional status, and such behavioral and developmental parameters as the degree of activity, gait, posture, coordination, and emotional state.

Physical appearance usually includes a description of the child's facial expression because this might give clues about a child who is in pain, extremely frightened, or happy. Symmetry and coordination of body movement also are noted, with attention to posture and types of body movement. A child might favor a painful body part, and movements might be stiff and awkward. A child who is fearful or ill might not physically interact with the environment, whereas a secure, happy child might play freely with the available toys or sit in a straight, upright, well-balanced posture.

Also important is the child's state of cleanliness or hygiene. The condition of the child's hair, nails, skin, teeth, and feet can give clues to the home environment. Appropriateness of dress can indicate the parent's knowledge of children's needs, as well as the family's financial resources.

General appearance also should include an impression of the child's nutritional status. The nurse observes body size and shape, noting the relationship between the child's height and weight. The nurse's impression of the child's nutritional state should be compared with the parent's history of feeding practices. Any discrepancy might be an indication for nutritional counseling.

An assessment of the child's behavior and elements of the child's personality encompasses the child's activity level, interactions with others, and response to new situations. These data are documented as part of general appearance but are part of a larger developmental assessment.

A complete developmental assessment should be included as part of every health assessment for well-child care, but general developmental impressions guide the nurse in sequencing the physical examination and provide clues to specific systems that might need further testing. For

TABLE 10-3 Approaches to Health Assessment During Childhood

Age	Preparation and position	Sequence of examination
Infancy (0–18 months)	In a warm examination room completely undress infant leaving only diaper on. Gain parent's cooperation in holding infant and keeping infant quiet and comfortable. For a young infant, examination can be done on parent's lap with infant supine or prone. As infants sits alone, examination can be done with child sitting on parent's lap or sitting on table with parent standing nearby. For uncooperative child, use appropriate restraints with the child lying on examination table.	With a quiet infant, begin with auscultation of heart, lungs, and abdomen. Palpate and percuss if infant remains relaxed. Proceed with a toe-to-head approach, examining each body system using gentle and then more invasive techniques. Terminate examination with the most traumatic procedures, such as examination of eyes, ears, and mouth (EENT). Neurologic assessment can be integrated into examination, left until the end, or done just before the EENT examination.
Early childhood (18 months–4½ years)	During history interview with parent, have child become familiar with environment by having appropriate play toys available. Before examination begins, allow child to see, feel, and play with stethoscope and otoscope. If this increases anxiety, proceed as quickly as possible. Some children might not become unduly upset by getting completely undressed; others might do better by having articles of clothing removed as that body part is examined. It is usually best to have child's underpants on throughout the examination.	Begin to observe child playing in the room during the history interview. Much of the musculoskeletal and neurologic examination can be done by astute observation of the child in play. Inspect and palpate as much as possible by playing with the child. Auscultate heart, lungs, and abdomen. Then proceed in a toe-to-head approach, palpating and percussing all remaining body parts. All traumatic procedures (such as the EENT examination) should be left until the end.
Middle childhood (4½–8 years)	These children often like to become involved and can be very cooperative when given responsibility for answering a few questions during history interview. It is usually best to let children undress themselves, leaving underpants on and putting on gown. *Briefly* explain each procedure while examining child, allowing child first to manipulate equipment if that seems to decrease anxiety. Younger children might still prefer to sit on parent's lap; older children might like to be examined sitting on table or standing next to parent.	This age group can be cooperative and allow examination to proceed in head-to-toe sequence, but it is often wise to leave ear and throat until the end.
Late childhood (8–12 years)	Older children usually do not mind getting undressed but often prefer to be left alone in the room to do so. Gowns should be provided; child usually prefers to keep underwear on. If females have begun to wear bras, these can be removed as the breast examination is to be done. Children of this age like to have everything explained to them and should be encouraged to be involved in the history interview and examination as much as possible. Some children prefer that their parents remain in the room; others (especially preadolescents) may prefer having their parents wait outside. It is best to discuss this with both parent and child.	Examination usually can proceed in head-to-toe sequence, with examination of the genitalia done at the end. If a neurodevelopmental exam is to be done, it is best done at the beginning of the process. Health education should be incorporated into appropriate sections by discussing knowledge of health behaviors (for example, skin care, diet, sports injuries, sexual development).
Adolescence (12–19 years)	Adolescents require privacy in undressing and in being examined. Often parents wait outside during the examination and sometimes during the history interview but both the adolescent and parent should meet with the clinician together to discuss appropriate health issues. Usually, adolescents are familiar with the equipment and procedures. Most important to them is the immediate feedback of the exam results. They like to know that everything is "normal."	Examination proceeds in head-to-toe sequence with genitalia usually left until the end, although some female adolescents often like to have the pelvic examination (if one is to be done) first. They should always be asked for their preference. Health education should be included. Adolescents are often receptive to anticipatory guidance on such issues as sexual maturity, drugs, and school behaviors.

example, a statement recorded about general appearance might be, "cooperative, smiling 3-year-old, well developed, well nourished, playing with toys, in no acute distress."

Skin

The skin protects the deeper tissues from injury and the invasion of bacteria, regulates body temperature, provides an avenue for excretion, and is involved in sensations of touch, heat, or cold. Physical assessment of the skin involves evaluating the skin's ability to perform these functions. The nurse assesses the skin systematically through inspection and palpation for color and pigmentation, turgor, moisture, texture, temperature, sensitivity, and the presence of any lesions. Hair, nails, and mucous membranes also are included in this assessment.

The skin is examined generally as a whole to assess the client's overall condition, then specifically as each body part is examined. For example, as the head and face are examined, the skin also is assessed, first by general inspection of the area, then more specifically as the scalp and areas of the face are assessed. Although the skin is assessed throughout the complete examination, the findings are recorded under one heading for skin.

Color and pigmentation Skin color varies from whitish-pink to shades of brown, depending on race; within a specific race, color variations are found. Dark-skinned children, such as those of American black, native American, Mexican, Mediterranean, Latin, or Asian descent, have various pigmentations from brown to red, bluish, and olive-green skin tones. For example, because of the yellow pigmentation of their skin, Oriental children might appear jaundiced when compared with white children. Black children might have a normal bluish pigmentation to their gums, buccal mucosa, and nail beds. Therefore, in making an accurate assessment, the nurse considers the amount of melanin genetically inherited among children of different races. If the child looks different from the parent, the nurse asks about the other parent.

Skin color also changes in response to the body's adjustment to heat and cold. Children might seem to have a reddish pigmentation when they are flushed from *hyperthermia* (fever). *Hypothermia* (lowered body temperature), which might be caused by excessive exposure to cold, can cause a child to look abnormally pale. The pallor associated with hypothermia can be difficult to distinguish from the pale appearance associated with nutritional anemia, which is a serious concern. Edema also decreases the skin tone and sometimes produces a false pallor. Skin color therefore is most reliably assessed in a well-illuminated, temperature-regulated room. The color of the examining room is important: yellow walls make a white child appear slightly jaundiced, and blue walls make the child appear slightly cyanotic. If the nurse suspects a change in skin color, the best procedure is to assess those areas of the body where the least melanin is produced: the sclera, conjunctiva, lips, palate, nail beds, and mucous membranes.

Turgor Tissue *turgor* refers to the amount of elasticity and recoil in the skin. Turgor is one of the best indications of nutrition and hydration in children. Normal skin turgor is elastic and taut. It is assessed by grasping the skin on the abdomen with thumb and forefinger, pulling it up and taut, and quickly releasing it. Skin with good turgor resumes its normal shape without residual marks. Depending on the amount of dehydration or malnutrition, the skin will maintain its pinched shape or fall back slowly onto the abdomen. Other causes of poor or decreased skin turgor are muscle disorders, excessive exposure to ultraviolet rays, and chronic disease.

Edema, which should be evaluated with turgor, is identified by pressing a thumb over the body surface that appears edematous. After releasing the finger, any sign of indentation that lasts several seconds indicates *pitting edema;* puffiness that does not remain indented is *nonpitting edema.* Both pitting and nonpitting edema are caused by excessive retention of water in the body tissues. Edema often is seen in the periorbital area of the face when it is due to crying, sleeping, allergies, or kidney disease. Dependent edema, seen in the buttocks and lower extremities, often indicates kidney or cardiac anomalies. The nurse therefore assesses the symmetry of the edema in the corresponding body part and the color of the edematous area.

Moisture Normal skin is slightly moist. Any increase in moisture is seen as clamminess or perspiration; any decrease in moisture, evidenced by dry, parchmentlike skin, should be evaluated. The nurse palpates all areas of the skin, assessing any variations in moisture from one body area to another. Dry skin only on the hands, lips, or genitalia might indicate a contact dermatitis, whereas generalized dry skin might indicate poor nutrition, overexposure to the sun, or overbathing.

Texture Inspection and palpation of the skin for texture assesses the quality and character of the skin surface. Normally, children's skin is smooth, not oily or clammy, and of even temperature. Skin that is rough and dry might indicate an endocrine problem or might be the result of overbathing, overexposure to the weather, or poor hygiene.

Temperature and sensitivity The nurse palpates the skin to evaluate temperature. Palpation is best done by feeling each body part on both sides, comparing each side with the other, and by comparing upper with lower body parts.

In assessing the sensitivity of a child's skin, the nurse needs to rely on both nonverbal and verbal clues to the child's discomfort. Any body area that has abnormal findings for color, turgor, texture, and temperature is assessed for pain or abnormal sensations such as burning, itching, tingling, or throbbing. If possible, the child should describe the feeling. Otherwise, the nurse documents the child's nonverbal responses while palpating sensitive areas. Children typically protect a painful area or pull away from the nurse, cry, or fuss.

Hair, nails, lesions Scalp and body hair is assessed for distribution, color, texture, amount, and quality. Children's scalp hair is usually soft, pliable, shiny, and strong. The scalp hair should be inspected for cleanliness and for lice. Genetic factors affect a child's hair and are responsible for curliness or coarseness, as well as for color and distribution. Some dark-skinned families have hairlines that normally extend down the neck and below the midforehead; this familial trait should be noted before attributing this hair pattern to cretinism. Hair that is dry, brittle, fragile, or depigmented might indicate a nutritional deficiency. Loss of hair, or *alopecia,* might be caused by hair pulling, the child's lying in the same position for an extended period of time, or disease.

Other types of hair that should be evaluated in addition to head hair include body hair, beard hair, axillary hair, and pubic hair. Eyebrows, eyelashes, and any hair on the face should be evaluated. Chest, axillary, and pubic hair should be evaluated as part of the assessment of the development of secondary sexual characteristics. The spine and buttocks should be inspected for hair tufts, which might be seen in children with spina bifida.

Nails are examined for color, shape, and condition. Such characteristics as clubbing of digits, curving, and spooning of nails are noted. Clubbing often is seen in children with congenital heart disease or chronic respiratory disease. Convex or concave curving might be hereditary or due to injury, poor nutrition, or infection. Cuticles should be assessed for intactness and smoothness, noting any signs of infection. The nurse also notes any evidence of nail biting, skin picking, or thumb sucking.

Any lesion noted on the skin is described in detail for size, shape, color, location, and surface characteristics.

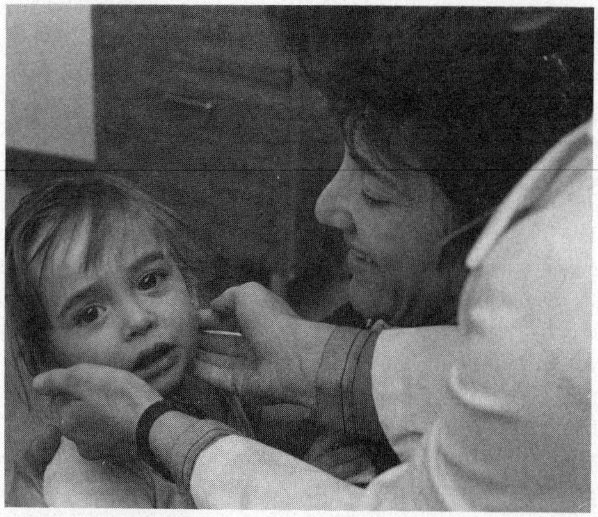

Lymph nodes are palpated gently, with a firm, circular motion.

Lymph Nodes

The lymphatic system—with its intricate network of capillaries that collect lymph from organs and tissues, of collecting vessels that carry lymph to the bloodstream, and of lymph nodes that act as filters for the collecting vessels—is a major contributor to the immunologic and metabolic processes of the body (Fig. 10-2). The lymphatic system is involved in the formation of macrophages and lymphocytes (cells involved in immunity and inflammation) and in the process of phagocytosis. In the physical examination of lymph nodes, the nurse assesses the presence or absence of *lymphadenopathy* (enlargement of the lymph nodes) because a single large lymph node or generalized lymphadenopathy might be the first sign of disease.

Lymph nodes are found in clusters or chains; they seldom occur singly. They are either in the subcutaneous connective tissue (*superficial lymph nodes*), or are beneath muscular fascia and in body cavities (*deep lymph nodes*). Lymph nodes are evaluted when the part of the body in which they are located is assessed. Normally, lymph nodes are not palpable; therefore, when nodes are felt the nurse documents this finding in the assessment.

Lymph nodes are palpated with the distal portion of the fingers (fingerpads) by gently but firmly pressing in a circular, rotary motion along the regions in which lymph nodes are normally present. Lymph nodes that are felt during the examination are described and assessed by noting the location, size, surface characteristics, firmness, mobility, tenderness, and temperature.

Head, Face, and Neck

Head The head is inspected and palpated for size, shape, symmetry, deformities, control, movements, and position. In infants, the head is also inspected for fontanelles and

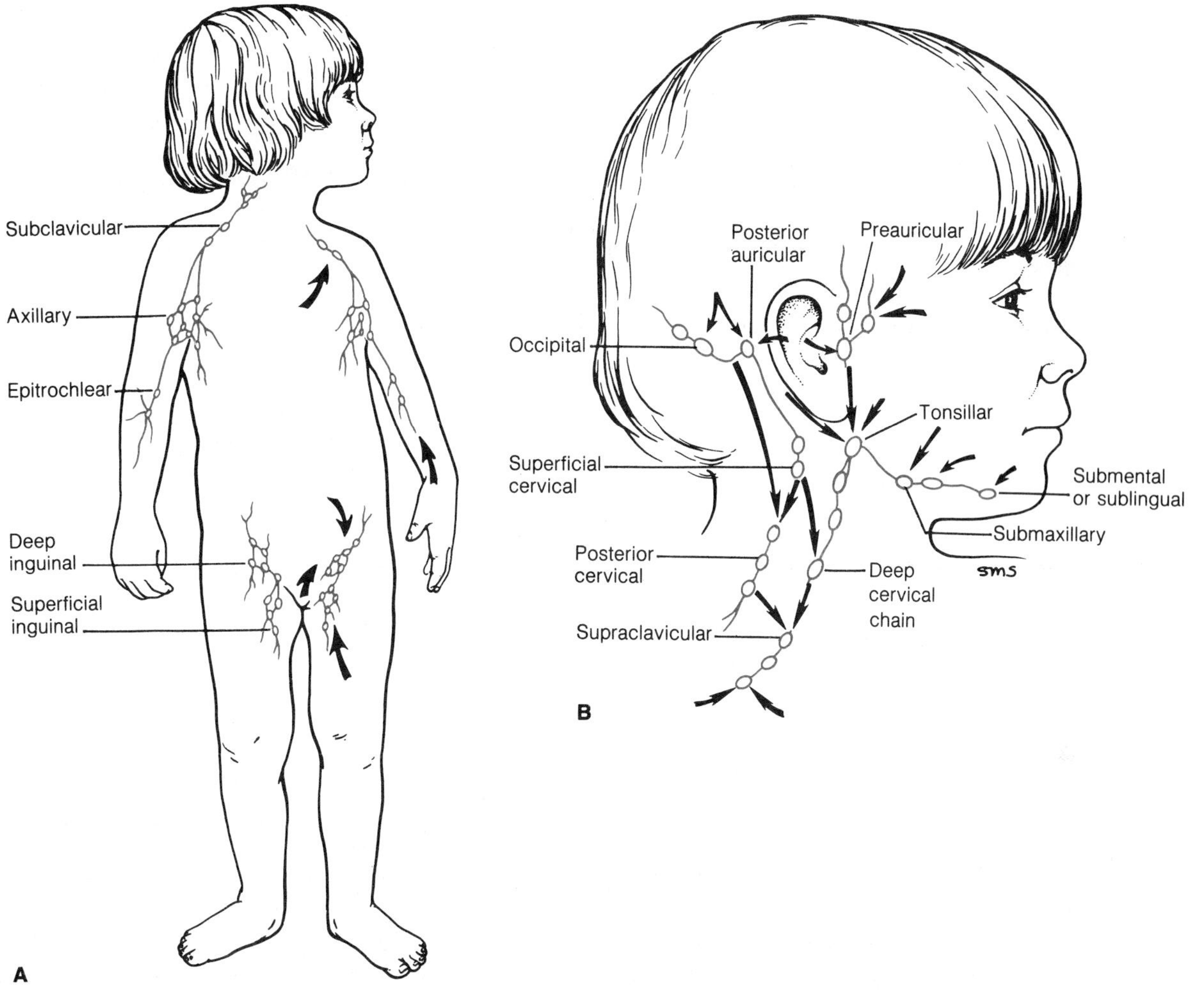

FIGURE 10-2
A. Location of lymph nodes. B. Direction of lymph flow.

sutures (spaces in the skull that are not yet ossified). Normal head circumference is between 32 and 38 cm at birth and is generally 1–2 cm larger than the chest until after the first year of life. Head size then approximates chest size, but chest growth begins to exceed head size during early childhood until the head is 5–7 cm smaller than the chest. Any significant discrepancy in head circumference as measured and plotted on the head circumference graph warrants further evaluation to rule out congenital neurologic defects.

The shape of a neonate's head may be asymmetric because of the birth process, but any prominent bulges or swellings should be noted. *Cephalohematoma* (bleeding below the periosteum of the skull bones, normally restricted to one bone) and *caput succedaneum* (edema that generally crosses suture lines) might be seen immediately after birth. Generally, however, heads are described as normocephalic. The range of norms is hereditary; thus, the child's normal head circumference and shape will be similar to the parents'.

A thorough examination for any asymmetry or deformities of the head involves inspecting the head from all angles. The nurse might be able to do this as the child sits on the parent's lap, or the child might need to stand up for clearer inspection. At the same time, the nurse can inspect head control and movements. Because infants attain head control from a lying to a sitting position by 4 months of age, significant head lag after 6 months of age signifies the need for referral to evaluate possible developmental delay or cerebral injury.

Range of motion of the head and neck is evaluated by asking the older child to look in each direction (up, down, and to either side) or by manually putting the child through each position. Infants can be shown a bright toy to follow

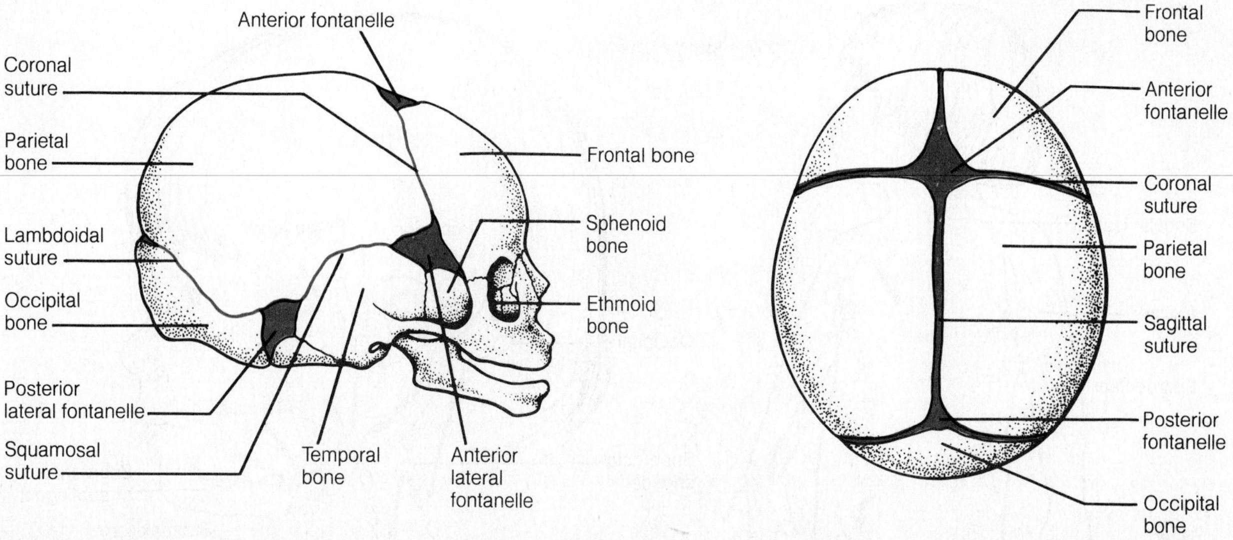

FIGURE 10-3

The bones of the skull showing the fontanelles and suture lines. (From Kozier B, Erb G: Fundamentals of Nursing, *3rd ed. Addison-Wesley, 1987.)*

horizontally from side to side. Any lateral limitations in head movement should be noted and referred for further evaluation.

In the infant the scalp is inspected and palpated for fontanelles and sutures, scaliness, infections, and ecchymoses. Infants are born with six fontanelles, but generally only the anterior and posterior fontanelles are palpated (Fig. 10-3). The fontanelles are assessed for size, pulsations, and tenseness (that is, bulging, flattened, or sunken appearance). The nurse notes whether the fontanelles are clean because some parents are afraid to touch them, having heard myths that doing so could cause brain damage.

The size of the anterior fontanelle is palpated and recorded as, for example, "anterior fontanelle 1.5 cm by 2 cm." This fontanelle generally closes between 9 and 18 months of age. Any premature or delayed closing warrants further evaluation and referral. The posterior fontanelle, which might not be readily palpable at birth or shortly after, closes by 3 months of age. Fontanelles are normally flat with slight pulsations. Any significant bulging, sunken appearance, or great pulsations when the infant is quiet require further evaluation and referral. Sutures, which because of the birth process may appear as prominent ridges at birth, usually flatten by 6 months of age and should not be palpable or overriding (overlapping).

In older children, the scalp is assessed for lesions, scaliness, cleanliness, evidence of infections such as those caused by ticks or lice, and signs of trauma such as ecchymosis or scars.

Face The face is inspected and palpated for symmetry, movement, spacing of features, color and texture, temperature, and tenderness. Looking at the child from several angles or observing the child laughing, frowning, and smiling allows the nurse to observe symmetry, movement, and the placement of features.

The eyes should not be widely set, a condition termed *ocular hypertelorism,* or unusually close together, a condition called *ocular hypotelorism.* The nose should be midline with symmetric nares; the mouth and lips should be symmetric. The child's ears should be located at the same level, and the top of the pinna should cross an imaginary line drawn from the occiput to the lateral corner of the eye (this is termed the *eye-occiput line*). Low-set ears might indicate renal anomalies or Down syndrome (Fig. 10-4).

Neck The neck is inspected and palpated for position, movement, size and shape, and the position of the trachea and thyroid gland and is auscultated for bruits or pulsations (Fig. 10-5). The neck should be symmetric from all angles. Observation of extra folds of posterior skin, or webbing, warrants further evaluation.

With the child's neck hyperextended, the neck is inspected to determine the position of the trachea and the presence of any masses. The larynx and the trachea are palpated. The nurse first locates the hyoid bone which lies just below the mandible. The thyroid cartilage, shaped like a shield, lies in the neck below the hyoid bone. The thyroid gland and isthmus are then palpated on either side just

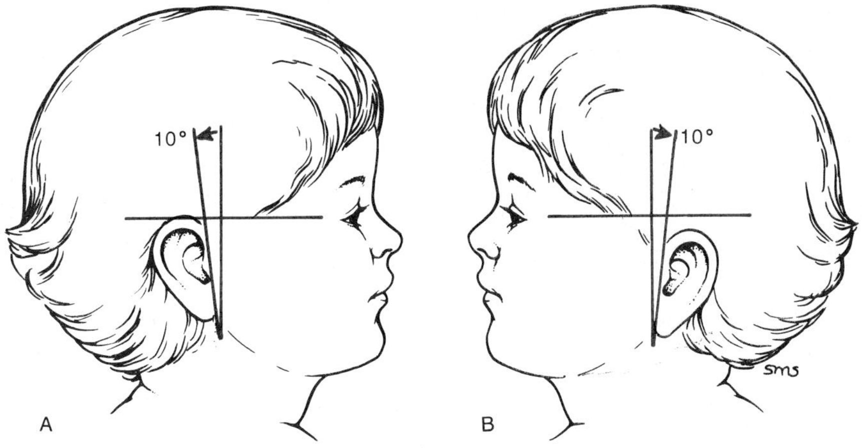

FIGURE 10-4

Alignment of ears. ***A.*** *Normal ears.* ***B.*** *Low-set ears.*

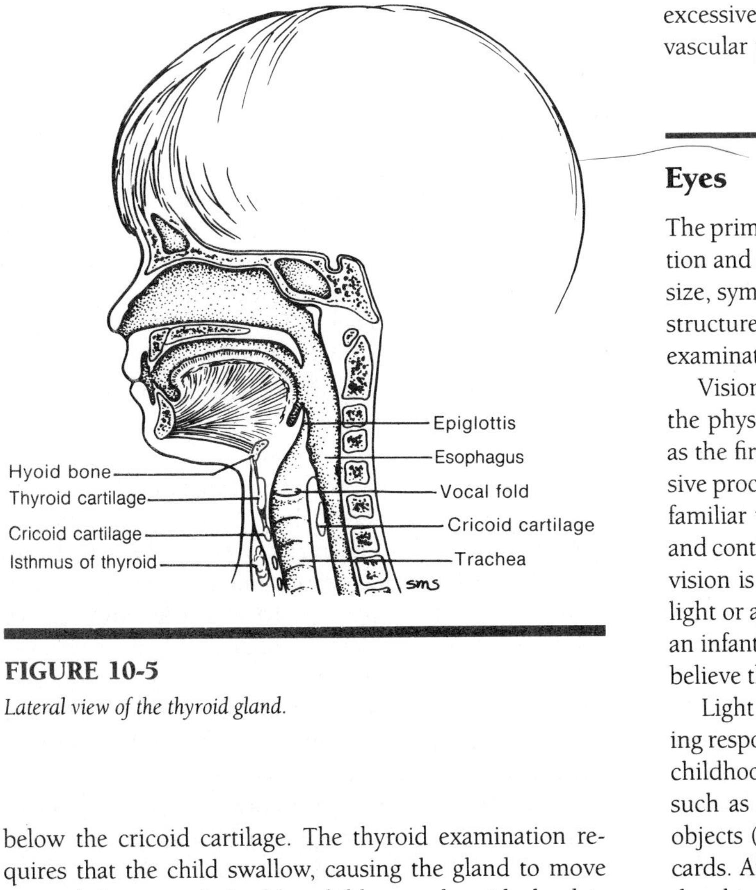

FIGURE 10-5

Lateral view of the thyroid gland.

below the cricoid cartilage. The thyroid examination requires that the child swallow, causing the gland to move upward. In normal, healthy children a thyroid gland is often not palpable.

The neck is auscultated to identify any bruits (soft rushing sounds), pulsations, or murmurs. The bell of the stethoscope is placed over the carotid arteries. Any bruits, excessive pulsations, or murmurs might be signs of cardiovascular problems.

Eyes

The primary methods for examining the eyes are (1) inspection and sometimes palpation of the external structures for size, symmetry, and color and (2) inspection of the interior structures to assess the retinal structures. A complete eye examination also includes a series of tests of visual acuity.

Vision screening often is done at the beginning of either the physical examination after measurements are taken or as the first part of the eye examination. It is the least intrusive procedure in the eye assessment, and children are most familiar with it. Vision screening should begin in infancy and continue throughout life at regular intervals. In infancy, vision is tested by observing the child's ability to follow a light or a brightly colored toy. Most parents are sensitive to an infant's sense of sight and should be asked whether they believe their child can see.

Light perception in neonates is tested by noting a blinking response as a light is shined into the child's eyes. In early childhood, visual acuity can be tested with a picture test such as Allen cards, which are black pictures of familiar objects (horse, birthday cake, house, and so on) on white cards. After ascertaining that the child can correctly name the objects, the nurse shows the cards while slowly moving away from the child. A 3-year-old should achieve a score of 20/40; a 4-year-old should obtain a score of 20/30 (that is, the 3-year-old should identify the pictures correctly at 20 ft that someone with normal visual acuity could identify at

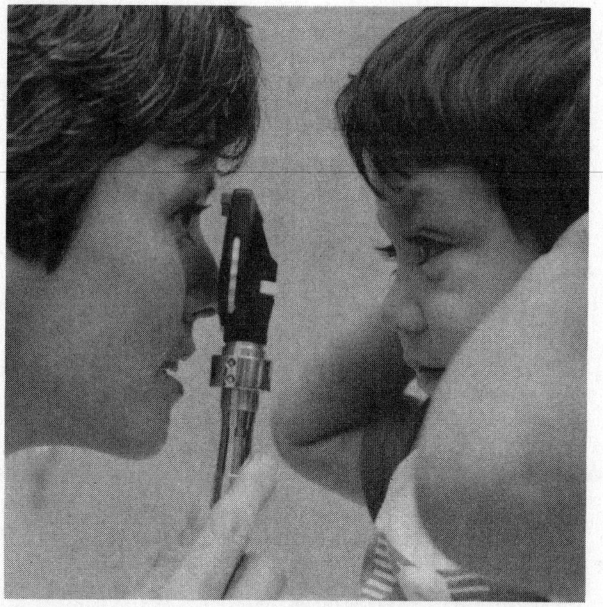

Inspection of the external eye. The child must keep both eyes wide open. Holding the ophthalmoscope 12 in. from the child and steadying it against the nose, the nurse uses the right eye to examine the child's right eye and vice versa.

40 ft). The fraction denotes the resolving power of the eye. A child who cannot identify the pictures or has a 5-ft difference between eyes should be referred for further evaluation. (Expected visual acuity for various ages is listed in Table 10-4).

Children who are unable to read letters, including those for whom English is not the first language, may have their vision tested with the Snellen E test. The child indicates which direction the E is pointing (up, down, right, or left) either by pointing a hand in the same direction or by identifying the direction by referring to concrete items placed in the environment (for example, table, door, ceiling, floor).

The Snellen Alphabet Chart is used for children and adults who can identify letters. Whatever test is used, the nurse must follow the directions correctly to ensure an accurate assessment. Adequate lighting is essential. There should be no glare, and the chart should be placed at the child's eye level. The child should be provided with a large paper cup, index card, or eye patch to help occlude the eye not being tested. The occluding object is placed against the midline of the child's nose, not directly against the eye or eyeglasses, if worn. Children often need to be reminded several times to keep both eyes open, even the eye that is covered. After the child clearly understands the procedure, the nurse tests the child's vision as far down the chart as the child is capable of reading. Reading more than half the letters is a passing score. The child should be started on line

TABLE 10-4 Visual Acuity at Various Ages

Age	Visual acuity
Birth	Fixates on objects 8–12 inches away; might follow object briefly if in alert, quiet state (20/600–20/800)
2–3 months	Fixates and follows objects in horizontal and vertical directions (20/300)
1 year	20/100
2 years	20/50
3 years	20/40
4 years	20/30
5 years	20/20

20/40 or 20/50 and moved up or down, depending on the results. The results are then recorded immediately in the child's chart. Any child who does not have age-appropriate visual acuity or a one-line difference between eyes should be referred for further evaluation.

Color vision also should be assessed in every child. Color blindness is hereditary; therefore, a positive family history warrants a careful examination of the child. Most 3- and 4-year-old children know their colors and can simply be asked to name the color of their clothing or of colored blocks or toys. The Ishibara Plates is a standardized color vision test that can be used with children who are able to discriminate among letters, numbers, geometric figures, and a figure background. A color-blind child and the child's parent will need counseling for such safety purposes as interpreting traffic signals.

External eye The external eye examination begins with the eyelashes. They should be assessed for distribution, direction of growth, and pigmentation. Lashes that turn inward can cause conjunctival irritation. The examination continues with the eyelids (Fig. 10-6). The lids are observed for edema, color, position, the presence of any exudate or infection, and the ability to open and close completely. Edema of the lids can be the result of systemic disease (for example, nephrosis) or a local response such as from an insect bite. Any ecchymosis should be noted.

The lids are inspected for proper placement on the eye. When the eye is open, the upper lid should fall somewhere between the upper iris and the pupil. Any deviation requires further evaluation. Neonates cry without tears. Infants usually begin to tear by 3 months of age, and the persistent absence of tears might indicate a blocked duct.

Epicanthal folds are vertical rolls of skin on the lid and often cover the inner canthus (Fig. 10-7). They give the

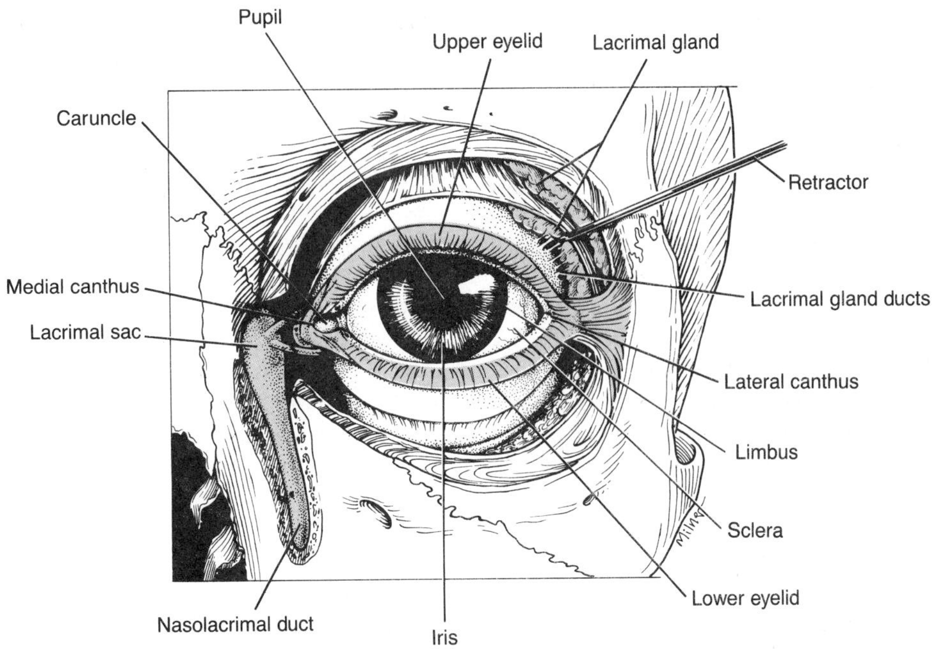

FIGURE 10-6

Structures of the eye with lacrimal retracted to show ducts. (From Spence AP, Mason EB: Human Anatomy and Physiology, *3rd ed. Benjamin/Cummings, 1987.)*

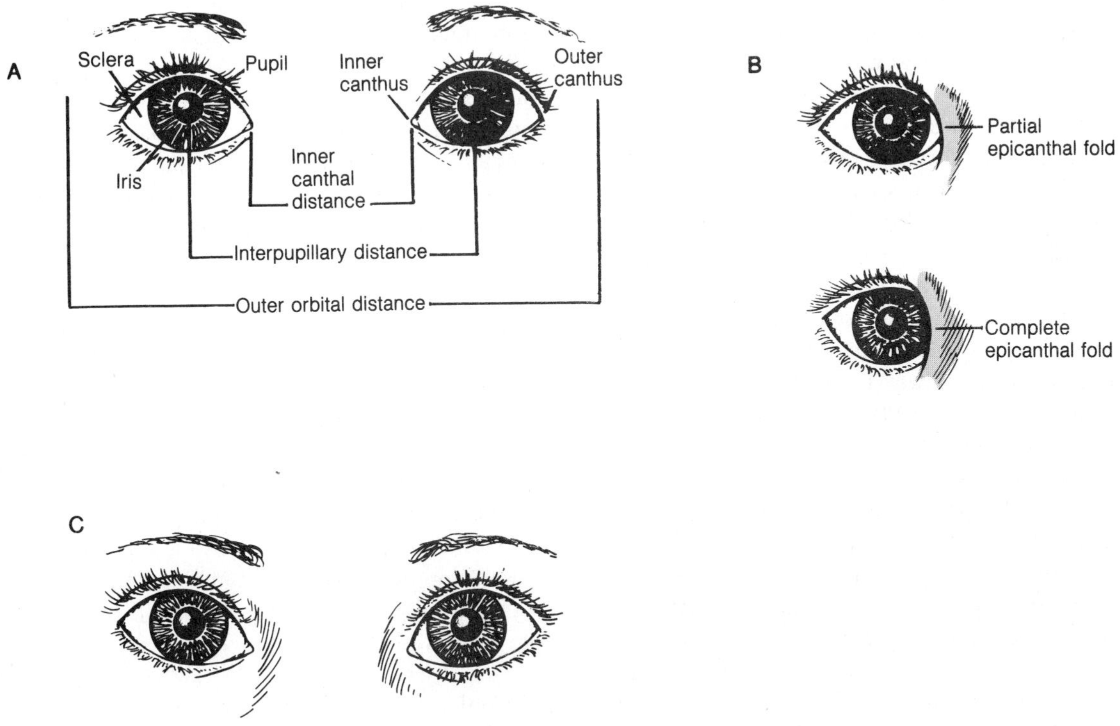

FIGURE 10-7

A. *Anatomic landmarks of the eye.* **B.** *Epicanthal folds.* **C.** *Upward palpebral slant ("almond-shaped eyes").*

child the appearance of "slant eyes." Epicanthal folds might be present in Asian children and some Caucasian neonates. They also might be a sign of Down syndrome and metabolic or renal diseases and are then seen with other physical characteristics of these conditions.

The nurse inspects the conjunctiva for color, hemorrhages, and inflammation. The *palpebral conjunctiva* is the lining of the lids. The upper conjunctiva is best examined by gently everting the lid as the child looks down. A cotton-tipped applicator can be placed over the upper lid and the lashes gently grasped and rolled over to expose the conjunctiva clearly. The lower conjunctiva is more easily inspected by gently pulling the lid down as the child looks up. Normal conjunctiva is pink and glassy. Inflammation of the conjunctiva, causing redness and often discharge, can be due to bacterial or viral infections, allergy, or chemical or mechanical irritations. A "cobblestone" appearance of the conjunctiva often is seen in children with severe or chronic allergies.

The *bulbar conjunctiva* covers the eye up to the junction of the cornea and sclera. It should be transparent, and the white color of the underlying sclera should be visible. Redness is due to dilation of blood vessels and might indicate eye strain, irritation, or bleeding disorders.

The *sclera,* or white covering of the eyeball, should be clear. Dark-skinned children might have tiny black marks, which are normal. The *cornea,* or covering of the iris and pupil, should be crystal clear, without any inflammation, ulceration, or opacity. The best way to test for abrasions is with staining, but they also can be seen by shining a light obliquely toward the cornea.

The iris is observed for color and inflammation. The permanent color of the iris is seen by 6 months of age in 50% of children and in all children by 1 year of age. *Heterochromia,* or irises of different colors, can be normal or associated with congenital syndromes or chronic low-grade infections of the iris. *Brushfield's spots* (a light or white speckling of the iris) might occur in normal children but is seen most often in children with Down syndrome or other syndromes associated with mental retardation.

The pupils are examined for pupillary response and size. Pupil size should be equal, and pupils should be responsive to light both directly and consensually. A pupil reacts to light directly if the pupil into which the light is shone constricts; it reacts consensually if it constricts when the light is shone in the opposite eye. Accommodation, or constriction when focusing on a nearby object, and dilation when looking into the distance also are tested. Difference in pupil size can be normal, but any sudden differences noted require a complete neurologic evaluation.

The lens should be evaluated with examination of the iris and pupil. Opacities of the lenses can be seen by flashing a light into the eye, preferably at an oblique angle. A red reflex should be visible. Any patient with a possible cataract or dislocated lens should be referred to an ophthalmologist.

The final part of the external eye examination is observation of extraocular movements (Fig. 10-8). The nurse assesses the child for nystagmus, strabismus, and peripheral vision. *Nystagmus* involves involuntary, rapid, jerky movements of the eye as the child is observed through the six visual fields associated with each eye. The direction of the nystagmus should be recorded. *Strabismus* involves deviation of one or both eyes. A paralyzed extraocular muscle or nerve causes paralytic (noncomitant) strabismus. Paralytic strabismus is present only in the field of action of the involved muscle or nerve. Nonparalytic (concomitant) strabismus occurs when the eyes do not move simultaneously in any quadrant. Strabismus that occurs only intermittently (for example, when the child is fatigued) is a *phoria;* an overt strabismus is a *tropia.* The movement of the eyeball is observed for deviation outward, *exo,* or deviation inward, *eso.* Therefore, a child with overt strabismus in which the eye deviates inward during examination of extraocular movements through the visual fields is described as having esotropia. Strabismus that remains undetected can cause *amblyopia* (reduction or dimness of vision) or even blindness.

Two screening tests used to detect phoria types of strabismus are (1) the corneal light reflex test and (2) the cover test. The corneal light reflex test is performed by shining a light at the bridge of the child's nose as the child looks straight ahead, fixating on an object. The light reflex normally should fall at the same point on the pupils; any deviation indicates strabismus. This test requires the cooperation of an older child who can follow directions. The cover test may be performed on younger children who can be kept in a quiet, alert state. The cover test is done by first getting the child to fixate on an object about 12 in. away, then quickly covering one eye, making sure both eyes remain open and observing any inward or outward movement of the uncovered eye. The occluded eye is then uncovered and inspected for any movement. The child with this condition should be referred for further testing to prevent the development of amblyopia.

Children who have wide nasal bridges or epicanthal folds may appear to have strabismus, a condition referred to as *pseudostrabismus.* Negative cover and light reflex tests rule out this condition.

Internal eye The internal eye examination involves assessment of the optic disk, retinal vessels, macula, and general background with an ophthalmoscope. This part of the eye examination requires patience to learn and a coopera-

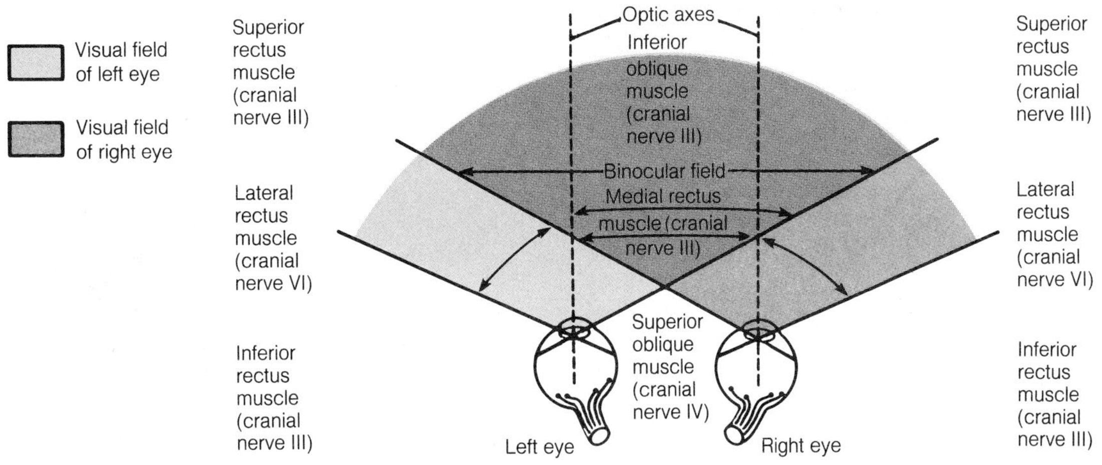

FIGURE 10-8

Visual fields of extraocular movement. If the child's eyes cannot move to a given position, dysfunction of a muscle or cranial nerve is indicated. (Adapted from Spence AP, Mason EB: Human Anatomy and Physiology, *3rd ed. Benjamin/Cummings, 1987.)*

tive child who can sit quietly in a semidarkened room. An ophthalmoscope has from 15 to 20 diopters in the black (positive lens) and in the red (negative lens). (A diopter is the refractive power of the lens with a focal distance of 1 m.) The refractive ability of the child's and the nurse's eyes determines the diopters to be used during the examination. The red numbers, or negative lens, compensate for nearsightedness, and the black numbers, or positive lens, compensate for farsightedness.

The ophthalmoscope generally is initially dialed to 0. At a distance of 12 in., the nurse centers the light on the child's eye and assesses the red reflex. Gradually moving closer to the child and turning the dial to the red negative numbers, the examiner assesses the cornea, aqueous chamber, lens, and vitreous chamber (Fig. 10-9). With the nurse's and child's foreheads almost touching, the nurse examines the fundus (back of the eye), arteries, and veins. The optic disk is then located and observed for size, shape, color, margins, and physiologic cup. Normally, the optic disc is creamy white to pinkish, 1.5 mm in diameter, and round to oval, with sharp, clear margins. A depression slightly temporal of the center is the *physiologic cup*.

The retinal vessels are observed for color, size, and regularity. Normal arteries are one-fourth the size of veins and brighter in color, exhibiting a light reflex from the center. Veins are darker and may pulsate near the optic disc. They should both be observed for any narrowing, dilatation, tortuosity, or nicking. Any abnormality warrants referral for further evaluation.

The *fundus,* or general background, is assessed for pigmentation and integrity. The color varies depending on skin and hair pigmentation but is normally an orange-red color and uniform throughout. The *macula* is a spot that lies near the temporal side of the fundus, two disc diameters away, and is one disc diameter in size. It is brighter than the optic disc, and the gleaming light in the center is the *fovea centralis.* This is the most light-sensitive part of the eye, and the nurse often can locate it by asking the child to look briefly into the light on the ophthalmoscope. This, however, might cause the child some discomfort, which is why it is the last part of the eye examination.

Ears

External ear The ear examination begins with an assessment of the position, size, shape, color, and symmetry of the ears (Fig. 10-10). Any lesions or deformities are noted. The pinna should be level with the eye. The pinna is inspected for the normal skin tone, color, and such structural anomalies as ear tags; it is palpated for nodules, lesions, or masses and for turgor. The *mastoid,* the bony prominence posterior to the earlobe, is observed for color, temperature, tenderness, and lesions.

The external auditory canal is observed for color, edema, discharges, amount and texture of cerumen (earwax), lesions, masses, or foreign bodies. (The nurse also notes

FIGURE 10-9

A. Internal structure of the eye. *B. Retinal nerve fibers of the internal eye as seen with fundoscopic (slit-lamp) camera. (From Spence AP, Mason EB:* Human Anatomy and Physiology, *3rd ed. Benjamin/ Cummings, 1987.)*

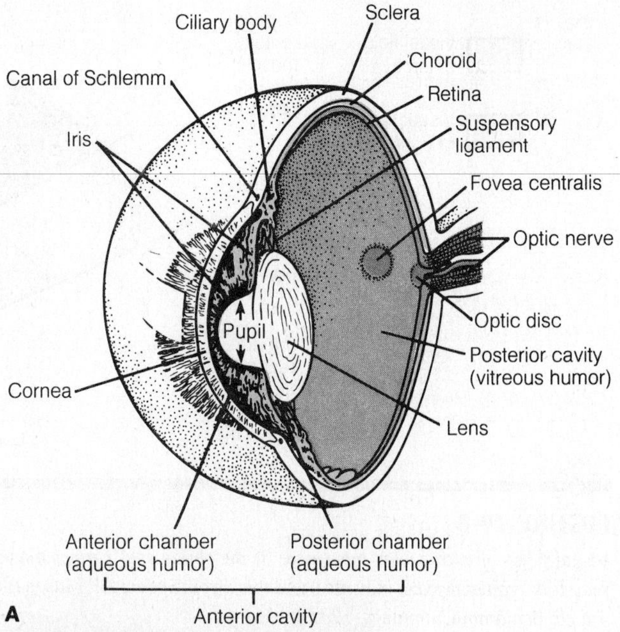

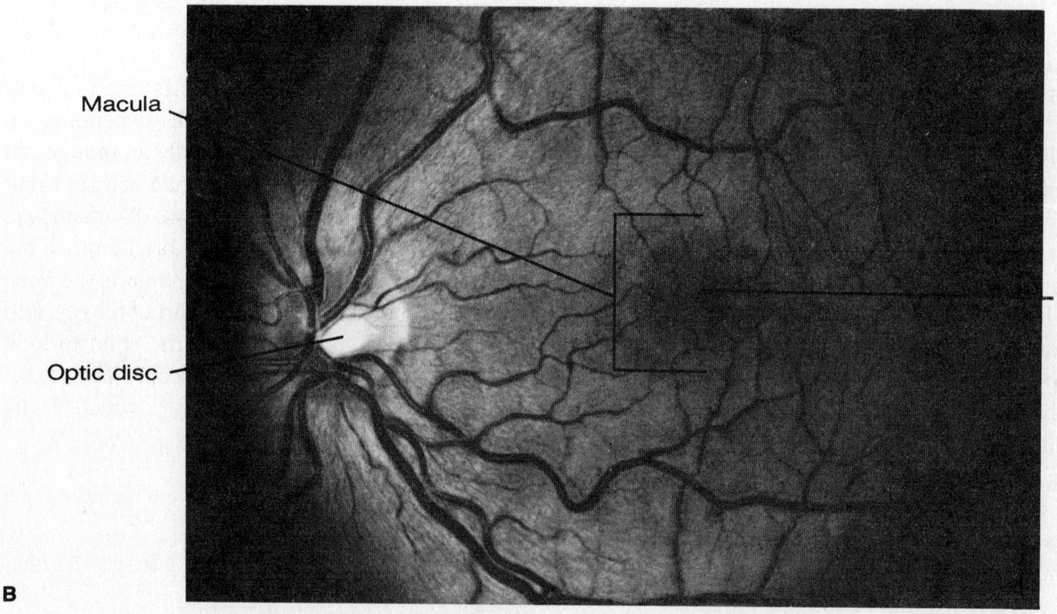

whether cerumen is fresh or old.) Any serosanguineous discharge may be from a perforated tympanic membrane, a foreign body irritation, or scratching. A purulent discharge usually means infection and needs to be referred to the physician.

Middle ear The middle ear is examined with an otoscope. The largest speculum that can comfortably fit in the child's ear should be used. The otoscopic examination generally is not painful unless there is an external otitis or furuncle in the ear canal. Children, however, become easily frightened and anxious during this part of the examination, although adequate preparation and a secure environment might alleviate these problems. Any child who cannot cooperate needs to be securely restrained to prevent traumatic damage to the ear during the examination.

Children who cannot be trusted to remain still should be restrained gently in one of two general positions. The first position is to have the child seated on the parent's lap, with the child's head resting securely against the parent and the

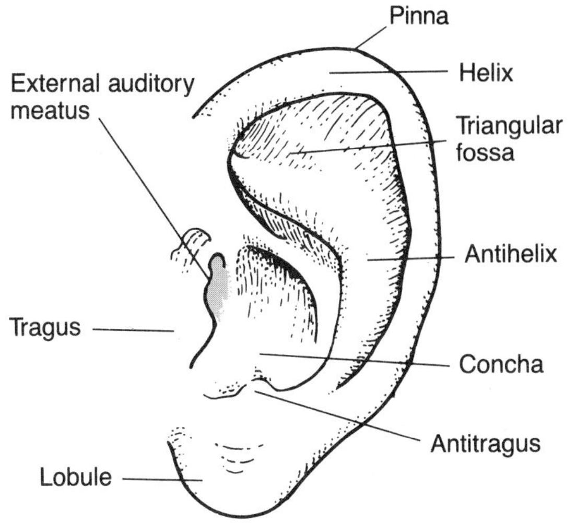

A

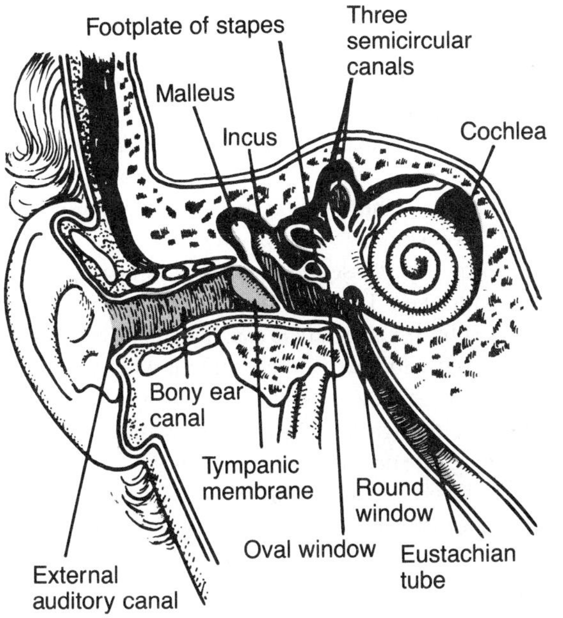

B

FIGURE 10-10

A. Structures of the external ear. *B. External auditory canal, middle ear, and inner ear.*

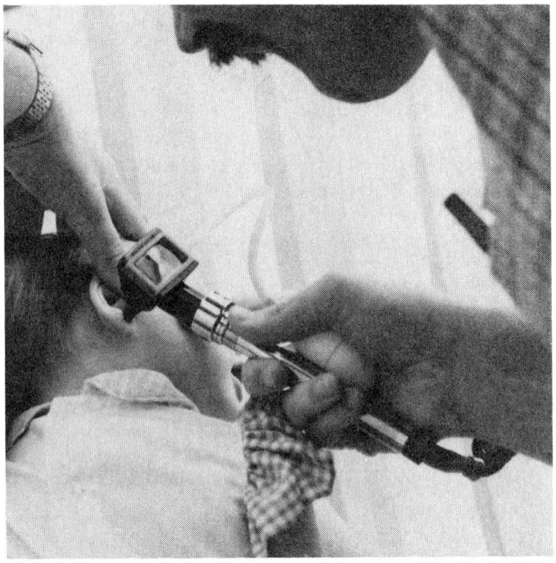

A

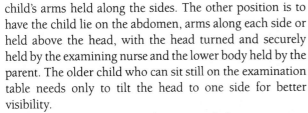

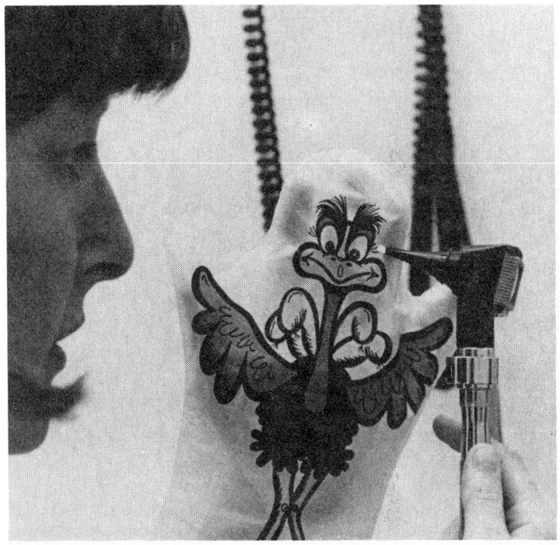

B

A. The infant's head is held against the mother while the ear is examined. (From Kozier B, Erb G: Techniques in Clinical Nursing. *Addison-Wesley, 1982.) B. During early and middle childhood, preparation for ear examination helps in gaining the child's cooperation.*

child's arms held along the sides. The other position is to have the child lie on the abdomen, arms along each side or held above the head, with the head turned and securely held by the examining nurse and the lower body held by the parent. The older child who can sit still on the examination table needs only to tilt the head to one side for better visibility.

Once the child is adequately restrained, the otoscope can be placed inside the ear canal. Ear canals of infants and young children curve upward, so the ear lobe is pulled gently down and out for visibility. Ear canals of older children and adults are longer and curve downward; therefore, the top of the pinna is grasped up and back (Fig. 10-11).

The external canal is then examined internally for any erythema ("swimmer's ear"), foreign bodies, or discharge. The amount, color, and texture of cerumen (earwax) is noted and described.

Examination of the middle ear consists of observation of the tympanic membrane and landmarks (Fig. 10-12). The tympanic membrane is assessed for color, light reflex, and

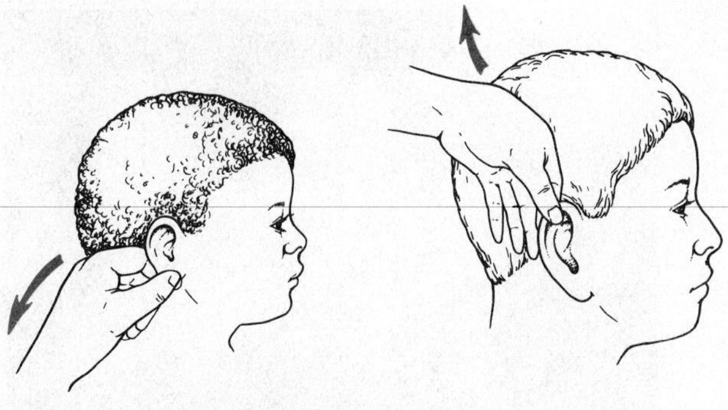

FIGURE 10-11

Straightening the external auditory canal for insertion of otoscope. **A.** *Infant.* **B.** *Adolescent.*

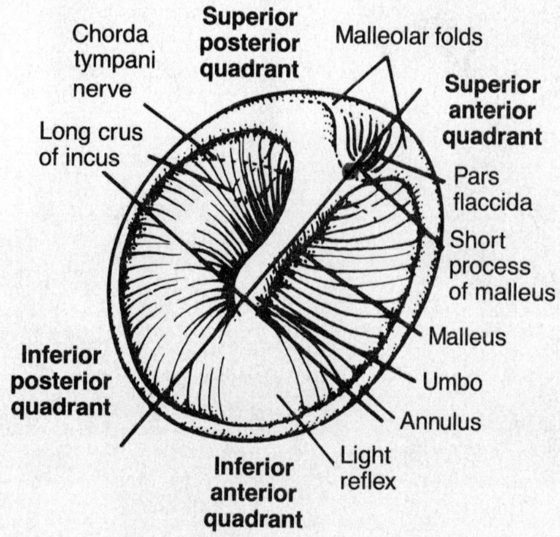

FIGURE 10-12

Anatomic landmarks of the middle ear.

mobility. Normally, it is pearly gray. An erythematous membrane indicates a middle ear infection but also might be seen in a child who is crying. A dull gray-to-yellowish color often is seen with serous otitis. The light reflex is a triangular cone of light located at the inferior anterior quadrant, to the right of the umbo. A diffuse, spotty, or absent light reflex indicates a middle ear disease. Mobility is then tested with a pneumatic bulb attached to the otoscopic head. Slight instillation of air will cause a normal tympanic membrane to move smoothly. Jerky, sluggish, or absent mobility is another sign of middle ear disease.

Landmarks assessed during the examination are the umbo, short and long processes, and cannulas. The pars flaccida and the anterior and posterior malleolar folds also are assessed, although these structures are not always clearly visible. In an acute suppurative ear infection, the landmarks might not be visible because of bulging of the eardrum. Serous otitis that causes negative pressure in the middle ear and retraction of the eardrum might cause the long process to appear more forward than normal or the malleus itself to be more accentuated.

The tympanic membrane is then observed for any perforations or scars. Perforations commonly are seen along the cannula; scars might be seen anywhere on the eardrum.

Hearing screening Hearing is an essential part of examining the senses and should be included in every well-child physical examination. The development of speech and language depends on adequate hearing.

Children who are at risk for hearing problems are those who have had multiple middle ear infections, have a familial history of congenital hearing impairment, had a cleft palate, were exposed prenatally to infections such as rubella, were premature, had birth anoxia, or who took ototoxic drugs during infancy (for example, neomycin, streptomycin). These children require early and periodic hearing evaluations.

Hearing is best assessed in infants by eliciting the startle reflex with a bell. The nurse also notes the infant's ability to localize sound. The parent is usually reliable in assessing an infant's ability to hear. Young children who can sit quietly and respond to directions such as "Give me the truck" most likely have no significant hearing problem. The child who seems to ignore parental requests or listens to the television or radio turned up loudly might need audiometric testing.

An audiometer measures the threshold of hearing for pure-tone frequencies and loudness. It determines both the severity of the hearing loss and the sound cycles involved.

Nose

The nose is responsible for temperature control of the air, humidification, and filtration of the first passageway to the respiratory tract. It is also the sensory organ of smell. Each of these functions depends on the patency of the mucosal lining of the nasal cavity. The nurse assesses the health and integrity of the nose and its structures principally by inspection.

The nose is examined for size and shape, patency of nares, color of mucous membranes, and the absence or presence of discharge, masses, or polyps. Although the size and shape of a child's nose may be determined by heredity, several unusual shapes need to be noted. A flat nose may indicate congenital anomalies (for example, cleft palate) or

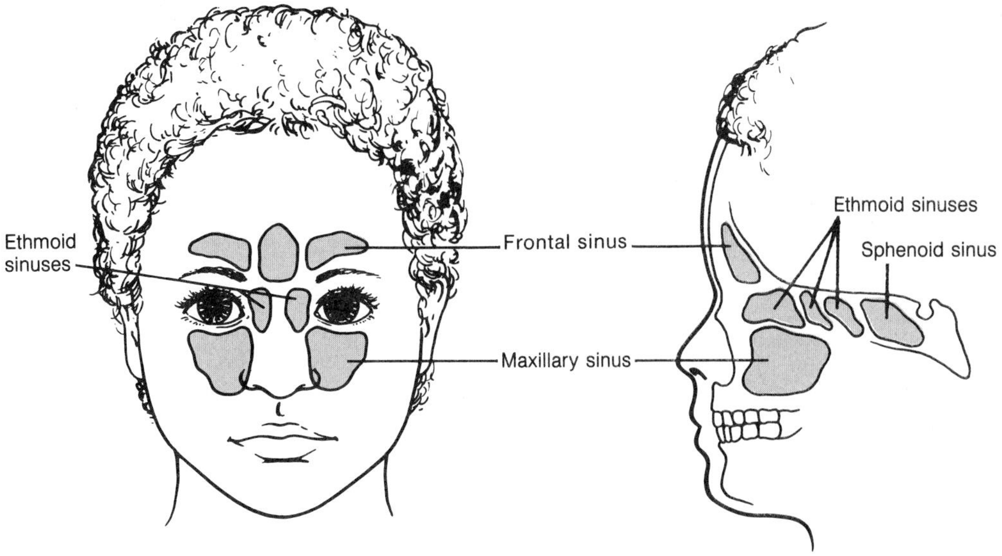

FIGURE 10-13
Front and lateral views of the facial sinuses.

other conditions. Children with chronic allergies develop a crease across their noses as a result of pushing up against the tip of the nose in response to itching or rhinitis.

Patency of the nares is assessed by placing the diaphragm of the stethoscope under one nare while blocking the other nare. As the child breathes, a film appears on the diaphragm. Infants are obligatory nose breathers. A child who breathes through the mouth might have enlarged adenoids, nasal polyps, allergies, or a deviated septum.

Internal examination of the nose requires either a penlight or a nasal speculum attached to the otoscope. Gently inserting the speculum, the nurse observes the color, integrity, and secretions of the nasal mucosa. Normal mucosa is pink, sometimes with a bluish hue, and moist. Reddened mucosa indicates infection or irritation; pale, boggy mucosa indicates allergies; and gray, swollen mucosa indicates chronic rhinitis. Watery discharge might be caused by allergies or upper respiratory infections. Purulent discharges are common with sinus infections or foreign bodies. Blood-stained discharge might indicate nasal bleeding occurring at the anterior tip of the septum. Allergy, trauma, a dry climate, nose picking, or blood dyscrasias will cause epistaxis (nose bleeding).

The vestibule of the nose is assessed for such lesions as furuncles. The inferior and middle turbinates are assessed for patency and discharges. The anterior portion of the septum is assessed for any septal deviation.

Palpation and percussion of the sinuses are also performed (Fig. 10-13). Normally, the sinuses cannot be felt, but a child with sinusitis might complain of pain or tenderness on palpation. The maxillary and ethmoid sinuses are the only sinuses developed at birth. By 7–8 years of age, the frontal sinuses develop; the sphenoid sinus develops after puberty.

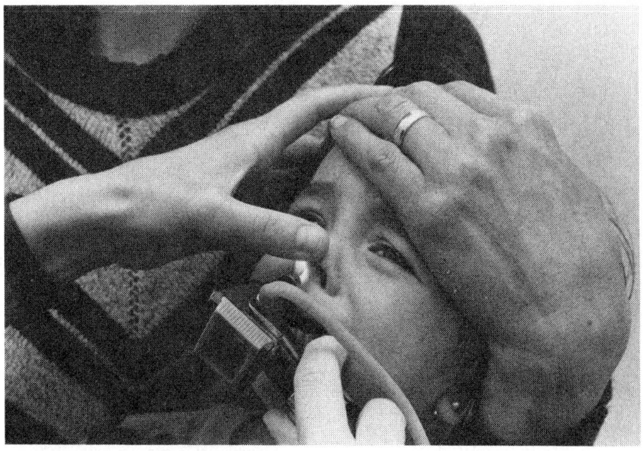

Inspection of the internal structures of the nose.

Mouth and Throat

Evaluation of the mouth and throat is best left until the end of the examination because it is often difficult for the child. With a cooperative child, almost the entire examination can

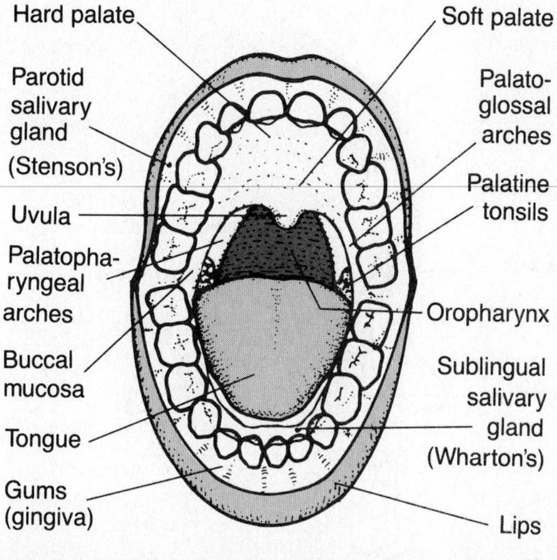

FIGURE 10-14

Internal structures of the mouth.

be done without a tongue blade. Playing games with the child, asking the child to open wide, and shining a penlight to examine the structures often suffices for a complete assessment. Infants and younger or uncooperative children, however, need adequate restraints. In addition, a tongue depressor and penlight usually are needed for viewing the structures.

The examination should proceed in an orderly manner from the external structures, from the lips to the gums, teeth, tongue, buccal mucosa, palate and oropharynx (Fig. 10-14). The lips are inspected for symmetry, color, moisture, the presence of any fissures or lesions, and edema. The surrounding area also is inspected for pallor or cyanosis.

Mouth odor also should be assessed at this time. Unusual odors might be present in children with poor oral hygiene; nasal obstruction due to allergies, foreign bodies, or polyps; metabolic disorders; and malnutrition.

Teeth are inspected for number, location, type (deciduous or permanent), malocclusions, color, caries, and hygiene. The first teeth erupt at about 6 months of age; all 20 deciduous teeth have erupted by 30 months of age. Permanent dentition begins at about 6 years of age and continues until all 32 teeth have erupted (Fig. 10-15).

Teeth with flattened surfaces might be due to bruxism (teeth grinding); notches might be due to trauma. Malocclusion can be caused by persistent thumb sucking or overcrowding of teeth in the mouth. Normal occlusion occurs when the upper central incisors just overlap the lower incisors. Teeth that are mottled or pitted are seen in children who have ingested an excessive amount of fluoride; green or black discoloration of the teeth is caused by antibiotic ingestion (for example, tetracycline) or iron ingestion.

The teeth also should be inspected for evidence of caries, and any dental work should be inspected for intactness. The nurse might want to incorporate dental hygiene counseling at this point in the examination. Children should begin to be exposed to dental hygiene by 2 years of age by being taught to hold a toothbrush to clean their teeth. Dental radiographs are contraindicated until 5 years of age.

The gums (gingiva) are inspected for color, inflammation, recession, swelling, bleeding, tenderness, and ulcerations. Gums might be affected by the ingestion of medications such as iron, anticonvulsants, and tetracycline, much as the teeth are affected. A black line might indicate lead poisoning, although this line might be normal in dark-skinned children. Inflammation, swelling, and bleeding might be secondary to infection, poor oral hygiene, or poor nutrition. Hypertrophied or receding gums should be noted.

The buccal mucosa is inspected for color, moisture, condition of the salivary ducts, and the presence of lesions and masses. Normal buccal mucosa is pink and moist, but brown or black areas might be seen in dark-skinned children.

The salivary glands, Stensen's duct (parotid gland), opposite the upper second molar, and Wharton's duct (submaxillary gland), at the base of the tongue on opposite sides of the frenulum, are assessed for patency. Any blockage or swelling could indicate an infection.

The tongue is assessed for color, texture, size, movement, position, and the presence of masses or lesions. The normal tongue is pink and has a normal configuration of papillae. A gray tongue with exaggerated grooves is called a "geographic tongue" and might be normal, or it might indicate allergies, fever, or drug ingestion. Vitamin deficiencies can cause a tender, red tongue. Excessive protrusion of the tongue, or *glossoptosis,* is seen in mental retardation or in children for whom the mouth cavity is too small for the normal-sized tongue.

The hard and soft palates and the pharynx are inspected and palpated for color, shape, position, condition of the tonsils, and the presence of exudate, lesions, and masses. Any cleft in the soft or hard palate is noted, and the height of the palatal area is assessed. An abnormally high arch might cause speech problems and is often associated with congenital disorders. *Epstein's pearls,* found in neonates, are white nodules in the midline of the palate and are insignificant.

The uvula is inspected for movement and symmetry as the child says "ahhh" or gags. The uvula should remain midline, and the soft and hard palates should rise upward symmetrically. Abnormal movement or absence of movement should be referred for further evaluation.

Tonsils, if present, are inspected for color, edema, size (noted as 1+ to 4+), symmetry, and the presence of exudate or crypts. (Tonsillar crypts are scars from past infections.) Tonsils are normally large during childhood but begin to shrink by the time a child reaches puberty. Red-

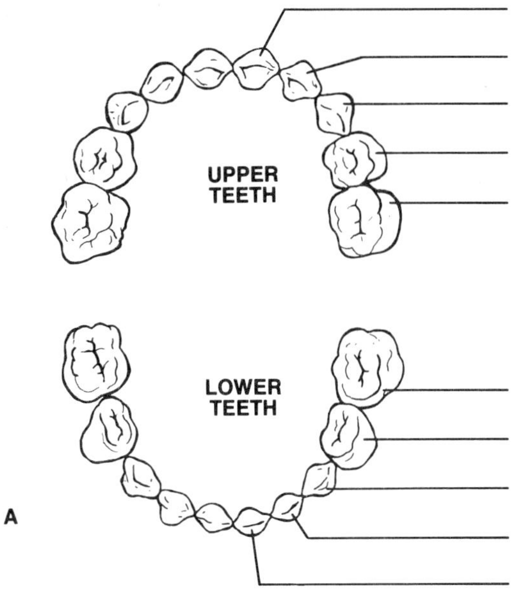

	ERUPTION (months)	SHEDDING (years)
Upper teeth		
Central incisor	8–12	6–7
Lateral incisor	9–13	7–8
Cuspid	16–22	10–12
First molar	13–19	10–12
Second molar	25–33	10–12
Lower teeth		
Second molar	23–31	10–12
First molar	14–18	9–11
Cuspid	17–23	9–12
Lateral incisor	10–16	7–8
Central incisor	6–10	6–7

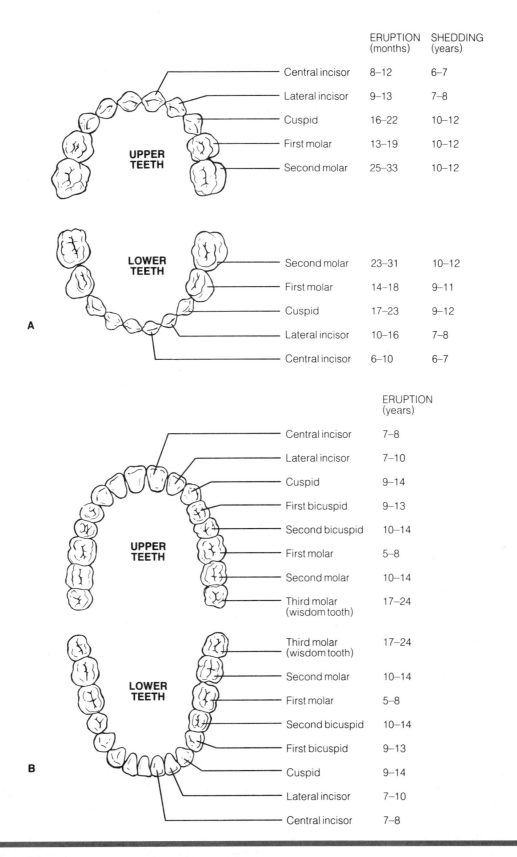

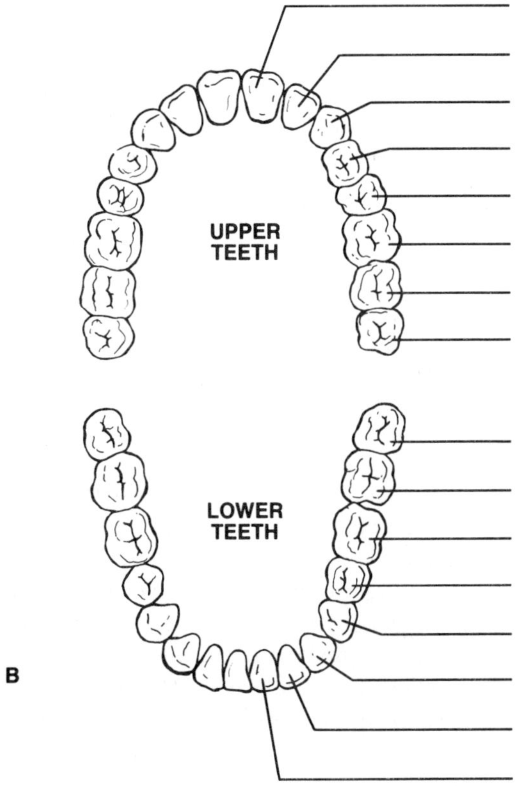

	ERUPTION (years)
Upper teeth	
Central incisor	7–8
Lateral incisor	7–10
Cuspid	9–14
First bicuspid	9–13
Second bicuspid	10–14
First molar	5–8
Second molar	10–14
Third molar (wisdom tooth)	17–24
Lower teeth	
Third molar (wisdom tooth)	17–24
Second molar	10–14
First molar	5–8
Second bicuspid	10–14
First bicuspid	9–13
Cuspid	9–14
Lateral incisor	7–10
Central incisor	7–8

FIGURE 10-15

A. Eruption and shedding of primary teeth. B. Eruption of permanent teeth.

dened, enlarged tonsils covered with exudate indicate infection.

The posterior pharynx is assessed for color, edema, and the presence of exudate, lesions, and petechiae. Enlarged adenoids may be seen as lymphoid hyperplasia; viral infections often cause petechiae, ulcers, or vesicles. Postnasal discharge might indicate allergy or sinus infection. At the end of the examination, the child's gag reflex may be tested by stroking the posterior pharynx with the tongue depressor.

Chest

The chest is examined by inspection, palpation, percussion, and auscultation. Knowing the landmarks of the thorax is important in identifying the underlying structures and describing the exact location of abnormalities. The lines of reference are the midsternal line; the midclavicular lines; the anterior, mid-, and posterior axillary lines; the scapular lines; and the vertebral lines. The landmarks used as points of reference are the manubrium and body of the sternum, the xiphoid process, and the scapula. The *angle of Louis,* just below the suprasternal notch, is an important landmark because the second rib articulates there and the trachea bifurcates into the right and left bronchi (Fig. 10-16). The 12 pairs of ribs (the first seven pairs articulate with the sternum; the next three pairs articulate with the ribs above them; and the last two pairs are floating with no direct attachment) can then be palpated laterally to the sternum, taking care to avoid the costochondral junctions (ribbon cartilage). The nurse needs to be familiar with locating and palpating each rib because ribs are anatomic landmarks for the underlying organs. The space beneath the second rib is the second interspace. Posteriorly, the tip of the scapula is at the sixth to eighth rib, depending on scapular deviation.

The chest is inspected and palpated for skin color, texture, and the presence of lesions and masses. Supernumerary (extra) nipples 5–6 cm below the nipples or on the milk line might be noted. Any scar should be described according to size, shape, and location.

The chest is inspected for shape. The neonate's chest is round with the anteroposterior diameter equaling the transverse diameter. With growth, the chest assumes a more oval shape, with the transverse diameter greater than the anteroposterior diameter. Marked disproportions in the chest are checked by measuring chest size and comparing it with head size. The relationship between the two will be altered by abnormal chest shapes, such as a barrel chest.

Any kyphosis or scoliosis (curves of the upper or lower spine), which affect the shape of the chest, are noted. Atrophy or hypertrophy of chest muscles should be further evaluated. Asymmetry of the chest might be caused by tumors, the congenital absence of some chest muscles, precordial bulging (enlargement of the heart), or pneumothorax (air in the pleural cavity). Abnormal chest structures may include "pigeon chest" (sternum protruding from the chest wall and with a series of vertical depressions along the costochondral junction), "barrel chest" (ribs forming circles), and "funnel breast," or pectus excavatum (depression of the sternum). The posterior chest wall also is inspected for symmetry of the scapulas; any deformities are noted.

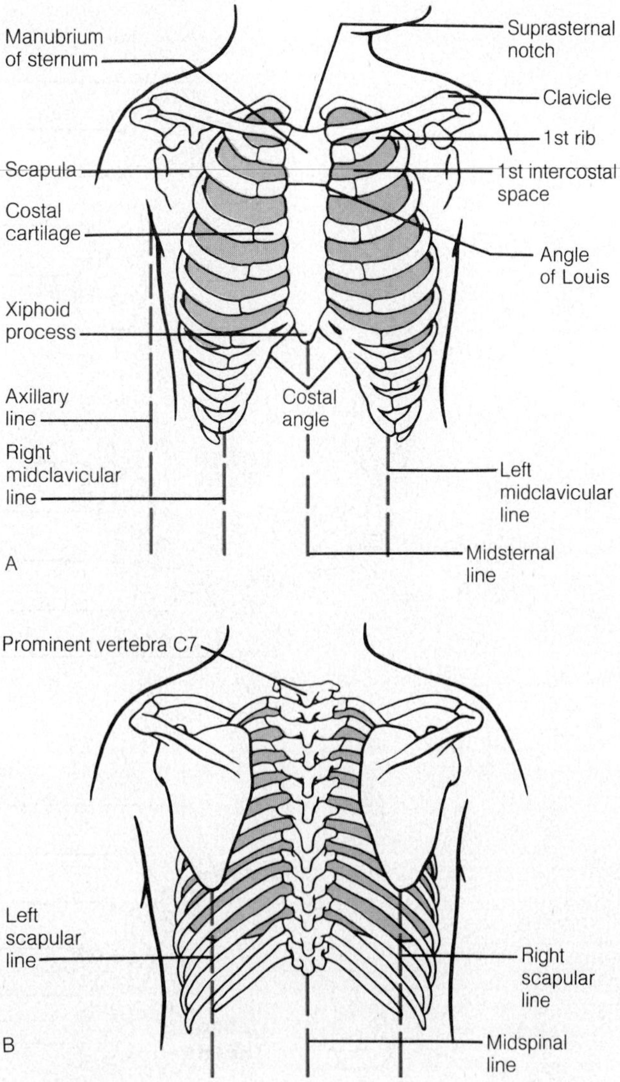

FIGURE 10-16

Landmarks for assessment of the chest. ***A.*** *Front.* ***B.*** *Back.*

Lungs The chest should be inspected and palpated during inspiration and expiration (Fig. 10-17). Respiratory

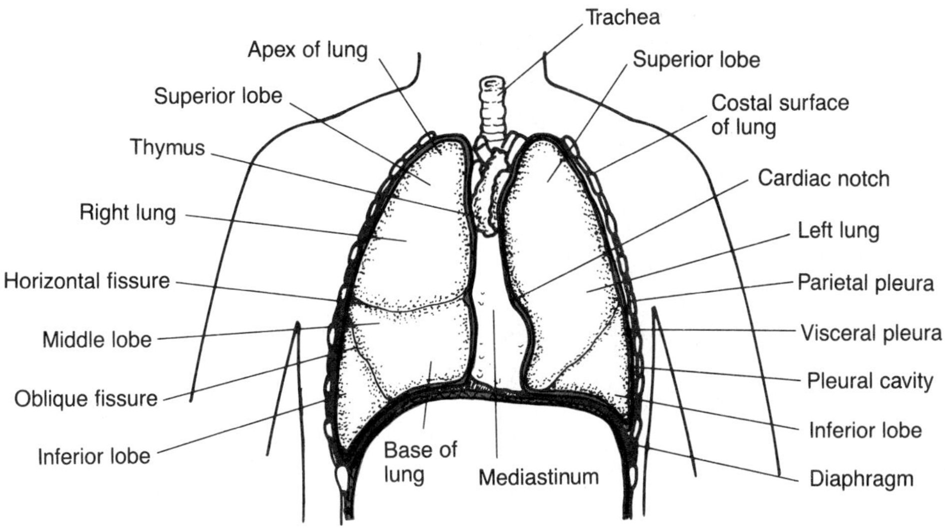

FIGURE 10-17
Internal structures of the chest cavity.

motion is observed during quiet and deep respiration. Important to note are the type, rate, rhythm, and depth of respiration. Any use of accessory neck muscles or the presence of retractions is described. With normal inspiration, the chest expands, the sternal angle increases, and the diaphragm descends. With normal expiration, the chest diminishes, the sternal angle decreases, and the diaphragm rises.

The nurse assesses respiratory excursion by placing the hands with fingers slightly spread out at the lower costal borders anteriorly or at the tenth rib posteriorly. During respiration, the nurse's hands will move with the chest wall. The nurse notes any asymmetrical movement of the thumbs on expiration.

In children under 6 or 7 years of age, respiratory movements are abdominal (diaphragmatic); in older children costal (thoracic) movements are observed during respiration. Abdominal breathing in an older child indicates respiratory problems that need further evaluation. Decreased movement on one side of the chest might indicate a pneumothorax, pneumonia, atelectasis (collapsed lung), or an obstructive foreign body. Retractions are noted, and locations are described as intercostal (between the ribs), suprasternal (above the sternum), substernal (below the sternum), or supraclavicular (above the clavicles).

The character of the respirations is noted and described as normal, unlabored breathing or as dyspnea (labored breathing). The nurse assesses respiration for a full minute because episodes of irregular respirations are normal during infancy. (Abnormal respirations should be described as listed in Table 10-5.)

TABLE 10-5 Various Respiratory Patterns

Pattern	Definition
Cheyne-Stokes respiration	Predictable pattern followed by a pause and then several breaths; hyperpnea, shallow breathing, apnea (may be normal in children)
Kussmaul breathing (hyperpnea)	Deep gasping, hyperventilation
Alkalotic breathing	Slow, shallow breathing
Bradypnea	Abnormally slow respirations, respirations less than normal
Tachypnea	Rapid respirations, faster than normal
Apnea	Cessation of breathing 15–20 seconds or more

Tactile fremitus, the palpation of voice conduction through the thorax, is felt as a vibration on the chest as the child speaks. With the palmar surfaces of the hand, the nurse palpates the child's chest wall, moving symmetrically on either side of the sternum anteriorly and the vertebral column posteriorly. As the child speaks the words "ninety-nine" or "blue moon," the vibrations are felt under the

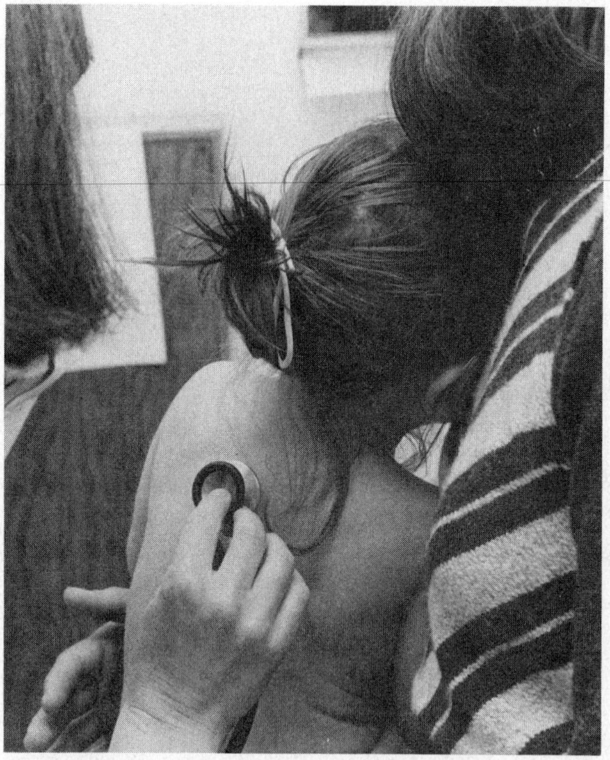

The chest and lungs are auscultated with the diaphragm of the stethoscope.

nurse's hands. Tactile fremitus normally is more palpable in infants, thin children, and at the regions of the thorax where the trachea and bronchi are closest to the surface. As the nurse's hands progress downward, the sound decreases and is least palpable at the base of the lungs. Absent or decreased tactile fremitus occurs in disease processes or conditions that cause bronchial blockage, such as asthma or aspiration of a foreign body. Increased tactile fremitus occurs when a solid mass is present as a result of pneumonia or atelectasis. *Crepitation,* which is actually a sound, is felt where the subcutaneous tissue contains air. It gives a coarse, crackly sensation.

The chest is percussed to determine the presence and location of air, liquid, and solid material in the underlying lung and to determine the position and landmarks of organs. The sound waves of percussion penetrate to a depth of about 5–7 cm, and the sound that emanates depends in part on the amount of muscle and fascia present. The indirect method of percussion, striking the examiner's finger placed on the chest, is best used to percuss the chest and should proceed in an organized, symmetric manner from side to side in sequence to compare the sounds, then slowly progressing downward. Anteriorly, percussion should begin at the apices of the lungs, between the neck and shoulder muscles.

Resonance, a low, loud, long sound, normally is heard over all lung surfaces. Dullness is normal at the fourth to fifth right intercostal space at the midclavicular line (because of the liver) and at the fifth left intercostal space medially to the midclavicular line to the cardiac borders. *Tympany,* a high, loud, long, musical sound, is normal at the sixth left intercostal space over the air-filled stomach. Any deviation from these expected sounds is noted and warrants referral.

Posteriorly, percussion begins at the shoulders and proceeds in the same symmetric manner. The posterior lung fields should be heard as resonance, with dullness of the diaphragm heard at the level of the eighth to tenth ribs. *Hyperresonance,* or a deep, dull sound in unexpected areas, warrants referral. Hyperresonance might indicate excess air in the lung tissue or an increase in density. (See Table 10-6 for a description of percussion notes.)

The chest and lungs are auscultated using the diaphragm of the stethoscope because most of the sounds are of high frequency. Auscultation is necessary to assess breath sounds, to identify any adventitious breath sounds, and to assess voice sounds. Breath sounds are evaluated for pitch, intensity, quality, duration, and location. (The types of breath sounds are listed in Table 10-7.) Breath sounds are caused by the motion of air through the upper respiratory tract, trachea, and main bronchi. These sounds are then filtered and altered as they pass through small airways and lung tissue. Therefore, breath sounds vary in healthy and disease states as the underlying lung is altered by the disease process.

Adventitious breath sounds (additional sounds not normally heard) are superimposed on normal breath sounds and are not alterations of normal breath sounds (Table 10-8). They are classified as either rales or rhonchi and, if noted, are described. *Rales* result from the passage of air through secretions present in the alveoli. *Rhonchi* are continuous sounds produced by the passage of air through edematous or spasmodic airways or through bronchi laden with secretions. *Wheezes* result from partial obstruction caused by the narrowing of the lumen of a respiratory passageway.

Children having adventitious sounds are referred for further evaluation. Absent or diminished breath sounds are always abnormal and also need further investigation. An obstructed airflow can be caused by a foreign body, fluid, air, or mucus.

Voice sounds also are part of the normal auscultation of the lungs. They are elicited in the same manner as tactile fremitus except that the nurse uses the stethoscope. Normal voice sounds or resonances are heard as muffled, indistinguishable sounds. Hearing clear, distinct words on auscultation is abnormal.

TABLE 10-6 Percussion Notes

Note	Description	Examples
Tympany	High pitch, loud intensity, long duration, musical quality	Gas-filled organs such as stomach or intestines
Hyperresonance	Deep pitch, loud intensity, prolonged duration	Overinflated parts of the lung
Resonance	Low pitch, loud intensity, long duration	Normal parts of the lung
Dullness	Medium pitch, intensity, and duration	Liver, spleen, mass density of an organ
Flatness	High pitch, soft intensity, very short duration	Bone

TABLE 10-7 Characteristics of Breath Sounds

Type	Description	Location
Vesicular 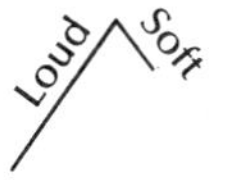	Medium-to-low pitch, low intensity; breezy, swishing, or rushing quality; inspiration three times longer than expiration, seen as 3 : 1 or 5 : 2 ratio	Periphery of lung fields except over sternum and scapulae
Bronchovesicular 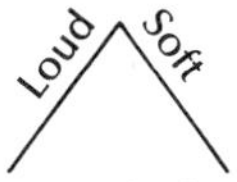	Medium-to-high pitch; moderate intensity; blowing, muffled sound; inspiration equal to expiration	Normally over upper one-third of sternum and intrascapular area, abnormal in areas where normal vesicular heard, usually indicates a mixture of aerated and consolidated lung
Bronchial 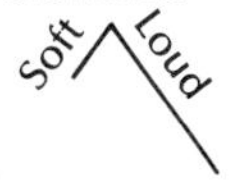	High pitch, loud intensity, harsh and tubular quality, expiration twice as long as inspiration and separated by a brief pause, seen as 2 : 1 ratio	Normally over trachea and manubrium, abnormal over lung periphery and heard in disease states

NOTE: Breath sounds in children seem louder than in adults because of the thinness of the chest wall.

Whispered pectoriloquy occurs when the child whispers and the nurse listens to the chest through the stethoscope. The nurse should not understand the child's whispered syllables. *Bronchophony* occurs when the nurse listens to the chest but the child speaks in a normal volume and tone. Any condition that causes increased fremitus also causes the spoken syllables to be clearly distinguishable.

Breasts The breasts should be examined in girls and boys as part of the routine well-child examination. The examination can best be incorporated into the inspection and palpation of the skin surface of the chest. If the nurse provides a relaxed and comfortable environment, most children, even pubertal-age children, will cooperate with the examination.

The nipples should be assessed for color, symmetry, spacing, and the presence of any lumps. The darker pigmented areola also should be assessed. Pubertal breast development usually begins in girls between 10 and 14 years of age. One breast might develop before the other, and the child might need to be reassured that this is normal. Precocious breast development in both boys and girls might be normal but requires further evaluation. In males, *gynecomastia* (female-like breast development) often causes anxiety and conflicts of body image. The nurse needs to explore the child's feelings and explain that the condition is temporary and that spontaneous regression usually occurs within a few months. The condition seldom lasts longer than two years. Delayed breast development should be evaluated along with the development of any other secondary sexual characteristics.

The breasts are assessed for size and symmetry, contour, skin color, temperature, tenderness, and the presence of masses or lesions. The breasts are palpated with the child in a supine position with the arm on the side to be examined under the head and a pillow under the shoulder. Proceeding from the nipple and progressing in a counterclockwise

TABLE 10-8 Adventitious Breath Sounds

Type	Description	Etiology
Rales		
Fine (crepitant)	High pitch, soft, crackling or popping noises, noncontinuous, heard at end of inspiration, located at periphery of lung fields	Pneumonia, early pulmonary edema, congestive heart failure
Medium (subcrepitant)	Medium pitch, loud, wet, moist, noncrackling, heard on early on midinspiration, clear with coughing, located in the bronchioles	Pulmonary edema, increased accumulated secretions
Coarse (bubbling)	Low pitch, loud, bubbling, heard on expiration, clear with coughing, located in the trachea or bronchi	Bronchitis, resolving pneumonia
Rhonchi		
Sibilant	High pitch, loud wheezing or musical, mid or late expiration, located in the trachea, bronchi, or bronchioles	Anatomic narrowing of respiratory tract, asthma
Sonorous	Low pitch, loud, snorelike, throughout respiratory cycle, cleared with coughing, located in the larger bronchi or trachea	Upper respiratory tract infections, bronchitis
Pleural friction rub	High pitch, moderately loud, jerky and leathery, most frequently at end of inspiration	Irritated or inflamed pleural surfaces
Wheezes		
Inspiratory	Either more sonorous or musical, heard during inspiration	High obstruction (for example, laryngeal edema or foreign body aspiration)
Expiratory	Whistle or sighing sound heard during expiration resulting from turbulence of airflow	Low obstruction (for example, asthma, bronchiolitis)

manner in concentric circles, the nurse palpates lightly with the fingertips in a rolling, circular motion. The entire breast and surrounding area up to the axillas should be palpated. The procedure is then repeated with the opposite breast.

Breasts should be examined in various positions: (a) with the child sitting with arms at the sides, (b) with the child sitting with arms raised above the head, (c) with the child sitting with arms on hips pushing down, and (d) with the child leaning forward with arms extended. With all of these positions, inspection for asymmetry, dimpling, masses, and discharge is possible.

Any palpable nodules are described according to location (by quadrant or clock method in centimeters from the nipple), size, shape (round or discoid, regular or irregular), consistency (soft, firm, hard), circumscribed or merging with surrounding tissues, mobility or fixedness, and tenderness.

During the breast examination, the nurse can use the opportunity to discuss sexual maturation and the importance of routine self-examination, especially in adolescent females who have reached sexual maturity. This includes demonstrating the palpation technique and the most appropriate time of the month to perform breast self-examinations (a few days following menstruation). Estrogen and progesterone hormones might cause benign palpable cysts during preovulatory and ovulatory periods, but these hormones are at their lowest level just after menstruation.

Heart The heart is examined using inspection, palpation, percussion, and auscultation. Percussion to outline the size and shape of the heart may be done using the direct or indirect method. Much practice is required to master either technique. Auscultation provides the most significant data on cardiovascular status and is a useful technique for nurses. Observations of cardiac functioning also include assessing for any clubbing of fingers, peripheral cyanosis, distended neck veins, edema, and bounding pulse pressures.

Overall cardiac assessment involves a comprehensive

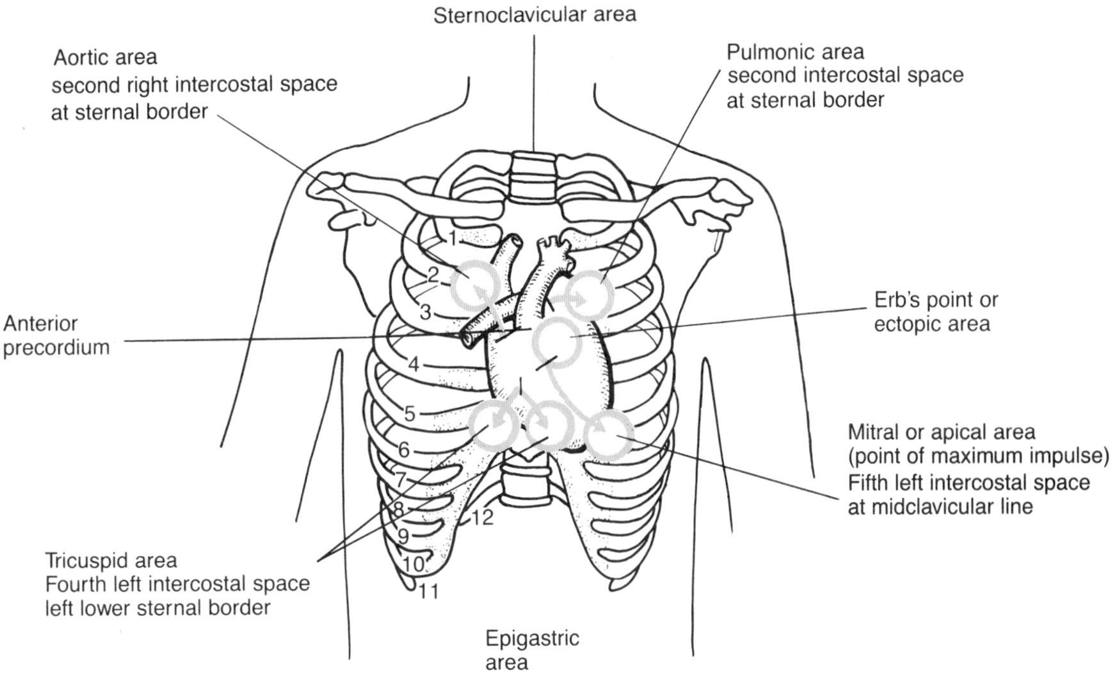

FIGURE 10-18
Sites of auscultation of the heart.

evaluation of the pulses, blood pressure, respiratory function, and general physical growth and development. The nurse therefore palpates the following pulses: superficial temporal, carotid, radial, bronchial, femoral, popliteal, and dorsal pedalis. (Normal pulse rates are listed in Appendix B.) A pulse that is abnormally rapid is referred to as *tachycardia;* an abnormally slow pulse is called *bradycardia.* A change in the rhythm of the heart rate during inspiration and expiration is known as *sinus arrhythmia.* This arrhythmia is usually normal. Other types of arrhythmias, such as a strong beat followed by a weak beat, should be referred for further evaluation. If a pulse is felt to be weaker on one side of the body than the other or if a pulse felt in a previous examination is no longer palpable, further evaluation is warranted.

The precordium (area of the chest wall over the heart) is inspected and palpated to assess precordial bulging, thrills, lifts or heaves, precordial friction rubs, and the point of maximal impulse (PMI). The normal chest is symmetric and quiet, but in thin children the PMI, or apical pulse, might be seen or felt as a slight pulsation. With children 8 years of age and above, this pulse usually is located at the fifth left intercostal space at the midclavicular line (Fig. 10-18). In younger children the PMI may be located higher and more medially because the heart lies slightly more horizontally with the apex to the left of the nipple line.

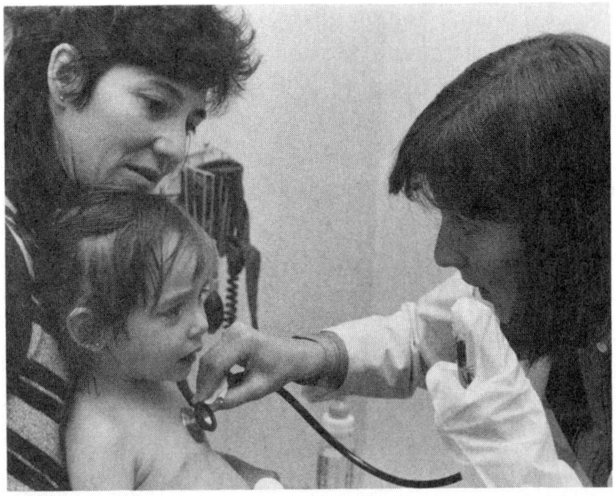

Auscultation of the heart includes the intensity, quality, duration, and location of heart sounds.

The PMI should be sustained throughout systole and should not be diffuse. As the nurse feels for the PMI, any vibratory thrills and precordial friction rubs are noted.

Thrills feel similar to the belly of a purring cat and are caused by forced blood flow from one chamber of the heart

TABLE 10-9 Heart Sounds

Heart sound	Cause	Location	Characteristics
S_1	Closure of the mitral and tricuspid valves, which occurs at the beginning of systole	Apex of the heart	Slight split may be heard as mitral valve closes slightly before the tricuspid and occurs simultaneously with carotid pulse
S_2	Closure of the aortic and pulmonic valves, which occurs at the beginning of diastole	Base of the heart	Split sound may be heard as aortic valve closes slightly before pulmonic valve. Normal "physiologic split" is wider on inspiration and narrower on expiration. A wide split or a "fixed split" (no variance with respiration) is not normal and is associated with atrial septal defect
S_3	Thought to be caused by rapid blood flow from atria to ventricle. Heard early in diastole	Near the apex of the heart with the bell in the left lateral decubitus	Referred to as "gallop rhythm." May be normal in children but also is a symptom of congestive heart failure
S_4	Heard late in diastole, just before S_1		May be normal in children but usually requires further evaluation

to another through narrowed or abnormal openings. *Precordial friction rubs* are high-pitched grating sounds that are not affected by changes in respiration. In children holding their breath, a precordial friction rub will not cease, whereas a pleural friction rub will stop.

The clinical appraisal of a child's cardiovascular status is based to a large extent on the findings made during auscultation of the heart. The heart sounds heard are produced by the opening and closing of heart valves and by the vibration of blood against the walls of the heart and vessels (Fig. 10-18). In an organized manner, using both the bell (low frequency) and the diaphragm (high frequency), the nurse assesses the auscultatory areas of the heart as follows:

Sternoclavicular area at the right and left sides of the sternum

Aortic area at the second right interspace adjacent to the sternum

Pulmonic area at the second and third interspaces next to the sternum

Anterior precordium

Erbs' point, or ectopic area, at the third, fourth, and fifth right interspace and sometimes to the left and directly over the sternum

Mitral or apical area at the fifth interspace at the midclavicular line

The nurse also auscultates the area around the left lower sternal border because this is often where functional murmurs are heard best. Auscultation should include assessment of the intensity, quality, duration, and location of the heart sounds. The point at which they are loudest and whether any splitting is present also should be noted. (Table 10-9 shows the categories of heart sounds.)

Under normal circumstances, only two sounds are produced during each cardiac contraction. The first heart sound (S_1), the "lub," is the result of vibrations transmitted from the area of the mitral and tricuspid valves as they close at the onset of ventricular systole.

This first heart sound is synchronous with the carotid pulse. The nurse can time the heart sounds by simultaneously palpating the carotid pulse and auscultating the apical pulse. The S_1 sound is normally louder at the apex and is long and low pitched. The mitral valve closes slightly ahead of the tricuspid valve but is not normally audible.

The second heart sound (S_2), the "dub," results from closure of the aortic and pulmonic valves (semilunar valves). Aortic valve closing occurs slightly ahead of pulmonic valve closing and may be audible. S_2 is shorter and higher pitched than S_1. With closure of the semilunar valves, blood flows into the aorta and the pulmonary artery.

The aortic valve closure is heard best in the second intercostal space to the right of the sternal border. The pulmonic valve closure is heard best in the second intercostal space to the left of the sternal border. The tricuspid valve is heard best in the fourth and fifth intercostal spaces to the left of the sternal border and also to the right of the sternum. The mitral valve is heard best in the fourth and fifth intercostal spaces just to the left of the midclavicular line.

The examiner should also listen over the carotid area in the neck, over and under the clavicle, along both the right and left sternal borders, and over the left anterior chest, the left lateral thorax, and the left and mid back. Auscultation should be done with the child in the upright position, the recumbent position, and the left lateral decubitus position.

The interval between S_2 and S_1 is the *diastole,* or heart relaxation. A split of these sounds in S_2 often is distinguishable as a widening of the sounds during inspiration because inspiration prolongs ventricular filling and delays pulmonary valve closure. It is considered normal in children and should disappear when children are asked to hold their breath. "Fixed splitting," in which the split in S_2 does not change during inspiration, is abnormal and warrants referral.

Two other heart sounds, S_3 and S_4, may be auscultated. S_3 is heard early in the diastole at the apical area and is the result of vibrations produced during ventricular filling. It is normal in children and young adults, especially in conjunction with a slow heart rate. S_4 is a presystolic heart sound caused by an audible atrial contraction as a result of ventricular overload. It is considered abnormal and requires further evaluation.

Murmurs are another category of heart sounds. The two categories of murmurs are innocent (functional) and organic. *Innocent murmurs* are generally systolic, of short duration, low pitched, musical, and not transmitted to other areas of the heart. They do not increase over time and vary according to position. They do not affect normal growth and development. (Organic murmurs are pathologic and discussed in Chapter 23.)

Abdomen

The abdomen usually is examined with a progression of assessment techniques, beginning with inspection and then proceeding to auscultation, percussion, and palpation. Depending on the age and cooperativeness of the child, the sequence may be altered. If the child remains quiet, auscultation frequently follows evaluation of heart and lung sounds. Inspection can occur whenever the child is undressed, and palpation might be left for the end of the examination, when the child is more comfortable with the nurse. A thorough abdominal evaluation requires that the nurse be familiar with the location of the abdominal organs and their normal size, shape, and consistency (Fig. 10-19).

In inspecting the abdomen the nurse observes abdominal movement, size, symmetry, contour, skin color and integrity, the umbilicus, and the presence of any masses. The umbilicus is inspected for position, herniation, inflammation, discharge, and odor. An *umbilical calculus* is a hard mass of debris that is the result of poor hygiene. A *granuloma* is a small, red, solid button deep in the umbilicus and

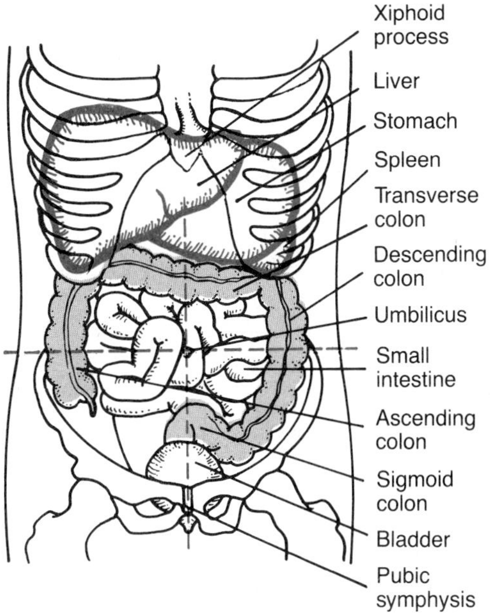

FIGURE 10-19

Abdominal structures.

is seen in neonates. Protrusion of the umbilicus might indicate a herniation. The nurse should palpate the size of the opening, document the findings, and refer the child for further evaluation. Drainage from the umbilicus should be assessed for odor, color, amount, and consistency. The periumbilical area also should be examined. Any drainage should be cultured and the child referred for further evaluation.

Because the respiratory pattern of the young child is abdominal, the nurse can observe movement of the abdomen with inspiration and expiration. Peristalsis is not normally visible and, if observed, might indicate an intestinal obstruction. Pulsations in the epigastric area might be normal aortic pulsations. These are especially evident in thin children but should be further assessed.

A child's abdomen should be symmetric, but the contour varies depending on the child's age, muscular development, and general nutritional status. The normal abdomens of infants and young children have a prominent "potbelly" appearance. By 4–5 years of age, this potbelly shape begins to disappear, and the child's abdomen has a flatter contour. A scaphoid (concave) abdomen is seen in children who are thin or undernourished. A large, prominent, flabby abdomen often is seen in obese children. Any protuberant abdomen needs to be evaluated for tumor, *organomegaly* (enlargement of an organ), ascites, feces, flatulence, or pregnancy. The abdomen should be inspected from all sides to determine the extent and location of the distension; it is then percussed and palpated.

The abdominal muscles strengthen with maturation and increased activity, especially walking. *Diastosis recti abdominis* (splitting of the rectus muscles of the abdomen), which leaves the central portion of the abdomen uncovered, is not uncommon. As long as the muscle is not herniated and only 1–2 in of width are bulging, this condition can be considered normal.

Auscultation follows inspection so that bowel sounds are not disturbed by percussion and palpation. Bowel sounds, the result of peristalsis, are the short clicks and gurgles heard through the stethoscope. They occur every 10–30 seconds, and their frequency is recorded as the number per minute (for example, five bowel sounds per minute). *Borborygmus,* or "stomach growls," the loud grumbling noises often heard without a stethoscope, can occur as frequently as 15–34 per minute. High-pitched, hyperactive sounds are heard in children with gastroenteritis, diarrhea, and intestinal obstruction. The absence of peristalsis might indicate disease, but bowel sounds might be irregular. Therefore, the nurse must listen for at least 5–10 minutes before judging that they are absent.

The frequency and character of bowel sounds should be auscultated in each quadrant. Various other sounds, usually vascular sounds, might be auscultated and are described for pitch, intensity, and location. Bruits, rubs, and hums warrant referral for further evaluation.

The abdomen is percussed to delineate the location, size, and contour of specific organs. With the child in a supine position, either on the examining table or on the parent's lap, the abdomen is percussed using indirect percussion. The nurse follows a pattern beginning on one side and proceeding around to all four quadrants. Liver dullness is percussed at the sixth interspace anteriorly, the midaxillary line, and the ninth interspace posteriorly. The lower border of the liver often is percussed 2–3 cm below the costal margin. The best technique for assessing the size of the liver is to percuss downward from lung resonance to dullness at the midclavicular and midaxillary lines and up from tympany in the lower quadrant to dullness of the lower borders.

The spleen generally is percussed between the ninth and eleventh interspaces in the left midaxillary line. An occasional tympanic note is percussed where the lung overlies the splenic flexure. Tympany generally is heard over the stomach and the rest of the abdomen. Any other percussed areas of dullness might indicate masses or excessive obstruction with feces and requires careful evaluation.

The final method of assessment is palpation. The two types of palpation are superficial and deep. Superficial palpation of the abdomen involves lightly palpating each quadrant, noting any areas of tenderness, assessing muscle tone, and noting the presence of any superficial lesions. Superficial palpation is best done by placing the examining hand flat onto the skin and using the fingertips as points of slight pressure. Tenderness elicited during superficial palpation might be caused by visceral pain, somatic pain, or rebound tenderness. *Visceral pain* is pain from an organic lesion or organ dysfunction. It is dull, poorly localized, and difficult to characterize. *Somatic pain* arises from involvement of somatic structures such as the peritoneum of the abdominal wall. It is a sharp pain and is well localized. *Rebound tenderness* is the phenomenon of pain occurring when the fingers are removed during palpation.

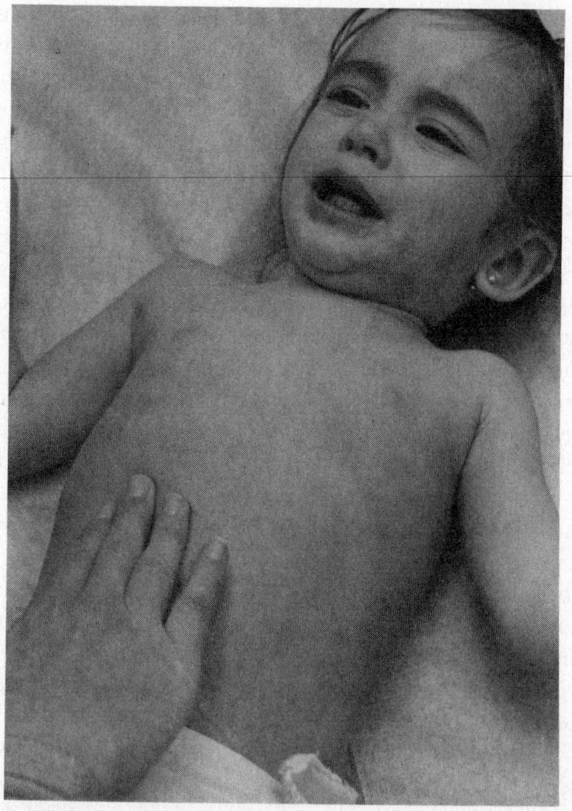

Superficial palpation involves lightly palpating the abdomen by using the fingertips as points of pressure to identify areas of tenderness, muscle tone, and presence of any lesions.

Deep palpation is performed to detect any organomegaly (of the spleen, liver, kidneys, or part of the colon) and any masses. Masses are described by their size, location, consistency, contour, mobility, and tenderness. Deep palpation usually begins in the lower left quadrant and then proceeds to the lower right quadrant and upward so that an enlarged spleen or liver is not missed. Deep palpation requires warm hands and a relaxed child. The nurse might find it helpful to have the child flex the knees to relax the abdominal musculature or to divert the child's attention by playing games or asking interesting questions.

Deep palpation is best done during deep inspiration and deep expiration. The nurse might use one hand to support

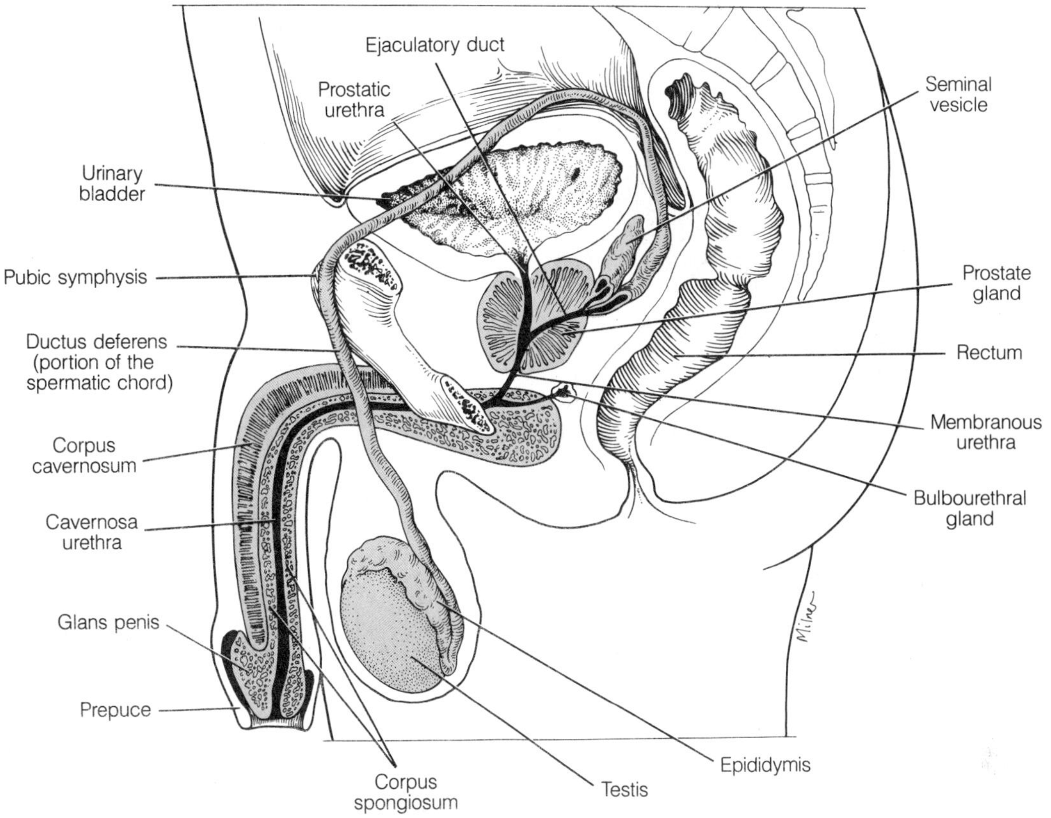

FIGURE 10-20
Sagittal section of the male pelvis. (From Spence AP, Mason EB: Human Anatomy and Physiology, *3rd ed. Benjamin/Cummings, 1987.)*

the posterior structures while placing the examining hand on the abdomen. Another method is to place one hand on top of the other to provide guidance and firmer pressure. If a child has complained of pain during superficial palpation, that area of the abdomen is deeply palpated last.

The spleen normally can be palpated 1–2 cm below the left costal margin in infants and young children. It often is not palpable in older children. Normally, only the tip of the older child's spleen is felt during inspiration as it descends into the abdominal cavity. *Ballottement,* or palpating for the spleen between two hands, one placed against the back and the other pushing frontward, is often useful in locating the spleen. Special care must be taken when inflammation of the spleen is likely (for example, in infectious mononucleosis or erythroblastosis) because it is possible to rupture an inflamed spleen.

The liver edge normally can be palpated 1–3 cm below the right costal margin in infants and young children. In older children the liver might not be palpable. It is best felt by palpation beginning below and easing toward the costal margin, pressing in and up as the child inspires or holds the breath in. Normally, the liver descends during inspiration as the diaphragm moves downward, and its sharp edge can be felt on the flat palpating fingers. Liver tenderness should be referred for further evaluation.

The kidneys are only significantly palpable in neonates. The kidneys are rarely felt at any other time because they lie too deep in the abdominal cavity. If they are palpable, only a normal lower pole of the right kidney is often felt. The bladder, if distended, is palpable above the symphysis pubis. Occasionally, the cecum, a soft, gas-filled mass, is palpable in the right lower quadrant. The sigmoid colon also might be palpated as a sausage-shaped mass that is freely movable and often tender, but not painful, in the left lower quadrant.

The inguinal canal should be inspected and palpated for masses, such as hernias, during the routine examination. Palpation for inguinal hernias involves sliding the little finger into the external ring at the base of the scrotum and following the spermatic cord (which comprises the ductus deferens and connecting nerves and vessels) (Fig. 10-20). A direct inguinal hernia bulges through the posterior wall of

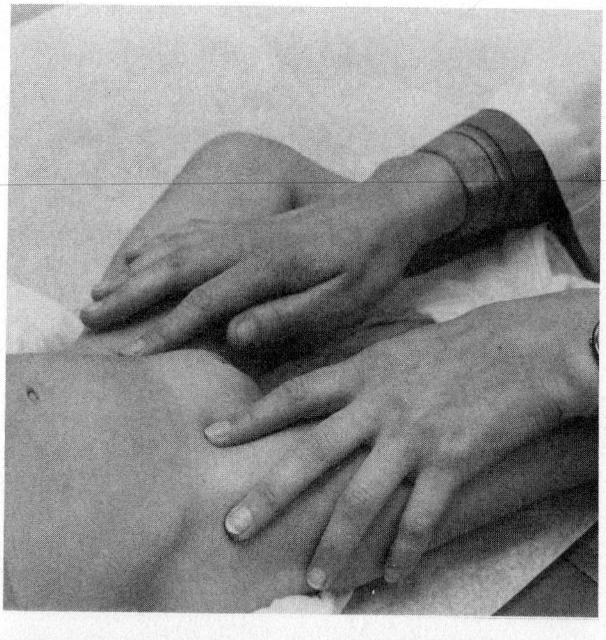

Palpation for a femoral hernia, which may be found about two fingerbreadths inside the femoral artery.

the inguinal canal, an area called *Hesselbach's triangle,* directly behind the external ring. A direct inguinal hernia is palpated as a bulge at the area of the inguinal canal. It is frequently an acquired hernia in males. A femoral hernia is found about two fingerbreadths inside the femoral artery and is common in females. It is palpable as a small, soft mass in the femoral canal, on the anterior surface of the thigh.

Genitalia

Male genitalia The genital examination of boys should proceed in an efficient, nonchalant, and relaxed manner (Fig. 10-20). Reassuring the child and parent that the findings are normal reduces anxiety and fearfulness.

The penis is assessed for skin color, texture, and integrity. An enlarged penis may be due to precocious puberty or disease and should be further evaluated. In uncircumcised neonates the foreskin remains tight and is not freely retractable until 1–2 years of age. After 2 years of age, the prepuce, or foreskin, of uncircumcised boys should be assessed for retractability. It normally retracts easily from the glans. Phimosis is present when the foreskin is not freely retractable and prevents observation of the glans and interior surface of the prepuce. Because of circumcision or traumatic retraction of a tight foreskin, adhesions sometimes are seen in males. Lesions palpated on the dorsomedial surface of the penis are described, documented, and referred for further evaluation.

The urethral meatus is assessed for position, shape, ulceration, and discharge. Normally, it is positioned centrally on the tip of the glans. *Hypospadias* is a condition in which the meatal opening is on the ventral side of the penis. *Epispadias* is a condition in which the meatal opening is on the dorsal side of the penis. If possible, the child's urinary stream should be observed, or information from the child or parent should be obtained on the strength and steadiness of the urinary stream.

The shaft of the penis is inspected for size and masses. The infant's penis is approximately 2–3 cm long. During puberty, the penile shaft enlarges to adult size, and pubic hair develops. Pubic hair should be described for its distribution, color, quantity, and quality.

The scrotum is inspected and palpated for size, symmetry, edema, masses, and lesions. The scrotum enlarges with the development of secondary sexual characteristics, and the number of rugae (ridges) increases. The scrotum may appear asymmetric because the left testis is generally lower than the right testis in the scrotal sac. Any lesions should be noted; firm, yellow-to-white, nontender sebaceous cysts frequently are seen.

The scrotum should be palpated bilaterally for the testes. The testes are evaluated for size, shape, and consistency. They should be equal in size, regularly smooth, freely movable, and slightly sensitive to compression. To palpate the testes, the nurse holds one finger over the inguinal canal, occluding it while palpating the scrotum with the other hand. The procedure is then repeated on the opposite side. The normal cremasteric reflex causes the testes to ascend into the inguinal canal, making them inaccessible to palpation. The absence of testes in the scrotum is called *cryptorchidism* and warrants referral.

Hernias also might be assessed as part of the genital examination. Assessment of femoral pulses and regional lymph nodes also should be included at this time.

Female genitalia Assessment of the female genitalia should be part of every routine well-child examination. It often follows the abdominal assessment while the child is still in the supine position. Adolescents, because of their concern and modesty, might request that the examination be done either at the beginning or at the end of the physical assessment. It is best to proceed quickly with the examination and to reassure both child and parent if everything appears normal. It is advisable for the nurse to wear examining gloves during inspection and palpation of the genitalia.

The external female genitalia are examined for any masses or lesions on the mons pubis (Fig. 10-21). The presence or absence of pubic hair is noted, and hair is

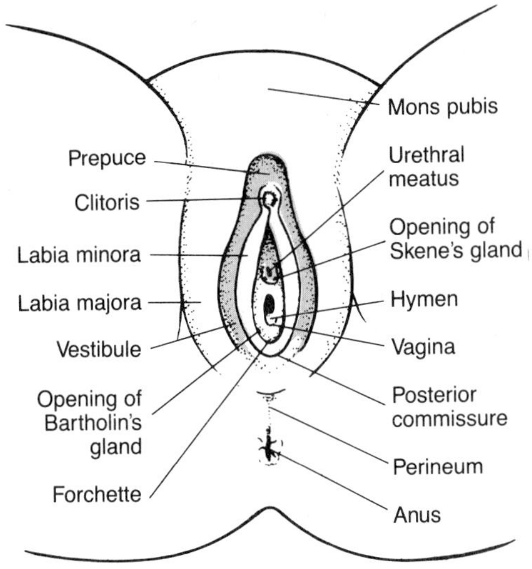

FIGURE 10-21

External female genitalia.

described according to its distribution, color, quantity, and quality. The labia majora and labia minora are inspected for skin integrity, color, size, and the presence of any masses. In infants the labia minora usually are larger than the labia majora. Any swelling and redness in an older child might signify an infection, masturbation, or foreign-body or sexual molestation. Any skin lesions are described, documented, and referred. The clitoris is assessed for size. Any enlarged clitoris should be further evaluated. Because of the presence of maternal hormones, the neonate often has an enlarged clitoris, which is considered normal.

The urethral meatus should be assessed for erythema, edema, and discharge. If Bartholin's and Skene's glands (mucus-secreting glands for lubrication during intercourse) are palpable, an infection (usually a sexually transmitted disease) is present and requires further evaluation. The vestibule should be inspected and palpated for lesions and masses. In sexually active adolescents the urethral meatus frequently is the site of venereal lesions.

The vaginal opening is assessed for size, adhesions, erythema, edema, and discharge. Congenital absence of the vagina or an imperforate hymen are noted if either condition is present.

An internal pelvic examination also is performed on sexually active adolescents, girls requesting oral contraceptives, older adolescents whose mothers received diethylstilbestrol (DES), and adolescents with primary amenorrhea. Younger children with histories of sexual abuse and trauma might require speculum examinations of the walls of the vagina.

Musculoskeletal System

The musculoskeletal system is responsible for the support of the body and movement as muscles attached to the bones shorten in contraction and lengthen in extension. The examination of the musculoskeletal system begins as the child is observed walking, sitting, rising from sitting, playing, and performing such tasks as dressing and undressing. The examination should proceed from general to specific inspection.

General inspection should include observations for general body alignment and symmetry of movements; the nurse notes any clumsy, awkward, or involuntary movements. Any deformities are often immediately obvious, and any shortenings or lengthenings of the extremities should be described. Unusual postures might be evident and should be assessed completely during the regional examination of the spine.

Every inch of the spine and extremities should be palpated to gather complete data. Bones are palpated for general shape and outline. Any thickening, abnormal prominences, or indentations are noted. The skin over the joints is palpated for temperature, tenderness, pain, and swelling. Both sides of the body should be compared. Active and passive motion of the joints should be assessed. Findings are described by normal range of motion, restricted motion, severe weakness, or paralysis.

Muscles are inspected and palpated for symmetry, mass, tone, strength, and any paralysis. Muscle tone normally is felt as slight resistance when a relaxed limb is moved passively. Muscle tone is described as normal, rigid, spastic, or weak. The strength and power of muscles are assessed with gravity, against gravity, and against resistance. A simple test is to place both the nurse's hands in the child's and ask the child to squeeze hard. Another test is to have the child attempt to pull away as the examiner firmly grasps both hands.

Inspection and palpation of the upper extremities begins with assessment of the head and neck. The clavicles and scapulas are palpated for size and symmetry, and any fractures or abnormalities are noted, especially in the neonate. The neck is placed through a range of motions, and any trapezius muscle spasm or neck swelling is noted.

The hands and wrists are tested for range of motion, and the joints are palpated for warmth, tenderness, redness, and bony enlargement. The length of the fingers is assessed as long, narrow, short, stubby, or clubbed. The number of fingers is counted and any deviation from normal is noted. The hands are inspected for the crease pattern of the palms (*dermatoglyphics*). The single palmar (simian) crease seen in individuals with Down syndrome and other chromosomal abnormalities also is seen in 5% of the normal population. It might be normal but is noted.

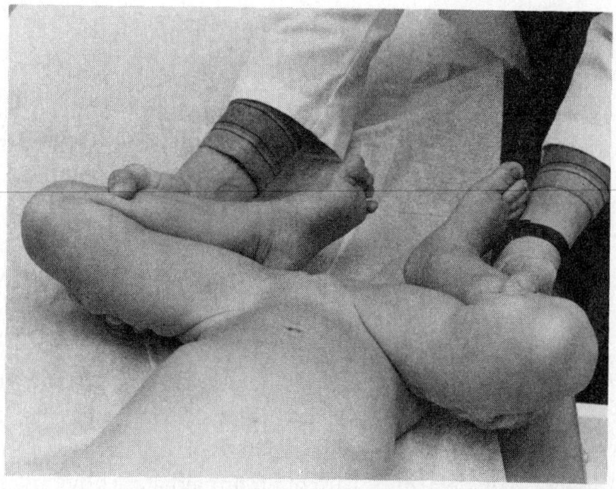

A

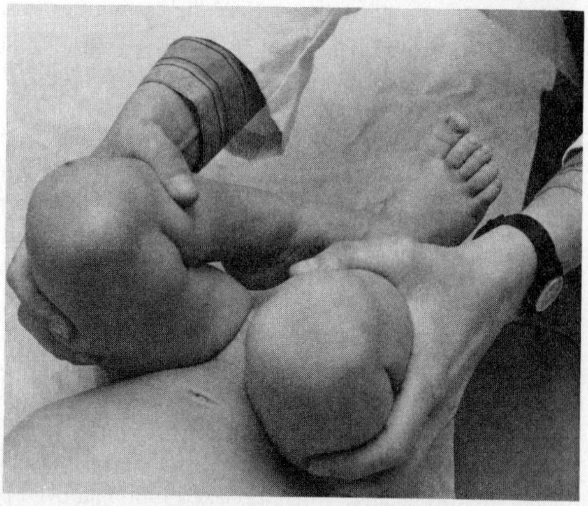

B

Testing for hip contractures and range of motion. **A.** *Abduction.* **B.** *Adduction.*

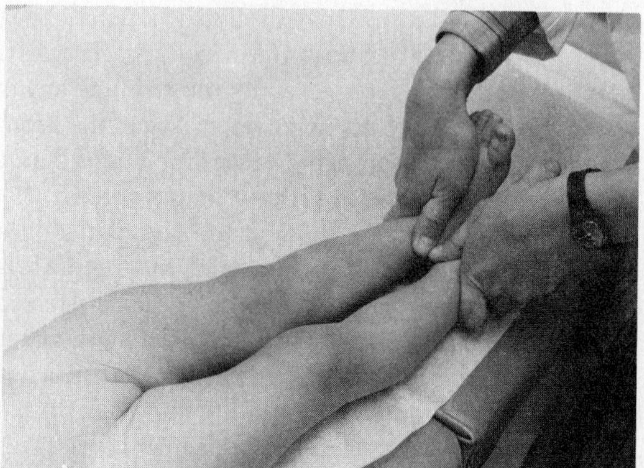

Measuring for equality of leg length.

The elbows are assessed for swelling, inflammation, tenderness, nodules, and the carrying angle. The arms normally form a smooth, continuous line of approximately 180 degrees. If the lower arm is bent forward, decreasing the angle, the child is said to have an increased carrying angle. The child's shoulders also should be assessed for pain and motion; the nurse attempts to push the child's arms down as the child resists by extending the arms in front.

The lower extremities are inspected and palpated, beginning at the hips. The range of motion of the hips is very important in childhood and must be assessed from the neonatal period throughout development. Undiagnosed hip contractures, which may be preventable, can cause lifelong disability. The neonate's hips are therefore assessed for adduction and abduction to rule out congenital dislocation or subluxation of the hip. *Ortolani's maneuver* is used to assess a neonate's hips. This test is done by placing the infant in the supine position. While flexing the infant's hips and knees to a 90 degree angle, the nurse's middle finger is placed opposite the lesser trochanter and the thumb is placed in the inguinal area. The infant's thighs then are moved into abduction while thumb pressure is applied forward and inward over the lesser trochanter. This maneuver will demonstrate dislocation of the hips if a palpable "click" is felt as the femoral head relocates in the acetabulum. The hips of older children can be tested for contracture (flexion deformity) by having the child lie supine and alternately flexing each hip by bending the knee and pulling it up toward the chest. If a hip flexion contracture is present, the hip opposite the bent knee will flex up also, which indicates a positive *Thomas test.*

The knees are inspected and palpated for normal hollows above the patella. Any loss of normal contours might indicate fluid in the knee. The knees also should be assessed for discomfort due to injuries or joint inflammation.

The legs are assessed for symmetry, shape, strength, and equality of length. *Genu varum,* or "bowlegs," is a lateral bowing of the tibia. It may be normal in infants and should disappear as the child begins to walk but might persist up to 3 years of age. If genu varum continues, the child should be further evaluated as persistent weakening of the bone might be indicative of rickets. Genu varum is present when, as a child stands, the medial malleoli are in opposition, and the knees are greater than 1 in. apart.

Genu valgum, or "knock knees," is seen if knees touch and when the medial malleoli are more than 1 in. apart from each other. Genu valgum appears between 3 and 4 years of age. If it persists beyond age 6, however, it should be further evaluated.

Tibial torsion, or abnormal rotation or bowing of the tibia, also might be seen in young children. The nurse may test for tibial torsion by having the child sit upright with legs hanging over the side of the examining table. Normally, an imaginary plumb line dropped from the middle of the knee

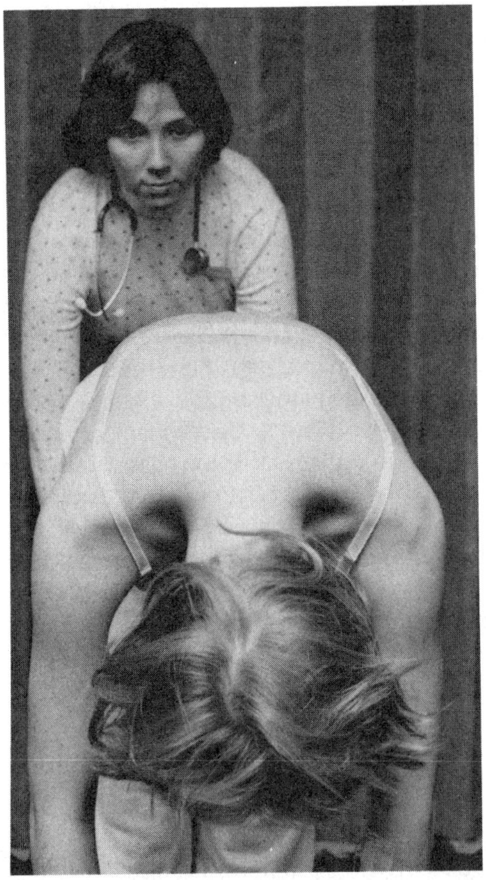

Inspection of the spine should indicate any curvature, which suggests poor posture or a skeletal disorder, such as scoliosis.

should intersect between the second and third toes. In addition, only the anterior edge of the lateral malleoli is seen. If one-half to three-fourths of the malleolar circle is seen or the tibial shaft appears curved in relation to the plumb line, bowing is present and the child should be referred.

The child's feet are assessed for *pes cavus* (high arch) and *pes planus* (flat feet). Both conditions might be normal, depending on the child's age, but referral is warranted if they are causing pain or problems with proper shoe fit. Normally, the nurse is able to place one finger under the child's medial arch as the child stands. An arch that does not allow the one finger is considered flat, and an arch that allows more than one finger is considered high.

The feet also are inspected for size and position. Clubfoot, or *talipes,* is described according to the position of the foot. *Talipes equinovarus* is the most commonly seen form of clubfoot. In talipes equinovarus, the foot twists inward, the forefoot is adducted, and the foot is in plantar flexion. Seen less frequently is *talipes equinovalgus,* or outward twisting with forefoot abducted. Either finding should be referred for further evaluation.

The spine is inspected and palpated for position, curvature, and lesions. As the child stands erect, the head normally is centered on the spine, so that if a plumb line is dropped from the occiput, it falls directly to the midline of the sacrum. The level of the shoulders should be equal and the scapulas should be symmetric, with a 3- to 5-in. distance between them. The hips and popliteal creases should be symmetric. The spine is observed for the normal cervical, thoracic, and lumbar curves. Any *lordosis* (exaggerated anterior convexity of the spine), *kyphosis* (exaggeration or angulation of the posterior spinal curve), or *scoliosis* (lateral curvature of the spine) is noted for further evaluation.

Posture should be observed from the front, side, back, and when the child is bending forward toward the toes. A spinal curve evident when the child is standing upright that disappears when the child bends forward is functional and usually indicates poor posture. If the curve does not disappear, the child might have idiopathic or congenital scoliosis and needs to be referred.

The child also is observed for gait and balance. The child learning to walk typically has a broad-based gait with poor balance. By 4–5 years of age, the gait is narrow and well balanced. Smoothness of movement and the position of the child's arms and legs should be noted as the child walks, runs, skips, and follows a straight path.

Neuromuscular Function

Neurologic assessment usually is integrated into the total physical examination as the nurse proceeds in a systematic manner. For example, as the child's face is being examined, the nurse may assess the cranial nerves, which supply sensory enervation, sensation, and muscle enervation to the head and neck. Vision, smell, taste, hearing, motion of facial and neck muscles, swallowing, and gag responses are all measures of cranial nerve intactness.

The nurse observes the child at play and assesses gross and fine motor functioning, balance and coordination, strength, and muscle tone. It is often necessary and appropriate, however, to perform a neurologic examination as a separate and complete element in a total health assessment. A neurologic examination consists of assessing the child's intellect and language ability, cerebellar function, motor function, sensory function, reflexes, and "soft" neurologic signs. "Soft" neurologic signs are signs whose significance is not understood fully but which tend to alert the nurse to possible difficulties in school, attention-requiring tasks, and coordination. These include such signs as clumsiness, hyperactivity, inconsistencies in perceptual development, language disturbances, balance disturbances, and mixed or confused laterality. Much research is being done in this area to ascertain whether these signs are predictive of future learning difficulties. If they are, early intervention when first noted is desirable.

Data from the health history help the nurse to determine whether a complete and separate neurologic exam is warranted. For example, any historical information that includes reports of seizures, headaches, vertigo, changes in visual acuity, changes or loss of hearing, loss of sensation, muscular weakness, or involuntary movements might be neurologically significant and indicate the need for a specific neurologic evaluation. In addition, any child with a history of behavioral, developmental, or learning problems should have a complete neurological examination and specific developmental and educational tests.

Because of the variability in maturation of the nervous system, assessment of neurologic integrity of the infant or young child requires modification of most testing approaches and interpretation of findings. Variabilities in physical endurance of young infants and children and in their abilities to cooperate requires a modified method for valid testing. A standard neurologic examination generally is not appropriate (or likely to be successful) before middle childhood.

The neurologic examination involves assessment of function in six major areas: the cerebrum, the cranial nerves, the cerebellum, the motor system, the sensory system, and reflex action.

General cerebral function The assessment begins with general observations of the child's appearance, posture, facial movements, speech, behavior, and movements. These observations are made by the nurse during history taking or examination of the other body systems. Marked variations are noted and guide the remainder of the examination and the choice of specific additional tests.

Assessment of general cerebral functions includes evaluation of the child's state of consciousness, intellectual performance, and mood. The older child can be examined for orientation to time, place, and person. While asking the child questions to assess these areas of cerebral function, the nurse keeps in mind the child's cognitive, speech and language, and general developmental levels.

Memory is another part of general cerebral function, and recall, short-term memory, and long-term memory are therefore evaluated. Immediate recall, the retention of an idea or thought for a brief time, is tested by having the child repeat numbers. A 4-year-old child usually can repeat three numbers (for example, 3, 2, 1), whereas a 5-year-old can repeat four numbers, and a 6-year-old usually can repeat five numbers. Recent memory is memory that lasts slightly longer than immediate recall and is tested by showing the child a familiar object. Later during the examination, the child is asked what object was shown earlier. Remote memory is memory for longer periods of time. To assess this, the child can be asked about projects that were done in school.

Specific cerebral function Three specific cerebral functions should be evaluated: (1) cortical sensory interpretation, (2) cortical motor integration, and (3) language. Many of the tests for cortical sensory and cortical motor evaluation can be presented as games to the child. The games are useful ways to establish rapport with the child and thereby elicit cooperation and trust.

Cortical sensory interpretation is the ability to recognize objects through the senses. The inability to do this is called *agnosia*. Tactile sensory interpretation, or *stereognosis*, is evaluated by placing a familiar object in the child's hand and asking the child to identify the object with eyes closed. Familiar objects used are often coins, keys, or paper clips. *Graphesthesia*, the ability to identify familiar shapes traced in the palm or on the back of the hand, is also tested. By middle childhood, children usually can identify numbers, especially 0, 1, 3, or 8. Younger children usually can identify geometric shapes such as circles or parallel lines.

Visual sensory interpretation is tested by asking the child to hand the nurse a familiar object. The child is instructed to retrieve the object from an assortment of three or four objects. Auditory sensory evaluation is tested by having the child listen, with eyes closed, and identify familiar sounds such as a bell or a whistle.

Cortical motor integration, the ability to perform responsive acts, is tested in several ways. One way is to have the child copy various designs. A 3-year-old child usually can draw a circle; a 4-year-old can draw a square; and a 5-year-old can draw a triangle. Older children usually can draw diamonds or more complicated forms. Another way of testing motor integration is to have a child of 6 years or older fold a piece of paper to fit and be placed inside an envelope.

The child's ability to use language, both receptively and expressively, also is tested. Screening tests for articulation and speech might be used. The nurse also tests the child's ability to follow directions, discriminate between two similar words, and repeat nonsense syllables.

Cranial nerves Evaluation of the 12 pairs of cranial nerves is the next component of the neurologic assessment. If a complete neurologic examination is not done, this evaluation can be integrated into the physical examination of the face, neck, eyes, and ears.

Complete assessment of the cranial nerves depends on the cognitive and developmental level of the child; the nurse can test only those functions that the child is able to understand and therefore is capable of performing in the testing. (See Chapter 31 for the complete assessment of cranial nerves.)

Proprioception and cerebellar function Tests for proprioception and cerebellar function assess posture, balance, and coordination. The nurse can assess these functions

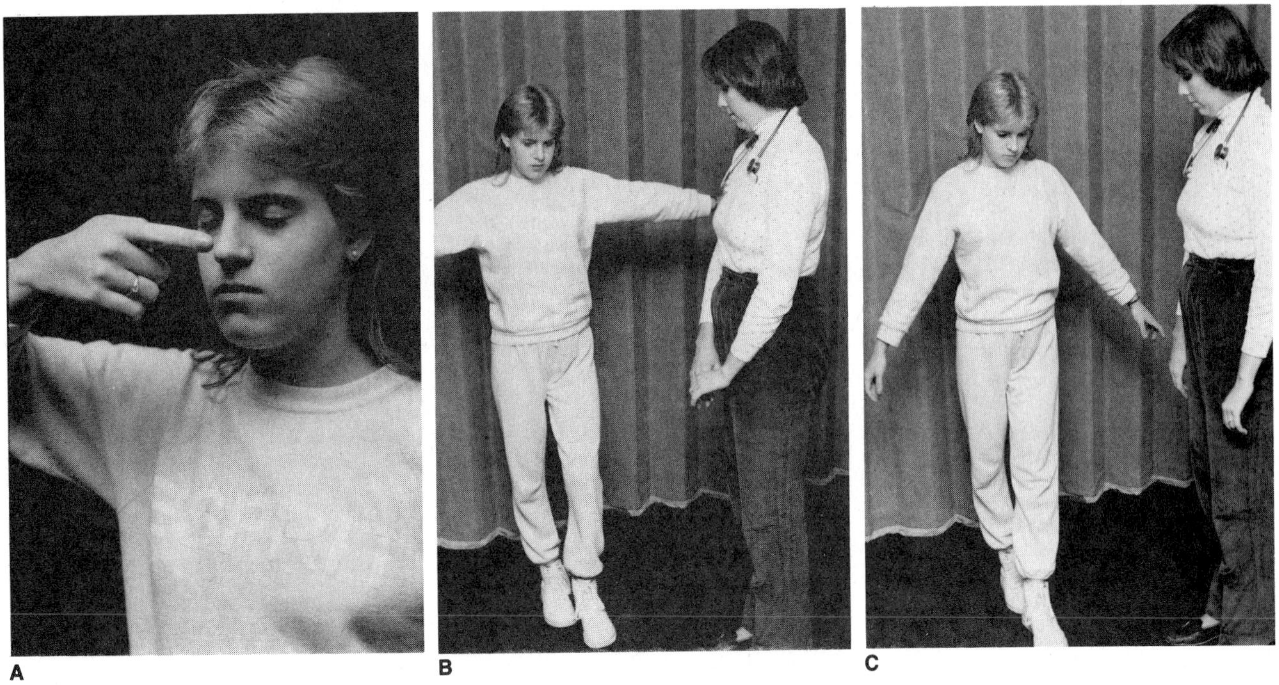

Neurologic function may be assessed by testing for coordination. ***A.*** *The child touches the nose with a finger.* ***B.*** *The child stands on one foot.* ***C.*** *The child demonstrates a heel-to-toe walk.*

through standardized developmental tests that evaluate gross and fine motor abilities, balance, and coordination. Knowing the expected developmental level of a child at any given age is necessary to interpret the child's abilities appropriately. For example, in early childhood the child usually can stand well balanced on one foot for 5 seconds; by middle childhood, the child can do so for 15 seconds and usually can hop on one foot while staying in place and maintaining balance. Younger children have more difficulty with hopping, usually until 4 or 5 years of age.

General cerebellar function begins with an examination of the child's gait. Gait is evaluated by having the child first walk normally and then walk a straight line by walking heel-to-toe. Balance is tested by having the child stand unsupported, feet together, eyes open and then with the eyes closed. This test of cerebellar integrity, the *Romberg test,* is positive if the child sways significantly, although a slight-to-minimal sway is normal. Safety measures, usually standing close to the child, should be taken to prevent injury if the child falls.

Coordination generally can be assessed by observing the child's ability to stack blocks, dress and undress, and throw and kick a ball. Specific tests for coordination are finger-to-nose, fingers-to-thumb, heel-to-shin, and rapid alternating motions such as supination and pronation of the child's hands. In the finger-to-nose test, the child is asked to touch the nose with the index finger first on one hand and then the other, first with the eyes open and then with the eyes closed. The child should be "on target," and any miss should be documented.

The fingers-to-thumb test is done by asking the child to touch each finger of one hand to the thumb of the same hand as rapidly as possible. The nurse observes the smoothness and accuracy of the responses, noting any misses between thumb and fingers or any additional movements elsewhere in the body, especially lip smacking, eye twitching, or facial grimaces.

In the heel-to-shin test, the child lies supine and is asked to place one heel rapidly down the shin of the opposite leg from knee to ankle. Any uncoordinated or inaccurate movements are documented. Rapid alternating movements are tested by asking the child to pat the knees with the palms of the hands and then the backs of the hands as rapidly as possible. Any clumsiness of movement or irregular timing is noted.

Motor function Evaluation of the motor system includes a gross examination of muscle size, tone, strength, and any abnormal muscle movements. Most of the motor system is evaluated during the musculoskeletal examination, but any abnormality is assessed in relation to both the neurologic and musculoskeletal systems.

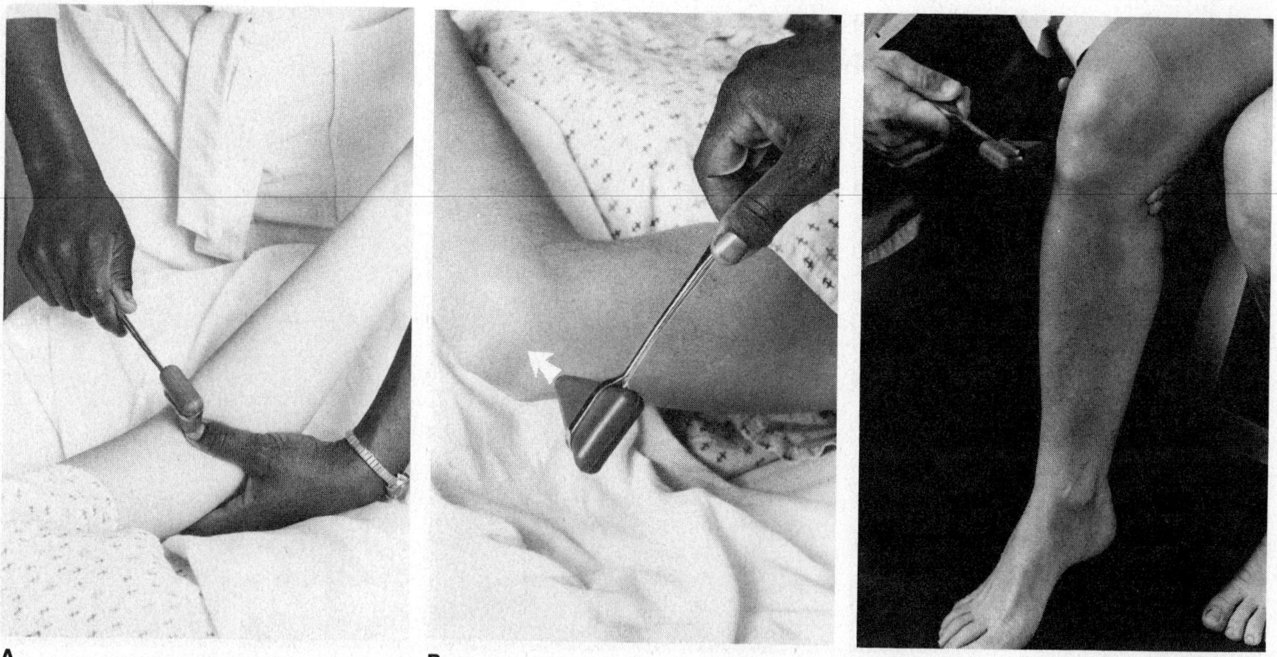

A B C

Assessment of deep tendon reflexes. **A.** *Biceps reflex.* **B.** *Triceps reflex. (From Swearingen PL:* The Addison-Wesley Photo-Atlas of Nursing Procedures. *Addison-Wesley, 1983.)* **C.** *Patellar reflex.*

Muscle size and tone are assessed for any hypertrophy, atrophy, and asymmetry. Muscle strength is assessed in upper and lower extremities and evaluated for any asymmetry or involuntary movement, when put through such stressful maneuvers as hand grasping or leg raising. Any twitching or tremors are abnormal.

Sensory function Assessment of the senses includes evaluation of superficial sensation (pain, temperature, and light touch) and deep sensation (vibration sense, position sense, deep pain, and discrimination). Assessment must be done on symmetric body parts for comparison. Any suspected sensory loss is mapped out from most affected to least affected area.

Superficial sensation is assessed by stroking body parts (for example, the face, trunk, arms, or legs) with a wisp of cotton and, with the child's eyes closed, having the child point to or verbally identify the area touched. Superficial pain is evaluated by using blunt and sharp tips of a safety pin on body parts and asking the child to identify the sensation from the pin as either dull or sharp. (This is often traumatic for a child and may be omitted if the sensation of light touch is intact.) Temperature sensation often is not evaluated, but if it is, the child is asked to indicate hot or cold sensations as they are felt in test tubes filled with cool and warm water.

Deep sensation is evaluated by testing vibration sense over long prominences such as the sternum, elbows, knees, and iliac crests. The child is asked to note when the vibrating tuning fork stops. The nurse tests the validity of the child's response by placing the tuning fork on the nurse's own corresponding body part. Position sense is tested by grasping the child's distal phalanx of the finger or toe digit on its lateral surfaces and moving it up or down. The child, with eyes closed, is asked to identify whether the finger or toe is in an up or down position.

Sensory discrimination is tested through stereognosis and graphesthesia. Another test for discriminatory sensation is one-point discrimination. One part of the body is touched, and the child is asked to point to that area. This can be done with a wisp of cotton and is easily integrated into the tests for primary sensation.

Reflexes Assessment of the deep tendon reflexes (DTRs) provides the nurse with information about the intregity of reflex arcs at known levels of the spinal cord. Deep tendon reflexes are really stretching reflexes that occur when a muscle is suddenly stretched by a brisk tap over the tendon of insertion. The DTRs evaluated are the biceps reflex, the triceps reflex, the brachio-radialis reflex, the patellar reflex, and the Achilles tendon reflex.

Superficial reflexes, such as the abdominal reflexes, the

TABLE 10-10 Assessment of Reflexes

Reflex	Test	Normal response
Deep tendon reflexes		
Biceps reflex	Hold child's arm by placing partially flexed elbow in hand with thumb over antecubital space. Strike own thumbnail with hammer	Partial flexion of forearm at the elbow
Triceps reflex	Abduct arm, supporting upper arm and let the forearm hang freely. Strike triceps tendon above the elbow	Partial extension of forearm
Brachioradialis reflex	With arm and hand in relaxed position, strike above the styloid process of the wrist	Flexion of arm at elbow and at forearm
Patellar reflex	With child sitting on edge of table or on parent's lap and with lower leg flexed at the knee and dangling freely, tap the patellar tendon just below the kneecap	Partial extension of lower leg
Achilles reflex	With child sitting on edge of table or on parent's lap and with lower leg flexed at the knee, support the foot lightly in one hand and strike the Achilles tendon with the hammer	Plantar flexion of the foot (foot pointing downward)
Superficial reflexes		
Abdominal reflex	In the upper abdomen, stroke the skin over the lower thoracic cage, from the midaxillary line toward the midline. In the midabdomen, stroke toward the midline at the umbilical level. In the lower abdomen, stroke from the iliac crest toward the midline of the hypogastrium	Ipsilateral contraction of the muscles in the epigastric abdominal wall, or umbilical deviation toward the stimulated side
Cremasteric reflex	In males, stroke the inner aspect of the thigh	Elevation of the cremaster with prompt elevation of the testis on the ipsilateral side
Plantar reflex	Scratch the sole of the foot near the lateral aspect, from heel to toe	Plantar flexion of the toes or entire foot (toes or foot pointing downward)
Superficial anal reflex	Stroke the skin or mucosa of the perianal region	Contraction of the external and anal sphincters

cremasteric reflex, the gluteal reflex, and the plantar reflex also are evaluated, as is the Babinski reflex. Reflexes usually are graded as follows:

4+ = brisk, hyperactive with clonus
3+ = brisker than normal
2+ = normal, active
1+ = low normal, slightly diminished response
0 = no response, absent

Reflexes are evaluated for strength and symmetry from side to side and from upper to lower extremities. In eliciting deep tendon reflexes, the tendon should be slightly stretched and briskly tapped with a reflex hammer. (Methods for eliciting the deep tendon reflexes and expected normal responses are listed in Table 10-10.)

The superficial reflexes are evaluated (see Table 10-10).

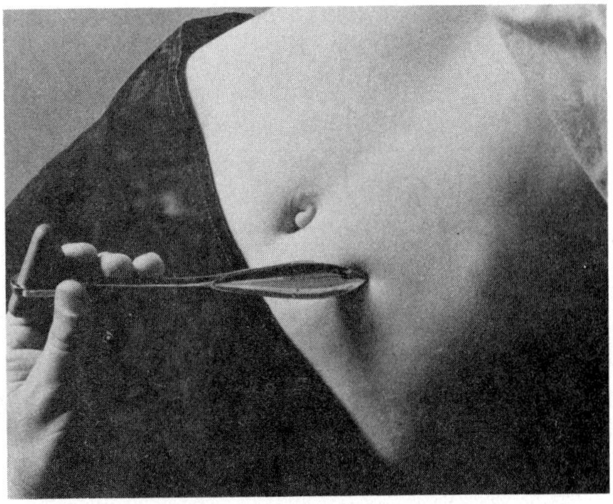

The abdominal reflex is elicited by stroking the abdomen toward the umbilicus so that the umbilicus moves toward the stimulus.

The abdominal reflex is elicited by stroking the four quadrants of the abdomen toward the umbilicus. A normal response is that the umbilicus moves toward the stimulus. The cremasteric reflex, present in males, is elicited by stroking the inner aspect of the thigh; the nurse then observes whether the testes move into the inguinal canal (a normal response). The gluteal reflex is elicited by stimulating the perianal area and observing for contraction of the anal sphincter. The plantar reflex is elicited by stimulating the lateral border of the sole of the foot, starting at the heel and continuing to the ball of the foot and then proceeding over toward the great toe. The normally observed response is flexion of all of the toes. The Babinski reflex can be tested by observing for dorsiflexion of the great toe and fanning of the other toes when the sole of the foot is stroked.

Essential Concepts

- Health-screening tools, principally physical measurements and laboratory tests, are useful in augmenting and validating assessment findings and in identifying children likely to have specific problems.
- The nurse plans the sequence of and health teaching associated with the physical examination according to the needs of both the parent and child.
- Essential skills for performing a physical examination include inspection, palpation, percussion, and auscultation.
- Physical examination begins with an assessment of the child's general appearance, which includes the nurse's impression of the child's nutritional status and developmental progress.
- Assessment of the skin, which includes hair and nails, might reveal evidence of injury, underlying disease processes, nutritional deficiency, or need for health teaching.
- Assessment of the lymph nodes proceeds throughout the physical examination and might reveal signs of infection or hypersensitivity reactions
- The head, face, and neck are assessed for symmetry, control, and movement.
- Eyes and ears are assessed for the level of function and any evidence of defects or infection; vision and hearing screening are important parts of the physical examination.
- The nose, mouth, and throat are examined for the degree of function and any evidence of abnormalities or infection.
- Assessment of the chest—lungs, breasts, and heart—includes examination of function, developmental progress, and any deviation from normal.
- Examination of the abdomen involves palpation of the abdominal organs and identifying any symptoms of dysfunction.
- Genitalia are examined for developmental progress and any evidence of malformation or disease.
- The musculoskeletal system is assessed for the level of function and for any developmental anomalies.
- Assessment of neuromuscular function involves a neurologic examination that includes the reflexes and sensory, cerebral, cerebellar, and motor functions.

Additional Readings

Alexander MM, Brown MS: Physical examination. Parts 1–17. *Nurs '73* (July, Aug, Sept, Oct, Dec) 1973. *Nurs '74* (Jan, Feb, April, July, Aug) 1974. *Nurs '75* (Jan) 1975. *Nurs '76* (Jan, Feb, March, April, June, July) 1976.

Anyan W: *Adolescent Medicine in Primary Care*. Wiley, 1978.

Barnard M et al.: *The Handbook for Comprehensive Pediatric Nursing*. McGraw-Hill, 1980.

Barness L: *Manual of Pediatric Physical Diagnosis*. 4th ed. Year Book, 1973.

Barrus DH: A comparison of rectal and axillary temperatures by electronic thermometer measurement in preschool children. *Pediatr Nurs* 1983; 7:424–425.

Bates B: *A Guide to Physical Examination*. Lippincott, 1974.

Britton CV: Blood pressure measurement and hypertension in children. *Pediatr Nurs* 1981; 7(4):13–17.

Brown M, Murphy M: *Ambulatory Pediatrics for Nurses*, 2nd ed. McGraw-Hill, 1981.

Chinn P: *Child Health Maintenance*. Mosby, 1974.

Chow M et al: *Handbook of Pediatric Primary Care*. Wiley, 1986.

Committee on Children with Handicaps: Vision screening of preschool children. *Pediatrics* 1972; 50(6):966–967.

DeAngelis C: *Pediatric Primary Care*. 2nd ed. Little, Brown, 1979.

Delancy VL, North C: Skin assessment. *Topics Clin Nurs* 1983; 5(2):5–10.

Delaney MT: Examining the chest. Part I. The lungs. *Nurs '75* 1975; 5(8):12–14.

Delaney MT: Examining the chest. Part II. The heart. *Nurs '75* 1975; 5(9):41–44.

Downs M, Silver H: The A, B, C, D's to H.E.A.R.—early identification in nursery, office and clinic of the infant who is deaf. *Clin Pediatr* 1972; 11(10):563–565.

Emans SJ, Goldstein D: *Pediatric and Adolescent Gynecology.* Little, Brown, 1977.

Eoff JJ, Joyce B: Temperature measurements in children. *Am J Nurs* 1981; 81:1010–1011.

Ferholt JDL: *Clinical Assessment of Children: A Comprehensive Approach to Primary Pediatric Care.* Lippincott, 1980.

Green M, Haggarty RJ: *Ambulatory Pediatrics.* Saunders, 1978.

Holland SH: 20/20 vision screening. *Pediatr Nurs* 1982; 8(2): 81–87.

Holland SH: Screening vision to detect eye disorders. *Child Nurs* 1984; 2(1):1–3.

Jarvis CM: Vital signs—how to take them more accurately and understand them more fully. *Nurs '76* 1976; 6(4):31–37.

Jarvis CM: Perfecting physical assessment. Parts 1–3. *Nurs '77* (May, June, July) 1977.

Lehmann J: Auscultation of heart sounds—where to listen, how to listen and what to listen for in the identification of heart sounds. *Am J Nurs* 1972; 72(7):1242–1246.

Malasanos L et al: *Health Assessment.* Mosby, 1977.

Moss JR: Helping young children cope with the physical examination. *Pediatr Nurs* 1981; 7(2):17–20.

Moss JR: Predicting young children's cooperation with the physical examination. *Pediatr Nurs* 1983; 9(3):188–190.

Murphy-Alexander M, Brown M: *Pediatric History Taking and Physical Diagnosis for Nurses.* McGraw-Hill, 1979.

Osborn LM: Group well-child care: An option for today's children. *Pediatr Nurs* 1982; 8(5):306–308.

Park M, Kawabori I, Guntherath W: Need for an improved standard for blood pressure cuff size. *Clin Pediatr* 1976; 15(9): 784–787.

Patient Assessment Program Instruction. *Am J Nurs* (Sept, Nov) 1974; (Jan, March, May, Sept, Nov, April) 1975; (Sept, Nov) 1976; (Feb) 1977; (Oct, Nov) 1978.

Recommendations of the task force on blood pressure control in children. *Pediatr* (Suppl):799–820.

Redman J, Bissada N: How to make a good examination of the genitalia of young girls. *Clin Pediatr* 1976; 15(10):907–908.

Roach LB: Color changes in dark skin. *Nurs '77* 1977; 7(1):48–51.

Saul L: Heart sounds and common murmurs. *Am J Nurs* 1983; 83(12):1679–1689.

Silver H, Kempe C, Bruyn H: *Handbook of Pediatrics.* Lange, 1973.

Thompson J, Bower A: *Clinical Manual of Health Assessment.* Mosby, 1980.

Visich MA: Knowing what you hear: A guide to assessing breath and heart sounds. *Nurs '81* 1981; 11(11):64–79.

Yoos L: A developmental approach to physical assessment. *Am J Matern-Child Nurs* 1981; 6(3):168–170.

III

Preventive Child Health Nursing: Strategies for Health Promotion

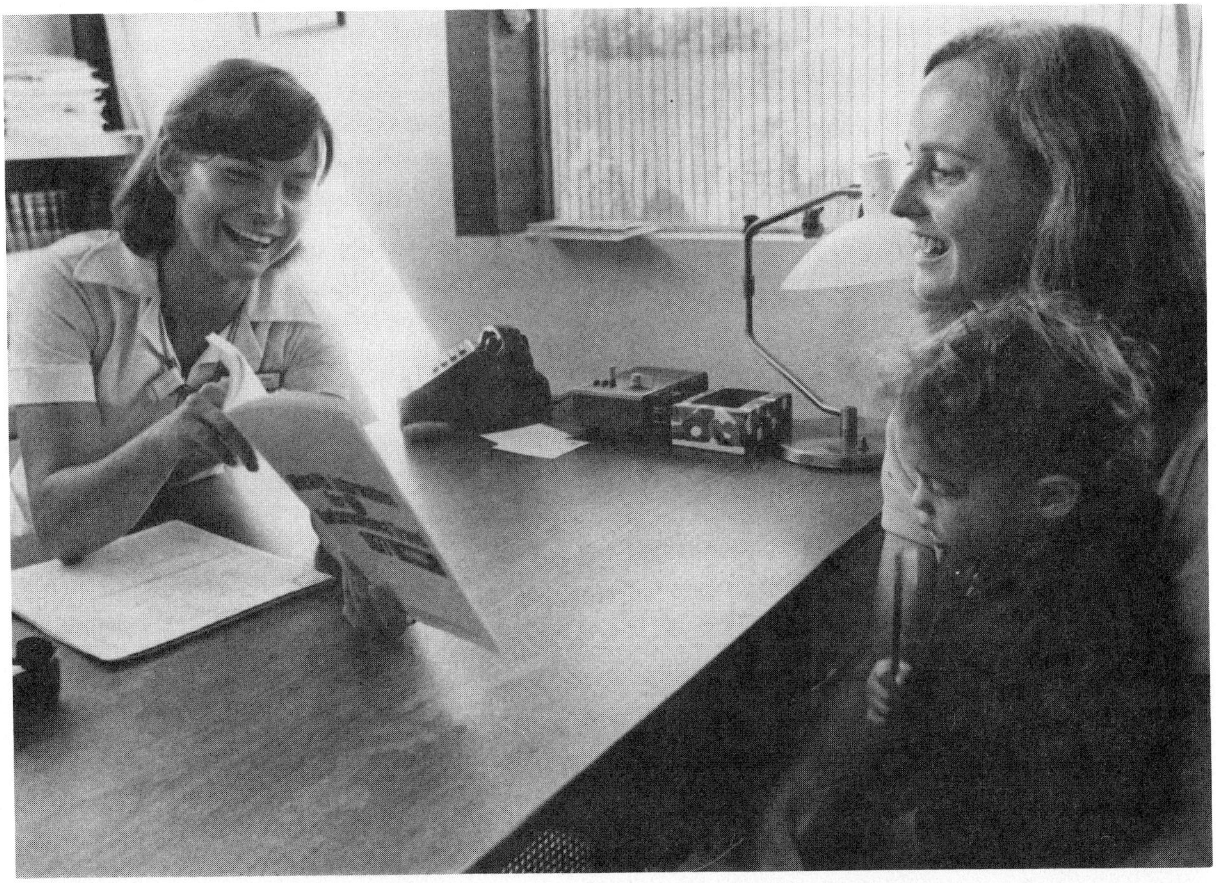

Chapter 11

Prevention of Illness

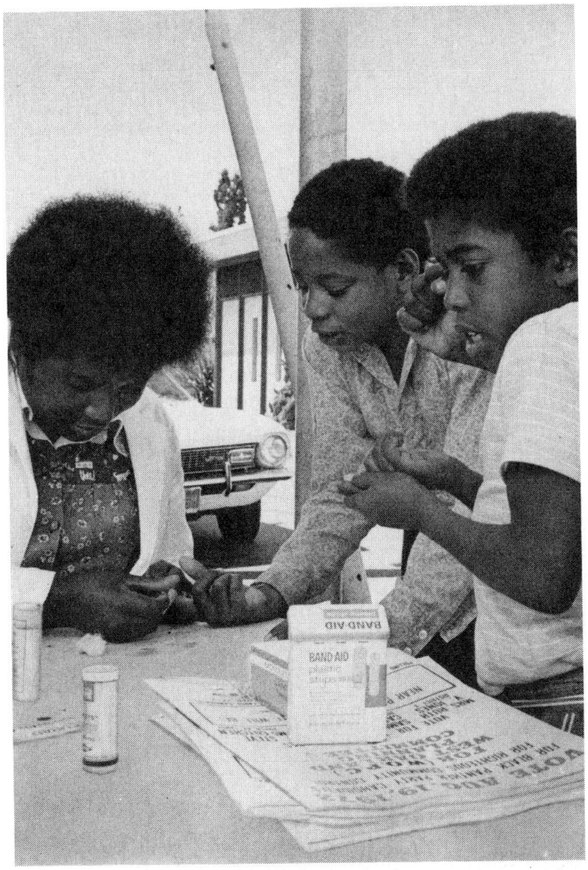

Chapter Contents

(Continues)

Objectives

- Discuss the concept of health within the context of an epidemiologic framework.
- Identify the nurse's role in health promotion, protection, and prevention of illness in children.
- Explain the data required for the assessment of the child, the agent, and the environment at the primary and secondary levels of prevention.
- List the nursing strategies related to consumer awareness, health education, and techniques for staying healthy.
- Illustrate health protection measures affecting the child as an individual and society as a whole.
- Discuss measures to reduce the severity of an illness or to contain its communicability.
- Explain strategies to prevent infection and to reduce the complications of illness.

The nurse's role in the promotion of health and the prevention of illness in children is increasingly important today, particularly since the responsibility for health is shifting from medical care systems to the individual. Children can learn to make positive health behaviors an integral part of their lives. Healthful living early in life will lower the risk of disease and the frustration of major lifestyle changes necessitated by a preventable health crisis.

Regardless of practice setting, nurses can make a great impact on the health of children. As a role model, the nurse can positively influence parents, teachers, children, community leaders, and other health care professionals. The nurse also can provide information about how to stay healthy and can promote the effective use of health resources to children and their significant others.

A holistic concept of wellness entails a respect for individuals, their heritage, and the corresponding variety of choices available to attain maximum physical, mental, and spiritual well-being. The nurse can encourage the child and family's active participation in the effective use of personal resources in the practice of health promotion. The nurse needs to identify the significance and purpose of cultural, social, familial, and economic factors and to include them in any teaching.

When changes or additions to lifestyle are necessary, it is essential to assess first the client's level of readiness for new information. Change can be difficult, requiring a period of adjustment as the client works on developing habits, attitudes, and beliefs that are positive and growth enhancing. The more positive, health-promoting habits the child establishes, the fewer negative behaviors will have to be changed when the child becomes an adult. Every nurse who comes in contact with children needs to bear this in mind.

The assessment of individual attitudes, beliefs, and lifestyle relating to health must become part of professional practice. The nurse can use personal experience to encourage health promotion. Successful practice results when the practitioner can cite examples that confirm the value of a healthful lifestyle as a practical reality.

Concepts in Illness Prevention

Health

Health implies the ability of the individual to maintain a state of balance between the internal and external environments. The World Health Association has defined health as "a state of complete physical, mental, and social well-being, and not merely the absence of disease" (Read, 1973).

Illness

Illness results from the failure of the individual to adapt to, or cope with, internal and external stressors. *Stressors* are factors that alter the physical, psychologic, developmental, or social balance of the individual. For example, a fractured femur might be a physiologic stressor, while a failing grade in school might represent a psychologic stressor. One stressor can result in the development of others. For example, a child with a fractured femur might experience the social stressor of isolation from a peer group.

Wellness

Wellness is a concept that includes both health and illness. As a continuum (Fig. 11-1) the concept ranges from high-level wellness at one end to premature death at the other. Throughout life, individuals move along the wellness continuum, depending on their state of well-being at any given point. A person's level of wellness is determined by the person's own perceptions, as well as by the perceptions of others. Wellness can change from day to day or minute to minute.

High-level wellness means more than just being in good health. It involves a conscious attempt to be aware of, to learn about, and to incorporate healthful practices into one's lifestyle. With this definition of wellness, an individual can have a disease or disability and still be considered well because the focus is on the individual's conscious choice to be self-directed and move toward achieving high-level wellness.

Illness occurs at a point on the wellness continuum, but illness usually is preceded by *signs*. Early signs of illness, such as fatigue, irritability, or depression might be unrecognized or ignored, thus preventing the individual from realizing high-level wellness. When warning signals are not heeded, the individual might develop symptoms of a *disease,* either physical or psychosocial. Lack of attention to symptoms might eventually result in a *disability* such as heart disease, arthritis, cancer, or psychoses. Further debilitation might result in premature death.

Children, with the help of their parents, need to decide on the focus for their life and choose behaviors that support their choice. With a goal of high-level wellness, a commitment to health includes a balanced lifestyle, with time for rest and relaxation, adequate diet, and regular exercise.

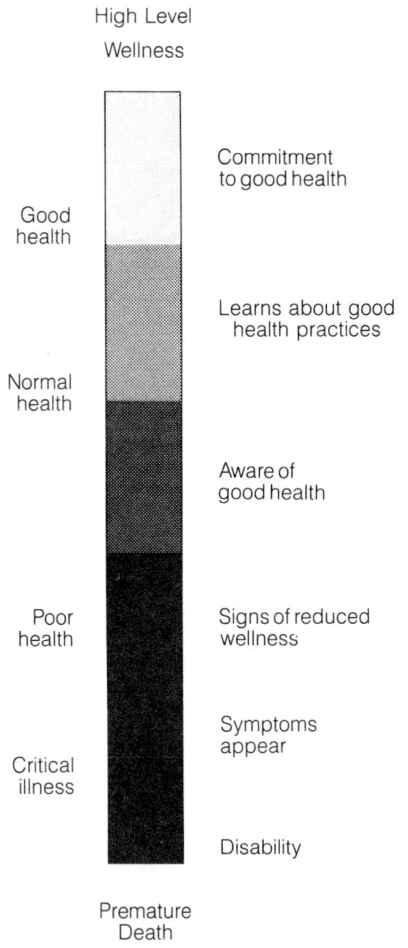

FIGURE 11-1

Wellness-illness continuum.

Stress

The concept of stress and its relationship to illness also is a factor in prevention of disease and disability. *Stress* is a general reaction pattern that occurs as a response to stimuli (*stressors*) confronted in the activities of daily living. The potential for stress is ongoing, and stress may act as either a constructive or a destructive force.

There are three general stages of stress:

1. *Alarm* The individual responds through biologic defense mechanisms (such as increased secretion of cortisone and epinephrine and the mobilization of the body's lymphatic defense system) and attempts to return to a balanced state.
2. *Resistance* The body attempts to adapt physically and psychologically to the stressor.
3. *Exhaustion* The individual who does not achieve balance becomes depleted and vulnerable. At this point the person is open to disease.

An important part of this process is that stressors can be either life-supporting or life-threatening. A positive reaction to stress depends on the person's ability to reachieve balance.

The process of regaining balance is called *adaptation*. Adaptation differs among individuals according to individual differences in perception, conditioning factors, and coping strategies. *Coping strategies* are thoughts and behaviors used to adapt to stress. The same stressor (for example, entering a new school) can produce opposite effects in different people (Fig. 11-2).

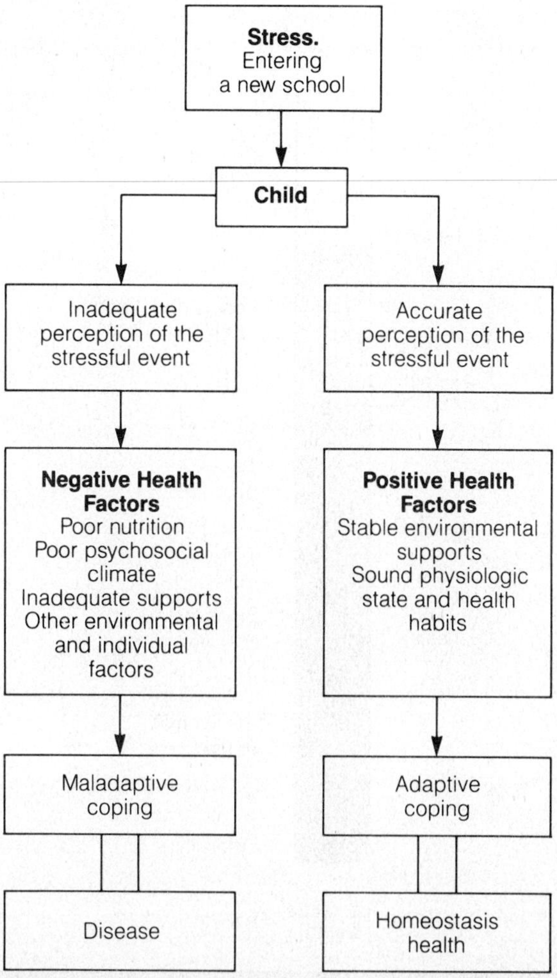

FIGURE 11-2

The process of adaptation and coping with stress. [Adapted from Smith M, Selye H: Reducing the negative effects of stress. Copyright 1979, American Journal of Nursing Company. Reproduced with permission from Am J Nurs (Nov); 79(11).]

Stress in childhood People tend to view childhood as a time of pleasure without the pressures of adulthood, but children also respond to the events in their lives. Stress and the need to adapt to it begins in childhood. The child can begin to develop insight about the source of stress, routine practices leading to good health, and a repertoire of positive coping strategies.

Events in the lives of children might be positive (for example, a family trip) or negative, such as the death of a parent. Both positive and negative events can produce stress in the child. In addition, a stressful event might create greater stress in a child of one age group than in a child of another. For example, a change to a new school might be more stressful to a seventh grader than to a preschooler, while a mother beginning to work might be more stressful for the preschooler.

Nursing implications of stress in children In addition to considering life events as stressors, the nurse considers the child's developmental crises and activities of daily living. A routine activity such as mealtime, toileting, bedtime, or naptime can be either a positive or negative experience for a child, depending on how it is handled by the parent.

For example, Amanda is a 5-year-old, well-adjusted kindergartener. Both of her parents work at jobs each finds challenging and demanding, but they are at work from 7 AM to 6 PM daily. Amanda attends a day-care center before and after school and has direct contact with her parents between 6 PM and 7 AM each weekday and all day on weekends. Much of Amanda's experience with mealtime and rest/sleep time has been dictated by her parents' work lives.

This family situation can be either a positive, growth-producing lifestyle or a negative, distress-producing lifestyle. If the family is able to make the time together special so that it contributes to growth as a family, Amanda will interpret home and family as pleasant and joyful. If the time at home is hurried, without a plan for meals, bedtime, and other routine health-promoting daily activities, Amanda might be in a stressful environment. Routinely hurried mealtimes and daily bedtime battles are in direct conflict with a lifestyle of minimal distress and hinder the teaching of positive health behaviors to children.

Constant exposure to stress results in a higher risk for the child to develop illness. Learning early in life to attend to the controllable behaviors is an important health promotion goal. (Specific techniques for teaching children positive ways to accomplish the necessary daily activities of life are discussed later in this chapter.)

Health Status of Children—Current Emphases in Child Health Care

Historically, the primary focus of child health has been on the physical and environmental factors influencing the morbidity and mortality rate in childhood. Current concerns about the health status of children have been expanded to include social and emotional perspectives as well as health promotion measures.

As children's problems from communicable diseases and poor nutrition have declined, the emphasis on child health care has shifted toward the promotion of wellness and elimination of the factors contributing to illness. *Health protection* and *health promotion* are terms used to describe activities that maintain and enhance health. These terms are distinct from one another with respect to the manner of choice and control exercised by the individual.

Health Protection

Health protection refers to action that focuses on controlling environmental factors, such as immunization, fluoridation of water, infectious disease control, and sanitation. In this category the responsibility is outside the individual's control and benefits the general population. The government legislates and regulates certain health protection measures. Whereas health promotion strategies benefit the individual directly, society at large benefits more from specific protection measures.

Health Promotion

Children and families can make the decision and assume responsibility for activities that relate to health promotion. These activities are most beneficial when they are an active part of living, performed prior to the presence of an illness.

Anticipatory guidance is a form of health promotion. The nurse uses anticipatory guidance to help parents with the process of anticipating child health problems and intervening before they occur. Anticipatory guidance is used as a tool to help parents learn what physical, developmental, and behavioral changes to expect in their children. The nurse teaches parents in a collaborative, supportive manner, allowing them to be active participants in child care.

The extent to which families maintain their functioning depends greatly on the childrearing methods practiced by the parents. Parents often express the need for affirmation or guidance in developing a flexible repertoire of skills that they can adapt to the unique qualities of their children. Nurses might, therefore, need to teach parents methods of discipline, management of normal developmental concerns (eg, toilet-training or temper tantrums), communication with children, and safety principles.

Other health promotion measures include promoting good nutrition, exercise, rest, and development of a healthy self-concept. Physical fitness programming, for example, is a health promotion measure. It advocates adoption of specific health behaviors that might result in maintaining a state of wellness in the child. Health promotion is internally chosen rather than externally imposed.

Promoting self-care Self-care, as a concept of health promotion, is a major personal characteristic that affects the commitment to wellness. Self-care is action taken by individuals to care for or cure themselves, whether acting alone or in consultation with a health care practitioner (Mattson, 1982).

Because of previous experiences and the relationship between the environment and the self, each person in a family thinks, acts, feels, and responds to health-related events in an individual manner. The goal of nursing is to assist each family member to attain the highest level of health possible according to personal definition, perspective, or ability.

The nurse interacts with the child and family in three major ways: "(a) helping people to make decisions about health; (b) substituting [providing] for health-seeking behaviors when necessary; and (c) helping people to promote, maintain, and restore health behaviors" (Lunney, 1982). In most situations the nursing action is some combination of the three methods. The nurse's intention in giving assistance is to interact with empathy to foster trust and encourage growth. One positive outcome of nursing intervention is an increase in the knowledge, skill, and coping strategies in health-related matters, so that parents and children can continue to provide for their self-care, including self-care behaviors related to illness.

Levels of illness prevention Illness prevention is a major focus of nursing today. To prevent an illness or disability saves the child and family from physical, psychologic, and financial stress and reduces society's burden of providing optimum quality of life. Strategies to prevent illness include health promotion and health protection measures.

Illness prevention strategies usually fall into three categories depending on the child's position on the wellness-illness continuum at a given time. These levels of prevention are *primary, secondary,* and *tertiary.* Strategies at the primary level are designed to prevent consequences that would require secondary strategies. Strategies at the secondary level prevent consequences that would place the child at the tertiary level. In planning nursing care, it is important to remember that although the child might require certain interventions at one level, strategies used at another level are not ignored. For example, the child might be hospitalized (a strategy at the secondary level), but the nurse still determines whether the child has had routine childhood immunizations (a strategy at the primary level).

Strategies at the primary level of prevention Nursing activities at the primary level of prevention are directed toward the prevention or elimination of stressors that can cause illness or injury. At this level, nursing care focuses on increasing the child and family's responsibility for self-care and decision making.

At the primary prevention level, the nurse uses data from the physical, nutritional, developmental, and activities of daily living assessments to identify what is needed. Strategies might include educating about health, providing resources to strengthen the child's resistance to stressors, or supporting coping behaviors. Specific protection measures such as immunization programs are strategies at this level, as well as many health promotional activities such as anticipatory guidance.

The goal of primary prevention is to help the child and family identify and practice activities that are beneficial to health and prevent disease. The nurse encourages parents to allow their children to make choices for health gradually, while educating them to make responsible decisions.

Strategies at the secondary level of prevention Most nurses function at the secondary level of prevention. Children requiring secondary-level strategies are those who might be experiencing temporary illness or dysfunction. These children might be hospitalized or cared for at home. Strategies at this level usually are directed toward interrupting or minimizing the consequences of the dysfunction. At this level, the nurse temporarily takes over or assists the child or the parent to perform certain aspects of self-care.

If the dysfunction is minor, the nurse might be able to teach the necessary adaptations in the activities of daily living that will support recovery. Many other times, however, the dysfunction or perception of the dysfunction prevents or limits self-care. The nurse provides treatment and care until the child once again regains the previous state of health.

Because the secondary level of prevention includes early recognition and treatment measures that interrupt or minimize the consequences of disease, certain screening procedures are considered secondary-level strategies. These might include vision and hearing screening and screening for certain diseases such as phenylketonuria (PKU) or anemia.

Strategies at the tertiary level of prevention The tertiary level of prevention frequently is described as rehabilitation. At this level, the nurse assists the child and/or family to modify the usual methods of functioning to compensate for a chronic dysfunction. The nursing emphasis is to promote the adaptation of self-care activities to enable the child to be as independent as possible. The interaction between the nurse and child focuses on ways to use internal and external resources in new combinations to offset those areas that are not fully functional. When this is accomplished, the child is able to be as actively involved as possible in performing self-care and maintaining a reasonable, adaptive level of functioning. The child and family can then use all levels of prevention to achieve wellness.

Integrating prevention strategies Once a family makes a commitment to a lifestyle that promotes wellness, its members choose behaviors in nutrition, exercise, sleep and relaxation, work and recreation, spiritual activity, and social relationships that will enhance and support their health promotion program. They will benefit from such protective primary prevention measures as obtaining proper immunization and drinking pasteurized milk and fluoridated water. Regular dental and vision screening and physical assessment will be part of their secondary prevention program. If a disability is present, attention will be given to measures designed to return the individual to an optimal level of functioning. These measures are then tertiary-level behaviors.

Primary Level of Prevention: The Nurse's Role

Nursing Contact with Children

Primary prevention involves manipulating those factors that can be altered to prevent illness from occurring. Nurses influence children's health through their contacts with them in the community and in the schools.

Primary health care nurse The nurse might be a child's only continuous health care professional throughout childhood. This continuity provides a unique opportunity for the child, family, and nurse to participate together in the growth process. The nurse might be an independent practitioner or part of a team. The focus of care is to help the child freely choose positive health behaviors. The child and the nurse not only share the goal but also work together to attain that goal.

For example, although most parents of young children cite good health as a goal, some parents' behavior might counteract progress toward that goal. Unstructured lifestyles, reliance on fast foods, irregular schedules that preclude regular rest periods, and inconsistent caregivers might be incompatible with the development of a physically and mentally healthy child. Although the stated goal might be health, the real priority in that parent's life might be economic well-being. The role of the nurse is to help the parent work out lifestyle patterns that will best meet the goal of economic security without compromising the goal of having a healthy child.

It is important for the nurse to consider the demands of work, family, and community and the need for personal satisfaction as they affect the parent and child. The flow of information and support must be interchangeable from client to nurse and from nurse to client. Each must view the other as a resource to be considered in meeting individual and common goals.

Regular health maintenance visits for children generally occur through 6 years of age. After this age, parents and children might not seek health counseling unless a problem exists. At this stage, health care can become fragmented, and health promotion can become less holistic. Health professionals might unwittingly contribute to the neglect of general health care by confining their contacts with the child to the issues central to their specialties. The tunnel vision that is sometimes part of specialized practice might hinder a view of the patient as a whole person. For example, lack of consideration for the total nutritional needs of a child might delay the healing after surgery.

When contact with the child is for diagnosis or treatment purposes, the effective primary health care nurse will take the opportunity to assess wellness and institute appropriate strategies for health promotion. Nurses can alert other health professionals to the need to encourage parents and responsible children to seek support for wellness behavior.

School nurse The most influential nurse from middle childhood through adolescence is the school nurse. The role of school nurses is comprehensive and includes health promotion, health teaching, health protection, and other strategies to prevent and control the spread of illness (see Chapter 1).

Nurses encourage the development of positive health behaviors in children through teaching in the classroom as well as in the office. Stress-reduction techniques; the hazards of drugs, alcohol, and cigarettes; and sex education are all areas where the school nurse can be an effective teacher and role model. School nurses are also role models for such self-care activities as nutrition, exercise, and preventive dental care.

School nurses promote children's awareness of health as a holistic concept. They support children in developing a personal health history. They emphasize emotional and spiritual health by helping children to clarify their values.

School nurses work with children, families, teachers, and the community to plan for the health needs of all. They are instrumental in helping both children with special needs and those who are chronically ill to enter the mainstream of school life. In addition, they can provide referrals for children needing more specialized follow-up care.

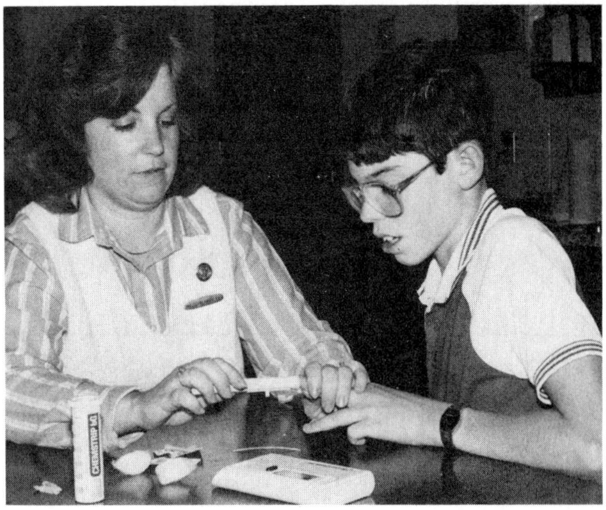

The role of the school nurse is comprehensive and includes health promotion, health protection, and other strategies to prevent and control the spread of illness. (Photograph by Judy Koenig.)

Assessment at the Primary Level of Prevention

Assessment at the primary level of prevention is directed toward determining the individual characteristics of children as they relate to the environment and the agents with which they come in contact. Assessment data indicate where the child and family fall on the wellness-illness continuum. In addition, assessment enables the nurse and client to formulate diagnoses and construct a health plan that will increase the child's level of wellness (Fig. 11-3).

Characteristics of the child Some characteristics of the child include prenatal "givens" (resistance and immunity to disease, genetic predisposition to disease, and so on), emotional state (temperament), understanding of wellness concepts, health habits, and developmental skills.

A major psychosocial factor affecting child health is lifestyle. The effects of stress and the ability of a child to adapt to the changes in daily life are important to consider. Unlike adults, children have not developed the coping strategies needed to deal with situational, societal, and personal changes (see Chapter 16 for a discussion of coping strategies). Children's understanding of wellness concepts plays an important role in developing positive health habits.

Self-care during infancy During infancy, the parents meet the self-care needs of their children. Parents respond to the basic needs of infants in general and to the specific

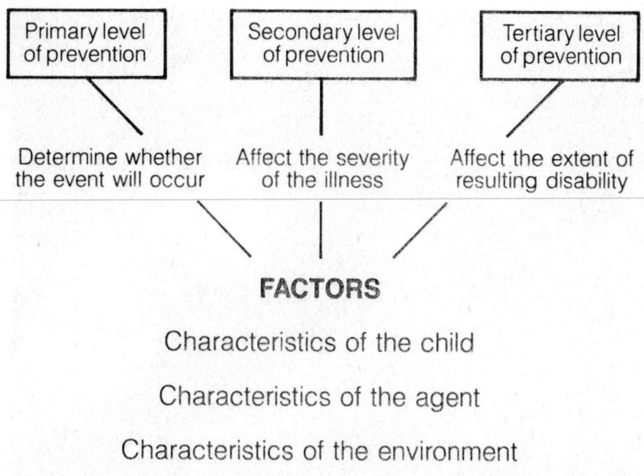

FIGURE 11-3

Levels of prevention.

cues given by their infants. By appropriately meeting the needs of infants, parents establish the groundwork for positive health behaviors in their children.

Self-care during early childhood In early childhood, emphasis is on the basic needs for social interaction, safety, and food. Because lifestyle patterns are developing in this period, special attention to habit formation is important. Establishing positive health behaviors for good nutrition, regular exercise, and adequate rest and sleep is essential.

A potential major health hazard is the nutritional status of children. Nutritional status includes eating habits as well as the amount and choices of food. Child health problems related to diet and nutrition begin prenatally and continue through adolescence and throughout life. Poor nutrition or excess food intake has been reported to have at least some causal relationship to obesity, high blood pressure, dental disease, heart disease, cancer, and diabetes. Childhood problems such as failure to thrive, delayed physical and mental growth, and learning disabilities also have been linked to poor nutrition.

Between the ages of 2 and 5 years, self-care increases rapidly. Children can articulate the desire for food and feed and dress themselves with assistance. Bowel and bladder control are developing, and complete self-care is possible by 4½ years of age. Meeting self-care needs for rest and activity is individualized. Some children lie down when they are tired, whereas other children need to be directed to do so.

Self-care during middle childhood The child in middle childhood exhibits a large measure of autonomy in most self-care activities, but special consideration must be given in the area of safety. Exposure to substance abuse begins at the end of this period. The role and influence of the school increases. Children at this age are able to initiate their own health care visits. Children whose parents emphasize self-care will cope with many health crises by themselves.

Self-care during late childhood and adolescence During late childhood and throughout adolescence, the predominant problem is safety. Because of increased participation in athletics and greater exposure to the hazards of substance abuse, the older child and adolescent are at risk for injury or illness. Although able to understand safety concepts, children at these ages need support from parents to cope with the increasing demands of peer groups, which sometimes involve unsafe or unhealthy practices.

Other characteristics of the child that the nurse assesses include the child's level of cognitive development, temperament, respect for self, spiritual and moral development, and commitment to wellness concepts, as evidenced by the presence of positive health habits.

Characteristics of the agent The *agent* is the means by which the child sustains an alteration in health. Assessment data relative to the agent include the (1) length of contact with the agent, (2) transmissibility of the agent, and (3) potential effect of the agent on the child's wellness level. Examples of agents are microorganisms, stress, abusable substances, and diet.

Microorganisms The destructive potential of a microorganism-caused disease depends on its effect on the child and its mode of transmission. The effect of microorganisms on a child's health is the result of a combination of the virulence of the organism, its ability to produce symptoms, and the magnitude of the immune response.

The modes of transmission of an organism also determine its destructive potential. Modes of transmission include:

1. *Contact transmission*—(a) direct, body to body (for example, sexually transmitted diseases), (b) indirect, object to body (for example, touching contaminated objects or substances and transferring the infection from hand to mouth), and (c) droplet, which is considered a form of contact transmission because infection spread occurs within 3 ft of a contaminated individual
2. *Airborne transmission*—transfer of extremely small organisms under certain environmental conditions (for example, influenza)
3. *Vehicle transmission*—transfer of edible substances and biologic products (blood) that convey organisms to a susceptible host (for example, botulism, hepatitis)
4. *Vector transmission*—transfer of disease-carrying arthro-

pods that infect the child by biting or by transferring organisms onto the food or the skin (for example, Rocky Mountain spotted fever)

Stress Other disease-causing agents, however, are entirely unrelated to organism transfer. Stress in particular can have an adverse effect on the body in that it breaches body defenses and contributes to disease. The action of stress alters physiologic processes, specifically neuroendocrine pathways and hormonal activity. Stress most likely alters the immune response, although the mechanism is still being studied.

Chemicals Certain chemicals produce illness. For example, asbestos, used for many years in buildings, is a known cancer-causing agent. A recent controversy over the effects of saccharin emphasized the uncertainty regarding agents in food. The list of suspected cancer-causing agents grows longer each year, creating problems for local and national regulatory agencies.

Not only food additives but also the foods themselves can contribute to disease—both in kind and in amount. For example, a diet high in cholesterol or low in iron can contribute to disease. Too many calories results in obesity—a known risk factor in cardiac disease. When left between teeth, food promotes bacterial growth, leading to dental caries.

Abusable substances Abusable substances, such as alcohol, drugs, and cigarettes, also can affect the wellness level and the occurrence of disease in the child. Alcohol, considered for years to be a socially acceptable substance, has known effects on the brain, circulatory system, and other body organs. Overuse of this substance affects the thinking processes and coordination. For this reason, alcohol is particularly dangerous in conjunction with driving. Alcohol-related deaths, particularly in adolescents, have increased dramatically. Many states in the United States have raised the drinking age to 21 and imposed mandatory jail sentences for drunk driving.

Children are exposed to alcohol at a young age, particularly if it is present in the home. Inadequate role modeling and other individual and environmental factors can lead to alcoholism in the young adult (see Chapter 13). The deleterious effects of alcohol on the fetus are beginning to be discovered.

Drug availability also has increased in the last 20 years. Substances such as marijuana, cocaine, amphetamines, and tranquilizers, among others, are commonly found in high schools. Drug use among elementary school students has increased. In addition to the detrimental effects these drugs have on physical performance, addictive behavior can affect all areas of children's lives, initiating a maladaptive cycle that is difficult to break.

Perhaps the most common, although no less dangerous, substance children are exposed to throughout their lives is cigarette smoke. Heavy smoking can contribute to many cardiovascular and respiratory diseases—lung cancer being one of the more serious. The effects of smoking are felt in utero, resulting in smaller-birthweight babies born to mothers who are heavy smokers. Children who themselves do not smoke can still exhibit respiratory problems from the amount of smoke in their environment. Fortunately, vigorous school health programs and public campaigns and the provision of nonsmoking areas in public locations have cut down the influence of smoking on nonsmokers.

Finally, environmental allergens are agents that can lead to disease occurrence in susceptible children. (See Chapter 25 for a discussion of allergens.)

Characteristics of the environment Environmental characteristics also affect the child's health status. Areas to assess include geographic factors influencing disease occurrence, facilities in the home, emotional climate, air and water quality, education of parents, and socioeconomic status. Prevention of the following health hazards is included in the US Public Health Service recommendations for national goals and objectives for child health promotion: exposure to hazardous chemicals, radiation, and lead; inadequate waste disposal; unsafe water, foods, and drugs; and accidents (US Department of Health and Human Services, 1981a).

Exposure to hazardous chemicals and radiation Exposure to hazardous chemicals and radiation is especially problematic during fetal development. Such chronic disorders as growth retardation, minimal brain damage, and altered immunologic response in very young children have been linked to exposure to noxious substances. Some public health experts attribute nearly all the major chronic diseases as well as some of the acute conditions such as poisoning, gastroenteritis, and seizures in the United States to exposure to hazardous substances.

A serious aspect of exposure to hazardous substances in childhood is the delayed effect. Sometimes the problems are not evident for 20 years (US Department of Health and Human Services, 1981a).

The Panel on Promotion of Child Health (US Department of Health and Human Services, 1981a) reports that 45% of radiation exposure to the general public is through medical and dental care, whereas the remaining exposure to radioactive materials is in the air, soil, and water. This panel has recommended the creation of national standards to limit medical- and dental-related exposure of pregnant women and the medical-related exposure of children under 1 year of age.

Exposure to pesticides is a problem that extends from fetal life throughout adulthood. The hazard includes exposure to dangerous chemicals in food and water as well as those in the atmosphere from aerial spraying. In children the effects are more dangerous because of the proportionately low body weight per exposure as compared with adults. This results in problems such as birth defects, stillbirths, infant mortality, and poisoning from contaminated breast milk.

Another environmental health hazard for children is exposure to lead. Elevated lead levels are associated with brain damage, poor school performance, and slow development. Both community and family efforts are necessary to combat this problem.

The issues surrounding the disposal of hazardous waste are embroiled in political and economic controversy. Health crises due to improper waste disposal have been reported in several states. One of the first major incidents, at Love Canal, New York, was discovered after the residents reported an unusually high incidence of spontaneous abortions and birth defects. Subsequent investigations resulted in the discovery of a chemical leakage from a waste disposal site. Citizen action and long periods of working with public and private agencies resulted in a solution. Numerous other sites around the United States are being identified, however, and the problems of who is primarily responsible and what to do remain unsolved.

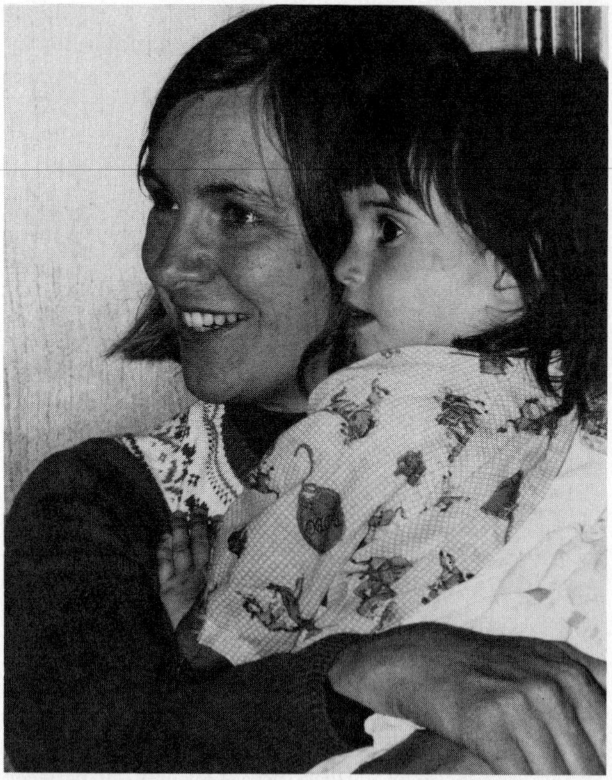

When parent and child "read" each other's signals correctly, there is a healthy parent-child fit. (Photograph by Judy Koenig.)

Social and affective factors Although difficult to measure, the effects of social and emotional factors on health status are receiving more attention. It is generally accepted that there is a connection between these factors and physical problems. In addition, the effects of physical illness on the emotional and behavioral aspects of living are becoming better understood.

Parent-child "fit" An important part of family functioning is *parent-child "fit,"* or the extent to which both parent and child meet and adapt to each other's needs. An imperfect parent-child fit might be the result of insufficient or deficient attachment early in infancy, or it might become evident later, as the child's developing personality fails to match the parent's expectations.

The nurse assesses the parent-child fit by asking the parent about the expectations concerning the child, whether reality and expectations are similar, and how well parent and child have adapted to each other. When the parent and child "read" each other's signals correctly, their responses are appropriate, and each feels competent.

For example, when observing the infant who is beginning to squirm and fuss, the parent changes the infant's position, provides a new toy, or spends a few minutes in play, feeling confident that those actions will satisfy the infant. The parent has learned to interpret correctly the infant's sounds and to respond in ways that are satisfying to both parent and child. Another mother has learned that when her young son whines and lays his head down on the table, it is better to give him a nap before the meal. He plays so hard that he is unaware of his fatigue until he sits down to eat. Her sense of competence in her ability to interpret her son's needs enables her to follow through with her decisions even when questioned or criticized by others.

At other times, a developmental history might reveal that the parent had anticipated a quiet, cuddly infant and instead had to contend with an infant who fussed a great deal and was difficult to console. The infant's temperament did not "fit" the parent's expectations. Normal development might therefore be compromised unless interventions can help the parent adapt to the behavioral pattern of the infant and experience positive reciprocal interactions with the child.

Socioeconomic status Poverty and educational status also affect attitudes about health. Parents who are unable to pay for preventive care might not consider health maintenance visits a priority. Even the availability of health care

Assessment at the Primary Level of Prevention: Prevention of Illness

Characteristics of the child	Characteristics of the agent	Characteristics of the environment
Prenatal "givens" such as temperament, resistance to disease, and health habits	Length of contact with the agent	Geographic factors influencing disease
Adaptation to stress	Transmissibility of the agent (such as in microorganisms)	Facilities in the home including both *physical,* such as condition of the house and sanitary facilities, adequate heat and humidity, home safety, and privacy, and *social-emotional,* such as education of parents, socioeconomic status, and positive relationships
Understanding of wellness concepts	Potential effect of the agent on the child's wellness level	Air and water quality
Commitment to self-care		Community resources
Development of positive health habits good nutrition, regular exercise, adequate rest		
Level of cognitive development		
Respect for self		
Spiritual and moral development		

facilities does not guarantee that they will be used. Historically, the poor have been crisis oriented toward health, using the emergency room as the primary source of health care. Health promotion and illness prevention have not been part of their lifestyle. Economically disadvantaged parents are reported to perceive their children's health as poor (US Department of Health and Human Services, 1981b).

Even for children who are above poverty levels, access to preventive health care is limited. Most third-party payments are made for the treatment of acute illnesses. Few insurance companies compensate for well-child visits, even under major medical coverage. The growth of health maintenance organizations is a partial answer to this problem, but these are not yet widespread enough to provide for the wellness needs of most families.

Results of a set of studies by the National Center for Health Services Research (US Department of Health and Human Services, 1981c) indicated that of the many environmental factors contributing to children's health, the mother's educational level was particularly significant as a health determinant. Children of mothers who had received more schooling tended to be healthier, particularly in the area of dental health. The factors influencing this appeared to include the development of positive health attitudes through education and the encouragement of preventive health care by these mothers. In addition, smaller families enabled parents to give more individual attention to the health needs of their children.

Conditions in the home contribute to the family's state of wellness. Emotional stability, spiritual and moral values, and positive relationships between family members reduce the level of stress. Physical aspects of the home environment are important in determining comfort and family safety as well as conditions conducive to disease transmission.

The nurse assesses the following characteristics of the home:

1. Age and type of the dwelling
2. Toilet and washing facilities
3. Provision of warmth and the type of heat
4. Humidification and insulation
5. Waste disposal
6. Home safety (see Chapter 12)
7. Adequate space for the number of family members
8. Presence of allergenic or adverse chemical substances
9. Room for privacy and play

Other important variables in the home environment involve cultural approaches to health care (see Chapter 2), positive childrearing practices, and adequate role modeling.

Interventions at the Primary Level of Prevention

After assessing the characteristics of the child, agent, and environment, nurses initiate strategies that alter negative health habits and promote wellness. Optimal health can be achieved through increased participation in the health care system (by consumer awareness) and in health education. Certain health protection measures also can be encouraged.

Consumer awareness Manufacturers of children's toys, cereal companies, and producers of television programs have recognized for years that children comprise a major portion of the consumer block. Clever advertising policies have encouraged children to demand products from parents. Competition among peers to possess these products adds fuel to an already large fire.

Unfortunately, health consumerism has not kept pace with commercialism. Recognizing that children are consumers in their own right challenges health care providers to use consumerism and marketing techniques to promote health. Children need to be taught from an early age that greater consumer participation in the health care system will improve the health care delivery to society as a whole.

Consumer awareness includes the right to health, the means to health, and the marketing of health. Health is a natural state. Everybody possesses a measure of health, regardless of the presence of a disability or an illness. Children do not think about their health because it is natural, it is given, it is expected, and that is as it should be. Individuals who do have a particular health problem are more likely to focus on their problem rather than on health in general. Individuals should recognize, however, that although health is a right and is natural, it is essential to make choices to maintain health and move toward optimal potential.

Three areas need to be considered in health and consumer awareness. First is the individual's responsibility to exercise the right to health. Second is society's responsibility to promote and protect the health status of everyone. Third is the responsibility of the health care professional, especially the nurse, to make services and information available to assist consumers to make choices that are best suited to their particular situation.

Individual responsibility The individual is responsible for making choices. A heightened awareness of one's personal health status might elevate health as a priority. Individual lifestyle is an important variable, which to a greater or lesser degree is affected by heredity, culture, income level, age, familial attitudes, personal beliefs, and educational level.

Behavior reflects belief. For example, the adolescent who lists health as a priority but eats primarily at fast-food restaurants, smokes, and doesn't exercise is in reality placing a higher value on peer acceptance than on health. The actions of this individual contradict the stated belief.

Societal responsibility What is society's responsibility for health promotion? The efforts of society must be aimed at health protection measures that allow the best possible environment for the individual to reach personal goals. For example, the individual has very little direct control over issues such as the disposal of hazardous waste, safe roads, protection against communicable disease, and unsafe drugs and food. It is the responsibility of the private and public sectors to meet their responsibilities through safe waste disposal, healthful work conditions, and the enforcement of health regulations.

The state of the economy is related to health and the quality of life. Funds for nutritional and well-child programs might be decreased during an economic crisis. Such changes can be instrumental in increasing the risk of morbidity and mortality.

Society has a responsibility to provide the possibility of choice. Risk-taking behavior is the right of the individual, but the options must be presented. The risk involved in smoking, for example, has been widely publicized, and most children and adolescents are aware of the hazards. Therefore, smokers are acting at their own risk. The societal issue of risk to nonsmokers exposed to smoke is receiving increasing attention. More nonsmokers are questioning the right of the individual to smoke versus the rights of nonsmokers who are subjected to this hazard.

Nursing responsibility Health education as a vehicle for information and the availability of health services as support systems are the means through which the individual can make choices. Nurses can be instrumental in health education both as consumers and as professionals by being positive role models.

The provision of health services is a means of promoting health to the consumer. Although economics is an issue in the use of health services, it is not always the major barrier. More often, the greater obstacle is lack of awareness of the concepts of wellness and health promotion on the part of the consumer. Important areas for nursing are assessment of knowledge deficits and education to make up the deficit. Parents need to be taught and supported to best fulfill their role as primary seekers of their children's health care. Attitudes and habits learned during childhood and seen practiced by the family are more likely to be retained when the individual becomes independent.

Children and adolescents also require direct information that is appropriate to their level of understanding and that relates to current concerns. There are times when they have specific questions that need to be answered, and the nurse is regarded as one who is knowledgeable and approachable. Generally, these children are oblivious of the concepts of wellness and health promotion and need to be "sold" on the idea that what one eats and how one lives does make a difference.

Active participation in the health care system is a goal for children to achieve to exercise their rights and responsibilities as health care consumers. One program designed to meet this goal is Project PACT, developed by nurses at the University of Colorado. Project PACT is a unique program that encourages children's participation in their health care. The purpose of the program is to increase children's abilities to communicate with health care professionals. Increased communication allows children's greater participation in their own care as well as health care that is individualized to the child's own needs.

Communication promotes the attitude that children are in control of their own health and health care. In addition, children who use these communication skills from an early age become articulate adults who are able to be critical consumers, thus improving health care delivery to society as a whole. The program encourages children to do the following:

1. Ask questions
2. Relay information about themselves
3. Express the need for health instruction
4. Cooperate with health professionals in decision making and constructing a health plan
5. Clarify their own self-care responsibilities (Igoe, 1980)

Programs such as this, together with creative marketing techniques, will create conscientious and informed health consumers.

Marketing health promotion The concept of marketing health promotion involves the same elements as the nursing process: assessment, planning, intervention, and evaluation. Successful marketing depends on providing the consumers with the product or service they need. Therefore, consumers need to be convinced that the information or service is appropriate in a personal way.

For children, efforts regarding nutrition, substance abuse, or lifestyle education need to take into account that the child or even the family might not understand or accept the need for such programs or services. For example, young children cannot understand the need to eat nutritious foods or establish regular eating habits in childhood to avoid the threat of illness in middle age. They want to know what difference it will make in running the race, learning to read, or making a snowman. It is just as difficult for children to comprehend the cause-and-effect relationship between their current lack of exercise and the development of illnesses and disease in later life. Adolescents might be aware of the negative effects of the use of alcohol, tobacco, and drugs, but the priority at that age usually is acceptance by the peer group rather than future health. The selling of health thus is a major challenge.

Television The media has a subtle but powerful influence on the beliefs and attitudes of children. The most obvious health-related effects are through the advertising of foods and drugs and the aggressive, sometimes violent television programming. Other influences of television on children have been noted as follows:

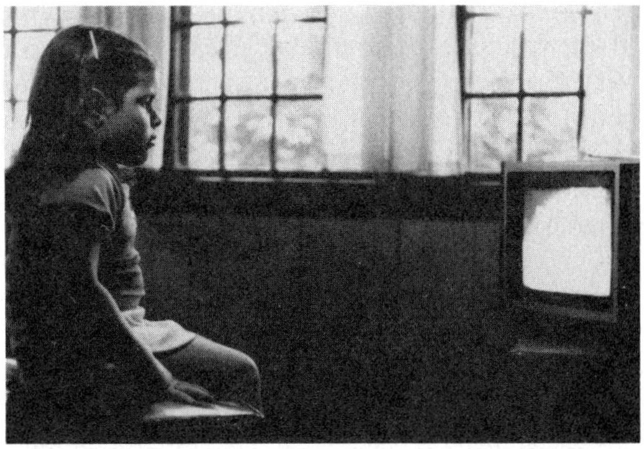

Television can have a positive or negative effect on the child's health, depending on the amount of viewing time and the type of programs seen. (Photograph by Paul Sabin.)

1. Programming on health issues presents health problems from an organic cause perspective rather than from the perspective that individual responsibility for prevention is necessary.
2. Health programming focuses on sensational issues, such as artificial hearts, rather than on the benefits of positive health behaviors at an understandable level for children.
3. Nurses as role models are downplayed by the media.

Television is a primary source of information in the American culture. It is reported to be the most influential source of information other than the parents. The average child spends 27 hours a week watching television. About 20% of television time consists of advertising (Samuels and Samuels, 1982). To date, several attempts have been made by both commercial and public television to air children's health programming. The efforts have been short-lived because they are not economically rewarding.

Television has a profound effect on children. Because of their great capacity for fantasy and their inability to scrutinize the information, children can be victimized by television. Some programming, such as *Sesame Street* and *Electric Company,* provides children with good self-care health promotion attitudes. Violent, aggressive behavior that is prevalent on television, however, is not a positive influence on children, although opinions differ regarding its long-lasting effects.

Because young children are hero worshipers, health segments are more effective if current heroes are incorporated. For example, children will respond better if Michael J. Fox tells them something about nutrition than they will to the words "Milk is a natural." Conversely, the widespread use of well-known athletes to advertise alcoholic beverages has an adverse health effect on children. Encouraging critical television viewing for children and families is a major nursing responsibility.

Other media The printed word, primarily magazines, and radio both influence children. The message in many songs and the words and actions of some public figures idolized by the young is to get "high" by using drugs, alcohol, and sex. One avenue for communicating the message of positive health behaviors to children is the public relations requirement of the Federal Communications Commission, which dictates that all stations must allow free public information programming. This obligatory time can be used for health promotion segments directed toward children.

A major obstacle to adequate health programming for children is its cost. One question related to cost is whether the taxpayer will be receptive to the public's being responsible for these programs. There might be less resistance to the cost of clean air, safe food and water, and immunization programs because these would clearly benefit all persons. The question still remains, though, how much responsibility each individual has for the health and safety of the whole group. The increased participation in and encouragement of creative media marketing of health by nurses will positively influence children's consumer awareness.

Although individual efforts are important, the private and public sectors also must be involved in the marketing campaign for health promotion. Environmental goals can only be met by large groups coming together and working toward a common goal.

Health education—teaching health to children

Children learn about health in many ways. Although the family is the primary teacher, the influence of peers, teachers, and media is increasingly significant as the child develops. Nurses and other health care providers also are important references and affect health behaviors through education, service, and role modeling. The world of children includes direct and indirect contact with people, active and passive learning about health, and the practice of health behaviors.

Parents Parents are the first model for the child. Mullen (1981) cited research on beliefs about food and disease in children and showed ways in which parents are the source of information. Behaviors such as smoking and the use of alcohol are more prevalent in children whose parents also exhibit these behaviors. In a study of child-initiated health visits to the school nurse, patterns reflected parental attitudes and beliefs about health. The study showed that behavior patterns were internalized by 12 years of age (Lewis, 1980).

The family plays an important role in the health education of children. Specifically, the role is as follows:

1. To set the health-related goals and objectives for the family
2. To identify the behaviors and habits that are consistent with the family's beliefs and attitudes
3. To seek information and consultation appropriate to the family's needs

Peers The influence of the peer group begins when children interact with other children outside the family. As early as nursery school, the ideas expressed by a young companion are considered and heeded along with the teachings of parents. Getting along with and being accepted by peers is a major developmental task during childhood and adolescence. At times peer pressure might outweigh the influence of the family.

During adolescence, the work of early health education reaches fruition. Peer group influence is particularly evident in an adolescent's choice to smoke. In a study of smoking behaviors among teenagers, the habits of their peer group, especially best friends, furnished the greatest incentive to smoke; parental examples were second. More information is needed on the role of the peer group in establishing positive health behaviors as well as how to counterbalance the negative influences of peer pressure.

Teachers Although the educational community is aware that it plays a role in health education and the modeling of positive health behaviors, these are not considered educational priorities. With the increasing emphasis on science, mathematics, and technology, curricula allocate cursory time to health and creative arts instruction. Despite the national objective of physical fitness for all children, physical education time might be nothing more than a glorified recess. Recognition that health is a lifelong process and is not limited to physical well-being is not always evident in the schools.

Personal health beliefs are communicated by the educator as well as the parent. Demonstrating positive health attitudes and behaviors is effective even when a health course is not established. Teachers often need the resources supplied by the school nurse to assist children in managing and finding answers to their health concerns.

The role of the school in health education is as follows:

1. To supplement the parents' role as the primary health educator
2. To provide instruction based on the needs of children
3. To offer supportive health services
4. To maintain a safe and healthy environment

Nurses Nurses have a professional mandate to promote health and teach positive health behaviors. Changes in attitudes and orientation have been developing in all areas of the human services. The terms holistic and wellness are evidence of these changes; however, the practice of these concepts and principles is not widespread. There is some resistance to these changes in attitude and the locus of responsibility. For many educators, for example, the response to physical or emotional distress in a student is a trip to the school nurse.

The primary role of the nurse is to assist the individual to promote, maintain, or restore health. The growing interest in holistic health and self-care affords nurses the opportunity to move into the forefront as health promoters. More research must be conducted on health promotion by nurses. Nurses need to become more visible in the media, teaching health and defining their role as health providers. Nursing activities such as speaking to parent groups, participating in career awareness programs, and counseling at health fairs will provide an avenue for defining roles.

Health education—techniques for maintaining health
Nurses have the opportunity to provide health education throughout the life span. Education begins during the prenatal period as the nurse assists the pregnant woman to define behaviors that will not only promote the good health of the fetus but also assist the woman with optimal postpartum recovery. Education continues throughout childhood to prepare the child for an adulthood of optimal wellness. Throughout the process, the nurse emphasizes the child's strengths and achievements and helps the parent identify the child's unique behavioral style.

Life is a process, and wellness is a continuum. Child health education requires an understanding of the development of both children and adults. Learning the skills to meet the goal of high-level wellness depends on the developmental stage of the individual. (Table 11-1 illustrates the teaching strategies for children at various developmental stages.)

Health education is directed toward staying healthy and preventing illness. When teaching children health promotion techniques, the nurse discusses both general and specific concepts. Health-promoting behaviors include techniques for meeting all the basic needs of humans. Health promotion measures also include primary and secondary prevention.

By understanding the child's temperament and behavioral style, the parent can approach each developmental stage in a way that is consistent and fosters growth. Parents whose expectations for their children's development are realistic come to appreciate each child's unique characteristics. Knowing developmental norms also allows the parent to promote development by providing appropriate stimulation.

For example, some 1-year-olds need special attention to verbal stimulation to help them practice language skills. Others need toys that provide opportunities to enhance gross motor development. The parent who has learned about developmental norms and who knows the child's behavior patterns, strengths, and weaknesses is more likely to be prepared for the child's developmental progress.

The nurse might need to remind some parents that children progress at different rates and that when most children concentrate on one or another area of development, they "plateau" or appear slower in the others. The nurse therefore explains that normal developmental milestones occur within a range and that a pace that might appear to be slow in some areas is not necessarily evidence of seriously delayed development. Some parents also might need to learn to accept their children's slower-paced development. The nurse then counsels the parents to focus on the child's strengths and to accept the child's need to learn skills at a slower pace.

When parents cite problems in feeding, sleeping, discipline, or dependence, the nurse's best response is usually, "What have you tried to do about it so far?" If the parent then describes a method that has failed, the nurse might ask, "Why do you think it didn't work?" As parents describe their responses, the nurse might discover that the parent did not give the method a chance or that the parent was not comfortable with the method chosen. Parenting styles and methods need to be suited to the parent as well as the child. For example, a parent who finds it difficult to allow an infant to cry unattended for a few minutes need not be encouraged to do so. The nurse might instead ask, "What would you like to do now?" and proceed to work with the parent to develop a plan for solving the problem. By helping the parent and child better understand their own selves and each other, the nurse can facilitate communication between them.

Because nursing roles overlap during some developmental periods, nurses should recognize the danger that some important information might not get to the child. This problem can be corrected through adequate communication between health professionals and families.

Basic concepts in health maintenance Nurses and clients need to understand both the basic concepts related to health promotion and their rationale. These concepts then become part of the plan of action for each health promotion technique:

1. Establish the need for the behavior to sustain life.
2. Identify the specific purpose or function of each need that, when integrated into lifestyle, helps to form a whole and balanced person.

TABLE 11-1 Developmental Approach to Health Education

Age	Developmental characteristic	Learning style	Teaching strategy
Infancy (birth to 18 months)	Dependent on others for meeting universal health care demands; beginning cognitive development, requires stimulation; expression of needs by crying, moving, and so forth; emotional—trust vs mistrust; beginning development of coping mechanisms	Sensorimotor (Piaget); stimulation for adequate growth; preverbal	Help parent clarify roles; encourage bonding; assist parents to meet universal self-care demands and foster a nurturing environment; teach parents health care measures—importance of regular well-child checkups, immunizations, and environment modification
Early childhood (18 months to 4½ years)	Tendency to demand; aggressive and protest behavior; fantasy and fears; focus on control of elimination; positive or negative attitudes learned from environment; self-protection decreased due to increased curiosity	Preconceptual; trial and error; use of fantasy and drama; short attention span requires varied presentation; needs repetition to learn	Teach parents importance of continuing immunization and well-child visits; continue environmental protection; teach cleanliness and safety by role modeling; encourage beginning responsibility for self-care—bathing, dressing, dental care; teach parents appropriate criteria for choosing child or day care; encourage positive self-image; coordinate teaching with periods of optimal wakefulness and attention; encourage regular rest periods
Middle childhood (5–8 years)	High activity level; increased emphasis on physical prowess; increasing intellectual development; increasing spiritual and moral development; emphasis on following rules; awareness of socially acceptable behavior; increasing identification with peers	Beginning to be a concrete thinker and problem solver; language skills improving; learns best by manipulating objects	Continue to emphasize well-child care; encourage participatory care and control over own health; teach rules of safety; encourage self-esteem by positive reinforcement; give clear, concise answers to questions regarding death and moral issues; explore values and how they relate to peers' values; encourage independence in meeting self-care demands; encourage parents to provide a wide variety of experiences and opportunities to solve problems; begin education in areas of sex, substance abuse, and child abuse; allow for questions; use humor as a teaching tool to gain and keep affection

TABLE 11-1 (Continued)

Age	Developmental characteristic	Learning style	Teaching strategy
Late childhood (8–12 years)	Increasing awareness of causes of disease might lead to psychosomatic complaints; peer group important; need to achieve competence in school and sports; beginning exposure to abusable substances; increased self-direction (eg, will initiate visits to school nurse)	Concrete, with beginning development of abstract conceptual thought; problem-solving capability; well-developed language skills	Focus on safety principles; use influence of peer group to alter health behaviors; encourage parental support and continued role modeling; utilize the media to encourage positive health habits; teach health education in the schools to continue fostering positive health habits and prevent substance abuse; use problem situations and discussion groups to teach health concepts and grapple with moral issues
Adolescence	Physical maturation; peer pressure most influential; accidents increase, particularly automobile; substance abuse; sexual activity—can lead to pregnancy or sexually transmitted disease; focus on social rather than healthful aspects of living	Abstract; problem solving; future oriented	Emphasize enhancing self-esteem; identify and reinforce positive behaviors; utilize peer counseling and alter group rather than individual behaviors; minimize the negative

3. Each of the needs should fit into a natural order or progression.
4. Commit to a regular practice of positive health behavior that will yield the desired result.

Proper diet exemplifies the first concept. The child who becomes aware of the need for food on more than an automatic response level begins to consider eating behaviors that are commensurate with meeting the goal of wellness, that is, nutritional snacks, fruits instead of candy, and so forth.

The second concept involves identifying the specific role the need plays in achieving a balanced personal life. For example, understanding that food is needed to sustain the body-mind system helps the individual to develop habits consistent with meeting that goal.

Third, all of nature works in an orderly way. The concept of order is difficult for humans to accept as a working principle. Relative to food, each nutrient is utilized in an orderly way to meet specific biologic needs and according to a natural timetable. When committed to changing dietary behaviors, the client needs encouragement to sustain the behavior until the desired result becomes evident.

It probably is most difficult for the client to practice health-promoting behavior with sufficient regularity to ensure results. Being committed to making the health behavior a regular part of the client's life is the only way that the goal can be achieved.

Specific concepts in health maintenance

Nutrition Clients need to understand the role nutrition plays in their lives as well as understanding why they eat and the function of food. Next, each client should choose the types of food that will promote optimal body, mental, and spiritual function. This includes the basic nutritional requirements for each person and specific dietary practices appropriate for individuals with special needs.

Understanding the relationship between food and illness helps in making positive choices if avoiding illness is a priority. Young children get their attitudes about food from adults. Food is used negatively in our culture as a pacifier, a time filler, or as an incentive. These negative uses of food

Objectives for School Health Programs

1. Continuing appraisal of each child's health status.
2. Understanding of each youngster's health needs.
3. Supervision and guidance of each child's health.
4. Development of the highest possible level of health for each child.
5. Prevention of defects and disorders.
6. Detection and referral of all defects and disorders.
7. Special health provisions for the exceptional child.
8. Reduction in the incidence of communicable diseases.
9. Positive health awareness and a desire for a high level of health in each child.
10. Development of wholesome health attitudes.
11. Development of healthful personal practices.
12. Acquisition of scientific and functional knowledge of personal and community health.
13. Development of an appreciation of aesthetic factors related to health.
14. Development of a high level of self-esteem in each child.
15. Effective social adjustment.
16. Hygienic mental environment at school.

SOURCE: Anderson, CL, Creswell WH: *School Health Practice*. Mosby, 1980.

can lead to obesity and subsequent development of disease. Certain types of cancer and heart disease, among other diseases, are linked to excessive consumption of an inappropriate nutrient balance. These negative dietary behaviors need to be replaced by positive ones.

Children need to be taught the basic uses of food, regardless of whether they have a food-related problem. For example, children who are obese first need to learn the principles of a basic diet and then the specific dietary practices that are related to obesity. A child who is a diabetic needs to know the basic food combinations and then learn to modify the diet to meet the specific needs for that disability. In teaching a child about nutrition, modeling is the most important technique. The use of too many facts should be minimized. The desired outcomes are as follows:

1. To understand the relationship between food and the body
2. To develop a sense of excitement and adventure in learning about food
3. To begin to develop a personal responsibility for food selection, understanding the consequences of the food choices made (Frankel, 1980)

Specific nutritional techniques for children include regular meals, nutritious snacks spaced between meals and at least 1½ hours before a regular meal, and beginning the day with a wholesome breakfast. Eating slowly and chewing completely increase enjoyment and promote effective digestion.

Parents need to study their own dietary habits and needs and be aware of how these habits are being learned by their children. They also need to be aware of the food intake of their children, especially in the school-age period when children are not home for each meal. Attention needs to be given to the school lunch program and after-school snacks and, in the case of working parents, breakfast for those children responsible for getting their own meal. Some unsupervised children eat food that can alter behavior and result in poor school performance. Being aware of the role specific foods play in special problems is important. Food plays a role in the following illnesses or maladaptive situations: dental problems, obesity and its sequelae, hyperactivity, allergies, and eating disorders.

Dental problems The prevention of dental disease related to food intake focuses on sugar intake. Decreasing the intake of sugar and removing the plaque buildup by proper brushing and flossing is primary dental prevention. It is not necessarily the amount of sugar consumed that causes plaque but is instead the pattern of intake. For example, eating a large amount of sweets all at one time followed by proper dental hygiene is more effective in preventing cavities than eating small amounts without brushing. Encouraging schools and other public facilities to eliminate cavity-causing foods from vending machines is another prevention method.

The avoidance of foods that commonly predispose the child to develop tooth decay is recommended. In addition to eliminating sugar-based sweets, prime offenders include sugared cereals and white bread. Milk products are not allowed to remain in the mouth without taking the appropriate dental hygienic measures because they stimulate bacterial growth, which leads to dental caries. For this reason, parents are encouraged not to give the infant a bottle in bed.

A diet high in calcium, phosphorus, and appropriate vitamins encourages the development of strong teeth. Oral fluoride preparations reduce the later incidence of tooth decay.

In addition to diet, individual self-care behaviors include brushing the teeth with fluoride toothpaste, using fluoride rinses, and taking advantage of routine dental care. Toothbrushing in early childhood helps the child begin good dental habits early in life. Because the early morning and evening routines might be hurried, children of working parents might need extra attention and reminders to brush their teeth.

Devices such as bathroom stools, special toothbrushes, and Water Piks® enable even small children to participate fully in their dental care. Routine dental prophylaxis is recommended throughout the life span.

Sleep Recognizing the effect of sleep on daily life is important. Children have regular sleep/wake cycles that are determined by the body's natural biorhythms. A regular bedtime and a rest schedule as close to the individual's biorhythms as possible will allow the body to rejuvenate. Children can be taught to become aware of their biorhythms and to rest and relax according to the cues they receive. Young children often follow rituals such as rocking themselves to sleep or having bedtime stories read to them around sleep time. The pleasure of having a story read, a soft cuddly animal, or a blanket should be respected. The environment for rest is important. The use of low music or night-lights can calm an upset child. Decreasing activity before sleep is helpful because many children need time to wind down.

Psychosocial factors affecting sleep include the quality of the relationship with the parents or siblings and fears. In the early childhood period, fears and separation anxiety are normal. Many children are afraid to go to sleep because they are afraid to be separated from their parents or afraid of "monsters." Sleep is not used as a punishment. When a child is threatened with bed for disruptive behavior, a negative reason is given for a positive health behavior.

Sleeping with parents has many implications, the primary one being sleep disruption for both parent and child. The underlying causes of this behavior might vary from overdependency in the child to loneliness in the parent. Some children initiate the behavior as a way to seek comfort during a nightmare or to obtain warmth. Unfortunately, sleeping with parents can become habit forming and cause stress between parent and child or between parent and spouse.

Each family needs to consider the needs of both parent and child when dealing with the behavior. The nurse needs to be alert for any unstated contributing factors such as single-parent loneliness, sexual rejection by a spouse, or limited space in poor families (see Chapter 5 for a more detailed approach to the problem).

Elimination Elimination is the body's natural mechanism for ridding itself of waste through perspiration, voiding, and defecation.

Generally, bowel elimination is regular and need not be assisted by laxatives. The individual differences depend on rhythm, exercise patterns, and the kind of food eaten. Attitudes toward elimination are important. To ignore such issues as readiness and the development of sphincter control or to use fear and coercion during toilet training will affect the child's attitude about defecation in the future. Certain culturally laden ideas about cleanliness and elimination must be considered in health promotion. Many children will hold their urine or bowel movement because they are unable to use a toilet outside their own home or at certain times of the day. They might have inaccurate ideas about unclean toilets and disease or embarrassment over odors.

Nurses need to encourage parents to approach toilet training in a calm, nonthreatening manner to encourage positive elimination habits in their children. Parents can assess readiness for toilet training and encourage regular elimination according to the child's own natural schedule (see Chapter 5). Children can be taught how to use public toilet seats properly to avoid direct contact with the seat itself.

Children of all ages should be encouraged to take the time for proper elimination and to be in tune with their bodies' needs. Adequate water and proper nutritional intake will help promote regular elimination.

Exercise The three major forms of exercise include aerobic exercises, which increase cardiovascular function, stretching exercises, which are important to muscle and bone structure, and body-building exercises, which are not essential. To derive the most benefit from exercise, the person should include exercises from both the aerobic and stretching groups in any exercise routine. Exercise needs to be fun so that it is incorporated more easily into one's lifestyle. For some people, exercise is a competitive activity. The competition, however, is secondary to the health benefits. Proper exercise needs to be regular, at least three to four times a week. The safety aspects of exercise are important, and supervision is essential. Warm-up and cool-down periods need to precede and follow any strenuous exercise.

Exercise programs in the schools need to be carried over to the home on weekends and during the summer. These programs should be part of the routine family activities. Family walks, hiking trips, and swimming and running together are also beneficial family activities. Many activities can be either group or solitary. Jumping rope and basketball are activities that can be done alone or with a group and can be performed from childhood through adulthood.

The rebirth in the interest in exercise and its role in health means that exercise is being used for everything from curing emotional problems to alleviating physical maladies. Children are happy when they are in motion, and they move naturally. Adults, from presidents to sports figures, are models for children for the positive use of exercise. Children need to be taught to extend exercise into adult life. They should know that regular exercise will affect health positively by preventing heart disease, reducing blood pressure, controlling weight, and increasing lung capacity. Exercise should be incorporated into the child's regular daily routine to establish healthful habits that will carry over into adulthood.

One danger of exercise is overuse of the body, which can result in structural or functional injury. Children therefore need to be provided with proper clothing and equipment, especially footwear, to prevent this occurrence. Stretching exercises and cool-down periods need to be components of all aerobic workouts to minimize adverse effects.

"Life sports," such as swimming, tennis, and biking need to be encouraged at an early age. Unlike team sports, these aerobic activities are enjoyable throughout the life span and provide optimal health benefits.

Physical care Clothing provides protection against exposure to extreme temperatures and foreign bodies. Clothing, to promote health, needs to be loose and clean. Attention needs to be given to the role of clothing in the development of self-esteem. The need to be part of the group is related to clothing fads and fashion. In adolescence, clothing gives an opportunity to develop individuality. Many children have their own style of dress. They should be allowed to experiment with the kinds of clothes and colors they enjoy.

The purpose of bathing is to prevent or protect from disease and to enhance appearance. It is also excellent for relaxation. Young children do not need to bathe every day. Twice a week and as necessary to remove visible dirt is sufficient. The face and hands need frequent washing, as well as the diaper area in infants. Too much bathing or extremely hot water can deplete body moisture. For dry skin, oils need to be replaced. For safety, the use of oil in the bath water of very young children should be monitored to prevent slipping. Parents need to be reminded to check the water level and water temperature and to supervise young children during bath time.

The notion of cleanliness as a preventive measure against disease is difficult for young children to understand. Handwashing can be taught as a habit before meals, after toileting, and after handling animals. As children move into school, they will learn the facts related to the spread of disease and begin to take responsibility for preventing the transfer of disease.

Children can be taught that their bodies are necessary for living, and they can develop the concepts for maximum use of the physical self. Caring for the body through cleanliness, safety, and protection against abuse are part of the proper use of the body parts. For example, maximum eye health requires attention to diet, safety, cleanliness, proper lights, and rest. Correct posture, proper nutrition, adequate rest, and exercise are essential for optimal body structure.

Respect for one's own body and the bodies of others is an important concept to be taught to children. Parents need to provide privacy for their children and encourage them to respect the privacy of others. Healthy respect for the self increases the child's feeling of importance and allows for appropriate relationships with others.

Health services Child health care includes a well-child health maintenance schedule (Table 11-2). A comprehensive health history encompasses both the present and past history. A family profile, the child's profile, a review of body systems, and a general care history (dietary, elimination, sleep and rest, and development) form the data base.

The assessment includes objective data in the form of a physical examination; necessary laboratory studies; screening procedures, such as vision and auditory screening; and

TABLE 11-2 Health Maintenance Schedule

Nursing activities	Ages
Assessments	2 weeks; 2, 4, 6, 9, 12, and 18 months; 2, 3, 5, 8, 11, 13, 15, and 17 years
Complete history and physical examination	First visit, interval history thereafter
Immunization (DTP—diphtheria, tetanus, pertussis; OPV—oral polio vaccine; MMR—measles, mumps, rubella; TD—tetanus, diphtheria)	According to schedule
Rubella serology	Prepuberty (unvaccinated girls)
Haemophilus b	24 months
Tuberculin (tine) test	1, 3, 5, 11, and 15 years
Hemoglobin/hematocrit	1, 4, 9, 12, 14, and 16 years
Lead screening	2 years
Urinalysis	6 months; 2, 3, 4, 5, 6, 9–10, 11–12, 13–15, and 15–18 years
Urine culture	3 and 8 years
Blood pressure	4 years and at each subsequent visit
Vision/hearing	1, 4, and 6 months; 1, 3, and 6 years and at each subsequent visit
Language	2, 3, and 5 years
Dental	6, 7–8, 13–15, and 15–18 years
Scoliosis	9–10, 11–12, and 13–15 years
Counseling (nutrition, physical care, psychosocial concerns, sex education, safety, family interaction)	Each visit

the plan of action based on the data collected, client's needs, and anticipatory guidance by the nurse.

Support for parents Family life has changed dramatically since the 1950s as families have been affected by technical, environmental, political, and economic forces. Children are now influenced by a variety of factors outside their families as they come in contact with television, day-care centers, government agencies, schools, and religious institutions. As all of these factors influence the family, they challenge parents to monitor these factors by being informed and selective about the influences to which their children are exposed. Parents then need to decide when to encourage or restrain their children's participation. In an increasingly complex world, some parents have difficulty teaching values, setting limits, and promoting development in ways that are consistent with the expectations of the family and the community at large.

Nurses in community-based health agencies, sometimes in collaboration with social services, might conduct parenting classes. In other settings the nurse intervenes to refer parents to educational sessions sponsored by churches, school systems, or private organizations. The nurse might, however, need to consider whether a family's financial resources make such a referral feasible or whether a social service agency can offer financial aid.

Another source of confusion for parents is the vast array of advice they receive. Relatives, friends, books, and other well-meaning advisors might offer conflicting solutions to problems and information about childrearing. Many parents need the nurse to help them sort through the advice and determine the solution to a specific problem or general parenting style that is most consistent with their values, cultural norms, parenting goals, and child's personality.

The nurse might find it useful to refer parents to books about parenting. An extensive body of literature is available in libraries and bookstores. Therefore, the nurse will want to be familiar with the family's needs and preferences before making specific recommendations. Printed materials also are best used in conjunction with counseling sessions to provide parents with opportunities to discuss their reactions. Books that describe "how to be a parent" can be helpful, but they also can confuse parents if the information is misinterpreted, inappropriate, or followed too rigidly.

Many parents also worry about leaving their children with others, whether with a babysitter occasionally or with a child-care center on a regular basis. They might express concerns about safety, nutrition, cleanliness, or the overall quality of attention given by child-care providers. The nurse often can help parents choose appropriate child care by providing information. Some parents need checklists of points to consider in selecting a sitter. Others need to know about options available for child care during the day.

Some parents need to know that child-care providers,

Guidelines for Picking a Sitter

1. *Recommendations:* Check with friends or relatives who have used the sitter previously. Discuss an adult sitter's qualifications with the agency or, if younger, with parents, teachers, or club leaders. Inquire about letters of reference or special classes in babysitting responsibilities.
2. *Age:* The sitter's age varies somewhat with the child's age and child-care need. Adults are preferred for extended periods of time such as weekends or for several days. Young infants require a sitter who is thoroughly familiar with infant care and demands—either an adult or an experienced high school student who has younger siblings. Elementary school children can care for young children for brief periods during the day. It is usually best if the babysitter resides in the neighborhood and his/her parents are at home. Older children might resent sitters who are close in age; it is best to have an adult in that situation.
3. *Experience:* It is best if the sitter has had previous experience with child care, including the care of younger siblings or relatives. If using an agency service, inquire about the sitter's employment history. If the sitter's experience is limited, begin with a short assignment.
4. *Experience with your child:* If the sitter lives in the neighborhood, evaluate interactions with the child in other situations, child's response to sitter, and sitter's ability to tend to the child's needs. If the sitter is unknown, it might be helpful to have the sitter come for an hour the day before to get acquainted with the child so that the child will view the sitter as a friend. If coming the day before is inconvenient, have the sitter arrive an hour earlier for the same purpose.
5. *Personal characteristics:* The sitter should be healthy, with no acute illnesses, have mature judgment, be responsible, and be knowledgeable about safety in general and specific safety for the child's age. The sitter should enjoy being with and playing with children and be patient. The sitter should follow the parent's directions about food, bedtime, television, clothing, and other routines and rules. The sitter should not ask to have personal friends of either sex over while sitting and should not use the telephone for social calls. The sitter should be told where the parent may be reached, if necessary; the expected return time; emergency telephone numbers; and where to put messages.

Guidelines for Selecting Day Care

1. *Facilities:* Should be clean; have safe, sturdy equipment inside and sturdy playground equipment outside; and be furnished according to the size and age of the children. Rooms should be bright and cheery, with no peeling paint or wallpaper. General safety measures should be observed (eg, wall plugs, fire extinguishers, no dangling cords, kitchen area gated, smoke detector alarms, and sprinkler system).
2. *Philosophy of care:* Should have organized activities and a structured day that includes independent, free play. Assess the tools and toys available for creative expression, supervision of interactions, and willingness to discuss the child's experience with objects and tools in the act of creating. A variety of play and learning experiences should be available. Observe the nature of the discipline practiced.
3. *Organization:* Note the age divisions of the groups, how many groups, and the space allotment. Evaluate how meals are served and feeding managed. Note the type of food served and its appropriateness. Note the provision for naps and willingness to adapt to each child's need for more or less rest.
4. *Policy for illness:* Evaluate the center's plan if the child becomes ill or injured at the facility. Inquire whether the center has a firm policy about children not attending when ill with a "cold." Does the center provide transportation to a primary health care agency?
5. *Ratio between staff and children:* Assess if each infant or child is provided with sufficient individual attention. Do time and staffing allow individual or small group play and teaching experiences?
6. *Recommendations:* Be sure the center is state-approved and licensed and passes all board of health and safety regulations and fire code requirements. Obtain references from friends or relatives who have used the center. Drop in unexpectedly at various times to check the operation.
7. *Child's response:* The best indicator is the child's reaction. Note whether the child is happy when picked up, reasonably happy to be attending, talks positively about the staff and other children, and whether the child seems to have a special or preferred staff person.

National Environmental Health Objectives

1. Control of toxic agents responsible for cancer, birth defects, respiratory disease, kidney disease, and other chronic diseases.
2. Decrease in the prevalence of lead toxicity.
3. Eradication of exposure to toxic chemicals that cause birth defects and miscarriages.
4. Reduction of the risk factors caused by toxic waste.
5. Increased air quality by emission control programs.
6. Protection of community water systems.
7. Safe toxic waste disposal for industrial residential waste.
8. Elimination of dangerous pesticides, fungicides, and herbicides known to be carcinogenic or mutagenic in humans.
9. Decrease in unnecessary diagnostic radiographs in medical and dental practice.

especially those who care for a child daily, also might require information about a specific child's developmental needs. For example, if an infant who is learning to crawl spends each day at a babysitter's home, the parent will need to assess that environment to determine whether the child's safety needs are being met.

Health protection measures—maintaining public health Health protection measures are directed toward both the general population and the individual. They prevent dental and infectious diseases as well as limit exposure to toxic agents, accidents, and injuries. Protection measures include fluoridation of water, immunizations, and other strategies that will achieve national environmental health objectives.

Fluoridation Fluoridation is a dental health protection measure. Its goal is to reduce the incidence of cavities in permanent teeth and to reduce gum disease. The use of fluoride in community water and in toothpastes and rinses and fluoride supplements are current practices. Fluoride has been used in community and school water systems and has reduced cavities up to 90% in children (US Department of Health and Human Services, 1981a).

Immunization The goal of immunization is to prevent the occurrence of an infectious disease by introducing an antigen or an antibody (see Chapter 25). Immunization programs may be started on any well child who is 2 months of age and weighs more than 10 lb.

TABLE 11-3 Recommended Schedule for Active Immunization of Normal Infants and Children

Recommended age*	Vaccine(s)†	Comments
2 months	DTP-1‡, OPV-1§	Can be given earlier in areas of high endemicity
4 months	DTP-2, OPV-2	6-week to 2-month interval desired between OPV doses to avoid interference
6 months	DTP-3	Additional dose of OPV at this time optional for use in areas with a high risk of polio exposure
15 months¶	MMR**, DTP-4, OPV-3	Completion of primary series
24 months	*Haemophilus b*	Can be given at 18–23 months for children at increased risk
4–6 years††	DTP-5, OPV-4	Preferably at or before school entry
14–16 years	Td§§	Repeat every 10 years throughout life

SOURCE: New immunization guidelines issued by the CDC. *Hosp Pract* (March) 1983; 18:1000.
*These recommended ages should not be construed as absolute; that is, 2 months can be 6–10 weeks, etc.
†For all products used, consult manufacturer's package enclosure for instructions for storage, handling, and administration. Immunobiologics prepared by different manufacturers might vary, and those of the same manufacturer might change from time to time. The package insert should be followed for a specific product.
‡DTP—diphtheria and tetanus toxoids and pertussis vaccine.
§OPV—oral, attenuated poliovirus vaccine contains poliovirus types 1, 2, and 3.
¶Simultaneous administration of MMR, DTP, and OPV is appropriate for patients whose compliance with medical care recommendations cannot be assured.
**MMR—live measles, mumps, and rubella viruses in a combined vaccine.
††Up to the seventh birthday.
§§Td—adult tetanus toxoid and diphtheria toxoid in combination, which contains the same dose of tetanus toxoid as DTP or DT and a reduced dose of diphtheria toxoid.

Immunizations have greatly reduced the worldwide incidence of diseases. Smallpox, for example, has been virtually eliminated as a result of vigorous immunization policies. Cases of poliomyelitis, rubella, and rubeola have decreased markedly since the development of vaccines against these diseases. One of the goals of the US Department of Health and Human Services is to have 90% of the nation's children properly immunized by the year 1990. As of January 1987 (85% immunized), the target appears realistic.

The national goals for immunization include adopting standard records, reviewing procedures to identify children needing immunization, and making the services available regardless of the ability of those needing immunization to pay (US Department of Health and Human Services, 1981). Although the incidence of communicable disease has decreased as a result of a vigorous immunization effort, the US government is still concerned with keeping the numbers of immunized people at a high level. The success of the immunization program has contributed to public apathy in this regard.

Nurses need to take responsibility for disseminating information about immunizations through the school curriculum, during health maintenance visits, and through day-care centers and other community forums. (The Centers for Disease Control's recommendations for childhood immunizations are listed in Table 11-3.)

Immunization Guidelines

1. Live viruses should be administered at least 1 month apart if not given on the same day.
2. There should be intervals of 2–3 weeks to 1 month between the administrations of an inactivated virus.
3. Live viruses and inactivated viruses can be given simultaneously at different sites or together orally.
4. Live viruses may be given in licensed combinations such as MR and MMR.
5. Killed viruses may be given simultaneously at different sites.
6. If immune serum globulin has been given, a minimum of 6 weeks must elapse before a live virus can be given. It is better to wait 3 months.
7. Vaccines associated with adverse local or systemic effects (for example, typhoid and cholera) should not be given simultaneously.

SOURCE: Adapted from Centers for Disease Control, 1983.

Contraindications and Precautions Related to Immunization

1. Do not immunize a child with an active infectious disease or one who has a febrile illness, with the exception of the common cold.
2. Do not administer a live-virus vaccine to a child who has a malignancy and/or is on radiation therapy, is receiving an alkylating agent or an antimetabolite, or is immune-depressed naturally or artificially.
3. Do not immunize a person who had a previous allergic reaction to the vaccine or an individual who has received a blood product within the past 8 weeks.
4. A child in a family with a known member who has an immunologic problem should not be vaccinated or immunized without consultation with a physician.
5. Although a pregnant woman should not receive rubella vaccine, susceptible children living with a pregnant woman should be vaccinated.
6. Extreme caution should be exercised in giving vaccines that are grown on fibroblast tissue cultures of chickens and ducks (such as measles, mumps, or influenza vaccines) to children with known allergies to feathers, eggs, chickens, or ducks.
7. Vaccines containing antimicrobial agents are contraindicated in people who are sensitive to antimicrobial drugs.
8. The administration of DPT vaccine to children with known neurologic problems might be contraindicated.

SOURCE: Williams L: Childhood immunization. *Pediatr Nurs* (Jan/Feb) 1982 8:18–22.

Recent publicity regarding adverse effects of the pertussis (whooping cough) component of the DTP (diphtheria, tetanus, pertussis) vaccine has lead the Centers for Disease Control to issue new guidelines regarding the administration of the vaccine. Children who exhibit the following reactions to the vaccine should not have the vaccine repeated: fever of 105°F or higher, shocklike episode, severe crying lasting 3 hours or an unusual high-pitched cry (within 2 days), convulsions (within 3 days), an allergic reaction, severe alterations in consciousness within 7 days (*Morbidity and Mortality Weekly Report,* July, 1985). The vaccine is contraindicated in children with certain neurologic problems such as epileptic seizures. Although the safety of the pertussis vaccine has aroused public concern, the benefit of the vaccine seems to outweigh the possible adverse consequences for most children. (A discussion of tetanus is found in Chapter 24.)

A vaccine newly recommended by the Academy of Pediatrics is the vaccine against *Haemophilus influenzae* type b (Hib). *Haemophilus influenzae* is a bacterium that, when it affects young children, can cause meningitis, epiglottitis, and joint infections, among other systemic diseases. Because diseases caused by Hib are contagious and young children are particularly susceptible to their adverse consequences, it is recommended that children of age 24 months receive the vaccine. A single dose confers the proper immunity. Possible side effects from the vaccine include redness and swelling at the injection site and fever, although the vaccine causes side effects in relatively few children.

Education and environmental protection Additional health protection measures include water supply protection through mechanisms such as chlorination, control of animals that carry diseases, and other public health policies such as pasteurization of milk.

Education is a powerful health protection strategy in dealing with infectious diseases. The educational process changes individual health habits and environmental practices. For example, individuals and groups need to be educated about sexually transmitted diseases such as gonorrhea, syphilis, herpes, and acquired immunodeficiency disease (AIDS). Children and their parents need information about sexually transmitted diseases to reduce the risk of contracting them. School-age children need to be educated and informed before and during the time of greatest risk of contracting sexually transmitted disease. Peer counselors are effective when working with adolescents. Mass training can be effective for health professionals and others. Health care professionals working in clinical settings and schools need training. Improved public awareness about sexually transmitted diseases and assurance of confidentiality, along with the help of the media, has made prevention and treatment more effective.

In addition to school-age children and adolescents, according to the Public Health Service, target populations for education and treatment related to sexually transmitted diseases are adolescents, homosexual groups, and women with pelvic inflammatory diseases (Hacker, Palchik-Allen, & Rosey, 1980). Prevention requires early detection and treatment. Community control of prostitution and the discouragement of sexual promiscuity are other protection issues in need of community support. (See Chapter 28 for information about detection and treatment of sexually transmitted diseases.)

Environmental protection includes dispersing information to schools and the private sector. Additional public health education facilitates disease control through safer water and food, increased technology for water sterilization, water treatment systems, and improved design of health care facilities (US Department of Health and Human Services, 1981c).

Health education regarding toxic substances needs to occur on both individual and group levels. The problems of industrial and institutional disposal of waste, air control, and air pollution associated with automobile emissions have implications for the private and public sectors. The individual has less control in this area but can be effective through political and community action. Parents need to be aware of the potential threat to the family's health from exposure to hazardous substances. Children can be taught by parents and through the school health curriculum to avoid vacant lots and abandoned buildings near industrial sites and also not to eat food or drink water from unsafe areas.

Secondary Level of Prevention: The Nurse's Role

The secondary level of prevention involves factors that determine the extent of illness once it has occurred. The nurse's role again involves assessing the characteristics of the child, agent, and environment and intervening to prevent the disease or dysfunction from becoming severe or being transmitted.

Assessment data obtained from the child, agent, and environment are similar to the data obtained in primary prevention. If symptoms of illness are apparent, these indicate that health promotion and protection strategies were ineffective. Nursing strategies at the secondary level of prevention are directed toward screening measures to detect and arrest health deviations, isolation and control of communicable disease, prevention of infection, and prevention of complications.

Assessment at the Secondary Level of Prevention

Characteristics of the child Assessment of the child includes determining such factors as psychosocial and emotional health, cognitive and developmental level, understanding of disease concepts and body functions, and self-care level. Physical bodily differences in children often determine the susceptibility to and extent of illness. For example, girls are more prone to develop urinary tract infections because their anatomic structure facilitates bacterial invasion.

Individual responsibility for cleanliness and positive health habits can arrest the extent of disease. Children who are reliable about hand washing after toileting are less likely to develop or spread diseases related to hand-to-mouth contact. Those children who cover their mouths when coughing or sneezing and who properly dispose of tissues can limit the extent of droplet-spread organisms.

Characteristics of the agent The nature of microorganisms and their modes of transmission affect disease occurrence and severity. (See "Assessment at the Primary Level of Prevention, Characteristics of the Agent" for an in-depth discussion of these agents.) The extent of illness also is affected by such factors as diet, stress, environmental chemicals such as lead, abusable substances, and allergens.

Because this level is determined by manifestations of illness, devices used to control the severity of a problem might be considered to be agents during this phase. For example, eyeglasses and hearing aids, although used to improve the functional quality of the senses, might actually be detrimental if not maintained properly.

Conservation of energy—sleep/rest—is an important variable in preventing complications of illness and as such becomes an agent during the acute phase. Other treatment measures used to alleviate disease or restore health also are considered to be agents.

Characteristics of the environment In addition to environmental factors such as air and water quality, socioeconomic status, parents' educational level, and conditions in the home, the acute phase also includes access to community resources and mechanisms for referral. Groups such as the Leukemia Society, the Arthritis Foundation, and the American Lung Association provide assistance to children and families (see Appendix D). This assistance might take the form of actual financial aid for medical costs or of providing group and individual support.

Efforts are directed toward minimizing disease consequences and disseminating information to increase public awareness. Nurses need to assess the availability of community agencies and other supports to make appropriate referrals for illness intervention.

Interventions at the Secondary Level of Prevention

Screening Although health screening certainly can be considered an aspect of child health promotion, specific screening procedures are performed to detect the presence of a deficit. Abnormal screening results indicate the need

TABLE 11-4 Vision Screening

Test	Age	Nursing implication
Direct observation for ocular pathology	All	Refer to physician if signs of inflammation; strabismus; opacities; foreign bodies
Visual acuity tests Snellen; Allen/picture cards "E" Game	Early to middle childhood and older	Refer for further testing children 3 years if greater than 20/50; 4 years if greater than 20/40; 5 years and over if greater than 20/30
Cover test	Older children able to fixate	Refer for evidence of strabismus
Corneal light reflex	Infants and younger children	Refer for evidence of strabismus
Hardy-Rand-Ritter; Ishihara	Late childhood	No referral for color blindness, but parents and teachers need to be aware of the problem

for intervention to prevent a further deficit. Screening is performed on a regular basis as part of the health maintenance schedule and as needed if problems are suspected.

Vision Complete vision screening includes tests for muscle coordination, ocular disorders, color vision, and visual acuity (Sprague, 1983). (The indications for referral are presented in Table 11-4. Specific vision tests are described in detail in Chapters 10 and 32.) Nursing strategies for limiting vision deficits include the following:

1. Encouraging children to wear eyeglasses if they are prescribed
2. Teaching children to avoid eyestrain by using proper light when reading
3. Encouraging the use of protective glasses when working with power tools or caustic chemicals
4. Teaching children not to rub their eyes, particularly when their eyes come in contact with a foreign object
5. Recommending plastic lenses for children who participate actively in sports
6. Teaching the proper care of contact lenses

Hearing Routine auditory screening is performed during infancy and childhood. Special considerations that warrant auditory screening of infants are as follows:

1. Family history of a childhood hearing deficit
2. Congenital perinatal infection such as cytomegalovirus or rubella
3. Anatomic malformations of the head and neck
4. Birthweight less than 1500 g
5. Hyperbilirubinemia (elevated blood bilirubin) at a level requiring an exchange transfusion
6. Meningitis
7. Severe asphyxia, including birth hypoxia (Downs, 1983)

Special indications for auditory screening during childhood include the following:

1. Children with a history of frequent episodes of otitis media (middle ear infection)
2. Inattention in the classroom
3. Apparent hearing difficulties in the home environment

(Table 11-5 lists the auditory screening tests and referral indications. Detailed descriptions of the tests are found in Chapters 10 and 32.) Interventions directed toward limiting hearing deficits are as follows:

1. Encourage prompt treatment of an otitis episode.
2. Teach proper ear care, including cleaning and the removal of cerumen.
3. Discourage loud radio, stereo, or television volumes.
4. Teach children not to insert objects into their ears, especially cotton-tipped swabs.

Tuberculosis Although the incidence of tuberculosis has decreased dramatically since the mid-twentieth century, children, particularly those from foreign countries where the disease is still endemic, are susceptible. Tuberculosis is spread by droplets, and the incidence increases in overcrowded environments.

The most common tuberculosis skin test is the tine test, which is administered at approximately 1 year of age and every several years throughout childhood. A positive tine test (2 mm of induration) warrants rescreening with purified protein derivative (PPD). Positive PPD necessitates a more comprehensive diagnostic workup, including a chest

TABLE 11-5 Auditory Screening

Test	Age	Nursing implication
Reflex elicitation	Birth to 3 months	Refer if reflexes absent in response to sound
Hearing and communication questionnaire	Birth to 12 months	No referral needed if parents report child's response to their vocalizations
Crib-O-Gram	Newborn	No response to stimulus of 90 dB peaking at 3000 Hz indicates referral
Tympanometry	6 months and older	Refer if there is abnormal middle ear pressure and absent acoustic reflex
Pure tone audiometry	3–5 years	Failure of child to respond to any one frequency (1000, 2000, 4000 Hz) at 25 dB indicates referral
Audiometry	Older than 5 years	Failure at any frequency indicates referral

radiograph and sputum examinations. It must be remembered that children who have been immunized against tuberculosis with the bacille Calmette-Guérin (BCG) vaccine will demonstrate a positive PPD.

Lead Sources of lead in the environment vary from lead paint to the atmosphere (see Chapter 12). Lead screening is routine during early childhood because children in this age group characteristically use their mouths to explore their surroundings. The screening procedure involves a fingerstick capillary blood sample, which is tested for lead and erythrocyte protoporphyrin. The normal lead level is below 25 μg/dL (micrograms per 100 mL of whole blood). Results in the 25–55 mg/dL range might indicate treatment depending on results of additional tests (*Morbidity and Mortality Weekly Report,* February 1985). Nurses need to encourage parents to keep children away from lead-based house paint, painted antique furniture and toys, and improperly baked earthenware—all sources of lead. Children exhibiting signs of pica (see Chapter 12) should be referred for special care.

Anemia Lowered hemoglobin and hematocrit levels might indicate iron deficiency anemia (see Chapter 26). A capillary blood sample reveals the following abnormal values:

Hemoglobin
- Infant < 11 g/dL
- Child (6–12 yr) < 11.5 g/dL
- Adolescent (male) < 13 g/dL
- (female) < 12 g/dL

Hematocrit
- Infant < 34%
- Child (6–12 yr) < 35%
- Adolescent (male) < 37%
- (female) < 36%

Interventions are based on teaching proper dietary practices to increase iron consumption. Encouraging compliance with taking prescribed medication is an important nursing strategy.

Scoliosis Posture screening is important for all children, but particularly for preadolescent and adolescent girls. The causes of scoliosis are varied, but if unchecked, scoliosis can lead to visible structural and functional deformities (see Chapter 30). Observation of the child includes visual inspection of frontal and dorsal posture. The nurse checks for uneven hip and shoulder levels as well as for muscular disproportion. In addition to the standing posture, the child should be seen while bending loosely from the waist as if to touch the toes. Again, visible curvatures or uneven muscular development are noted. Because poor posture is a contributing factor in scoliosis, nurses encourage proper posture and body mechanics in children. Schoolbooks or heavy objects should be carried in a backpack rather than on either hip.

Control of communicable disease Nursing strategies in controlling communicable diseases are directed toward containing the illness and preventing complications. Droplet-spread illnesses, such as colds, can be contained by teaching the child and family proper hygienic measures and disposal of contaminated articles. Children can be taught from an early age to cover their mouths while coughing or sneezing. Tissues that have been contaminated with nasal discharge are not left where other family members can come in contact with them. Children need to be encouraged to wash their hands frequently, particularly after coughing.

Strict isolation is not necessary, although close contact with other family members can and should be discouraged. Young children in particular need constant reminders to prevent droplet spread.

Personal and environmental cleanliness is an important deterrent to contact diseases. Among the contact conditions are impetigo, pediculosis, fungal and parasitic infections, and sexually transmitted diseases (see Chapters 18 and 28). Children should be advised to wash their hands thoroughly after elimination and not to share articles of clothing, particularly hats and underwear. Children need to be reminded continuously to develop these habits because they often feel there is too little time for such practices. In their enthusiasm they might swap baseball hats or combs, leading to the rapid spread of lice. Simple explanations of the dangers inherent in such actions will help establish positive behaviors.

Prevention of infection and its complications Measures taken at the secondary level of prevention will decrease the potential for disability resulting from unchecked illness. Simple prevention measures such as thorough cleaning of wounds and the application of antibacterial ointments will decrease the incidence of skin infection (see Chapter 24).

When children sustain abrasions, parents usually are informed and institute appropriate action. Nurses might need to make parents aware, however, that often the older child is too busy to stop playing to have an injury attended to. Untreated wounds might be noticed days later when the child complains of pain in the area. Nurses need to encourage parents to be observant of their children's physical state. Prompt and adequate treatment of illness and injury will prevent the appearance of more serious complications.

Essential Concepts

- Children can make positive health behaviors an integral part of their lives with the help of the nurse.
- Respect for individuals and their heritage, along with choices to attain one's physical, mental, and spiritual potential, provide a holistic concept of wellness.
- The concept of health is viewed in relation to the wellness-illness continuum.
- The health status of children has improved as a result of increased emphasis on prevention and individual responsibility for health.
- Health promotion and health protection strategies are directed toward the goal of preventing illness.
- Levels of illness prevention are primary, secondary, and tertiary, corresponding to factors that prevent the occurrence of an illness, reduce its severity, and limit complications.
- Data for nursing assessment and diagnosis arise from the examination of the characteristics inherent in the child, the agent, and the environment at all levels of prevention.
- Characteristics of the child include prenatal and hereditary factors, cognitive and developmental level, emotional state, understanding of wellness concepts, and health habits.
- Characteristics of the agent encompass the nature and action of organisms and the effects of stress, toxic chemicals, abusable substances, and diet on the child.
- Important environmental factors include air and water quality, socioeconomic status, education of parents, and conditions in the home.
- Nursing strategies for health promotion in children are directed toward increasing consumer awareness and health education.
- Children as health consumers assume control over and responsibility for their own health status.
- Influential factors for successful health education of the child are the parents, peers, teachers, and health professionals.
- Health education encompasses techniques for staying healthy and for reducing the severity and spread of illness.
- Health education is geared toward the developmental characteristics and age-related learning styles of children.
- Techniques are effective in specialized areas of nutrition, dental problems, sleep, elimination, exercise, and physical care.
- Adequate health maintenance requires regular health promotion and well-child monitoring.
- Health protection measures include fluoridation of the water supply, immunization, pasteurization, and other public health policies directed toward environmental protection and the control of communicable disease.

- Health education is a powerful health protection strategy.
- Interventions to reduce the severity of a child's deficit include visual, auditory, lead, anemia, tuberculosis, and scoliosis screenings.
- Nursing strategies for illness control encompass teaching an awareness of disease transmission and actions children can take to counteract communicability.
- The complications resulting from an illness can be reduced by prompt and adequate treatment and referral to appropriate community agencies.

References

Downs M: Early identification and intervention for auditory problems. In: *Detection of Developmental Problems in Children*. Krajicek M, Tomlinson A (editors). University Park Press, 1983.

Frankel R: It's never too early for nutrition education. *School Health* (Sept) 1980; 50(7): 387–391.

Hacker S, Palchik-Allen N, Rosey C: Factors influencing the success of a community VD program held in a university facility. *Public Health Rep* (May/June) 1980; 95: 247–252.

Lewis CE, Lewis M: Child-initiated health care. *J School Health* (March) 1980; 50: 144–148.

Lunney M: Nursing diagnosis: Refining the system. *Am J Nurs* (March) 1982; 82: 456–459.

Mattson PH: *Holistic Health in Perspective*. Mayfield, 1982.

Morbidity and Mortality Weekly Report. (Feb 8) 1985; 34(5): 66–68.

Morbidity and Mortality Weekly Report. (July 12) 1985; 34: 405–426.

Mullen PD: Behavioral aspects of maternal and child health; natural influences and educational intervention. In: *Better Health For Our Children: A National Strategy*. Vol IV. *Background Papers*. US Department of Health and Human Services. US Government Printing Office, 1981.

Read D: *The Concept of Health*. Holbrook Press, 1973.

Samuels M, Samuels N: *The Well Baby Book*. Summit Books, 1982.

Sprague J: Vision screening. In: *Detection of Developmental Problems in Children*. Krajicek M, Tomlinson A (editors). University Park Press, 1983.

US Department of Health and Human Services: *Better Health for Our Children: A National Strategy*. Vol 1. *Major Findings and Recommendations*. US Government Printing Office, 1981a.

US Department of Health and Human Services. *Better Health For Our Children: A National Survey*. Vol III. *A Statistical Profile*. US Government Printing Office, 1981b.

US Department of Health and Human Services. *Determinants of Children's Health*. NCHSR Research Summary Series. National Center for Health Services Research, 1981c.

Additional Readings

Anderson CL, Creswell WH: *School Health Practice*. Mosby, 1980.

Bauman E et al (editors): *The Holistic Health Lifebook*. And/Or Press, 1981.

Bellinger D et al.: Longitudinal analyses of prenatal and postnatal lead exposure and early cognitive development. *N Engl J Med* (Apr 23) 1987; 316(17): 1037–1042.

Blattner B: *Holistic Nursing*. Prentice-Hall, 1981.

Bonaguro A: PRECEDE for wellness. *School Health* (Sept) 1981; 51: 501–505.

Brown J: Child health maintenance. *Nurse Pract* (Jan/Feb) 1980; 33–43.

Choosing a day care center. *Child Today* (Oct) 1985; 9.

Clark CC: *Enhancing Wellness: A Guide to Self Care*. Springer, 1981.

Cochi SL, Broome CU, Hightower AW: Assessment of strategies for immunization of U.S. children with *Haemophilus Influenzae* type b polysaccharide vaccine: A cost-effectiveness model. *JAMA* 1985; 253: 521–529.

Coates T: Adolescence: The transition years. *J School Health* (May) 1982; 52: 293–294.

Doren L: Children's concepts of illness: Clinical application. *Pediatr Nurs* (Sept/Oct) 1984; 325–327.

Dwyer J: Nutrition education and information. In: *Better Health for Our Children: A National Strategy*. Vol IV. *Background Papers*. US Department of Health and Human Services. US Government Printing Office, 1981.

Granoff DM, Daum RS: Spread of *Haemophilus Influenzae* type b: Recent epidemiologic and therapeutic considerations. *J Pediatr* 1980; 97: 854–860.

Hollander A: *How to Help Your Child Have a Spiritual Life*. Bantam Books, 1980.

Igoe J: Project health PACT in action. *Am J Nurs* (Nov) 1980; 80: 2016–2021.

Jessor R: Problem behavior and developmental transition in adolescence. *J School Health* (May) 1982; 52: 295–300.

Johnson J: More about stress and some management techniques. *J School Health* (Jan) 1981; 51: 36–42.

Kilmon C, Helpin M: Update on dentistry for children. *Pediatr Nurs* (Sept/Oct) 1981; 7: 41–46.

Lamontagne L, Mason K, Hepworth J: Effects of relaxation on anxiety in children: Implications for coping with stress. *Nurs Res* (Sept/Oct) 1985; 34:289–292.

Liebow P: The new-look school nurse. *Psychosocial Nurs* (March) 1984; 22(3):37–41.

Lorenz KY et al: Toward a conceptual formulation of health and well-being. In: *Strategies for Public Health: Promoting Health and Preventing Disease*. Lorenz KY, Davis DL (editors). Van Nostrand, 1980.

Maheady D: Health concepts of preschool children. *Pediatr Nurs* (May/June) 1986; 12(3):195–197.

McKay R, Segall M: Methods and models for the aggregate. *Nurs Outlook* (Nov/Dec) 1983; 31(6):328–334.

Mitchell P, Mitchell A, Mandell F (editors): Update on the DPT vaccine. *Child Health Alert* (Sept) 1985; 5.

Mitchell P, Mitchell A, Mandell F (editors): Noisy toys—how loud is too loud. *Child Health Alert* (Oct) 1985; 1.

Mitchell P, Mitchell A, Mandell F (editors): Progress on a DTP vaccine. *Child Health Alert* (Oct) 1986; 4.

New recommended schedule for active immunization of normal infants and children. *MMWR* (Sept 19) 1986; 35(37):578.

Newacheck PW et al.: Access to ambulatory care services for economically disadvantaged children. *Pediatrics* (Nov) 1986; 78(5):813–819.

Peltola H et al.: Prevention of *Haemophilus influenzae* type b bacteremic infections with the capsular polysaccharide vaccine. *N Engl J Med* 1984; 310:1561–1566.

Perry CL, Murray DM: Enhancing the transition years: The challenge of adolescent health promotion. *J School Health* (May) 1982; 52:307–311.

Pontious SL: Practical Piaget: Helping children understand. *Am J Nurs* (Jan) 1982; 82:114–117.

Rhodes RL et al: *Elementary School Health, Education and Service*. Allyn and Bacon, 1981.

Ryan RS, Travis JW: *The Wellness Workbook*. Ten Speed Press, 1981.

Selekman J: Immunization: What's it all about. *Am J Nurs* (Aug) 1980; 80:1440–1445.

Selye H: Stress and the promotion of health. In: *Strategies for Public Health: Promoting Health and Preventing Disease*. Lorenz KY, Davies DL (editors). Van Nostrand, 1980.

Simons-Morton B, O'Hara N, Simons-Morton D: Promoting healthful diet and exercise behaviors in communities, schools, and families. *Fam Community Health* 1986; 9(3):1–13.

US Department of Health and Human Services: *Promoting Health/Preventing Disease: Objectives for the Nation*. US Government Printing Office, 1980.

Vipperman JF, Rager PM: Childhood coping: How nurses can help. *Pediatr Nurs* (March/April) 1980; 6:11–18.

Watts P: The whole person concept as a part of the elementary school health education program. *J School Health* (May) 1982; 286:90

Williams L: Childhood immunizations. *Pediatr Nurs* (Jan/Feb) 1982; 8:18–22.

Wood S: School-aged children's perceptions of the causes of illness. *Pediatr Nurs* (March/April) 1983; 9:101–104.

Wold SJ: *School Nursing: A Framework for Practice*. Mosby, 1981.

Wong D: Helping parents select day-care centers. *Pediatr Nurs* (May/June) 1986; 12(3):181–187.

Chapter 12

Prevention of Accidents and Poisonings

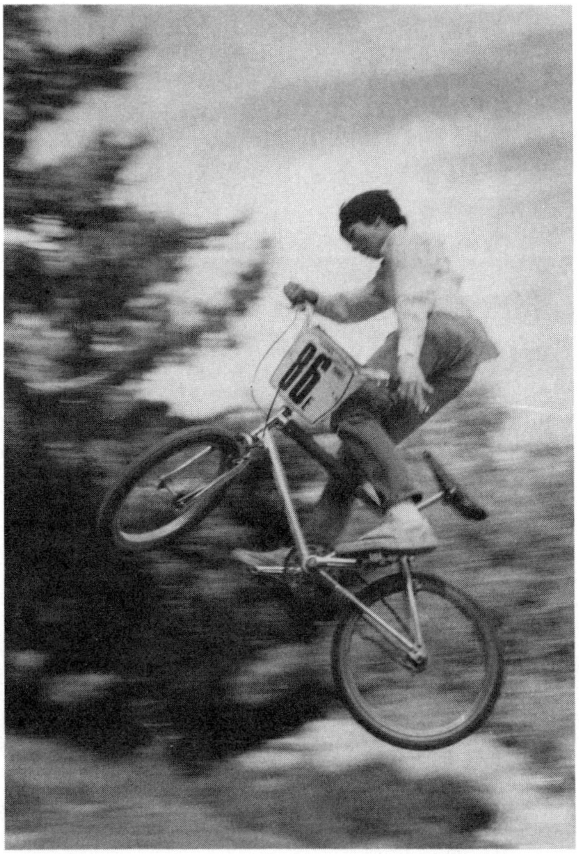

Chapter Contents

Cross Reference Box

To find these topics, see the following chapters:

Chemical burns	Chapter 24
Epistaxis	Chapter 18

(Continues)

Hydrocarbon ingestion	Chapter 22
Ocular emergencies	Chapter 32

Objectives

- Describe the nursing strategies for injury prevention.
- List the characteristics of children that predispose them to injury.
- List the characteristics of injurious agents.
- Identify the environmental characteristics that contribute to childhood accidents or poisonings.
- Relate the developmental characteristics of children to injury prevention strategies.
- List the components of a safe play area.
- Describe safety hazards in the home and environment and the prevention strategies to alter them.
- Describe safety education as it applies to specific injury and poison prevention.
- List the assessment criteria and nursing interventions to reduce the severity of an injury.
- Describe the general first-aid measures nurses need to teach parents to use in the event of a poisoning.
- Explain the nurse's role in the assessment and management of the acutely poisoned child.
- Describe the facets of the nursing care of children poisoned by specific agents.

Injuries are the single most important cause of childhood disease, disability, and death (Rivara, 1982). Injuries also are the leading cause of death among all persons between 1 and 38 years of age (Halperin et al., 1983). Motor vehicle accidents are the number one cause of death in children. Of these deaths, 25% are not the direct result of a collision but are instead the result of children falling out of a vehicle or falling against an object within a vehicle because they were not properly restrained (Nachem, 1984).

Burns and drownings account for most other deaths related to accidental injury. Although deaths from accidental household poisonings have decreased dramatically since 1962 as a result of poison prevention education and the Poison Prevention Act of 1970, accidental poisoning occurs in an estimated 2 million children in the United States each year. Of all poisonings 90.8% occur in the home, two-thirds of which affect children under 6 years of age (*American Journal of Nursing,* 1985). Bleaches, disinfectants, and detergents are the most frequent nondrug poisonings, followed by plants (philodendron and dieffenbachia). Acetaminophen is the most commonly ingested drug, followed by alcohol (Survey, *American Journal of Nursing,* 1985). Most poisonings occur between 10:00 and 11:00 A.M. and 5:00–7:00 P.M. Thirty-six percent of poison ingestions from prescription drugs were a direct result of grandparents leaving the drugs accessible to the child (US Consumer Product Safety Commission, 1985).

Deaths by any one of these causes can be prevented by proper education and safety promotion strategies. Routine well-child care therefore incorporates safety education at every level. *Injury prevention* is a topic of paramount importance.

Injury Prevention as a Nursing Responsibility

Children can learn to make safe health behaviors an integral part of their lives. Safe health practices will lower the risk of injury and the frustration of major lifestyle changes necessitated by a preventable health crisis.

Regardless of practice setting, nurses can make a great impact on the safety of children. As a role model, the nurse can positively influence parents, teachers, children, community leaders, and other health care professionals. The nurse also can provide information about safety hazards and can promote the effective use of health resources to children and their significant others. The nurse can use personal experience to encourage health promotion. Successful practice results when the practitioner can cite examples that confirm the value of a safe, healthy lifestyle as a practical reality.

Prevention at the Primary and Secondary Levels

The nurse's role in injury prevention requires accurate data collection at both the primary and secondary levels. The modification of factors that prevent or alter the severity of injury can only occur after thorough assessment and identification of nursing diagnoses. Interventions are directed toward both the individual and society. The goal then is to alter the factors that lead to an injury, either through health promotion or health protection (see Chapter 11).

For example, safety education promotes recognition of dangerous practices by the child or persons within the environment. Health protection includes legislation that alters agents and the environment for the benefit of society as a whole. Both safety promotion and injury protection measures can reduce the incidence of accidental injury.

Factors Affecting Injury Prevention

Everyone considers a fall from a tree, an automobile collision, or choking on a piece of food—and the injuries these cause—as "accidents." They are accidents, in that they are not intended. Injuries are not completely random occurrences, however. Predisposing factors contribute to both the actual event of an injury and to the severity of its physical consequences. Manipulating these factors at the primary or secondary level of prevention can help to prevent accidents or lessen the injuries they cause (Rivara, 1982).

Factors contributing to the occurrence of an injury can be grouped similarly to those causing an illness. These include characteristics of the child, characteristics of the agent, and characteristics of the environment.

Characteristics of the child Many characteristics of the child can influence the incidence, type, and severity of injury. These characteristics include age or developmental stage, sex, locomotor skill, activity level, cognitive ability, and peer influence, among others. The influence of age, for example, has been suggested by research that examined the different kinds of injuries most often suffered by children in different age groups. Whereas preschool children are most likely to be injured from poisonings, burns, and home injuries, older children are at greater risk of drownings, sports injuries, and motor vehicle collisions (Rivara, 1982).

Characteristics of the agent The agent of an injury is the means by which the child acquires the injury. For example, if a plant poisons a child, the plant is the agent. Other agents include hot water, motor vehicles, fire, bicycles, toys, and electricity. Agents of injury exist everywhere in the child's environment. Their complete elimination often is not possible. Being aware of how children interact with these agents and adjusting behavior accordingly are the strategies by which safety can be promoted and injury avoided.

Characteristics of the environment The elements of the environment that can affect the occurrence and severity of injuries are both physical and sociocultural. Physical elements include such factors as how the home is arranged and whether the child is protected from potential hazards. The conditions on public streets and whether they present unusual dangers to pedestrians are important for safety. Proper design, maintenance, and supervision of child and youth recreation areas—playgrounds, swimming pools, schoolyards, and the like—can prevent injury. Sociocultural elements in the environment also can affect child safety. Poverty, parenting style, family stress, the cultural emphasis placed on the values of aggression and competition, and governmental interventions, such as the 55-mph speed limit, have all been studied with regard to their effects on the frequency and severity of injuries.

Primary Level of Prevention: The Nurse's Role

Assessment at the Primary Level of Prevention

Assessment of the child involves identifying those characteristics that might lead to injury. Along with age, many other variables play important roles in determining the incidence of accidents and the type of injury that occurs.

Characteristics of the child

Curiosity Curiosity is a natural motivator for children as their senses develop. Children learn from their senses of touch, taste, sight, hearing, and smell as they explore the playground of new experiences outside their cribs. Parents therefore need to provide a safe but stimulating environment. All children, but especially adventurous children, need careful supervision. Children whose environment is unlimited often can find themselves in danger.

Whereas some children are adventuresome, and this spirit of adventure gets them into difficulties, other children need limits to feel secure in their environment. An environment that allows limitless freedom for exploration might result in an insecure child who takes extra risks as an attention-getting mechanism. This "stop me" behavior, although not conscious, by its very nature can lead to injury. Testing parental limits is something children do to validate parental caring. Without this validation, children will continue their attempts, sometimes finding themselves in situations beyond their control. For example, 3-year-old Bobby was allowed to roam the neighborhood at will. Eventually, he wandered out of his familiar surroundings and was seen by a family friend playing near a new house foundation. Fortunately, the friend recognized Bobby and brought him home before anything happened to him. The injury potential was high, however, because the child wandered out of his familiar environment.

Developmental stage The developmental stage of a child helps contribute to an increased tendency for accidental injury. For example, young children are insatiably curious and actively explore their environments. They might be attracted by patterns and shapes of plant leaves or the interiors of cabinets and drawers. Mouthing behavior of infancy and early childhood can lead to injury from accidental ingestion of poisons or to other injuries from sharp objects or electrical wires.

Children in middle or late childhood are most apt to be poisoned accidentally by materials used in play or craft activities. Sampling of unknown berries has resulted in emergency room visits. Children of this age group have increased freedom but often lack the judgment to avoid accidents.

In rare cases, young children have a condition called *pica.* Pica is manifested by a compulsion to ingest unusual substances such as dirt, matches, paint, and newspapers. Children with this condition do not merely put these substances in their mouths but actually swallow them. Pica seems to be related more to an emotional than a nutritional deficit, although many children with pica exhibit signs of nutritional deficiencies. Children with pica often manifest signs of lead poisoning.

Adolescents are exposed to an increasingly complex and readily available supply of psychoactive drugs. Poisonings occur when adolescents take these drugs and experience unexpected and dangerous effects. Alcohol is an extremely dangerous drug, not only because of its ability to poison but also because its effects on coordination and judgment lead to drunk driving and subsequent injury. Drugs and alcohol have been implicated in other common accidents of adolescence, such as drowning.

A discrepancy between the developmental skill level and the ability to manipulate toys results in injuries. Children try to operate playthings that are inappropriate for their level of motor skill development. (Table 12-1 lists further developmental characteristics that predispose a child to injury.)

Gender Gender is a determinant of injury incidence. Boys appear to have more accidents than girls. This might be due to behavioral differences. For example, boys might take greater risks in their play activities, climbing higher, riding faster, and performing complicated moves on bicycles and skateboards. Aggressive behavior, although certainly not exclusive to boys, is a proven injury risk factor.

Peer pressure Peer pressure contributes greatly to accident incidence. Competitiveness is exaggerated by peers and can lead to injury in children who try to "do one better" or succumb to taking dares.

Special needs Some children with special needs are at greater risk for injury. For example, children who are hyperactive or have high activity levels appear to be at risk. These children might be excessively stimulated by their environment. They react diffusively to stimuli, and their excessive activity can be random and without purpose. Their short attention span and inability to attend to directions leads them into accident-causing situations that they are not prepared to deal with appropriately.

Disabled children have special problems, and normal hazards become particularly dangerous for them. For children with disabilities affecting hearing and vision, additional precautions around traffic are necessary. Children with medical problems such as seizures, diabetes mellitus, cystic fibrosis, and asthma can be at greater risk for injury, particularly when participating in competitive sports. Keeping such children in a state of maximum health can reduce the injury potential.

Characteristics of the agent Assessment of the agent involves identifying those agents that are hazardous and that, if altered, can prevent injury from occurring. Agents of major importance include automobiles, bicycles, the child as a pedestrian, water, fire, toys, infant equipment, and poisons.

Automobiles Automobiles are the primary agents of injury in children and are the number one cause of death for children in some age groups (Nachem, 1984). Victims of motor vehicle accidents include not only children who are passengers but also children who are pedestrians, bicyclists, and automobile drivers.

There are two periods of impact in an accident. The first impact occurs when the automobile comes to a sudden stop in a collision. The second impact occurs when the occupant stops motion by hitting part of the car or the restraint of a seatbelt or car-restraint system. An unrestrained child in a motor vehicle is propelled forward during a collision at a speed and force comparable to a fall from a third-floor

TABLE 12-1 Developmental Approach to Accident Prevention

Developmental characteristic	Potential hazard	Preventive strategy
Infancy		
Age: 0–3 months		
Newborn is totally dependent on care given by parents; some head control and can move in crib; taste, sight, and hearing are developing	Can catch arms or fingers between loose-fitting mattress and frame of crib	Use crib sides and bumpers; stuff towels between mattress and crib side; cribs should have slats no more than 2⅜″ apart
	Suffocation in crib	Do not use pillows or excess blankets
	Automobile accidents	Infant car seats should be used from birth
	Sudden movement leading to falls	Do not leave baby alone on high places, particularly on an adult bed or infant seat; keep a hand on baby at all times, especially during bathing when baby is slippery with soap; on stairs, hold baby with two hands
	Burns and punctures from bathing and changing; poisoning from spoiled formula	Test bath water for lukewarm temperature; be careful of sharp points of diaper pins near baby's skin; store formula in cool, dry place; protect child from sunburn
Age: 3–6 months		
Good head control; can turn from stomach to back and can put hands in mouth; touch is used to learn about the properties of objects	Harmful objects within baby's immediate reach	Remove potential hazards such as hot coffee while baby is sitting on parent's lap; protect baby from hot faucet while bathing in sink; toys should have no removable parts or sharp edges that could be put in baby's mouth or eyes; do not allow access to plastic bags
	Sharp fingernails	Parents can cut baby's fingernails while baby sleeps
Age: 6–9 months		
Holds own bottle; beginning to drink from cup; might sit unsupported; can pull to standing position and has pincer grasp; transfers objects; some children begin to scoot or crawl—world expands beyond nursery; like to feed themselves crackers and finger foods	Glass breakage if dropped	Use plastic bottles
	Range of grasp increases with mobility	Cover electrical outlets and wind cords on appliances to keep them out of reach; lock lower cabinets or remove any dangerous objects (eg, glass jars, soap powders)
	Increased access to hazardous fixtures and furniture	Use gates to protect from stairways; fence off woodburning stoves and space heaters; supervise constantly when child is in walker, swing, jumper, or high chair; wastebaskets, plants, and household cleaners contain potential poisons and should be placed out of child's reach; remove hazardous machinery such as fans and humidifiers from floor level
	As teeth develop, babies enjoy teething biscuits	Supervise for choking; do not leave baby unattended while eating

(Continues)

TABLE 12-1 Developmental Approach to Accident Prevention *(Continued)*

Developmental characteristic	Potential hazard	Preventive strategy
Infancy *(Continued)*		
Age: 9–12 months		
Can pull self to a sitting position; creeps and cruises around furniture; exhibits purposeful behavior and can reach for objects out of their grasp; some children begin to verbalize; begins to eat finger foods	Mobility and range of grasp increase further	Turn pot handles in on stove; remove stove burner dials if within reach; remove dangerous objects from counters and tables
	Hazardous fixtures become increasingly accessible	Screen windows and use gates on stairways if not already done; use playpens with sides up and corrals with net siding
	Choking from small objects	Cut food into small pieces; no peanuts or popcorn; child should eat while sitting; easy to handle eating utensils; check toys for small pieces; keep money out of reach
Early childhood		
Age: 12–18 months		
Can walk alone and navigate stairs; can stoop and retrieve; has some fine motor skills and some verbal skills	Body control not highly developed, resulting in an unsteady walk; would rather run than walk	Keep furniture with sharp edges, glass coffee tables, and the like out of child's way; keep house clutter-free; lock up poisonous substances if not previously done; pull-toy strings should not be greater than 12" in length
	Bath—temperature of water and slippery tub	Lukewarm water at low level in tub; teach child not to stand in tub; never leave child unattended during bath time; run cold water first before mixing with hot
Age: 18–24 months		
Can run, jump, and stand on one foot; verbal skills expanding; taste, touch, and smell continue to develop	Accidents are more frequent when parents are preoccupied such as at mealtimes and in the morning	Parents can share responsibility for preparing meals and watching children; children's television programs can hold attention during meal preparation; parents should be alert to children's whereabouts
	Fire begins to be a hazard, especially charcoal fires in the summer	Parents should begin to educate children about danger of fire; place matches out of reach; teach fire safety
	Curiosity makes household and yard plants more interesting	Teach child not to put any plants, leaves, berries, etc in mouth
	Climbing accidents become more frequent, especially out of cribs	Parents can have child sleep with crib sides lowered temporarily until a bed is obtained
Age: 2–3 years		
Walks on tiptoe; enjoys imitating adults; enjoys riding toys; can learn simple prohibitions; uses many nouns and verbs in speech	Injury from riding toys	Parents should teach child about riding in streets or behind cars; plastic tricycles are lower to the street and slower than metal ones—but lower vehicles are harder to see by passing motorists
	Children are attracted to brightly colored objects such as pills	Child should be taught never to take pills unless given by parent; medicine should not be made to "taste good"
	Drowning—children who have been taught to swim might get careless in the water	Pools should be fenced; carefully supervise children at beaches; even children who swim should be observed

TABLE 12-1 ***(Continued)***

Developmental characteristic	Potential hazard	Preventive strategy
Early childhood ***(Continued)*** *Age: 3–5 years*		
Has good gross motor coordination; interested in action toys, "big wheels," and tricycles; loves to explore and experiment, especially on playgrounds	Injury from playground equipment	Safety teaching should include no walking in front of swings and no pushing and shoving off equipment
	Foreign objects in Halloween candy	Parents should check Halloween treats before allowing child to eat them; throw away any loose or open candy
	Choking	Teach children not to run with candy or other objects in their mouths
	Increasing freedom out of doors; contact with unleashed animals	Encourage cooperative play; teach street safety—looking both ways, crossing at corners, watching lights; teach children to avoid strangers and keep parents informed of their whereabouts; teach children to walk quietly near animals and to avoid approaching them if parents are not present
Middle and late childhood *Age: 5–12 years*		
Increased muscle tone; improved motor coordination enables increasingly difficult activities; sensitive to peer pressure; responds to rules; magical thinking leads to identification with superheroes	Imitates action seen on television	Parents should teach critical television viewing and talk to children about their favorite shows
	Dogs and cats	Teach child to avoid all strange animals, not to break up an animal fight even when own pet is involved, not to tease animals, and how to behave when encountering a strange animal (stand still, move slowly. Keep an eye on the animal)
	Skateboard misuse, particularly in populated areas	Caution children to remember street safety when on skates or skateboards; extra control is needed for downhill runs; discourage jumps
	Bicycle accidents are common	Teach bicycle safety
	Drowning—ice or water	Teach children water safety; do not allow skating unless ice thickness is proven safe; never swim or skate alone
	Sports injuries	Teach parents and children sports safety
	Automobiles	Require seatbelts at all times; teach child not to hide or play near cars
	Nighttime accidents increase as child is allowed more freedom	Parents should encourage children to be home before dark; wear light-colored clothing and reflective material when walking at night
	Vacant buildings, excavations, quarries, sand pits, house foundations	Teach children to avoid these areas and not to play around heavy machinery; tell child not to hide in refrigerators or piles of leaves

(Continues)

TABLE 12-1 Developmental Approach to Accident Prevention *(Continued)*

Developmental characteristic	Potential hazard	Preventive strategy
Middle and late childhood *(Continued)*	Flying objects—balls, darts, arrows, stones	Any target sport should be carefully supervised; targets should be in isolated areas or against walls; teach children not to throw objects at people or moving vehicles
	Abusable substances—effect of drugs and alcohol on coordination and judgment lead to accidental injury	(See Chapter 16)
Adolescence *Age: Older than 12 years*		
Conflict between dependence and independence; increased decision-making skills; peer influence more important than parental influence; increasing goal orientation	Abusable substances	(See Chapter 16)
	Vehicle hazards—cars, motorcycles	Driver safety; parents need to set firm limits on car use, particularly regarding drinking and driving
	Outdoor activities—swimming, jogging, boating, etc no longer under direct parental supervision	Encourage adolescents to do activities in a group so others can obtain help in case of injuries
	Firearms	Teach rules for hunting and proper care of firearms; keep firearms locked up and hidden away
		Parental role modeling regarding safety and hazards leading to injury can affect their children's safety practices; open communication between parents and children is a powerful preventive measure

NOTE: These ages are arbitrary. Parents should be taught to anticipate their children's development and take preventive action according to individual developmental patterns.

window. Head-first propulsion results from the child's body weight and distribution.

Automobile safety primarily involves use of seatbelts and child safety restraint systems. Seatbelts are proven to be effective in reducing injury and mortality from automobile collisions. It is said that for every 1% increase in seatbelt use, 172 lives are saved (Righi and Krozy, 1983). Effective January 1, 1978, Tennessee was the first state to legislate that children under 4 years of age or weighing less than 40 lb had to use a federally approved car restraint while riding in a car. Most states presently have laws governing car restraints, and many states have car safety education programs, although compliance with the law is low (Faber, 1986).

As of January 1, 1981, all car restraint systems manufactured after May 1980 are required to follow standards set by the Federal Motor Vehicle Safety Standards 213–80. These guidelines require that

1. All car restraint systems manufactured for infants and children be dynamically tested in frontal collision situations at 30 mph. The seats must protect and restrain the occupant adequately.
2. Sufficient force be required to open the harness to prevent children from accidentally releasing the clasp.
3. The directions for use be clear and visible.
4. The restraint be tested under a variety of conditions of improper use.

Lists of approved car seats are available in consumer magazines or from the US Department of Transportation.

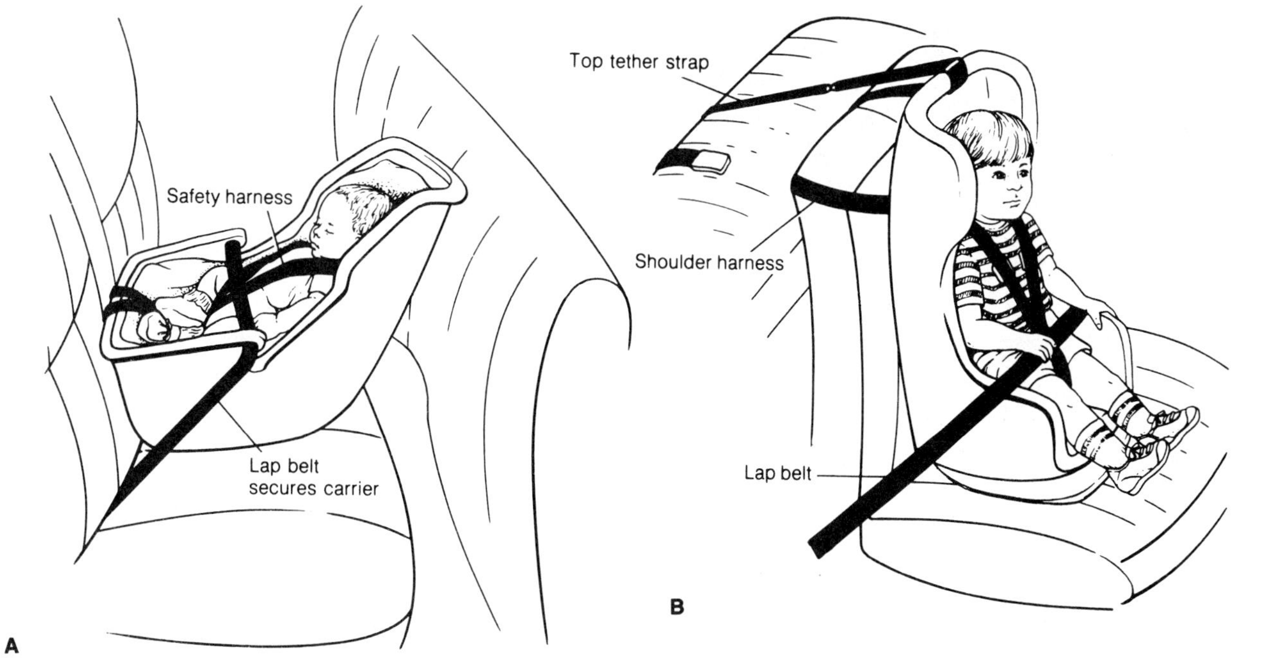

FIGURE 12-1
*Infant restraints. **A.** Infant carrier for the infant from birth to about 12 months of age. **B.** Anchoring the top tether of an infant carrier.*

Car seats are made of energy-absorbing material. They distribute pressure over the entire body and provide support for the head and neck. They are secured by the standard lap belt and often a tether (Fig. 12-1).

A safety-tested car seat is an integral part of the layette for the newborn. The infant's first experience in a car seat should be on the ride home from the hospital. The newborn will learn to associate the motion of the car with being fastened and secure. The seat allows the infant to be in a reclining position, secured with a regular seatbelt and a safety harness, and facing the rear of the car. Some car seats must be anchored to the body of the car (tethering) to prevent the seat from flying forward in a crash (Fig. 12-1B).

Early-childhood car seats are elevated so that the child can see out the windows. Again, tethering is often necessary to prevent forward motion in a collision. The child sits in an erect position facing forward. Many car seats provide safety shields to protect vulnerable chest and abdominal organs. Parents might be frustrated by children climbing out of car seats. Children should learn that the car only moves when they are restrained in their car seats. Children who are larger than 40 lb or 40 in may be safely restrained in regular seatbelts with cushions to keep the belts in position over their laps and to keep them from applying pressure over the abdomen.

In addition to assessing accessibility to child-restraint systems, nurses need to assess parental role modeling in relation to cars. If children do not see their parents "buckle up," they will not understand why they should be restrained. Also, parents' behavior in the automobile and while driving sets the standards for their children's later behavior.

Other problems with automobiles occur when cars are overcrowded or when children are playing near streets. Station wagons, which often are used to transport large numbers of children, are not safe when children are riding unrestrained in the back window area. Children riding in the backs of pickup trucks are at additional risk for injury. Not only are they unrestrained, but also, in the event of a collision, they will be propelled directly onto the street and might very well be run over by another vehicle. Children should not ride in a parent's lap because of the danger of being thrown forward and crushed by the parent during impact. Children also should not be allowed to play in or near parked cars.

Bicycles Since the late 1970s, bicycle accidents have accounted for 1.25 million accidents, 77% of which occur to children younger than 15 years of age (Betz, 1983). The greater percentage of accidents affect children in the 5- to

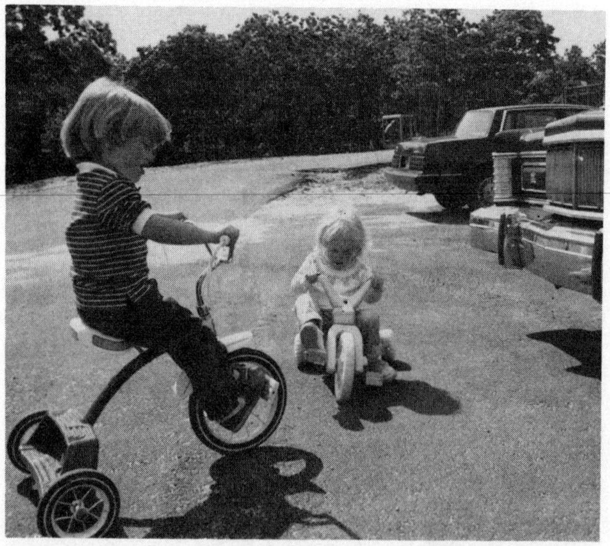

Minicycles are difficult to see by motorists. (Photograph by Judy Koenig.)

14-year-old age group, although 30% of accidents occurred to children under 5 years of age (Betz, 1983).

Structural factors in the bicycles themselves, such as mechanical defects, account for only a small percentage of accidental injury (Betz, 1983). Factors influencing the incidence of accidents are the style of the bicycle, the type of braking device, child and size mismatch, and type of child bicycle seat. Bicycle accidents can involve collision with a motor vehicle or an environmental obstacle. Other injuries are caused by falls and by limbs caught in wheel spokes.

Small children ride tricycles or minicycles. Although the small, plastic minicycles are more stable and slower moving than metal tricycles, they are quite low in height, making it difficult for passing motorists to see the child.

"High-rise" bicycles with long, thin seats and high handlebars are not suitable for beginning riders. They place the center of gravity over the rear wheel and do not give the necessary protection to the genital area. Hand brakes, which require that equal pressure be applied to both wheels, demand coordination not usually possessed by children until they are about 11 years old. Coaster brakes are the simplest and safest to operate.

Assessment of a safe bicycle includes asking the parent whether the child's bike has the following: slip-resistant pedals, a strong frame, handlebars that are low and in proportion to the seat height, the center of gravity over the center of the bicycle, a bicycle flag, and reflectors on the spokes and pedals. The bicycle should not be too large for the child's size.

Bicycle seats should be used by all children over 1 year of age who are passengers on a bicycle ridden by an adult. Children under 1 year of age are not stable enough in a seat to prevent injury. A safe bicycle carrier is secured tightly to the bicycle and is constructed of durable material. The seat needs to protect the child's lower body and needs to prevent foot and hand access to the spokes. The child is belted into the seat at all times while moving and is encouraged to wear a protective helmet.

A minibike is a bicycle with a small motor. Although licensing laws vary, children younger than driving age might have access to minibikes. Because of this, the potential for minibike accidents in children under 15 years old is high. Minibikes are not intended for on-street operation and are misused in many instances. Because minibikes are capable of speeds up to 30 mph, helmets are necessary to prevent injuries (Consumer Reports, 1981). Minibike riders should avoid traffic situations where automobiles are traveling at speeds greater than 40 mph.

Minibikes cause injuries in several ways. The exhaust pipes can burn the legs. Many children cannot apply adequate pressure to the brake pedal, and some of the braking systems are unsafe. Because of the small design and short wheelbase, minibikes can be unstable. Some children even have experienced hearing loss from the noise of the motor.

All terrain vehicles (ATVs) are a recent innovation in bikes. Unlike the minibike, the ATV has three wheels and has the illusion of greater stability. Like the minibike, the ATV is capable of attaining high speeds, there are no age requirements for driving, and helmets are not required. The number of accidental injuries from use of these vehicles in children appears to be increasing.

Walking and running Children often dart into traffic from between parked cars, contributing to accidental deaths caused by motor vehicles. These accidents often occur quite close to home and occasionally in the child's driveway.

Factors that contribute to the high number of pedestrian accidents in children include the child's natural curiosity, short attention span, and impulsiveness. These qualities often lead to poor judgments near the streets. Drivers have difficulty distinguishing and reacting to the sudden appearance of small moving objects. It is natural for children to be so immersed in a game that they automatically chase a ball into the street without thinking of the dangers involved.

Young children are so short that they are difficult for drivers to see. Children might be unaware of traffic signals or rules. They might be unable to judge the amount of time it will take to cross the street and either do not make it across or fall in their haste to do so.

Assessment of children as pedestrians involves ascertaining the child's knowledge of safety as well as the child's developmental level and temperament. In pedestrian accidents the child and the car as agents combine to produce the injury.

Water Water is an agent for both drownings and burns. Drownings occur as a result of contact with a variety of water hazards, including those in common household locations such as the bathtub or toilet. Most drownings occur from accidental entry into the water through falls, boating accidents, and accidents in the home.

Children at different ages are susceptible to different kinds of drownings. Infants less than 1 year old might drown when left unattended in a bathtub. Toddlers fall into private swimming pools and lakes. In middle and late childhood, children drown in pools and lakes while swimming. Adolescents take risks in large bodies of water. When learning to walk, children are unsteady on their feet, and extra caution is needed when they are near sources of water, particularly in the bathroom or outdoors.

Scaldings are the most common burns seen in all age groups, and children under 3 years of age are burned by hot liquids more than by any other agent. The temperature of the liquid and the duration of contact determine the degree of injury. Cooling the scald with cold water is an important immediate response. It takes only a couple of seconds for a severe burn to occur in a child exposed to hot water of a temperature found in some households (approximately 150°F). A pan of boiling water or freshly poured coffee is much hotter (212°F).

Very young infants are burned less frequently than those beginning to crawl or walk, but scalds do occur. An adult unwisely holding an infant while eating hot soup or drinking a hot beverage might spill some and cause a deep scald.

Typically, the older infant or toddler is burned when adults leave a cup of hot tea or coffee too close to a tabletop or counter edge. As the adult turns to replace the kettle on the stove or attend to some other task, the child reaches for the cup, upsets it, and sustains a significant scald burn. Pot handles protruding over the stovetop are another hazard, as are tablecloths and dangling electrical cords—anything a child can reach, grasp, and overturn. Common appliances such as electric coffee pots and frying pans are associated with major, disfiguring, and life-threatening burns.

Hot liquids must be kept out of reach, pan handles turned inward to the back of the stove, and electrical cords tied up and away from curious toddlers. Children should not be underfoot in the kitchen when meals are being prepared, particularly when parents are carrying pots of boiling liquids from the stove to the sink and countertops.

Bathroom tap water scalds occur when children are left unattended in or near the bathtub. The doorbell or telephone rings, and the parent leaves "for just a moment." The children might then try to climb into a tub where the water is untested and too hot or might experiment with faucets. The rules to follow include not leaving children alone in a bathroom, always running hot water well mixed with cold, and testing the temperature of the water before placing the child in the bathtub. Children need to be taught to turn cold faucets on first and then to mix in the hot water.

Child abuse with scalding tap water does occur and should be considered, especially when there are no splash marks and an even burn. For example, a burn over the "socks area" of the feet and ankles along with a buttocks burn suggests that the child might successfully have resisted further immersion. (The nurse's role in assessing child abuse is discussed in Chapter 13.)

A less frequent but often deep and disfiguring injury is an electrical burn caused by biting through the wire or chewing on the end of a cord. Saliva, primarily water, is an excellent conductor of electricity. Because water conducts electricity, children need to be taught not to bring televisions or radios into the bathroom with them and particularly not to touch an electrical appliance when they are wet.

Ice is a water hazard with a high injury potential. Children should not have small ice cubes in drinks since, if aspirated, the cube can occlude the child's airway. Also, they should be discouraged from running while eating popsicles or other frozen treats on sticks. (Ice skating is another hazard; see p. 344.)

Fire Fascination with and curiosity about fire starts at an early age, long before the child can competently handle matches, fireplaces, and stoves. As children grow, they imitate adult behavior and might attempt activities beyond their skills. For example, a 3-year-old girl watched her mother tightly wad newspaper to start a fire in the stove. She took a piece of paper herself, loosely crumpled it, and tossed it into the open flames, only to have it ignite quickly in her hands and then ignite her clothing. Flame burns are particularly serious because they almost always require skin grafting for wound closure (see Chapter 24).

Clothing does not protect the body from fire, although different fibers react differently to flame, and fabrics can be treated with flame-retardant chemicals. Synthetics melt, natural fibers (cotton, silk, wool) ignite, and combination fabrics both melt and support flames. The laws regulating the manufacture of childen's sleepwear (FF3-71, FF5-740) specify that sizes 0–14 must be flame resistant, meaning that the fabric is treated with a chemical that helps it resist continued burning when brought in contact with a source of flames. Sleepwear in stores has been treated to meet flame-resistance requirements. Parents need to follow laundering instructions and be advised to ask for flame-resistant materials if they make their children's pajamas or nightgowns.

In assessing fire hazards in the home, the nurse asks about provisions made for the proper handling and disposal of cigarettes. Naturally, children of parents who smoke are at greater risk because of the availability of matches or lighters. Matches need to be stored in metal containers and out of children's reach. Cigarette lighters are a particularly dangerous fire hazard because, depending on the type, less manual dexterity might be needed to light them than matches. Cigarettes should not be left in ashtrays within a child's reach, and they should be extinguished completely before disposal.

Gas stoves also can present a fire hazard to children. Many stoves have on and off dials within a child's reach, allowing for easy flame ignition. These dials can be removed to prevent accidental lighting. Wood stoves, radiators, heating grates, space heaters, barbeque grills, and discarded hot charcoal also can create fire hazards.

Toys Toys are a most important ingredient of a child's normal growth and development. They also can be instruments of danger when inappropriately manufactured or used.

Most toy-related injuries are caused by bicycles, but a large number of toy-related injuries occur from misuse of the toys rather than from the toys themselves. For example, most choking incidents can be traced to balloons (Toy safety, *MMWR,* 1984).

At any one time, thousands of a particular toy might be recalled because of manufacturing defects or use problems. Among the types of toys that might be recalled are stuffed animals whose facial features can be removed easily and are of choking size, toys with sharp points, or toys that can be strung across a crib or playpen and might cause the child to strangle were the child to sit or stand suddenly.

The Child Protection and Toy Safety Act of January 1970 was instituted to identify and remove hazardous toys from the market. The US Consumer Product Safety Commission is a federal organization with the authority to ban hazardous toys from sale. Unfortunately, mechanisms for establishing safety standards for all toys before they are marketed are not yet in place. The result, then, is that dangerous toys are recalled after they have injured children. The burden of providing safe toys rests, as it always has, with the parents.

Resources concerning toy safety include pamphlets by the US Consumer Product Safety Commission and the US Government Printing Office. Information regarding toy recalls can be found in consumer magazines and newspapers.

Toys need to be bought and maintained with injury prevention in mind. Nurses can assess parents' knowledge regarding toy purchasing according to the following principles:

1. Read all toy labels for age recommendations and information concerning the safety of the component materials.
2. Check all toys for sharp edges or points, small loose parts, adequate construction, loud noise, improper electrical wiring, and objects that can be propelled.
3. Avoid buying toys with flexible joints that can catch children's fingers.
4. Avoid baby-teething toys that are breakable or contain liquid. Even minute cracks can precipitate bacterial growth in the liquid.
5. Electrical and chemical toys, particularly those with heating elements, are recommended for older children only (over 8 years of age).
6. Check directions that come with toys to ensure they are legible, give step-by-step instructions, and state clearly how the toy is to be used.
7. Buy only nontoxic items for young children.
8. Encourage grandparents and others giving the child toys to follow these recommendations.

The proper maintenance and storage of toys is as important as proper purchasing. Toys need to be checked on a regular basis for breakage or excessive wear. Wooden toys can be resanded and repainted with nontoxic paint. If toys are irreparable, they should be discarded. All plastic wrappers should be disposed of immediately. Balloons are particularly hazardous when broken and have been known to cause obstruction of the airway. For this reason, they should not be used by young children without supervision. Parents need to use caution with toy chests because they can injure children's fingers or heads if the lid falls on the child.

The nurse also needs to assess the availability of toys in families with children of various ages. It might be necessary to recommend separate play areas if the age discrepancy between the children is too wide.

Infant furniture Prior to 1974, there were no uniform safety standards for infant cribs. As a result, many children were injured each year in crib accidents. Federal requirements for infant cribs were established, and all cribs manufactured after February 1, 1974 are required to comply with these standards. They include regulating the width of the space between crib side slats (no more than 2 3/8 in. at any point), standardizing the interior measurements (28 in. ± 5/8 in. in width and 52 3/8 in. ± 5/8 in. in length), requiring special latch release features, recommending standard mattress size and thickness, and regulating the height of the crib sides in relation to the mattress support height.

Nurses need to be aware, however, that many parents purchase older cribs and playpens at yard sales and are not knowledgeable about the safety standards. If cribs are found to fail these standards, especially in the use of lead paint or the slat space width, the nurse needs to recommend the use of full crib bumpers until a safer alternative can be provided.

More recent attention has focused on play space. As an alternative to the traditional playpen, many parents have been using expandable wooden "corrals" to confine children. The advantages of these corrals are that they allow the

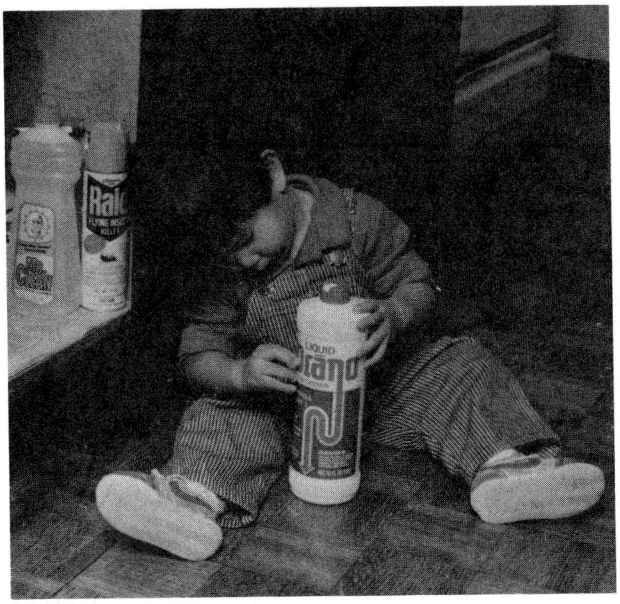

Household cleaners are a major cause of nondrug poisonings in children.

child greater play area and are more portable. Although generally stable, corrals have contributed to injury by providing openings for children to use as footholds for climbing. Some children have been injured by placing their heads through the openings and having the corrals collapse on them. Folding play spaces with net sides or playpens with side netting decrease this type of injury occurrence. The netting needs to be small enough that the child cannot insert objects through it or get buttons caught in it.

Playpens with net sides, however, are not without danger. Infants should not be left in these areas with one side left down. Placing an infant in a playpen with the side down increases the potential for the infant to suffocate from being caught between the playpen pad and the netting.

Poisons Modern society offers an almost limitless potential for toxic exposure. Over 58,000 chemical substances are manufactured, imported, or processed for commercial purposes in the United States (Environmental Protection Agency, 1982). These chemicals are combined into hundreds of thousands of products for use in industry and the home. Household cleansers, disinfectants, dishwasher detergents, pesticides, automotive supplies, art and hobby supplies, and perfumes are among the many common household products that can be toxic if used improperly.

A wide variety of pharmacologic compounds commonly are found in home medicine cabinets. Many of these medications are flavored and brightly colored, resembling candy. Adults often are unfamiliar with pediatric dosages, and chronic poisoning can occur if a child is given a slightly high dose over a period of several days. Poisoning also can occur if a child is given medication prescribed for another family member. Illegally manufactured psychoactive drugs are increasingly accessible to adolescents and in some cases younger children.

Not all poisons are manufactured by humans. Poisoning from food sources has been a concern since the beginning of recorded history (Temple and Mancini, 1980). Bites or stings from some insects, spiders, and snakes can cause serious illness. Many trees, plants, and mushrooms contain toxic compounds. The increase in the popularity of houseplants is reflected by a substantial increase in the number of accidental poisonings from plants.

In assessing a child's susceptibility to being poisoned, the nurse determines the parent's knowledge regarding frequently found household poisons. Is the parent aware that many decorative plants are poisonous? Does the parent keep perfume and other cosmetics out of reach? Parents need to be asked whether the child comes in frequent contact with a grandparent who might be taking prescription medications since 33% of poisonings related to prescription medications were grandparents' prescriptions (Consumer Product Safety Commission, 1985).

Characteristics of the environment If a child is an accident repeater or if the nurse notices a discrepancy between the child's needs and parental expectations, an environmental assessment is indicated. The assessment is geared toward identifying parental factors that might be contributing to accidents as well as assessing the relative safety of the child's physical environment. The assessment needs to be noncritical, with the nurse emphasizing concern about the child's safety to the parents while giving support and encouragement.

If the home is particularly chaotic and the child seems to be using accident behavior as an attention-getting mechanism, further counseling and family sessions are indicated. This might need to be followed by referral for special counseling. Factors in the environment that contribute to injury include parental factors such as inattention or fatigue, general developmental expectations of children, family stability, socioeconomic status, and physical environment conditions.

Family/parental factors Accidents increase at times of the day when the parent is paying less attention to the child. Among these critical times are the morning rush, when parents are getting off to work or children off to school, and meal preparation time. After a hard working day, parents tend to "tune out" their children while trying to unwind, thus becoming relatively unaware of what their children are doing.

Parental fatigue and worry can contribute to accidents, and the nurse therefore assesses the family's support systems. Do the parents have supportive relationships that enable them to renew their own strength? Caring for children all day can be an isolating experience for a parent. Play groups, mother's groups, and babysitting co-ops represent attempts to develop supportive networks to deal with these feelings. A parent who feels personally renewed has more strength for childrearing and an increased ability to attend adequately to each child.

Other factors also contribute to parental inattention. For example, illness of a family member, which requires parental attention and concern, also might contribute to parental inattention and greater potential for injury. Children in the care of a babysitter, particularly if the sitter is an older sibling, can increase their testing behavior, which might result in an injury. To prevent such occurrences, parents therefore need to caution babysitters to pay special attention to the younger children.

Developmental expectations Parental expectations should coincide with the child's actual developmental level. Expectations that are too low can increase risk of injury. For example, a mother reported that a real estate broker showing their house cautioned her to keep the crib side up because her infant was standing up in bed. The mother's response was, "My baby cannot stand yet!" Perhaps in the chaos of moving, this child's development was temporarily ignored, or perhaps the mother's expectations of the child lagged behind the child's actual development.

Expectations that are too high also can lead to injury by prompting children to attempt skills for which they are not ready. For example, a 3-year-old can learn to follow simple directions but is not able to cross a street alone or to play outside unsupervised. An infant is not ready to master steps on a steep, 14- to 20-foot stairway but can be taught on two-step plastic toy stairs. The challenge for parents is to provide a stimulating environment that not only promotes development but also protects from injury.

Family stability Parental discord or family stress can predispose children to injury because any instability can distract parental attention. Family events that can cause confusion might include moving, vacations, household company, or the addition of a new family member.

Divorce or separation creates disequilibrium within the family. Parents preoccupied by family disorganization can allow a young child to go unwatched. In some divorce situations, most notably those involving a custody dispute, children might increase acting-out behavior. In some instances this behavior leads to increased risk taking and subsequent injury.

A new child in the family causes similar family disequilibrium and decreased parental attention. Children who feel displaced often take risks to gain attention. Parents with a new infant are often exhausted and under stress and therefore not as vigilant as they might be ordinarily. Parental well-being is a significant variable in the prevention of injuries. Recognizing that parents are under stress and encouraging them to use support systems (family, friends, or babysitters) can give parents the necessary relief to cope.

Family relocation, either temporary, such as a vacation, or permanent, might contribute to accidental injury. Vacations often place children near unsupervised bodies of water or wooded recreational areas. The child's need to be supervised constantly might not allow parents much relaxation while on vacation. Drowning, boating accidents, fish hooks, camp fires, and sunburns, among others, pose hazards.

For a child, being lost in a strange neighborhood is a terrifying experience. When on vacation, parents need to redefine boundaries and rules immediately with their children. Some parents bring their babysitters with them from home so that their children will be watched while the parents have some free time. When moving to a new neighborhood, touring adjacent streets and learning the new telephone number and address can prevent a child from experiencing the trauma of being lost.

Parental/family values The style of childrearing affects the child's risk of injury. Particularly pertinent to this issue is the promotion of autonomy. From the early childhood years, becoming independent is a major developmental task. Some parents, however, encourage autonomy to such a degree that safety is jeopardized. Young children are allowed to wander at will, and some children in middle childhood are left at home unsupervised after school. Although children at this stage might understand safety concepts, they might panic and take inappropriate actions when confronted by a crisis, such as a fire.

The young child's decision-making skills are not highly developed. Parents need to recognize that young children are not capable of seeing all sides of an issue and need to be assisted to clarify issues and understand consequences. Children who are allowed complete freedom regarding decision making not only will feel insecure but also will increase their injury potential because they process data incompletely.

Some families value competitiveness and aggression, and children are encouraged to develop these characteristics at an early age. The child's primary outlet for aggression and a competitive spirit is athletic participation. Unfortunately, sports and fitness-related accidents account for more than 22 million injuries each year (Lee and Jacobsen, 1987). More than 55% of these injuries are related to supervised athletics. The following facts are related to sports injuries:

1. The majority of injuries are to the lower extremities.
2. The most common types of injuries are sprains, strains, contusions, abrasions, and lacerations (Lee and Jacobsen, 1987).

Assessment of an Athletic Program

Do coaches have a positive attitude and refrain from destructive criticism?

Is there less emphasis placed on winning and greater emphasis on learning skills, team participation, and having a good time?

Are there adequate playing facilities and safe, well-maintained equipment available?

Does the sport have penalties for injury-causing maneuvers (high sticking in hockey, for example)?

Are the teams divided according to size and maturation, not by age?

Do girls' sports equipment and clothing adequately protect and support breast tissue and the pelvic girdle?

Does the program require a preseason physical examination?

Are injuries attended to promptly by qualified personnel?

The prevention of accidents needs to be the focus of sports for children. An important decision for parents is to determine at what age their children can participate safely in competitive sports. Children begin to value competition at about 6 years of age. Young athletes require different rules, equipment, and coaching than adults because of the vulnerability of their growing bodies and their emotional health. For parents, both psychologic and physical considerations are relevant. Does the enjoyment of playing as part of a team outweigh the criticisms of organized competitive sports?

Socioeconomic factors Living conditions for people in lower socioeconomic groups can result in an increased incidence of accidents. The environment might be more hazardous and difficult to childproof. Trash and litter in houses or streets, dim lighting, faulty electrical wiring, steep or broken stairways, unscreened windows, or porches on second and third stories can create dangerous situations for small children. Bicycles in city traffic become very different toys from those used to ride on a country road.

Children often play or run into streets when yards or playgrounds are unavailable. For people in the lower socioeconomic groups, family vigilance and community activism are necessary for the child's welfare. Community groups can work toward better sanitation and improved lighting. They can put pressure on landlords to repair hazardous living conditions, thereby preventing accidents.

In a recent study (Wicklund and Mons, 1984) maternal education was found to be a determining factor in accident risk. Children whose mothers completed fewer than 8 years of school were found to have double the risk for accidents than those whose mothers completed high school.

Physical environment of the home The home can be one of the most dangerous places for a child if it is not properly childproofed. The challenge to parents is providing a safe environment without completely suppressing the child's curiosity and sense of adventure. If parents are reluctant to confine a child in a playpen, a playroom, which can be kept separate from the rest of the house by a gate, is a viable alternative. If the child is allowed to wander freely, the entire house needs to be made safe. The nurse's assessment of the home environment is directed toward room-by-room safety (Fig. 12-2 and Table 12-2).

The kitchen and the bathrooms need special attention because most dangerous substances are stored in these rooms. Devastating internal and external burns can occur when corrosive household products are left within reach. The exploring child can both spill and ingest these products. Drain openers, oven cleaners, electric dishwasher powders, and low-phosphate detergents contain corrosive alkalis. There are dangerous acids in toilet bowl cleaners, metal polishes, and swimming pool cleaners. All of these chemicals need to be stored high up and out of reach. Sometimes, if the child likes to climb, it is necessary to keep the chemicals under lock and key.

Food stored near the kitchen stove attracts young children. They climb close to the flame, intent only on getting to the cookies or candy. Matches or lighters left lying about might be too much of a temptation even for the child who "knows better" to resist. Other factors influencing the types of burns children receive are cultural practices such as cooking on the floor or ground, using open flames with small children about, or using popular products like the slow-cooking electrical cookery pot or the woodburning stove.

Bathrooms have their own particular hazards. In addition to the storage of cleaners, medications of all kinds are commonly stored in bathroom medicine cabinets. Children who can climb find these substances easily accessible. Other poisonous substances also are found in the bathroom. Many cosmetics can be poisonous if ingested, particularly astringents, which are primarily alcohol, and nail polish remover. Hairspray, if sprayed directly into the face, can cause eye injuries. Razors and razor blades are bathroom items that need to be inaccessible to children.

Basements and garages contain many hazardous substances such as pesticides, fertilizers, weed killers, paints, and paint-cleaning products. Tools also can be a safety hazard. Poisonous and caustic substances preferably should be located in a locked cupboard. All tools need to be kept out of reach. Lawn mowers should be disconnected to prevent accidental activation. Both basements and garages should be considered off limits to young children.

Young children also should be encouraged to stay away from sewing areas. Pins, needles, thread bobbins, and curtain weights are small enough to be ingested and cause internal damage.

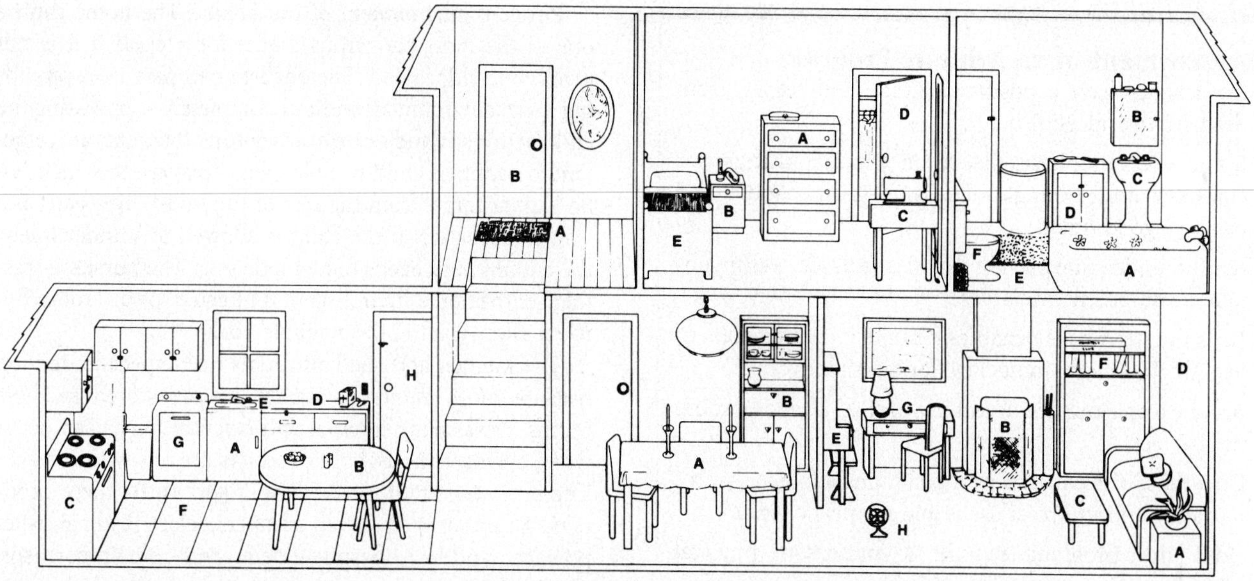

FIGURE 12-2
Childproofing the home: home safety check.

TABLE 12-2 Home Safety Check*

Room/object	Hazard	Prevention strategy
Kitchen		
A—lower cabinets and drawers	Poisonous and corrosive substances in cabinets or on counters, including spices and extracts used in cooking	Remove and place out of reach in locked cabinet
	Alcohol or liquor in lower cabinets	Place in upper cabinets with cabinet lock
	Sharp knives, scissors, or other dangerous articles in drawers	Place in upper cabinet with cabinet lock or use drawer lock
	Breakable bowls or pie plates in lower cabinets	Remove or use cabinet lock
B—kitchen table	Pills or medicine on kitchen table or window sills	Lock up with other dangerous substances; use childproof caps
C—stove	Stove dials easily accessible	Remove until needed
	Cookies or other attractive food over the stove	Remove to another location; have fire extinguisher available
	Stove turned on when not in use	Make sure burners are off and that gas pilot is working properly; keep matches in metal container covered and out of reach
D—countertop	Food processor on counter	Remove blades to make them inaccessible; keep processor unplugged to prevent accidental activation
	Other electrical appliances on countertops—toaster, coffee pot, etc	Keep unplugged; use short cord or wind and secure cord
E—sink	Accessible disposal	Keep covered to prevent children from sticking hand in

TABLE 12-2 (Continued)

Room/object	Hazard	Prevention strategy
Kitchen *(Continued)*		
F—floor	Wastebasket	Have a covered wastebasket to reduce curiosity; keep in closet or cabinet or in out-of-reach location
	Accessible stepstool might be used for climbing	Keep in kitchen closet; use plastic door handle covers to prevent entry
G—dishwasher	Knives within reach	Keep door closed and locked
H—door	Outside access available to children	Use simple door lock out of child's reach
Dining room		
A—table	Tablecloth hanging within reach	Remove cloth or use shorter cloth, particularly when lighted candles are on table
B—buffet with hutch	Breakables on buffet	Remove
	Glass and china items accessible in china cabinet	Use cabinet locks to prevent access
	Chafing dishes and hot trays	Keep unplugged until just before use
	Accessible wine rack	Move to higher location; keep bottles out of reach
Living room		
A—end table	Poisonous plants	Identify plants that are poisonous and remove or place out of child's reach
	Lighting fixtures	Make certain table lamps are stable and not easily displaced
B—fireplace	Fireplace or wood stove	Use fireplace screen; place gate around wood stove; dangerous fire-stoking equipment should be out of reach; do not heat water on wood stove; never cook with charcoal in fireplace; keep chimney damper open
C—coffee table and couch	Furniture edges	Sharped-edged furniture should be removed or padded
	Ashtrays	Keep ashtrays empty; dispose of cigarettes properly; keep matches and lighters out of reach
D—window	Curtains and draperies	Short draperies recommended with small children; if using long drapes, make sure drapery rod is securely fastened to wall
E—piano	Pianos and piano benches	Keep cover over keys when not in use
F—bookshelves	Stereo equipment	Stereo cabinet with locked doors recommended
	Games	Games with small pieces must be kept out of reach or in locked cabinets
	Books	Check that books cannot be pulled off shelves easily
G—desk	Desk accessories	Remove sharp objects, pencils, pens, paper clips, etc from desk top; lock drawers if possible
H—dehumidifiers and fans	Blades and motors	Check consumer magazines to purchase child-safe appliance; grates should be too narrow for little fingers
Hallways and stairs		
A—carpets	Slippery rugs	Use nonslip rug pad under rugs
B—closets	Attractive playing area	Use plastic door knob covers for all closets containing hazardous items

(Continues)

TABLE 12-2 Home Safety Check* *(Continued)*

Room/object	Hazard	Prevention strategy
Bathroom		
A—tub	Slippery surface, hot water	Apply decorative nonskid strips to bottom; use flexible plastic faucet cover; keep hot water heater turned down; keep shampoo, soap, and razors out of reach
B—medicine cabinet	Dangerous substances	All medicines need childproof caps and should be in a locked cabinet. Remove any cosmetics, hair dyes, nail polish, etc and keep in a locked bathroom closet
C—vanity and sink	Dangerous substances	Remove perfumes and powders from vanity top; electric shavers and toothbrushes should not be near water source; use outlet fillers for exposed outlets; use cabinet locks on vanity cabinets; store bathroom cleaners in locked bathroom closet; hairdryers, curling irons, and wastebaskets should be out of reach
D—linen closet	Dangerous substances	Closet should have a bolt lock or door handle cover to prevent entry. Use a locked storage box for dangerous items
E—floor	Space heaters	Floor coil heaters should not be available for child's use
	Rugs	All bathroom rugs should have nonslip backing
	Clothes hamper	Hampers with covers are recommended
F—toilet	Water and dangerous chemicals	Keep toilet cover closed; avoid continuous toilet cleaners
Bedrooms		
A—bureaus	Dangerous substances and small objects	Remove cosmetics and small pieces of jewelry from bureau top; put loose change away and out of reach; keep jewelry box locked; drawers should not be easily removable
	Fans	Keep fans and air conditioners unplugged; use only when parent is around and never in children's rooms; do not place fans on floor; keep all electrical outlets filled
B—night tables	Breakable objects	Remove breakables; telephones, radios, etc should be situated in middle to prevent being pulled off; keep a flashlight here for emergencies
C—sewing table	Electrical appliance; small, sharp objects	Keep machine unplugged until needed; keep bobbins, needles, and pins in inaccessible locations
D—closets	Dangerous substances, plastic bags	Remove any mothballs or other insecticides; do not use plastic cleaner bags to store clothing in closets that are unlocked; keep clothes hangers off floors
E—beds		Do not use too much bedding or pillows for young children; keep children in sleepers if concerned about the cold; discourage children from playing on bunk beds or bunk ladders; see information about crib safety

NOTE: Be alert for dangerous items in the home. Use a commonsense approach to safety.
*Read this table in conjunction with Figure 12-2.

Outdoor environmental hazards Outdoor hazards are plentiful. Parts of some common garden plants are poisonous (Table 12-3), and children need to be taught not to eat anything found outside without first checking with a parent.

Other outdoor environmental hazards that can injure children include air pollution, noise pollution, toxic substances, smoking chemicals, and carcinogens in drinking water. Testing and tracking devices used by nearby military bases can violate safe levels of radiation or noise pollution. Proximity to commercial airports can have the same effect.

Swimming pools, fresh and saltwater beaches, and farm ponds present unique problems. Young children can slip and fall into unfenced private pools. Older children can slip

TABLE 12-3 Some Common Poisonous Plants

Common name	Botanic name	Poisonous part
Houseplants		
Boston ivy	*Parthenocissus quinquefolia*	All parts
Caladium	*Caladium*	All parts
Dumbcane	*Dieffenbachia*	All parts
Emerald duke	*Philodendron hastatum*	All parts
English ivy	*Hedera helix*	Leaves, berries
Parlor ivy	*Philodendron cordatum*	All parts
Split leaf philodendron	*Monstera deliciosa*	All parts
Umbrella plant	*Cyperus alternifolius*	All parts
Outdoor plants		
Apricot	*Prunus armeniaca*	Stem, bark, seed pits
Azalea	*Rhodendron occidentale*	All parts
Castor bean	*Ricinus communis*	Seeds, if chewed
Chokecherry	*Prunus virginiana*	Leaves, seed pits, stems, bark
Daffodil	*Narcissus*	Bulbs
Foxglove	*Digitalis purpurea*	Leaves, seeds, flowers
Hemlock (false parsley, snake root)	*Conium maculatum*	All parts, root, and root stalk
Hens-and-chicks	*Lantana*	All parts
Hydrangea	*Hydrangea macrophylla*	Leaves, buds
Jimsonweed	*Datura stramonium*	All parts
Jonquil	*Narcissus*	Bulbs
Lily of the valley	*Convallaria majalis*	All parts
Mistletoe	*Phoradendron flavescens*	Berries
Morning glory	*Ipomoea violaces*	Seeds
Nightshade	*Atropa belladonna*	All parts
Oleander	*Nerium oleander*	All parts, including dried leaves
Rhododendron	*Rhododendron*	All parts
Rhubarb	*Rheum raponticum*	Leaves
Sweet pea	*Lathyrus odoratus*	Seeds, pods
Tulip	*Tulipa*	Bulbs
Wisteria	*Wisteria*	Seeds, pods

SOURCE: Adapted from San Francisco Bay Area Regional Poison Center: *Poisonous and Non-Poisonous Plant List*. San Francisco Bay Area Regional Poison Center, 1979.

and fall while running on pool decks. Neck and back injuries are caused by children diving headfirst into shallow water. Extra precaution is necessary when children are visiting grandparents or families with no young children. Although the pool might be fenced, the gate might be left unlocked.

Fresh and saltwater beaches can be hazardous if children are not supervised carefully. The numbers of people frequenting beaches, combined with the unfamiliar landscape, can result in disorientation and a lost child. Broken pieces of shells or glass lying buried in the sand can cause severe lacerations of the feet. Jellyfish and man-of-war can cause painful stings. At saltwater beaches, children need to understand safety in dealing with tides, undertows, and currents.

Boating carries the additional hazards of motors, capsizing, or being caught far from land. Although boating is thought to be a relaxing sport, children require special consideration. Constant supervision of children might inhibit a parent's pleasure.

Children always need to wear life jackets while boating. Parents should check weather forecasts before leaving shore and have a radio on board. Extra life preservers, extra oars, and fire extinguishers also should be stocked for emergencies. The engine should be turned off when boarding the boat. Anyone swimming should not be near the propellers of the motor. Children need to be taught how to move around in a boat and not to stand in small boats.

Farm ponds or local swimming holes frequently are used for recreational purposes. Farm ponds, which formerly were used as watering holes for animals, have been adapted for swimming by the addition of rafts, docks, and other aquatic equipment (American Red Cross, 1981). Because of uncertain depths and hazards from trash disposed of on the bottom, these areas are used with caution. These ponds should be fenced like private pools and the water tested frequently for bacteria content (American Red Cross, 1981).

Ice has accident potential, particularly when frozen ponds are accessible to children. Children should be allowed to skate only when the ice is proven to be thick enough to support the weight of a group—approximately 4 in. (American Red Cross, 1981). Local police departments usually will provide information regarding ice safety on local ponds. Children should skate close to shore and never skate alone. Ice rescue equipment, such as a ladder or a flat-bottom boat, needs to be available where water depths are sufficient for drowning. Cold weather clothes, such as long scarfs, must be used with care because they can easily get caught and accidentally strangle a child.

Assessment at the Primary Level of Prevention: Prevention of Injury

Characteristics of the child

Curiosity

Developmental characteristics such as mouthing behavior, uncoordination, lack of judgment

Gender

Peer pressure

Special needs

Characteristics of the agent

Automobiles—children not restrained

Bicycles—child-bike mismatch, falls, limbs caught in spokes, children not restrained in bike seats

Children as pedestrians—children hit by motor vehicles

Water—both drowning and scalds

Ice—choking and drowning

Fire

Toys—not appropriate for age, manufacturer's defects

Infant furniture—noncompliance with safety regulations

Poisons

Characteristics of the environment

Family/parental factors—fatigue, worry, illness, number of children

Developmental expectations

Family stability—moves, vacations, illness, death, divorce, new baby

Parental/family values—style of childbearing, emphasis on aggressive behavior, freedom

Socioeconomic factors—location of home, parent education

Physical environment of the home—childproofing

Outdoor environmental hazards—plants, air and water quality, pools, beaches, boats

Interventions at the Primary Level of Prevention

Anticipatory guidance Anticipatory guidance is a major nursing responsibility to prevent injury. During the safety assessment, the nurse listens for parents' assessment of their children's individual characteristics. The child's general activity level, responsiveness, degree of adaptability to change, and sense of independence and caution determine the need for improved safety. The nurse then can discuss the activity limits the parent is currently using and the effectiveness of these limits in light of the accident liability of the child. If the child is a risk taker and shows little sense of fear, parents might need to structure the environment more tightly.

Nurses can assist parents by providing instructional materials and helping parents assess their children's capabilities and limitations according to their developmental stages. Two children of the same age might have different levels and different needs. One child might require more structure and more safety education than another.

Safety education is most effective when it is directed specifically toward changing a single aspect of an agent or the environment rather than dealing with the whole problem all at once. For example, during an initial conference, the nurse might deal with the use of restraints, or safety gates, or fire drills. Nurses need to evaluate the effectiveness of their teaching strategies during each successive conference, while remembering that the psychologic and socioeconomic aspects of the environment are as important as the physical aspects.

Community resources (library, fire and police departments) are good sources of teaching aids for parents. Poison control centers have stickers and warnings for medicines and poisonous substances. Pamphlets are available that might interest parents (Table 12-4).

In each well-child visit the nurse includes discussion of the child's anticipated period of growth and development with a focus on the appropriate safety issues. Observing limit-setting situations and the parent-child interaction in the office can give the nurse valuable information.

During the process of growth, safety for children changes from protection of the young child to education of the older child. A difficult issue for parents is the fine line between overprotection and allowing the child to make choices and take risks, which encourages growth. Allowing a child to ride a bicycle to the store alone or permitting an adolescent to take the family car are issues that most parents face.

Parents learn to teach children to know their own limits and responsibilities as they grow. Consistent and understandable limits enforced in a gentle, firm manner eventually teach children to make safe judgments for themselves. Children need to understand parental expectations regarding rules for safety as well as comprehend the reasons for them. External limits that make sense to children gradually will be internalized by them when they are called on to make safety decisions in new situations.

Parents teach by example as well as by method. Children are keen observers, and young children tend to imitate what they see. Fastening seatbelts, looking before crossing a street, and safe driving habits are a few examples of safe practices children might imitate. All parents would like their children to learn moderation and good judgment. Conscientious role modeling will facilitate the development of these qualities.

Nurses can instruct parents about appropriate conditions for teaching. For example, nurses need to encourage parents to discuss safety issues with children in a calm, relaxed atmosphere. Parents can then encourage children to describe how they would handle unsafe situations, that is, what to do if they smell smoke, how to get help if a friend is injured, what to do if they are lost or if a ball rolls into the street. Children are in hazardous situations before entering school and need to be taught safety at an early age. Practicing family fire drills, learning how to reach an operator or how to dial home, knowing the home address and parents' names, and learning to ask a police officer for help are certainly useful tools for teaching children to manage crises. Indicating safe habits or safety principles to children during daily contact with them promotes safe behavior. For example, practicing crossing the street appropriately can be done every time a young child accompanies a parent on a walk. Most children will automatically incorporate these safety actions into their behavior patterns after the constant repetition and practice.

TABLE 12-4 Resources for Prevention of Injury and Poisonings

Media	Title and address
Film	Physicians for Automotive Safety: *Don't Risk Your Child's Life*. Communications Department. Rye, NY.
	Visucom: *The Perfect Gift for Tamie*. Redwood City, CA.
	National Safety Council: *Childsafe*. Chicago, IL.
	Film Loops, Inc.: *Do You Care Enough?* Princeton, NJ.
Pamphlet	Action for Child Transportation Safety: *Car Pool Survival Kit, Kids are Fragile, Protecting Child Passengers,* and *This is the Way Baby Rides*. Bothell, WA.
	American Academy of Pediatrics Transportation Hazards Committee: *Will You Give Your Child the Perfect Gift?* Inglewood, CA.
	Martens R, Seedfelt: *Guidelines for Children's Sports*. American Alliance for Health, Physical Education, Recreation and Dance, Washington, DC.
	A Toy and Sports Equipment Safety Guide. Young Children and Accidents in the Home. Home and Fire Safety. US Government Printing Office, Pueblo, CO.
	Child Safety for Injury Prevention. No G836. Ross Laboratories, Columbus, OH.
	Poison Checklist. Consumer Product Safety Commission, Washington, DC.
	We Want You to Know About Preventing Childhood Poisonings. US Food and Drug Administration, HF-88, Rockville, MD 20857.
	Common Poisonous and Injurious Plants. Superintendent of Documents, Government Printing Office, Washington, DC.
	List of Materials March 17–23, 1985. National Poison Prevention Week Council, Washington, DC 20013.

Environmental modification: childproofing A parent learns to adapt the environment to respond to the child's needs. These adaptations are called childproofing. Each room of the house needs to be made as hazard-free as possible for the specific child's developmental level and in anticipation of the upcoming levels. Devices such as safety gates for stairs, electrical outlet fillers, locks for drawers and cabinets, and plastic door handle protectors can limit the environment for an inquisitive child. Most toy stores carry child safety equipment, all of which is simple to install. The removal of the parents' favorite breakable items until the children can handle them carefully prevents parental distress and the resultant increase in pressure on the children.(Room-by-room childproofing is illustrated in Figure 12-2 and Table 12-2.)

Nurses might need to remind parents that the home need not be a fortress, nor should safety proofing limit the enjoyment of other family members. Young children are perfectly happy playing with household implements such as pots and pans and wooden spoons, and these should be accessible to them. Older children need to have space allotted to them where they can keep their own possessions out of reach.

Nurses can assist parents to create a stimulating, attractive, and safe play area for their young children. Brightly painted shelves or cupboards for toy storage should be within the child's reach. Large, covered plastic containers can be used to hold toys with multiple pieces to prevent loss and injury to a family member who might trip on them. Play spaces made of large cartons allow children to hide and promote imaginative play. They can be painted to look like a train or a zoo cage—great for the storage of stuffed animals. Tape recorders to play children's music are simple to operate and safer than record players. Colorful wall murals come in a variety of subjects and are not only attractive, but also promote learning. Equipment for activities that require parental supervision can be kept out of reach, in a closet. Riding toys should be stable and low to the ground. Provision should be made for safe climbing such as toy stairs or small wooden boxes in a step structure.

By creating an attractive and interesting play area for children, parents can reduce injury because children will tend to play in the area created for them. If at all possible, this area should be close to a part of the house where a parent spends the most time so the young child will not feel isolated and be tempted to wander into an unsafe area.

Safety education: specific hazards

Burn prevention In the early years children's motor abilities develop at a much faster rate than their ability to protect themselves and make judgments about safety. Instead, they rely on adults to keep their surroundings safe, depending chiefly on parental knowledge, attentiveness, and love.

Most burn accidents are preventable and they occur in predictable patterns for each age group. In young children, burns happen when there is a temporary lapse in parental attention or a lack of knowledge regarding growth and development. In older children, burns often are related to lack of proper parental supervision along with a minor knowledge, on the child's part, regarding the dangers of fire and flammable liquids.

House fires cause injury and death in all age groups, and it is important to plan with children what to do in case of fire. For example, escape routes; a common meeting place; crawling under smoke; and the stop, drop, and roll sequence if clothing ignites are important pieces of information.

The very young are vulnerable in house fires because they have neither the ability nor the knowledge to escape. They also might be innocent bystanders of another child's match play or victims in a motor vehicle accident involving fire. All too often a youngster is found crouched under a bed or in a closet, badly injured or dead, when a clear escape route was available or a window handy nearby to call for help.

Adults do not supervise children in late childhood as closely as younger children and might unwisely assign tasks such as stoking a wood stove or filling a gasoline-powered lawn mower to children who are unable to do these jobs safely. Many burns result from the careless use of or experimentation with fires and flammable liquids, most commonly gasoline. Adults, as well as children, often do not understand the dangers of gasoline. Vapors ignite, and using a flammable liquid near open flames is very hazardous. Adults need to demonstrate safe behavior such as storing gasoline only when absolutely necessary, using specified containers, using gasoline only in well-ventilated areas, pouring with a funnel to avoid splashes, and storing and using gasoline away from heat sources such as clothes dryers and water heaters. They need to teach their children the common dangers around the home and neighborhood.

Electricity fascinates youngsters, particularly children in late childhood. Electrical wires high above the ground are not insulated; and it is not even necessary to touch them to receive a burn because electricity arcs. Boys, especially, might climb trees and utility poles or trespass in areas where there are high-voltage wires. Electrical burns from this source result in deep damage to muscle and bone, often necessitating amputation of an arm or leg.

Clothing design sometimes is associated with types of burns. Long, flowing nightgowns worn near fireplaces, space heaters, or while cooking are dangerous. Some states allow children to have access to firecrackers. Children need to know how to handle them properly to prevent accidental explosion and injuries to the hands or face.

Parents or teachers might turn to the school nurse for

help when a child consistently plays with matches. Individual counseling with families and using visual aids such as simple posters, films, and samples of burned clothing is often sufficient to stop this behavior. A session with the family, however, might reveal deeper problems such as a troubled marriage, a disturbed parent-child relationship, or a history of repeated fire setting. On-going psychologic counseling might be necessary.

Nurses in primary care agencies need to include burn prevention measures in their home intervention strategies for parents. Some important points include (1) inspecting electrical appliances for frayed or dangling cords and exposed parts, (2) checking for accessibility of matches, lighters, flammable liquids, and caustic household products, (3) measuring tap water with a meat or candy thermometer, and (4) turning water heaters to a low setting. Each floor of the house needs a smoke detector, and every family member should know fire escape plans.

Local fire departments can help school and community nurses with home and school-based prevention projects. Educational materials are available for school nurses to present to children and parents. PTA meetings are a good forum. Project Burn Prevention and other agencies have filmstrips for children and adults that are designed to reach each age group. The burned clothing of children who played with matches can be a dramatic visual and tactile aid. Children as young as 3 and 4 years old can comprehend that the clothing did not protect the skin from burns. Nurses can learn more about children's perceptions by asking them to draw a picture after the film and by discussing the presentation. Older children often ask questions and share their own experiences. Information about first aid fits in well with burn prevention teaching. Practicing the stop, drop, and roll sequence for clothing ignition; rehearsing what to do in case of a house fire; and practicing dousing "pretend" scalds with cool water gives children concrete behaviors to rehearse that will help them in an emergency.

Prevention of drowning Children can be taught to swim and follow the rules of water safety by about 5 years of age. If appropriately instructed, children at even younger ages can be taught to remain afloat until help arrives after an accidental fall into water. Use of the survival float (face forward taking intermittent breaths) conserves energy and is an effective method of reducing the incidence of drowning. Children who live close to natural water or pools need to be taught to swim at the earliest possible age. Rules for water safety should be given with swimming instruction.

Infant swim programs have their own advantages and disadvantages. Young infants can be taught to float, but they cannot be taught safety rules. Therefore, they should never be left near the water unsupervised.

Nurses can become involved in discussing water safety with parents and children. They should be knowledgeable about local facilities that provide swimming and water safety instruction. Camp nurses assess the safety of the camp waterfront and the adequacy and competency of the lifeguards as they assess other aspects of camp safety. Rescue equipment is necessary at all recreational swimming areas.

Water safety rules that nurses need to emphasize include always swimming with a buddy; accurately assessing swimming capabilities; knowing the water depth before diving; swimming in supervised areas; not swimming during electrical storms; avoiding swimming near diving boards or diving platforms; avoiding a reliance on buoyancy devices to boost swimming ability; knowing the basic, safe, rescue techniques; and calling for help only when needed.

Motor vehicle and bicycle accident prevention Nurses need to reinforce the statistics that validate the need for car seats to parents. Lists of safety-tested car seats are available to help parents choose alternatives. The expense of the car restraint system ($20–$60) is minimal when compared with the costs of hospitalization for injuries. Parents, clubs, and community organizations often recycle car seats. Nurses need to know what resources their communities offer.

Magazines offer a multitude of ideas to distract small children on long car trips. Stops every 2 hours allow children to stretch their muscles and unwind. Parents need to insist on the use of seatbelts for all car occupants. Appropriately approved car restraint systems are used for the child under 4 years of age or weighing less than 40 lb.

Developmentally, most 6-year-olds can balance a two-wheeler bike. Many schools and neighborhoods have bicycle safety programs. School-age children enjoy participating and receiving a certificate or special recognition while learning safety.

Rules for bicycle safety to reinforce with parents include:

1. Ride with traffic.
2. When riding at night, wear light-colored clothes and have a light and reflectors on the bike and clothing.
3. Look to both sides when changing lanes.
4. Yield when entering a roadway.
5. Obey traffic signals.
6. Use appropriate hand signals for turns.

Street accident prevention Children can be taught, in developmental steps, to navigate traffic and to cross the streets. A 2-year-old can learn where to play and walk, that is, only in the yard and on sidewalks or grass. A 3-year-old can learn to listen for cars and be aware if they are coming or going. A 4-year-old can begin to learn to cross the street. When learning colors, a 5-year-old can learn about traffic

TABLE 12-5 Poison Prevention Education

Well-child visit	Items to be discussed with parents
1 month	Correct dosage—vitamins/iron
2 months	Dosing—antipyretics
4 months	Dosing—cold preparations
6 months	Put products out of reach. Ipecac/what to do in case of a suspected poisoning
9 months	Ipecac follow-up
1 year	Child resistant locks/storage
1½ years	Child resistant packaging
2 years	Review what to do in case of a suspected poisoning
3 years	Poison symbols/reminders to emphasize to the child not to eat anything found outdoors
4 years	Preschool education program
5–12 years	School education program

SOURCE: Gillies et al: Management of pediatric poisoning: Role of the nurse practitioner. *Pediatr Nurs* (Sept/Oct) 1980; 6:33–35.

signals. The American Automobile Association Early Childhood Traffic Bureau offers an excellent set of booklets reinforcing traffic rules for young children.

Parents need to set clear boundaries and rules for their children about crossing streets. They need to provide safe areas for children to play (especially in cities where children often play in the street). For young children, parents might make arrangements with other parents to cross children back and forth to friends' houses. They need to teach children safety habits for dealing with traffic, that is, learning to cross with the light, looking and listening before crossing, entering and leaving a car from the curbside, and not chasing a ball or toy into a street. Caution when entering or leaving school buses is also important to emphasize to children. Children need to be warned not to go under the bus for any reason.

Poison prevention The discussion of poisoning should be a routine part of well-child visits (Table 12-5). Early visits can be used to familiarize parents with the therapeutic use of drugs. The nurse also reviews the correct dosages of common over-the-counter medications and the danger of overusing medications or saving and sharing medications within the family.

Parents need to be informed of the dangers present in the environment and the developmental characteristics of young children that make them susceptible to toxic hazards. They need to be encouraged to go through their home room by room, on their hands and knees at the child's level if necessary, and remove and safely store all potential toxins. Parents are given a list of poisonous plants and encouraged to identify and in many cases remove all toxic plants from their home and garden. Parents must be helped to make home safety so automatic that even in times of stress their ability to protect their child will not be decreased.

The nurse also reviews the principles of poison safety.

Safety Guidelines for Poison Prevention

1. Keep all household products out of the reach of young children when not in use. When these products are in use, they should never be out of sight of adults—even if it means taking them along when answering the telephone or the doorbell.
2. Choose cleaning supplies with childproof or hard-to-open containers. Containers should be rinsed prior to discarding.
3. Items should be kept in their original containers. They should never be stored in food containers or soft-drink bottles.
4. All products should be properly labeled, and one should read the label before using.
5. Don't save medicine. Leftover medications should be discarded by flushing them down the toilet. Current medications should be stored separately from other household products, preferably locked up. Metal boxes with locks commonly used to store checks are difficult for a child to open and can be used effectively to store medications.
6. Return medication to safe storage immediately after using. Never leave any medication (including vitamins or aspirin) by the sink or on the dining table.
7. The light always should be on when giving or taking medications.
8. Adults should avoid taking medications in front of children because youngsters tend to imitate adults.
9. Medications should be referred to as "medicine" and never as "candy."
10. Safety packaging should be used properly and closed securely after use.
11. Ask the nursery for the botanic name of any new plant purchased and record it. Avoid planting or placing poisonous plants in areas easily accessible to young children. Alert family where potentially poisonous plants are already planted and supervise children carefully when they are in those areas.

Most poison control centers provide educational materials on request. For example, Mr. Yuk or other stickers can be placed on any poisonous articles, and the child is taught not to touch anything bearing the sticker. In addition, various materials are available to professionals and parents at a low cost.

In spite of the most conscientious program of home safety, accidental poisoning can still occur. It is vital that the nurse help prepare the parent for such an emergency. It is a terrifying experience for parents to walk into a room and discover that their child has eaten all of the children's aspirin or tasted the bleach. The nurse can help by encouraging parents to develop a plan of action before such an incident occurs.

The nurse discusses poison prevention at a child's annual physical examination at least until the child is 5 years of age. Discussion with the child and parent can help the nurse to assess the level of understanding and degree of cooperation with the suggested actions and identify areas where further teaching is required. Assessment of the family might indicate situational or stress-related factors that might increase the chances of a poisoning accident. These factors and their relationship to poisoning can then be discussed. As the child enters adolescence, a frank discussion of the problems associated with experimentation with drugs is indicated.

Injury prevention for the disabled For children with hearing and vision disabilities, increased precautions around traffic are necessary. Parents can request special signs advising motorists to watch for deaf and blind children. For parents, the patience required to teach disabled children safety can be overwhelming. The nurse needs to be aware of local organizations and support groups for disabled children and their families.

Health protection for injury prevention Society is extremely concerned about the health of children. Child health protection involves specific federal and state legislation enacted to increase children's safety. The child car restraint legislation, the law regulating flameproofing of children's sleepwear, and the Child Protection and Toy Safety Act are all health protection measures enacted to prevent injury. It is the responsibility of the nurse to keep abreast of new legislation regarding child safety and communicating the facts to parents and the community at large.

Secondary Level of Prevention: The Nurse's Role

For the injured child, the secondary level of prevention often involves assessment and interventions that are quick responses to emergencies. First aid is often needed to stabilize the child's condition and prevent more serious effects. For the poisoned child in particular, the nurse's preparation and timely interventions might save the child's life.

Assessment at the Secondary Level of Prevention

Assessment of the injured child When a child becomes injured, the severity of the injury often is related to the promptness and effectiveness of the initial treatment. Nurses in a variety of settings might be called on to administer first aid to an injured child. Accurate assessment of the child's condition combined with knowledgeable first-aid measures can reduce the severity of an injury or even save a child's life. (The major injury crises and the corresponding nursing actions are presented in Table 12-6).

Assessment of the acutely poisoned child Nurses might be dealing with poisoned children in an ambulatory setting or emergency room, or they might be giving information as members of a poison control center team. As in any other aspect of nursing care, care of the child who is the victim of an accidental poisoning begins with a thorough assessment. Time is often a crucial factor. The nurse must be skilled in obtaining the maximum amount of information in a minimum amount of time.

The phone number of the poison control center, the ambulance rescue squad, and the family physician should be kept in plain sight by the telephone. The parents should be encouraged to decide ahead of time which hospital they would go to and the shortest route to take. Parents should become familiar with the principles of first-aid management for poisoning, and a copy of the emergency guidelines should be posted in a medicine cabinet or on a closet door.

Every home in which small children live or regularly visit should have a 1-oz bottle of syrup of ipecac for each child under 5 years of age (see p. 355). Parents are instructed to use syrup of ipecac only on the advice of a poison control center or physician. The nurse reminds parents to check the ipecac regularly for expiration date. Because it is used so infrequently, this might be overlooked.

Parents need to be alert for the signs of accidental poisoning. The most obvious indicators would be presence of poisonous items such as pills, mothballs, or plant parts in the child's hand, mouth, or in the play area. Burns, blisters, or odor around the mouth are possible signs of ingestion. Open, empty containers in the child's possession are another cause for investigation.

Less obvious signs of poisoning occur as the child begins to develop symptoms. These symptoms might include alteration in consciousness and respirations or a sudden onset of gastrointestinal symptoms.

(text continues on p. 354)

TABLE 12-6 First-Aid Principles for Children

Category and criteria	Intervention	
Cardiopulmonary resuscitation		
Airway		
Child not ventilating; cyanosis of lips and nail beds	*Infant:* pinch baby's feet or gently flick the base of the sternum; place infant on a flat, hard surface with hand on forehead, gently extending the head; place your cheek near the infant's nose and feel for exhalation *Child (under 8):* tap or gently shake; ask if child is awake; tilt child's head back gently lifting chin to open airway; do this procedure on a flat, hard surface; observe for respiration *Child (over 8):* treat as for adult	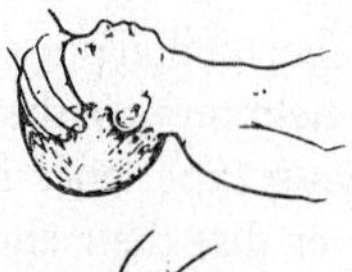 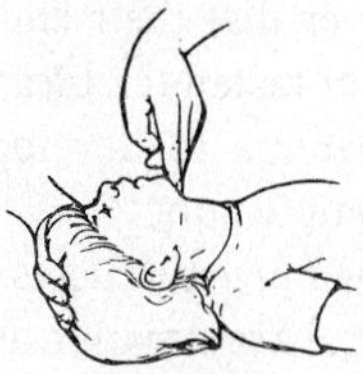
Breathing		
Child still not breathing after airway is opened	*Infant:* cover infant's mouth and nose with your mouth, creating a seal; give two slow breaths, allowing for exhalation between breaths; check for the spontaneous resumption of breathing; if infant not breathing, check pulse at the inner aspect of elbow; if pulse is present, continue with breathing only *Rate:* one breath every 3 seconds or 20 breaths/min *Child:* pinch the nose and make a seal over the mouth only; give two slow breaths allowing for exhalation between breaths; check the carotid pulse for 5 seconds; if pulse is present but child is not breathing, continue respirations *Rate:* one breath every 4 seconds or 15 breaths/min (one breath every 5 seconds or 12 breaths/min for child over 8 years of age) **NOTE:** Check to make certain of chest rise and fall; avoid getting air into stomach	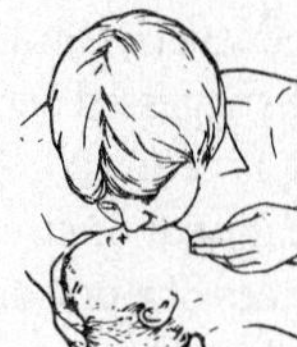 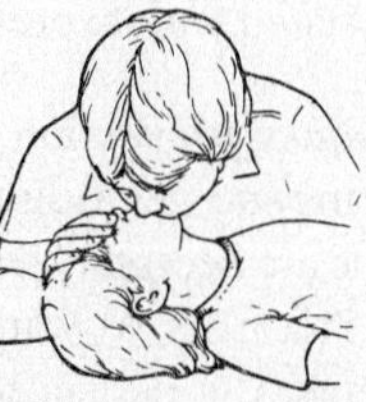
Circulation		
Absent pulse; cyanosis	*Infant:* place index finger and middle fingers one finger width below the nipple line; depress ½ to 1″ toward the backbone *Rate:* 100–120 compressions/min; give one breath for every five compressions; check for the resumption of cardiac rate for 5 seconds after each minute of CPR; **do not stop CPR for more than 5 seconds** *Child:* use the heel of one hand to compress sternum at the nipple line; depress 1 to 1½″ *Rate:* 80–100 compressions/min; give one breath for every five compressions, stop periodically to check for the resumption of circulation but not for longer than 5 seconds *Older child:* use two hands over lower portion of sternum, two finger widths from the xyphoid for compressions; depress 1½ to 2″ *Rate:* 80 compressions/min; give two breaths after each 15 compressions; stop periodically to check for the resumption of circulation but for no longer than 5 seconds *Two-person rescue:* 60 chest compressions with one breath after each 5 compressions	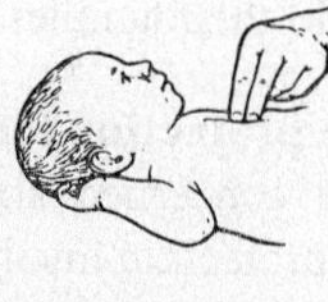 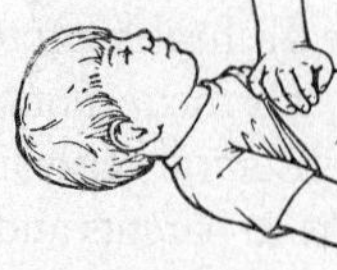

TABLE 12-6 *(Continued)*

Category and criteria	Intervention	
Choking		
Child appears distressed; unable to vocalize; cyanosis; older child will point to throat **NOTE:** if child is coughing and pink, WAIT and OBSERVE	*Infant:* turn infant upside down and administer four back blows between the scapula with the palm of the hand; if the object is not dislodged, turn the infant over and administer four chest compressions with index and middle fingers; continue alternating back blows with compressions until the object is dislodged	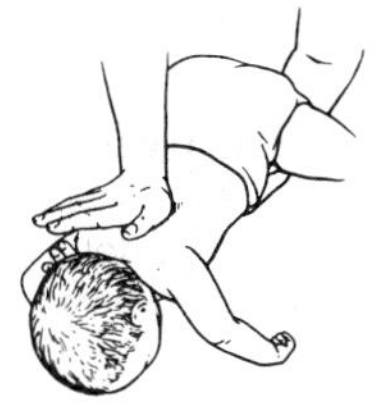
	Child: stand behind child, reach both arms around the child halfway between the sternum and umbilicus; make a fist with one hand (thumb inside); cover with the other hand and administer six to ten upward thrusts approximately 2 seconds apart **NOTE:** after object is dislodged, CPR might be necessary	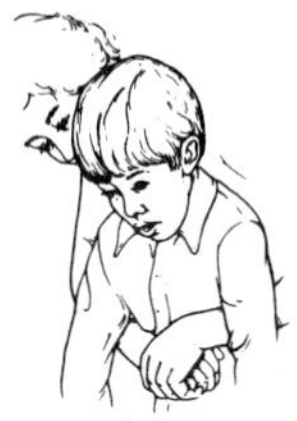
Bleeding		
Moderate bleeding from a wound	*Children of all ages:* cover the wound with a clean cloth or dressing and apply direct pressure with your hand over the dressing; if an extremity is affected, elevate it while applying the pressure; keep applying pressure for approximately 15 minutes *or* apply a pressure dressing with several layers of square pads held in place by gauze or other wrap; do not remove the dressing until medical advice has been obtained; if blood soaks through the dressing, add additional layers	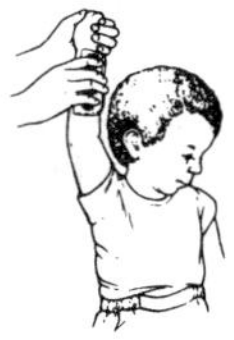
Severe bleeding from a wound that continues despite direct pressure and elevation; arterial bleeding; amputated limb	If direct pressure and elevation are unsuccessful in controlling bleeding, add pressure to pressure points with fingers and thumb; if the femoral artery is to be compressed, the heel of the hand should be used; treat for shock **NOTE:** do not use a tourniquet except as a last resort for bleeding that cannot be controlled by other methods	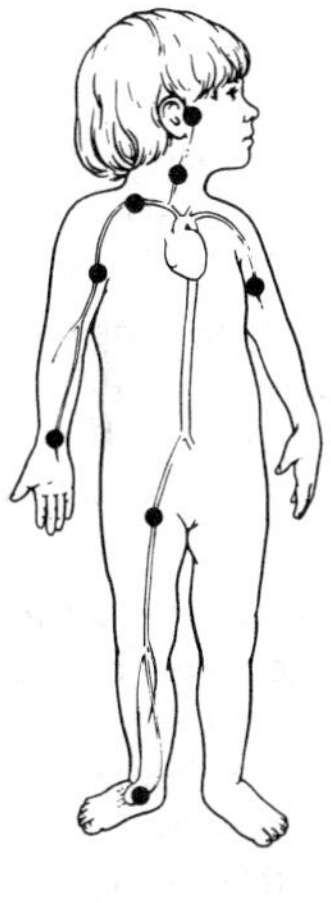
Head injuries		
Unconsciousness; contusion on the head; projectile vomiting; headache; disorientation; alteration in pupil size and reaction; convulsions; drainage from nose or ears; tense fontanelle	Differentiate unconsciousness from infant breath holding; apply ice to the contusion; allow the child to sleep but awaken at hourly intervals to check neurologic signs; encourage relaxation; head may be kept slightly elevated but never below level of the feet; seek medical consultation if there is a decrease in level of consciousness, convulsions, deterioration of neurologic signs, drainage from nose or ear, or bulging fontanelle	

(Continues)

TABLE 12-6 First-Aid Principles for Children *(Continued)*

Category and criteria	Intervention
Back and neck injuries	
Pain at site of injury; weakness, numbness, or paralysis below injury site; lack of movement in more than one extremity; decreased sensation in trunk or extremities	Prevent side-to-side movement of the child; preferably do not move; explain all actions to the child to ensure cooperation; if movement is necessary, the child should be secured to a firm, flat surface such as a backboard or door; pad the sides of the neck or head with rolled towels, newspapers, sneakers, etc to prevent movement; fasten the head to the board first, followed by the feet and the remainder of the body; enlist the help of several people to transfer the child to the board so as to maintain rigid alignment; if the child is injured in the water, CPR may be necessary 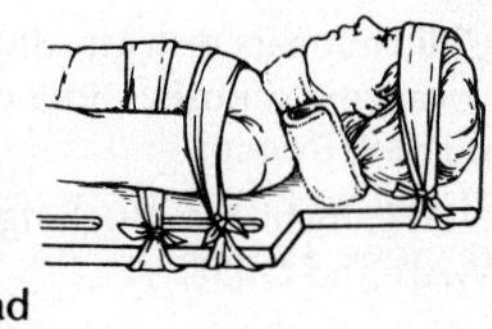
Drowning	
Child found floating just beneath the water or ice surface; cessation of respiration with associated cyanosis **NOTE:** time is a crucial factor; if resuscitation is initiated within the first 4 minutes of a drowning, sequelae from hypoxia will be reduced	Inflate the child's lungs with two slow breaths, then remove from the water if possible; continue artifical respiration or CPR as previously described; the child might vomit; turn the head to the side to prevent aspiration; institute artificial respiration even if the length of time in water is unknown; children who have drowned are known to have been successfully resuscitated after long periods of submersion due to a reflex that traps oxygen in the body and slows down body processes; a child who has been revived needs immediate medical attention for the prevention and treatment of complications
Burns	
Epidermis and part of dermis destroyed (partial thickness burns)—area is red, painful, edematous, and possibly blistered Dermal layer destroyed through subcutaneous fat (full-thickness burn)—area is pearly white, tan, brown, or black; not painful; tissue is dry *Criteria for hospital admission:* 1. Burns on children under 2 years of age unless minor and superficial 2. Electrical burns 3. Deep chemical burns 4. Burns complicated by fracture or soft tissue injury 5. Burns complicated by concurrent illness (eg, diabetes, renal disease, etc)	Stopping the burn process is the initial goal; smother flames by having the child do the stop, drop, and roll procedure or by wrapping the child in a blanket; douse clothing with cool water; cool down all burns from hot liquids; remove all nonadherent clothing; flush chemical burns with copious amounts of water for at least 20 minutes while en route to an emergency room; keep burned child warm because skin loss alters temperature-regulating mechanisms; if the burn is from an electrical current, switch off electricity before treating; initiate CPR as necessary and treat for shock 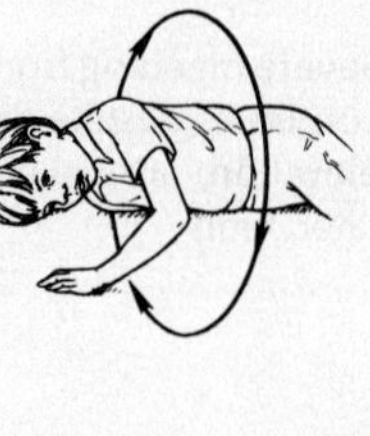
Frostbite	
Skin will be white, hard, numb, and cold	Immerse affected area in tepid water for approximately 20 minutes or until signs of warmth return; child might experience excruciating pain in the area as it warms

TABLE 12-6 *(Continued)*

Category and criteria	Intervention
Skeletal injuries	
Edema, discoloration, pain, and/or alteration of movement at injury site; extreme tenderness to the touch; numbness and tingling; appearance of bone through the skin	Radiography is the only method of accurately diagnosing a fracture; apply ice to the injury and elevate; if the bone protrudes, cover it with a sterile or clean dressing; immobilize to joints above and below injury location by the use of splints and/or sling; folded newspapers or magazines, barrel slats, etc can be used as splints; tape an injured toe to the adjacent toes to immobilize; consult physician when fracture is suspected or in cases of severe tissue swelling 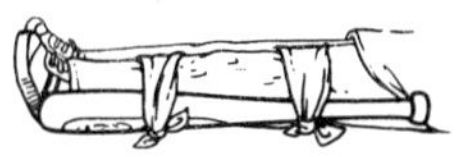
Anaphylaxis	
Generalized urticaria, bronchospasm, wheezing, laryngospasm, fainting, shock; history of recent exposure to an allergen—medication, insect sting, etc	If an insect sting, carefully remove stinger without rupturing the sac; apply a tourniquet proximal to a sting bite but do not completely close off circulation; if epinephrine is available, administer 0.2–0.5 mL of 1 : 1000 strength subcutaneously or into a sting site; this may be repeated in 20 minutes; antihistamines such as diphenhydramine also can be administered; treat for shock **NOTE:** this is a life-threatening crisis requiring immediate medical attention
Eye injuries	
Pain; watery eyes; conjunctivitis; visible object impaled in eye; blurred vision; light flashes or spots	Check eye for small foreign particles by having the child look up and down; lids may be everted and the particle, if seen, removed with a saline-moistened cotton-tipped applicator; severe pain in the corneal area should be checked by an ophthalmologist; the eyes can be patched for comfort; small objects impaled in the cornea must be removed by a physician; large objects (such as an arrow, pencil, etc) should be stabilized by surrounding them with sterile gauze pads; the other eye should also be covered; explain all actions to the child to increase cooperation and decrease movement from resistance; transport child to emergency room with minimal movement; if the eye has sustained a direct blow, observe the child carefully for signs of severe pain, blurred vision, and other signs of internal injury; consult an ophthalmologist 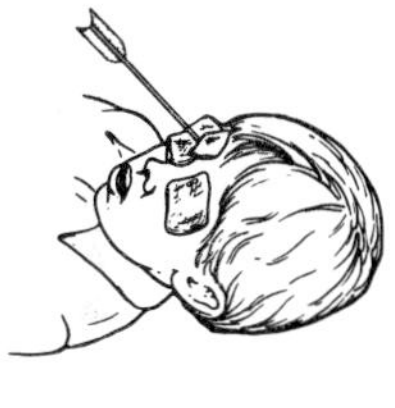
Bites	
Animal Laceration or avulsion tissue injury from dogs; puncturelike wounds from cats	Rinse the wound copiously with water, followed by washing the adjacent skin with mild soap; cover the wound and refer to a physician for additional treatment; prophylactic antibiotics might be required to prevent infection (appears in 24–72 hours); observe animal for 10 days for rabies; tetanus and rabies prophylaxis if indicated
Snake *Mild:* swelling, discoloration, pain and numbness at the site, weakness, nausea, dyspnea	Transport victim to medical facility immediately; immobilize the site lower than the heart; reassure the victim and treat for shock; if medical help is not within a 30-minute trip, place a ¾″ to 1½″ constricting band loosely above the site (2–4 in.); monitor the pulse (Thompson and Verbeek, 1984); provide the physician with a description of the snake if possible

(Continues)

TABLE 12-6 First-Aid Principles for Children *(Continued)*

Category and criteria	Intervention
Bites *(Continued)*	
Spider	
Brown recluse (yellow-brown, has violin shape on the head): pain, bleb formation, erythema, bruising, and tissue necrosis; might be associated with fever, chills, and other systemic manifestations	Cleanse wound; soak with cool packs; debridement might be necessary; treatment with steroids in some cases; surgery with grafting if tissue damage is extensive
Black widow (black, red hourglass-shaped mark on ventral surface): pinprick sensation followed by numbness, muscle aches, and cramping; paralysis, muscle rigidity, and pain are later symptoms; weakness, nausea, vomiting, pruritis	Keep victim quiet; clean bite with alcohol or peroxide; immobilize the affected area; transport to medical facility for antivenin; muscle relaxants and narcotics might be ordered for pain

History When a suspected poisoning occurs, it is essential for the nurse to obtain a good history. Nurses in doctors' offices, emergency departments, and poison control centers are often called by parents of children who have been exposed to poisons. Whether it is a minor ingestion or a serious emergency, the nurse needs to obtain certain basic information. In cases where the poisoning is severe or potentially severe, the patient's address is important so that emergency equipment can be dispatched.

In less critical situations the patient's name and telephone number needs to be obtained so that follow-up calls can be made if the patient is to be treated at home. It is important for a parent to post the home address and phone number when leaving a child with a babysitter. This ensures that the sitter gives the correct call-back number to the poison control center.

Basic information Specific initial information includes the exact name of the product, when the exposure occurred, the approximate amount involved, route of the exposure, evidence of exposure, current symptoms, and age, weight, and gender of the patient. The caller is asked if any treatment already has been instituted. Some treatments that used to be common can be more dangerous than the poison itself. Among these common remedies are neutralization and gagging with a finger down the throat.

Age and weight are necessary to assess the potential severity of an exposure. Knowledge of age-related differences in drug effects or metabolism and the amount of the exposure on a weight basis (that is, milligrams of drug ingested per kilogram of body weight) are necessary to manage the potentially poisoned patient appropriately. Close approximation of weight is especially important in dealing with children.

The initial assessment can then allow the nurse to determine whether life is in immediate danger, potential danger, or no danger.

Secondary information Further information might be needed before the final assessment and treatment plan are established. A secondary history clarifies the amounts involved (for example, counting pills and verifying the amount originally in the container). Other medication/products included in the exposure need to be ruled out. The patient's past medical history, general health, known allergies, and current medications are determined.

In cases of childhood poisoning, the nurse always suspects the possibility of sibling or playmate exposure. All too frequently, only the child "caught in the act" is considered to be at risk for developing toxicity. The possibility of shared adventures and of one child "feeding" another child should be considered.

Interventions at the Secondary Level of Prevention

Poisoning has no universal antidote. Contrary to popular belief, most poisons do not have any antidotes. Alleged antidotes such as tea and burnt toast are useless. Home remedies to induce vomiting, such as saltwater, mustard water, or a finger down the throat, are ineffective, often harmful, and cause dangerous delays in seeking effective treatment. Antidotes and first-aid information on product labels are often incorrect and sometimes dangerous.

Parents are instructed always to call the poison control center or their physician as soon as the exposure is discovered and before administering any antidote or emetic, including syrup of ipecac. If they are unsure if the exposure is dangerous, they should not wait for symptoms to appear but call for assistance immediately.

First aid for poisoning Once the history-taking process is complete, first aid for poisonings can be initiated. The most common routes of exposure are (1) ingestion, (2) inhalation, (3) ocular, and (4) dermal. Other less common routes are parenteral, rectal, and vaginal.

Preventing further absorption Preventing absorption of substances from the gastrointestinal tract, skin, and eyes is necessary to prevent toxic effects. Ocular exposure should be treated with copious irrigation for 15–20 minutes with normal saline or water. The best way to accomplish this task in children is to "mummify" or wrap them in a bath towel with their hands at their sides. The child is held over the sink, and pitchers of tepid water are poured over the eyes. It is not necessary to force the child's eyes open. Given reassurances, the child will relax and blink frequently enough to let the solution irrigate the eye (see Chapter 32 for further discussion).

First aid for dermal exposures is a 15- to 20-minute irrigation with water to the affected area. The nurse then assesses the exposed area for burns, particularly with caustic exposures (see Chapter 24 for further discussion).

For inhalation exposures, the victim is removed from the exposure site. Resuscitation is not attempted in the contaminated area. Respiratory status is assessed by monitoring respirations. Supportive care is given as needed.

The greatest number of poisonings involve ingestion. The parent or nurse immediately calls the local poison control center for a suspected poison ingestion. Numbers for the regional poison control center usually can be found inside the front cover of any telephone book.

Most regional poison control centers are open 24 hours per day, 365 days per year and answer calls from the public and from health professionals. The poison control center will give explicit directions for handling the child. This information might include instructions about emptying the stomach and administering resuscitation if needed.

The initial first-aid measure for any ingestion other than medicine is the administration of milk or water, as long as the child is awake and alert. Fluids are not given to the unconscious or convulsing child. Children should be given 6–8 oz of milk or water, whichever is readily available in the home. The American Association of Poison Control Centers has suggested that pills not be diluted by fluid intake because drug absorption might be enhanced. Neutralization, the concept of adding a strong acid to a strong base for caustic ingestions, is an outdated method of therapy. Neutralization produces an exothermic (heat-producing) reaction, which can be harmful. Milk is the preferable first-aid remedy for ingested caustic poisons, with water as an alternative.

Removing the poison

Gastric emptying Syrup of ipecac has been a nonprescription drug since 1966 in amounts of 30 mL or less. Because of its excellent safety record, no toxicity has ever been reported when the drug has been used in the recommended doses (Haddad and Winchester, 1983: 11).

Children should be given 15 mL of ipecac followed by 6–8 oz of water. If the child is young, the water might be given first, since the child is less likely to want to drink after tasting the ipecac (King, 1984).

If vomiting does not occur within 20–30 minutes, the dose of ipecac can be repeated once. It would be wise to call the poison control center prior to giving the second dose of ipecac. Recent evidence has indicated that ipecac can be safely given to infants as young as 9 months of age (Litovitz, 1985). This is not done, however, without direction from the physician or poison control center.

Ipecac is contraindicated in the following situations:

1. In the child who is comatose, has seizures, or has ingested a substance with the potential to cause rapid-onset seizures or central nervous system depression
2. In a child who has ingested a caustic substance (strong acid or base)
3. For some petroleum distillates (for example, mineral seal oil) in which the risk of aspiration outweighs the benefits of emesis (see Chapter 22 for discussion of hydrocarbon ingestion)

Gastric lavage Gastric lavage is indicated to empty the stomach if the child is unconscious, has seizures, or is expected to experience a decrease in consciousness. Gastric lavage is also indicated when the poison is rapidly absorbed. Endotracheal or nasotracheal intubation precedes the placement of an orogastric hose for airway protection. The patient is placed in a left-lateral, head-down position.

A large-bore (28 French Ewald) tube is safe in children over 1 year of age. Smaller tubes will not adequately remove the larger fragments of material (Haddad and Winchester, 1983: 11). Repeated washings are conducted until the returns are clear. Children should receive no more than 10 mL/kg per washing. Saline solution is recommended, and it

First Aid for Poisonings—Instructions for Parents

1. **Check breathing** If the child is not breathing, call for help and institute CPR.
2. **Call the poison control center** Be prepared to give the exact name of the substance from the container and the details of the exposure. Describe any plant if you do not know its name. Estimate how much was taken and how long ago. Give the age of the child and a description of symptoms if any. Save the container and any material that the child vomits.
3. **Follow the directions of the poison control center or physician** Do not make a person vomit unless instructed to do so. If ipecac is ordered and the child is young, give the water first. Do not attempt to give anything to an unconscious child or one who is having convulsions. Call the fire department or rescue squad.
4. **Call the poison control center back if the ipecac has been ineffective.**
5. **If there is no phone available, give milk or water and get help.**
6. **Ocular poisoning** Flush the eyes with lukewarm tap water poured from a cup or pitcher for at least 15 minutes. Do not use anything but water in the eye before talking to your poison control center or physician.
7. **Chemicals on the skin** Remove the clothing and flood the involved area with water. Then wash with soapy water and rinse. Call your doctor or poison control center.
8. **Inhalation** Move the victim to fresh air as quickly as possible. Call your poison control center or physician. Institute CPR if necessary.

is important to recover any lavage fluid that is instilled. When lavage is complete, the tube is kept in the stomach for activated charcoal and cathartic instillation. When the tube is no longer needed, it is pinched off and removed.

Whenever gastric lavage is performed, the patient should be on the left side and in the Trendelenberg position to minimize the risk of aspiration and maximize the return (Haddad and Winchester, 1983: 11). To ensure proper tube placement, air should be injected into the hose and a stethoscope used over the stomach.

Charcoal Activated charcoal is a fine black powder that is highly absorbent of most drugs and chemicals and is not itself absorbed through the gastrointestinal mucosa. Activated charcoal can be given either orally in a water slurry or through a nasogastric tube. It should be given to all overdose patients after the completion of a gastric emptying procedure. Activated charcoal should not be given with ipecac because the ipecac will be inactivated by the activated charcoal.

The recommended dose of activated charcoal in children is 15–50 g. A sweetener such as 70% sorbitol or cherry syrup can be added to the charcoal to make it more palatable for children.

Cathartics Cathartics usually are administered simultaneously with charcoal. Saline cathartics (sodium sulfate, magnesium citrate) are given in a dose of 250 mg/kg for a child and 30 g for adults.

Management of the acutely poisoned child Initial evaluation of the child's immediate danger and good supportive care comprise the basic management of any poisoned patient. Basic supportive care incudes:

1. Establishment and management of the airway. The patient is intubated if the gag reflex is lost, if seizures are present, or if the patient has lost consciousness. Oxygen is given as needed.
2. Cardiovascular stabilization. Shock is prevented and treated with fluids or vasopressors if necessary. Fluids are given to hydrate the patient, using caution with the amount given to prevent pulmonary edema.
3. Establishment and management of an acid-base and electrolyte imbalance.
4. Naloxone (Narcan) given in any overdose to rule out the presence of any narcotics.
5. Glucose administration as warranted.

Most poisoned patients can be managed by adhering to simple protocols such as gastric emptying, decreasing absorption, administration of charcoal and a cathartic, and basic life support. In certain poisonings, however, more specific management techniques might be indicated. For a child presenting to an emergency care facility several hours after ingesting a poison and exhibiting life-threatening symptoms, gastric emptying and observation alone might not be effective. More complex techniques such as hemodialysis and hemoperfusion might be indicated.

When a poisoning has occurred, parents often feel extremely guilty. They need support and understanding from the nurse. Their correct actions, such as calling for professional help immediately, should be praised. They have now seen firsthand how easily a poisoning accident can occur and are usually eager for help in preventing its recurrence.

Many poison control centers send poison information to callers as a way of following up on this concern. Nurses who

TABLE 12-7 Poisons Frequently Found in Households

Poison	Clinical effects	Poison	Clinical effects
Insecticides	*Initial:* anorexia, nausea, vomiting, sweating, diarrhea, salivation, tearing, dyspnea, wheezing *Intermediate:* muscle twitching, fatigue, generalized weakness *Late:* central nervous system signs, anxiety, headache, drowsiness, confusion, coma, death by cardiac arrest	Iron	Stupor, shock, acidosis, bloody vomiting and diarrhea, coma
		Caffeine	Convulsions, tremors, tachycardia, fever, vomiting and diarrhea, insomnia, restlessness, gastric bleeding, headache, photophobia
Cold and cough preparations		Alcohol	
Antihistamines	Tachycardia, urinary retention, dry mouth and skin, anxiety, delirium, hyperactivity, seizures, coma, respiratory paralysis, death	Ethanol	Nausea, vomiting, mental confusion, ataxia, muscle incoordination, hypoglycemia, seizures, breath odor, impaired vision and reflexes
Decongestants	Anorexia, nausea, vomiting, cardiac arrhythmias, tachycardia, and elevated blood pressure	Ethylene glycol (antifreeze, thinners)	Altered mental status, shortness of breath, rapid breathing, aciduria, respiratory distress, pulmonary edema, renal failure
Dextromethorphan	Hyperexcitability, drowsiness, dizziness, ataxia, stupor, coma	Methanol (wood alcohol)	Visual disturbances, malaise, dizziness, headache, weakness, metabolic acidosis, pain in eyes, abdomen, and back, seizures, coma
Multivitamins (fat soluble)	Nausea, vomiting, confusion, fatigue, headache, hypothrombinemia (vitamin A), renal tubular damage and hypercalcemia (vitamin D)	Camphor (mothballs)	Nausea, vomiting, central nervous system excitation followed by central nervous system depression, seizures, respiratory failure

come into contact with parents in an acute-care hospital or during a follow-up appointment need to discuss the poisoning with the parents, looking for the factors that influenced the incident and working together on a plan to prevent its recurrence. Occasionally, a poisoning accident signals the presence of more serious family problems. Nurses should be alert to this possibility and be ready to make the proper referral if their assessment indicates further action is needed.

Specific Poisonous Agents

Certain poisonous agents are commonly available and might be accessible to children in their homes. Information about these poisons can be used as a reference guide for nurses and as a resource for nurses to assist parents in the removal of poisonous agents from the home. (Common household poisons are listed in Table 12-7.)

Caustics Bleaches, disinfectants, and detergents are the most frequently seen nondrug poisonings in the home. Alkaline corrosives include lye, lime, Clinitest® tablets, electric dishwasher detergents, and low-phosphate detergents. Various household bleaches contain chlorine-active compounds, which are potentially caustic. Ammonia-containing products include cleaning and bleaching agents, liniments, and aromatic spirits of ammonia. Acids are found in hydrochloric (muriatic) and sulfuric acids and aqua regia (nitric and hydrochloric acids). Disinfectants, wood preservatives, and creosotes might contain phenols.

Clinical manifestations Alkalis and acids produce different clinical effects after ingestion. The main effect of alkalis occurs on the lips, tongue, oral mucosa, and esophagus. Esophageal burns might be present in the absence of burns to the mouth. Acids might produce mild to moderately severe oral and esophageal burns, with the more severe burns occurring in the stomach, mainly in the pyloric area.

Systematically, chlorine-active compounds can produce hypotension and coma. Convulsions, coma, and liver and kidney damage can result if ammonia is absorbed. In a phenol ingestion hyperactivity, marked diaphoresis, hyperkinetic activity, convulsions, and hepatic and renal toxicity can result.

Treatment Vomiting should not be induced after the ingestion of a caustic. The single most important action is to have the victim drink milk or water immediately. Acid or base substances should not be used in an attempt to neutralize the caustic. Emesis or lavage should be avoided. Children with symptoms should have nothing by mouth after initial dilution until after surgical consultation.

Surgical consultation is indicated if the patient has dysphagia, pain, excessive drooling, or oral burns. Esophagoscopy might need to be performed within the first 24 hours. Although controversial, steroids are started immediately if esophageal burns are present (0.1 mg/kg/day of dexamethasone [Decadron].) The steroids usually are given for 3 weeks and then tapered if burns are found or esophagoscopy is not done.

With an industrial-strength ammonia oral exposure, the patient is assessed for shock and pulmonary edema. A tracheostomy might be necessary for glottic edema. Steroids might help prevent stricture.

If there are burns in the mouth from an acid ingestion, the esophagus must be examined. The tube should not be passed into the stomach. If a gastrointestinal obstruction is present, parenteral fluids and hyperalimentation are given (usually for 3 weeks or longer).

Activated charcoal is given with a phenol and related compound ingestion. The patient is monitored for seizures and the acid-base balance. Baseline liver and renal tests should be obtained and followed if the patient is symptomatic.

The skin is decontaminated by removing the clothing and irrigating the skin with water for 20 minutes. The burns should be treated symptomatically.

If the vapors are inhaled, first-aid management is to remove the patient to fresh air. Oxygen should be administered for severe dyspnea or hypoxemia. The patient is assessed for oral or nasopharyngeal burns and monitored for chest pain, pulmonary edema, and pneumonitis. The patient's vital signs are monitored. If pulmonary edema develops, mechanical ventilation with positive end-expiratory pressure should be considered.

An eye exposure requires immediate irrigation with tap water or preferably sterile saline for 20 minutes. An eye examination should be performed if there is persistent pain, redness, irritation, or visual disturbances to determine if the eye has been damaged.

Acetaminophen More than 200 nonprescription acetaminophen preparations are available in tablet, suppository, capsule, liquid, and long-acting forms. Acetaminophen is often found in combination with other analgesic agents. It is used mainly for its antipyretic and analgesic effects. Acetaminophen ingestion is the most common drug poisoning agent in children.

Range of toxicity An amount of 140 mg/kg or greater in a child is considered potentially toxic. Severe toxicity occurs when the blood level reaches 150 μg/mL or greater 4 hours after ingestion.

Clinical manifestations Toxicity mainly affects the liver, resulting in cell necrosis and even death. During phase I (up to 24 hours after ingestion), the child might be asymptomatic or present with anorexia, nausea, vomiting, diaphoresis, and malaise.

In phase II (after 24 hours), right upper quadrant pain secondary to hepatic damage occurs. Abnormal blood chemistries and elevated liver function tests are seen. Other signs of liver damage appear in phase III (3–5 days after ingestion). Death related to hepatic failure occurs in 10% of cases of serious ingestion. Recovery occurs in the last stage.

Treatment Treatment is based on the time interval following ingestion and the history of co-ingested substances. If 100–140 mg/kg of acetaminophen has been ingested, emesis with ipecac can be induced at home. If a toxic blood level is obtained, the child is treated with N-acetylcysteine (Mucomyst).

If there is a mixed ingestion, which is potentially toxic, charcoal and a cathartic should be given if the patient is treated before approximately 10 hours after ingestion. Clinical judgment is important as to the time of ingestion and the potential outcome of co-ingestion. The charcoal should be lavaged out after 2 hours and prior to giving the loading dose of Mucomyst because the charcoal will bind the Mucomyst, rendering it ineffective.

Salicylates Aspirin is found in cold and allergy medicines along with antihistamines and decongestants. Sustained-release preparations are available, in which sustained high levels and prolonged absorption might be present. Methyl salicylate (oil of wintergreen) is almost 99% pure salicylate. It is absorbed quickly after oral ingestion, and the peak might appear sooner than with other aspirin products. Various sunscreen agents and topical creams for osteoarthritis also contain salicylate. Aspirin is used for minor aches and pains, arthritic and rheumatoid conditions, analgesia, antipyresis, and anti-inflammatory conditions. Children's aspirin is flavored and can appeal to children because of its taste similarity to certain candies.

TABLE 12-8 Aspirin Toxicity

Acute: single oral dose	Symptom	Treatment
Mild toxicity (therapeutic)—150 mg/kg	Nausea, vomiting, tinnitus	If less than 100 mg/kg, no treatment is necessary. If 100–150 mg/kg, a cathartic should be given
Moderate toxicity—150–300 mg/kg	Mild to severe hyperpnea, lethargy, and/or excitability; neurologic involvement	Emesis should be induced at home and a cathartic given. Patient should be followed by phone for 24 hours
Severe toxicity—300–500 mg/kg	Life-threatening metabolic acidosis, seizures, coma, and death	A physician should evaluate. Emesis or lavage should be performed and charcoal and cathartic administered. 6-hour salicylate level should be obtained
Potentially lethal—greater than 500 mg/kg	Potentially lethal cardiovascular and respiratory shut-down—death	Emergency room evaluation of salicylate level; dialysis might be indicated

Range of toxicity The pediatric preparations of aspirin contain 75–81 mg (approximately 1 1/4 grains) of aspirin per tablet, and the adult preparations contain 325–650 mg of aspirin. A blood level of 50–100 mg/mL is considered toxic. A single aspirin ingestion of 150 mg/kg can produce moderate toxicity in a child. For example, an average 2-year-old boy weighing 13 kg can experience toxicity with ingestion of 24 baby aspirin, 6 adult aspirin, or 3 extra-strength tablets.

Toxicity from chronic ingestion is believed to be obtained by 2 or more days of greater than 100 mg/kg/24 hours (Temple, 1981). Frequently in pediatrics, toxicity from salicylates can be the result of too frequent or too much aspirin administered for therapeutic purposes. Toxicity can also develop from therapeutic administration to a child who has a decreased fluid intake and urine output, resulting in a decrease in the excretion of salicylates. The diagnosis of a chronic overdose is often missed or delayed. Chronic overdose therefore should be ruled out in a patient presenting with altered level of consciousness.

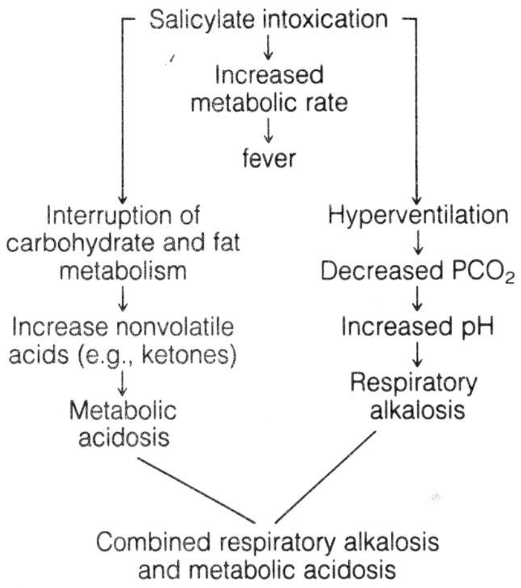

FIGURE 12-3

Primary physiologic outcomes occurring with salicylate intoxication.

Clinical manifestations The clinical findings rather than the drug levels should be used to assess toxicity. (In addition to prolonged bleeding time, the symptoms of salicylate toxicity are presented in Table 12-8 and Figure 12-3.)

Treatment Blood levels should be evaluated 6 hours after ingestion when the salicylate peaks (with oil of wintergreen ingestion, 2- and 6-hour blood levels should be obtained). Ingestion of a large amount of aspirin might cause a concretion to form in the stomach, and absorption might be delayed. Symptomatic patients with a low serum level could be the result of a chronic ingestion or of a concretion being absorbed continuously. A peak level from enteric-coated tablets might occur for up to 28 hours because of the erratic absorption.

Supportive care includes establishing respiration and hydration, monitoring electrolytes and arterial blood gases, and correcting acid-base imbalances.

Absorption can be prevented by emesis induced with ipecac or lavage; administration of charcoal and a cathartic are also indicated.

Promoting excretion is important in the patient with a salicylate overdose. The dehydration should be treated first with IV fluids and a good urine flow established. Bicarbonate is administered if the patient is acidotic. The nurse monitors hydration and the potassium level until the salicylate level is therapeutic. Alkalinization of the urine after rehydration (changing the urine pH from 5 to 8) appears to increase the excretion of salicylate but a pH of 8 might be difficult to maintain (Newton et al, 1987). Hemodialysis or peritoneal dialysis is considered for children with severe toxicity. Vitamin K might be administered for bleeding. Seizures are treated if they occur.

Carbon monoxide Carbon monoxide is a colorless, odorless gas that can cause poisoning in an insidious manner. It is produced by a variety of well-known sources: automobile exhaust, inadequately ventilated fireplaces, and malfunctioning gas appliances (furnaces, water heaters, stoves). Other causes include space heaters or charcoal grills that are operated improperly or with insufficient ventilation.

Carbon monoxide toxicity is due to the special affinity of the gas for oxygen. Carbon monoxide binds with the hemoglobin molecule with an affinity 250 times that of oxygen (Zimmerman and Truxal, 1981). This results in the formation of carboxyhemoglobin and ultimately prevents adequate oxygenation of all tissues of the body.

Low levels of carboxyhemoglobin (between 10% and 25%) produce minor shortness of breath on exertion, headache, nausea, and throbbing temples. Levels above 25% are toxic and can cause headache, dizziness, confusion, convulsions, coma, and death.

Following removal of a victim from the source of exposure, the carboxyhemoglobin level starts to diminish. When the patient breathes room air, the half-life of carbon monoxide is about 5 hours. Oxygen, the primary treatment for carbon monoxide poisoning, will reduce the half-life of carbon monoxide to 90 minutes at an FIO_2 of 100% (Zimmerman and Truxal, 1981). Oxygen competes with carbon monoxide for the hemoglobin molecule. In addition, oxygen is dissolved in the plasma for distribution to the tissues independent of the hemoglobin carriage mechanism.

Even more effective is the use of hyperbaric oxygen, which at 3 atm of pressure reduces the half-life of carbon monoxide to less than 30 minutes (Zimmerman and Truxal, 1981). Hyperbaric oxygen should be considered in comatose children or those with hypotension, acidosis, or electrocardiographic changes suggestive of ischemia. Actual improvement in morbidity and mortality with the use of hyperbaric oxygen awaits further research.

Chronic problems can be seen in children who have experienced carbon monoxide poisoning. These include behavior disturbances, neurologic disturbances, and learning deficits.

Lead Poisoning with lead (plumbism) remains a concern for the young child in today's world. Lead is present everywhere in the environment. Sources of lead include paint chips from lead-based paint, food contaminated by lead-based earthenware, fumes from leaded gasoline, colored newsprint or wrapping paper, and craft equipment such as that used in stained glass craft. Azarcon (a folk medicine), containing approximately 93.5% lead, is brought into the United States from Mexico and is another known cause of lead intoxication in children (FDA, 1983). The most frequent cause of lead poisoning in children, however, is the ingestion of paint chips from windowsills and frames painted with lead-based paint.

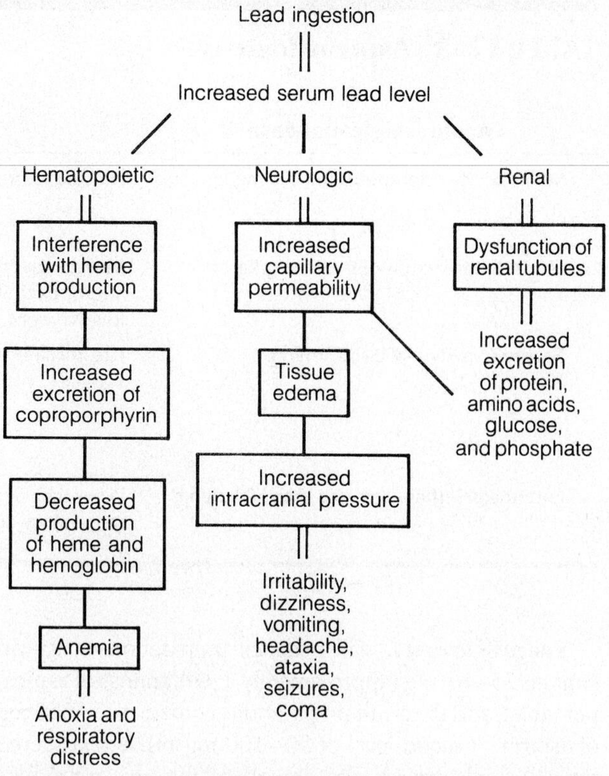

FIGURE 12-4
Physiologic effects of lead poisoning.

Range of toxicity Because the body absorbs lead poorly, multiple exposures are required to produce toxic effects. It takes a minimum of 3 months of exposure for symptoms to become evident.

Normal blood level is 20 μg/dL. Toxicity can occur at 34 μg/dL, and treatment is indicated for the child with serum levels of 25–55 μg/dL, depending on supporting tests (*MMWR*, 1985). A recent study (Bellinger et al, 1987) indicates that children can experience adverse effects from prenatal lead exposure (cord blood lead greater than 10 μg/dL).

Increased lead absorption alters body systems (Fig. 12-4). Lead interferes with the body's production of heme and its

STANDARDS OF NURSING CARE *The Child with Lead Poisoning*

RISKS

Assessed risk	Nursing action
Increased intracranial pressure	Observe the child for headache, vomiting, increased blood pressure, and other signs of increased intracranial pressure (see Chapter 31). Institute seizure precautions and monitor vital signs and neurologic status frequently. Restrict oral fluid intake and carefully monitor IV fluid intake if signs of increased intracranial pressure occur. Monitor serum lead levels. Provide a quiet, restful environment.
Hypocalcemia from chelation	Administer calcium, phosphorus, and vitamin D supplements. Increase calcium and phosphorus in the diet.
Renal dysfunction	Monitor urine output. Determine urinary status prior to chelation. Collect 24-hour specimens as ordered, and monitor urine coproporphyrin levels.

GUIDE FOR NURSING MANAGEMENT

Nursing diagnosis	Intervention	Rationale	Outcome
1. Activity intolerance related to imbalance between oxygen supply and demand	Monitor the child's respiratory status and have oxygen available at the bedside.	Increased respiratory effort might indicate lack of oxygen.	The child cooperates with plan to conserve energy. Hemoglobin and hematocrit return to normal levels.
	Monitor blood gases and hemoglobin and hematocrit levels.	These give an accurate picture of the child's oxygenation status.	
	Provide quiet activities that will allow the child to play but also conserve energy.	Conserving energy decreases oxygen demand.	
2. Alteration in comfort: pain related to multiple injections	Rotate injection sites.	Rotating sites decreases tissue damage and pain at one site when the child requires IM treatment rather than IV.	The child expresses relief of pain and sleeps and plays appropriately.
	Warm packs to the injection site.	Warm packs relieve pain.	
	Move painful areas slowly and gently.	Gentle movements prevent pain.	
3. Parental knowledge deficit related to incomplete understanding of environmental sources of lead and requirement to delead house	Explain the causes of lead poisoning to the parents and discuss with them the common environmental sources of lead—peeling paint from house walls or old painted furniture, paint on some imported toys, colored pages of newspapers, lead-based glazed earthenware.	Information increases understanding.	The parents can list the environmental sources of lead. The home is modified to eliminate sources of lead prior to the child's discharge. Referral is made to the public health nurse and appropriate social service agencies.
	Refer to social service or have the parents lead-proof the house if there are children under age 5 living there—all lead paint needs to be removed down to bare wood by an experienced professional to a level of at least 3 to 4 feet from the floor.	Only professionals can remove all traces of lead from wood. Young children are not allowed to return home until house is lead-free.	

(Continues)

STANDARDS OF NURSING CARE *The Child with Lead Poisoning (Continued)*

GUIDE FOR NURSING MANAGEMENT

Nursing diagnosis	Intervention	Rationale	Outcome
	Cover problem walls with coverings such as wood or masonite paneling that will totally prevent access to peeling paint.	Covering walls is less expensive and more easily accomplished than stripping.	
	Encourage regular checks of serum lead levels; refer the child with pica for counseling.	Regular monitoring prevents reoccurrence of poisoning.	
	Refer the family to a public health nurse for assessment and evaluation of the home.	Professional assessment helps parents clarify what needs to be done and ensures compliance.	
	Educate the public about the environmental dangers and sources of lead.	Education is the best form of prevention.	

subsequent use in the formation of hemoglobin. Coproporphyrin, a precursor of heme, is excreted in the urine. Lead alters renal tubule effectiveness and increases membrane permeability to cause fluid retention and increased intracranial pressure.

Clinical manifestations Initial signs of lead poisoning are nonspecific. When the lead level increases to approximately 50 μg/dL, signs of listlessness, irritability, vomiting, abdominal pain, clumsiness and ataxia become apparent. With a lead level greater than 70 μg/dL the child can experience encephalopathy, seizures, coma, and respiratory arrest. The child with chronic low level lead poisoning can experience learning delays.

In addition to elevated serum lead levels, urine tests show an increased coproporphyrin level of greater than 150 μg/24 hours. A complete blood count might reveal anemia. Lead deposits in bones can be evident on radiographs.

Because early manifestations of lead poisoning are easily confused with other illnesses, an accurate diagnosis of lead poisoning might be missed. Frequently, only intensive questioning by the physician or nurse will uncover the environment risk factors that warrant further diagnostic testing.

Treatment *Chelation* is a procedure that effectively interrupts or reverses the toxicity of lead by promoting its excretion. This is accomplished by the administration of specific chelating agents that bind with the metal, forming a complex that can then be eliminated by the bowel and kidneys. The chelating agents used for lead poisoning include BAL (British anti-lewisite) and $CaNa_2$-EDTA (edetate calcium disodium). Treatment regimens usually begin with a loading dose of BAL followed every four hours by BAL in conjunction with $CaNa_2$-EDTA. The serum lead level dictates the amount of the medications given (Piomelli et al, 1984). $CaNa_2$-EDTA can be given alone to children who are asymptomatic. BAL is given in a deep intramuscular injection, while the route of choice for $CaNa_2$-EDTA is either continuous or intermittent intravenous infusion. Chelation is carried out over a 3–5 day period. A second course might be necessary after a 5–7 day period of rest.

Adequate renal function must be established prior to administering $CaNa_2$-EDTA because of the increased load on the kidneys as the lead is eliminated. Intravenous fluids are given to establish renal function. In the child with lead levels above 70 μg/dL and who exhibits signs of increased intracranial pressure (severe headache, vomiting, increased blood pressure, irritability) intravenous fluids are contraindicated. The $CaNa_2$-EDTA is given intramuscularly to these children. Intramuscular injections of chelating agents can be painful and can cause underlying tissue necrosis.

Rotating injection sites and applying warm packs can alleviate discomfort.

Supplemental calcium, phosphorus, and vitamin D are helpful with removing lead from the blood and depositing it in bones where it becomes inactive. Increased calcium also is necessary for replacement of calcium lost through chelation and prevention of hypocalcemia.

Oxygen might be required for extreme anemia or for the child with respiratory distress. Anticonvulsants are given for seizures and seizure precautions are instituted (see Chapter 31).

Removing the child from the environment that contributed to the poisoning is essential. Children are at a greater risk for lead poisoning if they have a history of pica or reside in older homes (built prior to 1957) with peeling paint. A home assessment is indicated when a child has a diagnosis of lead poisoning. Siblings need to be screened if they are younger than age 6.

Parents need to be aware of environmental causes of lead poisoning, and appropriate environmental modifications need to be undertaken. Any walls containing lead paint need to have the paint professionally removed down to bare wood to a level of 4 feet from the floor. This includes all window sills. If paint removal is impossible, any peeling plaster can be covered with masonite or wood paneling. Baseboards and moldings need to be replaced if they are peeling.

Essential Concepts

- The incidence of accidental injury or poisoning can be reduced by the application of appropriate prevention strategies.
- Nurses assess the characteristics of children, agents, and the environment that contribute to injury.
- The characteristics of children that contribute to injury include curiosity, developmental level, sex, peer pressure, and disabling conditions.
- Injurious agents include automobiles, bicycles, children as pedestrians, water, fire, toys, infant furniture, and poisons.
- Agents can be altered to prevent injury (for example, the use of child car restraint systems).
- Environmental characteristics that contribute to injury are parental inattention and fatigue, improper developmental expectations, family instability, cultural values, socioeconomic status, and physical surroundings.
- Environmental aspects can be changed to reduce injury potential (for example, improved athletic facilities and equipment for children).
- Nurses can influence the childhood injury rate through anticipatory guidance and parent/child safety education.
- Childproofing in a home means creating a safe living environment for children by preventing access to hazards.
- Burns can be prevented by educating children in schools and at home and by practicing how to react in a fire.
- Drownings can be prevented by strict attention to water safety rules.
- Vehicle injuries can be reduced by the use of seatbelts in automobiles and by knowledge and practice of bicycle safety measures.
- Children can be taught pedestrian safety according to their developmental level.
- Discussion of poisoning should be a routine part of well-child visits, informing the parents of the characteristics of the child, agent, and environment that contribute to poisoning.
- Keeping syrup of ipecac in the house and having the poison control center telephone number easily accessible are important first-aid principles.
- Parents should call their nearest poison control center before treating any poison ingestion.
- Nurses should help the parents deal with their feelings of guilt following an accidental poisoning.
- Nurses need to be aware of health protection legislation and communicate the information to families and the community in general.
- Nurses can reduce the severity of injuries and poisonings by accurate assessment and effective interventions, using the principles of first aid.

References

American Red Cross: *Swimming and Aquatics Safety*. The American National Red Cross, 1981.

Bellinger D et al: Longitudinal analyses of prenatal and postnatal lead exposure and early cognitive development. *N Engl J Med* 1987; 316(17): 1037–1042.

Betz CL: Bicycle safety: Opportunities for family education. *Pediatr Nurs* (March/April) 1983; 9:101–111.

Consumer Product Safety Alert (March) 1985. US Consumer Product Safety Commission.

Consumer Reports. Motorized bikes and mopeds. (May) 1981; 46:260–261.

Environmental Protection Agency: *Toxic Substances Control Act Chemical Substances Inventory*. US GPO, 1982.

Faber M: A review of efforts to protect children from injury in car crashes. *Fam Commun Health* 1986; 9(3):25–41.

FDA Drug Bill. 1983; 13:1. Dept Health and Human Services.

Haddad LM, Winchester J: *Clinical Management of Poisoning and Overdose*. Saunders, 1983.

Halperin S et al: Unintentional injuries among adolescents and young adults: A review and analysis. *J Adolesc Health Care* 1983; 4:275–281.

King C: Dealing with poisonings. RN 1984; 47(12):45–48.

Lee EJ, Jacobsen JM: Accident reports: Survey of high school injuries. *Pediatr Nurs* 1987; 13(3):151–153.

Litovitz TL: Ipecac administration in children younger than 1 year of age. *Pediatrics* 1985; 76(5):761–764.

Nachem B: Children still aren't being buckled up. *MCN* (Sept/Oct) 1984; 9:320.

Newton M et al: Specific treatments of poisoning by household products and medications. *JEN* 1987; 13(1):16–25.

Piomelli S et al: Management of childhood lead poisoning. *J Pediatr* 1984; 105(4):523–532.

Preventing lead poisoning in the young child. *MMWR* 1985; 34(5):66–68.

Righi F, Krozy R: The child in the car: What every nurse should know about safety. *Am J Nurs* (Oct) 1983; 83:1421–1434.

Rivara F: Epidemiology of childhood injuries. *Am J Dis Child* 1982; 136:399–405.

Survey points up poison dangers. *Am J Nurs* 1985; 85(3):235.

Temple AR: Acute and chronic effects of aspirin toxicity and their treatment. *Arch Intern Med* 1981; 141:364–369.

Temple AR, Mancini RE: Management of poisoning. In: *Pediatric Pharmacology*. Yaffe SJ (editor). Grune & Stratton, 1980.

Toy safety. *MMWR* 1984; 33(50):697–698.

Thompson S, Verbeek D: When a snake bites. *Am J Nurs* 1984; 84(5):620–623.

Wicklund K, Mons S: Effects of maternal education, age, and parity on fatal infant accidents. *Am J Public Health* 1984; 74(10):1150.

Zimmerman SS, Truxal B: Carbon monoxide poisoning. *Pediatrics* 1981; 68(2):215–224.

Additional Readings

Allen C: The female athlete. In: *Issues in Comprehensive Pediatric Nursing*. McGraw-Hill, 1980.

A History of National Poison Prevention Week. Poison Prevention Week Council, 1985.

Berger LR, Rivara FP: Minibikes: A case study in under-regulation. *Business Soc Rev* (Summer) 1980; 34:41–43.

Carey RJ et al: Sports trauma management and the high school nurse. *J School Health* 1982; 52(7):437–440.

Carter JH: CPR: Breathing life back into a child. *Nurs '86* 1986; 16(10):54–57.

Conrad F: Tips for treating corrosive burns. *Nursing* 1983; 13(2):55.

Dershewitz RA: Home safety: Is anticipatory guidance effective? In: *Preventing Childhood Injuries. Twelfth Ross Roundtable on Critical Approaches to Pediatric Problems*. Ross Laboratories, 1982.

Drug Facts and Comparisons. Lippincott, 1985.

Eckelt K: A successful burn prevention program in elementary schools. *J Burn Care Rehabil* 1985; 6(6):509–510.

Feller I et al: Assessing the impact of flammability standards. Presentation to the Twelfth Annual Meeting of the American Burn Association. San Antonio, Texas, 1980.

Findlay JWA et al: Analgesic drugs in the breast milk and plasma. *Clin Pharmacol Ther* (May) 1981; 29:625–633.

Gilles C et al: Management of pediatric poisoning: Role of the nurse practitioner. *Pediatr Nurs* (Sept/Oct) 1980; 633–635.

Hazinski MF: New guidelines for pediatric and neonatal cardiopulmonary resuscitation and advanced life support. Part I. *Pediatr Nurs* 1986; 12(5):373–376.

Hodgeson C, Woodward CA, Feldman W: A descriptive study of school injuries in a Canadian region. *Pediatr Nurs* 1984; 10(3):215–220.

Jacobi A: Preschooler's discrimination of poisonous from non-poisonous household items as identified by the Mr. Yuk poison prevention sticker. *Child Health Care* 1983; 11(3):98–101.

Lacouture P et al: Emergency assessment of severity in iron overdose by clinical and laboratory methods. *J Pediatr* 1981; 99(1):89–91.

Lawson D: Priorities for motor vehicle occupant protection among children and youth. *Health Educ* 1984; 15(5):27–29.

National Clearinghouse for Poison Control Centers Bulletin. 1980; 24(10).

Pappas A: Children and sports. In: *Sports Health*. Southmayd W, Hoffman M (editors). Quick Fox, 1981.

Parker PR, Parker WA: Pharmacokinetic considerations in the haemodialysis of drugs. *J Clin Hosp Pharm* 1982; 7:87–99.

Pomerantz J, Schultz D: Safe and sensible play-things. *Parents* 1982; 57:88.

Rehm R: Teaching cardiopulmonary resuscitation to parents. *Matern-Child Nurs J* (Nov/Dec) 1983; 8:411–414.

Reinhard S: Nursing responsibility in infant car safety. *Matern-Child Nurs J* (Jan/Feb) 1980; 5:64–65.

Rich J: Action STAT: Snake bite. *Nurs '87* 1987; 17(6):33.

Rumack BH, Sullivan J, Peterson R: *Management of Acute Poisoning and Overdose*. Rocky Mountain Poison Center, 1981.

Russell FE: Page 254 in: *Snake Venom Poisoning*. Lippincott, 1980.

Scherger D et al: Ethylene glycol intoxication. *J Emerg Nurs* 1983; 9(2):71–73.

Schering Symposium on Sports Medicine. *Am J Sports Med* 1980; 5:370–384.

Sousa B: School emergencies—preparation not panic. *J School Health* 1982; 52(7):437–440.

Thorne B: A nurse helps prevent sports injuries. *Matern-Child Nurs J* (July/Aug) 1982; 7:236–239.

US Consumer Product Safety Commission: *For Kids' Sake*. US Consumer Product Safety Commission No. CPSC-75-630-9.

US Department of Health and Human Services: *Monthly Vital Statistics Report*. Vol 32. Government Printing Office, 1983.

IV

The Child and Family at Psychosocial Risk

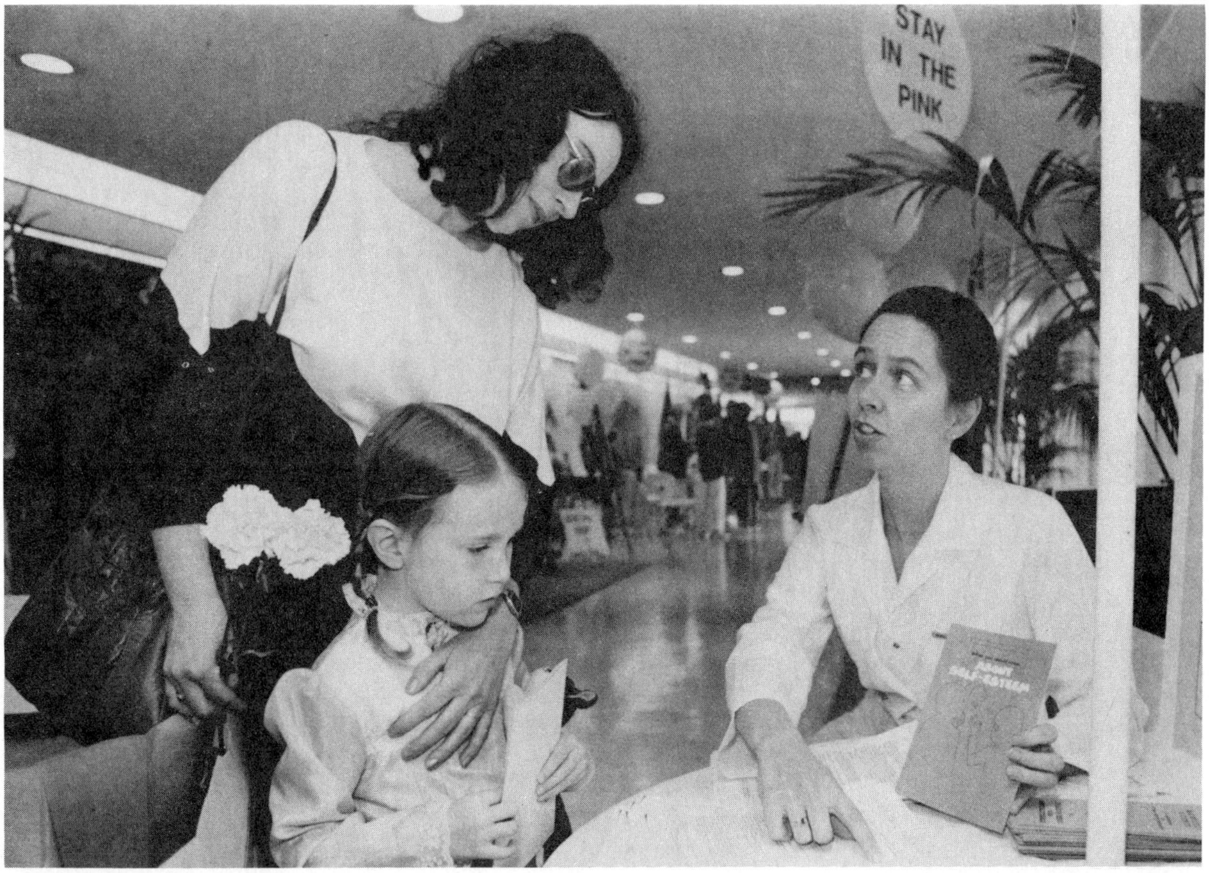

Chapter 13

Nursing Care of the Family at Risk

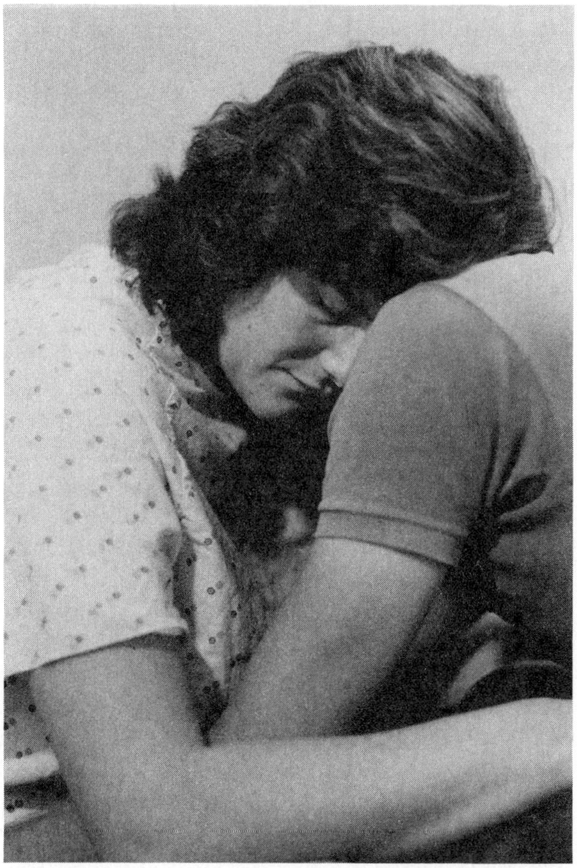

Chapter Contents

Objectives

- Define dysfunctional parenting.
- Describe the risk factors that indicate the potential for dysfunctional parenting.

(Continues)

- Explain the nurse's role in supporting adolescent parents.
- Describe the common needs and interventions for families prone to violence.
- Describe the common needs of multiproblem families.
- Explain the relationship among failure to thrive, delayed development, and dysfunctional parenting.
- Define the types of child neglect and abuse.
- Describe the process of reporting a case of child abuse and the possible legal outcomes of child abuse reports.
- Explain the nurse's role in preventing child abuse and neglect.
- List the possible community supports to which nurses might refer dysfunctional families.
- Explain the nurse's role in supporting dysfunctional parents and children in dysfunctional families.

When the development or life of a family member is threatened, the family might be described as a "family at risk." In such families individual members who are not able to function appropriately threaten the family as a whole. The family at risk is often a family characterized by *dysfunctional parenting,* which causes a disturbance in the parent-child relationship.

The extent to which a family is at risk depends on a complex series of characteristics and events. These are risk factors that suggest a potential for dysfunctional parenting. *Risk factors* are indicators, not predictors, of areas where the potential for unmet needs exists. They include developmental and situational stressors that historically have had a high correlation with dysfunction. Adolescent parenthood, for example, is commonly correlated with dysfunctional parenting, although specific stressors and parenting problems vary among families.

Because a risk factor is not a predictor of dysfunction, the nurse can never assume that the presence of one or more risk factors means that dysfunctional parenting exists. Before identifying existing or potential dysfunction, the nurse completes a thorough assessment that includes parenting risk factors along with other assessment data. A comprehensive analysis then allows the nurse to identify areas of unmet needs for which nursing intervention is required.

The number or severity of stressors and unmet needs places some families at high risk for dysfunction. For example, the pregnant adolescent is developmentally vulnerable both because of the stress of pregnancy and because of her own ongoing growth and development. Additional risk factors for this individual might include single parenthood without necessary material and personal support systems, limited experience and knowledge of child care, and social isolation. These combined developmental, sociologic, and psychologic factors create a situation of high risk for this family. The degree of risk is an important concern in planning nursing care.

Holistic nursing care looks at all aspects of the family. Knowing risk factors enables the nurse to identify potential dysfunction and to plan interventions that prevent disruptive effects on families. Nursing goals consist of identifying families at risk, preventing predictable dysfunctional behaviors, reducing disintegration, fostering positive relationships, and providing referrals to community resources and services.

Dysfunctional Parenting

Families are assumed to be loving and nurturing and are supposed to provide for the needs of their members. Many families, however, do not meet these goals. A family that is unable to provide physically and emotionally for the needs of its members is said to be a *dysfunctional family.* The dysfunctional family is one in which risk factors override family strengths. All families experience times when they function well and other times when they function poorly, some even to the point of disintegration. Determining whether the dysfunctional pattern is temporary, situational, or chronic is therefore a nursing goal for the family at risk.

High-risk families often are victims of accumulated stress and might be subjected to more than one stressor in a short period of time. Of these stressors, some are normal occurrences in daily living or in growth and development. Many individuals and families cope with these stressors and still maintain their equilibrium. Others, however, experience disequilibrium in response to stressors. When disequilibrium occurs, the individual or family experiences a *crisis* (Fig. 13-1).

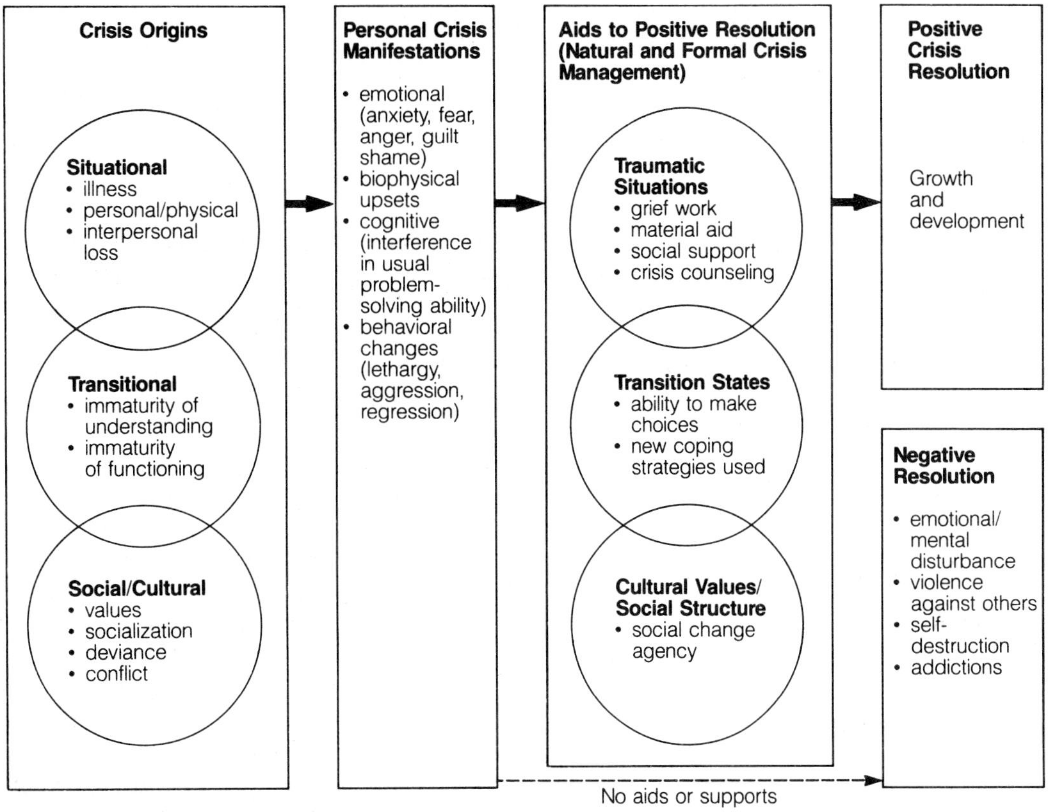

FIGURE 13-1
Crisis origins, manifestations, and outcomes. (Adapted from Hoff L: People in Crisis, *2nd ed. Addison-Wesley, 1984, p. 32.)*

Some families face continuous multiple stressors. Reactions to stress vary, but in the face of recurring pressures, family members experience a sense of powerlessness if the family simply cannot cope. Stressors might include illness, conflicts, role confusion, unrealistic expectations for family members, and the effects of poverty, housing problems, unemployment, and racial conflicts. In dysfunctional families most reactions are out of proportion to the threat. Minor stressors are viewed as major crises, and the energy expended to resolve the stress can be devastating. For example, the breakdown of a vacuum cleaner is a source of irritation to a functional family but a full-blown crisis to a family with limited resources and coping abilities.

The high-risk family is usually unstable and has many internal and external problems. When faced with multiple stressors, family members usually demonstrate predictable patterns of dysfunction. Stages in a family's developmental cycle, such as marriage, birth, entrance into school, puberty, career changes, and retirement, also tend to create periods of stress. The nurse who understands the family's developmental stage and supports the family at risk during situational stresses can do much to prevent further dysfunction.

When assessing the child and family, the nurse observes the parent-child relationship and notes any stressors that are affecting family members. Dysfunctional parenting frequently is associated with high social and economic stressors. Some parents survive multiple stressors and remain effective parents, whereas other parents have problems with parenting when faced with only mild or temporary stress. Evidence of dysfunctional parenting includes observed deficits in self-care, in judgments concerning child care, and in planning for the future.

Dysfunctional parenting might result when the parenting style has been affected negatively by one or more risk factors, often resulting in a parenting style that is marked by inconsistency or inflexibility. Inflexibility might be dysfunctional if a parent is unable to adjust expectations to match the individual needs of different children. Inconsistent parenting often takes its toll on selected children in a family, usually when a parent singles out one child as a scapegoat. Inconsistency also occurs when the same behavior receives very different responses depending on the parent's mood. The child never establishes a trusting relationship because care is not directed toward providing a consistent, nurturing environment to satisfy basic needs.

The nurse assesses the family dynamics in relation to the potential for crisis: (1) the origin of the stressor(s), whether situational, transitional, or social/cultural; (2) the personal reaction to the stressor as manifested by cognitive, biophysical, emotional, and behavioral responses; and (3) the support services and family resources available to facilitate coping and crisis management.

Risk Factors Associated with Dysfunctional Parenting

Inadequate communication Using clear, functional communication patterns is one way in which a parent interacts and expresses emotions with the child. An inability to communicate needs and feelings and a limited ability to use communication for solving problems or conveying ideas are risk factors. Patterns of communication might be haphazard because the parent has difficulty stating thoughts or beliefs. Frequently, feelings are overlooked or are not expressed either verbally or nonverbally.

Inadequate communication usually leads to inappropriate expectations among family members. The inability to meet these expectations robs members of opportunities for self-esteem through accomplishment. The adult who lacks interpersonal skills has a minimal capacity to support the emotional development of a child.

When family members fail to interact effectively, they create many problems in activities of daily living. Their sparse or irregular use of language might result in members' relying on nonverbal cues to convey messages. When family members fail to listen actively to each other, they do not share achievements and goals. For example, one boy decided not to bother to tell his mother about his first-place honor in the spelling contest and instead waited until she read about it. By then, however, his excitement over winning had passed. His mother worked at home and would scowl or ignore him if he interrupted her when she was concentrating. Her negative response occurred so frequently that he stopped sharing school events unless she initiated the topic. Although she was physically present when he returned home from school, she was emotionally distant and unable to provide consistent interaction or interest in his activities or accomplishments to support his development.

Many times dysfunctional parents communicate by responding only to negative behaviors in their children. Positive behaviors, though expected, are not recognized, thus conveying a sense of unimportance to the child. When enforcement of rules is sporadic, with compliance either demanded immediately or overlooked, the child becomes confused. Extremes in behaviors, which might be either overly permissive or overly rigid, thus rob the child of problem-solving experiences.

Restrictive communication to a child can have lasting effects. The child might conclude that language is unnecessary. The most serious effect is that the child might not have insight into feelings or the power of communication for solving problems. For example, one mother repeatedly told her daughter not to bore others with her idle chatter. If she had something important to say, she should say it as concisely as possible, but otherwise she should keep quiet. Constant reminders of this rule, which essentially allowed the communication of facts but not feelings, resulted in the girl's belief that her thoughts, questions, and ideas had little value. She gradually withdrew her attempts to solve problems verbally or to put feelings into perspective, sensing that there was something inherently wrong with her for attempting to do so in the first place.

Children who are thwarted in their attempts to express their feelings or who receive confusing and mixed messages from their families often have a mixture of unexpressed anger, aggression, resentment, self-pity, fear, and guilt. Helping the child to identify the existence of these feelings is the first step and takes time, patience, and empathy. Once identified, the reasons for the feelings should be uncovered.

Family members need help in voicing feelings to each other and in learning to share concerns. Because this kind of communication is often foreign, progress is usually slow and should be evaluated frequently to meet the family members' needs.

Role confusion among family members Adult roles include taking responsibility for one's own life, making sound judgments, and occupying a useful place in society. Parents who are unable to take on adult roles fail to provide for their children both economically and emotionally. Dysfunctional parents who experience conflict about their roles often have difficulty in providing for their dependent children. They might view children as little adults and in so doing expect too much development too soon. Because of their own unmet needs, some parents expect their children to become the parents they never had and so create a cycle of parental dysfunction.

If, in a two-parent family, either parent is competing with the children for love and attention, unhealthy relationships develop. The competing parent might feel deprived when the child is nurtured and vent anger and rage on the child rather than the spouse. Because children learn from their parents by imitation and identification, the child then learns inappropriate ways to express anger. Children need parents to assume authority, provide guidance, and make decisions. Any deviation from these expectations is confusing to the child and results in unhealthy relationships and developmental vulnerability. The child who is cast into an adult role prematurely might begin to compete with the parent, and the parent might in turn resent the child's taking over an adult role in the family.

In dysfunctional families, relationships among siblings usually mirror other troubled family relationships. Dysfunctional parenting usually causes normal sibling rivalry and competition to be far out of proportion and so intense as to be destructive. The siblings battle each other for recognition and for the limited amount of attention they perceive as being available from their parents. Parental attention is then more likely to be given for negative, even violent, behavior than for positive, empathetic behavior.

The role of scapegoat is also evident in some troubled families. One child usually is singled out because of temperament, appearance, birth order, disability, sex, or health status and is treated as the cause of all family problems. Much family activity then focuses on this child. Occasionally, scapegoating and other forms of role confusion are related to a parent-child mismatch, in which the child does not seem to "fit" the parents. This mismatch is sometimes the only plausible explanation for a certain child's differential treatment and might explain child abuse or neglect.

Family members who feel negative about their roles carry invisible scars. Their unmet needs for attention, love, and recognition interfere with the identification of others' needs. For example, a mother craving recognition for the output of energy and accomplishment of managing a home has a difficult time giving appropriate recognition and praise to the child's initial efforts to wash the windows. The nurse might need to help the mother identify times when her child's efforts need to be praised and provide guidance in ways to give sincere praise. The nurse, remembering that people with emotional scars need much support and praise in any new venture, then praises the mother for recognizing her child's efforts. Praise for progress, however small at first, is an important nursing intervention.

Identifying the parent who is the main decision-maker and the distribution of power in a family is helpful in planning intervention. If one parent is passive and the other is dominant, certain behaviors are interdependent and might hamper one member's progress. For example, a wife who is submissive to a dominant husband might wish to initiate change but also might feel that she needs permission from her husband before taking any action. A first step in planning interventions might then be to interest the husband in making the necessary changes so that accustomed family functions are not entirely disrupted.

Isolation Some families live in both physical and emotional isolation. Parents who have few friends often have difficulty forming close personal relationships. As a result of their aloneness, they seldom leave their homes. They make contacts rather than friends, have no meaningful interactions with neighbors and family members, and rarely join groups or organizations. They feel less than adequate in social situations and endure much loneliness. For parents, such isolation results in their having no outside outlets for tension and frustrations. Their apparent lack of interpersonal skills might be related to their own limited opportunities to learn as children.

If the family is isolated from the community, the lack of belonging and acceptance places the family at further risk. Because a problem or stressor is often lessened by knowing that others have successfully mastered the problem, isolation deprives family members of common problem-solving techniques. For example, sharing child-care skills and responsibilities is common in many cultures and communities and provides parents the opportunity to exchange both knowledge and services. An isolated family is denied this sharing and struggles alone to provide continual care.

Because isolation is likely to be both physical and emotional, lack of social skills might be misinterpreted as disinterest or snobbery and usually triggers behaviors that add to the problem. Efforts at friendliness might be missed, and mistrust becomes pervasive. Individual needs for acceptance and belonging go unfulfilled. Nurses who identify family isolation therefore might need to teach parents to break the bonds of isolation and learn to use resources.

The parent's experience as a child The type of parenting that a parent received as a child directly affects current parenting skills. The single most significant and predictable factor in all research is that parents who were significantly deprived, neglected, or abused are more likely to show dysfunctional behaviors toward their own children (Kempe and Kempe, 1978; Steele, 1975). In some families, dysfunctional patterns can be traced back three or four generations. This risk factor outranks all other data (such as race, age, religion, culture, environment, education, family structure, socioeconomic status, and psychiatric state).

Parents who were not properly nurtured as children do not measure their parenting against healthy norms. They lack the frame of reference that a functional family provides. Not having been reared to experience parenting as nurturing, these adults are unable to nurture their own children. The problem then becomes cyclic.

Unmet parental needs Parents who were made to feel guilty and inadequate as children lack confidence in their abilities to parent and are unable to identify the needs of their children. The parent's lack of secure feelings can result in insecurity and dependence, which then place the child at further risk. The insecure parent has difficulty understanding a child's cues and might become impatient when the child does not respond in an expected manner.

For example, an infant's cry is loud and annoying so that the dependent infant can communicate basic needs. To insecure parents, crying might be interpreted to mean that the child is "bad" or "spoiled" or that the parents have "failed"— attitudes that lead to more insecurity. In such instances, the child's failure to live up to a parent's distorted view of love only serves to release more feelings of parental inadequacy. Lacking confidence, such parents do not derive much pleasure from their children, a subtle clue to family problems that the nurse needs to investigate further.

Many dysfunctional parents also have had childhood experiences that taught them to mistrust others. For some parents, lack of nurturing or intermittent nurturing has caused feelings of insecurity at each developmental stage. Erikson's theory of development points out that when mistrust instead of trust characterizes initial parent-child relations, the lack of trust has repercussions throughout the developmental process. Anxiety typifies the child's interactions with others, especially adults, because the child never knows whether a particular behavior will be met with approval or disapproval. Repeated parental disapproval contributes to a subsequent sense of guilt and inferiority.

As an adult, this inability to trust others for fear of being betrayed limits any ability to provide a trusting environment for the child. The parent who has not experienced a trusting relationship cannot provide one. As one mother blurted out during a counseling session, "How can I be consistent with him; I have never known the meaning of consistency in my life? My mother practiced inconsistency to keep us girls on our toes and not take her love for granted."

The parent with unmet needs from childhood is greatly handicapped in providing effective parenting. The unmet needs cause the parent to desire dependence that is similar to that of a child. When two parents in a family have unmet needs simultaneously, the family might be in crisis because both parents attempt to manipulate the child to satisfy their own needs. The child is unprotected and vulnerable because both parents expect but are unable or unwilling to provide nurturing. The child's failure to gratify the needs of one parent or the other or to show favoritism are likely to result in criticism, punishment, and even abuse, thus repeating the cycle the parents had experienced in their own childhood.

The nurse's role Sometimes, assisting parents to identify available resources to meet some basic needs is the first step in altering dysfunctional parenting. "Parenting the parent" is thus one avenue of resolution. Parents often benefit from a temporary dependence on a multidisciplinary team member, someone who takes a special interest in the personal problems of childrearing, homemaking, or employment difficulties; who makes appointments and offers reminders and transportation to keep clinic appointments; who provides a phone number to call when a question or concern arises; and who calls periodically to check on the parent's welfare.

Nurses need to know that dysfunctional parents often are not aware that their family lifestyles are different or abnormal, although many dysfunctional parents do describe their own childhoods as chaotic and report deep feelings of rejection. Nurses also need to be mindful that an insecure parent seems to have a very low tolerance for criticism. Any advice or health teaching therefore should be stated positively, carefully, and slowly.

Marital problems In two-parent families the relationship between the parents also is closely intertwined with their parenting style. Dissatisfaction with any aspect of marital life, including sex, influences the parenting ability. If the parent feels rejected by the spouse, the lost love might be sought from the child by excessive demands for companionship or minimal tolerance for uncooperative behavior. Luckey and Bain (1970) noted that because companionship between spouses was low in unhappy marriages, these parents sought compensation from their children and identified them as the most satisfying aspect of the marriage. The nurse therefore assesses parent-child relationships in the context of other relationships within the family.

The emotional climate that marital strife creates is likely to have negative effects on children. If parents remain in an unhappy, unhealthy relationship "for the children's sake," the emotional climate in that family ranges from neutral to explosive. Children perceive nonverbal cues and often know about parental strife and problems despite parental efforts at concealment.

In two-parent families the history of the parents' marriage, especially their ages and the circumstances surrounding their decision to be married, is most helpful in assessment. If the parents married young to escape unhappy home situations or if the marriage was impulsive, each partner might have little knowledge of the other's strengths and weaknesses. For such families, the first severe stressor might result in turmoil and frustration. The family is at risk if the partners have not had time to grow together and learn about each other. If the first child arrives soon after the relationship begins, the family faces further risks. These partners frequently have not had time to establish a close positive relationship that permits intuitive understanding and meeting of each other's needs. They therefore do not have that "emotional buffer" needed to cope with a difficult infant or additional environmental strain such as an overcrowded apartment or tight finances.

The parents' own history of family life also provides clues to their potential coping strategies, available internal strengths, and external resources. Marital expectations, like many other behaviors, are learned from childhood experience. Seeing one's parents give and take teaches a child about the reciprocal nature of marriage.

Family dysfunction is seen more frequently when partners have stereotyped ideas of appropriate male and female or husband and wife roles and behaviors. A husband, believing that he should be the head of the household, for example, might make major decisions in an autocratic manner. He might consider housework and child care "woman's work" and of little importance. One partner's lack of respect for the other can, in this way, prevent the family from adapting to stressors.

Families that allow few deviations from expected roles have high degrees of dysfunction and even resort to violence. Women who get married believing in patriarchy (that is, accepting traditional values of the male as the controlling head of the household) assume that their primary responsibility includes all the tasks related to homemaking and childrearing. The performance of these tasks is a service to the husband and a symbol of commitment to please and remain subservient to him. When this mind-set prevails, poor or reluctant performance deserves punishment, thus justifying for both of them the husband's verbal and/or physical abuse. Unfortunately, many men who abuse their wives believe that they are enacting the standards promoted in Western civilization and the general acceptance of cultural norms espousing aggressiveness, male dominance, and female subordination.

The nurse who identifies marital tensions and disharmony from family assessment data encourages the parents to seek marital counseling. Counseling is often the first step taken by people attempting to gain insight into their relationship with each other. The nurse's knowledge of community resources is valuable in such cases. Open communication between parents is a long-range goal, and a mediator might be able to guide the husband and wife to listen effectively and discuss feelings as an alternative to force.

Parental separation If the parent who was the primary source of family disharmony chooses to leave the family, the remaining members might feel a sense of relief or a sense of guilt or anger. The remaining parent, however, must struggle to keep the rest of the family intact. Financial hardships, loneliness, sadness, denial, and detachment are only some of the risk factors associated with separation.

Reactions to a separation vary, just as each family varies, and to a large extent depend on the reasons and preparation for the separation. Most common is a period of mourning as family members struggle to cope with loneliness and loss. If the child is not helped to identify what is happening, the alternative is self-blame, which increases the risks for low self-esteem and dysfunction in a future family. In early childhood, for example, the child might view the separation as a penalty for being bad and might act in a manner that invites punishment.

The longer a separation lasts, the greater the tendency for family members to become ingrained in their new roles and be unwilling to surrender them if the original member returns. The stress of reconciliation also can be a risk factor for the nurse to consider. Family members might experience dysfunctional interactions and conflict over roles if underlying problems are not addressed.

Chronically ill parents Chronic illness in a parent has a profound and prolonged impact on all aspects of daily living. Family functioning is usually affected because of changes and pressure brought on by the altered lifestyle and ability of the parent to provide care. Parents with chronic illness are doubly challenged in that they must try to manage their personal, social, and occupational activities while continuing to be parents. Sometimes, the treatment regimen involves periods of discomfort, immobility, or pain. The illness itself might necessitate modifications in daily activities and routines, rearrangement of environment, and revised patterns of interactions. Parents who have limited socioeconomic resources, limited health knowledge, and unfavorable attitudes toward health care are less likely to continue long-term health supervision, which then affects the course of the illness. Parents with limited coping strategies, poor self-images, and dysfunctional relationships face enormous challenges in parenting as their fragile self-esteem is further challenged.

The multiple stressors associated with illness intensify the family's vulnerability for dysfunction. Financial responsibilities become a new burden if the illness affects a family wage earner. Overwhelming pressures can occur when the bills mount up and income decreases or disappears. Financial hardships place additional stress on all family members and might result in drastic changes in lifestyle. The family then might be forced to move to less expensive housing and leave familiar community support services and resources.

Children might resent ill parents who become the center of attention, or they might be so solicitous and concerned that they have little time for themselves. Some illnesses require frequent medical and clinic visits, expensive medicines, time-consuming treatments, and periodic hospitalizations. All these needs are changes that might require an older child to assume additional family responsibilities and all the children to limit their requests for material possessions.

Behavior during illness is usually consistent with past behaviors during frustration or crisis. If the family has limited coping strategies and is without the resources of an extended family, the risk for dysfunction usually is compounded. If the family was cohesive prior to the illness, the risks for dysfunction are lessened. Children's behaviors reflect the tensions and discomforts of their parents. If there is anger in the family, the child might withdraw to avoid unleashing new problems. If a parent withdraws, the children might misbehave or become loud and boisterous in an attempt to regain lost attention.

Large families with many children close in age Not all large families are at risk. Some large families have adequate resources, such as experience, motivation, health, and extensive external supports. Family health can be affected, however, by the number and spacing of children. When children are fewer than 15 months apart, the older child is still very dependent when the younger infant is born. Both infants present many demanding but different needs. If the family is experiencing other stressors such as poverty or unemployment, the multiple demands might result in diminished parental care to one or both infants.

Nutritional deficits might be found in large families, especially if the family income falls below the poverty level. Many such families have difficulty navigating through the forms to apply for supplemental food or food stamps. Dependent children take time to feed. One mealtime often runs into the next, leaving the parent no free time for personal care. The laundry for many children might seem monumental. When clothing is limited, washing becomes a daily necessity. Families without the resources of home laundry facilities are doubly stressed by being forced to trudge to the laundromat and pay for washing their clothes. The point at which resources become overtaxed and tolerable levels of stress are surpassed is the line separating the family's ability to cope with adversity and the potential for dysfunction.

Fatigue is a factor for parents with many small children. The parent's tolerance for normal developmental needs might be limited, especially when the child does not cooperate. For example, a parent with many children might demand early toilet training in an attempt to decrease the work load. The child's noncompliance combined with the parent's fatigue might lead to physical punishment.

All parents need time away from the multiple demands of parenting. The most motivated parent will feel entrapped if not given any free time. Chronic fatigue often is a major factor in feelings of entrapment. The nurse can help the parent identify such feelings by discussing the pluses and minuses of parenting. For example, the nurse might ask a parent to describe the routine chores of a day. As the tasks are reviewed, the nurse notes the physical stamina required of the parent. The parent who reports no free time or enjoyment with children can then be given special attention. Open-ended questions such as "How do you unwind?" or "What do you like to do to relax?" can assist parents in coming to terms with their own needs and feelings.

Families with limited resources might need assistance from social services if these parents are to have any child-care relief. Sometimes these parents need guidance in planning free time and assistance in discussing anxiety about being away from the children. The nurse can convey to the parent that this time is vital to the child because it will enhance the parent's health.

Single parents with inadequate supports Single parents assume all responsibilities and decisions traditionally shared by two parents. Factors such as age, personality, maturity level, emotional stability, financial status, and motivation need to be considered in determining the potential degree of risk that a single-parent family faces.

Problems of single parents Single parents are confronted with many problems and constraints. Society generally is geared to two-parent families and is slow to acknowledge alternative lifestyles. Some single parents feel their status to be a stigma, whereas others draw praise and recognition for their ability to function alone. The nurse does not equate successful childrearing with the number of parents in the home. Nursing diagnoses are formulated only after observing the emotional climate, level of family functioning, quality of child supervision, and family dynamics.

Financial strain usually heads the list of problems for single parents, especially women. A single income often is not enough to meet all the necessities of the family members, especially if day care is needed while the parent works. Financial worries detract from a parent's ability to be a good parent. A single parent who draws income from welfare assistance, for example, remains at the poverty level and has long-range financial worries about housing, food, and clothing. The responsibility of providing for the physical, social, and emotional needs of a child becomes an awesome task with no other parent to share the burdens.

Loneliness can have a crippling effect on the single parent. Dialogue with children can be fun, but it is limiting if the parent has no other adult contacts. Physical and emotional isolation, together with the frustrations and tensions of the household, can create a potentially explosive situation if the single parent has no outlets for the release of tension.

The nurse's role Single parents might need the opportunity to discuss normal stages of development and their children's behavior with other adults. Without another parent with whom to discuss their children's responses, single parents can misinterpret behavior. Problems in childrearing are then more likely to lead to self-blame, guilt, and a sense of failure. Occasionally, single parents attempt to compensate for their role by being overly permissive (hoping to secure the child's love) or overly strict (proving to the world it can be done).

Although for many single parents the basic need for income necessitates leaving children with other caregivers, separation caused by the parent's employment might lead to feelings of insecurity, loneliness, and despair in children. Children who feel neglected might misbehave just to get the attention that discipline requires. Single parents need to understand this phenomenon and also might need help to learn how to make the best use of time spent with their children.

The single parent might need assistance in identifying and cultivating new interests and friends with similar lifestyles. The nurse can refer clients to single-parent organizations, community groups, and church or school resources. The nurse often assumes the role of coordinator when making such referrals and then should follow up with the family to assess whether the referrals are meeting specified needs.

Parental substance abuse The use of mood-altering substances is now evident in all socioeconomic classes, in all ages, and in both sexes. Use is related to the need to satisfy curiosity, foster peer acceptance, relax, escape boredom and the realities of life, alleviate anxiety, enhance social situations, and produce pleasurable states of euphoria.

Alcohol Alcoholism is one of today's largest health and social problems. It is a progressive terminal illness characterized by uncontrollable drinking. Alcohol abuse affects all aspects of family life, including parenting.

Excessive intake of alcohol leads to physical dependence, which affects all body systems and creates major health problems for the abuser. If alcohol is used in combination with depressants, the effects are synergistic (that is, each drug increases the effectiveness of the other). The combination can be dangerous and even lethal. The physical symptoms of alcoholism include malnutrition and alterations in coordination. Because physical illness usually is perceived to be more acceptable, physical symptoms might lead family members to seek help. Because the client often minimizes the degree to which alcohol is used and the extent to which it controls the family, the nurse needs to be alert for subtle cues of alcohol abuse.

The effects of chronic alcoholism on family life depend on the length and severity of the abuse. The nurse cannot assume that all alcoholic parents abuse or neglect their children, nor can a causal link be made between alcoholism and abuse or neglect in situations in which both factors are present.

Chronic alcoholism has been divided into four stages for purposes of identifying family dysfunction (Tapia, 1980). The first stage is always denial. Drinking episodes are intermittent, and parents attempt to explain away early symptoms of dependence as normal social drinking. Denial both allows the drinking to continue and delays treatment. In the second stage the nonalcoholic parent attempts to solve the problem. Behaviors such as nagging, bargaining, hiding the liquor and/or money, and avoiding social situations involving drinking are common. In two-parent families "helping" the alcoholic often diminishes the energy left for parenting. Children instead might be called on to perform household tasks and care for younger siblings.

The third stage is disorganization and chaos. The family is disrupted because of the alcohol problem. The nonalcoholic parent begins to look for help outside the family and usually shows signs of marital problems, acute anxiety, severe financial hardships, and problems with the children. If children are caught in a struggle between parents, they become confused as the alcoholic parent alternately ignores, indulges, or abuses the children while the nonalcoholic parent becomes increasingly embarrassed and irritable. The children might, in a sense, be victimized by both parents and eventually have much difficulty trusting others (Hecht, 1973).

In the fourth stage the nonalcoholic parent assumes authority and responsibility for all family decisions and activities while the alcoholic parent takes on the role of the child. Families with parental alcoholism therefore show much role confusion. Parents often are unaware of their children's needs, so poor school performance, nutritional problems, and health deviations might go undetected. Occasionally, the school or health officials might be the first to identify a problem.

Current literature on alcoholism and its effects on the family stress three important aspects of treatment:

1. The whole family, including children over 5 years of age, need treatment. Alcoholism is a family problem.
2. Regardless of whether the alcoholic parent can be persuaded to seek treatment, the rest of the family needs specific supportive therapy (such as Al-Anon, Ala-Teen, Ala-Tot, Parents Anonymous). Any child reared in a family troubled by alcoholism is, by definition, at risk for emotional abuse and neglect.
3. In families with violence and alcohol problems, the alcoholism needs to be treated first for other therapies to have maximum benefit (Wheat, 1980).

Drugs Like the parent who abuses alcohol, the parent who abuses drugs causes many of the same problems within the household and family. Children are often neglected, confused, and cast into adult roles and responsibilities prematurely. If reliance on drugs is the parent's primary coping strategy, other coping behaviors rapidly will fall into disuse (Mitchell, 1986).

The mood swings that accompany drug use can be most uncomfortable for the drug abuser and family. Small children are especially vulnerable when parents are between the drugged and nondrugged states. Dependent children are most at risk because the family dynamics might focus on the drug problem rather than the children's needs.

The nurse's role Family life with a substance-abusing parent often requires child-care responsibilities to be assumed by extended family members without advanced planning. Sometimes, young children are left to care for themselves. Because a child's security needs are closely related to the stability of the environment, children of a substance-abusing parent must learn to expect unreliability, inconsistency, ineptitude, and general household disorganization as the norm and are unable to trust the environment. Nurses working with children need to recognize these clues and plan intervention with support services. For example, the school nurse assessing a student might be the first to identify the risk. Other public health agencies might provide additional data so that multidisciplinary management is made available to the family.

Alcohol and other drugs decrease the appetite and result in poor nutrition because meal preparation is sporadic and unplanned. Chaotic meal schedules place the children at risk for nutritional problems, so physical complaints often provide clues about the family disorganization. Health problems related to nutritional deficiencies might prompt the family's entry into the health care facility. A careful physical and nutritional assessment establishes the approximate intake of nutrients, which is compared with the Recommended Daily Allowances. If nutritional needs are identified, the nurse then assists the family in nutritional planning and any necessary referrals.

Adolescent parents The incidence of adolescent pregnancy has risen to epidemic proportions, especially among girls under 16 years of age. Young people are sexually active earlier but often lack information about the consequences and necessary precautions. About 20% of the total number of births in the United States today are to adolescent parents. Approximately 90% of these adolescent parents keep their infants, resulting in a double risk for both the infant and parent (Adolescent Perinatal Health, 1979).

Providing services and counseling to an adolescent parent requires a multidisciplinary team of health care providers, social service planners, and educators. Special emphasis must be given to health care, nutrition, education, and the developmental needs of both the parent and child. The family should be defined as broadly as possible. All motivated persons such as the father of the child, grandparents, and siblings should be included.

Adolescents are emotionally and intellectually immature and lack the physical, emotional, economic, educational, and social resources necessary for parenting. For most young people, the change from adolescent to parent is itself overwhelming. Most adolescent parents are faced with uncertainty, self-doubt, and inexperience. Their youthful energy does not entirely compensate for their lack of experience and skills.

Preparation for parenthood begins in childhood, but for the adolescent parent, the preparation time is abbreviated by the child's birth, and the younger the parent, the higher the degree of risk. Some adolescent parents willingly enter into an early marriage. Teenage marriages are very fragile, prone to divorce, and often a crisis in themselves. If an adolescent parent comes from a dysfunctional family, the risks for successful parenting are compounded.

An adolescent parent usually has a limited repertoire of coping skills, and the pregnancy itself might be both a symptom and a cause of conflict. Some adolescents use pregnancy as a means of escape from intolerable family situations. The pregnancy might be an unconscious wish to prove adulthood or to compensate for feelings of rejection and insecurity. Whatever the reason, the reality of the demands of parenting place the young family at risk for many problems and in great need of support.

Risks for adolescent mothers and infants Adolescent pregnancies occur at every social, economic, and intellectual level, and adolescents often complete rather than abort their pregnancies. For the adolescent from a low socioeconomic background, health care is a major concern. Health care for families that lack resources is apt to be episodic and crisis oriented. For pregnant adolescents, prenatal care frequently does not occur until late in the pregnancy. This pattern of seeking health care adds an additional risk dimension to the health of both parent and child.

The child born to an adolescent parent is usually at risk both during and after birth. The infant is often preterm and small for gestational age (SGA). The smaller the infant, the greater the potential health problems to be resolved and the longer the separation time while the infant is in intensive care. Lengthy separation from the infant is itself a risk factor for unsatisfactory parent-infant attachment. (Specific illness-related nursing care for these high-risk infants is discussed in Chapter 34.) The inexperienced parent also might misinterpret the constant demands of an infant. The small infant frequently is more demanding and less responsive than the average infant.

At a time when the new mother needs the most emotional support, she often gets the least. Her boyfriend might be frightened of the awesome responsibilities and turn away. Her family might voice disappointment or anger and refuse to assist in child care, thus creating an emotional detachment that serves to reinforce her feelings of unworthiness. Her peers are usually still in school. The adolescent mother often finds herself alone, without the support of family and friends. This emotional void is itself a crisis and often is a sharp contrast to the adolescent's fantasies. The infant is unable to provide the love and affection to erase the confusion and conflicts of adolescence. The reality of the infant's demands instead places the infant at risk for neglect or abuse.

Risks for adolescent fathers Although the major impact of adolescent pregnancy is felt by the mother, the adolescent father's life is affected as well. He might deny his involvement with the mother, resulting in feelings of guilt and anxiety, or he might make emotional commitments and offer support and financial aid. Financial assistance usually has long-range effects on his educational and career plans. If he drops out of school to support the child, he often has to settle for jobs that pay poorly. Those who work with adolescent fathers have found that they feel more responsibility and concern than is sometimes assumed. They too need someone to assist them to sort out confused and troubled feelings.

Developmental needs of adolescent parents Early adolescence is accompanied by a developmental need to accept the bodily changes associated with puberty. Pregnancy and motherhood bring about still greater bodily changes superimposed on the physical changes that might not have been resolved by the adolescent mother. Infants of young adolescents are most at risk if the mother perceives her pregnancy as a cause of changes in body image and consequently comes to resent the infant.

Adolescent parents face the developmental tasks of parenthood superimposed on the developmental tasks of adolescence. Accomplishing the developmental tasks of parenthood can be impeded by a lack of motivation, inadequate knowledge, and immaturity. Adolescence is itself a time of stress. Parenting is markedly influenced by the extent to which adolescents attain some of their own developmental milestones.

One of the greatest conflicts for the pregnant adolescent is her independence. For the adolescent who has not achieved independence prior to parenthood, problem-solving and decision-making abilities often are compromised as personal desires and needs get in the way of the infant's needs. Mothers under 16 years of age need follow-up and nurturing for themselves and their infants. The older adolescent is better able to nurture an infant if her immediate family and friends are supportive. She often has enough maturity to place the infant's needs ahead of her own.

When children have children, society pays the price. Both parents and children require services to maintain their health. The responsibilities of parenthood might interrupt education, thereby limiting skills and trapping them in low-income jobs or in need of social and financial assistance. Because of strained or absent finances, young parents might be forced to rely more heavily on their own parents, thereby increasing their dependence when they were struggling to decrease it. The resulting conflicts might be expressed in many ways; decreased motivation, anger, depression, and anxiety are but a few reactions.

Adolescence is a time for establishing identity and ego strength. The pregnant adolescent might have attempted to solve identity problems through sexual behavior. These mothers frequently express feelings of being unloved. Sexual intimacy often provides the experience of being loved, and a strong wish for a child can express a need for an object toward which to direct love. After birth, the mother might view the child as security against feeling unloved.

During the first ten months or so, the infant fulfills these needs for the mother. When the infant gets older and begins seeking autonomy, however, conflicts of interests and needs increase. The infant now is demanding more attention and time but does not provide more love or security to the mother. Coping strategies in general are strained during adolescence, with normal inconsistencies in behavior and thought plus rapid mood fluctuations. Emotionally volatile adolescents tend to develop strained relationships with others. Their children are most at risk if they are expected to conform to the moods of adolescent parents.

In general, adolescents find it difficult to focus on the needs of others. Many feel intense conflicts between a wish to grow up and a wish to hold onto childhood security and dependence. Consequently, some adolescents literally turn their infants over to their own parents while they assume the role of sibling to the child.

Adolescent parents need continual support services and much anticipatory guidance. The nurse can assist them in identifying their own needs, the needs of their child, and the relationship between these two sets of needs. Support services and education for parenthood should begin during pregnancy because if the mother emerges from pregnancy and birth with a feeling of dignity and self-worth, she will be better able to progress to parenthood. The type and extent of support services needed vary with each adolescent parent.

(text continues on p. 390)

STANDARDS OF NURSING CARE *The Dysfunctional Family*

RISKS

Assessed risk	Nursing action
Multiple family stressors	Identify situational stressors such as poverty, inadequate housing, financial strains, overcrowding, and multiple demands from dependent others. Tap community resources to help the family to meet basic needs for shelter, food, and clothing. Identify behaviors that place the child at risk. Listen actively to parents to identify needs and "cries for help." Identify resources to assist with family coping (eg, marital or personal counseling, employment counseling).
Inability to trust professionals related to unmet personal needs	Demonstrate caring for parents by attending to their needs. Discuss available resources for parental support as perceived by parents. Establish a means of parental support (eg, "lifeline") and encourage its use. Praise efforts toward positive parenting. Obtain services needed by the family (eg, homemaker or child care assistance). Involve family members in the evaluation process.
Lack of information or experience with normal child development and positive methods of discipline	Teach normal process of growth and development. Refer parent to parenting classes or establish support for parent in the home (eg, parent aide); provide for any secondary needs (eg, transportation or child care needed to attend classes). Role model positive parenting behaviors such as proper feeding, bathing, or comforting. Foster parent-child attachment by pointing out child's strengths and praising positive parenting behaviors. Discuss appropriate role enactment behaviors; praise parent when nurturing behaviors are performed and child is allowed to be dependent according to developmental level. Discuss parent's childhood experience and its reflection in parenting skills and expectations; provide appropriate means (parent aide, lifeline visitor) to meet the parent's needs for attention and approval.
Social isolation	Encourage expanded range of parent activities by suggesting possible child care alternatives. Introduce family members to local families with similar interests. Provide information about possible family activities (eg, school, church). Identify parent's interests, leisure activities, hobbies, and arrange time for parent to develop these and care for self as needed.
Role reversal—dependent needs of parents	Identify and reinforce the child's age-appropriate behaviors demonstrating independence. Identify and reinforce parental behaviors that demonstrate autonomy and self-confidence. Help parent and child learn how to verbalize their feelings and needs to each other and to resource personnel. Encourage honest discussion of feelings through open-ended questions. List problems and strengths as observed by staff and perceived by parents and share list with parents.
Substance abuse	Establish a contract that sets deadlines for behavioral changes. Identify behaviors that must stop (eg, leaving children unattended, substance abuse). Discuss various adaptive coping strategies to replace maladaptive behaviors of withdrawal, anger, or substance abuse.

STANDARDS OF NURSING CARE *The Dysfunctional Family (Continued)*

GUIDE FOR NURSING MANAGEMENT

Nursing diagnosis	Intervention	Rationale	Outcome
1. Ineffective parental coping: disabling related to personal vulnerability secondary to presence of life stressors	Discuss parent's usual pattern of coping with stress and assess whether parent shows a tendency to use force, power, or violence as a way to overcome frustration or settle arguments.	Individuals tend to employ patterned behaviors when coping with frustration, regardless of what precipitated the stress.	Parent demonstrates appropriate use of resources when stressed. Parent copes adaptively to stress, using new behaviors that enhance personal and family growth.
	Discuss parent's perception of personal ability to control emotions such as anger; be alert for comments that indicate exceptions (eg, "I usually act responsibly but . . .," "Sometimes I get so mad I lose it," or "I cannot tolerate being embarrassed publicly, otherwise I manage").	It is important to discover what the parent considers acceptable behavior and what situations trigger loss of control.	
	Have parent explain what is meant by vague statements indicating exceptions (eg, "What happens when you 'lose it'?").	Obtaining explicit definitions of vague words is necessary, otherwise meanings attached to them might differ between parent and nurse.	
	Encourage parent to describe events, behaviors, or situations that present coping difficulties.	By describing precipitating factors, the parent is helped to identify relationships between daily interaction and problematic behavior.	
	Have parent list stressors; as necessary, provide examples or verify whether some areas are or are not perceived as stressors (eg, employment, housing, fatigue, illness, irritability of child).	The parent often is experiencing multiple stressors, some of which have existed for so long the parent is unaware that they contribute to the felt pressure and frustration.	
	Discuss with parent ways to facilitate coping (eg, talking oneself down; counting to 100; using time out for the child, self, or both; planning ahead to avoid certain events; obtaining additional resources for basic necessities).	The parent will benefit from having a variety of appropriate coping strategies suggested, none of which use force.	
	Have parent identify a plan for coping with stress that seems most compatible to personality; contract with parent to have parent practice it for 1 week and then return to discuss the results.	Having the parent take responsibility for identifying a coping strategy that "fits" will enhance cooperation in practicing it.	

(Continues)

STANDARDS OF NURSING CARE *The Dysfunctional Family (Continued)*

GUIDE FOR NURSING MANAGEMENT

Nursing diagnosis	Intervention	Rationale	Outcome
	Discuss information with multidisciplinary team so that appropriate resources can be provided to alleviate stress.	If all team members know the plan, they can support each other and the parent in facilitating the plan.	
2. Alteration in parenting related to physical abuse secondary to history	Help parent to identify factors leading to and resulting in the child's injury.	It is important for the parent to identify the relationship between the parent's response to stress and the child's injury.	Parent demonstrates positive parent-child interaction and is able to employ effective discipline without anger or violence.
	Attempt to establish whether such factors are chronic or acute.	Interventions differ according to the extent that the behavior has become the usual response pattern.	
	Observe carefully the child's response to the parent, determining whether there is obvious fear or anxiety; document all objective behaviors and responses, being conscious to omit personally subjective analyses.	Child-parent interaction provides cues to relationship. An abused child might either ignore the parent or be overly anxious to please. It is important only to describe and not to interpret actions and conversations so as not to bias later observations.	
	Provide age-appropriate play for the child and note the child's use of materials; have available a variety of media, including clay, pencils, crayons, paper, a doll family, blocks, toy cars and trucks, and a dollhouse.	By providing the child with a variety of materials, the child might convey through play recent events, fears, questions, or family interactions that provide cues to the real-life situation.	
	Express interest and listen as the child talks about the pictures or plays with the toys; if beneficial, refer the child to a play therapist for a more extensive expression and an opportunity to work through feelings of anger, guilt, or betrayal.	Expressing interest will encourage the child to continue to play-out or describe events. Once feelings start to be expressed, the child needs support to work through these feelings and the guilt often associated with them.	
3. Parental knowledge deficit related to cognitive limitations secondary to inability to state the normal process of the child's growth and development	Determine what the parent knows about growth and development and temperamental differences, as well as what the parent's expectations are for the child's behavior.	Always begin a plan of care by determining the knowledge base of the parent. How in tune are the expectations with the child's developmental level and capabilities?	Parent has a realistic perception of the child's abilities. Parent's expectations of the child's skills and behaviors are age appropriate.

STANDARDS OF NURSING CARE *The Dysfunctional Family (Continued)*

GUIDE FOR NURSING MANAGEMENT

Nursing diagnosis	Intervention	Rationale	Outcome
	Review the aspects of growth and development that normally occur, especially those resulting in changes in mobility, learning, and autonomy.	Provide baseline information concerning general patterns of growth and development and how changes affect the abilities and behavior of the child.	
	Have the parent discuss personal perceptions of the child's behavior and note any misconceptions; listen for phrases that indicate a loss of power or violation of expectations (eg, "I thought all babies were cuddly, but mine wants freedom," "She was so cute as an infant, but now she is a terror," or "He does that because he does not like me").	It is important to learn how the parent interprets the child's behavior. Parental descriptions of the child provide insight into whether normal developmental processes are viewed positively or negatively.	
	Acknowledge the parent's frustration concerning the quantity and rapidity of changes that occur as the child develops.	Change always is difficult to accept; this is true in parent-child expectations and in need fulfillment as well. Important for fostering open communication is the ability to express empathy concerning this ongoing need for change in the relationship.	
	Clarify the aspects of the child's behavior that the parent finds difficult; provide anticipatory guidance and model appropriate interactions.	It is important to restate the specific behaviors that the parent finds problematic so that interventions can be focused on these and specific suggestions given for change.	
	Discuss and demonstrate for the parent ways to promote development through stimulation and realistic expectations.	To facilitate cooperation with altering specific behaviors, it is necessary to keep expectations reasonable and outcomes specific so that the parent can see results.	
	Refer the parent to appropriate resources for additional information; if beneficial, review the age-related standard assessment form with the parent as a guide for revising expectations.	Providing a resource guide will help the parent to compare child behaviors with so-called norms. For the parent with more advanced coping skills, the guide will encourage planning ahead for the next developmental behavior.	

(Continues)

STANDARDS OF NURSING CARE *The Dysfunctional Family (Continued)*

GUIDE FOR NURSING MANAGEMENT

Nursing diagnosis	Intervention	Rationale	Outcome
4. Parental knowledge deficit related to unfamiliarity with information resources secondary to inexperience and inadequate role models for learning parenting skills	Observe parenting behaviors, noting whether the parent talks to the child and the tone of voice used, whether parent answers questions addressed to an older child, how the infant is held (eg, closely, stiffly, supported adequately or not), amount of eye contact sought and maintained, and parental response to cues and bids for attention.	Verbal and nonverbal communication conveys how sensitive the parent is to the child's cues. Positive communication enhances responsiveness and needs to be supported. Negative communication encourages withdrawal and must be changed. Specific areas for change can be addressed only after careful observation.	Parent responds appropriately to the child's cues for attention or signals of distress. Parent describes a realistic perspective of the positive and negative experiences of parenting.
	Discuss with the parent the difficulty and demands of being a parent; note any comments that indicate disappointment or a deficit in personal need fulfillment.	Open-ended questions and statements conveying understanding of the parent's situation will facilitate trust and honest sharing of problems.	
	Help the parent to compare expectations concerning parenting before the child's birth with the realities of parenting since that time.	Comparison of expectations and realities often reveals areas of fantasy or specific disappointments and thus directs nursing interventions.	
	Discuss the parent's experiences as a chlid and how parenting was role-modeled during childhood.	Parents most frequently use their own parents as the standard for parenting. If the experience of being parented was deficient, it will influence present parenting ability.	
	Provide guidance for the parent in identifying parenting behaviors to emulate, especially if the parent's childhood experience includes abuse.	If supported, the parent can learn positive parenting behaviors from other models.	
	Discuss the influence of the parent's culture together with personal ideas or philosophy about discipline and its purpose, form, and desired results.	It is important to have plans for change coincide with parent's culture, values, and beliefs. If plans are in conflict with these, the parent is not likely to cooperate, and desired change is not likely to occur.	
	Provide anticipatory guidance for areas of parenting concern (eg, toilet training, self-feeding, tantrums, and manipulative behaviors such as screaming in public or threatening to run away).	Prepare parent for the next stage so it will not be a surprise, and the parent will have some idea about specific responses and strategies to use.	

STANDARDS OF NURSING CARE *The Dysfunctional Family (Continued)*

GUIDE FOR NURSING MANAGEMENT

Nursing diagnosis	Intervention	Rationale	Outcome
	Discuss alternative ways of disciplining that do not involve physical measures.	It is important to explore with parent ideas about other means of discipline and identify what is acceptable and viewed as effective before recommending anything specific.	
	Discuss the parent's needs, noting a need for "parenting the parent" or befriending the parent temporarily.	Acknowledging the parent's dependent needs for attention, praise, recognition, love, and care will help the parent to demand less and give more to the child.	
	Help the parent to express needs and discuss more appropriate ways of meeting them (other than through the child).	Personal growth results from need identification followed by suggestions concerning ways to meet the stated need.	
	Work with health team members to find ways to assist the parent in meeting personal needs.	Assisting a dysfunctional parent requires the combined input and resources of the multidisciplinary team.	
5. Disturbance in self-esteem of the parent related to unrealistic self-expectations	Point out and praise positive parenting behaviors and parent-child interactions.	Praise and recognition are positive reinforcers that promote repetition of behavior.	Parent expresses pleasure and pride in role performance as a parent.
	Help the parent describe a sequence of events and analyze why specific interactions illustrate positive parenting behaviors.	Involving the parent in relating specific behaviors with positive outcome reinforces the behaviors.	
	Help the parent identify nurturing behaviors and support their continued practice.	Parental knowledge of what behaviors provide nurturance is a first step toward performing the behaviors.	
	Discuss parental expectations of the parenting role and the parent's performance; determine whether expectations are realistic.	For a parent to want to work at performing the parenting role, the difference between expectation and reality must not be too great. Identifying the parent's expectations will direct nursing interventions.	
	Model positive, consistent parenting behaviors.	The new parent will learn parenting behaviors that are modeled by a respected person.	
	Teach the parent to identify positive feedback from the infant or child.	By identifying for the parent ways in which the infant shows pleasure (quieting, alerting, snuggling), the parent will relate infant-care activities with the infant's expressions of satisfaction.	

(Continues)

STANDARDS OF NURSING CARE *The Dysfunctional Family (Continued)*

GUIDE FOR NURSING MANAGEMENT

Nursing diagnosis	Intervention	Rationale	Outcome
	Help the parent to identify successful parenting actions; suggest keeping a diary of these examples for reference and positive feedback.	Supporting the parent in identifying additional positive responses from the infant encourages the parent to seek new ways of eliciting positive responses and provides an immediate self-reward.	
	Discuss ways to ignore or not reinforce the child's negative behavior.	Behavior that is ignored is not rewarded and tends to disappear after a brief time.	
6. Ineffective family coping: compromised related to emotional conflicts secondary to inadequate support or ineffective role performance	Discuss with the parent the typical daily routine; have the parent identify ways to improve it or compare it with the personal ideal; note areas that are incongruous and suggest ways to compensate (eg, home health aide, day care, parents' group).	Emotional conflicts decrease when the ideal and reality are similar. Discussion of these two assists the nurse in formulating a plan of intervention that increases the parent's ability to cope with reality.	Family members demonstrate satisfactory role performance and an ability to modify roles to help each other in times of need, thereby coping effectively with stress.
	Have the parent note significant people and discuss whether they are available for support; review the parent's history for recent losses by death, moves, or changes in commitment.	Helping the parent identify friends or relatives who could serve as supports will encourage the parent to request their help, especially if a recent situational crisis has intensified the parent's need for support.	
	Discuss the parent's knowledge and use of community or religious resources.	Knowledge of community resources is necessary before the parent can seek their services.	
	Have the parent identify who in the family performs household chores, childrearing tasks, and home management responsibilities; note whether distribution is a source of friction.	The gap between role expectation and role performance is sometimes the source of friction that interferes with all other aspects of parenting.	
	Discuss the parent's perception of personal role performance and (if applicable) the partner's role performance; have each family member identify who is blamed and who feels guilty for perceived incompetence.	Before effective parenting can be practiced, the parent must deal with and resolve feelings of guilt and anger about expected and actual role performance.	

STANDARDS OF NURSING CARE *The Dysfunctional Family* (Continued)

GUIDE FOR NURSING MANAGEMENT

Nursing diagnosis	Intervention	Rationale	Outcome
	Determine whether role performance meets the basic needs of the family; whether there is flexibility when needed; whether roles are ambiguous, overlapping, unfilled, or pejorative; whether role performers conflict or complement one another; and whether anyone occupies a dysfunctional role (eg, scapegoat).	Analyzing the adequacy of role performance and noting areas of discrepancy will give direction for planning nursing interventions.	
	Share observations and information with a multidisciplinary team.	Communication is essential for the functioning of the team.	
	Encourage the parent to participate in family therapy or a parents' group, as recommended.	The parent will benefit from group support and assistance in learning to cope with reality.	
7. Alteration in family processes related to situational crisis secondary to the arrival of a special child	Discuss with the parent the meaning attached to the child and why the child is special.	Before planning interventions, the nurse must know why the parent views the child as special.	Family members demonstrate equal concern for each other without any favoritism or blame directed to a specific member.
	Help the parent identify ways in which family life has changed since the child's arrival.	It is important to determine whether the changes are related to the child's arrival or to other factors.	
	Have the parent compare expectations for this child with those of other children.	Once the parent explains how or why expectations for this child are different than for the other children, the nurse can determine if the expectations are realistic or not and provide support accordingly.	
	Determine whether the parent is more or less patient, tender, demanding, or frustrated when interacting with the special child than with other children.	Observing the parent's interaction with this child will direct the nurse's plan of care.	
	Help the parent identify realistic expectations for the child and acknowledge the need for personal assistance to accomplish parenting tasks.	Many times parents view seeking help as a sign of failure; the parent might need support in making this decision.	
8. Altered growth and development related to inadequate caretaking secondary to dysfunctional parent-child interaction	Assess the child's developmental skills in physical, cognitive, affective, and social behaviors; compare with standard; note areas of delay.	A thorough developmental assessment reveals areas of delay and directs intervention.	The child's development is within normal parameters. The child and parent demonstrate adaptive changes in their interactions.

(Continues)

STANDARDS OF NURSING CARE *The Dysfunctional Family (Continued)*

GUIDE FOR NURSING MANAGEMENT

Nursing diagnosis	Intervention	Rationale	Outcome
	Provide child with a primary nurse.	A primary nurse will foster the child's sense of trust and provide stability.	
	Demonstrate acceptance of child, providing nurturing interactions and consistency in expectations.	For self-esteem to develop, the child must feel loved and accepted.	
	Provide age-appropriate stimulation to foster development in all areas.	For development to progress, the child must be stimulated to learn new, achievable skills.	
	Assist the child in learning acceptable and unacceptable ways to gain attention; keep responses consistent and affirm positive behaviors.	To learn social skills, the child must be given specific, direct guidelines concerning acceptable and unacceptable behavior.	
	Suggest the use of age-appropriate facilities (eg, day care, nursery school, or YMCA program) to provide time out for parent and stimulation for child after discharge.	Socialization occurs best in a nurturing environment with other children and supportive adults.	
	Refer family to public health, visiting nurse, or social service for continued supervision and support after discharge.	Learning new behaviors and ways to cope with stress is difficult and requires long-term support and assistance.	
9. Potential for disturbance in child's self-esteem	Observe the child's behavior and interaction with peers; note whether the child is overly aggressive or submissive; if the child is aggressive, provide time in a safe environment for the child to express feelings; discuss when aggression is appropriate and when it is not; provide guidelines and support the child in following them; offer positive feedback for evidence of control; if the child is submissive, support the child in gradual interaction with peers, beginning with one other child or small group in an activity that the child enjoys; provide positive feedback and affirm attempts at interaction.	The child who has been abused is at risk for developing a negative sense of self, including self-blame and guilt. This child needs professional help to work through these feelings and to establish a positive sense of self. The nurse who follows this family observes the child's interactions with others and affirms positive behaviors so they continue.	Child's behavior is age appropriate and demonstrates self-confidence in trying new skills and interacting with peers. Parent demonstrates support and affirmation of child's abilities.

STANDARDS OF NURSING CARE *The Dysfunctional Family* (Continued)

GUIDE FOR NURSING MANAGEMENT

Nursing diagnosis	Intervention	Rationale	Outcome
	Observe the child's response to questions about injuries; encourage the child to talk about positive experiences and happy times with the parent; acknowledge the child's feelings for the parent and validate the importance of parental care.	It is essential to help the child resolve feelings of ambiguity toward the parent and to assist in the development of trust.	
	Observe the child's reaction to the hospital environment to identify unmet needs.	Identification of unmet needs provides direction for planning both immediate and ongoing care.	
	Prepare for discharge with age-appropriate teaching about the treatment plan.	The parent needs specific guidance concerning age-appropriate expectations of the child. Specific suggestions for ways to stimulate development while not expecting more than the child can contribute must be provided	
10. Potential for injury	Monitor the home and family situation with respect to the likelihood for future injury to the child (or any siblings); use assessment tools as needed.	The home and family situation must be assessed and evaluated for basic safety provisions before the child is discharged.	The child experiences no further injuries from parent.
	Refer the family to assistance according to their perceived needs.	If the family is informed about available resources and are encouraged to use them when needed, they are more likely to take advantage of them.	
	Encourage parental cooperation in following through with family therapy; note any improvements in parent-child interactions.	Acknowledgment of improved relations provides positive feedback and encourages continuation with treatment plan.	
	Discuss with the parent the commitment to learn and practice nonviolent coping strategies.	Once the individual makes a commitment to learn a new behavior, the desire to succeed is stronger than if the commitment is not made. In many respects, commitment serves as a contract.	

Developmental Implications of Dysfunctional Parenting

Developmental delays Children who are nurtured sporadically make only sporadic developmental progress, leading to delays in the age-expected norms. Delayed development often is first evident when the child does not meet normal developmental skills and behaviors (see Chapter 9). Some developmental delays are related to family dysfunction. Problems with the parent-child relationship affect the child at each developmental stage. Some of the behaviors that the infant might demonstrate are feeding difficulties, such as being irritable and never satisfied or responding apathetically to all feedings. The irritability usually is accompanied by an annoying cry. In addition, the infant might be slow to turn over, reach out for toys, or sit. Social responses such as smiling and vocalizing might also be delayed.

As the infant matures, other delays become evident. The child might not show separation anxiety and might respond indiscriminately to new stimuli. The child might accept toys passively, not protest when they are removed, and exhibit little interest in exploring the environment.

Developmental delays during early childhood are evident during the child's play. The child might use toys in a primitive way and with a lack of interest. Lack of eye contact and much passivity are common. The child might have poor coordination, indicating delayed progress in both gross and fine motor development and poor muscle tone. Speech is usually delayed, with poor enunciation and vocabulary. The child usually is unable to express feelings or describe family members. The child with disturbed parent-child relationships has difficulty relating to people, shows a sense of mistrust, has a poor self-concept, and is preoccupied with many fears.

Whenever delayed development is identified, the nurse documents the child's gross and fine motor skills, language capacity, and ability to use toys in an age-appropriate way. The nurse frequently is the health provider who is responsible for assisting parents in understanding children and their needs. Many times the parents' fulfillment of their own needs interferes with their ability to use information to modify or learn new parenting skills. Therefore, simply teaching the parent about child development is not an adequate solution. Assessing parental learning readiness and motivation must be done prior to sharing information about the normal strivings children have to master developmental tasks. The nurse might discover that the parental needs are multiple and complex. Then it is best to refer the family for counseling.

Inorganic failure to thrive The term *failure to thrive* describes a syndrome, not a diagnosis. It is characterized by a lack of normal growth and development in children. The child's height and weight usually falls below the third percentile on standard growth charts. Slow physical growth is accompanied by lags in social, motor, adaptive, and language development (Table 13-1).

The etiology of failure to thrive is often difficult to identify. The syndrome must first be classified as organic or inorganic in origin. Children with organic failure to thrive have difficulty using nutrients because of neurogenic, metabolic, endocrine, enzymatic, or genetic disease. Inorganic failure to thrive has an environmental or social cause and often is seen in children from dysfunctional families. Children with inorganic failure to thrive predictably prefer distant social encounters and inanimate objects, whereas children with failure to thrive caused by medical problems

TABLE 13-1 Common Findings in Infants with Inorganic Failure to Thrive

Age	Findings
0–6 months	Prematurity
	Neonatal illness or anomaly necessitating early separation
	Feeding difficulties (eg, anorexia)
	Height and weight below third percentile
	Unresponsiveness and withdrawal
	Watchfulness, little smiling
	Delayed socialization and vocalization
	Irregular sleep patterns
	Developmental delays
6–12 months	Absence of stranger anxiety
	Rumination
	No displeasure at separation
	Apathy/passivity
	Delayed milestones as to sitting and standing
	Muscular hypotonia
12–18 months	Indifference to caregivers
	Small physical size
	Delayed dentition
	Little vocalization
	Little eye contact
	Intense watchfulness
	Repetitive self-stimulation behaviors (eg, rocking, head banging, rolling, intense sucking)

consistently respond more positively to close personal stimuli such as touching and holding.

Children with failure to thrive are usually thin, frail, and undernourished. They might show evidence of improper physical care, such as poor hygiene or open sores. Infants with failure to thrive frequently are hospitalized to document changes in weight and to rule out organic causes for growth failure. Children with inorganic failure to thrive might show a substantial weight gain while in the hospital and also show progress in developmental skills while receiving consistent nurturance from hospital personnel.

The behaviors of an infant and parent might provide clues to the cause of the disorder. When the parent-child relationship is problematic, both parent and infant demonstrate maladaptive behaviors. For example, the infant who is irritable, resists cuddling, and is unresponsive to initial attempts at nurturing often creates a response pattern in the parent that increases fears, anxiety, and avoidance behaviors. The parent responds with anxiety and tension to the infant who reacts with irritability and rigidity, and a vicious cycle of unmet needs is set in motion.

The parent who suffers from unmet needs or has multiple environmentally related stresses is likely to have problems providing care to an irritable, resistant infant. Failure to have parental needs gratified can trigger unconscious feelings of rejection. The new, inexperienced parent, the depressed parent, and the adolescent parent are especially at risk for having a child who fails to thrive. Failure to thrive is rarely the result of willful neglect but is more frequently a symptom of family dysfunction.

The family dynamics that lead to failure to thrive are stagnant. Members do not communicate, and a general feeling of helplessness pervades the family. Family members cannot identify what is happening. In their troubled, isolated lives, dysfunctional behaviors keep them from experiencing joy in living. Early identification and interventions with high-risk families are therefore crucial. Funding to accomplish this goal, however, never has been adequate. Breaking the complex cycle of dysfunction requires planning and interventions that incorporate the interrelationships among the child, family, and community.

Health-Threatening Parenting

Health-threatening parenting is a severe manifestation of family dysfunction. It occurs when the safety of a child is at risk and is generally classified as child neglect or child abuse. Heins (1984) reported 929,310 cases of child abuse and neglect nationwide. Twenty-six percent of these reports involved abuse, 43% neglect, and 19% combined abuse and neglect.

Child Neglect

Child neglect is the failure to provide a child with the basic necessities of life: food, clothing, love, shelter, supervision, and medical care. Neglect usually is associated with parental acts of omission. The neglect can be deliberate or unintentional, but in either instance the caregiver fails to provide the supports necessary for developing a child's physical, intellectual, and emotional capacities. Neglect is more commonly found in infants and young children, although older children are not exempt.

Child neglect is not easy to define. Most authorities agree that neglect is any form of substandard child care. Although professionals can reach some consensus about what constitutes minimally adequate child care, the right to intervene when parents neglect or provide poorly for their children is limited because laws protect families from intrusion. Child neglect is more prevalent than child abuse, and its emotional and physical sequelae have been demonstrated to be equally serious.

In some instances neglect has even been found to be lethal. For example, a parent might "forget" to feed an infant for several days, or a young child, when left alone in a house or apartment for extended times, might fall out of a window or down the stairs or ingest poisons.

Inadequate physical care Physical neglect might be evident in many ways. An infant, for instance, might be dirty or inadequately clothed, have evidence of chronic diaper rash, or appear unkempt, with a stale, urine odor. Nutritional neglect, which results either from lack of food or from a bizarre diet, frequently is manifested by signs of malnutrition. The child often has a decreased muscle mass and an appearance of gauntness, with prominent bones and little subcutaneous fat. Physical assessment might reveal a bald spot on the back of the head from the infant's lying alone and unattended in the crib.

Infant behaviors, however, give the most valuable clues to the inadequacy of care. The neglected infant is often listless, makes few demands, and does not respond to the stimulation of voices or friendly faces. The infant prefers to turn away from people and engages in little eye contact. With prolonged and severe neglect, infants often arch their bodies when they are picked up. Neurologic and neonatal examinations show developmental progression but not the increased capacity for orientation, self-consolation, and social responses that are characteristic of the normal neonate.

As neglected children grow, developmental delays become more apparent. Physical size often suggests a much younger child. The nurse therefore needs to identify the proper age and expected level of development for every child. Gross motor skills often are delayed because the child is reluctant to interact with the environment. Delays in eye-

Common Findings Related to Child Neglect

Child

- Height and weight below third percentile on growth chart
- Apathy—does not smile; appears solemn and watchful
- Stiff body that resists being held
- Suspiciousness and inability to trust adults
- Unkempt appearance—foul odor; ground-in dirt; ill-fitting clothing; clothing inappropriate for weather
- Restless sleep patterns
- Frequent absences from school
- Developmental delays
- Marginal communication skills
- Few coping skills
- Poor eye-hand coordination
- Poor dental care
- Chronic malnutrition; excessive intake of junk food
- Haphazard medical attention—late or missing immunizations
- Lack of safety (eg, in cars; has many "mishaps")
- Skin problems (eg, crusting, impetigo, scabies, rashes)
- Rumination
- Arrives early to school and stays late
- Tired and falls asleep in class

Parent

- History of inadequate parenting
- Use of denial and projection as coping strategies
- Poor performance in day-to-day activities
- Intense need to be cared for
- Limited ability to plan
- Few external resources
- Inability to use resources
- Inability to assess infant's needs
- Need for concrete direction in providing child care
- Diminished self-esteem
- Passivity; lack of warmth and tenderness
- Dissatisfaction with parenting role
- Little awareness of normal growth and development
- Little awareness or concern for child's progress or problems in school
- No attendance at any school programs or participation in parent-teacher conferences
- Minimal awareness of child's activities, interests, or friends

Family

- Marital discord, often with periods of separation
- Erratic habits (eg, no scheduled mealtime; little planning for food, rest, or recreation)
- Chronically unstable home environment
- Poverty
- Employment instability
- Substance abuse
- Children left unattended or in care of strangers
- Isolation, with minimal participation in any community activities
- Unhygienic environment—foul odor caused by accumulated garbage; bedding with urine odor; broken furniture; spoiled food
- Nutritional deficits in all members (eg, obesity, malnutrition)
- Lack of motivation to change
- Lack of emotional bonds among members
- Inconsistent or sporadic discipline
- Medical care only in emergencies

hand coordination frequently affect reading and writing skills and ultimately affect the child's self-confidence and self-esteem.

Language development also is frequently delayed in the neglected child because the infant needs to hear language to imitate it. Language skills are notably lacking from 2 years of age on, as children cannot name simple body parts or identify common objects within the home. Many neglected children speak only in phrases rather than in sentences and have limited vocabularies, although they frequently can repeat television commercials.

Interacting with strangers is especially difficult for neglected children because of their mistrust. When supplied with toys, neglected children often need to learn how to use them because they simply have not learned how to play.

In the older child, poor physical care might be apparent by ill-fitting clothing or clothing that is inappropriate for the weather. The child might smell dirty and have multiple layers of dirt and grime, suggesting infrequent bathing. Nutrition is poor, and the child has learned to eat whatever is available, including many snack foods that have minimal food value. School lunch programs provide most of the child's nutrients for the day.

In school, the child might be restless and irritable, have poor concentration, and daydream because of constant hunger. Fatigue is common because the child's sleep habits often are not supervised. Listlessness or falling asleep in class affects learning and leads to asocial behavior among peers.

Another sign of neglect might be a consistent lack of

supervision, either in allowing children to engage in dangerous activities or in leaving small children unattended. Unattended children are at risk for falling, causing fires, ingesting poisons or medicines, and playing with unsuitable companions. Parents often have no extra money for babysitters or day care and are forced to leave young children without supervision before and after school.

Another form of physical neglect is inattention to medical needs. The child might have bad teeth; lice; various skin rashes; a sporadic, incomplete immunization record; and few follow-up visits for health problems. If much parental time and energy are spent on day-to-day survival, it is difficult to plan ahead to make and keep a health visit appointment. Therefore, when the child does become ill, the illness is intensified because of poor nutrition, neglect, and multiple other problems within the family.

Inadequate emotional care Emotional neglect is an act of omission on the part of the parent or caregiver. Lack of positive emotional support and stimulation is not necessarily accompanied by inadequate physical care but usually is evidenced by few expressions of love and caring. Emotional neglect is difficult to identify early.

The parent who emotionally neglects a child tends to respond only to such behavior as crying or misdeeds. The parent seldom looks at, touches, or talks to the child. Such parents show little interest in their children and often leave them unattended. Limit setting is usually inconsistent because the parent has neither time, energy, nor interest to invest in the child. Any positive behaviors go unnoticed, and the child soon learns to increase the intensity of negative behaviors to get attention.

In the older child, emotional neglect is evident in poor self-concept. The child might be distant or disruptive in the classroom but typically wants approval and affection from teachers. Hostile, angry children also might alienate teachers just when they most need the teacher's care and affection.

Causes of child neglect Neglectful parents often were themselves victims of child abuse or neglect and might have had no positive role models for parenting. They often are not trying to hurt their children but merely are treating their children as they were treated. Neglectful parents also tend to report profound sadness over not having been loved or wanted by their own parents.

Many of these parents are constantly under stress, which interferes with their ability to spend time to enjoy their children, or much of their time and energy is taken up with the basic necessities of life, so they have little time and energy left for child care. Inadequate knowledge about children, parenting, and normal development is also common.

Neglectful parents also tend to be impoverished, isolated, and involved in fewer relationships with others. They are less able to plan, less confident about the future, and more plagued by psychologic and psychosomatic problems. The nurse often finds that the presence of multiple risk factors or the intensity of one or two risk factors so overwhelms the parents that they are unable to cope with the daily tasks related to child care (Table 13-2). Their personal repertoire of coping strategies is so limited that they need assistance to survive and provide for the family.

Child Abuse

Child abuse is "human-originated acts of commission or omission and human-created or tolerated conditions that inhibit or preclude unfolding and development of inherent potential of children" (Pelton, 1981). In the past 20 years, child abuse has been identified in epidemic proportions throughout the world.

Abuse is always complex. It is not a diagnosis but is instead a symptom of severe family dysfunction. Data now indicate that the social environment, as well as children and parents, shows many patterns of risk, but no single family configuration is most likely to cause child abuse. The focus for identification, treatment, and prevention must include the child, family, and life setting. When child abuse occurs, each member of the family is in some way a victim and needs help if the family is to achieve any degree of positive functioning.

Estimates of the incidence of victimized children and families are only crude measures because of the lack of uniformity in defining the problem and the hesitancy in reporting it. Some authorities place the figure at over 2 million cases of child abuse annually in the United States. Abuse of adolescents is often not included in these data, usually because adolescent abuse is called something else (such as adolescent-parent conflict, discipline problems, adolescent provocation, arrest). Some data might classify all adolescents in a separate category. Statistics also give only part of the picture because most abusers are repeating child-care patterns from previous generations. About 6000 children die annually from child abuse or neglect, more than from any disease (Ten Bensel and Berdie, 1976).

In the early 1960s, child protection became public policy. In 1962 the Social Security Administration amended its regulations to require states to plan the protection of children. In 1963 the Department of Health, Education and Welfare (HEW) developed a model mandatory reporting law for states to follow in writing their own regulations. Within 5 years, every state had laws mandating certain professionals to report abuse and established state agencies to receive and investigate all such reports. In 1973 the federal government passed the Child Abuse Prevention and Treatment Act. Public Law 93-247, also known as the Mondale Act, provided financial assistance for projects for preventing, identifying, and treating abuse and neglect. It also

TABLE 13-2 Risk Factors for Dysfunctional Parenting That Might Lead to Child Neglect or Abuse

Risk factor	Assessment finding
Lack of nurturing experience	Inadequate experience with parenting (eg, multiple foster homes)
	Parent neglected or abused as a child
	Parent expected to meet high demands of own parents as a child
Lack of knowledge of normal growth and development	Inability to read "cues" of child
	Impatience when child does not respond as expected; unreasonable discipline
	Unrealistically high expectations for the child
Isolation	Inadequate use of supports
	Inability to identify resources
	Unknown to others in community
Low self-esteem	Lack of trust, particularly of authority figures
	Expect rejection
High vulnerability to criticism	History of family violence in family of origin or in current family system (eg, spouse abuse)
	Low tolerance for frustration
	Impulsive
Many unmet needs	Feelings of being unloved or having unresponsive spouse, unstable marriage, or no marriage at all
	Youthful marriage, forced marriage, unwanted pregnancy
Multiple stressors	Poverty, unemployment, substandard housing, lack of job opportunities
	Inadequate clothing and insufficient food
Substance abuse	Abuse of alcohol or drugs
Role reversal	Emotional immaturity, lack of patience, inability to make judgments
	Preoccupied with self
	Depression
	Dependent on others

established a national center on child abuse and neglect, provided an information clearinghouse, and published annual summaries of research into abuse and neglect.

During the 1960s, early efforts at treatment emphasized detection and removal of abused children to foster homes. Initially, many families were lost to follow-up because few outreach programs were available. Trends revealed, however, that many dysfunctional parents who had more children repeated patterns of abuse. Clearly, society needed to assist the families in learning new parenting styles.

Patterns of child abuse Child abusers are found among all socioeconomic, religious, and ethnic groups. Some child abusers are irrational or even psychotic, but most are ordinary people who feel trapped in stressful life situations with which they cannot cope satisfactorily (Table 13-2). Many abusive parents are simply confused and overwhelmed by parenthood or by life in general and often vent their frustrations on their children. Because all parents have negative feelings about their children at one time or another, the difference between parents who abuse and those who do not is often only a matter of degree. All parents are at risk occasionally, but most parents are able to channel their frustrations and anger appropriately.

Child abuse is most likely to occur during times of crisis. The parent's loss of a job, for example, might be just enough to make the crying of a fretful infant unbearable. Some families hover on the brink of perpetual crises by living with constant changes that contribute to feelings of inadequacy. The magnitude of the crisis is not always in proportion to the abuse. Instead, the parental perception of the crisis coupled with the lack of available resources often leads to an abusive episode. A relatively minor crisis might be viewed as the "last straw" in an unhappy life situation.

Solving a crisis for troubled families is not enough if new crises and stressors merely reestablish dysfunctional patterns. Instead, the nurse teaches parents to develop their own coping strategies and to identify when and how to seek help. Parents who learn the problems inherent in isolation, for example, will then seek assistance when under stress and will avoid the patterns of behavior that cause them to abuse their children.

Types of child abuse Although physical abuse is the most obvious form of abuse, it is not the only type. The scars from emotional, sexual, and adolescent abuse might not be as visible, but the effects might be longer lasting and more damaging to the personal development of the child (Table 13-3).

Physical abuse Physical injuries might resemble those caused by accidents, but child abuse should be suspected whenever a child's injury has no explanation or plausible

TABLE 13-3 Types of Child Abuse

	Definition	Characteristics
Physical abuse	Nonaccidental injury of a child	Physical injury at variance with history or explanation given; repeated pattern of physical punishment with short- or long-term effects
Emotional abuse	Nonphysical, often verbal, assault on a child—usually critical, demeaning, and emotionally devastating	Attack inflicted by parent or other adult, often as part of a continuing pattern
Sexual abuse	Use of a child for sexual purposes, including incest, rape, molestation, prostitution, or pornography	Nonabusing parent or other family members often aware of the abuse (and might be criminally liable if they do nothing to stop it)
Adolescent abuse	Physical, emotional, or sexual abuse inflicted on an adolescent	Adolescent who runs away from home; abusing parent often considers abuse justified

reason (Table 13-4). Children who sustain many injuries should be considered possible victims of abuse. Fresh and old injuries together suggests a series of traumatic events rather than a single accident. Another important clue is the distance from the child's home to the treatment facility because parents might go to distant facilities to escape detection.

Physical abuse might be obvious if marks on the child's body are inconsistent with a traumatic injury. Some of the more common injuries include localized burns on the buttocks from being placed on a stove or radiator and circular extremity burns from immersion in hot water. The child might have slap marks resembling a handprint; welts from beatings with coat hangers, belts, or buckles; or circular abrasions on the wrists and ankles from being tied down. A particularly harmful practice is shaking the child vigorously, which can lead to a whiplash injury and even cause brain damage, especially in the young infant who has not developed good head control. Children who are thrown into a crib or against a wall might have signs of both fractures and dislocations because during infancy, the periosteum is less securely attached to the bone, allowing it to be stripped from the shaft by hemorrhage. Sometimes, the abused child will have a "paradox of clothing," which is the parent's attempt to hide the abuse by dressing the child in clothing such as a baptismal dress.

Physical abuse might result from overdiscipline or from punishment that is too severe. Some children are punished for behavior that is perfectly appropriate for the child's developmental stage but is not perceived as appropriate by the parent. For example, crying in the infant or toilet training in the toddler might precipitate abuse. Most parents who abuse their children have good intentions and really care about the welfare of their children. They might be trying to change the behavior of the child but overreact to stressors. Many abusive parents know that they need help but are afraid to ask for fear of losing their children to foster care.

Emotional abuse Emotional abuse is most difficult to define and diagnose because its scars are hidden and because both the victim and abuser might not recognize the behavior as dysfunctional. Variations in parenting styles and cultural norms compound the problem of defining and documenting the abuse. In most instances the child is called foul names, ridiculed, and made to feel stupid, hated, ugly, unlovable, or unwanted. The parent might blatantly reject the child and demonstrate a consistent lack of concern for the child's welfare.

Emotional abuse causes suffering and lasting effects on the development of the child's self-concept. Emotional abuse ultimately affects the child's future relationships with others. Because the scars are not obvious, its effects tend to be diagnosed only years after the event. The adult who was emotionally abused as a child has many unmet needs and is often filled with self-doubt and anger.

Most physical abuse is accompanied by some degree of emotional abuse, but the reverse is not always true. Some children receive only verbal abuse, but the sequelae can have far-reaching effects. These children often repeat the pattern when they become parents. The manifested results of emotional abuse typically are speech disorders, developmental delays, apathetic or hostile behaviors, or depression. Sucking, biting, rocking, sleep disorders, unusual fearfulness, and play disturbances are also common. Behaviors might vacillate between extremes, so the child might be both aggressive and apathetic.

The legal definition of emotional abuse varies. Legal intervention is often possible only if psychologic damage can

TABLE 13-4 Signs and Symptoms of Physical Abuse

Indication of abuse	Assessment finding
Bruises or welts on eyes, mouth, lips, torso, buttocks, genital areas, calves	Injuries might be in shape of object used to produce them (eg, sticks, belts, hairbrushes, buckles)
	Injuries located on parts of body not usually injured (normal bruises commonly appear on forehead, shins, knees, elbows)
	Injuries often in various stages of healing
Burns	Shape suggests type of burn
Immersion burns	Immersion burns have "socklike" or "glovelike" appearance
Pattern burns	Pattern suggests object used (eg, iron, stove grate, electric burner, heater); small, circular burns on feet, face, hands, chest, or buttocks suggest cigar or cigarette
Friction burns	Friction often caused by rope on legs, arms, neck, or torso and might be caused by child having been tied up
Fractures of skull, face, nose, long bones	Multiple or spiral fractures caused by twisting motion
	Evidence of epiphyseal separations and periosteal shearing
	Shaft fractures from direct blows
	Fractures might be in various stages of healing if earlier fractures went untreated
Lacerations or abrasions on mouth, lips, gums, eyes, genitals	Human bite marks, especially those of adult size, might be evident
Child's behaviors that indicate fear or apprehension	Extreme aggressiveness or withdrawal; wariness of adults; fear of going home; apprehension when other children cry
	Appears frightened of parents
	Vacant stare; no eye contact
	Surveys environment but remains motionless
	Stiffens when approached as if expecting punishment of a physical nature

Ideas for Informing Children About Sexual Abuse and Preventive Measures

1. A "good touch" is nice, like a hug, whereas a "bad touch" makes a person uncomfortable. Children need to be told, "Your body belongs to you; you can decide who touches it. Private areas are those covered by a bathing suit. If you are touched by someone and you don't like it, tell the person to stop, and tell someone else about it."
2. Secrets and surprises are not the same. Secrets sometimes are not fair to keep. Surprises are fun; secrets are not fun if they make you feel funny or uncomfortable.
3. Strangers can be dangerous. Never go with someone you don't know who says anything like, "Your mother is ill and sent me to get you," or "Will you help me look for my lost puppy in the woods?"
4. Do not let others undress you, even if they promise to give you something such as candy or new clothes.
5. Do not listen when an older person tells you that they are going to help you grow up by showing you what big people do.
6. If you feel uncomfortable with someone, do not allow yourself to be left alone with that person.

be demonstrated. Health professionals and agencies responsible for protecting children need to develop consistent, accepted legal criteria defining emotional abuse. In the process, nurses and other health professionals can take the following steps:

1. Contact the juvenile court and reach agreement on terms and guidelines.
2. Document the abuse and its impact.
3. Use expert witnesses such as psychiatrists and psychologists.
4. Evaluate previous interventions and results.
5. Educate the public to recognize and report emotional abuse.
6. Act as an advocate for children and intervene before a child's behavior becomes the issue.
7. Establish a network of community services to provide counseling to families with emotional abuse (Dean, 1979).

Sexual abuse *Sexual abuse* is the exploitation of a child for the sexual gratification of an adult. Statistics reflecting its incidence are not available. Because secrecy and social

TABLE 13-5 Myths and Reality of Sexual Abuse

Myth	Reality
The child seduces the adult	Blaming the child is blaming the victim. A child needs nurturance and closeness, not sex. Sex with children is always initiated to satisfy adult needs
Nonviolent intercourse is not emotionally traumatic because the child receives pleasure (some professionals tend to foster this belief)	Sex with a child is a violation of trust. The child feels both physical and emotional discomfort. The issue for the adult is power
Sexual abuse of children is done by "dirty old men" or "sex fiends." Children need to be aware of "stranger danger"	Offenders come from all walks of life. They usually are known to their victims. Many offenders are "good with children" and occupy responsible positions
Incest is less traumatic to the child than sexual assault by a stranger	The child feels betrayed by the person who should be protective. Strong sense of ambivalence to both parents results. Child exhibits high level of guilt, depression, and anxiety
Incest is limited to one or two incidents	Most incestuous relations continue for 3–5 years
Children are telling "stories"	Adults wish to deny

taboos prevent cases from being reported and recorded, a "conspiracy of silence" often keeps victimized children from telling adults about the abuse, and the denial of some adults further contributes to the secrecy. Sexual abuse of children is essentially a crime of power in which an adult exploits the child's vulnerability. The behaviors are sexual, but the intent is domination rather than intimacy (Table 13-5).

Sexual offenses against children fall into two general categories: (1) nontouching offenses and (2) touching offenses. Nontouching offenses include verbal sexual stimulation, obscene telephone calls, exhibitionism. Touching offenses include fondling; vaginal, oral, or anal intercourse or attempted intercourse; incest; prostitution; and rape. Some forms of sexual exploitation use children to enhance adult sexual pleasures for profit. "Kiddy pornography," for instance, is a lucrative illegal business.

Incest is a form of sexual abuse of a child by a family member. The adult might be a parent, stepparent, extended family member, or surrogate parent figure (such as a foster parent or common-law spouse). Incest always occurs within the family configuration. Most victims of incest are girls who are abused by older male relatives. Adults who commit incest often are family members in whom children have placed trust. The power of the adult over the child contributes to the enforced secrecy.

Incest can have serious, long-term consequences for the child. The child usually feels guilty for participating and is afraid of disrupting the family by revealing the incestuous relationship. Incest contributes to delinquency, substance abuse, prostitution, sexually transmitted disease, and unwanted pregnancies. Seventy-five percent of runaway children are said to be running from incest, and research suggests that 60%–90% of prostitutes claim to have been sexually abused as children (Densen-Gerber and Hutchinson, 1978).

Incest most often is a symptom of severe problems in marriage, family relationship, and life adjustment. Sometimes other family members might be aware of the incest but allow it to continue. If nonabusing adults in the family are passive, the child essentially is victimized twice, first by the abuser and then by any other adult who refuses to protect the child.

The child who is being sexually abused feels torn between telling and not telling someone. They are uncomfortable about what is happening to them, but they have promised an authority not to tell anyone about these "special times." Instead of verbalizing the discomfort, the child reveals it through subtle behavioral changes or various physical complaints. Adults such as school teachers, nurses, or club leaders must be alert to these changes in mood or behavior. The child might give subtle clues in statements such as, "Mr. Smith sure has funny underwear" or "I don't like Uncle Joe anymore" or "Daddy said it was our special secret, but . . ." If the child attempts to tell and is not believed, the child is unlikely to try to reveal the abuse again.

When a child does reveal sexual abuse, definite steps must be taken to protect the child. The child might be in immediate danger, and in some instances even the child's life is endangered. Either the child or the offender must be removed from the situation. Disclosure then puts the family in crisis, and the child needs reassurance about not having caused the crisis. The primary goals of treatment are to prevent further sexual abuse and to overcome any harmful

Signs of Sexual Abuse

Physical sign	Behavioral sign
Laceration of labia, vagina, or perineum	Discussion of or implied involvement in sexual activity
Irritation, pain, or injury to genital area	Expression of severe emotional conflict at home with fear of intervention
Hematomas in genital area	Reluctance to participate in sports, showers, changing of clothes
Vaginal or penile discharge	Sitting carefully because of injuries
Dysuria	Unusual interest in genital area (eg, "French kissing" or fondling of genitals)
Sexually transmitted disease in young child (on eyes, mouth, anus, or genitals)	Sleep disturbances (eg, nightmares, enuresis, fear of sleeping alone)
Pregnancy	Reluctance to participate in activities with a particular person or at a particular place
Itching, bruises, or bleeding in genital area	Increased number of new fears
Unexplained vaginal or rectal bleeding	Fear of being alone
	Poor peer relations
	Change in performance at school
	Vague somatic complaints

effects from the abuse that has occurred. The family needs intensive counseling, both as individuals and as a group.

The victim needs a complete history and physical assessment, with gentle questioning about the abuse. Encouraging the child to discuss the abuse can aid in working out feelings. The use of drawings and doll play is beneficial with the younger or intimidated child. If the examination is hurried or insensitive, the child might resort to silence and refuse to cooperate. The timing of the assessment therefore is crucial in winning the child's cooperation.

The reporting of sexual abuse always involves Child Protective Services and law enforcement agencies. Because sexual abuse is a crime, an investigation is mandatory. In some states the parent who fails to protect the child might be tried as an accomplice to the crime. Police, teachers, nurses, and physicians also might be held liable for not reporting sexual abuse.

Adolescent abuse The abuse of adolescents is a major social problem that is often caused by conflict and difficulty in parental regulation of adolescent behavior (Table 13-6). Conflict between parents and adolescents tends to involve the refusal to cooperate or the deliberate violation of parental values and cultural traditions in areas such as personal appearance; choice of friends; curfews; school performance; choice of books, television programs, movies, or music; sexual activity; alcohol or drugs; and responsibilities within the family.

Disciplining adolescents is often problematic to parents. Parents who discipline with physical force need to learn other methods of control. Because adolescent abuse might be part of a pattern of abuse throughout childhood, the nurse identifies the discipline methods used when the child was younger.

Behavior patterns are sometimes the only indications of abuse in adolescents. Some abused adolescents are identified only when they run away from home, thereby drawing the attention of teachers or other families in the community. Once abuse is identified, however, intervention by the interdisciplinary team is initiated. Available community resources are assessed, and families and adolescents are directed to those services that are best equipped to meet their needs for counseling, activities, and support.

Legal aspects of child abuse Child abuse is against the law in most industrialized countries. In the United States, reporting of child abuse and neglect is governed by federal standards and regulations, state laws, and local policies and procedures. Most state statutes define child abuse and neglect and specify who must report, the form and content of the report, and to whom the report is sent. Because of the diversity in laws and state statutes, the nurse needs a copy of the applicable reporting form, laws, or position papers. Many states do not record sexual abuse as a separate offense. Some state statutes do not cover sexual abuse, and definitions of terms vary from state to state.

The purpose of all child abuse legislation is to protect children and prevent further abuse or maltreatment; the

TABLE 13-6 Myths and Realities of Adolescent Abuse

Myth	Reality
Adolescents provoke their parents into abuse	Adolescents can be difficult, but the problem lies with the parents' problems, frustrations, and inadequacies
Adolescents usually deserve punishment	Who ever deserves abuse?
Adolescents can protect themselves and fight back	The vast majority of adolescents do not strike back. They usually submit to the assault or run away. Adolescents might still be emotionally and psychologically dependent on their parents
Adolescents are less likely to have serious injuries	Adolescents in the throes of identity crisis are vulnerable, especially to emotional abuse. Rejection has far-reaching sequelae as the adolescent internalizes the blame for problems

TABLE 13-7 Components of Report of Child Abuse or Neglect

Aspect of report	Example
Reason for suspicion or assessment of incident	Child's comments; nature or extent of injury
Behaviors observed and by whom	Teacher's report; circumstances of discovery (eg, "child found alone by police in car")
Quality of parent-child relationship (if observed)	Any comforting measure noted or lacking (eg, "father speaks in angry tones")
What family has been told (to assist in follow-up for all team members)	Purpose of Child Protective Services (if family is unaware of report, explain rationale)
What protection team should do first	Possible interventions (eg, assess home and risks to siblings; investigate and enlist possible community supports)

purpose is not to punish parents. Inherent in all laws is the assumption that the best way to help most children is to help their families. In essence, everyone is a mandated reporter. State laws mandate that suspicions of abuse and neglect be reported. No state requires the reporter to have proof of neglect or abuse, but incidents must be reported as soon as they are noticed. Sound nursing practice therefore means being honest with the family and reporting findings promptly. It is not wise to attempt to work with the family independently or to give family members a warning or second chance.

A report is not an accusation but is instead a request for an investigation. All persons who report suspected abuse or neglect are given immunity from criminal prosecution and civil liability if the report is made in good faith. Because anonymous reports are not as valuable as those that are signed, a reporter should give name, title, and reason for the report. Despite all the publicity and concern, many cases of child abuse or neglect still go unreported.

Documentation of child abuse In situations of child abuse and neglect, documentation of evidence is vital. Records provide the legal basis for intervening on behalf of the child.

At the onset, the nurse is careful to record all data. For instance, pertinent data include physical trauma or neglect, a factual description of the appearance and emotional state of the child and family, and any interactions observed between the child and family members (Table 13-7).

Behaviors are described in detail. For example, if the child is said to be hyperactive and clumsy, the nurse might note that the child was unable to sit still for more than a few minutes or that the child knocked over objects in the examining room. The nurse also records any of the child's at-

Common Behaviors at the Time of Injury

Parental behavior	Child's behavior
Hesitation to give information	Withdrawal, extreme passivity, evidence of fear
Illogical explanation	Does not cry when approached by a stranger
Inability to report the history of the injury	Little reaction to separation
Irritability or evasiveness when requestioned	Unwillingness to talk about the injury (although reactions vary)
Reluctance to look at or handle the child	Seeks to console the parent
Inability to comfort the child during painful or invasive procedures	Might express concern for siblings
Blaming the child for the injury	Little reaction to examination, including painful procedures
Little concern for the child's condition or course of treatment	Monotone answer to questions
Physical distance between the parent and child maintained	
Evidence of role reversal	
Leaving as soon as possible, with or without the child	
Infrequent visits to the hospitalized child	
Not keeping appointments with health care professionals	

tempts to play or any of the parent's attempts to assist the child. Any explanations by either the parent or child also should be recorded. If the child is out of parental care, either because of hospitalization or foster care, the nurse records the number of parental visits, the child's response, and the parent's behavior and attitudes.

In follow-up visits, medical treatment is recorded with notes about whether appointments were kept. The nurse clearly documents the purpose of each visit by listing goals. Also included in the notes are the names of family members present at the visit and any evidence of new members living in the household. Cooperation in meeting goals should be documented as well. In addition, it is noted whether or not the parent has been cooperating with any prescribed medical treatment for the child.

Investigations An investigation is a fact-finding process undertaken to determine whether child abuse or neglect has occurred. Each state has a designated agency that provides services on a 24-hour basis. Within 72 hours, services must be initiated. Agencies receiving abuse reports might include Child Protective Services, law enforcement agencies, juvenile courts, county health departments, and state or central registries.

Parents have the right to know that someone has reported suspected abuse or neglect, although exceptions might be made if the family has a history of violence. In such instances the child or children must be moved to safety before confronting the family. The child also needs to know what is happening. The child often is frightened by the process, especially if the child has revealed the abuse.

The child should be told what to expect. The child will be questioned, have a medical examination, have pictures taken, and perhaps experience police involvement (in cases of assault). The child needs gentle explanations, a private place for unhurried interviewing, and someone to act as an advocate. Discussions about guilt should be ongoing because repercussions might occur from parents, siblings, or others.

The initial investigation focuses on the risks involved, the family dynamics, the nature of the incident or injury, and the duration of dysfunctional parenting. The investigation consists of collecting data from separate interviews of the parents and children. Verification of abuse or neglect might occur through an admission by the parent or offender or through medical or other factual evidence. Supportive services might be provided to the family if abuse or neglect is verified. Court intervention might be necessary if the child has serious injuries, if the parent refuses to allow an investigation, if the child is in immediate danger, or if the risks do not diminish over time.

Long-term legal involvement After the investigation, legal interventions might require a program for treatment, which may be voluntary or involuntary.

Voluntary treatment is possible if (1) the parents are

willing to work on problems, (2) the reported injuries are not serious, (3) there is no continual history of abuse, and (4) the prognosis is favorable. In such cases services are slowly withdrawn when the home environment stabilizes and the danger to the child subsides. Involuntary treatment is likely, however, if (1) the parents are uncooperative, (2) the reported injuries are severe, (3) there is a history of past abuse, (4) the prognosis is poor, or (5) foster care or a termination of parental rights is indicated. Action then remains under the supervision of the court.

Questions of custody usually present the court with four options:

1. Leave the child with the parent but under court supervision.
2. Place the child with relatives under court supervision.
3. Place the child in foster care.
4. Permanently sever the parent-child relationship.

Interventions for Dysfunctional and Health-Threatening Parenting

By the nature of their work, nurses in a variety of settings collaborate with members of other disciplines in protecting children at risk and advocating care for both children and families. Because each family is part of a community, nurses also need to be aware of community resources. Early detection of child abuse and neglect is essential.

The American Nurses' Association (ANA) Division on Maternal and Child Health Nursing Practice has passed resolutions concerning child abuse and neglect that call for action on the part of the ANA, other organizations, and the government. The resolutions call for nurses to participate in ensuring that funding of programs and services for high-risk families is adequate and that preparation for nurses in this area is provided in nursing curricula.

Prevention

Because early recognition and reporting are crucial to preventing child abuse, primary prevention must be the ultimate goal of all who are involved with the well-being of children. Children who are abused or suspected of being abused must be protected until a thorough investigation can be conducted.

Usually, the child is admitted to the hospital for more definitive assessment of the family dynamics. An emergency, court-ordered, 96-hour hold might have to be obtained by the multidisciplinary team, thereby granting the institution temporary custody of the child. Safety of the child must be the primary objective of any treatment plan.

Primary prevention For the family at risk, primary prevention efforts are aimed at influencing parents before dysfunction occurs. The emphasis is on wellness and on identifying societal forces that affect parenting.

For example, child-care courses taught to high school students to orient them to the roles and pressures of parenting are primary prevention. These classes give adolescents direct access to information about the management of time, money, and resources to provide for the basic needs of shelter, food, clothing, and family maintenance. In addition, adolescents learn basic child-care skills and confront through discussion and role play some of the predictable childrearing challenges. This exposure to the realities of parenting and available sources for information about growth and development provides them with additional internal and external supports to cope with various life stressors.

Prenatal parenting classes provide another excellent opportunity for nurses to help parents prepare for the birth experience and for life as a parent. Listening carefully to parents' comments and observing their behaviors provide clues that help identify those individuals who might be at risk for dysfunctional parenting. The nurse can then spend extra time with the potential high-risk parent to foster trust and give support. The nurse might provide additional information or listen and respond to the parent's concerns, refer the individual to social services for assistance with supplying basic needs, or refer the parent to counseling or family therapy for assistance with marital or interactional needs.

Behaviors might indicate potential for dysfunctional parenting. Prenatal indicators include parental overconcern about the infant's gender; minimal support from the family; attempts to deny or terminate the pregnancy; maternal sadness or depression; the feeling that this pregnancy is "the last straw" of many stressors; isolated lifestyle; or multiple, unrealistic fears (Kempe, 1976).

Assessment of parent-neonate interactions following delivery and during postpartum hospitalization provides important information concerning the attachment process and the potential for dysfunction. (See Chapter 4 for a discussion of attachment.) The nurse performs a more thorough assessment and validates suspicions if indicators suggest a risk for dysfunction (Fig. 13-2). Behavioral indicators include lack of interest in the neonate, extreme awkwardness holding the neonate (such as stiff, outstretched arms or inadequate support for the neonate's head and neck), few if any attempts to make eye contact, disappointment about the gender or appearance of the neonate, an ill or deformed

	1	2	3	4
Pregnancy planning	Unplanned and did not want to be pregnant	Unplanned	Not really planned but wanted	Wanted and planned
Support systems	No friends or relatives nearby or poor relationship with parents	New in town, few friends or no phone	Relatives far away, has friends	Relatives nearby, has many friends
Adjustment to infant	Not important to change; no adjustment	Hasn't thought about changes	Must wait and see what changes needed	Made plans for rest, safety, child's room, babysitters
Marital status	Single or under 18	Has boyfriend or hopes infant will improve marriage	Happily married up to $1\frac{1}{2}$ years	Happily married over $1\frac{1}{2}$ years
Delivery style	Wanted to be asleep	Father does not want to participate	Wanted to be awake but could not be	Father present at birth
Infant's name	Unusual name or delay in naming	Name chosen for one sex only	Chose name; changed mind	Chose names ahead of time
Feeding	Finds breast-feeding distasteful/ too anxious to breast-feed successfully	Chose bottle-feeding	Undecided—will try breast-feeding	Breast-feeding successfully
Living arrangements	Unsure of living arrangements after discharge	Living with friend(s)	Living with parents	Has own home or apartment
Eye-to-eye contact	Never occurs	Only occurs one-third of time together	Occurs 35%–50% of time	Occurs 50%–100% of time
Acceptance	Expresses many frustrations—resentful	Occasional frustrations, disappointments with infant	Neither accepts nor rejects	Pleased and concerned about infant's progress
Physical closeness	Holds infant away from body or does not hold	Distorts or misses infant's cues	Somewhat aware of infant's needs	Notices and interprets infant's cues most of time
Touching	No affection, rough or little touching	Does necessary handling only	A little caressing of infant	Caresses and plays with infant
Vocalizing/ talking	Rude or demanding words to infant	Does not vocalize	Little vocalizing	Talks with inflection, coos

FIGURE 13-2
Parenting ability risk quotient. Many parenting behaviors and circumstances that correspond to the criteria in the first two columns indicate a need for further assessment and possible referral. (Adapted from Funke J, Irby M: An instrument to assess the quality of maternal behavior. J Gynecol Nurs *1978; p. 19–22.)*

neonate, enforced separation of the neonate and parent, minimal family support for the parent, little home preparation for the neonate's arrival, disgust expressed at changing diapers, or resentment about the time demands for feedings (Kempe, 1976).

Parenting concerns are ongoing. The nurse who includes a family update with every well-child visit is more likely to note characteristics that have the potential to become risk factors and plan interventions to prevent such potential from becoming reality.

For example, one mother questioned when to begin toilet training her 2-year-old. Further questioning revealed that the mother wanted the child to be toilet trained because an elderly parent had recently moved in with the family and the mother was busy caring for two dependent individuals. The nurse discussed with the mother the normal responses young children have when parental attention has to be shared—that regression and increased demands for affection are common. The nurse also empathized with the mother's situation and energy-draining responsibilities. Together, they planned to delay the toilet training and wait until the child and mother were both more ready. The nurse also arranged for a home-health-aid to assist the mother several times a week. Being sensitive to cues that parents provide and following up on them immediately enables the nurse to institute primary intervention.

Early identification of potential problems and referral to community resources, including the public health nurse or visiting nurse, are primary prevention. Gil (1974) stated that primary prevention includes a reaffirmation of the rights of children; the elimination of poverty, isolation, and alienation; and a rejection of the use of force. These changes would indirectly influence and enhance psychologic well-being, thus fostering improved parent-child interactions throughout society. Despite skepticism, public and professional resources are increasingly invested in such preventive programs. By being aware of the community resources and social and environmental conditions that affect parents, the nurse is able to advocate needed changes. Advocating changes that influence parents and children is an important role for the nurse.

Secondary prevention Secondary prevention for families at risk consists of services for individuals considered to be at risk for dysfunctional parenting. This level of prevention is more problem focused and identifies particular stressors. For example, because adolescent parents usually face multiple stressors, adolescent support groups are one example of secondary prevention. With support, the adolescent learns child-care skills and positive interactive behaviors.

Secondary prevention requires nurses to identify readily those families most at risk for dysfunction. Current practices, past life experiences, and societal problems are indicators that signal risks. The nurse can then recommend community services and supports to relieve stress.

Teaching parenting and homemaking skills Dysfunctional parents often have strong emotional needs that have to be addressed before they can assume child-care responsibilities. An empathetic listener can assist by discussing ambivalent feelings and attachment behaviors. Normal growth and developmental stages should be discussed along with realistic expectations for a child's abilities at each stage and level of development. Parents also need to know about negative responses and how these affect the relationship between the parent and child.

Classes in parenting skills are vital. Specific tasks of child care such as diapering, feeding, and burping an infant need to be discussed and practiced, especially with inexperienced parents. Using an infant rather than a doll during practice sessions is immensely valuable because an infant behaves spontaneously. Parents need to learn about infant stimulation and specific methods of accomplishing this. Emphasis should be placed on concrete behaviors and ways to increase parental sensitivity to the infant's cues. The nurse then serves as a role model for adaptive parenting.

For the nurse, dysfunctional parents are difficult to reach because the quality of parenting is a delicate issue to discuss. The nurse tries to establish trust by patiently forming a relationship of reliability and honesty and by strengthening and reinforcing positive parenting skills. Parents' unmet needs and defenses often get in the way of their ability to modify behaviors, and for parents who have been hurt before, trust comes slowly if at all.

Assisting the parent to develop communication skills enhances parenting. Focusing on the positive expression of feelings and ways to improve relationships has long-lasting benefits. When focusing on parenting skills, the nurse stresses the parent's vital role in the care of the child and looks for and capitalizes on strengths in the parent's ability. For example, remarks such as, "You're doing a fine job; the baby's gaining weight nicely" will do much to enhance a parent's self-confidence.

Dysfunctional parents require special attention to their parenting role. Arranging group sessions provides many benefits. Discussions with other parents can provide a new peer group for these parents that serves to offset isolation. The group allows parents to share feelings, frustrations, and home management difficulties. In addition, it can provide access to common problem-solving techniques. These sessions also might assist parents to increase feelings of effectiveness, which eventually strengthen the parent's self-concept.

Discussions of basic homemaking skills need to be incorporated into support services for dysfunctional parents. Wise meal planning and budgetary hints are important topics. Many of these parents have poor concepts of money and effective buying strategies. Many need to learn the pitfalls of time payments and charge accounts or how to balance a checkbook or plan a budget. Squabbles over money and bills are one of the largest factors in domestic quarrels, sometimes leading to violence, separation, or divorce. Knowledge of financial planning can do much to offset the risks.

Contraceptive counseling and services should be made available to all parents to prevent future unplanned pregnancies. Nurses cannot assume that parents are informed about sexuality and contraception. Many are hesitant to ask for information. Cost, availability, and acceptability are prime factors in contraception.

Parents need to know about their own physical and mental health, about the value of exercise and nutrition in promoting healthy bodies, and about the effective use of leisure time to promote hobbies and personal interests. Adolescent parents also need counseling and the support services necessary to complete their education.

An important nursing role in working with dysfunctional parents is identifying positive behaviors and providing praise. All parents need recognition during times of troubled identity and will respond to encouragement by trying to perform. Accomplishments might be small but always are significant.

Ongoing nursing support Resources for secondary prevention include telephone "hotlines" for specific needs, whether it is a personal call for help when a parent feels about to lose control or a plea for funds to obtain the basic necessities of food or fuel or available, low-cost health care, including services for mental health. Depending on the situation, the nurse might refer families to emergency and maintenance homemaker or child-care services; self-help groups; day-care programs; counseling and family or individual therapy programs; job retraining programs; welfare assistance; and before- and after-school child-care programs. The nurse's role varies according to the expressed need of the parent and the nurse's own experience and knowledge of community resources.

Before working with dysfunctional families, many nurses have to identify their own feelings about the family's practices. The culture, lifestyle, and experiences of an individual all contribute to personal beliefs and values. The nurse therefore puts into perspective the culture, ethnic group, values, and beliefs of the family. Although the nurse's values might conflict with those of the family, the nurse cannot let this conflict interfere with the goal of facilitating open, honest sharing.

Establishing mutually agreed-on goals is mandatory at the start of any working relationship. Goals must be clear and concise, citing specific outcomes and realistic deadlines. The nurse discusses specific maladaptive behaviors targeted for change or elimination with the parents. By agreeing to these goals, the parent essentially is agreeing to a contract. The criteria for evaluation also will aid the family in knowing what changes are expected. Family motivation and cooperation are the key factors in changing a dysfunctional family into a thriving family.

An early indicator of a desire to alter behavior might be the keeping of appointments. Later indicators include a willingness to take some personal responsibility for the dysfunction and not project blame onto others. The parent who can identify a problem and seek help is usually the one who will achieve success in behavior changes.

Tertiary prevention Tertiary prevention is offered to families after dysfunctional parenting has occurred. Tertiary prevention is essentially treatment of the child and family following the damage of abuse or neglect. It is preventive in that it seeks to stop future dysfunctional behaviors.

Tertiary prevention for dysfunctional parenting should begin as soon as the dysfunction has been identified. The goal is to prevent further trauma by having the parents change their childrearing habits. Efforts to involve the family in rehabilitation can be the first step in breaking the bonds of isolation.

Community Services Commonly Needed by Families Demonstrating Health-Threatening Parenting

Public housing
Welfare
Mental health centers
Emergency shelters
Subsidized child care
Homemaker services
WIC program
Food stamps
Free medical or dental care
Family and/or marital counseling
Vocational rehabilitation, employment services
Foster care
Parents Anonymous
Fuel assistance agencies
Child guidance centers
Child development clinics
Housing authorities
Alcoholics Anonymous, Al-Anon, Ala-Teen, Ala-Tot
Visiting Nurse Association
Juvenile authorities
DCYS (Division of Child and Youth Services)
Ambulatory care settings
Occupational health settings
Religious-affiliated groups

Assessment In all cases of suspected abuse or neglect, the nurse needs to ask the child and family members present the following questions:

1. How did the accident (or incident) happen?
2. When did the accident happen?
3. Where were the child and other family members at the time?
4. Who was caring for the child at the time?
5. Who saw the accident?
6. What did the child do after the accident?
7. What measures were taken by the parent?

After recording answers to these questions, the nurse proceeds with the physical assessment, noting the location, color, and characteristics of all cutaneous lesions. Photographs might be needed as legal evidence, and orthopedic, surgical, ophthalmologic, and gynecologic examinations also might be needed depending on the type of injuries.

To identify any treated or untreated fractures, skeletal radiographs should be obtained for all children under 5 years of age who are suspected of having been abused or neglected. If the child has unexplained bruising, tests for blood dyscrasias are needed. In cases of sexual abuse, evidence for legal proceedings must be gathered. This includes cultures for gonorrhea and other sexually transmitted diseases, microscopic examination for blood and sperm, pregnancy testing, and clothing examination for semen, blood, or pubic hairs. To have data the courts will accept, strict procedures must be followed in collecting evidence and specimens.

The most important determination to make is the risk of reinjury to the victim or injury to other children in the household. Assessment of family functioning, coping strategies, and current state of crisis provides valuable data for such determination. Sometimes, even when the injuries are not severe, hospitalization or foster home placement is necessary. Protection of the child (or children) is always the priority.

An interview is needed with parents or extended family members. Interviewing adult family members separately allows the interviewer to compare the facts and check the validity of the data. Determining who caused the injury might not be critical because the passivity of the other parent often contributes equally to the dynamics. In cases of severe injuries, however, police need to identify the guilty person to intervene legally.

The gathering of data is sometimes best accomplished over the course of several interviews. If the child is hospitalized, the hospitalization can be used as a "cooling off" time, during which the child is protected from further injury and the parent is relieved from the responsibilities of care. A home visit also might be necessary in gathering data about family structure and concurrent environmental stressors.

In assessing neglected or abused children and their families, the nurse considers the long-term ramifications of neglect and their possible effects on family cooperation in meeting goals. Some considerations in planning interventions are the following:

1. The parents' emotional ability to accept services
2. Communication patterns within the family
3. The range and availability of services
4. The family's use of services
5. Supportive counseling for all family members
6. Children's growth and developmental patterns
7. The parents' attempts to diminish isolation
8. The parents' responses to expectations to change behaviors
9. The quality of nurturance within the family
10. Family dynamics and other risk factors such as substance abuse or violence
11. Environmental stressors such as inadequate housing, hygiene, or nutrition

The first concern always is the safety of the child, but providing for the child's safety is often a dilemma. Temporary removal of the child from an unsafe home might be the beginning of a series of unsatisfactory foster home or state institution placements. Interventions therefore should be matched carefully to goals that reflect possible outcomes (Table 13-8).

A recorded history of dysfunctional behaviors and resistance to change present especially challenging situations to the nurse. Sometimes, pointing out past patterns of behavior can assist the parent to realize the need for change. Many parents report that making a contract to change specific behaviors is the first time anyone ever spelled out expectations.

Ongoing nursing support To provide ongoing evaluation, the nurse needs to see the family at regular intervals. Specific evidence of progress or failure is identified during these evaluative sessions. Informing the parents of the consequences of failure to meet expectations and deadlines is a delicate and crucial issue for the nurse because most nurses find it difficult to discuss removing children from the family. Parents must know, however, that children's safety and security are of primary importance. The parents' failure to meet goals indicates a need for more intervention. Otherwise, trust in the system would be compromised because the nurse also would be breaking the contract.

Correcting deficits is most successful if the family is willing to participate in planning care. For instance, the plan might involve role modeling of professionals, or it might involve patiently teaching parents about the long-range ramifications of neglect for normal growth and development.

If parents lack motivation, the nurse assesses their apathy and monitors their progress carefully, with special attention to specific behaviors and their duration. Dysfunctional behaviors are cited, documented, and addressed individually. The ego strength of each parent is an important criterion in predicting success for any plan of care because parents who feel self-confident about the prospects for change are more likely to cooperate with the multidisciplinary team.

TABLE 13-8 Evaluation of Interventions to Alter Dysfunctional Parenting

Goal for parental behavior	Evaluation
Identifies problems in the family system	Parent develops insight into the emotional climate of the family
Identifies factors that contribute to potential or actual abusive behaviors	
Demonstrates ability to meet own needs	
Finds positive alternatives to present coping strategies by first identifying external stressors	
Describes feelings toward self and children	
Demonstrates alternative coping strategies in stressful situations	
Demonstrates realistic expectations of children by identifying age-appropriate behaviors	Parent improves parenting skills
Identifies methods of discipline	
Demonstrates some consistency and appropriate use of discipline	
Identifies a person or agency to contact in a crisis	
Provides a safe environment for children by identifying an adequate caregiver during parental absence, identifying and correcting environmental hazards, providing ongoing health care for children	
Identifies family members and friends available for support	Parent establishes and uses a positive support system
Indicates frequency of visits to family and friends	
Identifies ways in which family, friends, community supports (church, school, etc) can be helpful	
Identifies ways in which health care system can be helpful	
Demonstrates appropriate use of health care system and other agencies by keeping appointments	
Earns income above the poverty level or receives and manages public assistance optimally (eg, food stamps used to buy food that is then allocated appropriately among family members)	Parent has adequate income to maintain family
Manages budget to purchase appropriate low-cost clothing for family members	
Provides adequate housing that meets minimal requirements (heat, electricity, cooking and refrigeration facilities, some furnishings)	
Remains at same residence without frequent moves	

SOURCE: Adapted from Christensen ML, Schommer BL, Velasquez J: An interdisciplinary approach to preventing child abuse. Copyright © 1984 American Journal of Nursing Company. Reproduced with permission from *Matern/Child Nurs J* (March/April); 84(2).

Multidisciplinary Management

Because many complex factors must be assessed in evaluating suspected or known cases of child abuse or neglect, no single professional group can best render services to a child or family. A multidisciplinary team approach is therefore best to aid in diagnosis, planning, and interventions. Teams can pool expertise from various fields and provide integrated planning and delivery of services.

A multidisciplinary team might be composed of a mental health worker, lawyer, nurse, social worker, police officer, physician, teacher, juvenile division worker, and hospital or ancillary personnel. Ancillary personnel might include receptionists, drivers, custodians, secretaries, nutritionists, homemakers, or child-care workers. Some are volunteers who might or might not have expertise and training. Most personnel working with abusive or neglectful families need orientation concerning typical behaviors that suggest mistrust of the system, lack of self-esteem, or hostility and anger.

Ancillary personnel can aid professionals in convincing dysfunctional families that change is worthwhile and that they are worth the team's efforts. Ancillary personnel also might provide additional insight and collaboration in a decision-making process. Because each team member brings a different range of experiences and knowledge of dysfunctional families and successful treatment, each is called on to define needs and, if necessary, find legal grounds for intervention. Team involvement offers planning coordination and a way to offset the frustration that professionals feel when nothing helpful can be done.

Usually, the various disciplines and agencies represented on a team can provide data about the child and family, support, expertise, and knowledge of various community resources. Multiple assessments of the family help to determine the likelihood of parental capacity for change and the likely length of time that the family will need services. Because Child Protective Services often are equipped only to handle crisis management, parent aides and others might be needed. Because of their understanding of planned intervention and health care delivery, nurses are essential to this process.

Each team needs a coordinator, a designated professional who is responsible for planning therapy, setting deadlines, and arranging team meetings. Because some families are mobile, much communication is required among social service agencies so that they are not lost to therapy. The coordinator therefore might invest a significant amount of time in charting the family's progress.

Supporting dysfunctional parents Providing parental supports to marginally functioning parents is preferable to removing the child from the home. Removing children is first of all traumatic, and most communities lack adequate foster care homes. Foster care is more expensive than maintaining the family and promoting positive change. Dysfunctional parents also tend to continue the cycle of dysfunctional parenting with other children in the family.

Dysfunctional parents are often angry, argumentative, obstructive, rejecting, and evasive. If isolation has been prolonged, with little previous contact with agencies, parents are mistrusting and difficult to reach. They usually fear criticism, rejection, and ultimate punishment. For some, the initial contact is their first experience with supportive help. Such parents have enormous needs for love, acceptance, and approval, and no treatment that seems rejecting, critical, or unreliable can be effective.

Five hours per month (or 60 hours per year) for each family is a minimally acceptable amount of time, and as much as 50 hours per month might be needed in some cases (Kempe and Kempe, 1978). The three distinct phases in the management of child abuse are (1) crisis management, which includes diagnosing the family situation and developing a long-term treatment plan for each family member, (2) implementation of the plan, and (3) evaluation of the results.

Working with neglectful and abusive parents is emotionally draining and disturbing for all people involved. Seeing a child victimized calls forth strong emotions, particularly among nurses, who might be required to provide nursing care during the time of the acute injury. The tendency is to protect the victim, the innocent child, and to punish the parent, who after all is the offender.

The nurse needs to recognize that the abusive or neglectful parent is also a victim—a victim of past experiences, present crises, and inadequate coping strategies. The etiology of abuse is complex and multifaceted. Parents "bring to the family and to their roles as parents developmental histories that may predispose them to treat their offspring in an abusive/neglectful manner. Stress-promoting social forces both within the family (eg, handicapped child, marital conflict) and beyond (eg, social isolation, unemployment) increase the likelihood that parent-child conflict will occur" (Belsky, Lerner, & Spanier, 1984, p. 175).

Nurses can avoid judgmental attitudes by first examining their own thoughts, feelings, and beliefs about poverty, neglect, alternative lifestyles, and different ethnic and cultural groups. Nurses need to understand the complex relationships among poverty, alienation, and neglect, not only to identify risk factors but also to recognize the social forces that keep some families locked in a cycle of dysfunction.

Helping parents cope with stressors A major nursing task is helping dysfunctional parents to understand the impact of stress and crises in their lives. The next step is learning the appropriate responses to these crises.

In a family that is providing only marginal child care, any stress, however small, might create a crisis. Illness, separation of a family member, or problems with housing, heating, cooking, or laundry might trigger further neglect or apathy in an already fragile parent. The nurse who identifies stress in dysfunctional families therefore needs to assess coping strategies.

Successful patterns of coping suggest growth and motivation. The nurse might be able to praise parents for positive coping behaviors or might need to teach appropriate ways to cope with stress. A family's reaction to stress is often a measure of the family's degree of strength.

Most parents need support services as they learn to develop new coping techniques. Group therapy often assists abusive parents by providing peer support. Finding others with similar problems minimizes isolation. The child health nurse might provide the necessary referral to initiate therapy. Nurse therapists can address and help parents verbalize common fears and misconceptions about parenting.

Many communities use public health nurses in the treatment of abusive parents so that care focuses on all family members and not just on the abused child. The nurse and family establish goals related to specific behavior changes. The nurse carefully monitors the family's commitment to achieving the established goals. If the nurse observes any additional risk factors or evidence of dysfunctional parenting, these are discussed with the family.

Support services for families Various innovative programs have been developed specifically for the treatment of child abuse and neglect. One of the earliest of these programs, SCAN (Suspected Child Abuse and Neglect) Volunteer Service, Inc., was organized in 1972. SCAN volunteers provide emergency intervention as well as long-term counseling and supportive services. Parents are offered the alternative of working with SCAN or facing law enforcement officials and possible foster placement of the child. Various other programs such as Homebuilders are modeled after SCAN and are intended to rehabilitate both the child and parent and to hold the family together (Haapala and Kinney, 1979).

The nurse's role In planning interventions, long-term goals are usually to rehabilitate the dysfunctional family and to support and encourage normal development. Short-term goals are best planned together with family members, but the developmental needs of children must be the nurse's prime consideration.

Interventions may be accomplished both in and out of the child's home. If the child remains at home and the child's primary nurturing figure remains the natural parent, that parent also receives support. Treatment at home might include play therapy, recreational activities, homemaker services, Big Sisters or Big Brothers, foster grandparents, and parent aides. In addition, the nurse makes arrangements for services for special needs such as dental, medical, nutritional, or remedial education. Other services might be provided outside the home while the child continues to live at home. The responsibility for care is then shared with the natural parent by crisis nurseries, day-care centers, respite care providers, and schools.

Homemaker services can provide cooking, cleaning, bed making, and laundry services as a step toward improving the child's standard of living. The homemaker also might be a role model, the confidante, and "friend" of the parent. Other intermittent services include special education, health care, and "emergency parents" for short-term crises or stressors such as illness within the family.

If the child is removed from the care of the natural parent, nurturance becomes the sole responsibility of a substitute caregiver. Additional social services are then necessary, particularly if the child has special needs. These services might include shelters, with temporary removal to a foster home or institution on a short-term basis; foster care; longer-term care oriented toward an ultimate return of the child to the original family; special care for physical disabilities or emotional disturbances; and guardianship or adoption, in which the child is permanently removed from the original home and custody is given to another caregiver.

Today, temporary foster care is intended to help rather than punish dysfunctional parents. Foster parents are taught about children's emotional needs so that children's feelings are incorporated into the treatment plan. When a child is in foster care, the focus of support to the foster family centers on helping the child understand the rationale for the change and facilitating the original parent's visits with the child. Foster care is designed to be temporary and thus conveys a lack of continuity and permanence, even though extended placements are much too common.

In the evaluative process, the input of all involved persons, including the children, should be sought. Professionals can express their views of the chances of family restoration; foster parents can report on behavioral changes, especially positive changes; original parents can report on progress or failure regarding the factors that led to the need for foster placement. A key behavior to evaluate is the way the original parent reacts to stress. Certain behavioral changes, such as moving from isolation to the ability to seek and use resources, are monitored in this way. The criteria for determining whether a home is safe for the child's return need to be specific.

Agencies for referral Child welfare agencies generally are involved in both the treatment and prevention of child abuse and neglect. Child Protective Services also has a vested interest in the effectiveness and accessibility of a wide range of resources in the community and usually takes the lead in working with the family and mobilizing resources.

A Child Protective Services office generally is located in a department of social services and is administered by county, city, or state. Its prime functions include receiving, investigating, and evaluating reports of child abuse and neglect and providing necessary services, either directly or through referral. Its goals are to prevent injury to children, promote the development of healthy children, preserve and enhance family life, strengthen and support parents and families, and provide for children to remain in their own homes and communities whenever possible.

Child Protective Services usually coordinates fiscal and technical support to community-based child protection teams. Coordinated services are thus designed to accomplish the following:

1. Maintain and improve the availability of community resources for the prevention and treatment of child abuse and neglect
2. Strengthen cooperative working relationships through interdisciplinary teams
3. Integrate clinical knowledge with child welfare practice
4. Educate the public and professionals about the prevention and treatment of child abuse and neglect

Self-help for parents Parents Anonymous is a self-help group that is especially effective for both the prevention and treatment of child abuse. The organization was founded in 1972 in California by Jolly K., who was both an abusive parent and an abused child who had lived in 35 foster homes. Meetings of Parents Anonymous are led by a parent, and participants are invited to share their feelings, concerns, and problems, but meetings are neither therapy nor classes in parenting. Members are often able to confront one another about parenting behaviors, especially if they have experienced the same problems, and they also can share possible solutions to family dilemmas.

All members are parents who need a support group to meet family stresses. Most attendance is on a voluntary basis, but some members are ordered to attend by the court system. Meetings usually are held once a week for 2 hours in accessible locations in the community. Professional sponsors who are present during the meeting are there as consultants rather than authorities. Members often exchange phone numbers to contact each other between meetings because Parents Anonymous suggests, "Reach for your phone instead of your kid."

Two studies of Parents Anonymous have found that physical abuse usually stops within 1 month of the parent's joining and that verbal and emotional abuse decline significantly and continue to decline as long as the parent participates (Nix, 1980). Formerly abusive parents often report increased self-esteem as they assist other parents in distress. Some continue to attend meetings long after their initial needs are met, and many parents report pleasurable relationships with their children for the first time in their lives.

Supporting the child If significant changes in the family are unavoidable, the child needs assistance in working through guilt feelings of having caused the changes. Siblings also need to be included in the treatment plan of an abused or neglected child. If the child is hospitalized, fears of pain or violence are intensified by the unfamiliar surroundings and people. The child is often confused, hurt, and frightened.

Nurses and other hospital staff therefore can identify pain, fear, and confusion and assist the child in discussing feelings. The child needs to be told what will happen in developmentally appropriate terms and be reassured, as much as possible (see Chapter 19). The fewer the number of caregivers, the more likely it is that the child will establish trusting relationships.

Children who withdraw from human contact must be allowed a reasonable period of time in which to grieve and appraise new people. If the child's behavior is not developmentally appropriate for the child's age, the behavior needs to be accepted. With time, the child can learn more appropriate behaviors.

Younger children are likely to need nurturing in the form of rocking, cuddling, and soothing. The child initially might appear to reject any comforting, however, and might become aggressive in response to overwhelming anxiety. The aggressive behaviors are learned responses to chaotic living and can become problematic if the child manages to manipulate many people. Team members therefore need to set consistent limits in a firm but kindly manner and assist the child in learning more acceptable behaviors. Aggressive children usually have feelings of deprivation, sadness, and loneliness and might believe themselves to be unworthy and bad. Such children have little faith in their ability to inspire approval and affection.

Children who have been severely abused or who have witnessed severe abuse in a sibling also need much support in developing future relationships that are free of fears, guilt, and anxieties. Children facing loss of separation from their parents need therapeutic assistance to handle the loss and time to mourn the loss.

Long-term follow-up of dysfunctional families has no set time frame for completion. In some instances services are required until the children reach adulthood. Periodic evaluation of parental progress and family growth includes monitoring the behaviors of the children, who might exhibit anger, anxiety, intense loneliness, or apathy. The children's progress in school also must be assessed, together with their response to authority figures. Dysfunctional behaviors suggest that the child needs individual attention. Communication and caring, although time consuming for the team members, does assist both parents and children in coping with the normal stress of development.

Essential Concepts

- Risk factors are indicators of potential dysfunction; they are not predictors, although their correlation with dysfunction is high.
- By knowing the factors that place a family at risk, the nurse is able to assess the potential for dysfunction and plan interventions to prevent dysfunction and its secondary effects.
- A family that is unable to provide for the physical or emotional needs of its members is said to be a dysfunctional family.
- Dysfunctional parenting characterizes the dysfunctional family and involves a disturbance in the parent-child relationship.
- Dysfunctional parenting is characterized by inadequate family communication, role confusion among family members, and isolation from community and other support systems.
- Risk factors that indicate a potential for dysfunctional parenting include the parent's experience as a child, parent-child role reversal, and multiple stressors, which might include marital problems, chronic illness in the family, or inadequate supports.
- Adolescent parents are at high risk because of the stress of their own developmental needs, the physical risks of pregnancy for both the mother and the infant, and the need for support from both family members and peers.
- The parent's experience as a child greatly influences parenting style and expectations of children.
- Dysfunctional parenting might lead to developmental delays and failure to thrive in the infant.
- Inorganic failure to thrive is a syndrome characterized by a lack of normal growth and development, physical symptoms that suggest malnutrition and lack of adequate care, and infant behaviors that show unresponsiveness and lack of trust.
- Child neglect is the failure to provide a child with the basic necessities of life, which might be physical or emotional.
- Indicators of child neglect include developmental delays, especially in social and language development; inattention to a child's safety, hygiene, or nutrition; and inadequate discipline and emotional support.
- Physical abuse, which is one type of child abuse, is the nonaccidental injury of a child.
- Indicators of physical abuse include a series of injuries in various stages of healing (especially a series of similar injuries), the family's delay in seeking treatment, use of multiple treatment facilities, and attempts to hide or minimize the abuse, sometimes with special clothing.
- Emotional abuse often is characterized by the parent's calling the child foul names, ridiculing the child, and making the child feel stupid, hated, ugly, unlovable, or unwanted.
- Sexual abuse is the exploitation of a child for the sexual gratification of an adult; incest is sexual abuse by a family member.
- When a child is sexually abused, the long-term goals are to prevent further abuse and help the child to overcome the psychologic effects of abuse.
- Adolescent abuse often is caused by conflicts in parental regulation of adolescent behavior.
- Prevention of child abuse and neglect involves early identification of risk factors and family dysfunction, education about parenting skills, and referral to appropriate community supports to improve family functioning and prevent further dysfunction.
- Child abuse is against the law, and suspected cases are mandated by law to be reported.
- The nurse documents evidence of child abuse by noting and describing parent and child behaviors in specific terms.
- Because a parent's childhood experiences are a strong influence and often an indicator of that parent's parenting style, the nurse teaches and models parenting behaviors, especially to new parents who are at risk.
- Cases of child abuse and neglect are best managed by a multidisciplinary team consisting of nurses, other professionals, health care workers, and volunteers.
- In cases of suspected abuse, the nurse questions the child and the family members present about the circumstances of the child's injury and collects data through physical assessment and parent-child interviews.
- In supporting dysfunctional parents, the nurse assesses and teaches adaptive coping strategies and refers the family to appropriate support services, which might include help with household tasks, family therapy or self-help groups, or foster care.
- Abused and neglected children need assistance in understanding that they have not caused the abuse or the changes occurring in the family. They often need to learn adaptive coping strategies to avoid dysfunctional behaviors.

References

Adolescent Perinatal Health. The American College of Obstetricians and Gynecologists Task Force on Adolescent Pregnancy. American College of Obstetricians and Gynecologists, 1979.

Belsky J, Lerner RM, Spanier GB: *The Child in the Family.* Addison-Wesley, 1984.

Dean D: Emotional abuse of children. *Child Today* 1979; 8(4): 18–20.

DeMayse L (editor): *The History of Childhood.* Harper & Row, 1974.

Densen-Gerber J, Hutchinson SF: Medical-legal and societal problems involving children—child prostitution, child pornography and drug-related abuse: Recommended legislation. In: *The Maltreatment of Children.* Smith SM (editor). University Park Press, 1978.

Gil DG: A holistic perspective on child abuse and its prevention. *J Sociol Soc Welfare* 1974; 2:110–125.

Haapala D, Kinney J: Homebuilder's approach to the training of in-home therapists. In: *Home-based Services for Children and Families: Policy, Practice, and Research.* Maybanks S, Bryce M (editors). Thomas, 1979.

Hecht M: Children of alcoholics are children of risk. *Am J Nurs* (Oct) 1973; 1764–1766.

Heins M: The "battered child" revisited. *JAMA* 1984; 251(24): 3295–3298.

Helberg JL: Documentation in child abuse. *Am J Nurs* (Feb) 1983; 83(2):236–239.

Kempe CH: Approaches to preventing child abuse. The health visitors concept. *Am J Dis Child* 1976; 130:940–945.

Kempe CH: A practical approach to the protection of the abused child and rehabilitation of the abusing parent. *Pediatrics* (April) 1973; 51(4):804–808.

Kempe CH, Helfer RE (editors): *Child Abuse and Neglect. The Family and the Community.* Ballinger, 1976.

Kempe RS, Kempe CH: *Child Abuse.* Harvard University Press, 1978.

Luckey EB, Bain JK: Children: A factor in marital satisfaction. *J Marriage Fam* 1970; 32:621–626.

Mitchell CE: The drug abusing parent. In: *High-Risk Parenting: Nursing Assessment and Strategies for the Family at Risk.* Johnson SH (editor). Lippincott, 1986.

Nix H: Why Parents Anonymous? *J Psychiatr Nurs* (Oct) 1980; 18:23–28.

Pelton LN (editor): *The Social Context of Child Abuse and Neglect.* Human Sciences Press, 1981.

Steele BF: Working with abusive parents—a psychiatrist's view. *Child Today* 1975; 4(3):3–6.

Tapia J: Fractionalization of the family. In: *The Process of Human Development: A Holistic Approach.* Schuster C (editor). Little, Brown, 1980.

Ten Bensel RW, Berdie J: The neglect and abuse of children and youth: The scope of the problem and the school's role. *J School Health* 1976; 46(8):453–461.

Wheat P: *The Standoffs—A Story About Touching.* Parents Anonymous Booklet, 1980.

Additional Readings

Aguilera DD, Messick JM: *Crisis Intervention Theory and Methodology.* Mosby, 1982.

Ainsworth M: *The Effects of Maternal Deprivation.* Public Health Paper 14. World Health Organization, 1962.

American Nurses' Association. *A Call for Action on Behalf of Children.* ANA Division of Maternal and Child Health Nursing Practice. Clark, A (chairperson). Publication No. MCH-11 ZM, (March) 1980.

Belsky J, Tolan W: The infant as producer of his environment: An ecological analysis. In: *The Child as Producer of Its Own Development: A Life-Span Perspective.* Lerner R, Busch-Rossnagel N (editors). Academic, 1981.

Belsky J, Robins E, Gamble W: The determinants of parenting: Toward a contextual theory. In: *Beyond the Dyad: Social Connections.* Lewis M, Rosenblum L (editors). Plenum, 1984.

Bonney A, Rowe LH: FACES aids formerly abused young adults. *Caring* 1983; 8(3):3–5.

Braden JA: Adopting the abused child: Love is not enough. *Soc Casework J Contemp Soc Work* 1981; 62:362–367.

Brodie B: Children: A glance at the past. *Am J Matern-Child Nurs* (July/Aug) 1982; 7:219–225.

Broek E: Protecting the family: A California act. *Child Today* 1981; 10(1):7–11.

Bruckman P, Ferguson L: Two steps forward and one back—familial patterns of child abuse. *Can Nurse* (May) 1981; 77:29–34.

Burgess AW, McCausland MP, Wolbert WA: Children's drawings as indicators of sexual trauma. *Perspect Psychiatr Care* 1981; 19(2):50–58.

Burgess AW et al: *Sexual Assault of Children and Adolescents.* Lexington Books, 1982.

Campbell J: Nursing care of families using violence. In: *Nursing Care of Victims of Family Violence.* Campbell J, Humphreys J (editors). Reston, 1984.

Campbell J: Theories of violence. In: *Nursing Care of Victims of Family Violence.* Campbell J, Humphreys J (editors). Reston, 1984.

Christensen ML, Schommer BL, Velasquez J: An interdisciplinary approach to preventing child abuse. *Am J Matern-Child Nurs* (March/April) 1984; 9(2):108–112.

Critchley DL: Therapeutic group work with abused preschool children. *Perspect Psychiatr Care* 1982; 20(2):79–85.

Curto JJ: *How to Become a Single Parent.* Prentice-Hall, 1983.

Davidson HA: The guardian ad litem: An important approach to the protection of children. *Child Today* 1981; 10(2):20–23.

Elbow M: Children of violent marriages: The forgotten victims. *Soc Casework J Contemp Soc Work* 1982; 63:465–471.

Fraley Y: The family support center: Early intervention for high-risk parents and children. *Child Today* 1983; 12:13–17.

Gentry R, Brisbane F: The solution for child abuse rests with the community. *Child Today* 1982; 11:22–25.

Gill D, Bogart K: Foster children speak out: A study of children's perceptions of foster care. *Child Today* 1982; 11:7–9.

Greenspan S: Developmental morbidity in infants in multi-risk-factor families: Clinical perspectives. *Public Health Rep* 1982; 97(1):16–23.

Groth AN: Patterns of sexual assault against children and adolescents. In: *Sexual Assault of Children and Adolescents*. Burgess AW et al (editors). Lexington Books, 1982.

Hall M, de la Cruz A, Russel P: Working with neglected families. *Child Today* 1982; 2(2):6–36.

Hayes P: The long-term treatment of victims of child abuse. *Nurs Clin North Am* (March) 1981; 16:139–147.

Heindl MC (editor): Symposium on child abuse and neglect—Foreword. *Nurs Clin North Am* (March) 1981; 16:101.

Heindl MC: Who is the victim? *Nurs Clin North Am* (March) 1981; 16:117–125.

Humphreys J: Child abuse. In: *Nursing Care of Victims of Family Violence*. Campbell J, Humphreys J (editors). Reston, 1984.

Humphreys J: Nursing care of abused children. In: *Nursing Care of Victims of Family Violence*. Campbell J, Humphreys J (editors). Reston, 1984.

Jackson PL, Runyon N: Caring for children from divorced families. *Am J Matern-Child Nurs* (March/April) 1983; 8(2):126–130.

Johnson SH: *High-Risk Parenting: Nursing Assessment and Strategies for the Family at Risk*. Lippincott, 1986.

Johnston K: Maintaining the family unit. In: *The Process of Human Development: A Holistic Approach*. Schuster CS, Ashburn SS (editors). Little, Brown, 1985.

Kauffman CK, Neill MK: The abusive parent. In: *High-Risk Parenting: Nursing Assessment and Strategies for the Family at Risk*. Johnson SH (editor). Lippincott, 1986.

Kufeldt K: Including natural parents in temporary foster care: An exploratory study. *Child Today* 1982; 11(5):14–16.

McKittrick CA: Child abuse: Recognition and reporting by health professionals. *Nurs Clin North Am* (March) 1981; 16:103–115.

McPherson KS, Garcia L: Effects of social class and familiarity on pediatrician's responses to child abuse. *Child Welfare* 1983; 62(5):387–393.

Medical News (editorial). *JAMA* 1984; 251(24):3201–3207.

Millor GK: A theoretical framework for nursing research in child abuse and neglect. *Nurs Res* (March/April) 1981; 30(2):78–83.

Munro JU: The nurse and the legal system: Dealing with abused children. In: *Nursing Care of Victims of Family Violence*. Campbell J, Humphreys J (editors). Reston, 1984.

Newberger EH (editor): *Child Abuse*. Little, Brown, 1982.

Newberger EH: When the injury is a symptom: Interrelations among the pediatric social illnesses. In: *Minimizing High-Risk Parenting*. Johnson & Johnson Baby Products, 1983.

Rosenkrantz L, Joshua V: Children of incarcerated parents: A hidden population. *Child Today* 1982; 11:2–6.

Ruger J, Wooten R: A developmental approach to helping families at risk. *Soc Casework J Contemp Soc Work* 1982; 63:3–14.

Sahin S: Physically disabled child. In: *High-Risk Parenting: Nursing Assessment and Strategies for the Family at Risk*. Lippincott, 1986.

Schuster C: The family with a disabled child. In: *The Process of Human Development. A Holistic Approach*. Little, Brown, 1986.

Sgroi SM: *Handbook of Clinical Intervention in Child Sexual Abuse*. Lexington Books, 1982.

Sherwen LN: Alternative parenting patterns: Clinical implications. *Top Clin Nurs* (Oct) 1984; 6(3) Entire issue.

Sink F: Child sexual abuse: Comprehensive assessment in the pediatric health care setting. *Child Health Care* (Fall) 1986; 15(2):108–112.

Sugar M (editor): *Adolescent Parenthood*. SP Medical and Scientific Books, 1984.

Tankson EA: The single parent. In: *High-Risk Parenting: Nursing Assessment and Strategies for the Family at Risk*. Johnson SH (editor). Lippincott, 1986.

Velasquez J, Christensen ML, Schommer BL: Intensive services help prevent child abuse. *Am J Matern-Child Nurs* (March/April) 1984; 9(2):113–117.

Yoos L: Taking another look at failure to thrive. *Am J Matern-Child Nurs* (Jan/Feb) 1984; 9(1):3236.

Chapter 14

Nursing Care of the Child with a Chronic Condition

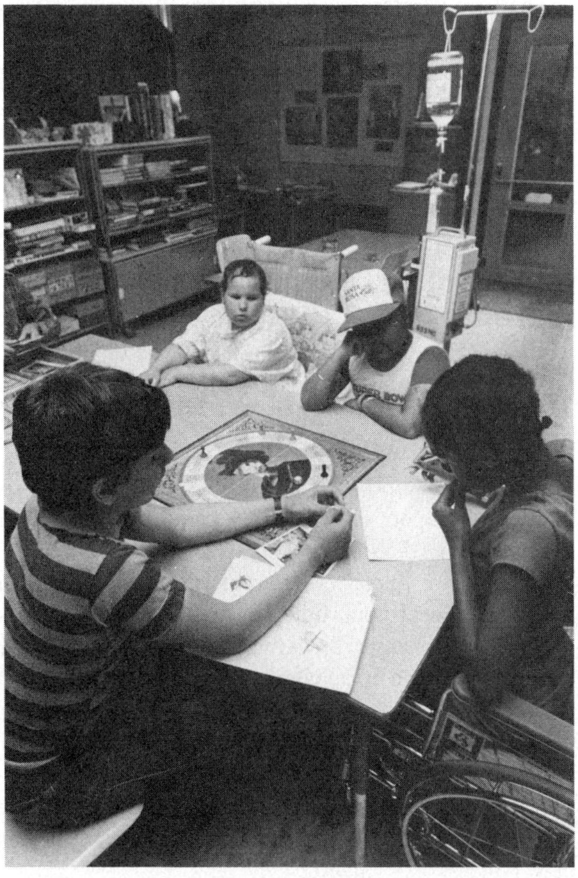

Chapter Contents

(Continues)

Objectives

- List the factors that affect a family's response to the diagnosis of a child's chronic illness.
- Explain the need for community resources in supporting the family with a chronically ill child.
- List common needs of parents with chronically ill children.
- Describe developmental changes in children's responses to chronic conditions and their limitations.
- Explain how temperament and social development affect the child's response to chronic illness.
- List the factors affecting siblings' responses to chronic illness in a child.
- Delineate principles of care and nursing goals common to chronically ill children.
- Present assessment criteria for both the family and the child with chronic illness.
- Compare expected outcomes in chronic care with expected outcomes in acute, short-term care.

Chronically ill children comprise 10%–20% of all children who are hospitalized. They are hospitalized not only for problems related to their chronic illness but also for diagnostic studies or treatment of acute problems. All treatments and illnesses affect and are affected by the child's disease or disability.

Chronically ill children have the same needs and developmental concerns of well children. Children with chronic illness, however, do need more frequent and more comprehensive health care than their healthy peers. For these children, contact with the nurse is not an isolated event. It is one of a series of contacts, each having potential to enhance or inhibit the development and optimal health of the child and family. Nursing care of a child during an acute episode or for routine primary care therefore requires planning for continuity of care. This includes not only the child's acute or wellness needs but also the child's special needs related to the chronic illness.

In children with chronic diseases or disabilities, three factors correlate with the development of secondary problems. These factors are (1) the age at onset of the condition, (2) the relative permanence of the disability, and (3) the severity of the condition. Experts in this area of study agree that the specific disease or disability is less important in predicting psychosocial outcomes than are these three factors.

The earlier the disease or disability is diagnosed, the more profound effect it has on the child's development. A chronic progressive disease with a poor prognosis is likely to cause depression in the child. Approximately one-third of all children with chronic conditions develop secondary emotional, functional, or learning problems. Some children develop all three. (Dysfunctional behavior in children is discussed in Chapter 16.)

Chronically ill children require continuous nursing care by nurses possessing the requisite knowledge and skills for coordinating health care from the time of diagnosis. This is a complex task, which includes providing nursing care during hospitalizations and managing resources to meet the health care needs of chronically ill children.

Impact of Chronic Illness on Children and Families

The Parent—Impact of the Diagnosis

Parents expect their children to grow and develop free of physical and emotional problems. When a child acquires a chronic illness or is born with a physical disability, this expectation is directly challenged. Parental responses to learning the diagnosis of a chronic illness in a child vary from severe emotional upheaval to a more moderate reaction. Most parents, however, suffer some sense of disequilibrium in the initial phases of the child's disease. Long-term reaction to the diagnosis cannot be predicted from the initial reaction, but parents of chronically ill or disabled children might well be at increased risk for development problems such as incomplete bonding and maladaptive coping behaviors. When these problems occur, the family itself is at risk (see Chapter 13).

❋ Anxiety related to perceived loss of a healthy child and threat of the diagnosis

Parents who experience the diagnosis of chronic illness in their children describe learning of the diagnosis as a crisis during which the first few hours and days are filled with anxiety, fear, and emotional upset. Some parents tend to block their feelings; others become overtly angry; still others cry. Regardless of their observable responses, these parents, siblings, and sometimes grandparents are in the midst of a crisis, and consequently, their usual individual and emotional coping mechanisms are affected.

For example, the families of two 12-year-old girls diagnosed as having diabetes reacted in far different ways. One family was interested and ready to learn about the condition, whereas for the other family the diagnosis was a tremendous blow. The child spent much of her time in bed as the family gathered around the bedside and spoke in low voices, openly grieving. Another family had been so upset when their son was born with a cleft lip that they told the boy when he was older that his surgical scar was related to an accidental fall he had had as an infant and were unable to talk with him about the defect.

❋ Anticipatory grieving related to loss of a healthy child

Parental grieving and guilt are often associated with the diagnosis of chronic illness, the birth of a premature infant, or the diagnosis of developmental disability. Grief responses vary among and within families, however, because the process of grieving is not necessarily a steady progression through identified stages. (See Chapter 17 for a discussion of grief.)

A family's response to a chronic condition also might be expressed in a variety of ways. In determining the family's definition of the diagnosis and its significance, the nurse considers not only family members' verbal messages but also their nonverbal cues. For example, the nurse notes whether the behavior of family members agrees with what they say. Often, parents do not express distress verbally, but body posture and other behaviors indicate extreme tension.

Although most people do not react violently to hearing distressing news, the nurse often needs to help family members express their feelings. Getting past the frightening feelings can facilitate better communication among all family members. The father who can admit to his son that he is scared of the diagnosis and that he is going to try to help in any way he can has, by example, permitted his son to talk about fears. Handled in this way, feelings become a topic, and family members can begin to communicate about the many issues they face.

Factors Affecting Parental Response

Nurses need to be careful not to attempt to predict which families and children are headed for trouble and which are going to do well. The overall outcome or impact of chronic illness on a child and family is the result of a complex set of interactions among the community, family, and child (Fig. 14-1).

Community resources The community in which a family lives reflects the shared values and attitudes of its members toward the institutions serving families. Providing health care and education for the disabled and chronically ill, for example, is a manifestation of a community's positive attitudes toward disability. Families are influenced both directly and indirectly by the community, and the child in turn is affected by the family-community interaction.

For instance, the health care system and educational institutions in the community have a direct impact on the child and family. Lack of such resources as early intervention programs might, for example, allow secondary effects of disability to become more severe.

The family's position in the community and its political affiliations also can affect the impact of chronic illness on the child. The relative ease with which the family can influence the community to provide needed resources, for example, increases or decreases the degree of stress that family members experience. The family that feels powerless and incapable of influencing positive change in the community experiences additional stress. These direct and indirect factors also affect family members' perceptions of available options. Thus the outcome for any child is much more than a direct result of the disease. It is instead a complex interplay among the child, family, and community.

❋ Potential for ineffective family coping

Fortunate indeed is the child who, in spite of disability, lives in a community that can support both family and child. Less lucky is the child born into a marginally functional family with minimal resources in an impoverished community. For example, 7-year-old John has parents and siblings who are able to travel 2000 miles to accompany him for a bone marrow transplant and remain with him during several months of hospitalization. Eight-year-old Robert, on the other hand, needs a bone marrow transplant, but his mother must work to support him and his 3-year-old brother and can visit the hospital only on weekends.

The first family, although away from extended family and friends, is together, not concerned about finances, and able to focus attention on caring for John and for each other. In contrast, Robert's mother struggles to provide the basic

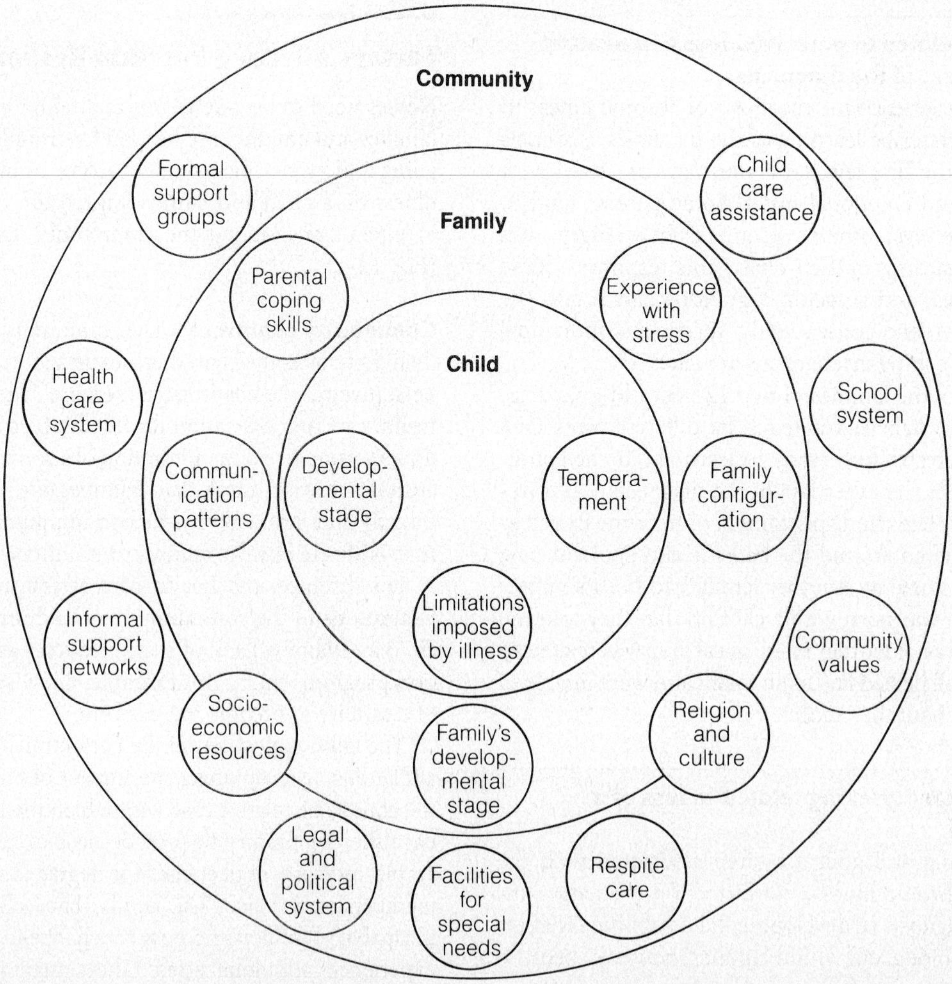

FIGURE 14-1
Factors affecting family and child adjustment to chronic illness.

necessities, is able to be with Robert only a short time each week during his hospital stay, and has few supports on which to rely. As a single-parent family facing additional stress, Robert's family is at greater risk for dysfunctional parenting (see Chapter 13).

Effects of long-term care In families with disabled children, dysfunction might appear as the child grows older. Parents might cope successfully with a disabled child during infancy and early childhood, when all children are dependent, but find that the physical and emotional exhaustion that comes with chronic care eventually taxes their resources. A child's normal growth and development also might be restricted by a treatment regimen or by physically restrictive equipment such as prosthetic devices for orthopedic problems. As the child must learn to adapt to physical and developmental differences from peers and siblings, the stress of adaptation can negatively affect the family's normal course of growth and development as well.

The nurse therefore watches closely for behavioral clues to family dysfunction. Even if interpersonal communication between parents is relatively poor, they might maintain appropriate social roles and might continue to show a united front to others. As stress builds for such families, nurses might need to help parents identify additional sources of support. Doing so serves to take the "spotlight" off the ill member and to create a more normal situation for all. Knowing about the many stresses and concerns these families must face, nurses can guide them in this process of normalization.

One type of service available to families to reduce the stress of caring for a chronically ill child is respite care.

Respite care is a type of care developed specifically to reduce family stress of caring for a person who is chronically ill. Respite programs train workers to enter homes and care for the ill person in order to provide a break for the family. If the family needs to get away for a few hours or even a weekend, respite care provides relief.

In spite of the extraordinary burdens of chronic illness, some families express heightened excitement about living and ascribe high value to interpersonal relationships because they are acutely aware of the transitory nature of life. For instance, a family with four children, one of whom was an adolescent with cystic fibrosis, derived great pleasure from each other's accomplishments and company. As the boy's illness progressed, the family seemed to draw closer together, not in a way that restricted the boy's contacts with peers but in a way that actually drew in supporting people in the environment. They simply enjoyed the minute-by-minute activities of each day together.

Experience with stress and crisis Other family resources include the parents' previous experience with resolving crisis and handling stress. Older families, that is, those in which the parents have been married for several years, might have had the advantage of working through problems as a couple. Together, they might have experienced the illness of their own parents, perhaps even the death of a loved one. Although the death of one's parents is not equated with the loss of a child, the experience, if faced and dealt with adequately, will provide a measure of maturity that those who have not had the experience will lack. Yet even parents who have encountered many problems and have handled them well describe the diagnosis of fatal disease in a child as the most serious problem they have ever faced (see Chapter 17).

In general, parents who have experienced and have coped well with problems prior to a child's diagnosis have the experience with stress that can protect them from family disruption. Nurses might therefore expect families that have experienced problems to accept a serious diagnosis better than a less experienced family learning of a less serious condition. Even "experienced" parents can, however, be overwhelmed by the specific problems they face. Previously successful coping strategies, which are part of the psychologic repertoire for any individual or family, are not invincible.

Stage of family development Related to the family's experience with stress and crisis is the family's stage of development. The family's developmental stage is an important factor in predicting family disruption. A family with an older child about to enter college might experience less stress than a family with a young child who has been newly diagnosed. The family with the younger child is likely to be a younger, less experienced family. Such families face many years of medical problems and disruptions in family life, whereas older families are more likely to share these responsibilities with older children.

❁ Potential alterations in parenting

A chronic condition is one of the many risk factors that can contribute to dysfunctional parenting (see Chapter 13). The parent's perception of the condition is also significant in the parent's adjustment to the disorder. The parent-child relationship can be adversely affected by a disability unless the parent is able to alter expectations to match the child's needs and capabilities. Two important factors in the parent's response are the child's gender and birth order.

The child's gender can place the parent at a particularly high risk for the development of secondary psychologic problems. One father reported that his hopes were dashed when his only daughter developed a seizure disorder. The fact that he had three healthy sons did not relieve his pain. He had hoped for a daughter but was crushed by her potentially significant health problems.

Another father was withdrawn and was described as depressed by other family members and neighbors. He had a diabetic first-born son but eventually realized that his hopes and aspirations for his son were only moderately altered and was able to talk about the disease with his son. If the father had not been able to accept his son's illness, both the family and the son's development would have been affected. An adolescent boy, cut off from effective communication with his father, might have blamed himself for causing his father's problems and the family's as well.

Parents of children who are at greater risk for developing a sex-linked disease might have psychologic problems at the birth of a male child. Sex-linked diseases, such as hemophilia, are genetically transmitted disorders that occur in males. (Modes of genetic transmission are described in Chapter 15.) For these parents, feelings of anxiety about the child can interfere with appropriate attachment and thus distort the parent-child relationship at its beginning.

The number and sex of children in the family can often affect parental reactions. In one- and two-child families, the intensity of the reaction might be greater than that in larger families. The father who described his hopes as "dashed" by the diagnosis of his daughter's seizures might not have had such an intense reaction to an infant son's diagnosis of the same condition. The father of the diabetic adolescent boy might have had an entirely different reaction to the diagnosis in one of his daughters.

Later-born children with chronic illnesses might not threaten a family as seriously as earlier-born children. A younger child with cystic fibrosis who has several older siblings, none of whom has the disease, might receive special attention from these older siblings. This not only takes pressure off the parents but can also give the siblings the pleasure of participating in the ill child's care.

To promote effective parenting, the nurse emphasizes the child's positive characteristics. For example, demonstrating handling of and social interaction with an infant helps the parent view the child positively and enhances parent-infant attachment.

Potential for spiritual distress

Parents can be helped to cope with chronic childhood illness by using religious supports. Religion plays a role in several ways. First, family members feel assisted when care and empathy are expressed by people in the religious community. Second, religion might help the family gain perspective on the situation by focusing attention toward new priorities that are more humanistic than materialistic. Some parents describe the child's illness as a kind of blessing that requires a redefinition of what is really important in their lives. Many describe themselves as living a day at a time and trying to get the most out of each day. They mention a heightened sense of the meaning of life and feel that they are not in control of life but that life itself is a gift.

Nurses also need to recognize that not all families use organized religion to work through the difficulties of chronic illness. Some who have drifted away from a religious orientation come back to it during times of stress; others do not. Furthermore, the research on this issue is scarce, so generalizations are at best cautious. What is not known is why families who have religious persuasions seem to do better, overall, than those who do not. This might be due not only to the perspective that religion can bring to the child's illness but also to the cultural benefits of family involvement and community support.

A family's cultural values also will influence the family's response to the diagnosis of chronic illness. For example, in families that prize athletics, the birth of a child with mild cerebral palsy but with no mental retardation will be hard to accept. As with religious values, the nurse needs to ascertain the ways in which cultural differences are likely to influence a particular family's acceptance of a child's disability.

The child

Child's health status The child's general development and health prior to the diagnosis are among the many contributing factors influencing a parent's reaction and adjustment to the child's diagnosis. A previously healthy child diagnosed with an incurable disease can be a psychologic blow, but the parent of a chronically ill child might experience a sense of relief when the medical diagnosis is finally determined. Some diagnoses are ironically relieving to parents.

For example, the parents of an adolescent boy who was subsequently diagnosed with cancer spent 9 months trying to convince health care providers and other authorities that a black-and-blue spot was not self-inflicted or the result of parental abuse. Needless to say, the diagnosis was a significant relief even though the sadness of cancer was itself nearly overwhelming. Developmental and health histories therefore provide critical information which the nurse uses to assess a family's response to the diagnosis of a child with chronic disease.

Child's prognosis While the specific disease does not generally determine a family's unity or dissolution, different diseases require different resources from families. A fatal disease, such as cystic fibrosis, is manageable in the child's early years, but if the disease advances, the demands on parents increase. Hospital stays become more frequent, home treatments intensify, restriction of the child's and often the family's activities increases dramatically, and family members are allowed little personal time for themselves. Even cancer, so threatening to so many, might also be relatively easy to live with in its early stages.

Chronic illnesses vary considerably in the amount of interference they impose on the lives and development of children. Although very little research has specified these differences, nurses do find that fatal illnesses generally are disruptive to families, producing fear in both parents and children. Living with a fatal illness further places all family members "on emotional hold."

Having a child with a life-threatening illness makes a family highly vulnerable and creates long-term implications for the family as a unit and for family members as individuals. Recognizing this vulnerability is a first step in planning nursing interventions, and it ensures consideration of the needs of all family members in the care plan. Parental adjustment is the keystone to the children's response and must be central in the plan.

Needs of Parents with Chronically Ill Children

Although families with chronically ill children differ in a multitude of ways, they do share common basic problems and needs that form a framework for nursing management. Because the availability of financial resources or of an adequate support system varies widely among families, these issues need to be addressed as the nurse tailors the care plan to the needs peculiar to a particular family.

Financial needs The impact of increased financial demands varies among families. Financial concerns constitute a serious threat for some families and minimal problems for others, depending on both the family's resources and the expenses of a particular condition. Over time, however, many chronic illnesses impose heavy financial burdens on families regardless of their financial stability. Concerns include insurance benefits, entitlement programs, and actual out-of-pocket expenditures. Many families might have insurance to cover doctor and hospital charges but have many indirect expenses not covered by insurance.

For example, families coming to a tertiary care center need to pay for transportation, lodging, and food, and provide chlid-care services for their other children. Often, these expenses are not covered by insurance or entitlement programs. Changes in US government policies regarding financial assistance for medical problems are resulting in higher and more direct costs to families. For some families, the availability or decreased availability of these resources might well influence their ability to carry out recommended treatments.

Potential for social isolation

Need for support Although some families tend to be isolated from kin and neighbors and are therefore more vulnerable to the disruption of chronic disease, other families experiencing childhood chronic illness might be part of supportive networks, extended families, surrogate families, or friendships. Such a family is fortunate because the support of family and friends is critical to preventing the physical, psychologic, and even financial stresses occurring from a child's chronic illness. The nurse therefore assesses the family's actual or potential support systems. A family that has recently moved into an area might have to rely more on professional services than one that has lived in an area for many years with an extended family available, an extensive number of friendships, or both.

The nurse needs to be cautious here, however, for even though a family might be well integrated into a community, the diagnosis of chronic illness might change family patterns, if not immediately then eventually. For example, the more restrictive the child's disability, the less time, energy, and money are available for the family to maintain friendships. Much depends on a particular family's creativity in dealing with the circumstances of the illness. The nurse can assist the family with devising creative ways to include the child in family activities, despite the child's disability.

Parents often form new friendships to replace those that cannot be maintained. Support groups composed of families experiencing similar problems often are effective because the issues faced in rearing a child with chronic disease are better understood by those directly involved. A health professional, however, needs to be available to these groups because parents may often be so overwhelmed with their own problems that they are unable to reach out and support others. The nurse might best direct parents to groups that include professionals who listen and guide discussion as appropriate to the situation. A sensitive health professional often is helpful to parents by relieving their guilt and providing them with needed emotional support.

Need for time away from care Chronic illness involves a constant and ever-present regimen of care that must be maintained, and many medical routines are time-consuming and inflexible. A child needing dialysis, for example, must literally live by the clock. Parents might become resentful because the regimen impinges on their personal time.

These families usually experience increased stress from the day-to-day burden of caring for the ill child. Depending on the disease, parental involvement in care can range from an additional 15–20 minutes per day to an extra 5 to 6 hours. Parents describe feeling frustrated and fatigued at being on call 24 hours a day, 7 days a week, year in and year out. A mother of an epileptic 4-year-old, for example, said she never had a waking moment when she was free from thinking about her child's safety. Another mother, one with a diabetic 4-year-old, said that diabetes affects everything in her life and in the functioning of her family.

Needs of Children with Chronic Conditions

The emotional impact of the diagnosis of chronic illness on a child is a highly complicated phenomenon. Just as each family has its unique strengths with which to meet stress and crisis, children have their own personal resources. Developmental stage, temperament, effect of the illness on social roles, and the nature of the illness itself determine a child's response to a chronic condition.

Potential for altered growth and development

A child's response to the diagnosis of a chronic condition depends on the child's age and developmental level. Although the nurse might ordinarily expect to gauge a child's reaction according to the child's age, the nurse needs to pay particular attention to developmental level in children with chronic conditions. Disease or disability can cause developmental delays (see Chapter 9). The child's response to the diagnosis of a condition or to associated procedures and treatments might not be age appropriate. For some children, referral for comprehensive developmental assessment is necessary.

Infancy Lacking the ability to understand the need for invasive procedures and treatments or having to be handled by strangers, an infant might show signs of developmental delay and stranger wariness. Infants might be highly irritable, might not sleep deeply, or might have basic physical rhythms disrupted. For example, because the infant with retinoblastoma (a malignant tumor of the eye) requires immediate treatment, the attachment process might be disrupted by repeated hospitalizations and separations from parents.

Reciprocal parental interaction might also be affected by parental feelings about the disease, especially its genetic implications. Blind infants, for instance, might be slower to develop cognitively if their caregivers do not learn to communicate effectively with them using the tactile and auditory routes. Infants with disabilities of the sensory and central nervous systems are therefore vulnerable to delays in cognitive, social, and affective development.

Early childhood The young child who develops a chronic illness or acquires a disability has difficulty understanding and accepting treatment and its limitations. For example, the 2½-year-old insulin-dependent diabetic child, who is typically establishing autonomy, often refuses to eat on parental demand and does not understand the need for injections. The child might also perceive injections as punishment for bad behavior. Parental understanding of child development, patience, and a positive attitude are essential qualities to help the young child through this difficult period.

Although children of this age group are developing language skills rapidly, they might demonstrate protest against procedures by shutting down communication or by simply not talking. They demonstrate their frustration in the extreme by becoming either rebellious against or totally compliant with adult requests. In early childhood, the younger the child at the time of diagnosis, the more the disease process interferes with development.

As young children attempt to comprehend their situations, they piece together available verbal and nonverbal cues from significant people in their lives. One 4-year-old told an interviewer that she could tell how serious her condition was by watching her mother's eyes as the mother talked to the doctors. The young child's conclusions are often accurate. Children whose parents have not discussed the seriousness or fatal nature of a disease with the child find that the child often learns of possible death by overhearing a parent discussing the issues with a sensitive and interested listener. An inherent danger, however, is that children might possess misinformation or reach the wrong conclusions with the correct information.

Middle childhood By middle childhood, cognitive development allows the child to grasp the reasons for treatment, and the child is less likely to see treatment as punishment for real or imagined misdeeds. Because these children still have problems separating fantasy and reality, however, parents need to be aware of their children's perceptions of illness, treatment, and limitations.

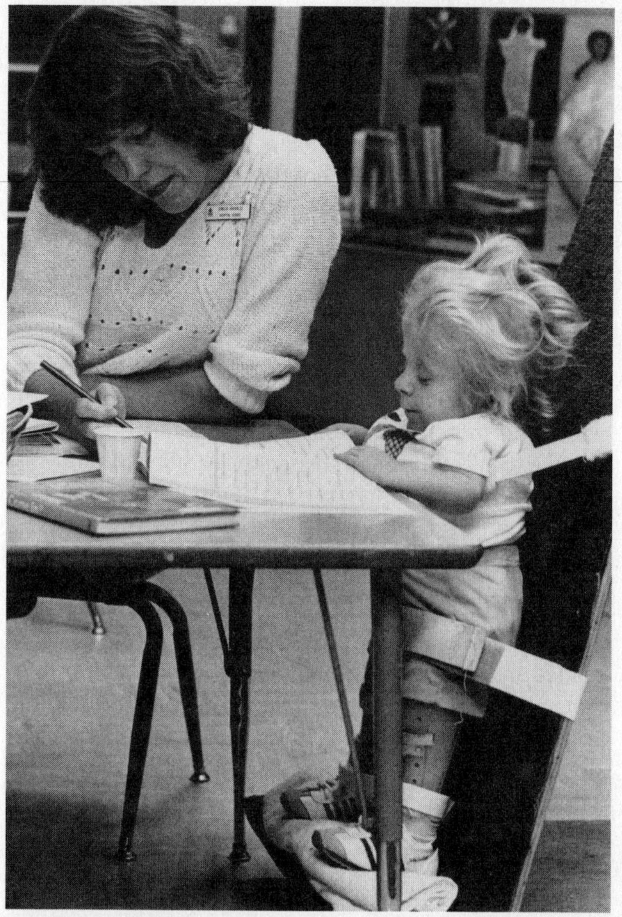

Children with chronic conditions require special attention, adaptation, and assistance from educators.

Because the child's attitudes toward school, learning, and social relationships are in a state of transition during the middle childhood years, chronic problems that interfere with developmental changes may, if poorly handled, have long-term consequences for the child. School requires increasing cognitive skills and greater application of learned principles. Social relationships are formed in school and in the many extracurricular activities offered to children of this age. Inability to function appropriately in a learning environment might therefore cause social isolation. Not only does the nature of the condition itself interfere with the developmental tasks, but long hospitalizations and lost contact with peers might also exacerbate the problem.

Incorrect classroom placement can inhibit learning. Incorrect placement might be caused by inaccurate perceptions of the child's learning potential rather than by genuine learning impairments. The nurse therefore helps teachers and administrators with an accurate assessment of the child's learning capabilities.

Late childhood By late childhood, appropriate cognitive development and a healthy self-esteem allow the child to understand chronic illness and accept responsibility for much of its treatment. At this stage the child is characteristically emotionally stable, so the diagnosis of chronic illness or disability, although traumatic, is not as upsetting as it might be for the younger child or the early adolescent.

Because a child in this stage faces many demands for academic and athletic achievement and peer group involvement, intense competition develops. Peer groups often include or exclude others on the basis of their physical attributes. Chronically ill or disabled children, who might already be developmentally delayed because of their conditions, tend to fall behind their peers during the late childhood years. For example, the child who is unable to sit still and listen in class now faces increasing classroom discipline and more homework.

Although chronically ill and disabled, children should be encouraged to participate in activities as much as possible. The child who cannot fully participate because of physically limiting conditions such as arthritis, spina bifida, or cerebral palsy has to develop a sense of industry and worth that is independent of the resources available to peers.

Because athletics and academic achievement foster industry and self-esteem, they also keep children in the mainstream with peers. The child lacking in both intellectual and athletic ability is in serious jeopardy for forming and maintaining needed friendships. Children who are separated from peers repeatedly or extensively for hospitalization or home care also are in danger of being excluded. Organizations outside school and sports, such as scouting and church groups, can help such children achieve at their own level and stay in contact with peers.

Adolescence Because early adolescence is characterized by physical and emotional changes that disrupt the child's social roles, this period is especially troublesome to children who are different from their peers. Being shunned by intolerant peers is devastating to adolescents because the peer group is the structure on which they rely for self-acceptance and emotional separation from parents. Older children, although better able to comprehend the disease and its therapy, might become anxious and depressed. Disabled younger adolescents might handle developmental tasks by denying them or by putting off required demands until later. Others rebel against the disease, either through denial or through inconsistent self-care. Some adolescents develop illness-related problems because of self-inflicted neglect.

The impact of the disease is modified by the extent to which the illness interferes with an adolescent's lifestyle. Adolescents with diabetes, for instance, might neglect to carry out their diabetic therapeutic regimen to show that they are truly able to live without insulin or to prove that they are actually just like their peers. Although these assumptions are not at all accurate, adolescents accept them as reality. The adolescent feels invincible and challenges reality by denying what is obvious to anxious parents and health providers. The adolescent might possess sufficient knowledge of the disease to write a quality term paper on the subject and at the same time behave in ways that contradict this knowledge.

When ignoring the disease becomes the means by which the adolescent expresses emancipation from parents, the family interactions can become strained. Parents who have invested much of themselves in the care of their children over the years find this seemingly destructive behavior intolerable. Some parents overreact, which makes the situation worse.

For example, Jenny, a 15-year-old with temporal lobe epilepsy, rebelled against her domineering mother by using alcohol and street drugs. Multidisciplinary treatment for chemical abuse involved the family and helped Jenny's mother develop parenting behaviors appropriate for an adolescent daughter. As the adolescent comes to terms with the illness and comes to be accepted by peers, better self-care is evident. This can take several years, however, so the adolescent's health is sometimes compromised.

Later adolescence requires not only emotional emancipation from parents but also financial and social independence. During late adolescence, developmental tasks include clarifying career or job decisions and establishing satisfying relationships with members of the opposite sex. Chronically ill adolescents and those with disabilities might be at a disadvantage in accomplishing these tasks.

Society is beginning to recognize the capabilities of the disabled and chronically ill, but often blocks the way. Issues such as inability to obtain health insurance, inaccessible buildings, and misperceptions of the disabled young adult's potential are barriers to independence. The nurse who works with adolescents therefore needs to be aware of the many problems they face in completing developmental tasks.

⊛ Potential for ineffective individual coping

The child's temperament, like the child's developmental stage, affects the process of coping with illness. Children respond to their diseases and their consequences much as they do to other stressors. Placid, easygoing infants might continue to make good developmental progress socially and emotionally because they are low-keyed and adaptable. A basically irritable infant who is quick to respond to any environmental change, however, has more difficulty with the stress of chronic illness. Easygoing children generally remain so, while irritable children exhibit additional psychologic and behavioral problems.

The nurse assesses a child's temperament to establish a baseline, since subtle changes in behavior can later indicate shifts in either the disease process or in the child's response to it. Without a baseline for assessing the child's temperament, the parent and nurse might have difficulty discriminating those behavioral responses caused by temperament from those related to the disease itself. Temperament also can be a predictor in determining a child's successful coping with chronic illness or disability.

⊛ Potential for impaired social interaction

Effect on social roles The disruption of the child's social roles can negatively influence overall adjustment. Helping a child continue actual participation with peers is critical, especially for children in late childhood and adolescence. These children need to maintain contact with friends during episodes of illness or hospitalization.

Although all responsible adults should encourage such contacts, the child's social interactions remain the immediate responsibility of the child's parents. Teachers can encourage schoolmates to write to or visit the child, if appropriate, since a class visit to the hospital could mean a great deal to the child. In addition, teachers might spend some time with classmates explaining the nature of the condition and its usual therapy, thereby preparing them for the child's return to the classroom. The child and family's preference in this matter should, however, determine the extent to which the illness is discussed. Some families do choose to protect the child by keeping information about the disease confidential. Physicians and nurses can facilitate the child's peer contact by emphasizing to the parents that it is an important aspect of treatment.

Parenting style As the child with chronic illness grows, parents develop a parenting style that affects the family's adjustment to living with chronic illness or disability. Although parents' feelings interfere somewhat with the way they would discipline the child, the goal is to develop a style of discipline that accounts for the child's limitations but is as normal as possible. If the child has siblings, discipline needs to resemble closely discipline given to siblings in order to incorporate the ill child fully into the family structure and prevent sibling resentment.

Parents readily let guilt affect common sense and fall into a trap in which the child lacks discipline. Guilt can allow parents to be overpermissive, overprotective, or resentful. The overpermissive parent allows the ill or disabled child essentially to run the family. The parent constantly accedes to the child's wishes and demands because giving in is easier than fighting or because the parental guilt is so great that the parent tries to make up for the child's disability. The child of overpermissive parents becomes a tyrant who manipulates the parents. Siblings become resentful because the disabled child is favored. The disabled child's self-esteem diminishes because parental caring lacks any constructive limit setting. The nurse who observes an overpermissive parenting style needs to intervene to preserve healthy family functioning. The nurse encourages the parents to set firm limits for the child and not to give in to manipulative behavior. The parent needs to regain control by reimposing limits gradually. Explaining to the child what the limits will be and adhering to them is the first step.

The overprotective parent is unable to allow the child to function independently within the child's developmental and physical capabilities. Overprotective parents do everything for the child or they set limits that are so restrictive that the child becomes fearful and unable to participate in care. Guilt is again the underlying mechanism. The parents feel so guilty about the child's disease or disability that they feel they must assume total care of the child to compensate for what the child lacks. The nurse encourages the overprotective parent to let go and encourages the child to participate in self-care. The nurse explains to the parent the child's capabilities and allows the child to demonstrate these skills. Allowing the parent to express fears and anxieties about the child helps in realistically assessing the child's potential.

Some parents, although feeling guilt, feel resentment at the changes to their lifestyle that a child with a chronic illness or disability brings. They might openly demonstrate anger or resentment for the child, thus greatly diminishing the child's self-worth. The nurse allows and encourages these parents to express anger and resentment openly but in ways that are not harmful to the child. The nurse demonstrates a caring attitude toward the child and emphasizes the child's positive characteristics. Working with the parents to incorporate the child's limitations as much as possible into the family's lifestyle is an important nursing function.

Needs of Siblings of Chronically Ill Children

When a brother or sister is diagnosed with a chronic illness, the lives of siblings are changed. As with both parents and ill children themselves, the initial impact of the diagnosis on the child's siblings is determined by several of the following factors. To plan care that addresses the needs of the entire family, the nurse assesses siblings' responses to a child's illness and its effect on family functioning.

Parental behavior toward siblings Among the most important factors is the parent's ability to recognize the siblings' psychologic needs. Although parents usually tell siblings about the disease and its probable implications for their brother or sister, parents sometimes fail to determine their level of comprehension. In addition, a common assumption is that if parents are secure in their roles as parents and as individuals, and if they are receiving support from family and friends, they will have energy not only to care for the ill child but also to care for their other children.

Frightened and anxious, parents of children often feel as if they've lost control to the professionals. Often they feel they are emotionally unable to meet the needs of the other children, especially those in crisis. Frequently, such parents are surprised by a healthy child's negative behavior toward them and toward the ill child. For example, a mother of 4-year-old twin daughters, one of whom was critically ill, was completely dismayed by the normal twin's regressive behavior. The ill sibling displayed maturity beyond her years while the healthy sibling rejected her mother's attempts to correct her behavior.

Parents who find sibling behavior difficult often ignore or deny the problem. Unfortunately, ignoring the behavior tends to increase the need for attention and further frustrates the sibling's attempts to cope constructively.

Siblings' responses The greater the number of demands placed on parents caring for ill children, the less likely they are able to provide physical or emotional care to the other children. This reality is intensified when parents must stay in an urban medical center many miles from their home. The siblings, who also are psychologically vulnerable, often find themselves without parental attention and must therefore cope with the stress of separation from parents, in addition to the other stresses they have incurred as a result of a sibling's illness.

When assessing siblings' reactions and adjustments to having a chronically ill child in the family, the nurse considers age, temperament, gender, and birth order. Younger children are more cognitively and emotionally vulnerable than older children. They are less able to understand a situation and less able to delay their own emotional needs. The other 4-year-old twin, whose mother's attention was focused on her ill sister, fantasized that her mother and sister were off at the hospital having a good time and not including her. She was accustomed to having her sister and mother available, and the hospital was a major barrier to contact during frequent hospital stays. This child responded by acting out her anger and frustration with her mother through wetting the bed and being generally noncompliant, ornery, and rebellious, much to her mother's consternation.

Siblings, like the child with the disease, react to situations according to the developmental stage they are in and thus with the emotional and cognitive faculties associated with this stage. Therefore, the 4-year-old who has become used to constant companionship with a sister and whose temperament might be a bit irritable will behave in a manner consistent with her usual reaction to stress.

Some children, keenly aware of parental discomfort but not understanding it, react by becoming overly anxious and withdrawn. Siblings express feelings of jealousy and anger toward the child with the illness and feelings of anger toward parents. They also report being very lonely and scared. Relationships among siblings can also affect and be affected by the family's response to a childhood illness.

Very young children are unable to accept their parents' giving extra attention to the ill sibling. Their feelings are expressed in many ways, from being aggressive toward the parent, to meeting parental demands unconditionally, to developing symptoms of the illness in an effort to gain attention.

Children in middle to late childhood are able to rationalize their parents' attention to the sick sibling, but they find it difficult to tell their parents how they are feeling. They "read" the situation quite well and try to cooperate, even when it means putting their own needs aside.

Adolescents appear to be less troubled by parental involvement with an ill sibling, but they might resent being expected to provide services at home that interfere with their social activities.

The nurse attempts to encourage effective communication between parents and children and among siblings. Advising parents to set aside a small amount of time each day to give exclusively to each child can be helpful. Even 5–10 minutes of uninterrupted attention can enhance a child's self-esteem.

Nursing Management for Children with Chronic Conditions

The Health Care System for Chronic Care

Nurses care for chronically ill children in a health care system designed for treatment of acute, short-term problems of adults and for medical cures rather than extended care. Chronically ill children have needs that contrast sharply with those of children who are temporarily ill. The health care system, with its advanced technology, is ill-suited to deal with such special needs. When a cure is not possible, the long-term goal of nursing care is to maintain physical function and address the adverse physical, social, and emotional effects of the disease process.

Health care services also are needed to accommodate the child's long-term requirement for medical intervention. Nurses working within the health care system are therefore pivotal in adapting the system to accommodate the needs of the child and family. Some health care providers and fami-

Basic Components of Assessment for the Chronically Ill Child

Child

1. Establish a trusting relationship with the child.
2. Determine basic information about the child's eating, sleeping, and elimination habits, either from the parents or from the child. (With older children it is preferable to obtain this type of information directly from the child.)
3. Perform a complete physical assessment (see Chapter 10).
4. Determine the child's ability to engage in self-care activities.
5. Determine the child's knowledge base regarding the illness.
6. Use standard assessment tools as necessary (see Chapter 9).
7. Analyze the child's current developmental level.
8. Determine the child's usual coping responses.

Family

1. Review the child's medical history prior to meeting with parents.
2. Create a "family tree" or genogram (see Chapter 15).
3. Determine how family members are dealing with their feelings.
4. Determine whether any family members are experiencing eating or sleeping difficulties.
5. Determine whether parents are able to share in the care of the affected child and the siblings.
6. Determine the parents's level of understanding of the child's condition.
7. Determine the reaction of the siblings.
8. Observe family communication, noting who is most verbal and who expresses feelings.
9. Determine the role of the extended family (grandparents and other relatives) in giving needed support.
10. Determine the family's involvement in community organizations that might be supportive emotionally or financially.

lies might become so well acquainted that they might be able to use the telephone to consult on simple, recurrent problems or for anticipatory guidance, which otherwise would require the family's visiting the facility. This can decrease the burden and stress of a chronic condition on the family. Such an approach enables the family and child to live without unnecessary intrusion from health care providers.

Principles of Care for Chronically Ill Children

The nurse considers the following principles in planning specific care for any child with a chronic illness:

1. Care is based on the child's cognitive, affective, and social development.
2. Procedures and treatments allow as much mobility and comfort as possible, so that the child and family have maximum control.
3. Separation from the family is minimized.
4. Both child and family are prepared for procedures to maximize cooperation and minimize trauma.
5. The child's dignity is respected at all times and in all situations.
6. Both child and family are included in planning care, so that medical treatment is carried out in the context of an overall care plan for the child.

Home-centered care Whenever possible, children should be cared for in their own environments but with careful monitoring of the family's capabilities. The advantages of home care include avoiding the separation of family members and allowing parents to carry on essential family routines for maintenance of the family unit.

Some families, however, might not be able to cope with sick members without respite care, especially when the emotional and physical drain proves overwhelming. Nursing management therefore includes both ongoing assessment of family dynamics and careful observation for signs of unmet needs and potentially dysfunctional parenting.

Provider continuity Continuity of care is essential in chronic illness, and although advocated by both physicians

(text continues on p. 429)

STANDARDS OF NURSING CARE *The Child with a Chronic Condition*

GUIDE FOR NURSING MANAGEMENT

Nursing diagnosis	Intervention	Rationale	Outcome
1. Ineffective individual coping related to personal vulnerability secondary to chronic illness	Observe the child's solitary play, art, interactions with others, and ability for and interest in self-care.	Direct observation of the child is an essential part of the assessment process.	The child verbalizes—or expresses through art or play—feelings of anger or depression.
	Encourage child to express feelings about self and the effects of illness on the child's life.	The ability to express feelings is essential to good emotional health.	
	Provide realistic reassurance through verbal communication, or role play the child's actions in response to siblings', peers', and adults' questions about the illness or its restrictions.	Helping the child anticipate uncomfortable situations will enable the child to realistically come to terms with the reality of the disability and the potential reactions of others.	The child participates in self-care activities and in the decision-making process.
	Encourage family and peer support.	Families and peers play a pivotal role in assisting the child in accepting the problems associated with chronic illness.	
	Observe the child for more severe psychologic alterations (see Chapter 16).	Chronically ill children are at risk for the development of secondary psychologic problems.	
2. Potential knowledge deficit (stressors: developmental cognitive limitations, unfamiliar material)	Ask the child to describe the illness and its causes.	Understanding the child's perception of the illness will guide the nurse in preparing a specific teaching plan.	The child either correctly repeats teaching or chooses correct information out of several choices. The child listens and participates appropriately in teaching sessions.
	Clarify misconceptions.	Part of the adjustment process for the child is to be presented with clear, concise, realistic information regarding the chronic condition.	
	Set mutual long- and short-term goals for learning.	Mutually agreed on goals are more likely to be implemented.	
	Implement a teaching plan at the child's functional developmental level, making use of drawings, stories, and games when possible.	A teaching plan that takes into consideration the child's developmental level will be accepted by the child more readily.	
	Share the teaching plan with other nursing staff members.	Quality nursing care must continue on a 24-hour basis.	
	Repeat and augment teaching as needed if evaluation indicates incomplete comprehension.	Repetition enhances the learning process and allows the information to be integrated by the child.	

(Continues)

STANDARDS OF NURSING CARE *The Child with a Chronic Condition (Continued)*

GUIDE FOR NURSING MANAGEMENT

Nursing diagnosis	Intervention	Rationale	Outcome
3. Potential health management deficit (stressors: incomplete understanding of treatment regimen, physical limitations, cognitive limitations)	Observe the child's level of self-care relative to hygiene, exercises, medications, diet, rest.	Direct observation is necessary to determine a need for additional teaching.	The child shows an interest in and participates in self-care. The child and parent identify problems and initiate reevaluation periodically or as needed.
	Set mutual goals with the child for increasing participation in self-care.	Mutually agreed on goals are more likely to be carried out.	
	Teach the child the appropriate skills, with sensitivity to the child's need to participate, observe, practice, and withdraw.	Timing is an essential element in the teaching of any skill.	
	Demonstrate enthusiasm and encouragement for any progress.	Success in any endeavor breeds confidence.	
	Repeat and augment as needed if evaluation indicates incomprehension or reluctance to perform skills.	Teaching of basic skills frequently requires repetition. Additional learning will be required as the chlid grows and adapts.	
	Plan any further learning necessary for proper care of condition (eg, special hygiene, medications, activity recommendations, or diet).	Not all teaching can and should be done in an initial endeavor.	
	Facilitate referral to community resources if needed.	Multidisciplinary management often is needed for chronically ill children.	
	Reevaluate when the child enters adolescence and whenever rebellion occurs.	Adolescence is a particularly dangerous time for lack of cooperation because rebellion against parental authority occurs frequently during that developmental stage.	
	Plan any treatments to coincide as much as possible with the child's lifestyle.	A child is more likely to cooperate with treatment if the treatment doesn't make the child feel different from peers.	
4. Potential for ineffective family coping: compromised (stressors: knowledge deficit, emotional conflicts, role changes, family disorganization)	Observe the parent for overt signs of anger, fear, depression, denial or guilt.	Anger, fear, depression, denial, and guilt are common coping reactions in parents whose children are diagnosed with chronic illness.	Parental response is within normal limits for the duration of the child's condition, the seriousness of the condition, and the child's current health status. Family interactions seem mutually supportive. Parent expresses interest in community support group.
	Listen to and note any verbally expressed psychologic needs of family members.	Appropriate use of communication techniques encourages expression of feelings from the parent(s).	

STANDARDS OF NURSING CARE *The Child with a Chronic Condition (Continued)*

GUIDE FOR NURSING MANAGEMENT

Nursing diagnosis	Intervention	Rationale	Outcome
	Actively elicit verbal expression of feelings from the parent.	The ability to express psychologic needs is an indication of positive emotional adaptation.	
	Observe family interactions and parental behavior for indications of maladaptive coping related to adjustment to the child's condition.	A change in the child's condition might precipitate a crisis and engender maladaptive coping.	
	Support the parent and provide reassurance.	Parents need to know from the members of the health team that they are doing a good job.	
	Reassess parental response before a hospitalized child is discharged.	A hospital stay might indicate that the child's condition has worsened or changed significantly, and the parents usual methods of coping will no longer work for them.	
	Facilitate referral to community resources or support services as parental needs and readiness indicate.	The care of the chronically ill child is multidisciplinary and members of the team will change as the needs of the child and family change.	
5. Potential parental knowledge deficit (stressors: unfamiliarity with information, anxiety, unrealistic perception of child's needs)	Elicit parental perception of the child's illness and observe for factors indicating readiness to learn: decreased anxiety, increased interest in and attention to the child's case, increase in appropriate questions.	Readiness to learn is an essential element in the teaching-learning process and can be evidenced by specific, objective behaviors.	The parent listens to teaching and explains care accurately. The parent properly carries out all physical care necessary for the child. The parent describes home changes needed because of the child's condition.
	Design an education plan for all aspects of the physical care regimen.	To be effective, a teaching plan needs to be inclusive of all elements of physical care of the child.	
	Using books, diagrams, and participation in care, as appropriate, provide teaching based on parental readiness.	To foster retention of learning, include as many senses in the process as possible.	
	Discuss changes in home routine or environment that might benefit child and family; discuss resources for acquiring adaptive devices if needed.	Planning needs to include home-based care as well as hospital-based care.	
	Communicate the teaching plan to other members of the nursing staff.	Quality nursing care continues on a 24-hour basis.	

(Continues)

STANDARDS OF NURSING CARE *The Child with a Chronic Condition (Continued)*

GUIDE FOR NURSING MANAGEMENT

Nursing diagnosis	Intervention	Rationale	Outcome
	Repeat and augment if necessary.	Repetition enhances learning.	
	Facilitate referral to outside resources as needed for appropriate follow-up and further teaching.	The care of the chronically ill child includes a multidisciplinary team.	
6. Potential alteration in parenting (stressors: knowledge deficit, stress, unrealistic expectations, perceived threat to personal goals)	Initiate discussion of the effects of the chronic condition on parental perceptions of the child and the child's needs.	Parental expectations might need to be adjusted when a child is diagnosed with a chronic condition.	The parent describes the child as growing, maturing, and needing the security of limits and the freedom of appropriate independence. The parent provides for alterations and special considerations necessitated by the child's condition. The parent expresses basic satisfaction with the ongoing parent-child relationship.
	Help parents decide appropriate parental behavior toward the child in relation to normal development, discipline, independence, involvement in the child's health care, school, and peer activities.	With the help of the nurse, parents need to make decisions regarding refinement of their parenting skills with their chronically ill child. Parents can tend to overprotect chronically ill children and not set appropriate limits for their behavior.	
	Plan for multiple follow-up discussions as the child grows.	Children change as they grow and adapt to their environment. They have different needs at different age stages.	
	Monitor for overt behavior indicating overprotection, resentment, overpermissiveness.	Overprotection, resentment, and overpermissiveness are all indications of maladaptive coping.	
	Facilitate referral to counseling if problems arise.	Caring for a chronically ill child can be emotionally overwhelming.	
7. Potential alteration in family processes (stressors: difficulty adapting to change, increased time demands to provide for ill child's needs, poor communication within family, emotional conflicts, fears, embarrassment)	Monitor siblings' reactions through direct observation and conversations and through active listening to parent and child.	Siblings play an important role in overall family adjustment to a chronic illness and their reactions and adaptation must be monitored.	The siblings discuss the causes and course of the ill child's disease or disability. The siblings express feelings, either verbally or nonverbally. Parents give each sibling at least 10 minutes of individual attention each day.
	Observe for fears, feelings of guilt, and jealousy; unmet needs; difficulty in coping.	It is not unusual for siblings to have unmet needs and difficulty in coping; nurses need to be aware of this and assess for it.	

STANDARDS OF NURSING CARE *The Child with a Chronic Condition (Continued)*

GUIDE FOR NURSING MANAGEMENT

Nursing diagnosis	Intervention	Rationale	Outcome
	Note siblings' reactions toward the ill child, particularly expressions of pity and anger.	A basic emotion underlying pity and anger toward the chronically ill child might be fear.	
	Observe for withdrawal, unhappiness, or acting-out behavior.	Maladaptive coping will lead to behaviors that are unacceptable and potentially dysfunctional, both physically and psychologically.	
	Clarify any misconceptions for siblings.	Siblings might not understand the true impact of the chronic illness, and a simple, age-appropriate explanation will aid in understanding.	
	Support siblings.	Siblings need emotional support in adjusting to the chronic illness as much as the child and parents.	
	Assist siblings and parent in plans to meet siblings' needs.	Once the needs of the siblings are identified, exhausted parents might need assistance in setting goals to meet the needs.	
	Facilitate referral to outside resources or counseling if needed.	Outside counseling or additional resources might be necessary if the parents are unable to meet the siblings' needs, regardless of the reason.	
	Encourage parents to give each child some undivided attention.	Demonstrated parental concern, even for a short period, minimizes behavior problems and maintains the child's self-esteem.	

and nurses, it is often ignored in favor of short-term expediency. Continuity assures coordination of care. When many professional people are involved in a child's care—a typical situation for chronically ill children—one person needs to serve as the family and child's "quarterback," or, if the professional is a nurse, the primary nurse. This arrangement is especially important for multidisabled children who are served by a variety of health care and other providers, such as educators and vocational and psychological counselors. Multidisciplinary management necessitates a designated coordinator who can identify needs and assure that services are not duplicated. The nurse is, with the family's permission, well suited to assume the role of coordinator. The continuity that a coordinator can bring thus compensates for an otherwise fragmented system of care.

Child participation The chronically ill child and the family might need encouragement to be as independent in the management of the condition as possible. This often involves teaching both the child and the family to use equipment designed for the child's needs (Fig. 14-2). The nurse works with other health care providers and parents to facilitate independence, while recognizing dependence as appropriate during periods of extreme stress or crisis. Nurses might encourage families and ill children to act as members of the health team, although this role cannot develop unless health care providers insist on it, create an atmosphere in which it is fostered, and reinforce it when the family and child demonstrate participation and self-care.

Participation begins as simply encouraging the child and parent to talk about their responses to treatment regimens. Many will give their opinions, thinking that health care personnel know what is best and must be aware of their problems. The child and family, on the other hand, might even withhold information important in planning further treatment. With an ongoing illness or condition, family participation in planning care is crucial. For example, an insulin-dependent diabetic failing to report incidents of hypoglycemia actually hinders appropriate insulin, diet, and exercise regulation.

From the beginning, the nurse invites the child to participate as much as possible in self-care. By requiring the child to participate, the nurse not only conveys respect for the child's ability but also implies that the child's participation is essential to recovery. A child must come to understand that neither parents nor health professionals "own" the disease and that the child can be an agent in or an obstacle to recovery. Using the child's responses to guide further conversation, the nurse then learns the child's perception of the illness and can use this initial contact to gather information on the child's psychologic as well as physical status.

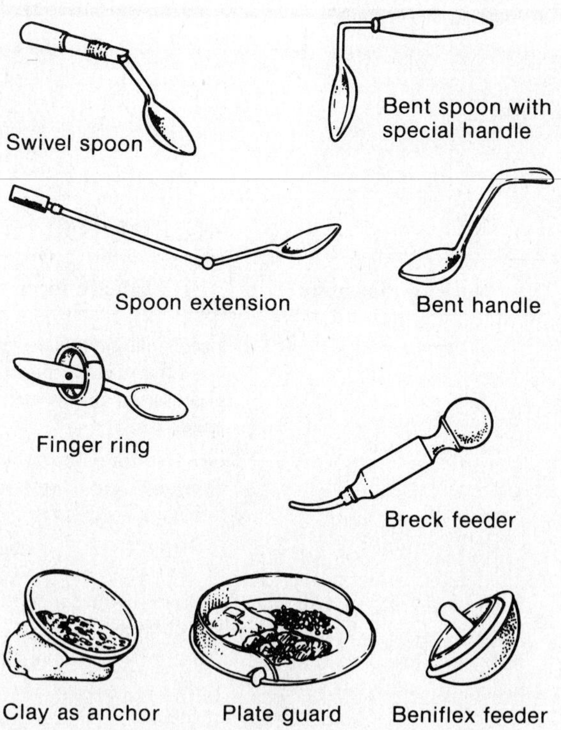

FIGURE 14-2
Eating utensils for disabled children.

Parent and child education is the means by which family members become part of the health care team. Family and child education is thus an essential component of any nursing care plan, and the nurse needs to view education as an intervention equivalent in importance to medical care.

Essential Concepts

- Parents view a child's diagnosis of chronic illness as a crisis that initially causes family disorganization and emotional upset.
- A family's perception of a chronic illness is affected by the child's condition, the child's gender, the family's religious and cultural background, the family's experience with stress and crisis, and the child's prognosis.
- The overall impact of chronic illness on a child and family is a result of interactions among three factors: community, family, and child.
- Families need to make psychologic and environmental adjustments for children with chronic illness, which in turn place a family with marginal coping skills at risk for dysfunction.
- Parents of chronically ill children commonly need assistance with financial burdens, resources for support, and ways of finding time away from the demands of constant care.
- The impact of the diagnosis on the child depends on the child's developmental stage, temperament, and current social roles.
- Adolescents are especially likely to rebel against the limitations of illness and treatment and need support in accomplishing developmental tasks.
- Siblings of children with chronic illness are affected by changes in family dynamics and communication patterns, by parental behavior toward them, and by fears of the illness.

- Because the health care system is designed for acute, short-term needs, nurses need to plan specific long-term interventions that provide continuity of care and participation for the child and family.
- Health care for the child with a chronic illness should be home-centered so that family functioning can be maintained as much as possible.
- The nurse's assessment of the family involves analysis of parent, child, and siblings as well as social contacts, relatives, and community.

Additional Readings

An annotated bibliography on respite care for children and families. *Child Health Care* (Winter) 1986; 14(3): 183–186.

Anderson S, Bauwens EE: *Chronic Health Problems.* Mosby, 1981.

Gliedman J, Roth W: *The Unexpected Minority: Handicapped Children in America.* Harcourt Brace Jovanovich, 1980.

Horner M, Rawlins P, Giles K: How parents of children with chronic conditions perceive their own needs. *MCN* (Jan/Feb) 1987; 12: 40–43.

Hymovich DP: Assessing the impact of chronic childhood illness on the family and parent coping. *Image* (Oct) 1981; 13: 71–74.

Ireys H: Health care for chronically disabled children and their families. In: *Better Health for Our Children: A National Strategy.* US Department of Public Health, 1981.

Johnson BH, Steele BB: Community networking for improved services to children with chronic illnesses and their families. *Child Health Care* (Fall) 1983; 12(2): 98–102.

Kempe H et al: *Pediatric Diagnosis and Treatment,* 4th ed. Lange Medical, 1976.

Kleinberg SB: *Educating the Chronically Ill Child.* Aspen, 1982.

Koocher G, O'Malley J: *The Damocles Syndrome: The Psychosocial Consequences of Surviving Childhood Cancer.* McGraw-Hill, 1981.

McKeever PT: Fathering the chronically ill child. *Am J Matern-Child Nurs* (Mar/Apr) 1981; 6: 126–128.

Menke E: The impact of a child's chronic illness on school-aged siblings. *Child Health Care* (Winter) 1987; 15(3): 132–139.

Miller M, Dias J: Family friends: New resources for psychosocial care of chronically ill children in families. *Child Health Care* (Spring) 1987; 15(4): 259–264.

Minuchin et al: *Psychosomatic Families.* Harvard University Press, 1980.

Montague JP, Rheba A: Use of parents' suggestions in evaluating a long-term care program for disabled children. *Child Health Care* (Summer) 1984; 13(1): 24. (Fall) 1983; 11(2): 74–77.

Pierce PM, Freedman SA: The REACH project: An innovative health delivery model for medically dependent children. *Child Health Care* (Fall) 1983; 12(2): 86–89.

Pierce PM, Giovinco G: REACH: Self-care for the chronically ill child. *Pediatr Nurs* (Jan/Feb) 1983; 37–39.

Reiss I: *Family Systems in America,* 3rd ed. Holt, Rinehart, & Winston, 1980.

Rodgers et al: Depression in the chronically ill or handicapped school-aged child. *Am J Matern-Child Nurs* (July/Aug) 1981; 6: 266–273.

Rutter M: *Changing Youth in a Changing Society.* Harvard, 1980.

Schilling R, Gilchrist L, Schinke S: Coping and social support in families of developmentally disabled children. *Family Relations* 1984; 33: 47–54.

Spinetta J, Deasy-Spinetta P: *Living With Childhood Cancer.* Mosby, 1981.

Steele S: *Nursing Care of the Child With Long-term Illness.* Appleton-Century-Crofts, 1977.

Stein R: A home care program for children with chronic illness. *Child Health Care* (Fall) 1983; 12(2): 90–92.

Steiner P: The well child and the hospitalized disabled sibling. *J Psychosoc Nurs* (Mar) 1984; 22(3): 23–26.

Wallace H, Gold E, Oglesby A: *Maternal and Child Health Practices.* Wiley, 1982.

Wallerstein J, Kelly J: *Surviving the Breakup.* Basic Books, 1980.

Yoos L: Chronic childhood illnesses: Developmental issues. *Pediatr Nurs* (Jan/Feb) 1987; 13(1): 25–28.

Chapter **15**

Nursing Care of the Child with an Inherited Disorder or the Child with a Developmental Disability

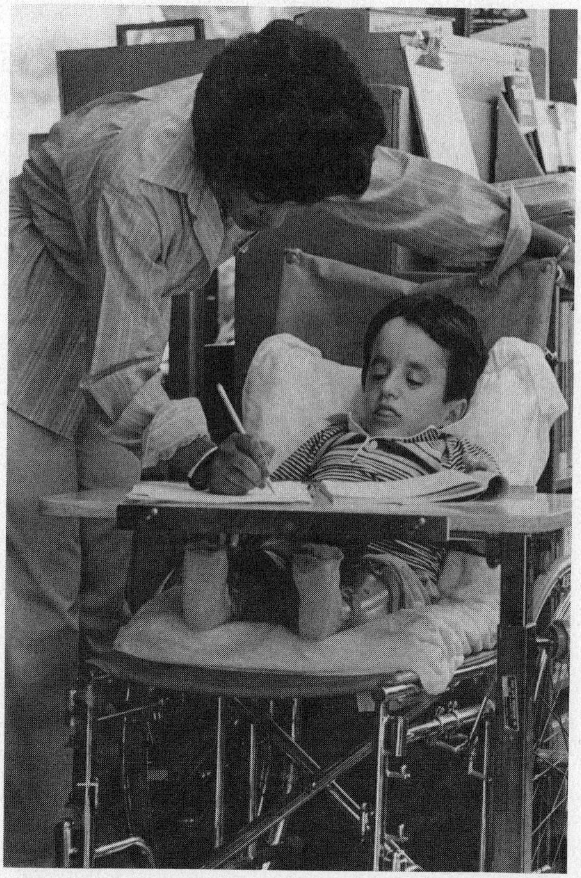

Chapter Contents

The Child with a Disorder Leading to Developmental Disabilities

Down's Syndrome (Trisomy 21)
Neonatal Infections Leading to Developmental Disabilities
Fetal Alcohol Syndrome

Cross Reference Box

To find these topics, see the following chapters:

Galactosemia	Chapter 29
Hemophilia	Chapter 26
Hyperactivity	Chapter 16
Learning disorders	Chapter 16
Neurologic impairments	Chapter 31
Phenylketonuria	Chapter 29
Sickle cell disease	Chapter 26

Objectives

- Describe the components of a cell that are directly involved in heredity.
- Describe the basic mechanisms of inheritance.
- Identify common examples of inheritance patterns.
- Discuss genetic aspects of biophysical development.
- Discuss the role of the child health nurse in caring for families at risk for genetic disorders.
- Distinguish between developmental disability and mental retardation.
- Define the terms used to classify retarded people.
- List risk factors associated with developmental disabilities.
- Discuss the role of the child health nurse in caring for the developmentally disabled child in both hospital and school settings.
- Describe overall goals for nursing care for both developmentally disabled children and their families.
- List issues that are likely concerns in the care of children with developmental disabilities.
- Describe nursing interventions related to nutrition, toilet training, behavior modification, sexuality, and independence, with regard to the developmentally disabled.

The pattern and progress of human development begins before conception. The mechanisms of inheritance that govern development have long fascinated scientists, health professionals, and parents. Investigations have ranged from rigorous genetic research to parental observations and informal exchanges. For example, geneticists examine the influence of chromosome number and arrangement on development; psychologists address such issues as birth order and environment; and parents look often to their own behavior and treatment of the child. In seeking to understand developmental influences, they all share a common goal—to identify factors that would support and enhance the developmental potential of any given child.

Both environment and heredity contribute to the normal development of the child. Environmental factors are physical as well as emotional. The health and the nutritional status of the mother prior to conception and during pregnancy influence the development of the fetus. Once born, infants require not only food but also love and affection for their progress to be normal. As the child becomes more mobile and social, opportunities to practice new skills are necessary. Without practice, reinforcement, and encouragement, the child's developmental potential might not be reached.

Genetic factors also can affect the child's potential for optimal development. Children born with chromosome aberrations that cause dysfunction often begin life with developmental limitations. Because child health nurses are responsible for promoting optimal childhood development, it is the nurse's responsibility to maximize the child's abilities. The nurse therefore works with both the child and the family to promote normal development within the limitations of dysfunction.

Mechanisms of Genetic Transmission

The mechanisms of genetic transmission depend on the information stored in genes contained in the nuclei of the body's cells. The *gene* is the basic unit of heredity. Each gene contains coded biochemical information that directs and determines some human characteristics. Genes are composed of chemical building blocks called *nucleotides.* Two strands of nucleotides arranged in a specific sequence form a molecule of deoxyribonucleic acid, or DNA.

The double-helix configuration of the DNA molecule looks like a twisted ladder (Fig. 15-1). The rungs of the ladder contain a series of four nitrogenous bases. The specific sequence of bases is part of the genetic code that determines a person's genetic traits.

Some of the genetic code is common to all human beings. For example, an infant's biophysical development always proceeds in a cephalocaudal, proximodistal direction, a pattern of growth that is genetically determined. Other aspects of the genetic code determine traits that distinguish one person from another. For example, eye color and height are individual characteristics that are genetically transmitted. Certain diseases, syndromes, and developmental disabilities also are genetic traits.

Genes are situated on larger structures called *chromosomes.* Chromosomes are formed by DNA molecules that wind themselves around protein molecules like thread around a spool. The human cell contains 46 chromosomes in its nucleus, half donated by the person's mother and half by the father. Twenty-two pairs of chromosomes are *autosomes,* which include all but the sex chromosomes. The *sex chromosomes* are the remaining pair and are designated X and Y. Each person has a pair of sex chromosomes designated either XX, which produces a female, or XY, which produces a male.

During cell division, individual chromosomes can be identified by their characteristic sizes, shapes, and banding patterns produced by biologic stains. Laboratory techniques can arrange the chromosomes of a cell into a karyotype (Fig. 15-2). A *karyotype* is a pictorial array of chromosomes used for analysis. It is especially useful for diagnosing diseases caused by an abnormal number of chromosomes.

Before a cell divides, chromosomes reproduce themselves, thus ensuring that the same genetic information is carried to each of the newly created cells (called *daughter cells*). The DNA molecules of each gene replicate themselves with the assistance of specific enzymes. Ribonucleic acid (RNA) acts as a primer during DNA replication. The DNA stays within the cell nucleus, and RNA moves out of the nucleus, carrying coded information to the cytoplasm of the cell. Because of this complex process of DNA replication and chromosome division, genes are precisely reproduced in each of the daughter cells.

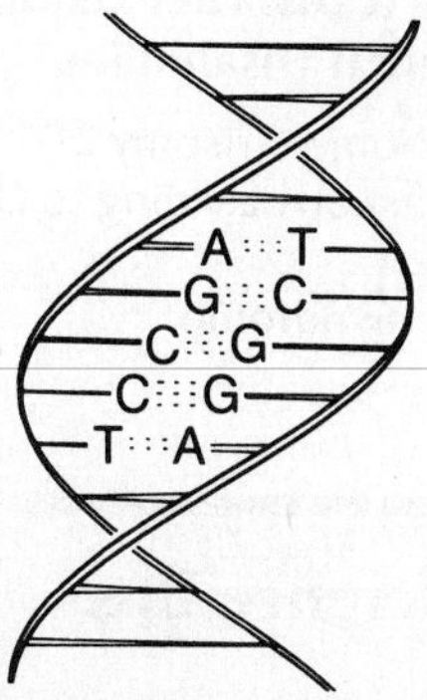

FIGURE 15-1

The structure of the DNA molecule. The sides of the "ladder" are sugars and phosphates, and the "rungs" are the nitrogenous bases. (From Jenkins JB: Human Genetics. *Benjamin/Cummings, 1983).*

Occasionally, a nucleotide in the DNA or RNA molecule is changed. Any such change (called a *mutation*) will be passed to the daughter cells, and the structure and function of the cell proteins will be forever changed.

Processes of Cell Division

The human organism begins as a *zygote,* a cell formed by the union of sperm and egg cells, which normally contains all the necessary genetic material. Shortly after fertilization, the zygote begins to undergo cell division through the process of *mitosis.* During mitosis, each daughter cell receives the same complement of genes as the zygote from which it has descended. The exception in number of chromosomes occurs in the *gametes* (sperm and ova), which develop later and have 23 rather than 46 chromosomes.

Gametes divide through the process of *meiosis,* which cuts in half the number of chromosomes in each cell. Meiosis is essential to reproduction. Without it, gametes would each contain 46 chromosomes, and the zygote would begin development with 92 chromosomes. Meiosis thus allows the number of chromosomes to remain the same for all human beings.

Modes of Inheritance

A trait is inherited as genes are passed on during fertilization. For a given pair of genes, one is contributed by the mother, and one is passed on by the father. Alternate forms

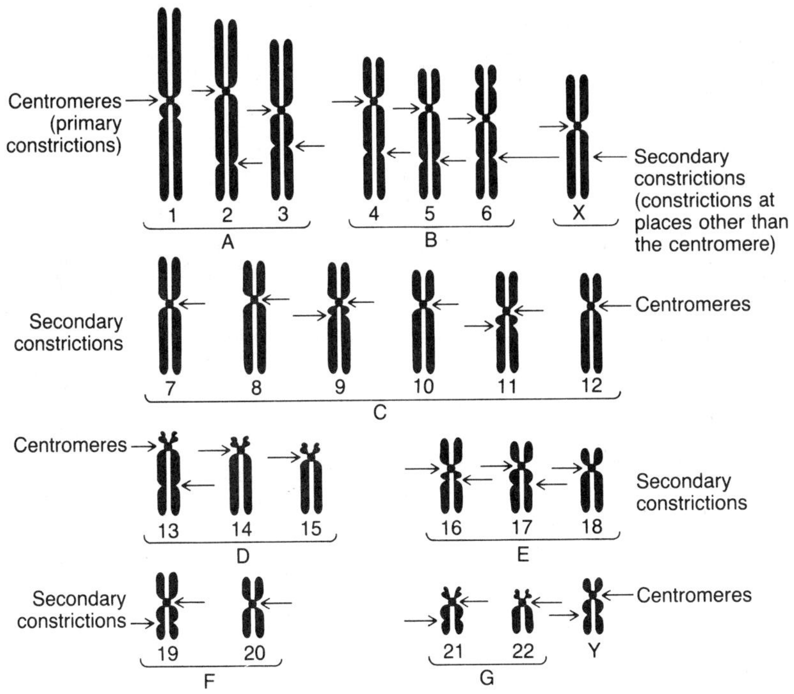

FIGURE 15-2

Representation of a normal male karyotype, showing chromosomal makeup. Chromosomes are numbered for reference. Only one member of each pair of autosomes (nonsex chromosomes) is shown. The X and Y chromosomes are grouped with the autosomes according to size and position of the centromere (constricted portion in the center). (From Jenkins JB: Human Genetics. *Benjamin/Cummings, 1983.)*

of each of the paired genes are termed *alleles*. If the two alleles for a given gene are identical, the person is said to be *homozygous* for that gene or the trait associated with that gene. If the alleles are different, the person is *heterozygous* for both the gene and the trait.

For instance, cystic fibrosis is an inherited trait. The gene for this trait has two alleles: *C*, the normal allele, and *c*, the allele that can result in the disease. If a person has identical alleles, either *CC* or *cc*, the person is homozygous for that gene. If the alleles are different, that is, *Cc*, the person is heterozygous for that gene.

The collection of genes that make up a person's entire set of chromosomes is called the person's *genotype*. Genotype is also the term used to designate an individual gene; for example, blood group A might be noted as genotype I^Ai. A person's genotype remains relatively stable throughout life. For some traits, the genotype determines whether or not a trait is expressed (ie, seen).

Traits that depend on the specific pairing of alleles are termed either dominant or recessive. An allele is *dominant* if its trait is expressed when only one copy is present in the genotype—I^Ai is a genotype for blood group A, I^A being the dominant allele. A trait is *recessive* when two alleles are required for its expression in the phenotype. For example, ii results in blood group O.

The sum of the traits characterizes a person and contributes to the phenotype. The *phenotype* is the actual expression of genes—the entire physical, biochemical, and physiologic makeup of an organism. The phenotype includes both a person's genetic inheritance and the person's interaction with the surrounding environment. Height, for example, is part of a person's phenotype. Although a tendency to be tall, short, or average is part of the genotype, environmental factors, especially nutrition, play a role in the height that a person actually attains.

Also important in identifying inherited characteristics are the concepts of penetrance and expressivity. *Penetrance* is defined as "the proportion of individuals (with the same allele) showing the expected phenotype" (Ayala and Kiger, 1984). *Expressivity* is the degree to which the trait is evident in the individual. For example, complete penetrance and full expressivity would result in all individuals with identical alleles expressing the trait in the identical manner—all individuals with I^Ai will have blood group A.

Autosomal inheritance The inheritance of traits that are controlled by genes located on autosomes is called *autosomal inheritance*. Autosomal inheritance can follow either dominant or recessive patterns. In the dominant pattern, the allele responsible for the trait is dominant, and the trait will be expressed regardless of the other allele. In the *recessive* pattern, the allele responsible for the trait will not result in the expression of the trait if the other allele in the pair is dominant. An autosomal recessive trait will be expressed only when the alleles specifying it are homozygous.

Genetic disorders caused by *autosomal dominant inheritance* are relatively rare. Examples are achondroplasia (dwarfism). Huntington's disease, neurofibromatosis, and

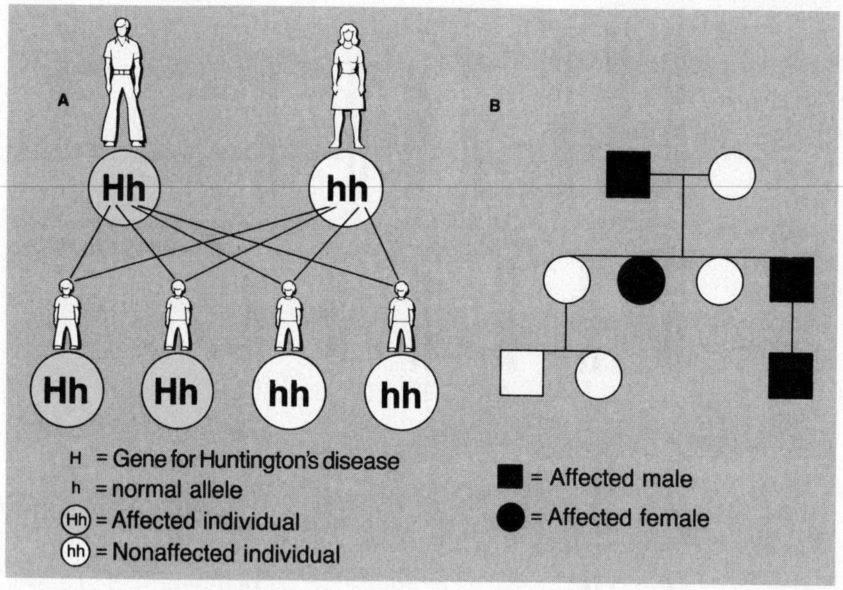

FIGURE 15-3
Autosomal dominant inheritance. The father in this diagram has a faulty gene (H), which is dominant for its counterpart (h). Each offspring's chance of inheriting the faulty gene for Huntington's disease (H) is 50%. (From Olds S: Maternal-Newborn Nursing, *2nd ed. Addison-Wesley, 1984.)*

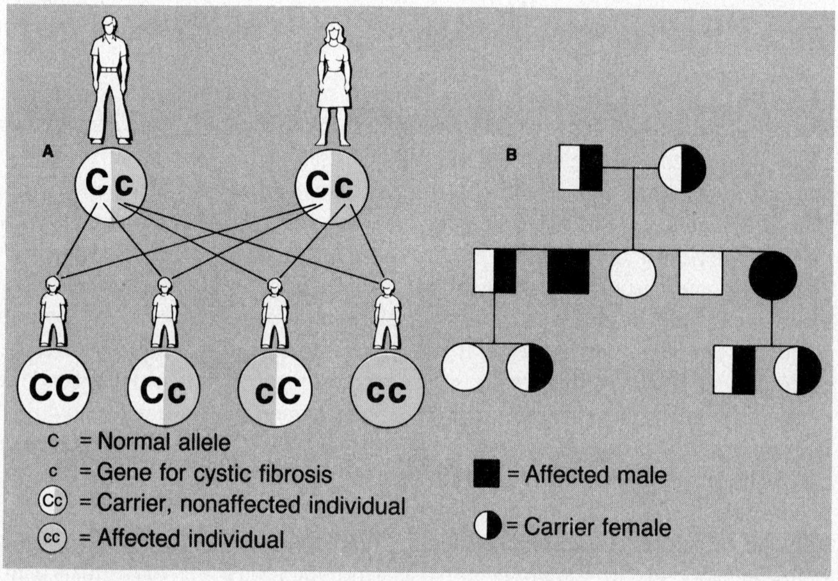

FIGURE 15-4
Autosomal recessive inheritance. Both parents in this diagram carry a normal allele for cystic fibrosis (C) and its counterpart, the gene for cystic fibrosis (c). Because the gene for cystic fibrosis is recessive (C), a child must inherit this gene from both parents to be affected with the disease. Therefore, each child has only a 25% chance of inheriting cystic fibrosis. Each does, however, have a 50% chance of being a carrier for the disease. (From Olds S: Maternal-Newborn Nursing, *2nd ed. Addison-Wesley, 1984.)*

osteogenesis imperfecta (Fig. 15-3). Some autosomal dominant defects occur as new mutations.

Autosomal recessive disorders (Fig. 15-4) include Tay-Sachs disease, cystic fibrosis, and phenylketonuria. When children have one of these disorders, they have inherited two copies of the deleterious allele, one from each parent. Each parent is a *carrier* of the trait because the parent's genotype contains the gene without expressing the trait.

Sex-linked inheritance Because most chromosomes contain more than one gene, genes are said to be linked together on specific chromosomes. The concept of *linkage* explains why certain traits are often inherited together.

Technically, *sex-linked inheritance* involves genes that are linked to either the X or the Y chromosome, although there are no traits yet determined to be linked to the Y chromosome. Therefore, sex-linked inheritance usually is defined as X-linked, or associated with genes on the X chromosome.

X-linked inheritance is significant because a number of diseases are inherited as X-linked recessive traits. These occur almost exclusively in males. When an X-linked dis-

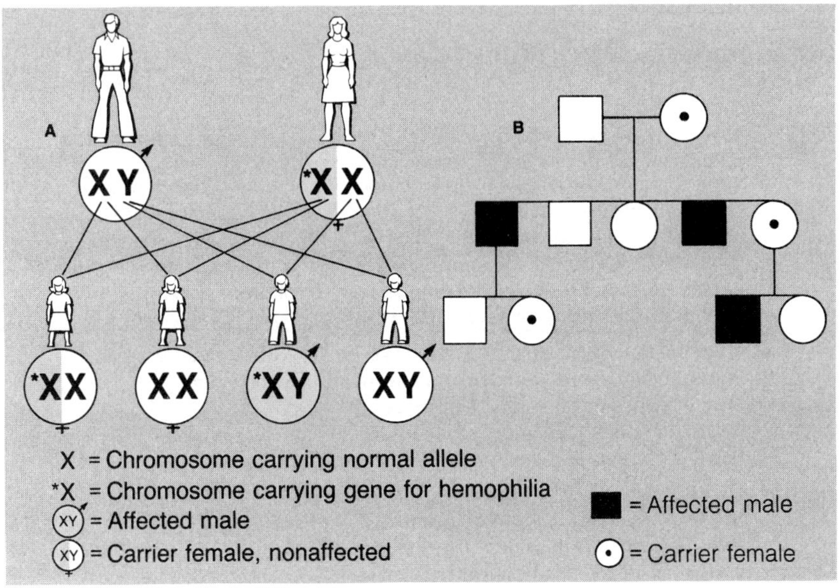

FIGURE 15-5

*Sex-linked inheritance. In this diagram the sex chromosomes of an unaffected mother carry one faulty gene (*X) and one normal gene (X). The father has normal X and Y chromosomes. Each male child then has a 50% chance of inheriting the disorder and each female child has a 50% chance of being a carrier for the disorder. (From Olds S:* Maternal-Newborn Nursing, *2nd ed. Addison-Wesley, 1984.)*

order is recessive, a person will express the trait only if (1) that person is homozygous for the trait (ie, has two genes for the disorder) or (2) that person lacks a corresponding normal gene that will be dominant over the recessive trait. The latter condition occurs in males, who have only one X chromosome (Fig. 15-5).

A male who inherits an X chromosome carrying a gene for a specific disease has no corresponding normal gene and will therefore express the trait. A female, who has two X chromosomes, will express the trait only if both chromosomes contain the abnormal gene (an occurrence that is statistically rare). Women who are carriers for X-linked disorders can thus transmit these conditions to their sons. Among the disorders transmitted through X-linked inheritance are factor VIII hemophilia, red-green color blindness, and Duchenne type muscular dystrophy.

Chromosome aberrations Deviations from the normal chromosome complement can be categorized into those involving a change in the number of chromosomes and those involving a change in chromosome structure. Numeric changes can affect the autosomes or sex chromosomes and result in more than or less than 46 chromosomes. Trisomy 21 (Down's syndrome) results from an extra number 21 chromosome. Turner's syndrome (XO) is an example of a numeric change affecting a sex chromosome. With Turner's syndrome, the total number of chromosomes is only 45.

Several factors are associated with an increase in the occurrence of numerical aberrations. Late maternal age is a major factor associated with trisomy 21, for example, and to a lesser extent with other trisomies. It has been suggested that paternal age over 55 years also is a contributing factor. Radiation exposure, neoplastic drugs, viruses, and chromosome abnormalities themselves are all associated with alterations in chromosome number.

Changes in chromosome structure include a loss, gain, or rearrangement of genetic material. The change can involve only a small segment of DNA, or it can involve the entire chromosome.

Chromosome aberrations are the cause of a range of genetic disorders (Table 15-1). All clinically significant abnormalities can be identified by routine cytogenetic (cell examination) techniques. For example, amniocentesis during the first trimester of pregnancy can provide information about the chromosome complement of the fetus. Amniocentesis involves the extracting of amniotic fluid, which contains fetal cells. A karyotype is then created so that all chromosomes can be identified (see Fig. 15-2). Recently an alternative to amniocentesis, chorionic villus sampling, has been used to obtain fetal cells. Chorionic villus sampling is less invasive than amniocentesis (a vaginal approach is used) and can be performed earlier in the pregnancy (ninth week).

Multifactorial inheritance *Multifactorial inheritance* (sometimes called polygenic inheritance) involves the interaction of both genetic and environmental factors. Multifactorial inheritance accounts for much of the normal variation in families such as in stature and intelligence. Intelligence, for example, is a trait that shows continuous variation in the general population. Intelligence is affected by environment and genes. Most of the differences among normal human

TABLE 15-1 Disorders Related to Chromosome Alterations

Disorder	Genetic alteration	Description	Nursing implication
Down's syndrome	Trisomy 21	Most common chromosome disorder, occurring in 1:600 to 1:1000 births. Phenotypic features include epicanthal folds, simian creases on palms, hypotonia, flat nasal bridge, protrusion of the tongue. Various degrees of mental retardation	Associated with other conditions such as cardiac disease and hematologic disorders, among disorders of other systems
Edward's syndrome	Trisomy 18	Mental retardation. Almost all organ systems affected. Appearance of small head, low-set ears, small features. Abnormal flexion of fingers. Only 13% of infants live beyond one year; most die within 10 weeks	Assessment for organ involvement
Pateu's syndrome	Trisomy 13	Most severe malformations of all chromosomal abnormalities. Mental retardation. Small head, small malformed eyes, spasmodic seizures, deafness, extra digits, split tongue. Only a few infants live longer than one year; most die soon after birth	
Cri-du-chat syndrome	Deletion of short arm of chromosome 5 (5p−)	Infants up to 1 year of age have a characteristic cry of a cat due to abnormal laryngeal development. Severe mental retardation, microcephaly, widely spaced eyes, broad nose, low-set ears. Congenital heart anomalies present in about 25% of cases. Children survive better than with trisomies, and some survive into adulthood	IQ is so low (less than 35) that institutionalization might be required
Klinefelter's syndrome	Additional X chromosome (47,XXY) Variants include XXYY, XXXY, XXXXY	Small testes, sterility, abnormally long legs; 50% of individuals develop breasts, female distribution of body hair. Slight mental retardation, though some individuals have IQ in the normal range	(see Chapter 29)
Turner's syndrome	Monosomy X (XO)	Failure to develop normal secondary female sexual characteristics at puberty. Low hairline. Wide chest with broadly spaced nipples. Narrowing of aorta. Puffy feet in newborns. High palate. No apparent mental retardation	(see Chapter 29)
XYY syndrome	Additional Y chromosome	Nearly all males with this karyotype are phenotypically normal. They tend to be taller than XY males but with lower muscular strength and poorer coordination and may be susceptible to severe acne. Sexual development is normal. IQ might be somewhat lower, but within normal range	
Wilms' tumor	Deletion of short arm of chromosome 11 (11p−)	A type of renal cancer in young children. Strong association with absence of irises in the eyes. Other physical defects affect the gastrointestinal and genitourinary systems. Some mental retardation	(see Chapter 33)

beings demonstrate continuous variation. The question is not a matter of having intelligence or not having intelligence but rather where one falls along a continuum.

Multifactorial inheritance also accounts for many common disorders and congenital malformations. Congenital hip dysplasia, pyloric stenosis, congenital heart disease, spina bifida, and cleft lip and palate are included in this category. Multifactorial traits and diseases tend to cluster in families, but there is no clear-cut, predictable genetic pattern in individual families.

In general, once a couple has had one affected child, the chance of having another child with the same defect is between 2% and 5%. After having two affected children, the risk increases again because the second birth indicates that the parents might have more predisposing factors than originally suspected. These risk figures can vary in different geographic areas and should be checked prior to counseling a couple regarding the risk of recurrence.

Genetic Effects on Biophysical Development

Inborn errors of metabolism Body homeostasis is maintained by regulatory mechanisms, some of which affect the biochemical pathways. A *biochemical pathway* is a series of steps in which a final chemical product depends on the successful completion of the previous step. Any alteration in this sequence will result in an abnormality. Genetically coded information directs the synthesis of enzymes that regulate these steps.

For example, in phenylketonuria (PKU) the gene that codes for the enzyme that converts phenylalanine into tyrosine is defective, and the enzyme is not produced. Phenylalanine accumulates in the blood and eventually causes brain damage. In this way, a single defective gene can cause multiple problems in the person's phenotype by interfering with biochemical pathways. In children with PKU, however, the severity of the disease (ie, its ultimate phenotype) is related to environmental factors. Early detection through neonatal screening can prevent brain damage if it is followed by nutritional therapy (see Chapter 27).

Other diseases classified as inborn errors of metabolism are galactosemia and Tay-Sachs disease.

Antibody function Genes play an important role in the proper functioning of the body's immune system. The study of the genetics of antibody formation and of the immune system in general recently has offered exciting insights into gene behavior. Although the various theories proposed are very complex, they all attempt to shed light on one question: How can genes coded to direct antibody function produce the rich diversity of antibodies of which the human body is capable? What is unquestionable is that genetic activity underlies the formation of antibodies and thus controls the function of the immune system itself.

Current research is uncovering many connections between disease, or susceptibility to disease, and the genetics of the immune system. Three areas in particular are the HLA gene complex, autoimmune diseases, and diseases of immunologic deficiency (see Chapter 25).

The Nurse's Role in Genetic Disorders

Prenatal screening Prenatal screening is now available to diagnose a number of genetic problems in utero, thus enabling a woman to make decisions regarding the best options for her particular situation. Amniocentesis, chorionic villus sampling, ultrasound, alpha fetoprotein determinations, and fetoscopy are a few of these available tests.

Women over age 35 are at greater risk for bearing children with chromosome alterations, and chorionic villus sampling or amniocentesis early in pregnancy are useful diagnostic tools. Some women, however, choose not to undergo these procedures. Reasons for choosing not to undergo a prenatal diagnostic procedure are many. Some might fear what will be discovered or the decisions involved in bearing a defective child. There might be a lack of knowledge about age-related genetic defects or a conscious decision to live with the consequences of defect, regardless of whether the problem is diagnosed in utero. Some women unconsciously avoid making any decision and consequently make a decision by default. Regardless of the reasons, nurses need to be accepting of personal attitudes regarding prenatal diagnosis, while encouraging prospective parents to be aware of what is available.

In many settings nurses are able to identify and refer for counseling families at risk for genetic defects. In acute-care settings, chronic-care settings, well-child clinics, or schools, child health nurses can identify families who would benefit from counseling.

Genetic counseling Underlying most parents' aspirations for a successful pregnancy is the ability to have a healthy child. Any threat to this normal expectation can result in a threat to the parents' self-esteem.

Parents sometimes seek genetic counseling when they are concerned about having a second child with an abnormality. Some seek advice when one or both parents are concerned about transmitting a defect. Nurses in a variety of settings are often asked to provide information or to refer the client for more extensive genetic counseling. Indications for referral for genetic counseling include:

1. Congenital anomalies, including mental retardation in child or family

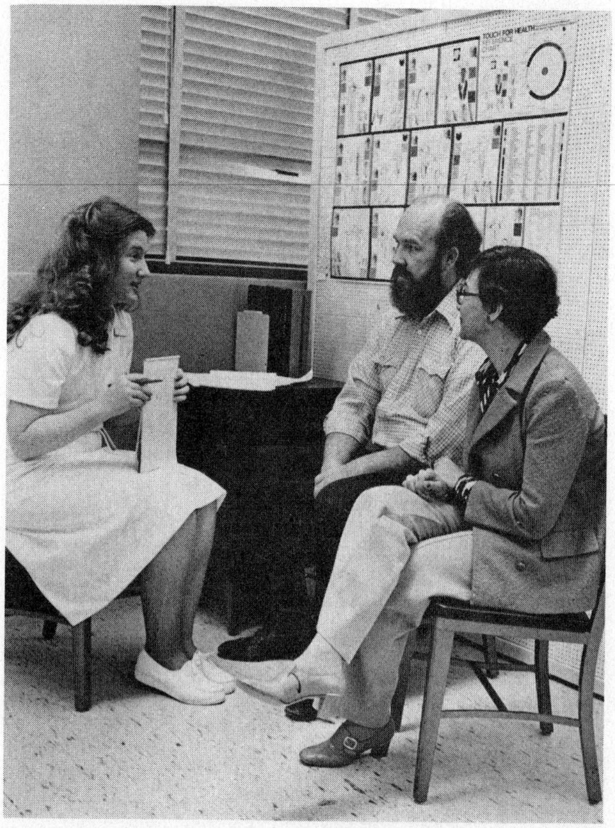

Knowing the mechanisms of genetic transmission and the modes of inheritance is important for the nurse involved in genetic counseling of families.

2. Familial disorders such as diabetes
3. Known inherited disease
4. Metabolic disorders
5. Chromosomal abnormalities

The nursing role in genetic counseling depends on the practice setting and the nurse's level of preparation. If the mode of inheritance is fairly straightforward (for example, PKU), the counseling can be done in the primary-care setting. For more complicated situations, referral to a genetic clinic is in order.

General roles for nurses are:

Assessing the couple's level of understanding of the genetic information. (Can parents explain the mode of inheritance? What recurrence risks were explained to them?)

Identifying how each parent interprets the information. (Do the parents view the recurrence risk as low or high? How will this information affect their decision regarding more children?)

Clarifying information and correcting misconceptions.

Identifying how the genetic component of the information has affected the feelings of each parent. (What is the meaning of "carrier"; does a parent feel stigmatized or guilty?)

Reassuring the parents that it is not their "fault," that each individual carries six to eight deleterious genes.

Assisting the parents with decision making as necessary. (Decisions related to genetic information might include changing to a more reliable birth control method, becoming pregnant again, adopting, or informing relatives who also might be at risk).

Finding resources that the couple might need (for example, prenatal diagnosis, artificial insemination by donor, additional counseling or therapy).

Educating the public for the early recognition and prevention of genetic defects.

One method for identifying an inherited disease pattern in a particular family is a genogram. A *genogram* is a diagramatic form of recording a family history using standard symbols (Fig. 15-6). The extent of the genogram depends on the disorder being considered. Minimally, the nurse includes the affected child through whom a family comes to the attention of the investigator, siblings, and preceding and succeeding generations. Consanguineous marriages (those between relatives) or multiple marriages are carefully documented. Information on each member includes age, health, live births, stillbirths, and miscarriages. If a member is dead, the age of death and the cause are documented. The place of birth or origin of a family also can be important. For example, the incidence of Tay-Sachs disease is higher in Ashkenazic Jews than in Puerto Ricans.

A well-constructed genogram can give clues to genetic etiologies and modes of inheritance. Knowledge of inheritance patterns permits health professionals to predict the risk that a particular trait or disorder will occur in offspring or other relatives.

A major nursing role in genetic counseling is to provide support to families who either have a defective child or who have predictable chances for having one in a future pregnancy. Inevitably, parents ask, "Will this happen to us again?" If they do not wish to have more children, they might be asking the question for healthy siblings or other relatives.

It is important that the health professional responding to this question be well versed in genetics. This means understanding the modes of inheritance, communicating scientific information to clients, and recognizing the impact that

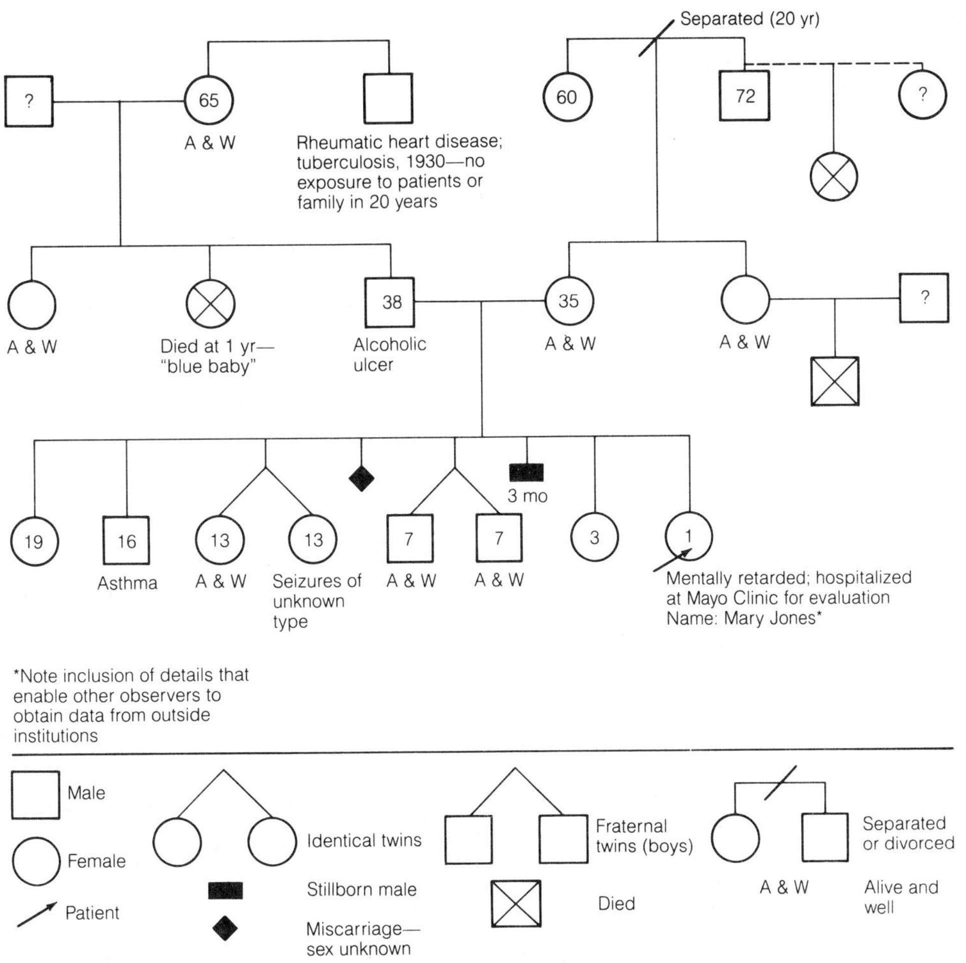

FIGURE 15-6

Genogram used to diagram a family history.

this information might have on the families. The counselor needs to have updated information on the disorder in question with regard to mode of inheritance, therapies, and prenatal diagnostic capabilities. Modes of inheritance for some disorders, such as diabetes mellitus, are not clear cut. The counselor also needs to be knowledgeable about procreative alternatives if the couple does not wish to risk another pregnancy themselves. Good interpersonal skills are therefore a necessity.

Fear of future pregnancies after the birth of a defective child suggests such ethical issues as birth control, abortion, sterility, and right to life. Anxiety regarding these issues must be expressed before any effective, genetically focused information is understood. Otherwise, important information might be lost because anxiety interferes with its processing. Parents who have given birth to defective children need to grieve before they can adequately prepare to plan for the future. (The process of grieving for children with chronic conditions is discussed in Chapter 14.) Children who are at risk for developing genetic disorders, such as Huntington's disease, later in life need to be given the opportunity to express their feelings and obtain supportive nursing care.

To provide support to parents, nurses need to have clarified their own feelings about the ethical issues involved. Nurses too have difficulty with some of these issues but need to understand their feelings before they can provide unbiased, professional nursing care. Learning that something in one's genes is responsible for a disorder in a child is very difficult, even when it is something that is clearly beyond the control of the individual. A knowledgeable, compassionate nurse can help these people accept genetic information and make realistic and appropriate decisions for future childbearing.

Developmental Disabilities and Mental Retardation

Developmental disabilities are associated with complex etiologies. Causal factors often are genetic, but the child's external environment also can play a role in the degree of severity of the disability. Developmental disabilities usually are defined by deficits in cognitive development.

Although some health and education professionals use developmental disability and mental retardation interchangeably, mental retardation actually is a part of the broad spectrum of developmental disability. The mental impairment associated with any compromised functioning, however, has come to be associated with mental retardation, but this is only a partial definition. The official definition published by the American Association of Mental Deficiency (AAMD) is

> Mental retardation refers to significantly subaverage, general intellectual functioning existing concurrently with deficits in adaptive behavior and manifested during the developmental period. The developmental period extends to approximately 18 years of age (Grossman, 1983).

Thus a diagnosis of mental retardation cannot be based on low intelligence alone but is also determined by the individual's capacity to adapt behaviorally to the environment (Fig. 15-7).

A diagnosis of mental retardation requires intelligence tests that have been standardized for large cross-sections of the population for which they are designed. The child then is assigned an intelligence quotient (IQ) computed by dividing the child's mental age by the chronologic age and multiplying the quotient by 100. Common intelligence tests include:

- Stanford-Binet Intelligence Scale
- Gesell Developmental Schedules
- McCarthy Scales of Children's Abilities
- Weschler Intelligence Scale for Children—revised (WISC-R)
- Weschler Preschool and Primary Scale of Intelligence for Children 4–6½ years (WPPSI)
- Slosson Intelligence Test
- Bayley Scales of Infant Development
- Catell Infant Intelligence Scale

To indicate mental retardation, behaviors must show significantly limited functioning. For example, an IQ test might show that a child is retarded, but an assessment of adaptive skills might show that the same child is normal. It is not unusual for some developmentally disabled children to exhibit impaired intellectual functioning but appropriate adaptive functioning. Such children might, however, be appropriately identified as mentally retarded if they exhibit functional limitations that require long-term intervention.

Adaptive behavior	Measured intellectual functioning: Retarded	Measured intellectual functioning: Not retarded
Retarded	Mentally Retarded	NOT mentally retarded
Not retarded	NOT mentally retarded	NOT mentally retarded

FIGURE 15-7

Classification based on measured intellectual functioning and adaptive behavior. A child is classified as retarded only if the level of intellectual functioning and the degree of adaptive behavior are both impaired. (From Grossman HG (editor): Classifications in Mental Retardation. *American Association on Mental Deficiency, 1983, p. 12. Reprinted with permission.)*

Etiology of Mental Retardation

Factors related to mental retardation closely parallel the social, economic, and health status of a society and the resources available for education, development, and employment. The incidence of mental retardation therefore is higher in countries lacking mass immunization programs, proper nutrition, hygiene and safe environment, and public health services for pregnant women and children. The incidence of mental retardation in the United States generally is estimated at about 125,000 births per year. The most widely quoted figure is 3% of the general population, or more than 6 million people.

More than 200 causes of mental retardation are known. Genetic causes, especially inborn errors of metabolism and genetic diseases continue to be identified. The complex relationship between genetic and environmental causes often suggests multifactorial inheritance. For child health nurses, more than 75% of the retarded children with whom they work have no definitive medical diagnosis or defect. Current knowledge about the role of prenatal, perinatal, and postnatal influences on mental function therefore can assist in identifying children at risk and providing preventive health care. (Risk factors associated with developmental disabilities are summarized in Table 15-2.)

TABLE 15-2 Risk Factors for Developmental Disabilities

Type of risk	Specific concerns
Prenatal factors	Maternal disease (diabetes mellitus, hypertension, infections, toxemia, anemia)
	Maternal malnutrition
	Maternal age
	Exposure to chemicals (environmental, drugs, alcohol, tobacco)
	TORCH infections (see p. 452)
	Exposure to high doses of radiation
	Metabolic disorders
Intrapartum factors	Prolonged or precipitous labor
	Fetal distress
	Interruption of oxygen
	Significant blood loss
	Encephalopathy from injury in utero
Neonatal factors	Low birthweight (premature or small for gestational age)
	Neonatal asphyxia
	Low Apgar evaluation
	Birth defects
	Sensory malfunction (eg, blindness or deafness)
Neonatal factors *(Continued)*	Disease (hypoglycemia, sepsis, respiratory distress syndrome, meningitis, hypothyroidism)
	Kernicterus
	Brain tumors
Social factors	Poverty
	Poor attachment between parent and child
	Over- or understimulating environment
	Severe emotional neglect
Genetic factors	History of mental retardation, learning problems
	Genetic disorders, birth defects in blood relatives
Factors in older child	Serious illness (such as meningitis)
	Head trauma
	Chronic illness
	Lead poisoning
	Psychologic trauma (eg, abuse, separation, multiple losses)
	Malnutrition (decreased protein intake, skim milk intake during first 6 months of life, inadequate caloric intake for bodily needs)

Classification of Mental Retardation

The 1983 AAMD classification system developed by the AAMD Committee on Terminology and Classification reflects current efforts in proper terminology to identify developmental disabilities and mental retardation.

The categories of mental retardation and their corresponding IQ ranges are:

Term	IQ range
Mild mental retardation	50–55 to approximately 70
Moderate mental retardation	35–40 to 50–55
Severe mental retardation	20–25 to 35–40
Profound mental retardation	Below 20 or 25

The category of borderline intelligence (a 70–84 IQ) was once included but has been eliminated to avoid classifying among the mentally retarded those individuals whose dysfunction might be caused by socioeconomic deprivation.

Children in the mild category are estimated to comprise 75%–90% of the retarded population and are termed "educable" in the educational system. They are expected to learn to read, write, and do basic computations up to a third- to sixth-grade level. Estimates of the number of moderately retarded people range from as low as 6% to as high as 17%–21% (Thain, Castro, & Peterson, 1980; Blackman, 1983) of the mentally retarded population.

These children can learn to care for themselves, develop social skills, and perform simple routine tasks. They rarely learn to read and write but can recognize important words and do basic counting. A program of training throughout childhood might enable a moderately retarded person to participate in structured employment such as a sheltered workshop. Moderately retarded adults might be able to live in communities in group homes or in individual households with varying degrees of supervision. The more retarded a child, the sooner that child will be noticed.

Severely retarded children frequently have detectable disabilities at birth, including physical handicaps. A child with physical abnormalities, particularly those involving the face and head, is usually evaluated at an earlier age.

The nurse therefore is valuable in providing support to the parents at this time. In addition to extremely low cognitive functioning, severely retarded children have minimal adaptive skills. Some learn to walk and acquire language skills. Most learn adaptive skills and are trainable to varying degrees.

Profoundly retarded children require ongoing nursing care to improve disabilities, prevent further difficulties, and maintain life. Many of these children develop life-threatening illnesses and die early in life from complicating illnesses. They need general care as well as protection. The severely and profoundly retarded comprise about 4% of the retarded population.

Assessment of the Hospitalized, Developmentally Disabled Child

1. Health history
   a) Pertinent prenatal and postnatal events
   b) Allergies to food or medication
   c) Number and length of previous hospital stays
   d) Child's reaction during and after hospital stays
2. Physical examination
   a) Muscle tone and skin turgor
   b) Height, weight, and head circumference
   c) Sensory function—visual, auditory, tactile, gustatory, olfactory, and kinesthetic responses
   d) Dentition and oral integrity
   e) Reflexes, postural patterns
3. Nutritional status
   a) Dietary intake (including calories and volume)
   b) Level of feeding skills
4. Health care history
   a) Availability of routine pediatric supervision
   b) Specialists (therapists, nurses, or others) who have evaluated, referred, or treated the child
5. Developmental assessment
   a) Milestones accomplished (gross and fine motor skills, toilet training, self-care abilities)
   b) Ability to understand and follow directions
   c) Methods of communication (sign language, special signs, speech)
   d) Ability to interact with others, especially strangers
   e) Comfort measures and routines used
   f) Necessity to continue special program of exercise or stimulation
6. Environmental assessment
   a) Place of residence
   b) Primary caregiver(s)
   c) Special equipment used
   d) Usual program of daily activities

The Role of the Nurse Caring for Developmentally Disabled Children

Settings for Nursing Practice

Nurses care for developmentally disabled children in a variety of settings. These include the home, acute- and chronic-care facilities, and alternative living arrangements. Child health nurses are most likely to encounter mentally retarded children in the hospital, where the child might be admitted for acute care, or the school, where the school nurse might be involved in monitoring and coordinating a child's care plan.

Hospital Mentally retarded children often are hospitalized for recurring infections and chronic illnesses. Common problems include immature immune response systems; failure to thrive; organically based behavior problems; and correction of neuromotor, metabolic, and nutritional problems.

Hospital staffs might be unprepared to meet the needs of the developmentally disabled child. Prior planning reduces the fear experienced by the child and the anxiety felt by the parent. A nurse familiar with the child can assist the parent in writing a description of the child's behavior. The parent explains how the child makes needs known; how physical needs are provided; what routines are expected; any special adaptive equipment and chairs required for motor control, feeding, or toileting; and types of toys enjoyed. Portable items unavailable at the hospital but used at home are brought when the child is admitted. Simple instructions about any special behavior management programs also are included. All of this information can be incorporated in the nursing care plan for the child.

The nursing care plan includes structured plans for the child's free time, especially when the child has difficulty using long periods of unplanned time constructively. Close supervision is necessary, with a variety of carefully selected leisure activities based on the child's skill level in reading, counting, and fine motor control. Health teaching for both child and parents can occur during these unstructured time periods.

The child's admission process documents the child's level of functioning, and the process should involve the child as much as possible. Gestures and facial expressions help the child understand what is being said. Maintaining eye-to-eye contact, touching the child's arm or face, and calling the child by name helps to maintain the child's attention. Repeating information and having the child repeat it back to the nurse verifies that the child has understood.

School Mentally retarded and developmentally disabled children once were placed in separate schools and institutions. These children are now integrated in educational settings with normal children, and school nurses have an integral role on the educational team. As a consequence of Public Law 94-142, the Education for All Handicapped Children Act of 1975, school children include those with deafness, orthopedic and neuromuscular impairments, vision impairments, learning disabilities, mental retardation, emotional disturbances, and behavioral impairments.

School nurses working with the developmentally disabled are involved in health promotion that is essentially primary prevention.

Goals for Nursing Care

In recent years nursing has extended involvement in the care of the mentally retarded to encompass nursing practice in the home, community, and institutions. Nursing goals generally include

1. Providing guidance to families in the areas of infant care and stimulation
2. Helping parents accept and adjust to the birth of retarded children
3. Screening for symptoms of developmental problems
4. Planning and implementing programs with other health and education professionals concerned with preventive health care (for example, exercise and weight reduction programs, sex and family life education, and maintenance of adaptive skills)
5. Providing family support for management of retarded children in the home and guidance in seeking respite care
6. Managing medical problems of children in acute-care hospital facilities and supervising daily care of retarded children in institutions and residential programs.

Multidisciplinary management Like other aspects of nursing, nursing care for the developmentally disabled involves collecting and analyzing data, making a nursing diagnosis, and planning interventions. The overriding goals are ensuring optimal development and preventing further disability in the developmentally disabled child. Depending on educational preparation and experience, nurses are involved in providing direct care or acting as case coordinators to develop plans for treatment.

Nurses collaborate with physicians to provide follow-up for medical treatment, drug therapy (for example, in managing seizures or hyperactivity), and nutritional management (for example, in dietary counseling for PKU, galactosemia, and obesity). Nurses also support and coordinate with other health professionals, including social workers and mental health therapists, to help parents cope with stress and use appropriate community resources. Community supports include agencies for health maintenance; child-care facilities; developmental programs; physical, occupational, and speech therapy; pediatric psychologists; early intervention programs; and organizations for respite care and planning for long-term placement.

Care of the family The nurse's role with the developmentally disabled is focused primarily on the needs of the child, but like other aspects of child health nursing, the nurse's scope of practice includes the entire family.

Impact of the diagnosis Having a developmentally disabled child is a crisis that requires special coping abilities if the parent is to accept the child. Identification and acceptance of disabilities are difficult for many families, and developing ways to promote optimal development and include the child in the family requires joint adaptation by all family members. This process is assisted by nurses in contact with the infant and family at the time of delivery; in the nursery; during the postpartum period; and in the weeks, months, and years following the diagnosis.

Reactions of parents and other family members to the arrival of a retarded child vary according to a great many factors. Religious orientation, the degree to which the child was wanted in the first place, the parent's previous experiences with crisis, the nature and degree of the problem, the parent's inner coping mechanisms and self-esteem, the family's socioeconomic resources, the child's similarity to other family members, and the quality of professional support are all important. (See Chapter 14 for further discussion of the impact of chronic conditions on families.)

Parent teaching In establishing contact with the family, the nurse first clarifies the nursing role. A preliminary goal during this initial contact is to foster acceptance by the child and family. The nurse therefore views a client's behavior as a response to the nurse's actions and attitudes.

If the nurse is to foster acceptance, nursing interventions need to communicate basic respect, or positive regard, for the client. Communicating basic respect involves demonstrating consideration for the child's feelings, both verbally and nonverbally. The nurse also can demonstrate caring and respect while providing for the child's physical needs.

Another goal of nursing intervention is helping parents recognize the normal aspects of their disabled children's development and behavior. Parents usually have to learn to distinguish behaviors that are healthy or expected from those that are real problems. For example, the nurse teaches parents to differentiate normal motor development from abnormal reflex activities. With careful explanations from the nurse and other health professionals, most parents can become astute observers and managers of their child's special needs.

Many parents also need advice about handling problems of daily care, such as sleep, feeding, and temperament, that are common to all children. The special problems presented by the disabled child's vulnerability to acute illness might require more than the ordinary measures.

The day-to-day responsibilities also can be taxing and stressful. Because nurses might be the most frequent health care contacts, providing guidance and health supervision, they are likely to be alerted first to family stresses and crises. Developmental disabilities are risk factors that cause children to be mistreated, neglected, or abused (see Chapter 13).

Parents of severely disabled children often are faced with such health problems as seizure disorders, abnormal reflex activity and abnormal body posturing, and episodes of acute illness. The nurse acting as coordinator might either provide care or provide access to specific programs for handling the child at home.

Issues in the Care of Developmentally Disabled Children

Nutrition and feeding Nursing interventions related to nutrition for developmentally disabled children are planned to inform parents about appropriate developmental skills and feeding tasks, to teach parents to feed children with motor impairment, and to teach parents about maintaining adequate levels of nutrition.

Children with developmental disabilities sometimes have brain damage that causes feeding problems, which in turn can cause alterations in nutritional status. Nursing diagnoses might include

Alterations in nutrition: less than body requirements related to feeding difficulties and decreased intake

Alterations in nutrition: more than body requirements related to increased intake and decreased mobility

Dietary planning Diets of many severely disabled infants are deficient in calories, nutrients, bulk, and fluids. This deficiency presents a threat to adequate growth. Minimal ingestion of solids during the first year becomes an even greater problem later in life and contributes to other areas of health concerns, including dental hygiene, lower resistance to disease, and elimination problems (Zelle and Coyner, 1983).

Calorie intake is affected by degree of severity and motor involvement. The developmentally disabled child whose condition reduces mobility tends to need fewer calories. Thus, mentally retarded children with motor impairment may need fewer calories and smaller quantities of most nutrients.

Some developmental conditions, such as Down's syndrome, are associated with weight gain and obesity. Some retarded children are sheltered by their parents and lead sedentary lives with fewer opportunities for active games and exercise. Obesity and fatigue then become established patterns. Parents who fail to see ways to express affection to their retarded children might overindulge their children with food, thus establishing a pattern leading to obesity.

Nurses can suggest and demonstrate appropriate expressions of affection and can reinforce acceptable behavior that does not involve food. Because parents and health professionals necessarily are concerned about intake and weight gain in these children, weight gain can be a hopeful sign of progress, causing a tendency to overfeed the child.

Many developmentally disabled children have additional organ defects of the heart and neuromuscular system. Those children who have neuromuscular characteristics of fluctuating muscle tone and athetosis (slow, involuntary movements) need more calories to compensate for frequent muscle activity. When abnormal oral motor problems involving tongue thrusting, muscle rigidity, and muscle tone severely interfere with feeding, the increased risks to the child's health can be life-threatening. Gavage or tube feeding then might be necessary (see Chapter 27).

Infant feeding Parents expect their infants to have pleasant feeding experiences, which are essential to the establishment of basic trust. Infants who show no interest in eating do not participate in the reciprocal process and so do not reinforce parenting behaviors.

Mothers who had planned to breast-feed their babies might automatically assume that a child with problems must be bottle-fed. Breast-feeding, however, is a desirable choice for feeding developmentally disabled infants. The nursing staff can encourage mothers to breast-feed. Breast-feeding disabled infants who have oral motor problems promotes development of the oral muscles. Infants with structural anomalies of the mouth and palate or with muscle tone abnormalities, however, do better with special nipples. For these infants, nurses can guide parents in choosing among commercially available nipples.

When the mechanics of eating cause problems, parents need guidance in choosing the appropriate time in the child's development to offer solid foods. Poorly controlled tongue movements, abnormal posture and tone, and gagging and biting problems can present difficulties. Many parents feel pressured to offer solid foods early because of an infant's poor weight gain or fussiness related to neuromotor immaturity and dysfunction (Zelle and Coyner, 1983).

Feeding skills The mentally retarded child learns feeding skills in much the same way as the normal child but at an unpredictable and slower pace. Nevertheless, parents can identify times to promote progress by teaching more advanced feeding skills.

A primary goal is to help developmentally disabled children become as independent in their feeding skills as possible. Self-feeding, however, depends largely on the degree of motor impairment. When the developmentally disabled child has a motor dysfunction in addition to retardation, the ability to follow the normal sequence of feeding behaviors might be altered. Some children achieve only very low levels of self-feeding. Because it is much less time consuming for a parent to feed the child, parents need much encouragement in remaining patient as their children learn.

Children also are not left to struggle unaided for too long, or they become discouraged by failure. The nurse teaches the parent to show the task to the child and then help the child to perform the movements. After a number of trials the child might be able to imitate the parent's behavior or at least to offer minimal resistance. At this point the parent should gradually withdraw effort, particularly at the end of a sequence, so that the child completes the feeding task independently.

The challenge of learning to eat solid foods also encourages development of self-help skills and enhances the child's self-confidence. Feelings of self-worth also can help the child maintain a desired food intake and hence a desired weight.

Parents of developmentally disabled children sometimes subtly prevent their children from maturing, often because the child remains an infant and dependent in the parent's mind. Such children might be fed strained or junior foods even when the cues indicating readiness for unstrained foods are present. Because of a child's oral hypersensitivity to textures, the transition from strained to unstrained foods can be upsetting. The child might refuse to eat, and weight loss might result. A program of desensitization often increases a child's tolerance of textures.

Retarded children sometimes develop inappropriate, negative behaviors associated with feeding. Behaviors such as spitting, purposeful gagging, vomiting, ruminating, and throwing food can overwhelm parents. The nurse helps parents understand that disruptive behaviors should not be tolerated or reinforced. In such instances the nurse might teach behavior modification techniques, so that negative behaviors can be extinguished in favor of functional feeding patterns.

Anxiety over feeding sufficient quantities of food can lead a parent to choose foods high in calories, carbohydrates, and fats but deficient in nutrients. Parents therefore should be advised to make good choices in the quality of food and to feed smaller amounts more frequently, rather than offering a nutritionally poor selection of foods that seem more pleasing to the child's taste.

⊛ Self-care deficit: toileting related to developmental delay

Achievement of toileting is a step that parents of retarded children, like those of normal children, eagerly await. Toileting signals a major milestone in the retarded child's self-care. Managing personal care is a demanding task for a parent. It is often unrewarding when the child is large and difficult to handle or when negative behaviors such as encopresis or smearing of feces are associated with elimination.

Toilet training for the mentally retarded child requires patience and time. Rarely is it easy. Success, however, has been demonstrated with all levels of retarded children, including the profoundly retarded.

The age for management of toileting varies among retarded children. Some learn at the same age that normal children are toilet-trained, whereas others might never reach any degree of control in taking care of their own toileting needs. In some instances, neurologic impairments or organic conditions such as cerebral palsy, neural tube defects, and constipation make it more difficult to manage the smaller steps that make up the toileting task.

Parents usually are anxious to start working on toileting. Nurses can help them recognize signs of readiness in the child by assessing the child's general developmental status in self-help, motor, and communication skills. Some maturity is necessary in those areas before the child indicates readiness. Bowel training is easier to initiate first because sphincter control is obtained earlier than bladder control. Generally, girls train more easily than boys, but no child should be compared to another.

Observation of the child's defecating around the same time each day signals the parent to put the child on the training potty. The goal is to establish a schedule. Sitting on a potty can be a tense and upsetting experience for some children at first, so this alone might be viewed as an achievement. Therefore, the nurse explains the need for preliminary steps in the toileting process. These might be getting the child to feel comfortable while sitting on the potty and gradually increasing the time until the child understands the purpose of the toilet and what is expected.

The parent can encourage cooperation by engaging the child in a pleasant, relaxing activity such as looking at a picture book or listening to a story or to music. Comfort is enhanced when the feet are flat on the floor or on an elevated box or stool, the trunk is balanced, and the child has something to hold. Balance and support give a sense of security. Once the child is comfortable on the potty, toys and other play items need to be removed gradually so that the child is able to concentrate.

Parents should not be discouraged when the child produces immediately following removal from the potty. Regression too is common in the early stages of toilet training. This is frustrating for parents, so nurses are often needed to lend a supportive ear and to offer hope and reassurance. Accidents are frequently mixed with successes.

Mastering small steps therefore marks progress toward independence in self-care, and nurses need to help parents recognize small successes. The child's clean and dry periods should be rewarded with praise. Mentally retarded children look forward to pleasing their parents and are eager to receive praise following any success.

Nurses also are expected to guide families in selecting specific equipment, aids, and procedures that might be required. Some of the aids are disposable pads and sheets, waterproof pants, disposable bedding, mattress covers, urinals, raised commode seats, toiletries, and deodorants. For children with bladder dysfunction, special equipment is helpful.

Pictures of devices and guidance about using adaptive equipment help parents determine what to purchase. Special potty seats and devices for children with cerebral palsy, for example, are commercially available. A little ingenuity, however, often can be used to improvise special equipment with household items when commercially designed devices are not comfortable or stable.

⊛ Potential knowledge deficit regarding behavior modification as a useful form of discipline

Principles of behaviorism are used to discipline retarded children. Behavior modification, a series of techniques based on behaviorism, is commonly used to bring about changes in the child's behavior. (Behaviorism and behavior modification are discussed in Chapter 3.)

The principal goals of behavior modification are to encourage behaviors that do not occur often enough and to weaken (or extinguish) behaviors that are excessive or undesirable. Molding the behavior of retarded children makes care more rewarding for parents and is a way of teaching self-care. If basic self-care skills such as feeding, dressing, and bathing are not learned, the child does not attain greater independence and is less likely to engage in other activities inside and outside the home. Outside experiences in turn enhance learning.

If behavior modification programs are to be successful, nurses need to believe that retarded individuals can be influenced to achieve positive behavioral outcomes. Behavior programs that are improperly planned and carried out can result in little or no behavior change or in the addition of new and undesirable behaviors.

Time to work with the child and caregiver is vital to observing the behavior in context. In such observations, the nurse notes the behaviors that occur immediately before and after the behavior in question. The nurse is also needed to model positive reinforcement and to monitor progress.

Retarded children often develop inappropriate behavior patterns simply because they are inactive, bored, or lacking in models of normal behavior. Even after the most carefully planned behavior modification program is executed by the most conscientious nurse, the child's family or caregiver needs to be able to carry out the program. The nurse collaborates with caregivers in analyzing the behavior and planning the program. Participation is essential.

Program failure is unavoidable when caregivers are uncommitted or when family dysfunction prohibits adequate follow-through. When behavior modification does fail or is inappropriate for a particular family, the nurse assesses the availability of community support systems. Community resources can help the family cope with the child's day-to-day care and behavior problems.

⊛ Altered sexuality patterns related to the stigma associated with developmental disabilities

Sexuality comprises the ways in which people use gender as a part of their roles, relationships, values, and customs. For developmentally disabled children, sexuality involves understanding and enjoying one's body and gender in ways that are consistent with levels of understanding, function, responsibility for self-care, and cultural norms.

Nurses and other professionals working with the families of retarded children need to examine their own conscious and unconscious attitudes toward developmentally disabled persons as sexual beings. Misconceptions that retarded individuals were sexually aggressive, dangerous, and incapable of heterosexual relationships, whether sensual or platonic, were once commonly accepted assumptions.

Nurses working with parents who are resolving sexual issues plan care to provide anticipatory guidance and education to dispel misinformation. They show respect for parents' values and beliefs, help prevent problems related to sexuality or sexual behavior, and counsel or arrange counseling when the therapy required is beyond the scope of nursing. Above all, a parent needs reassurance that the quality of the child's life is the nurse's primary goal.

Social development In some families the sexual needs of a developmentally disabled child are ignored. Mentally retarded children are often raised in protective environments where they are deprived of many experiences and peer interactions that form the basis for heathy, fulfilling friendships in later years. Some parents of retarded children even tend unconsciously to deprive these children of sensory input and experiences in infancy that enhance normal sexual development. For example, many parents fail to hold, caress, or handle these infants as normal infants are usually handled.

Body awareness Like the normal infant, the developmentally disabled infant learns that the body's senses produce good feelings about oneself through sensual experiences involving the eyes, ears, nose, mouth, and skin. Caressing, stroking, and other behaviors are a part of the bonding process that promotes this awareness.

In learning to discriminate among sensory stimuli, children learn which body parts are most pleasurable and so learn that they can exert control to promote pleasant experiences with their bodies. Parents can facilitate children's sense of control by referring to body parts by name, just as they would for normal children. They also can provide sensory feedback through expressions of happiness, sadness, disappointment, embarrassment, or anger. For example, retarded children frequently are not taught or even permitted to learn physical skills that lead to a sense of mastery of the environment.

Some children grow up lacking basic skills that lead to strategies for making choices or for expressing feelings of pleasure appropriately. Acknowledging feelings and modeling appropriate expressions of emotion are ways to teach control of sensory experiences. Some parents fail to acknowledge that retarded children grow up, even when their children's levels of intelligence are adequate for some of the developmental tasks of normal children.

Sexual behavior When children are severely retarded, many parents and professionals contend that any attention to sex is inappropriate because these children are incapable of learning sexual behavior. When the sexually retarded child masturbates, for example, the parent might be astounded and might want to know where the child learned the behavior. Such parents fail to recognize that natural and instinctive sexual needs are present from birth. A parent's denial of sexual maturation encourages attitudes that the retarded person is sexless and remains a child forever.

As with normal children, discussion of sexuality occurs prior to physical maturity and in the context of other body functions. Sexuality is not an isolated subject. Nurses can help parents understand that young developmentally disabled children should learn about their bodies and how to appreciate them. Parents often need to know that expressions of feeling promote a positive self-image and gender identity. Teaching about privacy to younger retarded children, often through role modeling, encourages the children to learn about sex roles and about the types of behaviors and expression of emotions that are acceptable in private but not in public.

Adolescence Although the physical development of many developmentally disabled adolescents is slower and secondary sex characteristics are acquired much later than normal, these adolescents and their parents have concerns about sexuality and sexual development. Many parents recognize the need to deal with sexual issues in their children but hold back because of insecurity and anxiety. To provide effective management of sexual issues, nurses therefore are required to anticipate the needs of the child and parent.

Sex education For developmentally disabled adolescents, issues surrounding sexuality are similar to those for normal adolescents. The difference lies in the disabled person's lack of appropriate information about physical and emotional changes. Developmentally disabled adolescents need to be taught in simple terms about how male and female bodies work, how they are alike and different, how they grow and mature, how one becomes a mother or father, and how babies are made. When talking about their bodies, developmentally disabled children need to discuss and examine their own bodies, since they often have difficulty applying what they see in drawings and pictures.

Nurses can help parents understand that what their developmentally disabled adolescent needs to know about sexuality can be taught in the context of differentiating self from others, learning about health and hygiene, and developing self-care skills. Sex education thus includes cultural mores, male and female roles, appropriate touching and showing of affection to family members and to others, and heterosexual friendships.

Pubescent girls need preparation for the onset of menstruation so that they know that this is normal. Preparation prevents fear of menstruation and the tendency to try to hide its occurrence from parents or caregivers. Preparation includes teaching about the use of sanitary pads or tampons and special hygiene during the menses. Severely retarded girls might have trouble handling their own care, and in such instances, caregivers usually manage this along with other areas of personal care.

Masturbation As they mature physically, some mentally retarded adolescents experience erotic sensations that they do not understand. As a result they often act out these feelings with inappropriate public display of such behaviors as masturbation. Masturbation is normal, unharmful, and can be gratifying and fulfilling at any age. It is, however, a private matter and can be a problem at an inappropriate time or in the presence of others.

Nurses often need to reassure parents that providing privacy does not encourage masturbation; privacy merely protects the feelings of others and should be ensured regardless of the child's age or functional level. Providing a private place can be difficult in institutional settings where the child's own bedroom is rarely available for privacy, but the masturbating adolescent can be taken to the bathroom and given time alone.

For some adolescents, excessive masturbation might be an indication of boredom and a need for other kinds of stimulation. Parents and caregivers then can provide recreational and enjoyable activities for the retarded child who lacks the ability to choose a variety of gratifying leisure activities.

Interaction with peers For retarded adolescents, friendships with nonretarded adolescents also are extremely important. Such contact provides opportunities for mature role models with appropriate behavior patterns. The developmentally disabled adolescent who is physically handicapped also might have fewer opportunities for what other adolescents experience on their own. Warm, caring, nonintimate friendships enhance social development and help prevent loneliness for the retarded adult. Nurses can explore community groups such as churches, scouting, and civic groups such as the YMCA and YWCA where programs often are designed to integrate the retarded and normal peers in social activities. Helping parents recognize and accept signs of sexual maturity in developmentally disabled adolescents enables parents to dress, groom, and choose personal items appropriate for this developmental stage.

Retarded adolescents experience much of the internal conflict and turmoil of normal adolescents. One sign of this turmoil is moodiness. Retarded adolescents, however, usually lack the verbal skills to describe their emotions. For these children, parents can model and label feelings, pointing out that other people are happy, unhappy, sad, or excited and then pointing out these same emotions when they are experienced by the retarded child.

Parents might fear their child's interest in the opposite sex as a desire for a loving relationship that can lead to sexual intercourse. Nurses can reassure parents that, for the mentally retarded, sexual needs are often not synonymous with sexual intercourse. Retarded adolescents often attend school with normal children, however, and are not protected from the influence of peers, the media, and other environmental factors stressing sexual behavior. When they face peer pressure to engage in intimate relationships, retarded children are known to be compliant, which makes them vulnerable to promiscuity and sexual exploitation.

Reproduction Both parents and society in general often fear reproduction in retarded persons. For many developmentally disabled persons, reproduction is impossible because of hereditary defects associated wth mental retardation or physical disabilities that make reproduction less likely. Infertility in retarded individuals is most common when the level of retardation is severe to moderate (Craft and Craft, 1983). Males with Down's syndrome, for example, are rarely capable of reproduction. Nurses often are asked to refer parents to doctors who will perform hysterectomies or tubal ligation for sterilization. (Parents usually are more concerned about sterilization of retarded girls than boys.)

Today parents can petition the courts for permission to have retarded children sterilized. Some parents believe they should have retarded girls sterilized when they are incapable of caring for their menses, cannot make responsible decisions concerning sexual behavior, and could not care for any children they might have. In these cases some states require that the medical opinions of more than one physician be obtained and that a legal guardian be appointed by the court to act in behalf of a retarded person. Laws governing criteria for deciding such cases, however, vary.

When sterilization is sought solely to prevent an unwanted pregnancy, nurses can inform parents of the various methods of contraception and clinics where contraceptive counseling can be obtained. Retarded persons require diverse solutions to their contraceptive needs. Many factors need consideration when helping retarded persons or their families choose the most appropriate contraceptive method. Some of these factors are individual needs; personality, including degree of motivation and amount of supervision required; other medication taken regularly; and convenience (Craft and Craft, 1983).

⊛ Alteration in family processes related to child's achievement of independence

Some degree of independence is often possible for developmentally disabled adolescents who are functioning with a mild to moderate level of retardation and approaching adulthood. Parents, however, might express ambivalence that their children show readiness to live independently. An adolescent's interest in dating and relationships that can lead to marriage often causes parents to feel uneasy.

Nurses provide support to parents who are in turmoil about letting go of their children. Providing information about supervised group living situations is often a first step. In some communities, retarded young adults live together with relative independence and opportunities to visit indi-

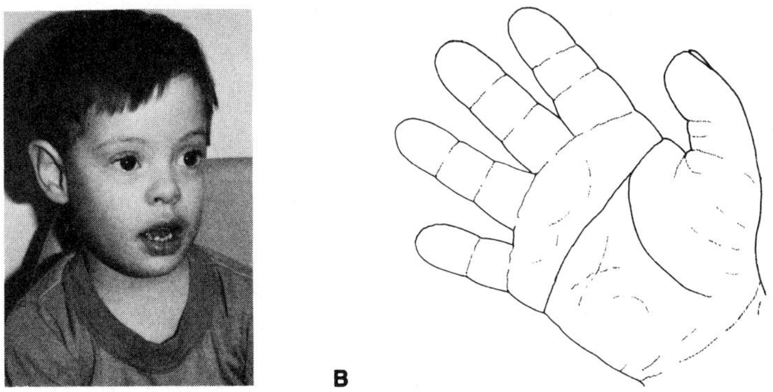

FIGURE 15-8

Down's syndrome (trisomy 21). ***A.*** *The face of a child with Down's syndrome.* ***B.*** *Handprint showing the simian crease, found in the midpalm in about two-thirds of children with Down's syndrome and in those with other congenital disorders. (From Jenkins JB:* Human Genetics. *Benjamin/Cummings, 1983.)*

viduals of the opposite sex who are in similar facilities. This allows greater chance to form heterosexual friendships that indeed might lead to marriage for those who are responsible enough to make decisions and support their families.

The Child with a Disorder Leading to Developmental Disabilities

Down's Syndrome (Trisomy 21)

Down's syndrome, also known as trisomy 21, is the most frequently seen chromosomal aberration. The condition is estimated to affect 5%–10% of all retarded people. Children with Down's syndrome range in cognitive functioning from mild to severely retarded, although most are moderately retarded. With early intervention, many children with Down's syndrome are educable.

Down's syndrome can be detected through prenatal diagnosis. A karyotype of the child's chromosomes shows an extra chromosome number 21. The defect can be the result of errors in the sperm or ovum, causing the zygote to receive an extra chromosome, or it can be the result of an error in cell division.

Down's syndrome is also caused by chromosome translocation. Translocation occurs when an arm of one chromosome abnormally attaches itself to the arm of another. Down's syndrome caused by translocation is genetically transmitted, and the risk for future offspring is much greater than in Down's syndrome caused by trisomy 21.

Children with Down's syndrome usually have characteristic manifestations. These include inner epicanthal folds, simian palmar creases, fifth digits that are short and curved, short necks with loose skin folds, tongues that are thick and protruding, small noses with low bridges, and generalized hypotonia (Fig. 15-8). If amniocentesis has not been performed, a chromosome analysis can confirm the diagnosis.

A number of congenital anomalies also are associated with Down's syndrome. Cardiac defects and subsequent respiratory problems are the most common. Other associated anomalies include renal agenesis, intestinal anomalies, and visual difficulties. The child health nurse who cares for a child with Down's syndrome in the hospital is likely to encounter one of these associated problems. In addition to caring for the child with an associated anomaly, nursing care for the child with Down's syndrome is similar to care for any child with developmental disabilities.

Neonatal Infections Leading to Developmental Disabilities

TORCH infections are intrauterine infections that can have serious effects on the fetus. TORCH is an acronym for toxoplasmosis, other (such as syphilis), rubella, cytomegalovirus, and herpes. Although several of these infections are asymptomatic in the mother, the consequences in the child can be immense. Consequences can include prematurity or small for gestational age (SGA) infants, microcephaly, seizures, liver dysfunction, eye defects, thermoregulatory dysfunction, rashes, hypotonia, abnormal spinal fluid, and associated anomalies. Some of these children are mentally retarded, whereas others might have severe learning disabilities.

The extent of organ damage from intrauterine infections depends on the stage of organ development at the time of infection. (Herpes and syphilis are discussed in Chapter 28. See Table 15-3 for toxoplasmosis, cytomegalic inclusion disease, and congenital rubella.)

TABLE 15-3 TORCH

Infection	Etiology	Clinical manifestation	Nursing consideration
Toxoplasmosis	*Toxoplasma gondii.* Cats are a reservoir and communicate the organism to humans through fecal/oral contact. Spreads to the fetus through the placenta	Inflammation of the choroid and retina, SGA, failure to thrive, liver dysfunction, lymphadenopathy, hypotonia, intracranial calcifications, abnormal spinal fluid, hydrocephaly	Advise pregnant women to avoid strange cats and contact with cat litter. Thorough cooking of meat will kill the organism
Cytomegalic disease (CMV)	Cytomegalovirus. Human reservoir. The virus is shed in secretions, urine, and breast milk. The fetus acquires it via ascending infection from the vagina or through the placenta	Prematurity, SGA, microcephaly, seizures, failure to thrive, liver dysfunction, bleeding tendencies, thermoregulatory dysfunction, rashes, hypotonia, meningitis, severe learning disorders from deafness, mental retardation	Pregnant women need to avoid exposure. Isolate infants who are actively shedding the virus. CMV can remain in the nasopharynx and urine for a number of years
Rubella	RNA virus of the togavirus group. Spread by droplet or congenitally through the placenta	SGA, seizures, failure to thrive, liver dysfunction, inflammation of the choroid and retina, cataracts, pneumonitis and altered immunoglobulins, rash, hypotonia, congenital heart disease, severe disabilities and mental retardation	Childhood rubella immunizations prevent transmission. Pregnancy is contraindicated for 3 months after vaccination. Blood titer elevation indicates exposure

SOURCE: Kohl S: Infection in the newborn. In: *Infectious Diseases of Children and Adults.* Pickering LK, DuPont H (editors). Addison-Wesley, 1986.

Fetal Alcohol Syndrome

Fetal alcohol syndrome (FAS) affects 1–2 infants per 1000 live births and is the leading preventable cause of congenital defects and mental retardation.

Estimates suggest that there are 2.5 million female alcoholics of childbearing age in the United States. Studies indicate that a pregnant woman is at risk if she drinks 3 oz or more of absolute alcohol (100% alcohol) per day. This is equivalent to about six to eight average-size drinks. Intake of ten drinks per week increases the risk of birthweight below the tenth percentile. (Care of infants who are small for gestational age is discussed in Chapter 34.) Infants of mothers who smoke and have only five drinks per week also are at increased risk for low birthweight.

Infants with FAS have varying degrees of retardation and low birthweight. Anomalies include prenatal and postnatal growth deficiency; small head size; and facial anomalies, including droopy eyelids, a wide space between the nose and upper lip, a thin upper lip, and, occasionally, cleft palate and congenital heart disease.

Even when they do not show signs of FAS, infants of drinking mothers might be at high risk for neonatal respira-

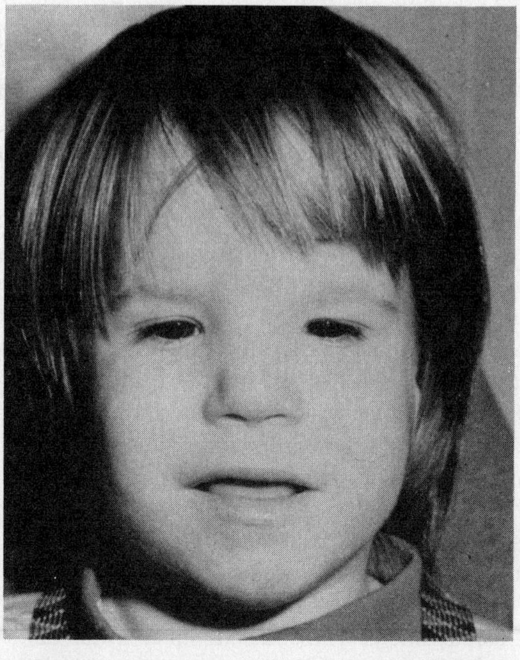

A child with fetal alcohol syndrome (FAS) has distinctive facial characteristics that will vary with the severity of the disability.

NURSING CARE PLAN *The Infant with Fetal Alcohol Syndrome*

Assessment data: Karena is an 8-month-old infant who is being seen in the clinic upon referral from the public health nurse. She is brought in by her mother. Mrs. M tells the clinic nurse that Karena is a very difficult baby to care for. She cries all the time and feeds poorly, spitting up after almost every feeding. Mrs. M's other two children were not like this as babies. Mrs. M appears quite impatient and disorganized and expresses feelings of helplessness with this baby.

Karena was a full-term, small for gestational age infant, weighing only 4 lb 11 oz. She stayed in the newborn nursery a total of 10 days for weight gain and observation. In the nursery, she was noted to be jittery, have features of microcephaly, small eyes, flat midface with a thin upper lip, hypoplastic nails on the fifth toes, and thick hair on the face and extremities, all signs of fetal alcohol syndrome.

Karena is a small infant (fifth percentile for height and weight), fretful, and uninterested in cuddling. Developmental assessment revealed milestones at approximately a 4-month level. Physical examination revealed features similar to those noted at birth.

The family consists of Mr. M, 27 years old; Mrs. M, 26 years old; and two other children, aged 3 and 5 years. Mrs. M did not work during the pregnancy, and her obstetric history reveals that she admitted to "only occasional alcohol intake." She states she drank two 12 oz cans of beer each night with Mr. M and three cans a day on weekends. She consumed two 4-oz glasses of dinner wine when she and her husband went out for their weekly Friday night dinner together. At her husband's office Christmas party, she recalled having drunk three mixed drinks and two glasses of wine, but denies being intoxicated.

The Ms live in a small neighborhood with relatives about a hundred miles away. Mrs. M has no close friends and few social outlets. Mr. M is a partner in an insurance business and works long hours.

Nursing diagnosis	Intervention	Rationale
1. Alterations in parenting related to the child's unresponsiveness to nurturing attempts	Encourage the mother to explore her feelings about Karena's fretful and unresponsive behavior; determine how she reacts to situations when this behavior occurs.	Defining a pattern of response is essential to determining a plan of action.
	Observe with Mrs. M times of the day when Karena seems less irritable.	Nurturing activities might be rewarded if they coincide with times the child is less irritable.
	Encourage Mrs. M to cuddle Karena after feedings and to persist for a while even though Karena might resist; gradually increase the cuddling time.	Cuddling provides security and assists with the development of trust. Children who react adversely to being touched can learn to accept it if exposed to it in a gradual fashion.
	Observe Mrs. M's nurturing behaviors toward her younger children; discuss how she could improve behaviors if problems exist.	Both siblings might have been neglected when Mrs. M was drinking.
	Observe Mr. M's relationship with the infant and with other children in the family.	Nurturing might be assumed by the father of the family; however, if the father is absent most of the time, it is unlikely he assumes a nurturing role and might need encouragement to do so.

Outcome: The parents will be able to verbalize their children's need for physical and emotional nurturing. Parents will identify nurturing behaviors and begin to use them with their children.

(Continues)

NURSING CARE PLAN *The Infant with Fetal Alcohol Syndrome (Continued)*

Nursing diagnosis	Intervention	Rationale
2. Alterations in family processes related to the mother's alcohol consumption and her lack of supports	Explore with Mrs. M her present drinking patterns; have a nonjudgmental attitude while listening.	A trusting nurse-patient relationship is the first step toward helping Mrs. M face denial of her drinking problem. Nonjudgmental attitudes avoid provoking guilt.
	Strongly recommend to Mrs. M that she be referred to an outpatient facility for counseling to assess her alcohol consumption and to determine an appropriate treatment plan—inpatient or outpatient.	Denial and projection are the two main defenses of persons with alcohol-related problems; Mrs. M needs to be presented with the reality of the situation.
	Determine Mr. M's understanding of his wife's pattern of alcohol consumption.	Denial also is the main coping mechanism of spouses of persons with alcohol-related problems.
	Encourage Mrs. M to make more frequent contact with her extended family and use them actively for support.	Having frequent contact with an extended family can prevent isolation and reduce the emotional need for alcohol.
	Explore her interests with Mrs. M and encourage her to join community activities that reflect her interests.	Developing outside interests provides additional supports that can assist Mrs. M and decrease her social isolation and opportunities for drinking.
	Discuss alternate activities to eating out that Mr. and Mrs. M can do together.	Avoiding restaurants decreases the social opportunities for alcohol consumption.

Outcome: Mrs. M will acknowledge her dependence on alcohol and will seek appropriate treatment. Mrs. M will begin to develop a support network outside of her immediate family.

Nursing diagnosis	Intervention	Rationale
3. Altered growth and development related to inadequate nutrition, possible maternal inattention, and sequelae of FAS	Observe Karena at feeding time and record intake for 3 days to compile assessment of nutritional status; observe Mrs. M's feeding technique.	A record of dietary intake is a very effective means of monitoring caloric intake.
	Collaborate with a nutritionist to find ways to increase Karena's intake of nutrients.	Calories over and above the required amount might be required to promote weight gain in Karena.
	Measure linear growth and weight monthly.	Measurement of growth at selected intervals is a reliable, objective indicator of utilization of nutrients.
	Teach mother ways to attempt reducing Karena's spitting up—burping frequently, cuddling in an upright position, feeding solids slowly.	Karena might be losing considerable calories when spitting up and this can become habitual.
	Design an infant stimulation program to teach Mrs. M appropriate play activities that will decrease Karena's resistance to touch while promoting acquisition of new skills.	Infant stimulation programs are essential in assisting mentally retarded children to grow and develop.
	Coordinate services to the family and discuss Karena's progress with her primary health care providers and other professionals who are closely involved in her care. Make a recommendation of referral for a comprehensive developmental evaluation for some specific time in the future.	Because FAS is irreversible, further developmental assessments are necessary as Karena grows.

Outcome: Karena will gain at least 2 pounds in the next month. Karena's mother will understand the principles of good infant nutrition and will be willing to cooperate with methods for increasing caloric and nutritional intake. Karena's development will show steady improvement as determined by monthly assessment.

tory depression, small stature, attention deficit disorders, and poor school performance. A small percentage of children are diagnosed with FAS in the nursery, but most are not identified until late infancy or early childhood. Some are not identified at all.

Nursing care for the child with FAS is similar to care for any child with developmental disabilities. The nurse gives special attention to the emotional and social problems of the mother. An important nursing responsibility is prevention of FAS through community education.

Essential Concepts

- The influence of heredity on the developing person is complex and often cannot be isolated from environmental factors.
- Genes, the biologic units of heredity, are reproduced by DNA replication and chromosome division.
- Any genetic defect occurring in the embryo will affect proper growth and function of the system involved.
- The genetic makeup of an organism—genotype—is expressed in the phenotype—the sum of observable traits.
- Traits are inherited through various modes, including autosomal, sex-linked, and multifactorial.
- Nurses need to be aware of the genetic role in development to intervene appropriately with families at risk for genetic defects.
- The child health nurse can intervene by identifying and referring high-risk families for appropriate counseling, as well as by educating the public regarding the importance of prevention.
- Mental retardation is part of a broad spectrum of developmental disabilities and is distinguished by intellectual deficits and concurrent lack of adaptive behaviors.
- Mental retardation is classified according to degree, from mild to profound.
- Diagnosis of mental retardation includes intelligence testing and measurements of adaptive behavior.
- Child health nurses are involved in the care of developmentally disabled children in both hospital settings and school settings.
- Nursing care for developmentally disabled children is usually part of a multidisciplinary collaboration that might include physicians; social workers; mental health therapists; physical, speech, and occupational therapists; and community agencies.
- Overall nursing goals in the care of developmentally disabled children include screening for disabilities, assisting parents in adjusting to the birth of a disabled child, planning and implementing programs that promote optimal child and family functioning, and managing acute care for children with medical problems.
- Nursing care of the developmentally disabled child is directed toward providing adequate nutrition, promoting appropriate sexual development and expression of sexuality, and encouraging independence in activities of daily living.
- Down's syndrome, fetal alcohol syndrome, and TORCH infections are conditions that commonly cause developmental disabilities in children.

References

Ayala FJ, Kiger JA: *Modern Genetics,* 2nd ed. Benjamin / Cummings, 1984.

Blackman JA: *Medical Aspects of Developmental Disabilities in Children Birth to Three: A Resource for Special Service Providers in the Educational Setting.* The University of Iowa, 1983.

Craft A, Craft M: *Sex Education and Counseling for Mentally Handicapped People.* University Park Press, 1983.

Grossman HJ: *Classification in Mental Retardation.* American Association on Mental Deficiency, 1983.

Thain WS, Casto G, Peterson A: *Normal and Handicapped Children: A Growth and Development Primer for Parents and Professionals.* PSG Publishing, 1980.

Zelle RS, Coyner AB: *Developmentally Disabled Infants and Toddlers: Assessment and Intervention.* Davis, 1983.

Additional Readings

Applewhite S, Busbee D, Burgaonkar D (editors): *Genetic Screening and Counseling in Multidisciplinary Perspective.* Thomas, 1981.

Casey P, Bradley R: The impact of the home environment on children's development. *J Dev Behav Pediatr* 1982; 3: 146–152.

Dickey RP: *Managing Contraceptive Pill Patients,* 3rd ed. Creative Informatics, 1983.

Elder JO, Magrab PR: *Coordinating Services to Handicapped Children: A Handbook for Interagency Collaboration.* Brookes, 1980.

Evard J R: Fetal alcohol syndrome. In: *Providing Care for Children of Alcoholics: Clinical and Research Perspectives.* Lewis O, Williams C (editors). Health Communications, Inc., 1986.

Fibison WJ: The nursing role in the delivery of genetic services. *Issues in Health Care of Women* 1983; 4:1–13.

Gilbert W: Gene sequencing and gene structure. *Science* (Dec 18) 1981; 212:1305–1312.

Hatcher RA et al: *Contraceptive Technology,* 12th revised ed. Irvington, 1984.

Haynes U: *Holistic Health Care for Children with Developmental Disabilities with Special Reference to Young Children with Neuromotor Dysfunctions.* University Park Press, 1983.

Herr SS: *Rights and Advocacy for Retarded People.* Lexington Books, 1983.

Jenkins JB: *Human Genetics.* Benjamin / Cummings, 1983.

Keele DK: *The Developmentally Disabled Child: A Manual for Primary Physicians.* Medical Economics, 1983.

Kopelman L, Moskop JC: *Ethics and Mental Retardation.* D. Reidel, 1984.

Kozlowski BW: *University Affiliated Facilities' Collaborative Study of Nutritional Status of Developmentally Delayed Children.* University Research Foundation, 1981.

Krajicek MJ: Developmental disability and human sexuality. *Nurs Clin North Am* (Sept) 1982; 17:377–378.

Krajicek MJ, Tearney Tomlinsin AI: *Detection of Developmental Problems in Children: Birth to Adolescence,* 2nd ed. University Park Press, 1983.

Levy-Shiff R: Mother-father-child interactions in families with a mentally retarded young child. *Am J Ment Deficiencies* 1986; 91(2):141–147.

Marx J: Antibodies: Getting their genes together. *Science* (May 29) 1981; 212:1015–1017.

Matson JL, Breuning SE: *Assessing the Mentally Retarded.* Grune & Stratton, 1983.

Maxwell BM: The nursing role in the Special Olympics. *J School Health* (March) 1984; 54:131–133.

McKusick V: *Mendelian Inheritance in Man,* 6th ed. Johns Hopkins University Press, 1982.

Menolascino FJ, Newman R, Stark JA: *Curative Aspects of Mental Retardation: Biomedical and Behavioral Advances.* Brookes, 1983.

Mertens TR, Hendrix JR, Morris M: Nursing educators: Perceptions of the curricular role of human genetics/bioethics. *J Nurs Educ* (March) 1984; 23(3):98–104.

Miezio PM: *Parenting Children with Disabilities: A Professional Source for Physicians and Guide for Parents.* Marcel Dekker, 1983.

Olds S: *Maternal-Newborn Nursing,* 2nd ed. Addison-Wesley, 1984.

Parker G: Incontinence services for the disabled child. Part 1: The provision of aids and equipment. *Health Visitor* (Feb) 1984b; 57:44–45.

Parker G: Incontinence services for the disabled child. Part 2: The provision of information and advice. *Health Visitor* (March) 1984a; 57:86–88.

Payne JS, Patton JR: *Mental Retardation.* Merrill, 1981.

Scarr S, Kidd K: Developmental behavior genetics. In: *Mussen Handbook of Child Psychology.* Haith M, Campos J (editors). Wiley, 1982.

Scheerenberger RC: *A History of Mental Retardation.* Brookes, 1983.

Smithells RW et al: Further experience of vitamin supplementation for prevention of neural tube defect recurrences. *Lancet* (May 7) 1983; 8332:1027–1031.

Stephens CJ: The fetal alcohol syndrome: Cause for concern. *Matern-Child Nurs J* (July/Aug) 1981; 6(4):251–256.

Stephenson SR, Weaver DD: Prenatal diagnosis—a compilation of diagnosed conditions. *Am J Obstet Gynecol* 1981; 141:319.

Strauss S, Munton M: Common concerns of parents with disabled children. *Pediatr Nurs* 1985; 11:371–375.

Summer G, Shoaf C: Developments in genetic and metabolic screening. *Fam Community Health* (Feb) 1982; 4:16–27.

Tishler CL: The psychological aspects of genetic counseling. *Am J Nurs* 1981; 81:733–734.

White J: Special nursing needs of hospitalized children with learning disabilities. *Am J Matern-Child Nurs* (May/June) 1983; 8:209–212.

Wikler L, Keenan MP: *Developmental Disabilities: No Longer a Private Tragedy.* National Association of Social Workers, 1983.

Williams DN: Becoming a woman: The girl who is mentally retarded. *Pediatr Nurs* (Mar/Apr) 1987; 13(2):89–93.

Williams J: Genetic counseling in pediatric nursing care. *Pediatr Nurs* (July/Aug) 1986; 12(4):287–289.

Chapter 16

Nursing Care of the Child with a Psychosocial Disorder

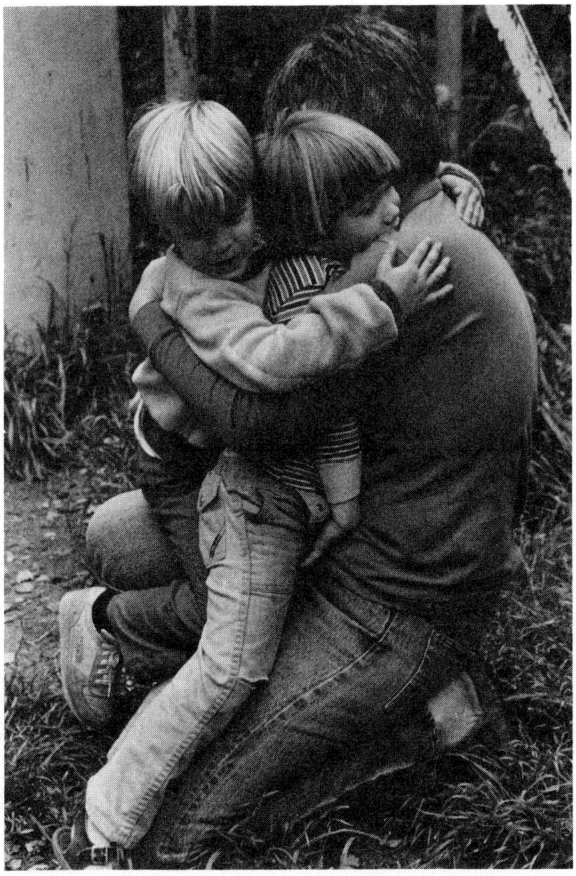

Chapter Contents

(Continues)

Objectives

- Define the types of coping behaviors that children use to adapt to stress.
- Identify the factors that influence coping strategies.
- Define the principal coping strategies used by children.
- Explain how the styles of coping change as the child matures.
- Define basic techniques that can assist children in learning to cope.
- Describe dysfunctional behavior as an outcome of maladaptive coping.
- Describe the role of the nurse in identifying psychiatric disorders in children.
- Identify factors that contribute to psychiatric disorders in children.
- Explain the *Diagnostic and Statistical Manual of Psychiatric Disorders* (DSM III) and its applicability to child health nursing.
- Describe assessment criteria and nursing management of children with selected behavioral, emotional, physical, and developmental disorders.

Childhood is a period of rapid biophysical, affective, cognitive, and social development. It is a time that requires children to adjust to demands made by family, schools, churches, the legal system, peer groups, and other social networks. Adjusting to these demands is one of the child's primary developmental tasks. The complex process of development and the problems related to establishing social relationships, however, often make this task difficult to achieve.

The child's mental and emotional health is evident in the behaviors exhibited at each developmental stage. The nurse considers these behaviors during a developmental assessment. The nurse's observing and noting age-appropriate behaviors enables parents and others responsible for the well-being of children to identify and seek early intervention for children at risk.

With a projected increase in the number of children who enter the health care system each year, nurses in a variety of child health care settings can expect to find children exhibiting behaviors that indicate some degree of developmental risk. Indeed, the majority of children and adolescents seen for mental health assistance present problems due to conflicts or faulty life experiences.

Coping as Adaptation

Throughout childhood, children use specific behaviors as ways of achieving growth and equilibrium. These behaviors are strategies by which the child learns to cope with maturational and situational stressors and to manage the world more effectively. *Coping strategies* are therefore learned behaviors that are influenced by the child's prior experiences, stage of development, environmental demands, areas of vulnerability, and significant role models. Coping strategies are specific behaviors the child uses to deal with challenges, threats, or problems (Table 16-1).

For example, 5-year-old David was always well behaved in school until his parents adopted a baby. Suddenly, he became aggressive, pushing and hitting other children to be first in line or closest to the teacher. He appeared to feel that the baby had taken over first place in his parents' affections. For David, the aggression was a coping strategy. Releasing his anger at school allowed him to cope with the stress of a new baby at home. The behavior was a normal, age-appropriate response to a perceived threat.

Normal children at any age use a variety of behaviors to

TABLE 16-1 Specific Coping Strategies

Strategy	Definition	Example
Displacement	Strategy that shifts emotional energy from the stressful object or situation to one that is less threatening	The adolescent who is angry at a parent punches a door rather than the parent
Regression	Return to a behavior used in a previous stage of development in order to cope with a threatening situation	A toilet-trained three-year-old who returns to wetting or soiling to cope with the introduction of a new baby in the home
Denial	Suppression of an awareness of people or events that could be threatening	A child who tells about success in schoolwork to avoid acknowledging difficulties
Projection	Placing negative feelings and qualities in others while denying they originate in self	The child who uses a doll or puppet to express fears or anxieties that the child actually has
Rationalization	The development of a false justification of behavior to hide an anxiety-provoking situation	Children afraid they might fail in team sports claim they are too busy to join the team. "The other kids made me do it" is a common rationalization of childhood
Sublimation	Behavior that focuses attention on a substitute for an unacceptable feeling	The child who expresses anger or fear through artistic expression
Attack	Verbal or physical aggression in response to fear	The child who attempts to take equipment away from the examiner during a physical examination or who screams or hits
Identification	A socialization process by which a child takes on or internalizes characteristics of another	A child who identifies with a parent, teacher, or other authority figure by dress or speech
Temper tantrums	Screaming, kicking, or pounding in response to frustration, fears, or difficulty with self-control	The two-year-old who screams every time the parent says "no"
Fantasy	Imaginary role change used by children to conquer fear, act out aggression, avoid stressful situations, and try out new roles. Fantasy is a form of play	Children who pretend to be astronauts, princesses, mothers, fathers, and superhuman beings
Daydreaming	A form of fantasy that is a method of obtaining omnipotence so that one can cope with feelings of vulnerability	A child who imagines inventing an important piece of scientific equipment

reduce stress. These strategies can be classified into three major categories:

1. Strategies that allow the child to seek help from others
2. Strategies that allow the child to ignore the threat or to diminish its importance
3. Strategies that allow the child to deal with the threat before it actually happens (Pearlin and Schooler, 1978).

In some instances, coping strategies are *defense mechanisms,* behaviors that defend the child's ego against situations of severe stress. Defense mechanisms are indirect ways of coping with a stressor. They give the child time to organize resources to deal with the stress.

Factors Influencing Coping

A variety of interacting factors influence the coping behaviors of children and adolescents:

Developmental stage Each stage brings its own stressors with which the child must cope, and each stage involves its own normal coping behaviors. For example, temper tantrums, which are normal coping strategies during early and middle childhood, become abnormal as the child's cognitive development permits the child to internalize anger and cope intellectually.

Temperament Each child has a behavioral style when

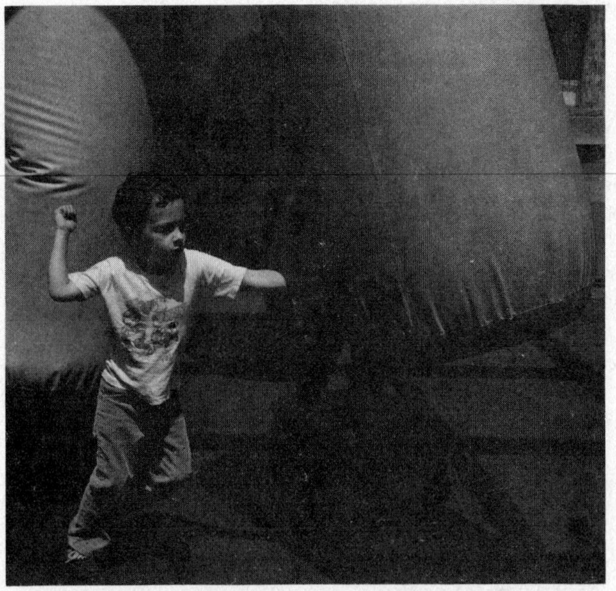

The releasing of a child's feelings of aggression may be channeled into less harmful and more acceptable directions.

TABLE 16-2 Process for Problem Solving

Step	Characteristics
1. Establishing a set	1. The child's orientation to the problem, which includes strengths, weaknesses, and innate and learned resources
2. Defining the problem	2. The child's ability to identify and set priority for the problem objectively
3. Identifying resources	3. The child's accumulation of all available information about resources that might be used to solve the problem
4. Generating solutions	4. The child's generation of as many solutions as possible
5. Implementing solutions	5. The child's attempt to initiate solutions
6. Evaluating outcomes	6. The child's determination that solutions are effective

reacting to stress. The child's style depends on immediate environment and genetic factors. Temperament changes as the child grows, thus changing the child's coping style.

Previous experiences The long-term effects of stressful events are related to the ways in which the child has dealt with stress previously and whether the child coped successfully then.

Role models Support and example of parents and peer group can influence the way children cope with stress. Personal success in coping at home and in other settings helps children to develop the self-esteem needed to cope with stressful life events.

Techniques for Learning Coping Strategies

Solving problems effectively Stressful events can be viewed as both times of danger and opportunities for growth. In adapting to the stress, the child can grow, effectively and cognitively, by learning to solve problems posed by the stressor.

Perhaps the greatest challenge to children is to develop effective problem-solving skills appropriate to each phase of development. Even small children use rudimentary problem-solving skills in their activities of daily living. For example, the child might learn to withdraw from play situations when not successful at each attempt. Withdrawal is the child's way of coping with being unsuccessful, yet it allows the child to observe the activity and to learn how to do it successfully.

Problem solving is a six-step process (Table 16-2). Coping strategies are adaptive when problem solving is effective and assists the child in interacting with the environment. The child's ability to solve problems, perceive threats, and use effective coping strategies grows in direct relation to developmental progress. In this way, coping and adaptation continue to be linked to the child's developmental stage.

Reducing stress A child can learn to cope with stress by relaxing rather than fleeing from the source of the stress. Children learn to reduce stress by responding actively to it. Parents and others can teach children to minimize negative reactions to stressful events. Some cognitive coping strategies include the following (Davis, Shelmar, & McKay, 1980):

Preparation for stress	Confronting stress
There's nothing to worry about	Stay organized
I'm going to be all right	Take it step by step; don't rush
I've succeeded with this before	I can do this; I'm doing it now
What exactly do I have to do?	I can only do my best
I know I can do each one of these tasks	I can get help if I need it
It's easier once you get started	It's OK to make mistakes

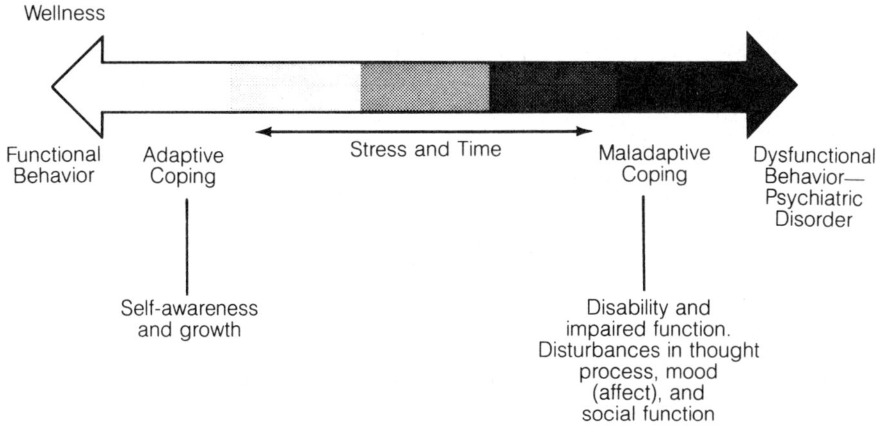

FIGURE 16-1
Adaptive-maladaptive continuum.

Dysfunctional Behavior as Maladaptive Coping

Learning to cope with situational and developmental stressors promotes effective problem solving. Coping strategies, however, offer only a temporary means of dealing with problems. When the child does not learn effective long-term strategies for dealing with stress, the child becomes vulnerable to maladaptive coping. *Maladaptive coping strategies* are ineffective behaviors that a child uses over time to deal with real or perceived threats or stressors. Maladaptive coping results in dysfunctional behavior.

Dysfunctional behavior is characterized by deficient problem-solving skills and increased vulnerability to stress. Because coping is maladaptive, the child has difficulty interacting with the external environment, which in turn generates more stress. Over time, the dysfunctional behavior can prevent interpersonal growth and inhibit social development.

Dysfunctional behavior threatens the child's mental health and developmental progress and therefore requires nursing interventions. The child health nurse needs to conduct systematic assessments over a period of time before identifying a pattern of behavior that is maladaptive. Assessment of behavior in children begins by comparing a child's affective and social development to normal ranges for each developmental stage (see Chapters 3–8). The child health nurse then analyzes the assessment data with attention to areas of developmental vulnerability. Areas of concern include:

- Developmental delays: physical and psychologic
- Developmental progress
- Illnesses of childhood
- Immunizations
- Peer relations
- Parent-child interactions
- School/play activities
- Temperament
- Significant losses
- Separations from significant people

Once identified, developmental vulnerability indicates a lowered resistance to stress.

Adaptive-Maladaptive Continuum

Behavior and adaptation can be viewed as a continuum (Fig. 16-1). At one end of the continuum lies functional behavior, correlated with adaptive coping strategies. At the other end lies dysfunctional behavior, correlated with maladaptive coping strategies. As the child's behavior becomes increasingly dysfunctional, developmental vulnerability also increases.

Viewing the child's behavior as part of a continuum aids the nurse in a holistic assessment of the child's developmental progress. Identifying patterns of dysfunction and degrees of adaptation helps the nurse in determining the extent of disability and the type of intervention required. The child who exhibits habitual dysfunctional behavior or coping strategies that are clearly maladaptive is at psychosocial risk. The nurse might then need to refer the child to the appropriate specialist for further evaluation.

Nursing Care for the Child with Dysfunctional Behavior

Providing for the psychosocial needs of children with severe dysfunctional behavior presents the child health nurse with a challenge. Children with severe problems typically expe-

FIGURE 16-2
Factors that contribute to psychiatric disorders in children.

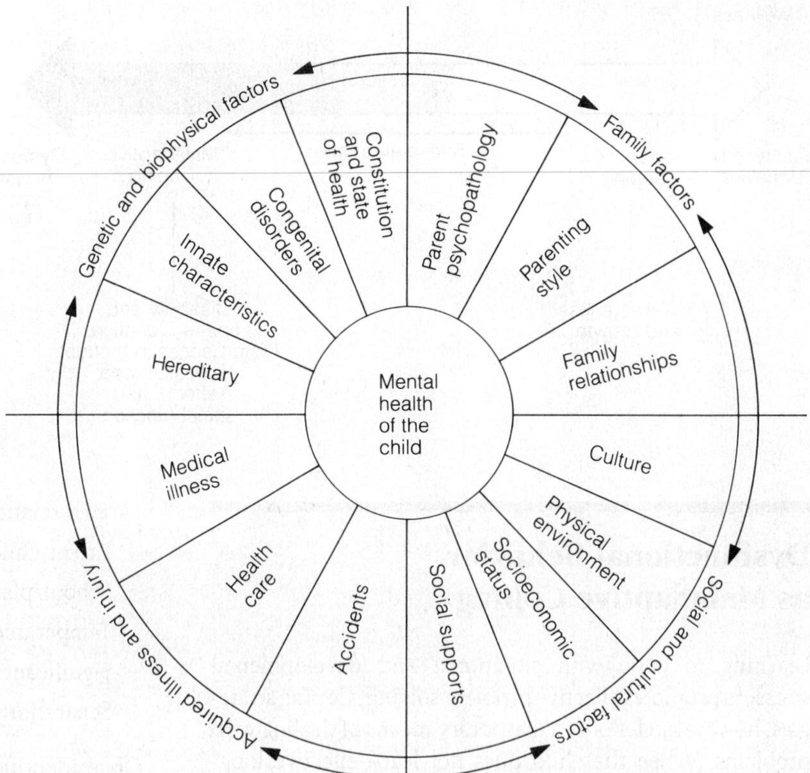

rience difficulties functioning with their families, schools, and communities. They tend to exhibit developmental delays, which cause them to lag behind their peers. They might experience somatic (physical) problems, communication difficulties, or confused sense of reality.

Identifying dysfunctional behavior in children is difficult because of the lack of a reliable, objective system for classifying emotional and behavioral problems. The difficulty is compounded by the differences across developmental stages, each of which poses a distinctive set of norms. Some underlying principles, however, are useful to the child health nurse:

1. Assessments are not limited to isolated behaviors and traits but identify patterns of maladaptive behaviors over time.
2. Assessments of dysfunctional behavior are made relative to expected developmental norms for age, gender, environment, developmental tasks, and level of function.
3. Dysfunctional behavior can be transitory. Current problems do not mean that the child has exhibited dysfunctional behavior in the past, nor do they predict dysfunctional behavior in the future.
4. Certain physical factors such as toxic substances, therapeutic regimens, lead poisoning, degenerative brain disease, and drug and alcohol ingestion can produce dysfunctional behavior that is not necessarily a result of maladaptive coping.

Assessment Nurses frequently encounter children with psychosocial problems, therefore they assess the child's psychologic functioning. Child health nurses also provide care for children with psychiatric disorders, a process that requires planning and communication with the child's other health care providers.

Factors influencing mental health Because of the many causes of dysfunctional behaviors and psychiatric disorders in children, the child health nurse considers a number of factors that might influence the mental health of the child (Fig. 16-2). The primary etiologic factors generally fit the following four categories:

1. Genetic and biophysical factors
2. Social and cultural factors
3. Family factors
4. Acquired illness and injury

For any particular child, however, it is not possible to isolate specific factors leading to a dysfunctional behavior or a

TABLE 16-3 Areas for the Assessment of Psychologic Functioning in Children

Child	Parent
General appearance	Developmental history
Grooming	Health history
Hygiene	Description of typical day in child's life
Orientation—time, place, person	Behavioral concerns—frequency, severity
Motor behavior—fine, gross	Digestion and elimination
Ability to relate/socialization	Sleep
Peers—best friend/ages	Appetite
Adults	Motor activity
Ability to separate from parents	Speech
Activities	Vision and hearing
Interests, hobbies	Mannerisms
Groups	Aggression—toward self and others
Chores	School history
Ability to have fun	Family
Speech/language	Structure
Expressive language	Developmental stage
Receptive language	Parent-child interaction—warmth, empathy, spontaneity, physical nurturing
Content	Activities
Mood (affect)	Discipline
Behavior—skills and activities of daily living	Social supports
Attitudes	History of psychotropic drugs
School—teacher, homework, performance	Dose
Hospitalization or other health care	Duration
Family—parents, siblings, significant extended family	Effect on mood, activity
Self-concept and body image	Side effects
Behavior	Child's extrafamily relationships
Aggression, fears, ability to follow limits	Peers
	School
	Antisocial behavior

psychiatric disorder. Mental health professionals tend instead to view the causes of any dysfunction as an accumulation or interaction of factors.

Child health nurses base assessments on an understanding of diverse etiologic factors and normal processes of growth and development. Data are then validated with parents or primary caregivers (Table 16-3).

The therapeutic relationship Accurate psychosocial assessment depends on effective data collection. The nurse-parent and nurse-child interview is the vehicle by which data are acquired. Therefore, regardless of the severity of the psychosocial problem and resultant dysfunctional behavior, the therapeutic relationship begins with the first interaction. The setting might be a well-child clinic, school nurse's office, or acute-care unit. Common to all settings is the child health nurse's awareness that the child does not seek intervention, might not be aware that behavior is problematic, and might not perceive parental distress. Therefore, a positive initial contact with parent and child is essential to establish trust between parent, child, and child health nurse. (Table 16-4 provides an overview of techniques that facilitate communication and enhance the assessment process.)

Nursing management Nurses intervene with children who are at risk for dysfunctional behavior related to maladaptive coping and with children who have psychiatric disorders. Child health nurses intervene directly at all levels of prevention (Table 16-5), although tertiary prevention requires the skills of nurse specialists in child psychiatry. Child health nurses in many settings, however, frequently encounter children with suspected psychiatric problems and therefore need to assess psychologic functioning.

For children with existing or potential problems causing dysfunctional behavior, the child health nurse might be

TABLE 16-4 Effective Communication with Children and Parents

Child health nurse behaviors	Rationale
Maintain neutral position in attitudes and comments	Awareness of a positive relationship between nurse and parent by the child facilitates the child's trust
Reassure and support parents in initial contacts	Allowing parents to discuss successes and frustration at coping with the child's behavior enables parents to gain confidence in the parenting role
Provide opportunities for parents to describe problems	Clarification of parental perceptions of the problem enhances their potential to help the child
Maintain a nonjudgmental position when gathering information from each parent	Parental trust is gained when positive feedback and reinforcement is provided
Assess the need for the child to have the parent(s) participate in the interview	Children move slowly into new relationships and might require the presence of someone to ease the transition
Modify nonverbal communication when attempting to communicate with a child	Modifying one's gestures according to the child's tempo facilitates the child's comfort in a new situation
Assess the child's tolerance for physical touch	The use of touch when establishing a relationship with a child is an important nonverbal communication to be used with care
Assess the degree to which encouraging the parent to assume the parental role is therapeutic	Encouraging the parent to resume the parental role to develop satisfaction in the parent-child relationship is essential

SOURCE: Adapted from Beck, Rawlins, & Williams. *Mental Health Psychiatric Nursing, A Holistic Life Cycle Approach.* Mosby, 1984.

TABLE 16-5 Levels of Prevention and Child Health Nursing Interventions

Level of prevention	Nursing intervention
Primary prevention: Maintain wellness and prevent onset of dysfunctional behavior	1. Observe prenatal factors (ie, acceptance of pregnancy, age of parents, number of children in the family) 2. Provide anticipatory guidance throughout the child's development: ■ Observe parent-infant attachment ■ Observe parenting skills ■ Teach parent about normal development and realistic expectations ■ Provide support and refer to other services if necessary
Secondary prevention: Prevent disability through early diagnosis	1. Observe and monitor behavior that differs from established developmental norms 2. Refer for diagnostic evaluation and treatment a child whose behavior is a cause of parental or others' concern
Tertiary prevention: Provide rehabilitative activities that promote the highest level of function	1. Establish a therapeutic milieu 2. Teach parent about the child's social and emotional development 3. Function as a child advocate 4. Function as a child and/or family therapist

TABLE 16-6 Disorders First Evident in Infancy, Childhood, and Adolescence

Intellectual disorders	Behavioral disorders	Emotional disorders	Physical disorders	Developmental disorders
Mental retardation Mild Moderate Severe Profound	Attention deficit disorder With hyperactivity Without hyperactivity Conduct disorders Aggressive Nonaggressive Socialized Undersocialized	Anxiety disorders Separation anxiety disorders Avoidant disorder Overanxious disorders Reactive attachment disorder Schizoid disorder Elective disorder Oppositional disorder Identity disorder	Eating disorders Anorexia nervosa Bulimia Pica Rumination disorder Stereotyped movement disorders Chronic motor tic Transient tic Tourette's disease Disorders with physical manifestations Stuttering Functional enuresis Functional encopresis Sleepwalking disorder Sleep terror disorder	Pervasive developmental disorders Infantile autism Childhood-onset pervasive developmental disorder Specific developmental disorders Reading disorder Arithmetic disorder Language disorder Articulation disorder

NOTE: Other disorders also can affect children. Substance use, for example, can induce a variety of conditions termed *organic mental disorders*. Substance use also can cause specific forms of drug abuse and dependence.

SOURCE: Adapted from the American Psychiatric Association: *Diagnostic and Statistical Manual of Mental Disorders*. 3rd ed. The American Psychiatric Association, 1980.

called on to plan interventions with the child and family. For these children, nursing goals are to minimize the dysfunctional behavior, to alleviate the stressors that lead to maladaptive coping, and to promote optimum development.

Psychiatric Diagnoses in Children

Classifying psychiatric disorders in children is difficult because children are very different from adults and differ drastically from each other according to developmental stage. Scales attempting to measure such child-specific behaviors as cognition, conduct, mood, and attention are being developed. Eventually, these will enable clinicians to tailor diagnostic categories and behavioral descriptions to the problems that children experience.

Although it is as yet an imperfect tool to be used for classifying disorders in children, the *Diagnostic and Statistical Manual of Mental Disorders* (DSM III), published by the American Psychiatric Association, is useful. The DSM III describes dysfunctional behavior according to observed behaviors rather than according to psychologic theory. The DSM III method for classifying childhood disorders, outlined in a section entitled "Disorders First Evident in Infancy, Childhood, and Adolescence," divides childhood disorders into five groups: intellectual, behavioral, emotional, physical, and developmental (Table 16-6).

Within the framework of the DSM III, nurses can extract the basis for making nursing diagnoses. Nurses diagnose and treat human responses to actual and potential health problems. Depression, for example, is a health problem characterized by disturbances in thinking, feeling, and acting. The human response is to the actual health problem (depression), and the nursing diagnosis might be *dysfunctional grieving and potential for self-injury.* Nursing interventions are then focused on prevention of injury and not on the medical diagnosis of depression.

TABLE 16-7 DSM III Diagnostic Criteria for Attention Deficit Disorder

Criteria	Behavior
Inattention (at least three behaviors)	Often does not complete activities Often does not seem to listen Is easily distracted Has difficulty concentrating on schoolwork or other activities requiring sustained attention Has difficulty maintaining a play activity
Impulsivity (at least three behaviors)	Often acts before thinking Shifts excessively from one activity to another Has difficulty organizing work (not due to cognitive impairment) Needs much supervision Frequently calls out in class Is impatient
Hyperactivity (at least two behaviors)	Runs and climbs excessively Fidgets easily, does not sit still Moves about excessively in sleep Is always "on the go"; acts as if "driven by a motor"

SOURCE: Adapted from American Psychiatric Association, DSM III, 3rd edition, 1980.

TABLE 16-8 Problems Associated with the Teaching-Learning Process

Deficits	Language-processing problems
Receptive deficits	Poor verbal memory Poor auditory comprehension Inability to understand rapid verbal messages
Expressive deficits	Word finding problems Syntactical errors Difficulty organizing verbal messages Dysfluency
Short-term memory deficits	Poor recall of recent data Recall in wrong order
Dyslexia (reading disability)	Disorder in naming, comprehension, imitative speech, and sound discrimination Blending and coordination deficits with normal receptive language Visual-perceptual deficits Difficulty in ability to read, spell, and write

The Child with a Behavioral Disorder

Attention Deficit Disorder

Attention deficit disorder refers to childhood behavior that is inappropriate for mental and chronologic age. Labels formerly used to identify this disorder are hyperkinetic syndrome, minimal brain dysfunction, and minimal brain damage. These inaccurate and nondescriptive terms have for the most part been eliminated from the nomenclature.

Attention deficit disorder is characterized by patterns of behavior observed in the child and often reported by parents, caregivers, and teachers. Although a variety of behaviors may be observed, they generally fall into three broad categories: (1) inattention, (2) impulsivity, and (3) hyperactivity (Table 16-7). These and other behaviors adversely affect the teaching-learning process and are collectively known as *learning disabilities*. Learning disabilities do not, however, include cognitive weaknesses associated with primary visual, hearing, and motor impairments or social/cultural deprivation (Table 16-8).

The major developmental task of middle to late childhood is industry, or mastery of skills that enhance independence. Industry requires that the child develop self-control, cooperation, and the ability to compromise. Therefore, attention deficit disorder, along with conduct disorder (a disorder characterized by the child's repeated violations of accepted norms), interferes with the child's development. The resultant social and learning problems might eventually become occupational problems.

Assessment Typically, attention deficit disorders become apparent prior to age 7 and peak around age 10. The pattern of behavior established over time, at least 6 months, is an important variable to consider when assessing these problems. Although parents or the child health nurse may identify many of the behaviors at some point in the child's development, it is necessary to distinguish truly dysfunctional behavior from age-appropriate and stress-related overactivity.

It is also important to note any conflict in the identification of the child's behavior. In such instances, consideration should be given to reports offered by individuals familiar with age-appropriate developmental norms. In fact, many behaviors become apparent when the child undertakes activities requiring concentration and/or when the child is under stress, such as in the classroom.

For the child with a learning disability, behavior problems cause conflict and failure in social and academic activities. These children are often poorly understood by family, peers, and teachers. Children with learning disabilities generally have the innate ability to learn but do not. Intervention allows the child to use existing potential to achieve success. Careful design of the educational plan and specific teaching methods are often necessary. Behavioral counseling, family education, and adjunct medication therapy might be indicated in selected situations.

Comprehensive evaluation of the child's cognitive, language, perceptual, and motor skills and of social and emotional strengths might be necessary to determine the degree of dysfunction. Members of the evaluation team might include the nurse, psychologist, special educator, speech and linguistic therapists, social worker, physician, and physical therapist. Data are generated by these professionals from history, interview, observation, and standardized tests.

Diagnostic evaluation for attention deficit disorder involves a complete child and family history and a complete physical and neurologic examination. The history includes information about behavior, health, school, and social interactions. Attention to prenatal, perinatal, and significant family problems can provide clues about the disorder. The physical examination is carried out to detect any underlying medical problem. A neurologic examination might uncover signs of developmental delays, signaled by immaturity for the child's chronologic age or signs of borderline dysfunction.

The neurologic examination might, for example, indicate left-right confusion, fine motor incoordination, or problems with rapidly alternating movements or "mirror" movements between opposite extremities. These behaviors suggest neurologic immaturity. Borderline neurologic signs include choreiform (twitching) movements, mild asymmetry of reflexes or muscle tone, and mild tremors. Depending on findings from the history, and from the physical and neurologic examinations, additional diagnostic tests might be indicated.

Possible nursing diagnoses related to the child with an attention deficit disorder include:

Ineffective individual coping related to decreased self-control

Altered development related to interference with learning and social development

Social isolation related to inappropriate social behavior and lack of cooperation

Potential for ineffective family coping

Potential for injury from lack of judgment

Potential self-esteem disturbance

Nursing management Multidisciplinary management of the child with an attention deficit disorder and the family involves nursing interventions in a variety of settings. The nurse initially might detect problem areas and refer to the family for further evaluation. As the treatment plan is developed, the nurse participates in health care management, family guidance, and behavioral therapy. The nurse plays a vital role in coordinating medical and educational programs to provide an integrated approach.

The nurse often acts as liaison between the family, school, and specialized treatment settings. In the community, the nurse helps families to cope with their children's needs through long-term involvement in home management. Parents are guided in making environmental adjustments to provide safety for their children and to help them experience success. They are taught about their children's needs and helped to understand the factors that aggravate or improve their children's behavior. The principles of behaviorism (defined in Chapter 3) may be employed in a specific program of reinforcements. Parents are encouraged to use praise as well as criticism and to set realistic goals.

Pharmacologic treatment for both attention deficit disorders and conduct disorders alters the child's behavior through *paradoxical* response to selected medications. For example, methylphenidate hydrochloride (Ritalin) and pemoline (Cylert) are central nervous system stimulants but have a calming effect on the child's behavior, while decreasing hyperactivity and prolonging attention span. (Medications used in the treatment of both attention deficit disorders and conduct disorders are outlined in Table 16-9.)

For optimal results, medication treatment must be monitored closely. Communication with school staff and parents is essential to determine the child's response and recognize adverse effects. Often, a behavior checklist is a helpful way for school staff and family to note changes in the child's attention span, activity level, and impulsivity. This approach provides documentation for assessing medication treatment and aids in communication. If adverse effects develop, the dosage or time of administration can be adjusted. Usually, stimulant medication is given once a day (in the morning) or in the morning and again at noon. If the stimulant is given later in the day, the child frequently experiences insomnia.

The child with learning and behavior problems requires long-term and sensitive care to foster strengths and a positive self-image. Both the child and the family will encounter frustrations and setbacks along the way, which can be discouraging. Helping parents to feel competent in their parenting skills, providing anticipatory guidance, and being a supportive listener are valuable nursing interventions (Hahn, Oestreich, & Barkin, 1986).

Conduct Disorders

Children with conduct disorders exhibit a pattern of behavior that violates either the basic rights of others or major age-appropriate societal norms or rules. Like attention defi-

TABLE 16-9 Drug Treatment of Attention Deficit Disorder and Conduct Disorder

Drug	Dosage	Adverse effects	Nursing considerations
Methylphenidate (Ritalin)	Children over 6 years 5 mg before lunch and breakfast; may be gradually increased to 5–10 mg weekly. Dosage should not exceed 60 mg	Central nervous system irritability, dizziness, headache, anorexia, nausea, rash, weight loss, and cardiac arrythmias	Might lower the seizure threshold Evaluation of child and family knowledge about medication, indications, schedule, and adverse effects
Pemoline (Cylert)	37.5 mg in morning. Dose may be gradually increased by 18.5 mg/day until desired effect is achieved. Therapeutic dose is 56.25 mg–75 mg/day, not to exceed 112.5 mg/day	Sleep disturbances, seizures, headache, dizziness, irritability, anorexia, weight loss, jaundice, and growth inhibition	Due to growth inhibiting effects, assess child's physiologic development for deviations from child's premedication growth pattern

SOURCE: Hahn, Oestreich, & Barkin. *Mosby's Pharmacology in Nursing*. 16th edition, 1986.

TABLE 16-10 Degrees of Aggressive Behaviors

Nonaggressive	Mildly aggressive	Moderately aggressive	Severely aggressive
Self-protective and manipulative lying	Bullying	Physical aggression	Serious, repeated physical aggression, mugging, beating, gang fighting
Whining, demanding, temper tantrums	Cruelty toward peers	Reckless driving	
Bed-wetting	Abusive language	Breaking and entering	
Stealing	Vandalism	Extortion	
Truancy		Car theft	

cit disorders, conduct disorders can be identified in a variety of ways. The distinctive feature of a conduct disorder, however, is that the behavior always brings the child into conflict with parents, peers, school personnel, and others in the social environment. Intervention is imposed by those in the social network to protect the safety and property of others.

Although *juvenile delinquency* is the term used to describe the variety of behaviors associated with aggressive and undersocialized behavior, this is a legal term and not descriptive of the child's psychosocial impairment. *Juvenile* refers to the age at which an individual is considered a child by the judicial system.

Conduct disorders, according to DSM III, are divided into four categories based on the presence or absence of aggressive, nonaggressive, socialized, or undersocialized behavior. The range and severity of dysfunction caused by aggressive and antisocial behavior vary from mild to severe (Table 16-10). Socialized children are found to have more age-appropriate relationships and emotionally healthy experiences, thus enabling them to develop a greater capacity for empathy, affection, and social skills. Undersocialized children, however, are unable to develop and maintain lasting peer relationships and have few close friends. Relationships tend to be opportunistic, and the child shows little guilt or remorse for the misfortune of others. Intervention is difficult because the child seems to have little conscience and exhibits impaired moral development.

Assessment Regardless of the etiology or type of conduct disorder, the child has a poor self-concept. Beyond the negative, defiant, manipulative, and frequently hostile behavior, the child health nurse might assess depressive feelings, including self-hatred and hopelessness. Gellar et al. (1985) found that antisocial behavior usually begins after the onset of depressive disorder. The child tends to direct feelings to the individuals and institutions within the social network. The nurse assessing the child must therefore con-

TABLE 16-11 Nursing Management of Antisocial and Aggressive Behavior

Approach	Rationale
Setting firm, consistent limits	Limits provide the child with a sense of security
Time out	For younger children, time out is a nonpunitive method that enables the child to regain self-control. The child is placed in a neutral environment for a specified time
Behavior modification techniques	These provide positive reinforcements for desired behaviors
Encouraging verbalization	Verbalization is a more adaptive way to express angry feelings

sider that the cause of depression might also be the source of the behavior problem.

Anger is the predominant emotion expressed by the child and is a necessary coping strategy. When given opportunities to express anger in appropriate ways, the child learns to solve problems in more effective ways, thereby learning to deal with the limitations imposed by the real and imperfect world.

Nursing diagnoses that might apply to children with conduct disorders are:

Social isolation related to the inability to develop and maintain lasting relationships

Self-esteem disturbance related to self-hatred, hopelessness, and anger against society

Potential for violence

Nursing management Children with conduct disorders react toward others with anger and provoke angry responses from those working with them. It is useful for the child health nurse to remember that the child has a poor self-image and is usually angry at personal shortcomings. Therefore, intervention strategies provide greater success when directed to early identification of conflict and referral to individual, family, and behavioral therapy.

The child's verbal interaction tends to invite the nurse to retaliate in a manner that seems to direct anger at the child, thereby confirming a suspicion that the child is not worth caring about. If the nurse uses basic knowledge about communicating with an angry child, however, intervention will be effective (Table 16-11).

The Child with a Physical Disorder

The general category of physical disorders includes problems where the psychosocial dysfunctional behavioral pattern is characterized by physical manifestations. Among these are enuresis, encopresis, anorexia nervosa, and bulimia. Enuresis and encopresis are the primary problems of elimination for which parents seek professional intervention. Anorexia nervosa and bulimia are related eating disorders that have become more prevalent in recent years.

Nursing diagnoses for children with physical disorders differ depending on the disorder involved. Specific nursing diagnoses might include:

Potential alteration in family processes

Body image disturbance related to perceived imperfections

Alteration in urinary elimination: incontinence related to no known physical cause

Alteration in bowel elimination: incontinence related to diminished self-worth and stress

Alteration in nutrition: less than body requirements related to anorexia or purposeful vomiting from anxiety or stress

Enuresis

American culture places heavy emphasis on cleanliness and personal hygiene, and failure to achieve or maintain bowel or bladder continence is a major stressor for both child and family. Failure to resolve this stress typically results in additional stressors and feelings of inadequacy.

Functional enuresis is described in the DSM III as repeated involuntary voiding of urine during the day or at night, after an age at which continence is expected, that is not due to any physical cause. *Nocturnal enuresis,* the passage of urine only during sleep, is the most common type. *Diurnal enuresis* refers to the passage of urine during waking hours. The child health nurse should be aware that the child might experience both phenomena.

Assessment In assessing the child with enuresis, the nurse looks for three diagnostic criteria: (1) repeated involuntary voiding of urine during the day or night, (2) involuntary voiding that occurs at least twice a month in children from ages 5 to 6, and (3) lack of an organic cause.

The family is usually the source of information concerning incidence of enuresis and toilet training. The nurse therefore usually questions the parent to obtain baseline data. Categories for assessment of enuresis, as identified by Maizels and Ferlit (1986), include:

1. Perinatal complications
2. Developmental and physical disorders
3. Toilet-training history
4. Voiding pattern (diary of number of daily voids)
5. Micturition pattern (length of voiding time, description of urine stream)
6. Defecation pattern
7. Urinary tract infection
8. Food sensitivities

Assessment data and evaluation of structural abnormalities of the urinary tract by appropriate specialists must be analyzed. Structural problems therefore will not be overlooked, even in the presence of severe psychosocial problems.

Nursing management A variety of techniques can be helpful in managing the child with enuresis. For nocturnal enuretics, providing a nightlight or a stuffed animal, restricting fluid intake, and even scheduling bathroom trips at night are among the methods that can be effective. Incidence of spontaneous remission and subsequent relapse is high among enuretics, so establishing exact causes of remission is useful, although difficult.

If treatment is indicated, motivational or behavioral conditioning techniques have proved to be an effective approach to enuresis. The nurse in the clinical setting can make use of an intensive procedure that achieves initial success in one day. The nurse requires the child to urinate in the toilet in order to receive a reinforcer (eg, snacks, hugs, praises). The child might need to consume a large amount of liquid to ensure a successful number of trial episodes. In the process, the nurse teaches the child the sequence of going to the bathroom, removing clothing, voiding, cleaning, and redressing, and the nurse rewards the child for dryness. "Accidents" are treated without punishment or disapproval, but the child is required to attend to all self-cleaning by removing soiled clothes and linen, disposing of them properly, and replacing them.

Another frequently used conditioning technique is the buzzer or bell method. The technique involves a urine-sensing pad connected to an alarm system placed on the child's bed. When the child urinates, the alarm is activated because the urine acts as an electrolyte. The alarm then awakens the child, inhibiting urination. To avoid being awakened by the alarm, the child learns to delay urination or to awaken when bladder tension is increased. These pad and alarm units are available commercially and, combined with behavior modification, have proved effective (D'Epiro, 1985).

Medications, such as tricyclic antidepressants (imipramine hydrochloride, Tofranil) and anticholinergic medication (oxybutynin hydrochloride, Ditropan), have been used with marginal success in short-term management of enuresis when behavior modification fails. Evidence suggests (Shapiro, 1985) that results derived from medications are temporary at best and that side effects and complications render such drugs unpleasant or dangerous.

Throughout the period of assessment and intervention, the child health nurse needs to be supportive of the family as they attempt to cope with a child who exhibits enuresis. Pothier (1976), points out that a period of exploration takes place when the parents have an opportunity to deal with their responses to having a child who manifests a behavior that is disapproved by society. It is important that the nurse encourage parents and the child to verbalize feelings of embarrassment so that specific strategies to alter the undesirable behavior will be identified. The child health nurse assists parents to acknowledge their child's distress and explain that they want the child to feel better and, most of all, that they want to assist in the process.

Encopresis

Functional encopresis is repeated voluntary or involuntary passage of feces of normal or near-normal consistency into inappropriate places. This disorder is differentiated from *retentive encopresis,* which results in involuntary oozing or seepage of stool due to chronic constipation and/or mechanical obstruction of the colon or alteration in external sphincter activity of the rectum during defecation (Loening-Baucke, 1986).

By DSM III criteria, encopresis begins by ages 4 through 8. The degree of psychosocial dysfunction depends on the child's self-esteem, the responses of peers, and the degree of anger and rejection expressed by caregivers.

Although the etiology of encopresis remains unclear, psychodynamic interpretation has suggested that encopresis is an unconscious process involving independence and control. This theory has been much questioned. Abrahamian and Lloyd-Still (1984) report, however, that severe psychologic problems are present in many children with this disorder. Children with encopresis do tend to feel a diminished sense of self-worth, feel less in control of life events, and express a desire to change their behavior, therefore suggesting that encopresis is a response to stressors (Landman et al., 1986).

Assessment Assessment of the child begins with attempts to rule out organic causes of the encopresis such as gastrointestinal pathology or nutritional deficiencies and food intolerances. Endoscopy (direct examination of the upper gastrointestinal tract by means of a fiberoptic flexible scope), proctoscopy (examination of the anus and rectum), and sigmoidoscopy (examination of anus, rectum, and lower colon), along with stool analysis, allow the clinician to identify any parasites, ova, or other explanations for the child's soiling behavior. The nurse conducts a nutritional history to identify any dietary factors and gathers information about how toilet training was conducted and at what age, if ever, the child mastered bowel control. Family expectations, knowledge, and any traumatic training techniques are identified in this way. The nurse discusses stressors affecting the family, such as separations, deaths, illnesses, or births of siblings.

Like enuresis, encopresis is often a regressive symptom in the face of a real or perceived threat. Family interactions and parenting styles need close evaluation because encopresis is at times used as a means of defiance or control of others. Observing parent-child interaction in the clinical setting and monitoring the child's pattern of resistance or cooperation often sheds light on potential causes of difficulty.

Parents usually are willing to provide information about the child but resistant to sharing information about their own behavior and methods of dealing with the problem. Clinical observations seem to indicate that parents at times see themselves as "victims" of the child's behavior. Children with encopresis often attempt to conceal their soiling by hiding stained linens, throwing soiled clothes away, or defecating into shoes, closets, or showers. Supervision and observation are important in detecting episodes of encopresis. To encourage an accurate assessment, the nurse neutrally acknowledges the impact of the problem on family members, caregivers, and the child.

Nursing management Determining whether or not the child has retentive encopresis and whether encopresis is caused by anxiety or failure to master bowel control during toilet training is important to planning interventions. Retentive encopresis is generally treated with laxatives, stool softeners, and enemas until the bowels are empty and bowel retraining can begin. Careful monitoring of the child's nutritional status and fluid and electrolyte balance are necessary during treatment with laxatives and enemas. Normal intestinal flora can be eliminated and thereby trigger malabsorption syndromes or diarrhea. In small children, diarrhea can cause fluid and electrolyte imbalances and related complications. Bowel retraining involves gradually allowing the colon and anal vault to return to a more normal capacity and reestablish the defecatory reflex (Loening-Baucke, 1986).

Behavioral techniques similar to those used for enuresis are useful for facilitating toilet retraining. The nurse first fosters a sense of security in the child by removing the anxiety associated with toileting tasks and then teaches the family to foster this security by making the toileting behaviors both desirable and rewarding to the child.

Working through the young child's sense of anxiety and guilt over incontinence is best achieved through play. Puppet or doll play or use of drawing materials with a relatively structured theme allows the child to express concerns. Mutual story telling and other story-telling techniques communicate in a nonthreatening way that the child's concerns are shared by others. Building trust is a priority in dealing with such an emotional subject as elimination. Methods of minimizing anxiety therefore are essential interventions.

Eating Disorders—Anorexia and Bulimia

Although not necessarily indicative of depression, dysfunctional eating patterns can be linked to anxiety and maladaptive coping in children. Eating behavior is a sensitive barometer of the child's emotional state and parent-child interaction. Misuse of feeding in an attempt to solve or camouflage family problems can take the following forms: failure to thrive, obesity, excessive finickiness, and protracted mealtime struggles (Satter, 1986). Any of these conditions might indicate that the family is at risk (see Chapter 13). When these problems are identified, the nurse and other health care providers plan interventions that will improve functioning for the entire family.

Anorexia nervosa and bulimia are extreme maladaptive responses involving self-image and self-control. These problems require the family and child to learn new patterns of behavior and ways of managing stress. Problems common to young people with eating disorder(s) result from the relentless pursuit of thinness, preoccupation with food, and dysfunctional attitudes about eating (Garner and Garfinkel, 1985). Although some research suggests a hypothalamic-pituitary dysfunction as the explanation for eating disorders, cultural, social, familial, and psychologic causes also are being explored.

Children with anorexia nervosa willfully limit food intake to reduce body weight. They do not experience loss of appetite from any organic cause. In identifying indicators of anorexia nervosa, the nurse might need to distinguish this condition from loss of appetite associated with medications or procedures that make the child nauseated. Essential features of anorexia nervosa include:

- Intense fear of becoming obese
- Refusal to maintain normal body weight
- Amenorrhea (absence of menstruation)
- Disturbance of body image (seeing oneself as fat, although thin in reality)

Although a distinct entity, bulimia is characterized by cyclical binging on enormous quantities of food, followed by purging oneself with laxatives or by vomiting (Fig. 16-3).

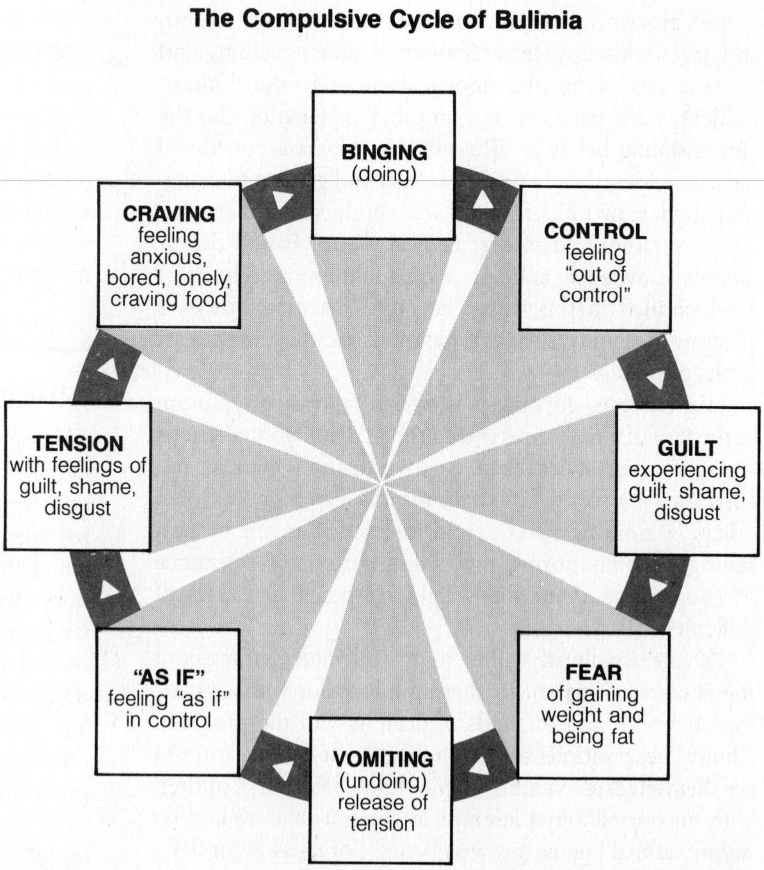

FIGURE 16-3

The compulsive cycle of bulimia. (From Edmands MS: Overcoming eating disorders. J Psychosoc Nurs *1986. 24(8):22. With permission of the author.)*

Inducing vomiting by ingestion of large quantities of syrup of ipecac (several 30 mL vials per day) is a phenomenon widely reported in the literature. Palmer and Guay (1985) report that ipecac abuse is attractive to people with eating disorders because it is readily available, inexpensive, and very effective. Ipecac abuse can cause severe muscle weakness and even death.

Although binge eating followed by purging is generally attributed to bulimics, anorexic young people occasionally engage in similar behavior in addition to restricting their food intake. *Bulimarexia* is a starvation-purge syndrome where the young person might be of normal or near-normal weight. In bulimarexia, the dysfunctional eating pattern might follow an episode of anorexia or any period of deliberate dieting (Bauer and Hill, 1986).

Additionally, bulimics often have histories of anorexia. Features of bulimia include:

- Episodic binge eating followed by an awareness that the eating pattern is abnormal
- Fear of inability to stop eating voluntarily
- Depressed mood and self-deprecating thoughts following the episode
- High-caloric food binges that are secret or inconspicuous
- Binging that usually is terminated by abdominal pain

Assessment The young person, usually an adolescent girl, comes to medical attention when significant weight loss from self-starvation causes serious physical complications. Although a psychiatric assessment is necessary to confirm the diagnosis of eating disorder, the child health nurse may suspect anorexia nervosa or bulimia in the adolescent who has no explanation for an emaciated appearance. Because the adolescent often attempts to deny or conceal the problem, the nurse might have difficulty obtaining accurate information regarding the amount of weight loss, psychologic stressors, or the duration of weight loss.

Objective data that can validate the nurse's suspicion include height and weight, which are compared with norms, and abnormal lab values for serum electrolytes, complete blood count, and urinalysis. Of particular importance are urinalysis ketone levels that suggest self-imposed "starvation." Whenever a state of starvation exists, fats are metabolized with subsequent elevation of ketone bodies in the urine. Abnormally low glucose, sodium, or red blood count values also suggest a threatened nutritional status indicative of anorexia nervosa. Physical symptoms of anorexia nervosa and bulimia include:

1. Weight loss to 25% of original body weight
2. Dehydration and electrolyte imbalances
3. Bradycardia, hypotension
4. Low body temperature
5. Amenorrhea
6. Dry skin
7. Lanugo hair
8. Cold extremities, cyanosis of hands and feet

Observations of behaviors such as hiding food (particulary high-carbohydrate foods), refusing food (either by turning down offers of food or by disposing of food secretly), or vomiting also suggest anorexia or bulimia. Young people who are anorexic tend to look frequently in mirrors, as if to make sure that they have not been gaining weight. They also tend to talk constantly about food, food preparation, and eating. Often they are observed encouraging others to eat or preparing meals for others.

Young people with bulimia tend to exhibit fluctuations in weight. They also can exhibit poor impulse control comparable to their difficulty in controlling their eating behavior. Eating binges might be pleasurable but are followed by self-criticism and feelings of depression (Edmands, 1986). Complications associated with bulimia include dehydration, malnutrition, electrolyte imbalance and dental enamel erosion.

Nursing management Children with anorexia who are severely emaciated (40% below their ideal body weight) usually are hospitalized, often against their will. For the child in an acute-care setting, sensitive and consistent nursing management is the most essential component in the plan of care. Though weight gain and physiologic improvement are necessary, these are an insufficient foundation for sustained recovery.

Improvement depends on treatment, which focuses on the interaction of psychosocial factors. The long-term goal of care is to restore weight with adequate nutrition and to provide a supportive environment to ensure cooperation. Included in the treatment plan are specific measures to monitor and reduce the physiologic effects of starvation, vomiting, and laxative abuse. The process of weight restoration is initiated slowly, preferably with a balanced 1200-calorie, salt-limited diet. Calories are gradually increased to promote a weight gain of approximately 2 pounds each week (Williams, 1985).

Weight usually is measured daily and is measured at the same time with the patient wearing the same clothing. Patients should void before being weighed because they might attempt to increase weights by drinking large quantities of fluid. To promote weight gain, activity should be restricted to a minimum. In some cases bed rest might be necessary.

Eating after prolonged periods of starvation can lead to edema, abdominal distension, and constipation. The nurse monitors such potential problems, keeping in mind that children with anorexia frequently complain of feeling "bloated" after meals because of psychologic discomfort with eating. Gradually inviting more patient control over issues related to food and body image can reinforce positive eating behaviors.

In the acute-care setting, the nurse is supportive but firm during mealtime to assure that a significant portion of the meal is consumed. Although power struggles with patients are certainly not desirable and tend to limit their control over their own eating behavior, the first nursing goal is to decrease the potential for nutritional deficiency in the patient who is nutritionally compromised. If the patient refuses food, liquid protein supplements with equivalent caloric amounts can supplement uneaten food portions. Ideally, the patient should be observed while eating and closely monitored after meals for at least 1 hour to ensure that food is not regurgitated. Refusal of all oral intake might necessitate nasogastric tube feedings or, in extreme cases, hyperalimentation (parenteral nutrition).

Care of a child with anorexia nervosa is a challenge to the child health nurse. Most patients resist treatment efforts after an initial sense of relief that the treatment team has assumed responsibility for their decisions. Although patients with anorexia nervosa are usually not engaging in conscious efforts at suicide, they are overwhelmed with fear of gaining weight. The patient experiences anxiety, guilt, and panic after eating because of the distorted belief that all food is "bad" and will lead to excessive weight gain. This belief leads to such desperate behavior as hiding food during meals or vomiting afterward.

The difficulties that arise around eating might be surprising to the staff in light of the patient's pleasing, cooperative facade in other areas of interaction with the nurse. In some instances the nurse begins to feel angry and avoids the patient because of the apparent refusal to accept treatment. The nurse therefore needs to remember during this stressful time that patients with anorexia are not malevolent in their attempts to sabotage efforts of the staff. They are instead clinging to the security of their symptoms.

If the nurse uses a firm, matter-of-fact approach about eating, power struggles with the patient about particular foods and portions are more easily avoided. The critical factor is a consistent approach from all staff members. Coordinated efforts, often with the consultation of a psychiatric nurse specialist, ensures that one nurse is not identified as stricter or more lenient than another.

NURSING CARE PLAN *The Adolescent with Anorexia Nervosa*

Assessment data: Jane is a 5′4″ 17-year-old high school junior admitted to the pediatric unit for severe weight loss (from 120 lb to 80 lb), excessive fatigue, amenorrhea, pallor, and cyanosis of the feet. Her admitting diagnosis is starvation as a result of anorexia nervosa. Several months prior to admission, Jane began a diet to lose some weight for a wedding she was to be in. Her mother, always weight conscious, had told her she needed to lose a few pounds. Since beginning the diet, Jane has found that she has not had enough energy to participate in school extracurricular activities and has slowly withdrawn from her usual social contacts. She still sees herself as being fat, and her major complaint is not the weight loss but the associated lack of energy.

Jane's parents are very concerned about her condition and express frustration that they have not been able to convince her that she has lost too much weight. Her mother feels particularly guilty that she encouraged the diet in the first place and allowed Jane's older brother to tease her about having large hips.

Jane is to be started on a 1200-calorie diet and will be monitored closely to ensure she receives adequate nutrients.

Nursing diagnosis	Intervention	Rationale
1. Alteration in nutrition: less than body requirements related to refusal to eat	Provide a 1200-calorie diet.	A 1200-calorie diet is sufficient for Jane to gain weight gradually and includes meals of a size that will not appear overwhelming.
	Find out from parents what foods Jane liked prior to beginning her diet; consult with the dietician to include these foods if possible.	Including foods the adolescent likes might encourage her to eat what is required.
	Allow food only at prescribed meal times (8 AM, 1 PM, 6 PM, or according to hospital schedule); monitor Jane for at least one hour after each meal.	Allowing food at any other time gives too much emphasis to the food and might prevent adequate nutritional intake at meals. Close monitoring prevents secret regurgitation.
	Weigh daily; have Jane void prior to weighing, weigh first thing in the morning, and make sure Jane is dressed in a hospital gown.	Daily weights monitor progress. A full bladder and different clothing can add weight artificially.
	Monitor Jane's elimination patterns.	Adequate elimination is confirmation of adequate intake.
	Develop a reward system (eg, reduced observation or increased activity) to reward positive nutritional behaviors.	Rewards encourage repeat of positive behaviors and successful accomplishments enhance self-esteem.
	Recommend hyperalimentation or nasogastric tube feeding if Jane consistently refuses to eat.	The primary goal when the adolescent is first admitted is to restore nutritional deficiency.

Outcome: Jane will gain 2 pounds a week. Jane will eat the prescribed quantity of food and liquids. Jane will begin to choose some of her own food.

Nursing diagnosis	Intervention	Rationale
2. Body image disturbance related to distorted weight perception	Encourage Jane to verbalize her fear of food and of gaining weight.	Encouraging verbalization allows the adolescent to express her fears and allows the nurse to examine the adolescent's unrealistic perceptions of food and weight gain.
	Emphasize Jane's positive traits—that she has pretty eyes, that she is a fine athlete.	Emphasizing positive traits enhances self-image.

NURSING CARE PLAN *The Adolescent with Anorexia Nervosa (Continued)*

Nursing diagnosis	Intervention	Rationale
	Encourage Jane to use make-up and to dress when allowed out of bed.	Promoting self-care enhances self-image.
	Talk to Jane about her interests and encourage her to continue her schoolwork.	Talking about other things decreases the emphasis on food and fear of excessive weight gain.
Outcome: Jane will demonstrate an increased interest in her appearance. Jane will talk less about food and how fat she is and more about her other interests. Jane will participate in self-care.		
3. Activity intolerance related to poor nutritional status	Maintain bed rest; have her get up for meals only.	Bed rest conserves energy.
	Allow only a gradual return to activity.	Exercise uses more calories and can prevent attainment of weight goal.
	Promote quiet activities—Jane enjoys crewel embroidery.	Quiet activities conserve energy while keeping the mind off food.
	Encourage peers to visit on a regular basis; caution them not to comment on her weight.	Encouraging peer visits allows her to reinitiate social contact.
Outcome: Jane will verbalize understanding of why activity restrictions are necessary. Jane will comply with activity restrictions. Jane will suggest other quiet activities that interest her.		
4. Alteration in family processes related to conflict between Jane and parents	Observe and record family interactions and communication patterns.	Identification of family coping and interaction patterns alters the focus from the child problem to a family problem.
	Allow the parents to express their guilt and frustration about dealing with Jane.	Allowing verbal expression can decrease guilt and frustration by placing factors in a more realistic light.
	Explain to the family the nature of the eating disorder and what behaviors to expect.	Family understanding ensures cooperation.
	Give the parents a realistic view of treatment measures such as limit-setting and the reward system.	Parents can feel the treatment is punitive if they do not understand the basis for the treatment.
	Encourage the parents to participate in the treatment.	Encouraging participation increases the parents' sense of control and decreases guilt.
Outcome: The parents will be able to verbalize their guilt and frustration at watching Jane refuse to eat. Both parents participate in the treatment by enforcing limits, decreasing the emphasis on food, and emphasizing Jane's positive traits.		
5. Potential for impaired home maintenance management (Stressors: insufficient knowledge about reasons for treatment regimen, possible manipulation by the child)	Explain to Jane and her parents the diet and activity regimen Jane will be on after discharge; include information about how to handle Jane's potential refusal to eat; inform parents of weight guidelines and at what weight it would be necessary to contact the physician; encourage the family to gain follow-up care.	Specific information given to the adolescent and family prevents relapses and ensures adequate home management.
Outcome: Jane and her parents will explain the treatment to be continued in the home. They will make an appointment for follow-up care.		

In general, firm limits coupled with genuine sensitivity and support are most helpful. Patients need encouragement to explore their feelings about eating, without being given false assurances. Limits might be defined by using such behavior modification techniques as granting privileges (for example, reduced observation, increased activity) if the patient meets a weight goal.

At the same time, the nurse needs to be aware that the child's parents might inadvertently interfere with treatment. For example, the patient might complain that nurses are cruel and punitive and might lead parents to believe that the child should be discharged before home care is medically safe. Parents need to be forewarned about the behavior and encouraged to discuss it with the nurse. Parents should also be told not to discuss eating and weight with the anorexic child but to let the staff handle this aspect of care.

Although dysfunctional family interactions might be contributing to the development of eating disorders, the nurse cannot sit in judgment of families of these patients but needs to remain sensitive to their problems. The parents might have been struggling for many months to force the child to eat, and the distress of watching one's child willfully starve might be enough to cause chaos in the household. The parent is likely to feel guilty, ineffective, and depressed about the situation and needs support from the nurse to address these feelings.

Weight maintenance, resolution of psychosocial conflicts, and improved parent-child communication are desired outcomes. Bryant and Kopeski (1986) describe a useful approach to discharge planning from inpatient or community treatment settings. Assisting the child to develop a self-assessment "survival plan" will allow the child to develop awareness of strengths and coping strategies before returning to the stressful home situation. The plan enables the child to demonstrate readiness for discharge by identifying behaviors associated with eating disorders, identifying personal strengths, recognizing support systems, describing a personal danger signal indicating the need for further support, and identifying and verbalizing personal feelings discovered during treatment.

The Child with a Substance Abuse Disorder

Substances used to modify mood or behavior might be acceptable in a given culture. Alcohol, caffeine, and to some extent nicotine are used by a great many Americans. These substances, as well as certain drugs, can induce symptoms that DSM III terms organic mental disorders. DSM III also refers to a category of disorders whereby use, abuse, or dependence on a substance that alters central nervous system function might lead to physical deficits and behavioral changes resulting in social and occupational impairment.

The degree of impairment varies according to substance used and the intensity and duration of use. DSM III distinguishes nonpathologic substance use from substance abuse by three criteria:

1. The presence of a pattern of abuse
2. Impairment in social or occupational (school) functioning caused by the pattern of pathologic use
3. Duration of impairment due to pathologic use throughout one month

The fiscal and human cost of dysfunctional behavior induced by dependence on selected substances is high. Estimates attribute millions of deaths, injuries, loss of productivity, and crime to substance abuse. Many substances are illegal when used in unauthorized ways by various age groups, but it is the *pattern* of use rather than the actual substance that results in dysfunctional behavior and physical dependence.

Patterns of Substance Use

Of children in various developmental stages, the adolescent demonstrates the most vulnerability to patterns of substance use. Indeed, research is directed toward understanding the etiology and antecedents of drug use and abuse during the teen years (Newcomb et al., 1986). The environment in which the drug is ingested, together with the expectations of the user, can also affect the response. For children and adolescents, the effect of the peer group is as significant as the drug itself. Because the peer group serves as both a learning source and a competitive arena, the adolescent's reliance on this social group promotes abuse when peers are using substances.

The intensity of substance nonuse, use, and abuse can be represented by a point on a continuum (Fig. 16-4). As the substance user begins to abuse a substance, associated health problems become more prevalent. If use continues, the substance abuser might become dependent. *Substance dependence* refers to a more serious form of substance abuse. It is marked by physiologic dependence as evidenced by tolerance and withdrawal. *Tolerance* refers to the marked increase in the amount of substance that is required to achieve the desired effect. *Withdrawal* is a syndrome that follows abrupt cessation of a specific substance. Physiologic responses related to withdrawal include fatigue, anorexia, chills, sweating, cramps, nausea, and elevated vital signs.

For many substance users, *habituation,* or psychologic

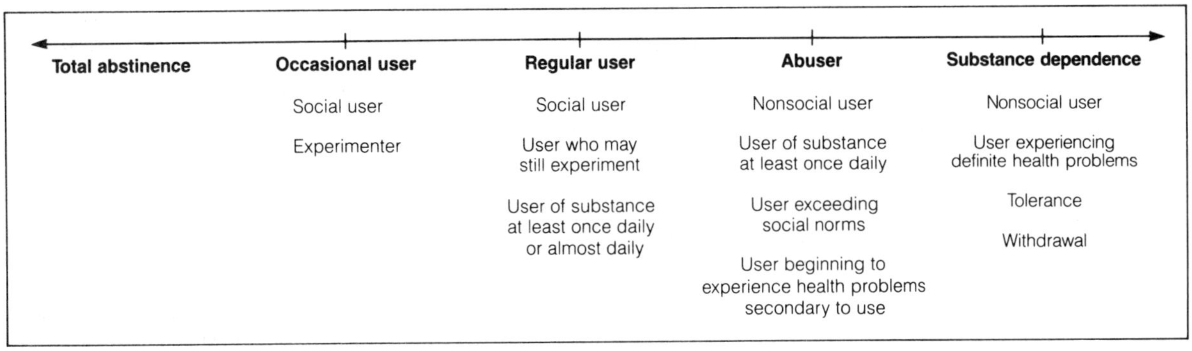

FIGURE 16-4

Intensity of abuse without interventions. The degree of abuse might be represented by a point on a continuum.

dependence, occurs because of the individual's vulnerability to the drug's effects. Continued substance use does not necessarily lead to habituation, but all substances can become habituating. In many instances psychologic dependence causes a compulsive need to use the abused substance. The degree of dependence is related to the psychologic needs of the user.

Five general classes of substances are associated with abuse and dependence:

1. Alcohol
2. Central nervous system (CNS) depressants
   a. barbiturates or similarly acting sedatives or hypnotics
   b. opioids (narcotics)
   c. cannabis (marijuana, hashish) and similarly acting hallucinogens
3. Central nervous system stimulants or other similarly acting sympathomimetics (amphetamines, cocaine, or "crack")

Some of these drugs, such as opioids and barbiturates, have legitimate medical uses. Otherse are cultivated or manufactured in illegal laboratories and are strictly "street drugs." (A selection of commonly abused drugs and their possible effects is outlined in Table 16-12.)

Nursing Care Associated with Substance Abuse

Assessment Child health nurses in all settings eventually deal with children experiencing conditions or traumas directly related to nonmedical drug use. Drug abuse usually is only one of a variety of behaviors exhibited by the child during a given time. Truancy, runaway behavior, sexual promiscuity, or conduct disorders also are associated with substance use and can be observed in many combinations.

Adolescents and young children under the acute influence of drugs, alcohol, or both have tragically sacrificed everything through suicide or have suffered fatal injuries, often from driving under the influence of drugs or alcohol. Still others, because of chronic drug or alcohol use, have destroyed their health by neglecting their bodies' basic needs. Some young people, because of substance abuse, have withdrawn from society and have given up any opportunity to be freely involved in the world.

Assessment relies on accounts given by parents, school, and criminal justice system representatives. Newcomb et al. (1986) identified the following risk factors to correlate positively with adolescent vulnerability to substance use:

Poor academic achievement
Low religious commitment
Early alcohol use
Low self-acceptance
Psychopathology or emotional lability (depression, irritability)
Poor or deteriorating relationship with parents
Antisocial behavior
Sensation seeking
Peer drug use
Drug use by adults in immediate social network

These findings demonstrate that the number of risk factors was associated with increased percentage of drug users, frequency of drug use, and drug abuse.

TABLE 16-12 Commonly Abused Substances

Drug name	Effect and use
Central nervous system depressants—barbiturates	
Amobarbital sodium (Amytal, blue birds, blue devils, truth serum)	Depresses all areas of the central nervous system, although many enhance pain sensation; used as hypnotics, sedatives, anesthetics, and anticonvulsants
Butabarbital sodium (Butabell HMB, Quibron Plus, Tedral-25)	
Sodium pentobarbital (Nembutal, yellow jackets)	
Phenobarbital (Luminal, Antrocol, Bronkolixir, Quadrinal)	
Secobarbital sodium (Seconal; Tuinal, tooeys, reds, rainbows)	
Central nervous system depressants—miscellaneous	
Antihistamines: Actifed, Benadryl, Chlor-Trimeton, Comtrex, Dimetap, Isochlor, Nyquil, Phenergan, Rondec, Sudafed, Triaminic	Used in prescription and nonprescription cold preparations for upper-respiratory symptoms; also found in sleep aids. Antihistamines exert an anticholinergic effect that results in drying of mucous membranes and sedation. These medications are also used for the treatment of motion sickness and parkinsonism and frequently are used in the management of allergic reactions
Central nervous system stimulants—amphetamines	
Dextroamphetamine (Dexedrine)	Stimulates the central nervous system and is commonly used in treatment for exogenous obesity and narcolepsy
Methamphetamine (Desoxyn, speed, crystal, meth)	
Racemic amphetamine (Benzedrine, uppers, bennies)	Those used in obesity treatment are called anorectics
Amphetamine complex (Biphetamine, black beauties)	
Central nervous system stimulants—miscellaneous	
Cocaine hydrochloride (cocaine, coke, blow, snow, lady, powder)	Cortical stimulant used to elevate mood, enhance alertness, and provide local anesthesia. Route of administration varies, but inhalation is most popular
Central nervous system stimulants—miscellaneous *(Continued)*	
Crack (pure form of cocaine)	Crack is rapidly addicting; reactions are similar to those from cocaine but intensified due to the relative purity of the drug
Caffeine (No-Doz, cola beverages, coffee, Anacin)	Central nervous system stimulant found in a variety of common over-the-counter products
Hallucinogens	
Lysergic acid diethylamide (acid, blotter acid, crystal, microdot, windowpane)	Alters mood, thought, behavior, perception, sensation, and often creates hallucinations
Psilocybin (mushrooms)	Overt psychosis is common
Mescaline (mescalito, white line, peyote)	Oral route of administration most common although marijuana and its derivatives are typically inhaled
Methoxyamphetamine (MDA)	
Phencyclidine (PCP, angel dust, horse tranquilizer)	
Cannabis (marijuana, grass, pot, tea, Acapulco gold, Maui wowie, Tai sticks, Colombian, hemp, weed)	
Hashish (knot, tar, oils)	
Opiates and synthetic opiates	
Morphine sulfate	Affects the central nervous system, alters mood, and provides analgesia; clinically used as an analgesic in postoperative and terminal cases
Oxycodone (Percodan)	
Hydromorphone (Dilaudid)	
Meperidine (Demerol)	
Methadone (Dolophine)	
Propoxyphene (Darvon)	
Pentazocine (Talwin)	
Butorphanol (Stadol)	
Heroin (smack, horse, junk, skag, zap)	

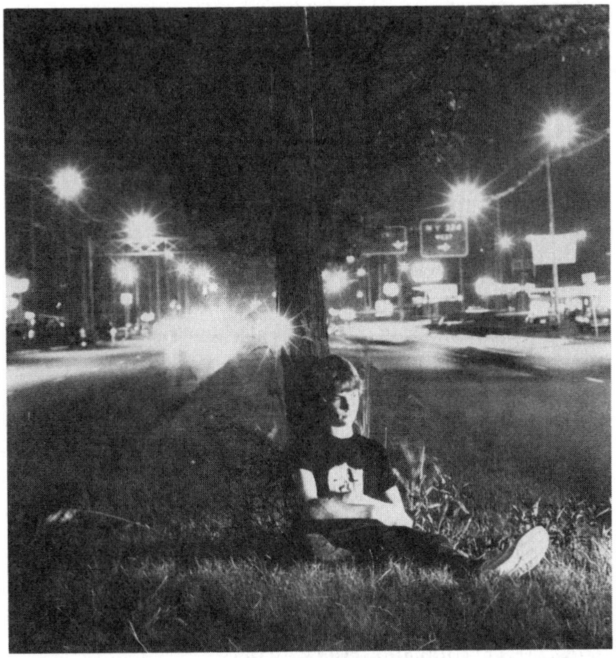

Truancy or runaway behavior can be associated with the adolescent who abuses substances.

By observing specific behaviors, the nurse might identify signs of drug use. Indicators include

1. Increasingly poor adjustment and deteriorating function at home or school or among peers
2. Emotional lability with rapid mood swings but with increasing depression, irritability, and restlessness
3. Secretive behavior, longer periods of time spent alone, longer periods of time away from home
4. Deterioration in personal hygiene or dress
5. Alterations in schedule (for example, sleeping longer, tardiness, truancy)
6. Existence of drug paraphernalia (for example, needles, syringes, pill containers, bottles)
7. Disappearance of family money or valuables, large amounts of money found in the child's possession
8. Bizarre behavior or behavior that seems inappropriate to a specific occasion or a particular context

The drug user also is at risk for drug-related conditions. These risks include increased susceptibility to disease, particularly to hepatitis or acquired immune deficiency syndrome (AIDS) if adolescents are injecting drugs. Drug sensitivities may develop with resultant organ damage, seizures, and possible death. Drug abuse often results in increased risk-taking behavior, changes in perception, disturbances in judgments and decision making, and poor impulse control. Of special concern are the growing number of "polyabusers," those who are dependent on a combination of alcohol and drugs or on more than one chemical substance.

The many risk factors and conditions associated with substance abuse suggest a great range of assessment findings. Nursing diagnoses resulting from this assessment might include:

Ineffective individual coping related to substance dependence

Potential for injury

Potential for infection

Alteration in family processes related to ineffective communication among family members

Potential impaired thought processes

Potential cognitive impairment

Nursing management Nursing management of substance abuse, dependence, and related dysfunctional behaviors encompasses all levels of prevention with obvious attention to primary prevention. With the many risk factors for substance abuse, prevention programs should focus on reducing exposure to risk factors while attempting to modify the factors already present.

Adolescents and school-age children are becoming increasingly well-informed about the health hazards of such substances as tobacco, caffeine, alcohol, and drugs. The goal for educational efforts by health and school personnel is to encourage responsible, informed decision making. As with other psychosocial problems, the emphasis is on prevention of dysfunctional behavior. Swett (1984) uses a three-tiered model of substance abuse prevention:

Primary prevention activities to reduce the occurrence of substance abuse among the general population and to encourage healthy lifestyles (including balanced diet habits, regular exercise, positive family interactions, satisfying academic and social experiences)

Secondary prevention detection of early warning signs and appropriate intervention to deter further abuse

Tertiary prevention restoration and treatment of individuals with abuse disorder

The "gateway theory" developed by Kandel and Logan (1984), suggests that prevention, through use of anticipatory guidance, is an effective way to reduce drug use and abuse by young people. The gateway theory demonstrates that a predictable sequence of drugs exists: milder legal substances (tobacco, then beer and wine) progress to harder substances (distilled liquor), and then to illegal drugs (marijuana and others). Even though the sequence of drug use may vary, research indicates that earlier and later initiation of drug use (younger than age 15 or older than age 24) tends to result in the most dysfunctional behavior patterns (Jones and Bell-Bolek, 1986).

Primary prevention Primary prevention for substance abuse might include multidisciplinary education efforts directed toward health care providers, parents and teachers, together with educational programs for children. Even those in middle childhood need basic information about available substances and ways to cope with peer pressure.

Six basic approaches to school-based primary prevention programs have been identified by the National Institute on Drug Abuse (1984):

1. *Drug abuse education* providing information about drugs, possibly through fear or scare tactics
2. *Affective training* teaching decision-making skills (values clarification, analysis of choices, and selection of alternatives)
3. *Alternative programs* focusing not on drugs but on engaging young people in activities designed to reduce alienation (i.e., risk factors)
4. *Psychosocial approaches* teaching specific techniques for resisting social pressures
5. *Social skills training* emphasizing the development of adaptive coping skills
6. *Cognitive-developmental training* focusing on physiologic reactions to drugs and user perceptions, particularly to assist junior high school children to make decisions about tobacco use

Educational programs for primary prevention must be geared to the cognitive and psychosocial development of the child, the child's values, and the need to develop decision-making skills. Education for parents, school personnel, and health care providers should include information about drugs, jargon, indications of use, and paraphernalia.

Secondary prevention Secondary prevention occurs in routine health assessment and in emergency settings. All adolescents should be asked to describe their pattern of drug and alcohol use, including nonmedical and medical use. Physical examination sometimes reveals puncture sites, needle tracks or skin-popping ulcers in regular users of injectable drugs. Reddened conjunctivae are sometimes associated with marijuana use. Slurred speech, decreased attention span, and inappropriate affect may indicate use of central nervous system depressants. Nasal and bronchial irritation may be seen with smoking or inhaling of any drug. Additionally, the child health nurse may observe a poorly nourished, poorly groomed young person who should be assessed, in a nonthreatening manner, for indications of existing or potential drug use.

Emergency care is sometimes necessary to intervene in severe physical and psychologic reactions caused by drug ingestion. Although subjective data provided by parents and family might suggest a drug reaction, objective data from laboratory tests [thin-layer chromatography (TLC) and gas-liquid chromatography (GLC)], detect drugs in blood and urine. Drug overdoses also cause central nervous system depression. If the child is disoriented or uncoordinated, the nurse monitors the child's state of consciousness. When the child is conscious but disoriented, the nurse intervenes to calm the patient and prevent panic. Controlling the environment and providing continual reassurance help to reduce stress and remind the child that the hospital is safe. The constant presence of one nurse adds to the child's sense of security. Clear directions in a calm tone of voice and accurate descriptions of what will happen enhance cooperation and reduce anxiety.

Tertiary prevention Tertiary prevention includes preventing the long-term effects of drug dependence and dysfunctional health practices and coping behaviors. Peer counseling, group treatment on a residential or community basis, and individual therapy provide the child with opportunities to abstain from the abused substance, thus allowing the development of effective problem-solving skills.

The family is an essential component of any prevention or intervention strategy. All too often, the child's drug use and related behavior has caused disruptions in the family's organizational structure long before parents are willing to admit that a problem exists. Regardless of the root causes of the drug abuse, the behavior communicates a strong message that there is a problem in the family. Intervention is therefore oriented around the famliy to demonstrate that the child's problems are shared by all and solutions require the collective power of the entire unit. With support and guidance, the family finds strength to hold the adolescent accountable for the consequences of drug-related behavior. Disruptive behavior is rejected and appropriate adaptive approaches to problem solving are supported.

Tough Love is a community-based support group in which parents of troubled children come together to help each other learn to look at problems and change responses to the child's behavior. Developed by Phyllis and David York (1982) from their personal struggle with a troubled child, Tough Love assists families to live together in a caring way. Tough Love's philosophy can be described with the following beliefs:

Family problems have roots and supports in the culture.

Parents are people too.

Parents' material and emotional resources are limited.

Parents and adolescents are not equal.

Blaming keeps people helpless.

Child's behavior affects parents; parents' behavior affects the child.

Taking a stand precipitates a crisis.

From controlled crisis comes positive change.

Families need to get support in their own communities in order to change.

The essence of family life is cooperation, not togetherness.

Family intervention in adolescent drug abuse is designed to eliminate disruptive behavior and facilitate organizational change in the family. With appropriate guidance, parents determine the goals for behavioral change, the methods by which change will be accomplished, and the ways in which responsibility will be shared. It is through this process that the family is empowered to solve its problems and ensure that the child's needs are met (Jansen, 1986).

The Child with an Emotional Disorder

The tasks required for successful development involve the emergence of the child's individual personality and sense of self. The process of development creates periods of disequilibrium—times when the child is vulnerable to external and internal stressors. During these times, the child tests personal abilities and demands of authority, attempting to master new interpersonal and intellectual skills.

Typically, the child approaches these transitional periods with varied amounts of anxiety and often with a desire to withdraw to an environment that offers familiarity, security, and comfort. When the external environment facilitates adaptive coping with the stressors of daily life, the child begins to take control of stressful situations. By learning problem-solving skills, the child learns to make decisions that enhance the pursuit of industry, autonomy, and identity.

DSM III identifies a group of conditions broadly categorized as emotional disorders. Anxiety, the feature common to all these conditions, is defined by Doona (1979) as a subjective experience involving tension, restlessness, and apprehension in response to real or perceived threats to self-esteem. Anxiety can interfere with the normal processes of affective and social development. Attempting to avoid discomfort, the child's coping strategies become maladaptive, and behaviors become dysfunctional.

Assessing the child's behavior might indicate a variety of ways in which the child is exhibiting maladapative coping strategies. Such an assessment might lead to any of the following potential nursing diagnoses:

Ineffective individual coping

Disturbances in body image and self-esteem

Social isolation

Impaired verbal communication

Alterations in parenting

Ineffective family coping: compromised

Separation Disorder of Childhood

Separation disorder of childhood is a condition related to the anxiety of growth and development. Underlying the problem is the chlid's excessive anxiety when faced with separation from parents. DSM III identifies the following behavioral criteria, which must be documented over a 3-week period to be considered significant:

1. Unrealistic worry about significant others
2. Fear of abandonment
3. Unrealistic worry that a catastrophe will cause separation from parents
4. Persistent refusal to go to school in order to stay home with parent
5. Persistent refusal to go to sleep
6. Somatic (physical) complaints on school days
7. Excessive distress on separation or when anticipating separation

Assessment Anxiety and maladaptive coping often are correlated with the experience of separation, which might occur during a serious illness, after the death of a significant person in the child's life, or during times of intense family stress. When a child is experiencing separation, school can impose social, academic, and personal demands that threaten the child. Parents also might unknowingly encourage maladaptive coping by permitting dysfunctional behavior to continue and allowing the child to avoid the problem.

The nurse might observe any of the following behaviors, which are characteristic of persistent anxiety:

1. Unrealistic worry about future events
2. Preoccupation with the individual's past behavior
3. Excessive concern about competence (school, social, athletic)
4. Excessive need for reassurance
5. Somatic complaints (for which no physical cause can be established)

6. Excessive self-consciousness
7. Excessive susceptibility to embarrassment
8. Excessive tension and/or inability to relax

Using knowledge of age-appropriate norms, the child health nurse identifies dysfunctional behavior patterns and determines their severity. In addition, a complete physical and psychologic evaluation may be needed to establish baseline data and define related physical and learning problems. Observations of parent-child interactions may reveal overprotective or anxious behavior in the parent, indicating dysfunctional parenting (see Chapter 13).

Nursing management Effective management of anxiety and avoidance behavior allows the child opportunities for development and promotes affective and social growth. Controlling the behavior helps the child learn to control the environment. The nurse might therefore suggest or participate in planning a behavior modification program that rewards the child for functional behavior in which problems are managed and not avoided. For such a program, the child health nurse enlists the cooperation of parents and school representatives in determining the specific interventions.

Depending on the degree of dysfunction, additional treatment may be indicated. Modalities might include family, marital, and individual therapy. In general, however, the child with a separation disorder benefits from the following strategies:

- consistent cooperation of parents and teachers
- visual tools such as a star chart or calendar that marks attendance with stars or other stickers to track goals and achievements
- specific reminders of goals through positive reinforcers in behavior modification
- support for parents as they develop new interests and pursue activities away from the child
- referral to other therapeutic modalities that allow parents to separate their concerns from the child's concerns
- provision of opportunities for parents to express feelings about the child

Depression in Children and Adolescents

Alarming statistics, including the fact that in 1984 more than 5000 young people in the United States committed suicide, have precipitated concern and study of suicide. Suicide is the third highest cause of death among adolescents, suggesting that this renewed concern is well founded.

Additional data concerning accidents among children in early and middle childhood suggest that the incidence of self-inflicted accidents is high. Indeed, because of inaccurate reporting of cause of death in children, the exact measure of self-inflicted and intentional injury might never be known (Finn, 1986). Clearly, the causes of suicidal behavior are a problem of great magnitude.

Because many children who have suicidal thoughts are also depressed, these two concepts are linked together. Childhood depression, however, with or without suicidal thoughts, is different from depression in adults. Increasingly, clinicians are finding that the criteria outlined to identify depression in adults does not correlate well with features of depression observed in children and adolescents. For those in early childhood, health care providers can use a variety of psychologic assessment tools that are now available for identifying depression.

The most common type of depression seen by the child health nurse is *secondary depression*. This is sadness that occurs in response to a particular situation or event. The situations include the trauma of hospitalization, surgery, or separation from a family event. Children might become depressed secondary to medical disorders, such as diabetes mellitus, asthma, cardiac anomalies, or to cognitive and behavioral problems. Children with learning problems and specific learning disabilities frequently become depressed because of their frustration with school, particularly if the disorder is not recognized or special academic assistance is not provided.

Depression that is not a response to the stress of an event is termed *primary depression*. Primary depression is a depressive syndrome with identifiable symptoms. Its etiology, however, is not clearly understood.

Childhood depression might be caused by grief. Grief reactions in children are not well understood. A prolonged grief reaction extending beyond 6 months generally is considered pathologic in adults. The timing of extended grief that should be considered pathologic in children is not defined and might vary across the developmental stages. Children also might rework grief reactions when they enter new developmental stages. Some children with major life changes, such as parental divorce or a move to a new community, fail to make adjustments within a reasonable amount of time. In addition to difficulties in adjustment (such as not making friends or a decrease in school performance), the child might be sad. These situations, however, usually are not viewed as primary depression because the sadness is secondary to adjustment problems.

No biologic or genetic factor has been identified as a sole determinant of depression. Any factor or accumulation or interaction of factors might predispose a child to depression. So far, little conclusive work has fully described the interaction among genetic-biologic and sociologic-

TABLE 16-13 Symptoms of Depression in Children

Type of symptom	Example
Mood	Depressed feelings (verbal) Depressed feelings (nonverbal) Irritability Weeping
Somatic symptoms	Appetite—increase or decrease Sleep—initial, middle, or terminal disturbance Excessive fatigue Psychomotor retardation—slow activity and/or tempo of speech Physical complaints (nonorganic)
Subjective symptoms	Decreased self-esteem Guilt Morbid ideation Suicidal ideation
Behavior	Anhedonia Social withdrawal Schoolwork impairment

SOURCE: Adapted from Poznanski E et al.: Diagnostic criteria in childhood depression. *Arch Gen Psychiatry.* © American Medical Association.

psychiatric factors. Preliminary studies of family histories of depressed children appear to show trends similar to those uncovered in adult studies. A higher incidence is found in the relatives of depressed children (Geller et al., 1985).

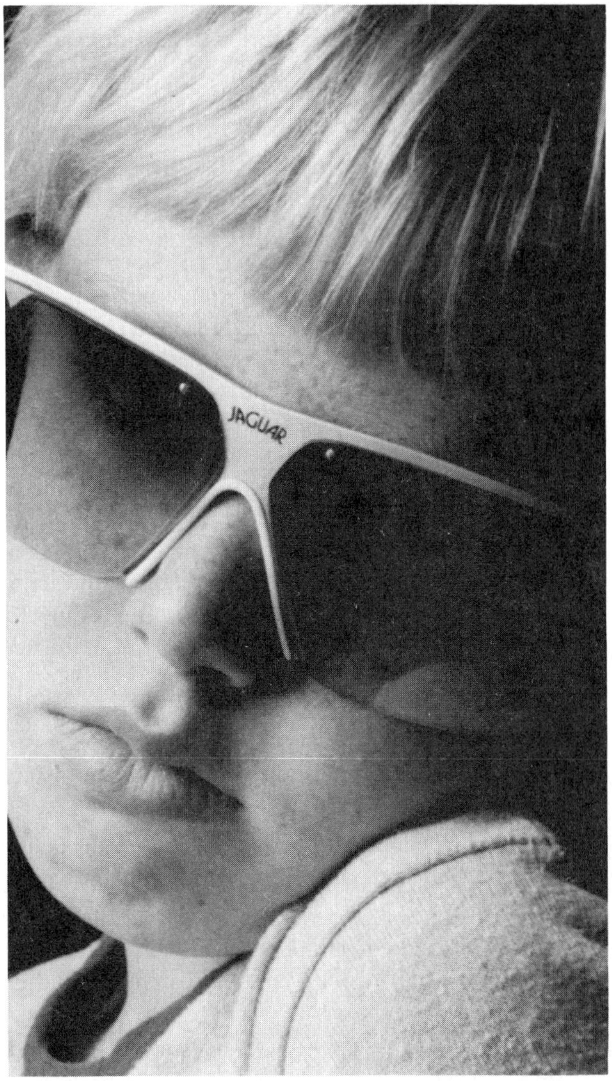

Depressed children can be socially withdrawn.

Assessment

Behavioral manifestations of depression Although childhood depression is different from depression in adults, children manifest some of the same depressive symptoms. (Behaviors associated with depression are outlined in Table 16-13.) Generally, these symptoms involve changes in activity level, social relationships, eating, and elimination patterns. Accurate assessment requires that the child health nurse use multiple sources of data, including interviewing parents and child (Mullins et al., 1985).

Verbal and nonverbal expressions of sadness are assessed along with indications of *anhedonia,* or inability to enjoy oneself. The child may not appear to be very sad, but verbal descriptors such as gloomy, bored, bad, empty, and "not being able to stand it," along with displeasure or concern about activities of prior interest, should alert the child health nurse of possible depressed feelings. Social withdrawal may be identified but must be differentiated in a child who has never developed positive peer relationships. Many depressed children had good peer relationships at one time but now report that "I have no friends" or "The kids don't like me." The withdrawn child might reject opportunities to play with other children or watch other children play.

Associated symptoms of depression include irritability, weeping, and somatic complaints. Irritable children are those who are easily bothered by the smallest event. Some depressed children cry more than their peers, feel like crying frequently, or appear to be about to cry. Depressed children might complain of minor aches and pains that have no organic cause.

Schoolwork often is impaired when a child is depressed, even though the child might previously have done well in school. The impaired schoolwork might be the result of the general apathy, an inability to concentrate, or distraction by internal stimuli.

An important distinction is the difference between the child who has depressive feelings and the child who has a depressive syndrome. Many children feel sad at some point in the day, but the sadness does not last all day or for several days. For example, in an interview with a nurse clinician, one 10-year-old girl described feeling sad but said that the sadness went away when she talked to her mother or when she woke up the next day. Unlike this child, truly depressed children have sad feelings that persist for 1–4 weeks. One depressed child reported to the nurse clinician that she could not remember the last time she felt happy or had a good time.

For young children whose language skills are rudimentary, the nurse cannot rely on verbal cues as a principal source of data. Current research by Kashani et al. (1986) concludes that depression in young children is associated with the following characteristics:

1. Parents and school personnel might identify depressed symptoms in preschoolers, although data are insufficient to diagnose the symptoms as depression.
2. Anger or irritability rather than sadness might be the predominant components of depression in young children.
3. Parents of children with depressive symptoms tend to report more stressful life events than parents of children without such symptoms.
4. Teachers and other care providers are important sources of data for the identification of depressive behavior.
5. Interviewing the young child, as well as using multiple sources of data, allows for more accurate diagnosis.

When interviewed, depressed children and adolescents often are able to identify some of the reasons for their depression. When asked about what makes them worry or feel sad, children describe family problems, school problems, and lack of friendships. A nursing perspective on depression considers the problem in youth as an interaction of biopsychosocial factors.

Indicators of suicidal risk Professionals and parents must acknowledge that children do think about and try to kill themselves. Nurses need to be aware of the factors that place children at risk for suicide, including the following:

1. Drug and alcohol abuse
2. Depression with prolonged helplessness
3. Conduct disorders, especially impulsive behavior
4. Emerging psychosis (thought disorder)
5. Losses (particularly close peers with adolescents and dependency relationships with children)
6. Changes in the child's usual pattern of behavior related to peers, school activities, academic performance, increased irritability, withdrawal, overt sadness, sleeping habits, somatic complaints, preoccupation with death

Children who are depressed often are preoccupied with morbid thoughts, which typically are about themselves or others dying. For example, one child drew himself in a family drawing as if he were thinking of his grandmother who had died 2 years earlier. Suicidal thoughts, plans, or actions also are reported by depressed children. One 7-year-old girl tried to jump out of a car on a busy expressway. Her mother also had been depressed and suicidal following the imprisonment of the child's father, who had committed several violent crimes.

School health nurses, school personnel, and other community resource people (coaches, scout leaders, and child-care workers) need to be aware that any threat of suicide should be taken seriously and evaluated by appropriate clinicians. Although the behaviors, etiology, and results are similar, the suicidal behavior manifests in different ways (Table 16-14). Covert suicide and cluster suicide are two suicide related phenomena receiving attention in the literature.

Covert suicide is described as "those forms of self-destructive behavior that involve a deliberate threat to life but are not typically recognized as suicide attempts" (Molin, 1986). These attempts may include drunken-driving incidents, accident proneness, some forms of substance abuse, and dieting to the point of starvation. The key feature of covert suicidal attempts is denial by the child. The family might unknowingly contribute to this behavior by failing to set limits, ignoring the signals of suicidal risk, providing access to the car, or allowing excessive time alone. Intervention in covert suicidal attempts focuses on getting the family to acknowledge the danger to the child and accepting responsibility to protect the child.

Cluster suicide is a recent and alarming trend in which several young people commit a series of self-destructive acts. Usually, an initial suicide appears to trigger self-destructive behavior by other children. Clinicians theorize that this phenomenon might be coincidental or that it might be a self-dramatizing attempt to derive sympathetic responses similar to those that followed the initial death (Leo, 1986).

Diagnosis and treatment The diagnosis of depression in children is made on the basis of extensive psychiatric evaluation of both parents and child. The essential feature of

TABLE 16-14 Definitions from a Scale Used to Measure Suicidal Behavior in Children

Tendency	Manifestation
Nonsuicidal	No evidence of suicidal ideas and/ or behavior that could have caused self-injury or death
Suicidal ideation	Thoughts or verbalization of suicidal intention. Examples: "I want to kill myself"; auditory hallucinations commanding the child to kill himself or herself
Suicidal threat	Verbalization of an impending suicidal act and/or a precursor act which, if fully carried out, could have led to self-harm. Examples: a child says, "I am going to run in front of a car"; a child puts a knife under the pillow in preparation to kill himself or herself; a child stands near an open window and says he or she will jump out
Mild suicidal attempt	Actual self-destructive act that realistically could not have endangered life and did not necessitate intensive medical attention. Example: a child ingests a few nonlethal pills, following which the child's stomach is pumped
Serious suicidal attempt	Actual self-destructive act that realistically could have led to the child's death and might have necessitated intensive medical care. Example: a child jumps out of a fourth-floor window; a child hangs himself or herself

SOURCE: Adapted from Pfeffer CR et al: Suicidal behavior in child psychiatric inpatients and outpatients. *Am J Psychiatr* (June) 1986. 143 : 6.

this evaluation is that the child is seen over a 1- to 3-week period so that the persistence of depressive affect can be evaluated. Additionally, physical disorders are ruled out. Depression can coexist with other psychopathologies, such as conduct disorders, atteniton deficits, or separation disorder, and these also must be diagnosed.

The treatment of depression in children is preceded by a thorough discussion of the disorder with the parent. Depression does not have the stigma of some other childhood disorders such as autism and schizophrenia, and the parent therefore is often able to accept the diagnosis. In fact, parents might suspect the diagnosis because of their own depression or a history of depression in the family.

Currently, treatment tends to be carried out by child psychiatrists because of issues concerning psychopharmacology. Some drugs used to treat depression can cause adverse side effects and children need to be monitored closely during any period of pharmacologic therapy for depression. It is recommended frequently that children receive individual therapy with a professional who specializes in psychiatric disorders of children (such as the child psychiatrist, child psychiatric nurse, or child psychologist). The focus of treatment is to build a relationship with the child and to provide an opportunity for the child to deal with conflicts and feelings through play and verbalization.

For example, one 7-year-old girl with major depression spent almost 6 months in therapy with a psychiatric nurse. Play therapy stimulated the child to verbalize the violent threats her father had made to her mother, sibling rivalry, acting out in school, deliberate accidents, and role confusion. The nurse then worked with the mother to deal with the boundaries related to the child's role and with school personnel to help them understand the child's behavior in the context of her life situation.

Family or marital therapy might be recommended in conjunction with individual psychotherapy for the child or as the primary method of treatment. This method is indicated when the child's depression appears to be a manifestation of such family dysfunction as child abuse, neglect, intense sibling conflicts, and noninvolvement of a parent. Some psychodynamically oriented clinicians believe that family therapy is contraindicated when a family member is depressed, because the depressed member is thought to be unable to engage in family treatment, but rather needs individual therapy. Only recently have clinicians begun to realize the family's contribution to and maintenance of individual depression.

The administration of antidepressant medication in prepubertal children is controlled by the Federal Drug Administration so that only a small number of physicians can prescribe them.

Nursing management Throughout the child's treatment, it might be appropriate for the child health nurse to be involved in parent education and counseling. This should be done only in collaboration with the child's therapist. Education and counseling can include such areas as development, limit setting, discussion of symptoms, and ways to support the child when the child is feeling sad or bad about self.

The most effective treatment for children with depression is generally a treatment plan that involves more than one method of intervention. Parents can be encouraged to seek group activities for their child in the community because many depressed children are socially withdrawn. Depressed children typically are somewhat sedentary. Parents need to be educated about the mild antidepressant effect of

Guidelines for Suicide Prevention and Intervention

1. Recognize early warning signs: LISTEN.
2. Take every complaint or threat seriously.
3. Evaluate the seriousness.
4. Ask direct questions about the child's thoughts about suicide.
5. Beware of reassurances from the child that the crisis has passed.
6. Be affirmative but supportive.
7. Evaluate the child's internal and external resources.
8. Give the child specific direction—a plan.
9. Obtain appropriate assistance.

exercise because they might tend to excuse the child from physical activities.

Children who have major depression and conduct disorders might become involved in serious delinquency as adolescents and require residential treatment. Hospitalization might be indicated for depressed children with psychotic symptoms or children who require psychopharmacologic treatment. Hospitalization for the child who is exhibiting suicidal thoughts is critical to the child's safety. In the event that parents do not agree to this plan, suicide precautions should be planned for the home (such as constant supervision and the removal of medicines). Nurses have a role in facilitating the implementation of a suicide prevention plan in the hospital or home. Most pediatric units are not prepared to deal with suicide prevention, but pediatric and psychiatric nursing collaboration can result in the implementation of a program for the prevention of suicide in a child.

Cluster suicide and covert suicide behavior have precipitated community concern and involvement. School systems are instituting suicidal prevention programs that join three components in the helping process: students, school personnel, and parents. Through education and training, individuals prevent suicide through recognition of individuals at risk and referral to appropriate resources.

In addition to established mental health resources for suicide intervention, the Samaritans are volunteers specifically trained in suicide prevention. The group maintains local 24-hour telephone hot lines to befriend and talk with people who are considering suicide or with families or others who are concerned that a person might be considering suicide.

In the event that a child or adolescent is successful in commiting suicide, the parents and other survivors will require support. Toder (1986) describes losing a child as one of the most intolerable emotional experiences. The suddenness and finality of separation does not allow an opportunity to resolve differences and leaves the family with guilt and grief. Survivors of suicide are themselves at risk because they tend to isolate themselves from the family and grieve individually. Self-help, professional intervention, and support groups [Compassionate Friends and LOSS (Loving Outreach to Survivors of Suicide)] enable survivors to respond to the experience in an adaptive manner. The grief work for the family includes open grieving; reordering life goals and priorities; regaining family equilibrium; and moving on to new experiences, thoughts, and relationships.

Schizophrenia

Schizophrenia is a severe emotional or psychotic disorder that is characterized by moderate to severe impairments in thought, language, behavior, and social adaptation. Schizophrenic disorders involve delusions (false beliefs about oneself and others), hallucinations (distorted perceptions of reality), or certain disturbances in the order of thoughts. Individuals with schizophrenia have periodic difficulty coping with tasks of everyday living.

The etiology of schizophrenia is still in question. Research continues to explore genetic, behavioral, and biochemical theories to explain this complex disorder. Schizophrenia is rare in children, although it can be seen occasionally in adolescents. The child health nurse might encounter an adolescent with schizophrenia who has been hospitalized for another health problem.

Assessment The assessment of schizophrenia requires an extensive, multidisciplinary diagnostic evaluation with a child psychiatrist, child psychologist, and clinical nurse specialist. The evaluation includes clinical interviews and observation with the child, parent interviews, and psychologic testing. Psychologic testing is needed to rule out mental retardation because retarded children can demonstrate some of the same behaviors as psychotic children. A complete pediatric and neurologic evaluation is indicated to rule out an organic process or drug intoxication.

Treatment The adolescent with schizophrenia is likely to require simultaneous treatment modalities or a series of modalities. These include promoting activities of daily living, socialization, community activities, and parent education and counseling. Education is a key component of the treatment program. Educational settings include therapeutic day schools and classrooms for emotionally disturbed children in public schools.

NURSING CARE PLAN

Assessment data: Ken, 8½ years old, was admitted to the pediatric unit to be observed for suicidal behavior and to begin a regimen of antidepressant medication. Ken lives with his parents and is an only child. Both parents work. The family is socially isolated, and the majority of their outside contacts are with extended family members. Two months previously, the maternal grandmother, with whom the family was very close, died after a long illness. Ken was frequently at the hospital and at the grandmother's house. Ken's problem began 6 weeks prior to admission when he had gone to emergency rooms several times with complaints of severe stomach pains. A negative gastroenterology workup prompted the physician to refer Ken to a child psychiatrist.

Ken was evaluated extensively in an outpatient clinic and was diagnosed as having a major depression and separation disorder. Ken's depression was evident by his description of his sadness, sad and unkempt appearance, inability to have fun, social withdrawal, impaired schoolwork, sleep difficulty, and morbid and suicidal thoughts. He exhibited severe anxiety and refused to go to school. Desipramine has been prescribed as an antidepressant.

Nursing diagnosis	Intervention	Rationale
1. Dysfunctional grieving related to the loss of the grandmother	Note and record changes in mood or suicidal behavior.	Accurate observation is essential to prevent a suicide attempt.
	Encourage verbal expression of thoughts and feelings; use role play or storytelling if verbal expression is difficult for Ken.	Verbalizing feelings helps view them in a more realistic light. Often children have difficulty talking about feelings so storytelling or other play situations might be more helpful.
	Offer empathetic statements about Ken's worries (eg, it must be difficult to concentrate in school when you miss your grandmother).	Empathetic statements indicate caring as well as validate what the child might be actually feeling.
	Avoid pressuring Ken for verbal performance.	Pressure increases anxiety.
	Encourage Ken to share his wishes, fears, or thoughts about harming himself.	Verbal expression of suicidal thoughts allows the nurse to evaluate the seriousness of the suicidal tendencies.
	Reinforce the seriousness of the suicidal threats to his parents.	Often parents don't take suicidal threats seriously, thinking the child is saying things to gain attention but will never actually carry the plans out.

Outcome: Ken is able to express verbally or through play his feelings of loss or thoughts about suicide. Ken appears less depressed and sad and more interested in his surroundings. The parents are able to tell the nurse why any threat of suicide should be taken seriously.

Nursing diagnosis	Intervention	Rationale
2. Potential for injury (stressors: expressed wish to kill himself, expression of morbid thoughts)	Provide constant supervision.	Children who have the potential to injure themselves often do it when they feel they are not being observed. Close observation of the child provides a measure of security for him.
	Remove all potentially dangerous items such as ropes or cord-type items, sharp objects or toys, chemicals or other poisons from the room.	The child might act on impulse to injure himself and use what is readily available.
	Explain the precautions to Ken and his family.	Explaining the precautions can reassure the child and family that the child is receiving the maximum protection to prevent injury.

(Continues)

NURSING CARE PLAN *The Child Exhibiting Suicidal Behavior* (Continued)

Nursing diagnosis	Intervention	Rationale
Outcome: Ken and his family can explain the need for safety precautions. The parents can identify what objects are unsafe.		
3. Total self-care deficit related to decreased energy, poor self-esteem, and depression	Provide encouragement for health and personal grooming efforts.	Interest in personal appearance decreases when a child is depressed.
	Encourage self-care activities and participation in play opportunities on the unit.	Independence and self-care increases self-esteem. Play activities provide contact with other children whose positive feedback can increase self-esteem.
	Encourage Ken to eat appropriately—his favorite foods are pizza and ice cream.	Anorexia is frequently seen in depressed children.
	Encourage physical activity within the restrictions of the unit.	Exercise is a mild antidepressant.
Outcome: Ken will actively dress, feed himself, and perform other activities of daily living. Ken will increase the time he spends in the playroom and in contact with peers. Ken's unkempt appearance will improve.		
4. Ineffective family coping related to emotional conflicts secondary to Ken's refusal to attend school and the family's social isolation	Provide the opportunity for the parents to discuss their anger and frustration.	Allowing parents to express anger reduces frustration and allows for problem solving.
	Encourage parents to develop interests outside the home—adult education classes, volunteer activities, pursuit of a hobby.	Broadening social contacts will provide a wider base of support as well as help the parents remove themselves from problems in the home temporarily.
	Discuss an alternate temporary school schedule such as tutoring for Ken.	One-on-one schooling might help Ken's ability to concentrate and prevent feelings of failure and diminished self-worth.
	Determine with the parents a series of rewards (such as a story immediately after school or a special trip) for regular school attendance.	The child's positive behavior is rewarded, resulting in greater compliance and reduced tension at home. Parents will feel more in control.
Outcome: Ken will be able to increase his concentration while studying. Ken will gradually move back into the school setting with diminished sense of failure. Ken's parents feel more in control of the situation as evidenced by their ability to state and try various approaches to the problem.		
5. Potential knowledge deficit regarding home management (stressors: inadequate understanding of medication administration, anxiety)	Teach the parents about medication administration, including correct dose, side effects, storage, safety precautions, and dangers of sudden withdrawal.	Compliance with the medication regimen is essential for positive treatment outcome.
	Tell the parents to check Ken's mouth after administering the medication.	Children sometimes hide the medication instead of swallowing it and spit it out later.
	Encourage the parents to be aware of any mood change or suicide threats; give them the number for the local suicide prevention hot line.	The parents need to know where they can get help fast if they need it and how to determine whether help is needed.
Outcome: The parents can describe changes in mood that might indicate Ken is having trouble. The parents can demonstrate correct medication administration and can list side effects and precautions. The parents have the hot line number readily available and know who to contact in an emergency.		

Children with schizophrenia seem to do better clinically when they live at home, but even children who remain at home might need to be hospitalized in inpatient units during acute episodes. Pharmacologic management is not widely used because data on the effect of antipsychotic medication on children are limited.

Nursing management Consistency and structure are key elements in the care of the adolescent with schizophrenia, although the child health nurse is not responsible for interpreting psychotic symptoms. Documentation of symptoms, however, is valuable.

Adolescents with schizophrenia tend to isolate themselves and, when hospitalized for treatment of a medical condition, might isolate themselves further. The nurse might need extra persistence to make contact with the child.

Because children with schizophrenia are particularly vulnerable to life stresses, the stress of an illness can precipitate a psychotic episode (symptoms of hallucinations, delusions, or thought disorders). In the event that an acute psychotic episode occurs, the child's care on a pediatric unit needs to be carefully planned and managed through the collaboration of the pediatric and psychiatric nursing staff. The child's safety and that of others needs to be ensured. Parents need to be prepared and supported if the child regresses.

Parents of children with schizophrenia need ongoing counseling to deal with their feelings toward their children, to understand their children's behavior and development, and to plan management at home. Parents can be trained in behavioral management and assisted to develop a behavioral program for the home. Parents are encouraged to assess and build on their child's strengths. As adolescents grow older, interventions are geared toward group, community, and work activities.

The Child with a Developmental Disorder—Infantile Autism

Infantile autism is rare but is one of the most serious psychiatric disorders of childhood. Autism can be detected in the earliest stages of development and is characterized by withdrawal, self-absorption, and unresponsiveness. Child health nurses may encounter these children in the prediagnostic period when well-child visits indicate developmental problems. Acute child health care settings along with community health settings may offer opportunities for child health nurses to care for these exceptional children.

Autistic behavior includes language retardation with impaired cognition, unusual responses to the environment, self-stimulation, resistance to change, and inappropriate attachment to objects. The autistic child's perceptual dysfunctions severely distort personal experiences. Thus, the autistic child's behaviors can appear to be bizarre to individuals who do not share this unique reality.

One sensitive father's description of his autistic son provides some insight into the mannerisms and world of the autistic child:

> The rocking back and forth on the leverage of his own eternity. The soft and gentle retreat to the outside perimeter of our world. The spinning and fixed state. His great agility and his hypnotic fascination with inanimate objects. The self-stimulating smile and repetitious motion of his fingers against his lips. The pushing away of people and the silent aloneness. When Raun turned to you, he turned through you as if you were transparent. And then there was the keen awareness that he did not use language. Not just a slow talker, he offered no communication by sound or gesture, no expression of wants, likes or dislikes. Almost one and a half years old, Raun, a new creature in a strange land (Kaufman, 1976).

Knowledge of age-appropriate developmental norms is the key to identifying autistic behaviors. A team approach to evaluation is essential to ensure accuracy in diagnosis. Members of the team may include a physician, nurse, psychologist, social worker, occupational/physical therapist, special education teacher, speech and language pathologist, and other necessary resource people. Comprehensive evaluation may rule out such disorders as mental retardation, sensory impairment, and childhood schizophrenia.

Although no cure for autism exists, early intervention and appropriate management can benefit children and parents. Zoltak (1986) identifies five major areas for child health intervention:

1. Maintaining a trusting relationship between care providers and the child
2. Communicating instructions and information in brief, clear phrases (eg, "look at me")
3. Assessing effectiveness of prescribed medications and evaluating adverse or toxic effects
4. Supporting parents in their attempt to cope with the triumphs and setbacks of the child
5. Facilitating parental efforts to attain a regular and appropriate educational program for their child

Institutionalization for autistic children is not always necessary when appropriate community-based services are available. Although the prognosis is guarded, early detection can enhance the family's ability to cope and in some cases can provide direct care for the child.

Essential Concepts

- Coping strategies are learned behaviors that the child uses to adapt to stress.
- Coping behaviors that are age-appropriate and that help the child adapt to the environment are a normal part of development.
- Although specific coping strategies are evident across developmental stages, patterns of coping do change with the child's development.
- A child's coping behaviors are influenced by age, temperament, and the role models and experiences to which the child has been exposed.
- Children can learn adaptive coping strategies through such techniques as relaxation and problem solving.
- A knowledge of psychiatric symptoms allows the nurse to facilitate psychiatric referrals and intervene to prevent the manifestations of psychiatric disorders.
- Manifestations of psychiatric disorders vary according to the child's developmental stage.
- The most common classification for psychiatric disorders is the *Diagnostic and Statistical Manual of Mental Disorders,* or DSM III, published by the American Psychiatric Association, which applies a disease model to psychopathology.
- Nursing management for the child with learning, attention, and activity disorders is part of a multidisciplinary effort that may involve diagnostic evaluation, behavioral counseling, educational programs, medication, and support for the child and family.
- Nursing care for children with conduct disorders involves consistent limit setting and teaching appropriate ways to express feelings.
- Managing children with elimination disorders includes promoting self-image, use of behavior modification, and anxiety reduction through therapeutic play.
- Nursing care of children with eating disorders is directed toward promoting their self-image and self-control and preventing further nutritional deficiencies. Most important is to gain the family's cooperation and participation in the plan.
- Nursing management for substance abusers involves education at the primary prevention level, emergency and acute care at the secondary level, and referral for rehabilitation at the tertiary level.
- Nursing care for depressed children might involve social skills training, family therapy, suicide precautions, and psychopharmacologic therapy.
- Nursing care of children with severe emotional problems requires providing a safe, consistent, and structured environment; setting limits; and communicating in concrete terms.

References

Abrahamian FP, Lloyd-Still JD: Chronic constipation in childhood, a longitudinal study of 186 patients. *J Pediatr Gastroenterol and Nutr* (June) 1984; 3(3):460.

Bauer BB, Hill SS: *Essentials of Mental Health Care.* Saunders, 1986.

Bell CS, Battjes RJ (eds): *Prevention Research: Deterring Drug Abuse Among Children and Adolescents.* NIDA Research Monograph 63. DHHS Pub. (ADM) 85–1334, US GPO, 1985.

Bryant SO, Kopeski LM: Psychiatric assessment of the eating disorder client. *Top Clin Nurs* (April) 1986; 8(1):57–66.

D'Epiro P: Enuresis: The role of alarms and drugs. *Patient Care* (Jan) 1985; 19(1):75–78, 83, 87.

Doona ME: *Travelbee's Intervention in Psychiatric Nursing.* 2nd edition. Davis, 1979.

Edmands MS: Overcoming eating disorders. *J Psychosoc Nurs* (Aug) 1986; 24(8):19–25.

Finn PA: Self-destructive behavior in school age children: A hidden problem. *Pediatr Nurs* (May/June) 1986; 12(3):198–199.

Garner D, Garfinkel P: *Handbook of Psychotherapy for Anorexia and Bulimia.* Guilford Press, 1985.

Geller B et al: Preliminary data on DSM III associated features of major depressive disorder in children and adolescents. *Am J Psychiatry* (May) 1985; 142(5):643.

Hahn, Oestreich, Barkin: *Mosby's Pharmacology in Nursing. 16th edition.* Mosby, 1986.

Jansen DP: Benefits of a family oriented approach in adolescent treatment. *J Contemp Social Work* (Sept) 1986; 67(7):410–417.

Jones CL, Bell-Bolek CS: Kids and drugs: Why, when and what can we do about it. *Child Today* (May/June) 1986; 5–10.

Kandel DB, Logan JA: Patterns of drug use from adolescence to young adulthood: Periods of risk for initiation, continued use, and discontinuation. *Am J Public Health* (July) 1984; 74(7):660–665.

Kashani JH, Holcomb WR, Orvaschel H: Depression and depressive symptoms in preschool children from the general population. *Am J Psychiatry* (Sept) 1986; 143(9): 1138–1143.

Kaufman BN: *Son-Rise,* Harper and Row, 1976.

Landman GB et al: Locus of control and self-esteem in children with encopresis. *J Dev Behav Pediatr* (April) 1986; 7(2): 111–113.

Leo J: Cluster suicide. *Time* (Feb 24) 1986; 127(8): 59.

Loening-Baucke VA: Abnormal defecation dynamics in chronically constipated children with encopresis. *J Pediatr* (April) 1986; 108(4): 562–566.

Maizels M, Ferlit CF: Guide to the history in enuretic children. *Am Fam Physician* (April) 1986; 33(4): 205–209.

Molin RS: Covert suicide and families of adolescents. *Adolescence* (Spring) 1986; Vol. XXI. No. 81: 177–184.

Mullins LL et al: Cognitive problem solving and life events: Correlates of depressive symptoms in children. *J Abnorm Psychol* (June) 1985; 13(2): 305–314.

National Institute on Drug Abuse. *Report to Congress on Drugs and Health,* 1984.

Newcomb MD et al: Risk factors for drug use among adolescents: Concurrent and longitudinal analyses. *Am J Public Health* (May) 1986; 76(5): 525–531.

Palmer EP, Guay AT: Reversible myopathy secondary to abuse of ipecac in patients with major eating disorders. *New Engl J Med* (Dec 5) 1985; 313(23): 1457–1459.

Pearlin L, Schooler G: The Structure of Coping. *J Soc Behav* (March) 1978; 19(3): 2–18.

Pothier PC: *Mental Health Counseling with Children.* Little, Brown, 1976.

Satter EM: Childhood eating disorders. *J Am Dietetic Assoc* (March) 1986; 86(3): 357–361.

Shapiro SR: Enuresis: Treatment and over treatment. *Pediatr Nurs* (May/June) 1985; 11(3): 203–207, 214.

Swett WE: Helping young people to survive in a chemical world. *Fam Community Health* (Aug) 1984; 2(7): 63–73.

Toder F: *When Your Child is Gone: Learning to Live Again.* Capital Publishing, Sacramento, CA, 1986.

Williams SR: *Nutrition and Diet Therapy.* 5th edition. Times Mirror/Mosby, 1985.

York D, York P: *ToughLove.* Doubleday, 1982.

Zoltak BB: Autism: Recognition and management. *Pediatr Nurs* (April/May) 1986; 12(2): 90–94.

Additional Readings

Acee A, Smith D: Crack. *Am J Nurs* (May) 1987; 87(5): 614–617.

American Psychiatric Association: *Diagnostic and Statistical Manual of Mental Disorders.* 3rd edition. American Psychiatric Assoc., Washington, DC, 1980.

Arboleda C, Holzman PS: Thought disorder in children at risk for psychosis. *Arch Gen Psychiatry* (Oct) 1985; 42(10): 1004–1013.

Beck CB, Rawlins RP, Williams SR: *Mental Health—Psychiatric Nursing: A Holistic Life-Cycle Approach.* Mosby, 1984.

Biederman J, Jelinek MS: Current concepts in psychopharmacology in children. *N Engl J Med* (April) 1984; 310(15): 968–972.

Davis ME, Shelmar E, McKay M: *The Relaxation and Stress Reduction Workbook.* New Harbinger Pub., 1980.

Hofman AD: *Adolescent Medicine.* Addison-Wesley, 1983.

Nelms BC: Assessing childhood depression: Do parents and children agree? *Pediatr Nurs* (Jan/Feb) 1986; 12(1): 23–26.

Pfeffer CR et al: Suicidal behavior in child psychiatric inpatients, outpatients and nonpatients. *Am J Psychiatry* (June) 1986; 143(6): 733.

Pothier PC: Child psychiatric nursing: The gap between need and utilization. *Pediatr Nurs* (July) 1985; 23(7): 18–23.

Pozanski EO et al: Psychotic and depressed children: A new entity. *J Am Acad Child Psychiatry* (Jan) 1985; 24(1): 95–102.

Rhyne MC et al: Children at risk for depression. *Am J Nurs* (Dec) 1986; 86(12): 1379–1382.

Chapter 17

Nursing Care of the Dying Child

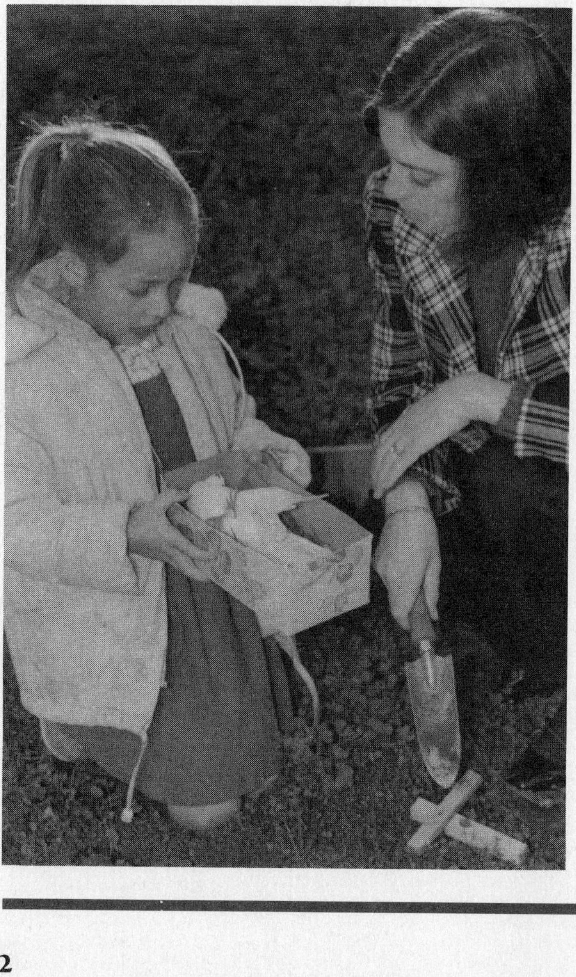

Chapter Contents

Peer Support
Settings for Terminal Care
Evaluation and Follow-Up

Objectives

- Explain why nurses need to prepare both cognitively and emotionally for the experience of dealing with dying children and their families.
- Distinguish the characteristic perceptions of and responses to death of children at various developmental stages.
- Discuss the factors of timing and level of awareness that affect a child's experience of death.
- Identify the most common coping strategies and emotional responses of dying children.
- Discuss the effects of the child's dying on the family.
- Anticipate the nurse's possible responses to the experience of caring for dying children and their families.
- List the principles of nursing care for dying children and their families.

The death of a child is a traumatic event for health care providers as well as for families. A child's death is relatively rare, and mortality rates for children have decreased dramatically in the twentieth century. Because death in children is now rare, the death of a child causes more intense emotional reactions than the death of an adult. Nurses working with dying children do not necessarily escape this emotional involvement because of more frequent contact with death.

Health care professionals need to prepare themselves to handle the experience of death. The most important preparation is psychologic. Nurses need to become acquainted with the personal feelings triggered by this experience and to identify the feelings that help and those that hinder the process of nursing care. Nurses also need to recognize common responses to death in both children and their families. Although death in children is never "normal," the nurse can identify patterns of response and understanding. Knowing these patterns can help the child, family, and nurse cope with the crisis of dying.

The Child's View of Death

A child's level of cognitive development plays a major role in that child's perception of death. A 3- or 4-year-old child, for instance, has a very different concept of death than an older child or adult. Whatever the child's age, however, questions about death and dying should be answered frankly and in a manner appropriate to the child's level of understanding. The adult responds to what the child asks and does not simply talk about what the adult thinks the child ought to know.

The work of Nagy (1948) is central to an understanding of the child's developmental views on death. Although most of Nagy's research was with child victims of war, her findings have proven to be consistent with those of subsequent researchers. (Table 17-1 presents children's concepts of death and implications for communication.)

Although nurses and health professionals might understand the feelings of the dying child and family, perhaps nobody is more of an expert on death than the child who is dying. Siblings experiencing the situation from moment to moment are also children in crisis. Both the dying child and the siblings can be the nurse's greatest teachers and most valuable sources of information for assessment.

The experience and process of dying is universal, although the pace varies. Identifying the moment when a child is close to death is often difficult, but health professionals can assume that the pace of dying is increased in children with certain illnesses. Illnesses with no known cure progress especially quickly.

Dying is also an individual process because each child views life in a unique way. Researchers have identified some common threads, however, and these can help professionals understand the child's experience of dying and death. Because the pace of dying is accelerated in children with terminal illnesses, most of the data have come from this source.

TABLE 17-1 The Child's View of Death: Implications for Communication

Common concepts of death	Representative behaviors and responses	Implications for communication
Infancy		
No concept of death. Reacts to all separation in a similar way	Experiments with object permanence and separation with "throwaway" and "peek-a-boo" behaviors	Understand the strategies appropriate to deal with separation anxiety. Focus communication on other family members
Early childhood		
Concept of death begins to form. The child responds to other people's reactions to death. Death is viewed as temporary, gradual, and reversible (that is, as a kind of sleep or absence). Popular media (for example, television) and magical thinking reinforce the child's belief in the reversibility of death	The child retains a sense of the dead person's being. Might be concerned that the corpse can sense cold or discomfort or might worry about how it goes to the bathroom. Might look forward to the dead person's return or to a visit from the dead person. Might carry on imaginary conversations with the dead person	Assess the need to correct the child's misconceptions, which might be either functional or dysfunctional depending on the circumstances
Middle childhood		
Begins to understand that death is permanent. Uses fantasy to personify death. The child is likely to believe that wishes, misbehavior, or unrelated actions can be responsible for death	Imagines death as a skeleton, bogeyman, or grim reaper. Might engage in burial rites or other enactments of death with dolls or small pets. Might want to touch the corpse to see what it feels like	Use fantasy figures, pets, or other elements of the child's experience as points of reference in achieving an understanding appropriate to the child's developmental level
Late childhood		
Understands that all people die eventually. Begins to understand the mortality of self. Might show an interest in questions of an afterlife. Fear of death also might surface	Uses rituals to decrease anxiety; reckless behavior to demonstrate invulnerability; and humorous or tough demeanor to hide fearfulness	Allow the child to verbalize fears and help the child to accept them as normal. Discuss the realistic consequences of reckless activity
Adolescence		
Reaches an "adult" perception of death but might be emotionally unable to accept it. Might still hold over concepts from previous developmental stages, depending on actual experiences with death in childhood. Might still view death, for instance, as the result of mere intention, punishment for wrongdoing, or confirmation of evil character	Anxiety on the subject of death might be particularly acute because body image and emerging self-concept are threatened. Withdrawal might be the preferred coping strategy	Avoid assumptions of an adult understanding by assessing the adolescent's specific perceptions. Reactions might resemble those of an adult, but the nurse should be alert to additional feelings of guilt or hostility associated with confusion of wishes, wrongdoing, or bad character with the actual cause of death

Perceptions of Illness and Death

The child's perceptions of illness and death differ according to developmental stage. Perceptions also change throughout the dying process. A child's perceptions depend on cognitive development, but five distinct stages can be identified in children of all ages beyond infancy:

1. The child realizes that the illness is serious, that the doctor is involved, that the family is worried, and that something bad is happening.
2. The child begins to understand and can describe the names of drugs, their effects, and each drug's side effects. Children in this stage realize they are seriously ill but believe they will get better.
3. The child begins to understand and is able to talk about the purposes of treatments and procedures such as drug therapy and radiation. In this stage children are always ill but still feel they will eventually get better.
4. The child sees disease as a series of relapses and remissions but does not yet recognize that death is the final outcome. Children in this stage realize that they will experience some pain, discomfort, and perhaps hospital stays but believe that they will eventually be able to go home. They feel ill, however, and expect that they will always be ill.
5. Children in this stage realize that they are dying and that eventually a time will come when there will be no more remissions (Bluebond-Langner, 1975a, 1975b, 1976, 1977).

Reactions to Dying

In addition to considering the child's perceptions of the process of dying, the nurse needs to be concerned about the child's reactions to the process. Elizabeth Kubler-Ross's work with dying people enabled her to describe five stages of grieving that individuals experience during the process of dying: denial, anger, bargaining, depression, and acceptance (Kubler-Ross, 1969). These stages are not, however, a "curriculum" that a patient, with the help of the nurse, must "get through" in sequence. The grieving process is not one of moving through separate and distinct stages. Nurses need to recognize that the child and family might experience these feelings and conflicting emotions all at the same time. It is also possible that child and family might move back and forth through various emotions without demonstrating any "progression."

The nurse identifies all these possibilities as normal. Using the word "state" instead of "stage" further enables the nurse to use the insights of Kubler-Ross without the pitfalls of viewing the five emotions as steps through which the child and family must be guided in sequence. The nurse remembers that each of these reactions can be an adaptive coping strategy and that a key priority is to communicate with the child and family according to their particular state of mind. In this way the nurse can acknowledge the pain, offer assistance, and deal with the child and family as they are.

⊛ Potential knowledge deficit

Intellectualization is the focus on facts and reason at the expense of emotion. Older children, adolescents, and parents might well use this method to skirt or deny the painful feelings they must face. This response might occur whether or not the child has been raised in an intellectual environment.

One form of intellectualization is to learn as much as possible about the illness and treatment. Indeed, many dying children and family members become mini-experts on the disease from which the children are suffering. This knowledge might lead to hostile interactions with the nurse, physician, or other health care staff who do not demonstrate a similar expertise with this specific malady. The nurse is particularly sensitive to some people's need for information and others' need to protect themselves from information. By far the biggest complaint received from children and families, however, is that they are not given enough information about the disease entity and its progress.

⊛ Fear of dying related to inability to control the event

Brantner (1970) has described three fears related to dying: darkness, pain, and the fear of being alone. Nurses sensitive to these fears can help to alleviate and in some cases eliminate them. For example, a 9-year-old girl who was dying asked her sister to do a special favor for her. She had always been afraid of a darkened room, and her concern had been transferred to fear of a dark casket. She asked the sister to put a nightlight in her casket after her death. It was unimportant that the nightlight could not be plugged into the casket. The sister was honored to pick out a nightlight and place it in the dead girl's casket.

The fear of dying alone is common to old and young alike. Such fears are related to the process of dying, concern about an afterlife, and a basic fear of the unknown, extinction, or nothingness. One person reported, "I am not afraid of death itself, but I am afraid of dying."

To alleviate some fear, the nurse can talk to the child

Don't Be Afraid

Don't be afraid of what you don't understand—
There's always a reason.
Don't be afraid when your neighbor takes your hand—
Love is always in season.
If someone's lonely outside your door
Say "Come on in, we have room for more."
Don't be afraid to let love come into your life.

Walkin' along, walkin' along the street.
There's people all over.
Singin' a song, singin' a song so sweet.
You're lookin' them over.
For all God's children there's room to grow.
A stranger is a friend that you don't know.
Walkin' along, singin' a song of love.

Don't be afraid of the feeling in your heart—
Be willing to wear it.
Love is so warm you will want to pass it on
Knowing others can share it.
The world is waiting to hear your song
So sing out loud and we'll sing along!
Don't be afraid to let love come into your life!

SOURCE: From the album, *Music, Laughter and Tears*, by Deanna Ed
Reprinted by permission of Epoch Universal Publications, 10802 N. 2
Phoenix, Arizona 85029 © 1978.

about the fear of being alone. Simple measures such as always keeping the call light within the child's reach, stopping by frequently to talk, and assuring the child that people are nearby help to reduce fear. Anxiety about death and fears associated with death-related objects affect the dying child. Death terrifies most people. The first step to overcoming terror is to define and examine the fears that surround it. Because imagination is almost always worse than reality, knowledge and understanding can do a great deal toward helping dying children and their families cope with their fears.

The fear of pain might be associated with the fear of dying in some children. Sensitive pain management and comfort measures become priorities for nursing care (see Chapter 20).

⊛ Potential for spiritual distress

Belief in an afterlife is determined not only by religious faith but also by cognitive development. The child who fears punishment or rejection after death or feels that the illness is a punishment will have a seriously impaired ability to cope.

The nurse needs to work with both the child and the family to help them express feelings about reward or punishment after death. The child whose cognitive development suggests that illness itself is a punishment is especially vulnerable. (Children's reactions to illness and hospitalization are discussed in Chapter 19.) Referral to appropriate clergy might be beneficial.

⊛ Potential for ineffective individual coping

Regression Regression usually involves becoming dependent and childlike in activities of daily life. Children who regress might retreat to much earlier levels of development and become even more helpless. Although this might appear to be a poor adaptive measure to many caregivers, regression may be an extremely appropriate method of coping for some children and might even be the only one possible. The nurse assists the child to become more independent in ways that do not threaten the child's self-esteem and supports the child during the search for effective coping strategies, whatever the child's developmental level.

Many children fear regression. Adolescents in particular might fear the surrender of autonomy and the return to a former, more childlike state. Lonely and in need of understanding, the adolescent might simultaneously seek the care and concern of others, especially parents, and might resent and reject this support when it is offered. Perhaps because older adolescents have a more mature concept of death on both a cognitive and an emotional level, they might not fear the threat of regression as acutely as the younger teenager. More secure in their self-image and less fearful of a childlike dependence, they might not need to struggle against parental love and comfort.

Denial Denial also is a useful coping strategy when the child feels overwhelmed by what is happening. When a child has shown full awareness and openness and then slips into denial, health care personnel and the family might feel that they should discourage this retreat. Nurses need to be sensitive to children's need for periodic retreats from the dying process. Allowing them to use denial as a coping strategy when the need arises is a part of nursing care.

Anger Most children feel at least some anger against God or fate for having selected them to die young. This anger might be coupled with resentment toward others whose very lives are a reminder of the child's own imminent demise. Anger also might be expressed toward nurses and health care personnel for their power and importance in dealing with the life-threatening condition.

Anger can be a common reaction among children in late childhood and adolescence because these children have begun to appreciate more concretely the possibilities of their thwarted adulthood. Teenagers in midadolescence, for instance, have just developed new self-confidence and a sense of mastery over life. A life-threatening illness can provoke anger and rage as the fulfillment of their life's promise is taken from them.

Guilt Guilt is a natural reaction to dying for many children and families. Guilt might occur in survivors who ask, "Why did this happen to this person I loved and not me?" Parents also might feel somehow responsible for the death.

Many adolescents do in fact die as a result of some transgression of society's rules regarding drugs, alcohol, and automobiles. Their behavior might have stemmed from a wish to test limits and explore their power. To them, the resultant injury and emotional trauma for themselves and their families might well seem to be deserved punishment and lead to feelings of intense guilt.

Parents also can feel guilty about not having given the child "enough"—love, understanding, material things, attention, and the like—during the child's short lifetime. If unresolved conflicts exist between the parents and child, the burden of guilt becomes compounded.

Regardless of whether the feelings of guilt are reasonable or have any basis in fact, they should be acknowledged and worked through. Parents and children need to be told that such feelings are normal. In helping families acknowledge and deal with such feelings, the nurse can help to identify adaptive coping strategies to handle the grief process.

Shame Shame is another common reaction to dying. Bodily exposure, incontinence, and the inability to care for oneself often cause the child to feel shame, warranted or unwarranted.

Adolescents in particular are concerned with body image and peer approval. They have been in the process of disengaging from parents and family and identifying more closely with their peer group. A life-threatening condition, especially if there are drastic alterations in physical appearance, might seem to be an insurmountable barrier to continuing participation in the peer group. The teenager's peers might in fact feel threatened by the dying person's situation. Death negates their own feelings of vitality, hope, and potential. Because of these feelings, peers might not be available for emotional support, thus reinforcing the dying teenager's sense of rejection, isolation, and shame.

Caregivers need to be alert for shame, which is a common reaction. Nurses need to be careful that their behavior and attitudes, as shown by facial expressions and gestures of withdrawal, do not increase the child's sense of shame. Nurses also can help to alleviate the sense of shame by actively providing acceptance and support.

Potential for anticipatory grieving

Grief is an inevitable emotion for the dying child and the family. The dying child grieves over the loss of the future, and the family and caregivers grieve over the loss of the child. Regardless of the child's developmental level, the child will focus feelings of loss and grief on particular aspects of life. For younger children it might be a favorite activity or, more often, the relationship with family and friends. For the older child and adolescent, the focus of grief might be future plans and goals that must now be given up.

Communication with the child Children undergo anticipatory grief in response to impending death and might come to accept the inevitability of death before their parents do. Occasionally, this can cause a problem of withdrawal from family and caregivers. As long as the parent and child remain open to each other, the danger of a premature leave-taking can be avoided. On the other hand, the benefit of participating in the grief experience with the child while the child is still alive can be a more fulfilling and satisfactory resolution of the parent-child relationship. For the parents, grieving then includes the child's own perspective and feelings, leaving fewer sources of doubt and reproach for the survivors.

Whatever the specific emotions that constitute the child's reaction, however, the child always perceives the seriousness of the disease. Through the experience of dying, the child develops a more defined and accurate concept of death than would seem normal for the child's stage of cognitive development. Caregivers and parents usually notice this development as an extremely rapid maturing process on the part of the dying child. Nurses who are open to this wisdom can help parents appreciate these changes. This acceleration in development affects the communication and caregiving process. The nurse needs to be able to assess and keep pace with the child's growing understanding and interpret it to the family if needed.

Active preparation for death Although children do not often have financial affairs to settle before they die, there can still be a good deal of emotional "business" to attend to. Relationships with family members or friends might contain problems that need resolution.

A child can demonstrate an acceptance of impending death by actively preparing for it. Giving away a favorite toy, writing letters to loved ones, planning the funeral arrangements, or talking about the afterlife are all forms of active preparation. The reactions of others can create an atmosphere of open communication and make this active preparation a successful growth experience for the child.

The Family's View of Death

Almost all the emotions that normally can be experienced by the dying child—fear, denial, anger, guilt, shame, and grief—are also part of the normal spectrum of reactions for family members. Parents, siblings, and nurses, however, often have different reasons for experiencing these emotions. For instance, whereas the dying child might feel shame about an alteration in physical appearance or exclusion from the peer group, a parent might feel shame over a perceived failure in parenting, and a nurse might be ashamed of the apparent failure to provide effective care as the child's condition declines and the family's grief intensifies. It is important that the nurse not only identify the emotions felt by those around the dying child but also explore factors that underlie these emotions for each individual.

Type of Death

The reactions of the child and others to the dying process and death depend in large part on whether the death is sudden or expected, swift or lingering, or painless or painful. Often called the trajectories of death (Glaser and Strauss, 1968), the type of death determines reactions to it. For example, the adolescent that dies from an automobile accident can die suddenly and swiftly, leaving parents and other family members in severe shock. With sudden, swift death, the child and family have little or no time to become anxious about death, to deepen understanding, or to ask questions. The potential for personal guilt among the survivors is high, and support and counseling will be needed.

Reactions to a lingering death can depend on whether the death is expected and accepted. The family of a child with a chronic illness, for example, expects death in the future but has time to prepare and can learn to enjoy the child while the child is alive (see Chapter 14 for a discussion of the child with a chronic illness). Therapies for certain diseases might allow partial or complete remission, but the remission encourages the parents and child to believe that the disease will not reoccur. Parents and children will need to be gently coaxed into accepting the temporary nature of the remission and the need to follow any prescribed medical regimen. The nurse walks a tightrope between supporting this necessary reality orientation while simultaneously supporting hope that death can be forestalled.

A painful death is much more difficult for a family to accept than one that is painless. In a child, painful death generates fear of personal suffering in relation to one's own death. This fear can carry over into actually experiencing suffering when the child is suffering. Parents also experience a high degree of guilt for being powerless to control their child's pain. Siblings might fear retaliation because of some imagined fault for the child's pain, suffering, or death. Nurses need to be aware of these feelings and be willing to explore them with the family members.

Awareness of Death

Degree of awareness of the impending death helps determine the family's reaction to it. Awareness depends in part on the philosophy of the health care institution and its personnel. Many traditional hospitals are still unwilling to recognize the need for an open acceptance and awareness of death. In such settings, personnel do not speak of death or define death even though people are dying around them.

In some situations the family chooses to keep information from the dying child. Everyone pretends that the child is not dying and talks about everything but the death, which is most important for them to share. Nurses feel uncomfortable in this situation, as they do when they suspect that a child is dying, but the physician has not confirmed such a judgment or made enough information available to confirm the suspicion. In both cases, the child knows that something is clearly wrong but cannot validate the suspicion. The nurse's communications with the child necessarily become superficial.

Children are able to understand and deal with what is happening to them. They have the right to believe that their nurses, physicians, and parents are being honest. They should not have to worry that their caregivers will withdraw from them in a time of extreme need. Only when openness encourages the child and family to talk about death and deal with feelings and thoughts about death will the child's fears be allayed.

To encourage open communication, the nurse provides as much information as possible about the child's condition and what to expect. The nurse also supports the family if the dying process does not follow the expected course. Families want to know, as far as it is possible, how soon death will occur. This way, the family can prepare and help the child to finish any unfinished business. In many cases, however, the time of death cannot be predicted with any accuracy. The nurse's behavior is, to a certain extent, influenced by this uncertainty because concrete support might be more difficult to offer in the face of many unknowns. Even when the time of death cannot be accurately predicted, however, support is essential for the child and family. Open communication allows the uncertainty to be acknowledged by all concerned.

Parents

Potential for powerlessness

The overriding emotions that parents feel at the death of a child are powerlessness and guilt. Parents might feel that the illness was their fault—through insufficient love, attention, or understanding. Guilt might be particularly strong if a genetic component is suspected in the child's illness.

Denial is also common—a means to protect the parent from overwhelming anxiety. As a means to limit the emotional burden to what the parent can bear, denial can be an adaptive coping mechanism, but if the parent persists in denial long into the course of the child's illness, important lines of communication will break down even as the need for clear and honest communication increases.

Anger is another common reaction for the parent of a dying child. Parents might be angry at the injustice of the tragedy, at their own helplessness, at the threat to their future plans for the child, or at the disruption in their lives caused by the illness. Very often, this anger is directed at the staff, who must recognize the roots of the parents' emotions. Staff members cannot become caught in responding to a perceived personal attack. Instead, health care providers accept the parents' rage and help them to deal with the feelings of impotence underlying the anger.

Guilt, denial, anger, and depression can be particularly acute and felt for a longer time in cases of sudden unexpected death (such as the death of an infant from sudden infant death syndrome, or a child from suicide). In such cases parents feel that they should have offered more protection. The greater intensity of these reactions also is related to "the fact that there is simply more with which to cope in a relatively shorter period. Problems also derive from the absence of the opportunity of anticipatory grief" (Gonda and Ruark, 1984).

Potential alteration in family processes

More than hospitalization and chronic illness, a child's dying severely disrupts normal family functioning. "In many instances, the pattern of family life will be changed from the initial period of diagnosis until some time after the [child's] death, when a reorganization of family roles takes place. In some cases, the family may be completely and permanently disrupted through divorce or separation of the parents" (Waechter, 1979). The emotional, physical, and financial strain of long-term hospitalization, emergency measures, or life-support systems can be staggering and, in the absence of community or other outside resources, can increase the family's vulnerability to other problems. Even if no visible disruption takes place, the family will be altered permanently by the empty space created by the lost child.

> January 25, 1983
>
> **Say Olin**
>
> The time of concern is over.
> No longer am I asked how my wife is doing.
> Never is the name of our son mentioned to me.
> A curtain descends. The moment has passed.
> A life slips from frequent recall.
> There are exceptions: close and compassionate friends,
> Sensitive and loving family.
> For most, the drama is over.
> The spotlight is off. Applause is silent.
> But for me the play will never end.
> The effects on me are timeless.
> Say Olin to me.
> On the stage of my life he has been both lead and
> supporting actor.
> Do not tiptoe around the greatest event of my life.
> Love does not die.
> His name is written on my life.
> The sound of his voice replays within my mind.
> You feel he is dead.
> I feel he is of the dead and still he lives.
> He ghostwalks my soul, beckoning in future welcome.
> You say he was my son.
> I say he is.
> Say Olin to me and say Olin again.
>
> SOURCE: Hackett D: *Saying Olin to Say Goodbye*. Old Cedar Publications, 1986.

Many clinicians have focused on the particular disruptive effects on the mother. Wong (1980) coined the phrase "empty mother syndrome" to depict the particularly disruptive effects the child's death has on the mother. While the child is dying, the mother might have severed many social relationships, postponed her career, grown somewhat apart from older children who are less dependent on her, and seen her husband withdraw into work to avoid prolonging the pain of the loss. All of these responses can result in a sense of having lost the mothering role, particularly for those mothers without additional, career-oriented roles ouside the home. "While the other family members picked up their lives as they were before the child's death, the mother was left in the lonely, empty house without her sick child to care for, or to visit, if he had been in the hospital" (Wong, 1980).

Fathers experience the same guilt, emptiness, and diminished self-esteem as mothers. The nurse therefore needs to remember that cultural prohibitions might prevent a father from expressing the loneliness and desolation he feels at the death of his child. Although work is often a retreat for the father, the pain he feels can disrupt work. Colleagues are often unable to give the support and assistance needed, and the father can easily become isolated.

Potential for social isolation

One of the results of a child's illness and death can be a sense of isolation, both for the family as a whole and for each family member. Family members experience isolation both from the community and from each other. Isolation from the community is a natural result of the time and energy devoted exclusively to the care of the dying child. Friends and neighbors, even if they wish to be supportive, might not be sure how best to express their concern and might fear that their efforts to help will be considered intrusions. Community members also might fear the pain that emotional involvement in the family's crisis might bring and refrain from offering the support that would lead to that involvement.

Parents also might drift apart from each other in the face of the child's dying. The intense grief that each parent feels individually can obscure the fact that the other parent is also in great pain. If the parent's coping strategy is to avoid sources of pain as much as possible, withdrawal from the other partner might be an important, although unconscious, need.

The ongoing stress of the family's crisis also can throw up barriers—such as overloaded schedules, emotional turmoil, fear of another pregnancy, guilt about feeling pleasure, or simple fatigue—to the couple's sexual intimacy, thereby reinforcing each parent's sense of isolation. In fact, for parents, "the ability to again enjoy intimate relations seems to be one milestone in resolving grief" (Wong, 1980).

Siblings

Nurses need to be aware of the reactions of siblings to a child's death. Nursing care means dealing not only with the dying child's feelings but also with the interactions of all family members.

Children frequently see death on television as a result of guns, bombs, or other forms of violence. A sense of unreality sets in, however, because the aftermath of death and its effect on the family rarely are shown on television. Children get used to seeing their favorite actors and actresses or cartoon characters "die" and instantly reappear or show up in other programs. Consequently, they develop a sense of unreality about death and cannot believe that it will strike them personally or strike someone they love.

Just like the dying child, the sibling understands death in a way that is related to the level of cognitive development. The dying child, however, quickly learns a fuller and more mature concept of death. Even children who are not told about the nature and extent of their illness gain an awareness they are reluctant to share in the presence of adult fears. Without this firsthand experience, siblings of the dying child are more likely to continue understanding death in age-appropriate ways. The nurse keeps this disparity in mind in adjusting the style and content of communication to the needs of the various children in a family. Siblings also need counseling, comfort, and care in the face of a crisis.

Siblings often experience a deprivation of parental time. They also might be aware of economic and other pressures that have resulted from a brother's or sister's illness. Siblings might be left in the care of extended family members. In their preoccupation with the sick child, parents might neglect the routine needs of the siblings. Older children might be assigned additional household tasks, or the dying child might be granted a special request, such as a trip, which the siblings also might desire.

All of these possible reactions often cause jealousy and resentment in siblings—feelings that seem natural but also tend to cause guilt. Surviving siblings in early or middle childhood might feel guilty if they believe their own destructive wishes were selfish or contributed to the dying child's death. Even older, seemingly mature children are capable of believing their wishes or actions in some way contributed to the death of another.

In addition to feelings of guilt and jealousy, siblings might respond to parental deprivation with dysfunctional behavior, including hostility toward the ill child and acting out in ways that cause discipline and performance problems at home or in school. Nurses who are sensitive to these possibilities can gain insight into the sibling's problems, help the sibling express and accept the feelings, and work with others, such as the school nurse or teacher, to develop a support system for the sibling.

Another reaction common to the siblings of the dying child is to feel left out, vulnerable, and caught up in their own grief. Often, they are at home attempting to live as normally as possible with one or both parents absent. Both their routines and their emotions are in turmoil, however, and they need a great deal of support from parents and the health care team.

Health professionals need to recognize that siblings, too, can play a supportive role in the child's dying. The siblings should be given time together with the child before death occurs. Siblings should not be made to feel helpless but should be encouraged to develop feelings of strength and support. The nurse therefore gives siblings the opportunity to participate in the process of the child's dying and to help ease the child's death in whatever ways they can. Nurses can work with parents to help siblings maintain their connection to the dying child. Creating vehicles to collect memories while the child is still alive—a photo album or other collaborative project, for instance—is a tangible way to maintain the siblings' relationship. Siblings also need to be allowed to participate in funeral arrangements and the service itself, if they wish to. The nurse can make an invaluable contribution by helping siblings to find their own way of saying good-bye.

The Nurse's View of Death

Nursing education does not make nurses exempt from experiencing human emotions. The nurse's reactions to the death of a child are influenced by culture, background, professional training, and personal and religious philosophies. Adams (1984) suggested six variables that also play an important part in nurse's reactions to dying patients:

- The length of time the child has been hospitalized
- The frequency of admissions
- The role of the family
- The condition of the child when admitted
- The child's coping style
- The role of the nurse's subconscious

For example, extended involvement with a terminally ill child might make the nurse's grieving more intense than it would be for a child who died quickly in an emergency room. This more intense grief might allow the nurse, on the one hand, to empathize more fully with the family members, or it might be so self-absorbing as to block the nurse's emotional availability to the survivors in need of care. The nurse who is able to identify and cope with normal responses of grief is more likely to experience personal growth through the process of caring for dying children than the nurse who is too overwhelmed by grief.

One of the ways to cope successfully with grief when working with dying children is to understand normal coping responses. Mandel (1981) identified some concerns that nurses experience when dealing with dying patients. These include: (1) being overwhelmed by grief, or taking a child's death as a personal failure; (2) overidentification, or attempting to assume some of the child and family's grief as well as one's own (often called the *surrogate sufferer syndrome*); and (3) avoidance, or becoming immune to personal feelings and reactions.

Nurses who recognize these pitfalls and learn to deal positively with the experience of death can experience a powerful and rewarding sense of personal growth. Through working with dying children, nurses might restructure their priorities and develop stronger value systems. Human relationships can become more precious, and the nurse's ability to communicate honestly can become enhanced.

Elements of Nursing Care for Dying Children and Their Families

As with other facets of the care of children, the nurse may assume a variety of roles in terminal care, including primary care provider, child and family advocate, patient teacher, and counselor. The nurse is often of increasing assistance to the child and family as medicine and technology have less to offer. The nurse is also in an excellent position to make referrals for the family and identify community resources such as support groups and community-based health services.

With a child who is expected to die, the nurse's goals shift in focus from the restoration of health to the promotion of comfort. The first priority is attention to the child's physical needs. If the nurse cannot adjust to this modification of goals, feelings of helplessness, frustration, anger, and guilt can result. Recognizing and overcoming these feelings can free the nurse to pursue the primary goals of providing comfort and hope for the dying child and the family.

Assessment

The nurse's assessment of the dying child and the family covers a broad range of concerns:

1. *The child's understanding of the illness, treatment, and prognosis as well as the child's concept of death.* This information is gathered as a baseline that underlies all other assessments. Information may come from the child or family or both.
2. *The normal coping strategies and support systems of the child and family.* Discussing feelings surrounding difficult procedures affords an opportunity to explore the family's ability to cope with the larger crisis posed by the child's severe illness.
3. *The specific details of family functioning and any special risk factors, as well as the effects of the child's condition on the family.* Examples of additional risk factors include single parents, families who live elsewhere, families with another ill member, and families with other young chil-

dren or infants (Williams, Rivara, & Rothenberg, 1981). The initial assessment of the family therefore should include attention to these points:

- financial resources of the family, measured against the costs of the child's illness
- marital stress
- medical or psychosocial problems in family members other than the dying child
- the family's usual support system in other crises and its effectiveness
- the community resources used by the family
- the potential resources and supports available to the family
- the openness of communication between parents or between parents and other family members
- the parent's predominant reactions such as denial, anger, or guilt
- whether the parent tends to become isolated from other family members, social support systems, or other potential sources of help

4. *The family's cultural perspective.* Any religious and moral beliefs that might affect the family's experience of illness, death, and grief should be assessed and taken into account so that the comfort, guidance, and support offered by the nurse can be presented in a way that is most likely to be accepted.

Communication

The complex and intense emotions that surround the dying child and family can make communication difficult among all the people involved—child, family members, and health care workers. It is precisely in this situation, however, where honest and sensitive communication skills are most needed. The hospital setting can be rushed, chaotic, and distracting, causing the child and family to feel more bewildered and fearful than they are already. Nurses and other health care professionals can work to create a relatively relaxed and unpressured atmosphere when dealing with patients. Such an atmosphere reduces the stress on children and families and allows them calm moments in which to come to grips with their situation and resolve unfinished emotional business.

The time imposed by a terminal illness is especially limited; therefore poor communication between the child and family can delay the necessary resolution of family problems and relationships until it is literally too late. Over and above the normal grief that survivors can expect to feel, an added burden of guilt and regret can result from unexpressed feelings or unresolved conflicts. Poor communication between the nurse and child or between the nurse and family also can have the following undesirable consequences (Gonda and Ruark, 1984):

- Mistrust
- A sense of powerlessness
- Anger
- Feelings of isolation and abandonment
- Failure to attend to important business

Verbal communication Sometimes the failure to communicate fully, openly, and honestly might stem from a wish to protect the child. Children should not be sheltered more than necessary, however, from either the fact of death or the feelings of grief that surround it. The clinical facts might be difficult for the nurse to communicate or for the child to bear. Reassurance is therefore important to the child who needs emotional security and physical care from the parent or other caregiver. The child needs to know that care will not cease because of the crisis. Attempts to protect clients from the truth might in any case be ineffective because children and parents both will sense the nurse's true feelings, even if the nurse wishes to disguise them. Honesty is thus an important component of effective communication for both nurses and parents.

In communicating with the child about death, Gonda and Ruark (1984) proposed three guiding principles: (1) avoid lying, (2) let the child determine how much to say at a particular moment, and (3) tailor the content of the communication as closely as possible to an accurate assessment of the child's concept of death. Nurses also can provide parents with guidelines for discussing death with children. Two specific guidelines to emphasize are (1) do not say death was the will of God or some other superior being because this might engender hostile feelings toward the deity, and (2) do not associate death with sleep because children might learn to fear going to bed and falling asleep (Sheer, 1977; Hutton, 1981).

Reflecting the child's and family's feelings is an important communication technique. In reflecting feelings the nurse paraphrases the feelings of the child or family. The paraphrase should be based on specific verbal and nonverbal cues and not simply a wild guess. The nurse should in any case phrase the reflected feelings in such a way as to allow the child room to clarify or correct the nurse's interpretation.

Hearing one's feelings reflected provides a sense of validation. Judicious use of reflection can also clarify feelings that the child might have denied or failed to identify and encourage the child to explore feelings without fear that the nurse is sitting in judgment.

Nonverbal communication Conversation is not the only useful medium of communication, especially with younger children, whose cognitive development might not support verbal skills to express the experience through which they are living. Various activities, including play and reading aloud, can provide the context and direction for an open exploration of the child's feelings and concerns. (Play for hospitalized children is discussed in Chapter 19.)

Music can be another way of expressing emotions and communication for the child. Because our society tends to deny death and pain, popular music does not often deal with the problems of dying. If the nurse is uncertain about a child's readiness to accept or understand the illness, a tape can be given to the child containing a variety of songs, including songs about dying. The songs the child listens to often and comments on will most likely reflect that child's readiness. Dying children who have strong adult support systems usually cultivate lively senses of humor and startlingly candid outlooks. Experiences in music therapy can help a child feel free to express laughter and tears.

Art is another invaluable mode of communication in working with dying children. One funeral director, for instance, makes sure he has crayons and paper in his funeral home for grieving children to explore their feelings. Dying children should be given frequent opportunities through painting, drawing, and sculpting to express their feelings. As the child develops art into a form of communication, the nurse or therapist might need to respond to the child in the same language. The sensitive pictures nurses draw for children can be a very helpful form of communication.

The use of touch can comfort the child and family. Often a quiet hug indicates acceptance of emotion and might allow the child to put feelings into words.

April 1, 1983

In the smallest ways, through the most common sights,
I remember you.
In the simple joys we shared, in the little things you loathed,
I remember you.
When I drink Pepsi instead of Coke,
I remember you.
When liver is served without your bacon and eggs,
I remember you.
As Burger King taunts MacDonald's,
I remember you.
Listening to the pool pumps gurgling behind the house,
I remember you.
Gazing at pruned trees, sealed with daubs of black tree paint,
I remember you.
Discovering a candy wrapper under a couch cushion,
I remember you.
Going to bed with no background music next to our bedroom,
I remember you.
In seeing dark haired boys with deep brown eyes,
I remember you.
In gnarled, thorny rosebushes, clinging to life,
I remember you.
In countless situations, in numberless ways,
The ordinary parts of life proclaim our time together,
And I remember you.

SOURCE: Hackett D: *Saying Olin to Say Goodbye*. Old Cedar Publications, 1986.

Assisting with Grieving

Especially when death is known to be inevitable, assisting the child and family with grieving is a most important nursing intervention. Nurses can facilitate the grieving process by providing opportunities for the expression of emotions, helping children and parents to anticipate and master these emotions, and providing an objective presence when these emotions become overwhelming.

Nurses can reassure the child and family and help them handle guilt or aggressive feelings such as anger and rage appropriately. The nurse provides outlets for the child's rage and reaffirms the child's self-control and worth. Reassurance is offered that such feelings are a normal part of the grieving process and will become manageable with the passage of time.

At critical moments, grief might become especially acute, and the hospital can provide a special room where feelings can be expressed without restraint. Particularly at the time of the child's death, the family's privacy is ensured while members attempt to deal with the shock and emotions the child's death causes. Grief, however, is a lifelong process. Although families do regain their equilibrium and precrisis level of functioning, they never cease to miss the dead child or mourn the loss in some way.

The death of an infant can pose special obstacles to the grieving process because the family might feel a vacuum as a result of not completing attachment. Detachment from the dead infant can be problematic when the attachment process was incomplete. Nurses can encourage the family to have as much contact as possible with the infant both while alive and after death, in order to cope with the loss. Parents of terminally ill infants need to be given a chance to do the following:

- Touch and hold the infant while alive
- Photograph the infant before or after death
- Discuss funeral arrangements
- Be present at the time of the infant's death
- Touch, hold, and even bathe the infant after death

Peer Support

For all those involved in a child's dying—the child, family members, and health professionals—support by other people is important. Others who are experiencing or have experienced similar situations can provide a kind of emotional assistance that cannot be obtained from any other source.

Support groups of parents who have lost their children can help newly bereaved parents express their grief, share it with others who will understand, and eventually put it in perspective. Nurses can be instrumental in referring parents to these support groups.

Parents need not assume that their friends and neighbors are unwilling to help or incapable of doing so. Some friends and relatives are too uneasy around the circumstances of dying to offer any real help. Others might only be waiting for a signal that an offer of help will not be perceived as an intrusion on the family's grief. Some might go so far as to ask the advice of health professionals who are in a position to note the family's special needs. The nurse might be able to suggest to a concerned neighbor, for instance, the need for an afternoon of child care for a young sibling of the dying child or for assistance with housekeeping or cooking. Such concrete assistance often is a welcome substitute for the awkwardness of "not knowing what to say" and can bolster parents by letting them know that their friends, relatives, and neighbors are there for them.

Support for siblings and other peers of the dying child is an important nursing concern. Especially for the dying child whose illness is in remission, interacting with healthy children is a way to continue living in a supportive environment. Classmates in the school setting can be part of the child's life, although these healthy children need to be informed and supported as they watch their friend die. Helping them learn to support each other is a primary goal. Coordination with the school nurse or community health nurse is an obvious strategy to achieve this kind of peer support.

The dying child also can benefit from interacting with other seriously ill children. Roommates of similar ages and interests can help meet each other's social needs. Children with the same disease can develop close bonds based on their common experiences, fears, and frustrations. Nurses will wish to monitor such relationships as they develop, not only to measure the psychosocial benefits to each child but also to watch for any health risks such as possible exposure to respiratory and other infections.

Nurses also need peer support and cannot neglect their own self-care needs. Mutual support and collaboration among health professionals are essential for maintaining an appropriate level of emotional involvement without losing sensitivity. Such support can be formalized into regular group meetings of concerned staff members to discuss the various issues, frustrations, and problems that they face. Regular peer support can lead to greater awareness, reassurance, and emotional resiliency for the nurse. Professional relationships based on mutual trust and support also will help to keep channels of communication open among the various health care team members, resulting in more organized and effective care for the child and family.

Support Resources for Children, Parents, and Nurses *

American Cancer Society: 777 Third Avenue, New York, NY 10019; (212) 371-2900.

The Candlelighters Foundation: Suite 1011, 2025 Eye Street NW, Washington, DC 20006; (202) 659-5136.

The Compassionate Friends, Inc.: PO Box 3696, Oak Brook, IL 60522; (312) 323-5010.

Concern for Dying: 250 West 57th Street, New York, NY 10019; (212) 246-6962.

Council of Guilds for Infant Survival: 923 Central Park Avenue, Davenport, IA 52804; (319) 322-4870.

Make Today Count: National Office, PO Box 303, Burlington, IA 52601; (319) 753-6521.

National Hospice Organization: 1901 North Fort Mier Drive, Suite 402, Arlington, VA 22209; (703) 243-5900.

Parents of Murdered Children: 1739 Bella Vista, Cincinnati, OH 45237; (513) 242-8025.

Resolve, Inc.: PO Box 474, Belmont, MA 02178; (617) 484-2424.

SHARE: St. John's Hospital, 800 East Carpenter Street, Springfield, IL 62769; (217) 544-6464.

* For a directory that describes organizations that help bereaved families, please consult Part II of Donnelly KF: *Recovering From the Loss of a Child.* Macmillan, 1982.

Settings for Terminal Care

Home care One option for terminal care that parents might wish to consider is caring for the child at home. Home care offers many advantages, but the choice is not for everyone. The nurse will have to help each family to make the best decision for them. This in turn means giving the family as much information about home care as possible and supporting whatever decision is reached.

Many of the advantages of home care stem from having the family physically in one place rather than dividing them between the hospital and the home. The isolation and separation that this division causes are thus diminished. Siblings can have more of their normal needs taken care of by parents instead of others, and their responses to the situation can be observed and discussed more frequently. In this way, normal feelings of resentment or guilt are less likely to become destructive.

Home care allows the entire family to participate more fully in the care of the ill child, thus lessening the physical burden on any one individual. The greater amount of time spent together in the familiar environment of home can give family members more opportunities to resolve unfinished emotional business, to deepen their relationship with the child, and to adjust their role relationships in response to the child's illness and eventual death.

Home care also allows the child and family a greater sense of independence and responsibility, thereby reducing feelings of helplessness. Parents and other family members can reassert their control over their disrupted routines and environment, thus creating a more normal atmosphere. The ill child can assume a greater role in self-care activities such as feeding and administering medications. This sense of self-reliance can be particularly important for adolescents.

In addition, home care can significantly affect the family's readjustment following the child's death. One study (Lauer et al., 1983) suggested that parents who provide home care for the child are less likely to need professional mental health services or to develop pathologic grief reactions involving feelings of denial or guilt. Parents who care for the child at home appear better able to confront the realities of the situation and work through their guilt feelings. Marital relations, instead of deteriorating, often are enhanced by the experience of caring for the child together because many parents find that the home care experience "deepened their respect for each other, facilitated communication by causing fewer separations, and enabled them to recognize each others' strengths more fully" (Lauer et al., 1983).

Home care does not, however, mean an end to professional involvement in the child's care. On the contrary, home care requires careful coordination among community and hospital-based professionals to provide the backup, consultation, and additional personnel needed to implement a plan of care at home. Full medical support, 24-hour access to nursing services, spiritual counseling, and lay support from relatives, friends, or hospice volunteers are all important components of a viable home care program. The parents must be clear about exactly what services they can rely on so that they can pursue the tasks of caring with as much confidence as possible. They also need to be aware of the option of rehospitalization should the physical or emotional stress, especially in the final stages of the child's life, prove too much to bear. Every nurse has the opportunity to encourage home care for those families who find it appropriate.

Hospice care Although home and hospice care are by no means synonymous, they share a humanistic, supportive philosophy. A hospice can refer to a group of people, a place, or an idea. Regardless of the structure of a particular hospice, the philosophy of hospice is to provide complete spiritual, emotional, social, and physical care to the dying and their families. The primary features of hospice care reveal much that is similar to the goals of home care:

1. Both the family and patient constitute the unit of care and caregiving.
2. Comfort, referring to the alleviation of physical, emotional, psychologic, and spiritual pain, is a primary goal.
3. A multidisciplinary team that includes the child and family plans and implements care. Medical backup is particularly important because the psychosocial care offered to the client might be ineffective if physical care needs are not attended to first.
4. Support is made available to the client at all times.
5. Trained volunteers may assist in achieving hospice goals.
6. Bereavement and follow-up care are provided.
7. Support for care providers themselves is an important part of the concept (MacElveen-Hoehn and McIntosh, 1981).

A hospice program can take a variety of forms, one of which is a physical place, with a staff that offers inpatient residential care (Burne, 1984). Other programs offer home care exclusively to terminally ill patients and might include nurses as part of a multidisciplinary staff. Nursing personnel also might be contacted through home health agencies. Some hospitals have developed their own hospice programs and choose to designate a unit or a number of beds for this purpose. Other hospitals have formed multidisciplinary teams that function as resources for terminally ill patients throughout the hospital (MacElveen-Hoehn and McIntosh, 1981).

Hospice can be a way of making home care possible, especially when the family is subject to other stresses, such as single parenthood, other young children, or other ill family members. The support provided by a hospice program can extend the family's physical, emotional, and spiritual resources to meet the demands of terminal care. Even if only providing respite care for the parents—managing household responsibilities so that the parents can run other errands or attend to their own self-care needs—hospice can render a vital service to the entire family.

Evaluation and Follow-Up

Nursing care does not end with the death of the child. The surviving family members will continue to grieve. In the absence of the ill child as a focus for their attention, family members sometimes manifest this pain in new ways that are dysfunctional.

After the child has died, the family will feel the need to begin reestablishing normal routines and resume their former activities, both at home and in the workplace. Picking up on interrupted social contacts might be one of the most difficult aspects of this effort. Well-meaning expressions of sympathy, sometimes accompanied by such presumptive statements as, "I know how you feel," might prove irksome to parents wishing to resume their normal lives. Some report that sympathy even causes them further anguish and anger.

Families need time not only to work through their grief but also to become accustomed to the child's absence. Parents might continue to sense the child's presence for a period of time after death. Mistaking strange children on the street for their own child or hearing doors slam, the teenager's record player, or the infant's cry are common reactions. Parents should be reassured that this is normal and not a sign of insanity or some other pathologic process.

Family relationships, particularly marital bonds, might suffer further disruption after the child's death. Some studies have shown a 50%–70% incidence of marital problems and divorce in families in which a child died from cancer (Lauer et al., 1983). Parents might feel that they no longer have a common bond. They might project their own feelings of guilt on to each other to give the death a cause, however unfounded. Each parent might feel that the other is a reminder of grief and not a consoling presence and begin to engage more intensely in activities that exclude the other parent. An inability to understand the other parent's grieving style or a need to "be strong" for the spouse also can reinforce each parent's individual isolation. As with other aspects of the grieving process, open and honest communication is the best preventive care individuals can provide for themselves and their family.

Various changes in parent-child interactions might take place with the surviving siblings after the death of a child. The surviving siblings might become scapegoats, the objects of projected guilt and idealization of the dead child. The parents might overprotect the surviving siblings in the hope of preventing a similar fate, or they might place the siblings in the role of substitute for the dead child. They might feel incapable of making decisions regarding the care of the siblings if their confidence in their parenting ability has been shattered by the child's death.

Grieving parents also might try to seek relief by deciding to have another child immediately. Such a decision, made in an intensely emotional climate, is often the prevailing wish of one parent. The nurse encourages parents to reach a mutual decision and to realize that no other child can truly fill the void left by the dead child.

How well survivors cope depends on the strengths of the family's normal support systems. Support can come from the immediate family, extended family members, friends, and neighbors. The role the dead child played in family function while alive and the parents' relationship with each other and with the other children also affect each family member's readjustment and new role functions. Readjustment also can be affected by the family's degree of involvement in the terminal care of the child, whether in the hospital or at home. Greater involvement with the child's care can assist the resolution of guilt feelings and enhance family relationships strained by the crisis of losing a family member.

The nurse can assist the family's adjustment by promoting a climate of full and open communication both to identify individual feelings and problems and to reveal any changes in family role relationships that have taken place silently. Feelings of helplessness on the part of all family members can be addressed by encouraging them to engage in activities that renew their sense of purpose and usefulness. These are as likely to be new activities as they are those that occupied the person before the bereavement.

Most importantly, the nurse should make sure that the primary health caregiver, whether primary nurse or physician, contacts the family at some interval after the child's death. The period of time may range from 10 days to 1 month and will depend on the family's own needs, desires, and religious mourning practices. "At this time the family can be observed for such normal grief reactions as somatic complaints, anger, preoccupation with the dead image, depression, guilt, and changes in normal daily patterns" (Williams, Rivara, and Rothenberg, 1981). Nurses also take this opportunity to extend themselves in offering sympathy, sharing their own memories of the child, and assuring the family that the support of the health care team remains available to them. The aftermath of a child's death is a critical time for the family—one of nursing evaluation, follow-up, and collaboration with other health professionals. The community health nurse can be a key factor in the family's ability to return to a normal state of functioning.

Difficult as it might be to believe, there are joys in caring for a dying child. One of the most important nursing tasks is helping the child to discover joy in the short period of life that remains. Nurses who feel continuously drained, depleted, and hurt when working with dying patients might decide that they are temperamentally unsuited to this role or might wish to deepen their insight into their own feelings and expectations.

The nurse who works with the dying child is one of the most significant persons in that child's life. Not only do nurses have one of the most clearly defined opportunities to serve and give, but they also have one of the most significant opportunities to receive. To minimize the pain and maximize the comfort in death are the ultimate privileges in the nursing experience. Nurses who take joy in their work will grieve at the loss of every single patient but also will feel a great fulfillment in being able to help others achieve the final goal of their lives.

Essential Concepts

- Nursing care of the dying child is an intense emotional experience, requiring personal preparation.
- A child's responses to death and dying are influenced by more than chronologic age. The nurse also assesses the child's developing view of death. Rapid cognitive development is common in children who are dying.
- To understand the child's experience of dying, the nurse considers several factors, including the child's understanding of the illness and its progression toward death.
- The behavioral and emotional reactions to the dying process do not occur in a progressive sequence of stages but can be used as coping mechanisms in any order. The nurse refrains from imposing an "agenda" on the child or family member to move them through a sequence of stages.
- The nurse and the dying child's family also can experience the common coping reactions of the dying child, although usually for different reasons.
- Reactions to a child's death can differ according to whether the death is sudden or expected, swift or lingering, painless or painful.
- In addition to the common coping reactions, parents often experience disruption of their personal and marital lives and isolation from the society of friends and neighbors as a result of the child's dying.
- The reactions of the dying child's siblings are too often ignored and can include jealousy and hostility toward the ill child, as well as the other reactions of grief.
- In addition to other normal grieving reactions, nurses need to be aware of other responses that they themselves often experience. Common responses include feeling overwhelmed, overidentifying with the dying child and/or family, and avoiding emotional involvement with the dying process.
- Cultural differences influence both the perception of death and the expression of grief and should therefore be taken into account as the nurse interacts with the dying child and family.
- Assessment of the dying child and family includes the child's understanding of death and illness, the normal coping strategies of the child and family, the specific details of family functioning (including special risk factors), and the famly's cultural perspective.
- Communication skills that foster an open atmosphere for communication are essential contributions the nurse can make to the care of the dying child, family, and other health care professionals.
- The nurse is also instrumental in supporting feelings of grief and initiating and promoting peer support for the child, family members, and other nurses.
- Home care is a terminal care option that can strengthen the bonds between the child and family, minimize family disruption, and positively affect the family's readjustment after the child's death. The nurse then continues to play a strong role in support, counseling, and the coordination of services.
- The hospice concept has much in common with the goals of nursing and of home care, with its focus on the family as the unit of care and caregiving.
- Follow-up and evaluation, especially with the family after the child has died, is an essential nursing role.

References

Adams FE: Six very good reasons why we react differently to various dying patients. *Nurs '84* (June) 1984; 14(6):41–43.

Bluebond-Langner M: *Awareness and Communication in Terminally Ill Children: Pattern, Process, and Pretense*. Unpublished doctoral dissertation, University of Illinois, 1975a.

Bluebond-Langner M: Meanings of death to children. In: *New Meanings of Death*. Feifel H (editor): McGraw-Hill, 1977.

Bluebond-Langner M: *Field Research on Children's and Adults' Views of Death*. Field Notes, 1976.

Bluebond-Langner M: *Meanings of death to children. In: New Meanings of Death*. Feifel H (editor): McGraw-Hill, 1977.

Brantner J: *Death and the Self* (Audiotape). University of Minnesota Center for Death Education and Research, 1970.

Burne SR: A hospice for children in England. *Pediatrics* (Jan) 1984; 73(1):97–98.

Glaser BG, Strauss AL: *Time for Dying*. Aldine, 1968.

Gonda T, Ruark J: *Dying Dignified: The Health Professional's Guide to Care*. Addison-Wesley, 1984.

Hutton LM: Annie is alone: The bereaved child. *Am J Matern-Child Nurs* (July/Aug) 1981; 6:274–277.

Kubler-Ross E: *On Death and Dying*. Macmillan, 1969.

Lauer ME et al: A comparison study of parental adaptation following a child's death at home or in the hospital. *Pediatrics* (Jan) 1983; 71(1):107–112.

MacElveen-Hoehn P, McIntosh EG: The hospice movement: Growing pains and promises. *Top Clin Nurs* (Oct) 1981; 3(3):29–38.

Mandel HR: Nurses' feelings about working with the dying. *Am J Nurs* (June) 1981; 81(6):1194–1197.

Nagy MH: The child's view of death. *J Genet Psychol* 1948; 73:3–27.

Sheer BL: Help for the parents in a difficult job—broaching the subject of death. *Am J Matern-Child Nurs* (Sept/Oct) 1977; 2(5):320–324.

Waechter EH: The adolescent with a handicapping, chronic, or life-threatening illness. In: *Perspectives on Adolescent Health Care*. Mercer RT (editor). Lippincott, 1979.

Williams HA, Rivara FP, Rothenberg MB: The child is dying: Who helps the family? *Am J Matern-Child Nurs* (July/Aug) 1981; 6:261–265.

Wong DL: Bereavement: The empty mother syndrome. *Am J Matern-Child Nurs* (Nov/Dec) 1980; 15:385–389.

Additional Readings

Arnold JH, Gemma PB: *A Child Dies: A Portrait of Family Grief*. Aspen, 1983.

Chitwood L: A lesson in living. *Nurs '84* (Jan) 1984; 14(1):55–56.

Corr CA: Books for adults: Coping with dying or with bereavement as they relate to childhood. *Issues Compr Pediatr Nurs* 1985; 8(16):367–371.

Corr CA et al.: Pediatric hospice care. *Pediatrics* (Nov) 1985; 76(5):774–780.

Cushing M: Whose best interest? Parents vs. child rights. *Am J Nurs* (Feb) 1982; 82(2):313–314.

Dailey A: Hospice care and the role of Children's Hospice International. *Caring* (May) 1985; 4(5):66–67.

Edwardson SR: The choice between hospital and home care for terminally ill children. *Nurs Res* (Jan/Feb) 1983; 32(1):29–34.

Grollman EA (editor): *Explaining Death to Children*. Beacon Press, 1967.

Henretta CB, Van Brunt PF: Sudden pediatric death: Meeting the needs of family and staff. *Nurs Educ* (Winter) 1982; 7:13–16.

Jones KW: Support for grieving kids. *Home Health Nurs* (July/Aug) 1985; 3(4):22–27.

Khoury MJ, Erickson JD, Adams MJ: Trends in postneonatal mortality in the United States. *JAMA* 1984; 252(3):367–372.

Kubler-Ross E: *On Children and Death*. Macmillan, 1983.

Mandell F, McAnulty EH, Carlson A: Unexpected death of an infant sibling. *Pediatrics* (Nov) 1983; 72(5):652–657.

Miles MS: Emotional symptoms and physical health in bereaved parents. *Nurs Res* (Mar/Apr) 1985; 34(2):76–81.

Miller JK: Pediatric hospice program. *Kentucky Nurses Assoc Newsletter* (Feb/March) 1982; 30:26–27.

Ross HM: Societal/cultural views regarding death and dying. *Top Clin Nurs* (Oct) 1981; 3(3):1–16.

Schowalter JE: Twenty years of pediatric thanatology. *Child Health Care* (Winter) 1986; 14(3):157–162.

Smith ML: When a child dies at home. *Nurs '82* (Aug) 1982; 12(8):66–67.

Thomas N, Cordell AS: The dying infant: Aiding parents in the detachment process. *Pediatr Nurs* (Sept/Oct) 1983; 9(5):355–357.

Walker KL: Easing the pain of bereaved parents. *Nurs '86* (April) 1986; 16(4):49–50.

Woods JR: Death on a daily basis. *Focus Crit Care* (June) 1984; 11(3):50–51.

Wooten B: Death of an infant. *Am J Matern-Child Nurs* (July/Aug) 1981; 6:257–260.

V

The Impact of Illness on the Child and Family

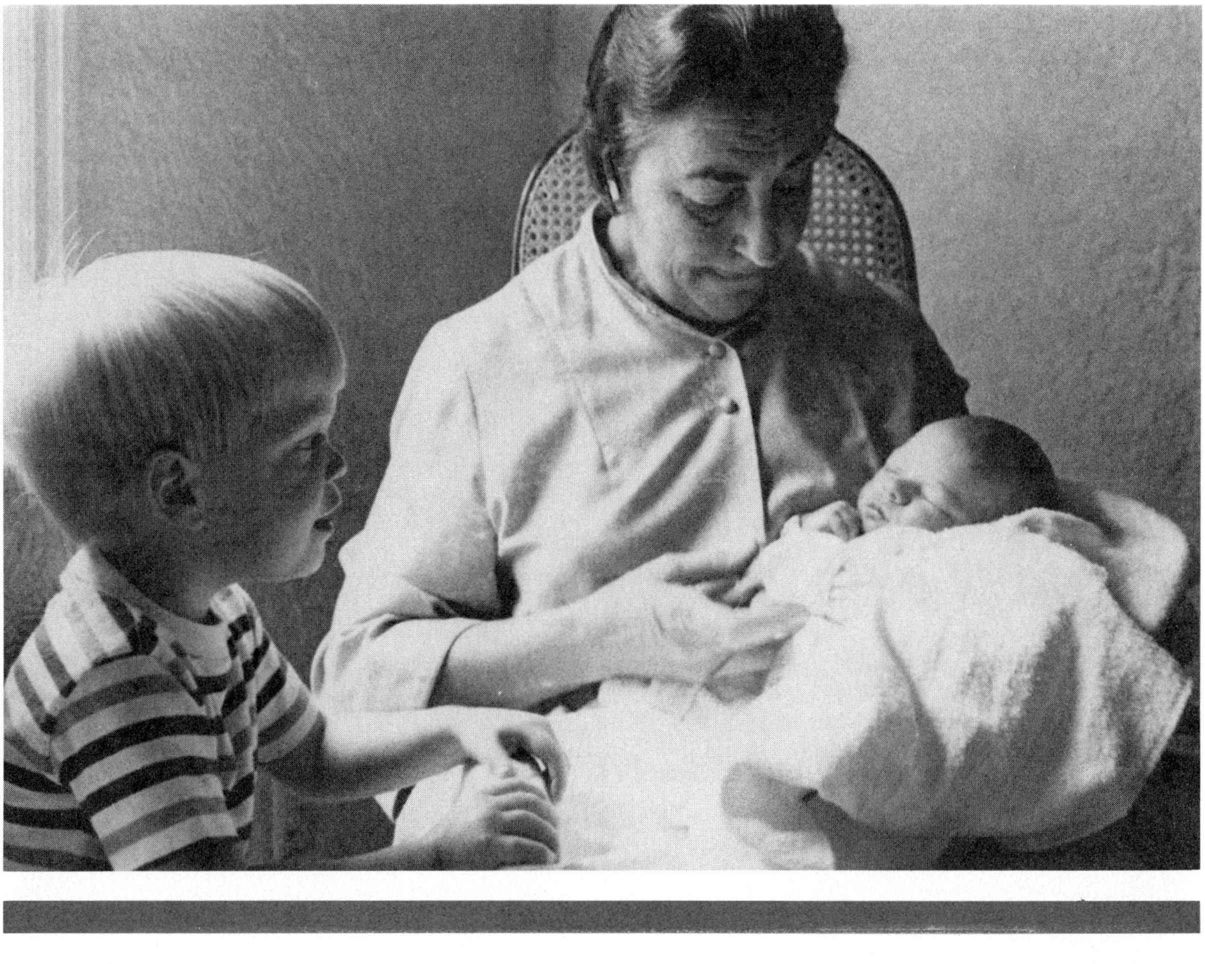

Chapter 18

Home Care of the Child with an Acute Illness

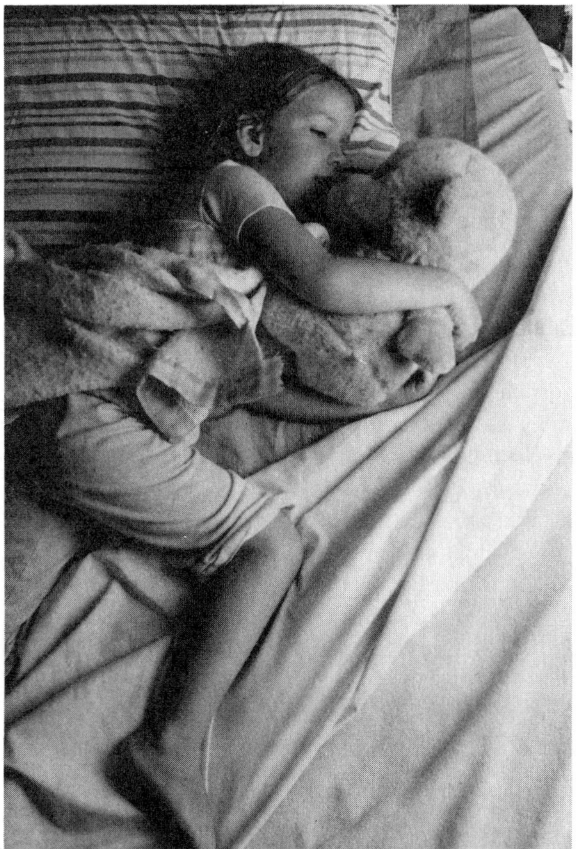

Chapter Contents

Cross Reference Box

To find these topics, see the following chapters:

Acne vulgaris	Chapter 24
Allergies	Chapter 25
Cradle cap	Chapter 4

(Continues)

Croup	Chapter 22
Diaper dermatitis	Chapter 4
Eczema	Chapter 24
Impetigo	Chapter 24
Otitis media	Chapter 32
Pharyngitis	Chapter 22
Pneumonia	Chapter 22
Severe gastroenteritis	Chapter 21

Objectives

- Explain the rationale for the care of the acutely ill child at home.
- Describe the nursing process as it applies to home care.
- Assist parents to make decisions regarding their capabilities to provide appropriate care in the home.
- Provide parents with criteria to assist them in making decisions regarding medical consultation.
- Explain the home care involved with frequently seen acute illnesses.

The recent trend away from hospitalization of the acutely ill child means that many ill children are now cared for in the home. This trend has important implications for nursing because the nurse is likely to be the professional to whom the parent turns for advice in caring for an ill child. The physician also might rely on the nurse once the diagnosis has been made to help determine whether the child can be cared for at home. The nurse almost certainly will communicate instructions to the parent regarding home care of the child.

Rationale for Home Treatment

For most childhood illnesses, home care is preferable to hospitalization, although hospitalization is occasionally necessary for many chronic diseases and some acute illnesses. Major emergencies, life-threatening conditions, and potentially crippling illnesses necessitate hospitalization. Certain psychosocial situations in the home also might make hospitalization preferable for some children. Hospitalization does, however, present additional risks, including the long- and short-term effects of separation, financial stress on the family and community, exposure of the ill child to the infections of other children or adults in the hospital, and undermining of the parents' confidence in their abilities as caregivers. Health professionals need to consider these risks and the potential that an acute illness will be further complicated when choosing how best to care for an ill child.

For the young child, the hospital is an unfamiliar, and potentially frightening place. It is filled with strange people and unusual, confusing routines. The home, on the other hand, is a familiar place where the child can be surrounded with personal possessions and where some of the child's normal routine can be maintained. The child who is cared for in the home does not have the stress of adjusting to an unfamiliar environment added to the stress of an acute illness.

With the recent approval of prospective payment legislation [see Chapter 1 about diagnosis-related groups (DRGs)], children are admitted to the hospital for serious conditions only. Procedures such as oxygen therapy, intravenous medication administration, total parenteral nutrition, and peritoneal dialysis once required the child to remain in the hospital for long periods of time. Current practice now allows children requiring these therapies to remain at home.

Flexibility is the key to optimal discharge preparation (discussed in Chapter 19). If parents or caregivers are unable to take care of the child in the home on a consistent basis, an arrangement might be made to keep the child in the home during the day, while overnights are spent in the hospital. Regardless of the type of home care provided, the goal is to promote the growth and development of children in a way that is best for each individual child (Feetham, 1986).

Settings for Nurses' Contact with Patients

Early discharge of children to the home is a direct result of the escalating costs of health care. Children might be sent home from the hospital requiring procedures such as complicated dressing changes, tube feedings or parenteral nutrition, and oxygen therapy. Frequently, nurses are responsible for decision making regarding the feasibility of home care. Hospital home care coordinators, many of whom are nurses, work closely with local visiting nurses and home care nurses to assess the child's home as a potential setting for care. Both coordinators and visiting nurses plan for care and evaluate the child's progress toward recovery or toward achieving optimal status.

In rural areas, where physician involvement might be limited, nurse practitioners are primary providers of care. In many instances they are fully responsible for making recommendations regarding feasibility of home care or necessity for hospitalization of the ill child. These decisions are complex because in many rural homes, accessibility to appropriate water and sanitation facilities is a problem.

Nurses working in ambulatory settings, such as physicians' offices, schools, camps, and clinics, frequently are the professionals who direct the parent initially regarding the care of common childhood illnesses and emergencies. Furthermore, in social situations any nurse is subject to questions from family, neighbors, and friends. Requests for assistance in deciding whether additional medical consultation is necessary are commonplace.

The Nurse's Role in Home Care

The nurse, with a thorough knowledge of pathophysiology, sociology, psychology, and family dynamics, is in a unique position to provide appropriate and accurate advice to parents and other health professionals. The nurse is capable of assessing the home setting to determine the family's ability to care for an ill child. Through the nursing process, the nurse helps the family to plan, implement, and evaluate home care. The nurse also is the one member of the health care team who is continually available to evaluate the effectiveness of home care.

The five steps of the nursing process are an integral part of home care for the acutely ill child. In the assessment phase the nurse appraises both the child and the family to determine the potential for home care. This includes an assessment of the nature and seriousness of the illness as well as the interest and capability of the family to cope with the illness or disease and care for the child in the home. Once the assessment is complete, the nurse works with the family in formulating a care plan that considers the unique needs of child and family. Implementation of the care plan is largely the responsibility of the family when the child is cared for in the home. The thoroughness with which the nurse and family develop the plan, however, will determine the potential effectiveness of its implementation.

Although the family carries out the plan, the nurse is still responsible for evaluating and reassessing the child's response to treatment. It is the nurse who decides whether the child is improving and whether continued care at home is feasible. This evaluation, although the last step of the nursing process, does not signal the end of the nurse's role. The nursing process is dynamic. Evaluation leads to reassessment and possibly to a new care plan. It is this dynamic nature of the nursing process that establishes a format for caring for the ill child in the home.

Assessment Assessment for home care is twofold. The nurse first needs to determine the particular needs of the individual child and family. The nurse then proceeds with a systematic assessment that provides the data needed to establish an individual plan of care. A detailed home assessment is performed when early discharge from a hospital is probable or when medical facilities are at a great distance from the home.

A major aspect of assessment for an acutely ill child is determining whether the family is able to care for the child. The nurse therefore assesses the seriousness of the illness, the home setting, and the family's support systems for each child to determine whether the child can be cared for at home. (Table 18-1 outlines the criteria used to assess the home and family to determine whether home care is feasible.)

Once the assessment data have been collected, analysis determines whether secondary care, or hospitalization, is indicated or whether home care is a viable alternative. (To illustrate how the decision is made, two situations are presented in Table 18-2. The background data are similar, but they differ in important areas that assist the nurse to make a judgment regarding the feasibility of home care for the individual child.)

Nursing diagnosis Once the decision for home care has been made, the nurse and family sit down and discuss the plan. Potential nursing diagnoses the nurse considers with any family undertaking home care of a child include:

Potential knowledge deficit regarding treatments or procedures to be performed in the home

Potential for injury to the child from inadequate safety preparations of the home

Potential for ineffective family coping

Potential alteration in family processes

Potential noncompliance with home care regimen

Potential for social isolation

Potential for impaired home maintenance management

Additional diagnoses might be identified, depending on the child's condition.

TABLE 18-1 Assessment Criteria for Home Care

Assessment questions	Rationale
Seriousness of the illness	
Is the illness self-limiting?	Certain illnesses such as the common cold, gastroenteritis, minor traumas, and some communicable diseases of childhood can usually be cared for in the home setting
What are the potential complications? Are they life threatening? Are they potentially debilitating?	More serious diseases such as croup, pneumonia, fractures, and concussion can have serious consequences, therefore the home setting must be carefully assessed
Is the child very young (less than 1 year)?	Infants are sometimes more susceptible to developing complications than older children with the same disease (eg, dehydration from gastroenteritis). Older children require less supervision when ill than infants
Is the disease communicable?	A person such as an infant or elderly person might be more susceptible to complications from communicable disease, which might preclude caring for the child at home
Is the child toxic? Is the oral temperature greater than 101° F? Has the child had a convulsion? Recently? Did the child have convulsions with a fever during a previous illness? Is the child dehydrated? Are complications present?	Potential complications require more careful assessment of whether the parent or caregiver is able to provide the necessary care
Support systems	
Is there an adult available to stay with the child who knows the child and the home? A parent? A grandparent or aunt if both parents work? An older sister or brother? A neighbor or friend?	A good support system will greatly improve the potential for the family caring for the ill child at home. A familiar adult needs to stay with the child, monitor the progress of the disease, administer the appropriate medication, and provide needed rest, nutrition, and diversion
Does the person who is to care for the child understand the instructions for care?	Instructions need to be written and in a language the caregiver can understand for home care to be successful
Are resources available for Obtaining needed equipment? Appropriate nutrition? Transportation (private automobile; public transportation, taxi or bus)?	The necessary equipment needs to be available to provide optimal care. The family needs to know where equipment can be obtained and the proper use and maintenance of all equipment. Some conditions require special dietary modifications
If needed, are visiting nurses and other support systems available in the community?	The family needs access to transportation to the health care facility. If transportation is not available, a visiting nurse or public health nursing agency can provide the needed therapies and care. Community emergency vehicles provide rapid support in emergency situations. Families feel more secure knowing consultation and help is available
Potential for home care	
Is the physical condition of the home appropriate for the care of an ill child? Is the source of water adequate? Acceptable? Are toilet facilities adequate? Indoor? Outdoor? City sewer system? Septic tank? Are bathing and washing facilities adequate? Hot water or heating facilities? Dishwashing facilities? Is a separate bed available for the ill child? Is heating adequate if the weather is cold? Are windows screened if the weather is hot? Can the child be isolated if the disease is communicable?	The home needs to be in good repair with adequate protection from the elements to prevent worsening of the child's condition. Not all these conditions are required for home care, but the home needs to have facilities to promote recovery and prevent the spread of disease to others.

TABLE 18-1 *(Continued)*

Assessment questions	Rationale
Potential for home care *(Continued)*	
Can the home be changed to make it appropriate for home care?	If minor changes can be made to make the home acceptable for home care, it might be preferable to make them rather than to keep the child in the hospital
Is the necessary equipment available? Thermometer—oral or rectal? Cleen sheets and bedding? Soap? Hot water? Dishes and means for sterilizing (ie, dishwasher or pot and stove for boiling water)? Refrigeration for medications?	Certain equipment is needed to adequately care for the child and prevent spread of communicable disease. The type of equipment needed depends on the child's condition
Do the parents have adequate financial resources To purchase the prescribed medication? To purchase analgesics? To purchase necessary equipment?	Often the family might not have enough money to purchase needed supplies and medications in which case arrangements can be made to help. The nurse needs to determine whether the family cannot afford the supplies or just will not purchase them or administer medications because of some cultural or personal objection
Do the parents have the psychic energy necessary to care for an ill child at home? How many other family members live in the home? Is there a current family crisis, death, separation, or divorce? Do any other family members have a physical or emotional illness? Is there a special need or handicapped child in the home?	Recent crises in the family, such as divorce, death, birth of a new baby, might contraindicate home care. If the care appears to be long term, relief for the primary caregiver is essential to conserve physical and psychic energy
Is there reasonable assurance that the parent or designated caregiver will follow through in implementing a plan of care for the ill child?	The parent or designated caregiver must be willing to implement the care plan in the home setting and must agree to the plan of care before the nurse can be reasonably assured the child will receive the needed care
Are any cultural or religious beliefs likely to interfere with the care plan? Are these customs or beliefs a potential threat to the health of the child?	Home remedies or methods for treating illness that have been handed down from generation to generation might interfere with adequate home care. Harmless remedies usually do not interfere with and can enhance the care plan. Some remedies can contribute to complications
Is there a history of noncompliance with prescribed treatment regimens?	Cultural beliefs concerning medication therapy can result in noncompliance with the medical regimen, and alternatives need to be considered for medication administration

Planning Planning helps to determine priorities among the identified problems. Planning requires the nurse, child, and family to determine mutual objectives or outcomes of care. Including both the child and the caregiver in the development of the care plan increases the potential for cooperation with the prescribed regimen.

In planning care, the nurse considers all aspects of the child's illness: the causative agent, communicability, severity or seriousness, expected progress, and potential complications. The primary goals of care should be to promote recovery in the shortest possible period while preventing any complications. These goals can best be achieved when the nurse, caregiver, physician, and child all work together as a team in planning and implementing the care plan.

The resources that the caregiver has available are an important consideration in the development of a plan of care. If necessary equipment or supplies are not available, the parent might need assistance in developing alternatives. This might include borrowing, renting, or purchasing the needed equipment.

If space in the home is a problem, the nurse can suggest alternative arrangements to create the necessary space for the patient. Physical problems in the home might be corrected with assistance from community resources. Family

TABLE 18-2 Determining the Feasibility of Home Care by Analyzing Data

Patient data: Name: Susan Age: 8 years Medical diagnosis: probable streptococcal pharyngitis

Assessment data	Nursing considerations
Situation 1	
Self-limiting disease with potential complications	Potential cardiac complications from improper treatment or resistance to prescribed treatment regimen
Highly communicable problem, especially in crowded conditions	Potential for communicability to other family members
Oral temperature of 103° F. No signs of dehydration, convulsions, or other complications	Discomfort from fever and pain; potential dehydration caused by decreased fluid intake from the sore throat
Both parents work all day. Child is alone because older siblings attend school. No close family or friends nearby; however, the mother's employer is amenable to her taking sick time to care for child	Potential for inadequate support for home care
Five people living in a three-bedroom, five-room apartment. Child shares a room with older sister. Child's brother has his own room. Bathing and toileting facilities are adequate. Family owns sleeping bags	Potential inability for the child to be isolated
Equipment necessary for home care is present. No dishwasher	Potential spread of disease through inadequate handling of dishes
Family is covered under a comprehensive health plan	
No history of failure to cooperate with medication regimen. Parents do not feel that once symptoms have disappeared, the medication can be discontinued	
Analysis leading to the decision for home care: Assessment factors indicate a strong probability that Susan can be cared for at home if the nursing considerations are addressed in the plan of care. For example, the isolation problem can be solved if the patient is put alone in the brother's room and the brother uses a sleeping bag on the floor of one of the living areas.	
Situation 2	
Self-limiting disease with potential complications. Patient's sister has history of rheumatic fever	Potential for complications is increased in patient because of family history of rheumatic fever. Potential for sister to become ill related to infectious characteristics of streptococcal pharyngitis and her own history of rheumatic fever
The disease is highly communicable in crowded conditions	Potential for communicability to other family members
Oral temperature of 103° F. No signs of dehydration, convulsions, or other complications	Discomfort from fever and pain; potential dehydration caused by decreased fluid intake from the sore throat
Mother will stay home to care for the child all day. Adequate supports	
Eight people living in a five-room apartment (three bedrooms). Patient shares a bedroom with two sisters	Inadequate rest; no way to isolate the patient
Equipment necessary for home care is present. No dishwasher	Potential spread of disease through inadequate handling of dishes
Family is covered under a comprehensive health care plan	
History of failure to cooperate with medication regimen. Parents discontinue the medication when the symptoms disappear	Knowledge deficit regarding germ theory leading to failure to cooperate with prescribed treatment regimen
Analysis leading to the decision for home care: Although the assessment data indicate similar problems to situation #1, home care in this situation might be contraindicated. The crowded living conditions are not easily modified, and the risk of the occurrence of rheumatic fever is increased because of inability to isolate the patient and the family history. The conclusive nursing diagnosis is that there is an increased risk for the development of complications because of personal and environmental factors.	

TABLE 18-3 Planning Phase of the Nursing Process Related to Home Care

Nursing diagnosis	Plan and intervention
1. Potential for non-compliance with the antibiotic regimen	Teach the parents the principles and importance of antibiotic therapy, effects of medication, and necessity to finish the prescription
Outcome: Susan will not experience any complications as a result of inadequate medication administration. The parent can explain the reasons for completing the prescribed dose of antibiotics.	
2. Knowledge deficit related to incomplete understanding of the potential complications of the disease	Teach the parents and/or caregiver to recognize the signs of complications—increased fever, fatigue, pain in one or more joints, tachycardia
Outcome: The parents can state and describe warning signals of complications. The parent knows who to contact if complications occur.	
3. Potential for infection in parents and siblings	Encourage the family to consider alternative sleeping arrangements, such as having the brother sleep in a sleeping bag in the living room, so that the child can temporarily have her own room; teach the family the importance of hand washing and the proper disposal of tissues Recommend the use of paper plates and plastic cutlery if affordable, or make certain that all dishes and silverware are washed thoroughly with detergent and very hot water Suggest using the same set of dishes for Susan at each meal
Outcome: Susan and her parents can identify measures to prevent the spread of the disease to others in the home.	
4. Potential fluid volume deficit	Teach parent to provide moderate amounts of cool liquids frequently (including Jello and Popsicles)
Outcome: Susan's urine output will be sufficient for her age and weight. Susan will not exhibit signs of dehydration.	

members will need assistance in budgeting their time to prevent fatigue while caring for the child at home. (Table 18-3 carries the case presented in Table 18-2 into the planning phase of the nursing process.)

During planning, the nurse identifies the person or persons responsible for resolving each problem and also identifies specific methods and steps to take to solve the problems. This information is compiled in a written care plan that is to be given to the child's primary caregiver. A written care plan provides a comprehensive plan of action to care for the ill child in the home or hospital, and it provides a reasonable assurance that the needs of the patient will be met.

Intervention Once the plan of care has been developed and agreed on by the nurse and caregiver, it is time to put the plan into action through nursing interventions. When the ill child is cared for in the home, the parent or designated caregiver is responsible for implementing the plan of care. The nurse's responsibility, however, does not end with planning. The nurse is also responsible for seeing that the plan is implemented properly. This can best be accomplished through teaching proper care, supporting the parent's efforts to provide care, coordinating the services of other health professionals, and, if necessary, referring the child to other health care providers or services.

Before sending the ill child home with a care plan, the nurse determines whether the parent fully understands the plan and knows how to implement it in the home setting. Instructions are given, and, if necessary, correct procedures are taught before the parent and child leave the office or clinic. If, for example, eardrops must be instilled at home, the parent needs to know the correct way to do this and might need to practice with supervision. If a special diet is needed, it is given in writing and reviewed orally by the nurse with the parent or designated caregiver to ensure understanding.

The nurse needs to be certain that the parent or caregiver

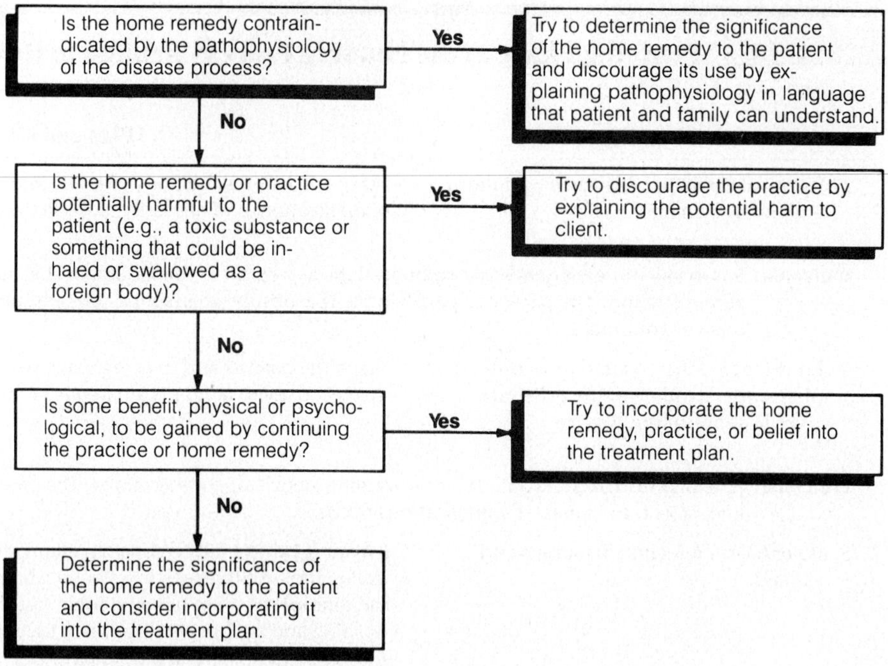

FIGURE 18-1
Home remedies and the nursing care plan.

has the information needed to care for the ill child at home and then fills information gaps with appropriate teaching. In teaching or explaining procedures to the caregiver or parent, the nurse applies the principles of teaching, gears the instructions to the parent's or caregiver's educational level, and avoids complicated medical terminology as much as possible. (Principles of teaching are discussed in Chapter 19.)

Once the parent has taken the child home and the care plan has been implemented, the nurse maintains contact with the family to provide support, encouragement, and any needed direction. This important contact can be done either through a telephone call or a home visit. Many parents, unfamiliar with disease entities, need to be reassured that they are doing the right things and that the child is progressing satisfactorily. The nurse therefore calls the family or visits the home 48 hours after the initiation of the treatment plan.

More information can be gathered during a home visit, but this is not always economically possible or time efficient. During the call or visit, the nurse gathers sufficient information to determine whether the care plan is being properly implemented. By questioning the parent or caregiver with careful reference to the written care plan, the nurse can determine whether the outcomes are being met, can monitor the progress of the child, and can identify any possible complications that might have developed. If the child is progressing satisfactorily, the parent needs positive reinforcement and encouragement to continue caring for the ill child as planned. If the child is not progressing satisfactorily or if complications have developed, the parent might need emotional support because guilt feelings or feelings of failure can interfere with care.

Evaluation Evaluation determines the patient's response to the treatment plan and whether the mutual objectives have been met. Evaluation is helpful to update or modify a plan of care.

After determining whether the outcomes have been achieved, the nurse decides whether home care is still a viable option. (The assessment criteria described in Table 18-1 are useful for evaluation as well.) If the objectives have not been met, the reasons need to be explored. The nurse therefore determines whether the parent or designated caregiver will be able to adapt to achieve the desired outcomes. When the health of the child might be compromised, alternatives to home care are indicated.

Referral of the Ill Child

Occasionally, the parent of an ill child will consult the nurse for help in determining whether medical attention is needed. The child usually has been receiving some treatment at home and either is not improving or is getting worse. In addition to determining whether the home remedies and treatment being administered are appropriate (Fig. 18-1), the nurse determines whether additional treatment is needed.

If the nurse can complete a history of the illness and an assessment of the child, objective data on which to base a

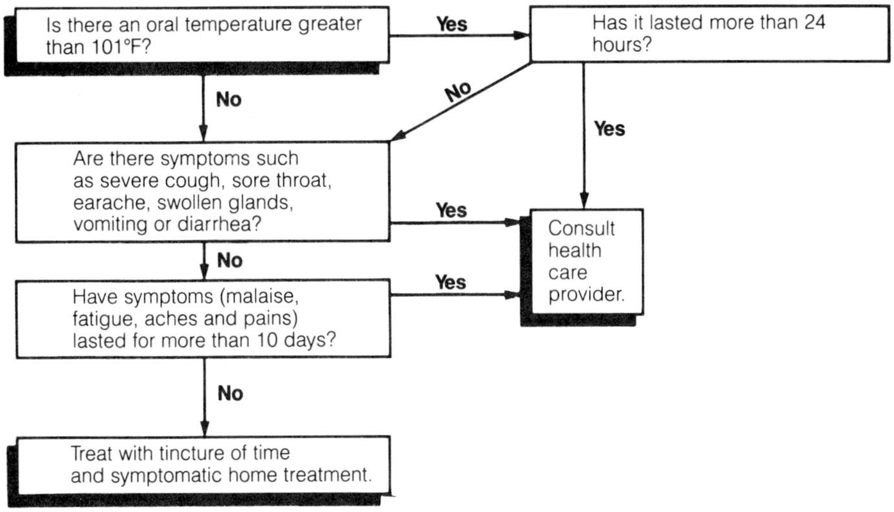

FIGURE 18-2

Parent decision: when to seek medical attention for a sick child.

decision are available. This might not be possible, however, because nurses often are asked these questions over the phone or in an informal setting such as the grocery store. In such cases it is usually best for legal and ethical reasons to recommend that the parent seek medical attention.

The nurse can assist the parents in determining when medical care is indicated for an ill child by assessing the status of the illness (Fig. 18-2). Did the illness occur suddenly? Many acute illnesses have a rather dramatic sudden onset of fever. Most illnesses that occur gradually over several days or weeks are less acute and usually do not require immediate referral to a health care provider. If the child had a sudden onset of high fever that has lasted for 24 hours and has not responded to antipyretic (anti-fever) treatment, the child needs to be referred for medical attention.

The age and general health of the child also needs to be considered when recommending to parents whether to seek medical care. A child with a chronic illness might need to seek medical attention early in the course of any illness to prevent possible complications. If a child has been ill for an extended period (more than 10 days), a medical provider should be consulted. Only a thorough assessment can determine whether an extended illness is serious and if medical treatment is needed.

Acute Illnesses Amenable to Home Care

When the home is chosen as the care setting for an ill child, the parent or caregiver will need the support of the health care community until the illness resolves. Questions about when to seek additional medical attention are prime concerns in caring for the ill child at home. (Figure 18-3 gives some guidelines to help the parent determine when further medical attention is needed after the initial treatment has been started.)

Disorders of the Respiratory System

Disorders of the respiratory system include those that affect the upper respiratory tract—the ears, nose, and throat—and those that affect the lower respiratory system—the trachea, bronchial tubes, and lungs. Most disorders of the respiratory system are amenable to home care. Only the more severe, serious, or complicated cases require hospitalization. Children who might require hospitalization are those whose illnesses cause deprivation of air exchange, in which oxygenation of the tissues is jeopardized, and those who develop complications. An accurate assessment of the seriousness or severity of a respiratory disorder is essential to determining the treatment setting.

The child with a respiratory disorder might demonstrate a variety of symptoms depending on age and the pathophysiology of the disease. All children with respiratory complaints need to receive thorough evaluations, including a history and assessment of the entire respiratory system. The nurse needs to be familiar with growth and development as well as the pathophysiology of each disease to assess the child with a respiratory disorder.

Otitis externa Otitis externa, inflammation and infection of the external auditory canal, can be caused by an abrasion or by a decrease in cerumen. (Cerumen is the waxy substance that coats the external ear canal.) Otitis externa often is called "swimmer's ear," because it can be caused by repeated removal of cerumen by water. Removal of the cerumen allows organism growth.

FIGURE 18-3

Parent decision: when to seek further medical attention for an ill child after initial treatment.

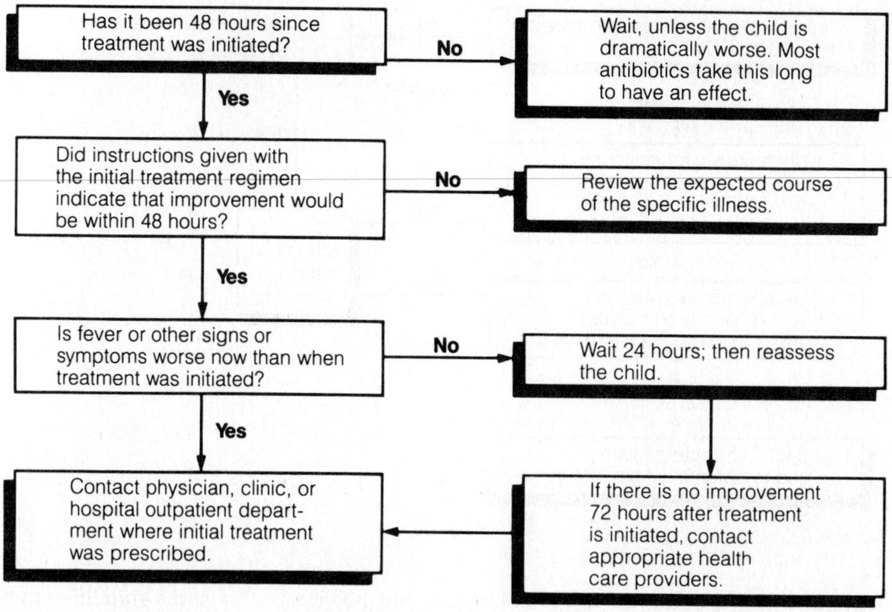

Organisms involved in the infectious process include bacteria, viruses, and fungi. The most common complaint is pain with movement of the aurical, decreased hearing, a feeling of fullness in the affected ear, purulent discharge from the ear canal, and a low-grade fever. The usual treatment involves oral antibiotics and antibiotic eardrops with or without corticosteroids.

Home care of the child with otitis externa involves the administration of oral antibiotics and the instillation of the prescribed eardrops. In giving instructions to the parent for care of the child at home, the nurse emphasizes the importance of administering all of the prescribed medication, even though the child might begin to feel better after taking only a few doses. Furthermore, the parent is cautioned not to use corticosteroid eardrops for longer than the prescribed period (usually 5 days) because of potential side effects.

The parent is taught how to instill eardrops (see Chapter 20). The parent is instructed to keep the child's head tilted to one side after the drops are put in so that the medication is in contact with the affected ear for as long as possible.

The prevention of future infections of the external ear canal is one of the goals of care. In this regard the nurse plays a major role in teaching the parent and child proper ear care. This includes avoiding cleaning the ears with hair pins, cotton-tipped swabs, keys, and other objects. The child is strongly discouraged from inserting anything in the ear. Recalling the physiology of the ear, the nurse can explain how the cilia, the small hairlike structures in the ear, normally keep the wax cleared from the canal. Very few people experience wax buildup of sufficient proportions to require professional ear cleaning. Otitis externa sometimes masks otitis media (middle ear infection) because of exudates that block the ear canal; therefore, the importance of follow-up care is emphasized in child and parent teaching (Fig. 18-4).

Rhinitis Rhinitis is inflammation of the mucous membrane of the nose. It is manifested by a nasal discharge and is almost always associated with an underlying disturbance. The most common causes of rhinitis are allergy, the common cold, infected adenoids, chronic sinusitis, foreign body aspiration, and various congenital anomalies. Besides nasal discharge, symptoms can include foul breath and disturbances of taste and smell.

Rhinitis is treated by correcting the underlying problem. Emphasis is placed on eradicating any infections. Medications that provide symptomatic relief are used with mixed results. Children are to be encouraged not to blow their noses with any force because the altered pressure from blowing can lead to middle ear infections.

Allergic rhinitis Allergic rhinitis (hay fever) occurs as a result of exposure to an allergen to which the child is sensitive. Symptoms include watery eyes, sneezing, runny nose, and occasionally a mild sore throat. In allergic rhinitis, mucous membranes are pale and boggy. Nasal obstruction is common and often cyclic. Symptoms are similar to those of the common cold but differ in some respects (Fig. 18-5).

The condition usually is self-limiting, and symptoms disappear as the pollen count decreases. Treatment is generally symptomatic and involves the use of an appropriate antihistamine. The nurse consults with the physician before recommending a particular medication to a parent because antihistamines can produce varied and annoying side

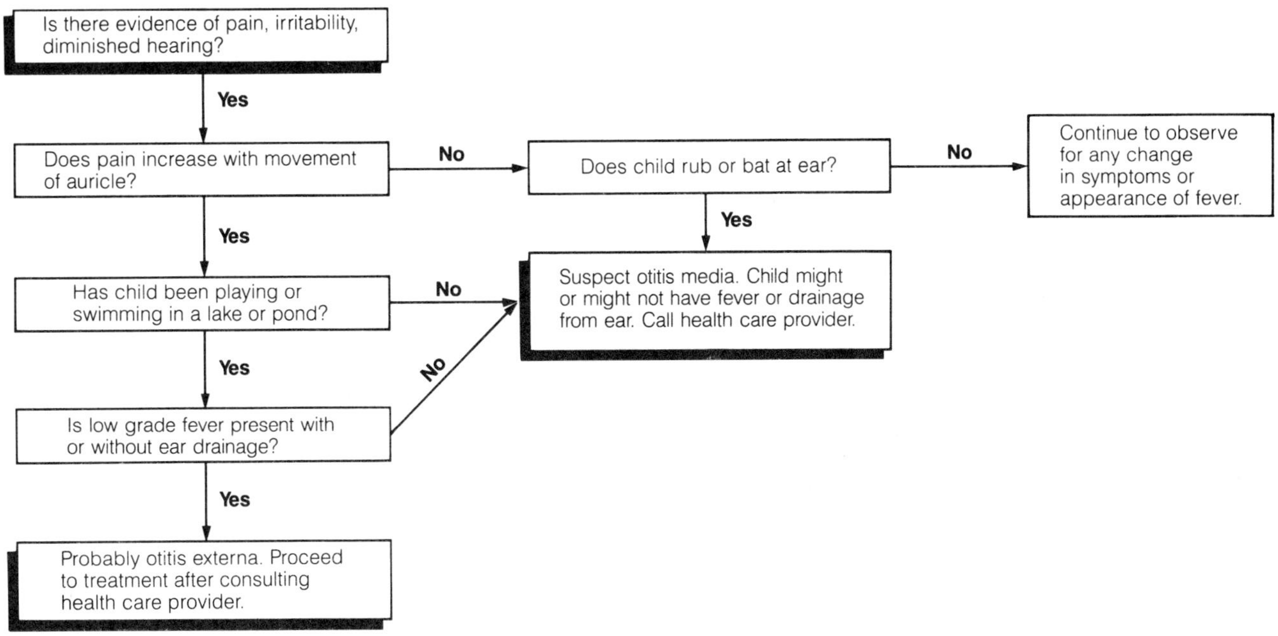

FIGURE 18-4

Parent decision: otitis.

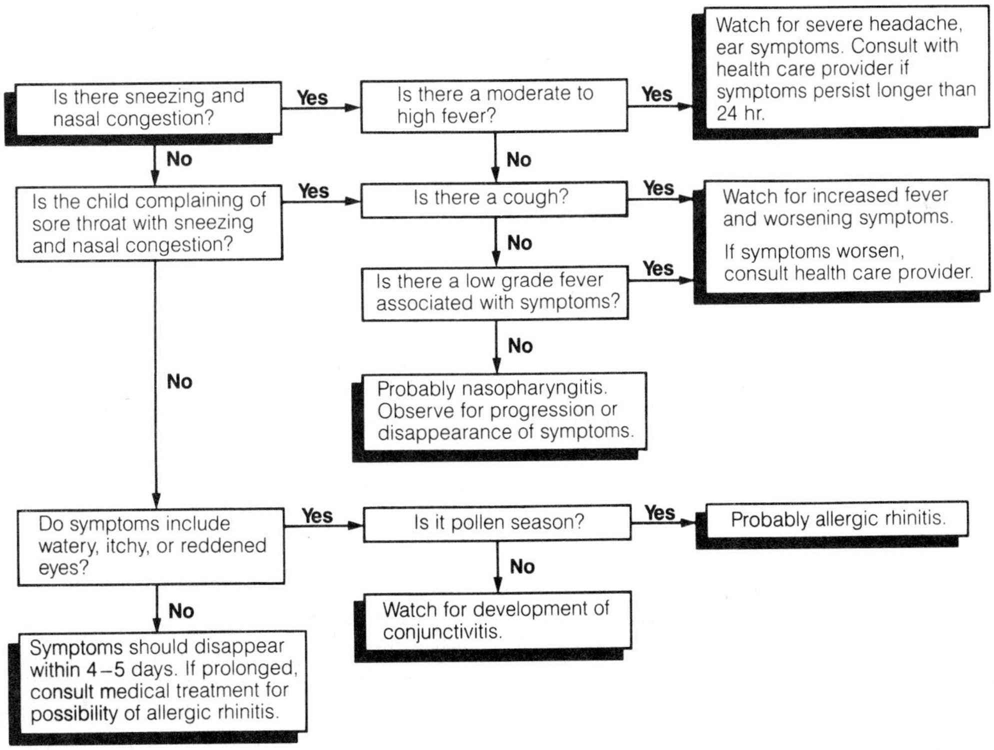

FIGURE 18-5

Parent decision: rhinitis.

effects in children. Parents might be bewildered by the number of over-the-counter antihistamines available and need to be cautioned not to experiment with these medications without professional advice.

Many children have periodic episodes of allergic rhinitis. Most of these children will be cared for in the home without seeking professional health care. Frequently, however, the parent of a child with allergic rhinitis will contact the nurse for advice and help in deciding whether the child needs professional attention. Parents are instructed to seek immediate medical attention if the child has difficulty breathing or swallowing. If the child develops an earache or fever or if rhinitis symptoms persist, medical consultation is indicated.

Acute nasopharyngitis Most children will experience one or more episodes of acute nasopharyngitis (the common cold) each year. Very few of these children will ever seek medical attention. Acute nasopharyngitis can be caused by numerous viruses. It usually includes symptoms of nasal stuffiness, sneezing, sore throat, nonproductive cough, and low-grade fever. Acute nasopharyngitis usually is self-limiting and will resolve in 4–5 days without specific treatment.

Because most antibiotics do not appear to be effective against viruses, antibiotic therapy usually is contraindicated for children with nasopharyngitis. Parents need to have information about why antibiotics are not effective against viral illnesses and information regarding the potential for developing antibiotic-resistant infections if antibiotics are not used judiciously.

The nurse encourages the parent to provide adequate rest, nutrition, and symptomatic treatment for the child with a cold. Acetaminophen can be given for fever symptoms. Fluids such as fruit juice and cold drinks need to be offered frequently to maintain adequate hydration. If nasal congestion is severe, the parent might want to consult the physician regarding the use of antihistamines for symptomatic relief. The parent needs to be cautious about administering over-the-counter cold preparations. Some of these preparations contain aspirin, which has been implicated in the occurrence of a rare, but dangerous disease—Reye's syndrome (see Chapter 31).

Measures need to be taken to prevent the spread of the cold to others by keeping the child home if possible, instructing the child to cover the mouth and nose when coughing or sneezing, and sterilizing dishes in a dishwasher or with very hot water. Parents are advised that if complications such as ear involvement, high fever, or productive cough develop or if the cold persists for more than 1 week, medical attention needs to be obtained.

Infectious mononucleosis Mononucleosis is a syndrome that occurs primarily in older children and adolescents. Although caused by the Epstein-Barr virus (EBV), its symptoms are seen in other diseases such as toxoplasmosis and cytomegalovirus infections.

Mononucleosis is characterized by lethargy, extreme fatigue, low-grade fever, mild pharyngitis (sore throat), rash, and generalized lymphadenopathy (lymph node enlargement). More severe manifestations include spleen and/or liver enlargement.

Laboratory serum tests reveal an elevated atypical lymphocyte count (greater than 10%) (see Chapter 25). Antibody to the EBV becomes positive approximately 2 weeks after the onset of the disease and is helpful in making a positive diagnosis (antibody function is discussed in Chapter 25). Specific blood titers for EBV can pinpoint the onset of the infection (Pickering and DuPont, 1986).

Infectious mononucleosis is transmitted to a susceptible child through saliva. It is a self-limiting disease, usually resolving in several weeks. Relapses can occur if the child returns to vigorous activity before the condition is appropriately resolved.

Mononucleosis rarely requires hospitalization, although hospitalization might be indicated if signs of complications are evident. Peritonsillar abscess, upper airway obstruction, and potential splenic rupture are the complications most often seen. Abnormal liver function tests might indicate impending difficulties (see Chapter 27).

The symptoms of mononucleosis can closely resemble those of a streptococcal pharyngitis. For this reason, a throat culture is performed routinely on any child with mononucleosis syndrome who complains of a sore throat. Treatment with appropriate antibiotics is indicated for a positive throat culture.

For individuals with mononucleosis, adherence to a home treatment regimen is essential. Because older children are most frequently affected, they need to be included in the development of the treatment plan, which usually involves rest, adequate nutritional intake, and increased fluid intake. The nurse emphasizes the importance of diet and rest to both the child and the parent because these are absolutely necessary for optimal recovery. The required therapy is, however, atypical of the usual behavior of adolescents, and it might be difficult to enforce the regimen. The child and parent need to understand that recovery might be gradual and that lack of adherence to the treatment plan can prolong the recovery period.

Occasionally, a child will not adhere to a treatment plan regardless of parental cooperation. In these instances, hospitalization might be the only viable treatment option. The parent needs to be encouraged to seek medical assistance if the child complains of excessive pain in the throat, exhibits any signs of respiratory distress, or complains of epigastric or abdominal pain.

Disorders of the Gastrointestinal System

Disorders of the gastrointestinal system include those that affect the mouth, esophagus, stomach and intestines, colon, anus, and rectum. These disorders might be bacterial, viral, or parasitic in origin. In some instances, disorders of the gastrointestinal system appear to be idiopathic (no known cause), although emotional disturbances might trigger their development.

Disorders of the gastrointestinal system occur in children almost as frequently as disorders of the respiratory system. Many disorders are amenable to home care if a competent parent or caregiver is available, if cooperation with a prescribed treatment regimen can be assured, and if the child is not exhibiting signs of dehydration or hemorrhage.

Thrush Thrush, often referred to as oral moniliasis or oral candidiasis, is a superficial fungal infection involving the oral cavity. It is caused by *Candida albicans* and might be a result of overgrowth from antibiotic therapy, contamination from an infected person, or contact with infected objects. The incidence seems to be higher in infants, with neonates acquiring the condition from the mother during birth.

There generally are no symptoms of thrush, although if the infection is severe, the child might have pain with swallowing. The child usually is brought to the physician following the appearance of white, tenacious plaques on the oral mucosa. These plaques resemble milk curds but are difficult to remove and bleed when removal is attempted.

Treatment is with an antifungal agent, such as Nystatin oral suspension, which is instilled into the mouth three or four times daily for 1 week. The nurse needs to teach the parent to drop the suspension on the lesions and into the front of the mouth slowly so that the medication will be in contact with the lesions for as long as possible. Sterilization of baby bottles and nipples is recommended to prevent reinfection. If the infant is breast-fed, the mother is advised to wash her nipples with soap and water after each feeding.

The parent is advised to bring the child back if the infection does not clear up or if it recurs. The nurse teaches the parent to recognize the signs of dehydration, particularly when oral discomfort prevents adequate fluid intake. A simple method for observing for dehydration is to have the parent watch for infrequent urination or a marked decrease in the number of wet diapers, dry skin, dry lips and tongue, and sunken fontanelles in an infant. Recurrent infection with *Candida albicans* warrants further investigation to rule out any underlying systemic diseases.

Acute gastroenteritis The child with acute gastroenteritis (inflammation of the stomach and intestines) usually experiences diarrhea or vomiting or both. Causes of gastroenteritis can be viral or bacterial (Table 18-4), although in most cases the causative organism is unknown.

Fever might or might not be present and, depending on the severity of the vomiting and diarrhea, the child might be dehydrated. Dehydration and the resultant electrolyte imbalance (see Chapter 21) might contraindicate home care for the very young infant with gastroenteritis.

If the origin of the acute gastroenteritis is nonspecific, it generally is treated with dietary restrictions. The parent is instructed that no specific therapy other than dietary control is available. Because of the potential side effects, the nurse discourages parents from using antidiarrheal and antiemetic medications unless specifically prescribed by the physician.

The child is removed from the current diet and is given clear fluids for approximately 12 hours. As the child improves, the amount of liquids is increased gradually. If the diarrhea and vomiting continue to improve, easily digested foods such as gelatin, dry toast, and crackers can be added to the diet. If improvement continues, the parent can give cereal without milk, bananas, and broiled meat to the child after 48 hours. Milk, eggs, cheese, and other milk products are not included in the diet until the child has been asymptomatic for 24–48 hours because temporary lactose intolerance frequently occurs following diarrhea.

If the vomiting and diarrhea fail to improve within 24 hours after dietary restrictions are initiated or if the child shows signs of dehydration, additional medical consultation is indicated. The nurse needs to be certain that the parent understands and will follow the dietary instructions and that the parent knows how to observe for dehydration (Fig. 18-6). If the nurse has any doubts about parental cooperation, alternatives to home care might be indicated.

Intestinal parasites Many children with intestinal parasites will be asymptomatic, but vague abdominal discomfort, rectal bleeding, anorexia (loss of appetite), weight loss, or anemia might be present. Infestation with intestinal parasites is frequently seen in school-age children and should be a consideration in all children with vague abdominal complaints. Fortunately, intestinal parasites are easy to eradicate with antiparasitic agents. Usually, however, it is necessary to treat the entire family. Unfortunately, because of the pathophysiology and life cycle of the parasite, reinfestation is likely.

Oxyuriasis (infestation by pin worms), the most common parasitic infection of children in the United States, is caused by *Enterobius vermicularis*. The child complains of rectal itching, and the parent occasionally might see the adult pinworm in the stool. The mature pinworm looks like a short piece of white thread. Diagnosis is made by the brief application of cellophane tape to the perianal region at

TABLE 18-4 Causative Agents of Diarrhea in Children

Causative agent	Incubation period	Clinical symptomatology: Fever	Nausea and vomiting	Abdominal pain	Other	Site and mechanism of action	Stool characteristics: Color	Odor & consistency	Pus	Mucus	Blood	Medical treatment	Comments
Bacterial causes													
Shigella *S. sonnei* *S. flexneri* *S. dysenteriae*	24–72 hours	Yes	Rare	Crampy	Seizures Rectal prolapse	Colon, sigmoid colon, rectum Produces an exotoxin that kills tissue and causes massive fluid loss	Yellow green or colorless	Watery	Yes	Yes	Yes	Usually self-limiting; stools clear in 7–10 days without antibiotics. Antibiotics—ampicillin or chloramphenicol (Chloromycetin)—used only in cases of severe disability, in high-risk children, or in infants or young children who are dehydrated	Seizures most common in young infants. Toxicity more common in infants than in older children. Bacteria may survive on linen for up to several weeks. Stool precautions necessary if child is hospitalized
Salmonella *S. paratyphi* *S. typhi*	8–72 hours	Occasionally low grade	Yes	Colicky	Septicemia Osteomyelitis in children with sickle cell disease	Small bowel and cecum Causes local inflammation with high fluid, sodium, and chloride loss in stools	Green	Rotton egg odor Slimy Watery	No	Rare	Rare	Children are treated only if they are immune suppressed. Antibiotic therapy appears to prolong excretion of the organism in the stool; ampicillin is the drug of choice	Severe cases might lead to septicemia. Debilitated children and children with certain chronic diseases might develop osteomyelitis, abscesses, or meningitis. Often found in contaminated foods and water, especially eggs, poultry, milk, and shellfish. Transmitted by animals
Staphylococcus aureus	1–5 hours	Rare	Severe	Acute, crampy	Acute onset	Small bowel Invades small bowel wall Produces an enterotoxin	Varies	Watery	No	Yes	Yes	Treatment is symptomatic; symptoms usually self-limiting within 24 hours	Severe dehydration might occur in infants. Most often transmitted through contaminated foods
Enteropathic *Escherichia coli*	24–72 hours	Rare	Vomiting in infant	Occasionally	More common in children under 2 years of age	Colon Produces possible enterotoxin Causes loss of fluid and electrolytes	Green	Slimy Watery Foul odor	No	Yes	No	Treatment is symptomatic, but antibiotics are often used in young children (neomycin, colistin, and ampicillin)	Transmitted through contaminated foods or through contaminated fomites. Most common in young infants
Viral causes													
Parvolike virus Rotavirus Others	Varies	Yes	Occasionally	Occasionally	Possible upper respiratory tract infection simultaneously	Small bowel?	Green	Watery	No	Rare	Rare	Treatment is symptomatic; child maintained NPO with fluid and electrolyte replacement	Often highly contagious, particularly in newborn nurseries, hospitals, and day-care centers. Often occurs in conjunction with upper respiratory tract infection. Stool precautions necessary if the child is hospitalized

TABLE 18-4 *(Continued)*

Causative agent	Incubation period	Clinical symptomatology: Fever	Nausea and vomiting	Abdominal pain	Other	Site and mechanism of action	Stool characteristics: Color	Odor & consistency	Pus	Mucus	Blood	Medical treatment	Comments
Protozoal causes													
Amoebae *Entamoeba histolytica*	Varies: may be present in nonsymptomatic carrier state	Rare	Varies	Varies	Liver abcess Brain abcess	Large bowel Invades large bowel wall Can invade ileum, liver, lungs, brain	Varies	Varies	No	Clear mucus	Occasionally in infants	Antiprotozoals such as diiodohydroxyquin, paromomycin, metronidazole (Flagyl) are used. Repeat stool examinations until clear	Transmitted person to person or through contaminated food and water. Family members should be tested to allow for treatment of asymptomatic carriers
Giardia lamblia	Varies	Varies	Varies	Varies	Intermittent diarrhea Malabsorption syndrome	Duodenum and jejunum Parasites act on bowel lining	Varies	Varies but may be watery in infants	No	Varies	Varies	Quinacrine, metronidazole (Flagyl) are used	Often transmitted through contaminated water supplies or foods. Family members should be tested to allow for treatment of asymptomatic carriers. Can be transmitted in swimming pools

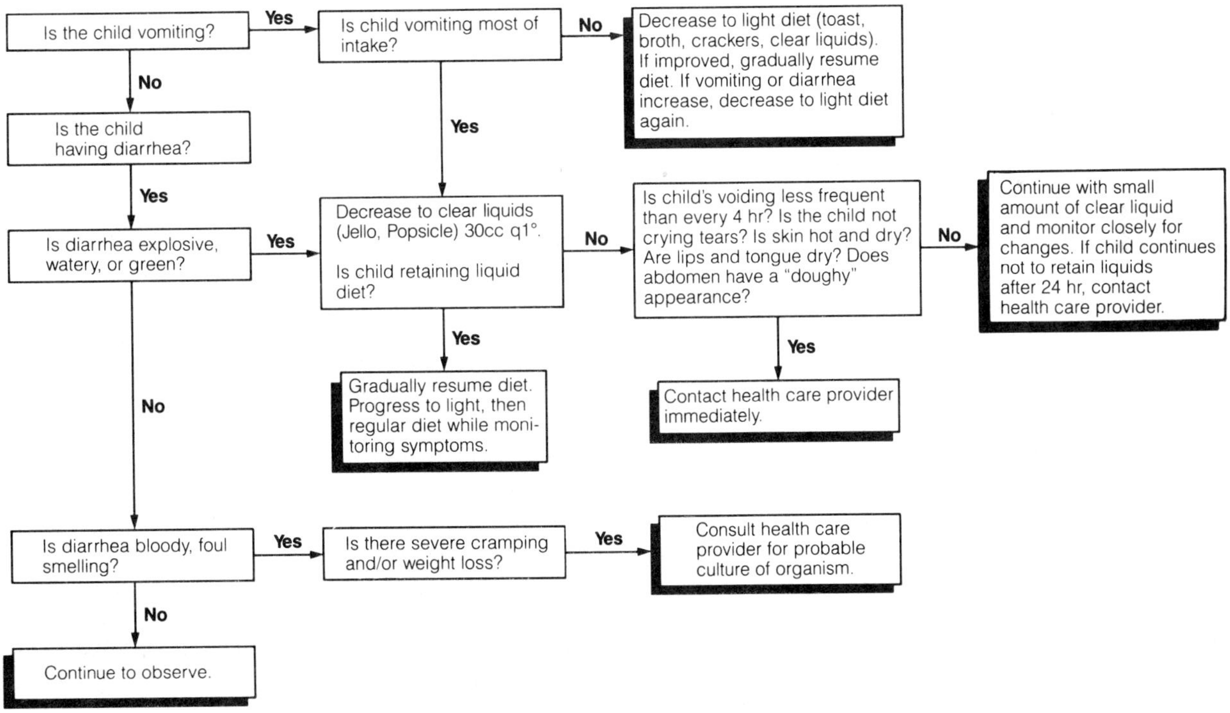

FIGURE 18-6
Parent decision: gastroenteritis.

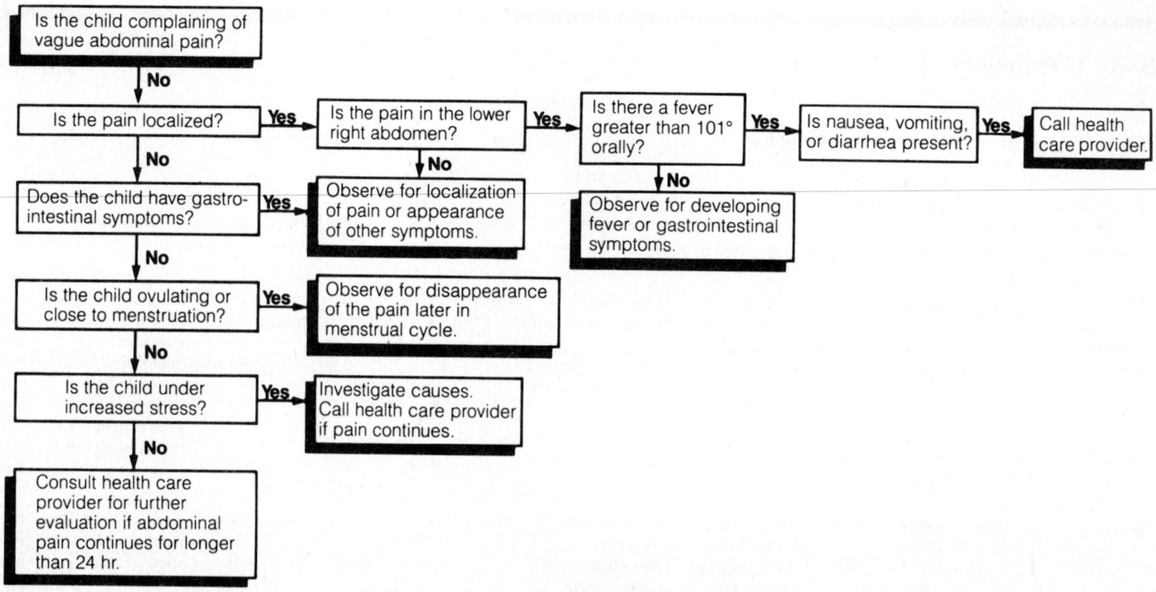

FIGURE 18-7

Parent decision: abdominal pain.

night and subsequent examination of the tape for the presence of eggs. Infestation usually occurs as a result of the ingestion of eggs by the anus-to-mouth route from contaminated articles. If one member of a family is infested, it is likely that other members are also infested. Therefore, all family members are treated simultaneously with an antiparasitic agent such as mebendazole or pyrantel pamoate.

In addition, it is necessary to launder thoroughly all underclothing, bed sheets, night clothes, and towels in hot water to destroy the eggs. The nurse explains to the parent the route of transmission of the parasite and explains the importance of cleaning the clothing and sheets and treating all family members simultaneously. The parent is encouraged to use good hygiene, including hand washing before eating and after using the toilet, and to see that the child also does so.

Ascariasis (roundworm) is an infestation of *Ascaris lumbricoides,* large, round worms, which can be asymptomatic or produce only vague abdominal discomfort. This organism is more common in warm climates, where the egg from an infected person might survive for weeks in the soil before being ingested. The life cycle of the ascaris worm begins with the ingestion of the eggs from contaminated soil. The eggs develop into larvae in the intestine and penetrate the intestinal wall, eventually migrating to the liver, heart, and lungs. If many larvae are present, the child might develop symptoms of atypical pneumonia at this stage. The child is usually asymptomatic, however, until the larvae ascend to the glottis and are swallowed. After being swallowed, they become established in the small intestine, where they can produce symptoms of vague abdominal discomfort. Nausea, vomiting, and weight loss can occur with heavy infestation.

The treatment for ascariasis is the same as for oxyuriasis. All family members need to be treated simultaneously, and the prevention of reinfestation requires good personal hygiene. As with oxyuriasis, the parent needs to launder towels, sheets, underclothing, and night clothing. The parent needs to scrub toilet facilities and should wash the hands thoroughly after using the toilet and before meals. Rarely do children with intestinal parasitic infections need to be hospitalized, but extremely heavy infestations might result in partial bowel obstruction, necessitating hospitalization.

Nonspecific, or functional, abdominal pain Children frequently will complain of vague abdominal pain for which no organic cause is apparent. These children need to receive a complete and thorough evaluation to rule out all possible pathologic processes. If no pathologic condition is found, the child's environment, family, and progress in school should be evaluated. Functional abdominal pain often has a psychologic origin; therefore, a psychologic consult needs to be considered (Fig. 18-7).

Constipation Constipation is a disorder of a society that is overly concerned with bodily functions. The emphasis on a regular, daily bowel movement has led parents to interfere with their child's individual bowel schedule in a misguided attempt to prevent constipation.

True constipation is rare in a child. The truly constipated child has infrequent bowel movements that are hard and dry and usually painful to pass. Constipation is treated with dietary measures, including whole-grain cereals, fresh fruits and vegetables, and large quantities of fluids. Dietary fiber is increased to levels that keep the stool soft (up to 10 grams a day). Laxatives and enemas usually are not necessary and might be harmful. In severe cases a natural laxative or glycerine suppository might be given under the physician's direction.

Occasionally, a child withholds bowel movements as a form of rebellion against the parent. This is especially likely if the parent has been overly concerned about early toilet training. The nurse can then assist the parent in developing a relaxed attitude toward toilet training and letting nature take its course. The parent can be sure the child receives an appropriate diet that is high in fresh fruits and vegetables, whole-grain cereals, and liquids and low in sugar and starches. Breast-fed infants often might go several days without a bowel movement. Parents can be assured that this is normal as long as the stool appears soft.

Foreign body ingestion Infants and young children are constantly putting inappropriate materials in their mouths, most common of which are small objects such as buttons, coins, and marbles. Invariably, if a child puts foreign objects in the mouth, some of them will be swallowed. Smooth objects that reach the stomach without lodging in the esophagus usually will pass through the gastrointestinal tract without difficulty, but sharp objects such as open safety pins, hairpins, and straight needles or pins might perforate the gastrointestinal tract and must be removed either by gastroscope, if the object is in the stomach, or by surgery if the object has passed out of the stomach. Occasionally, a smooth object might not pass the pylorus or will become lodged in the intestine, necessitating surgical intervention.

The physician initially will want to know what the child has swallowed and might want radiographs to locate the object in the gastrointestinal tract. If surgical intervention is not indicated, the child will be sent home to be cared for by the parent. No special care is indicated. The child continues a regular diet, and the parent needs to examine the stools daily to determine whether the object has passed. Parents can accomplish this by macerating the stool with a tongue depressor if the object is not readily visible. If the child is 6–8 years old or older, helping to search the stool for the foreign object might be a deterrent for placing foreign objects in the mouth in the future.

Recent incidences of children's swallowing small watch batteries or curtain weights have increased awareness of the hazards of leaving such objects within the child's reach. These objects, when broken down in the gastrointestinal tract, can have severe adverse effects. It is important for the nurse to review safety principles with any parent of a child who has swallowed a foreign object (see Chapter 12).

Communicable Diseases

The development and widespread use of vaccines has greatly reduced the incidence of many communicable diseases once common in childhood. Immunizations are available for such childhood diseases as rubeola (measles), rubella (German measles), mumps, pertussis (whooping cough), diphtheria, tetanus, polio, and *Hemophilus influenzae* (see Chapter 11). In most parts of the United States, immunizations are required for public school attendance. Parents need to be urged, however, not to wait until a child is of school age to begin the immunizations.

The nurse occasionally might be confronted with a child who has a preventable communicable disease. Such cases appear because most vaccines used for immunizations are about 90%–95% effective, leaving a margin of ineffectiveness. In addition, there is still a population of children who remain unimmunized, either because of religious beliefs, financial hardship, or lack of parental health education.

One of the goals in caring for a child with a communicable disease is to prevent the spread of the disease to others. Therefore, the child usually is cared for at home. Another goal of care is preventing complications from the disease. The nurse's responsibility is to assist the parent in planning and implementing nursing care to meet this goal.

Communicable diseases usually occur in phases. The first phase is called a *prodrome,* which is the period of time directly preceding manifestation of active symptoms of the disease. Prodromal symptoms often are nonspecific and can include fatigue, anorexia, nausea, vomiting, and occasionally a fever.

Following the prodromal symptoms, many communicable diseases produce a skin rash. (Table 18-5 lists the characteristics of the common skin rashes and should help to differentiate one from another.)

Rubeola (measles) Rubeola is an acute viral disease that begins as an upper respiratory disorder with fever, sore throat, and cough. The typical red, blotchy rash usually appears 4–5 days after the onset of symptoms. The diagnosis is based on the presence of *Koplik's spots* in the mouth. These spots have grayish centers with red, irregular outer rings. They are characteristic of measles.

Measles progresses in stages, from an incubation period

TABLE 18-5 Rashes Associated with Communicable Diseases in Children

Communicable disease	Prodromal symptoms	Appearance of rash	Progression of rash	Supporting clinical data
Measles (rubeola)	Fever of 101–104° F (higher before rash erupts)	Irregular, macular erythema that coalesces into larger red patches; lasts 4–7 days	Begins on face and behind ears; spreads to trunk and extremities	Cold symptoms; Koplik's spots on buccal mucosa; light sensitivity
Rubella (German measles)	Fever rarely over 101° F; possible malaise	Discrete macular rash	Appears first on face, then on trunk and extremities	Posterior cervical lymphadenopathy
Chickenpox (varicella)	Minimal fever; might be preceded by headache, nausea, and/or vomiting	Crops of lesions progressing from macular to papular to vesicular to pustular	Begins on trunk and clusters there with some lesions on extremities; few lesions on face and scalp	Fever might be high in adolescents
Roseola	High fever (to 104° F) for 1–5 days before the rash appears	Diffuse macular rash appears when fever subsides	Primarily confined to trunk	Possible mild pharyngitis
Erythemia infectiosum (fifth disease)	Usually none	Red coalescent macules that are raised and warm	Appears first on cheeks, then spreads to extremities	Usually none
Scarlet fever	Fever of 102° F or higher	Diffuse erythematous rash that fades with pressure except in the antecubital area	First noticed in areas of warmth and pressure; spreads to trunk and extremities	Sore throat with exudative pharyngitis and lymphadenopathy; strawberry-colored tongue; desquamation of palms and soles of feet as the disease resolves

that lasts for 7–14 days to a prodromal period that might last for 3–5 days before the rash appears. The child will be very ill during the prodromal stage, with a fever as high as 104°F, cough, coryza (runny nose), photophobia (sensitivity to light), and possibly conjunctivitis (inflammation of the conjunctiva). Koplik's spots appear on the buccal mucosa toward the end of the prodromal stage, a few days before the rash appears.

The eruptive stage begins with a dull reddish maculopapular rash on the face and neck, which descends progressively to the trunk, arms, and legs. The child is considered contagious and must be isolated from the onset of the prodromal period until 5 days after the eruptive stage begins. Convalescence usually requires 7–10 days, depending on the severity of the illness and the development of complications.

Most children with measles are cared for in the home. The parent needs to understand that the child's symptoms might worsen through the prodromal stage but that once the eruptive stage is complete, usually on the sixth or seventh day, marked improvement will occur. Treatment is symptomatic. Acetaminophen is given for fever; the child should rest in a dimly lit room to prevent eye discomfort, and increased fluid intake is necessary to maintain hydration. If the child has a cough, it is helpful to humidify the air with a cool-mist vaporizer. The child needs to be isolated at home until 5 days after the rash appears, and parents should try to protect unimmunized persons from exposure.

The complications of measles include otitis media, pneumonia, myocarditis, or encephalitis. The parent is told to contact the physician if earaches, productive cough, difficulty in breathing, chest pain, or a headache occurs. The

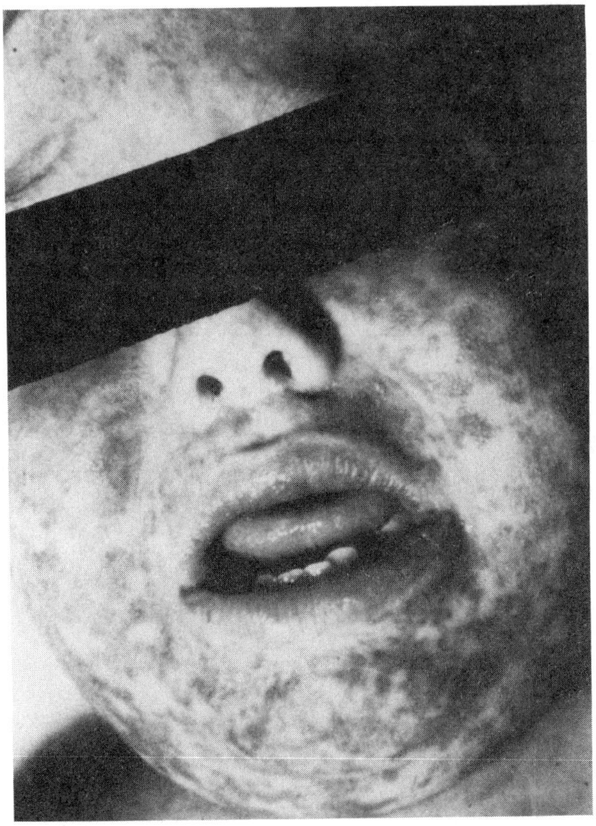

The erythematous, maculopapular rash in a child with measles. (From Pickering LK, DuPont HL: Infectious Diseases of Children and Adults. *Addison-Wesley, 1986.)*

child should not be brought to the clinic or hospital without first checking with the physician to avoid exposing susceptible persons.

Parotitis (mumps) Parotitis is a viral disease that is characterized by painful enlargement of the parotid gland. The child with mumps usually will have swelling of one or both sides of the face, fever, malaise, and pain behind the ear with chewing or swallowing. *Orchitis* (inflammation of the testicles) occurs in 20%–30% of infected postpubertal males (Thomson, 1982).

Treatment is symptomatic and involves analgesics to relieve pain, ice packs to reduce swelling, and rest. If orchitis is present, the physician might prescribe cortisone. Because of the weight of the swollen testicle or testicles, it might be necessary to suspend the scrotum in a sling or suspensory to prevent discomfort. Because mumps is a contagious disease, the child needs to be isolated at home until the parotid swelling is gone, usually 7–10 days.

Encephalitis is the most severe potential complication that can occur with mumps. The parent is advised to observe the child for any signs of mental confusion, sudden severe headache, projectile vomiting, stiffness in the neck or back, or a sudden dramatic increase in fever up to 105°F. The physician needs to be contacted or the child brought to the clinic or hospital if any of these symptoms develop.

Immunization is available now for mumps. Preventing mumps not only prevents encephalitis but also prevents male infertility caused by severe cases of orchitis.

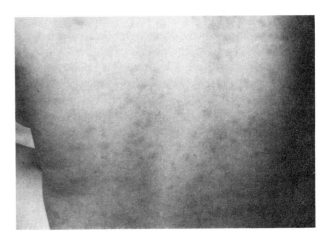

Pinkish, red, discrete, maculopapular rash of rubella. (From Pickering LK, DuPont HL: Infectious Diseases of Children and Adults. *Addison-Wesley, 1986.)*

Rubella (German measles) Rubella, a viral infection, usually is manifested as a discrete macular rash beginning on the face and spreading rapidly to the trunk, arms, and legs. Symptoms include lethargy, anorexia, a slight temperature elevation, and general lymphadenopathy, but these symptoms might be mild and might not be recognized.

Rubella is a mild disease that lasts only 3–5 days and requires no specific treatment. If contracted during pregnancy, the infection can, however, affect the fetus, causing severe congenital anomalies such as cardiac defects and cataracts. Thus, the major goal of treatment is to isolate the child at home to prevent the possible exposure of pregnant women. A rubella titer to determine susceptibility to the disease might be advisable for preadolescent girls who have not been immunized. Nurses might need to advise parents of preadolescent girls to have their children immunized to prevent congenital anomalies should they be exposed to rubella when they are pregnant.

Pertussis (whooping cough) Pertussis is a bacterial respiratory infection caused by the gram-negative bacillus *Bordetella pertussis*. Pertussis is transmitted from person to person by droplets or by contact with soiled articles from someone infected with the disease. The incubation period is from 7 to 10 days, and the child is considered communicable from 1 week before to 3 weeks after the onset of paroxysms of coughing.

Although a vaccine against pertussis has been available since 1950, approximately 2000 cases are still reported each year in the United States. Half of these cases occur in children under 1 year old, and parents who delay in beginning immunizations for their infants leave them unprotected against the disease. The pertussis vaccine is not, however, as effective as some of the other vaccines, and the immunity it provides declines rapidly. Few adults, even those immunized in childhood, are immune to pertussis (Baraff, 1981). Recent advances in the pertussis vaccine have reduced the side effects and ideally will reduce cases of pertussis in children whose parents have withheld the vaccine because of fear of side effects (see Chapter 11).

Pertussis begins with symptoms of an upper respiratory infection: fever, runny nose, sneezing, and cough. Within 2 weeks, however, the cough becomes paroxysmal (spasmodic) with a series of coughs followed by a deep inspiration that produces the characteristic whoop from which the disease gets its name. Periods of cyanosis might occur as a result of severe paroxysms of coughing in the very young child. Coughing spasms might cause vomiting in infants and very young children, resulting in problems with nutrition and hydration. These problems might contraindicate home care for the very young child with pertussis, but when an appropriate caregiver is present, older children can be cared for at home.

Home care goals include symptomatic care and the prevention of complications. Although antibiotics probably do not affect the course of the disease, an oral antibiotic, usually erythromycin, might be prescribed for 10 days to prevent pulmonary complications and shorten the period of communicability. Because many children vomit with the paroxysmal coughing, the parent needs to offer frequent small feedings and observe the child for signs of dehydration. Aspiration of the emesis also is a concern. The most common serious complication is pneumonia. The parent is advised to maintain a quiet environment for the child because excitement can precipitate a coughing spasm.

The parent needs to be advised to observe the child for symptoms of respiratory distress between the paroxysms of coughing. These symptoms include rapid respirations and cyanosis (blue skin color). If these occur or if the child develops a fever, further medical attention is necessary.

Varicella (chickenpox) Chickenpox is an acute communicable disease caused by the herpes zoster virus. The incubation period is from 11 to 21 days but can be as long as 25 days. The child is considered to be communicable from up to 5 days before the skin eruptions occur until the lesions are dry.

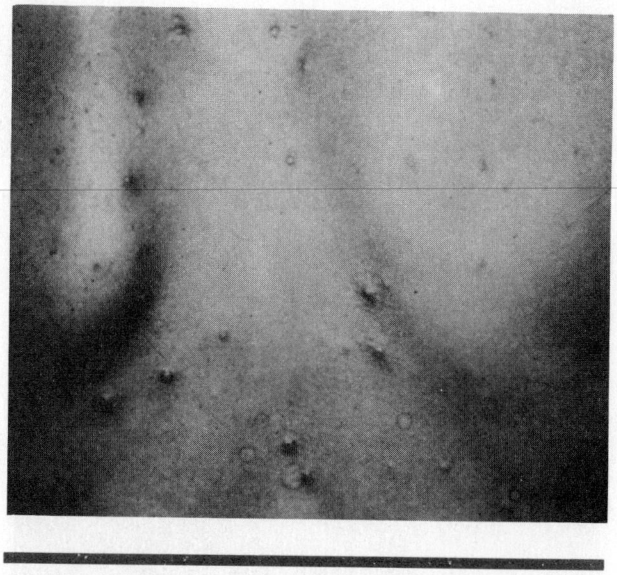

An adolescent with varicella. (From Pickering LK, DuPont HL: Infectious Diseases of Children and Adults. *Addison-Wesley, 1986.)*

A slight prodrome of fever might precede the appearance of skin lesions, which tend to erupt in crops. The lesions begin on the neck or the trunk and spread to the face, scalp, mucous membranes, and extremities. The lesions first appear as small, flat, red blotches that progress to raised vesicles. Crust formation occurs over a period of 2–4 days. Pruritus (itching) might be severe, and the prevention of secondary infection from scratching is a major goal of care. (See Chapter 24 for measures to treat pruritus.)

Isolation at home is necessary to prevent nonintentional exposure of susceptible adults and persons with altered immunologic status. Prevention might be undesirable in children, however, because chickenpox often is more severe in adulthood. Children receiving corticosteroid therapy need to be referred to a physician immediately if exposed to chickenpox.

The goal of treatment is to prevent complications and relieve symptoms. The parent is advised to cut the child's fingernails short and have the child wear gloves if necessary to prevent scratching and secondary infection. Antihistamines or antipruritic medications might be prescribed to be given orally to relieve pruritus. Also helpful are calamine lotion or a mild anesthetic ointment applied to the lesions. Tepid sponge baths seem to relieve the pruritus, and an antiseptic soap reduces the risk of secondary infection.

Complications from chickenpox include encephalitis and abscess of secondarily infected vesicles, but these complications are unusual, and the child usually can return to school in 1 week if there are no new lesions. Reye's syndrome, a sometimes fatal neurologic disease (see Chapter 31), has been linked to the occurrence of varicella, and the nurse needs to advise parents to contact a physician immediately if signs of fever, severe vomiting, abrupt behavior change, and changes in the level of consciousness appear.

Roseola Roseola (exanthem subitum) is an acute febrile illness in infants and young children that is believed to be caused by a virus. The mode of transmission and incubation period are not known. It is characterized by a high fever of 101–104°F that lasts from 1 to 5 days and is followed by a faint rash as the fever subsides. The rash first appears on the chest and trunk and spreads to the face and extremities. It is a discrete maculopapular rash that might last from 2 to 48 hours. Roseola is a mild disease lasting only a few days and is usually treated at home. The principal complication is febrile seizures from the extremely high temperatures. Treatment usually is symptomatic, with rest and acetaminophen for fever. Tepid sponge baths can be given if the fever is not controlled by acetaminophen.

Erythema infectiosum (fifth disease) Erythema infectiosum is a mild, contagious viral disease that is characterized by a rash similar to the rash seen with measles. The incubation period is from 7 to 14 days. The child is afebrile and might be asymptomatic. A rash appears first on the cheeks as red coalescent macules that are raised and warm. It spreads to the extensor surfaces of the extremities on the second day and over the next several days to the flexor surfaces and trunk. Often the rash is described as a "lace curtain rash" because the pattern resembles the pattern of a lace curtain. The palms and soles usually are not involved. The rash might last 3–7 days and can recur after 7–10 days. It tends to occur in epidemics and requires no special treatment, but a careful differential diagnosis is indicated to rule out other causes of childhood rashes.

Scarlet fever Scarlet fever is caused by a systemic reaction to a toxin from the *Streptococcus* bacterium. Scarlet fever is not communicable, but the streptococcal pharyngitis that causes it is communicable. Scarlet fever occurs most frequently in children under 10 years old and is characterized by a rash that appears 12–18 hours after the onset of fever.

The rash appears first in areas of pressure and warmth, such as the neck, axilla, and groin, and spreads to involve the trunk and limbs. It is a diffuse red rash that fades with pressure, although transverse areas of rash at the antecubital (forearm) area do not fade with pressure (a manifestation called *Pastia's sign*). The tongue might take on a beefy, red, raspberry appearance. Desquamation (peeling) of the skin might occur in the second week. Peeling of the fingertips, palms of the hands, and soles of the feet is significant diagnostically. The treatment for scarlet fever is the same as for streptococcal pharyngitis, and the same complications might occur.

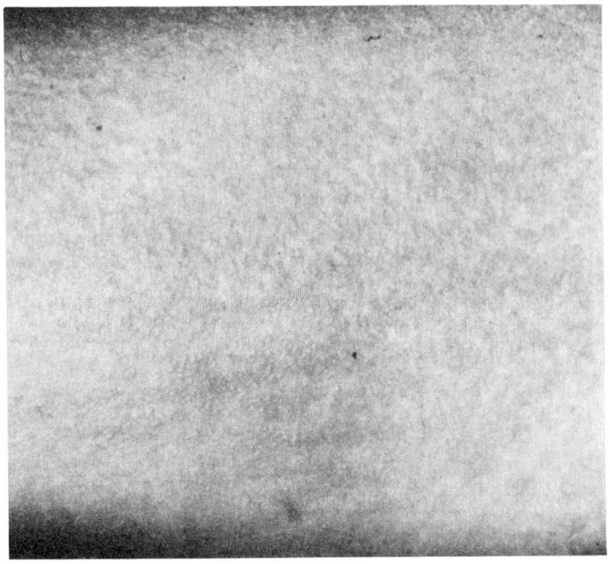

The characteristic rash seen in children with scarlet fever is an erythematous rash with tiny papules that feel like sandpaper. (From Pickering LK, DuPont HL: Infectious Diseases of Children and Adults. *Addison-Wesley, 1986.)*

Vector-borne Diseases

Communicable diseases that are transmitted from humans to humans or from animals to humans by an arthropod intermediary such as mosquitoes, fleas, or ticks are called vector-borne diseases. Many of the vector-borne diseases, such as yellow fever and malaria, are endemic to tropical countries and are seldom found in temperate climates.

Prevention of vector-borne diseases includes avoiding exposure to potentially hazardous arthropods and destroying any breeding grounds near inhabited areas.

Rocky Mountain spotted fever Rocky Mountain spotted fever (RMSF) is caused by a rickettsial organism that is transmitted to humans by infected ticks. It occurs most frequently in the spring and summer months in the southern United States, along the Atlantic coast, and in the Rocky Mountain region.

RMSF is characterized by a prodrome of nonspecific symptoms, including fever, restlessness, headache, and anorexia. One to 5 days later, a pale, discrete maculopapular rash appears, beginning first on the wrists, ankles, soles of the feet, or palms. Later symptoms include edema and central nervous system manifestations.

Treatment includes antibiotic therapy, which is most effective if begun early in the course of the disease. Tetracycline or chloramphenicol are the drugs of choice (Pickering and DuPont, 1986). If treatment is delayed or if nausea and vomiting are present, intravenous antibiotic therapy will be necessary, which requires hospitalization of the ill child.

If the disease is mild and therapy is initiated early, the child can be cared for in the home. The nurse needs to explain to the parents the importance of taking the prescribed medication and contacting the physician or bringing the child to the clinic should nausea or vomiting develop. Complications include pneumonia, otitis media, dehydration, myocarditis, and neurologic disorders. Children with complications need to receive immediate medical attention, possibly including hospitalization.

Because the infected tick must be imbedded in the child for 4–6 hours before the organism causing RMSF is transmitted (Thompson, 1983), frequent tick checks are an effective preventive measure. Ticks inhabit trees and long grass. Therefore, the nurse advises parents to check their children for ticks at least twice a day if they play in wooded or grassy areas. Ticks are found most frequently on the child's head or at the beltline. Removal of an imbedded tick can be a difficult task because complete removal, including the head, is essential. The preferred method of removal is to extract the tick by grasping the tick as close to the skin as possible with tweezers and pulling straight out with a steady pull. If fingers are used to remove the tick they need to be protected with gloves, paper towel, or tissue because it is possible for rickettsiae to enter the body even when there is no opening in the skin.

Once the tick is removed, the child's wound and the parent's hands should be washed thoroughly, preferably with an antiseptic solution. Tick removal can be an unpleasant task for the parent and child. If the parent is unable to remove the tick, professional assistance needs to be sought.

Other vector-borne diseases Diseases other than RMSF are associated with ticks. These include *tick toxicosis,* an ascending paralysis that resolves after tick extraction; *Lyme disease,* a syndrome that resembles arthritis and is caused by *Ixodes dammini* carried by the deer tick; and *babesiosis,* a disease also transmitted by the smaller deer tick (Thompson, 1983).

Other organisms also cause vector-borne diseases, although many of these are rare. The severity of symptoms associated with *equine encephalitis* (transmitted by mosquitoes from infected horses) and *plague* (caused by *Yersinia pestis* infection and sometimes transmitted by lice) necessitates hospitalization.

Disorders of the Skin

Skin disorders usually are not acute illnesses. They are almost always cared for in the home setting. If not appropriately treated, however, many skin disorders can lead to complications. It is therefore important for the parent or caregiver to have complete, accurate information regarding the appropriate prescribed treatment.

Congenital birthmarks The most frequently seen congenital birthmarks are *nevi,* or abnormally pigmented marks on the skin. There are several types of nevi that differ according to their color and pattern.

Mongolian spots, which appear mainly on the coccyx, are seen often in darker-skinned infants. The spots are dark blue and discolored and often disappear spontaneously. *Vascular nevi,* or *hemangiomas,* include port-wine stain, strawberry nevus, and salmon patch. The *port-wine stain* (nevus flammeus) appears as a flat, red patch that increases in size as the child grows. As the child matures, the port-wine stain might assume a cobblestone appearance. Treatment is not indicated, and cosmetics are useful in covering the lesion.

The *strawberry nevus* resembles a strawberry and generally appears on the head and neck of the infant. It will disappear by the time the child reaches school age with no treatment. *Salmon patch* is characterized by a macular, pink patch. It appears on the nape of the neck and eyelids of the infant and disappears by the end of the first year without treatment.

Tinea capitis, corporis, pedis, and cruris *Tinea* infections are caused by fungi. *Tinea capitis* (ringworm of the scalp) is seen frequently in school-aged children. It is characterized by patches of alopecia (hair loss) that begin as small papules at the base of the hair follicle. The hair loses its pigmentation, and the scalp becomes scaly and red.

Ringworm of the body and the feet is not as common in children as ringworm of the scalp. In *tinea corporis* (ringworm of the body), multiple lesions are evident, which are ringed with scaly edges. The lesions spread outward and are usually itchy. Lesions on the feet (*tinea pedis*) can be located between the toes, on the instep, and on the soles. This condition often is referred to as "athlete's foot." *Tinea cruris* (ringworm of the groin) generally is an eruption of papules and scales. Tight-fitting clothes and obesity are possible contributing factors.

The nurse can instruct the parent to scrub the lesions with tincture of green soap to remove scales and crust. A topical fungicidal agent, which is ordered by the physician, is then applied, usually twice a day for about 2 weeks. Parents and children are alerted to continue the treatment

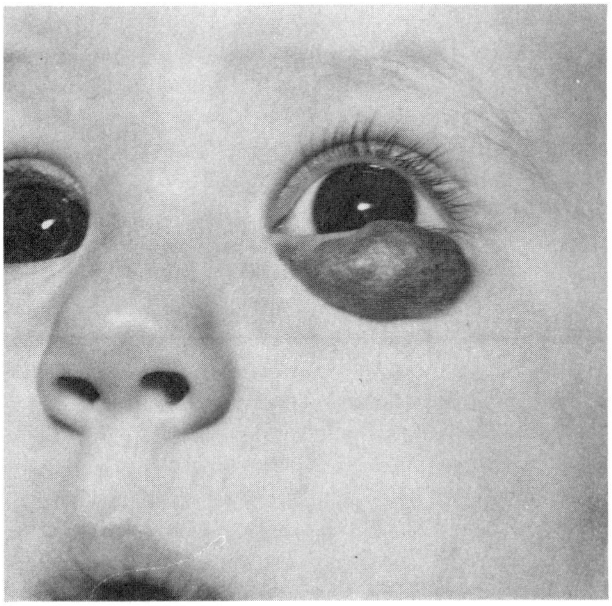

Nevus flammeus. (From Binnick SA: Skin Diseases: Diagnosis and Management in Clinical Practice. *Addison-Wesley, 1982.)*

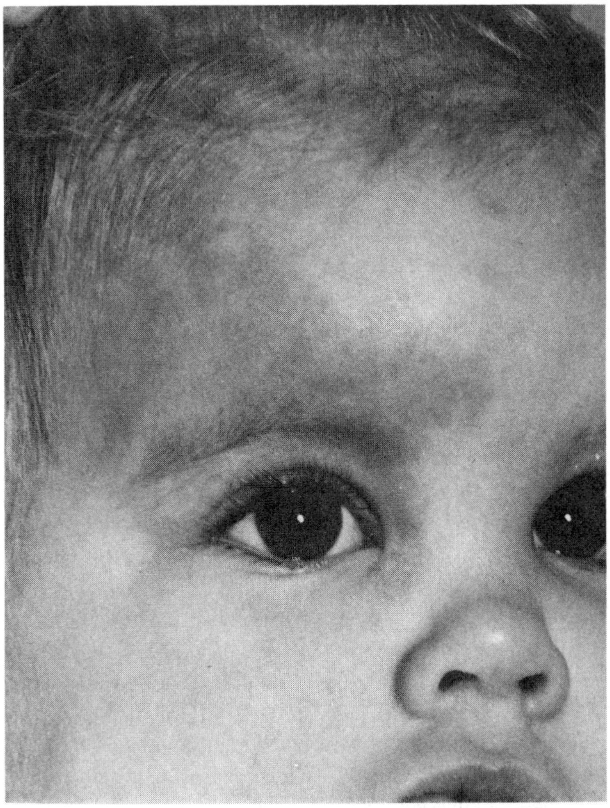

Capillary hemangioma. (From Binnick SA: Skin Diseases: Diagnosis and Management in Clinical Practice. *Addison-Wesley, 1982.)*

for at least 2 weeks after healing. An oral fungicide preparation, such as griseofulvin, 5–11 mg/kg/day for 2 weeks to 1 month, might be given to eliminate the fungus and promote the growth of healthy tissue.

The oral fungicide will likely be given if the condition responds poorly to topical therapy. The nurse informs the child and parent that the drug should be taken with meals containing milk or other fats or should be taken shortly after meals because fat enhances its absorption. In addition, the child needs to avoid prolonged exposure to sunlight and needs to be monitored for hematologic alterations.

Fungal infections are enhanced by moisture and heat. Therefore, infected areas must be kept dry. A talcum powder applied twice daily helps to keep the area dry. If the lesions are inflamed, with blisters and exudates, warm water compresses might help. These are applied about four times a day until the lesions are dry.

Viral warts *Plantar warts* appears like small, shiny grains of sand embedded under the skin of the foot. The condition is caused by viral penetration. It is believed that a break in the skin allows the virus to enter. The nurse encourages children to wear shoes or other coverings for their feet and not to go barefoot. Plantar warts may be painful. The use of adhesive foam for padding in the shoes might help to alleviate the pain.

Common warts most frequently are seen on the hands, fingers, and knees. They may be single or multiple. The biggest danger of these warts is that children pick them off. The nurse informs children that picking warts off is not good because of the risk of viral infiltration into other tissue. Often, a wart will disappear spontaneously if left alone. If infiltration occurs, medical treatment is necessary.

There is no known treatment for common warts. Removing warts often is accomplished through surgery, topical administration of liquid nitrogen or a blistering agent such as cantharidin, or chemical destruction. Chemical destruction is used most often in children with multiple warts because it is painless. Home treatment might include the use of Duofilm, a chemical that can be placed on the wart at bedtime with a toothpick or an applicator. Salicyclic acid (40%) ointment is another chemical means of removing a wart at home. Formalin, 10%, increases the potency of the salicylic acid ointment. Extreme caution must be used to avoid getting these preparations on healthy skin.

Juvenile warts are flat, slightly raised, smooth, brown lesions that appear mainly on the face and hands. They tend to be asymptomatic. *Genital warts* are classified as a sexually transmitted infection. They might coalesce into a cauliflowerlike growth on the genitals. Treatment of all of the types of warts varies from nothing to curettage to keratolytics to surgical removal. The treatment of choice depends on the dermatologist. Mechanical removal of dead wart tissue requires a pumice stone, the tip of a metal nail file, and curved scissors. Following a bath to soften the tissue, the pumice stone is used, after which the tip of the nail file is used to loosen the skin and dislodge the dead wart tissue. The scissors are then used to cut away the dead wart tissue.

Warts often disappear spontaneously. Occasionally, this phenomenon can be related to an emotional event in the child's life. This might account for the effectiveness of superstitious remedies for curing warts, such as scaring the affected child.

Children can be very embarrassed by warts, particularly those that occur on the hands. Many children's games involve holding hands, which leaves an affected child open to teasing. The nurse can assure the child that the warts will disappear eventually. If the child is particularly upset by the warts, removal might be indicated.

Pediculosis Pediculosis (head lice) causes intense pruritus, which is usually the first symptom. The nape of the neck is most frequently the site of the initial infestation of this easily transmitted infection. The lice are very difficult to find, but the eggs, or nits, are readily identifiable. They are small, translucent, white ovals attached to the base of the hair shaft approximately ¼ to ½ in. from the scalp. They are literally glued to the hair shaft by the female louse and are difficult to remove. Occasionally, secondary infection or excoriation might be caused by scratching.

Lice epidemics are becoming more prevalent among school-age children (McLaury, 1983), although they are not exclusive to this population. They are highly communicable from child to child, usually through sharing hats, combs, and articles of clothing that contact the head. If pediculosis is discovered by the school nurse, affected children will be sent home for treatment and not readmitted until they are appropriately cared for. The nurse's sensitivity to this issue is important because lice infestation historically has been associated with unsanitary conditions.

Nurses need to instruct parents carefully regarding the appropriate management of pediculosis. If a secondary infection is present, it should be cleared prior to initiating treatment for the infestation. A variety of pediculocide shampoos are presently available: gamma benzene hexachloride (*Lindane*), malathion, and pyrethrin are most commonly used. Although Lindane is more convenient to use because of its shorter time on the scalp, central nervous system and hematologic complications recently have been found to be associated with its use (Clore, 1983; McLaury, 1983). Lindane should not be applied to infants or pregnant women.

Treatment involves applying the shampoo according to directions, being careful not to get the shampoo in the child's eyes. Should the shampoo accidentally contact the eyes, they should be rinsed with large amounts of water. After rinsing the shampoo from the hair, it is necessary to comb out the nits with a fine-tooth comb or individually by hand. This procedure is essential because the shampoo is not guaranteed to kill all the eggs. Parents need to repeat the treatment in 7–10 days to kill any lice that might have hatched since the initial treatment.

Control of lice in the home includes laundering all contaminated articles with hot, soapy water or putting them through a 20-minute hot cycle in a clothes dryer (McLaury, 1983). Parents need to remember to include outdoor clothing and dress-up clothes. Combs and brushes can be soaked in the pediculocide. Thorough vacuuming eliminates any lice harbored in furniture or carpets. Clothing or blankets that cannot be laundered or dry cleaned can be stored in a sealed plastic bag for 10 days (McLaury, 1983).

Parents need to check their children's heads frequently by parting the hair with two Popsicle sticks or tongue depressors. Preventive measures include not sharing such objects as hats, combs, brushes, or scarves. The nurse explains this to both the parent and the child.

Scabies The itch mite, *Sarcoptes scabiei,* is the causative agent of *scabies*. The mite burrows under the skin, causing a fine papular rash and intense pruritus that is sometimes worse at night. The mite leaves a telltale burrow under the skin, which is occasionally visible between the fingers and in the axillary and cubital regions. Lesions are rarely found on the face.

Burrows might be overlooked in young children because they can be distributed on the head, palms, and soles of the feet. Finger webs, nipples of females, and the penis and scrotum of males seem to be target areas. Most parts of the body, however, can be affected. Scabies appear as gray-white, very thin lines. The mite may appear as a tiny white dot at the end of the thin line. Papules, pustules, wheals, and bullae may also be present. These lesions do not contain mites. A burrow that has not been excoriated is likely to contain the mite.

Feces from the mites are thought to be the cause of the itching. Itching, which is worse at night, is the major complaint of a child infected with the scabies mite. Clean, hygienic persons, contrary to many people's thinking, can also have scabies. They probably will not have as many burrows and the burrows might not be as easily seen. Poor hygiene and close living quarters increase the susceptibility to the infection.

Treatment is with gamma benzene hexachloride lotion, which is applied at bedtime, left on for 12–24 hours, and then washed off. The lotion is applied over the entire body from the neck to the feet. Retreatment might be necessary after several days. Again, caution is exercised to prevent complications from Lindane. The bed linens and clothing should be washed in hot water at the time of treatment, and all affected family members should be treated simultaneously.

Secondary infections from scratching are common in children with scabies. If a secondary infection is present, it must be treated and cleaned prior to using the gamma benzene hexachloride lotion because open lesions will cause potentially harmful levels of the medication to be absorbed. If a secondary infection is not present, measures such as cutting the fingernails and scrubbing with soap and water should be used to prevent this complication from developing.

Emotional Disturbances

Many emotionally disturbed children are cared for in the home. Most emotional disorders are chronic, but acute exacerbations might occur. A careful assessment of the home is as necessary before selecting a treatment setting for the emotionally disturbed child as it is for the child with a physical disorder. The nurse participates in decision making and treatment planning with the cooperation and participation of those who will be responsible for the child's care. (The implications of chronic illness are covered in Chapter 14. The implications of dysfunctional behavior are discussed in Chapter 16.)

Minor Accidents and Emergencies

Parents intervene in most minor accidents and emergencies in the home setting, and the child might never see a health professional. If the parent is in doubt about whether to seek professional care, however, the nurse might be consulted. The nurse therefore needs to know the accidents and emergencies that can safely be cared for at home, acceptable home treatments, and signs that indicate referral for further medical care.

Epistaxis Epistaxis is a spontaneous hemorrhage from the nose as a result of a ruptured blood vessel in the nares. It might be caused by a blow to the head or nose, by picking the nose, or by a foreign body or object inserted into the nares. It occurs most frequently in the winter months when the air is dry, causing the nasal mucosa to become fragile and dry.

Treatment of epistaxis consists of applying pressure to the site of the bleeding by pressing the nares together. The child is instructed to breathe through the mouth. Sitting upright and leaning slightly forward will prevent blood from going down the throat. Compression of the nostrils needs to be continued for 15 minutes, and the child should rest quietly for 15–20 minutes after the bleeding stops. If the bleeding cannot be controlled by compressing the nares together for 15 minutes, further medical consultation is indicated.

Children who have recurrent episodes of epistaxis need to be instructed in preventive measures. A cool-mist humidifier is used in the child's room during the winter months to humidify the air. The child is discouraged from picking at the nares, and if the nares are dry, a water-soluble lubricant (such as K-Y jelly) can be rubbed on the septum two or three times a day. If episodes of epistaxis are frequent or difficult to control, an evaluation to rule out anemia or hemorrhagic disorders might be indicated.

Contusions A contusion is an injury caused by a blunt blow to the body in which the skin is not broken. A contusion causes the rupture of small blood vessels beneath the skin, which results in swelling and discoloration (bruise) at the site of the injury. The treatment for contusions is to apply ice for 48 hours to reduce swelling. Applications of heat are indicated in 48 hours if significant swelling is still present.

Parents need to observe children with contusions of the head for cerebral concussion for 12–24 hours following the injury. A *concussion,* which involves alterations in cerebral function, is suspected if there is any loss of consciousness, headache, apathy, irritability, or vomiting. Tense or bulging fontanelles in an infant might indicate increased intracranial pressure. If concussion is suspected, the parent needs to seek immediate medical attention for the child.

Lacerations A laceration is a regular or irregular cut or tear of the skin. Children who are active by nature seem to be forever falling, jumping, and bumping into objects that cause lacerations. Minor lacerations usually can be treated at home. Major lacerations—those that are deep or involve tendons or nerves—require medical attention. A minor laceration does not penetrate the subcutaneous tissue (Fig. 18-8).

Home treatment of lacerations includes cleansing the wound with soap and water, making certain that all dirt and foreign objects are removed, and bandaging the wound with a sterile dressing. The bandage needs to be kept clean and dry and should be changed if it becomes wet because bacteria multiply rapidly in warmth and dampness. Decisions about suturing lacerations need to be made within 6 hours of the injury because a longer time interval will jeopardize the success of the procedure.

The parent needs to be taught to watch for signs of infection. Any redness, heat, or purulent drainage in the wound indicates the need for medical consultation. Red streaking from the site is a dangerous sign. The nurse as-

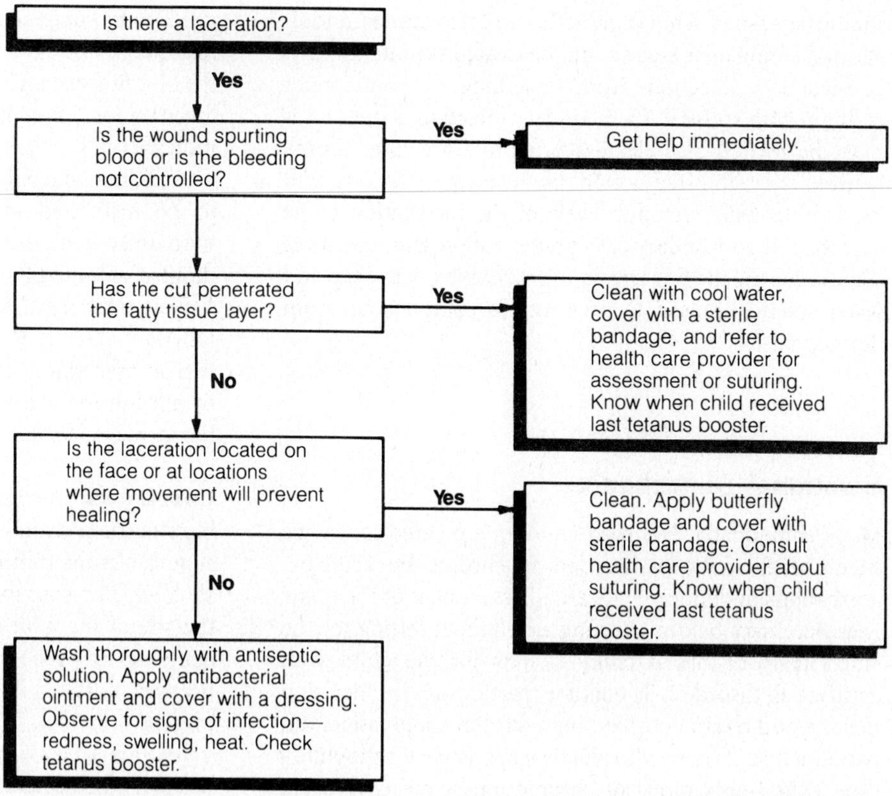

FIGURE 18-8
Parent decision: lacerations.

sesses the immunization status of any child with a laceration, and tetanus prophylaxis is administered if indicated (see Chapter 24).

Sunburn Sunburn is a common complaint in young children, particularly at the beginning of the summer months when the skin is most sensitive because of lack of exposure to the sun. Mild sunburn can cause discomfort, whereas severe sunburn with blistering can result in additional complications. Treatment for sunburn involves the application of cool compresses and/or an anesthetic lotion or spray such as Solarcaine or Noxema. The child needs to be protected from further exposure to the sun. If blistering occurs over an extended area, the parent should be encouraged to call the physician.

Sunburn can be prevented by gradual exposure, avoidance of the midday sun, protection of sensitive areas by covering with hat and clothing, and the use of sunscreens. The parent needs to remember to reapply the sunscreen after the child has been swimming. Some children exhibit allergic reactions to certain ingredients in sunscreens. Should this occur, the parent might try a sunscreen with alternate ingredients.

Essential Concepts

- Many childhood illnesses can be treated successfully in the home.
- Given appropriate home conditions, home care of the child can pose fewer risks than hospitalization.
- Nurses in ambulatory care settings, rural areas, communities, and hospitals are uniquely suited to assess for and recommend home care.
- The nurse's role in home care includes the five steps of the nursing process.
- Assessment provides data that enable the nurse and

parent to decide whether home care is feasible, as well as data that provide a basis for the home care plan.

- Nursing diagnosis focuses on the potential risk for complications and the nursing care problems identified by the assessment.
- The written care plan provides a comprehensive plan of action to care for the ill child at home and involves providing reasonable assurances that the child's needs will be met.
- Although it is the parent's or caregiver's responsibility to implement the care plan in the home, the nurse is responsible for overseeing its proper implementation.
- Changing circumstances in the child or in the home require constant evaluation and restructuring of the home care plan.
- The nurse is an important resource for parents in deciding whether the child needs referral for medical evaluation.

References

Baraff: Pertussis (whooping cough). In: *Current Therapy*. Conn H (editor). Saunders, 1981.

Clore E: Lice: Ancient pest with new resistance. *Pediatr Nurs* (Sept/Oct) 1983; 9:347–350.

Feetham S: Hospitals and home care: Inseparable in the '80s. *Pediatr Nurs* (Sept/Oct) 1986; 12(5):383–386.

McLaury P: Head lice: Pediatric social disease. *Am J Nurs* (Sept) 1983; 83:1300–1303.

Pickering LK, DuPont HL (editors): *Infectious Diseases of Children and Adults*. Addison-Wesley, 1986.

Thompson S: Summertime ticks. *Am J Nurs* (May) 1983; 83: 768–769.

Thomson W: No need to report. *Nurs Mirror* (Sept) 1982; 155:49.

Additional Readings

Baylor K: Bacterial diseases of the skin. In: *Current Therapy*. Conn H (editor). Saunders, 1981.

Clinical News: Will chicken pox bite the dust? *Am J Nurs* (Aug) 1984; 84(8):978.

Edwardson S: The choice between hospital and home care for terminally ill children. *Nurs Res* (Jan/Feb) 1983; 32(1): 29–34.

Gardner P, Charles D: Infections acquired in a pediatric hospital. *J Pediatr* 1982; 81:1205–1210.

Gutierrez K: Home is where the care is. *Nurs '85* (Nov) 1985; 15(11):49.

Harkess C: Clearing the occluded auditory canal. *Pediatr Nurs* (Jan/Feb) 1982; 8:23–25.

Henderson G, Primeaux M: *Transcultural Health Care*. Addison-Wesley, 1981.

John RL: Giardiasis and amebiasis. *RN* (April) 1981; 44(4):52–57.

Mitchell PL (editor): Whooping cough epidemic in Oklahoma. *Child Health Alert* (June) 1986:2–3.

Morris E: Home care today. *Am J Nurs* (March) 1984; 84:340–345.

Selekman J: Immunization: What's it all about? *Am J Nurs* (Aug) 1980; 80(8):1440–1445.

Todd B: Twenty-seven reasons why people don't take their meds. *RN* (March) 1981; 44(3):54–57.

Chapter 19

The Child's Adjustment to Hospitalization

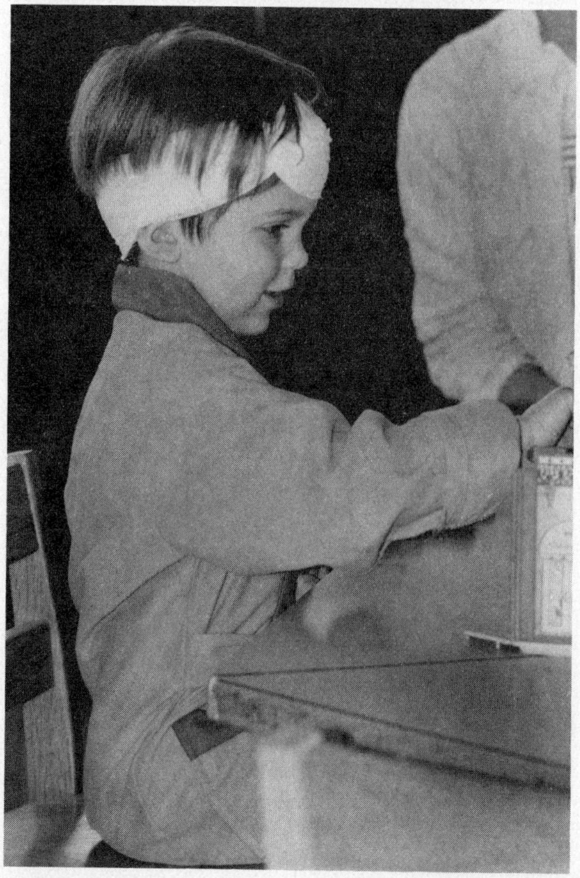

Chapter Contents

Objectives

- Define the components of both stress and crisis for families with hospitalized children.
- Relate coping behaviors to children's developmental stages.
- List the assessment criteria for identifying levels of stress and anxiety.
- Explain the developmental changes in the child's understanding of illness and its causes.
- Describe the common stressors related to hospitalization.
- Explain the developmental changes and age-appropriate needs for coping with the separation imposed by hospitalization.
- Explain the developmental changes in the child's experience of body image, function, and control.
- List the factors that affect the parent's perception of the child's illness.
- Describe the possible effects of the child's hospitalization on the family's day-to-day functioning.
- Compare the assessment criteria and possible interventions associated with the variety of family configurations.
- Describe the common needs of both the parents and the siblings of hospitalized children.
- Describe the nurse's role in facilitating the child's coping with and learning about the hospital environment.
- Explain the purpose of play for the hospitalized child.
- Distinguish between play therapy and therapeutic play.
- Relate the purpose of play in the hospital to each developmental stage.
- Define the role of the nurse and the play therapist in the hospital setting.
- Explain the ways in which the child uses play to cope with the experience of hospitalization.
- Describe ways to provide play for the immobilized or isolated child.
- List guidelines for parent and child teaching.
- Describe specific methods for preparing the child and family for hospitalization.
- List principles for preparing children for procedures and treatments.
- Explain the components of discharge preparation and specific considerations for teaching families and children.

Hospitalization during childhood is an experience with lasting effects. Approximately 4.5 million children are hospitalized annually. Of these children, 90% are treated in general hospitals, which might or might not have pediatric units and specially trained staff (Azarnoff and Hargrove, 1981). Nurses therefore need to examine the events of hospitalization to predict its long-term effects for the child. Will the hospital stay result in physical and emotional health, or will the ultimate outcome be emotionally traumatic for the child and family?

The hospitalization of a child is a major stressor for both child and family and, as such, hospitalization can be a major cause of stress. Stress is a physiologic and psychologic condition that develops in response to a stressor (see Chapter 11). Stress causes discomfort for the child and family and triggers the use of stress-reducing measures, or coping strategies (see Chapter 16). If the usual coping behaviors are strained beyond the child's or family's ability to manage, a crisis might develop.

The stress of hospitalization does not necessarily lead to a crisis for the child or family. If the stress of the hospitalization becomes overwhelming, however, a crisis is inevitable. When a child is hospitalized, the amount and effects of stress depend primarily on the child's and family's perceptions of the seriousness of the illness and its treatment. For example, to children—and often to their families—any illness or condition is considered major and any surgery threatening. To a young child, hospitalization seems endless, regardless of its length.

The current trend to avoid hospitalization for children,

and thus avoid additional stress, is based on a sound principle. Research findings have shown conclusively that children who are ill, frightened, fatigued, or in pain need the support of their primary caregiver (usually the mother and/or father) to make pyschologically healthy adjustments to these stressors (Prugh, 1953; Robertson, 1970; Triplett and Arneson, 1970; Kunzman, 1971; Johnson, Kirchhoff, & Endress, 1971; Meng, 1980; Azarnoff and Woody, 1981; Tesler and Savedra, 1981). The younger the child, the truer this principle.

In most instances the child is brought to a physician's office or to the hospital emergency room when the child's family becomes convinced that an illness will not respond to home cures or culturally derived healing methods. If they are admitted to acute-care facilities, many of these children enter general hospitals that might not have pediatric units and whose staffs are not specially trained in either the physical or the emotional care of children.

Because the staff in a general hospital might not be attuned to the needs of children, the hospitalization might appear more threatening than it would be in a more sympathetic environment, such as a children's hospital. Furthermore, hospital regulations sometimes require the child to be separated from the primary caregiver, increasing the risk of additional stress and crisis.

Because children and families often perceive hospitalization as threatening, regardless of the setting, nurses planning holistic care need to recognize and accept this perceived threat. What might seem insignificant to health care personnel might be a major obstacle to full cooperation with treatment plans and hospital routines.

When forming and implementing nursing care plans, nurses need to remember to listen and to identify the perceptions and feelings of others. The nurse who has assessed the attitudes of both the child and the family and who spends time listening to concerns can communicate respect. In this way, nurses can better bridge the gap between feelings and routine nursing care. Teaching children and families to cope with the stress of hospitalization and their feelings of helplessness can assist the child and family to minimize stress, avoid crisis, and regain control of their lives.

Assessing Stress Levels in the Ill Child

- Does the child have frequent visits from supportive, close relatives?
- Does the child express emotions appropriately? (For example, does the 3-year-old protest the mother's leaving or appear apathetic?)
- How frightened does the child become during required procedures or separation?
- Does the child attempt to socialize with children of the same age in the hospital unit?
- Does the child attempt to cooperate with health care staff?
- Is the child's sleep seriously disrupted?
- Does the child seem unusually irritable, anxious, or depressed?
- Does the child continually test the limits imposed by the parent or staff?

Assessing family relationships with the ill child

To whom does the child turn for comfort when upset? ____________

Who stays with the child in the hospital? ____________

How does the child interact with this person? ________

Who is significant to the child? ____________

Responses of Children and Families to Hospitalization

Crises, such as hospitalization, present families with circumstances that can draw family members together or tear them apart. Much depends on the nature of family relationships before the crisis occurs and the quality of support available to the family during the crisis. For example, the single parent with an ill child and no immediate family close by might be more vulnerable to the crisis of hospitalization than the large family with an ill child and an extended family close by to help with babysitting and cooking at home.

In assessing the impact of stress and crisis on the family and child, the nurse determines whether the child's and family's usual coping behaviors and adequacy of supports are sufficient to meet the stress of illness and hospitalization. If a number of behaviors indicate stress, the nurse notes that the child's or family's ability to cope might be jeopardized and that a crisis might be developing. The family's increased vulnerability to stress and crisis signals the need for support from the health care team.

Stress and Coping in Children

Coping behaviors are psychologic mechanisms the child uses to reduce stress (see Chapter 16). Coping behaviors are only temporary measures of dealing with the stress of hospitalization. They give children time to use problem-solving techniques to deal effectively with the threat they perceive.

General coping behaviors that nurses might expect to see include:

1. Direct expression of emotion such as crying, anger, and anxiety
2. Behavioral expressions such as hitting, stamping the feet, withdrawing, or engaging in delinquent behavior
3. Somatic complaints such as headaches
4. Cognitive expression such as talking about the stress and exploring alternatives

If the stress of hospitalization cannot be reduced through the use of coping behaviors, long-term consequences, such as chronic illness and adjustment problems after discharge, can result.

The stressors of illness and hospitalization differ according to the individual child. Certain stressors, however, are common in all children. These include separation, loss of function and control, and altered body image and pain. (Responses to these stressors are summarized in Table 19-1.)

Certain stress-related behaviors are also common in hospitalized children. *Regression,* the child's reversion to a previous level of development, is a typical response to stress. Regression can occur in affective, cognitive, biophysical, or social development. For example, the 4-year-old who generally is independent at home might demand constant help from the caregiver. The previously trained 3-year-old might experience toileting accidents.

One way to determine whether the child is using regression as a coping mechanism is to compare the child's age to assessment data about the child's usual behavioral characteristics. If the child's behavior in the hospital reflects a developmental stage that differs from the usual behavior, the child is probably using regression to cope with stress.

Because hospitalization and separation from friends and family normally produce regression in children of all ages, the nurse also determines whether a child's behavior in the hospital is consistently immature. If this is the case, the nurse needs to find ways to help the child to cope constructively, usually by providing more support and lessening stressors the child faces. This process involves not only the nurse and health care team but also those family members who can be supportive to the child. For example, the 3-year-old who feels anxious about toileting accidents needs reassurance that such accidents are all right in the hospital. Parents might then need to be told that regressive behavior is normal and that the child should not be made to feel ashamed or anxious about these behaviors.

The multiple stresses of hospitalization can indeed be the origins of a crisis for the child. By calling on the strengths of the child and by applying skilled nursing care, together with the support of the child's family, a positive resolution is possible. Without carefully planned interventions, a child might experience a detrimental outcome to the hospital stay (see Fig. 13-1).

Factors influencing coping with illness and hospitalization

Development, temperament, and past experiences An individual child's coping behaviors in response to the stress of hospitalization depend on the child's developmental stage, temperament, and past experiences. For example, aggressive behavior is an age-appropriate response in early and middle childhood. Cognitive expression is normal coping in adolescence.

Children who have been hospitalized many times bring with them expectations about hospital routines and procedures. If their past experiences have included adequate explanations about procedures and some measure of control over daily routines, they are likely to respond with age-appropriate coping behaviors. If their past experiences have left them afraid of the unfamiliar setting and afraid of invasive procedures, they are more likely to exhibit maladaptive or regressive coping.

The child's understanding of illness In addition to developmental stage, temperament, and previous hospital experiences, children's understanding of illness plays an important role in their adjustment to hospitalization. Research shows that many children associate illness with punishment, guilt, and self-blame (Beverly, 1936; Williams, 1979; Wood, 1983). Other factors that children believe cause illness include injury, "germs," and environmental phenomena such as heat, cold, and rain. Children's perceptions of illness differ depending on their cognitive development. In general, children do not understand illness logically until about 10 or 12 years of age.

With hospitalized children, the emotional effects of separation from parents and peers often cloud their notions of illness and its causes. For example, when healthy 6-, 8-, and 10-year-olds were asked about their understanding of illness, they did not see illness as punishment, but children of the same ages who had experienced repeated illnesses and hospitalization tended to perceive illness as punishment (Bibace and Walsh, 1980). Although the reasons for these different notions of illness have not been explored, possible reasons include cognitive regression associated with stress and a more limited exposure to general information.

The parent's perceptions The parent's views of a disease and its outcomes are among the factors that most influence the child's responses and ability to cope. Parents' emotions cannot be hidden from their children, and a parent's attitude therefore can have a positive or a negative effect on the child. Conditions or treatments that cause changes in physical appearance, such as amputation or baldness, usually cause some emotional response in the child's parent. Even

TABLE 19-1 Behavioral Responses to the Stress of Hospitalization

Developmental stage	Stressor: Separation	Stressor: Loss of function and control	Stressor: Altered body image and pain	Nursing management
Infancy				
Trust vs mistrust: child develops trust through close association with primary caregiver, responds to external environment, begins to explore	Separation anxiety: protest, despair, detachment Anxiety, grief, anger shown by crying, screaming, looking for parent, rejecting stranger, physical activity Withdrawal, inactivity, disinterest in the environment Easy distractibility in early infancy Physical resistance to restraints and procedures in late infancy	Lethargy with increased dependence Emotional distress associated with immobility	Emotional distress with body injury, especially if bleeding occurs Protest with repeated painful experiences	Provide consistent nursing care with primary nurse, if possible Sing and talk to infant Touch, hold, and rock infant and continue to interact during procedures Provide pacifier or bottle or allow finger sucking Encourage interaction with parent: rooming-in, parent's talking to child and saying good-bye when leaving Allow security objects, mobiles, toys
Early childhood				
Autonomy vs shame and doubt, initiative vs guilt: child learns new skills for mobility and communication, continues to develop attachment to family and caregivers, explores the environment, and begins to perfect fine motor skills	Separation anxiety: protest evident in crying and angry outbursts, physical attacks, clinging to parent; despair evident in lack of communication, loss of newly learned motor skills, disinterest, detachment evident in superficial adjustment to hospital environment	Feelings of failure associated with loss of recently learned skills Nightmares and fears of the dark, strangers, people in uniforms, and those who administer treatments Regression in areas such as toileting, independence in eating, thumb sucking Vigorous protest and anxiety associated with physical restraint	Upset by changes in body image, especially those associated with bleeding Fears of invasive procedures, including injections, especially when painful	Encourage parental presence, especially during painful invasive procedures Keep favorite toys from home with child Maintain maximum contact with a few nurses, introduce nurse in parent's presence, allow child to meet nurses before receiving treatment Facilitate visits from siblings Determine skill levels in such areas as toileting, and plan care to promote acquired skills

TABLE 19-1 *(Continued)*

Developmental stage	Stressor: Separation	Stressor: Loss of function and control	Stressor: Altered body image and pain	Nursing management
Early childhood (*Continued*)				Explain regression to parent and communicate acceptance to child Use restraints minimally Allow child as much freedom of movement as possible during and after procedures Give child chance to express fears and anxiety in play Facilitate parent's rooming-in Assist child in camouflaging body changes
Middle childhood Industry vs inferiority: child establishes new relationships with peers and friends outside the family, learns to coordinate skills to complete projects, applies fine motor skills, develops physical abilities	Ability to understand reasons for separation but might still require much parental presence Concern over separation from school routines and classmates	Anger and frustration evident Prolonged immobility associated with withdrawal, boredom, hostility Fear of losing emotional control, embarrassment over crying during treatments Fears of dependence and immobility	Fears of body disfigurement and mutilation evident in hesitation to look at apparatus or incision Ability to manage mild pain through diversion Particular fear of surgery involving genital region	Set and enforce limits on behavior Encourage parents to plan visits and share plans with child in advance Plan contact with teachers and classmates Plan play activities that allow as much mobility as possible Make environment predictable and explanations precise Allow choices within acceptable limits (eg, child might choose injection site) Provide ways for child to help with treatments and reward cooperation

TABLE 19-1 Behavioral Responses to the Stress of Hospitalization *(Continued)*

Developmental stage	Stressor: Separation	Stressor: Loss of function and control	Stressor: Altered body image and pain	Nursing management
Late childhood				
Industry vs inferiority: child develops problem-solving skills, learns to control emotional responses, develops sophisticated motor and social skills, learns to cooperate within peer group	Parental presence important but need not be continual Separation from school and peers often a major concern	Fears of dependence and loss of emotional control evident in attempts to be "brave" during procedures Concern about appropriate expression of feelings, fears of embarrassment associated with overt behavioral responses Need to discuss illness and hospitalization	Fears of death or long-term disability often more acute than fear of pain Fears associated with changed appearance and attitudes of peers Concern about procedures involving genital region and exposure of genitals	Monitor behavior to determine emotional needs, especially in withdrawn or unresponsive child Explain all procedures in detail, including information about the body and its needs if the child is interested Encourage visits from peers as well as family, if possible Discuss responses to questions about illness and bodily changes, using role play if helpful Provide time for child to discuss feelings, frustrations, and fears Set appropriate behavioral limits and discuss with parents Allow choices in daily routines and planned procedures Allow child to participate in planning treatment regimen and activities Ensure privacy for all procedures, especially those involving the genital area Follow child's wishes for parental presence or absence during procedures and explain to parents if necessary

TABLE 19-1 (Continued)

Developmental stage	Stressor: Separation	Stressor: Loss of function and control	Stressor: Altered body image and pain	Nursing management
Adolescence				
Identity vs role diffusion: child develops new ways to interact with family and peers, learns gender-related roles and works to establish new social roles, develops problem-solving skills, learns independent functioning	Separation from school and friends more significant than separation from parents Withdrawal from peers, especially outside the hospital, associated with fears of changed appearance	Fear of loss of independent functioning Difficulty admitting need for physical or emotional assistance evident in anger, frustration, or withdrawal	Serious anxiety associated with changes in body image, fear of others' responses to changed appearance, concern about being teased Lack of cooperation with treatment regimen associated with fears of body image changes Particular concern associated with alterations that threaten normal development of sexual identity and gender-related roles	Facilitate planning daily activities that include interactions with peers Explain to parents that child needs some independence as well as parental attention Monitor behavior for cues that child wants to talk Provide props, games, and other activities to facilitate discussion Provide time to listen and discuss concerns outside the child's hospital room Role play responses to other's reactions Provide detailed teaching about procedures and treatments, especially those involving the genitals Ensure privacy for all procedures

children who are far too young to realize that their appearance differs from the norm sense and react to the parent's feelings. In this way, the family's response to stress has a profound effect on the child.

Stress and coping in infancy

Separation Being separated from the people who are the child's usual sources of support causes the child to feel more anxious about the unfamiliar environment of the hospital. Separation from attachment figures during frightening or painful procedures deprives the child of needed comfort. Furthermore, the child's inability to understand the temporary separation and the reasons for the parent's absence frequently results in feelings of abandonment.

Separating infants from their caregivers and having them cared for in the hospital by many strangers is a far from optimal arrangement. If hospitalization deprives the infant of human interaction, developmental delays might result. Separation further deprives the infant and the parent of the essential interactions that form the basis of the parent-infant attachment. Both lack of contact with the primary caregiver, who is sensitive to the child's cues, and the care given by multiple caregivers in the hospital interfere with the development of trust. If, however, the nurses who care for infants are sensitive to each infant's need for reciprocal interactions and if they provide cuddling, rocking, and other soothing care, brief hospitalization usually is not overwhelmingly stressful.

In infancy and early childhood, children typically experience *separation anxiety,* a painful reaction to the threat of or actual separation from a loved one. Until they are able to understand that the parent will return, separation is equated with loss. As the notion of object permanence develops and the child's sense of self emerges, the stress of separation during illness and hospitalization becomes easier for the child to withstand.

For the infant who is old enough to differentiate the primary caregiver from others, the main response to hospitalization often is related to separation from the primary caregiver. By 9 months of age, developing attachment to the primary caregiver and the sense of dependence on the parent-child relation usually is evidenced by anxiety in the infant.

Bowlby (1953) demonstrated that the separation of infants and young children from their primary caregivers usually produces a distinct series of responses. The first stage in the infant's response to separation is protest. Protest is then followed by despair and withdrawal and finally by detachment and disinterest in forming close relationships.

Protest In the stage of protest, the child cries, screams, and might hit and kick in apparent outrage, grief, or anger. This behavior occurs when the parent is leaving or returning or when another adult approaches the child in the parent's absence.

The nurse or parent might question this behavior in a child who previously was happy and playful in the parent's presence. To the child, the parent's leaving and absence, especially the nurturing parent on whom the child relies most, is devastating. Protest is a healthy response of the young child to separation from the all-important parent.

Despair Despair might begin within an hour to days following separation. Infants and children who despair feel that their loved ones have left and that no amount of protest will cause them to return. They then become sorrowful and uncharacteristically quiet and seem to be grieving a loss. These children are not interested to the usual degree in the activities and people around them. They might suck their thumbs, refuse to make eye contact, turn away from anyone approaching, and fail to cuddle or reach when picked up. They might not enter into play activities and sometimes will not eat. These children are literally grieving for the lost person.

The parent's return during this stage might be marked by the young child's return to the stage of protest. With protest, the child expresses grief and anger and regains faith in the possibility of the parent's return. This reaction is clearly healthier than depression.

Detachment In the phase of detachment or denial, the child has given up expecting the loved person to return. Children protect themselves from the pain of separation by denying the importance of the loved person and by pretending that being left by that person does not matter.

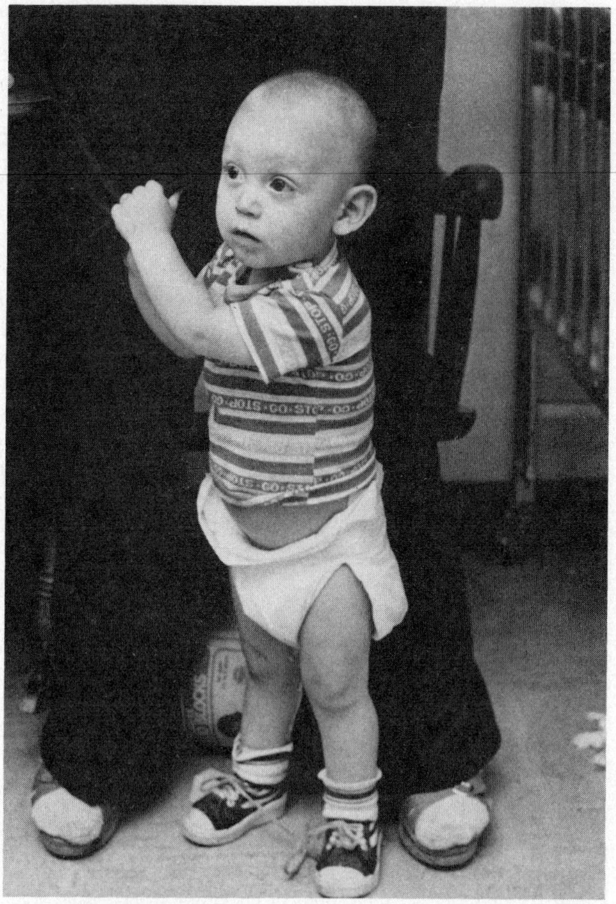

In infancy and early childhood, children typically express separation anxiety by clinging to parents.

In this stage the child might seem to have recovered from the parent's absence. The child relates to the surroundings and plays quite naturally. When the parent visits, this same child, who previously seemed to have a close, warm relationship with the parent, protested the parent's leaving, and grieved in the absence, now ignores and might not even seem to recognize the parent's presence.

The nurse might be relieved when the infant's or young child's protests or depression cease because the child becomes much more pleasant and less demanding. Rather than indicating that the child is making a good adjustment to the separation, however, this response suggests the opposite. Repeated angry demands, irritability, inconsolable crying, and shrieks of rage are more typical and adaptive responses for infants and young children who are coping with separation.

Dealing with the signs of separation anxiety is difficult for the parent. Parents usually are very upset when their children cry. They might wish to avoid tears on separation and can be devastated when their children cry at a parent's

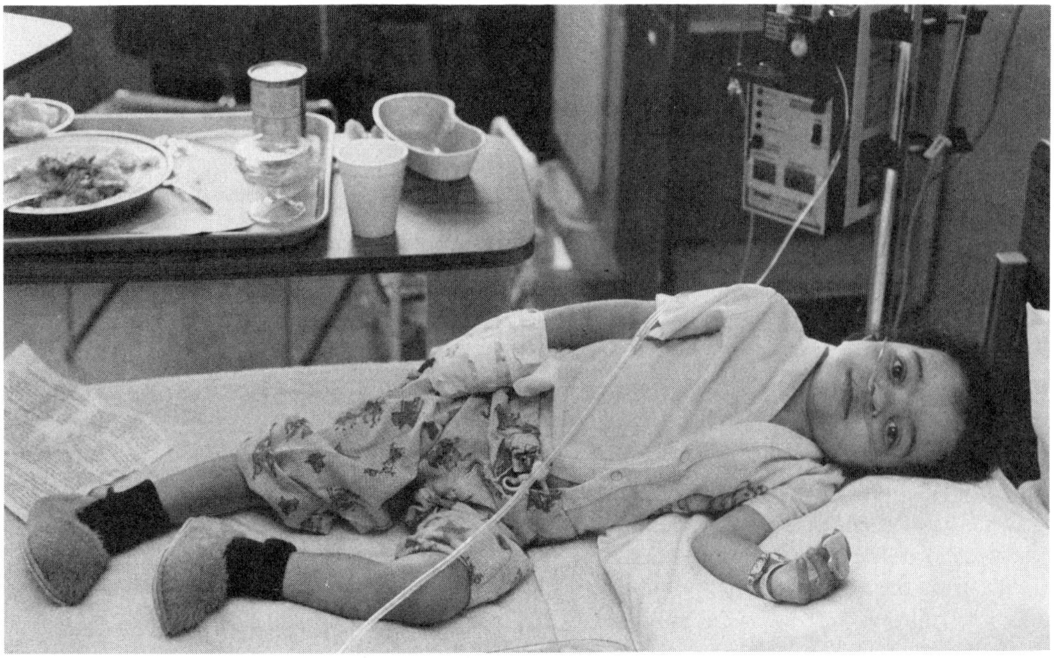

Children experiencing separation anxiety express despair through withdrawn behavior and lack of responsiveness.

return to the hospital. The lack of responsiveness evident during the stage of despair is no easier to withstand. The parent might feel that the child no longer cares to have the parent near. Some parents are so hurt by their children's reactions that they leave the children alone.

Even more difficult might be the stage of denial. The child's seeming to do quite well without the parent, particularly if the nursing staff does not see the behavior as a problem, might cause the parent to feel replaced and then to withdraw. After a period of separation, infants and young children tend either to cling to or to reject the parent. These behaviors, too, are difficult for the parent.

Parents require explanations of their children's behavior. Nurses therefore need to discuss separation anxiety and the child's responses to it. Parent teaching in such instances might require persistence on the nurse's part because some parents are so hurt by the separation and the child's behavior that they have difficulty listening. The parents also need to protect themselves, particularly when they are experiencing the stress of their children's illness and hospital stay. Some parents do this by talking about how much needs to be done at home, giving themselves an excuse to leave the hospital quickly.

Loss of function and control The lethargy that often accompanies illness increases the child's dependence on others. Until 9 months of age, this poses little threat to the child's development, but after the infant begins to sit and crawl, the loss of mobility can result in emotional distress. Restraints on the arms, legs, or hands or confinement to a crib or a small room can produce considerable stress.

The nurse thus keeps restraints to a minimum and encourages movement and activity. A mobile and other crib toys are stimulating to the infant and might offset some of the effects of limited mobility. Bringing the child to the playroom or placing the child in the playpen, crib, or play table outside the hospital room is very helpful.

Altered body image and pain Infants have only a vague perception of body image. With the development of motor skills such as crawling, the infant discovers body boundaries and forms a rudimentary knowledge of the body. As children become more aware of their bodies, they are concerned with changes in appearance, such as scratches or disfiguring trauma. Any lesion of the skin therefore might upset the child, especially if bleeding occurs. The child might look at the injury at first with a stunned expression. This quickly might develop into a quivering lower lip, wailing, and showing the injury to the parent.

Painful associations also add to the child's anxiety. In infancy the color of the nurse's uniform can become associated with the administration of painful procedures, and the infant might cry every time someone wearing that color comes into view. This response to color is less likely to occur when nurses wear colorful smocks or tops than when nurses wear uniforms that are all white.

Sensations in the mouth and genital areas are especially significant to the psychologic development of the infant. The infant might gain much comfort from sucking on a finger, bottle, or pacifier, thus helping to alleviate the stress caused by separation, loss of mobility, altered body image, or pain. Holding, cuddling, quiet talking, or singing to the infant also gives comfort. The attention of the infant's primary caregiver is, however, usually the most important factor in comforting the hospitalized infant.

Stress and coping in early childhood In early childhood the direct expression of emotion, such as crying, angry outbursts, and sadness, is a healthy coping strategy for children confronted with the stress of hospitalization. Because crying and other emotional expressions are a means by which children can express feelings and cope more readily with stress, the nurse acknowledges the child's emotions and avoids belittling or scolding the child for this behavior.

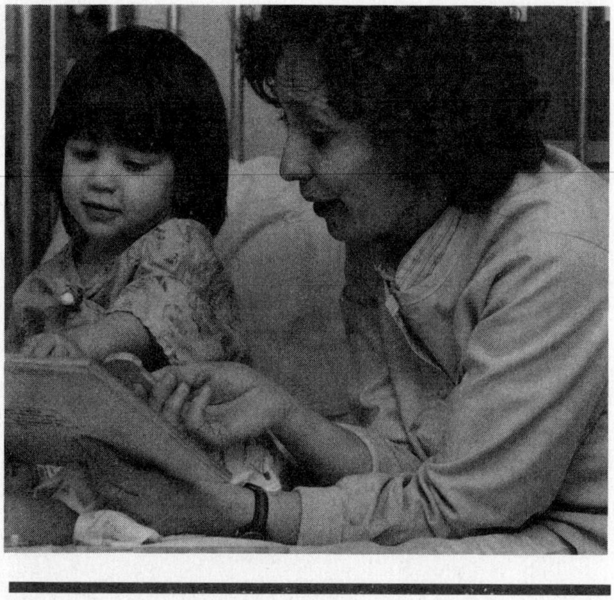

The presence of a parent and the parent's continued interaction with the child are ways to diminish separation anxiety in early childhood.

Separation In early childhood the most powerful force in the young child's life continues to be the parental relationship. The child derives security, comfort, and stability from the parent's presence while striving increasingly for independence and growth. During early childhood, children fear separation and might not understand that they are not being abandoned when their parents leave the hospital. These children continue to benefit from the reassuring presence of the parent, especially during painful or invasive procedures.

When the child is regressing during hospitalization, the nurse encourages the parent to remain with the child in the hospital. The nurse also talks with the parent about ways to explain hospitalization to the child and encourage the child to master this unfamiliar environment. The parent might bring favorite toys to the hospitalized child and play familiar games. In early childhood family support in remaining with the child as much as possible, participating with the nurse in explaining procedures, and obtaining the child's cooperation are powerful means of combating hospital fears.

The child at this age has a limited memory; therefore, visits from and reminders of siblings also help to ease the pain of separation from home. Siblings sometimes can visit the child in the hospital. If they are not allowed in the child's room, the child might be able to meet siblings in the hospital playroom, lobby, or cafeteria. Pictures at the child's bedside also serve as a reminder of those at home, and the nurse and parent can talk about brothers and sisters by name.

These children often have nightmares, and their vivid imaginations can cause them to be frightened by monsters, ghosts, and other aspects of the unknown. Consequently, they frequently are afraid of the dark, strangers, people in white clothes, and people who give bad-tasting medicines. Playing a tape of a parent's voice might help relieve these fears.

When nurses must temporarily become primary caregivers, the child does best with a few consistent nurses who devote a great deal of time and attention to the child. The nurse must not be discouraged if the child screams when the nurse approaches. Children, especially between 18 months and 3 years of age, might need to observe the nurse for half an hour or more before feeling comfortable with the nurse's being in proximity or actually caring for the child. This time can be shortened considerably if the child becomes familiar with a nurse in the presence of the parent.

Parents need to say goodbye or tell their children when they are leaving. Despite the pain of tears, screams of protest, and pleas to stay, it is far better to acknowledge leaving than to sneak away. Confronting the issue conveys respect and faith in a child's ability to cope with separation.

Loss of function and control Learning motor and cognitive skills in early childhood is important to the child's emerging self-concept. The child therefore might experience a sense of failure if newly mastered skills cannot be exercised. Children who are learning to run, talk, dress, and use the toilet need to practice these skills. Loss of function in these areas can cause true lack of confidence.

In early childhood children usually are just mastering specific developmental tasks, and their mastery of these skills might be fragile. The child might, for example, be in the initial phases of toilet training. The stress of hospitalization often results in the loss of this newly gained skill, and this loss might be very upsetting to both the small child and the parent. Some children return to thumb sucking, whine, become withdrawn, or refuse to eat.

For young children, restraints can cause anxiety because gross motor activity is the primary means by which the child releases tension. Holding the child still for a procedure, such as a rectal temperature, or applying a four-point restraint to arms and legs causes anxiety and fear. If restraints need to be applied (such as hand restraints for a child with an intravenous infusion), the nurse determines whether the benefit of restraints is worth the cost in anxiety. If the child needs to be held immobile for a procedure, the nurse should keep the time and extent of immobilization to a minimum. Perhaps the child's arms can remain free during a rectal temperature and the child be allowed to walk or run as soon as possible after the procedure is over.

Altered body image and pain Children from early childhood on often feel uncomfortable about changes that treatment, injury, or disability cause in bodily appearance or function. They might fear facing others and might not wish to look at themselves. A 3½-year-old boy, for example, whose head had been shaved for craniofacial surgery was outgoing and gregarious as long as he wore a baseball cap. He appeared embarrassed and became withdrawn the moment he took off his cap.

Invasive and painful procedures are stressful for children of all ages. Such procedures therefore require age-appropriate preparation to facilitate coping. During early childhood and thereafter, children learn to associate pain with specific procedures such as drawing blood samples, aspirating bone marrow, or changing dressings.

Injections, especially if painful, cause anxiety for children of all ages. A 4-year-old child who receives repeated painful injections for lead poisoning, for example, might not be able to understand and might feel attacked by hurtful people. The child uses kicking and fighting to cope with this apparently purposeful injury. The experience can be very traumatic if some trusted person is not present to comfort and reassure the child.

Stress and coping in middle childhood Middle childhood is a time when children tend to act out their stress if they are not so ill that their mobility is limited. Such behavior might include hitting, wheelchair racing, battling with the laboratory technician who wishes to draw a blood sample, and unwillingness to hold still. All of these behaviors are ways in which children diminish their anxiety. At this stage, as with younger children, restraints or immobilization can cause greater anxiety.

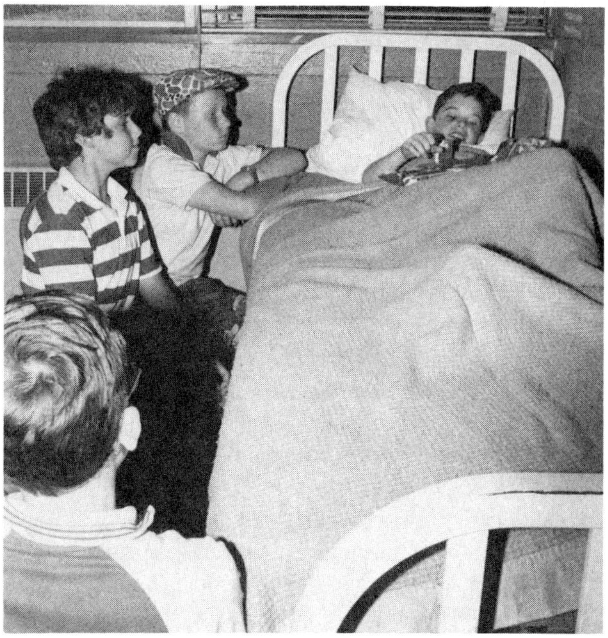

Siblings and peers should be encouraged to visit the ill child to reduce the adverse effects of hospitalization. (Photograph by Judy Koenig)

Separation As children grow older, they are better able to understand why separations occur. They also can comprehend when they are told how long separations will be. Thus, from middle childhood on children can anticipate when they will see their loved ones again. At this stage, for example, the parent can tell the child they will visit together after the child has had lunch. By middle childhood, the child is increasingly able to use developing cognitive skills to understand that a parent's leaving is sometimes necessary and that the parent will return.

At this stage, the child often is able to tolerate separation from parents for longer periods of time, but careful preparation of children requires that parents tell children when they will be coming back. These children might feel comfortable in the hospital without continual parental presence, but the stress of illness requires that parents and other supportive people in the child's life be present frequently.

Because children are increasingly influenced by the environment outside the home during this stage, separation from school routines and from friends and teachers becomes important. Even children who claim not to like school express concern about missing school activities. The child facing a prolonged separation from school routines thus benefits from planned contact with peers and teachers.

Loss of function and control From middle childhood on, a threat to the child's self-esteem is likely to result in feelings of frustration, anger, and even depression. If the child feels that hospitalization has caused the loss of a valued skill or activity, the reaction is likely to be extreme. These children often fear losing emotional control and might be embarrassed if they cry during frightening procedures.

Children who are learning to be independent fear dependence on others and need to be able to control, to an appropriate extent, the events affecting them. They also need to feel secure in knowing that the adults around them are powerful enough to impose limits for their protection. This delicate balance between allowing the child to make some choices and imposing limits on unacceptable behavior is difficult to maintain. To meet the child's developmental needs, the nurse might, for instance, allow the child to choose which juice to drink or whether an injection will be in the right or left thigh. A principal nursing goal is to make the child feel secure by creating a predictable environment. Giving the child opportunities to exercise control over that environment enhances the child's sense of security.

Explanations of illness and treatment should diminish the child's fear and enhance the child's sense of control. For example, the nurse might explain what the child can do to make a procedure go well. The 5-year-old who is having an intravenous infusion started might be told, "If you will try to hold your arm still, that will help me to put the needle in exactly the right spot. You may say anything you like, and you may move any of the rest of your body the way you want to, but it is important for you to hold your arm still." The child's parent or some other person can assist the child by saying, "If you want me to help you to hold your arm still, I can put my hand right here to remind you to hold still." The nurse needs to remember to give the child choices whenever possible. The nurse also plans activities that encourage creativity and allow physical movements.

Altered body image and pain By middle childhood, children might be able to find some diversion from pain through games and activities, although distraction might not work if the pain is severe. It is not unusual for a child on the first postoperative day to require no analgesic when playing games or hearing a story but to need medication when left alone for adequate rest.

Even as children comprehend procedures and learn to cooperate, they dread body disfigurement. In middle childhood body mutilation is a major, although usually unspoken, fear. Children frequently cannot look at mutilated body parts and might, for instance, be afraid to view a Penrose drain or an incision. Surgery involving the genitals is particularly threatening.

Nurses can first help children to learn about these changes and then encourage them to look at themselves by talking about changes, treatments, and the progress of recovery. The nurse can say something like, "Your incision looks wonderful. It's really healing well." Then saying, "It doesn't look good to you, perhaps" usually allows the child to express an inner thought or fear. The nurse also might ask the child to describe how something looks as a step toward helping the child adjust to tubes, traction, or injuries.

Stress and coping in late childhood In late childhood, growth and adaptive coping are more apt to involve the child's increasing ability to understand reasons for the limitations caused by illness and hospitalization. Understanding and problem solving are themselves coping strategies for older children, who are learning to cope with their fears as they strive for independence.

Separation In late childhood, parental presence is still crucial to the child's feeling of well-being. Parents must, however, give older children some distance and freedom to be independent while listening to their concerns.

Although children at this age might not wish to express their emotions openly, they need to have someone with whom they can discuss their feelings and concerns. By late childhood, coping behaviors are less likely to be aggressive and immediately obvious to the nurse. Older children might be withdrawn, unresponsive, or disinterested in social activities. Because they are striving for independence, they might not ask the nurse for help or support, and thus the nurse needs to monitor the older child's behavior to assess emotional needs.

As children become increasingly influenced by the environment outside their families and less dependent on their parents for support, separation from peers and school activities is likely to be a major source of concern. The nurse's encouraging continued contact with friends and other important people helps support the child.

Children often fear the responses of friends or any person with whom they have temporarily lost contact to their illness. Suggesting some responses the child can give and simple answers to questions they might be asked enhances their self-confidence. The nurse also can role play these questions and answers so that the child has a more concrete idea of what might be encountered and can practice possible responses.

Loss of function and control As they attempt to become less dependent on parents and more "grown up," older children come to equate control of their emotions with adult behavior. Consequently, these children might fear loss of self-control as much as they fear treatment or pain. Older children are likely to grit their teeth, act brave, or pretend that a procedure does not hurt. They do not want to look frightened or childish to their peers and might feel embarrassed if they express their feelings. In fact, these children frequently are so brave that others assume that they are not upset by hospitalization and have no fears.

Nurses can help by giving older children opportunities

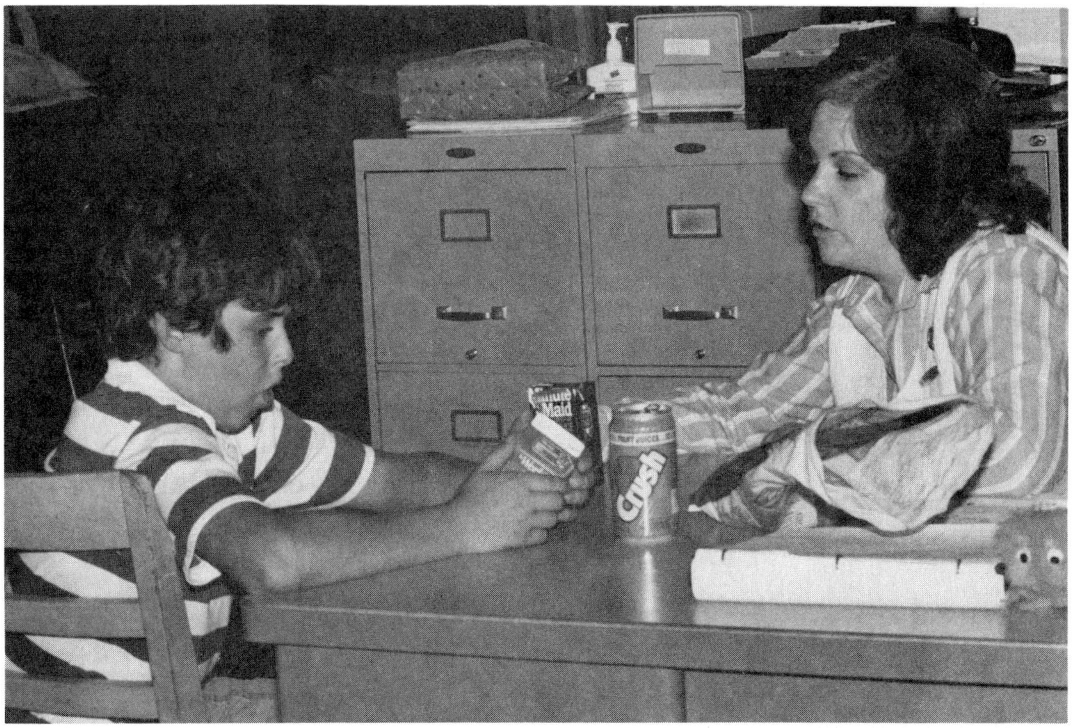

Late childhood is a time when the child needs to be involved with choices and developing a plan of care. (Photograph by Judy Koenig)

to discuss their feelings and express their frustrations. If the child learns to view the nurse as a trustworthy and supportive person, the nurse can help the child to express emotions appropriately and maintain self-control.

Children who have been model patients with the staff and other children sometimes unleash much anger and hostility when their own parents arrive. They blame their parents for all their difficulties, so that the parents then wonder why they came to visit. This behavior is difficult to understand and manage. The child usually feels sure of parental love and thus feels free to express feelings and frustrations. Hospital staff and parents sometimes assume that this is maladaptive coping and immature behavior and that the parent's presence is not very helpful to the child. The behavior is, of course, immature, but parents need to know that it is very necessary to the child's well-being.

The parents might not be able to see beyond the child's tantrum and recognize the child's deeper frustration and fears. The nurse often can help the parent both to understand and to deal with the child. Although verbal abuse must not be tolerated, the parent needs to listen through the words to hear the deeper meanings the child, often unknowingly, is trying to convey. Some parents can do this easily or can quickly be helped to listen to the child. Other parents err by being either permissive or inappropriately strict.

Some parents allow their children's rudeness to go far beyond the level they would tolerate at home, which tends to breed resentment in the parents. It also incorrectly teaches the child that these behaviors, actually unacceptable in the family's culture, are tolerable. Other parents expect their children to be polite and alert to the world around them, as if the child were not hospitalized. The nurse can talk with parents about their children's needs for both discipline and loving attention. The parent can then feel less guilty for disciplining when needed or less embarrassed about the child's behavior.

The child regains control and self-esteem through knowledge about hospitalization and illness and through participation in the plan of care. Because children at this stage are better able to understand the details of the illness, procedures, and their bodies' needs, teaching can be quite sophisticated and intellectual. This is an excellent opportunity to involve the child in the care plan because the child can, when given limits, make many decisions concerning the mechanics of carrying out the care plan. The child might plan walks and activities to meet ambulation needs and might readily drink fluids when the goal for ingesting the type and quantity of fluids is clear. The child needs to be given as many choices in daily care as possible. This is also an appropriate time to teach the child about wellness and remaining as healthy as possible.

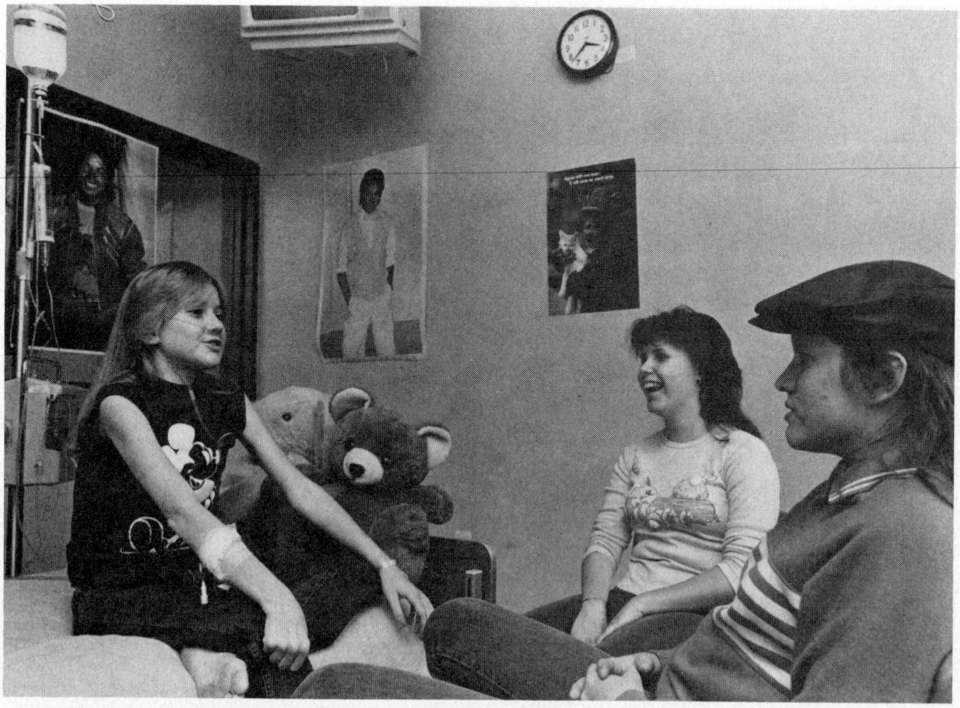

When adolescents are able to meet each other, they benefit from the support that interaction with peers provides.

Altered body image With cognitive development comes an ability to understand the seriousness of an illness and the consequences of treatment. By late childhood, children are more likely to fear long-term disability or possible death than pain and invasive procedures. They usually want information, and it is important that procedures and their rationale be explained carefully. Unlike younger children, who fear the strange environment and apparatus, they need to know what will happen, for example, during surgery and what they will find when they awaken.

Older children also are concerned about procedures that affect the genital area. As they approach adolescence, their awareness of sexual functioning makes them especially vulnerable to real or perceived threats to body image. Any procedure, including routine physical assessment of the genital area, also might violate the child's sense of privacy. Some children choose not to have their parents present during such procedures. Careful explanations and reassurance are important to these children.

Stress and coping in adolescence By adolescence, cognitive development allows children to understand abstract ideas and complex causes for illness and recovery. Adaptive coping is facilitated by the nurse's recognition of the child's individual preferences and interests. As adolescents grow increasingly independent from parents, they actually might achieve a sense of mastery when allowed to cope with procedures and treatments without much parental assistance.

Separation Adolescents are much influenced by their peers and might be concerned with prolonged separation from their friends. They need to participate in planning day-to-day care that includes contact with peers. Some adolescents prefer to minimize contact with their friends outside the hospital, especially if disability is a threat to the adolescent's role in a particular peer group. Isolation from peers, however, might leave an adolescent without adequate support systems. For these patients, contacts within the hospital might be an important part of care.

For example, in one hospital adolescents with cystic fibrosis were grouped together. They were free to decorate their areas as they wished and often made close friends. The girls washed and set each other's hair and did each other's makeup, and the boys worked on model airplanes together. The group held meetings and established rules for their unit. Outside activities were planned periodically so that hospitalization was less boring.

Loss of function and control Illness for the adolescent poses special difficulties because independent functioning might be impaired at a time when psychologic independence from parents is highly significant. This often makes it hard for the adolescent to admit to needing assistance, either physical or emotional. Adolescents therefore need the nurse to listen and acknowledge their perceptions of illness and the limitations it brings.

Some adolescents respond to the threat of dependence with anger or frustration, whereas others react by withdrawing. If adolescents are to use appropriate problem-solving skills, they need to feel comfortable in talking about their problems with a supportive, accepting adult. The nurse therefore assesses the adolescent's sources of support and intervenes if there is no one to whom the adolescent can honestly express feelings and perceptions of the illness. Adolescents often are better able to talk outside the hospital setting or at least ouside their rooms or units. Talking with adolescents in a teen room, hospital cafeteria, on the grounds of the facility, or even in the unit hallway is more likely to facilitate conversations than talking in their rooms.

Adolescents who cannot leave their rooms need to maintain some control over and privacy in conversations. The nurse can look for cues that the child wishes to talk. Sometimes the child will ask several seemingly small questions or make minor requests. "Do you like this song?" (or television show, etc.) can be an invitation to sit down and talk. Many adolescents will find it easier to talk with props such as a game or other simultaneous activity because in this way they can maintain control over the intensity and direction of a conversation.

Altered body image By late childhood the peer group has become essential in the child's socialization. Illness that causes an adolescent to be viewed as different from peers therefore affects the adolescent's ability to cope with the stress of a changed body image. These children might fear the responses of others, are often self-conscious, and worry about being teased.

As with slightly younger children, role playing is very effective in preparing for questions from peers and others. When illness causes a change in lifestyle or physical appearance or simply an absence from school and activities, the nurse can listen and learn how the child feels about seeing friends again. It might be very helpful to the worried or hesitant adolescent to pose possible questions and help think through potential answers.

In adolescence, changes in body image that deviate from the socially acceptable norm are likely to cause embarrassment. It is not uncommon for an adolescent to be hospitalized as a result of failure to take prescribed anticonvulsant medication or maintain a diabetic diet. Because sexual functioning and the attainment of adult roles are important to adolescents, illnesses or conditions that threaten the normal development of these roles also cause stress. A pelvic examination, for example, is stressful even for a well-prepared adolescent girl.

Nursing management for minimizing the stress of hospitalization Hospitalized children have the same needs to develop, learn, and grow that healthy children have, but hospitalization places a great deal of stress on the child and limits many natural avenues for development. The nurse needs to be alert to each child's thoughts and fears. For example, unresolved negative experiences can resurface in the older child, causing regression.

Because interventions need to meet the needs of each child, the nurse assesses cognitive development, emotional maturity, social skills, and coping behaviors prior to developing a plan. Interventions planned to enhance coping with hospitalization have the following desired outcomes:

1. The child will develop optimally within the limitations imposed by the illness.
2. The child's and family's self-esteem and hope will be enhanced.
3. The child and family will be able to express their emotions within a supportive, nurturing environment.
4. The child and family will be able to describe accurately the medical condition and the options for treatment.
5. Family communication patterns and positive interactions with the health care team will be enhanced.
6. The child and family will state they have been adequately prepared for any threatening events they are likely to encounter during the hospitalization and illness.

These outcomes can be achieved by planning interventions that improve communication with child and family, promote independence, and address social and emotional needs.

Communicating with the child In communicating with a child, the nurse first builds a trusting relationship that will help the child work through some of the feelings that accompany hospitalization. The therapeutic relationship developed between the nurse and child aids in providing emotional care. The nurse might be one of the few people who is in frequent contact with the child and can talk about fears and answer questions. In this way, the nurse provides consistency, sensitivity, and individuality to the child's care.

Nurses cannot underestimate the significance of communication because it is the key that unlocks the private world of fantasy, the feelings of guilt or helplessness, and the imagined purpose or results of treatment. Through age-appropriate communication, the nurse can help children to understand their feelings as well as the purpose of various treatments.

Children might be unable, for example, to look at skeletal traction, drainage tubes, or incisions because they are unattractive or frightening. Children need opportunities to express these feelings to someone who can sympathize with their concerns and answer their questions honestly. The nurse who is attentive to their concerns and willing to invest time and energy when they need it lays the foundation for a trusting relationship. Once trust is established, children are more willing to discuss their concerns and to learn about themselves, their treatments, their personal responses to treatment, and the need for treatment.

An important aspect of care is assisting the child to understand the reality of a situation. Although this is difficult and potentially alienating at first, it is more important to tell the child the truth than to obtain the child's cooperation through deception. Facts need to be reinforced, and the child must have consistently honest answers from all of the staff. This helps the child to accept reality and work through feelings.

Promoting independence The better children are able to manage their own care, the greater their sense of independence and self-confidence. Although nurses often find it easier to do things themselves than to teach, support, or even insist that children do the tasks for themselves, nurses do encourage independence by teaching about hospitalization and treatment.

Children need to understand what is happening to them and what their role is in the process. Nurses also can teach children the techniques that will aid in recovery. For example, a 9-year-old child might need to remain inactive and on bedrest after a particular eye injury to facilitate the recovery process. The nurse can then explain the purposes of these restrictions so that the child understands that they are temporary. Older children can learn that getting up and about after surgery is necessary, despite their not wanting to do so. As treatment goals become clear, children are better able to cooperate and become independent within the limits imposed by the condition. Giving the child the opportunity to make controlled choices also enhances the child's self-esteem.

Children and nurses need to agree about what is acceptable and unacceptable behavior. This understanding helps to prevent conflict, which is preferable to experiencing conflicts and then having to work through them. Specific expectations and discipline for the child help to encourage independence by enhancing feelings of security and self-worth.

Illness often is perceived as a threat because it inhibits independent functioning. The nurse or parent who supports the child's striving for independence, no matter how difficult or frustrating it might be, is enhancing learning and self-esteem by limiting regression, discouragement, and helplessness.

Addressing emotional needs

Providing sensory stimulation Because of separation, hospitalization for the infant is generally stressful. The parent's voice is a source of stimulation to the infant. Parents characteristically raise the pitch of the voice when talking to infants, and their voices tend to have a singsong quality. The positioning of the infant in the parent's arms so that the infant's trunk is cuddled next to the parent's trunk is another characteristic behavior that provides appropriate tactile stimulation. The infant's contact with the caregiver's body actually might be one means by which infants establish early perceptions of their own body's boundaries. As the parent rocks the infant, this stimulation is thought to develop the infant's kinesthetic perceptions further.

By the time they reach early childhood, children learn by doing, by exploring their environments, and by experimenting with and manipulating objects. The hospital, regardless of whether the child is technically immobilized, places the child in a restricted environment in which sensory deficit or overload is likely. Nurses therefore need to be attuned to each child's need for stimulation.

Nurses can encourage sensory stimulation as well as links to family and friends by having the child decorate the bed and room area. Large bulletin boards by each bed are good areas to put up cards, pictures, and posters. Some facilities allow walls and windows to be decorated. Frames and parts of mist tents provide additional space for get-well messages and seasonal decorations. The longer the hospital stay, the more homelike the child's area can become and the more significant the accumulated possessions become.

The child needs a balance between activities with others and quiet, solitary activities. Nurses might easily overwhelm some children with too many stimulating toys or activities. Structuring the days with some degree of regularity benefits everyone. It gives the family a routine to follow and helps to prevent the child from being overstimulated and fatigued or understimulated and bored.

Rooming-in Rooming-in is a very effective way to meet the young child's needs for consistency, security, and continued contact with the parent. Many institutions now allow or even encourage the parent to stay with the child 24 hours a day if the parent wishes. This policy is remarkable indeed because in the recent past, parents were confined to very restricted visiting hours. In some institutions the parent was not able even to see the child between admission and discharge. Accommodations for parents vary widely. Some institutions lack space but allow the parent to sleep on a cot in the hall or a chair at the bedside or even in the hallway or lounge. Others provide a bed in the child's room. Parents need to know in advance what facilities to expect.

Through infancy and early childhood, the continued presence of the parent is a critical factor in the child's emotional well-being. The child old enough to protest and be

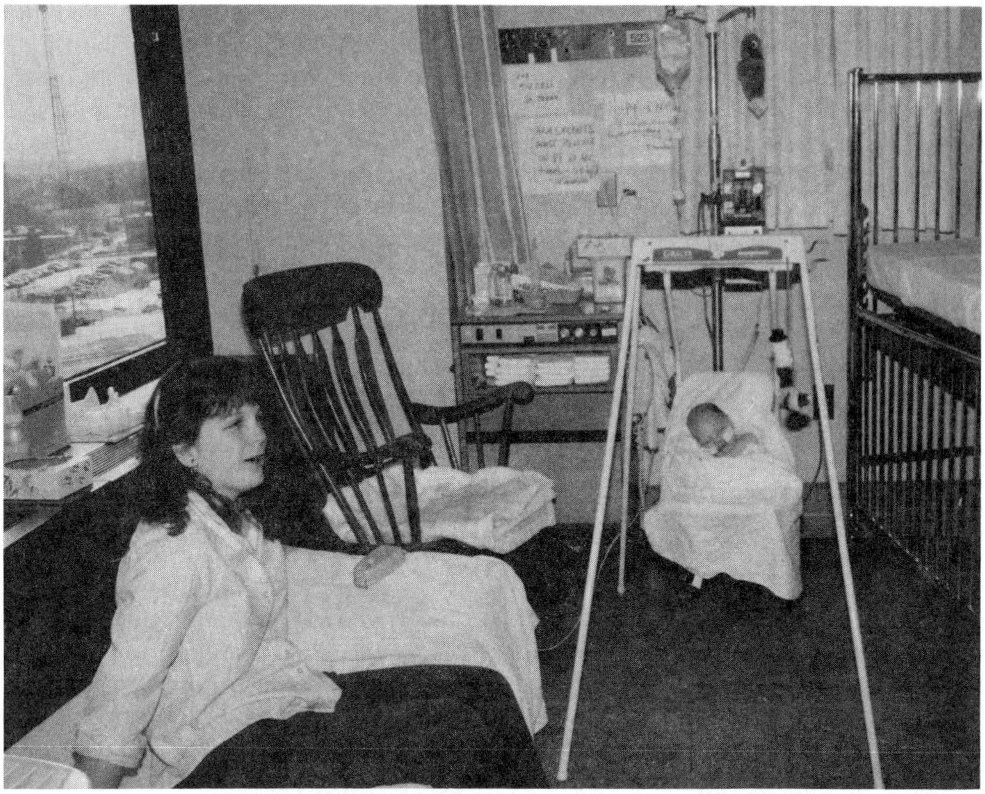

Rooming-in is a very effective way to meet the young child's needs for consistency, security, and continual contact with the parent. (Photograph by Judy Koenig)

deeply distressed by separation from the parent does not have to experience the distress of separation for extended periods of time. In middle childhood, the child is better able to tolerate separation, and rooming-in is not as necessary, although some children still benefit from the presence of a parent. By late childhood and adolescence, the child usually benefits more from consistent visiting than from rooming-in. The child's developing need for independence from parents can even make separation a beneficial experience.

Promoting socialization Maintaining social contacts aids in meeting developmental tasks. From infancy through adolescence, children need opportunities to interact with peers and adults. Not only is companionship beneficial, but the encouragement and stimulation of companions also help children to grow in all aspects of development. Companions help to provide the child with the impetus to keep striving toward health.

The infant's social behavior is learned from reciprocal interaction, first with the parents and later with siblings. Infants gradually learn to smile responsively, to seek the company of others, and to play such games as peek-a-boo. Some young children develop particularly close relationships with caregivers other than their parents. In such instances, whoever has a close enduring relationship with the child should be allowed to visit during the hospital stay, and plans for the child's care should reflect the importance of this relationship to the child.

All children, unless critically ill, also benefit from changes in the environment. The use of the playroom or solarium and trips to other parts of the hospital are helpful. The area around the nursing station is a gathering place on some hospital floors. The nurse, however, is often called on to keep friends, relatives, and visitors informed about a child's capabilities and restrictions so that they can reinforce treatment goals. Having parents and friends help with treatment assumes that they feel comfortable with both the treatment plan and the goals.

As much as possible, the child should remain a part of family activities. Celebrations such as birthdays should occur, at least in part, wherever the child receiving treatment is located. The closer the family ties, the more difficult it is for the hospitalized child not to be a part of family rituals and events.

Children who are hospitalized make many new friends, some of whom recover quickly and return home, whereas others require extended time and therapy before being able to leave the hospital. Close attachments among these children are beneficial. Helpful relationships can form between children who are mobile or further along in therapy and those who are just beginning treatment or are immobilized. Peer support and explanations of approaching events help in the development of coping strategies that sometimes make illness and hospitalization tolerable. Children who have gone home often return to visit friends still in the hospital. This contact with friends who have "made it through" is encouraging for children in various phases of treatment and recovery.

Stress and Coping in Families

Serious illness, whether acute or chronic, affects every member of the family. To a greater or lesser extent illness also alters family members' roles, daily routine, and expectations of each other and the ill child. The emotional upheaval of acute illness, the financial pressures of hospitalization, and the individual grief of family members place the entire family under stress. If relief and help are not available, family members might cope by escaping into work, withdrawal, alcohol abuse, or separation and divorce. Other children in the family also might act out their hostility at having to sacrifice for the ill sibling.

A nurse's attitudes and expectations often can influence the family's ability to cope with the child's problems. Furthermore, assisting the family is an important nursing responsibility, whatever the nurse's personal views of the family's situation. In case of child abuse or neglect or fetal alcohol syndrome, for example, nurses might feel that the child's parents should feel guilty, and the nurse might therefore have difficulty communicating and planning care with these parents. These parents do, however, need assistance in changing the factors that have led to the child's disorder. Nurses can assist parents in understanding their role in caring for their children.

The family's experience of illness The extent to which a person perceives a threat corresponds directly to that person's level of anxiety. Therefore, assessment of anxiety in both children and parents is most important. High levels of anxiety, intense expressions of emotions, changes in appetite, insomnia, and lack of personal hygiene are indicators of disruption. The nurse might note an impaired ability to manage the day-to-day tasks of living. Other children in the home might not attend school because the household is too disorganized for them to be fed, dressed, and transported as usual. Meals might not be prepared. Parents might cry uncontrollably in the presence of their children.

Anxiety should be most evident when the child faces the danger of loss or harm. If the nurse finds that family members or an older child do not show signs of anxiety when facing a threatening diagnosis or threatening information (for example, for a child who requires open-heart surgery), the nurse might correctly conclude that family members do not recognize or allow themselves to recognize the threat in the situation. Such a family might be using denial as a coping mechanism to reduce the anxiety level.

Impact of the diagnosis When children are diagnosed as having serious illnesses, their parents often feel an element of injustice. For many parents, it seems almost inconceivable that their child might become seriously ill, die, or experience serious limitations. Parents often say that they would do anything in the world to change places with the child. The impact of the diagnosis depends on several factors:

1. *Onset of the illness:* If a disease has a gradual onset, the family can gradually recognize the symptoms and their implications and might be better able to deal with the diagnosis. If the illness has a sudden, unexpected onset, however, families often are totally unprepared and might not be able to cope with the sudden development of a disorder.
2. *Seriousness of the illness:* Seriousness is ultimately defined by the family, not the nurse. A family might view as very threatening an illness that health professionals consider minor. For example, to nurses accustomed to caring for children undergoing renal dialysis and transplant, the diagnosis of undescended testicles (cryptorchidism) might seem insignificant. To the child, surgery on the genitals can be terrifying, and to the parents, it might seem major. Parents react more severely to illnesses that permanently limit their children's potential and are usually less threatened by conditions, such as mild asthma or milk intolerance, that are outgrown or do not permanently limit the child's growth and future capabilities.
3. *Course of the illness:* Some families are better able to cope with illnesses beyond their control than with a condition they might have prevented. Parents might be overwhelmed and feel guilty about sepsis from an infection not treated promptly. Other parents might feel sorry about a child with juvenile arthritis but still find that they can cope well with the condition.

Nurses sometimes find that even after careful explanation of a child's condition, parents do not always comprehend information that is too overwhelming to be accepted readily. Given support and consistent presentation of this reality, however, families and children usually can face painful facts and begin to use appropriate problem-solving strategies.

Effects on family functioning The parent is concerned not only with the child's illness but also with the wider impact of the illness on the entire family. The parent might be very concerned about other children in the family and their reactions to the child's hospitalization. The nurse frequently finds that family members are able to discuss these concerns, feelings, ideas about the illness, and beliefs about its causes when they participate in the child's care.

Patterns of communication The nurse notes any dysfunctional communication patterns within the family and plans interventions accordingly. The nurse determines whether family members discuss their feelings and concerns openly and frankly with each other. Can parents and siblings support the child? If family members are able to talk with and draw comfort from each other during the child's illness and if they are able to explain to and comfort the child and siblings, the ill child will perceive that the illness can be managed and that loved ones will be available to help with the unknowns the illness presents.

Serious illness and prolonged hospitalization might result in uncontrollable emotional responses. One parent, for example, might blame the other for the child's illness and feel that the child was supervised inadequately and that this caused the illness. In other cases the parent might be so unable to overcome the first emotional response to the child's hospitalization and illness that subsequent information cannot be grasped fully. Any lack of information in the initial stages of illness or unfavorable reports might then produce further feelings of anger, desperation, helplessness, and guilt. These responses can then interrupt family communication patterns.

The emotional responses of each parent to the child's illness or limitations are individual; seldom do two parents progress through their emotions in concert. One parent might be concerned about the technologic aspects of a child's treatment plan while the other is concerned for the child's suffering. Therefore, although those close to the child need to express their feelings openly, they must at some point also listen and try to understand other people's feelings. If the parents have great difficulty in resolving their feelings about the ill child's problems, these feelings might result in distortion of the parents' relationship with each other, with their other children, and with the ill child. This in turn negatively affects communication patterns.

Parents might direct their anger toward the nurses and physicians who deal with them. Family members also might make angry accusations toward each other. Nurses sometimes find it difficult to recognize that anger comes from parental pain and grieving. The nurse needs to recognize the inappropriately directed anger, listen to the parents' concerns, and continue to care for the child and family.

Family roles A child's illness and hospitalization can cause a shift in family roles. When the child faces a long hospital stay and recovery, the impact on family life can be serious. For example, a mother of a hospitalized infant might take a leave of absence from her job so that her child does not experience the emotional trauma of a long separation. In another family the expense of therapy might cause a parent to take an extra job.

The nurse assesses the significant persons in the child's life to determine who best can alter the daily routine to care for the ill child. Any changes in routine should be carried out with the least possible disruption in family structure. Can the family sustain the effort required to treat and care for the child for the required period of time? If adequate diversions, recreations, and opportunities for self-fulfillment are continually denied family members because of the child's illness, exhaustion and treatment failure are likely to occur.

The nurse and family therefore need to form a plan based on information and consultation from health professionals. The plan should take into account how each member will be able to change day-to-day activities and schedules to meet the specific goals for the ill child's therapy. If this can be accomplished, the whole family is on the road to coping successfully with problems. Chronic or life-threatening illness in a child quickly exhausts the family, however, and much outside support might be needed to relieve the family members of seemingly unending treatments and postponement of rest and recreation. (The effects of chronic illness are discussed in Chapter 14.)

Siblings Siblings' cognitive reactions to illness are much the same as the reactions of ill children. Siblings' understanding of illness is limited by their cognitive development, and fears and anxieties can interfere with understanding, much as they can with an ill child. Siblings might have unrealistic concepts of the illness. They might fear acquiring the illness themselves or fear that the illness is more serious than it actually is. Young children who have resented a younger sibling might feel responsible for the ill child's condition. As much as possible, siblings need age-appropriate information about the illness.

For example, one usually happy and well-behaved 4-year-old girl became increasingly difficult to manage when her infant brother became ill. When she was quite out of control, spinning herself around and screaming, it occurred to her mother that the girl might feel she was responsible for her brother's illness. The mother stopped the girl's spinning, held her by the shoulders, looked straight in her eyes and said, "It's not your fault that the baby is sick." The child's behavior immediately changed. She visibly relaxed and went off to play by herself.

Siblings also might fear the ridicule of peers, who might taunt them with jeers such as, "Your sister is retarded." Siblings then might reject the ill child or become overprotective and not allow an ill or disabled sibling to do things unaided.

A response common to children of all ages is jealousy. If the hospitalized child receives the lion's share of attention from parents and other family members, jealousy might be a way to demand attention. Behavioral problems in siblings often are bids for attention, but if the children at home misbehave more frequently than usual, this is yet another source of stress for the family.

The honest, open expression of such emotions as sadness, grief, despair, anxiety, anger, confusion, and depression that usually accompany serious illness and hospitalization of children is healthy and adaptive. If the adults and older siblings in the family can talk together about problems and express their feelings, acknowledging that it is all right to cry and feel angry, this is a step in the right direction. After the more mature family members have dealt with their own feelings, they can be more comforting to the younger children, whose verbal skills might not be sufficiently developed to allow them to comprehend the severity of the problem.

The other children in the family are often ignored in the stress of sudden, serious, or chronic illness in their sibling. They need to be reassured repeatedly that the illness is not their fault and that they are loved. The nurse can be helpful in planning for the child's needs so that the stress of the sibling's illness is not overwhelming. Siblings should be encouraged to visit the ill child as frequently as possible. Communication between the ill child and siblings can be maintained by phone and letters.

Family configurations

Nuclear families The nurse assesses the parents' relationship to determine the extent of support and identify any stress. Does one parent blame the other for the child's illness? Does one parent accept blame? Does one parent have a realistic view while the other denies reality? Are the parents able to talk about the child's condition and prognosis together? Do they have similar or differing views about the long-term consequences of the child's illness? Nurses often find that in times of crisis parents might view a crisis in different ways.

Single-parent families Single parenting, usually with a mother or grandmother as the head of the household, is the norm in approximately one-third of American households today. The stress of illness and hospitalization is greater on these families, but most single parents are able to rise to the occasion and cope successfully. The nurse therefore determines whether or not the stress level is inordinately high and refers the parent to appropriate resources as needed.

Single parents often feel guilty both because the child is ill and because the child does not have the company of the second parent. Poverty often is a stressor, as approximately 60% of households headed by a female live at or below the poverty level. Even when not impoverished, the family experiences the financial burden of hospitalization because women's earning power is usually less than that of men, and the woman's work may prevent staying with the hospitalized child. Other supportive relatives or a hospital volunteer (with parental permission) might be able to help the parent and support the child.

Divorced or separated parents In some families, conflict, disharmony, and competition mark the relationship between separated or divorced parents. Such relationships cause stress and conflicting loyalties in the well child and put additional strain on the ill or hospitalized child. The nurse therefore assesses separately the child's relationship with each parent and the parents' relationship with each other. Can the parents discuss the child's illness realistically and work together toward the child's recovery? Do they agree on the child's treatment? Is one parent going to assume the responsibility for the child's recovery? Will both parents visit and support the child? How will visiting be handled—together or separately? Are the parents civil and polite when together? It might be difficult but necessary to intervene and call on both parents to act in the best interests of the child. Are any stepparents supportive? Do any other relatives or family friends support the child and need to be included in the care plan? The nurse might need to monitor visitors carefully. The child needs adequate rest as well as support.

Nursing management to assist families in coping with hospitalization Parents need some relief from the constant stress and anxiety caused by a child's illness and hospitalization (Table 19-2). They need to deal with the tension, restlessness, and fear that high anxiety generates. Intense, prolonged anxiety can cause behavioral and emotional breakdown. Multiple stressors compounded by the illness of a child also can place parents at risk for dysfunctional parenting (see Chapter 13).

Communicating with families If family members are highly anxious, their ability to retain information is limited, and they might not be able to focus their attention while information is being given. For this reason, the nurse plans to review with family members their understanding of the child's situation and treatment. The nurse might need to repeat this information throughout the course of the child's hospitalization.

The nurse's discussions focus on the concerns of the family and child because family members will not see the nurse as helpful if their concerns are not sought each time they interact with the nurse. When family members are informed about the child's illness and treatment, medical procedures, and hospital policies, the nurse provides this information at a level the family is able to grasp.

Because parents frequently are disorganized, confused, and unable to comprehend events, the nurse makes every effort to communicate clearly and to present to the family a coherent picture of the child's condition and treatment.

TABLE 19-2 Nursing Management for Parents of Hospitalized Children

Need	Intervention
Support	Encourage open expression of emotions by parents, siblings, and extended family members. Help find solutions to immediate problems. Determine needs and plans that provide for care of siblings
	Ascertain status of family meal preparation, housekeeping chores, transportation. Encourage parents to seek needed assistance from extended family and friends. Provide support by listening. Provide one person to be available to the family throughout the child's illness
	Assist in accomplishing necessary tasks. Provide relief in staying with child to allow parents to eat and rest. Encourage use of supports such as food stamps, counseling, other supportive services as needed. Coordinate activities of supporting agencies
Information	Provide accurate information about child's reactions to illness, condition, and treatment to parent, siblings, extended family as needed. Determine level of understanding. Repeat and review information periodically. Communicate clearly. Provide information as requested
Participation	Encourage participation in child's care to extent family is able. Negotiate care to be given by families on day-to-day basis. Determine person(s) most appropriate to participate in particular child's care. Revise plans for parental participation as child's condition and treatments change. Relieve family of responsibilities of care as child's condition and parental needs require

When family members are highly anxious, the nurse intervenes to diminish anxiety. The nurse either is available to answer the family's questions or makes some other person available. Other health professionals, such as a social worker, might be able to give family members the time they require.

The nurse assesses the changing nature of the family's ability to understand both the broader picture of the child's illness and prognosis and the many details of therapy. Some families want to know only the broad aspects of the child's condition, whereas others tend to focus on minor details.

Some parents actually cope better when all their detailed questions are answered, even if the nurse thinks they are focusing unduly on minute changes in laboratory values and technical information. Such parents actually might be seeking reassurance that the nurse understands their child's complex care, or they might be coping through intellectualization. If their questions are answered consistently and without defensiveness, the parents might begin to focus on larger matters after a time.

Family members often become anxious when the nurse withholds requested information. For those families who focus almost exclusively on minute details, the nurse can repeat the broad picture of the child's condition as often as necessary. If the assessment indicates that the family has a limited understanding of the child's illness, treatment, and prognosis, even after repeated explanations over several days, the nurse might need to arrange a conference involving those health care professionals who interact with the family so that plans can be made to present the family with a clear picture.

Helping families participate in care Families need to continue to interact with their hospitalized child, both for the child's sake and for their own sense of security and need to see progress. Family members should be allowed to take part in the child's care to the extent that they are able. This process of caregiving by family members should be negotiated on a day-to-day basis, with initial and continued input from the family into the child's care plan.

A parent's involvement in care, which provides both a welcome continuity in routine and a sense of close caring for the child, does not mean that the nurse turns over responsibilities to the parent. Even when a parent becomes adept at meeting an ill child's physical needs, the nurse needs to relieve the parent of the full responsibilities for care. Nurses also need to provide parents with the required rest time away from their children and a sympathetic ear for the parents to express their own needs. Many parents must be reminded that the nurse can and will stay with a child so that the parent can eat or relax without the constant pressure of meeting the child's needs.

Principles of Play for the Hospitalized Child

Each child's care plan needs to incorporate play activities. These provide hospitalized children with opportunities to accomplish the normal tasks of development and with out-

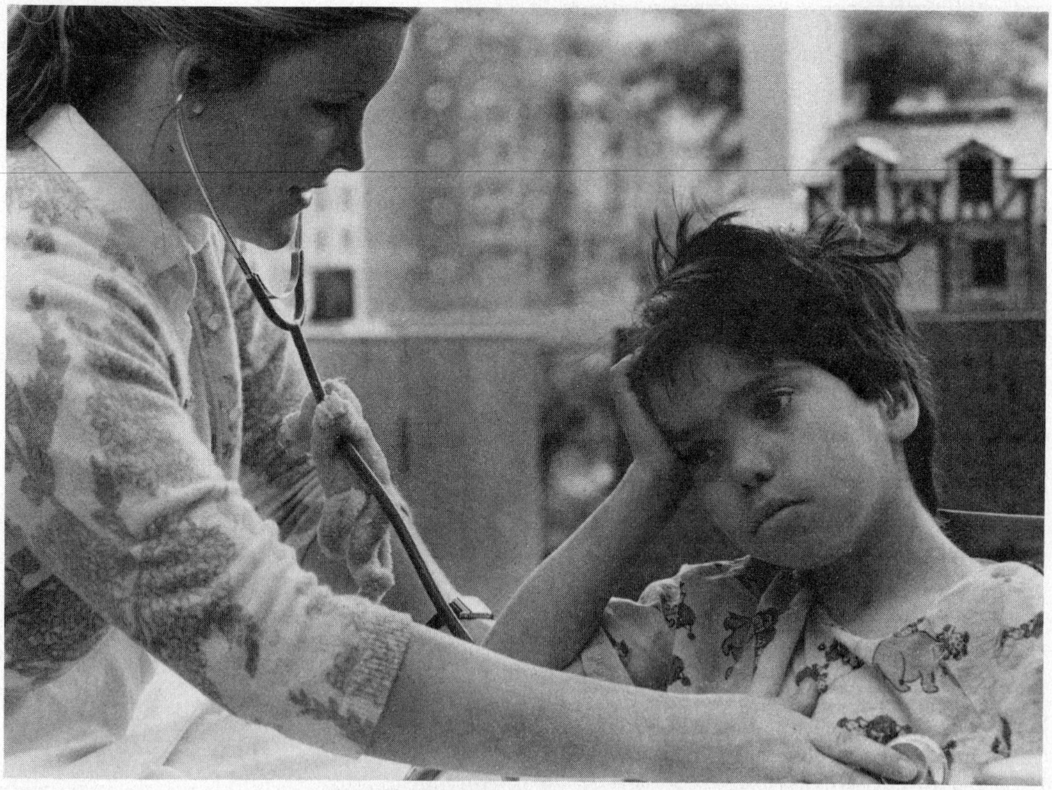

Performing procedures or treatments in a playroom can undermine the function of the play area as a child's sanctuary from stress.

lets to deal with stress, fears, anxiety, frustrations, and anger about their hospitalization and illness. Age-appropriate play is a tool for realizing both medical and developmental objectives.

For the hospitalized child, play increases the capacity for laughter and reduces the incidence of tears. It provides an opportunity for the child to work through questions, fears, and concerns about the injury, illness, treatment, and hospital environment. Play can also make the hospital stay a learning experience. The result can be more constructive parent-child interactions and more realistic perceptions of events related to illness or injury. Play provides the freedom to express emotion and allows the child a sanctuary from stress. Through play the child can continue behaving normally in the midst of coping with unpleasant experiences.

Play is essentially therapeutic. Children need help dealing with their fantasies, fears, and anxieties. During play the child is often more physically active and uses muscle groups that enhance biophysical development and might facilitate recovery. Play is a permissible way of releasing aggression and is a medium that satisfies the child's very basic need to learn to get along with others.

Therapeutic Play Versus Play Therapy

Therapeutic play and play therapy are not the same thing. *Play therapy* is a form of psychotherapy used by the psychiatrist, psychologist, or psychiatric nurse-practitioner. Its goal is to promote the child's insight into behavior and feelings. Play therapists work with children for several months or years. They can be either directive or nondirective, but they practice a specialty distinctly different from therapeutic play.

Therapeutic play helps the nurse and other staff members gain insight into the child's thoughts or feelings, likes or dislikes, wants or needs. The child often can tell the nurse, through either actions or words, about fears and concerns. Although children themselves can gain insight through play activity, the nurse does not interpret or discuss the meaning behind play. The nurse can, however, use understanding gained in play sessions to clarify a child's misconceptions and concerns. (Types of therapeutic play are described in Table 19-3.)

In some facilities, a play therapist designs, implements,

TABLE 19-3 Types of Therapeutic Play

Type of play	Therapeutic value
Getting ready	Aprons, plastic sheets, newspapers, paper towels, sponges, and wise supervision are crucial to success with art materials. At first, some children cannot accept simple aprons. Often, the apron can be slipped on unobtrusively when painting is in progress and an earlier attempt has failed
Play-Doh® or clay	Although clay has qualities that surpass Play-Doh®, it also requires closer supervision and special storage. Play-Doh®, therefore, is a nice substitute that is safe for bed play and table play, opening the way for the children to spend long periods of time squeezing, pounding, rolling, and stretching the Play-Doh® just for the fun of it
Sand play	Sand play is not as free but affords the same quality of fun as Play-Doh®. Cornmeal may be substituted for sand, poured in a plastic-lined box 4 ft by 4 ft and 6 in. deep
Water play, bubble blowing	Children of all ages love blowing bubbles and watching them float or pop. Soap or color added to the water enhances its interest
Fingerpainting	Fingerpainting is not as simple as water play. It is somewhat more exciting, requiring skillful supervision, and is satisfying and therapeutic
Doctor play	By acting out situations, children come to understand them. As they understand and act out what the doctor does, they control and lessen their fear of medical procedures and personnel
Playthings with moving parts	A substitute for real activity is a game that children can operate and make move
Crafts	During times of stress, children might be temporarily unable to socialize because the things on their minds are too frightening to talk about. During long periods of convalescence, crafts of all types are useful to help the hours pass happily
Mealtime	Meals might be served in a play setting for a group of children. Music is helpful, or a story might create a relaxed atmosphere conducive to eating, a natural activity that happy children enjoy
Board games	Games extend from solitaire, checkers, and Clue® to Monopoly® and even more complicated games. A simple game might act as a tool to help the shy, quiet child come to know the nurse
Video and computer games	Whether played to win or for the fun of watching and moving the characters on the screen, video and computer games are popular with children of all ages
Creative art expression	Voluntary art activity that is individual and personally expressive is therapeutic for children in stressful situations
Dramatic play	Through pretending, acting, or playing dress-up, children accomplish many therapeutic ends. They can escape from the present and find relaxation in a happy make-believe world
Punching, pounding, cutting, breaking down	Aggressive activities provide safe outlets for pent-up feelings. It is important to supervise closely because few children can tell when they are getting overexcited, and hysteria might be too close to the surface for comfort
Throwing games	Throwing can be casual, friendly, forceful, angry, or skillful, serving many purposes in therapeutic play. The child who is allowed to choose the target will find the game most therapeutic and might want to let off steam or make friends, using the game to do so
Balloons	Anxiety and tension accompany new experiences, treatments, and restrictions. Balloons can be freely thrown or punched, and they bounce right back for more, delighting a child on bed rest who needs activity and fun. Ambulatory children can also toss or kick balloons safely. (Broken balloons must be removed because children might put the pieces in their mouths and inhale them)
Cooking	Sociable occasions where nurses, children, and parents cook and eat together are a great success. When children cook a favorite food such as pizza, hamburgers, or brownies, not only are they caught up in the fun, but they also enjoy generally improved appetites as well

(Continues)

TABLE 19-3 Types of Therapeutic Play *(Continued)*

Type of play	Therapeutic value
Trips in the hospital	Trips within the hospital fight boredom and depression because they can be talked about before, during, and after they occur. Surrounding patients benefit as a happier child returns refreshed and talkative
Group activity	Children socialize among themselves, often relating to each other in ways that differ from their contacts with adults. Constructo straws encourage group activity and are fun for all ages. They can provide the base for colorful, eye-catching mobiles, which are a pleasure to watch as they slowly revolve
Parties	Party occasions provide a time of relaxation as well as a time to be remembered. Word games, guessing contests, and simple carnival stunts can lure children into happy participation
Music	Music has many advantages, and nearly every child will respond to some type of music. Strongly rhythmic songs often catch their interest. Many children who don't want to talk will join in with a rhythm band. Even teenagers join in the fun, especially if the adult in charge steers clear of teaching and sets a permissive, happy atmosphere.
Music *(Continued)*	A community sing-along also can grow out of music. Simple song sheets with words of favorite songs encourage participation. The child in isolation particularly needs stimulation to help combat depression
Hairdressing	Young people in the hospital still care about their appearances. A shampoo and blow dry by a friendly nurse ranks high on the list of therapeutic activities
Blocks	Building with blocks, either small or large, brings to a child a sense of skill and control. Individually or in group play intricate constructions can be formed and destroyed and reformed in new designs
Bowling	Bowling with a styrofoam set in a controlled area affords active children necessary physical play
Busy box or picture books	A busy box with dials to turn, knobs to slide, and doors to open can be used with younger children to provide movement, distraction, and learning. A loving story with lots of pictures also can help prevent depression and give the child a time of relaxed happiness

and directs the play program. Depending on the institution, this program might be called by various names, including child life, children's activities, and recreational therapy. The play therapist provides valuable guidance to all members of the health care team regarding space for a play area, age-appropriate equipment and toys, and the most effective use of resources to promote children's adaptation to the stress of hospitalization (Tables 19-4 and 19-5).

Play as a Tool for Nursing Management

Nurses who work with children need to incorporate age-appropriate play into their interactions. Observing the child at play enables the nurse to collect a wealth of data related to a child's growth and development. In addition, the knowledgeable nurse can be a valuable resource to children and their families by providing guidelines for the selection of materials and activities that promote a child's learning and self-esteem. Parents often need to be told that anger and frustration are normal responses to the restrictions of the hospital. The child might therefore need help in dealing with these emotions both at home and in the hospital.

In selecting any activity, the nurse considers the child's individual needs. Children do develop at their own paces, reflect their cultural environments, and have their own preferences and styles. Generalizations about age groups might be accurate, but they do not necessarily apply completely to each particular child. Among many children, tremendous differences are usually evident in maturation, skills, interests, and needs.

A child's gender and cultural background also play roles in the child's preferences for play. Girls tend to mature at a

TABLE 19-4 Age-Appropriate Playroom Activities

Age group	Play activities
Infants under 18 months	Toys that are bright, clean, and too large to be swallowed (everything the child holds is tasted) Dropping toys to be retrieved may be tied to the side of the bed, chair, or stroller so that the child can pull them back People watching Constant mobility and investigation requires close supervision
Two- and three-year-olds	Blocks Stacking toys Push and pull toys Balls Soft toys Stories Music Simple puzzles (fewer than six parts) Free play
Older three- and four-year-olds	Real-life play Puzzles Play-Doh® Bubbles Imitative play Music Stories Simple games Group play with adult supervision
Four- and five-year-olds	Real-life play Games (with an adult to help follow rules) Tearing and pasting (if handling scissors is difficult) Plain paper to color (coloring books require a separate page for each child) Paper bag puppets Paper bag masks Paper plate crafts
Five- to ten-year-olds	Structured games Group play (but with adult attention) Games or crafts Puppet shows Wooden construction sets Musical instruments (eg, rhythm bands) Magic tricks Video games
Ten-year-olds through adolescence	Games Crafts Conversation Music Complicated models Sewing Long-term or group projects Video games Ping pong or pool

faster rate than boys, until approximately 11 years of age. After that, boys catch up. Cultural variations and adult expectations affect some of these differences.

Play for expression of feelings and perceptions Children who do not easily express themselves in words often benefit from doll play or art activities such as painting and drawing. For example, the repetitive putting on and taking off of a "cast" on a doll or favorite stuffed animal might reassure the young child that the appearance or size of the arm or leg does not change while it is in the cast. A nurse talking with the child about this activity can identify some fears and fantasies that the child needs to explore. Simply reassuring the child that the arm or leg is okay is not adequate.

From early childhood through adolescence, art is often an effective means of identifying the emotional needs of children. Art, both nondirected and directed, allows children to express feelings through clay, paper, or other media. As the nurse encourages the child to talk about drawings, the interaction helps the child to understand that the nurse is interested in the child's thinking and concerns. This interest alone often opens the door to more therapeutic conversation.

When children are more easily able to discuss their thoughts and feelings, having the child talk about the content and colors of the pictures or tell a story about the drawing might give the nurse some insight into the child's perception of the environment.

Having older children write about their experiences and thoughts is another means of encouraging expression. These writings can be collected, printed, and distributed in the form of a hospital "newspaper." Sometimes, they are put in a scrapbook or on a bulletin board in the playroom

TABLE 19-5 Play Materials for Types of Play

Activity	Materials

Construction toys	Blocks
	  Sponge
	  Wood
	  Put-together (Lego®, Loc Blocks®)
	Tinker Toys®
	Lincoln Logs®
	Models

Sociodramatic play	Dolls Cars, trucks Dress-up clothes and props Kitchen set-up, dishes Doll beds, furniture Doll houses and family Cardboard boxes Stuffed animals Puppets
Aggression-release toys	Drums Styrofoam blocks Beanbags Hammer and nails Pegboard, pegbench Cymbals Xylophone
Art-related toys	Paper (various colored, construction, plain white) Pencils, crayons Markers Paints (water, tempera, finger) Glue Scissors Scraps of material, yarn, ribbon Macaroni shapes for collage Cotton balls Popsicle sticks or tongue depressors
Hospital play	Stethoscope Blood pressure cuff Tongue depressor Reflex hammer Intravenous tubing and soluset Band-aids Tape, gauze Tape measure Syringe without needle Gown, mask, surgery cap, and booties Dolls—nurse, doctor, children Other equipment appropriate to child's situation

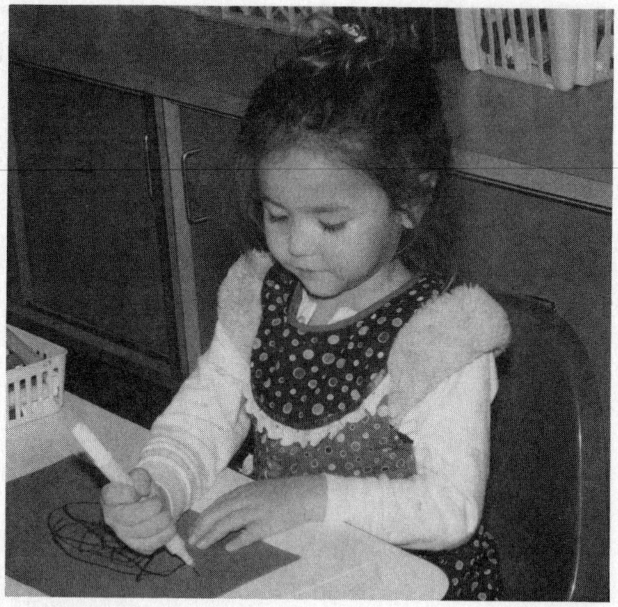

Art allows children to express feelings through a variety of media. (Photograph by Judy Koenig)

for other children with similar problems and treatments to read. This activity helps individual children to work through their concerns and makes them feel they are contributing to the understanding and mental health of other children.

Playing out ideas and emotions also might be done through fantasy. An idea or event precipitates the initial form and direction of this play. As the play activity unfolds, however, the child adds associations from memory and from previous games and experiences. Suggestions from other children or adults also aid in the effort to discover the child's notions about events so that these events can be understood.

Dolls, stuffed animals, and puppets can be used for expressive play as well as for teaching and learning. Allowing children to manipulate equipment, either miniature equipment used for dolls or apparatuses similar to and the actual size of these being used in their treatment, reaps enormous benefits. Fantasy play allows a child to recognize ideas and feelings and to comprehend them. Children move in and out of fantasy play. One moment they completely identify with the characters and happenings in the fantasy creation, and the next moment they are fully aware of the pretend nature of the play.

Children of all ages use fantasy. Older children and adolescents might daydream about what their lives would be like if they did not have certain illnesses or injuries, if they

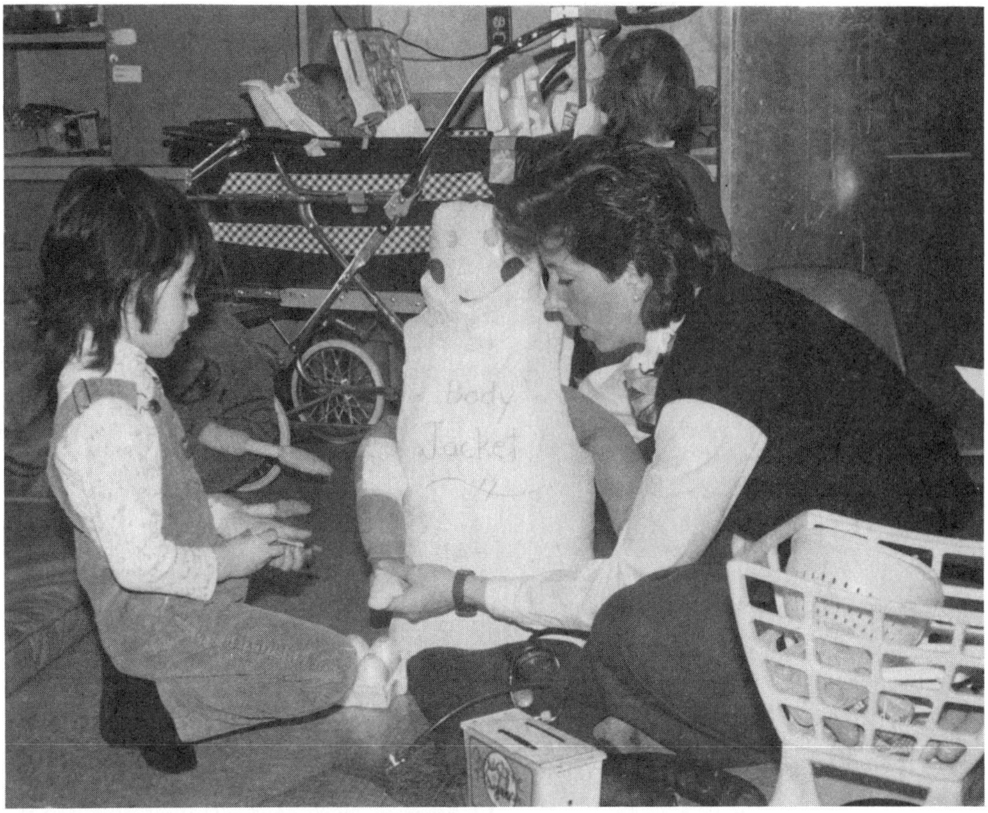

Play is a useful means of communication and teaching for the nurse and child and can help prepare the child for stressful procedures and treatments. (Photograph by Judy Koenig)

were doctors or nurses instead of patients, or if they won some contest and the prize was a glamorous vacation or new car. Fantasy play gives some insight into children's understanding or lack of understanding. Communicating in this manner, the child effectively is telling the nurse about the personal significance of events. Being alert to what might be expressed in this way enables the nurse to provide additional information and encourage the child to discuss the hospital experience.

The nurse might need to make it clear that no question is too trivial and no fear too ridiculous to be shared. The nurse can communicate this best by entering the child's role-play. For example, having a doll or animal ask questions or talk about what it is like to have a cast is a nonthreatening way to communicate with a young child.

Play for the movement-restricted child Some children cannot be moved to the play area. They might be in isolation rooms or on bed rest that prohibits moving the bed. These children are beset by the same threats of illness common to all hospitalized children, and their stress is compounded by separation from peers, greater immobility, and increased sensory deprivation. For them, play must be adapted to the immediate environment at the bedside or in the room. Activities might include the following:

- Scrapbooks, cloth or vinyl books (for younger children)
- Tracing
- Card games (appropriate to age)
- Musical instruments
- Paints: water, finger, or felt-tip markers
- Pegboard and hammer
- Clay or Play-Doh®
- Puppets
- Puzzles
- "Explore" or "Sunshine" box
- Beading (size of beads depends on the age of the child)
- Art materials
- Camera (for older child)

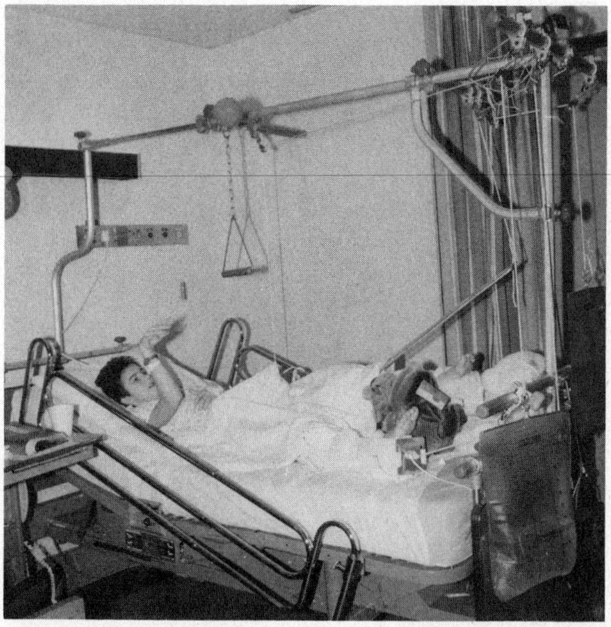

Velcro or Nerf® games are useful for the movement-restricted child. (Photograph by Judy Koenig)

Tape recorder
Aquarium
Dolls (type depends on age but might include baby dolls or older dolls such as Barbie™ and Ken™ dolls)
Stuffed animals
Collections
Sponge balls, blocks
Velcro-related games
Hospital-related toys and equipment
Toys with wheels

Pictures, mobiles, posters, plants, and even pets (those confined to safe places) can change a hospital room into a personal space. Walkie-talkies, tape recorders, and telephones provide communication opportunities. A window in the isolation room might provide a play space for the isolated child and a peer to play games such as checkers or tic-tac-toe. Water-soluble markers often work well for this because the game can be drawn on the glass and later washed off without leaving permanent markings.

Creativity in adapting play materials provides alternatives for regressive behavior or for an aggressive reaction, which immobile children often exhibit in response to the deprivation inherent in restricted movement or isolation. The Velcro-related games, which involve various degrees of vigorous arm movements, are popular. Some of these games use darts; some use balls; and some involve characters. The object is to throw the Velcro-backed object toward a special board and score points or make a bull's-eye. Nerf® basketball is another safe and popular game that meets a variety of needs for the immobile child.

Sharing in the planning of a playroom event or previewing a movie can transform the isolated child into a privileged individual. The child in an immovable traction bed will regain some sense of power and control if designated the starter or caller of such group activities as games of lotto or bingo. Such a child also might be the director of puppet shows put on within the room for other children to watch. The nurse uses every opportunity to reinforce these children's sense of self-esteem, thus assuring them that their developmental needs will be met.

Principles of Parent-Child Teaching

Teaching is a major role of the child health nurse and a necessity for helping the child adjust to the new and unusual environment of the hospital. Preparing the child for specific procedures, tests, and surgery and promoting the child's growth and development are part of the nurse's responsibility. Hospitalization can be a marvelous opportunity for ongoing extended interactions with the child and family. The nurse can establish a relationship of mutual respect and can use this for an assessment of the child's life at home. The nurse can then provide encouragement and support in the difficult areas of a child's and parent's growth and include anticipatory guidance, as needed, concerning the child's development.

Teaching should not, however, follow a formula. Even when family members need to learn specific information, such as administering home hyperalimentation to a child, the teaching plan needs to be individually designed. Individualized teaching is most effective because the child and family learn more and then feel more in control of their lives and their medical and nursing care. Teaching is individualized when the approach, pace, and content of the teaching plan are geared to the specific child and family.

Guidelines for Teaching

When preparing a child for admission, examinations, or procedures, it is often helpful to do so, at least in part, through play. In this way passive listening becomes active participation. Play usually increases the child's coping abilities and gives the child a sense of control, promoting cooperation in the process. Teaching formats, play materials, and the vocabulary to use for explanations depend on the age and specific needs of the child.

Establishing a baseline First, and perhaps most important, the nurse finds out from the parents and child what information they have received about the admission, examination, or procedure; what they understand; and what their response is to this information. Teaching plans have become so much a part of nursing practice that it might seem simplistic and obvious to say that teaching must be geared to what a child and family need to know. Yet many nurses proceed with a teaching plan without first obtaining this baseline information.

The nurse therefore finds out what the child and family already know, or feel a need to know, and are ready to learn. The nurse listens carefully to their questions and acknowledges their anxieties and then clarifies these areas of concern first, even though these very same topics may be covered later. Unless these questions are answered first, the anxiety level often is not reduced sufficiently for the family to hear any other information. A good rule to follow is to answer their questions first but then reiterate that same information in its usual sequence when teaching.

Identifying coping strategies The nurse also identifies the child's and parent's usual patterns of coping and the effectiveness of these patterns. If the child has been given any prior information about the anticipated experience, the nurse discusses the child's response to the information, behavior changes, and questions asked.

Children normally manifest anxiety when confronting a new experience, so nurses need to learn each child's expression of this anxiety. For example, after being told that he would be going to the hospital so the doctor could help him not to have so many sore throats and high temperatures anymore, one little boy ritualistically played "doctor" with his stuffed animals. Immediately on waking every morning, he took the animals to the "hospital," gave them medicine or operations, and sent them home. Only after completing this sequence was he willing to eat breakfast and get dressed for the day. Some accounts of children's reactions to impending hospitalization noted that all children experienced increasing anxiety that peaked on the admission day (Meng and Zastowny, 1982).

Children and parents often use denial as a coping behavior. The nurse therefore needs to determine what children and parents truly do not know and what information they may be denying. Nurses can do this by being specific and personal with questions. Rather than asking, "What do you know?" or "What have you been told?" a nurse might ask, "What do you think will happen to you?" or "What do you like or dislike about this?" For younger children, it is often helpful to discuss the situation by using a story such as *Curious George Goes to the Hospital* or one of the other books about a child's hospital experience. In this manner, children can hear about what is or will be happening to them.

While conversing with children, the nurse can assess their responses, their acceptance or denial of information, any increased need for parental support, and any signs of regression or anger. Once the coping behaviors and their applications are known, the nurse can adapt teaching to the individual not only to include information but also to facilitate beneficial coping strategies. Play and personal information thus enhance children's mental health.

Providing honest explanations Honesty is an essential part of preparing a child for medical or nursing interventions. Nurses need to be specific about what will and will not happen and what parts of the body will and will not be involved in such interventions. Children learn about and relate to events through their senses. They need to know what they will be hearing, seeing, feeling, touching, tasting, and smelling. For example, it is better for the child to know that an injection will hurt than to deceive and temporarily pacify the child by stating that it is like a mosquito bite. The child might perceive a big difference between the brief pain of an injection, which is often acute and burning, and the repeated itchiness of a mosquito bite.

Establishing limits A nurse does not give choices when, in reality, there are no choices. For instance, it is not a good idea to ask whether the child is ready for the treatment. The answer may be "no," and it may continue to be "no," but the treatment still has to be done. Disregarding the child's decision while having offered a choice jeopardizes a trusting relationship. When the nurse did not listen earlier, why should the child trust the nurse at a later time? When the child is receiving an injection, for example, it is better for the nurse to say something like, "I am going to count to five; tell me at what number to start." That way, the child has a choice and can maintain some control. The treatment will begin when the chosen number is reached; the child is not given a choice in accepting the treatment and stalling is limited.

Teaching for understanding of purpose The nurse reassures the child that an examination, procedure, treatment, or hospital admission is not punishment. Children often feel that they are to blame for their illnesses or that treatment is the result of some misdeed they committed. Parents and professionals therefore need to be aware of how children interpret certain admonitions. The child who had been told, "Wear your hat, boots, or jacket or else you will get sick" naturally concludes that any disobedience in this regard caused the current illness.

The nurse who tells the child to drink fluids or take medicine to get better is also conveying the message that if these orders are not followed, the child might become sicker. The nurse instead states why the child should drink and how fluids will help restore health. The nurse can tell a child to take the medicine so it can help the germ fighters in the body work better or that the germ fighters need supplies and the medicine provides the supplies. This helps the child understand why the medicine is important and how it works. Likewise, explaining to the child that fluids help to wash bad germs out of the body just as water washes dirt off hands gives both a rationale for drinking and a concrete example of its benefits. The child might need repeated assurances that germs were the cause of an illness or that drinking fluids or taking medicine is not a punishment for becoming sick.

Choosing words carefully The nurse uses words the child understands. Nursing has a vocabulary all its own, and it is easy to mystify the child and parents with complex technical words. The nurse who takes time to explain what a phrase or word means whenever a quizzical or confused expression is observed will ease both the child's and the family's anxiety. For example, the family and child might not know the meaning of the sign "NPO after midnight" taped to the bed. They need to be told specifically that the child is not to eat or drink anything after midnight and that this means no breakfast because it is necessary for the stomach to be empty for a procedure. After it is over, the nurse then tells them when the child can start to drink and eat again.

Words that have multiple meanings are confusing for children, and nurses therefore need to avoid using idioms. Pontious (1982, p. 115) lists the following words whose dual meaning might provoke unnecessary anxiety in children: cut, incision, take, fix, organs, test, and dye. It is less confusing for the child to hear "I want to listen to your heart and count how many times it makes a sound" than "I want to take your pulse"; it is better to hear "I want to count how many times you breathe when you are sitting quietly" than "I want to take your respirations."

Sometimes it is best to find out what a particular word means to the child before using it. In an effort to choose words carefully during preoperative teaching, the nurse told 6-year-old Susie that the doctor was going to repair her heart. She immediately asked whether the doctor planned to use glue, staples, tape, thread, or string for the repair.

Children want to know how an event will affect them, what will change, and what will be the same. As they get older, their concerns change from body integrity to body image, but the emphasis is still the preservation of self. This needs to be the emphasis of preparation, not a technical explanation of the procedure but how it will affect the child and what the results will mean. Puppets and doll play are good ways to prepare a child for these changes.

Proceeding from simple to complex Material presented to the child should proceed from simpler ideas, facts, and concepts to those that are more complex and difficult to understand. In this way, the child can retain interest in the subject and can feel a sense of mastery over the material presented. The nurse obtains feedback from the child as the teaching progresses and makes certain that the material is understood. When simpler material is mastered, the nurse can proceed. Presenting complicated material later helps avoid confusion and anxiety.

Spacing teaching The nurse spaces information over several sessions, depending on its complexity, and needs to be sensitive to signs of restlessness and inattention, which indicate the child needs time to absorb what has been discussed. Interposing information with play allows expression of feelings. Allowing the child to play with the doll and props used for explanations diminishes the anxiety associated with the unknown. Repeating material willingly and as often as requested helps to establish trust. Questioning the child about information given previously helps the child to review and clarify ideas.

Adjusting teaching to developmental level The nurse often faces a situation where assessment of developmental stage does not coincide with a child's chronologic age. Many children are anxious when hospitalized and might regress in their behaviors and in their abilities to learn. Other children, because of mental retardation or developmental delays, have not reached a mental or emotional level expected for their age (see Chapter 15). Whatever the cause of the discrepancy, nurses need to treat children as they present themselves.

So that a child understands, teaching is geared to developmental stage rather than to chronologic age. An anxious child will need a more concrete, slower, simpler explanation than would be necessary if the same child were relaxed. A retarded child or emotionally disturbed child also needs teaching that is understandable. When teaching, the nurse continually seeks evidence of understanding. Can the child repeat explanations? Does a child demonstrate through play an understanding of hospitalization and treatments?

When evaluating teaching effectiveness with children who are performing below their chronologic ages, the nurse uses criteria appropriate to each child's developmental stage to assess understanding. For example, perhaps a 16-year-old retarded girl will repeat preoperative teaching by demonstrating on a doll what she thinks will happen to her. She might also enjoy reading *Curious George Goes to the Hospital*.

Some children are not able to respond in ways that are easy for nurses to understand. Some cannot speak or do not have the organized thinking and motor control necessary for demonstrating what they learn. Many of these children, however, do understand and benefit from teaching. The nurse working with such children can plan simple teaching exercises with much repetition of facts and concepts. Often, someone accompanying the child is attuned to fine alterations in the child's behavior and can interpret the effects of teaching on the child.

Children often understand more than nurses think or can know. One 12-year-old comatose boy resisted a nurse's holding his arm. When she told him that she was going to give him a shot and it would hurt less if he held still, the child appeared to relax and did not move his arm.

Some children are gifted. Nurses need to give truthful, accurate answers when such children ask seemingly endless questions. In following the rule of going from the simple to the complex, nurses sometimes find themselves presenting very complex information and can forget that they are talking to children. Nurses thus need to remember that, despite the intelligence of such children, their logical thinking and emotional development need time to mature. The 7-year-old who is self-taught and adept at long division and simple algebra is still only 7 years old. The child still has the fears and fantasies of a 7-year-old.

Gifted children might already suffer from peer interaction problems because their vocabularies, interests, and activities often do not match those of their age mates. They need protection from feeling a need to act as if they were adults. Nurses can help by speaking to their fears and anxieties as well as answering their questions.

Providing reinforcement for learning At times, rewards are appropriate. When a child cooperates with a teaching plan and with care and changes necessitated by hospitalization, the natural rewards are feeling better and seeing progress in recovery. The nurse therefore points out such rewards to a child and family. Many times, however, a child does not immediately seem better and might, in fact, not show signs of recovery from an illness. The nurse then tells both parent and child, as specifically as possible, the ways in which they are contributing to recovery or health. When a parent follows the treatment plan and, for example, offers fluids very slowly to a postoperative child, despite the child's complaints of a dry mouth, the parent is told that this helps to ensure the child's comfort and to decrease the chance of nausea and vomiting in the early postoperative period. When parents encourage necessary fluid intake despite their child's protests, the parent is told how much this is truly helping the child.

When children cooperate as necessary with their treatment plans, the nurse encourages such cooperation by offering such rewards as a trip to the hospital cafeteria or coffee shop, where the change of scene and different food might be very satisfying. Children often need rewards for appropriately participating in their treatment plans. These rewards can be anything safe and reasonable that serves to encourage children. A child might want something to keep, such as a sticker or star. A chart of a child's accomplishments might be a reward for which a child enjoys working. The nurse might give attention to a child by playing a game or reading a story. Attention might be withheld by leaving a child's room, or other appropriate limits might be established for deviant or negative behavior. With the goal of helping children to help themselves, nurses use many of the same strategies used in effective parenting.

Preparation for Specific Procedures and Treatments

Most children who are properly prepared are cooperative during routine procedures. For many of these procedures—blood tests, radiographic examinations, and physical examinations—children have prior experience or have observed someone else's experience. Blood tests nonetheless are disliked and feared by children of all ages.

The child needs careful preparation before undergoing a test no matter how many times it has been done previously. In fact, the child's previous experiences with routine procedures are important factors in determining the current level of anxiety about a procedure. For example, discomfort from blood tests closely resembles that from injections or IV insertion. If a child has experienced either of these previously, the reaction to a blood test might be more severe. Because of a child's earlier traumatic experience, routine procedures, treatments, or tests often produce the most anxiety. (Age-specific interventions to prepare children for procedures are summarized in Table 19-6.)

Radiographs are used frequently in medical diagnosis and follow-up of hospitalized children. All children, especially younger children, need honest explanations and support before these procedures. Large machinery and the experience of being left alone while a radiograph is taken might be very frightening. The nurse emphasizes that the child must hold still during the procedure; otherwise, the repeated attempts can become tiring and frustrating. Some children cooperate better if a parent or nurse wears a protective lead apron and stays with the child. The child should also be protected from radiation as much as possible, and gonads should be shielded.

For examinations involving the injection of contrast material, preparation includes explanations of the procedure for injecting the dye or air and the sensations this causes.

(text continues on page 574)

TABLE 19-6 Age-Specific Preparation for Procedures

Nursing management	Rationale
Children under age 2	
Prepare parents carefully with details of procedure	Parents are often deeply upset when an infant or small child undergoes procedures. Parents' feelings are communicated to child
Prepare child at the time of the event	Ability to understand explanations and understand event is very limited
When possible, encourage primary caregiver to stay with child	The infant's sense of self is closely tied to the parents. The child derives comfort from their presence. Extreme distress results from separating the older infant from the parents
Approach child slowly and calmly. Have nurse familiar with child perform or assist with procedure	Stranger anxiety occurs during the first year of life. Young children might need 20 to 30 minutes in nurse's presence before accepting nurse
Use face-to-face position, from 1 to 2 feet, when talking to and touching infant before procedure	The very young infant shows a preference for the parent's face. The deliberate use of touch, voice, and *en face* position helps communicate the nurse's feelings and helps to identify the nurse as different from the parent
Talk calmly, quietly, and directly to child	Word repetition is calming to the younger child. Tone of voice is significant in communicating feelings and assisting the child in developing a sense of trust
Give simple explanations of procedures as events unfold. Use common words such as "ouch" or "owie" right before a painful aspect of procedure	Verbalization is beginning. Many older infants truly understand words and to a degree can anticipate events
Use gentle movements. Touch, hold, and cuddle child when possible	Child understands caregiver's feelings through touch
Touch area where child will feel pain or discomfort (for instance at site of IV insertion or injection) in addition to words	The child might understand specific as well as general communication through touch
Use transitional object such as security blanket or favorite toy. Give to child during and/or after procedure	Child derives true comfort from these objects. They aid the child in coping with the procedure
Provide bottle or pacifier (if child uses these) during and/or after procedure	Sucking is a means of coping for young children. It helps them settle themselves and thus gain some control
Hold and cuddle child after procedure	Assists in child's coping with stress. Helps reestablish relationship and sense of trust
When surgery or painful procedures are anticipated, the older infant (over 9 months or 1 year) can play with the equipment to be used or playact before the event. Allow child to hold equipment. Play peek-a-boo with surgical mask	Tactile familiarity with equipment might help decrease fears. Peek-a-boo helps child deal with separation issues
Children ages 2–3½	
Keep primary caregiver near child, especially during times of preparation for procedures. Have caregiver present and involved in procedures in comforting role, if possible. If procedure is done elsewhere, tell or show child where caregivers will be waiting	Separation from primary caregiver is even more a major trauma than the illness
Use play as means of explanation, with puppets' telling what is to be done, telling what it will feel like, and asking questions concerning the event; a story about a similar event; or dolls and hospital equipment that depict the event. Talk about how the puppet or doll might feel and what they might be thinking	Imagination and fantasies are intertwined with reality thinking

TABLE 19-6 *(Continued)*

Nursing management	Rationale
Children ages 2–3½ (*Continued*)	
Have the child's support systems available, usually parents or primary caregiver. Give the child specific things to do such as squeezing someone's hand, crying, or holding onto some object. Observe the child's rituals and maintain continuity with them. Have security objects such as stuffed animals, blankets, or pillows with the child during procedures or times when parents are not there	Coping skills are limited
Use single-meaning words in explanations. Avoid words that the child will not understand or have previous experience with; substitute simple words or use their definition	Interpretation of words is literal; child imitates words without understanding true meaning
Expect vague feelings of anxiety and anger, confusion, and frustration. Use play to help child express these. Have aggressive toys such as blocks, soft balls, beanbags, punching balloons available for child's use	Expression of feelings is nonspecific
Allow child to be involved in play and explanations; leave props with child for further exploration and play	Child learns through trial and error, imitation and play
Keep discussion short and use play and visual aids to encourage attention	Child's attention span is short
Use play to distract; when possible, have someone to play with the child while the second person does the procedure, such as taking vital signs. When lying still is required, distract the child with stories, puppets, talking, or books. Use restraints as minimally as possible; have child help by holding still while directing attention elsewhere. Be positive; explain to the child that the nurse will gently hold or touch the involved extremity as a reminder to hold still	Child protests strongly whenever something is disliked, especially when the child is being restrained
Emphasize the helping and healing purpose of procedures. Reassure child that there is no relation between procedures and punishment; it is often helpful for the doll or puppet to ask that question so the nurse can clarify any misconceptions	Child is unable to comprehend intentional pain
Children ages 3½–5	
Use play and help child to prepare for events by having doll or stuffed animal enact event with actual equipment or replicas of equipment. Have equipment proportional to size of doll or animal to lessen fears that equipment is overwhelming	Understands only what is seen, unable to conceive of events logically. Thinking depends on perception
Allow child time to play and use equipment before actual procedure. To enhance understanding and clarify misconceptions, use role playing where child can be the doctor, nurse, or patient	Child is involved in trial-and-error learning. Taking an active role encourages mastery of events
Give child complete explanations about what part of the body is and what parts are not involved. Have child point to the part that is involved. Specify whether the procedure takes place inside or outside the body and what the outside will look like when the procedure is over (eg, presence of bandage or tubing). Demonstrate on doll or stuffed animal, including immediate appearance and later appearance when ready for discharge	Child's fears of body mutilation are common
Watch child play out events both before and after actual procedure to observe perceptions, beliefs, and feelings about what happened. Clarify and further explore as needed	Child vacillates between reality and fantasy in thinking because of vivid imagination, which is sometimes an asset and sometimes a deficit in understanding explanations. Fears might be increased because fantasy and imagination take over and exaggerate events
Answer questions simply and directly. Provide information at the child's level of understanding. Emphasize the helping, healing purpose of procedures and medical personnel	World is ordered by asking questions. Incessant questioning helps child to learn about the world and roles of people in the world. All questions must have an answer; child is not concerned about the logic or correctness of the answer but that the question has an answer

(Continues)

TABLE 19-6 Age-Specific Preparation for Procedures *(Continued)*

Nursing management	Rationale
Children ages 3½–5 (*Continued*)	
Have primary caregivers present for stressful events and times. Follow child's rituals and provide continuity. Have security objects present and affirm their value. Familiarize the child with the event and equipment beforehand; encourage child to play with equipment to learn its properties	Coping behaviors are limited; child relies on primary caregivers
Give the child specific directions on what can or cannot be done (eg, state that "crying is okay but hold the leg still"). Have the child hold or squeeze a nurse's hand, hold tape or dressing package, count to ten, or recite the alphabet. Give honest praise for the child's performing the task; be specific and relate to the initial request with such statements as "You held your leg very still just as I requested; you really did a good job"	Child is becoming more social and wants to please others, especially adults
Incorporate time for play and expression of fears and feelings following explanations for procedures. Have available toys that facilitate expression of aggressive feelings	Expression of feelings is limited
Discuss events according to activities of daily living. Explain when an event will take place by relating it to mealtime, bedtime, or another part of the routine	Understanding of time is limited
Children ages 5–8	
Use simple medical terminology that is defined and illustrated during explanations	Child has improved language skills and is interested in new words and their meanings
Use anatomic drawings, dolls, or models to demonstrate procedures. Use these also to clarify thoughts about how the body functions, where organs are located in general	Child is beginning to understand body functions
Illustrate and give specific information about what body part or parts will be involved as well as what areas will not be involved	Child is concerned about body integrity and fears body mutilation or change in appearance
Give the child opportunity to play out experience both before and after its occurrence. Allow child to manipulate hospital-related equipment; use equipment or its facsimile on doll or stuffed animal	Child is helped to master situations through play
Provide child with a degree of control and give choice as much as possible. Allow child to help with procedure as much as possible by doing tasks such as holding dressing or tape package. If procedure is repeated, keep methodology the same	Coping behaviors are increased; child is more self-directive but parents are very important for support. Maintaining self-care is important to the child. Ritual behavior is a frequent coping mechanism
Reassure child that the experience is not a punishment for some misdeed. Relate events to body function and ways that procedures assist the body to recover or assist the doctors and nurses to identify the problem so the child can be helped and then return home	Child is beginning to sense right and wrong and needs reason to justify experience. Child tends to view hospitalization as punishment
Emphasize the helping, caring nature of the procedure. Spend time with child following the procedure doing a favorite activity such as playing a game or reading a story	Child is beginning to separate intent from conclusion
Children ages 8–11	
Prepare child for procedures on one-to-one basis when peers are not likely to be present. Reassure child of the appropriateness of asking questions, that questions will not be shared with others, and that it is okay to talk about fears and concerns and to cry. Praise the child's actions instead of the child so child can relate to the specific act when determining its appropriateness	Peer group and "being brave" in front of friends is important
Teach by demonstration on anatomic model or by diagram illustrating body parts and functions. Encourage child to participate in recalling the explanation and demonstration. Use art or writing as means of communication and working through experience	Child is concrete thinker and judges actions by logical effect. Intent is important and understood as separate from behavior

TABLE 19-6 (Continued)

Nursing management	Rationale
Children ages 8–11 (*Continued*)	
Give basic explanation, using and defining medical or technical terms. Discuss how to prevent certain illnesses and accidents	Child has increasing interest in body parts, functions, and relation of disease and health
Support coping behaviors. Facilitate expression of concerns, fears, and anger through appropriate play and equipment. Accept some regression and help child identify feelings; reassure their normalcy. Use of rituals and participation in procedures helpful	Increased coping skills and self-reliance but regression and overt expression of feelings common under stress
Prepare well in advance and include time involved for event and for recovery	Good concept of time relative to past and future
Include illustrations about body appearance after intrusive event, length of time in recovery, and final effects. Discuss implications of major change in appearance. Encourage daydreaming, writing, and playing out event with hospital-related characters and equipment	Child is concerned about body image, both immediate and future
Respect child's need to be independent and explain events with or without parents, according to child's choice. Assist parents to accept and understand child's need to be independent	Child shows increased independence from parents yet needs their understanding and support
Discuss relation of events leading to hospitalization and the rationale for care. Reassure child that hospitalization is not punishment, that discomfort and pain are not inflicted as discipline but as efforts to achieve recovery	Child has strong sense of justice. Child still might interpret hospitalization as punishment
Spend time with child to develop trust. Discuss common fears and events while child is absorbed in other activities such as playing a game, working a puzzle, or doing a craft to allow think time and reflection as well as to decrease the stress of having to respond	Child is able to verbalize some fears; others are more difficult to conceptualize (eg, fear of death)
Children ages 11–18	
Respect need to be like peers and to maintain their respect. Do procedures in private so as not to restrict adolescent's expression of feelings in order to "save face." Sometimes, it is beneficial for experienced person to discuss procedure with the one anticipating it	Peer group is extremely important; child is dependent on peer group
Use anatomic drawings and illustrations to describe event. Discuss procedure and its purpose in correcting problem that necessitated hospitalization	Child basically understands body parts and functions
Include all aspects of changes in body image, both temporary and permanent, caused by the procedure. Discuss and illustrate how to cope or adapt to permanent ones. Anticipate expressions of anger and grief when discussing changes in body image	Child is concerned about body image and long-range implications and procedures
Provide opportunity to express feelings of anger, disappointment, and frustration through crafts and games. Anticipate regression and accept it without judging or inferring loss of respect. Encourage participation and asking of questions to clarify events; give choices whenever possible to aid in sense of mastery	Child's coping behaviors are well established, but regression is common when experiencing stress. Independence, growth, and mastery are encouraged by participation and increased control over events
Review what the individual thinks will happen so that misconceptions and fears can be corrected. Child often finds it helpful to talk with someone of similar age who has experienced the event positively and helpful to talk about feelings and sensations during the event	Child is able to conceptualize and think in abstract
Encourage discussion of fears. Explain roles of people involved in procedures. Respect fears; never belittle them	Child is better able to verbalize fears
Promote positive sense of self-esteem in achieving independence. Discuss procedures and perform them in private. Respect ability to make decisions and give options as appropriate	Child is in the process of becoming independent of adults and parents

The timing of the explanation depends on the child's developmental level and specific needs. Some children need more time to learn than others. Honesty must prevail in all discussions, so that the child learns to trust the nurse and has time to react with appropriate coping strategies. The parent also needs to feel comfortable about the procedure and its purpose. Parents then can communicate strength and reassurance to their children.

The preparation of children for specific tests or treatments constituting the diagnostic or therapeutic regimen should be individually designed. The most effective preparation involves several members of the health team. Information about the child, which has been gathered by team members, is combined with facts that relate to the specific procedure. The nurse, play therapist, and others can then determine how best to prepare the child. For all children, regardless of age, play is a component of the preparation plan. At times, play is used for the explanation of the procedure and at other times as a means of expression about the experience. No matter how benign or simple a procedure seems to the nurse, that same procedure may be awesome and feared by the child and family. The nurse thus uses the information obtained from the assessment process and adapts the explanation or teaching accordingly.

The teaching approach most likely to diminish anxiety focuses on the sensations the child will experience and the reasons for that particular experience. The way that something will feel, smell, sound, and look is crucial information for the child. Knowing that a medication stings when injected, hearing the sound of a cast saw before it is used, knowing a cleansing solution is brown and will feel cold on the skin—these bits of information help immeasurably in reducing the child's anxiety and helping the child successfully cope with an experience. The child also needs to know what will happen and when this will occur. (Details concerning specific tests and ways in which to prepare children are included in Chapters 21–33.)

Preparation for Hospital Experiences

Ideally, preparation for hospitalization begins well before hospital admission. When family members first know that a child needs to go to the hospital, they must be as fully informed as possible, Parents, along with the referring source and the hospital to which the child will go, need to plan what, how, and when to teach the child. Timing, words, and the complexity of teaching vary with a child's age, stage of development, personality characteristics, and plan of care expected in the hospital. By late childhood, most children benefit from several weeks of preparation. They need to know about, learn reasons for, obtain details about, talk about, and act out ideas and feelings concerning an upcoming hospital stay. This time can be well used to teach and work through the older child's feelings so that the child is mentally and emotionally ready for hospital admission. Children in middle childhood need less preparation time. A few days to a week is ample time for introducing the idea of hospitalization and for allowing the child to play through feelings and fantasies. A child in early childhood may be introduced to the idea of hospitalization within a few days of admission, since the child's cognitive and verbal abilities do not allow for teaching about and playing out the experience until it is about to happen. A still-younger child can also be prepared when the experience is close at hand or is occurring.

Preparation begins with the referring source (doctor's office, clinic, emergency room). Nurses prepare parents of young children so that the parents in turn can prepare their children. With the older child, the nurse prepares both the child and the parent. Often the parent is not ready to take on the responsibilities of preparing the child.

Parents who have worked through fears, misconceptions, and guilt feelings of their own, however, have less of a problem helping their children work through fears and misconceptions about an upcoming hospital stay.

Parents need to be emotionally ready to support and teach their children. They also must know what to teach and have some understanding of usual reactions to the anticipated experience for the age and developmental level of their child. To help parents know what to teach, many hospitals and referring physicians have teaching protocols they can give to parents before a child is admitted to the hospital. These are invaluable in assisting a parent and child to know what to expect from the hospital experience.

Play and parental reinforcement of teaching is a real aid to the child. A parent can, for example, allow a child to play with makeshift or actual hospital equipment. This may be introduced and used in a nondirective way, presenting hospital equipment and allowing the child to use it as the child wishes. Equipment can also be used to teach or demonstrate procedures. Puppet or doll play can be used to help a child talk through fears and concerns and ask questions.

Hospital preadmission programs can help bridge the gap between children's fantasies and reality. Programs vary among hospitals. Some make use of commercial films and materials; others are designed by the individual facility. All programs should reflect the hospital as accurately as possible, both visually and in the policies and procedures described. The film might even describe a particular condition or procedure if the hospital population warrants this.

Programs are best designed for a particular age, so that cognitive level, common fears and concerns, and attention span are addressed. Dolls, puppets, models, and actual hospital equipment are excellent props for these programs.

Books to Help Prepare Children for Hospitalization

A Child's Visit to the Hospital, B. Lovelace and J. Delaney, Stanford University Hospital, Palo Alto, Calif.

A Child in the Hospital, Lutheran General Hospital, Park Ridge, Ill.

Curious George Goes to the Hospital, M. and H. Rey, Houghton Mifflin Company

Doctors and Nurses—What Do They Do? C. Green, Harper & Row Junior Books

Emergency Room, B. and D. Wolfe, Carolrhoda Books, Inc.

The Hospital Book, J. Howe, Crown Publishers, Inc.

A Hospital Story, S. Stein, Walker & Company

Johnny Goes To the Doctor, A. Fazio and M. C. Ritota, Dorrance & Company

Melissa Has Her Heart Fixed, Children's Hospital Medical Center, Oakland, Calif.

Michael's Heart Test; Margaret's Heart Operation, Children's Hospital of Philadelphia, Pa.

My Hospital Coloring Book, Children's Hospital Medical Center, Oakland, Calif.

Richard Scarry's Nicky Goes to the Doctor, R. Scarry, A Golden Book

The Team that Runs Your Hospital, M. P. Lee, The Westminster Press

Why Am I Going to the Hospital? C. Ciliotta and C. Livingston, Lyle Stuart, Inc.

Your Child Goes to the Hospital: A Book for Parents, H. Love et al., Charles C Thomas, Pub.

A book to take home helps reinforce learning for both parent and child.

Hospital Admission

Allaying fears On the day of admission, the members of the staff who oriented the child to the hospital (for example, nurse, play therapist) should, ideally, greet the child and family within a few minutes of arrival. This reassures the child and family that continuity of care is important to the staff and that they do have a support person in the hospital.

Not every child and family can prepare for hospitalization, and preparation might not, in fact, lessen fears, concerns, and fantasies. It would be a mistake to assume that a family who has been through preadmission preparation has no remaining concerns. Parents and children might not have benefited from preadmission preparation; furthermore, many children come to the hospital on an emergency basis. The nurse is making a mistake in assuming that a child who has had preadmission teaching and a tour has had all questions answered and misconceptions clarified.

Familiarity does not always remove fear. For example, the child (or adult, for that matter) who has experienced multiple hospital admissions and multiple surgical procedures might bring unresolved fears to the new hospital stay. A child who is returning to the hospital might be more afraid than the child hospitalized for the first time. The child therefore might know what to expect and might fear and anticipate specific situations. Depending on the child's age and level of development, these fears might express themselves as fear of separation; fear of doctors, nurses, or all people in white; fear of anesthesia; or fear of pain. For instance, a 10-year-old boy admitted for one of a series of many minor surgical procedures asked, after the admission interview had been completed, whether he could leave the floor to go to one of his favorite areas of the hospital. He was told that he would have to wait for the anesthesiologist to see him. He immediately said with obvious feeling, "Anesthesia . . . they put you to sleep . . . *really* to sleep." This statement from a poised, hospitalwise child could have been ignored, but instead it alerted the nursing staff to his unresolved fears and allowed the nurses to listen carefully and give the child a means to express himself. Because of this open communication, he was better prepared to face surgery the next day.

Orienting child and family to the environment Many hospital admissions are due to acute illness or injury. For these, preadmission preparation is possible only in the general sense of the child's receiving health instruction, health promotion, and information about hospitalization given by school or children's organizations. Specific preparation occurs as the child is admitted, after admission, and after the acute phase of illness or recovery from surgery. Therefore, because children and parents might still be worried or even uninformed despite preparation and because some cannot be prepared, all children and their families need assessment for learning and emotional needs. All families and children then need plans of care established to meet their needs.

Whether or not a child first comes to the hospital unit from the admissions department or from the operating room through the recovery room, each child and family needs an introduction to the unit. The hospital environment is, of course, new to the child and family. They have left their familiar surroundings, where they have possessions, routines, security, and control, for an environment where nurses and physicians control and determine the routines.

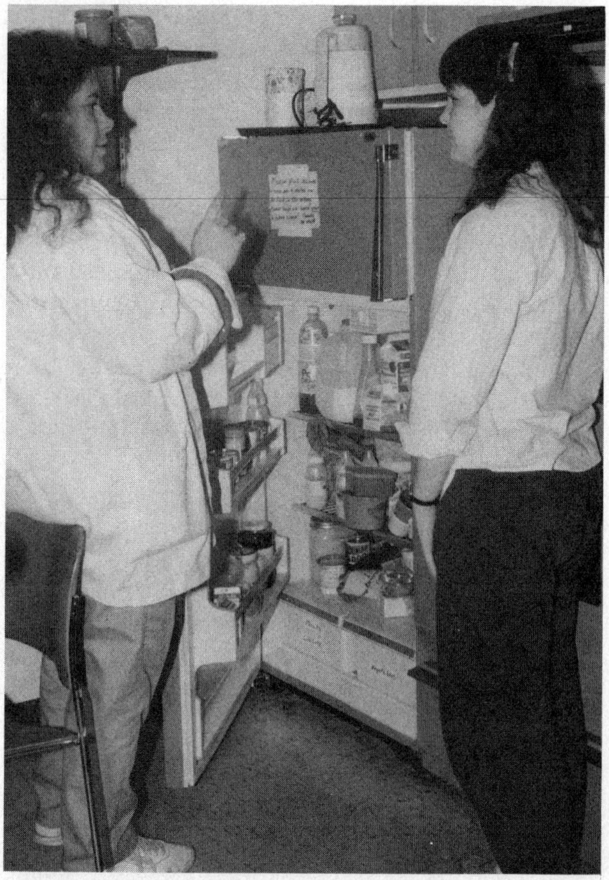

No matter what the route of hospital admission, each child and family needs an introduction to the hospital unit. (Photograph by Judy Koenig)

In the hospital they do not own anything except what they bring with them from home, and they often cannot use what they have brought from home because of the child's condition or because of hospital policy. For example, they will probably have to relinquish medicines brought from home, and children might have to wear hospital clothing to accommodate physical needs and care.

As soon as possible after admission, the family and child need to have a space of their own. The child's bed or crib space and bedside table often comprise the extent of the family and child's "territory" in the hospital. They need to be shown this space, and anything else that will be theirs during the child's hospital stay needs to be "given" to them. There might be a chair that can remain at the child's bedside, and sometimes there is a locker or closet for clothes or a private bathroom. The family also should see the equipment that will remain in the bedside stand for the child's use.

In addition to creating a personal physical environment for the child and family, the nurse protects the small home environment that the child and family have brought with them. Toys, clothing, and other possessions from home might not need much special attention if a child has enough space for them and if the possessions will remain at the bedside. But if a favorite blanket or toy will accompany a child to tests or surgery or if clothing or blankets could end up in the hospital laundry, these will have to be protected from loss. Nurses need to understand that these objects are the child's link to home and family and that they probably provide the child with a sense of security.

A hospital bracelet identifying the child and carrying a hospital number or a label with such information usually saves a stuffed animal or toy from loss, but greater care needs to be taken with a security blanket or article of clothing. If these are inadvertently placed in the hospital laundry, they are frequently not recovered. New, brightly colored garments or blankets might find their way back to a child in time, but security blankets are usually well used and "well loved." Although worth their weight in gold, they might look like old rags, especially if only one blanket or one corner of one blanket provides comfort. The staff thus takes great care to protect these precious and often irreplaceable items. Not only should such objects be labeled but their existence also should be noted in a child's records so that all staff will know about and care for these objects.

By showing a child and family the space that belongs to them and by caring for their possessions, a nurse is giving them a small degree of control over their lives during the hospital stay. Nurses are in this way giving them the privacy, respect, and territory that are essential for their security and growth. As much as possible, this space must be respected. Nurses need to knock before entering a room, announce their presence before opening a curtain around a bed, and try not to disturb a child's belongings on a bed or bedside stand. These courtesies are often forgotten in caring for a child, but they help create an atmosphere of respect and cooperation—an atmosphere in which children can begin to take on as much responsibility as possible for their health and well being.

During admission the nurse also assesses, listens, and learns as well as teaches. A formal written assessment needs to be a part of each child's hospital record. This includes the chief complaint, a history of the current illness, a description of the child's coping mechanisms, and emotional and developmental needs. Care is then based on this assessment. The nurse also obtains a physical and developmental history and does an appropriate examination. The nurse records as much as is known about the family's needs and their plans for participation during their child's hospital stay. (A sample admission guide is shown in Appendix E.)

The next part of the admission process is often the introduction of the child and family to the entire unit. If a tour is not possible because of the child's condition, it is postponed until the family and child are ready. A tour of the unit should include all areas that the family or child will use and those areas that will otherwise be important to them. Where are the children's bathrooms? Where is the kitchen, and can family members help themselves to food? Where is the playroom, and what are its guidelines for operation? Where can family members get linen if the child or parent wishes to participate in some aspects of care? What parts of the unit are noisy and might startle or disturb the family? (For example, the child might be shown an ice machine and told that it makes a good deal of noise when it is used.) How do bathroom fixtures work? When are meals served, and where can parents eat, use the bathroom, and make telephone calls? How can the child or family call for a nurse? How can they arrange to ask questions of the physician?

Preoperative Preparation

Preparing the child for surgery and describing what will happen postoperatively reduces fear and anxiety. Parents—and sometimes other family members—need to be included in the teaching session regarding their children's surgery. Children need not only the security of parental support but also the assurance that their parents share their concerns and understand and approve of the activity. A nonthreatening presentation of a potentially frightening event provides an opportunity for parents to understand both the event and their child's response. At a time when their normal roles are altered, it is imperative to reassure parents of their importance to their children and members of the health care team.

Because surgery is a very personal event in a child's life, teaching is done at least partially on a one-to-one basis. Group teaching is supportive for hospital admissions and perhaps for some aspects of surgery, but the child and family need the attention and support that can be given only when the nurse can spend undivided time with them. It is essential that they feel comfortable enough to voice any questions or concerns at any time during teaching sessions.

The use of dolls and puppets for preoperative preparation is particularly well suited to children in early and middle childhood. Drawings, diagrams, and anatomic illustrations in addition to discussion are usually most effective for older children and adolescents. Other teaching tools specific to the child's experiences can supplement teaching. Anatomically correct dolls can assist explanations. Other dolls or stuffed animals can demonstrate proposed changes in body image. The nursing unit could have on hand, for example, dolls with various casts applied, or the nurse could correctly apply the same type of cast to a doll as the cast the child is to have applied.

In presenting information the nurse is also able to assess the child's and parents' response to the situation. The nurse can then provide support and understanding to lessen the trauma. When the child can deal with the potentially threatening experience of surgery, as indicated by the response to the simulation with dolls or puppets, mastery can then be transferred to the child's experience.

Rehearsing an event can also lessen anxiety. Therefore, the teaching session might be followed with a tour of the surgical facilities. Encouraging children to operate the elevator controls on the way to surgery or allowing children to open the door to surgery and to meet some of the personnel

What Children Need to Know About Surgery

Preoperative scrubs and cleansing procedures—how many to expect and how they will feel

Child will have nothing to eat or drink after a specific time

Preoperative medications—how they will make the child feel (sleepy, dizzy, dry mouth) *

Ride to surgery—kind of transportation, how long it will take, whether it will include an elevator ride

Preanesthesia room—what staff and equipment will look like

When parent will leave child

Where parent will wait for child

Child will be asleep and not feel anything during surgery

Child will wake up as soon as surgery is finished—operating room personnel will be wearing gowns and masks

Child will wake up in the recovery room

Specifics of dressings, treatment devices, tubes (demonstrate as appropriate)

Return to hospital room or other planned location—what child will be expected to do (eg, cough, breathe)

Preoperative injection *

* Preoperative events should be described in order, but the injection should be left until last. Many children become anxious after learning to expect an injection and do not hear the rest of the preoperative teaching.

who will be providing care (who will often give a child surgical hats, gloves, etc.) reassures children of their importance and the concern that the hospital staff shares for their ultimate recovery.

Postoperative Teaching and Play

Equally significant for the child's recovery and emotional health is the opportunity to complete the experience with directed postoperative play. Children who are normally very active find the various constraints placed on them because of surgery and recovery difficult. For many, their coping behavior was some form of physical activity that is now denied. One therapeutic alternative is art in all its various forms. The nurse might need to protect such things as a cast or surgical dressing with a plastic cloth, but the child should then be allowed full expression of feelings with paints, clay (Play-Doh®), or crayons (see Table 19-3).

Other forms of expressive and aggressive play can be used as well. Art, however, is often the only means of communication for the child concerned with the surgical experience. The child might discuss the picture drawn or figure created, but if that is too difficult, much can be conveyed nonverbally through using the materials that lend clues to the child's impressions and ability to handle this recent experience.

Even though the child is well prepared for surgery and the postoperative phase, the reality of the experience is often quite different from what was expected. Actually coping with the strange sights, smells, and noises; the pain and limitations; and alterations in body integrity is much more difficult than thinking about having these problems occur in the future. The younger the child, the fewer the coping strategies and the less able the child is to conceptualize the changes and what they will mean. Fantasies and fears increase, and the child's reality becomes increasingly distorted. Younger children become convinced that this experience can only be justified as retribution for some wrong they committed. As a result, they might become passive and compliant or angry and anxious.

It is essential that the nurse be sensitive to the behavioral changes of children following surgery and various procedures. Behavior such as increased irritability, crying, regression, temper tantrums, nail biting, bed wetting, nightmares, passivity, withdrawal, and dependence are the child's way of asking for assistance to cope with the demands and traumas of hospitalization.

Parents need to be included in discussions about the child's behavior and possible reasons for the changes in response to surgery. The parent who understands why the child is expressing fears and concerns in certain behaviors and understands that the child's perception of these events is governed by developmental stage is able to be more supportive and can help the child cope. The nurse can offer suggestions on ways to incorporate therapeutic play into daily activity. Over time, therapeutic play will give the child an opportunity to express the fears, concerns, feelings, and fantasies that were and often continue to be overwhelming. Nurses might initially need to serve as role models for the parents in using games, puppets, art, or other forms of expressive play to facilitate communication.

Children who are helped to cope with events after they happen and are prepared for them beforehand are less anxious and better able to mobilize their energies toward recovery. Postprocedural play and teaching sessions as well as preprocedural teaching therefore should be a part of each child's hospital experience. Teaching sessions help to maximize growth by reducing stress and encouraging mastery of the experience.

Discharge Preparation

Preparation for returning home begins when the child is admitted. The initial assessment provides information about the family such as composition and roles, strengths, previous experiences with illness or hospitalization, understanding of the rationale for treatment, and fears and beliefs about health and illness. Using this as a guide, the nurse begins to plan the teaching and learning activities needed and begins to assess those who will need to be involved as teachers and as learners.

Some of the teaching can be accomplished by discussing a treatment or procedure and its rationale with the family while giving care. For example, when changing a dressing that will need to be changed again after discharge, the nurse's talking about what is done and why it is done begins to involve everyone in this aspect of routine care. By including the family from the beginning, learning takes place gradually and at a pace more accommodating to the needs of the learner.

This gradual process also creates an atmosphere conducive to asking questions. The family members feel more comfortable about mentioning their concerns or asking about some aspect of care. They have the opportunity to observe and to think through their management of care when the child returns home. The transition from hospital to home will be much smoother for all concerned if there is this time to anticipate the changes that will have to occur in daily routines.

Teaching plan In addition to this informal teaching, the nurse needs a structured plan. Information needed by the family regarding the child's care should be identified, and

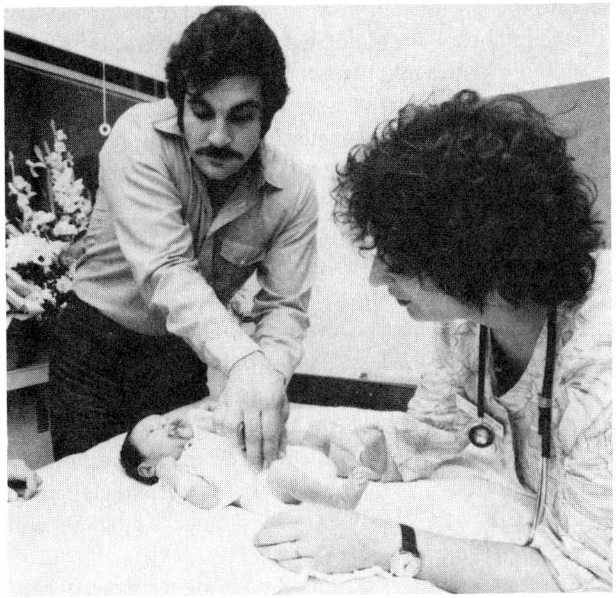

In supervising a return demonstration, the nurse teaches the primary caregiver to assume responsibility for the child.

someone, ideally the nurse responsible for planning care, organizes and coordinates the teaching. This teaching plan is adapted to the family and made specific to the family's situation and learning needs.

Included in the teaching plan are all of the physical, psychosocial, and developmental aspects of care the child requires. Beginning with observation, written information, and discussion of any procedure and then advancing through a step-by-step presentation and return demonstration, the family begins to assume responsibility for various aspects of care. When one procedure is well learned, another can be introduced. In this way, the family assumes more and more of the care for the child until family members feel confident and well prepared to continue at home.

If family members have had previous experience with necessary procedures, they should be encouraged to continue doing them during hospitalization. The nurse assesses their performance, compliments them, and, if necessary, adds suggestions or corrections.

Physical aspects of discharge preparation Physical aspects of discharge preparation might include dressing changes, cast care, and assessment of complications or recurrence of illness. Provision for changes in the activities of daily living is another aspect of physical care that has implications for teaching. Some children have an increased need for assistance in doing things formerly self-managed such as bathing, hair care, dental hygiene, and dressing. Safety factors and any adaptations according to activity restriction need to be taught. Sometimes the child's room needs to be changed if negotiating stairs or reaching a bathroom is a problem; at other times rearranging furniture and redirecting traffic flow are needed.

The nurse guides the family in thinking through these details and thereby facilitates the transition from hospital to home and lessens potential frustrations, surprises, and aggravations. Some families need the help of outside resources to meet the child's physical needs. The nurse carefully assesses requirements and plans for referrals where outside help is needed after discharge.

The nurse also reminds the family to include the child in family activities once the child has returned home. Family members should eat together, if this is their pattern, and should spend some time socializing, whether it be playing a game or talking. If the child is unable to join family members where the family usually eats, the nurse might suggest that the family or a family member eat with the child wherever this is possible. If the child has dietary restrictions, all members of the family might wish to adopt, at least temporarily, the new diet.

Discussing the child's nutritional needs and providing for them in a way compatible with the family lifestyle and individual food preferences is a nursing responsibility that should be addressed as soon as these needs are known. It is, of course, very difficult for the family to insist on good nutrition at home if a child has been allowed to eat "junk" foods at the hospital.

Psychosocial aspects of discharge preparation Providing for the child's needs presents a challenge if activity is retricted for a period of time. Sometimes special arrangements need to be made with the school for a home teacher. Some children need additional tutoring before reentering the classroom, and some are able to reenter without difficulty.

Immobilized children become bored easily, and planning activities and diversions for them at home demands forethought and creativity. Children who feel well but must refrain from usual activities present a special challenge. Arranging for release of energy in constructive ways that include a child's hobbies and pastimes is essential for emotional health. Nurses need to discuss these facts with the family, to provide ideas compatible with the child's interest that can be managed by the family, and to give the family information about resources in the community such as transportation aids, bookmobile availability, or children's programs.

Arranging for peer group contact and activities is another area for which plans should be made before discharge. The family needs answers to questions about a child's restrictions and the feasibility of having friends and relatives visit. How many at a time, what time of day or evening, and for how long are among the questions that should be discussed with the family and answered before discharge. In warm weather, it might be possible to have the child spend time outdoors, which facilitates peer group involvement. If restriction is minimal, the child might be able to join the activities of peers. Safety becomes a primary concern in determining what might or might not be an appropriate activity.

Developmental aspects of discharge preparation After discharge, children often show reactions to their hospital stays. With pain, with such frightening experiences as invasive procedures and surgery, and with separation and possible misinterpretation of intentions and actions of staff and parents, children experience after-effects of hospitalization. These reactions can be annoying, frightening, or confusing to parents. Children's reactions then need to be handled in a manner conducive to growth.

Parents should understand that the infant's patterns of feeding, napping, and waking are often disrupted by hospital routines. The child who previously slept through the night is likely to awaken for a time following hospitalization. Stranger anxiety might be more pronounced, and separation fears can increase. A child might seem overly dependent and constantly seek the reassurance of parental presence. Leaving the child with a sitter might meet with tremendous protest. Children might regress in toilet training or weaning from bottle to cup, behaviors that are upsetting to parents. A child's behavior tends to be either more negative and disruptive or quiet and withdrawn.

The child who interpreted hospitalization as punishment might feel wronged or afraid of again being "bad" and thus repunished. Children feeling wronged by their hospitalization tend to punish parents for causing or allowing the seemingly unjustified hardships of hospitalization. They might be aloof and hesitant to allow parental closeness and affection. They might seem angry and might talk back to parents. Parents need to understand these reactions so that they remain loving and available to the child. They can teach by their actions and words that hospitalization was not a punishment. They can try to reteach the reasons for the child's hospitalization. Such reassurances also help the children who thought they were "bad." When minor transgressions seem to evoke excessive fear of punishment or when children are uncharacteristically weepy, hearing and understanding the real reasons for hospitalization will often have dramatic effects.

Similar reactions occur with siblings of hospitalized children. Particularly vulnerable are children in early or middle childhood whose younger siblings have been hospitalized. These children often believe that thoughts cause events. They might have had less-than-loving thoughts about sharing their parents and home with the new baby, or they might have wished out of the way the younger sibling who disrupts their play and life. If this younger child then suffers illness or injury, older siblings might feel responsible and guilty. Reassurance that the child's illness was not the sibling's fault relieves the guilt.

The better prepared parents are for the reactions of children after hospitalization, the better they can deal with the situation. The family can avoid unnecessary tension and can help the child use hospitalization as an experience that leads to growth and development. The family that knows the care plan and has anticipated and planned for possible events is well prepared for the child's discharge. The more confident the family is in knowledge and ability to provide for the child's needs, the fewer problems family members will encounter.

Although most children adjust to treatments and supportive nursing interventions, some do not. They might require the help of counseling or therapy to cope and grow through the experience. In addition to careful teaching, the nurse gives the family several resources that can be contacted if a question or problem arises. Resources might also be needed for the purchases of any supplies or appliances or the rental of equipment. Providing families with written instructions and diagrams and telephone numbers of resources to use when questions arise adds to their security and self-confidence. Including the child, when appropriate, in the plans for home care also aids in cooperation and provides a healthy perspective about recovery.

Essential Concepts

- Illness and hospitalization are stressful for the child and family and might lead to a crisis in which previously learned coping strategies are not adequate for dealing with the perceived threat.
- The indicators of stress and coping in children include regression, somatic complaints, direct expression of emotion, expressive behaviors, and cognitive approaches.
- The extent to which a child's coping strategies are adaptive rather than maladaptive depends on the child's developmental stage, previous experience, and perception of the threat posed by the illness.

- Rooming-in of parents, especially when the hospitalized child is in infancy or early childhood, can help to offset the effects of separation.
- The indicators of ineffective family coping include anxiety, family disorganization, inadequate communication, and inadequate support systems.
- Children progress from viewing illness as punishment in early and middle childhood to understanding infectious agents and exposure in late childhood to recognizing a variety of interrelated factors in adolescence.
- Separation anxiety is an extreme reaction to the perceived loss of a parent and is most common in infancy and early childhood, until the child learns that the parent will return.
- Without appropriate interventions, separation in infancy progresses through three distinct stages, leading to withdrawn behaviors and lack of interest in human contact.
- In later infancy and early childhood, the child's developing mobility and sense of autonomy are greatly threatened by restraints or confinement.
- Infants and young children fear painful procedures and associate people, colors, or surroundings with pain.
- In early childhood the child's mastery of new skills often is threatened by hospitalization and normal regression.
- In middle childhood children are uncomfortable with changes in body function or appearance and often become anxious about invasive procedures and procedures involving the genital area.
- From middle childhood on, children learn to use developing cognitive skills to cope with separation from family, school, and peers.
- In middle to late childhood, children fear body disfigurement and might react with anger, frustration, or depression when faced with loss of control.
- In late childhood children use cognitive skills to control emotions and cope with separation and loss of function; therefore, nursing interventions focus on providing opportunities for discussion and problem solving.
- Older children and adolescents are especially fearful of long-term disabilities, possible death, and procedures that affect the genital area.
- Older children and adolescents might react to separation from peers as much as from parents and therefore might benefit from contact with friends outside the hospital and with other patients.
- The need for independence makes change of body image and function especially threatening for the adolescent, who often depends on the norms of a peer group to reinforce self-concept.
- Nursing care for children of all ages involves providing as much independence as possible, monitoring sensory needs, planning opportunities for learning, and maintaining social contacts, both with family members and with others.
- Nursing interventions are planned to enhance coping by facilitating understanding and age-appropriate expression, enhancing family communication, and preparing the child and family for the real or perceived threats of illness.
- Parental perception of a child's illness depends on its onset, likely outcome, extent of long-term limitations for the child, and possible feelings of guilt or anger.
- In assessing the effect of a child's illness on the family, the nurse observes family interactions and communication, family roles, and changes in the family's usual level of functioning.
- The nurse assesses the parents' relationship with each other and adapts interventions to the assessment criteria and to the family configuration.
- Parents need accurate, consistent information and might need to hear it repeated until they are ready to comprehend it.
- Family participation in the care of an ill child helps to maintain family functioning and to provide siblings with as much involvement as possible, which helps to offset the jealousy that siblings often feel.
- For hospitalized children, play is a way of coping with fears and anxieties, exerting some control over the environment, learning about treatments and procedures, and communicating concerns to the staff.
- In the hospital setting, play facilitators might include the play therapist, who is responsible for designing and directing a play program, as well as the nurse, who makes use of play in the process of nursing care.
- Therapeutic play is the means by which the child communicates fears and concerns; it is distinctly different from play therapy, which is a form of psychotherapy designed to promote the child's insight into behavior.
- In the process of therapeutic play, the nurse observes the child's use of materials, looks for recurring themes, analyzes the child's comments, validates conclusions, coordinates care, plans interventions, and evaluates results.

- Play activities during hospitalization should be fun, age appropriate, similar to play at home, and matched with the child's abilities during the hospital stay.
- Play in the hospital should provide the child with diversion, creative outlets, expression of feelings, and opportunities to learn about procedures.
- In observing the child's choice and expression of play, the nurse can identify areas of concern and plan interventions to address the child's emotional needs.
- Expressing feelings about treatments, procedures, equipment, and hospital staff provides the child with a way of controlling the experience and resolving fears.
- For children who are immobilized, the nurse looks for opportunities to adapt play activities to provide the child with a sense of control.
- Child and family teaching need to be individually planned to facilitate adjustment to hospitalization and to promote health after discharge.
- The first steps in child and family teaching are assessing what the child and family know and determining what they need to know, discussing what most concerns them, and identifying usual coping strategies.
- Teaching for both parents and children requires honest explanations, appropriate limits, a stated purpose, carefully chosen words, time between sessions, adjustment for developmental stage, and reinforcement of learning.
- Preparation for specific procedures or treatments should be individually designed, include opportunities for play, and describe the sensations the child will experience.
- The timing and content of preadmission teaching should be age appropriate and specific to the hospital and should involve as much parental participation as possible.
- Because preadmission teaching does not always bring reassurance, nurses need to assess anxiety levels and identify specific needs for additional preparation and emotional care.
- Hospital orientation includes touring the facilities on the unit, acquainting the child and family with the space allotted to them, and respecting their needs for personal possessions and privacy.
- Parents should always be included in preoperative preparation and postoperative care and might choose to take part in preoperative play and age-appropriate explanations of procedures and anticipated bodily changes.
- Discharge preparation requires assessment of physical, psychosocial, and developmental needs.
- In preparing the child and family for discharge, the nurse's teaching plan may include step-by-step demonstrations; recommended changes in the home environment; and adjustments in nutrition, behavioral expectations, and activity patterns.

References

Azarnoff P, Hargrove C (editors): *The Family in Child Health Care.* Wiley, 1981.

Azarnoff P, Woody PD: Preparation of children for hospitalization in acute care hospitals in the United States. *Pediatrics* (Sept) 1981; 68(3): 361–368.

Beverly B: The effects of illness upon emotional development. *J Pediatr* 1936; 8: 533–543.

Bibace R, Walsh ME: Development of children's concepts of illness. *Pediatrics* (Dec) 1980; 66(6): 912–917.

Bowlby J: Some pathological processes set in train by early mother-child separation. *J Ment Sci* 1953; 99: 265–272.

Johnson JE, Kirchoff KT, Endress MP: Altering children's distress behavior during orthopedic cast removal. *Nurs Res* 1975; 24: 404.

Kunzman L: Some factors influencing a young child's mastery of hospitalization. *Nurs Clin North Am* 1971; 18: 625.

Meng AL: Parents' and children's reactions toward impending hospitalization for surgery. *Matern-Child Nurs J* (Summer) 1980; 9: 83–98.

Meng A, Zastowny T: Preparing for hospitalization: A stress inoculation training program for parents and children. *Matern-Child Nurs J* 1982; 11: 87–94.

Pontious SL: Practical Piaget: Helping children understand. *Am J Nurs* (Jan) 1982; 82: 114–117.

Prugh DG et al: A study of the emotional reactions of children and families to hospitalization and illness. *Am J Orthopsychiatry* 1953; 23: 70–106.

Robertson J: *Young Children in Hospital.* 2nd ed. Tavistock, 1970.

Tesler M, Savedra M: Coping with hospitalization: A study of school-age children. *Pediatr Nurs* (March/April) 1981; 7: 35–38.

Triplett J, Arneson S: The use of verbal and tactile comfort to alleviate distress in young hospitalized children. *Res Nurs Health* 1970; 2: 17–23.

Williams PD: Children's concepts of illness and internal body parts. *Matern-Child Nurs J* (Summer) 1979; 8(2): 115–123.

Wood S: School-aged children's perceptions of the causes of illness. *Pediatr Nurs* (March/April) 1983; 9: 101–104.

Additional Readings

Adom D, Wright A: Dissonance in nurse and patient evaluations of the effectiveness of a patient-teaching program. *Nurs Outlook* (Feb) 1982; 30:132–136.

Algren CL: Role perception of mothers who have hospitalized children. *Child Health Care* 1985; 14(1):6–9.

Alterescu V: What do you teach the patient? *Am J Nurs* 1985; 85(11):1250–1253.

Atkins DM: Evaluaton of a preadmission preparation program: Goals clarification as the first step. *Child Health Care* 1981; 10(2):48–52.

Beckemeyer P, Bahr JE: Helping toddlers and preschoolers cope while suturing their minor lacerations. *Am J Matern-Child Nurs* (Sept/Oct) 1980; 5:326–330.

Betz CL: After the operation—postprocedural sessions to allay anxiety. *Am J Matern-Child Nurs* 1982; 7(4):260–263.

Betz CL, Poster EC: Incorporating play into the care of the hospitalized child. *Issues Compr Nurs* 1984; 7(6):343–355.

Birchfield ME: Nursing care for hospitalized children based on different stages of illness. *Am J Matern-Child Nurs* (Jan/Feb) 1981; 6:46–51.

Bolig R, Fernie D, Klein E: Unstructured play in hospital settings: An internal locus of control rationale. *Child Health Care* 1986; 15(2):101–107.

Craft MJ: Validation of responses reported by school-aged siblings of hospitalized children. *Child Health Care* 1986; 15(1):6–13.

Cummette BD, Mills HH, Beale AV: One latency-age child's coping with hospitalization. *Matern-Child Nurs J* (Fall) 1984; 13(3):167–175.

Denholm CJ: Hospitalization and the adolescent patient: A review and some critical questions. *Child Health Care* (Winter) 1985; 14(2):109–116.

Dorn LD: Children's concepts of illness: Clinical applications. *Pediatr Nurs* (Sep/Oct) 1984; 10(5):325–327.

Ellerton ML, Caty S, Ritchie J: Helping young children master intrusive procedures through play. *Child Health Care* 1985; 13(4):167–173.

Erikson, E: *Childhood and Society*. Norton, 1950.

Etzler CA: Parents' reactions to pediatric critical care settings: A review of the literature. *Issues Compr Nurs* 1984; 7(6):319–331.

Gohsman B, Yunck M: Dealing with the threats of hospitalization. *Pediatr Nurs* (Sept/Oct) 1979; 5:32–35.

Hahn K: Therapeutic storytelling: Helping children learn and cope. *Pediatr Nurs* 1987; 13(3):175–178.

Hansen BD, Evans ML: Preparing a child for procedures. *Am J Matern-Child Nurs* (Nov/Dec) 1981; 6:392–397.

Hunsberger M, Love B, Byrne C: A review of current approaches used to help children and parents cope with health care procedures. *Matern-Child Nurs J* (Fall) 1984; 13(3):145–165.

Huth MM: Guidelines for conducting hospital tours with early school-age children. *Pediatr Nurs* (Nov/Dec) 1983; 9:414–415.

Klein C: Going home. *Pediatr Nurs* (Sept/Oct) 1980; 6:59–60.

Knafl KA, Dixon DM: The participation of fathers in their children's hospitalization. *Issues Compr Nurs* 1984; 7(4–5):269–281.

Kubly LS, McClellen MS: Effects of self-care instruction on asthmatic children. *Issues Compr Nurs* 1984; 7(2–3):121–130.

Lambert SA: Variables that affect the school-age child's reaction to hospitalization and surgery. *Matern-Child Nurs J* (Spring) 1984; 13(1):1–18.

La Montagne L: Children's preoperative coping: Replication and extension. *Nurs Res* 1987; 36(3):163–167.

Lentz M: Selected aspects of deconditioning secondary to immobilization. *Nurs Clin North Am* (Dec) 1981; 16:729–737.

Mather PL: Serendipitous findings from a pilot project on preparation of healthy preschoolers. *Child Health Care* (Fall) 1984; 13(2):82–84.

McLeavey KA: Children's art as an assessment tool. *Pediatr Nurs* (March/April) 1979; 5(2):9–14.

Meer P: Using play therapy in outpatient settings. *MCN* 1985; 10:378–380.

Miles MS, Spicher C, Hassanein RS: Maternal and paternal stress reactions when a child is hospitalized in a pediatric intensive care unit. *Issues Compr Nurs* 1984; 7(6):333–342.

Nelson M: Identifying the emotional needs of the hospitalized child. *Am J Matern Child Nurs* (May/Jun) 1981; 6:181–183.

Parish L: Communicating with hospitalized children. *Canad Nurs* (Jan) 1986; 82(1):21–24.

Petrillo M, Sanger S: *Emotional Care of Hospitalized Children*. 2nd ed. Lippincott, 1980.

Piaget J: *Play, Dreams, and Imitation in Childhood*. Norton, 1952.

Pidgeon J: Functions of preschool children's questions in coping with hospitalization. *Res Nurs Health* 1981; 4:229–235.

Pidgeon V: Children's concepts of illness: Implications for health teaching. *Matern-Child Nurs J* (Spring) 1985; 14(1):23–35.

Puskar K: Structure for the hospitalized adolescent. *J Psychiatr Nurs* (July) 1981; 19(7):13–16.

Rager PM, Vipperman JF: Childhood coping: How nurses can help. *Pediatr Nurs* (March/April) 1980; 6(2):11–18.

Riffee D: Self-esteem changes in hospitalized school-age children. *Nurs Res* (Mar/Apr) 1981; 30(2):94–97.

Riserchia EA, Bragg CF, Alvarez MM: Play and play areas for hospitalized children. *J Assoc Care Child Hosp* 1982; 10(4):135–138.

Ross DM, Ross SA: Teaching the child with leukemia to cope with teasing. *Issues Compr Nurs* 1984; 7(1):59–66.

Rothenberg MB: The unique role of the child life worker in children's health care settings. *Child Health Care* 1982; 10(4):121–124.

Rumfelt JJ: How five-year-old children perceive the role of the nurse. *Matern-Child Nurs J* (Summer) 1980; 9(2):13–27.

Savedra M, Tesler M: Coping with hospitalized children. *Pediatr Nurs* (March/April) 1981; 7(2):35–38.

Schmeltz K, White G: A survey of parent groups: Prehospital admission. *Matern-Child Nurs J* (Summer) 1982; 11(2):75–86.

Schuster CS, Ashburn SS: *The Process of Human Development*. Little, Brown, 1980.

Smith FB: Patient power. *Am J Nurs* (Nov) 1985; 85(11): 1260–1262.

Waidley E: Show and tell: Preparing children for invasive procedures. *Am J Nurs* (July) 1985; 85(7):811–812.

White JE: Special nursing needs of hospitalized children with learning disabilities. *Am J Matern-Child Nurs* (May/June) 1983; 8:209–212.

Youssef MHS: Self-control behaviors of school-age children who are hospitalized for cardiac diagnostic procedures. *Matern-Child Nurs J* (Winter) 1981; 10(4):219–277.

Zurlinden J: Minimizing the impact of hospitalization for children and their families. *MCN* 1985; 10(3):178–180.

Chapter 20

Principles of Nursing Care for the Hospitalized Child

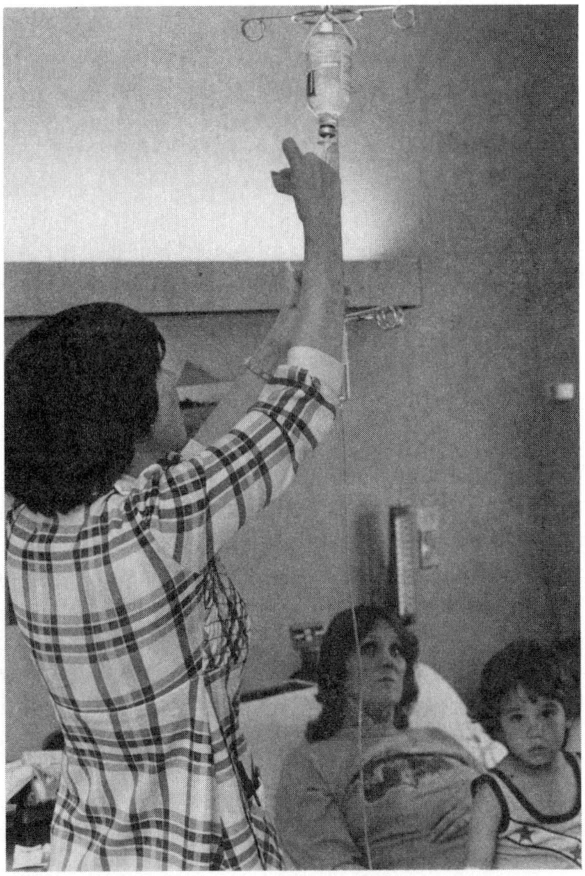

Chapter Contents

(Continues)

Objectives

- Describe potential threats to safety that hospitalization poses for a child.
- Define types of restraints and indications for their use.
- Describe principles of nutritional management for hospitalized children.
- Describe nursing care appropriate for the child who has an order for nothing by mouth.
- Explain methods of feeding hospitalized infants.
- Describe methods of increasing and limiting oral fluid intake.
- Delineate potential difficulties in elimination posed by hospitalization and nursing interventions that address these difficulties.
- Describe nursing care to promote sleep and rest in the hospital.
- List potential complications of immobility and nursing interventions to prevent them.
- Explain criteria for assessing pain in a child.
- Describe nursing care for pain relief in children.
- Describe nursing measures to manage the child with a fever.
- List criteria assessing for color, sensation, and motion assessment.
- Describe methods of collecting urine, stool, and blood specimens from children.
- Identify types of IV equipment and common sites for IV infusion.
- Explain the possible complications, safety considerations, and developmental needs associated with IV infusion.
- Compare the physiologic differences affecting dosage calculations in adults and children.
- Define dosage formulas used for medicating children.
- Describe methods of oral, topical, rectal, intramuscular, and intravenous administration of medications.
- Explain the components of psychosocial management in administering medications to children.
- Describe components of nursing care for children placed in isolation.
- Describe principles of postoperative care that are specific to children.

Nursing care to meet physiologic needs of hospitalized children is critical to both their emotional well-being and physical well-being. A child receiving optimal physical care is, within the limits of the child's condition, free to grow, express, develop, explore, and learn. The child has the opportunity to cope with and experience some mastery over the various stresses of hospitalization. The parent is freed from excess worry, frustration, or even anger and can deal more effectively with the stresses of the child's illness and need for support. As the nurse attends to the child's physical needs and thoughtfully carries out procedures, the parent is better able to use the nurse as a resource and for support.

All nursing care requires a careful assessment of the child's and family's physiologic and emotional needs. Nursing goals are to assist the child and family to regain health and maximum independence. Care is based on a thorough knowledge of the child and family before hospitalization, the child's physiologic problem, and the child's and family's responses to hospitalization. This care is far more likely to meet the needs of the child and family than care routinized for a child of a particular age or with a particular diagnosis. General principles of caring for the ill child provide a firm theoretic base that enables the nurse to assess the unique characteristics of individual children and their families.

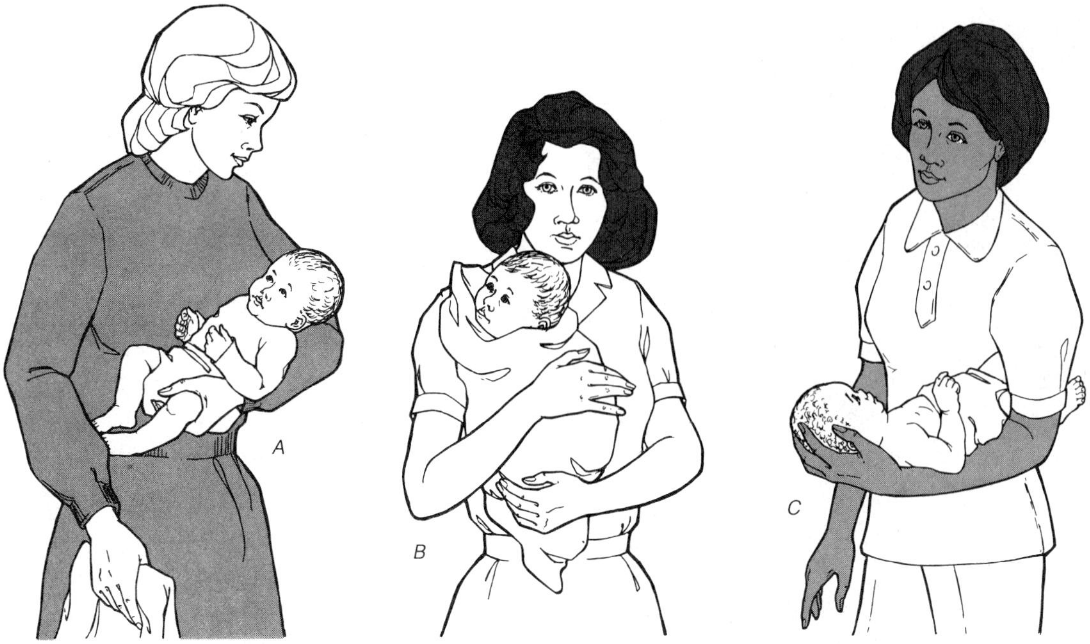

FIGURE 20-1
*Positions for holding an infant. **A.** Cradle hold, **B.** upright hold, and **C.** football hold. (From Ladewig PA et al:* Essentials of Maternal-Newborn Nursing. *Addison-Wesley, 1986.)*

Physiologic Needs of Hospitalized Children

Safety—Potential for Injury

Although safety is always important for adults who are responsible for children, the hospital presents special considerations. Whenever children are hospitalized, they are, by definition, removed from their familiar, usually comforting environment and are exposed to stress. These two factors alone make the child susceptible to accidents. The hospital environment also adds several obvious hazards for the child. In addition to the safety principles the nurse follows for any hospitalized person, certain safety considerations apply particularly to children.

Holding Because very young infants are unable to hold their heads erect, the nurse takes extra precaution to ensure that the head and neck are supported at all times to prevent injury. An infant is picked up from a lying position gently, making certain that head, shoulders, and neck are supported with one hand and the buttock with the other. By 4 months of age, an infant can hold the head erect with little effort. The nurse continues to be careful, holding and carrying all infants securely to prevent accidental falls.

The infant is carried close to the body, generally in one of three positions (Fig. 20-1). Infants with therapeutic equipment (eg, intravenous lines, oxygen cannulas, casts) might be carried more easily in the cradle hold, depending on the location of the equipment. The cradle hold allows for eye contact and provides a feeling of security. This hold allows the nurse to observe the infant's color and respiratory status easily and is the hold used most frequently for bottle-feeding.

The upright position is frequently used for burping the infant as well as for transporting from one location to another. The infant is cuddled closely, and because the hold requires two hands, the infant is very secure.

In the football hold, the infant is held securely, close to the nurse's hip. This hold might be favored for breastfeeding mothers because it permits relative freedom of the other hand, while providing security for the infant. The nurse uses this hold while washing the infant's hair. Like the cradle hold, it allows the nurse to observe the infant's status clearly.

Bathing Safety principles are important when bathing a child, to prevent burns, inadvertent water aspiration, and accidental falls. Infants can be immersed in bath water after

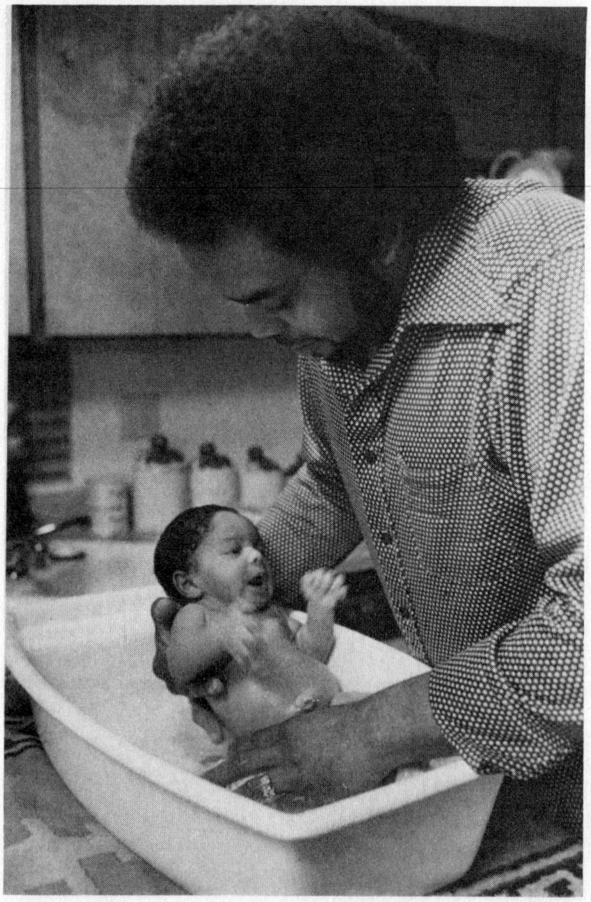

When bathing the infant, it is important to support the infant's head. (From Ladewig P et al: Essentials of Maternal-Newborn Nursing. *Addison-Wesley, 1986.)*

the cord has fallen off and healed (at approximately 2 weeks of age). The water temperature needs to be comfortably warm but not too hot. Water temperature that is comfortable to the wrist or elbow usually is a safe temperature for the infant or child.

The tub is filled with approximately 2–3 inches of water and placed on a firm, stable surface. The water level is sufficient to keep the infant warm while bathing but shallow enough to prevent aspiration should the infant squirm out of the nurse's or parent's grasp.

The infant is supported in the tub at all times with the nurse's forearm under the infant's head, neck, and shoulders and the nurse's hand holding the infant's upper arm. This position supports the infant's head, while ensuring a secure hold during the bath.

Older infants and toddlers can be bathed in large plastic tubs or in full-sized bathtubs on the unit. Children are assisted in and out of tubs and are encouraged to step over, rather than on the edge of the tub. Non-skid strips can be placed on the tub bottom to prevent slipping.

The nurse stays with all but the most responsible of children during the bath to observe the child's condition and prevent accidents. Bathtime can be fun for the child because it allows for limited water play. Safety, however, is the first consideration. After the bath, the child is wrapped in a warm towel, dried, and dressed immediately to prevent chilling.

Beds Cribs in the hospital are usually higher than they are at home. A young child able to climb out of the crib at home might have had the crib side rails left down to make climbing out relatively safer, or the child might have graduated to a bed. In the hospital this child might have to be placed in a crib with the side rails up to prevent roaming within or even out of the hospital. The child might be frustrated by the unaccustomed restraint to mobility and might try to climb over the raised side rails. A resultant fall onto the hard hospital floor could cause considerable injury. Children whose axillae come above the top of the side rail can pull up and tip themselves over the side of the crib. These children need to be protected from falls.

Infants learn to roll over suddenly, although within a predictable time period. Even when a parent seems certain that the infant is safe with the crib side left down, the nurse acts on the premise that the child could choose that moment to roll over for the first time. Even very young infants move about in their cribs. The nurse therefore protects the child by raising the crib rail to a stable position high enough to prevent the child from falling.

The most careful of parents have had their children roll off a surface when the parent either thought the child could not yet roll over or assumed that the child was too far from the edge to fall. For example, two parents were standing so as to block the open side of their child's crib and turned to talk to the nurses wheeling another crib into their child's hospital room. The child chose that moment to roll, rolled off the crib right between the parents, and landed head first on the floor. The child was immediately seen by a physician, had radiographs taken, and was carefully observed by the nursing staff. She was unharmed, but other children have not been as lucky. For this reason, the nurse keeps a hand on an infant whenever a crib side is lowered fully. Nurses also instruct parents to do the same both in the hospital and at home.

Beds on children's units are often high off the floor to facilitate nursing care and are frequently nonadjustable, preventing children from playing with their beds and incurring injury. A child either has a very big step when getting out of bed or has the use of a stool or chair as an aid. Either of these options is a new experience for the child. A child might forget when getting out of bed unassisted that it is

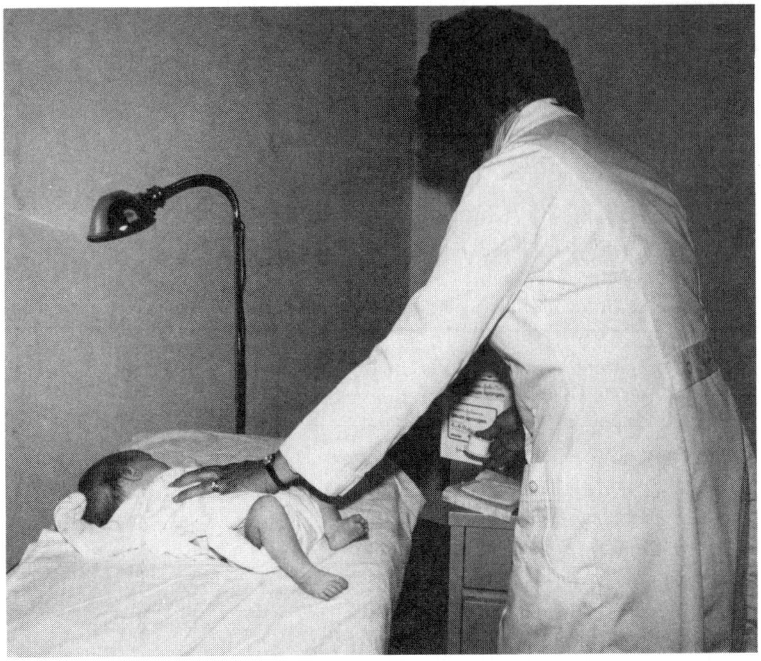

The nurse or parent keeps a hand on an infant whenever siderails are lowered or absent. (Photograph by Judy Koenig.)

necessary to take a large step or to step in the middle of the chair or stool. In either case, many children are prone to accidents at points in their hospital stays unless they accept help in an activity that is totally independent for them at home. They need to be carefully taught to keep themselves safe in the hospital. They also need to be assured of their independence in other areas and need to feel that the assistance is temporary.

Medications and equipment Medications and equipment present special hazards in the hospital. Medications or small objects left in a bedside stand can be taken out and left within reach of a child by other staff members, parents, other children, or the child. In one instance, a hospitalized 4-year-old was given a dime, and the dime was put away safely in the bedside stand. The next time the dime was seen, it was wedged between two of the child's back teeth. Luckily, the dime was not lodged in the child's airway, and with considerable effort it was safely removed.

The reach of children is much longer than it seems to be, and nurses cannot assume that something is safely out of reach merely because the child appears to be a safe distance away. Whenever introducing a child to an area and especially when leaving a child unattended, the nurse thoroughly checks the area for all the elements of safety. The same principles apply whether the child is in bed for a nap or in bed for the night.

When a child is out of bed, the nurse needs to be aware of all safety hazards in the general environment. Making a children's unit "child-proof" is difficult enough, but many children are hospitalized in locations with no specific unit for children. A few additional questions are then in order. Are all external and cleansing solutions out of reach? Are medications, syringes, and needles either locked away or constantly supervised? Are electrical outlets covered when not in use? Anything that must be left plugged in should ideally be locked in so that little fingers cannot unplug equipment. Are laundry chutes supervised or locked? Are treatment rooms accessible? Can the child open doors, such as bathroom doors, when necessary?

Intravenous administration and oxygen therapy equipment pose special problems. Use of IV equipment requires nursing attention to safety and mobility (see p. 611). Oxygen therapy involves special equipment and specific acute-care needs (see Chapter 22).

Restraints Many different kinds of restraints are used to help ensure the maintenance of necessary therapy and the safety of children. Although restraints interfere with a child's freedom, mobility, and independence, they are sometimes necessary. Most nurses and parents intensely dislike restraining a child, and young children often find the loss of control stressful.

As long as the child's safety can be maintained without restraint, this is preferable by far. If a child leaves an IV or nasogastric tube alone as long as a parent or nurse is by the crib or bed or if a child will not try to climb out of bed when someone is nearby, then the child can play and rest unre-

TABLE 20-1 Methods for Restraining Children

Restraint/Use	Procedure	Rationale	
Mummy			
Infants For comfort, scalp vein IV, NG tube	Arms in anatomic position as blanket/sheet is wrapped around each shoulder and arm, lower portion allows for leg extension, position on side allows for oral drainage	Prevents undue discomfort and strain on arms and joints Maximizes mobility within the restraint while still providing comfort of close wrapping Secretions or vomitus could be aspirated if child's position prevents drainage	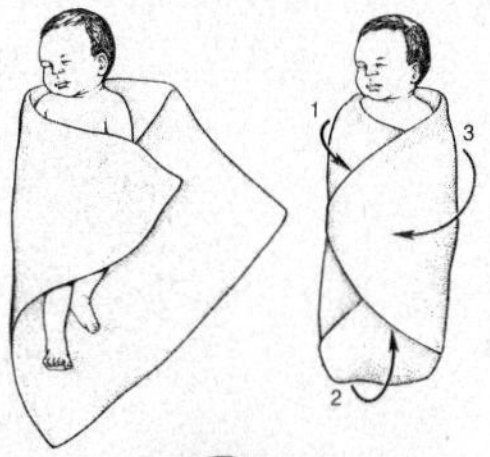
Safety straps			
Child of any age Prevents child's falling from a cart, chair, or frame	Folded sheet or strap firmly secured Large hospital gown may be used over clothes Ends of straps tied in back of a chair (high chair or stroller) Child checked very frequently	Child might climb or fall from go-carts, guerneys, high chairs, infant seats, feeding tables, orthopedic frames Child might slip within restraint, endangering airway or circulation Child might fall	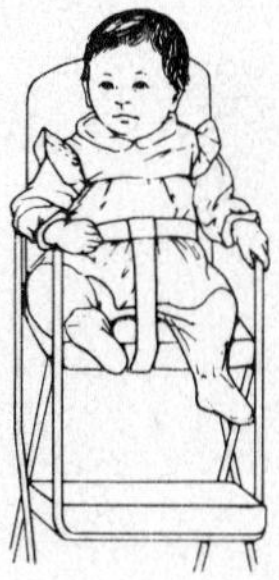
Bed cradle			
Older infant and child Protects lower part of the body from pressure of bedding and from child's hands	Cradle padded with a sheet or bath blanket secured with pins Hospital gown may be spread over the cradle and pinned to cover	Protects child from metal of bed cradle and provides some privacy Keeps gown off the child's body and provides privacy Pinning gown may be enough to keep child's hands from touching surgical site or from scratching irritated skin	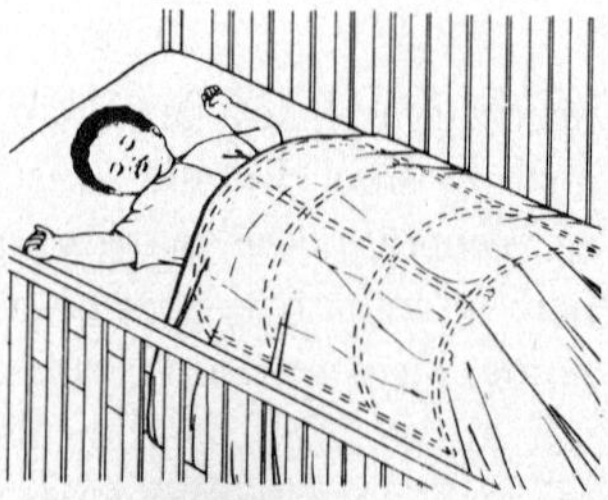
Elbow			
Child of any age Prevents flexation of elbows and thus touching of face, scalp, IV and other tubes, cleft lip or palate repair, skin conditions of face and upper trunk	Sleeves must fit well Restraint must be secured with pins or straps Color, sensation, and motion of fingers must be checked frequently Restraints must be removed frequently for range of motion	Prevents flexion of elbow Keeps restraint in place Nerve damage is possible from pressure of restraint on the brachial area	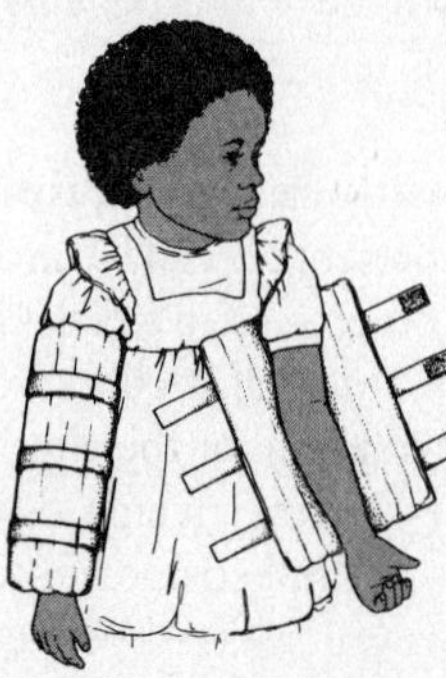
Bubble top and net-top crib			
Older infant and younger child Prevents falling and climbing out of crib	Bubble secured to ends of crib with clamps Net tight and secured to frame and legs of crib Side rails all the way up and secure	Firm attachment to frame of the crib allows child mobility and play without danger of dislodging the crib top With crib rails up and crib top tightly in place, child cannot climb out under the restraint	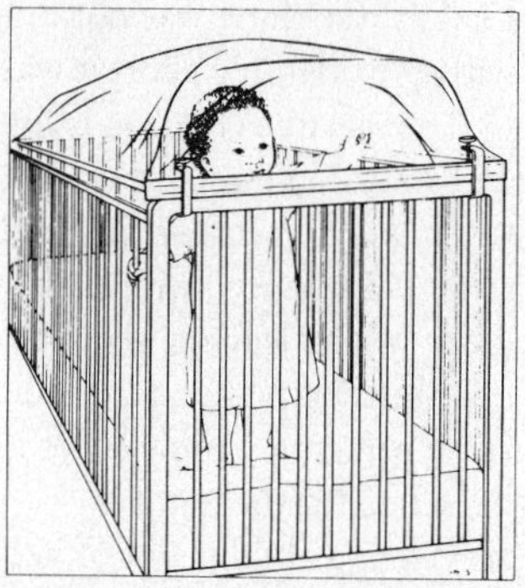

TABLE 20-1 *(Continued)*

Restraint/Use	Procedure	Rationale
Clove hitch		
Child of any age For restraining one or more extremities; for IVs, NG tubes, and other tubes; for prevention of self-injury	Extremity must be padded under each restraint	Restraint could irritate skin without padding
	Knot used must be a clove hitch	Knot will not tighten as the child pulls against the restraint (other knots could tighten and reduce circulation)
	Nurse checks to see whether the knot will tighten with a child's resistance or pulling	
	Restraint attached to frame of crib or bed with a slip knot	In emergency, nurse must be able to release the restraint quickly with one hand
		No pressure applied when side rail is lowered
	Limb distal to the restraint checked every 15 minutes and restraint released frequently—all at once or one extremity at a time	Prevents circulatory compromise

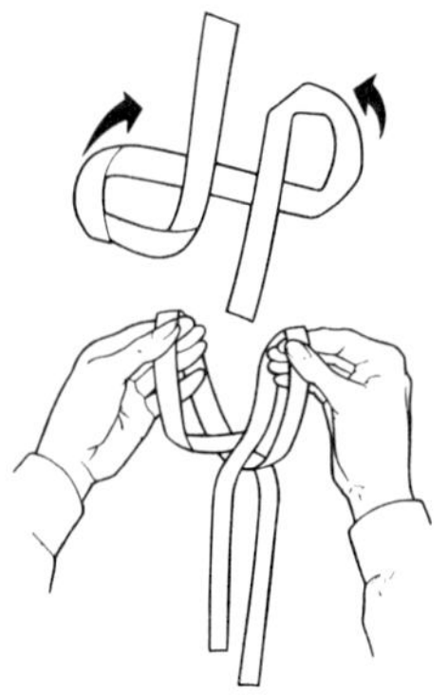

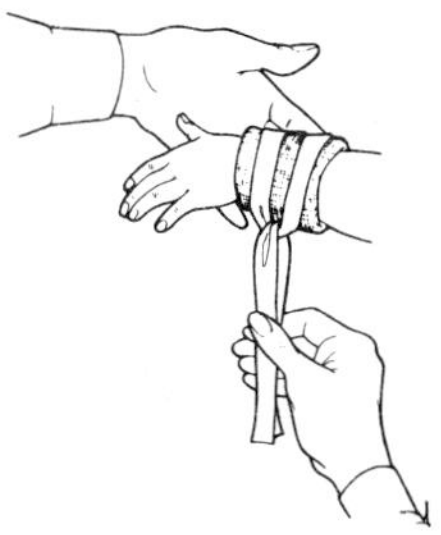

strained for part or all of the hospital stay. Unfortunately, a child is sometimes in danger if mobility is unrestricted. In these instances, some kind of restraint is needed. (Table 20-1 summarizes the characteristics of various restraints.)

Nutrition—Potential for Alterations

Many factors make eating and mealtimes difficult for hospitalized children. The first is the lack of routine and familiarity, which are critical to the young child's comfort. The food might also be quite different from food at home, either because of cultural variations or because preparation and selection differ.

Children hospitalized for illness and surgery often do not feel well enough to eat or drink what they need. They are frequently upset by hospital procedures and tests, and their feelings interfere with appetite and eating. Children who are ill or hospitalized lose control of much of their environment and lives. A child might need to control food intake as a means of feeling more whole and healthy, even when desire and refusal interfere with physical well-being.

For these reasons, nursing care for the nutritional well-being of the hospitalized child is many directional and multifaceted. Meeting the needs of the whole child and family in areas seemingly unrelated to food can help to ensure optimal food and fluid intake during a child's hospital stay.

The nurse first needs to obtain a thorough history of a child's and family's eating habits and preferences. In this way, nurses can better duplicate, whenever possible, a child's familiar and comfortable routine.

Mealtime itself provides an opportunity for assessment. The nurse can observe the child's eating habits, the foods the parent encourages, and the degree to which a parent allows a child developmentally appropriate independence. A child might regress when ill and in the hospital but might, on the other hand, be ready and anxious to help with self-feeding. A parent sometimes does not recognize or allow this development. The family's culture might allow or even encourage dependence of the ill child on others, and the nurse therefore talks with the parent to understand more fully the reasons for feeding methods. If families need and are ready to learn about children's capabilities, nurses can demonstrate these and encourage the parents to allow the children to develop further.

Nurses strive for optimal nutrition of the hospitalized child both for health and healing and for teaching sound nutritional practices to children and their families. Hospitalization can be a time to demonstrate principles of good nutrition and meal planning. Many times, however, diets of hospitalized children must be altered to ensure that food and fluids are easily assimilated or to encourage fluid intake. A child might be on a diet to meet short-term goals that would be unacceptable for growth and nutrition in the long run. A diet rich in juices, carbonated beverages, Popsicles, gelatin desserts, and ice cream might be easy for a child to accept and digest. It might also serve as a stepping stone from going without food and fluids to ingesting a regular diet, and it might be used to increase fluid intake in a child who needs large amounts of fluids. The reasons for the "unbalanced" diet must be explained to the child and family, lest they learn a negative lesson about the proper diet for a child.

The child who has nothing by mouth Mealtimes in the hospital are particularly significant and uncomfortable for one group of children—those who cannot eat. Some children have nothing by mouth (NPO) for a short period of time, as when they are awaiting surgery. Other children remain NPO for days or months while they are in the hospital. Watching, hearing, and smelling the preparation of food and the pleasant aspects of mealtime can be extremely painful for these children.

The child missing a meal because of impending surgery might be at least as upset as a child remaining NPO for an extended period of time. Many children have IVs started after anesthesia is induced, so thirst- and hunger-relieving fluid is withheld prior to surgery. A child on the children's unit waiting for surgery until 2 or 3 o'clock in the afternoon has truly suffered while surrounded by children, parents, and even staff eating and discussing food.

Many worries about impending surgery can become displaced on food. Although it may occasionally be helpful to distract children's attention from their upcoming surgery, it is usually preferable to deal directly with worries about surgery and distract attention from the discomforts of going without food.

Whether or not a child remains NPO for a morning or for months, the nurse assesses the effect of going without food on a child's physical and mental well-being. Children who are NPO need good mouth care. Some children can be trusted to brush their teeth and rinse their mouths without swallowing water. Others will need to have their mouths swabbed by the nurse with a damp washcloth or a prepackaged swab to ensure their not drinking any fluid.

Many children are upset when watching others eat. Some can be taken from their hospital rooms or even from their floors during mealtime. A nurse can wheel a bed to a playroom and engage a child in an art project or game or take a child for a walk in the hospital. For children who telephone out of the hospital to speak with family or friends, suggesting that they place a call during mealtime can help ease discomfort.

For the infant who must remain NPO, a major pleasure source and coping mechanism is thwarted. These children can be helped by being held and stimulated at regular intervals no fewer than if they were being fed. The child is allowed to suck on a pacifier unless there are medical contraindications. If a commercial pacifier is not available, one can be fashioned from a nipple stuffed with cotton or gauze and closed securely at the back with tape. Care must be taken to burp the NPO infant at intervals to allow the escape of any air sucked in from around the pacifier.

Feeding infants in the hospital The hospitalized infant's diet and feeding regimen are usually very similar to those at home. Formula and solid foods, if any have been introduced, will remain the same unless changes are indicated for therapeutic purposes, as when a child is recovering from anesthesia, has a gastrointestinal problem, or is not tolerating formula. If a child has been growing well and has remained healthy on the home diet, hospitalization is not the time to make a change.

A careful history shows what foods a child has been given and generally how the child has tolerated these foods. Because new foods should be introduced slowly and carefully during infancy so that parents can recognize allergies and ease the infant's adjustment to the change in taste or texture, no new foods should be introduced for taste or convenience when an infant is hospitalized. The nipple and bottle used need to be the same type as that used at home. This enhances feelings of familiarity for the child, encourages fluid intake, and also reinforces a parent's choices for the child.

A feeding period should not extend beyond 30 minutes because after 30 minutes the child fatigues and fluid intake is minimal. The time that the feeding ends also should not approach too closely the beginning of the next feeding.

Encouraging the hospitalized infant's growth and development during feedings mirrors what would be done at home. An infant is much more likely to be successful in holding a plastic bottle than a glass bottle. Formula can therefore be transferred from the glass bottle usually supplied to a disposable or sterilizable plastic bottle. When children can have some solid food, they can gain much pleasure in holding a biscuit or cracker during the feeding. They should never be left alone with the biscuit or cracker, however, because of the danger of choking. Older infants can sometimes use a spoon if they have considerable help.

After a feeding, an infant can, unless contraindicated by the condition, be bundled and placed on the right side to facilitate the rising of any air in the stomach. The chance of having food above the air is therefore minimized. Infants can also be placed in infant seats. The chair is helpful to the child who remains awake after feedings and can benefit from stimuli in the environment. It is also helpful and indicated for the child who regurgitates or vomits after a feeding. A child can at times be placed on the stomach after feedings, but to prevent aspiration in case of vomiting, a child is not left on the back.

The breast-fed infant Hospitalization can threaten the continuation of breast-feeding. Feedings might be missed, routines interrupted, and stress and fatigue can result in the mother's inconsistent eating and drinking. If a mother is planning to continue breast-feeding, the nurse can play a major role in its success. First, a mother needs to recognize and express her true feelings about breast-feeding. A nurse can sit with and listen to the mother as she talks about what the child's illness and hospitalization mean to her, what breast-feeding has meant to her, and what her plans for breast-feeding were before the child became ill.

The mother might wish to stop breast-feeding, and in most instances this will not adversely affect the child. Sometimes, however, a child needs to continue with breast-feeding if at all possible because of difficulty tolerating various formulas or the need for the security of minimal changes in routine. Often, mothers wish to continue breast-feeding but think this is difficult or impossible. A mother might need special provisions for privacy, ranging from assurance that she can nurse behind a curtain without being interrupted to the privacy of a special room in which to nurse. Although privacy is a rare commodity in the hospital, a suitable arrangement can usually be found.

Hospitalization of an infant, because it frequently shakes parental confidence and often leads to parental guilt, might undermine the assurance and ease crucial to successful breast-feeding. Helping the mother regain confidence facilitates breast-feeding. A nurse can assist the parent to resume care of the child. Showing parents how to pick up children who have scalp vein IVs, helping a parent hold a child with a burn, teaching about the reasons for and method of packing a wound, and pointing out the child's attachment to and recognition of the parent can all help with the continuation of breast-feeding.

The mechanics of breast-feeding are, however, difficult to maintain when a child is ill. A mother needs to drink, eat, and be rested, and the child needs to suck enough to maintain a somewhat steady demand for milk production. These criteria are rarely met when a child is hospitalized.

The nurse can help a mother recognize whether or not she is tired, hungry, or thirsty. The nurse can offer to keep a child close by or look in on a child more frequently so that the mother can take a break for the rest, food, and fluids she needs. It is helpful to ask a mother whether or not she has eaten, how much she is drinking, and whether she is rested. The mother might talk about any concerns with lowered milk production and, often for the first time, understand the connection between her health practices and production of milk. This realization tends to decrease dramatically worry and concern over her ability to produce enough milk for her baby.

When a child cannot suck to ensure continued milk production, the nurse can teach and/or provide the equipment for the mother to pump her breasts. Most women find an electric breast pump easier to use than a nonelectric model. One or more electric pumps may be in the hospital, especially if the hospital has a neonatal intensive care unit or a maternity division. The nurse can tell nursing mothers where these pumps are located and when the mother may use them.

For mothers who are unable to be at the hospital for every feeding but who wish their children to receive breast milk, an electric pump can be rented. Milk is pumped at home, frozen, and kept in the hospital for feedings when the mother is unable to be there. With lowered anxiety and such aids for expressing milk, most mothers who wish to continue breast-feeding their children can do so.

Women who choose to stop breast-feeding need to do so gradually whenever possible, phasing out one feeding for a few days or longer before stopping other feedings. Thus breast engorgement is kept to a minimum, and both mother and child have an opportunity to adjust. Ending breast-feeding is, for some women, a difficult emotional transition. Anything that the nurse can do to help breast-feeding continue during hospitalization can help reduce the stress of hospitalization for most mothers and children.

The bottle-fed infant The bottle-fed child also requires some special considerations when hospitalized. Some children, when at home, are left in their cribs with their bottles. This is an established pattern in certain households, although it is a questionable health practice because it encourages dental caries. Children in the hospital who are without the security of home and routine frequently do not receive sustained attention from their usual caregivers. For these reasons, children are held whenever possible while they are being fed through a bottle. Children can also be held when they are fed solid foods, though older infants usually prefer being placed in a high chair or at a feeding table.

Burping the hospitalized infant can be done using the upright hold or with the child sitting sideways on the nurse's lap. In this way, the child can be continually observed. As the infant is held on the lap, the chin and trunk are carefully supported with one hand and arm, and the nurse runs two fingers along either side of the spine with the other hand. This support of the chin and trunk allows a clear passage of air from the stomach. The fingers rubbing slowly but firmly up either side of the spine tend to make even very young infants' trunks straighten, thus encouraging the escape of air. An infant is burped frequently, at least

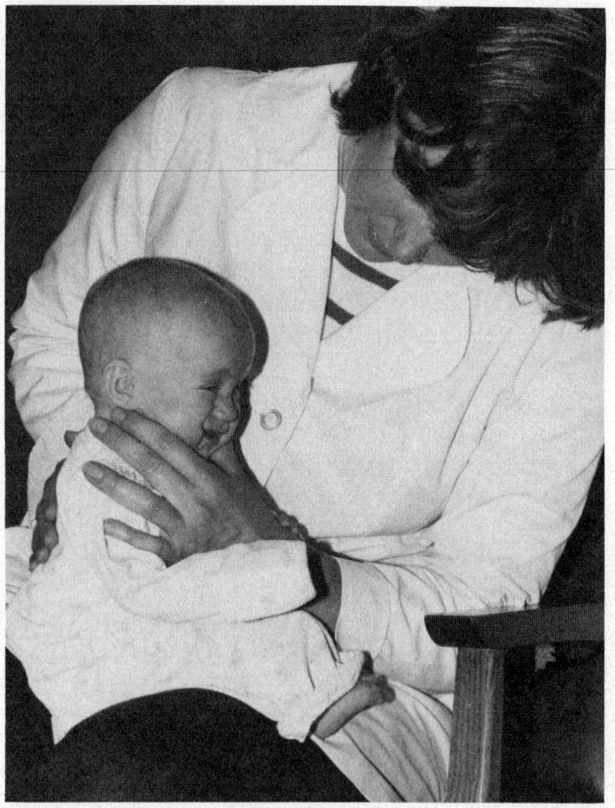

The infant is burped frequently to allow escape of air from the stomach and promote retention of the feeding. (Photograph by Judy Koenig.)

once midway through the feeding and again after the feeding, to prevent regurgitation.

Nutrition and the older hospitalized child The more similar mealtime in the hospital is to mealtime at home, the more likely a child is to perform as independently as possible and to eat the optimal quality and quantity of food. Appropriate independence and proper nutrition aid the child's physical and emotional well-being, the child's emotional and physical growth, and the child's physical healing. (Table 20-2 presents nutritional principles and nursing management for children.)

Companionship during meals is one of the most effective measures for encouraging children to eat. Arranging a child's food at a table where other children are eating; pulling some beds close together so that children on bed rest have company; or having parents, friends, or a nurse sitting with a child can bring dramatic changes in the child's attitude toward meals and food consumption. Talking with a child and creating a pleasant atmosphere with children and parents can help to diminish a family and child's anxiety. Creating a more homelike atmosphere thus helps a child to eat.

Sometimes, a child will eat better if there is a promise of an enjoyable activity after the meal. "We'll read a story after you finish" or "We'll play that game (or do a puzzle or draw a picture or go to the playroom) after you eat" are specific promises that might encourage the child.

The child and family need to know the consequences of a child's drinking or not drinking. If it is honest to say that an IV will remain in or that a child will not be discharged from the hospital until oral intake reaches a certain level, the child and family should be told this. Such statements are not threats or punishments if they are honest and presented without anger. Intravenous fluids are sometimes continued or restarted when a child's oral fluid intake is low. Children, especially after throat surgery, might not be discharged until they demonstrate that they can drink enough to meet their fluid needs. Child and family deserve to know the importance of fluid intake.

If the child is on intake and output measurement, all food and fluid is recorded immediately after meals and snacks. A sheet should be provided at the bedside. Recording exact quantities of fluids and liquid foods, measured in milliliters, is important. If the child is being monitored for solid food intake, the description of amounts needs to be accurate (eg, two cookies, one-half cup carrots).

Any meal should be appropriate to the developmental level and physical condition of the child. It should be easily reached and presented in appropriate portions, and all containers should be opened. The nurse needs to ensure that the food given to the child corresponds to any dietary restrictions or developmental considerations.

Limiting oral fluid intake For some children, the nurse helps restrict, rather than increase, fluids. Children starting fluids after surgery usually start with small amounts and progress to optimal fluid and calorie intake as their physical conditions allow. Some children cannot mobilize fluids well. The child with cardiac or renal problems, for example, might have a restricted fluid intake. Some children's gastrointestinal systems are unable to handle large amounts or even maintenance amounts of fluids.

Nursing management for these children will vary with the developmental level of the child. Despite a child's and family's understanding, accepting, and participating in the treatment plan, this aspect of the plan can be difficult to follow. The nurse can plan with the child and family when and how the child will be allowed fluids. The family then must not offer more than the child should have at a particular time.

Infants who are limited to 1 oz of fluids should be given a bottle containing only 1 oz of fluid. If more fluid is in a bottle or cup, a vigorous suck or momentary inattention to the amount consumed could mean that the child obtains too much fluid. This will risk overloading the gastrointestinal, renal, or cardiac system. In the same way, an older

TABLE 20-2 Interventions for Increasing Food and Fluid Intake in Children

Nutritional principle	Intervention
The eating environment needs to be as much like home as possible	Allow children to eat in high chairs, feeding tables, or at the table whenever possible. Make sure they are securely fastened into high chairs. Avoid feeding children in areas associated with pain. Encourage the parent to participate in feeding whenever possible
Children are more likely to eat foods that coincide with food preferences and choices	Allow children to choose meals from the menu. Have popular items such as peanut butter, bread, and jelly on the unit and available. Make ice cream milkshakes for children unable to eat and whose diets allow, in order to improve intake of protein and calories. Allow parent to bring in some food from home if the child has difficulty eating hospital food (be sure the food corresponds with the child's diet). Encourage jello, pudding, ice cream, frozen yogurt, and liked fluids when increased fluid intake is necessary ("forcing fluids").
Foods and fluids are more likely to be consumed if attractively served	Use decorated placemats, paper plates, or cups. Encourage the child to find the surprise picture at the bottom of a bowl, visible when all the food is gone. Cut sandwiches into decorative shapes. Use a child's tea set and allow the child to pour for everyone. Allow the child to use a straw. Flavor the milk if the child's diet permits.
Children are likely to eat more if food is served in small portions	Put small portions on a medium-sized plate and encourage seconds when the food is eaten. Fill drinking glasses only halfway and encourage the child to eat before drinking large amounts, unless increased food and fluid intake is crucial. Encourage the child to eat dessert after the meal, unless the dessert is particularly nutritious like custard or fruit. Bring small amounts of a variety of fluids to the child at frequent intervals during the day to increase fluid intake
Allow the child to eat independently	Allow the older infant to hold a cracker or spoon while being fed. Feed young children finger foods—small crackers, raw fruits and vegetables, small pieces of meat. (Cut hot dogs lengthwise first to prevent choking on round pieces.) Encourage children who are learning to eat to use utensils. Stay close by to observe or assist. Cut portions for the older child who is unable to do so, while acknowledging to the child that the help is temporary

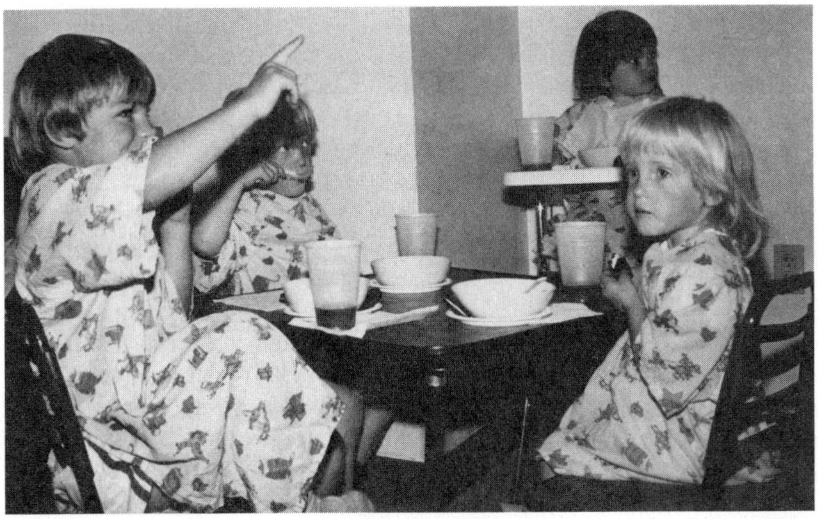

Companionship during meals is one of the most effective ways of encouraging children to eat. (Photograph by Judy Koenig.)

child should be offered no more than the child is allowed to drink. To offer more is tempting the child to rebel against the treatment plan and is truly unkind. It would emphasize what the child cannot have, whereas offering fluids that the child can finish emphasizes the positive aspects of following the plan. Children in late childhood and adolescence can usually plan their own fluid intake when they are given specific guidelines. Many will enjoy making charts outlining how they hope to meet their fluid goals.

Rewards for a child's appropriate restriction of oral intake are many. A child might notice feeling better, having increased activity tolerance, or exhibiting less edema if fluids are appropriately restricted. Some children will find cooperation easier with additional rewards. Spoken praise for a job well done, a star for reaching each small goal, a special food, or a special time with the nurse all encourage a child. Sometimes, withholding something is also appropriate. One nurse caring for an adolescent boy who was struggling to finish a liquid meal through wired jaws intercepted his mail and then gave him a letter for each significant amount he drank. It was effective in this particular situation in turning a pleading session into a joke and game for both child and nurse.

Elimination—Potential Alterations

The elimination patterns of children can be altered during hospitalization. The change might be related either to the stress of hospitalization or to the child's illness. Nursing care for these alterations reflects what is appropriate for the child's developmental stage and physical condition.

Needs of the younger child Many hospitals now supply disposable diapers for the infant, and most infants can use these without difficulty. Children who have developed rashes when disposable diapers have been used will, however, need cloth diapers. Usually these children have no difficulty if the nurse uses a cloth diaper to line a disposable diaper, making sure that the disposable diaper does not touch the child's skin. This practice protects the child's skin, and the outer plastic of the disposable diaper helps keep the child's bed from being changed as frequently as would be necessary if a cloth diaper were used alone.

Diaper rash is a common difficulty for any infant, hospitalized or not hospitalized. The nurse can use treatment measures that the child's parents have found helpful or can institute new practices when necessary (see Chapter 4). The nurse keeps the child as dry and as clean as possible, by frequently checking and changing the diaper and by carefully cleaning fecal matter from the child's skin. The child also benefits from having the affected area exposed to air when possible. This is easily done by putting the child in the prone position on an open diaper. When the anterior perineal area is irritated, the open-to-air method can still be used with a girl placed supine on an open diaper and a boy placed on his side with the diaper draped so that it will be likely to intercept urine.

Children are sometimes admitted to the hospital when they are in the process of being toilet trained or when bowel or bladder control have recently been achieved. The stresses of hospitalization cause many children to regress and temporarily to lose any recently acquired skill. A child who was previously dry and clean might, for example, begin to wet and soil. Because toilet training is an important milestone to both child and parent, any regression usually is very upsetting to the entire family. The nurse can help the family by supporting the child in maintaining as much continence as possible and by reassuring the child and teaching the parent that regression is common in such a situation.

Supporting a child's skills requires detailed knowledge about these skills, as obtained from assessment data. A child wearing diapers and a child wearing pants on admission might both be in the process of toilet training. Any child accustomed to using a toilet or a potty chair needs to know where these are located in the hospital and should know how to ask to use them.

Because the child's verbal skills and vocabulary are usually quite limited at the age of toilet training, the nurse learns from the parent and records on the nursing care plan the words the child uses to express toileting needs. Many parents help children in toileting by placing a child on the toilet or potty chair at specific times or after special cues from the child. If nursing staff can continue the parental practices, they will help to prevent unnecessary regression with its guilt and frustration for children and families.

Many children, despite support in toileting from family and nurses, do regress during hospitalization. The family needs to know that children frequently regress in skill levels when they are sick and hospitalized. After hospitalization, children will resume training when physically and emotionally ready. The child also needs to understand this problem. The nurse avoids scolding and making an issue of incontinence. Children needing diapers are told that diapers are all right for now and that they will wear pants again when they are able.

Needs of the older child Older children, secure in their urinary or bowel continence, also have difficulties with toileting during hospitalization. In various stages of development, children are very modest about toileting needs, words, and actions and are resistant to any exposure of their genitals. Many children in the hospital have their urine measured, need to give specimens of urine or feces, need to use a bedpan, or are asked whether they have had a bowel movement and to describe it.

Those who can use a bathroom unassisted have some privacy, although on many children's units the bathroom is off the main hall and even has a door that remains open. Many children cannot, for medical or safety reasons, use a bathroom independently. Some are too unsteady or groggy because of illness, medication, or recovery from anesthetic, and these children need the nurse's or family's assistance to ambulate to the bathroom. Asking for, waiting for, and accepting help can all be difficult. Once in the bathroom, some children need help to remain safely seated on the toilet.

Assisting while giving the child all possible privacy is a difficult task for the nurse. Nurses can physically support but look away from children; they can tell children that they are looking elsewhere; they can chat while assisting, which serves to distract a child and to assure with actions that the nurse is not concentrating exclusively on the child's toileting.

Many children are unable to get out of bed and use a toilet, and learning to use a urinal and bedpan is not always easy or natural for them. One 15-year-old boy had to remain in bed on the day of surgery and had not yet voided postoperatively. He told his nurse he did not need to void, but when he was asked to tell the nurse how to use the urinal, it was obvious that he did not know, was embarrassed to ask, and was afraid of wetting his bed. Repeated, simple, careful teaching about positioning the urinal and reassurance of privacy during voiding enabled this boy to void. For whatever reason—fatigue, effect of medication, pain, embarrassment—the child had not learned from previous teaching.

Some hospitalized children require catheterization or enemas. (Catheterization of the child is discussed in Chapter 28, and the procedures for enemas are discussed in Chapter 27.)

Sleep and Rest—Potential Disturbances

The hospitalized child has an obvious need for sleep to promote growth and restore health. Obtaining needed sleep and rest, however, is often difficult in the hospital. The hospital environment is new, different, often noisy, and without the usual security of home and routine. Most hospitalized children feel physically drained and uncomfortable even if they are not in actual pain, and sleep and rest are thus more difficult than usual. Children who are anxious or afraid find it difficult to trust the hospital environment.

The very inactivity of most hospitalized children is a dramatic contrast to their normal routines. A child used to burning off energy through vigorous physical activity rarely has the ability or opportunity to be as active in the hospital. Sleep comes slowly and sporadically to the child who is not physically tired.

Nurses sometimes overlook some simple areas for nursing management when planning care. One helpful intervention is to follow the child's bedtime routine as closely as possible, although several factors can interfere with this. For instance, nurses might find themselves ready to put children to sleep for the night and realize that they do not know the child's routine. A careful history is thus crucial on admission. The nurse might also find that the home routine is in some way contraindicated in the hospital. For example, a child accustomed to having a bottle before going to sleep cannot be allowed to follow this routine if the child has had oral surgery, is to receive limited fluids, or is NPO.

A nurse also might not feel it is possible to spend the time and energy needed to follow a child's bedtime routine. Many children are put to bed at home with a quiet story read or told to them or with a private conversation with someone they love. The nurse might feel far too busy to stop for any of these activities, but it is often more efficient to stop and read a short story than to quiet fretful, crying children who keep themselves and many other children awake. Furthermore, if children have felt somewhat secure at bedtime, obtain adequate rest, and feel more trusting of the hospital environment, they are likely to be more cooperative with nursing care.

The easiest and usually most satisfactory way to ensure close adherence to the child's bedtime routine is to have a parent available to the child. With young children, rooming-in is very beneficial. For the older child and those for whom rooming-in is not possible because of hospital policy and facilities or other demands on the parent, having the parent available to the child up to bedtime can provide the continuity that a child needs to relax and obtain needed rest. In middle childhood, children often appreciate the parent's presence, perhaps a kiss and being tucked in, and a story before going to sleep. Even in late childhood and adolescence, a child often appreciates the parent's being nearby.

To prevent injury from hard or sharp objects, only soft toys should remain in a child's bed or crib at bedtime. All objects purposefully removed from a child's bed must, of course, be truly out of reach. A child should be as comfortable as possible before going to sleep for the night. A high temperature or pain would ideally be relieved before bedtime. It might be possible to time an analgesic so that it will reach its peak when a child needs to sleep. Although nursing care does not mean withholding medication, a child might find adequate relief from noninvasive pain relief measures during waking hours, and it might be possible to time a medication for its effect at bedtime or naptime.

A child's feeling trustful rather than fearful is crucial to adequate rest. Nursing management to assist the child includes much that goes on at times other than bedtime. A child's preparation for procedures and ability to play out fears and fantasies aid the child's ability to rest. Keeping the child's sleeping area as nonthreatening as possible is also important, so that the child can use the space for rest. Painful or frightening procedures should, whenever possible, be done away from the child's bed. Finally, the nurse can attempt to plan the child's waking activities so that the child is tired at bedtime. This involves a creative use of play for the hospitalized child.

Immobility—Potential Complications

Immobility has multiple effects, both physiologic and psychologic, on a child. One of the most prominent characteristics of immobilized children, however, is their mobility. Many children confined to bed are hardly immobile. They scoot and slither, bounce and jump. Children asked to rest quietly can frequently be seen running, playing, and shouting with total abandon. Children in leg casts, for example, have climbed trees. Unless paralyzed or extremely developmentally delayed, either physically or emotionally, the immobilized child is to some degree mobile.

The general antidote for immobility is, within the confines of medical treatment plans and safety, mobility. Participation in self-care is one of the best ways to encourage increased activity. Activity should be purposeful and physically therapeutic and should encourage and stimulate self-respect. All activity encourages movement, with decreased pressure on the skin, increased muscle tone, increased lung expansion and venous return, and improved gastrointestinal and genitourinary function. These contribute to better health and faster recovery. Play, whether it be for fun and pleasure or expression and learning, also provides activity and growth. (See Standards of Nursing Care, the Immobilized Child.)

Pain—Alteration in Comfort

Any parent who has inadvertently jabbed a healthy infant with a diaper pin can attest to the child's immediate reaction of apparent outrage. Contrary to long-standing belief, research has shown that infants and children do feel and react to pain. Indeed, children might actually be less able than adults to tolerate pain.

Pain is experienced in two phases, depending on the nerve impulses generated. An immediate reaction to a painful stimulus in response to impulses is carried on myelinated nerve fibers. More prolonged pain is generated by impulses on unmyelinated nerve fibers (Franck, 1986). Infants and children, who have a high proportion of unmyelinated nerve fibers, clearly can experience prolonged pain.

Children's pain has emotional and developmental as well as physical components. Fear, anxiety, and deeply missing home and family are stressors that can increase the sensation of pain. Children often see pain as harmful or negative and they often fear bodily harm. Their thinking about pain tends to be immature, and they are unable to see pain as a helpful signal that something is wrong (*Children in Pain*, 1984). The child's experiences, therefore, contribute to pain, and pain then affects the whole child and the child's behavior.

Nurses need to keep an open mind about children's pain. Fears or misunderstandings that nurses have had about pain in children have resulted in less than optimal nursing care. Fears that children will be addicted to pain relievers administered on a short-term basis generally are unfounded. Inability to "read" the child's pain signals have led nurses to confuse pain with other sources of upset for the child. For example, the nurse might assume the child is crying in response to a parent's leaving, in response to hunger, or in response to other sources of discomfort.

Distraction is a powerful pain reliever, and children's reactions to distraction can confuse nurses. The effectiveness of distraction ceases, however, when the distraction ceases. Those children who can play wholeheartedly, even when experiencing postoperative or other pain, do attain temporary relief in this way. Nurses might forget, however, that the child needs additional pain relief measures when the distraction is over.

Assessment of pain To manage pain in children adequately the nurse needs to assess its presence accurately. Many children are unlikely to tell the nurse when they are in pain because they fear the nurse will give them an injection or because they're trying to be brave. Children see injections as additional sources of pain, and because the medication takes a while to become effective, young children cannot associate pain relief with the injection. Other children might not know they are actually in pain until the pain is relieved. In these children, the onset of pain is so gradual that the child is unaware of it (Eland, 1985).

Nonverbal cues Because children often cannot verbally express when they are in pain and might not be able to describe the location or severity of pain, the nurse needs to look at additional cues. Children who are experiencing mild to moderate pain might appear irritable, restless, and uninterested in activities. They might complain of the pain or just might become quiet and listless. Severe pain can cause withdrawal, loss of appetite, decreased social interaction, crying, depression, and inability to sleep. Facial grimacing is frequently seen. Increased pulse and respirations are initial signs of pain. To manage the pain, the child in severe pain focuses energy inward and is not easily distracted.

(text continues on p. 602)

STANDARDS OF NURSING CARE *The Immobilized Child*

GUIDE FOR NURSING MANAGEMENT

Nursing diagnosis	Intervention	Rationale	Outcome
1. Potential for impaired skin integrity (stressors: pressure on areas resulting in decreased circulation; decreased oxygenation to tissue)	Turn every 2–4 hours. Position in a functional position so body weight is off reddened areas and bony prominences and circulation is not restricted.	Turning relieves pressure on the skin and contributes to improved circulation to the skin, particularly where bony prominences press against the skin.	The child's skin shows no signs of redness over bony prominences. The child does not complain of skin discomfort. The child is free of skin breakdown.
	Massage skin over bony prominences; wipe from the skin any excess lotion used; give back care.	Gentle massage stimulates circulation to the skin, provides comfort to the child, and enables the nurse better to assess skin condition. Lingering redness is an indication that circulation is not yet adequately restored and that tissue damage has occurred. Lotion, although useful in reducing friction during massage of the skin, contributes to skin maceration if it remains on the skin.	
	Observe overall skin condition with special attention to elbows, knees, heels, ears, if a child is paralyzed or unconscious; has poor nutritional status or thin fragile skin; or is obese.	The paralyzed child cannot move and sometimes cannot feel an area with decreased circulation; the unconscious child cannot complain of discomfort. Skin is more friable in the undernourished child. Skin folds in the obese child are more likely to retain lotion and excess moisture.	
	Place the child on sheepskin or special mattresses (eg, air, water, Egg crate®).	These devices equalize pressure and avoid too much pressure in one area.	
	Use folded blankets, trochanter rolls, or pillows on legs, arms, hands, feet, and ankles.	These ensure proper positioning of the child.	
2. Impaired physical mobility related to decreased strength and endurance	Plan developmentally appropriate play activities that require use of various muscle groups and are compatible with treatment plan (eg, Nerf® games, clay, Velcro games).	Use of play activity in plans helps encourage the child's participation in the planning and implementation of the care.	The child's muscle strength and joint range of motion are increased. The child engages in developmentally appropriate play that will also increase muscle tone. The child and parent can demonstrate exercises and joint range of motion.
	Turn the child prone. Perform or supervise range-of-motion exercises; teach muscle-setting exercises when particular joint movement is not advised. Elevate any edematous body parts as compatible with treatment plan.	Immobility can result in loss of muscle tone, leading to tissue atrophy. Without proper activity, collagen fibers become thick, fibrous, and resistant to stretching. Joint movement and muscle-setting exercises help stem loss of muscle tone and strength and joint range of motion. Edema can interfere with motion.	

(Continues)

STANDARDS OF NURSING CARE *The Immobilized Child* (Continued)

GUIDE FOR NURSING MANAGEMENT

Nursing diagnosis	Intervention	Rationale	Outcome
3. Potential ineffective airway clearance (stressors: pooling of secretions from lack of mobility; position not conducive to adequate lung expansion)	Encourage the child to deep breathe every 2–4 hours; utilize blowing games such as blowing a paper tissue for young children and an incentive spirometer for older children.	Decreased lung expansion during inactivity results in decreased movement of air during inspiration and expiration. This discourages adequate movement of respiratory secretions.	The child's lung sounds remain clear. The child is able to use games to increase lung expansion.
	Encourage the child to inhale deeply and not to exhale more air than is inhaled.	Although blowing does encourage lung expansion, blowing that exceeds inhalation can cause atelectasis. Children's pain, fear, or the pressure of treatment devices such as casts can add to the effects of immobility and further decrease lung expansion.	
	Place the child in an upright position several times daily if compatible with treatment plan. Turn the child every 2–4 hours.	Changing the child's position increases lung expansion.	
4. Potential alteration in bowel elimination: constipation (stressors: sluggish gastrointestinal tract; reduced food intake and inadequate roughage)	Provide fluids at or above the child's maintenance level, if not contraindicated by the child's condition. Encourage foods high in roughage: raw vegetables, fruits, prune juice (usually more palatable if served over ice).	Fluids and foods high in roughage provide moisture and bulk, which promote peristalsis. The gastrointestinal tract is sluggish with decreased mobility of gastrointestinal contents. Accelerated breakdown with resultant negative nitrogen balance during inactivity, lowered energy needs of the inactive child, and the child's feelings when inactive contribute to the child's decreased appetite and food intake.	The child is free of abdominal distension and discomfort. The child has a soft bowel movement once a day or according to the child's individual pattern.
	Encourage food intake by providing companionship during mealtimes and foods familiar to the child. Allow the child all possible choices in foods. Maximize convenience of food for the child (cut foods as necessary, arrange meal tray for child). Position the child for ease of eating independently (sitting, prone, or on side, as allowed). Encourage meals at regular hours and discourage empty calories at snack or meal times.	Decreased food intake interferes with mass peristaltic waves in the colon. Irregular intake interferes with regularly timed peristaltic activity.	

STANDARDS OF NURSING CARE *The Immobilized Child (Continued)*

GUIDE FOR NURSING MANAGEMENT

Nursing diagnosis	Intervention	Rationale	Outcome
	Offer bed pan (or take the child to the bathroom, if allowed) at regular intervals. Ensure the child's privacy when toileting.	If the child cannot sit while defecating, thigh pressure on the abdomen and downward pressure on the rectum are lacking. Children might be embarrassed to use the bedpan or to get assistance to use the bathroom and might ignore the defecation reflex.	
	Encourage allowable activity at specified times throughout the day.	Encouraging proper nutrition and elimination habits and encouraging activity decreases the risk of constipation.	
5. Potential for infection (urinary tract) (stressors: urinary stasis from immobility; decreased fluid intake)	Provide fluids at or above maintenance levels if allowable with the child's condition.	Urinary stasis in the renal pelvis can result from lack of upright positioning. Urinary retention can result from failure of perineal muscles to relax and from reduced muscle tone in the bladder. Increased fluid helps prevent stasis.	The child passes clear urine. The child voids amounts appropriate for age and weight. The child does not complain of frequency, urgency, or painful urination.
	Encourage fluids and foods that help acidify urine (such as cranberry juice).	Alkaline urine might result from increased calcium excretion associated with immobility and inactivity.	
	Monitor the child for signs of urinary tract infection and renal calculi; measure urinary pH and specific gravity every 8 hours; report elevation in specific gravity or alkaline urine.	Although not common in children, renal calculi can form with the combination of increased mineral excretion and urinary stasis. Urinary stasis increases the risk of infection.	
6. Potential for altered growth and development (stressor: temporary physical disability that interferes with completion of normal developmental tasks)	As appropriate to the child's development and condition, encourage the child to help plan daily routines, including treatment regimens (within allowable choices), menu, fluids, and play and rest periods. Include both child and family in nursing unit activities as desired.	Giving allowable choices helps lessen feelings of dependence and loss of control, enabling the child to feel more helpful and less restricted.	The child demonstrates interest in participating in care. The child can explain the rationale for activity restrictions. The child maintains interest in activities that interested the child prior to the immobilization.
	Adapt unit and playroom activities to the child's restrictions (eg, use prism glasses, role of scorekeeper in games, ball games with soft ball). Arrange the child's immediate surroundings to maximize independence (have games and other activities within reach, arrange meal tray conveniently for the child, keep call bell within the child's reach).	Allowing the child as full participation as possible helps to maintain developmental level while providing relief from boredom.	

(Continues)

STANDARDS OF NURSING CARE *The Immobilized Child (Continued)*

GUIDE FOR NURSING MANAGEMENT

Nursing diagnosis	Intervention	Rationale	Outcome
	Provide activities to facilitate the child's coping strategies (acknowledge negative emotions, have the child throw or squeeze a soft ball, shape clay, provide privacy, provide diversion and acceptable outlets for frustrations). Alter the child's physical environment as much as possible (move bed into different area, allow child to use wheelchair or go-cart, have child display personal pictures and decide arrangements of objects in immediate environment).	Providing an appropriate role for the child in activities helps encourage participation and increase acceptance of immobility.	
7. Potential for ineffective family coping (stressors: anxiety; feelings of guilt; financial strain; family disorganization)	Encourage the parent to discuss concerns, guilt, fears, and frustrations and the child's immobility. Explain rationale for the child's immobilization and specific restrictions to the parent.	Understanding leads to increased parental feelings of control and competence.	The family can explain the rationale for the child's restrictions. The family demonstrates increased independence and participation in the child's care.
	Discuss with the parent reasons for and ways to encourage the child's independence. Involve the parent in decisions concerning the child's treatment plan. Encourage the parent to help the child develop coping strategies compatible with activity restrictions.	Parental support and encouragement is crucial to most children's acceptance of and comfort with a treatment regimen, particularly when cooperation is as difficult as it can be with immobilization.	

The child might favor the part of the body that is in pain. A limp, for example, might indicate pain in the leg or hip. Holding an arm, or shoulder close to the body might indicate pain in these areas. Refusing to put pressure on a painful area can be an indicator of pain.

Because they do not have verbal skills, infants pose difficulties for nurses assessing pain. Infants can show increased motor activity in response to pain. Crying and irritable behavior is frequently seen. The infant might "swipe" or pull at the area of the body where the pain is located (Franck, 1986).

Verbal cues In an attempt to assess a child's pain more accurately, the nurse first establishes an open line of communication. The better the nurse-patient relationship, the more open the child might be to describing sources of pain. The nurse conveys interest by sitting with and listening to the child.

Supplying descriptive words helps a child describe pain. For example, pain might be described as sharp (like a pinprick or sting), pounding, or pressure (like a squeeze). Even with help, children find it difficult to describe pain in the same manner as an adult. The nurse who listens carefully to a child's description of pain might find, however, that children's descriptions accurately correspond to the way they feel. To understand accurately what the child means, the nurse needs to question and clarify statements the child makes.

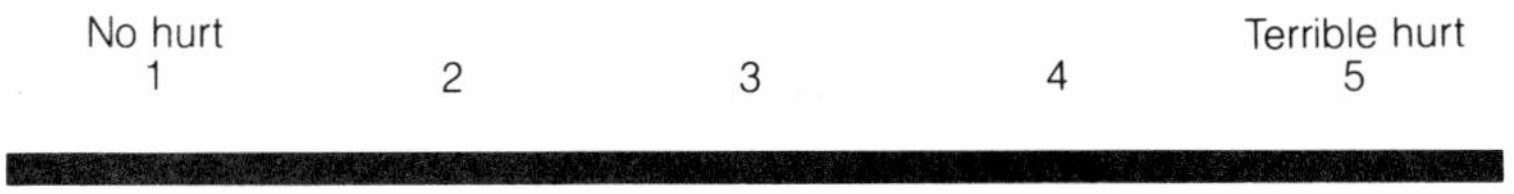

FIGURE 20-2
Pain intensity scale.

Assessment tools Assessment tools are available that help to determine the location and intensity of a child's pain. Asking a child to point to the place on the body where the hurt is helps localize the painful area. Having the child point to the painful area on an outline of a child's body accomplishes the same thing. Use of a rating scale to determine intensity of the pain is a simple assessment tool (Fig. 20-2). The Eland Color Tool is a reliable tool for assessing both location and intensity of pain. Different color crayons represent different degrees of pain. The child uses the crayons to locate on a body outline the sources of pain. The tool has identified pain in children before clinical symptoms have appeared (Eland, 1985). Other tools, such as the *Oucher* (Beyer and Aradine, 1986) have been tested for content validity.

Play can help in the expression and description of pain. A young child might respond to a story of a child or animal who goes to the hospital. The nurse can start the story describing circumstances that parallel the child's. The child can fill in some details as the nurse asks what happened to the character in the story. "What did it feel like? Did it hurt?" Some children share their feelings when the nurse tells a story in which the main character has pain. Such questions as "Does this sound right? What do you think is happening?" might elicit responses from the child and help in pain diagnosis.

Nursing management of pain

Choosing pain relief measures Remembering children's responses to painful procedures helps guide the nurse in choosing appropriate pain relief measures and in individualizing an approach for the child. Children try to avoid pain. They ask the nurse to be gentle, not to hurt. They want to postpone or avoid the procedure. "Maybe I'll have it later. Let me just finish watching this television show." They might go off the unit when a dressing change is needed. They might hit or kick the nurse. Maintaining a stream of conversation tends to postpone procedures for a short time. A nurse might go into a child's room, find the child "napping," and be tempted to leave the sleeping child alone.

In view of these tactics and the child's understandable reluctance to experience pain, nurses need to stand firm in their assessment. If analgesia would help a child perform necessary activities such as postoperative ambulation and deep breathing, if it would free the child to interact with others and to play, and if it would allow the child to sleep soundly instead of intermittently, then it is needed. Because not every pain relief measure is invasive, the least intrusive measures are used whenever possible. Medication, whether by mouth, rectal suppository, or injection, is not always necessary.

Noninvasive measures for pain relief Because anxiety works with physical stimuli to intensify the sensation of pain, any measure to diminish anxiety will help make the child more comfortable. General teaching to increase a child's understanding will help. To the best of their abilities, nurses also need to teach children about their pain and about what they are experiencing and why.

Knowledge is power in this case—power over the unknown. In the same way that preparation for childbirth can lessen the discomfort of contractions, children can benefit from knowing what sensations mean. Nurses can emphasize that postoperative pain is temporary. They can remind the child that the skin itches as it heals.

Other pain relief measures include involving the family and other significant people in a child's care. Familiar objects from home make the child feel comfortable. Telephone calls from family and friends help. A child's assisting, when possible, in a treatment or procedure helps return control to the child and can reduce the sensation of pain. For example, a child might help remove tape securing an IV or a dressing. Some children want to watch painful dressing changes or scrubs; others can be involved extensively in this care. All the measures that nurses use to decrease anxiety and enhance development also help to decrease pain.

Specific noninvasive techniques for children are the same as those used for adults. With children, however, nurses have an advantage not applicable to adults in that children will willingly participate in many games and new ideas. Much of nursing care with children involves distraction, and this is a powerful pain relief measure for the period in which it is used. Play for entertainment purposes distracts the child from fears, from focus on the self, and from pain.

Nurses can talk to children and can change a child's environment by bringing a child to the playroom, to another part of the hospital, or simply out into the hallway. Children often play together when encouraged and will then distract each other. The nurse can also help distract the child during specific painful experiences. Holding the child's hand and talking during an injection or dressing change is one example of the use of distraction.

Some children can easily be helped to relax by using imagery. They can think of themselves doing some enjoyable, restful activity such as floating on their backs in the water. Although the nurse frequently uses distraction or imagery at the spur of the moment, the nurse and child can plan to use these during painful experiences of relatively short duration. Children are more likely to feel supported and in control of themselves when interventions are planned.

Cutaneous stimulation is another noninvasive measure. Nurses frequently hug and rock an infant or a young child; the older child might receive a back rub. Other measures can be used, usually with the child's knowledge of their purpose. Rubbing an injection site or rubbing the side opposite the part of the body that hurts might help some children.

Humor can be an effective distraction technique. Laughter can ease mild or moderate pain by relaxing tense muscles and taking the child's mind off the source of the pain. Some evidence suggests that laughter can physiologically alter the effect of painful impulses by releasing endorphins that act on the central nervous system to inhibit pain (Smith, 1986). Telling funny stories or jokes or playing silly games such as peek-a-boo with the young child cause the child to laugh. Strenuous laughter can be contraindicated, however, for some children, particularly if they have had serious abdominal or chest surgery (Smith, 1986).

A combination of pain relief measures usually is more helpful to the child than either noninvasive or invasive measures used alone. If the nurse keeps a flow sheet that includes vital signs, time of pain relief measures, and the child's response, pain management can be improved. The nurse can then begin to assess the child's experience of pain more accurately and initiate interventions that prevent adverse consequences of pain. (Nursing management of chronic pain is discussed in Chapter 33.)

Fever—Potential Alteration in Body Temperature

Fever is one of the body's responses to an invading organism. Fevers are triggered by the body's immune response (see Chapter 25), and they assist the body in fighting disease. Former practice was to reduce any fever greater than 38.3°C (101°F) with antipyretic medication. Fevers higher than 40°C (104°F) called for tepid sponges in addition to the medication. It is now felt that fever might actually be beneficial in helping the body's defense. Fevers as high as 39°C (102°F) can go untreated as long as the patient is not uncomfortable or there is no history of seizures related to fever.

Children are likely to develop high fevers more readily than adults. It is not unusual to see body temperatures greater than 39.4°C (103°F) in ill children. A high fever in a child might not produce the severe fatigue, flushing, and chills that might accompany a moderate (38.3°C, 101°F) fever in an adult. Seizures associated with a high fever (febrile seizures) are seen in some children under age 5 (see Chapter 31 for a discussion of febrile seizures). Fever control is particularly important in children with a history or family history of seizures.

Assessment of fever A child's body temperature is taken by one of the three usual methods. Oral temperatures can be taken on children older than 6 years of age who are alert and not subject to seizures. The rectal method is used with infants and unconscious children. After lubrication, rectal thermometers are inserted gently with the child in a side-lying position, top leg forward. Infants can be supine, while the nurse raises both legs by the ankles up and back to expose the anal opening. It is necessary to insert the thermometer only slightly beyond the bulb (approximately 0.5 in. depending on the child's size) for an accurate temperature reading. The nurse holds the exposed end of the thermometer for the entire time the thermometer is inserted.

The preferred method for taking a young child's temperature is axillary. The thermometer is inserted into the dry axilla and the child's arm is held tightly to the chest. Axillary temperatures are less precise but far less invasive than rectal. The nurse can cuddle the child while taking the temperature and perhaps read a story to the child while the 5 to 10 minutes pass.

Nursing management of fever Once the fever has been documented, antipyretics (fever-reducing medications) might be ordered to manage the fever. Aspirin generally is a more effective antipyretic than nonaspirin products. Because of a possible link with an often fatal neurologic disease (Reye's syndrome), however, aspirin usually is avoided in children, especially when chickenpox or influenza is suspected. Acetaminophen has become the drug of choice for pharmacologic management of fever. Acetaminophen comes in chewable tablets, liquid, and infant drops. All are flavored to make them more appealing to children.

If tepid sponges are required, the child is undressed and placed on an absorbent towel. Towels, facecloths, or cloth diapers are saturated with tepid (98.6°F) water and placed on and around the child's extremities, abdomen, and chest. As the cloths become warm, they are removed and replaced. The nurse continues the procedure for 15 to 30 minutes or until the body temperature reaches the desired level. The nurse observes the child closely for excessive chilling. After removing the sponges, the child is dressed in light clothing, or the clothing remains off except for a diaper, and the child is covered with a light cotton blanket.

Pediatric Adaptations of Common Procedures

Color, Sensation, and Motion Assessment

The nurse obtains baseline data for color, sensation, and motion of an extremity to determine nerve function and circulatory status. This is a necessary assessment in conditions in which surgery or tissue swelling might impair circulation or damage nerve function. Constriction of an extremity can occur with cast application, bandaging, suspension, and restraint.

The nurse notes color and temperature of the affected extremity and compares these data to the child's unaffected extremity. Coolness and pallor might be related to impaired circulation. When a portion of the skin is lightly squeezed and released, the skin should blanch and normal color should then return immediately (capillary refill). A rapid return of color indicates tissue perfusion, whereas delayed or slow capillary refill means restricted circulation.

The nurse can assess sensation in a child over age 10 with normal emotional and cognitive development by asking whether the child has feeling in the affected extremity and whether the feelings are unusual (eg, numbness, tingling, foot asleep). The nurse touches a toe or finger and asks the child to state which toe or finger was touched. The nurse then notes how much pressure had to be applied before the child felt the sensation.

Children younger than age 10 might not be reliable enough to give accurate data. Therefore, in a younger or developmentally delayed child, a nurse proves sensation by observing the child's facial or withdrawal reaction to a light pinch or prick.

Motion can be assessed by watching the child's physical reaction to being touched or by asking a child capable of responding to try to move the affected fingers or toes.

Urine and Stool Specimen Collection

Collecting urine and stool specimens from a child, although frequently more difficult than collecting them from an adult, is a routine aspect of nursing care. Urine specimens are obtained on the admission of a child to the hospital. They are also needed when there is suspicion of infection, when assessing urine specific gravity or pH, and when the child is to undergo surgery. Among other purposes, stool specimens are needed in testing for occult blood, culture, and ova and parasite identification and in assessing products of digestion.

Although reasons differ among children of various ages, most feel private and embarrassed about their bodies' excrements. Many children state that the urine specimen container feels wet, despite the fact that it is dry. The temperature of the sample combined with the child's embarrassment probably account for this sensation. The nurse's reassuring the child that the container is dry, if it is, or that it is perfectly all right and easily remedied if it is wet, will help the child feel more comfortable in the hospital setting.

A child might need more assistance with giving a urine or stool sample than that needed for basic toileting. A toilet-trained 2-year-old cannot hold a cup in place to obtain a specimen. This child can sit on a toilet where a container for collecting urine has been placed under the seat. A boy might wish to stand while voiding but might not be able to hold a cup or specimen container. In this instance use of a urinal might be indicated.

Urine collection with the incontinent child A specimen can be obtained in various ways from an infant or an incontinent child. In some facilities, plastic wrap can be used as a diaper, especially for premature infants. The urine is collected easily in the plastic, and the nurse can quickly determine whether the infant has voided. The plastic should not remain too long in place, however, as it could contribute to skin breakdown. The crib mattress is placed in Fowler's position to aid the collection of urine in the loose part of the diaper. After the child voids, the diaper is removed and the specimen collected.

Applying a collection bag A pediatric urine-collecting device that fits over the perineal area of the child commonly is used (Fig. 20-3). The open end has an adhesive backing that adheres to the skin. In the most experienced of hands, however, the collective device sometimes fails to adhere adequately, and the desired urine specimen is found in the child's diaper. Unless the skin in the perineal area is broken down, the bag can be reapplied. Several steps and precautions will help prevent trauma to the skin and the child from unnecessary reapplications. These are described in Table 20-3.

Urine collectors are available in various sizes in clean or sterile packaging. For collecting a 24-hour urine specimen, collectors come with tubes extending from them. The tube may either be drained at intervals or, when urine flow is moderate to large, they may be connected to a closed-drainage system.

Determining specific gravity To test for specific gravity on an incontinent child, the nurse can use a sample obtained from a pediatric urine-collecting bag. Some nurses have use of a refractometer on their units, and only a few drops of urine are needed for the test. A *refractometer* is a

TABLE 20-3 Application of Pediatric Urine-Collecting Bag

Procedure	Rationale
Clean and dry the skin before application	Aids adherence of device
Place child supine with hips abducted	Provides clear access to perineal area. Stretches skin and helps eliminate skin folds
With girl, position lower center of opening in perineal area below urinary meatus. With boy, position penis inside collecting device	Proper positioning helps ensure collection of specimen and comfort of child
Remove paper backing from lower portion of bag and apply smoothly from back to front	Smooth application helps prevent wrinkles through which urine can leak
Remove paper backing from upper portion of collecting device and continue to apply without wrinkles	(See above)
Inspect for any loose areas	Reinforcement or immediate reapplication can save discomfort and delay
Tape may be used to reinforce bag if necessary	Pressure of urine filling the bag might loosen adherence
Diaper, if applied at all, either should be loose around the device or should have a hole made with the bag extended through the hole	Tight diapering will encourage the bag's overfilling at the upper portion and coming loose from the skin. When diapering is loose, the bag is exposed to less pressure from the diaper. When bag extends through the diaper, the child's voiding can be observed and the bag removed immediately

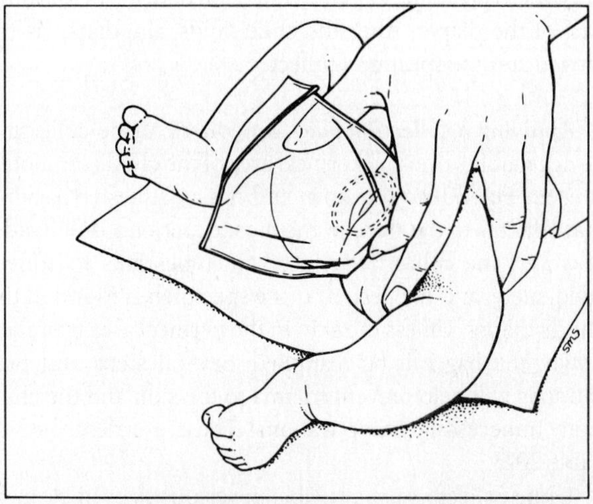

FIGURE 20-3
Application of a pediatric urine collector.

lighted device that can give an accurate specific gravity reading with a minute amount of urine. Withdrawing urine from a wet diaper by using a syringe without a needle has been found to give an accurate specific gravity value in tests with a specific brand of disposable diaper (Pampers) (Strohbach and Kratina, 1982). Nurses can repeat the study on the brand of diaper used in their facility. Aspirating urine from a child's diaper for specific gravity determinations saves the child the discomfort of urine bag applications and relieves the nurse of a time-consuming procedure. There is a possibility that the gel used in extra-absorbant disposable diapers can interfere with an accurate assessment of specific gravity. If frequent specific gravity readings are required, regular absorbancy diapers are recommended.

Urine collection with the continent child For a continent child, the nurse works in a more cooperative way with the child or parent in obtaining a specimen. The child needs an age-appropriate explanation concerning the purpose and method of obtaining the needed sample. Some children can voluntarily give a urine sample, even when only partially toilet trained. One mother, on learning that a urine sample was needed from her 18-month-old hospitalized child, asked the child to "tinkle" in a specimen container. The child had been wearing a diaper in the hospital, but within a minute and with no tears or protest, the child was able to give the sample.

Stool specimens A stool specimen is usually easy to obtain from an incontinent child. Scraping a soiled diaper with a tongue blade to obtain a specimen is all that is needed in most cases. When a stool specimen cannot be contaminated with urine, the nurse will have to observe the diaper carefully to determine whether or not the specimen can be used. A continent child can use a bedpan placed on either a bed or a toilet seat. A child will usually be embarrassed about giving the sample to the nurse or telling the nurse about the sample. Children need to understand, as well as they are able, the rationale for collection of the specimen. They might need help dealing with their feelings about the odor and about viewing the shape and color of the stool. The nurse's casual, straightforward handling of the situation will help the child accept the procedure as a necessary but minor part of the hospital care.

Blood Specimen Collection

Blood is collected from children in a variety of ways, most considered to be invasive measures. Children react adversely to any thought of "needles," and their fear of pain can make them less than cooperative when blood specimens are required. One of the major fears of childhood is that the child's insides will leak out of any opening in the body. The child expects to lose most of the blood from a puncture site and often becomes anxious and vocal about covering the site quickly. Preparation time for the procedure will vary according to the age of the child, but the nurse keeps in mind that fear can increase uncooperative behavior and that preparing a child too far in advance can increase fear.

Because children's veins can be very small and easily missed during a venipuncture, it is essential that the child remain as still as possible during the procedure. An older child or adolescent, if properly prepared, often can cooperate and keep the arm extended as directed. Younger children will need to be restrained with the arm held very still. The nurse reaches under the child and stabilizes the child's selected upper arm with one hand. With the other hand, the nurse holds the child's hand. In this way, little motion is likely during the procedure and the likelihood of missing the vein is decreased (Fig. 20-4). By reaching under the child's shoulders, the nurse effectively prevents the child's free hand from getting in the technician's way, and at the same time the nurse can face the child to offer comfort.

The femoral area is used frequently to obtain specimens in children. The child is positioned on the back with the knees in a frog-leg position. Standing at the child's head, the nurse restrains the child by placing arms on the child's arms. One hand is placed in the diaper area of the leg to be used to stabilize the area and retract the diaper slightly from the puncture site. The other hand is placed above the child's knee (Fig. 20-5). The diaper remains on the child to prevent urine contamination during the venipuncture.

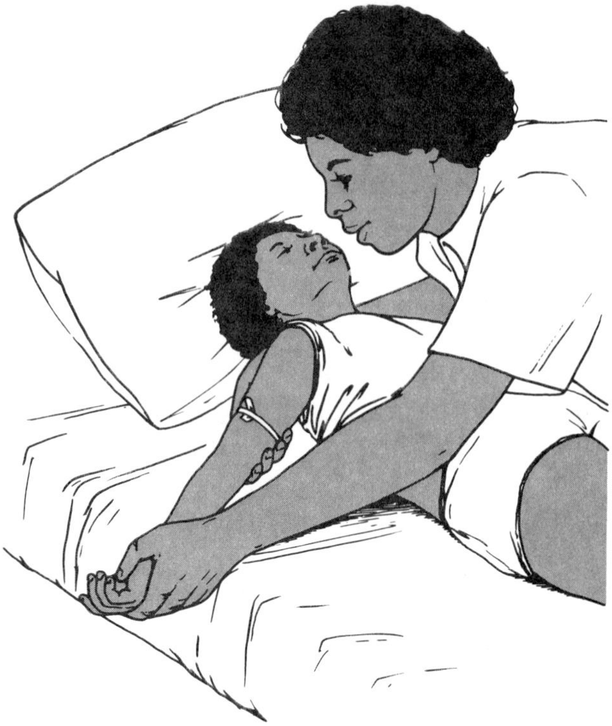

FIGURE 20-4
Position for a venipuncture.

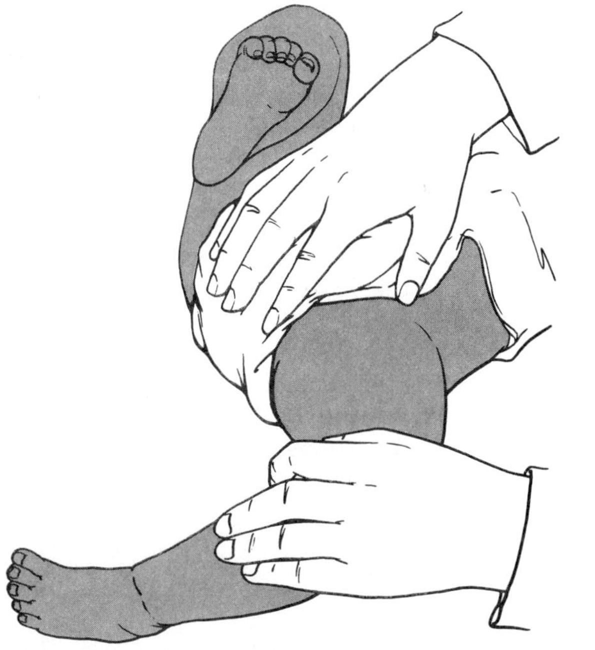

FIGURE 20-5
Position for a femoral venipuncture.

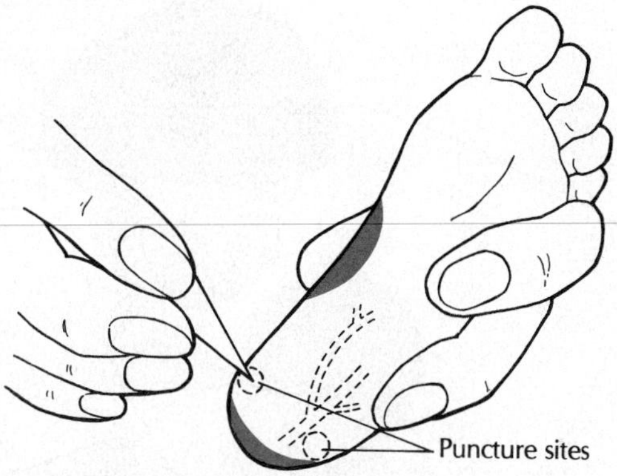

FIGURE 20-6

Puncture sites for a heel stick. (From Ladewig PA et al: Essentials of Maternal-Newborn Nursing. *Addison-Wesley, 1986.)*

The jugular vein can be used in children, but specimen collection from the jugular can be particularly frightening. The child is required to extend the neck and turn the head to the side to expose the vein. The advantage to the jugular site is that the vein is large and appears prominent when the child cries.

After a venipuncture, the nurse keeps pressure on the area or applies a pressure dressing to the puncture site. For a jugular or femoral puncture, finger pressure is applied for 3–5 minutes or until bleeding stops.

For some blood tests a capillary specimen is all that is necessary. Capillary specimens are obtained from the finger, earlobe, or heel (Fig. 20-6). If either the heel or finger is used, the nurse wraps it first in a warm cloth for 5 minutes to increase the capillary fill in the area. The earlobe is rubbed gently with a small piece of gauze. By doing this the nurse can increase the blood flow to the area, ensure an adequate specimen, and reduce the chance of the child needing a repeat stick.

The use of a lancet device such as a Monojector™ for finger and heel sticks not only is faster than the conventional lancet but also accurately controls the depth of the puncture. Adhesive strips (Band-Aids) are important for the child's peace of mind. Decorative Band-Aids are available that appeal particularly to children.

Intravenous Infusions

Intravenous infusions are used to supplement fluids and electrolytes when the child's oral intake is compromised, as it is in cases of vomiting or in preoperative and postoperative situations. Intravenous infusions also are needed for purposes of medication or anesthesia administration and to keep a vein open (KVO) for transfusions of blood or blood products. Most IV lines are short term until fluid and electrolyte balance is restored. In some instances, however, long-term therapy is required. Intravenous medications often present one such instance. Total parenteral nutrition presents another (see Chapter 27).

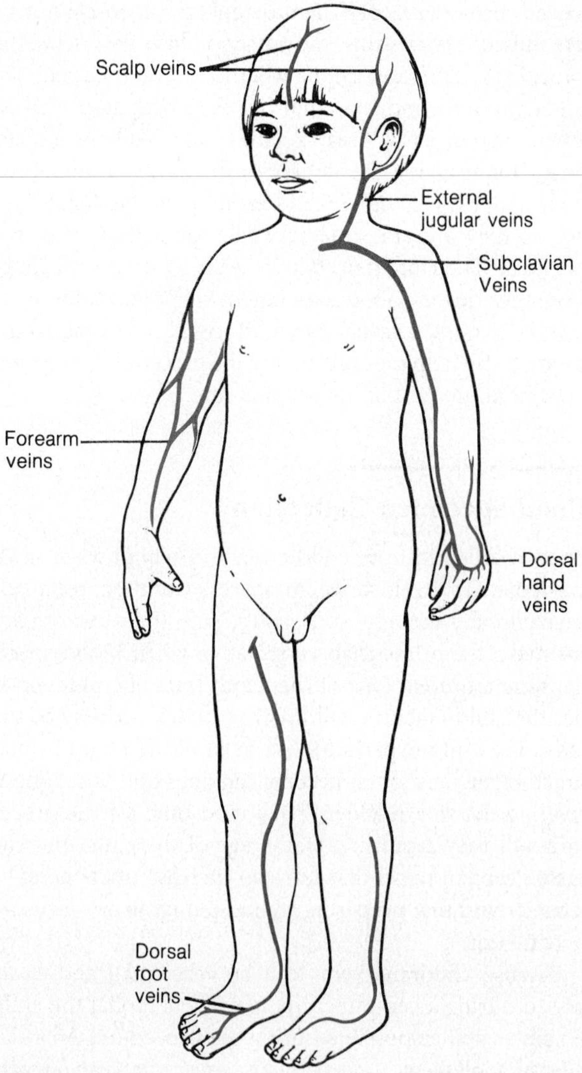

FIGURE 20-7

Common sites for intravenous infusions in children.

Intravenous sites The site used for an IV infusion in the child should allow for both protection of the IV and maximum mobility of the child. (Figure 20-7 illustrates the most commonly used intravenous sites in children.) Infusion sites frequently used for children include the back of the hand, the forearm, the dorsum of the foot, and the scalp for infants. These sites offer some natural restraint for protection of the IV because they are not usually very close to points of flexion; therefore, additional restraint of the child can be minimized.

With the hand or forearm, the nondominant side of the body should be used since even the infant can be highly dependent on sucking one particular thumb. The dorsum of the foot is a less desirable site for an ambulatory child because the child must not walk on the affected foot. It can be an adequate site for the infant, however, and sometimes must be used with the older child. Scalp veins are often used with infants. Many young infants derive pleasure from being bundled, which is the preferred method of restraint when the infusion site is a scalp vein. Some infants require additional restraints to protect their IVs.

The antecubital fossa and neck veins are sometimes used as a last resort for a peripheral IV. Either site is difficult to immobilize in the child, however, and the immobilization is restrictive. Both sites demand close nursing observation for signs of complications. The child has relatively good use of the arm when a forearm or hand vein is used, but when the elbow is extended and restrained, use of the arm is restricted. Although a neck vein may be used for a peripheral IV during surgery, it is difficult to maintain when a child regains consciousness and becomes somewhat active.

Intravenous equipment A variety of needles or catheters is available for IV administration to children. The *butterfly* (Fig. 20-8A) is a needle attached to a winged plastic piece and catheter. It allows for accurate control during IV insertion, especially with infants. Butterfly needles are approximately ½ to 1¼ inches long and come in various gauges—the larger the gauge number, the smaller the lumen of the needle. Infants and young children might require a 23 g or 25 g butterfly because their vein lumens are so small. Butterflies also are used with older children, especially when the IV is short term.

Intravenous catheters are often used for the older child or adolescent (Fig. 20-8B, C). These provide stability for the IV because the catheter passes approximately 2 inches into the vein. Like the butterfly, the catheter has a lumen that is inversely related to the gauge number. For long-term therapy or administration of blood products, a larger-lumen needle is most effective. Under some circumstances, it might be necessary to thread a long catheter into the vein. This procedure, called an IV cut-down, is performed by a surgeon (see Chapter 21).

Drip control chambers, or burettes, are used with children's IVs. Burettes permit very accurate determinations of fluid infused because they are marked in 1-mL gradations. They also have a mechanism for preventing air from entering the IV tubing and thus entering the child. They facilitate administration of IV medications.

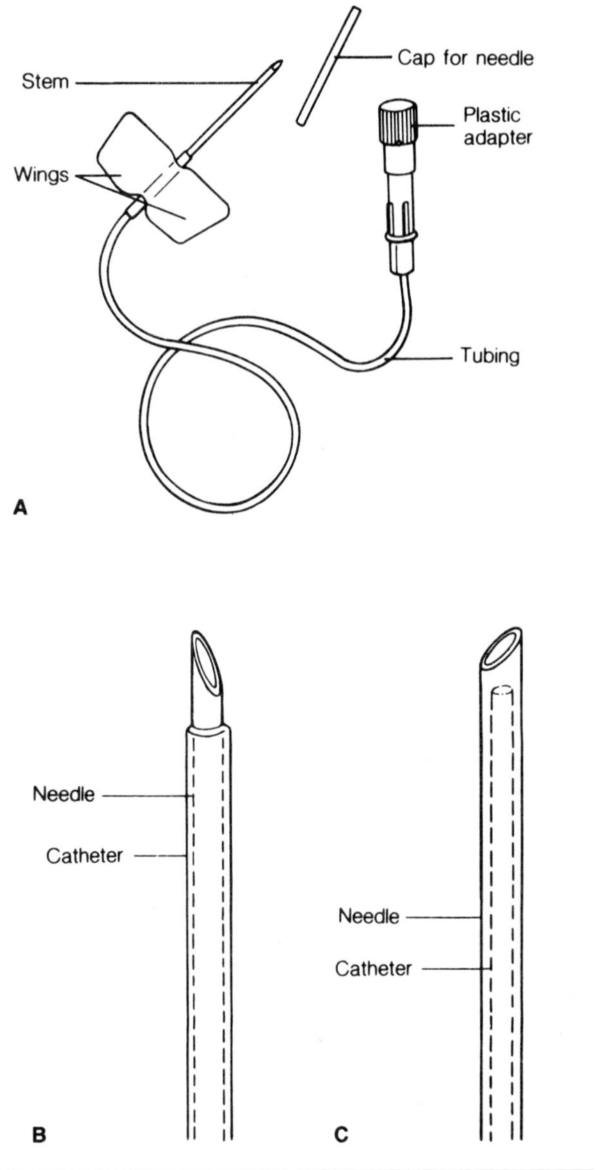

FIGURE 20-8

Intravenous needles and catheters: ***A.*** *An IV butterfly needle,* ***B.*** *an over-the-needle catheter. After insertion in the vein, the needle is removed, and the plastic catheter remains in place.* ***C.*** *An inside-the-needle catheter (intracatheter). The plastic catheter is threaded through the needle after the venipuncture. (From Kozier B, Erb G:* Fundamentals of Nursing, *3rd ed. Addison-Wesley, 1987.)*

Burettes also help prevent fluid overload in the child by limiting the amount of fluid to the amount in the burette. If the flow rate inadvertently increases, as it might with position changes, the fluid infused is limited to that in the burette instead of the entire IV bottle. To prevent fluid overload effectively, the burettes themselves must not contain

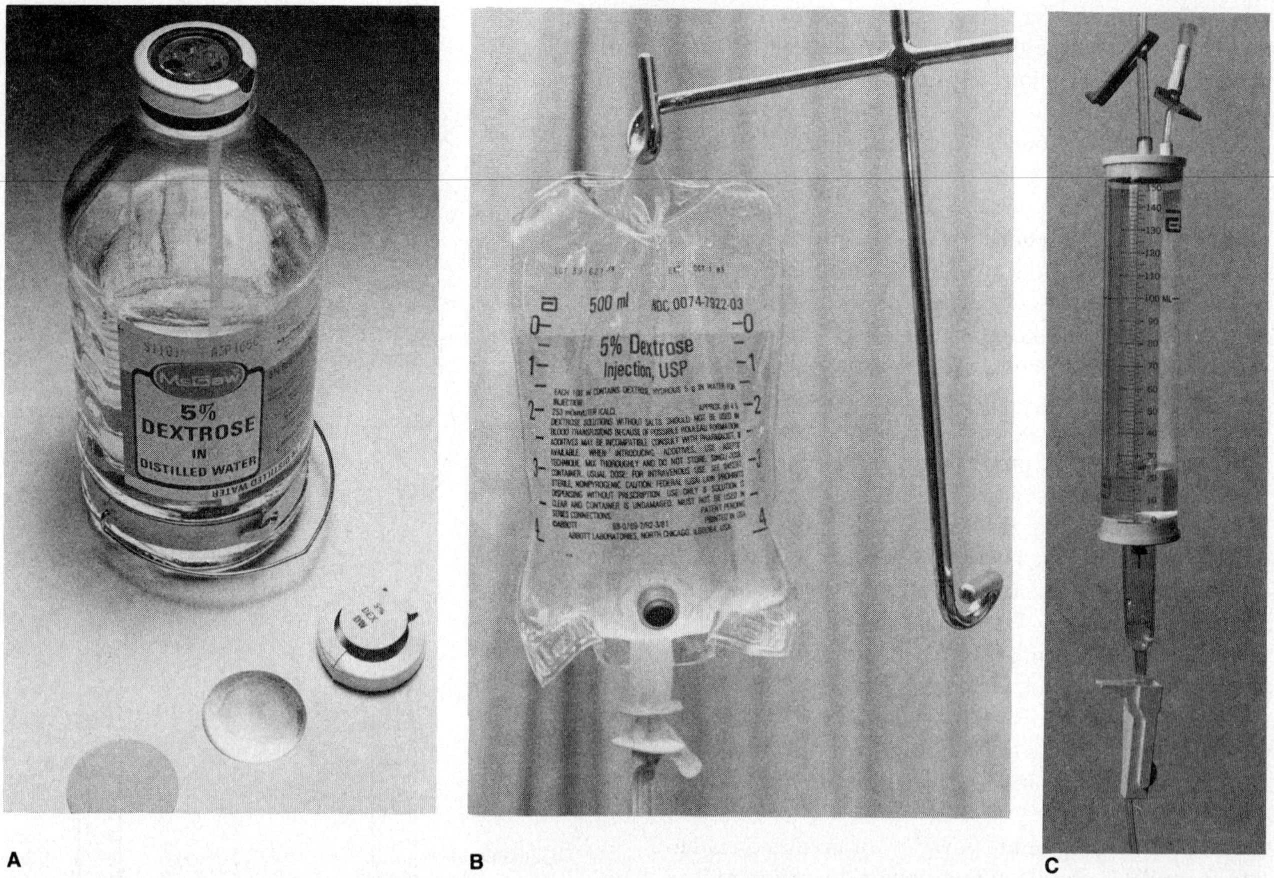

Intravenous equipment for children can include ***A.*** *an intravenous bottle or* ***B.*** *an intravenous solution bag, and* ***C.*** *a burette. (From Kozier B, Erb G:* Fundamentals of Nursing, *2nd ed.* Addison-Wesley, *1983.)*

excess fluid. The burette should contain a maximum of 2 hours' worth of fluid and even less with infants or children at risk for imbalance.

Most IV administration sets used for children are calibrated to flow at 60 drops per milliliter (60 gtt/mL), and since there are 60 minutes in an hour, the number of drops per minute (gtt/min) equals the number of milliliters to be delivered per hour. In a gravity administration set, the flow rate slows or stops with increased resistance, which occurs when fluid enters the tissues instead of the vein. Therefore, even with controlled infusion, the nurse's hourly observations of drip rates and amount of fluid infused are essential.

In addition to gravity administration sets, infusion pumps and syringe pumps are used to deliver a specified amount of fluid in a given period of time. The syringe pump is useful for small amounts of fluid. Either pump delivers fluid at a standard infusion rate despite any resistance, such as changes in a child's activities or a needle or IV catheter that is resting against the wall of a vein.

Infusion pumps are usually accurate to within 2%, but this very accuracy can give the nurse a false sense of security. Pumps do malfunction, and the nurse therefore determines the amount of fluid actually infused in a given period of time. Also, as pumps continue to work against pressure, they can pump fluid into the tissues when an IV is infiltrated (although with some pumps an alarm will sound if flow is actually obtructed). Thus an infusion pump, if not carefully monitored, could produce a serious infiltration with potential for tissue damage.

For intermittent administration of IV fluids or medications, a heparin lock might be indicated. A *heparin lock* is a small-lumen needle (usually 23 g) attached to a catheter with a latex stopper. The needle is inserted into the vein, usually in the forearm, and is secured in place with tape. Introduction of dilute heparin-saline solution through the stopper keeps the vein patent. Patency is preserved by injecting the heparin-saline solution after each infusion of IV medication or fluid. A heparin lock allows the child to be mobile while still receiving IV therapy.

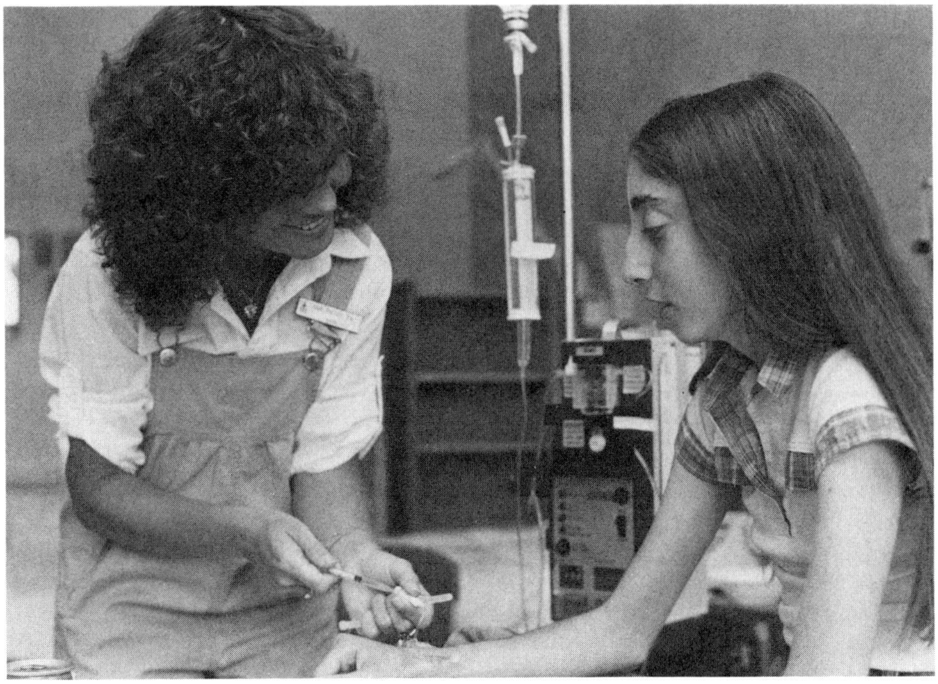

Intravenous administration by means of an infusion pump with a heparin lock.

Nursing management for intravenous infusion Three major aspects in the nursing care of the child with an intravenous infusion are (a) preventing complications, (b) maintaining safety, and (c) providing for developmental needs.

Complications of intravenous infusion Intravenous therapy can cause complications (listed in Table 20-4). Nursing interventions to prevent such complications center on frequent thorough checks of the IV insertion site and the entire administration set. The less the site is encumbered by tape, dressings, or protective devices such as trimmed-to-fit-the-area cups, the more easily the nurse can make observations and the earlier a complication might be determined. Some compromise needs to be struck, however, between ease of observation and protection of the IV.

If the nurse suspects a complication but is unable to confirm it, the nurse gently removes the tape and gauze to expose the needle insertion area. Minimal movement of the IV site is essential to preserve the fragile IV insertion.

To decrease the risk of inflammation, strict aseptic technique is necessary when the IV is inserted and when IV dressings are changed. Policies concerning dressings, the length of time a needle or IV catheter remains in place, the frequency with which IV tubing is changed, and the routine for changing solution bottles or bags vary with the facility. Because of the emotional trauma and physical difficulties of IV insertion in children, some facilities do not change IV needles or dressings for a peripheral IV. The IV is removed when it is no longer needed or when signs of infiltration or phlebitis are present. The IV solution and often the tubing are changed every 48 hours.

The nurse carefully monitors the infusion for rate and the child for both adequate therapeutic effect and possible fluid overload. To maximize therapeutic effect, the nurse checks the IV at frequent intervals, every 15–30 minutes, and records fluid intake hourly to determine whether or not the gravity system or pump is delivering the proper amount of fluid. When too little or too much fluid is infusing, the IV rate is adjusted appropriately. If the incorrect rate has been infusing for more than 1 hour, some adjustment often can be made. With too rapid an infusion, it is necessary to slow the rate, perhaps so that it is just enough to keep the vein open. If the rate has been too slow, the nurse carefully evaluates the child's needs and the method and desirability of "catching up." When a child is not a neonate and is free from cardiac, renal, or other fluid utilization difficulty, the IV rate can be increased slightly for a number of hours until the child's intake meets fluid requirements.

Safety and intravenous infusion The child's physiologic need for fluids or electrolytes requires the nurse's being concerned for the IV's safety. Restraining the child is therefore sometimes necessary. Use of a scalp vein for an infant allows some limb mobility, but the child still needs to be positioned so that head and limb movements are not likely to disrupt the IV. When the child is not being held, mummy

TABLE 20-4 Complications of Intravenous Therapy

Objective sign(s)	Intervention
Infiltration	
Swelling around site (possibly extending further up from site)	Discontinue infusion
Poor or absent flow rate	Remove angiocatheter or needle
Poor blood backflow	Apply warm, wet compresses to site
Cool to cold skin at site	
Thrombophlebitis	
Tenderness or pain at site	Discontinue infusion
Warm or red site	Remove angiocatheter or needle
Fever, leukocytosis	Apply warm, wet compresses to site
Possible hardness of vein	
Possible swelling at site	
Poor or absent blood flow	
Fluid overload	
Increased blood pressure	Slow infusion to keep vein open (KVO) rate
Increased urinary output	Place child in semi-Fowler's or Fowler's position
Tachycardia	Monitor vital signs as needed
Possible neck vein distension	Give oxygen as needed
Respiratory signs—tachypnea, dyspnea, orthopnea, rales	Monitor edema, intake, output and urine specific gravity
Edema, particularly periorbital	Monitor fontanelles in infants
Bulging, tense fontanelles in infant	Notify physician
Air embolism	
Signs of shock—tachycardia, hypotension, loss of consciousness	Turn child on left side
	Give oxygen if needed
	Inspect IV system for disconnections
	Notify physician

or extremity restraints might be necessary. The young child with an IV in any site might, when unattended, need to have extremities restrained. Some children can be helped to understand the importance of the IV and might not need restraints. Any restraints are periodically removed and the infant or child held to provide comfort, security, and tactile stimulation.

With the fear and fascination that IVs hold for children, and with their precarious positioning, IVs are prone to failure and require further safety considerations. Both infants and older children have been found changing the flow rates of their IVs or even removing the IV. Older children, after they have become accustomed to their IVs, sometimes try to use their portable IV poles as skateboards in the hospital corridors.

To prevent a child's reregulating an IV, the clamp can be slid up on the tubing so that it is far away from the child but still within reach of the nurse. Infusion pumps should be placed out of the child's reach. An IV must be secured against direct interference by the child so that it has as little positional variation in flow rate as possible. The amount of taping and restraint needed to protect a child's IV will vary with the site of the IV, the age and development of the child, and the child's ability to understand and cooperate with the treatment. An explanation of the need for and care of the IV and the nurse's help as the child learns to be mobile with an IV are enough for many children from age 4 and older.

Other aspects of safety include knowledge of compatibility of medications and maintenance infusions. An infusion line might need to be flushed before and after a medication with a maintenance solution and a solution compatible with the medication. The medication can then be "piggybacked" and infused with the compatible solution.

Developmental needs during intravenous infusions Play and the active manipulation of the environment are paramount for the cognitive and motor development of the child. Intravenous therapy restricts the child's mobility, therefore the nurse needs to consider the restrictions imposed when a vein is selected for IV therapy. Choosing the nondominant hand and avoiding the foot for a child who needs to walk are among the ways that nurses can address children's developmental needs. Likewise, choosing a scalp vein for an infant facilitates close contact with caregivers.

The older child can maximize mobility and control of restrictions by choosing, within acceptable limits, the IV site. The child also needs emotional support during IV insertion and removal and needs help in expressing feelings. As with all procedures, explanations for child and family need to be realistic and understandable.

Medicating a Child

Medicating children differs from medicating adults in many ways. First are the physical differences, beyond the obvious difference in height and weight, between the small child and the adult. Second, the mechanics of administering medications must be adapted to the child's changing characteristics and capabilities. Third, in teaching and other measures, the nurse takes into account the child's cognitive level and emotional needs.

Physiologic differences between adults and children If children were simply small but with the body composition and function of adults, pediatric dosages could be converted from adult dosages and based on a child's weight. Although dosages are often estimated in this manner, the differences between child and adult are far more complex.

Physiologic differences are many. Particularly in the neonatal period, the immaturity of body systems renders the effects of medication administration less predictable and riskier for the child. This is less true of the child over 2, as many body systems then function at close to adult levels. Differences are related to the following factors:

Diluting effect—The distribution of the child's body fluids combined with an increased metabolic rate and the infant's inefficient concentration of urine leads to a diluting effect with some medications. The result is that children require a higher dose than one ordinarily would expect.

Permeability of membranes—Increased permeability of skin and blood-brain barrier allows for greater absorption of certain medications with the resultant danger of systemic toxicity.

Absorption of oral medications—Immaturity of the gastrointestinal system increases the transit time, thus decreasing absorption in the gastrointestinal tract.

Dosage formulas Information about recommended medication dosages for a child of a particular age and weight are available to the nurse. Most pediatric medications are prescribed in milligrams per kilogram of body weight per 24 hours. A hospital formulary or other pharmacologic reference is a reliable source of information to aid the nurse in evaluating the safety of a dose. The hospital pharmacy can help clarify questions of dose and medication compatibility.

With the stated qualifications and precautions, the nurse also needs to be familiar with formulas for calculating pediatric dosages. No formula can accurately and consistently determine safe and effective medication dosage for the child, but the following methods give the nurse a rough guide to the safety of a dose. These formulas are for use with the child over age 2.

1. *Clark's rule.* Clark's rule for young children uses body weight of a child in comparison with the recommended adult dosage and the average adult weight (assumed to be 150 pounds).

$$\text{Estimated child's dosage} = \frac{\text{weight (lb) of child}}{150\text{ lb}} \times \text{adult dosage}$$

2. *Body surface calculation.* Body surface area is considered to be a more accurate means of calculating pediatric dosages. Body surface area is estimated when the child's height and weight are plotted on a nomogram (Fig. 20-9). Nomograms are found in most standard pediatric medical and nursing texts. The average adult is considered to have a body surface area of 1.7 square meters.

$$\text{Estimated child's dosage} = \frac{\text{surface area of child (m}^2\text{)}}{1.7\text{ m}^2} \times \text{adult dosage}$$

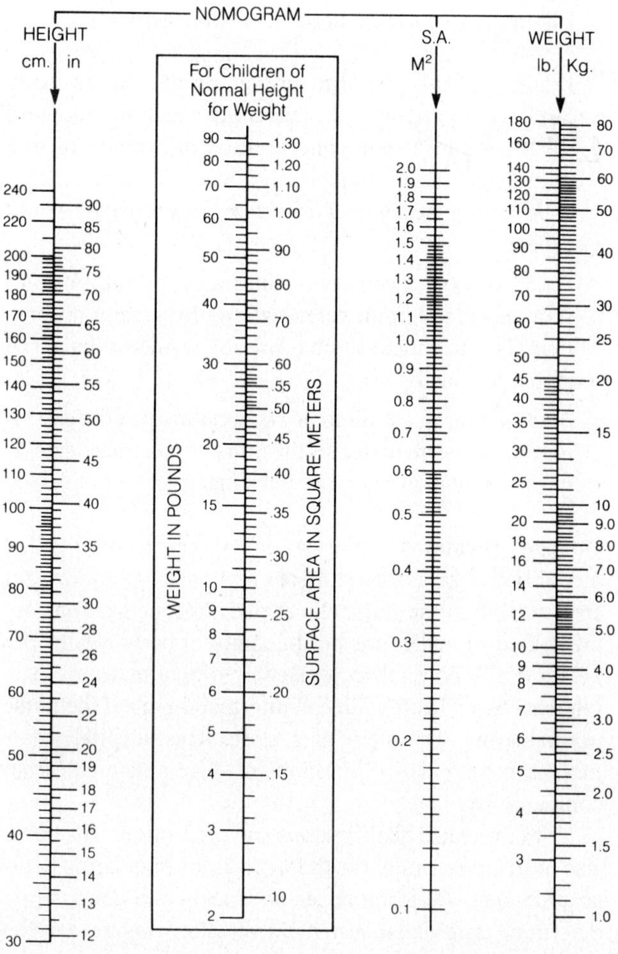

FIGURE 20-9

Nomogram with estimated body surface area. A straight line is drawn between the child's height and weight. The point at which the line intersects the surface area column is the estimated body surface area. (Source: Behrman RE, Vaughn VC: Nelson Textbook of Pediatrics, *12th ed. Saunders, 1983.)*

Administering oral medication Special considerations for oral medications center around the child's abilities to suck, drink, and swallow and around the small measurements necessary for liquid medications. Some children may take liquid medications from a small cup or spoon. Many infants and children need to have a medication placed directly into the mouth. This can often be accomplished with a syringe. The medication is drawn up in a syringe without a needle.

The child should be held in an upright or semi-upright position, and the tip of the syringe should be placed midway back at the side of the child's mouth. By using this position, the child is less likely to gag when the medication is administered or to expel the medication from the mouth. The child also is less likely to aspirate.

When an infant will suck from a nipple, the nipple can be placed in the child's mouth, and as the child begins to suck, the liquid medication can be placed into the nipple from a needleless syringe. This is a very simple, pleasant way to administer liquid medication to an infant. Despite the convenience, however, another method should be used for unpleasant tasting medication, so the infant will not associate the unpleasant taste with the nipple.

Measurement of liquid medications must be accurate and performed with a standard measurement source. A graduated medicine cup is acceptable if the markings match the amount of medication needed and no estimation is necessary. Measurement of small amounts of liquid medications can be accurately performed with some graduated cylinders or with a syringe. Some facilities have use of less expensive, nonsterile oral syringes for this purpose.

Measuring spoons specifically made for accurate medication measurement and administration are commercially available, and many parents find these useful. The nurse does not use a household tableware teaspoon or tablespoon and so instructs parents to follow the same principle. These household spoons vary in their actual size, and their use could lead to overmedication or undermedication of a child. Standard measuring spoons are appropriate for medication administration in the home.

Some oral medications do not come in a liquid but are instead in tablet or capsule form. Some very young children can and will swallow pills, whereas many older children and adolescents have not mastered the skill. A careful history usually identifies the child who can safely swallow pills and capsules. If such a history is not available, the nurse can show the medication to the child and ask the child whether swallowing it is possible. Liquid medication might be available for the child who needs it, but often the nurse can alter the form of a pill or capsule so that a child can swallow it.

Some medications have an enteric coating to prevent irritation to or deterioration in the child's stomach. These medications must be swallowed whole. The nurse needs to request another form of the medication for the child unable to swallow them. If the medication does not have an enteric coating, a child may choose to chew or the nurse may crush or dissolve the medication. Crushed medication can be placed in food or drink with which it does not adversely react.

Medication is mixed with the smallest possible amount of food or fluid to help ensure the child's taking the entire dose. Despite attempts to make the mixture palatable, it is likely to retain some of the medication's taste, and even a hungry or thirsty child would have difficulty consuming a moderate or large amount. The altered medication must be presented to the child honestly and not as food or a treat.

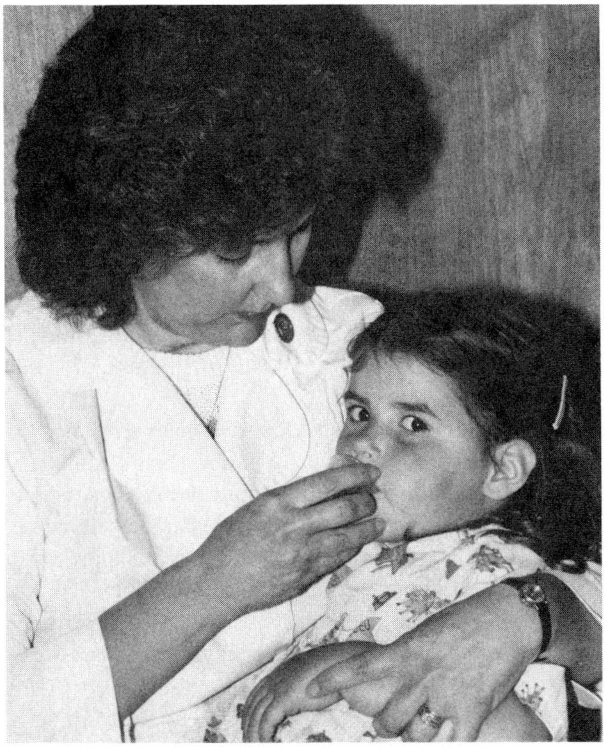

Oral medication is given when the child is in an upright or semi-upright position. (Photograph by Judy Koenig.)

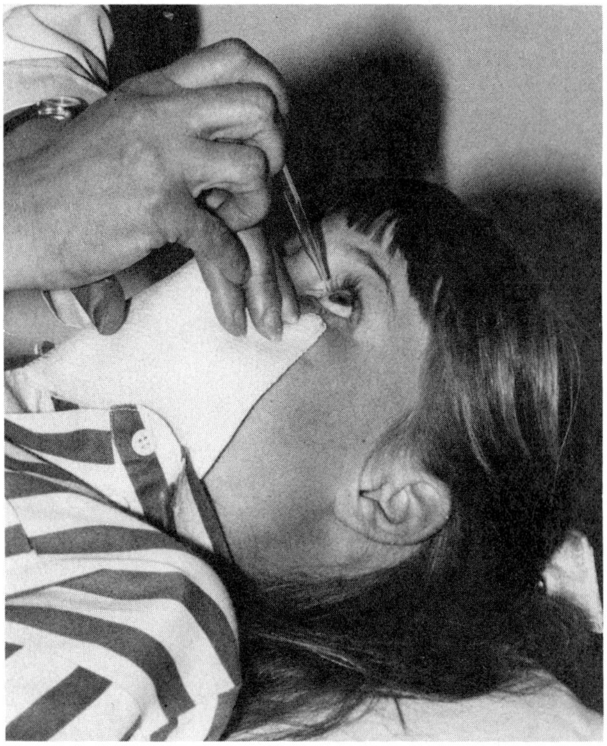

The child is positioned with the head tilted back for eye drop instillation.

It is important to remember that the child should be in an upright or semi-upright position while oral medication is administered. The nurse cautions the parent not to pinch the child's nostrils or perform other threatening movements while giving oral medication to children.

Administering topical medication When any medication is administered from a dropper or tube, the nurse is careful not to touch the child with the applicator. Such contact could cause injury or contamination to the child or applicator.

Ophthalmic instillations Eyedrops are administered to children as they are to adults. The child is positioned either lying or sitting so that the head is back. The child looks up while the nurse gently retracts the lower conjunctival sac. Moving the dropper from the outside below the child's line of vision might help prevent the child's blinking. As the drops are instilled, the dropper is held 1–2 cm above the middle to outer portion of the conjunctival sac. The nurse applies pressure for several seconds to the nasolacrimal duct at the inner corner of the eye to prevent medication from being lost through the nose. Absorption is increased if the child's eyes remain closed and the child doesn't blink. After the medication has bathed the eye, the child can resume activities.

Ophthalmic ointment is applied in the same manner with 2 cm of ointment squeezed from the tube onto the conjunctival sac. The child may then close the eyes and in so doing will spread the medication. When a child will not hold the eyes open, the nurse can place a liquid medication on the inner corner of the closed eye. Then when the eyes are opened, the medication spreads across the eyes.

Otic instillations Solutions for the ear are administered with the child's head on the side so that the affected ear is uppermost. For the child under the age of 3, the pinna is gently pulled down and back, thus straightening the external auditory canal. With a child over the age of 3, as with the adult, the pinna is pulled up and back.

The child remains with the head to the side for several minutes after the instillation of medication to help ensure the medication's bathing the entire external canal and reaching the eardrum. To aid in the spread of the medication, the nurse can apply gentle pressure and massage the outer ear after medication is instilled.

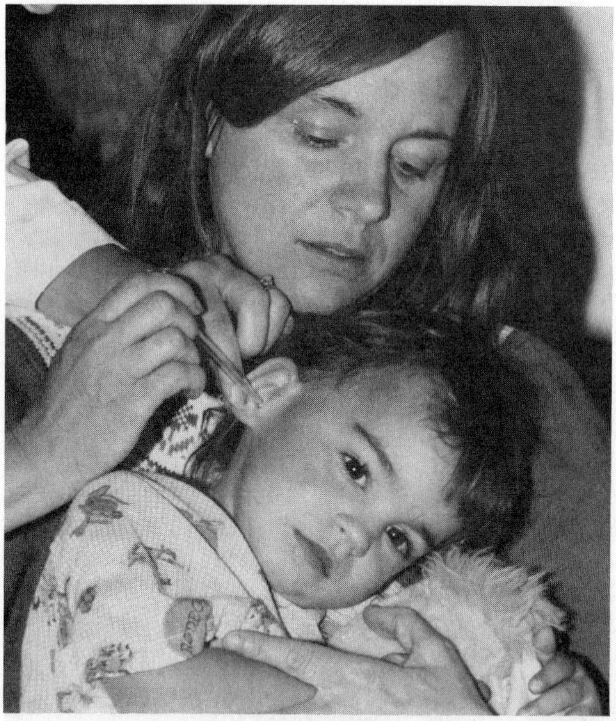

A

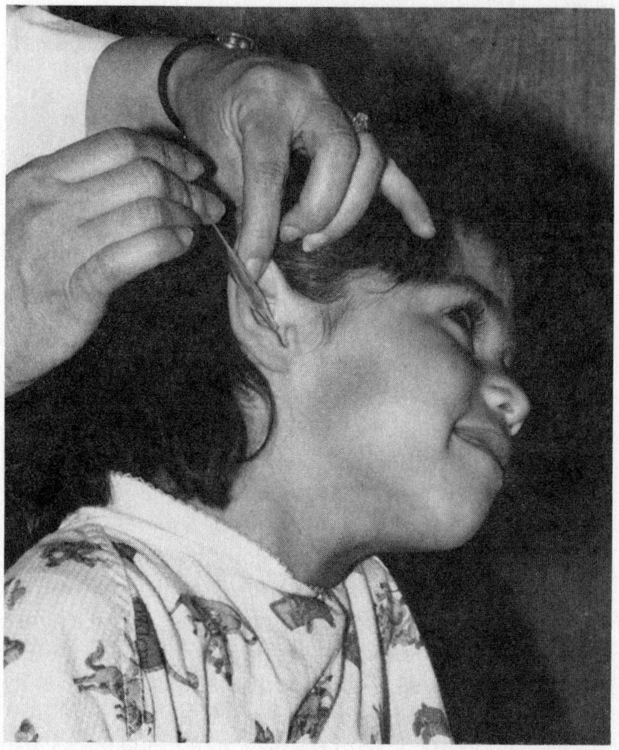

B

A. For the child under age 3, the pinna of the ear is pulled down and back for administration of drops. B. For the child over age 3, the pinna is pulled up and back. (Photograph by Judy Koenig.)

Nasal instillations Before nasal instillations, the nasal passages are cleared by the child's blowing the nose or the nurse's using a bulb syringe.

The head is hyperextended. With an infant or young child, the child's head can be positioned over one of the nurse's arms, with the arm and hand also used to restrain the child as necessary. Holding the infant's or young child's head in a lateral, though lowered, position can help prevent swallowing, with resultant increased absorption of the medication. After nasal drops are instilled, the child should keep the head back for 5–10 minutes for the medication to be effective.

Dermatologic administration Dermatologic medication administration is similar with children and adults. Because the young child's skin is more permeable, there is increased risk for medication absorption and resultant systemic effects. The nurse is especially careful to apply a thin layer of medication and confine it to those portions of skin where it is essential. The nurse assesses the child for signs and symptoms of systemic effects of the medication.

Administering rectal medication The rectal route of medication administration is very useful in children. Rectal administration often means subjecting a child to an injection is avoided and needed medication is provided when fluids are not well tolerated, as is the case preoperatively, postoperatively, or when a child is vomiting.

Medication blood levels subsequent to rectal administration might vary somewhat from those after other routes. Blood levels could be higher, it is thought, because medication absorbed into the venous system of the rectum does not pass through the liver before entering the systemic circulation (Hahn, Barkin, & Oestreich, 1982). A medication's absorption could be inhibited if it is embedded in feces in the rectum or expelled before being absorbed.

The child needs to be well prepared emotionally as well as physically. The rectal route is invasive and often embarrassing to the child. To decrease fantasies and increase understanding, the nurse also explains how the medication will feel when being inserted and what the child can do to facilitate the procedure and increase personal comfort. If the child knows the sensation of a suppository's insertion resembles a bowel movement and realizes relaxation will decrease discomfort, the child has increased control over and opportunity for mastery of the situation.

For insertion of a suppository, the child assumes a side-lying position with the upper leg flexed. A very young child may be supine with both legs flexed. With a gloved finger, the nurse inserts the lubricated rounded end of the suppository past the rectal sphincter and positions it along the wall of the rectum. The suppository is inserted to a depth of 5 cm (2 in.) or less for a small child and as much as 10 cm

(4 in.) for a fully grown child. The finger can then be removed and the child's buttocks gently held together until the child no longer strains or indicates the urge to expel the medication. Suppositories might need to be divided to administer a child's correct dose. To increase precision, the nurse can longitudinally split the suppository.

Administering intravenous medication The intravenous route has definite advantages for medication administration in children. Intravenous administration of antibiotics, for instance, allows therapy free from repeated painful intramuscular injections. Because IV medications are absorbed quickly, medication effects can be very rapid and serum levels high.

Concerns related to intravenous infusion The route is not without difficulties, however. Many children fear any manipulation of their IVs. Although the child will generally not experience any altered sensation when a medication is given intravenously, the nurse needs to prepare the child for the experience. Some children do mention having a sensation, such as a slight burning, when there is a change in the IV solution, as when medications are added or the maintenance IV is continued after a medication. Children's IVs are often delicate, and placement might be close to the small vein wall. Any movement can dislodge the needle or vary the flow rate of the IV.

The initial IV insertion is painful and traumatic to most children, and if the IV fails during the course of treatment, the child might have to have another. It is possible, from medication infusing directly into tissues instead of the vein, to cause tissue damage that can be extensive and result in deformity. The nurse therefore assesses carefully for inflammation, infiltration, and patency of the IV before administering any intravenous medication.

Methods of intravenous administration There are various methods of intravenous medication administration. Some medications, such as vitamins and electrolytes (for example, potassium), might be added to the child's IV bottle or bag. Frequently, medication is directly added to the child's maintenance IV burette. The medication must, in this case, be compatible with the child's maintenance IV solution.

When a medication is incompatible with the child's maintenance IV, a compatible solution with its own calibrated burette and tubing may be piggybacked into a portal in the maintenance IV. After the new IV is attached, it is started and the maintenance solution is stopped during the entire course of the medication administration. The tubing must be flushed with the new solution before and after medication, so as to avoid incompatibility of medication and solution.

The nurse also needs to be aware of how much a medication should be diluted and at what rate it can be safely infused. Medication generally will need to be infused over time of an hour or less, thus ensuring the medication's administration at the hour required and at its greatest potency. For medication to infuse, it must clear both the calibrated burette and the IV tubing. The tubing contains at least 10 mL of fluid and, with extensions, might contain 15 mL or more. When the burette functionally empties (some solution usually remains after solution ceases to drip), fluid must be added and then infused to flush the medication from the tubing. This fluid must be added and begin to flow immediately to prevent clotting of the IV needle at the infusing site. The amount of fluid added depends on the length of the IV tubing and generally ranges from 10 to 15 mL. The principle is that the child receives the full dose of medication at the appropriate time. If a child receives two or more medications consecutively, each medication might need to be flushed before the next is added. This creates a buffer of solution between medications.

For the very young infant or fluid-restricted child, the fluid required to flush the IV medication might place too great a strain on the child's fluid balance. Low-volume IV tubing, which contains 3 mL rather than the usual 10 mL, reduces the amount of fluid delivered to the child (Zenk, 1986).

Retrograde injection is a method by which IV medication is administered with little increase in fluid volume. The diluted medication is injected through a portal close to the child. The tubing close to the child is pinched momentarily, and the injection of medication is directed backward toward the IV burette. The medication is diluted and infuses more slowly than if it were injected toward the vein or if the tubing were not clamped.

Another method of reducing fluid volume during IV medication administration is the use of a retrograde administration set. A *retrograde administration set* is a system that allows medication to be added to the child's IV without any increase in fluid volume. Through use of stopcocks and low-volume tubing attached to the tubing between the child and the IV, the volume of the medication displaces an equal volume of IV fluid. The drug to be given is diluted in an amount sufficient to infuse over 30 minutes (1.5 mL for 3.0 mL/hour rate) (Zenk, 1986).

Administering intramuscular medication Although the actual technique used with children receiving intramuscular medication is the same as with adults, variations are needed depending on the child's size and muscle development. Because of children's smaller size, an intramuscular injection is often done with a shorter needle; a 1-in. needle is a common choice. Because of underdevelopment of the posterior gluteal muscle in a child who has been walking for

FIGURE 20-10

Sites for intramuscular injection. A. Deltoid muscle, B. dorsogluteal muscle, and C. vastus lateralis.

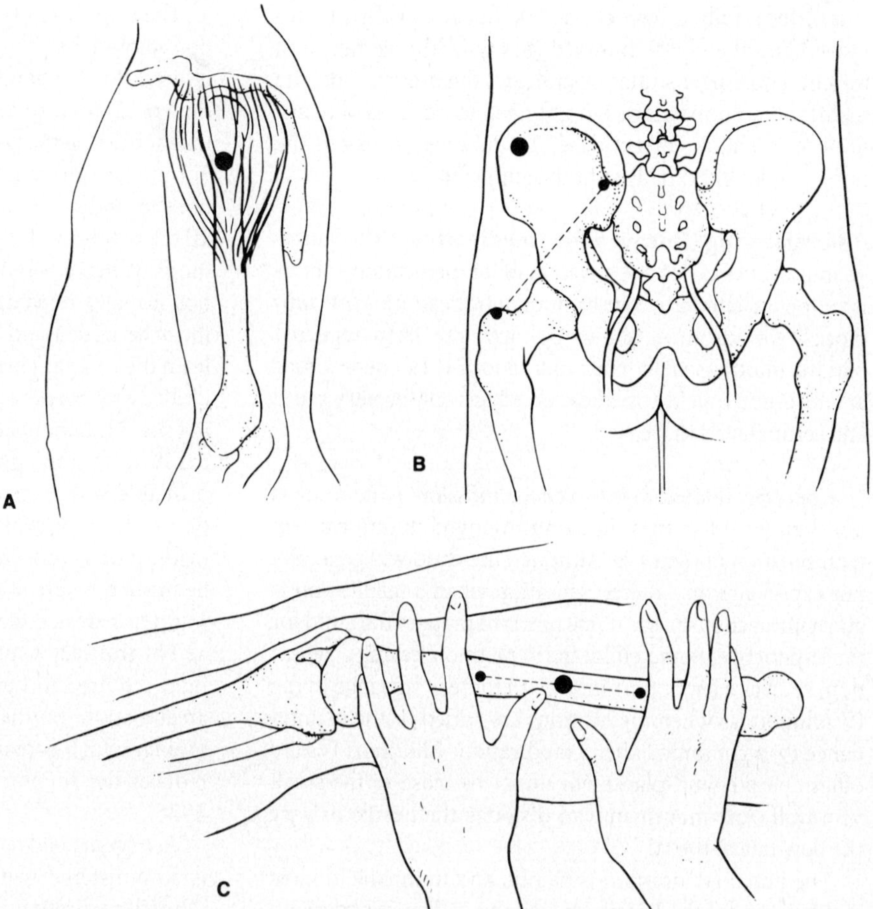

less than a year, this site is usually avoided in the infant and young child. Its use risks injury to the sciatic nerve. It should not be used in the child under the age of 2 and is preferably avoided until the child is over age 4.

Preferred injection sites in the young child are the thigh and the deltoid muscle. The vastus lateralis on the lateral aspect of the thigh or the rectus femoris on the anterior aspect are the usual choices. These are large muscles, and medication is generally well absorbed. Using the thigh as an injection site is not, however, without controversy. Multiple injections in the quadriceps group of the thigh have been linked to quadriceps contracture (Drehobl, 1980). Sites are always rotated when a child needs repeated injections, and the nurse carefully assesses the tissue perfusion and general condition of the skin.

The deltoid muscle is small but its use has some advantages. Children will sometimes feel it is less invasive than the thigh, and medication is absorbed most quickly from this site. This makes it ideal for giving medication in an emergency or analgesics for the child who is already feeling a high degree of pain. Medication is absorbed somewhat less quickly from the quadriceps of the thigh, and most slowly from the buttocks. (Site identification is reviewed in Fig. 20-10.)

Because of vast differences in size, muscle mass, and subcutaneous tissue, it is especially important to note bony prominences as landmarks for intramuscular injections in children. The muscle mass of the deltoid can be used for aqueous, nonirritating medications. The vastus lateralis can be used for most medications, except those that stain or are particularly irritating. The dorsogluteal can be used for any intramuscular medication, as long as the child has a well-developed gluteal muscle.

If the muscle mass chosen for an injection is small, either the needle used must be 1 in. or less or the muscle mass is supported and lifted slightly with one hand during needle insertion. Often it is necessary to use a short needle and to lift the muscle gently to ensure the needle's adequately penetrating the muscle while not striking bone.

The injection and any restraint necessary are first explained to the child. The child is gently but firmly restrained. The injection site is carefully chosen and the area cleansed. Allowing the alcohol to dry helps slightly to minimize the pain of the injection both by eliminating the sting of alcohol as the skin is pierced and by reassuring the child the nurse's goal is to make the injection as painless as possible.

The skin is quickly pierced with the needle at 90° for an intramuscular injection. The nurse aspirates to clear the needle (0.2 mL when a 1½-in. needle is used) to rule out the needle's having entered a blood vessel. Medication is injected at a moderate rate, and then the needle is withdrawn. Except when contraindicated, as with an irritating or anticoagulant medication, the skin should be massaged after the injection. This encourages absorption of the medication and distracts and reassures the child. The nurse and/or parent then must provide appropriate comfort measures.

The entire injection procedure should be as rapid as possible so as to minimize fear, anxiety, and restraint of the child. The nurse, however, cannot sacrifice technique for speed. The nurse carefully teaches and explains, selects the appropriate site, and uses such necessary methods as the Z track with irritating medications. Some of the most important nursing measures are then comforting, reestablishing a relationship with the child, and providing a means for the child's working through the experience.

Psychosocial management of administering medications Preparing children and adolescents for medications requires the same concepts that the nurse applies to parent and child education. The nurse first needs to be honest in explaining the purpose and necessity of medications. Will the medicine help control infection? Will it reduce pain or fever? The nurse then describes, as accurately as possible, any sensations the child might experience. Does the drug leave a bitter taste in the mouth? Does it hurt and sting as it is injected? An ophthalmic ointment, for example, makes vision blurry for a while. A rectal suppository's insertion feels somewhat as if a bowel movement is taking place. A child prepared for blurry vision will not be as frightened by it. A child prepared for the sensations of having a suppository can relax more during and after its insertion.

Children prepared for a bitter taste can gain an appropriate mental set before drinking a medicine and will be less likely to spit out or refuse to finish a dose. The child then can be ready to wash away the taste with a pleasant-tasting food or drink. Children understanding that a medication stings but that an injection itself hurts very little have more mastery over the situation and might better cooperate.

The timing and complexity of preparation depend on the situation as well as the developmental stage of the child. With injections, most older children can be prepared in advance. Young children, however, do better with an explanation immediately prior to the injection.

Even an infant can be prepared for a medication. The nurse automatically looks at, talks to, and touches an infant when giving an oral or topical medication. For an injection, the nurse also needs to remember to talk to and touch an infant. Going through a very simple explanation, such as saying that the infant is going to get a shot and that it will hurt, as the skin is cleansed will do no harm, and this kind of intervention might in fact help the child relax.

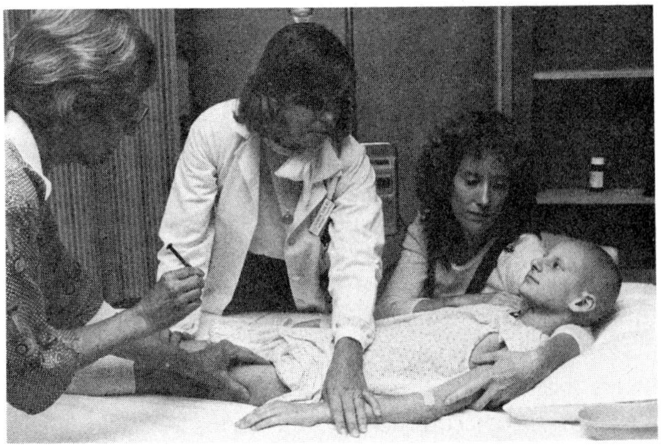

The child is gently but firmly restrained for an intramuscular injection. (From Kozier B, Erb G: Fundamentals of Nursing, *3rd ed. Addison-Wesley, 1987.)*

Using therapeutic play When time allows, a child benefits from age-appropriate therapeutic play before the experience. When therapeutic play is not possible prior to the injection, it is needed afterward so that the child can work out feelings and is able to clarify thoughts about a medication. Playing and talking through the experience also can improve a child's coping skills by allowing expression of fears and feelings, thus turning a passive situation into an active one. The nurse can use these sessions to teach children more effective coping mechanisms. A child can then practice positive coping behaviors such as squeezing a hand instead of hitting the nurse or such as saying "ouch" rather than screaming.

Setting limits For some children, medication is a way of life, and very little is demanded of the nurse either in preparation or in setting limits. For other children, even drinking an oral medication is traumatic. After an appropriate explanation, the nurse might need to set firm, though gentle, limits on the child. The 2-year-old almost always offers the proverbial "no" to any suggested activity. The child around age 4 is particularly adept at offering countless, seemingly plausible excuses to delay or prevent medication: "It doesn't hurt at all now. I need to go to the bathroom. Right now!" Although an anxiety-raising experience can cause a child to feel the need to void and there are rare occasions when a nurse should allow the child to do so before being medicated, a child can almost always be medicated first. Delay simply serves to raise a child's anxiety level even further. Preparation time then becomes lengthy, and the confusion causes the child to question who is the adult. The nurse's setting appropriate limits helps control the child's fears as well as the situation.

Children need a role in the medication process, and they can have a degree of independence and make decisions. The 4-year-old who shouldn't be allowed to use the bathroom before receiving an injection can choose, within appropriate limits, the injection site. A child can tell a nurse to give a shot on the count of 3 and can do the counting. A child can hold a medication cup or have a parent actually give an oral or dermatologic medication. An older child or adolescent might be able to help plan the timing of medications so as not to interfere with rest or activities. Oral medications are not forced on the totally uncooperative child. This is prohibited because of the danger of aspiration. It is also harmful to the child's relationship with the nurse and encourages feelings of helplessness and rebellion. The nurse can reteach and prepare the child and can search for new, creative nursing approaches. Perhaps a child will take medication if it is offered by a parent or if the nurse will read a story afterward. As a last resort, the nurse can attempt to have the route of administration changed.

Ensuring safety For parenteral administration of medications, the nurse frequently needs the assistance of another person or other persons to restrain the child safely. The child needs to remain still, with hands not interfering, and the injection site must be immobilized. So as not to be overwhelming, as few people as necessary should approach the child. A child's parent or other visitor should never be asked to restrain a child. Many are very upset seeing their child receive an injection or any treatment causing pain. Some do not wish to stay in the room and watch, and some will even leave the unit during painful procedures. Asking to restrain and thus help with the injection unnecessarily exposes them to anxiety and a guilt-producing experience.

If parents or other visitors wish to stay with a child and if the child so desires, they can stay near the child's head, hold a hand, and comfort the child. Many will repeat the nurse's teaching, encouraging the child to hold still and reassuring the child that the injection is necessary and will soon be over.

Establishing trust The last and perhaps most important nursing measures in medicating a child are comforting, building self-esteem, and establishing or reestablishing a trusting relationship after medication administration. In a developmentally appropriate way, the nurse comforts the child. This is very important following all pain-causing interventions. The nurse picks up, hugs, talks to, and perhaps rocks the infant and young child. Even an adolescent might need and enjoy a hug. Holding the child's hand and perhaps expressing unhappiness at causing pain can help.

Despite the importance of specific teaching and play techniques, it is the relationship between the child and nurse that to a large degree determines the child's acceptance of and cooperation with necessary medications and treatments. The nurse's expressing personal feelings, learning about the child's feelings, and spending time with the child—time beyond that needed for physical nursing care—forms a basis for a healthy relationship.

Isolation Procedures

Although recommendations concerning isolation in the hospital have been revised recently (Jackson and McPherson, 1986), isolation is still required for some children (Table 20-5).

Adaptations for isolation techniques center around variations in children's developmental levels; their abilities to understand and cooperate with isolation procedures; and the feelings, fears, fantasies, and needs brought about by these procedures.

Meeting sensory needs When isolation is prescribed, a child is likely to experience, and in fact suffer from, extreme sensory alteration. Most common is sensory deprivation. Children often cannot leave their rooms or beds and so cannot join in group activities or natural socialization available to them on the unit. The difficulties, time, and energy involved in gowning and gloving are not great, but they tend to discourage frequent, short visits from nurses and thus reduce opportunities for talk and play. Nurses need to guard against appearing at the child's bedside only for treatments, procedures, and necessary hygienic care. They need to plan time for other aspects of a child's care and allow time for reading, playing with, or simply being near the child.

Providing age-appropriate explanations For isolation practices, children need explanations geared to their developmental levels. Rather than telling children that cooperation with the treatment plan will make them "better," they can hear that such actions will make them well so that they can go home and play as they did before. Ultimately, nurses need to rely on the overall relationship with a child to reassure, comfort, and clarify that illness and isolation are not punishments. The nurse first observes the child's general behavior as well as specific responses to words, explanations, and teaching. Play can then greatly assist the nurse

(text continues on p. 624)

TABLE 20-5 Recommended Types of Isolation and Precautions

Type of isolation	Purpose	Private room	Gowns	Masks	Gloves	Articles
Strict	To prevent the transmission of pathogens spread both by contact and by airborne sources	Necessary; door must be kept closed	Must be worn by all persons entering room	Must be worn by all persons entering room	Must be worn by all persons entering room	Discard or wrap before sending to central supply for disinfection or sterilization
Respiratory	To prevent airborne infection from respiratory droplets that are coughed, sneezed, or exhaled	Necessary; door must be kept closed	Not necessary	Must be worn by all persons entering room	Must be worn for direct contact with secretions	Discard or disinfect articles contaminated with secretions
Enteric	To prevent transmission of pathogens in the feces	Necessary for children only	Must be worn by all persons having direct contact with the patient	Not necessary	Must be worn by all persons having direct contact with infected area or articles contaminated by fecal material	Disinfect or discard articles contaminated with urine and feces using special precautions
Wound and skin	To prevent the transmission of pathogens transmitted by direct contact with wounds or articles contaminated by wounds (eg, dressings or linen)	Desirable	Must be worn by all persons having direct contact with the patient	Not necessary except during dressing changes	Must be worn by all persons having direct contact with the infected area	Special precautions are necessary for instruments, dressings, and linen
Blood	To prevent the transmission of organisms carried by blood or blood products	Depends on disease entity	Depends on disease entity	Not necessary	Must be worn for direct contact with blood or needles	Dispose of all needles in a box clearly labeled as precaution. Extreme caution needed to prevent accidental skin puncture. Label specimens for laboratory
Secretions	To prevent the spread of organisms transmitted through saliva and mucous secretions	Depends on disease entity	Not necessary	Depends on disease entity	Necessary when handling linen, tissues, suction apparatus, and other contaminated articles	Special precaution necessary for all tissues, linens, and other articles that come in contact with body secretions

NOTE: For all types of isolation the hands must be washed on entering and leaving the room.

SOURCE: Adapted from Garner JS, Simmons BP: CDC guidelines for isolation precautions in hospitals. *Infection Control* (July/Aug) 1983; 4(4): 258–260.

STANDARDS OF NURSING CARE *The Postoperative Child*

RISKS

Assessed risk	Nursing action
Postoperative hemorrhage	Check incisional site and dressing for bright red bleeding. Monitor vital signs for increased pulse and decreasing blood pressure. Note any skin pallor, restlessness, or thirst. **Ear, nose, and throat surgery:** Observe for blood oozing from the nose. Observe for frequent swallowing and examine the back of the throat using a flashlight (do not use a tongue depressor). **Genitourinary surgery:** Observe for clots and obvious occult blood in the urine. **Gastrointestinal surgery:** Observe for blood in the stool or vomitus. **Orthopedic surgery:** Outline any cast staining and observe for a spreading stain. **Neurologic surgery:** Observe and monitor neurologic status.
Alteration in gastrointestinal function—nausea, vomiting, and possible paralytic ileus	Insert nasogastric tube as ordered for severe vomiting. Measure abdominal girth to monitor for abdominal distension. Place an indelible ink mark on the child's abdomen to indicate the placement of the measuring tape. Observe for returning gastrointestinal motility by listening for return of bowel sounds and observing for flatus and frequency of postoperative stools.

GUIDE FOR NURSING MANAGEMENT

Nursing diagnosis	Intervention	Rationale	Outcome
1. Potential for ineffective breathing pattern (stressors: anesthesia and presence of pain)	Observe for patent airway.	Child might show signs of a deepened anesthesia effect even after return from the recovery room. Aspiration after vomiting is possible.	The child's breath sounds are clear in all lobes. The child's respiratory rate, temperature, and blood pressure are within normal limits for age.
	Monitor quality of respirations for adventitious sounds and for depth and symmetry.	Pooling of secretions can lead to pneumonia. Inadequate air exchange is possible because of pain and inactivity; atelectasis can occur.	
	Monitor vital signs.	Increased respiratory rate can indicate respiratory distress or infection. Increased temperature in the first few days after surgery usually indicates respiratory infection.	
	Encourage adequate and frequent deep breathing (at least every hour). Time pain relief measures so that the child is as comfortable as possible before attempting deep breathing and coughing.	Deep breathing encourages adequate air exchange and loosens secretions. A slightly elevated temperature will often decrease after adequate deep breathing.	
	Have the child splint the incision line during deep breathing.	Splinting the incision line reduces the pressure exerted on it during breathing and reduces the pain incurred.	

STANDARDS OF NURSING CARE *The Postoperative Child (Continued)*

GUIDE FOR NURSING MANAGEMENT

Nursing diagnosis	Intervention	Rationale	Outcome
2. Potential for fluid volume deficit (stressors: fluid loss during surgery; maintenance of NPO status)	Provide optimal parenteral fluid intake by monitoring the IV. Encourage oral fluids when the child is taking p.o.s.	Fluid needs vary with age and weight of child. Because of postoperative sequestering and diuresis of fluids and immaturities in newborn and infant body systems, postoperative fluid needs for the infant may be considered to be 100 mL/kg body weight for 24 hours.	The child voids in amounts appropriate for age and weight and at least 1 mL/kg/hour. The child has normal skin turgor and moist mucous membranes.
	Monitor urine specific gravity and laboratory values (see Chapter 21).	In the absence of cardiac or renal disese, specific gravity is an excellent indicator of hydration status.	
	Measure urine output.	Urine output, in the absence of cardiac and renal disease or urinary retention, mirrors circulating blood volume and hydration status, and lowered output can be an early indicator of impending shock.	
	Be alert for signs of overhydration subsequent to replacement fluid therapy.	A child can become overhydrated from parenteral or oral fluids, and the infant is especially prone to fluid and electrolyte imbalances. Children are prone to imbalances, particularly to metabolic acidosis, and close, careful assessment is necessary.	
	Begin oral fluids very slowly when they are permitted; start with easily assimilated fluids such as water followed by bland clear fluids (flat carbonated beverages or ice pops).	Slow introduction of fluids might prevent or lessen postoperative nausea or vomiting.	
	Hold apple juice or strained orange juice until fluid intake is well established. With signs of nausea, vomiting, distension, or diarrhea, return child to NPO status or to a more bland diet.	Apple and orange juice might not be well accepted with some children and can lead to cramping or diarrhea.	
3. Potential alteration in urinary elimination pattern (stressors: anesthesia, preoperative medications)	Measure first voiding after surgery. Monitor total output. Monitor voiding pattern and signs of urinary retention. Observe for patency of drainage tubes after genitourinary surgery.	Anesthesia and other medications can lead to retention of urine. Inadequate volume of void can be a sign of urinary retention with overflow.	The child exhibits no sign of bladder distension. The urine specific gravity is within normal limits and the child is voiding appropriately for age and weight.

(Continues)

STANDARDS OF NURSING CARE *The Postoperative Child (Continued)*

GUIDE FOR NURSING MANAGEMENT

Nursing diagnosis	Intervention	Rationale	Outcome
	Position the child as close to normal voiding position as possible and provide privacy. Turn on running water so the child can hear it.	These measures are noninvasive measures to encourage voiding.	
	Catheterize as ordered for bladder distension and urinary retention.	Catheterization is necessary when noninvasive methods fail.	
4. Potential for impaired physical mobility (stressors: pain, surgical incision)	Provide range-of-motion exercises and other activities within treatment restrictions. Have the child ambulate as soon as possible.	Early ambulation promotes gastrointestinal and genitourinary mobility, muscle strength, and venous return. Formal range-of-motion exercises are not always needed with temporary immobility.	The child is mobile within the treatment plan restrictions and practices muscle activities that will decrease the effects of immobility. The child's joints remain flexible.
5. Impaired skin integrity related to the surgical procedure and immobility	Observe skin in general and its redness, quantity and nature of drainage, or excessive warmth in particular. Immediately report dehiscence (separation of the suture line) or evisceration (protrusion of the internal organs through the suture line).	The child, as well as the adult, might have red, irritated areas, and skin breakdown can occur. Wound infections or complications must be evaluated as quickly as possible. An increase in temperature after the first few postoperative days is usually indicative of a wound infection.	The child's incision is intact and healing. There are no signs of redness or purulent drainage at the incision site. The child's body temperature does not become elevated.
	Change dressings as ordered using sterile technique.	Sterile technique prevents the entry of organisms. Postoperative dressings are removed totally after a few days to enhance healing of the incision.	

in understanding the impact of isolation on the child and in teaching the true meaning of isolation.

Meeting social needs Both visitors and children need appropriate explanations. Many parents resist the imposed barriers of gown, gloves, or mask between them and their children because they are accustomed to and often highly value close physical contact and direct touch with the child. When a child has a medical condition or treatment that the parent considers serious (for example, a bone marrow transplant or an extensive burn), the parent might freely and eagerly cooperate with these restrictions. When a child has a condition the parent does not consider serious, cooperation might be less complete. The nurse attempts to learn the parent's perceptions of the child's illness and isolation. Denial and guilt might be contributing to a parent's lack of cooperation with isolation measures. Teaching the necessary components of and reasons for isolation might need to be repeated frequently.

Postoperative Care

The adaptations of postoperative care for children depend on psychologic as well as physical differences. An operation, regardless of its extent, alters a child's body image. An incision exists; a child moves from a relatively independent to a dependent condition. The nurse focuses on increasing a child's independence and encouraging expression of feelings.

Many children do not fully understand preoperative teaching until they are required to participate in postoperative nursing interventions. The child needs a repetition of preoperative teaching and preoperative play opportunities. Postoperatively, the nurse might need to reteach the purposes of the IV, deep breathing, catheters, tubes, and other postoperative care measures. The nurse needs to reemphasize their use and thereby defuse feelings of punishment, anger, helplessness, and dependence.

Children's postoperative play is adjusted to individual feelings, responses to suggestions, and opportunities for play. Many children in the early postoperative period need rest and quiet companionship. Play then centers around entertainment and activities familiar to the child. Soon many children are ready for expressive, creative play. Paints and clay are usually well accepted, as these give a child opportunities to work out frustrations and anger. Many children do not draw in the postoperative phase of hospitalization, but they can be encouraged to express themselves through other art media, stories, and dramatic play. Many of these same children express themselves through drawing when they are seen for follow-up care.

Some hospitalized children do make good use of drawing. For instance, a 5-year-old girl was unavoidably not visited by her family from the day of surgery until discharged from the hospital after her tonsillectomy and adenoidectomy. The day after surgery, she was very withdrawn and expressed little emotion. She was not able to talk about her surgery and didn't seem to listen to reassurances. She did not play and would not accept oral fluids. Her nurse asked her to draw a picture with available materials: a tray, place mat, and pen. The child drew her family, and she left herself out of the picture. Nursing reassurances could then be focused. She was assured that her parents missed her and would soon come to take her home. The child was then better able to play and drink, and when her parents did arrive, she cried and eventually laughed and smiled.

Physical care for the child after surgery includes the same optimal care measures used for the adult. (Several considerations specific to children's physiologic immaturities are illustrated with Standards of Nursing Care, the Postoperative Child.)

Essential Concepts

- Safety in the hospital presents special considerations for children, including proper holding, bathing, and use of beds, cribs, and restraints.
- Hospitalization can provide an opportunity for a thorough nutritional assessment and appropriate child and family teaching about temporary changes in nutritional needs.
- Children who have nothing by mouth require special nursing attention during mealtimes.
- Feeding patterns for a hospitalized infant should, as much as possible, approximate feeding patterns at home.
- Mothers often need encouragement and assistance to continue breast-feeding hospitalized infants.
- The mealtime environment should be as homelike as possible and is best located away from rooms and equipment associated with painful procedures.
- For young children who are learning toileting skills, the nurse supports the child's and family's efforts and explains that any regression is normal and temporary.
- Older children who need assistance with toileting might require special attention to their needs for privacy and modesty.
- The nurse can help a child to sleep by following the child's accustomed bedtime rituals, when possible, and by managing pain relief and activity to promote comfort and rest.
- Complications of immobility that the nurse addresses include alterations in activity, respiratory status, elimination, and skin integrity.
- Immobilized children need an environment that allows them some measure of control and feelings of independence.
- Assessment of pain includes observing for verbal and nonverbal cues and using simple pain assessment tools.
- Nurses cannot allow children to avoid necessary painful procedures, such as injections for pain relief.
- Diminishing anxiety, explaining the cause and temporary nature of pain, and planning activities that distract children from attention to their pain are all possible noninvasive measures for pain relief.
- Medication for pain relief is best tolerated if the child knows what sensations to expect when the medication is administered.
- Fevers of 39°C (102°F) can assist the body to fight disease.

- Nurses can administer antipyretics and tepid sponge baths, if ordered, to children with high fevers.
- Color, sensation, and motion assessment are necessary in determining the vascularity and innervation of body parts.
- In providing urine and stool samples during hospitalization, children often need nursing assistance that includes matter-of-fact, age-appropriate explanations with words the child understands.
- For the incontinent child, urine may be collected by means of a collecting bag or by properly withdrawing urine from a wet diaper.
- Venipunctures can be particularly threatening to children because a common fear of childhood is that the body insides can come out through a puncture in the skin.
- The choice of a site for IV infusion is determined by accessibility, type of solution, likely duration of the infusion, and age and condition of the child.
- Intravenous fluids may be delivered by gravity administration and by infusion and syringe pumps, all of which need to be carefully monitored for accuracy.
- Nursing care for the child receiving an IV infusion is planned to prevent complications, provide for developmental needs, and maintain safety.
- Medicating a child requires painstaking attention to dosages.
- Oral medications require careful measurement and sometimes require combining the medicine with food or drink if the child finds swallowing a pill or capsule difficult.
- Intramuscular administration of medication for a child is similar to that for an adult, although the size of the needle and preferred sites of injection vary depending on the child's size and muscle development.
- Playing and talking about unpleasant procedures and sensations are effective in helping children to cope with these experiences.
- Parents might choose to leave the room when their children must undergo painful procedures, although some parents are willing or able to assist the nurse in restraining or consoling their children.
- Children who are placed in isolation need age-appropriate explanations to assure them that the treatment is not a punishment and that they will eventually rejoin normal activities.
- Postoperative play is extremely valuable in helping children express and resolve their feelings of anger, helplessness, and violation of body integrity.

References

Beyer J, Aradine C: Content validity of an instrument to measure young children's perceptions of the intensity of their pain. *J Pediatr Nurs* (Dec) 1986; 1(6): 386–395.

Children in pain. (Pain consult.) *Am J Nurs* (Feb) 84: 247.

Drehobl P: Quadriceps contracture. *Am J Nurs* (Sept) 1980; 80: 1650–1651.

Eland J: The child who is hurting. *Semin Oncol Nurs* (May) 1985; 1(2): 116–122.

Franck L: A new method to quantitatively describe pain behavior in infants. *Nurs Res* (Jan/Feb) 1986; 35(1): 28–31.

Hahn AB, Barkin RL, Oestreich SJK: *Pharmacology in Nursing,* 15th ed. Mosby, 1982.

Jackson M, McPherson D: Infection control: Keeping current. *Nurs Educ* (July/Aug) 1986; 11(4): 38–40.

Kozier B, Erb G: *Fundamentals of Nursing,* 3rd ed. Addison-Wesley, 1987.

Smith D: Children's health care: Brief report using humor to help children with pain. *Child Health Care* (Winter) 1986; 14(3): 187–188.

Strohbach ME, Kratina SH: Diaper versus bag specimens: A comparison of urine specific gravity values. *Am J Matern-Child Nurs* (May/June) 1982; 7: 198–201.

Zenk KE: Administering IV antibiotics to children. *Nurs '86* (Dec) 1986; 16(12): 50–51.

Additional Readings

Abu-saad H: Cultural group indicators of pain in children. *Matern-Child Nurs J* (Fall) 1984; 13(3): 187–196.

Alexander D, White M, Powell G: Anxiety of non-rooming-in parents of hospitalized children. *Child Health Care* (Summer) 1986; 15(1): 14–19.

Arthur G: When your littlest patients need IVs. *RN* (July) 1984; 47(7): 30–35.

Bailey LM: Pain consult: Music's soothing charms. *Am J Nurs* (Nov) 1985; 85(11): 1280.

Beyerman K: Flawed perceptions about pain. *Am J Nurs* (Feb) 1982; 82: 302–304.

Birdsall C: Clinical savvy: What suction pressure should I use? *Am J Nurs* 1985; 85(8): 866.

Birdsall C, Pizzo C, Muller B: Clinical savvy: What are orthostatic BP changes? *Am J Nurs* (Oct) 1985; 85(10): 1062.

Black CD, Popovich NG, Black MC: Drug interactions in the GI tract. *Am J Nurs* (Sept) 1977; 77: 1426–1429.

Bordeaux BR: Television viewing patterns of hospitalized school-aged children and adolescents. *Child Health Care* (Fall) 1986; 15(2): 70–75.

Bradshaw C, Zeanah PD: Pediatric nurses' assessments of pain in children. *J Pediatr Nurs* (Oct) 1986; 1(5): 314–321.

Broome M: The relationship between childrens' fears and behavior during a painful event. *Child Health Care* (Winter) 1986; 14(3): 142–145.

Burrows C: IV needle selections. *Nurs '84* (Dec) 1984; 14(12): 32–33.

Burson JV, Brannigan CN: The use of play in the nutritional support of hospitalized children. *Issues Compr Pediatr Nurs* 1984; 7(4–5): 283–289.

Crowshore TM: Postoperative assessment: The key to avoiding most common nursing mistakes. *Nurs '79* (April) 1979; 9: 47–51.

D'Apolito K: The neonate's response to pain. *Am J Matern-Child Nurs* (July/Aug) 1984; 9: 256–257.

Dickmann JM, Smith JM, Wick JR: Wound care forum: A double life for a dental irrigation device. *Am J Nurs* (Oct) 1985; 85(10): 1157.

Erlen JA: The child's choice: An essential component in treatment decisions. *Child Health Care* (Winter) 1987; 15(3): 156–159.

Evans ML, Hansen BD: Administering injections to different-aged children. *Am J Matern-Child Nurs* (May/June) 1981; 6: 194–199.

Fernald CD, Corry JJ: Empathic versus directive preparation of children for needles. *Child Health Care* 1981; 10(2): 44–46.

Funk MJ, Mullins LL, Olson RA: Teaching children to swallow pills: A case study. *Child Health Care* (Summer) 1984; 13(1): 20–23.

Galligan AC: Using Roy's concept of adaptation to care for young children. *Am J Matern-Child Nurs* (Jan/Feb) 1979; 4: 24–28.

Griffin J: Fever: When to leave it alone. *Nurs '86* (Feb) 1986; 16(2): 58–61.

Hawley DD: Postoperative pain in children: Misconceptions, descriptions and interventions. *Pediatr Nurs* (Jan/Feb) 1984; 10: 20–23.

Infante MC, Mooney NE: Interactive aspects of pain assessment. *Orthop Nurs* (Jan/Feb) 1987; 6(1): 31–34.

Jacox AK: *Pain: A Source Book for Nurses and Other Health Professionals*. Little, Brown, 1977.

Jerrett R: Children and their pain experience. *Child Health Care* (Fall) 1985; 14(2): 83–89.

Long S, Henretiq F: Fever in children. *Pediatr Consult* 1987; 6(1): 1–8.

McCaffery M: Patients don't have to suffer: How to relieve pain with injectable narcotics. *Nurs '80* (Oct) 1980; 10: 34–39.

McCaffrey M: Relieving pain with noninvasive techniques. *Nurs '80* (Dec) 1980; 10: 55–57.

McCaffrey M: Undertanding your patient's pain. *Nurs '80* (Sept) 1980; 10: 26–31.

McCaffrey M: When your patient's still in pain don't just do something: Sit there. *Nurs '81* (June) 1981; 11: 58–61.

McCarron K: Fever—the cardinal vital sign. *Crit Care Quarterly* (June) 1986; 9(1): 15–18.

McGrath PJ: Psychological aspects of pain management in burned children. *Child Health Care* (Summer) 1984; 13(1): 15–19.

McGuire L, Dizard S: Managing pain in the young patient. *Nursing* (Aug) 1982; 12: 52–55.

Mitiguy JS: A surgical liaison program: Making the wait more bearable. *MCN* (Nov/Dec) 1986; 11: 388–391.

Russell H: *Pediatric Drugs and Nursing Intervention*. McGraw-Hill, 1980.

Schumann D: How to help wound healing in your abdominal surgery patient. *Nurs '80* (April) 1980; 10: 34–40.

Sciarillo WG: Using Hymovich's framework in the family-oriented approach to nursing care. *Am J Matern-Child Nurs* (July/Aug) 1980; 5: 242–248.

Schmeltz K, White G: A survey of parent groups: Prehospital admission. *Matern-Child Nurs J* (Summer) 1982; 11: 75–85.

Scott JG, Rigney-Radford K: Factors affecting the management of pain. *Am J Matern-Child Nurs* (July/Aug) 1984; 9: 253–255.

Shepherd MJ, Swearington P: Z-track. *Am J Nurs* (June) 1984; 84: 746–747.

Sheredy C: Factors to consider when assessing responses to pain. *Am J Matern-Child Nurs* (July/Aug) 1984; 9: 250–252.

Siaw S, Stephens L, Holmes S: Knowledge about medical instruments and reported anxiety in pediatric surgery patients. *Child Health Care* (Winter) 1986; 14(3): 134–141.

Stevens B, Hunsberger M, Browne G: Pain in children: Theoretical, research, and practice dilemmas. *J Pediatr Nurs* (June) 1987; 2(3): 154–166.

Tesler M, Savedra M: Coping with hospitalization: A study of school-age children. *Pediatr Nurs* 1981; 7: 35–38.

Thomas DO: Fever in children. *RN* (Dec) 1985; 48(12): 18.

Zollo M: Management of pain in critically ill children. *Am J Matern-Child Nurs* (July/Aug) 1984; 9: 258–261.

VI

Nursing Care of the Ill Child

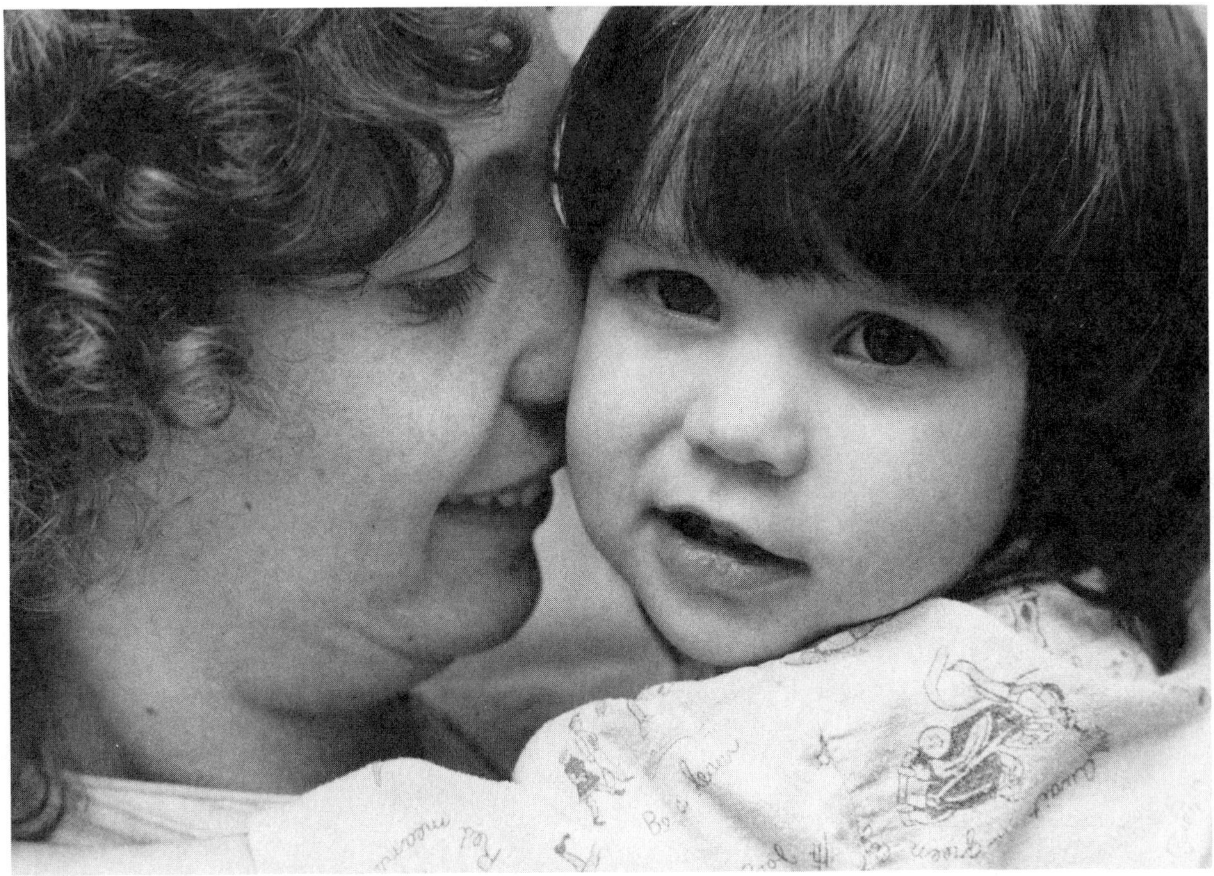

Chapter 21

Fluid and Electrolytes

Implications of Imbalance

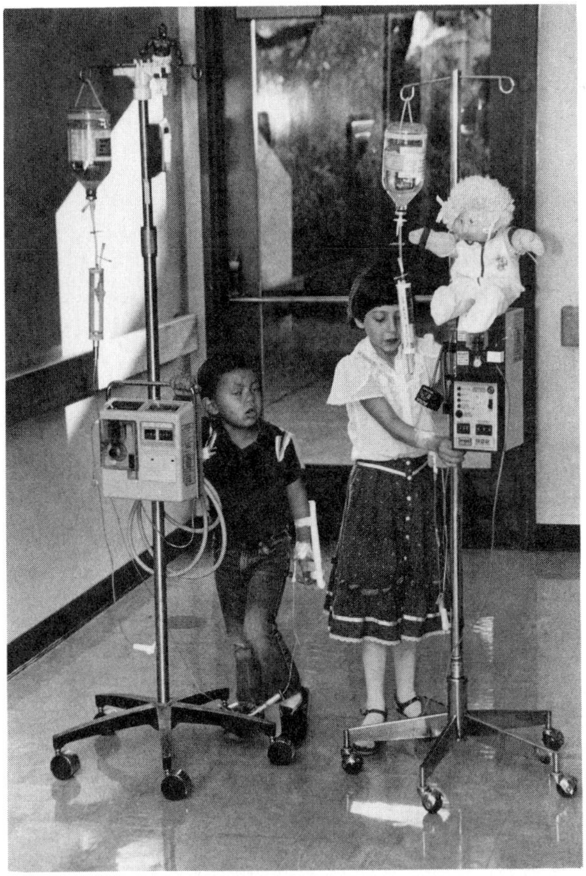

Chapter Contents

(Continues)

Cross Reference Box

To find these topics see the following chapters:

Burns	Chapter 24
Hyperalimentation	Chapter 27
Intravenous therapy	Chapter 20
Mild gastroenteritis	Chapter 18
Pyloric stenosis	Chapter 27
Salicylate poisoning	Chapter 12
Toxic shock syndrome	Chapter 28

Objectives

- Identify the components of extracellular and intracellular fluid.
- List the factors that affect water balance.
- Define the regulatory mechanisms that maintain fluid and electrolyte balance.
- Explain the nursing care measures associated with oral fluid therapy and intravenous administration.
- Describe methods of output measurement associated with monitoring fluid balance.
- Describe the physiologic dysfunction, assessment criteria, and nursing care associated with imbalances of major electrolytes.
- Explain the physiologic processes that control acid-base balance.
- Describe the physiologic dysfunction, assessment criteria, and nursing care associated with acid-base abnormalities.

ESSENTIALS OF STRUCTURE AND FUNCTION
Fluid Balance

Water performs a major role in the physiologic functioning of any cell. Cellular nutrients and waste products travel to and from the cells through water. Water regulates body temperature and is essential in the maintenance of intravascular (blood vessel) volume and thus, blood pressure. Body water contains many of the electrolytes necessary for cellular activity.

To maintain a state of body fluid balance, water intake must closely approximate water output over a 24-hour period. The body obtains water from (a) oral fluids (50%), (b) water contained in solid foods, and (c) oxidation (metabolism) of food substances (carbohydrates, fat, and protein).

Water output is primarily regulated by the kidneys (see Chapter 28). Water also is lost from the gastrointestinal tract and through insensible loss from the skin and lungs (through sweat and respiration).

Glossary

Acidosis Disturbance in acid-base balance from either increased acid accumulation or marked loss of bicarbonate resulting in lowering of blood pH.

Alkalosis Disturbance in acid-base balance from increased presence of alkalies or loss of acid or chloride from the blood resulting in raising the blood pH.

Body fluids Portion of the body made up of water (solvent) and substances (solutes) such as chemicals and protein molecules. Body fluids are located in two major body compartments—extracellular and intracellular.

Buffer systems Chemical processes in the body that help stabilize the pH concentration of body fluids. Buffers combine with hydrogen ions to counteract acidosis and release hydrogen ions to counteract alkalosis.

Electrolyte Substance that, while in a solution, carries an electrical current. Small particles (ions) that comprise electrolytes are positively (+) or negatively (−) charged. Electrolytes figure prominently in maintaining effective physiologic function (see figure showing major electrolytes).

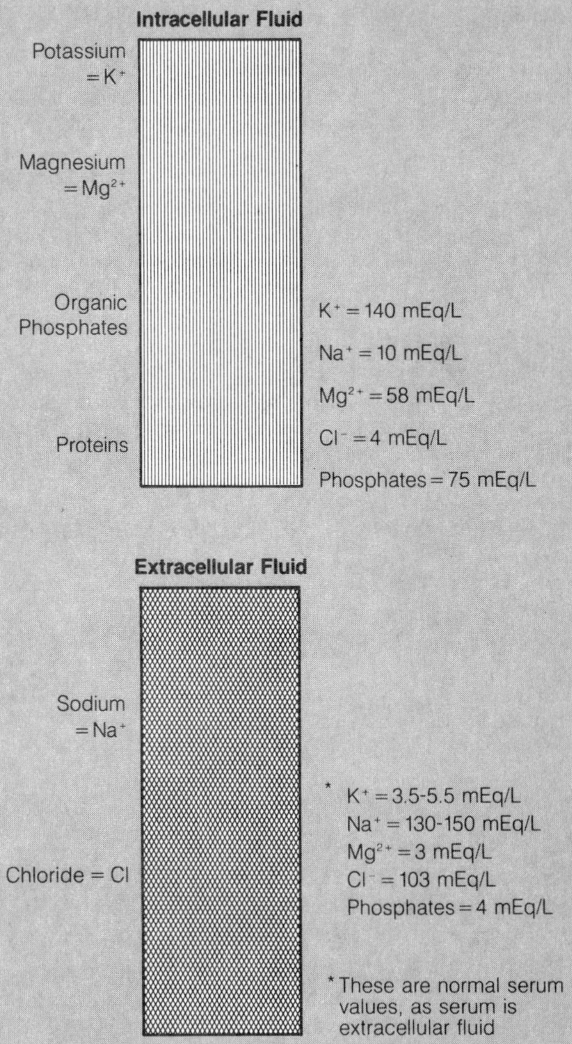

Extracellular compartment Fluid outside of body cells that transports nutrients to cells and waste products from cells. Includes interstitial fluid (the fluid environment surrounding the cells), plasma, and transcellular fluids such as saliva, sweat, urine, and certain secretions.

(Continues)

ESSENTIALS OF STRUCTURE AND FUNCTION *(Continued)*
Fluid Balance

Fluid Transport Mechanisms in Body Cells

Mechanism / **Physiologic example**

Diffusion A random dispersion of molecules caused by the normal motion of matter. The rate of diffusion is increased when the concentration of molecules differs, the size of the molecules is small, the distance the molecules must travel is short, the body temperature is increased, or when the difference between the electrical charge of opposite-charged ions (+ or −) is great.

Diffusion of inhaled oxygen into the lung capillaries.

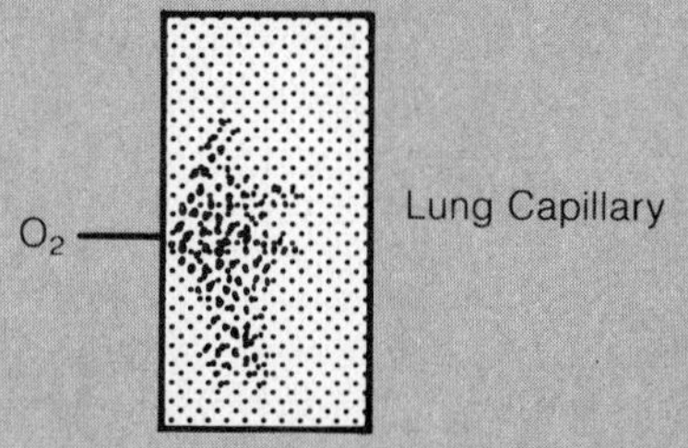

Osmosis The movement of water across a semipermeable membrane when concentrations on either side of the membrane differ. Osmotic pressure is the force exerted against the osmosis in an attempt to keep the water on the original side of the membrane.

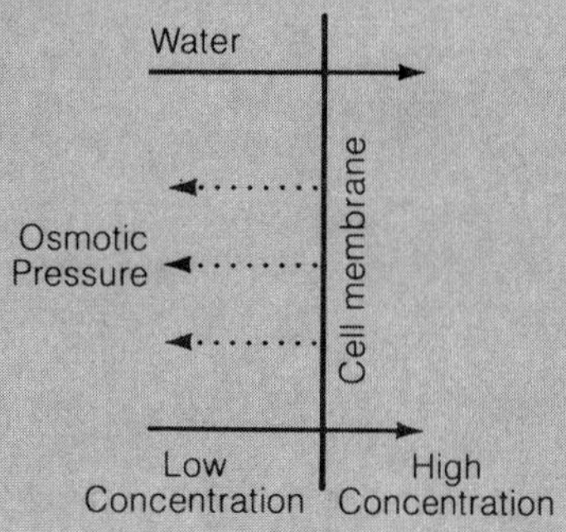

Capillary membranes are permeable to osmosis of plasma substances but not of plasma proteins. Plasma proteins (albumin and globulin) hold water in the capillary space by osmotic pressure, thus maintaining normal blood volume.

Hydrostatic pressure Causes the movement of water and solutes through a permeable membrane from an area of high pressure to an area of lower pressure—essentially caused by the pumping action of the heart.

Hydrostatic pressure causes fluid transfer from the glomerular capillaries into the interstitial fluid and then into the renal collecting tubule.

Active transport Energy (in the form of adenosine triphosphate, or ATP) moves solutes in opposition to solutions of greater concentration.

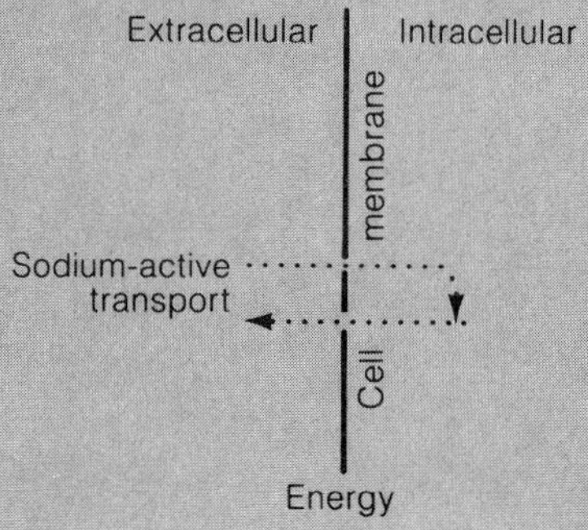

Greater concentration of sodium in extracellular fluid would normally diffuse into intracellular fluid because of the lesser concentration there. Active transport forces the sodium ions back into the area of greater concentration. Electrolytes, amino acids, and glucose cross cell membranes by active transport.

Fluid transport systems Mechanisms by which water and solutes cross cell membranes (see table of fluid transport mechanisms).

Intracellular compartment Fluid located within cells that promotes physiochemical function of each cell.

Osmolarity Concentration of solutes per liter of solution. Solutions can be *isotonic*—having the same tonicity as body fluids, *hypertonic*—having a higher concentration of solutes than body fluids, or *hypotonic*—containing a lower concentration of solutes than body fluids. Hypertonic solutions can pull water out of cells causing cellular crenation (shrinking). Hypotonic solutions can cause water to move into cells causing cellular edema (swelling). Certain dysfunctions can cause body fluids to become hyper- or hypotonic. The effects on the cells are the same regardless of the cause of the change in tonicity.

pH Measure of the amount of hydrogen ion (H^+) in a solution. Excessive H^+ results in an acidic solution and a resulting low pH measurement. Low H^+ results in an alkaline environment and a high pH measurement. The pH of body fluids can range on a scale from 0–14 with 7 indicating a neutral state. The pH of arterial blood, for example, is 7.4.

Regulatory mechanisms External and internal mechanisms that regulate fluid balance. These include osmolarity (tonicity) of body fluids, thirst, hormones (eg, antidiuretic hormone [ADH], aldosterone), and the renin/angiotensin mechanism of the renal system (see Chapter 28).

Total body water (TBW) The total amount of water in the body, usually stated as a percentage of the body weight. In infants the TBW is approximately 77% of the total weight, whereas in adults TBW is 40%–60% of weight (see figure showing water distribution).

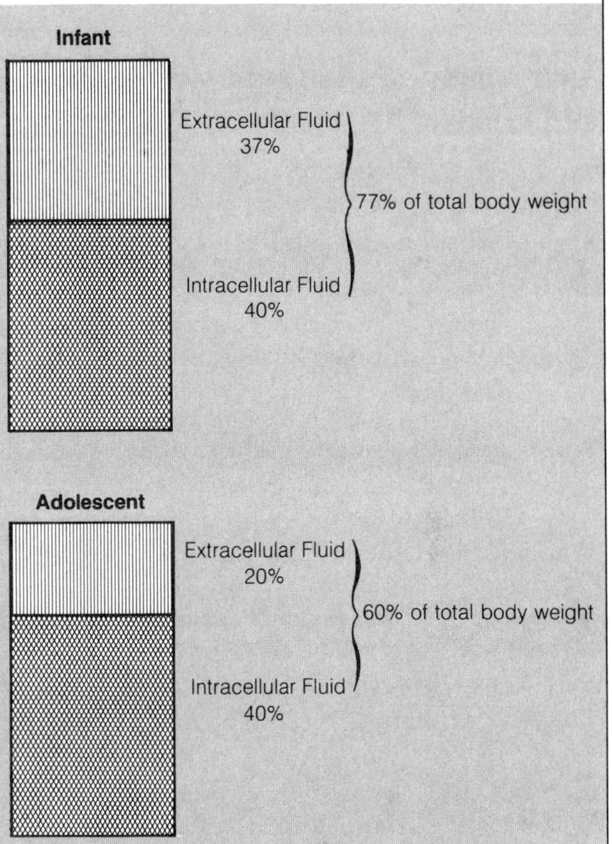

Distribution of total body water in the infant and adolescent.

The child's body is composed of fluids and solid masses within a structural frame. Health and homeostasis (balance) rely on maintenance of the appropriate proportion of fluids and solids within the body and its physiologic systems. Any marked change in the fluid volume with its associated change in electrolyte distribution can cause corresponding, serious changes in the child's internal environment. These changes include, but are not limited to, alterations in cardiovascular, renal, and respiratory function, and in the body's ability to provide nourishment for growth.

Clinical symptoms rapidly become apparent in the child suffering from an imbalance of fluid and electrolytes. Body water, electrolytes, and acid-base balance (for example, pH) need to be regulated within narrow limits to maintain proper physiologic functioning. Because of the high proportion of water contained in the child's body, the child is particularly vulnerable, even to slight shifts in body fluid, electrolytes, and arterial pH.

Because any alteration in function has the potential to upset the delicate fluid and electrolyte balance, knowledge of the physiologic processes involved in maintaining fluid and electrolyte balance is vital to a complete assessment of a child's health status.

Assessment of the Child with a Fluid and Electrolyte Imbalance

Differences Between Young Children and Adults

Infants and young children are at greater risk than older children and adults for fluid and electrolyte imbalances. These risks are related to the following factors:

1. The young child's total body water (TBW) is a higher percentage of body weight than an adult's (77% versus 40%–60%).
2. The young child has a larger percentage of fluid located in the extracellular compartment (37% versus 20%). Since extracellular fluid is lost more quickly, the higher percentage loss from an infant or young child causes more severe complications.
3. The young child's kidneys cannot concentrate urine as well as the older child's or adult's because of immaturity of the young child's renal system.
4. Infants and young children have a higher metabolic rate that results in a high daily exchange of body water. Infants can exchange (intake and output) half of their extracellular fluid per day, whereas adults might exchange one-seventh. Additionally, urea, the principal end product of metabolism, requires water for excretion. Therefore, any condition causing an elevated metabolic rate (for example, fever) increases the amount of water needed for elimination.
5. Infants and young children have a higher ratio of surface area to weight than older children and adults. Thus, insensible fluid losses through the skin and respiratory tract are proportionately higher.

Physical Examination

For any child with a suspected fluid imbalance, the following areas are particularly emphasized:

Weight
Skin quality
Vital signs
Respiratory rate and quality
Intake, output, and urine specific gravity
Changes in orientation and sensorium
Changes in laboratory data—sodium, potassium, chloride, hematocrit, blood gases, bicarbonate
Symptoms of the underlying condition precipitating the imbalance

Weight Weight is one of the most important indicators of fluid shifts in infants and children. After an initial weight loss during the early neonatal period, infants and children usually gain weight at a regular pace if they are properly nourished. Because a high proportion of an infant's weight is fluid and because a high proportion of this fluid is located in the extracellular space, an abrupt shift of weight in an infant can be attributed to fluid shift rather than to a change in body mass.

Approximately 1 g of weight is the equivalent of 1 mL of body fluid. A weight loss or gain of 1 kg (2.2 lb) in 24 hours represents a 1 liter fluid loss or gain. Because fluid shifts in infants and young children are so critical to their body function, a 50 g/day shift in an infant or 200 g/day in the older child requires notification of the physician (Hazinski, 1984).

Children are weighed at the same time daily, preferably prior to breakfast. Care is taken to remove clothing or to keep the clothing consistent from day to day. Infants need to be weighed without a diaper on an infant scale. Because weight in infants is such an important measurement, any item that might add even a small amount of weight is taken into consideration. This would include IV armboards or bulky dressings (Hazinski, 1984).

Skin quality Skin color, turgor (elasticity), temperature, and moistness can indicate the child's state of hydration. For example, the child's skin characteristically becomes cool and dry as a fluid deficit increases, but if a deficit is related to fever, the skin might be warm and moist with perspiration.

Skin turgor can reflect fluid loss or gain. Without a fluid deficit, the skin immediately returns to its normal position after being gently pinched to test the turgor. *Tenting* (elevation) of the skin occurs when there has been fluid loss (Fig. 21-1). Skin turgor is most accurately assessed on the skin of the abdomen or inner thigh.

In some instances tenting is not a reliable sign. For example, when a child has a fluid loss in excess of a sodium loss, some fluid leaves the cells and enters the extracellular spaces in an attempt to maintain a balance in osmotic pressures. The skin then is rubbery or leathery to touch and tenting is less important than would be expected for the child's fluid loss.

Skin turgor also will suggest underestimated fluid loss in the obese child or the child with abdominal distention. With the malnourished child, loose skin is related to loss of subcutaneous tissue as well as acute fluid loss and thus may be too sensitive a sign for the child's actual fluid loss. Under normal circumstances skin shows some signs of tenting with a mild loss of approximately 3%–5% of body weight.

The nurse inspects the mouth to assess the moistness of a child's mucous membranes. This inspection, too, can be deceptive, for mouth breathing causes the tongue and mouth to become dry with or without fluid volume deficit. The area where the gums and cheek meet, however, provides a differential assessment site as it remains moist during mouth breathing. The nurse therefore inspects this area to be certain a dry mouth is related to fluid volume deficit. Longitudinal wrinkles on the tongue are an excellent indicator of dehydration. Thirst is a good indication that fluid deficit exists, but the nauseous child might not wish to drink, despite fluid loss. Absence of tears in all but the very young infant can indicate fluid deficit.

In an infant under eighteen months of age the appearance of the fontanelles provides data relative to fluid loss. Sunken fontanelles, particularly the anterior fontanelles, might indicate dehydration in an infant. Tense or bulging fontanelles indicate possible cerebral edema and fluid retention.

Vital signs Blood pressure and pulse rate can give clues to the status of the child's fluid balance. Fluid loss can be associated with a rapid, thready pulse and a falling blood pressure. Fluid retention or edema might be associated with an increase in blood pressure and a bounding pulse. Alterations in rhythm and rate also are associated with certain electrolyte imbalances that occur during fluid shifts.

Increased respiratory rate is associated with both fluid loss and fluid retention, but the breath sounds of the child who is retaining fluid will be moist (rales). The child might experience some respiratory distress (see Chapter 22).

Intake, output, and specific gravity The child's total fluid intake within a twenty-four hour period should roughly be equal to the amount the child excretes. If the figures are not equivalent, the child might be experiencing some problems related to fluid balance or failure of regulatory mechanisms.

Intake Children of different ages require different amounts of fluid to maintain hydration. Sources of fluid intake include oral, intravenous (regular drip plus any fluid needed for medication administration or flushing IV lines), nasogastric instillations, and water produced by metabolism. All these need to be included when the nurse calculates the amount of fluid the child needs to receive daily.

To ensure adequate fluid intake, the nurse calculates the child's daily fluid maintenance requirement. Whereas an adult needs approximately 40 mL of fluid intake per kilogram of body weight per day, infants and children need far more. (Maintenance fluid requirements for infants and children of various ages and weights are presented in Table 21-1.)

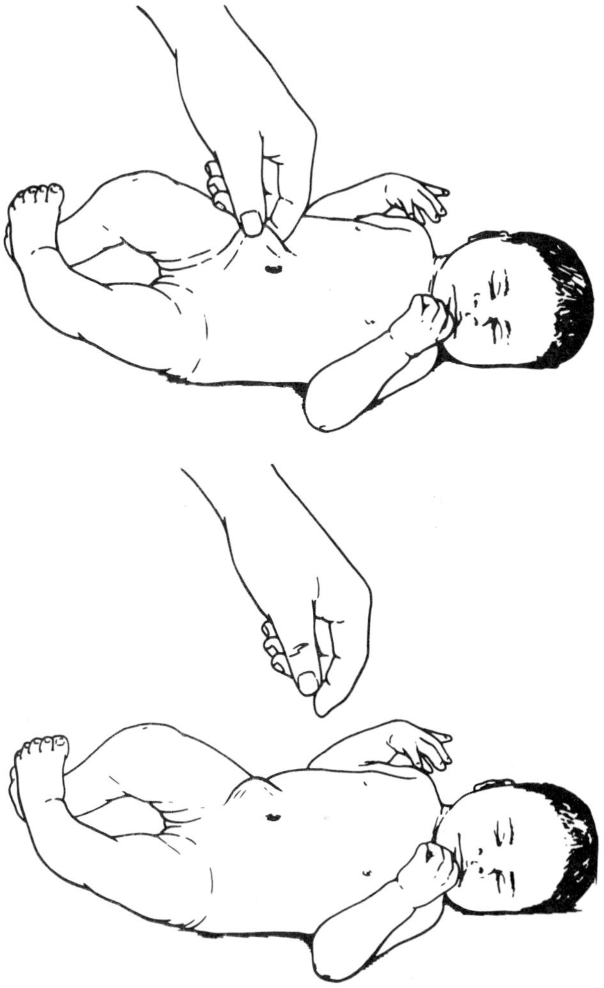

FIGURE 21-1

Testing for skin turgor—tenting.

Output To assess fluid balance, the nurse monitors all sources of output. Output includes urine, vomitus, loose stools, nasogastric drainage, blood, and insensible fluids. Daily insensible fluid loss in children is estimated to be 300 mL/m^2 of body surface (Hazinski, 1985). Thus, in a 1-year-old child insensible fluid loss might equal 135 mL (300 mL times 0.45 m^2) (see Table 21-1). Insensible water loss increases during fever or other dysfunction, and this needs to be considered for fluid replacement. In very small infants, the amount of blood removed for blood specimens

TABLE 21-1 Fluid Maintenance Requirements for Infants and Children

Age	Kg weight	Body surface area (m^2)	Fluid requirement (mL/24 hours)	Approximate hourly fluid rate (mL)	Formula
Newborn (less than 72 hours)	3.3	0.2	198–330	8–15	60–100 mL/kg body weight
1 week	3.3	0.2	330	15	100 mL/kg (can be increased if no renal or cardiac difficulties)
2 months	5.0	0.25	500	20	
6 months	8.0	0.35	800	35	
12 months	10.0	0.45	1000	40	
3 years	15.0	0.60	1250	50	1000 mL for the first 10 kg plus 50 mL/kg for each kg over 10 kg
5 years	20.0	0.80	1500	60	
8 years	30.0	1.05	1750	70	1500 mL for the first 20 kg plus 25 mL/kg for each kg over 20 kg
13 years	60.0	1.70	2050	85	1750 mL for the first 30 kg plus 10 mL/kg for each kg over 30 kg

needs to be added to the total fluid output, since even small losses can alter the infant's fluid balance.

Generally, a child is considered to be in fluid balance if urinary output equals 1 mL/kg/hour. Sharp decreases in this amount can indicate fluid volume deficit. A decreased urinary output, however, can be a sign of fluid retention. Therefore, any decrease in urinary output needs to be compared with data from weight, skin quality, and vital signs to make an accurate assessment.

Interpreting certain signs of fluid and electrolyte imbalances requires extra caution. For example, the character and frequency of the child's stools might directly reflect a fluid volume deficit. The dehydrated child frequently is constipated, having small, dry, hard stools. A primary cause of dehydration in young children, however, is related to diarrhea. Stools are then loose, frequent, and might have noticeable free water, seen easily in the diapered child as a ring of liquid feces surrounding any solid stool. The nurse accurately measures and records the frequency and amounts of loose stools as part of the measurement for fluid loss.

The nurse monitors fluid intake and output closely. At least every four hours (and more often if the child has cardiac or renal dysfunction), the nurse totals the intake and output and compares it to the maintenance intake for the child's age and weight. This ongoing assessment enables the nurse to keep a constant check on the child's fluid status.

Specific gravity Urine specific gravity (value 1.003–1.010) in most instances can be an excellent indicator of fluid balance. A high specific gravity can indicate concentrated urine and fluid volume deficit. In infants, specific gravity is a less accurate measure of fluid balance. The immaturity of the infant's renal system decreases the infant's ability to concentrate urine. Thus, an infant might be experiencing a fluid volume deficit although the specific gravity remains within normal limits. Specific gravity also can be dramatically increased with protein or glucose in the urine, so again, the nurse needs to consider other factors along with specific gravity for a total assessment.

Changes in orientation and sensorium Children who exhibit signs of fluid volume alterations often exhibit behavioral changes as well. They might become initially irritable, but this can be followed by lethargy and passivity. In severe cases the child can become comatose. Children with fluid retention that causes cerebral edema (swelling in the brain) can exhibit severe headache, vomiting, restlessness, irritability, and convulsions.

ASSESSMENT GUIDE *The Child with a Fluid and Electrolyte Imbalance*

Assessment questions	Supporting data
Is there any alteration in the child's weight compared to the pre-illness weight?	Weight loss from vomiting or diarrhea. Fruity odor to the breath. Weight gain and generalized edema
Does the skin appear dry or clammy, cold or warm, pale or flushed? Does it appear to have normal elasticity?	Poor skin turgor with tenting. Firm, rubbery, skin
Are there any alterations in vital signs?	Increase in rate or depth of respirations suggest acidosis; depressed respirations suggest alkalosis. Hypotension or hypertension. Arrhythmias, bradycardia, or tachycardia. Fever
Is there any alteration in urinary output?	Oliguria, polyuria, hematuria
Does the child complain of thirst and dryness of the mouth?	
If yes:	Sunken eyeballs, dark circles around eyes, tearless cry (child over three months of age). Dry mucous membranes, longitudinal furrows on tongue. Depressed fontanelle. Restlessness, alterations in neurologic state—irritability, crying, lethargy
If no:	Bulging fontanelle. Periorbital edema. Headache, restlessness, irritability

Additional data: Muscle weakness or cramping, tetany, hypotonicity, symptoms of the underlying disease causing the imbalance

Validating Diagnostic Tests

Observation of blood chemistries and electrolytes can give the nurse clues to the child's fluid status. For example, decreased serum sodium along with increased serum potassium might indicate a fluid and electrolyte shift from the intracellular to extracellular compartments as a result of extracellular fluid loss. An increase in the hemoglobin value might indicate increased viscosity (thickness) of blood from fluid loss. (Normal serum values for electrolytes are presented in the tables accompanying the discussion of the specific imbalances.)

Principles of Nursing Care

Acute Care Needs

Nursing care of the child with an imbalance of fluid regulatory mechanisms is directed toward restoring balance and preventing further disequilibrium. Generally, nursing interventions include ongoing observation of the child's status, accurate recording and reporting, and facilitating medical interventions.

Fluid volume deficit related to excessive body fluid loss or to electrolyte shifts

Parenteral fluid therapy Children with severe fluid and electrolyte deficits usually are hospitalized for intravenous fluid and electrolyte replacement. The type and amount of solution ordered will depend on the dysfunction and the type of associated imbalance. Intravenous solutions can be hypertonic, hypotonic, or isotonic (Table 21-2).

Administration of isotonic fluid is most frequently seen in the clinical setting, although other fluids might be ordered depending on the physiologic condition underlying the fluid loss. Dextrose in water can be given to children in very small amounts but is used with extreme caution. Although it is an isotonic solution, in large amounts it can alter the extracellular osmolarity, resulting in cerebral edema. Because electrolyte shifts accompany fluid shifts in many circumstances, a solution containing various electrolytes might be ordered.

Children, especially infants, who require intravenous fluid replacement lasting several days, present special nurs-

TABLE 21-2 Tonicity and Physiologic Consequences of Intravenous Fluids

Tonicity of solution	Example	Consequence
Isotonic	0.9% saline 5% dextrose in water	No cellular changes
Hypotonic	0.45% saline Water	Cellular edema (hemolysis)
Hypertonic	3% saline 10% dextrose in water	Cellular crenation (shrinking)

ing problems (see Chapter 20 for general care of a child with an IV). Their veins are so small that the IV position is precarious at best. In a matter of minutes a well-functioning IV might infiltrate, requiring an additional venipuncture. Frequently, the infant's usable sites are quickly depleted, making it extremely difficult to replace the fluid losses adequately. In these circumstances the physician might order an intravenous cut-down.

The IV cut-down is performed by a surgeon. An incision is made at an appropriate site (usually the dorsum of the foot), so that a vein is visible. A thin catheter is threaded into the vein and sutured in place. After the catheter is attached to the infusion set and checked for proper function, the incision is partially sutured, then covered with a dressing. Nursing care of a child receiving an IV infusion by cut-down is similar to the general principles of caring for any child with an IV. The dressing is checked frequently, and the nurse observes for signs of complications of phlebitis or infiltration. If the dressing appears wet, the physician needs to be notified, as the catheter might have slipped out of the vein.

A Six-Point IV Check

- ✓ type of solution and expiration date
- ✓ hourly fluid rate and regulate drip rate accordingly
- ✓ burette, tubing, connectors, and other administration equipment for proper functioning
- ✓ position of the body part used and position for uninterrupted flow
- ✓ for complications—infiltration and phlebitis (see Chapter 20)
- ✓ record shift total of intake and output

Because, in infants, the catheter can nearly obscure the vein in which it is placed, venous return to the extremity can be compromised. The infant might exhibit signs of decreased tissue perfusion in the area, including edema, pallor and coldness of the skin. The nurse observes and reports any signs of decreased perfusion.

Oral fluid therapy In addition to parenteral therapy, children might be receiving oral fluids at a prescribed rate. The child who is dehydrated, for example, might have oral fluids initiated after a perod of parenteral therapy. An oral electrolyte solution (for example, Lytrin or Pedialyte) might be prescribed, or other clear fluids (such as water, flat ginger ale, or diluted jello) might be introduced gradually. An accurate record of oral intake is as important for fluid measurement as recording intravenous fluids. The nurse considers oral fluid intake as well as parenteral intake in providing the daily fluid requirements for the child.

Fluids are administered initially in small amounts, often as small as 30 mL (or 1 oz) an hour. Patience is required when administering the fluids, as many children become resistant to taking them, particularly if they are irritable from the fluid loss. The nurse tries to provide fluids the child likes and uses play to encourage the child to drink. If the child retains the fluids, the amounts are gradually increased to resolve the fluid deficit. If the child appears adequately hydrated (no weight loss, stable vital signs, good skin turgor, urine output appropriate for age and weight), the amount of parenteral fluid is decreased as the oral intake is increased. When the child is tolerating fluids well, and the underlying condition causing the imbalance is corrected, the physician will order the parenteral therapy discontinued.

If the child does not tolerate fluids, that is, if vomiting or diarrhea recur with a fluid increase, the nurse decreases the intake to a previous level and notifies the physician that the child is not tolerating the fluid increase.

Output measurement An accurate record of output is as important as a record of intake. Major fluid loss can occur through urinary excretion, liquid bowel excretion, emesis, and nasogastric tube drainage. In cases of fluid imbalance, all of these need to be measured and recorded accurately.

In an older child who can use the bathroom, accurate measurement of urinary output presents little difficulty, although the nurse needs to encourage cooperation with the procedure. The child needs to use either a urinal, a bedpan, or a plastic "hat" that fits tightly under the seat of the toilet.

Output measurement for the child who has not been toilet trained becomes more of a problem, as accuracy can be compromised. The use of pediatric urine collectors is common practice in many institutions, but their accuracy depends on correct application and constant vigilance to detect voiding. A young infant might need to be catheterized if small alterations in urine output are critical.

The preferred method for accurately assessing urine output in diapered children is simply to weigh the wet diaper. Weight in grams corresponds to the volume voided. The dry diaper weight is subtracted from the wet diaper weight, and the difference equals the volume in milliliters voided. For example, if a dry diaper weighs 68 g and the wet diaper weighs 85 g, the urine output is 17 mL. Many of the disposable diapers have fairly standard weights for each of the types and sizes manufactured by the company. This method is acceptable when approximate rather than strictly accurate output records provide the necessary information concerning fluid balance. Urine aspirated through a syringe from the diaper also can be used for testing and measuring specific gravity.

If possible, emesis and liquid stools should be measured and recorded. If the nurse cannot obtain an accurate measurement, an estimate should be made as closely as possible. Again, diapers can be weighed for liquid stool measurement.

Because nasogastric drainage itself can alter electrolyte balance, careful monitoring of drainage amounts and quality is necessary. Most physicians replace gastric drainage loss volume-for-volume with parenteral electrolyte solution.

⊛ Potential alteration in fluid volume: excess

Because fluid shifts in the young child can occur so rapidly, the nurse needs to be particularly careful when replacing fluid. Fluid administered at too fast a rate can cause fluid overload if not corrected immediately. Often, infusion pumps are used to give an accurate hourly fluid amount, but pumps are not foolproof and need to be monitored frequently. Regardless of the method of IV administration, the nurse checks the IV every 30 minutes and keeps an hourly running total of the fluid administered and the child's output.

Signs of fluid overload include weight gain, generalized edema, decreased urine output, decreased specific gravity, dyspnea (difficult breathing), and moist breath sounds (rales). If any of these signs are recognized, the nurse slows the IV and reports immediately to the physician.

⊛ Potential sensory-perceptual alterations

The child can experience any of a number of sensory-perceptual alterations depending on the fluid imbalance involved. The child who is experiencing fluid deficit is irritable, cries frequently, and can become lethargic. The nurse plans care to allow the child maximum rest while ensuring fluid replacement. Vital signs, IV checks, diaper changes, and oral fluid encouragement can be performed at one time, thus allowing long periods of uninterrupted rest between periods of care.

Children with cerebral edema from fluid shifts will be irritable and restless from the increase in intracranial pressure. They might complain of headache, nausea, and vomiting. Convulsions are a distinct possibility, and the nurse needs to ensure the child's safety during any convulsive episode. Safety measures include padding the child's bed and keeping suction and oxygen at the bedside (see Chapter 31 for further discussion of the child with increased intracranial pressure).

Other sensory-perceptual alterations are manifestations of electrolyte disturbances and might include numbness and tingling in the fingers and toes, dizziness, and muscle cramping or twitching. These alterations usually are resolved when the appropriate electrolyte is replaced.

Nutritional Needs

⊛ Potential alteration in nutrition: less than body requirements

Depending on the cause of the fluid imbalance, the child might be NPO. In addition to considering fluid replacement, the nurse considers calorie replacement in children who are not receiving fluids or foods orally. Even though ill, the child still needs calories for metabolism and growth. Fever increases calorie expenditure because it increases metabolism.

For short-term fluid therapy, calories are provided through the use of 5% glucose solutions. The glucose keeps the child from being hungry and provides enough calories to prevent protein and fat breakdown. For long-term therapy, total parenteral nutrition (TPN) might be considered (see Chapter 27).

All children whose oral intake is restricted or who have nasogastric tubes need special mouth care for comfort. Frequent brushing of teeth and use of water or mouthwash for rinsing the mouth is helpful for the older child. Lemon and glycerine swabs frequently are used for younger children. If the child is allowed ice chips, this minimal amount of fluid should be recorded.

Emotional Needs

⊛ Potential for ineffective individual coping

Many children who are hospitalized for treatment have an IV. For young children and infants, this also means that the child will be restrained to preserve the IV site. Infants and children can become agitated and upset by restraints and often struggle against them.

The nurse removes the restraints frequently to provide range of motion and to meet the child's emotional needs. Sources of gratification and comfort for infants are associated with sucking and food. Because the infant's usual sources of gratification are removed during IV therapy, the nurse ensures that at least some of these needs are met. The nurse cuddles the child as often as possible, making certain that the IV site is protected. A pacifier can be given to provide satisfaction through sucking, but the child needs to be burped frequently to expell swallowed air. Familiar toys or blankets can be given to the child for comfort. Bright mobiles can provide a source of interest to the restrained infant, and a familiar television program might keep the young child relaxed.

To ensure cooperation in older children, the nurse explains the purpose of the IV. Children need to understand the purpose of the therapy so that they do not view the IV as a punishment. Every effort needs to be made to allow the child to choose the most comfortable site for the IV, usually leaving free the child's dominant hand.

Potential for ineffective family coping

As with any child who is ill, parents are concerned and anxious about the child's condition. They might experience some guilt that they did not recognize signs and symptoms early enough. The nurse supports the parents by encouraging them to express their feelings and ask questions. The nurse explains the purpose of the IV and other procedures and keeps the parents informed about the child's status.

Encouraging the parents' participation in care is an important nursing action. The parent can give the child oral fluids at the prescribed rate. In many instances, the child will take the fluid better from the parent than from the nurse. This gives parents the satisfaction that they are doing something active to improve the child's health status. The nurse encourages parents to hold and cuddle their children as much as possible and teaches parents to protect the IV site while doing so. Prior to discharge, the parents are taught to recognize warning signs of fluid alterations, such as excessively dry skin and mucous membranes, irritability, excessive thirst, and decreased voiding (see Chapter 18).

The Child with a Fluid and Electrolyte Imbalance

Although certain signs and symptoms characterize specific fluid and electrolyte imbalances, there is great variation in the clinical picture for any one child. Because of the disease process underlying the imbalance, a child's other conditions, and the age and size of the child, various signs might be apparent. Seldom is an imbalance a disturbance of only one electrolyte. Most imbalances are instead a mixture of electrolyte disturbances. For example, chloride usually is gained or lost with sodium, and sodium usually is lost with water.

The nurse considers two major principles when looking at fluid and electrolyte imbalances in children:

1. Signs of imbalance vary with a condition's rapidity of onset. The more rapid the onset of an excess or deficit, the more dramatic the signs might be and the more serious the imbalance for the child. An infant experiencing explosive diarrhea, for example, tends to show signs of extracellular fluid volume deficit quickly. The infant might not show such serious signs, however, if the same degree of dehydration had resulted from a gradual loss of fluid.
2. A young child is better able to handle a deficit than an excess. For example, hypernatremia (elevated blood sodium) can be caused by either excess sodium intake or fluid loss in excess of sodium loss. The young child's kidneys are better equipped to handle the deficit than the excess. Therefore, the excess produces more severe signs and has more serious implications for the child.

The nurse needs to check and recheck the child's laboratory values. Compensatory mechanisms such as fluid shifts and the movement of potassium between intracellular and extracellular fluids can create rapid changes in the laboratory values as the underlying illness is treated. As one problem is corrected, another might arise needing treatment. For example, an elevated serum potassium level in acidosis might become a serum deficit as acidosis is treated and potassium returns to the intracellular fluids.

Sodium and Fluid Imbalances

Sodium is the major cation (positive ion) within the extracellular fluid. Its most important function is to maintain water distribution through the fluid compartments of the body. Sodium controls water balance by maintaining osmotic balance between the intracellular and the extracellular fluid. Other functions of sodium include (a) maintaining intravascular (within the blood vessels) volume, (b) controlling muscle contractility (especially cardiac contractility), (c) assisting in nerve impulse conduction, (d) maintaining neuromuscular irritability, (e) acting as a buffer base, and (f) increasing cell membrane permeability.

TABLE 21-3 Types of Osmolar Dehydration

	Hypertonic (osmolar) dehydration	Hypotonic (osmolar) dehydration
Cause	Water decrease in excess of sodium due to decreased intake or increased output from conditions such as diarrhea, diabetes insipidus, fever, and conditions causing polyuria. Water (ICF) leaving the intracellular space to balance increased extracellular concentration causes cellular shrinkage (Figure 21-2A).	Extracellular sodium decrease in excess of water loss (hyponatremia). Occurs from decreased sodium intake or excess output as from diuretics, cystic fibrosis, burns, diarrhea, or vomiting. Water leaves the extracellular compartment and enters the intracellular space to balance the concentration. Blood volume is depleted from the shift of extracellular fluid and hypovolemic shock is a great risk (Figure 21-2B). Cerebral edema can result from cell swelling
Blood chemistry	$Na^+ > 150$ mEq/L (normal: 130–150 mEq/L)	$Na^+ < 130$ mEq/L
Clinical manifestations	Decreased blood pressure and increased temperature; tachycardia and tachypnea; flushed, dry, rubbery dry mucous membranes and tongue; thirst; soft sunken eyeballs and depressed fontanelles (infant); oliguria and increased urine specific gravity; irritability, restlessness, eventual coma; elevated hemoglobin	Muscle fatigue and weakness; irritability; oliguria; slightly dry mucous membranes; poor skin turgor; nausea, vomiting, abdominal cramps; decreased blood pressure and rapid thready pulse might indicate impending shock; severe headache, seizures might indicate cerebral edema
Treatment	Replace fluid losses gradually by saline-free IV solution and treat the underlying condition. Provide potassium replacement when kidneys are functioning properly. Give sodium bicarbonate for associated acidosis	Rapidly initiate electrolyte and fluid replacement to restore ECF volume
Nursing management	Strictly monitor intake and output, weight, and urine specific gravity. Observe for stabilization of vital signs and improvement in skin characteristics. Monitor laboratory values, particularly sodium and potassium levels. Protect and regulate IV to ensure fluid replacement (See Standards of Care for additional interventions)	Strictly monitor intake and output and IV. Monitor vital signs frequently (as often as q 15–30 minutes) to detect signs of shock. Monitor laboratory values for return of sodium level. (See Standards of Care for additional management)

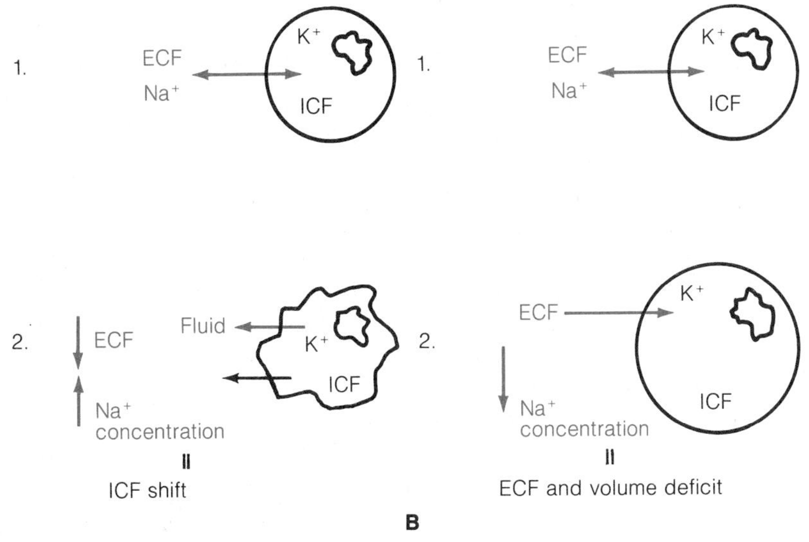

FIGURE 21-2
A. Hypertonic dehydration causes cellular shrinkage. B. Hypotonic dehydration causes cellular edema and extracellular fluid (ECF) volume deficit.

Because water imbalance affects sodium balance and sodium imbalance in turn affects water balance, the relationship between these two constituents needs to be considered in the child with fluid and electrolyte imbalance. The two types of sodium and water imbalances are *osmolar imbalances* (differences in the concentration of solutes between intracellular and extracellular fluids) and *volume imbalances* (differences in the amount of water between the extracellular and intracellular compartments).

When body fluid osmolarity is disturbed (eg, when the concentration of electrolytes is altered), water moves from an area of lesser osmolarity to an area of greater osmolarity. Thus the water distribution between fluid compartments changes. Osmolar imbalances result in cellular changes because water moves either into or out of cells. Some associated electrolyte changes also might occur, such as a potassium shift from the intracellular fluid to the extracellular fluid.

If water and sodium levels change together, the concentration of the fluids remains constant. This is termed *isotonic imbalance*. Volume disturbances will develop; however, cellular changes do not occur.

Osmolar dehydration A major consequence of fluid and electrolyte disturbance in the child is dehydration. The type of dehydration depends on the type of fluid and electrolyte shift that has occurred. (Osmolar imbalances causing dehydration are presented in Table 21-3.)

Regardless of the cause of the dehydration, a major nursing responsibility when caring for the child who is dehydrated is to determine the extent of the dehydration. Infants experience signs of dehydration when they have experienced approximately a 5% (3% in children) weight loss from their pre-illness weight. Symptoms of mild dehydration occur with a 5%–9% weight loss, moderate dehydration with a 10%–14% weight loss, and severe dehydration with a weight loss of 15% or greater (see Table 21-4).

Nursing management of the child who is dehydrated includes the general principles of care for the child with a fluid imbalance. Careful monitoring of the child's fluid and electrolyte status is essential to determine whether the dehydration is resolving.

Osmolar overhydration Shifts in sodium and water can cause overhydration. *Hypernatremia* (excess sodium in the extracellular fluid) can be caused by increased dietary salt intake or salt water dehydration. It results also from excessive solute loads, such as from IV saline solutions or improperly mixed infant formula. Water is retained in the extracellular space, but the increased sodium concentration there attracts additional fluid from the intracellular compartment. Fluid moves out of the cell into the extracellular space causing increased extracellular fluid volume (Fig. 21-3A).

Symptoms of edema, weight gain, and increased blood pressure with bounding pulse are related to hypervolemia. Hemoglobin levels are decreased because of the expanded extracellular water volume (dilutional hypervolemia). Neurologic manifestations such as confusion and coma are related to cerebral cellular shrinking.

Water intoxication occurs when the concentration of sodium in the intracellular fluid is higher than that in the extracellular fluid (Figure 21-3B). Unlike hypotonic dehydration, water intoxication involves no water loss but instead involves excessive water intake or decreased water output. Because of the concentration imbalance, water moves from the extracellular to the intracellular space, causing cellular edema.

Causes of water intoxication include increased water intake without corresponding electrolytes, such as in tap water enema administration and freshwater near-drowning.

TABLE 21-4 Assessing Dehydration

Degree of dehydration	Clinical signs
Mild	
Weight loss: 5% (infants) 3% (older child)	Pale, cool skin; slightly decreased urine output; increased pulse; thirst (in child)
Moderate	
Weight loss: 10% (infants) 6% (older child)	Greyish, cool skin with tenting; severely decreased urine output; decreasing blood pressure; increasing pulse; beginning signs of shock
Severe	
Weight loss: 15% (infants) 9% (older child)	Poor peripheral circulation with pale or mottled, cool skin; poor capillary refill; hypotension; tachycardia; very dry mucous membranes; sunken fontanelles (in infants); beginning signs of renal shutdown

SOURCE: Reilly MD: The renal system. In: *Pediatric Critical Care*. Smith JB (editor). Wiley, 1983.

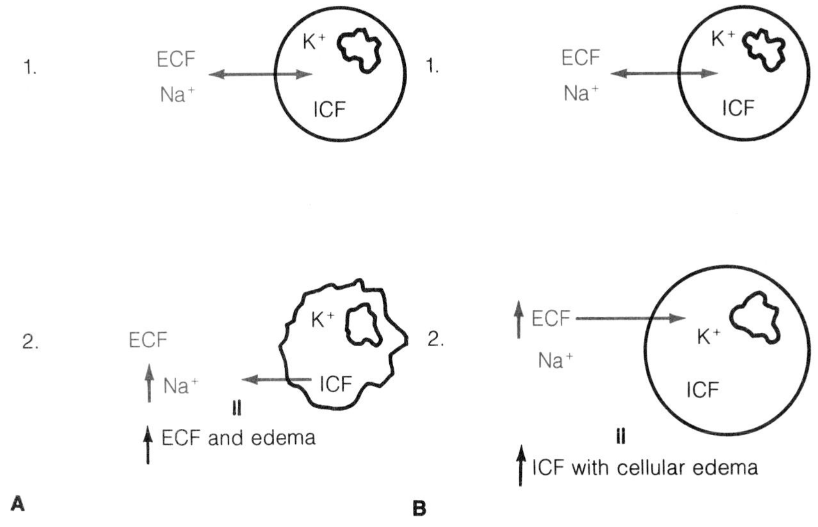

FIGURE 21-3

A. Hypernatremia causes cellular shrinkage with increase in extracellular fluid (ECF) volume and edema. B. Water intoxication causes water to shift to the intracellular space causing cellular edema.

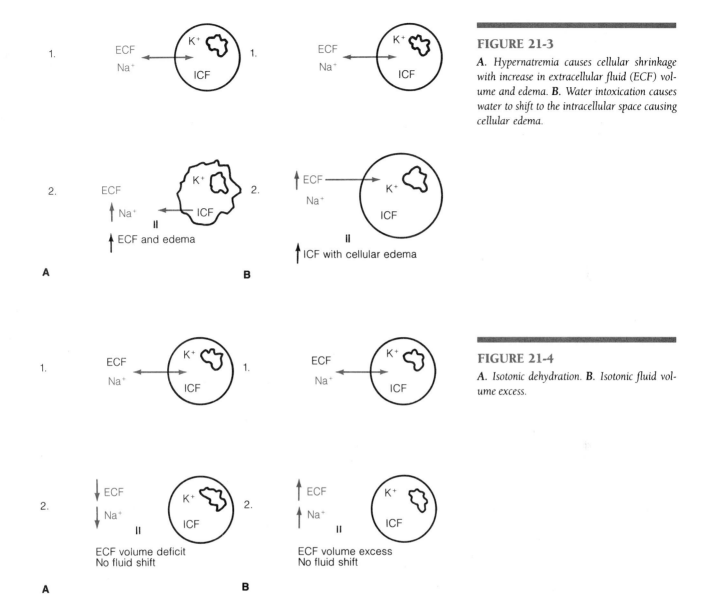

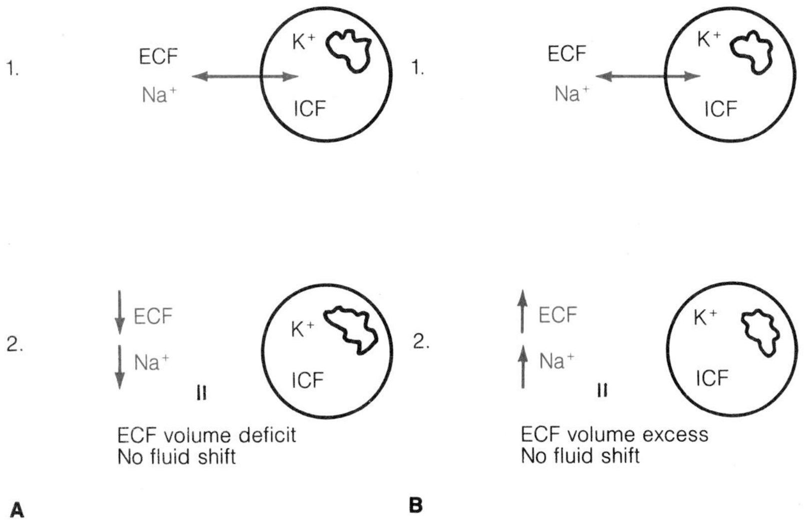

FIGURE 21-4

A. Isotonic dehydration. B. Isotonic fluid volume excess.

Overhydration also can occur with renal, cerebral, or cardiac dysfunction. Signs of overhydration include weakness, irritability, headache, disorientation, bulging fontanelles in infants, and other signs of cerebral edema (see Chapter 31). There might be sudden weight gain, nausea, anorexia, vomiting, and absence of thirst.

Treatment includes strict fluid intake restrictions. A hypertonic saline solution might be administered intravenously to increase the extracellular concentration. An osmotic diuretic such as mannitol might be given.

Nursing management includes maintaining strict intake restrictions, observation of neurologic condition with seizure precautions, daily weight monitoring, accurate observation of urinary output, and monitoring laboratory values.

Volume Disturbances

The term volume disturbance, or *isotonic disturbance*, implies that sodium and water increase or decrease proportionately (Fig. 21-4). Because this does not disturb osmolarity, cellular changes do not occur with these disturbances.

Extracellular fluid volume deficits create circulatory collapse with resultant dehydration. Such decreases are caused by hemorrhage, burns, fever, and excessive vomiting. Diarrhea is the most common cause of extracellular fluid volume deficit. Isotonic dehydration is the most frequent type of dehydration seen in children.

TABLE 21-5 Findings in Extracellular Fluid Volume Excess and Extracellular Fluid Volume Deficit

	Extracellular fluid volume deficit	Extracellular fluid volume excess
Skin	Poor turgor Dry mucous membranes	Diaphoresis Edema (periorbital)
Cardiac	Blood pressure decrease Weight loss	Congestive heart failure Blood pressure increase Weight gain
Pulmonary	No severe changes	Pulmonary edema Dyspnea Cough Rales
Renal	Oliguria Anuria Acute tubular necrosis	Increased output Eventual decrease in output as congestive heart failure progresses
Laboratory data	Normal Na^+ Increased hematocrit Increased protein Increased urine specific gravity	Normal Na^+ Decreased hematocrit Decreased protein Decreased urine specific gravity

Circulatory overload with resultant edema occurs in conditions causing an extracellular fluid volume excess. Such conditions include congestive heart failure, renal disease, and hepatic failure. Because the intracellular fluid volume is not increased (as in water intoxication), cerebral edema is not a complication.

Clinical manifestations Specific manifestations occur in volume disturbances. (Table 21-5 compares these subjective and objective findings.)

Nursing management Management of volume disturbances primarily involves assessment and interventions related to fluid and sodium therapy. The nurse assesses the child with a fluid volume deficit and determines the degree of dehydration (see Table 21-4). The child with an extracellular fluid volume deficit is treated with infusions of isotonic solution and correction of the underlying dysfunction such as controlling hemorrhage or diarrhea. Nursing management is directed toward these goals.

The child with an extracellular fluid volume excess is treated with fluid restriction, diuretic therapy, or sodium restriction, or all three. Specific data recorded for such children include

- Vital sign trends
- Daily weight and hourly intake and output measurements
- Respiratory status—rate, quality, abnormal breath sounds, thoracic excursion
- Cardiac status—heart rate, quality of pulse, peripheral pulses, extra heart sounds
- Skin color, temperature, turgor
- Laboratory findings—hematocrit, serum protein and serum sodium levels, urine specific gravity

Potassium Imbalances

Potassium, the dominant cation of the intracellular fluid, is critical to several physiologic functions. These include (a) regulation of intracellular osmolarity and electroneutrality, (b) conduction of nerve impulses, (c) energy

TABLE 21-6 Potassium Imbalances

	Hyperkalemia (excess)	Hypokalemia (deficit)
Cause	Conditions such as acute renal failure that cause potassium retention in body fluids; potassium ion release into the ECF from severe injuries, burns, and dehydration; excessive K^+ from inappropriate IV administration; acidosis	Low potassium intake; gastrointestinal tract losses by such problems as vomiting and diarrhea; excessive renal loss from renal dysfunction, diuresis, or burn healing; alkalosis
Blood chemistry	$K^+ > 5.5$ mEq/L (normal: 3.5–5.5 mEq/L)	$K^+ < 3.5$ mEq/L
Clinical manifestations	Cardiac irregularities with ventricular fibrillation and arrest; oliguria, anuria; muscle weakness and irritability; flaccid paralysis including respiratory muscles; nausea and intestinal colic	Cardiac irregularities; decreased blood pressure; muscle weakness or irritability; diminished reflexes; polyuria and decreased gastrointestinal function
Treatment	Medical emergency. Promote potassium excretion through potassium ion-binding medications such as Kayexalate®. Limit oral potassium. Start dialysis if renal failure exists	Replace potassium and correct the underlying dysfunction
Nursing management	Monitor laboratory values and ECG frequently. Strictly monitor intake and output. Monitor respiratory, cardiac, and neurologic status hourly. Monitor arterial blood gases (see Chapter 22) for signs of respiratory acidosis	Provide oral or parenteral potassium replacement. Begin potassium only after the child voids twice to determine adequate renal function. Monitor intake and output strictly, particularly nasogastric output if applicable. Monitor laboratory values and ECG

production by means of enzyme systems used in cellular work, (d) cellular growth, and (e) myocardial activity.

Potassium is easily absorbed from the gastrointestinal tract. Normally 10%–20% of ingested potassium is excreted in the feces, and almost 90% is excreted in the urine. Because the body does not have a sophisticated means of conserving potassium, daily consumption of potassium must approximate the daily amount excreted in the urine. (Potassium imbalances are presented in Table 21-6.)

The child does not usually experience cardiac effects of potassium imbalance until the level becomes less than 3 mEq/L or greater than 8 mEq/L (Hazinski, 1985). ECG manifestations of hyperkalemia include a tall, peaked T wave and flat P wave. Hypokalemia is evidenced by a flat T wave, a possible U wave, and a prolonged S-T segment.

Prevention of potassium alterations is a goal of nursing care. The nurse is especially cautious when replacing potassium. Because the major portion of potassium is excreted in the urine, the child must exhibit adequate urinary output, or potassium can be retained and hyperkalemia can result. The nurse does not administer potassium IV until the child has voided in adequate amounts at least twice.

Calcium Imbalances

Along with sodium and potassium imbalances, calcium imbalances are the most frequently seen electrolyte imbalances in children (Hazinski, 1985). Ninety-nine percent of calcium is concentrated in bone. The rest is distributed in other tissues and in extracellular fluids.

The cardiac, the skeletal, and the neuromuscular systems depend on calcium. Calcium is a positive inotropic agent, that is, it increases the strength of muscular contractions. Calcium, therefore, enhances myocardial contractility and decreases neuromuscular irritability and capillary permeability. Calcium also is essential for growth of normal bones and teeth. It is essential also for normal muscle contractility, for normal coagulation, and for the proper transmission of nerve impulses.

A normal serum calcium level depends on the availability of vitamin D, the intake of calcium in the diet, the serum phosphorus level, and the functioning of the parathyroid glands. Calcium is excreted in the urine. (See Table 21-7 for calcium imbalances.)

(text continues on p. 651)

TABLE 21-7 Calcium Imbalances

	Hypercalcemia (excess)	Hypocalcemia (deficit)
Cause	Excessive intake of calcium or vitamin D; immobilization; hyperparathyroidism; decreased calcium excretion by the kidneys; other conditions causing calcium imbalance	Low dietary intake of calcium or vitamin D; excessive loss with conditions such as diarrhea; hypoparathyroidism; excessive transfusions of stored citrated blood
Blood chemistry	$Ca^+ > 5.7$ mEq/L (normal: 4.5–5.7 mEq/L)	$Ca^+ < 4.5$ mEq/L
Clinical manifestations	Bone pains, fractures, growth failure; symptoms of kidney stones; lethargy and muscle weakness; anorexia, nausea and vomiting leading to coma; arrhythmias, bradycardia (slow pulse)	Tetany (violent muscular spasms); abdominal and skeletal muscle cramping; numbness and tingling in fingers and mouth; laryngospasm; arrhythmias and cardiac arrest
Treatment	Decrease calcium intake. Administer isotonic saline or corticosteroids. Correct underlying condition	Medical emergency. Administer calcium salts orally, IM, or IV (calcium chloride or calcium gluconate). Administer vitamin D to assist calcium absorption
Nursing management	Closely monitor the IV. Monitor the ECG for arrhythmias. Encourage reduction in calcium-containing foods such as milk products, leafy green vegetables, and legumes. Observe for renal, gastrointestinal, and neurologic alterations	Monitor for respiratory dysfunction. Have a tracheostomy set and calcium gluconate at the child's bedside. Institute seizure precautions (see Chapter 31). Monitor the cardiac monitor for arrhythmias. Monitor serum electrolytes

STANDARDS OF NURSING CARE *The Child with a Fluid and Electrolyte Imbalance*

GUIDE FOR NURSING MANAGEMENT

Nursing diagnosis	Intervention	Rationale	Outcome
1. Potential for fluid volume deficit (stressor: underlying dysfunction)	Compare current weight with the child's pre-illness weight; weigh daily.	Weight loss reflects fluid loss. 1 mg is equal to 1 mL. Weight is one of the most important indicators of hydration status.	The child's hydration status is improving as indicated by improved skin turgor, stabilization of weight or weight gain, moist mucous membranes, and urinary output at 1 mL/Kg/hour with specific gravity within normal limits. The child's electrolyte values become normal. The child retains oral fluids.
	Test skin for turgor; note color and temperature. In infants, observe fontanelles for depression. Observe for sunken eyeballs and dark circles around eyes. Describe condition of mucous membranes and degree of dryness. Note presence or absence of thirst or tears.	Characteristics of skin turgor and mucous membranes assist with the assessment of a child with a fluid volume deficit. The thirst mechanism will be activated in response to fluid loss or hemorrhage.	
	Monitor vital signs, particularly pulse, blood pressure, and respiratory status.	Decreased blood pressure and increased pulse might indicate hypovolemic shock. Respiratory rate increases or decreases with acid-base imbalances.	

STANDARDS OF NURSING CARE *The Child with a Fluid and Electrolyte Imbalance (Continued)*

GUIDE FOR NURSING MANAGEMENT

Nursing diagnosis	Intervention	Rationale	Outcome
	Begin oral fluids if ordered; give flat ginger ale or electrolyte solution 1 oz an hour; advance diet if fluids are retained.	Frequent, small amounts of fluid are more likely to be retained.	
	Calculate daily fluid requirements; regulate IV replacement carefully.	Careful monitoring and recording of fluid intake prevents fluid overload. A running intake and output record helps the nurse monitor the hydration status.	
	Monitor output hourly and record; report any signs of oliguria. Measure urine specific gravity.	Adequate hourly output in a child is 1 mL/Kg of body weight. A marked decrease in urine output can indicate dehydration or beginning fluid retention, as well as impaired renal function. Increased specific gravity can indicate dehydration.	
	Monitor laboratory values; place the child on a cardiac monitor for any alterations in K^+, particularly if any arrhythmias have been noted. Replace K^+ if ordered; determine adequate renal function first.	Hypo- or hyperkalemia can alter cardiac rhythm. Monitoring values can tell the nurse whether the child has developed a metabolic alteration along with the fluid alteration. Hyperkalemia can occur if the K^+ is not excreted properly by the kidneys.	
2. Potential alteration in fluid volume: excess (stressor: volume shift)	Compare current weight with the child's pre-illness weight; weigh daily.	Any abrupt gain in weight can indicate fluid volume excess and fluid retention.	Edema decreases. The child's weight returns to pre-illness levels. The child's respiratory effort decreases and other vital signs return to normal.
	Restrict fluids as directed; administer hypertonic IV fluids and osmotic diuretics as ordered.	Oral fluid restriction is necessary to decrease the volume overload. Hypertonic IV fluids pull fluid from the cells and decrease cellular edema. Osmotic diuretics promote fluid excretion.	
	Monitor output accurately and record hourly.	Accurate monitoring of output can provide indication of the child's hydration status.	
	Monitor vital signs; facilitate the child's respiratory effort by elevating the head of the bed and by changing the child's position frequently.	An increased blood pressure with a decreased, bounding pulse can indicate fluid overload. Respiratory effort is increased because of the additional load on the heart and the potential for pulmonary edema and congestive heart failure (see Chapter 23).	
	Monitor laboratory values.	Hemoglobin and hematocrit levels might be decreased, reflecting excess fluid in the extracellular compartment.	

STANDARDS OF NURSING CARE *The Child with a Fluid and Electrolyte Imbalance (Continued)*

GUIDE FOR NURSING MANAGEMENT

Nursing diagnosis	Intervention	Rationale	Outcome
3. Potential sensory-perceptual alterations (stressor: underlying dysfunction)	Describe changes in sensorium and report any worsening symptoms.	Restlessness and irritability can indicate impending shock. Lethargy and passivity are signs of dehydration. Progressive drowsiness and coma are associated with severe acid-base imbalance.	The child responds appropriately for age. The child demonstrates increasing ability to cope with environmental stimuli.
	Describe and report any muscle twitching, cramping, weakness, or hyperirritability.	Neuromuscular symptoms can signal electrolyte imbalances.	
	Monitor the child for signs of increasing intracranial pressure—increased blood pressure, headache, vomiting; institute seizure precautions (see Chapter 31).	Fluid shift into the intracellular space can cause cerebral edema resulting in increased intracranial pressure.	
	Plan nursing care to allow the child maximum rest; provide a quiet environment.	Rest helps the child conserve energy. Too much stimulation can trigger muscle spasms and cramping and can exacerbate headache in the child with cerebral edema.	
4. Potential impairment of skin integrity (stressor: decreased skin turgor or acidic secretions)	Observe child's skin for evidence of redness or breakdown.	Decreased skin turgor can cause reduced blood flow to pressure areas making them susceptible to skin breakdown. Edema also can contribute to skin breakdown.	The child is free of skin breakdown and experiences no excoriation from diarrhea.
	Provide meticulous skin care to perineal area if the child has diarrhea—wash and dry the area with every diaper change, apply protective ointment, leave exposed to air; give heat lamp treatments if ordered.	These measures prevent skin excoriation from stools.	
	Remove any restraints at least every 4 hours.	Removing restraints frequently allows improved circulation to the area and prevents skin breakdown.	
5. Potential alteration in oral mucous membranes (stressor: dehydration)	Provide mouth care and oral hygiene every 4 hours; lubricate dry lips with ointment or water soluble jelly; brush teeth gently or use lemon and glycerine swabs.	Mouth care alleviates the discomfort of dry mouth and prevents cracking of lips from dehydration or NPO status.	The child has intact oral mucosa.
6. Potential for ineffective individual coping (stressor: restricted movement)	Remove any restraints frequently; observe the child carefully while restraints are off.	Removal of restraints allows the child movement. Movement in children is essential for emotional health and restraint causes the child to become upset and struggle.	The child appears relaxed and comfortable in the hospital setting. The child demonstrates an interest in diversional activities.
	Cuddle the child frequently.	This gives the child a feeling of security.	

STANDARDS OF NURSING CARE *The Child with a Fluid and Electrolyte Imbalance (Continued)*

GUIDE FOR NURSING MANAGEMENT

Nursing diagnosis	Intervention	Rationale	Outcome
	Provide a pacifier to infants who are NPO; burp frequently.	Infants get emotional gratification from sucking. Without feeding, another source of this gratification is needed.	
	Give the child familiar toys or blankets.	Having familiar toys available helps the child cope with a new situation.	
	Provide age appropriate stimulation.	Stimulation within the confines of the child's limitations can distract the child. Play helps a child cope with an unfamiliar environment.	
	Explain to the older child the reasons for the IV.	Some children view the IV as punishment.	
7. Potential for ineffective family coping (stressor: hospitalization of the child)	Encourage the parents to express any feelings of anxiety or guilt; encourage them to ask questions.	Verbal expression helps families to deal with feelings.	The parents feel more in control of the situation and express confidence in their abilities to handle the child's dysfunction should it recur. The parents assume increasing responsibility for the child's care.
	Explain the purpose of any tests, procedures, or treatments.	Understanding what is occurring clarifies the parents' perceptions of the child's condition.	
	Encourage the parent to participate in the child's care by allowing the parent to give fluids, help monitor output, and cuddle the child frequently.	Allowing participation increases the parent's feeling of control and promotes effective coping.	
	Prior to discharge, teach the parent how to recognize signs of fluid alteration and how to prevent spread of infection.	Providing the parent with information about how to handle the child should the dysfunction recur increases confidence in the ability to cope in the future.	

The Child with an Acid-Base Imbalance

Hydrogen ions (H^+) are found throughout the body and contribute to the chemical reactions that power body functions. Hydrogen combines with some ions to form acids and others to form bases. For example, hydrogen ions in the stomach combine with chloride ions to form hydrochloric acid (HCl), which assists with food metabolism.

When the hydrogen ion concentration of the blood is higher than normal, the blood is considered to be acidic (a condition termed *acidemia*). When the hydrogen ion concentration is lower than normal, the blood is considered to be basic (a condition termed *alkalemia*). Each state is injurious to health.

Blood pH is a measurement that reflects the hydrogen ion concentration. The normal blood pH is 7.35–7.45. When dysfunction occurs such that the hydrogen ion concentration in the blood is decreased (such as in severe loss of HCl by vomiting), the arterial pH increases. When a dysfunction results in an increase in hydrogen, the arterial pH decreases. Because acid production is a natural by-product of metabolism, the body constantly attempts to reduce the

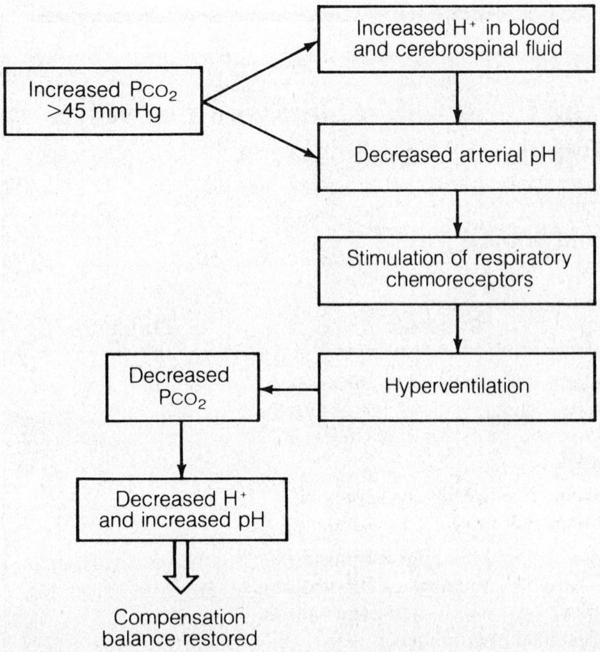

FIGURE 21-5
Mechanisms of pulmonary compensation for an acid-base imbalance.

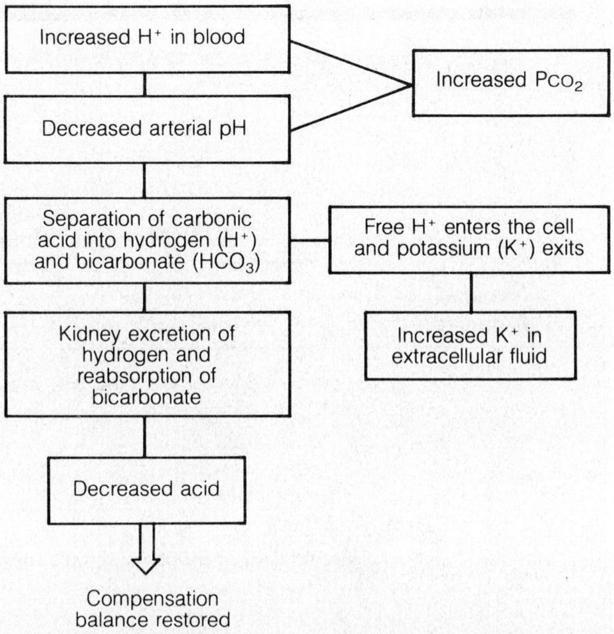

FIGURE 21-6
Mechanisms of renal compensation for an acid-base imbalance.

buildup of acid in body fluids, thus maintaining balance and a normal blood pH.

Buffer systems in the body handle initial alterations of blood pH. A *buffer* is a mechanism that acts as a "shock absorber." The buffer lessens the force of any drastic change in the pH by neutralizing the buildup of strong acids or bases in body fluids. Blood buffers function in both the extracellular and intracellular fluid compartments.

When acid or base increases become too much for the blood buffers to handle, the body attempts to compensate through the respiratory and renal systems. (These mechanisms for compensation are summarized in Figs. 21-5 and 21-6). The respiratory system works rapidly to compensate for acid-base imbalances, whereas the renal compensatory system is slower.

Acid-Base Abnormalities

Acid-base imbalances result from failure of the body's compensatory mechanisms. *Respiratory acidosis* is caused by retention of carbon dioxide that increases blood acidity. *Respiratory alkalosis* occurs when too much carbon dioxide is lost through the lungs, causing the blood to become basic. *Metabolic acidosis* results from a loss of base and buildup of acid through diarrhea or a buildup of acid from excessive catabolism (breakdown) of fats. *Metabolic alkalosis* occurs from a loss of acid from vomiting or retention of base. Potassium shifts are associated with both metabolic acidosis and metabolic alkalosis. (Causes, clinical manifestation, treatment, and nursing management of acid-base imbalances are summarized in Tables 21-8 and 9.)

Gastroenteritis

Gastroenteritis is a problem frequently seen during infancy and childhood and is characterized by varying degrees of diarrhea, vomiting, and abdominal cramping. Mild gastroenteritis associated with colds or gastrointestinal viruses is easily managed at home (see Chapter 18).

Children who are moderately dehydrated (more than 5%–8%) should be hospitalized for management of the dehydration. Children who are severely dehydrated might require intensive care, although this depends on age, cause of diarrhea, and type of dehydration. Causative agents of severe diarrhea in children are classified as bacterial, viral, and protozoal. (These are discussed in Table 18-4.)

Vomiting alone can produce a state of metabolic alkalosis in the child. The severe loss of gastric acid (HCl) causes

TABLE 21-8 Causes and Clinical Manifestations of Acid-Base Balance (Respiratory)

	Respiratory acidosis	Respiratory alkalosis
Cause	Hypoventilation and retention of CO_2 resulting from obstructive pulmonary disease (eg, asthma, cystic fibrosis); dysfunctions restricting chest expansion (eg, trauma, burns); atelectasis; central nervous system alterations	Hyperventilation and loss of CO_2 due to anxiety, salicylate intoxication, or dysfunction that overstimulates the respiratory center
Blood chemistry	pH < 7.35 (normal: 7.35–7.45) $Pco_2 > 46$ mm Hg (normal: 35–45 mm Hg)	pH > 7.45 $Pco_2 < 34$ mm Hg
Clinical manifestations	Restlessness, apprehension leading to disorientation and coma; rapid pulse; diaphoresis (sweating); cyanosis if critical	Deep, rapid breathing; anxiety, fear; tingling of hands and face; dizziness
Treatment	Correct underlying physiologic problem	Correct underlying physiologic problem
Nursing management	Monitor the child as often as hourly for respiratory distress. Perform chest physiotherapy and other actions to increase ventilation and gas exchange (see Chapter 22). Check vital signs and neurologic status q2h	Encourage the child to voluntarily decrease respirations. Allow the hyperventilating child to breathe into a paper bag to increase CO_2 content of inhalations. Monitor serum values and electrocardiogram

TABLE 21-9 Causes and Clinical Manifestations of Acid-Base Balance (Metabolic)

	Metabolic acidosis	Metabolic alkalosis
Cause	Loss of base through diarrhea; increased acids; excessive catabolism of fats (diabetes mellitus); hypoxia resulting in lactic acid accumulation	Loss of acid through vomiting; retention of base; hypokalemia
Blood chemistry	pH < 7.45 (normal: 7.35–7.45) $CO_2 < 22$ mEq/L (normal: 22–26 mEq/L) $HCO_3 < 25$ mEq/L (normal: 21–28 mEq/L)	pH > 7.45 $CO_2 > 32$ mEq/L $HCO_3 > 30$ mEq/L
Clinical manifestations	Lethargy leading to drowsiness, stupor, coma; fruity odor to breath; anorexia, nausea, vomiting; diarrhea; hyperventilation in attempt to compensate; increase in urine acidity as kidneys excrete more H^+ and reabsorb bicarbonate	Confusion, irritability; hypertonicity of muscles; tetany, tremors; restlessness; nausea, vomiting; diarrhea; depressed respirations
Treatment	Administer IV fluids with sodium bicarbonate to increase blood pH. Correct the dysfunction causing the acidosis	Replace lost fluid and electrolytes. Correct the underlying dysfunction
Nursing management	Frequently monitor Pco_2 and bicarbonate levels (at least once a shift). Perform hourly neurologic checks (see Chapter 31). Provide nursing management associated with the underlying disorder. Administer and record fluid and electrolyte replacement. Monitor serum electrolytes. Observe for ECG changes from hyperkalemia	Monitor vital signs and neurologic status. Closely observe ECG changes from hypokalemia. Monitor laboratory values. Administer and record fluid and electrolyte replacements

increased blood pH, increased serum carbon dioxide and retention of bicarbonate. Diarrhea without vomiting can cause metabolic acidosis from the loss of fluids high in base. Most frequently, infants and young children experience both vomiting and diarrhea. Some children experience chronic diarrhea, that is, diarrhea persisting from 3–6 weeks.

Clinical manifestations Frequent liquid stools, usually initially associated with vomiting, are the first signs of gastroenteritis in children. Since the frequency and consistency of stools varies with each child, an important factor is the degree of change in the child's usual bowel habits or in the appearance of the stool. The appearance of the stools in the child with diarrhea varies according to cause. The stools most frequently are green, watery, and foul smelling. There might be vomiting, possible abdominal cramping and abdominal tenderness on palpation, and tenesmus (involuntary bowel straining). Other changes associated with gastroenteritis are:

Change in sensorium. The child might appear tired, listless, lethargic, irritable, drowsy, or possibly confused.

Fever.

Change in cardiovascular status. The child might have decreased blood pressure, tachycardia (due to dehydration and deficient intravascular volume), or signs of dehydration (poor tissue turgor, sunken eyeballs, dry tongue and mucous membranes).

Change in renal functioning. Oliguria (diminished urine output) is common as dehydration progresses. Acute renal failure is possible.

Diagnostic evaluation Changes in laboratory values might reflect metabolic acidosis. These might be an elevated hematocrit (due to volume loss), normal serum sodium levels (because the loss usually is isotonic), and normal serum potassium levels, which might rise gradually as the glomerular filtration rate decreases. The BUN (blood urea nitrogen) increases as the glomerular filtration rate decreases, and there might be leukocytosis (elevated white blood cell count). Stool cultures might be positive for organisms or parasites.

Treatment Gastroenteritis caused by some bacteria and parasites is amenable to drug therapy (see Table 18-4). Most cases of acute childhood diarrhea are viral and self-limiting, requiring treatment for dehydration and electrolyte imbalances.

Treatment for severe gastroenteritis is directed toward (a) restoration of body fluid volume (both intracellular fluid and extracellular fluid), (b) restoration of electrolyte balance, and (c) restoration of normal renal function. Fluid and electrolyte solutions are infused intravenously to replace losses. Isotonic solutions usually are prescribed to restore fluid volume. Often potassium chloride is added to the IV to replace potassium losses. These might be followed by solutions containing various other electrolytes. Sodium bicarbonate might be required to restore acid-base balance in children with acidosis. In cases of extreme intravascular depletion and circulatory collapse, protein solutions (for example, plasma or serum albumin) are administered to expand plasma volume.

Nursing management Assessment findings for the child with gastroenteritis vary with the severity of the diarrhea and vomiting. The nurse observes and records signs and symptoms, noting carefully the amount and characteristics of stool and urine output. The nurse needs to be alert for signs of dehydration or other fluid and electrolyte imbalances. Continued assessment of vital signs, monitoring of laboratory reports, and accurate intake, output, stool, and emesis records are essential nursing actions.

Perineal skin care needs to be meticulous to prevent perineal excoriation due to enzyme- and acid-rich stools. Frequent diaper changes are essential. The perineum is washed with every diaper change and dried thoroughly. If the child's perineal area appears to be excoriated, the buttocks can be left exposed to the air.

A heat lamp treatment might be ordered for the child with severe skin breakdown. The infant or young child is restrained to prevent accidental touching of the lamp. A gooseneck lamp with a 60-watt bulb is positioned over the child's buttocks at least 18″–24″ away from the child. The treatment can last from 5 to 15 minutes depending on how the child tolerates the heat. The nurse preferably stays with the child, but always checks the child's skin for reddening at least every five minutes. Children have sensitive skin, and the nurse needs to prevent any burning.

Infection control measures for diarrhea are instituted according to the suspected causative agent. In some cases, hospitalized children might be isolated on enteric precautions (see Chapter 20). In any case, strict hand washing is essential. The nurse explains infection control procedures to families to prevent the spread of diarrhea among family members. Family members of children diagnosed with *Shigella, Salmonella,* and amoeba infections will need to submit stool specimens so infected individuals can be treated in a subclinical carrier state. Some infections require follow-up stool cultures by the state health department until child or family members demonstrate two or three negative cultures taken more than twenty-four hours apart.

Infants who remain NPO for long periods need to be

provided with a pacifier if the parents are agreeable. This allows the infant self-comfort through sucking. Older children require frequent mouth care. Mouthwashes can aid in dislodging thick oral secretions, and lubricant can be applied to the lips to prevent drying or cracking.

Oral fluids might be allowed depending on the child's state of hydration. The child might receive only sips of water or ginger ale, approximately 1–2 tbsp every half hour, for the first 12 hours. An electrolyte solution such as Pedialyte might be used in the place of the ginger ale if electrolyte replacement is necessary. As the child improves, the amount of liquids is gradually increased over the next 12 hours. Fluid intake is carefully monitored in light of the child's daily maintenance fluid requirements.

Prior to discharge, the nurse reviews good hygiene measures with the child and family and methods to prevent any spread of disease. Signs of dehydration are reviewed with the parent to ensure that the problem is recognized in the future and hospitalization is prevented.

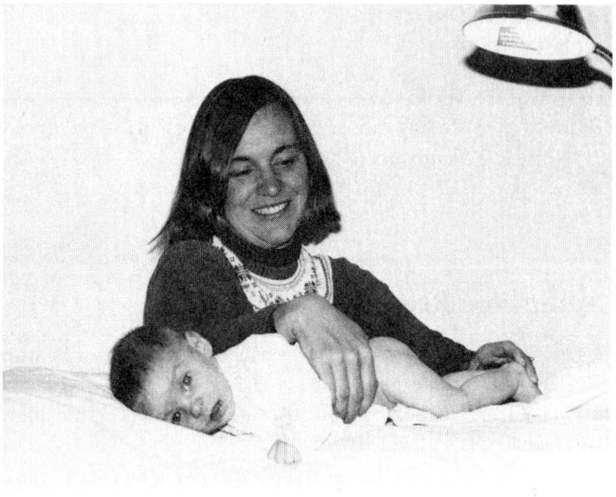

The child receiving a heat lamp treatment for excoriated skin. (Photograph by Judy Koenig.)

Essential Concepts

- Body fluid is contained in two compartments: intracellular and extracellular.
- Water is transported between the intracellular fluid and the extracellular fluid by the processes of diffusion, osmotic pressure, hydrostatic pressure, active transport, and vesicular transport.
- Fluid and electrolyte balance is regulated by thirst and by antidiuretic hormone (ADH), aldosterone, and the renin–angiotensin mechanism of the renal system.
- The fluid and electrolyte status of the child is more precarious than that of an adult for five major reasons: (1) total body water as percentage of body weight is higher, (2) a larger percentage of fluid is located in the extracellular space, (3) metabolic rate is higher, resulting in a high daily exchange of water, (4) the kidneys are immature, and (5) there is a higher ratio of surface area to weight.
- Nursing care for the child with a fluid imbalance is directed toward restoring the balance and preventing further disequilibrium.
- Assessment of a child's fluid status involves accurate observation of daily weight, skin quality, vital signs, intake and output, changes in orientation and sensorium, changes in laboratory data, and symptoms of the underlying condition.
- Because a high proportion of an infant's or young child's weight is fluid and because a high proportion of the fluid is in the extracellular space, an abrupt shift of weight can indicate fluid loss or gain.
- Skin turgor, color, temperature and moistness, along with changes in weight, intake and output, and vital signs, can indicate the child's state of hydration.
- Acute care needs for a child with a fluid imbalance might be related to fluid volume deficit, fluid volume excess, and potential sensory-perceptual alterations.
- Nutritional needs of a child with a fluid imbalance might be related to nutritional alterations providing less than body requirements.
- The child with a fluid and electrolyte imbalance and the family might require interventions related to ineffective individual and family coping.
- The major imbalances seen in children include imbalances of sodium and water, potassium, and calcium; each of these requires nursing interventions related to maintaining fluid volume, replacing any lost electrolytes, ensuring the child's safety, and assisting child and family to cope.
- The infant or young child with gastroenteritis can exhibit symptoms related to fluid and electrolyte loss and alterations in acid-base balance.

References

Hazinski MF: *Nursing Care of the Critically Ill Child.* Mosby, 1984.

Hazinski MF: Nursing care of the critically ill child: A seven-point check. *Pediatr Nurs* (Nov/Dec) 1985; 11:453–461.

Rielly MD: The renal system. In *Pediatric Critical Care.* Bloedel Smith J (editor). Wiley, 1983.

Additional Readings

Aperia A: Salt and water homeostasis during oral rehydration therapy. *J Pediatr* (Sept) 1983; 103(3):364–369.

Arant BS, Jr: Fluid therapy in the neonate—concepts in transition. *J Pediatr* (Sept) 1982; 101(3):387–389.

Boh DM, VanSon AR: The water load test. *Am J Nurs* (Jan) 1982; 82(1):112–113.

Callery P: Nursing care study—hypocalcaemia: Mother and child reunion. *Nurs Mirror* (Feb) 1982; 154(6):38–39.

Driggers DA: Managing the dehydrated child. *Am Fam Phys* (Nov) 1982; 26(5):189–194.

Filston HC et al.: Estimation of postoperative fluid requirements in infants and children. *Am Surg* (July) 1982; 196(1):76–81.

Finberg L et al.: *Water and Electrolytes in Pediatrics: Physiology, Pathophysiology, and Treatment.* Saunders, 1982.

Ghishan FK, Roloff JS: Malnutrition and hypernatremic dehydration in two breast-fed infants. *Clin Pediatr* (Aug) 1983; 22(8):592–594.

Golden SM, Steenbarger J, Monaghan WP: Osmolality and oncotic pressure of volume-expanding fluids for newborn administration. *Crit Care Med* (Dec) 1982; 10(2):863–864.

Greco A: Fluids, electrolytes, and nutrition. In: *Pediatric Critical Care Nursing.* Vestal KW (editor). Wiley, 1981.

Janusek LW: Metabolic acidosis. *Nurs '84* (July) 1984; 14(7): 44–45.

Kahn A et al.: Controlled fall in natremia in hypertonic dehydration: Possible avoidance of rehydration seizures. *Eur J Pediatr* (Feb) 1981; 135(3):293–296.

Martof M: Part 1: Fluid balance. *J Nephrol Nurs* (Jan/Feb) 1985; 10–15.

Martof M: Part II: Electrolyte balance. *J Nephrol Nurs* (March/Apr) 1985; 49–55.

McFadden EA, Zaloga GP, Chernow B: Hypocalcemia: A medical emergency. *Am J Nurs* (Feb) 1983; 83(2):227–230.

Meeuwisse GW: High sugar worse than high sodium in oral rehydration solutions. *Acta Paediatr Scand* (March) 1983; 72(2):161–166.

Nash MA: The management of fluid and electrolyte disorders in the neonate. *Clin Perinatol* (June) 1981; 8(2):251–262.

Nursing 81 Books: *Managing I.V. Therapy.* Intermed, 1981.

Okstein CJ: Patient tampering with electronic intravenous fluid regulators. *Pediatrics* (Feb) 1984; 73(2):250–251.

Press S, Setzer N: Profound acidosis in infancy. *South Med J* (Aug) 1983; 76(8):1070.

Pickering LK, DuPont HL: Infectious diarrhea. In: *Infectious Diseases of Children and Adults.* Pickering LK, DuPont HL (editors). Addison-Wesley, 1986.

Ree GH, Clezy JK: Simple guide to fluid balance. *Trop Doct* (Oct) 1982; 12(4, Part 1):155–159.

RN Master Care Plan: Preventing electrolyte imbalances. *RN* (Nov) 1984; 47(11):32–33.

RN Master Care Plan: Correcting acid-base imbalance. *RN* (May) 1985; 48(5):39–40.

Sack DA et al.: Risk of hypernatremia with oral rehydration. *Pediatrics* (July) 1982; 101(1):154–155.

Santosham M et al.: Storing oral rehydration solution. *Lancet* (April) 1982; 1(8275):797.

Santosham M, Carrera E, Sack RB: Oral rehydration therapy in well-nourished ambulatory children. *Am J Trop Med Hyg* (July) 1983; 32(4):804–808.

Sinclair HC: Babies and children: Fluids in balance. *Nurs '80* (May) 1980; 10(4):574–575.

Snyder JD: From Pedialyte to popsicles: A look at oral rehydration therapy used in the United States and Canada. *Am J Clin Nutr* (Jan) 1982; 35(1):157–161.

Sugijanto Abbas N: Edema in oral rehydration. *Paediatr Indones* (Nov/Dec) 1981; 21(11–12):229–234.

Suh KK: Care of infants and children. *Int Anesthesiol Clin* (Spring) 1983; 21(1):117–125.

Tejani A, Dobias B, Mahadevan R: Osmolar relationships in infantile dehydration. *Am J Dis Child* (Nov) 1981; 135(11):1000–1005.

Toto KH: When the patient has hypokalemia. *RN* (March) 1987; 38–41.

Vaughan A: *Nelson Textbook of Pediatrics.* Saunders, 1983.

Vick RL (editor): *Contemporary Medical Physiology.* Addison-Wesley, 1984.

Wildblood RA, Strezo P: The how to's of home IV therapy. *Pediatr Nurs* (Jan/Feb) 1987; 13(1):42–46, 68.

Wink DM: Fluid-induced hyponatremia in infancy: A preventable problem. *Am J Nurs* (May) 1983; 83(5):765–767.

Chapter 22

Oxygenation

Implications of Airway Obstruction and Infection

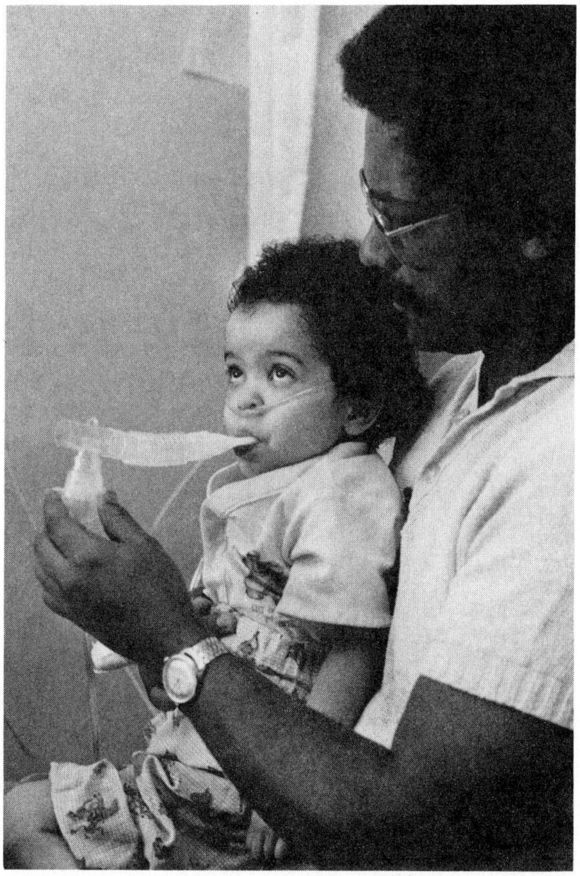

Chapter Contents

(Continues)

Developmental Needs
Altered growth and development related to disease limitations
Emotional Needs
Anxiety related to the acuity of the respiratory dysfunction
Potential for ineffective family coping
Health Maintenance Needs
Potential knowledge deficit regarding home management

The Child with an Acute Respiratory Infection

Tonsillitis and Pharyngitis
Acute Spasmodic Croup
Laryngotracheobronchitis
Epiglottitis
Bronchiolitis
Bronchitis
Pneumonia

The Child with Tuberculosis
The Child with an Acute Noninfectious Respiratory Problem

Foreign Body Aspiration
Aspiration Pneumonia
Near-Drowning

The Child with a Chronic or Noninfectious Respiratory Disorder

Asthma
Cystic Fibrosis

Objectives

- Describe the structure and function of the respiratory system.
- Describe how to obtain data from the history, physical examination, and associated clinical findings for a child with suspected respiratory dysfunction.
- Describe nursing actions associated with diagnostic tests for respiratory dysfunction.
- Describe the nursing care required in providing oxygen therapy and chest physiotherapy.
- Describe nursing responsibilities relative to care for the child with an artificial airway.
- State nursing diagnoses applicable to children with respiratory dysfunction and their families.
- State the chief nutritional deficit likely in the child with respiratory dysfunction.
- Describe the nursing diagnoses and interventions to meet the developmental, emotional, and health maintenance needs of the child with respiratory dysfunction.
- Identify common viral and bacterial respiratory tract infections and classes of drugs used to treat them.
- Describe the nursing management for a child with an infection of the respiratory tract.
- Describe the management of the child with a noninfectious respiratory tract dysfunction.

ESSENTIALS OF STRUCTURE AND FUNCTION
The Respiratory Tract

Glossary

Bronchi Branches of the trachea that lead directly to the lungs. The right bronchus is larger and straighter than the left. Bronchi branch and decrease in size in the lungs, becoming bronchioles. Bronchioles terminate in respiratory units.

Control of respiration Neural system (pons, medulla, and spinal cord) controls respiratory rate and depth according to nerve impulses generated in the lung. Chemical control depends on changes in serum carbon dioxide partial pressure (Pco_2) and oxygen partial pressure (Po_2). An increase in Pco_2 stimulates increased ventilation, while a decrease in Pco_2 causes decreased ventilation.

Larynx "Voicebox." The larynx is formed by nine cartilages and its superior opening is covered by a flap of cartilage known as the *epiglottis*. The epiglottis covers the larynx and prevents swallowed food from entering the respiratory system.

Lungs Two organs that occupy the thoracic (chest) area, one on either side of the *mediastinum* (cardiac area). The right and left lung each are divided into lobes, with the right having three and the left having two. Lungs are surrounded by membranes called *pleura,* which facilitate expansion during respiration.

Mechanics of Respiration

Phase I Inspiration (air in)

1. Intercostals and diaphragm contract causing an increase in the thoracic cavity.
2. The diaphragm flattens to allow maximum expansion (see the figure showing diaphragm position).
3. As lung volume increases, gases expand causing decreased gas pressure and increased air movement into the lungs.
4. Movement of air stops when intrapulmonary pressure equals atmospheric pressure.

Phase II—Expiration (air out)

1. Inspiratory muscles relax, causing elastic recoil of the lungs, which begins to force air out.
2. Increasing density of gas molecules increases intrapulmonary pressure and forces more air out until the pressure inside and outside the lungs is equalized.
3. The diaphragm returns to its original dome-shaped position. Pressure within the pleural spaces remains negative, preventing lung collapse.

SOURCE: Marieb EN: *Essentials of Human Anatomy and Physiology*. Addison-Wesley, 1984, pp. 251–252.

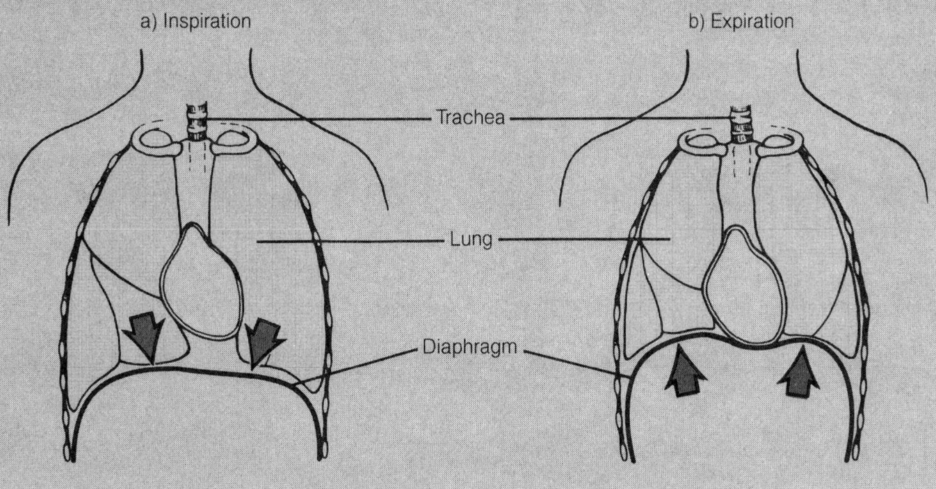

Diaphragm position during ***A.*** *inspiration and* ***B.*** *expiration. (From Marieb EN:* Essentials of Human Anatomy & Physiology. *Benjamin/Cummings, 1984.)*

(Continues)

ESSENTIALS OF STRUCTURE AND FUNCTION *(Continued)*

The Respiratory Tract

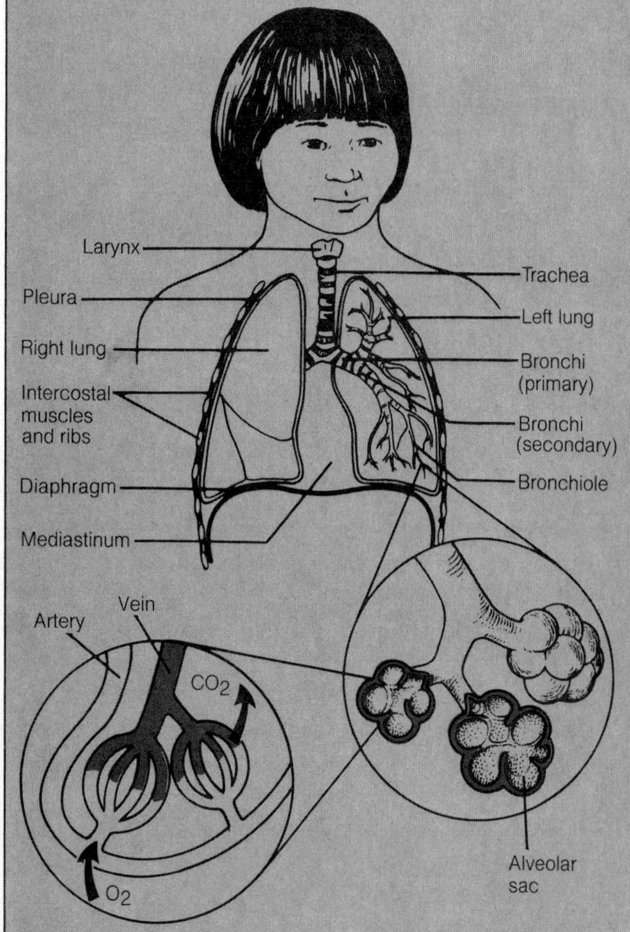

The respiratory unit.

Respiration The mechanism by which the lungs oxygenate arterial blood (inspiration) and remove carbon dioxide from venous blood (expiration). Air exchange is called *ventilation*. Gaseous exchange is accomplished by diffusion of gases across the alveolar membrane to the lung capillaries and from the capillaries to the alveoli. Oxygen is combined with hemoglobin molecules in the red blood cells and is carried to body tissues.

Respiratory units Consist of terminal bronchioles, alveolar ducts, and alveoli. They are the location of gas exchange. Cells in alveolar lining produce surfactant. (See figure showing the respiratory unit.)

Surfactant A phospholipid protein complex that reduces the surface tension of the alveoli, preventing their collapse at the end of each expiration.

Trachea Extends from the larynx to the division of the right and left bronchi. The trachea is structured of cartilage rings and covered by smooth muscle.

Functional development of the respiratory system occurs at 28 weeks of gestation. An infant born prior to 28 weeks of gestation has surfactant production inadequate to keep the alveoli inflated and experiences respiratory distress syndrome (see Chapter 34). The neonate is at risk if the upper and middle airways fail to develop normally. Any developmental abnormality that prevents normal respiration requires immediate relief in the delivery room.

All the cells and organs of the body rely on the respiratory system for their supply of oxygen and for removal of carbon dioxide. Anything that interferes with the functioning of this system threatens life itself. Obstruction of airflow, restriction of normal lung mechanics, and impaired gas exchange can result from infection, trauma, or physical abnormality. Any of these disturbances alone or in combination interfere with respiratory function.

Lung growth and development continues from birth through young adulthood. Airways and blood vessels increase in length and diameter, and the number of alveoli increases tenfold by age 3. The pharynx is proportionately smaller in the neonate and infant than in the adult. This occurs because the maxilla and mandible of the infant are short, while the soft palate is proportionately large. In conjunction with the narrow posterior nasooropharynx, the infant's tongue is large and might occlude the pharynx. Infants are obligatory nose breathers. Any upper respiratory tract infection that blocks nasal passages is a cause for concern about potential airway occlusion. This situation is corrected by growth during early and late childhood.

Assessment of the Child with Respiratory Dysfunction

History

The history provides valuable data for assessment and nursing diagnoses related to present or potential respiratory dysfunction. It is important to encourage the child to supply as much information as possible. If the parent of an older child supplies most of the health history, the nurse is alert to the child's possible inappropriate dependence on the parent. The parent might have assumed too much responsibility for the child's illness, particularly if the illness is a chronic and life-threatening one. Because any pulmonary disease can be life threatening, the nurse might decide to defer taking the history if the child's condition is unstable.

The family's health history is important. Some diseases of the lungs are inherited. Others have both genetic and environmental causes. For example, it is believed that certain individuals are genetically predisposed to asthma (a respiratory disease of allergic origin), particularly if they have a family history of atopy. *Atopy* is the inherited tendency to produce antibodies to environmental antigens and can be manifested by asthma, rhinitis, hay fever, infantile eczema, and urticaria (hives) (see Chapter 25).

Reviewing the general health status of family members also can help identify pulmonary disease caused by exposure to infectious or physical agents in the environment. A particular microorganism might cause gastrointestinal symptoms in a parent or older sibling and upper or middle respiratory tract infection in a young child. Smoking in the home can cause symptoms of respiratory dysfunction in the patient and other family members.

Neonatal history Information about the child's neonatal health and health during early infancy can help differentiate among disease processes. Infants who had neonatal respiratory distress syndrome (RDS) frequently have later respiratory difficulties.

Recurrent symptoms of upper, middle, or lower tract infections require further assessment. If the child has had chest radiographs in the past, they can be compared with current radiographs to evaluate the chronicity and progression of disease. It is helpful also to elicit information from the family about both successful and unsuccessful prior treatments.

History of the present illness The history of the present illness includes information about the child's cough, mucus production, dyspnea (difficult breathing, or "air hunger"), *orthopnea* (difficult breathing except in an upright position), wheezing, or pain. The nurse notes any recent exposure to irritants or infection, fatigue, decreased exercise tolerance, changes in weight or height, or gastrointestinal problems.

Cough Coughing is a protective reflex of the respiratory system. The nurse records information about the onset, frequency, duration, pattern of recurrence, sound, and productivity of the cough. Information about when the child or parent first remembers hearing the cough can provide clues to its cause. The nurse asks the parent and child what prompts the cough and whether it is intermittent, occasional, recurrent, or increasing or decreasing in frequency.

The time of day the cough typically occurs is important. Children with some chronic respiratory conditions might typically cough more in the early morning and on awakening. Some children have no cough symptoms at all during the night but awake coughing and cough continuously for several hours thereafter. It is sometimes helpful to have the parent fill out a daily report sheet to keep track of the times of day when the cough occurs, how long the coughing episodes last, and the number of coughing episodes a child is having. The parent can note also the child's activity prior to a coughing episode.

Information about the sound of the child's cough and its productivity also indicates possible causes. For example, infection might be considered likely in a child whose parent reports a loose-sounding cough productive of yellowish-white mucous as opposed to a child having a dry, nonproductive cough.

Sputum The nurse asks the child and parent to describe the child's sputum: the consistency of sputum as viscous (thick) or nonviscous; its color as clear, green, yellow, white, or blood-tinged; and the amount expectorated as small, moderate, or large. Some mucus also has an odor and this can be described.

Respiratory pattern Very young children are not able to describe dyspnea, and so the nurse looks for clues in the history. The parent might report the child's decreased exercise tolerance or shortness of breath with exercise. Orthopnea, retractions, grunting, or nasal flaring are all signs of dyspnea. A child experiencing some dyspnea might be described as quiet, inactive, and lacking interest and enthusiasm for normal play. Infants can demonstrate dyspnea by refusal to eat and irritability. Withdrawal and loss of interest in play are additional signs of dyspnea in an infant.

A child who is uncomfortable breathing except in a semisitting or standing position has orthopnea. Children with pulmonary edema or asthma might demonstrate orthopnea by propping themselves up and resting their weight on their arms, which they extend behind them. Retractions are frequently seen in children with airway obstruction or other dysfunction causing respiratory distress. *Retractions* are caused by the pulling in of the soft tissues surrounding the bone of the thoracic cavity. They occur mainly in the middle and upper intercostal spaces (intercostal retractions), in the sternum (sub- or suprasternal), and in the jugular notch, supraclavicular, and infraclavicular spaces.

Grunting and nasal flaring most frequently are seen in children with severe respiratory distress (see Chapter 34 for assessment of respiratory distress in the neonate). *Grunting* is an expiratory grunt heard as the child strives to force air past a partially closed glottis. This maneuver helps to maintain some pressure at the alveolar level and prevents complete collapse of alveoli with each expiration. *Nasal flaring* is enlargement of both nares (nostrils) during inspiration. It is a sign that the accessory muscles of respiration are needed to breathe.

Quality of respirations Audible wheezing, which can occur on inspiration or expiration, is noted in the history of the present illness. Wheezing is caused by air passing through swollen mucous membranes, over thick secretions, and through contracted bronchioles, all of which create a partial obstruction in the bronchi or bronchioles. The vibration of the edematous membranes or secretions causes the characteristic high-pitched whistle (sibilant sound) or low-pitched snore (sonorous sound). The nurse gathers information about the onset, duration, and severity of any wheezing. Whether the wheezing is on inspiration or expiration is important to note also.

Pain Chest pain is frightening at any age, and it might be the chief complaint. The neonate or infant can react to chest pain with crying, irritability, withdrawal, changes in vital signs, and loss of interest in food, fluid, and play. Very young children are apt to indicate their discomfort in general terms (for example, "It hurts"), but they are seldom able to give more specific information about the location, intensity, nature, duration, frequency, and events surrounding the occurrence and relief of the pain.

The older child might describe chest pain as being sharp or dull, or constant or occurring only when breathing deeply or coughing. The child might describe the pain as tightness of the chest or might be able to pinpoint the exact source of the pain.

Exposure to infectious agents or irritants The history of the present illness includes information about possible exposure to infectious microorganisms and irritants. If infection is suspected, the nurse seeks data about possible contributing factors, such as inadequate nutrition, unsanitary living conditions, or delays in obtaining routine immunizations. If tuberculosis is suspected, the nurse discovers whether the child has been exposed to active bacilli and obtains records pertaining to immunization and results of tuberculin skin tests. Information about whether the child has traveled recently, and where, is helpful.

The nurse asks about recent cold or influenza symptoms of other family members. Many agents that produce respiratory infections are airborne and easily passed throughout the household. If the child is being assessed for asthma, the nurse seeks information about possible irritants in the child's home environment that might be worsening respiratory symptoms. The nurse also inquires about local industrial pollutants, air quality, pets and animals at home, the type of vegetation in the area and home, toys and bedding in the child's room, and heating and cooling systems used in the home.

It is important also to ask whether anyone smokes in the home. Studies have indicated that children of parents who smoke might later exhibit adverse effects. They can experience increased tendencies for respiratory infections (Mitchell, 1986). Adolescents are questioned in private about smoking because they might be hiding this behavior from their parents.

Alterations in weight and height Often, one of the earliest indications of chronic lung disease is the failure to gain weight. If the disease continues unchecked, weight loss and subsequent failure to gain height follow. If the child's weight and height have been recorded since birth, the nurse plots these measurements on a standard growth chart to help determine when the altered growth pattern began.

Gastrointestinal symptoms The nurse also questions the child and family about the onset, severity, frequency, and duration of gastrointestinal signs and symptoms of fatigue. Acute or chronic infection invariably produces lethargy, anorexia, vomiting, and abdominal pain, which further interfere with growth. Nausea, vomiting, and resultant poor intake of food can be problems for children who swallow mucus. The nurse also questions the child and family about any changes in the child's stools. A history of frequent, foul-smelling, bulky gray stools and associated abdominal pain might indicate a malabsorption.

Physical Examination

Respiratory arrest or the inability of the respiratory system to oxygenate the blood and remove carbon dioxide can result from acute or chronic dysfunction. In either case, the child's life might depend on the nurse's rapid and accurate clinical assessment and ability to initiate emergency interventions within moments. Table 22-1 lists the clinical signs and symptoms most often associated with impending or frank respiratory failure.

Cyanosis *Cyanosis* is a bluish color of the skin and mucous membranes of children experiencing *hypoxia* (poor tissue oxygenation). Although cyanosis is listed in Table 22-1 as a sign of respiratory failure, it is not always a reliable sign in children. Anemia masks cyanosis, for example, and the child with vasoconstriction or the chilled neonate might have cyanosis despite adequate oxygenation. If cyanosis persists despite oxygen administration, the child might have multiple right-to-left cardiac shunts (see Chapter 23).

While inspecting the nail beds for cyanosis, the nurse also looks for clubbing. *Clubbing* of the fingers and toes is evidenced by lateral and longitudinal spreading of the nail base. The fingernails and toenails appear shiny and bulbous. The exact cause of clubbing is unknown, but it is always significant. It usually is associated with diseases involving some degree of hypoxemia (decreased blood oxygen) over a period of time. Clubbing can be reversed if the disease process is reversed.

Thoracic shape A change in the shape of the thorax is another indication of chronic disease. Children who have chronic respiratory diseases might develop *pectus profundum,* or barrel chest. This is caused by chronic obstruction. Barrel chest is normal, however, in infants and young children and, in some cases, is hereditary. A nurse following a child with chronic obstructive lung diseases in a clinic might plot measurements of chest diameter serially on a graph at each visit to help assess response to therapy or the course of the disease. (Assessment of other skeletal deformities is discussed in Chapters 10 and 30.)

Deformities of the sternum, ribs, or spine can interfere with respiration. The nurse observes for symmetry of thoracic expansion during inspiration. If one side of the thorax does not expand as fully as the other or lags behind, the child might have a fractured rib, chest trauma, *pneumothorax* (air in the pleural cavity), or a skeletal deformity.

Vital signs The physical examination includes obtaining baseline vital signs. Alterations in vital signs provide significant data concerning the child's response to the disease process or its treatment. For example, temperature might be significantly elevated with a bacterial infection but only slightly elevated or normal with a viral infection. Hypoxia can cause an increased pulse rate and increased blood pressure. *Hypercapnia* (increased serum CO_2) can cause decreased blood pressure. Bronchodilators, theophylline, and other medications given to children with respiratory dysfunction can cause changes in pulse and blood pressure.

TABLE 22-1 Criteria for Diagnosis of Respiratory Failure in Infants and Children with Acute Pulmonary Disease

Clinical	Physiologic
Decreased or absent inspiratory breath sounds	$P_{CO_2} \geq 75$ mm Hg
Severe inspiratory retractions and use of accessory muscles	$P_{O_2} \leq 100$ mm Hg in 100% oxygen
Cyanosis in 40% ambient oxygen	
Depressed level of consciousness and response to pain	
Poor skeletal muscle tone	

NOTE: Three clinical symptoms and one physiologic symptom must be present to confirm the diagnosis of acute respiratory failure.

SOURCE: Downs JJ et al: Acute respiratory failure in infants and children. *Pediatr Clin North Am* (May) 1972; 19(2):429.

Information is needed about what medications the child might have been taking at home.

Respirations Four aspects of the child's respirations are assessed: rate, depth, ease, and rhythm. The nurse counts the child's resting respiratory rate for 1 minute for two reasons. First, normal respirations do not occur at a consistent, regular rate. Both depth and interval can vary. Periodic deep breaths are normal and help prevent *atelectasis* (incomplete expansion of small airways). Second, the margin of error increases proportionally with a decrease in the length of time respirations are counted. (Normal resting respiratory rates for children are listed in Appendix B. Abnormal respirations are defined in Chapter 10.)

After an initial assessment of the child's ability to sustain respiration and a general assessment of the child's color, thoracic movements, vital signs, and character of respirations, the nurse begins the "hands on" part of the physical examination: palpation, percussion, and auscultation. Breath sounds are an important indicator of respiratory function. Adventitious (acquired) breath sounds include rales, rhonchi, and wheezes (see Table 10-8 for a description of adventitious breath sounds). It is important to note the presence and description of any adventitious breath sounds.

TABLE 22-2 Diagnostic Studies for Respiratory Dysfunction

Test	Normal values	Alteration/clinical significance
Po_2 Partial pressure of oxygen—reflects amount of O_2 diffusing through pulmonary membrane into blood	Sea level: 80%–100% Altitude > 5000 feet: 65%–75%	*Increased:* Excessive administration of oxygen *Decreased:* Hypoxemia from pulmonary or cardiac disease
Pco_2 Partial pressure of carbon dioxide reflects tension exerted by dissolved carbon dioxide in blood	Sea level: 35%–45% Altitude > 5000 feet: 32%–38%	*Increased:* Breathing more shallow or slower than normal; occurs in respiratory acidosis (asthma, upper or lower airway obstruction, respiratory depressants) *Decreased:* Breathing deeper or more rapid than normal; occurs in respiratory alkalosis (incorrect ventilator settings, anxiety, high altitude, mild hypoxia)
pH Measures the chemical balance in the body	7.35–7.45	*Increased:* Alkalemia *Decreased:* Acidemia
Base excess Quantification of total base excess. The sum of the concentration of buffer ions in whole blood	Sea level: −2–+2 Altitude > 5000 feet: −4–+2	*Increased:* Metabolic alkalosis; deep, rapid breathing, weakness, shortness of breath, disorientation, coma; related to vomiting, gastric drainage to high suction, rapid infusion of $NaHCO_3^+$, ingestion of alkali *Decreased:* Metabolic acidosis; shallow, slow respirations, hypertonicity of muscles, tetany; related to ketoacidosis, salicylate poisoning, renal failure, hypoxia, diarrhea
Blood bicarbonate (HCO_3) Primary buffer union in whole blood, accounts for about half of the total buffer anions	Sea level: 22–26 mEq/L Altitude > 5000 feet: 18–26 mEq/L	*Increased:* Metabolic alkalosis *Decreased:* Metabolic acidosis
Oxygen saturation Measures actual O_2 content of hemoglobin compared to the maximal potential of O_2 carrying capacity	Sea level: 95%	*Increased:* Excessive administration of oxygen *Decreased:* Hypoxemia from pulmonary or cardiac disease
Pilocarpine iontophoresis (sweat chloride test)	Sodium < 70 mEq/L Chloride < 60 mEq/L Potassium < 60 mEq/L	*Increased:* Cystic fibrosis
Cultures Throat Sputum		*Growth of pathogens:* Upper or lower respiratory tract infection or contamination of specimen
Radiologic examinations Anterior-posterior lateral views	Normal appearance	*Abnormal appearance:* Congenital or acquired defects of rib, spine, thoracic cavity, sternum; abnormalities of diaphragm; chest expansion; pneumothorax; mediastinal shift; certain cardiac abnormalities; abnormal density of lung tissue; hyperinflation; atelectasis
Assisted inspiratory-expiratory radiograph	Normal and equal lung expansion on both sides	*Hyperexpansion of one side of chest:* foreign body aspiration
Barium swallow	No evidence of reflux	*Reflux of barium from stomach into esophagus:* Gastroesophageal reflux

TABLE 22-2 *(Continued)*

Test	Normal values	Alteration/clinical significance
Pulmonary function		
Tidal volume	Varies with age, sex, height, weight	*Decreased:* Restrictive lung disease
Expiratory reserve volume		*Decreased:* Restrictive lung disease
Inspiratory reserve volume		*Decreased:* Restrictive lung disease
Residual volume		*Increased:* Obstructive lung disease
Capacities		*Decreased:* Obstructive or restrictive lung disease
Flow rates		*Decreased:* Obstructive lung disease
Diffusion		*Decreased:* Alveolocapillary membrane defect
Tuberculin skin test (Mantoux, PPD)	No reaction	Wheal > 9mm in diameter indicates exposure to tuberculosis

Validating Diagnostic Tests

Table 22-2 summarizes some of the diagnostic tests used in assessing respiratory status. Serum immunoglobulins and complete blood count are required for additional data. An elevated white blood cell count can indicate a respiratory infection, while serum immunoglobulins are used to assess immune deficiency and allergy (see Chapters 25 and 26 for values).

Arterial blood gas studies are done to assess oxygenation and the acid-base balance (pH) of the body. Arterial gas determination is preferred to venous sampling in infants and children because it is more accurate. Because the vessels in infants and young children are so small, however, venous blood by capillary stick can be used to determine oxygenation and acid-base status. Diagnostic information can be obtained through an anterior-posterior and a lateral radiograph. The inspiratory-expiratory radiograph is taken from an anterior-posterior view at the end of expiration. It is used to demonstrate air trapping in children with suspected foreign body aspiration. A lung scan can be done to pinpoint an area of pathology in the lungs.

Cultures Throat cultures are done to isolate and identify pathogens from the throat and blood cultures are done to isolate pathogens causing generalized infections. Sputum cultures are difficult to obtain from children. It might be helpful to have the child rinse the mouth with a warm saline solution before the nurse performs percussion and postural

Pulmonary Function Tests

Explain the reasons for the test to parents and child; tell them that the tests will evaluate the ability of the lungs to perform adequately the functions of breathing and gas exchange.

Children of all ages should be taught to perform the maneuvers required, although children under age 5 years might not be able to perform them well. The tests will not hurt.

The child will be taken to a room with special equipment that will measure various aspects of pulmonary function.

The child will be asked to breathe a mixture of oxygen and air through a mouthpiece. Depending on the respiratory volume being measured, the child might be asked to forcefully inhale or exhale or hold the breath.

The child might be asked to breathe in as much as possible, hold the breath briefly, and then force the breath out for at least 3 seconds. Practicing this maneuver can be done by having the child blow bubbles or blow a Ping-Pong ball across a table.

To measure proper gaseous diffusion, a mixture of helium and carbon monoxide might be used.

The nurse encourages the child to rest following the test since the tests can be very tiring.

ASSESSMENT GUIDE *The Child with a Respiratory Problem*

Assessment questions	Supporting data
Is the child having difficulty breathing? (**Note:** any signs of respiratory distress need to be reported immediately)	Crowing sound on inspiration or associated with cough, stridor, or excessive drooling. Signs of increased respiratory effort—tachypnea, retractions, nasal flaring, expiratory grunt, pallor, cyanosis, extreme fatigue, apnea
Is the child complaining of a cough? Describe frequency, type (dry, loose, productive, non-productive), time of day it most frequently occurs, and color of sputum	Presence of adventitious breath sounds—rales, ronchi, wheezing. Diminished or altered breath sounds. Asymmetrical chest movements. Chest pain
Does the child prefer to be in a particular position—sitting up, leaning forward, stooping?	Clubbing of the fingers. Inability to handle oral secretions. Changes in vital signs—increased pulse, alteration in blood pressure, fever
Is the child complaining of hoarseness, sore throat, or runny nose?	Sneezing, fever, itchy eyes, dark circles under the eyes
Have the child, or family members, had a history of recurrent respiratory problems or allergy? Does the child have a history of respiratory distress syndrome (RDS), or foreign body aspiration? Has the child been exposed recently to any respiratory infection?	

Additional data: Signs of dehydration (see Chapter 21), anorexia, abdominal pain, vomiting, loose bulky stools, failure to thrive, alteration in neurologic signs indicating hypoxemia (eg, drowsiness, lethargy, confusion, numbness, tingling, coma)

drainage to stimulate the child to expectorate sputum. Secretions from the child's posterior pharynx also can be aspirated into a special collecting device, or trap. Because accurate sputum cultures require a deep specimen collection, and this is difficult in children, gastric washing (lavage) can be performed to obtain a specimen of swallowed sputum. The nurse records the color and character of the sputum.

Pulmonary function tests Pulmonary function tests indicate the lungs' ability to perform mechanical ventilation, deliver oxygen to the cardiovascular system, and remove carbon dioxide from venous blood. These tests measure lung volume, capacity, and air flow rates during inspiration and expiration. Normal values for lung volume, capacity, and flow vary according to the child's age, sex, and height. Generally, volume and capacity diminish with lung disease. Flow usually diminishes in obstructive lung disease and is normal in restrictive lung disease.

Nurses are often responsible for helping children learn to perform the maneuvers required for pulmonary function testing. Many of these maneuvers are difficult for children to perform so practice before the procedure is helpful.

Additional tests Exercise testing is used to assess overall respiratory function in response to exertion and is particularly useful for children who experience exercise-induced bronchospasm (spasm of the bronchi). Visualization and manipulation of the larger branches of the tracheobronchial tree are possible through *bronchoscopy,* or the insertion of a flexible fiberoptic tube into the bronchial tree. This procedure is ideal for the removal of aspirated foreign objects, frequently seen in children. When prolonged serious lung disease cannot be diagnosed by less invasive means, open lung biopsy might be necessary. Lung biopsy is performed under general anesthesia in children and routine preoperative and postoperative nursing care is required.

Nursing Management for Procedures and Treatments

Oxygen Therapy

Indications The indication for administration of supplemental oxygen is arterial hypoxemia, which leads to tissue hypoxia. *Hypoxemia,* which is a decreased blood oxygen level, is evidenced by an increased respiratory rate, pallor, headache, tachycardia, cyanosis, and alterations in blood gas values. Severe hypoxemia causes mental confusion.

Administration Equipment used to give supplemental oxygen includes hoods, isolettes, masks, cannulas, and catheters. The mode of delivery depends on the child's age and the percentage (concentration) of supplemental oxygen required.

The delivery of high concentrations of oxygen (above 40%) requires an isolette with ports blocked, a hood, a face tent, or a nonrebreathing mask. For lesser concentrations, nasal cannulas are the most efficient and best-tolerated mode. Cannulas are now available for infants.

Because keeping the cannula or catheter in place is difficult in infants and young children, placing squares of stoma adhesive on each cheek and then taping the cannula or catheter to the adhesive stabilizes the cannula and prevents skin breakdown. The stoma adhesive is not removed until it falls off, and the cannula tape can be replaced as needed. An oxygen tent is seldom used for infants or children unless they are being treated for croup, in which case the tent's primary purpose is to deliver mist, not oxygen. Oxyhoods might be used, however, to deliver high concentrations of oxygen.

The nurse can use a number of oxygen-concentration analyzers continuously or intermittently to monitor supplemental oxyen delivery by hood, isolette, or mask. It is most difficult to measure the oxygen concentration delivered by cannula or catheter. Oxygen delivery by these means is best monitored through blood gas values or transcutaneous oxygen monitoring.

Transcutaneous monitoring (TCM) of oxygenation is a technique that measures oxygen concentration through use of a monitoring transducer probe secured to the skin so that air cannot leak into the area of skin-probe contact. A heating element warms the small area of skin to 43–44.5°C (preset and age-dependent). As the skin temperature rises, the capillary bed in the skin dilates and arterializes. Oxygen molecules diffuse across to the probe membrane. The pressure of the oxygen is then measured and recorded.

In a well-perfused child, transcutaneous measurements can correlate very closely with actual arterial oxygenation. With underperfusion, however, the transcutaneous values might indicate only trends, not accurate oxygenation status. As long as it is known that trends are being monitored, transcutaneous monitoring is very helpful.

In some small infants, hypoxemia causes diminished cardiac output and perfusion, and the transcutaneous monitoring might suddenly drop to the 20–30 range without obvious clinical signs of cyanosis and tachypnea. This drop is an important indirect reflection of oxygenation and must not be disregarded. It is a dramatic demonstration of the cardiovascular response to even brief hypoxemia in young infants.

There is usually a desired Po_2 value for any infant or child receiving supplemental oxygen. The oxygen concentration needed to achieve that Po_2 is prescribed by the physician. In acute conditions, Po_2 might be determined as frequently as every 15 minutes. Continuous, long-term administration of oxygen generally is low-flow and is monitored much less frequently. For example, an infant receiving oxygen therapy at home might be assessed monthly.

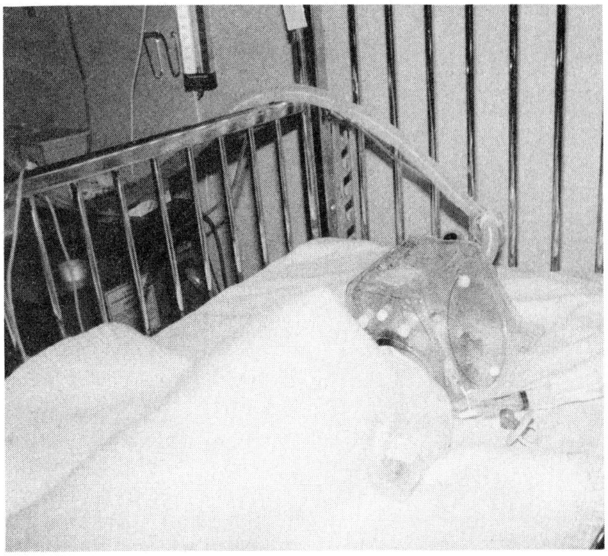

An infant in an oxyhood. (Photograph by Judy Koenig.)

Complications Oxygen administration must be monitored; administration of too much or too little oxygen can cause adverse effects. In preterm infants, administration of too high a concentration (Po_2 reaches 100 mm Hg) can injure the eyes, causing retrolental fibroplasia and blindness (see Chapter 34). Whenever the long-term delivery of high concentrations of supplemental oxygen is needed for infants, it can cause bronchopulmonary dysplasia, or chronic lung disease of infancy. Too little concentration of oxygen can lead to pulmonary vascular constriction, airway constriction, hypoxia, coma, and death.

Inhalation Therapy and Humidification

In inhalation therapy, drugs in liquid form are atomized by a nebulizer into a mist of fine particles, which are inhaled by the child. Prefilled, hand-held, freon-propelled units (for example, Medihalers) are used at home. The device chosen for a particular child depends on the medication to be delivered and the ability of the child to cooperate with treatment.

An aerosol needs to be inhaled deeply for maximum benefit, and so patient education is important. Particularly

STANDARDS OF NURSING CARE *The Child Receiving Oyxgen Therapy*

GUIDE FOR NURSING MANAGEMENT

Nursing diagnosis	Intervention	Rationale	Outcome
1. Potential for impaired gas exchange (stressor: dysfunctions that impair alveolar ventilation)	Check for correct O_2 liter administration (O_2 concentration between 1–5 liters per minute) at least every hour.	Incorrect administration of oxygen can result in complications and possibly in insufficient oxygen to improve gas exchange.	The arterial blood gases are within normal limits. The child does not exhibit any signs of hypoxia or hypercapnea.
	Closely monitor oxygen concentrations by O_2 analyzer or by transcutaneous oxygen monitoring. Correct the liter flow to achieve the oxygen concentration ordered.	Therapeutic results can be obtained only with the correct amount of oxygen being received by the body tissues. Transcutaneous monitoring can correlate well with arterial oxygenation.	
	Monitor blood gas values; in acute conditions as often as every 15 minutes.	Blood gases give an accurate picture of oxygenation.	
	Encourage the child to breathe through the nose if child is old enough to cooperate.	Increased amounts of oxygen can reach the blood if the child with a nasal cannula breathes through the nose instead of through the mouth because more of the oxygen reaches the lungs.	
	Maintain slightly elevated head position.	Elevated position facilitates lung expansion by decreasing pressure on the diaphragm.	
	Observe the child's vital signs and note any signs of respiratory insufficiency—increased or labored respirations, increased pulse, retractions, nasal flaring, cyanosis.	Signs of respiratory distress can indicate inadequate oxygen administration.	
2. Potential for impaired skin integrity (stressors: irritation from the nasal cannula, drying quality of oxygen, type of oxygen equipment used)	Attach oxygen flow meter to the humidification reservoir containing distilled water; keep the reservoir filled to the marked line.	Humidity administered with oxygen prevents drying of the mucous membranes and thus cracking or fissures.	Mucous membranes appear intact and moist. There are no signs of cracks, fissures, or ulcerations. The skin beneath the catheter or tubing appears intact. There are no signs of breakdown in diaper area or other body area.
	Use a nasal cannula of proper size.	The correct size cannula decreases nasal irritation.	
	Change nasal cannula or catheter at least every eight hours.	Providing a clean cannula or catheter decreases the chance of organisms entering compromised mucosa.	
	Apply water soluble jelly frequently (q4h) to nares and dry lips.	Water soluble jelly keeps lips and nares moist and is not a hazard for use with oxygen, as is petroleum jelly.	

STANDARDS OF NURSING CARE *The Child Receiving Oyxgen Therapy (Continued)*

GUIDE FOR NURSING MANAGEMENT

Nursing diagnosis	Intervention	Rationale	Outcome
	Give frequent (q4h) mouth care.	The drying effects of oxygen can dry oral membranes, making the child uncomfortable and susceptible to mucosal irritation. Mouth care increases moisture to the area and provides comfort.	
	Encourage the child's favorite fluids.	Fluids keep the mucous membranes hydrated and promote comfort. They also liquefy secretions in the lungs.	
	Secure stoma adhesive to the child's cheeks and tape the catheter or cannula to the adhesive.	The stoma adhesive protects the child's skin and prevents skin breakdown from frequent removal of tape used to secure the cannula.	
	Check the skin around the cannula and on the cheeks frequently for signs of irritation or breakdown.	Early recognition of problems allows for early intervention.	
	Keep the child who is in an oxyhood or O_2 tent dry by changing the bed linens, diapers, and pajamas frequently.	Linens get damp quickly in the humid environment of a tent. Damp clothing against the skin can contribute to skin breakdown and can be a medium for organism growth.	
3. Potential for injury (stressor: the gaseous properties of oxygen)	Prohibit smoking in any room where oxygen is administered; place a warning sign at the child's bedside.	An open flame can spread rapidly in the presence of oxygen.	The family and staff can state the regulations and safety hazards associated with oxygen administration and can abide by them.
	Make sure all electrical equipment is properly grounded.	Ungrounded electrical equipment can cause sparks that ignite a fire.	
	Do not allow the child to use any toys or bed linens that might cause static electricity, such as nylon or wool stuffed animals; nurses should wear antistatic fabrics.	Static electricity can cause sparking that would ignite a fire.	
	Do not use petroleum jellies, alcohol, or other flammable substances when giving nursing care to the child.	Oxygen supports combustion.	

(Continues)

STANDARDS OF NURSING CARE *The Child Receiving Oyxgen Therapy (Continued)*

GUIDE FOR NURSING MANAGEMENT

Nursing diagnosis	Intervention	Rationale	Outcome
4. Potential for ineffective individual coping (stressors: isolation in an oxygen tent, anxiety, separation from parent)	Frequently cuddle children receiving oxygen therapy.	Tactile stimulation decreases the sense of isolation and anxiety.	The child appears comfortable receiving the oxygen. There are no signs of anxiety or of respiratory distress. The child demonstrates appropriate coping mechanisms.
	Provide appropriate developmental stimulation such as allowing for play opportunities, contact with peers, and changes in location; child can be brought to the playroom with portable oxygen and appropriate supervision.	Children can feel isolated when enclosed in a tent or when restricted by a treatment. Providing appropriate stimulation decreases isolation and sensory deprivation.	
	Give the child in an oxygen tent appropriate toys; maintain verbal contact frequently.	Verbal contact provides auditory stimulation and helps the child feel less isolated.	
	Encourage the young child to pretend the tent is an exciting place such as a space ship or a tent in the woods.	Using play helps children to cope appropriately with treatments and decreases anxiety level.	
	Double check that the crib or bed rails are up when a child receives oxygen by tent.	It occasionally happens that, because the child is in a tent and secure, attention to crib safety lapses. The plastic tent can become untucked allowing the child to fall.	
	Teach parents how to care for the child in a tent and encourage them to participate in the child's care.	Maintaining tactile and verbal contact with the parents decreases the child's feelings of isolation and anxiety, and assists the child to cope with the method of treatment.	

important is reminding the child to hold the breath for several seconds after inhalation to keep the medication in contact with the respiratory passages for as long as possible. Making a game of deep inhalation followed by breath holding can help the child get used to the procedure required. For example, the child can be told to pretend the lungs are balloons. To fill the balloons, the child has to breathe in instead of out and try to keep the balloon filled for as long as possible. Any nebulizers can be used with children, but the nurse's close observation and stimulation is required to encourage deep breathing.

Because dry air irritates the airways, humidity (moisture) is added to dry air to prevent respiratory irritation. This is particularly important during oxygen administration or whenever the natural pathway of ventilation is bypassed, as with an artificial airway.

Houses often are dry in the winter when the heat is in use. If a child experiences repeated upper respiratory infections during the winter, the parent might want to consider humidification. Providing humidity in the home can be accomplished by general humidification, which is expensive, or with a cool-mist humidifier placed in the child's room. Steam vaporizers are to be avoided. If a cool-mist humidifier is not available, taking the child to the bathroom, closing the door, and running a warm shower provides humidity.

Artificial Airways

A variety of artificial airways are used in infants and children, usually as emergency measures to prevent or treat airway obstruction. Nasal or oral intubation ensures airway patency and provides a means for artificial ventilation. Nasal or oral intubation is used only when short-term ventilation is needed. If artificial ventilation is required, a cuffed tube is preferred because it is more stable, although a cuffed tube is used rarely in children under 8 years of age.

To prevent tracheal irritation, the nurse checks cuff pressure periodically (every 3–4 hours). The cuff need not be inflated sufficiently to prevent all leaks. A small leak does not interfere with ventilation and lessens chances of pressure necrosis.

A tracheostomy is usually done if an artificial airway is going to be a long-term requirement for ventilation or for removal of secretions. It is a surgical procedure. Tube size depends on age and size of the child and the reason for placement.

Nursing considerations The nurse's main responsibilities in caring for the child with an artificial airway are:

1. Making sure the tube does not inadvertently come out. The child might have to have elbow restraints if it appears the airway is likely to be removed by the child.
2. Monitoring cuff pressure, if a cuffed tube is used.
3. Suctioning accumulated secretions through the tube as necessary to maintain a patent airway and providing extra breaths of oxygen both before and after suctioning (hyperoxygenation, because oxygen is removed during suctioning).
4. Providing skin and stoma care to prevent breakdown and infection.
5. Changing the tape on the tube as needed to keep it dry and secure. If the child has a tracheostomy, the nurse changes wet ties to prevent neck irritation or dislodgment of the tube. Ties are tied on the side of the neck to prevent confusing them with ties on the hospital gowns. The ties need to be tight enough to stabilize the tube but loose enough for comfort (one finger slipped under the tie tests for appropriate tension). Gauze is not placed under the flange of the tube because it prevents observation of the site and does not allow the skin to dry.
6. Relieving the child's anxiety. The intubated child is unable to talk or cry audibly, which is very frightening. It is necessary to reassure the child frequently and place the call light within easy reach. Giving the older child paper and pencil for communicating eases frustration. Pantomime often assists with communications with the younger child.

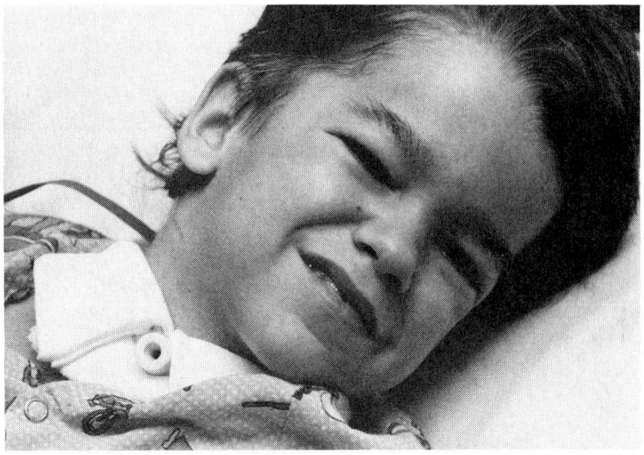

Tracheostomy tube secured in place.

Chest Physiotherapy

To perform postural drainage, the nurse or physiotherapist positions the child so that gravity enhances removal of secretions from specific lobes of the lungs. Postural drainage is usually done in conjunction with percussion and vibration. The purpose of all three procedures is to stimulate productive coughing. The nurse schedules postural drainage procedures before feedings or meals to avoid inducing vomiting.

Percussion is done by clapping a cupped hand over the area to be percussed. The wrist and arm remain relaxed, while the cupped hand is clapped on the child's body firmly enough to cause a popping sound. If the patient is a premature or very small infant, the nurse can use an infant-sized mask, rather than the cupped hand. Percussion is not done over bare skin, the sternum, the spine, the stomach, or the kidneys. Usually, percussion is done for 1–2 minutes in each postural drainage position.

Vibration, which is often done in addition to percussion, can be performed with a mechanical vibrator or manually. To perform manual vibration, the nurse or physiotherapist places the hands, one on top of the other, over the area to be vibrated, tenses the arms, and creates a vibrating motion that travels from the arms to the child's body. Vibration is done only during expiration to enhance the child's respiratory effort.

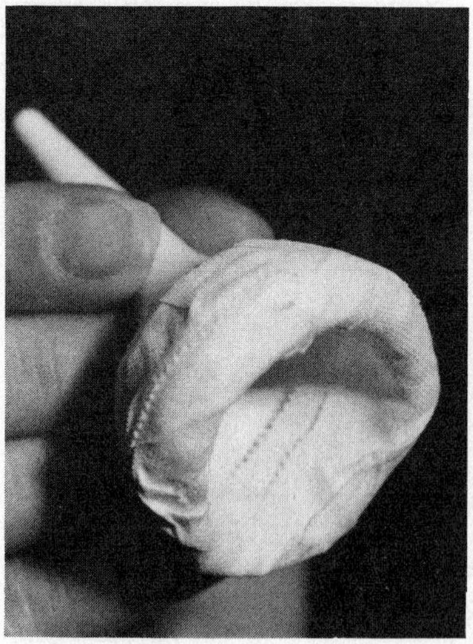

A Bulb syringe adapted for an infant too small for hand percussion. The bulb is cut in half and the edges padded with tape. The nurse percusses while holding the nozzle of the syringe.

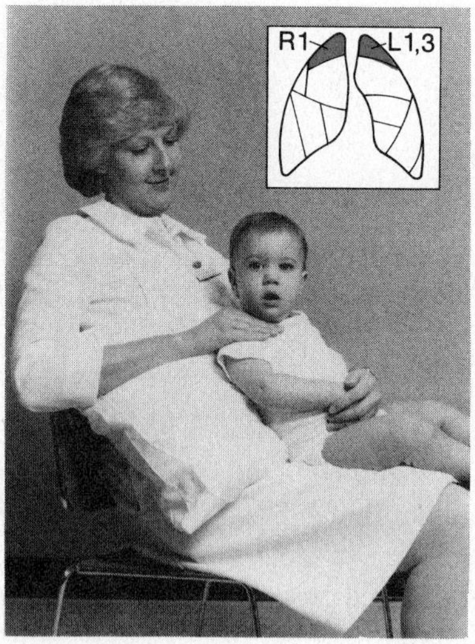

B Drainage apical segments of upper lobes. The child reclines at a 30° angle while the nurse percusses and vibrates segments between clavicles and scapulae.

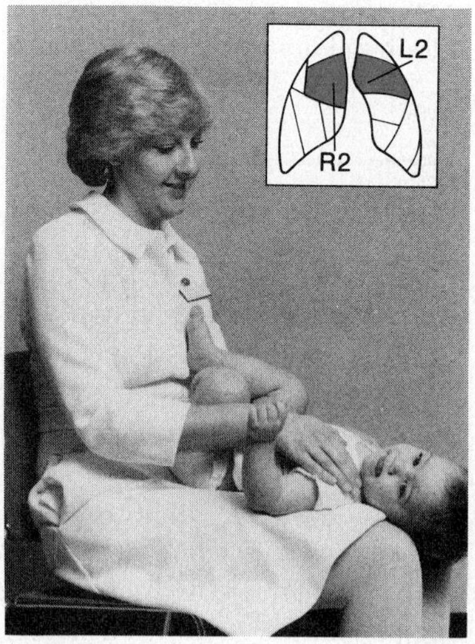

C Draining anterior segments of the upper lobes. The child lies supine while the nurse percusses and vibrates segments between clavicles and nipples.

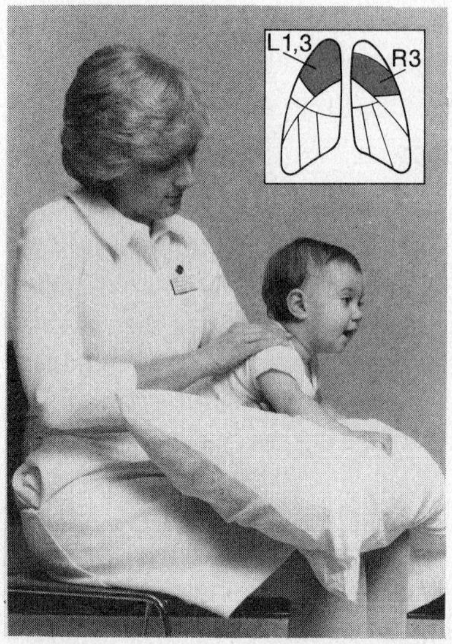

D Draining posterior segments of upper lobes. The child is propped at a 30° angle while the nurse percusses and vibrates the upper back on both sides of the spine.

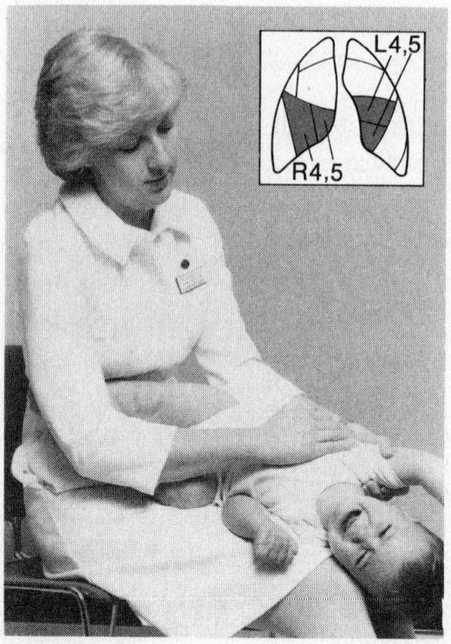

E Draining lateral and medial segments of the right middle lobe. The child lies on the side with head down 30°. The nurse rotates the child a quarter turn to the back and percusses and vibrates over the uppermost nipple. To drain lingular segments of the left upper lobe, the nurse turns the child to the corresponding position on the opposite side and repeats over the uppermost nipple.

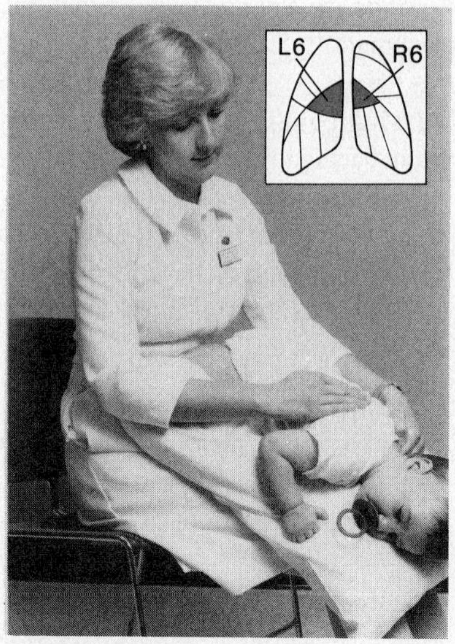

F Draining the superior segments of the lower lobes. The child lies prone with head down 15° while the nurse percusses and vibrates on both sides of the spine, below the tips of the scapulae.

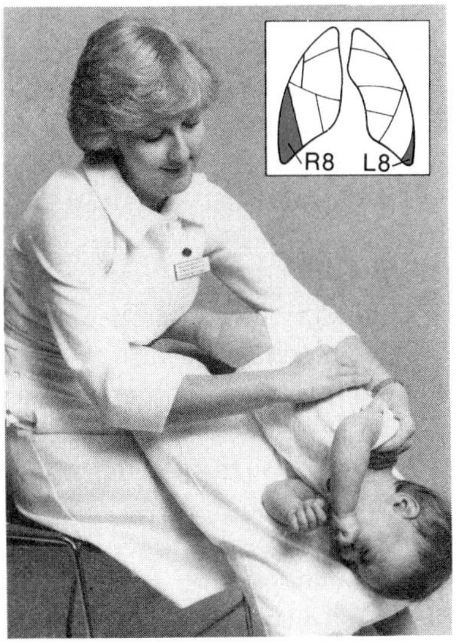

G Draining anterior basal segments of lower lobes. The child lies on the side with head down 30° on the nurse's extended legs. The nurse percusses and vibrates over the lower ribs beneath the axillae, then turns the child and repeats on the opposite side.

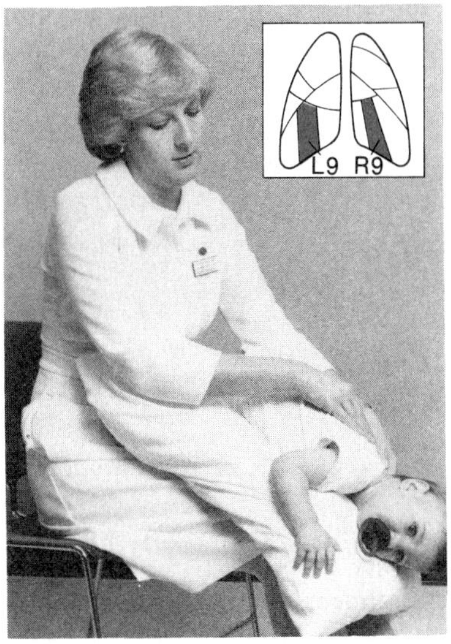

H Draining the lateral basal segments of the lower lobes. The child lies prone with head down 30°. The nurse rotates the upper half of the child's body a quarter turn toward the side and percusses and vibrates over the lower ribs, then turns the child to the opposite side and repeats.

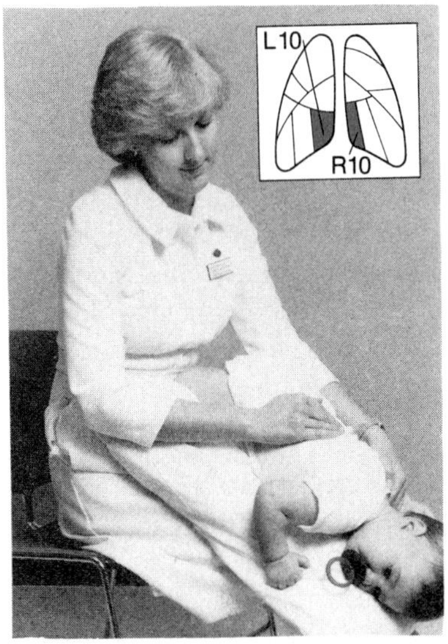

I Draining the posterior basal segments of the lower lobes. The child lies prone with head down 30° while the nurse percusses and vibrates over the lower ribs on both sides of the spine, avoiding the area over the kidneys.

Postural drainage procedures for an infant. (From Swearingen PL: The Addison-Wesley Photo-Atlas of Nursing Procedures. *Addison-Wesley, 1984, pp. 364–366, with permission.)*

Principles of Nursing Care

Acute Care Needs

The acute care needs of the child with respiratory dysfunction depend on whether the dysfunction is obstructive, restrictive, or caused by inefficient gas transfer. Any of these dysfunctions can lead to development of one or both of the others, and all three can lead to respiratory failure.

⊛ Potential for ineffective airway clearance

Obstructive lung disease is characterized by increased resistance to airflow. Pulmonary function tests indicate decreased flow, with normal or slightly decreased volumes. Blood gases are normal unless the obstruction is prominent, in which case the child will have respiratory acidosis. Wheezing, rhonchi, retractions, coughing, tachypnea, and dyspnea are all characteristic of obstructive lung disease. Clubbing and cyanosis occur if obstruction is chronic or severe. Obstruction can occur at any level of the respiratory tract and can be due to structural or functional anomalies, aspiration of foreign bodies, infection, tumors, or bronchospasm caused by allergens or irritants.

Interventions related to airway clearance include administering percussion and postural drainage, providing oxygen if blood gases indicate respiratory compromise, encouraging fluids to liquefy mucus secretions, and frequently observing vital signs, especially signs of respiratory distress.

⊛ Potential for ineffective breathing pattern

Restrictive lung disease is characterized by impaired lung expansion. This can be related to loss of lung volume, decreased elasticity, or a chest wall disturbance. A typical cluster of signs and symptoms might include decreased lung volumes demonstrated by pulmonary function testing, poor exercise tolerance, fatigue, shallow respirations, increased respiratory effort, and nasal flaring. The child might have an infection, congenital or neonatal anomalies, or a chest deformity that interferes with respirations.

Nursing interventions include observing for changes in respiratory status that might indicate respiratory failure. Oxygen and chest physiotherapy might be required if alterations in respiration adversely affect blood gases. The nurse encourages slow deep breathing and teaches the child relaxation exercises to use when breathing becomes difficult. Making a game of lung expansion exercises promotes cooperation by the child. Bubble blowing, particularly with the giant bubble frames, blowing pieces of paper with a straw along a small table racetrack, or use of an incentive spirometer are examples.

⊛ Activity intolerance related to increased respiratory effort

The nurse plans care so the child obtains adequate rest. Adequate time is allowed for procedures and treatments to avoid increasing the child's respiratory effort in response to increased activity. Quiet games, reading, and puzzles can conserve energy while providing distraction. Increases in activity levels are introduced gradually. The nurse might allow the child to perform one or two activities of daily living. After determining that the child can tolerate the activity, greater independence can be allowed.

⊛ Potential for impaired gas exchange

Inefficient gas transfer Inadequate alveolar ventilation or any defect that impairs diffusion across the alveolocapillary membrane results in inefficient gas transfer. Inadequate ventilation can be the result of a defect in the respiratory control mechanism. Inefficient gas transfer from this cause is manifested by signs of central nervous system depression such as confusion, sensory changes, decreased levels of consciousness, and coma.

Inefficient gas transfer related to a defect in diffusion can cause signs and symptoms of dyspnea, cyanosis, and blood gas values that indicate respiratory acidosis and hypoxemia. There might be dullness on percussion and bronchial breath sounds heard on auscultation. Restlessness, confusion, and other signs of hypoxia and hypercapnia also might be present. Disorders that impair gas transfer include pulmonary edema, pulmonary embolism, anemia, and hemorrhage, among others.

Treatment is focused on maintaining the alveolocapillary surface area, maintaining red blood cell and hemoglobin levels (see Chapter 26), and maintaining an intact respiratory control center (see Chapter 31). Nursing interventions are supportive. Nursing goals are to help conserve the child's energy, prevent infection, preserve pulmonary function, and prevent pulmonary crippling by maintaining an optimum level of activity. Positioning to promote adequate ventilation is important as is encouraging the child to breathe deeply. Infants can be placed in an infant seat to elevate them. Elevating the head of the bed is appropriate for children. The nurse ensures that the child's position is maintained, since it is easy for the child to slip down or bend over in the middle, thus placing pressure on the diaphragm. Frequent monitoring of blood gases can provide data about oxygenation.

Respiratory failure Respiratory failure can be related to obstructive disease, restrictive disease, or inefficient gas transfer. Respiratory failure can have an abrupt or an insidious onset, and the cause can be an acute or chronic dysfunction. Whatever the cause, respiratory failure results in hypoxemia and hypercapnia.

Hypoxemia and acidemia (acid accumulation in blood) lead to pulmonary capillary and arteriolar constriction, which can cause clots to form as blood flow through these vessels is restricted. Increased pulmonary pressure occurs, which leads to right cardiac ventricular enlargement and finally to right ventricular failure (Fig. 22-1). The nurse who is caring for a child with respiratory dysfunction watches for early signs of respiratory failure and is prepared to intervene. (The clinical signs of respiratory failure are listed in Table 22-1.) Acute care for the child with respiratory failure includes mechanical ventilation. Respiratory arrest calls for the rapid initiation of cardiopulmonary resuscitation (CPR), which is discussed in Chapter 12. Immediate intervention is mandatory because cardiac function continues only a few minutes after breathing stops.

Nutritional Needs

⊛ Alteration in fluid volume: deficit related to increased respiratory rate

The nature of body fluid composition and metabolism in infants and young children makes them much more susceptible than adults to rapid depletion of body stores of water and electrolytes (see Chapter 21). Anorexia, vomiting, diarrhea, and fever are characteristic of acute infections of the respiratory system, and so dehydration is always a risk. Dehydration also results from an increased respiratory rate. Approximately two-thirds of the child's total daily water loss normally occurs through the respiratory tract lining. The amount lost increases in direct proportion to increases in the respiratory rate. Thus, the faster the child breathes, the more fluid is lost.

Dehydration can cause mucus to become too dry or too viscous and difficult for the child to expectorate. Therefore, adequate hydration is a priority for a child whose disorder

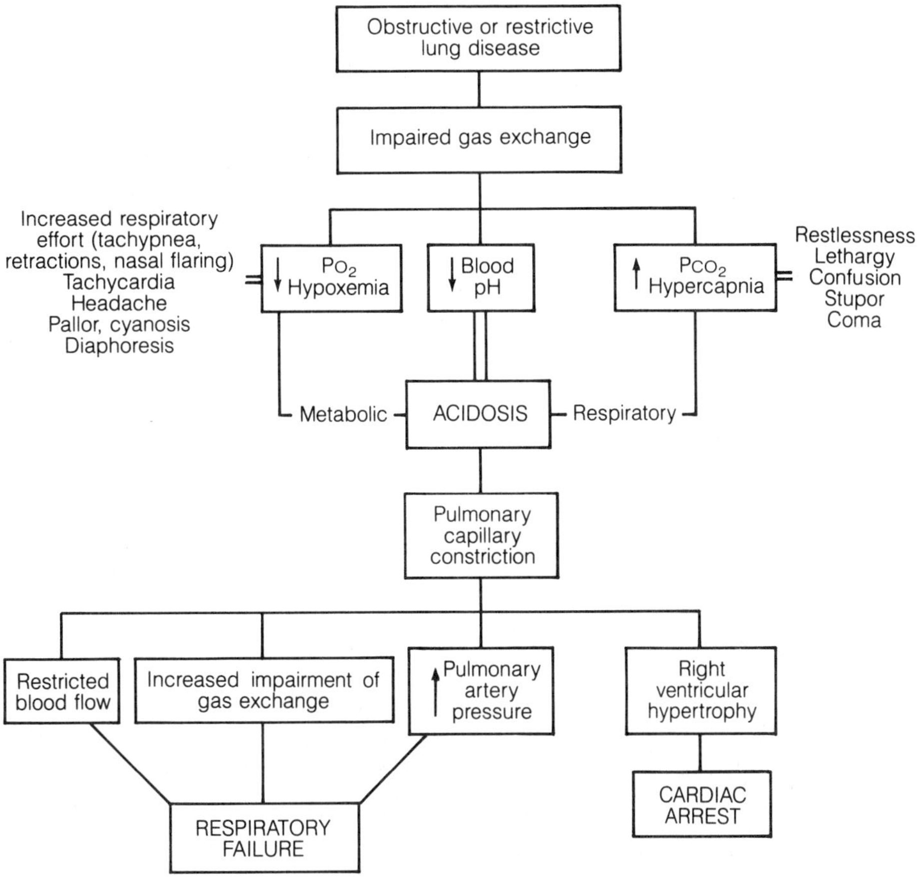

FIGURE 22-1
Mechanisms leading to respiratory failure.

causes mucus production. To prevent dehydration, the nurse offers small amounts of the child's favorite fluids at frequent intervals. Milk and milk products such as ice cream or puddings are avoided since they can increase the thickness of the mucus secretions preventing expectoration.

Unless the respiratory illness is chronic, it does not compromise the child's nutritional status. The nurse offers favorite foods as much as possible. High-calorie liquids, such as soda pop or fruit juices, can provide calories and prevent dehydration for the child who is having difficulty swallowing solid foods. If the child has had vomiting or diarrhea, the nurse can offer commercially prepared fluids that contain electrolytes.

If fever is the cause of dehydration, the nurse institutes measures to reduce the fever. Acetaminophen is the antipyretic of choice, as aspirin has adverse side effects including possible association with Reye's syndrome, especially when given during an infection (see Chapter 31).

(text continues on p. 679)

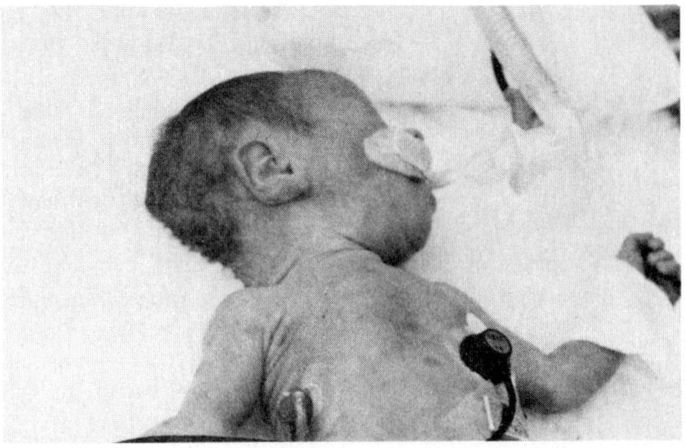

Child with substernal and intercostal retraction.

STANDARDS OF NURSING CARE *The Child with a Respiratory Problem*

GUIDE FOR NURSING MANAGEMENT

Nursing diagnosis	Intervention	Rationale	Outcome
1. Ineffective airway clearance related to accumulation of mucus in the respiratory passages	Assist child to cough productively. Tell child not to suppress cough or waste energy on weak coughing.	Coughing with expectoration clears respiratory passages.	Child clears respiratory passages of mucus and breathes through the nose without difficulty. The child's mucous membranes are moist, and skin turgor is good. Urine output is appropriate for age.
	Monitor fluid intake; measure and record intake and output accurately; maintain intravenous flow at appropriate rate; observe for signs of dehydration.	Increased respirations increase fluid loss causing dehydration.	
	Offer small amounts of favorite fluids frequently. Avoid ice-cold fluids.	Fluids, except milk or milk products, liquefy secretions and decrease potential for obstruction. Cold fluids can trigger bronchospasm.	
	Provide humidity. Keep child in mist tent or room with vaporizer.	Humidity helps liquefy secretions, which can then be expectorated to clear the airway.	
	Change child's position at least every 2 hours and encourage activity as tolerated.	Changing position and increasing activity enhances lung inflation and prevents pooling of secretions.	
	Note presence and character of nasal discharge; note quantity and quality of sputum or presence of mucus in vomitus.	A description of the quantity, quality, and color of mucus helps in evaluating interventions.	
	Provide chest physiotherapy (percussion, vibration, and postural drainage) as indicated; use games or diversion to encourage child to cooperate; listen to breath sounds before and after chest physiotherapy.	Chest physiotherapy loosens secretions and promotes expectoration. Clearing breath sounds indicate effective treatment.	
	Suction nasopharyngeal area to remove thick secretions or vomitus. (Remember that too-frequent suctioning stimulates mucus production.)	Suctioning keeps the airway clear when the child is unable to clear it effectively.	
	Teach and practice breathing exercises with child—use of incentive spirometer, paper bag breathing, and games with straws or blowing that require maximal inspiration.	Breathing exercises assist with airway clearance and lung inflation and prevent lower respiratory tract obstruction.	

STANDARDS OF NURSING CARE *The Child with a Respiratory Problem (Continued)*

GUIDE FOR NURSING MANAGEMENT

Nursing diagnosis	Intervention	Rationale	Outcome
	Support child in upright position and monitor closely for signs of upper airway obstruction (orthopnea, inspiratory stridor, hoarseness, barky cough, drooling, refusal to swallow).	An upright position facilitates respiratory effort by decreasing pressure on the diaphragm.	
	Prepare child and family for possible intubation or tracheostomy; have tracheostomy kit at the bedside.	Preparation can reduce anxiety, thus facilitating respirations. In order to avoid increasing anxiety, the nurse emphasizes that the procedure would be used in emergencies only and for purposes of maintaining the airway.	
	Remain calm and offer reassurance to child and family.	Remaining calm reassures the child and the family and decreases anxiety. Anxiety can contribute to respiratory difficulties by contributing to bronchospasm or tensing the respiratory musculature.	
2. Impaired gas exchange related to respiratory dysfunction	Observe for signs of hypoxia, tachypnea, tachycardia, elevated blood pressure, restlessness, and anxiety.	These are signs of impending respiratory failure.	The child appears alert and free of restlessness or anxiety. Blood gases are within normal limits. The child's skin color is pink, and vital signs are within normal limits.
	Observe for cyanosis: note mucous membranes, nail beds, periorbital area. Monitor arterial blood gases.	Cyanosis occurs with hypoxia. Blood gases provide data about oxygenation.	
	Monitor vital signs and listen to breath sounds every 30–60 minutes.	Respiratory failure can occur quickly and can be fatal if intervention is not rapid.	
	Provide oxygen therapy as ordered.	Oxygen therapy increases the amount of oxygen in the circulation and thus in body tissues.	
	Provide rest to reduce oxygen requirements; plan periods of undisturbed rest; group scheduled procedures together; observe closely for signs of fatigue.	Rest reduces the body's need for oxygen by decreasing metabolic needs.	
	Administer medications as ordered.	Bronchodilators can open the airway allowing greater amounts of oxygen to reach the lungs for exchange.	

(Continues)

STANDARDS OF NURSING CARE *The Child with a Respiratory Problem (Continued)*

GUIDE FOR NURSING MANAGEMENT

Nursing diagnosis	Intervention	Rationale	Outcome
3. Ineffective breathing pattern related to respiratory dysfunction	Observe and record the type and depth of retractions and whether the child is using accessory muscles for breathing.	Increased respiratory effort can lead to respiratory failure.	The child has a regular respiratory rhythm and rate within normal limits for the child's age. The ratio of inspiration to expiration is appropriate.
	Observe the chest for symmetry of movements during respiration.	Atelectasis or pneumothorax of one lung can cause uneven chest expansion.	
	Note length and character of inspiratory and expiratory phases of respiration.	The length of expiration is usually two times the length of inspiration. Prolonged expiration can be indicative of dysfunction.	
	Elevate the head of the child's bed.	Elevation allows for increased lung expansion and facilitates respiration by decreasing pressure on the diaphragm and accessory muscles.	
	Teach the child to relax and breathe slowly during times of altered breathing pattern.	Anxiety can worsen the breathing pattern by contributing to hyperventilation. A calm approach decreases anxiety and facilitates respiratory effort.	
4. Alteration in comfort: chest pain related to increased respiratory effort or position	Observe for signs of dyspnea, such as shallow breathing or chest splinting.	Dyspnea can cause chest pain by contributing to forced respiratory pattern.	The child is able to resume activity without discomfort.
	Listen to breath sounds to detect areas of absent or greatly diminished ventilation.	Alteration or absent ventilation in one lung can indicate atelectasis.	
	Observe child's posture in lying, sitting, and standing positions for signs of painful respiration.	If one posture is more painful, it can be avoided.	
	Ask child to describe pain: when it began or first occurred, whether it is sharp or dull, episodic or continuous.	The child's description of the pain can give clues to underlying pathology.	
	Demonstrate to child how to support or hold painful area with pillow or hand.	Splinting can decrease pain.	
	Administer analgesics as ordered.	Analgesics provide pain relief.	

Developmental Needs

The developmental and psychosocial needs of the child who is chronically ill or hospitalized are discussed in Chapters 14 and 20. Specific needs relative to respiratory disorders are covered in this section.

⊛ Altered growth and development: related to disease limitations

Using exercise to promote development Age-appropriate exercise is essential for the child's healthy development and the development of social relationships. Moderate exercise not only improves ventilation but also allows the child to participate in activities consistent with the peer group, thus promoting peer relationships. Children with chronic lung disease, particularly asthma, need to exercise at a level consistent with endurance. Medications can be taken prior to exercise to prevent exercise-induced bronchospasm. If the child has become increasingly sedentary to avoid dyspnea or bronchospasm, a carefully planned exercise program is needed to gradually increase stamina and muscle mass. Exercise can stimulate coughing and help the child raise and expectorate sputum. Swimming or bicycle riding are excellent exercise for children with chronic lung disorders because they require breath control and exercise several muscle groups.

Children who have been bedridden for extended periods or who have been mechanically ventilated also benefit from appropriate exercise training. A training schedule is developed that gradually increases the child's amount of exercise in accordance with the child's increasing tolerance. Any exercise program for children needs to be creative, needs to use play, and needs to provide appropriate incentive. For example, a child could use dance as an exercise, starting out at a slow tempo and gradually increasing the tempo as tolerance develops. Children love to be competitive, so timing exercise and encouraging the child to beat the previous time can motivate the child.

Promoting independence Children with chronic respiratory dysfunction, like children with any chronic illness, can experience problems with development related to the inability to assume self-care activities. The nurse observes parent-child interaction and determines whether the parent allows the child to participate in care according to the child's age and normal developmental expectations. Because respiratory distress can be so anxiety provoking and serious, parents often become overprotective of their children. In other cases, children can manipulate parents into providing for their every request by playing on guilt parents might be experiencing. The nurse talks with parent and child and attempts to establish with them a plan to facilitate the child's independence and assumption of self-care. (See Chapter 14 for additional nursing interventions for the child with a chronic illness.)

Emotional Needs

⊛ Anxiety related to the acuity of the respiratory dysfunction

A child who is admitted to the hospital with sudden onset of an acute respiratory condition has had little or no preparation for admission. The nurse can use principles of crisis intervention to help the child and family cope with their anxiety in a positive way. Parents and children often are anxious because the child seems so seriously ill and the equipment is unfamiliar and threatening. The nurse clarifies parental understanding of the dysfunction and explains the purpose of all equipment used. The parent is encouraged to cuddle a crying child and participate with the nurse in helping ease the child's respiratory effort.

Further assessment might lead to a nursing diagnosis of compromised family coping. The parent might be afraid the child will die. This overwhelming fear might cause the parent temporarily to be unable to provide effective support, comfort, and assistance. Instead, the parent might be preoccupied with reactions of guilt and anger. Nursing interventions include helping a parent express feelings of guilt and anger, reducing anxiety by being calm and supportive, and helping the parent gain a better understanding of the disease process, its usual treatment, and the prognosis.

⊛ Potential for ineffective family coping

Chronic illness creates chronic stress and often a series of crises that occur throughout the child's life. The first crisis occurs when the child and family learn the diagnosis. The immediate response is intense anxiety. Information given to the family at this time is kept brief, and any instructions are written out, since high levels of anxiety interfere with learning. The nurse helps the family express feelings and handles the situation as an acute crisis.

The nurse's assessment of the family's strengths, prior experiences in coping with crisis, and concurrent stressors begins with this initial contact with the family. The child's developmental level, sex, and prior coping abilities also affect the family's and child's ability to cope emotionally with chronic illness.

A child's fear of dying is one of the most difficult emotions for parents and health professionals to deal with and the nurse intervenes to meet their emotional needs (see Chapter 17).

Health Maintenance Needs

Potential knowledge deficit regarding home management

The child who is hospitalized for treatment of an acute or chronic respiratory dysfunction usually requires home care or follow-up after discharge. (Home care for the child with an acute illness is discussed in Chapter 18.) Home care for the child with a respiratory disorder frequently involves home administration of oxygen, inhalation therapy, and physiotherapy aimed at mucus clearance. A prescribed exercise regimen or breathing exercises also might be continued at home.

The parents of children who are sent home with inhalation therapy or oxygen therapy equipment need to practice using the equipment with the nurse several times prior to the child's discharge. The parent learns proper techniques for cleaning nebulizers, which can harbor infectious microorganisms. The nebulizer and the mask are washed daily with soap and water and soaked twice weekly in a weak solution of vinegar and water. The nurse gives the parent detailed written instructions about aerosol treatment schedules, doses, and precautions.

If oxygen equipment is to be used at home, rental of oxygen tanks and regulators is arranged before the child is discharged. The nurse teaches the parent how to use the equipment and reviews the safety measures listed in Table 22-3.

Even if the child is being discharged on the same home care regimen that was carried out before admission, the nurse reviews all aspects of home care with the child and family to be sure that incorrect procedures have not inadvertently become habitual. The nurse also can use this opportunity to increase the child's and parent's understanding of the disorder and its treatment.

If the child has been admitted for foreign body aspiration or near-drowning, the nurse discusses safety and well-child issues with the parent, being careful not to add to any guilt that the parent already might feel. If it is possible to make a home visit after discharge, the nurse works with the parent to identify safety hazards in the home. The nurse also recommends that the parent learn CPR and emergency maneuvers for managing airway obstruction by foreign bodies. If the child has been admitted for an acute infection or inflammation, such as acute spasmodic croup or laryngotracheobronchitis, the nurse reviews with the parent the signs and symptoms that indicate the need for immediate medical attention.

It is extremely important for the child, parent, and nurse to plan details of emergency care before discharge. All children who are old enough to use the telephone should learn who and how to call for help in an emergency. The emergency care number should be placed on the telephone, and each child should practice dialing the number, stating the nature of the emergency, and giving name, address, and telephone number.

TABLE 22-3 Safe Use of Oxygen at Home

Safety guideline	Rationale
Secure oxygen tank in upright position	Oxygen tanks are highly explosive. If a horizontally positioned tank explodes, the rapid release of oxygen can catapult it through walls and into people
Keep oxygen tanks at least 5 feet from heat source and electrical devices (that is, space heaters, heating vents, fireplaces, radios, vaporizers and humidifiers)	Heat can increase pressure inside the tank, causing it to explode
Ensure that no one smokes in the room or area of the oxygen tank	Smoking increases the risk of fire, which could cause the tank to explode. Escaped oxygen would feed the fire
Use lemon-glycerin swabs to relieve dryness around the child's mouth. Avoid oil- or alcohol-based substances (for example, petroleum jelly, vitamin A and D ointment, baby oil)	Alcohol and oil are both flammable and increase the risk of fire
Have the child wear cotton garments	Silk, wool, and synthetics can generate static electricity and cause fire
Keep a fire extinguisher readily available	It is necessary to put out fire immediately
Turn off both volume regulator and flow regulator whenever oxygen is not in use	If the volume regulator is on when oxygen is turned on, the child might receive a rapid, forceful flow of oxygen in the face that could be frightening and uncomfortable
	Oxygen leakage, which might not be detected because oxygen is odorless, can cause fire

Most parents appreciate knowing when the next follow-up contact will occur. It is helpful to arrange the time of the next visit before discharge so that parents have plenty of time to arrange their schedules to keep the appointment.

The nurse prepares the parent for any changes or deterioration in the child's condition that are expected. For example, the parent of a child with asthma might be warned that the upcoming cold weather could predispose the child to more frequent infections and therefore to exacerbations of asthma. The nurse also discusses age-appropriate reactions to stress with the parent. The nurse might say, "It is common for young children to lose interest in taking their respiratory treatments correctly after they return home. You will need to set firm limits." This helps prepare the parent for "posthospital syndrome." The longer the child has been hospitalized, the more difficult it will be to return to the home care routine. The nurse encourages the parent to plan routines with the child and to allow the child some choices. Medications and treatments need to be non-negotiable issues, but the child's interests need to be considered when determining types of exercise.

The nurse identifies sources of parental support in the community, such as mental health workers, psychiatrists, psychologists, social workers, community health nurses, and clergy. Other parents who have had similar problems with chronic illness can provide the unique support that comes through experience. There are many cystic fibrosis and asthmatic parents' groups throughout the country. The American Lung Association and the Cystic Fibrosis Foundation are good sources for information about these groups.

The Child with an Acute Respiratory Infection

Tonsillitis and Pharyngitis

Infections of the tonsils and throat (pharynx) can be viral or bacterial. Nonbacterial exudative tonsillitis generally is a mild disease requiring little medical intervention. The onset is gradual and is typified by low-grade fever, mild headache, and loss of appetite. Sore throat, hoarse voice, and a productive cough are common symptoms. Causative organisms include coxsackievirus, adenovirus, and herpes simplex. Treatment includes comfort measures, acetaminophen for pain, and oral fluids. The disease is self-limiting. Complications are rare.

Clinical manifestations The symptoms of bacterial tonsillitis and pharyngitis can be dramatic. Group A beta-hemolytic streptococcus is the most common bacterial cause. Fever (38–40°C) usually is the first symptom. Generalized signs of muscle aches, headache, and nausea develop within 18–24 hours. The severity of pharyngeal pain varies. In its early stages, bacterial infection often is difficult to diagnose, and a second throat culture might be needed to determine whether the causative agent is viral or bacterial.

The throat appears inflamed, with varying amounts of exudate. There might be associated lymphadenitis (inflamed lymph nodes). The incidence of streptococcal pharyngitis increases during the winter and spring, and the disease is more commonly found in children who live in crowded environments. The disease is self-limiting; however, if untreated, it can cause serious sequelae in children.

The sequelae of streptococcal infection sometimes include skin rashes (scarlet fever). Extension of the disease can result in peritonsillar abscess, sinusitis, middle ear infection (otitis media), and involvement of the mastoids or meninges. Late sequelae, although rare, might include rheumatic fever.

Treatment A throat culture is done to rule out a bacterial cause. Throat cultures presently are available that can give accurate results within minutes. Thus, treatment can be more accurate than when cultures took twenty-four to forty-eight hours.

If the culture is positive for group A beta-hemolytic streptococcus, an appropriate antibiotic is prescribed. This is generally a 10-day course of penicillin (or a derivative) or, if penicillin is contraindicated, erythromycin. Comfort measures for the child with bacterial pharyngitis include bed rest until the fever is absent for 24 hours, fluids, acetaminophen, and warm saline gargles for throat pain.

Nursing management It is important for the nurse to assess the parent's understanding of the need to administer the entire amount of the prescribed medication. If failure to cooperate with the antibiotic regimen is a potential problem, intramuscular rather than oral medication is considered. Intramuscular penicillin is effective in one dose, as opposed to the 10-day oral dosage schedule. However, because the injection is painful, the oral route is less traumatic and is the treatment of choice when cooperation is assured.

The nurse instructs the parent to seek additional medical attention if the child develops a rash, swollen joints, stiff neck, periorbital edema, earache, or temperature above 101°F that cannot be controlled with acetaminophen. A careful assessment of the home setting is important if the child with streptococcal pharyngitis is to be cared for at home; vigorous antibiotic therapy and measures to prevent sequelae and the spread of the disease must be instituted. Nursing management includes teaching the parent how to humidify the air with cool mist; to increase the child's fluid intake; to relieve discomfort with gargles, lozenges, or hard candy; to prevent the spread of infection to other family members; and to observe the child for possible complications.

Many upper respiratory infections can be prevented if the child avoids close contact with infected individuals, washes the hands correctly, and disposes carefully of tissues contaminated with upper airway secretions. The affected child should have a room alone if possible.

Tonsillectomy Children with chronic enlargement of the tonsils or adenoids, which interferes with swallowing or breathing; a history of four or more documented episodes of group A beta-hemolytic streptococcal infections; recurrent otitis media; peritonsillar abscess; retropharyngeal abscess; or in rare instances a tonsillar tumor are candidates for tonsillectomy, adenoidectomy, or both. Although tonsillectomy and adenoidectomy (T and A) were done frequently in the past, surgeons and pediatricians are more selective about performing the procedure now. The lymphoid tissue of which tonsils and adenoids are composed is one of the body's lines of defense against infection. Also, a normal shrinking of the lymphoid tissue occurs during middle childhood, which resolves many of the problems related to enlargement.

If the procedure is necessary, it is rarely done before the child's own immune system is functioning, at around two years of age. The surgery is not performed during times of acute infection or if the child has a bleeding disorder or cleft palate.

Parents need to be cautioned that the procedure will not guarantee fewer infections, increased appetite, or increased growth. It might lessen snoring during sleep and improve nasal speech.

Preoperative nursing management Preoperative nursing care and teaching for a child undergoing a T and A is the same as for any child undergoing surgery. The nurse needs to know the results and implications of the bleeding and clotting studies done since postoperative bleeding is a frequent occurrence. The child also needs to understand, either through doll play or through verbal instructions, that although the throat will be very sore postoperatively, it is necessary to drink plenty of fluids.

Children sometimes have a difficult time understanding how the tonsils can be removed when told that the doctor uses a special instrument that can take the tonsils and adenoids out through the mouth. Some children also need reassurance that nothing will happen to their voice and they will be able to talk after surgery.

Postoperative nursing management Postoperatively, these children require close observation for bleeding during the first 24 hours. The child should lie prone with the head slightly lower than the chest to decrease the likelihood of swallowing blood from any active bleeding sites during the initial postoperative phase. Frequent throat and nasal checks with a flashlight are done to note the location of clots and to check for any signs of bleeding, such as bright red blood trickling down the back of the mouth from the nose. Any increase in the frequency of swallowing is investigated because often it is an indicator of active bleeding. Vital signs, including blood pressure, are monitored frequently. An increase in pulse rate or restlessness that might or might not be accompanied by decreased pulse quality or lowered blood pressure also indicates active bleeding. Since sutures seldom are used and since needed hemostasis (clotting) is obtained by pressure, there is a risk for bleeding until the clot is well formed. In many hospitals, routine postoperative care for a child following a T and A includes vital signs and throat checks every hour for the first four hours and then every 2–4 hours for the next 24 hours or duration of hospitalization.

Other nursing care measures include ensuring an adequate fluid intake to promote healing of the operative site and to maintain hydration. Ice chips are offered as soon as the child is fully awake. If tolerated, tepid water is offered and then other clear liquids. Hot or very cold fluids should be avoided, and it is best to withhold full liquids until the next day. Because the child's throat is sore, considerable nursing ingenuity might be required to convince the child that drinking is important. Hydration status is monitored by accurate records of intake, output, and urine specific gravity. If a potential for dehydration exists, intravenous therapy might be necessary.

Measures to prevent bleeding need to be observed, such as no straws, forks, or sharp-pointed toys available to be placed in the mouth. Aspirin in any form, including gum, should not be given because it prolongs bleeding time.

Pain control measures are utilized as needed. An ice collar applied postoperatively is an effective pain reliever. Mild analgesics such as acetaminophen (liquid) or mouth sprays also provide relief. The child usually is more willing to drink fluid following an analgesic.

It is not unusual for the child to vomit once or twice and sometimes even more, often as a result of having swallowed blood during surgery. There is little concern as long as the emesis contains old, dark red, or brown-colored blood. If an appreciable amount of bright red blood appears, it probably is an indicator of the presence of active bleeding. Because vomiting is distressful and the retching painful, antiemetics might be given for comfort as well as for reduction of emesis. Oral rinses with tepid water can be helpful in rid-

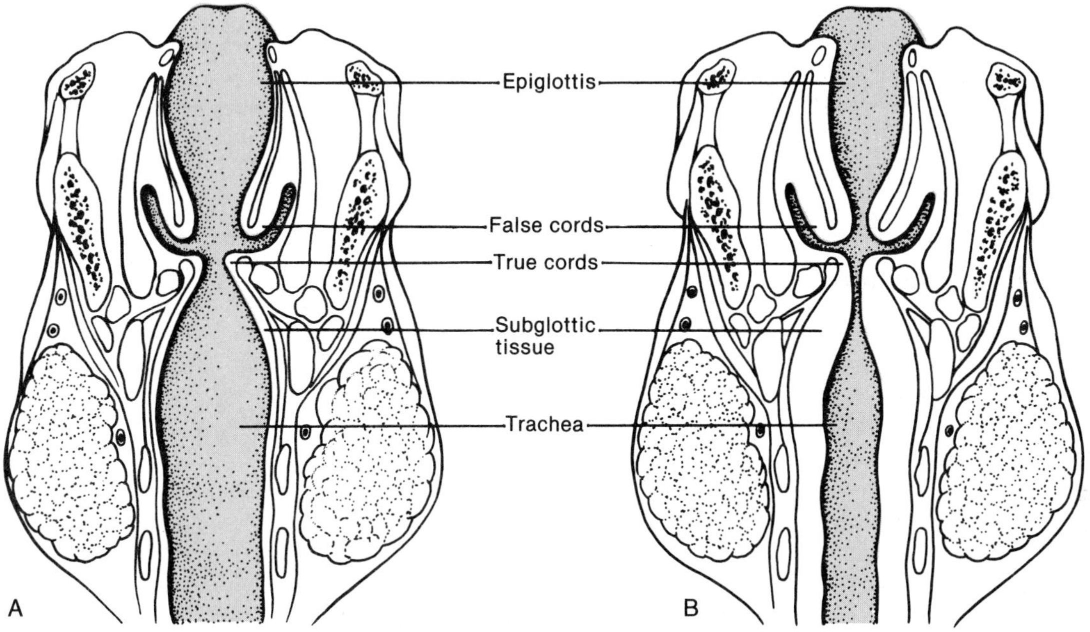

FIGURE 22-2

A. Normal larynx. B. Obstruction and narrowing caused by the edema of croup.

ding the mouth of the bad taste after vomiting. The child should be cautioned not to gargle but only to swish the water around in the mouth.

Most children are discharged the day after or even the evening of surgery. The parents are given discharge instructions, which include:

The child should engage only in quiet activity for the first week.

Give a soft diet—bread but no toast; eggs but no bacon; mashed potatoes but no french fries; and no spicy, rough, or coarse foods in general for the first 7–10 days.

The child should drink plenty of fluids—1–1/2 quarts a day as a minimum; tepid fluids or slow-melting fluids (ice chips, frozen fruit juices) are usually tolerated best.

Do not give the child any straws, forks, or sharp-pointed toys because putting them into the mouth might injure the operative site.

Use actaminophen for pain relief; do not use any form of aspirin.

Halitosis (bad breath) is common for 10–14 days and can be relieved with mouth rinses.

Call the physician if there is any bleeding, fever, or complaint of earache (potential for bleeding 5–7 days postoperatively when the operative site membrane begins to slough).

For 1–2 weeks after surgery, avoid crowds or contact with anyone known to be ill.

The child may return to school 1–2 weeks postoperatively.

Make a surgical follow-up appointment 2 weeks after the operation.

Acute Spasmodic Croup

Acute spasmodic croup, commonly known as croup, is an obstructive narrowing of the larynx thought to be due to viral infection, genetic predisposition, or emotional upsets (Fig. 22-2). Its chief symptom is inspiratory stridor (high pitched, crowing, or blowing sound). Acute spasmodic croup is common in young children. Its onset is sudden, usually during the night. Symptoms are relieved by humidity and cool air. The parent is instructed to take the child into a steamy bathroom or out into cooler and more humid night air. If these measures are unsuccessful, the child is seen in the emergency room. Acute spasmodic croup usually occurs in an otherwise healthy child and is resolved quickly.

Laryngotracheobronchitis

The signs of obstruction caused by laryngotracheobronchitis (LTB) are similar to signs of acute spasmodic croup, but LTB develops more slowly and is less quickly resolved than acute spasmodic croup. Other conditions such as foreign body obstruction, epiglottitis (inflammation of the epiglottis), and diphtheria present with symptoms similar to laryngotracheobronchitis. The nurse therefore needs to be sure that the child who presents with these symptoms is carefully assessed (Table 22-4).

LTB is a viral infection of the larynx, trachea, and bronchi and can be associated with an upper respiratory infection. Inflammation causes edema of the mucosa and submucosa of the airway, resulting in narrowing. In severe cases, vocal cord spasm can cause airway obstruction. Because of the infant's small airway size, particulary in the subglottic area, any narrowing is significant, and respiratory distress might result.

Parainfluenza 1, 2, and 3 viruses; respiratory syncytial virus; and rhinoviruses are the most common causes of LTB. Rarely, primary or secondary bacterial infections are the cause. The disease occurs throughout childhood, but incidence peaks at 18 months. The typical age range is 6 months–4 years. Like many other respiratory diseases, LTB occurs more frequently in boys than in girls.

Clinical manifestations The onset of LTB is gradual. Typically, it develops over several days in conjunction with upper respiratory infection and rhinorrhea. Initial symptoms of LTB include a harsh, croupy, or barky cough; hoarse voice; inspiratory stridor on exertion; low-grade fever; and continuing cold symptoms. The signs of increasing obstruction that require hospitalization and close observation include stridor and retractions at rest, tachypnea (respiratory rate greater than 60 breaths/min at rest), tachycardia (pulse rate greater than 140 beats/min at rest), restlessness, and circumoral and circumorbital cyanosis. Late signs of obstruction that require immediate intubation are listlessness, decrease in stridor, bradycardia, cyanosis, and retractions without clinical improvement.

Treatment Inhalation therapy with an aerosol preparation of racemic epinephrine is presently the treatment of choice for LTB. Epinephrine can be given with a hand-held nebulizer. Racemic epinephrine is not used in outpatient therapy since close observation and repeated treatments are required. Antibiotics are not prescribed unless the child has a secondary bacterial infection, such as otitis media. Treatment with steroids is still controversial (Cleary and Pickering, 1986).

Low concentrations of oxygen (less than 30%) can be given to relieve mild hypoxia. Greater concentrations of oxygen might mask signs of obstruction and therefore are avoided. Because adequate hydration is important to decrease the viscosity of secretions, fluid intake might be maintained by intravenous infusion.

If signs of moderate hypoxia develop, intubation is carried out immediately. A tube one size smaller than usual is chosen to decrease the risk of subglottic stenosis (narrowing). Either oral or nasotracheal intubation is acceptable, but the latter is often more comfortable for the child. Generally, the nasotracheal tube remains in place for 3–5 days. It is removed when the child can breathe and cough around the tube and is afebrile.

Nursing management Nursing management for a child with LTB includes conserving the child's energy, humidifying with cool mist, and monitoring vital signs and intake and output. The nurse observes the child's color, respiratory effort, and evidence of fatigue to detect impending respiratory failure. Administration of medications and fluids and measures related to possible intubation for respiratory failure or obstruction are additional nursing actions. Through all phases of nursing management, explanations and a reassuring manner are needed to reduce the anxiety of parent and child.

The nurse plans care so as to disturb the child as little as possible. Anything that disturbs the child causes hyperventilation, which increases airway obstruction and oxygen consumption. Hands-on nursing care and examination is minimal. Direct examination of the epiglottis is done only by skilled personnel in a facility where immediate intubation can be done, since examination can precipitate spasm and total obstruction. For the same reason, throat cultures are not taken by the nurse if the child is acutely ill. Cool, large-particle mist is the mainstay of treatment for LTB because cool mist decreases edema in the subglottic area. In the home, hot water vaporizers are not used because of the risk of spilling the water and burning the child. In the hospital, croup rooms or large, clear plastic tents that envelop the whole bed are best because the child need not be restrained.

Close observation by skilled nursing personnel is essential. Knowledge of normal growth and development and responses to illness are keys because the downward course of LTB is often subtle and rapid. The nurse frequently checks pulse rate, respiratory rate, color, activity, and

TABLE 22-4 Characteristics of Acute Infections Resulting in Croup Syndromes

Acute spasmodic croup	Laryngotracheobronchitis (LTB)	Acute epiglottitis
Age of child		
1–3 years	6 months–4 years	3–7 years
History of present illness		
Sudden symptoms in otherwise healthy child, usually at night History of repeated episodes	Preceded by acute upper respiratory tract infection; respiratory distress frequent at night	Preceded by mild upper respiratory tract infection Severe, sudden onset of respiratory distress
Clinical manifestations		
Laryngospasm Mucosal edema in subglottic area	Edema and inflammation of vocal cords and tissue below vocal cords, including bronchi	Edema and inflammation of epiglottis and surrounding area above vocal cords, large red epiglottis
	Laryngospasm	
Anxiety, restlessness	Anxiety, fatigue, apprehension, restlessness	Anxiety, restlessness, fear
Dyspnea	Dyspnea	Dyspnea
Inspiratory stridor	Inspiratory stridor, prolonged inspiratory phase	Deliberate inspiratory stridor, mouth breathing with hyperextended neck, insistence on an upright position
Hoarseness	Hoarseness	Sore throat
Barky, metallic cough	Barky cough	Muffled voice, dysphagia (difficulty swallowing), drooling of saliva
No fever	Fever, usually low-grade	Fever greater than 38.5° C
Mild or moderate supraclavicular, suprasternal, substernal retractions	Moderate to severe supraclavicular, suprasternal, substernal retractions	Mild to moderate suprasternal and substernal retractions, use of accessory muscles of respiration
Respiratory rate 45–55	Respiratory rate 45–60	Respiratory rate 45–50
Pulse 140–160	Pulse 140–160	Pulse less than 160
No adventitious breath sounds	Rhonchi, coarse rales	Usually wheezy breath sounds
	Nasal congestion	Paleness, sallowness, or cyanosis
Occasional mild cyanosis	Paleness or cyanosis	Rapid, progressive worsening of distress
Etiology		
Unknown, but thought to be viral, emotional, or familial predisposition	Usually viral, but occasionally bacterial	Bacterial, usually *Hemophilus influenzae*

quality of stridor and retractions to detect early signs of hypoxia.

The adequacy of oral fluid intake is assessed through urine specific gravity, which should be maintained between 1.008 and 1.015. Both overhydration and dehydration should be avoided. Intravenous fluids are given only if adequate oral intake is not possible.

Parents can handle a child with LTB at home if they are capable of recognizing worsening symptoms and can seek treatment immediately. The parent can bring the child outside for 10 or 15 minutes at the onset of croup. Moist night air has been known to relieve symptoms by stimulating mechanoreceptors, which decrease the respiratory rate and facilitate airway opening (Wilson, 1984). The parent must maintain the child's hydration, and extra creativity will be needed to encourage fluids when the child is having difficulty breathing.

The most important consideration is that the parent know when to seek emergency care. Parents need to be taught the signs of respiratory distress. If the symptoms worsen, if the child exhibits restlessness and anxiety and prefers a sitting rather than a reclining position, or if the child becomes febrile, emergency treatment is indicated. Immediate transportation should be available for this possibility. Parents should be discouraged from administering cough or cold preparations to the child because the drying effect of the preparations might exacerbate symptoms.

Epiglottitis

Epiglottitis is a bacterial infection of the epiglottis that can obstruct the airway. It is less common than laryngotracheobronchitis, but its course is rapid. Without prompt diagnosis and treatment, severe airway obstruction can result in death. The causative microorganism is *Hemophilus influenzae* type B or, rarely, a beta-hemolytic streptococcus. The incidence of epiglottitis has little seasonal variation. The patient's usual age range is 3–7 years and peaks at 3.1 years.

Clinical manifestations The clinical picture is typified by sudden onset of fever (generally above 38.5°C or 101°F) and lethargy. The parent often reports that the child has had a minor upper respiratory infection for a day or so. During the next 2–4 hours, difficulty in breathing increases. The child's voice has a muffled quality, but rarely is there a cough. Drooling and refusing to eat or drink because of an intensely sore throat are classic signs of epiglottitis. The child usually insists on being upright.

The signs of increasing obstruction are restlessness, tachycardia, thready pulse, and orthopnea manifested by the desire to sit up and breathe through the mouth. The characteristic breath sounds are wheezy inspiratory stridor and a snoring expiratory sound, depending on the degree of obstruction. Some children have a "crouplike" appearance on initial assessment. Late signs of hypoxia due to obstruction are listlessness, cyanosis, bradycardia, bradypnea (slow breathing), and decreased inspiratory and expiratory sounds.

The history of the illness and the clinical appearance of the child enable the physician to make a tentative diagnosis. To confirm the diagnosis, a visual examination of the epiglottis can be done. This is dangerous, however, because it can precipitate obstruction. Visual examination must be done in a controlled situation where intubation, oxygen, and suction equipment is available. If visual inspection is deemed inadvisable and the diagnosis is in doubt, the physician might order neck radiographs. Lateral neck views are preferred to visual inspection of the epiglottis by many physicians. The physician or nurse remains with the child and parent during the radiographic examination, since the procedure is disturbing to the child and anxiety can lead to further closure of the airway, causing total obstruction.

Treatment and nursing management Treatment for acute obstructive epiglottitis is relief of obstruction with a nasotracheal tube and intravenous administration of antibiotics. Prior to intubation, the nurse helps the child sit up and position the head comfortably. This position is often referred to as the "sniff" position.

Oxygen can be given through a face mask a few minutes prior to intubation as a safety measure. The nasotracheal tube can be removed after 3–5 days or when the swelling has decreased. In general, the more rapid the onset of the disease, the more rapid is remission.

Appropriate antibiotics are started as soon as intubation is done and an intravenous line is in place. Chloramphenicol is given until the organism is identified because it is effective against *H. influenzae,* the most usual cause. If the organism is susceptible to ampicillin, the chloramphenicol is discontinued, and ampicillin is initiated because of chloramphenicol's serious side effect of bone marrow depression (Cleary and Pickering, 1986). With the advent of the new vaccine against *Hemophilus influenzae* type B (see Chapter 11), cases of epiglottitis would be expected to decrease.

Bronchiolitis

Bronchiolitis is a widespread inflammation and obstruction of the bronchioles that is sometimes difficult to distinguish from acute asthma of infancy and bronchopneumonia (see Table 22-5). The prognosis of bronchiolitis is generally good, although several studies have shown that 50% of infected infants develop subsequent episodes of wheezing associated with allergies. Some researchers think that infants with a strong family history of allergy are susceptible to bronchiolitis in infancy or that bronchiolitis might trigger the development of asthma (Behrman, Vaughan, & McKay, 1983).

Respiratory syncytial virus is the most common cause of bronchiolitis, but it is also caused by parainfluenza virus and rhinovirus. Bronchiolitis is characterized by inflammation of the small airways or bronchioles. Inflammatory edema and increased mucus production in the bronchioles contribute to obstruction of the bronchiole lumina. Plugs of mucus and cell debris cause atelectasis and collapse of alveoli. The partial obstruction of the bronchioles causes inadequate ventilation to the alveoli and subsequent hypoxemia. There is air trapping in the alveoli that causes hyerinflation of the lungs. The clinical manifestations of broncheolitis are listed in Table 22-5.

Usually, respiratory distress becomes more severe during the first 24–72 hours of hospitalization. Cyanosis, pallor, listlessness, and sudden diminution or absence of breath sounds indicate impending respiratory failure.

TABLE 22-5 Characteristics of Bronchiolitis and Pneumonia

Bronchiolitis	Pneumonia
Age of child	
2 years or less	Any age, higher incidence during first 5 years of life
Etiology	
Viral infection, usually respiratory syncytial virus	Viral, bacterial (for example, *Klebsiella, H. influenzae,* staphylococcal, streptococcal, pneumococcal, or *Mycoplasma pneumoniae* infections)
	Aspiration of food, fluid, medication, poisonous substances (for example, hydrocarbons), powders
	Hypostatic (related to immobility, or postoperative accumulation of secretions)
History of present illness	
Accompanies or follows upper respiratory tract infection	Follows upper respiratory tract infection
Gradual onset over 1–3 days	Acute or gradual onset
Clinical manifestations	
Fatigue, anxiety, irritability	Fatigue, irritability, anxiety, lethargy
Dyspnea, shallow respirations	Dyspnea, shallow respirations
Paroxysmal, dry, harsh cough	Productive or congested harsh cough
Clinical manifestations *(Continued)*	
Mild to moderate intercostal, subcostal retractions	Mild to moderate intercostal retractions
Fever (low grade) or hypothermia	Fever
Respiratory rate 60–80	Tachypnea
Cardiac rate 180–200	Tachycardia
Rales, expiratory wheeze, expiratory grunt	Rales, rhonchi, wheeze, expiratory grunt, pleural friction rub (sometimes heard)
Prolonged expiratory phase	Respiratory lag on affected side
Increased anterior-posterior dimensions of the chest (barrel chest)	
Nasal flaring	Moderate respiratory distress with pneumococcal pneumonia
Cyanosis	Circumoral cyanosis with pneumococcal pneumonia
Obstruction present from trapped air	Pain with respirations
Barely audible breath sounds if very severe	Decreased breath sounds
Diminished appetite	Diminished appetite, vomiting (in young children)
	Great variation in signs and symptoms among patients

Treatment Treatment consists of oxygen therapy, fluid and electrolyte replacement, and antibiotic therapy if a secondary bacterial infection is identified. Bronchodilators are only rarely beneficial. Infants who have not responded to epinephrine might respond to aminophylline. Sedatives are avoided because they are respiratory depressants. In 1% of infants with bronchiolitis respiratory failure develops. Intubation and ventilatory assistance can be required for several days.

Nursing management Nursing management consists of measures relative to oxygen therapy, hydration, and chest physiotherapy. Humidified oxygen is given through a hood, face mask, tent, or nasal catheter. Supplemental oxygen concentrations are based on arterial blood gas values. Any infant receiving oxygen concentrations greater than 40% requires arterial blood gas or transcutaneous oxygen monitoring. Mist is not beneficial and can make some infants worse.

Nursing care includes frequent observations of respiratory status, particularly observations for respiratory failure during early hospitalization. Respiratory isolation is maintained throughout hospitalization, since the mode of transmission of respiratory syncytial virus is by droplet.

Dehydration due to increased insensible fluid losses and feeding difficulties is assessed early in the child's care. Oral

TABLE 22-6 Types of Infectious Pneumonia

Type/Organism	Treatment
Pneumococcal/*Streptococcus pneumoniae* Occurs in children under 4 years of age. Can be located in a single lobe (lobar) or segment of lung	Penicillin G or V orally; procaine penicillin parenterally
Mycoplasmal/*Mycoplasma pneumoniae* Occurs in children 5–19 years old. Patchy infiltrates in more than one area of the lung. Symptoms of dry cough, headache, low-grade fever, and fatigue are nonspecific and can be confused with other illnesses. Diagnosis is confirmed by throat culture	Erythromycin orally
Staphylococcal/*Staphylococcus aureus* Occurs primarily in infants. Chest radiographs can show the classic picture of lung cavities and herniations of lung tissue (pneumatocele). Empyema (pus in the pleural cavity) can be a complication	Parenteral penicillinase-resistant synthetic or cephalosporin
Other (eg, respiratory syncytial virus) Symptoms similar to those of mycoplasmal pneumonia. Onset usually is insidious. Fatigue, cough, and low-grade fever might be present. Lungs show patchy infiltrates	Viral pneumonias often are not treated. Some physicians treat with antibiotics to prevent secondary bacterial invasion

feedings and unnecessary handling tire the acutely ill infant and increase the risk of aspiration. Intravenous therapy to replace fluids and electrolytes is initiated early if there is any feeding difficulty. Initially, the nurse checks the infant's hydration status, including urine specific gravity every time the infant voids. As the infant recovers, specific gravity is checked every 8 hours. The urine specific gravity is maintained between 1.008 and 1.015, since fluid overload can increase the work of the cardiovascular system and cause pulmonary edema.

Elevation of the head of the bed decreases compression of the diaphragm and aids in ventilation. An infant seat is used if the infant can maintain the head in the midline. Any extreme flexion or hyperextension of the neck is avoided because the infant's poorly supported large airways become compressed very easily, increasing the work of breathing.

The infant with moist-sounding rales and minimal hypoxia might benefit from percussion with postural drainage. The moderately to acutely ill infant often cannot tolerate this procedure, and extra handling is kept to a minimum to prevent tiring. Postural drainage is postponed until toleration is improved and moist rales are present.

Bronchitis

In childhood, bronchitis often occurs in conjunction with other respiratory diseases. It is a transient inflammation involving the trachea and large bronchi. The primary symptom is a productive or dry cough. Rhinovirus is the most frequent cause of acute bronchitis, though parainfluenza, adenovirus, and respiratory syncytial virus have also been isolated.

The onset is usually gradual, with such cold symptoms as a runny nose and a productive cough developing over 3–4 days. Rales and wheezing are frequently present. Symptoms usually subside in 7–10 days. Chest radiographs are usually normal. If symptoms persist, secondary infection is suspected.

Treatment consists of adequate fluid intake and rest. Antibiotics are not necessary unless a secondary bacterial infection develops. Sedation and cough suppressants are contraindicated for bronchitis, as they are for most respiratory diseases in children.

Pneumonia

Pneumonia is defined as an inflammation of the lung. A relatively common condition of childhood, pneumonia is caused by a variety of infectious agents such as bacteria, viruses, fungi, and others (for example, mycoplasmas, chlamydiae) (see Table 22-6). Pneumonia also can be caused by aspiration.

Most childhood pneumonia is described as bronchopneumonia, that is, a combination of disseminated lobular pneumonia (patchy areas of infiltrates in both lung fields and surrounding the bronchi) and interstitial pneumonia (diffuse bronchiolitis with exudate evident in alveolar walls but not alveolar spaces). Bacterial pneumonias more often cause lobar or lobular (respiratory unit) involvement, whereas viral pneumonias cause inflammation of interstitial tissue.

Clinical manifestations Clinical manifestations of pneumonias are diverse (see Table 22-6). The classic picture of the child with pneumococcal pneumonia includes fever, cough, and chills, accompanied by chest pain. The child appears seriously ill, unable to eat, and excessively fatigued. There might be dyspnea, tachypnea, and other signs of respiratory distress. Auscultation reveals rales and decreased breath sounds in the area of lung affected. Other pneumonias have a similar clinical picture; however, the onset might be more insidious and the symptoms less severe. Young infants and children with chronic respiratory conditions are more likely to be severely affected.

Treatment Treatment of pneumonia is related to causative organism and presenting symptoms. If a bacterial agent is suspected, either intravenous or oral antibiotic therapy is instituted. Oxygen is ordered as needed to maintain normal arterial blood gas levels. Fluids are provided to meet daily requirements and to compensate for the additional fluid lost through rapid, shallow, difficult breathing. In addition, vigorous pulmonary hygiene measures are ordered. Progress is monitored by the patient's response to therapy and a follow-up chest radiograph. Rarely, an infant requires intubation or chest tube insertion to treat pneumothorax. The child with staphylococcal pneumonia might require a chest tube insertion to drain empyema (pus).

Nursing management Nursing management includes close observation of the child's respiratory status, color, required effort, and cardiovascular status. Vital signs including auscultation of breath sounds are monitored frequently (every 1–2 hours initially). Hydration status is assessed, and the child is encouraged to drink fluids. If fluid intake is inadequate, intravenous infusion will be necessary because fluids prevent secretions from becoming too viscous. An environment that provides mist therapy either by means of a mist tent or by a face mask also helps to loosen secretions. This increased humidity is combined with frequent position changes and chest physiotherapy to loosen and remove secretions further.

Percussion, vibration, and postural drainage are done every 4–6 hours, with particular attention to areas of consolidation as noted on chest radiographs. Oxygen therapy is used as indicated. When oxygen is used, the nurse monitors the concentration of the oxygen in the tent or hood as well as the child's arterial blood gases.

Oropharyngeal suctioning sometimes is needed when the infant or young child is unable to remove secretions effectively. Suctioning is done carefully and with discrimination; too-frequent suctioning irritates the mucosa and causes increased mucus production.

Fever control measures are instituted whenever the child's temperature is elevated. Good skin care and frequent linen changes are needed to keep the child dry in the high-humidity environment. Changing the child's position every 2 hours, while maintaining a semi-Fowler's position, facilitates respiration and pulmonary drainage.

Promotion of rest is an important nursing function. Nursing care is planned to allow the child maximum uninterrupted rest. Diversional activities need to involve little effort in order to conserve the child's energy. Whenever possible, the parent should be involved in the child's care. It is not unusual to observe a parent sitting inside a mist tent reading stories or playing games with the child.

Children with pneumonia frequently can be treated at home. The age of the child, the severity of the disorder, and the potential for cooperation with a treatment regimen are critical indicators of the potential for home care. The child might have to take antibiotics for 5–10 days depending on the cause of the pneumonia. In addition, rest and increased fluid intake will be necessary, along with analgesics for fever. It might be helpful if the air in the child's room can be humidified with a cool-mist vaporizer. Parental understanding of the treatment regimen and cooperation are essential if the child is to be successfully treated at home. Respiratory complications or failure to improve within 24 hours after treatment is initiated indicate that hospitalization needs to be considered as an alternative to home care.

The Child with Tuberculosis

Tuberculosis in children has decreased dramatically in many countries but remains a significant problem in the world today. Immigration to the United States of persons from countries where tuberculosis is still common brings an occasional child with tuberculosis to the clinic or hospital. The causative agent is *Mycobacterium tuberculosis,* an acid-fast, red rod. Tubercle bacilli can survive and remain virulent for many months if kept in the dark but die if they are exposed to ultraviolet rays (for example, direct sunlight) or are boiled for 1 minute.

The most common mode of transmission of tubercle bacilli is by droplet. Consequently, the most common site of primary lesions is the lung. The body's response to primary pulmonary tuberculosis is healing, but lesions might spread to and involve surrounding tissue. In acute miliary tuberculosis, tubercle bacilli are disseminated (carried) to various organs of the body through the bloodstream or by way of regional lymph nodes and the thoracic duct. Complications of primary tuberculosis usually occur within the first year of infection.

In its early stages, tuberculosis usually causes few if any symptoms. Consequently, any child who has a history of contact is tested 2–10 days after the contact. If a tuberculin skin test is positive, chest radiographs are taken. Tuberculosis is confirmed by cultures of gastric contents obtained by repeated gastric lavage. Acid-fast tubercle bacilli are found in gastric washings from a child with tuberculosis because the child swallows some sputum rather than expectorating it.

Treatment and nursing management involve early detection, vigorous chemotherapy, respiratory isolation of the patient, and serial radiographs to monitor the course of infection. Attention is also given to nutrition, vitamin supplements, rest, and protection from other infections. Tuberculosis of the lungs is treated with isoniazid, streptomycin, para-aminosalicylic acid (PAS), ethambutol, or rifampin. For older children, the usual regimen consists of 1 year of isoniazid and rifampin therapy. A third drug is added if immediate response to treatment is inadequate. The child is no longer considered communicable when sputum and gastric secretions are free of the tuberculin bacillus.

Home care of a child with tuberculosis is a challenge for parents. The child needs to be isolated from others who are susceptible to tuberculosis, which requires that the child be given a single room. In the home setting parents need to dispose carefully of tissues used by the ill child, preferably by incineration. The dishes the child uses need to be disposable (burnable) or sterilized, and the child must have adequate rest, nutrition, and a place to sleep and play where exposure to other persons will be minimal.

It is rare for one member of a family to have active tuberculosis without other family members having at least a positive tuberculin test. Public health departments usually are involved in the follow-up care of families with children with active tuberculosis and will determine what family members might be at risk of developing the disease and therefore need chemoprophylaxis. Public health departments usually make some effort to identify the person from whom the child contracted tuberculosis and make certain that that person receives treatment. Laws vary from state to state, but in most states it is mandatory to report new cases of active tuberculosis to public health officials.

Prevention of tuberculosis is the goal of most public health officials. Basic principles of prevention include the administration of isoniazid for 1 year to household contacts of tuberculosis patients. Bacille Calmette-Guérin (BCG) vaccination increases resistance in children living with an adult who has infectious tuberculosis. BCG vaccine is also recommended for children who live where the incidence of tuberculosis is high. Unfortunately BCG vaccine does give a person a positive tuberculin test and chest radiographs would be necessary for further screening.

The Child with an Acute Noninfectious Respiratory Problem

Foreign Body Aspiration

Aspiration of foreign material is most common in children from 6 months–6 years of age and results in more than 2000 deaths per year. The objects most frequently aspirated include popcorn, peanuts, balloons, round toys such as small balls, hot dog portions, and teething biscuits. Aspiration might not be witnessed, so awareness of its potential in the identified age group and knowledge of the common symptoms are crucial to diagnosis. Symptoms depend on the material aspirated and where in the respiratory tract the object lodges. A large object is likely to lodge in the trachea, resulting in complete obstruction. A smaller object could lodge in a mainstem bronchus, causing obstruction to one lung. A very small object could merely obstruct one segment of a lung.

Clinical manifestations A foreign body aspirated into a mainstream bronchus or smaller airway causes immediate severe coughing, which usually subsides in minutes. Therefore, if aspiration is not observed or reported, it can be missed for hours, days, or even months. Eventually, such secondary symptoms as wheezing or chronic coughing occur. Symptoms can be similar to those of croup. These symptoms might accompany infection, which is likely to develop if the foreign body has been lodged in an airway for a significant period. Other complications include atelectasis, bronchiectasis, and, rarely, erosion of the airway.

It is not difficult to recognize the signs of complete obstruction caused by aspiration of a large object. Emergency measures need to be performed immediately, since complete obstruction can cause death within minutes. (These measures are described in Chapter 12.) If obstruction is not complete, and if aspiration was not witnessed, the diagnosis is based on a well-taken history, physical examination of the chest for signs of uneven excursion or inspiration, and an inspiration-expiration radiograph. Even if assessment provides no evidence of foreign body aspiration, it should not be ruled out if the child is in the typical age range and has the classic symptoms.

Treatment If an object is thought to be lodged beyond the trachea, bronchoscopy is performed to locate and remove it. This might mean transferring the child and delaying removal of the object. Because a foreign body lodged beyond the trachea is not life threatening, delay in removal of the object is reasonable and probably wise.

After removal of the foreign body, treatment consists of inhalation therapy with an aerosol bronchodilator and chest physiotherapy.

In some circumstances it is reasonable to attempt postural drainage and percussion to dislodge a foreign body. If aspiration is suspected but the history and initial examination are negative, then a limited trial of percussion and postural drainage at home or in the hospital is warranted to attempt dislodging the object before performing a bronchoscopy.

Nursing management Nursing care following the removal of a foreign body from the airway involves keeping the child NPO until the gag reflex returns and then providing sips of water while observing the child's ability to swallow. Once satisfied that the child can manage fluids, the nurse gradually advances the diet. Nursing care also includes administering an inhaled bronchodilator and performing percussion and postural drainage every few hours for the first 12 hours or so. The child who is doing well after 24 hours usually is discharged. The nurse instructs the parent to carry out postural drainage procedures 2–3 times daily for a specified number of days. The nurse also instructs the parent about measures that can be taken to prevent foreign body aspiration in the future (see Chapter 12 for discussion of prevention).

Aspiration Pneumonia

Swallowing disorders and gastroesophageal reflux are the primary causes of aspiration pneumonia in infants. Severely retarded children continually aspirate oropharyngeal secretions, causing irritant and bacterial pneumonias. Other causes of aspiration pneumonia are accidental aspiration of liquids or solid food, hydrocarbon poisoning, aspiration of environmental agents such as talcum powder, and near-drowning.

Clinical manifestations The degree of lung response to aspirated substances is related to the concentration of the substance, rather than its volume. For example, very highly concentrated fluids can cause fulminating pulmonary edema. Most commonly, though, aspirated material causes widespread infiltrates, particularly interstitial. Signs and symptoms are similar to those of any pneumonia.

The type of hydrocarbon and the presence of additives such as camphor, naphthalene, heavy metals, nitrobenzene, or trichloroethane affect the degree of toxicity and injury in children who have ingested hydrocarbons. Hydrocarbons' low surface tension, low viscosity, and high volatility cause them to move rapidly over tissue and migrate into distal airways. The higher volatility of hydrocarbon makes it easy to inhale.

Respiratory symptoms usually occur within 30 minutes after inhalation. A nonproductive cough, tachypnea, dyspnea, grunting, retractions, and cyanosis are typical early signs. Continuation of the nonproductive cough usually indicates severe involvement. Oil absorption by the lung causes parenchymal damage. Defenses against secondary infection can be altered by the injury.

Generally, pulmonary effects peak by 24 hours, remain severe for several days, and start to subside within 2–5 days. Respiratory symptoms might persist for several weeks. Severely affected survivors of hydrocarbon inhalation can have persistent wheezing and frequent lower respiratory tract illnesses.

Diagnostic evaluation Diagnosis of aspiration pneumonia is made with chest radiographs and a history of episodes of sudden coughing and color change. More important, however, is diagnosis and correction of the cause of the aspiration.

Swallowing disorders are identified by direct observation of the infant during a feeding session and follow-up with studies of swallowing coordination (see Chapter 28 for discussion of tracheoesophageal fistula and gastroesophageal reflux). Diagnosis of hydrocarbon inhalation is made by the history of hydrocarbon ingestion and rapid onset of respiratory symptoms. Abnormal arterial blood gases and radiographic evidence of chemical pneumonitis confirm that inhalation injury has occurred.

Treatment Treatment consists of correcting the cause of aspiration. Special feeding techniques are used for children who aspirate due to inadequate swallowing.

Emergency treatment for hydrocarbon ingestion is controversial. Some clinicians prefer to use ipecac and induce vomiting, provided that the child is conscious and alert. This treatment is based on the belief that the neurologically intact child will not aspirate during emesis. Ipecac is given only in the hospital and never to a child who is comatose or convulsing or who has signs of central nervous system depression.

Gastric lavage (washing and pumping stomach contents) is the treatment of choice in children with central nervous system depression. An endotracheal tube is inserted prior to the lavage. Some clinicians prefer not to initiate vomiting unless there is a toxic additive or heavy metal mixed with the hydrocarbon.

Supportive care of the child starts with immediate attention to hypoxemia. Mechanical ventilation might be necessary if pulmonary edema or respiratory failure occurs. Steroids are prescribed in some instances.

Nursing management Nursing care of the child with aspiration pneumonia is similar to that of a child with any lower respiratory infection. The child with hydrocarbon inhalation will likely be seen first in the emergency room to remove the poison, if necessary, and to stabilize neurologic and respiratory status. Support is given to the parents, who will be anxious and might be feeling guilt. Prior to the child's discharge, poison prevention methods are reviewed with the parents (see Chapter 12 for prevention of poisoning).

Near-Drowning

Hypoxemia is the major concern in near-drowning. The degree and duration of hypoxemia depends on the length of time the child has been submerged, whether the child has aspirated water, and water temperature. The child who is submerged in cold water can survive longer because cold reduces the metabolic rate, which in turn decreases oxygen demand by the brain. Water is generally swallowed, but aspiration might be prevented (until death occurs) by reflex laryngospasm (mammalian reflex).

Blood volume is altered in both fresh- and salt-water drowning but by different mechanisms. This is not what kills. Death occurs from severe hypoxemia and acidosis. Therefore, the primary goal at the site of near-drowning is to oxygenate the victim. The quickest and most effective way to oxygenate the child is by CPR (see Chapter 12), which must be started immediately and continued until the child revives or a physician determines that death has occurred. The stomach is evacuated as soon as it is possible and safe to do so. This prevents vomiting and aspiration. Complications of near-drowning include hypoxic brain damage, aspiration pneumonia, pulmonary edema, and infection.

Care of the child who is recovering from near-drowning includes monitoring arterial blood gases to determine the need for artificial ventilation in addition to supplemental oxygen, and monitoring and correcting blood pH and electrolytes. Bronchospasm, which can occur due to the irritation of aspiration, is treated with bronchodilators. The nurse also observes for signs of infection. Appropriate antibiotics are prescribed once an infection is identified. The child is hospitalized and observed for a minimum of 28 hours after the event so that treatment can be given if untoward reactions occur. Prior to discharge, methods of preventing such an accident are discussed with the whole family.

The Child with a Chronic or Noninfectious Respiratory Disorder

Asthma

Asthma is a reversible obstructive respiratory disease that occurs in about 26 of 1000 children. Asthma probably is the most frequently seen chronic disease of childhood. It affects children of all ages and both sexes with boys in a slight majority. It is classified as *extrinsic* (caused by environmental factors) or *intrinsic* (caused by internal body mechanisms). Asthma also can be intermittent or chronic, and mild, moderate, or severe. It is a complex disease process, affected by a multitude of factors, both physical and emotional.

Asthma is characterized by bronchospasm (smooth muscle contraction in the bronchi) causing air trapping in the bronchioles. Bronchial narrowing increases as the mucosa lining the bronchial passages becomes edematous and produces increasing amounts of thick mucus (see Fig. 22-3). Closure of the bronchioles causes air trapping in the alveoli with hyperinflation and the inability to rid the alveoli of carbon dioxide without severe respiratory effort. The child has difficulty breathing, particularly on expiration due to the air trapping. The buildup of carbon dioxide interferes with gas exchange, causing hypoxemia, hypercapnia, and respiratory acidosis.

Asthma can be precipitated by a variety of stimuli. Physical factors include allergic responses, hormonal alterations, cold temperatures, and exercise. Emotional stress also can precipitate an attack. It is important to note, however, that although asthma might occur initially in response to an allergen, subsequent attacks are not usually without other influences.

Inhalant irritants (eg, pollen, mold, mildew, animal dander) are most frequently implicated in asthma. Rarely is asthma caused by a food allergy.

Theories suggest several factors that contribute to the occurrence of asthma attacks in the child:

1. An allergen directly irritates the respiratory mucosa. This triggers the immune response resulting in the production of the antibody IgE (see Chapter 25). The antibody attaches to white blood cells (basophil mast) and causes their destruction. As they are destroyed, they release chemicals (mediators) that cause bronchospasm, edema, and increased mucus production. The tendency to produce increased levels of IgE seems to be inherited, which is why it is not uncommon to find more than one child in a family with asthma.

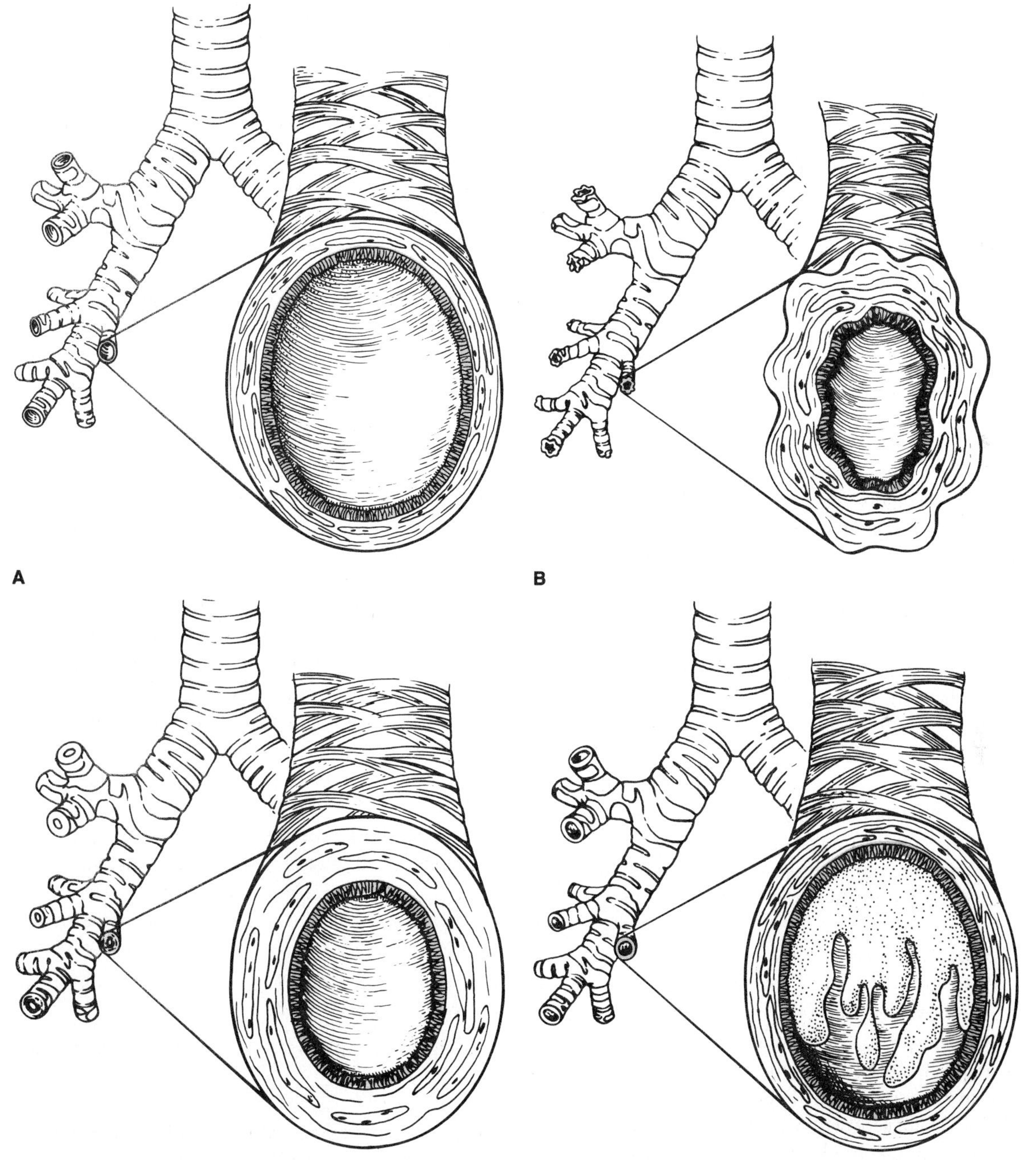

A B C D

FIGURE 22-3

Bronchial changes that decrease lumen size occur during an asthma attack. **A.** *Cross-section of a normal bronchial tube.* **B.** *Bronchospasm. Smooth muscle surrounding the bronchus contracts.* **C.** *Bronchial edema.* **D.** *Increased mucus production.*

2. Increased or sudden stress, such as from abrupt changes in temperature from warm to cold; excessive physical activity creating fatigue; and emotional stressors such as anxiety or fear can trigger bronchospasm and the development of an asthma attack.
3. Viral infections of the upper respiratory tract can precipitate an attack by their effect on the bronchioles.

Clinical manifestations Initial symptoms of an impending attack might be a feeling of tightness in the chest and an audible expiratory wheeze. As bronchial smooth muscles contract, airway wall edema and mucus production increase respiratory effort. As wheezing and chest tightness continue, they might be accompanied by fatigue, tachypnea, coughing, dyspnea, retractions, cyanosis, and diaphoresis (excessive sweating).

If the child is not treated promptly, status asthmaticus can result. *Status asthmaticus* is asthma that does not respond to the usual treatment within a certain period, usually several hours. It is an indication for hospital admission and treatment because prolonged attacks can lead to increased respiratory distress and possible respiratory failure. Respiratory failure can be seen more frequently in children younger than 6 years old because of the immaturity of their airway development and immune systems (Wabschall, 1986).

Diagnostic evaluation Diagnostic tests for asthma include chest radiographs, immunologic assays (see Chapter 25) to determine the level of IgE, a complete blood count (including an eosinophil count), and pulmonary function tests. A sweat chloride test might be performed to rule out cystic fibrosis.

The child's response to an aerosol bronchodilator needs to be assessed through pulmonary function testing. If the bronchodilator improves pulmonary function, asthma is the likely diagnosis. Response to epinephrine can differentiate asthma in young children from bronchiolitis.

Blood gases in the child with a moderate to severe asthma attack can change depending on the amount of hypoxemia. During a moderate attack it is not unusual for the Pco_2 to increase, the Po_2 to decrease, and the blood pH to decrease.

Following a tentative diagnosis of asthma, skin sensitivity tests might be performed to identify the causative allergen. Usually, more than one allergen is implicated in children with asthma (see Chapter 25 for explanation of skin testing).

Treatment Treatment depends on whether the asthma is mild, moderate, or severe. In mild asthma, attacks are episodic (no more than once a week) and of short duration if treated with bronchodilators. Between attacks, the child carries on a normal life free from medication. If the attack begins at home, the child is placed in a humidified environment. The parent encourages the child to drink fluids, promotes rest, and helps the child to use relaxation techniques. If the child has prescribed medications, they are taken (see Table 22-7). Usually, these methods reverse the attack.

In the child with moderate asthma, attacks occur more frequently than once a week. Between episodes, the child might have a chronic cough or wheeze, especially at night. The child might miss school or other activities due to illness and require constant bronchodilator therapy.

Children with severe asthma demonstrate continuous wheezing punctuated by more severe attacks. Attacks frequently need to be treated in the hospital. The child usually requires steroid therapy in addition to routine medications. Respiratory difficulties and airway obstruction are more difficult to reverse with conventional treatment.

Whether the child has mild, moderate, or severe asthma, if the usual measures fail to alleviate an attack, the child is treated in the emergency room. Initially, the child is given epinephrine injections at 20-minute intervals for an hour. An intravenous line is started if epinephrine fails to resolve the attack. The physician administers an initial dose of theophylline, which is followed by a constant infusion. If the child has severe respiratory distress, theophylline administration can be augmented by the administration of a steroid. Oxygen is administered if indicated.

If the physician fears respiratory failure is imminent, intubation and mechanical ventilation might be necessary until drugs alleviate symptoms.

Indications for admission to the hospital include:

1. No response after three doses of epinephrine or two doses of terbutaline
2. Three emergency room visits within 24 hours for treatment of an attack
3. Vomiting or no appropriate supervision at home (Wabschall, 1986)

The child is admitted often to the hospital intensive care unit depending on the severity of the symptoms.

Nursing management

Acute phase During the acute phase of an asthma attack, the nurse assists with oxygen administration, subcutaneous or intravenous injections of bronchodilators or corticosteroids, aerosal therapy, and postural drainage to provide immediate relief of the child's symptoms. Oxygen can be given by nasal cannula or mask, depending on the child's preference. The nurse should be prepared to assist with intubation if the child is in severe respiratory distress. Rapid-acting bronchodilators are frequently given via

TABLE 22-7 Drugs Used to Control Asthma

Generic name (brand name)	Action	Usual dose	Side effect
Epinephrine (Adrenalin)	Smooth muscle relaxant to relax bronchioles and promote bronchodilation	0.01 mg/kg body weight subcutaneously. Can be repeated for status asthmaticus in 20 minutes, up to 3 times	Palpitations, tachycardia, increased blood pressure, tremors, nausea and vomiting, headache, pallor
(Sus-Phrine) Contains both rapid-acting and slow-release epinephrine preparations. Immediate action and sustained release up to 8 hours	Same as adrenalin	0.005 mL/kg body weight subcutaneously	Same as for adrenalin
Theophylline Theophylline (Theo-Dur, Slo-Phyllin, Somophyllin, Theolair, Aminophylline, Quibron, Theospan, Choledyl) Duration of effect varies depending on preparation used	Relax bronchial smooth muscles, opening the airways	Varies depending on form used and route of administration. A serum level of between 10 and 20 μg/mL is desirable. Toxicity occurs at levels greater than 20 μg/mL	Stomachache, nausea and vomiting, loss of appetite, abdominal cramps, headache, dizziness, nervousness, tachycardia, pounding in chest, trouble sleeping
Adrenergics Metaproterenol (Metaprel, Alupent) Effective for 3–4 hours	Relax bronchial smooth muscles	1–2 teaspoons 3–4 times a day	Tachycardia, pounding in chest, nervousness, tremors, nausea and vomiting, drowsiness, bad taste in mouth
Isoetharine (Bronkosol, Bronkometer) Effective for 3–4 hours		3 to 7 inhalations by hand nebulizer. 1/4–1/2 mL diluted with saline and administered with O_2 flow of 4–6 L/min over 15–20 min	
Albuterol (Proventil, Ventolin) Effective for 4–6 hours		2 inhalations. Not recommended for children under 12 years	
Terbutaline (Brethine, Bricanyl) Effective for 3–7 hours		2.5 mg orally TID for children over age 12 years. Not recommended for younger children. 0.25 mg subcutaneously	
Antihistimines Cromolyn sodium (Intal)	Prevent release of histamine, lessening response of the lungs to allergenic triggers of asthma. Blocks exercise-induced asthma	20 mg by inhaler	Coughing, wheezing

nebulizer. The nurse observes the child for adverse effects (see Table 22-7).

A child receiving intravenous aminophylline is observed carefully for signs of toxicity (nausea, vomiting, headache, dizziness, restlessness, hypotension). The goal is to reach a therapeutic level (10μg–20μg/mL blood level) of aminophylline without having the child experience any toxic effects. The intravenous rate needs to be accurate. With children, an infusion pump is used to ensure accuracy and to deliver the medication at a steady rate. Signs of toxicity are reported to the physician immediately. If the child's response to the continuous administration of aminophylline is slow and dyspnea and wheezing persist, the physician might order a bolus of aminophylline. This is a "booster" dose given over a short period of time (usually 30 minutes) in addition to the continuous infusion of aminophylline. The child receiving IV aminophylline is placed on a cardiac monitor, since arrhythmias are associated with toxicity. The nurse monitors the serum aminophylline levels closely.

The nurse notes and reports any signs of increasing respiratory distress, including alterations in blood gases or changes of consciousness. Vital signs are monitored frequently. The child is placed in an optimal position for promoting comfort and facilitating ventilation, usually a semisitting position. The nurse monitors the child's hydration status and encourages the child who is alert and cooperative to drink clear fluids.

Maintaining a comfortable room temperature to decrease metabolism and thus heart rate and promoting rest are important nursing actions. The child might be excessively fatigued from loss of sleep or from increased respiratory effort. All nursing interventions are carried out in a calm, reassuring manner to promote rest and allay the child's anxiety.

Early Warning Signs of Asthma Attack

"Funny feeling" in the chest
Headache
Dry mouth
Itchy chin
Itchy throat
Changes in breathing pattern
Moodiness
Fatigue
Paleness
Glassy eyes
Sadness
Nervousness
Runny nose
Dark circles under the eyes

Recovery phase When the child is in the recovery phase, the medication schedule is changed from intravenous to oral. The nurse monitors the continued effectiveness of medications by observing improvements in respiratory status and noting decreasing episodes of wheezing and the resolution of signs of respiratory distress. If the physician orders chest physiotherapy, the nurse either remains with the child or performs the procedure.

Before the child is discharged from the hospital, the nurse discusses prevention and early intervention measures with the child and parent. Once precipitating factors are identified, the child can learn to avoid them. Allergens can be identified by subcutaneous or intradermal skin tests and eliminated from the child's environment if possible.

If the history of the attack shows that it might have been triggered by emotional upset or exercise, the child and family need to learn how to minimize reoccurrence. The nurse teaches the child and family to watch for the early warning signs of asthma attack and to intervene immediately to minimize the severity of the attack. At the first sign of an impending attack, the child needs to slow down, rest, relax, and do abdominal breathing. Sometimes this can prevent an attack. Even if it does not, it provides the child with some energy reserves.

To this end, several programs have been developed to promote relaxation and avoid an attack. For example, a program in self-management of asthma called "Airwise" has reduced significantly the number of emergency room visits by children with asthma (McNabb et al., 1985). The American Lung Association has developed a program for elementary-school-age children with asthma called *Superstuff*. It is a packet of play activities designed to teach asthmatic children to know the symptoms of their disease, recognize the precipitators, initiate their own treatment, and practice tension-reduction techniques. Developing responsibility for one's disease is the underlying principle.

Included in this packet is advice and assistance for parents. Situations are presented that promote parental decision making and teach the parents how to break the overprotectiveness cycle. Perhaps the most important fact emphasized is that rewards should be given for progress in assuming responsibility and independence. Rewards given for illness only encourage manipulative behavior (American Lung Association, 1981).

Stress can activate the autonomic nervous system, resulting in the "fight or flight" mechanism. This can cause bronchospasm that will exacerbate an asthma attack. Practicing relaxation techniques during times of stress can promote muscle relaxation and prevent spasm.

Regular exercise is vitally important for the child with asthma. Exercise increases lung function and allows the child contact with peers. Exercise and sports that allow periods of rest, such as tennis and baseball, are preferred to those that require extended periods of exertion. Swimming and cycling, however, are sports that do not seem to have an adverse effect on the child with asthma. Depending on the exercise and the child's condition, medication might be required before the child engages in any exercise. This is especially important with exercise-induced asthma.

The family life of a child with asthma might be disrupted when the child is diagnosed. There can be financial burdens. The long-term nature of the disease can place strain

(text continues on p. 701)

NURSING CARE PLAN *A Child with Severe Asthma*

Assessment data: Chad is a 5-year-old boy accompanied to the emergency room by his mother. Chad's mother appears very anxious and keeps repeating, "My baby can't breathe; someone help him before he dies."

Chad weighs 20 kg (44 lb), and he is 114 cm (44.5 in.) tall. He is diaphoretic and has circumoral and nail bed cyanosis. Inspection of Chad's chest reveals substernal and intercostal retractions. Auscultation reveals audible wheezing on inspiration and expiration, with prolonged expiration. Chad does not respond to epinephrine.

Because of hypoxemia and altered blood gases, Chad is admitted to the children's unit. He is placed on oxygen by mask. An IV with theophylline drip is started.

This is Chad's second asthma attack in a month. Chad is an only child and lives at home with both parents. His father works for the Merchant Marine and is out to sea for six months out of the year.

Nursing diagnosis	Intervention	Rationale
1. Ineffective breathing pattern related to increased mucus production and narrowed respiratory passages as indicated by audible wheeze	Identify factors contributing to the attack, such as anxiety, allergic reactions, infection, excessive activity, emotional stress.	Information is needed about contributing factors to better plan for treatment and prevention of future attacks.
	Assist the child to a position that facilitates an open airway—sitting upright, relaxed shoulders, and use of accessory muscles of breathing.	Position, posture, and correct use of muscles will improve ventilation. Use of abdominal muscles forces trapped air from lungs.
	Teach Chad to relax and concentrate on one aspect of breathing by doing breathing exercises with the nurse.	Bronchospasm is less likely to worsen a relaxed child who is concentrating on moving air from lungs.
	Encourage practice of breathing exercises by using games such as blowing bubbles through a straw and pretending to blow out candles on a birthday cake.	Children are more cooperative and results more apparent if children enjoy the exercises.
	Offer the child sips of favorite clear fluids. Chad likes apple and cranapple juices and all sodas.	Sipping is a simple diversion that will help the child to relax.

Outcome: Chad attempts to slow his breathing rate and ventilate more effectively. Chad becomes free of respiratory distress as evidenced by disappearance of retractions, return to normal color, and stabilization of vital signs.

Nursing diagnosis	Intervention	Rationale
2. Impaired gas exchange related to ventilation-perfusion imbalance	Administer aminophylline drip as ordered; use an infusion pump; monitor serum theophylline levels.	Aminophylline relaxes smooth muscles causing bronchodilation. Because aminophylline is toxic, the blood level is critical.
	Monitor effects of medications, particularly changes in pulse and blood pressure; auscultate breath sounds when taking vital signs (initially 1/2–1 hr); place child on cardiac monitor.	Dosage might need to be adjusted if signs of ineffectiveness or toxicity such as hyperalertness, agitation, tachycardia, arrhythmias, or hypotension occur. Auscultating breath sounds helps to define air movements and restrictions as evidenced by wheezing and rhonchi.
	Administer oxygen by mask at 5–6 liters (see Standards of Nursing Care for interventions related to oxygen administration).	Oxygen reduces hypoxemia and corrects blood gas alterations.

(Continues)

NURSING CARE PLAN *A Child with Severe Asthma* (Continued)

Nursing diagnosis	Intervention	Rationale
	Monitor Chad's response to therapy by observing for cyanosis, monitoring arterial blood gases, and noting evidence of return to normal respiratory pattern.	Monitoring status provides data for evaluating the effectiveness of the treatment.

Outcome: Chad's respiratory distress decreases. His arterial blood gases return to normal limits for his age.

Nursing diagnosis	Intervention	Rationale
3. Ineffective airway clearance related to increased mucus and dyspnea	Administer Bronkosol as ordered by oxygen nebulizer with flow set at 6 L/min; encourage Chad to breathe deeply during the therapy.	Bronkosol relaxes smooth muscles, allowing for increased ventilation and more effective airway clearance. Aerosol therapy is effective only when the child inhales deeply to bring medication into the lungs.
	Provide percussion and postural drainage subsequent to the aerosol therapy.	Expectoration of mucus is more easily accomplished when the airways are clear and bronchospasm is decreased. Removal of secretions from the lungs permits better movement of air.
	Teach Chad how to cough effectively and how to expectorate mucus from lungs; note whether mucus is expectorated or swallowed.	Direct inhalation of bronchodilator is an effective means to reduce bronchospasm and dilate airways.
	Explain to Chad the importance of telling the parent or nurse whenever breathing becomes difficult, there is tightness in the chest, or he is unable to take a deep breath.	Early reporting of breathing difficulty enables prompt intervention and avoidance of further distress.
	Encourage Chad's mother to remain calm while Chad is having difficulty breathing; teach her how to regain control by demonstrating how she can help Chad.	Reducing parental anxiety reduces the child's anxiety and allows for maximum airway clearance; demonstrating how the mother can assist the child by positioning him and breathing with him helps her calm down and regain control in an anxiety-producing situation.

Outcome: Chad cooperates with breathing exercises and aerosol therapy. Improvement in airway clearance is evidenced by a decrease in respiratory rate, disappearance of cyanosis, normal breath sounds, and the child's ability to expectorate excess mucus.

Nursing diagnosis	Intervention	Rationale
4. Potential for fluid volume deficit	Observe Chad for signs of dehydration—changes in vital signs, poor skin turgor, dry mucosa, sunken eyes, decreased urine output or elevated urine specific gravity.	Insensible fluid loss increases during an asthma attack. Adequate hydration makes respiratory secretions less viscous and easier to clear.
	Offer Chad frequent small amounts of his favorite clear fluids; set goal of 100 mL of fluid each hour.	Small amounts are more likely to be consumed by the child; goal is compatible with total fluid requirement for age and weight.
	Monitor intake and output.	Accurate recording is necessary to determine fluid demands, adequacy of intake, and hydration status.

Outcome: Chad appears adequately hydrated as evidenced by moist mucous membranes, good skin turgor, urine output adequate for age, and urine specific gravity within normal limits.

NURSING CARE PLAN *A Child with Severe Asthma (Continued)*

Nursing diagnosis	Intervention	Rationale
5. Anxiety related to the strange environment	Maintain a calm and relaxed manner when dealing with child and family.	The nurse's manner will have a calming effect on the child.
	Allow Chad to use his He-Men® to act out feelings; give him nebulizer equipment and other hospital equipment to use on the He-Men®; incorporate the mask into the play.	Observing the child's play enables the nurse to assess child's feelings about therapy. Play gives the child an opportunity to express fears.
	Give Chad choices, if possible, about modes of treatment.	Participation in self-care fosters feelings of control, which make the child less anxious.

Outcome: Chad demonstrates a decrease in anxiety as evidenced by calm, relaxed appearance, the ability to focus on play, and the ability to obtain adequate sleep.

Nursing diagnosis	Intervention	Rationale
6. Knowledge deficit related to limited understanding of immediate and continuing management of asthma attack	Review with child and parent the signs and symptoms of an attack (chest tightness, wheezing, dyspnea, cough, anxiety, diaphoresis).	Understanding and knowing the early signs and symptoms of an attack will enable the parent and child to take appropriate action and not to panic.
	Teach Chad and his mother proper use of aerosol therapy, the importance of taking deep breaths during an attack, and the importance of holding the breath for ten seconds after each inhalation from the inhaler.	Proper use of aerosols can limit progression of attacks; holding the breath for ten seconds after each inhalation allows maximum contact of the medication with the respiratory passages.
	Use a doll with exposed lungs to explain the mechanisms of an attack.	Visual aids assist with understanding.
	Discuss with Chad and his family measures to control an impending attack—relaxation exercises, slow breathing, pulmonary therapy, other anxiety-reducing measures, encouraging fluids, medications.	Knowledge of what to do during an attack provides control for the child and family, reduces anxiety, and can prevent hospitalization.
	Provide written instructions to Chad's mother delineating measures to be taken for immediate treatment when an attack occurs—medication to be taken, breathing exercises, positioning, indications for hospitalization.	Knowing what to do and having written directions helps the parent remain calm and initiate appropriate action.

Outcome: The child and parent can explain the mechanisms of an asthma attack, can demonstrate appropriate procedures for dealing with an impending or actual attack, and can state the indications for hospitalization.

Nursing diagnosis	Intervention	Rationale
7. Ineffective family coping related to the child's hospitalization	Help Chad to express feelings about the illness and facilitate this expression through use of clay, pounding toys, or art.	Expression of feelings through creativity allows the child to deal appropriately with them.
	Explain Chad's feelings and coping mechanisms to the parent and allow the parent to verbalize any feelings of anxiety, fear, or helplessness.	If a parent is able to understand how the child is feeling, the parent can more easily deal with the child's and parent's feelings.

(Continues)

NURSING CARE PLAN *A Child with Severe Asthma (Continued)*

Nursing diagnosis	Intervention	Rationale
	Encourage the parent to participate in Chad's care.	Encouraging participation in care increases the parent's self-esteem and ability to cope.
	Explore with the mother whether she has close family or friends to rely on for help when Chad's father is at sea; encourage her to join a community organization to help her develop outside interests and friends.	Support systems provide needed encouragement and support for families of hospitalized children.

Outcome: Chad and his mother are able to verbalize their feelings, or express them in other acceptable manners (such as play or art). The mother demonstrates support of the child and participates readily in the child's care.

Nursing diagnosis	Intervention	Rationale
8. Knowledge deficit related to limited understanding of home management of the child with asthma	Assist the family to identify precipitating factors, including such factors as stress, allergens, or other child or family dysfunction.	Reducing precipitators of asthma attacks reduces their occurrence.
	Explain how to allergy-proof the home if necessary.	Allergy proofing reduces environmental allergens (see Chapter 25).
	Describe desensitization.	Desensitization can be used to minimize the effect of environmental allergens by gradually increasing the child's tolerance to them.
	Demonstrate use of hand-operated inhalers, including effects and side effects of the medication and care of inhalant equipment.	Correct operation and care of inhalation equipment facilitates treatment.
	Encourage Chad to participate in age-appropriate activities, including regular exercise and sports that facilitate lung expansion, such as swimming or biking, while not overloading the respiratory system.	Regular lung expansion improves respiratory health by maintaining adequate air exchange and promoting effective airway clearance.
	Discuss overprotectiveness with Chad's mother. Teach Chad's parents not to be overprotective but to use a common-sense approach to limit-setting and providing for his health-maintenance and developmental needs; encourage them to allow Chad independence and self-care according to his developmental level.	Overprotectiveness can result in stress that can precipitate an attack. This can start a cycle of manipulation that is detrimental to child and parents.
	Refer Chad and his parents to the American Lung Association or the Asthma and Allergy Foundation of America for assistance if needed.	These organizations provide support and information to families with asthmatic children.

Ease up . . .
Ease up . . .
You can be cool and so free
Let the worries go by
Let the tensions all fly
Relax, it's the best way to be . . .

Ease up, ease up
Let breathing be gentle and deep
Don't be uptight
Just relax and feel right
And you'll put your fears
all to sleep . . .

Ease up . . .
Ease up . . .
Help your worries slip past
You're breathing with ease
Just relaxed as you please
You're breathing the smart way
at last . . .

From *Superstuff*, "Ease Up Relaxation Record," American Lung Association. Reproduced with permission.

on the family's ability to cope. Nursing interventions are similar to those for any child with a chronic condition (see Chapter 14).

Allergens need to be eliminated from the environment, including cigarettes and possibly a favorite pet. The emotional upset that might result from such changes needs to be addressed. Attention might be focused on the identified patient, perhaps to the exclusion of the other children. The nurse addresses these concerns and refers the child and family to appropriate community resources if necessary.

Patient teaching also includes instructions related to medications the child will be taking at home to prevent attacks. The parent and child will need to know when to administer the medication, how frequently, and how many times it can be repeated. They also need to be specifically instructed to get medical attention if the prescribed medication does not relieve the asthmatic symptoms. The nurse discusses compliance and teaches methods of administration. In addition, expected side effects and signs of toxicity are explained to the family.

Cystic Fibrosis

Cystic fibrosis is a syndrome characterized by widespread dysfunction of the exocrine glands. It occurs in from 1 of 1600 to 1 of 2500 live Caucasian births. The incidence of cystic fibrosis in other racial groups is considerably less. The disease is transmitted to the child as an autosomal recessive trait. Carriers have no symptoms and cannot yet be identified by any reliable test. If both parents are carriers, there is a 25% chance with each pregnancy that the infant will have cystic fibrosis.

Until recently, cystic fibrosis could not be diagnosed by amniocentesis. Recently, however, researchers have found reduced levels of certain proteases in amniotic fluid of fetuses with cystic fibrosis (Ladewig, London, & Olds, 1986). Additionally, a genetic marker has been found that will help researchers discover on what chromosome the defective gene for cystic fibrosis might be found. This will improve the likelihood for accurate prenatal diagnosis of cystic fibrosis in the near future.

The severity of symptoms varies greatly. Some children have minimal involvement, while others have extensive involvement resulting in limited growth and development and death before adolescence. Median age at death is 18–20 years, though some patients die in infancy and others live until 40 years of age.

All exocrine glands are affected to some extent, but 95% of deaths from cystic fibrosis are due to abnormal mucus secretion and fibrosis in the lungs. Mucus secreted by the mucous glands of children with cystic fibrosis is abnormally viscous, sticky, and tenacious. It adheres to the walls of the glandular ducts and eventually obstructs them entirely. Obstruction causes fibrosis of the glands themselves. This process occurs in many of the body systems. Most affected are the respiratory and gastrointestinal tracts (Fig. 22-4). In the gastrointestinal tract, the pancreas, small intestine, and biliary system are especially affected. The reproductive system becomes involved at puberty. Integumentary involvement causes the sweat glands to produce sweat containing four times the normal concentration of sodium chloride.

Clinical manifestations

Respiratory The child is born with healthy lungs. Usually, pulmonary evidence of cystic fibrosis appears gradually as the bronchi become hypertrophied in response to abnormal mucus production. As mucus clogs the bronchi and bronchioles, the child becomes increasingly susceptible to respiratory infections. Bronchitis, bronchiolitis, and pneumonia often become chronic. *Pseudomonas* and *Aspergillus* are the most common causes of infection. Except in the lungs, the child's general immunity and ability to produce antibodies are within normal ranges.

Cough, which might be dry and hacky or loose and productive, often is the first sign of pulmonary involvement. This occurs usually during infancy and is intermittent at first. The cough becomes progressively worse, especially

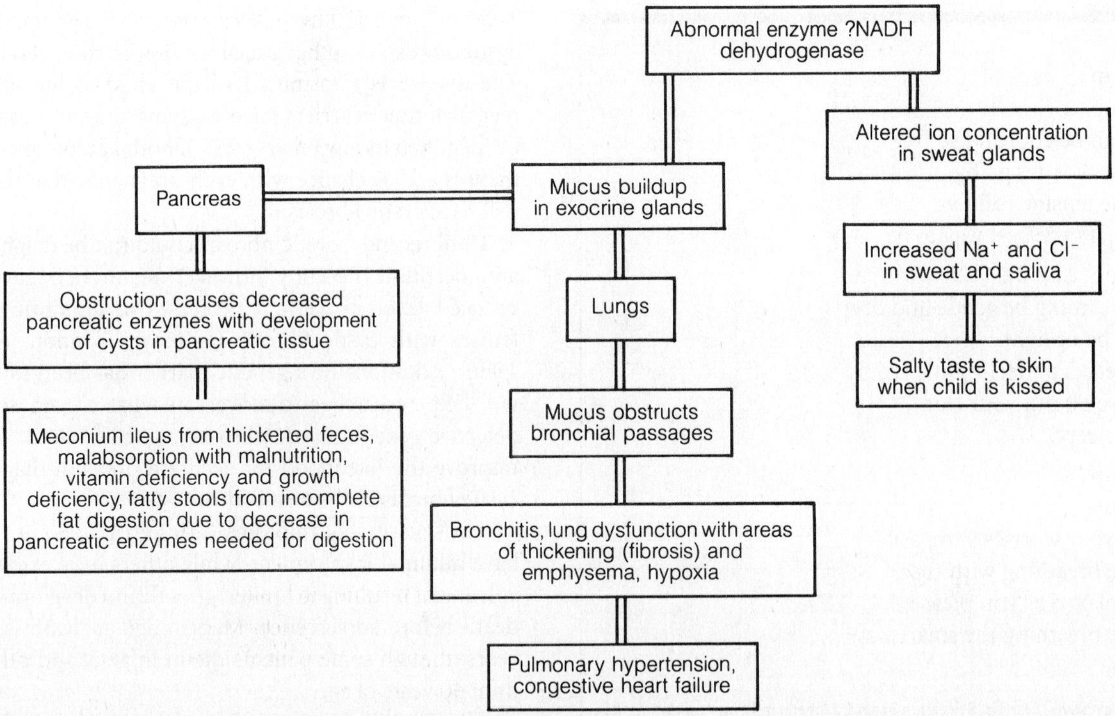

FIGURE 22-4
Etiology and manifestations of cystic fibrosis.

during periods of illness, when dyspnea makes excessive secretions more difficult to manage. Over time, the child develops clubbing of the fingers and a barrel chest. Pulmonary complications can include cor pulmonale, pulmonary hypertension, and pneumothorax.

Gastrointestinal Early symptoms in infancy are failure to thrive; frequent, foul-smelling stools; and voracious appetite. More rarely, the child presents with *meconium ileus* (5%–10% of affected infants), which is ileal obstruction from thick, tenacious meconium. Many infants and older children with cystic fibrosis develop rectal prolapse, which occurs most commonly when the children have been passing large quantities of bulky stool (steatorrhea) or have been straining at stool. If reduced quickly, it poses no hazard to the child.

The dysfunction of the mucous-producing glands contributes to the development of multiple gastrointestinal absorption problems. The thick mucoidal secretions block the pancreatic ducts, leading to formation of cysts within the pancreas. These cysts are later replaced by fibrotic tissue. This ductal obstruction and continued fibrosis prevents the secretion of the digestive enzymes. The absence of trypsin, lipase, and amylase in duodenal fluid causes the malabsorption of fats and proteins. The dietary fats remain undigested, and the fat-soluble vitamins A, D, E, and K are not absorbed efficiently. Unabsorbed food fractions are then excreted in the stool, resulting in steatorrhea. The stools are bulky and foul smelling, might appear greasy, or might float in the toilet.

The loss of vital nutrients and fat-soluble vitamins contributes to the classic picture of failure to thrive. Poor skin healing and easy bruising can result from the malabsorption of fat-soluble vitamins.

The islet cells of the pancreas can be affected, and glucose intolerance can develop as the child grows older. Insulin supplementation is rarely needed, and ketoacidosis does not occur. Cystic fibrosis also can contribute to the development of biliary obstruction and fibrosis.

Increased flatus, thinness, cough, stature, and delayed puberty can present psychosocial problems for the child. Thickened cervical secretions in girls and sterility in boys can cause reproductive difficulties as the child reaches adulthood.

Diagnostic evaluation Diagnosis is by pilocarpine sweat iontophoresis (sweat chloride test). Over 60 mEq/L of sodium and chloride is diagnostic. Because infants under

3 months of age might not sweat sufficiently, the sweat chloride test might be unreliable. Family history of cystic fibrosis, presence of reducing substances in the stool (see Chapter 28), or reduced or absent pancreatic enzymes support the diagnosis.

Treatment

Respiratory The goals of treatment are to maintain airway patency and control lung infection. Airway patency is maintained by chest physiotherapy (percussion and postural drainage), inhalation therapy with aerosol bronchodilators and humidified oxygen if needed, breathing exercises, and an appropriate exercise program. Mucolytics are rarely used. Infection is treated with appropriate antibiotics, particularly the aminoglycosides (amikacin, gentamicin, and tobramycin) and the semisynthetic antipseudomonal penicillins (carbenicillin, ticarcillin, azlocillin, and piperacillin). Increased salt intake is prescribed during prolonged hot weather or febrile periods because children with cystic fibrosis are prone to electrolyte imbalances that, if not corrected, can lead to heat prostration and circulatory collapse.

Gastrointestinal Medical management of gastrointestinal involvement in cystic fibrosis is directed toward promoting absorption of nutrients. The infant is given predigested protein formula (Pregestimil), and medium-chain triglycerides (MCT) can be used as a calorie supplement.

Older children might require a high-protein or a low- or limited-fat diet, although some can tolerate a normal diet. Individual response to a regular diet should be determined before automatically limiting a child's diet. Those children requiring a low-fat diet can use MCT oil as a supplement for cooking oil. Foods that are high in salt or additional salting of foods might be necessary in warm weather.

Pancreatic enzymes are given to replace enzymes not available due to pancreatic involvement. The amount of enzyme given is based on the individual response to diet therapy. Supplementation might not be needed for those with early-stage disease or those with limited pancreatic involvement. If needed, however, enzyme capsules, tablets, or powders (for example, Pancrease, Cotazym, Viokase) are given with all meals or snacks.

In addition to enzyme supplementation, water-soluble supplements of fat-soluble vitams A, D, and E are necessary. Vitamin K supplements are indicated if hypoprothrombinemia occurs.

Other complications are treated symptomatically. Bowel obstruction might require surgery. A prolapsed rectum can be reduced by exerting gentle pressure against the everted portion with a lubricated gloved finger. The child's buttocks are then taped together to prevent immediate reprolapse.

Nursing management

Pulmonary Nursing management for the child with pulmonary effects of cystic fibrosis includes promoting effective airway clearance by administering aerosol bronchodilators and performing or supervising chest physiotherapy. Chest physiotherapy, breathing exercises, and inhalation therapy (with aerosols) are done 2–3 times daily and more frequently during acute illness. If these treatments are carried out at home, the nurse instructs the child and family about correct procedures.

The nurse also instructs and encourages the child to perform appropriate breathing exercises and advises the child and family about the positive results of participation in physical activity and certain sports. The child with cystic fibrosis can benefit from an activity such as swimming, which requires breathing control and enhances correct posture. Activity promotes coughing, which, if done effectively, helps to clear the respiratory passages.

The nurse advises the child and family about avoiding people with upper respiratory infection. If infection occurs in the child, the nurse administers prescribed antibiotics or instructs the child and family about their use at home.

Oxygen therapy also might be part of hospital or home care. Close follow-up in a recognized cystic fibrosis center is very important in the early detection of lung changes that require hospitalization for a thorough pulmonary clean-out and reassessment of the maintenance regimen to be continued at home.

Gastrointestinal Parent and child teaching also includes dietary information. The nurse or nutritionist provides the parent with information regarding the preparation of a high-protein, low-fat diet. The nutritionist might provide appropriate meal plans, snack suggestions, and helpful hints to assist the family and the child to adjust to the sudden changes in diet. In any foods requiring cooking oil, MCT oil might be used, or it can be used as a calorie supplement in infant formulas.

The parent also needs to learn the appropriate use and type of supplemental enzymes that the child will be using. If the infant requires enzymes, a powdered form can be mixed in pureed fruit, or the pancrease capsule can be opened and the powder mixed with pureed fruit. Because direct contact with enzymes can contribute to skin breakdown, the parent needs to clean the face and lips of the child after feeding.

Older children can use capsules or tablets and need to remember to take enzymes with all meals and snacks. Vitamin supplementation usually is necessary and usually includes vitamins A and E and often vitamins D or K as well. Some children also require iron supplementation.

Emotional care Cystic fibrosis is a chronic disease that causes many physical and psychosocial problems throughout the child's life. Parents of a newly diagnosed infant might express feelings of guilt or might attempt to blame each other for causing the disease. Genetic counseling might identify problems that will affect future pregnancies or might alter parental expectations for their intended family.

Because of the limitations forced on the family, stress can become overwhelming for parents, siblings, or the affected child. Families might find they are unable to dine out or travel as before because of dietary restrictions or the need for frequent respiratory therapy. Siblings can encounter many questions from peers regarding their "sick" brother or sister.

The affected child might also encounter continual questions or might become an object of ridicule by peers because of the marked delay in growth and development. Adolescents with cystic fibrosis usually experience delayed sexual development, and girls can be amenorrheic or lack breast development. The wasted appearance together with a chronic cough can also cause impaired body image or decreased self-esteem.

There might be problems with peer relationships. Older children or adolescents might fear that the disease is contagious or might be repelled by the continual coughing and expectoration of mucus encountered in children with pulmonary involvement.

The nurse provides psychologic support necessary to deal with these chronic problems as they affect both the child and the family (see Chapter 14). In addition, family support groups consisting of families of children with cystic fibrosis are a great help to parents of a newly diagnosed child because group members are familiar with the stress and practical concerns and difficulties encountered by affected children and their families. They can offer information for meeting day-to-day needs and are of great help when parents must cope with an acute illness or approaching death of the child.

Essential Concepts

- Ventilation of the lungs, diffusion of gases to and from capillary blood, and perfusion of body tissues by capillaries are necessary for adequate respiratory function.
- Physical examination of a child with a suspected respiratory dysfunction includes observation for signs of hypoxia and dyspnea; assessment of the rate, depth, ease, and rhythm of respiration; palpation; percussion; and auscultation.
- Pulmonary function tests are done to measure the volume of air normally inspired and expired, the capacity of the lungs to inspire and expire more than the usual volume, and the rate of flow in and out of the lungs.
- Supplemental oxygen is administered to correct hypoxemia (insufficient oxygenation of arterial blood), which is assessed by arterial blood gas studies and manifested clinically as tachypnea, tachycardia, headache, pallor, cyanosis, and mental confusion.
- In inhalation therapy, aerosols are atomized into fine mist by a nebulizer and inspired by the patient.
- Humidity is added to air inspired through an artificial airway and to supplemental oxygen to prevent drying and irritation of the respiratory mucosa.
- Postural drainage, percussion, and vibration are done by the nurse or physiotherapist to enhance clearance of respiratory secretions or an aspirated foreign body.
- Acute care needs of the child with a respiratory dysfunction include airway clearance, regular breathing patterns, and appropriate gas exchange. The nurse provides optimal rest and performs activities of daily living until the child is able to resume self-care.
- Nutritional needs of the child with a respiratory disorder involve careful attention to hydration status with correction of any fluid volume deficit.
- The nurse addresses the developmental needs of children with respiratory dysfunction by promoting normal development within the disease restrictions and encouraging the parents to allow the child independence and self-care appropriate to developmental level.
- Anxiety related to the acuity of the disease and the potential for ineffective family coping are emotional problems the nurse considers when caring for a child with a respiratory dysfunction.
- Health maintenance needs of the child with a respiratory disorder might include teaching related to home therapy involving oxygen equipment, nebulizer-delivered aerosols, chest physiotherapy, exercise regimens, prevention and management of emergencies, and follow-up care.
- The child with an acute respiratory infection might experience inflammation and infection of the pharynx (pharyngitis), the larynx (croup, laryngotracheo-

bronchitis, epiglottitis), and the respiratory unit (broncheolitis).

- Lower respiratory tract infections can result in pneumonia, which can be viral or bacterial. Pneumonia also can be caused by aspiration.
- For the child with tuberculosis, nursing care involves instituting isolation measures, administering medications, teaching patients about compliance with the drug regimen, and monitoring the course of infection.
- The child with a chronic, noninfectious respiratory dysfunction might experience asthma or cystic fibrosis.
- Nursing care of the child with asthma involves administering medications that promote airway clearance, providing oxygen for sufficient gas exchange, promoting rest, encouraging fluids to prevent dehydration, providing anxiety relief, teaching child and family home management of this chronic condition, and addressing stressors that might precipitate attacks.
- Nursing care of the child with cystic fibrosis is directed toward relieving gastrointestinal as well as respiratory symptoms. This might include dietary management, vitamin supplementation, and administration of pancreatic enzymes as well as promotion of optimal lung function and prevention of infection. Nursing interventions also might be directed toward helping the family adjust to a chronic illness and, possibly, adjusting to impending death of the child.

References

American Lung Association: *Superstuff,* 1981.

Behrman RE, Vaughan VC, McKay RE: *Nelson Textbook of Pediatrics.* Saunders, 1984.

Cleary TG, Pickering LK: Upper respiratory tract infections. In: *Infectious Diseases of Children and Adults.* Pickering LK, DuPont HL (editors). Addison-Wesley, 1986.

Ladewig P, London M, Olds S: *Essentials of Maternal-Newborn Nursing.* Addison-Wesley, 1986.

McNabb W et al.: Self-management education of children with asthma: Airwise. *Am J Public Health* (Oct) 1985; 75(10): 1219–1220.

Mitchell P (editor): Harmful effects of passive smoking on children—the evidence intensifies. *Child Health Alert* (Sept) 1986:5.

Wabschall J: Nursing management of children during a mild to moderate asthma attack. *JEN* (May/June) 1986; 12(3): 134–141.

Wilson J: Pediatric emergency! Croup and epiglottitis. *Can Nurs* (March) 1984; 77:25–29.

Additional Readings

Ahrens TS, Rutherford KA: The new pulmonary math: Applying the a/A ratio. *Am J Nurs* (March) 1987; 87(3):337–340.

Castiglia PT, Aguilina S: Streptococcal pharyngitis: A persistent challenge. *Pediatr Nurs* (Nov/Dec) 1982; 8(6):377–381.

Dawson A, Simon R: *The Practical Management of Asthma.* Grune & Stratton, 1984.

Dean JM, Kaufman ND: Prognostic indicators in pediatric near-drowning: The Glasgow coma scale. *Crit Care Med* (July) 1981; 9:536–539.

Do day-care centers pose excessive health risks to children? *Pediatr Alert* 1983; 8(2):5–6.

Ellmyer P, Thomas NJ: A guide to your patient's safe home use of oxygen. *Nurs '82* (Jan) 1982; 12:56–57.

Emami CL, Delbianco LM: An improved technique for securing nasoendotracheal tubes. *Am J Matern-Child Nurs* (Sept/Oct) 1981; 6:337–340.

Hartsell MB: Noninvasive oxygen monitoring. *J Pediatr Nurs* (Feb) 1987; 2(1):64–65.

Hartsell MB: Chest physiotherapy and mechanical vibration. *J Pediatr Nurs* (April) 1987; 2(2):135–137.

Jennings C: An alternative: Nasal cannula oxygen therapy for infants who are oxygen dependent. *Am J Matern-Child Nurs* (March/April) 1982; 7:89–92.

Kendig EL, Chernick V (editors): *Disorders of the Respiratory Tract in Children,* 4th ed. Saunders, 1983.

Kennedy AH, Johnson WG, Sturdevant EW: An educational program for families of children with tracheostomies. *Am J Matern-Child Nurs* (Jan/Feb) 1982; 7:42–49.

Larter N: Cystic fibrosis. *Am J Nurs* (March) 1981; 81:527–532.

Metaproterenol (Alupent) now available without prescription. *Pediatr Alert* 1983; 8(7):25–26.

Moozam F, Talbert JL, Rogers BM: Foreign bodies in the pediatric tracheobronchial tree. *Clin Pediatr* 1983; 22:148–150.

New formulations and devices for administering asthma medications. *Pediatr Alert* 1983; 8(2):7–8.

Ng L, McCormick KA: Position changes and their physiological consequences. *Adv Nurs Sci* (July) 1982; 4(4):13–25.

O'Neill E: Cystic fibrosis. Pages 58–83. In: *Chronic Obstructive Pulmonary Disease.* Sexton DL (editor). Mosby, 1981.

Patton A, Ventura J, Savedra M: Stress and coping responses of adolescents with cystic fibrosis. *Child Health Care* (Winter) 1986; 14(3): 153–156.

Petty TL (editor): *Intensive and Rehabilitative Respiratory Care*, 3rd ed. Lea & Febiger, 1982.

Petty TL: Drug strategies for airflow obstruction. *Am J Nurs* (Feb) 1987; 87(2): 180–184.

Pinney M: Foreign body aspiration. *Am J Nurs* (March) 1981; 81:521–522.

Rachelefsky GS: Asthma self-management programs for children. *Child Care Newsletter* 1984; 3(2): 5–8.

Schuler PM, Cloutier MM: Chronic cough in children. *Pediatr Basics* (April) 1984; 38: 10–14.

Simkins R: Asthma: Reactive airways disease. *Am J Nurs* (March) 1981; 81:522–526.

Simkins R: The crises of bronchiolitis. *Am J Nurs* (March) 1981; 81:514–516.

Simkins R: Croup and epiglottitis. *Am J Nurs* (March) 1981; 81:519–520.

Stepdesign Inc: Pulmonary function tests in patient care. *Am J Nurs* (June) 1981; 80: 1135–1161.

Stratton CW: Bacterial pneumonias—An overview with emphasis on pathogenesis, diagnosis, and treatment. *Heart Lung* (May) 1986; 15(3): 226–244.

Stullenbarger B et al.: Family adaptation to cystic fibrosis. *Pediatr Nurs* (Jan/Feb) 1987; 13(1): 29–31.

Traver GA (editor): *Respiratory Nursing: The Science and the Art.* Wiley, 1982.

Wade JF: *Respiratory Nursing Care: Physiology and Technique.* Mosby, 1982.

Chapter 23

Circulation

Implications of Abnormalities in Structure and Function

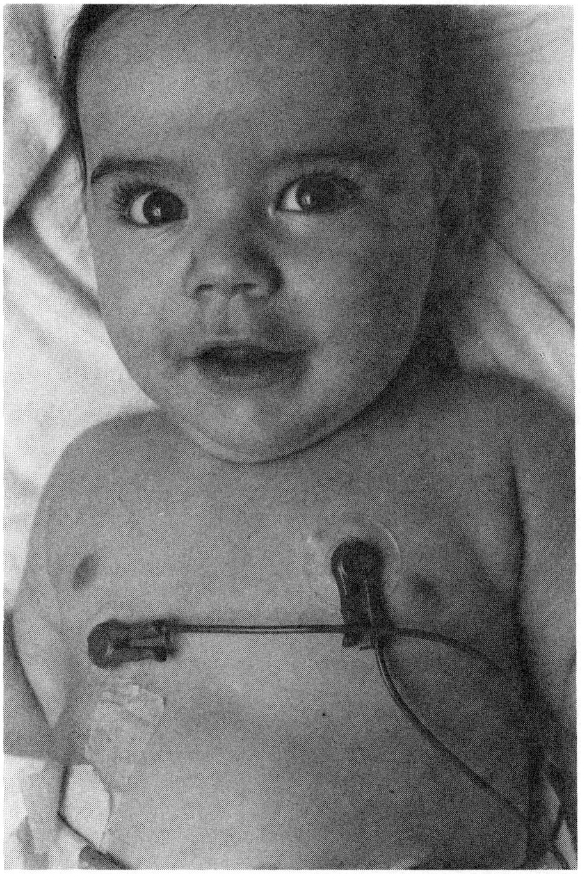

Chapter Contents

(Continues)

Alteration in nutrition: less than body requirements related to inadequate intake

Developmental Needs

Altered growth and development related to effects of physical limitations

Altered growth and development related to environmental and stimulation deficiencies

Emotional Needs

Potential alteration in family processes

Anxiety related to perceived threat to the child's health status

Potential body image disturbance

Health Maintenance Needs

Potential for impaired home maintenance management

The Child with Complications Related to Cardiac Dysfunction

Congestive Heart Failure

The Child Undergoing Cardiac Surgery

The Child with Subacute Bacterial Endocarditis

The Child with Hypertension

Cross Reference Box

To find these topics, see the following chapters:

Cardiopulmonary resuscitation (CPR)	Chapter 12
Kawasaki disease	Chapter 25
Acute rheumatic fever	Chapter 25
Shock	Chapter 25

Objectives

- Describe the structure and function of the heart, arteries, veins, and cardiac conduction system.
- Explain how prenatal circulation differs from postnatal circulation.
- Explain the physiologic effects and changes in circulation caused by left-to-right shunts, right-to-left shunts, and obstruction defects.
- Identify assessment criteria and diagnostic tests pertinent to history taking and physical examination of the child with suspected or diagnosed cardiac disease.
- Explain nursing care common to procedures and treatments that involve the cardiovascular system.
- Describe the acute-care, nutritional, developmental, emotional, and health maintenance needs of the child with cardiac disease.
- Describe nursing management and parent teaching involved in the administration of diuretics, digoxin, and prophylactic antibiotics.
- Describe the major acyanotic cardiac defects and their general clinical manifestations, treatment, and nursing management.
- Describe the major cyanotic cardiac defects and their general clinical manifestations, treatment, and nursing management.
- Describe preoperative and convalescent nursing management for the child experiencing cardiac surgery.
- Identify the causes, signs and symptoms, and nursing management of the child with congestive heart failure.
- Describe assessment and nursing management for the child with subacute bacterial endocarditis.
- Discuss the management of the child with hypertension.

ESSENTIALS OF STRUCTURE AND FUNCTION
The Cardiovascular System

The Heart, Arteries, and Veins

The heart is a muscular organ consisting of two atria, two ventricles, and four valves that pumps blood throughout the body (see figure showing normal circulation).

Glossary

Aorta A great vessel that conducts oxygenated blood from the left ventricle of the heart to the organs of the body. The aorta has three major branches: (1) the *innominate artery,* which subdivides into the *right subclavian* (blood to right arm) artery and the right common carotid artery, (2) the *carotid* arteries, which supply blood to the head, and (3) the *left subclavian* artery, which supplies blood to the left arm.

Atrioventricular node Passes impulses to the *bundle of His,* a collection of specialized tissue that divides into right and left bundle branches along either side of the ventricular septum. The bundle branches terminate in *Purkinje fibers,* which conduct impulses to stimulate ventricular contraction.

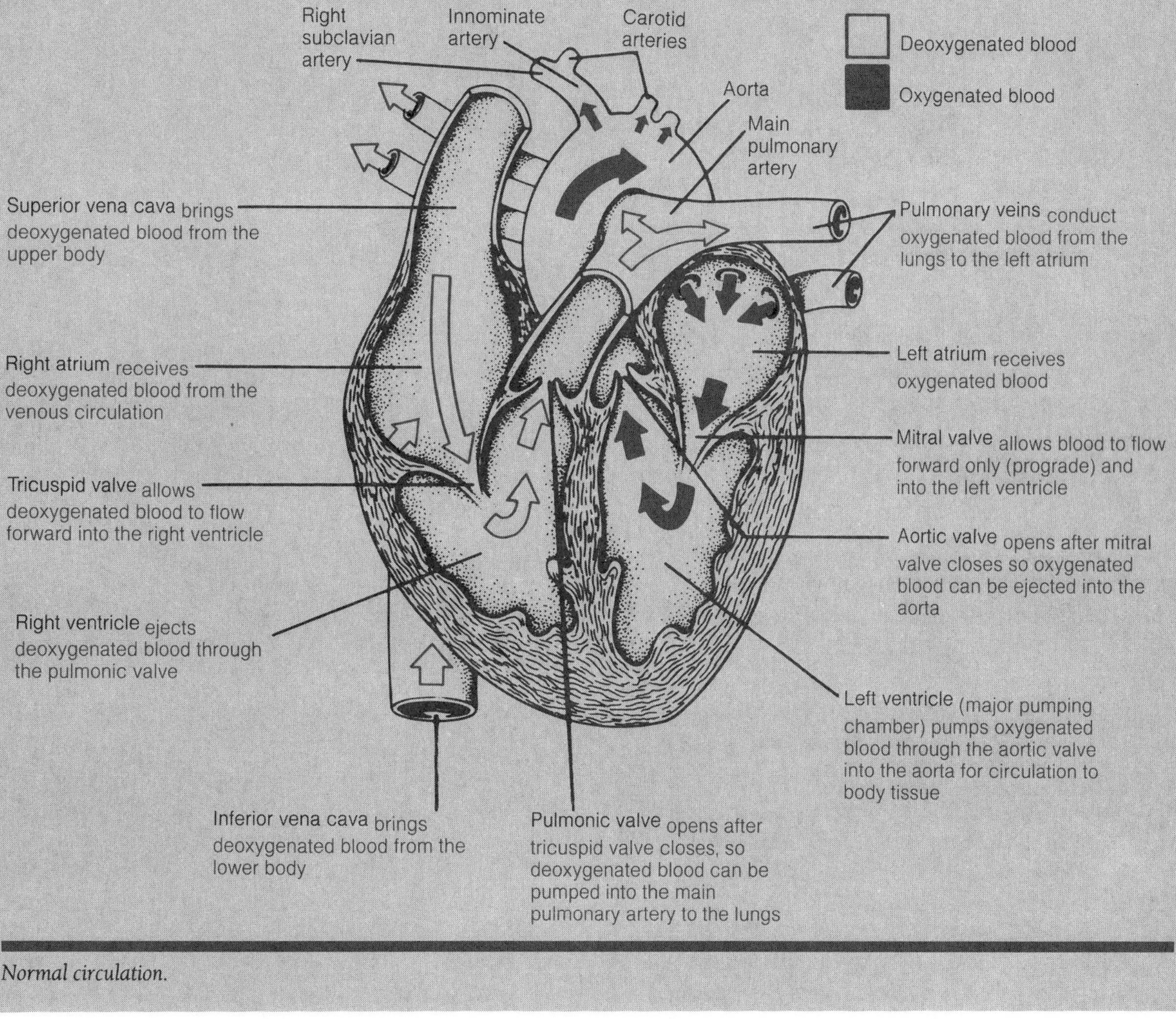

Right subclavian artery
Innominate artery
Carotid arteries
Aorta
Main pulmonary artery
Deoxygenated blood
Oxygenated blood
Superior vena cava brings deoxygenated blood from the upper body
Pulmonary veins conduct oxygenated blood from the lungs to the left atrium
Right atrium receives deoxygenated blood from the venous circulation
Left atrium receives oxygenated blood
Mitral valve allows blood to flow forward only (prograde) and into the left ventricle
Tricuspid valve allows deoxygenated blood to flow forward into the right ventricle
Aortic valve opens after mitral valve closes so oxygenated blood can be ejected into the aorta
Right ventricle ejects deoxygenated blood through the pulmonic valve
Left ventricle (major pumping chamber) pumps oxygenated blood through the aortic valve into the aorta for circulation to body tissue
Inferior vena cava brings deoxygenated blood from the lower body
Pulmonic valve opens after tricuspid valve closes, so deoxygenated blood can be pumped into the main pulmonary artery to the lungs

Normal circulation.

ESSENTIALS OF STRUCTURE AND FUNCTION *(Continued)*
The Cardiovascular System

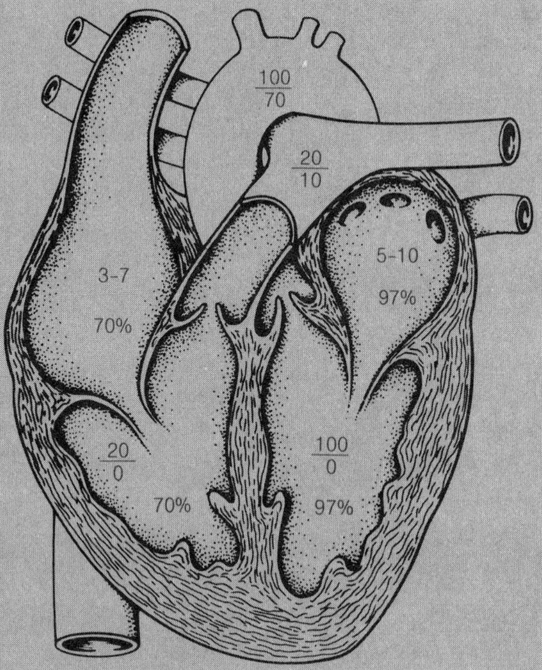

During diastole, pressure in the right ventricle (0) is lower than that of the right atrium (3-7 mm Hg) so blood flows through the tricuspid valve from the atrium into the ventricle
During systole, pressure in the right ventricle increases to 15-25 mm Hg. The tricuspid valve is closed and the pulmonary valve opens as blood is ejected from the right ventricle into the pulmonary artery (pressure=15- 25 mm Hg)
100/70
20/10
3-7
70%
5-10
97%
20/0
70%
100/0
97%
Pressure in the left atrium is higher (5-10 mm Hg) than that of the left ventricle during diastole so blood flows through the mitral valve to fill the ventricle
During systole, pressure in the left ventricle rises to 90-140 mm Hg and ejects blood into the aorta (100-120 mm Hg). During systole the mitral valve is closed and the aortic valve opens

Oxygen saturation (percentage) and pressures during diastole and systole.

Atrium A thin-walled muscular chamber that receives blood.

Cardiac output The volume of blood ejected by the left ventricle and expressed as liters of blood per minute. It is the heart rate times the volume of blood ejected by the left ventricle during each heartbeat.

Coronary arteries The first branching of the aorta, immediately distal to the aortic valve and consisting of vessels that supply blood to the heart muscle itself.

Coronary sinus The opening of the coronary veins into the right atrium.

Diastole Relaxation of the cardiac muscle.

Main pulmonary artery Divides into right and left pulmonary arteries and conducts deoxygenated blood from the right ventricle into the lungs.

Oxygen saturation The percentage of hemoglobin that is combined with oxygen. Deoxygenated blood (oxygen-poor blood returning to the heart from the body) has an oxygen saturation of 70%–75%. Oxygenated blood (oxygen-rich blood circulating from the heart to the body) has an oxygen saturation of 95%–98%.

Pulmonary veins Return oxygenated blood from the lungs to the left atrium.

Sinus node The normal pacemaker of the heart. It is a microscopic collection of specialized myocardial tissue, which generates electrical impulses that stimulate atrial contraction.

Systole Contraction of the cardiac muscle.

Valves Thin flaps of tough but flexible fibrous tissue that allow blood to flow forward but not backward. Two types of valves are (1) the *atrioventricular valves* consisting of the *tricuspid valve* between the right atrium and ventricle and the *mitral valve* between the left atrium and ventricle and (2) the *semilunar valves* such as the *pulmonic valve* between the right ventricle and the pulmonary artery and the *aortic valve* between the left ventricle and the aorta.

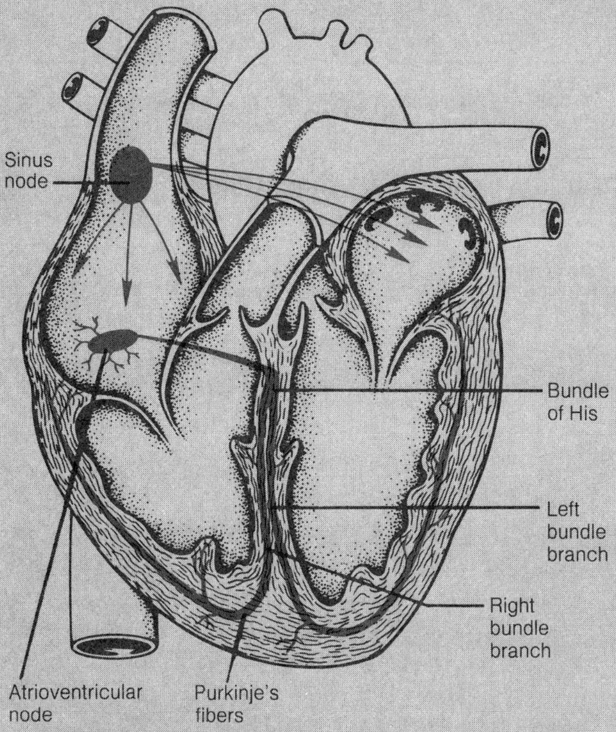

Cardiac conduction system.

Vena cavae Great vessels that return venous blood from the body into the right atrium. The superior vena cava conducts venous drainage from head, neck, and arms and upper portions of the thorax. The inferior vena cava conducts blood returning from areas below the diaphragm and lower portions of the thorax.

Ventricle A thick-walled muscular chamber that forcefully ejects blood.

Because the heart is a pump intended to propel blood in one direction, the movement of blood by the heart obeys the laws of hemodynamics. In essence, blood (or fluid) flows from a high-pressure to a low-pressure area. Systemic venous blood returns to the right atrium propelled by the force of gravity (from the head and neck) or assisted by the pumping action of skeletal muscles, especially in the legs and one-way valves in the veins. Pressurement, which varies considerably from person to person and among persons of different ages (see Appendix B; see also the figure showing internal cardiac pressure).

The Electrical System

The heart contracts when it is stimulated by rhythmic electrical impulses that originate in the sinus node. From the sinus node, the electrical impulse travels in concentric waves throughout the left and right atria, causing atrial contraction. From the atria the impulse reaches the atrioventricular node which is the bundle of His (collection of Purkinje fibers prior to dividing). At the atrioventricular junction, the Purkinje fibers form two bundle branches. The impulse then travels down the bundle branches and to the cells in the ventricles, causing ventricular contraction. (See the figure showing the electrical conduction system.)

Embryonic Development of the Cardiovascular System

The heart is one of the first organs formed, and the cardiovascular system is the first system to function. Its developmental sequence is important, for it allows the embryo to receive an adequate supply of nutrients and to dispose of wastes, thus facilitating rapid growth. The primitive heart is a fairly straight tube consisting of only two chambers. Between the second and seventh week of gestation, however, this tube undergoes a series of rotations and partitionings, thereby creating a four-chamber heart and its great arteries. The table that follows shows the embryonic development of the heart.

At approximately the twenty-first day after conception, the blood begins circulating, and the heart begins beating. The lungs cannot exchange gas in utero, so gas exchange takes place in the placenta. Maternal and fetal blood remain separate in the placenta, which functions as an interface for gas, nutrient, and waste exchange between the two separate circulatory systems. (Refer to the illustration of fetal circulation.)

After birth, the lungs expand, and the umbilical arteries and veins are severed. The neonate's lungs take over the role of oxygenating the blood. Now, blood from the right ventricle, which in utero had passed through the *patent ductus arteriosus,* perfuses the lungs. The ductus arteriosus is no longer necessary, and it closes functionally by 48 hours of age and structurally by 6 weeks of age. The *ductus venosus* likewise obliterates, becoming the *ligamentum venosum.* The *foramen ovale* closes as a result of pressure on the valvelike opening from decreased pulmonary resistance, lowered right atrial pressure, and increased atrial pressure.

(Continues)

ESSENTIALS OF STRUCTURE AND FUNCTION *(Continued)*

The Cardiovascular System

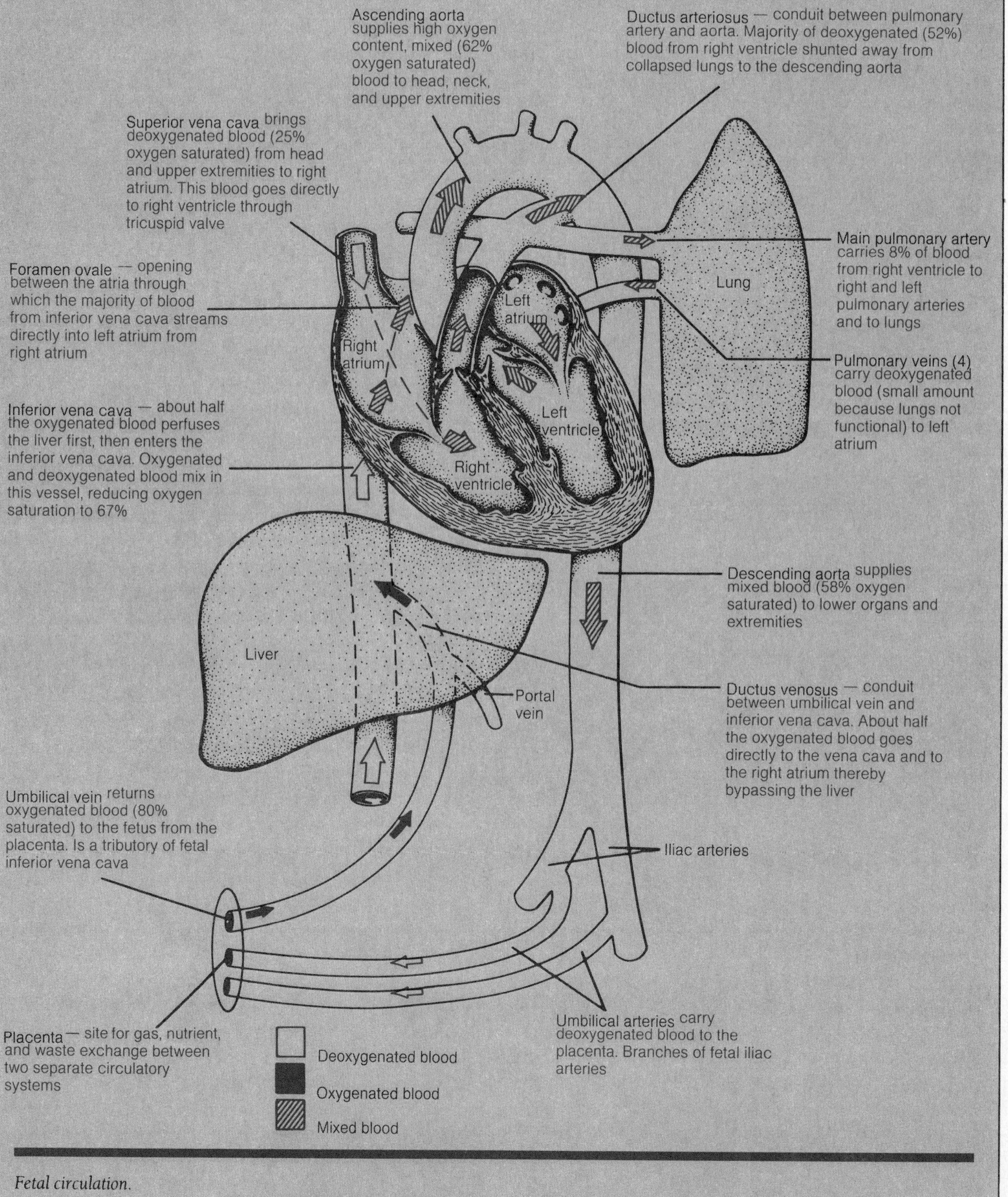

Ascending aorta supplies high oxygen content, mixed (62% oxygen saturated) blood to head, neck, and upper extremities
Ductus arteriosus — conduit between pulmonary artery and aorta. Majority of deoxygenated (52%) blood from right ventricle shunted away from collapsed lungs to the descending aorta
Superior vena cava brings deoxygenated blood (25% oxygen saturated) from head and upper extremities to right atrium. This blood goes directly to right ventricle through tricuspid valve
Main pulmonary artery carries 8% of blood from right ventricle to right and left pulmonary arteries and to lungs
Foramen ovale — opening between the atria through which the majority of blood from inferior vena cava streams directly into left atrium from right atrium
Lung
Left atrium
Right atrium
Pulmonary veins (4) carry deoxygenated blood (small amount because lungs not functional) to left atrium
Inferior vena cava — about half the oxygenated blood perfuses the liver first, then enters the inferior vena cava. Oxygenated and deoxygenated blood mix in this vessel, reducing oxygen saturation to 67%
Left ventricle
Right ventricle
Descending aorta supplies mixed blood (58% oxygen saturated) to lower organs and extremities
Liver
Portal vein
Ductus venosus — conduit between umbilical vein and inferior vena cava. About half the oxygenated blood goes directly to the vena cava and to the right atrium thereby bypassing the liver
Umbilical vein returns oxygenated blood (80% saturated) to the fetus from the placenta. Is a tributory of fetal inferior vena cava
Iliac arteries
Umbilical arteries carry deoxygenated blood to the placenta. Branches of fetal iliac arteries
Placenta — site for gas, nutrient, and waste exchange between two separate circulatory systems
Deoxygenated blood
Oxygenated blood
Mixed blood

Fetal circulation.

Embryonic Development of the Heart and Potential Abnormalities

Conversion of the heart tube to final form	Example of defects
Rotation	
Shift of primitive structures to adult relationship to left ventricle	Dextroversion—heart rotated to the right plus anomalies such as transposition of the great arteries or ventricular septal defect and pulmonary stenosis
Partitioning or separation	
Division of the atrioventricular canal into mitral and tricuspid orifices	Endocardial cushion defects Atrial septal defect primum and mitral insufficiency or incomplete atrioventricular canal
Formation of the proximal ascending aorta and the pulmonary trunk from the truncus arteriosus	Truncus arteriosus, persistent Defects in semilunar aortic or pulmonary valves
Formation of the right and left ventricular outflow tracts	Defects in position or competency of outflow tracts such as double outlet right ventricle
Formation of the muscular portion of the ventricular septum	Ventricular septal defect
Formation of the atrial septa	Atrial septal defect, secundum Atrial septal defect, primum

Changes in pressure and resistance also occur in pulmonary and systemic circulation after birth. After delivery, as the neonate's lungs expand, oxygen in the precapillary vessels causes dilatation of the pulmonary vasculature, and pulmonary resistance to blood flow drops markedly. Simultaneously, as the umbilical cord is cut, systemic vascular resistance increases. Thus blood from the right ventricle flows to the pulmonary system; shunting across the fetal structures decreases; the structures begin to close; and by 6 weeks of age, the structures should be closed completely.

These postnatal changes in resistance and blood flow explain why some types of heart disease might not be recognized in the neonatal period. Symptoms of heart disease might not be present until the fetal structures are closed.

The cardiovascular system consists of a pump (the heart) and a series of conduits (arteries and veins) that move blood to and from organs for the purpose of supplying the metabolic needs of the organs and removing metabolic products. Because its function is essential to life, any dysfunction of the cardiovascular system is serious and often life threatening.

Treatment for cardiovascular disorders often requires surgery, extended periods of hospitalization, and long-term follow-up care. The stress of a child's cardiac condition can also place the family at risk for dysfunction. (The implications of chronic childhood conditions are discussed in Chapter 14.)

Assessment of the Child with Cardiovascular Dysfunction

Physiologic Effects of Cardiac Defects and Disease

To understand and be able to assess the acute-care needs of the child with cardiovascular problems, the nurse needs to understand the physiologic effects that occur most commonly as a result of cardiac disease. Not all of these effects occur with each type of cardiac problem. In general, cardiac defects are defined as alterations in blood flow and in pressure related to the presence of shunts or obstructions.

Shunts Blood always flows from an area of high pressure to an area of low pressure and takes the path of least resistance. Blood flow through an abnormal communication between the right and left sides of the heart is called a *shunt*.

Left-to-right shunts Normally, pressures in the left side of the heart are significantly higher than the pressures on the right side of the heart. Therefore, if there is an abnormal opening in the septum between the right and left sides, blood flows from the left to the right. If the abnormal opening (called a *septal defect*) is small, only a small amount of blood flows or shunts through it. If the septal defect is large, a large volume of blood flows left to right, creating a left-to-right shunt.

This type of shunt usually does not cause significant *hypoxemia* (decreased arterial oxygen saturation) and *cyanosis* (blue-tinged skin caused by hypoxemia). The workload of the right side of the heart is increased because the right ventricle must pump its normal volume of blood plus the extra volume shunting from the left side. The heart responds by pumping at a faster rate (causing tachycardia) and by pumping more blood with each contraction. This increased workload causes the myocardial fibers to enlarge and the right ventricle to dilatate, resulting in *cardiomegaly* (cardiac enlargement).

The lungs normally receive blood from the right ventricle under relatively low pressure. With a left-to-right shunt, the lungs are exposed to an increased volume of blood under high pressure. Tachypnea, dyspnea, and pulmonary edema might result. Blood pools in the lungs and creates conditions that promote bacterial growth. Recurrent respiratory infections occur. In an attempt to protect the lungs from the increased volume and pressure, *hypertrophy* (thickening) of pulmonary arterial walls develops. Hypertrophy increases the resistance of blood flow to the lungs, causing pulmonary arterial hypertension. Although this is a helpful short-term response, severe restriction of pulmonary blood flow might occur over time. If not treated, the changes become irreversible. Because they do not directly cause hypoxemia and cyanosis, septal defects that result in left-to-right shunting are among the *acyanotic heart diseases*.

Under certain circumstances, a left-to-right shunt might reverse direction so that blood flows from right to left. This usually occurs when pressure in the pulmonary circulation increases. It might occur as the lungs are subjected to high volumes and pressure from a left-to-right shunt over time, causing pulmonary hypertension, which might reach a point at which the pressure in the right ventricle exceeds pressure in the left ventricle, so that the shunt reverses.

Right-to-left shunts In some types of defects, the pressure in the right side of the heart might be greater than in the left side of the heart. This might occur if resistance in the lungs is abnormally high or if the pulmonary artery is constricted. If a septal defect is also present, deoxygenated blood from the right side of the heart shunts to the left side and out into the body (blood from the right side normally goes to the lungs). Significant right-to-left shunting might be due to any of a number of defects known collectively as *cyanotic heart disease*.

Hypoxemia in the systemic circulation results in *hypoxia* (decreased tissue oxygenation). Secondary polycythemia (increase in red blood cells) develops as the body attempts to compensate for hypoxemia by producing more red blood cells. Although secondary polycythemia enables the blood to carry more oxygen, it has important negative effects. The viscosity of the blood increases significantly, thus creating resistance to the blood flow, making the heart pump harder to overcome the resistance. Circulation becomes sluggish, and the risk of thrombus, or clot, formation increases.

A right-to-left shunt also causes a portion of the blood to bypass the filtering system of the lungs. Bacteria or emboli might pass through the shunt and go to the brain, causing a stroke or brain abscess.

Chronic hypoxia might also result in metabolic acidosis, which might be partially compensated. In normal metabolism, pyruvic acid is converted into carbon dioxide, water, and energy in the Krebs cycle. This process requires oxygen. If sufficient oxygen is not available, pyruvic acid is anaerobically converted to lactic acid, which collects in the tissues and causes acidosis. The body can compensate for mild acidosis, but severe acidosis, if not promptly treated, leads to death.

Obstruction defects In *obstruction defects* the forward progress of the blood is impeded by a narrowing or blockage in the valves or great vessels. Obstructive lesions generally create elevated pressure proximally and decreased pressure distally. Congestive heart failure might occur as a result of obstructive lesions.

History

Children with heart disease often have histories of decreased tolerance for exercise. They might become excessively fatigued or short of breath with normal activity because of hypoxemia, inadequate myocardial function, or obstruction to cardiac outflow. The parent might first become aware of this when the infant becomes fatigued and breathless during feedings, taking only limited quantities of milk before needing to rest. Infants with heart disease also might have weak cries and hypotonic or flaccid postures. The older child might be unable to keep up with siblings and peers, might need to stop and rest at intervals, or might consciously select quiet, more sedentary activities.

The nurse inquires about changes in the child's skin color, because children with heart disease often have unusually pale or mottled skin or varying degrees of cyanosis, ranging from a mild blue tinge of the lips during exercise to severe cyanosis at rest. The nurse asks the parent whether the child has experienced dizziness, syncope (fainting), diaphoresis (profuse perspiration), congested cough, edema, rapid respirations, or repeated respiratory infections. A tendency to assume a squatting posture might also be a sign of heart disease. Hypoxic spells are assessed for frequency, severity, precipitating factors, and family management. In addition, the nurse refers to the child's medical record or asks the parent about any delays in physical growth and development.

Any of the child's symptoms are then further assessed according to severity, frequency, chronology, aggravating and alleviating factors, setting, associated symptoms and changes, and impact on the child and family. If the child is known to have heart disease, the nurse documents when the diagnosis was made, the course of the disease, and the management thus far.

The nurse also explores the health of the mother during pregnancy. Any illness, particularly infectious illness, should be noted. Several viral infections (rubella and infections due to cytomegalovirus, coxsackie, and herpes hominis B viruses) are known to be associated with congenital heart disease. Maternal diabetes, alcoholism, and poor nutrition also have been associated with heart disease in the infant. Any medications taken by the mother are noted. Folic acid antagonists, anticonvulsants, progesterone, estrogen, and warfarin are thought to be related to heart defects. Exposure to radiation also might be a cause of congenital defects.

The nurse ascertains whether any intrapartum or postpartum complications were present. Low birth weight, prematurity, congenital infections, cyanosis, respiratory problems (respiratory distress syndrome, apneic spells, hypoxic spells), and heart murmur might all indicate an increased risk of heart problems.

The nurse inquires about previous or concurrent conditions that might be associated with cardiac disease. Several genetic syndromes have congenital heart disease as one manifestation. Streptococcal pharyngitis is an antecedent to rheumatic fever and rheumatic heart disease. Repeated respiratory infections might be related to congestive heart failure. Subacute bacterial endocarditis and Kawasaki disease (see Chapter 25) might lead to chronic cardiac disease. Myocarditis is a rare complication of certain viral diseases.

The nurse further inquires about congenital heart disease or genetic disorders in any blood relative. A history of atherosclerosis, hyperlipidemia, hypertension, stroke, myocardial infarction, or arrhythmia in a family member indicates that the child is at increased risk for acquired heart disease.

Although most children with heart disease have normal intelligence, children with certain genetic defects (such as Down's syndrome) or histories of severe hypoxia might be mentally disabled. A thorough developmental assessment of all children with cardiac disease thus is essential. Even the child with cardiac disease and normal cognitive development might show significant physical developmental delays, and delay in one area of development potentially affects performance in other developmental areas. (Developmental disabilities are discussed in Chapter 15.)

Because cardiac disease might have an impact on the child's nutritional status, the nurse explores the child's feeding behavior and diet history. Exercise intolerance might limit the amount of nutrients an infant is able to ingest. Anorexia might be a side effect of medications or congestive heart failure caused by liver and bowel edema. The nurse also notes the occurrence of fatigue, dyspnea, cyanosis, or diaphoresis during feeding. If the child is to be hospitalized, specific feeding routines used at home should be recorded and integrated into the plan of care. If the child is on a special diet (for example, a high-calorie or low-sodium diet), the nurse determines how the family has managed the diet.

Physical Examination

The physical examination of the child with a suspected cardiac disorder is similar to that for any child (see Chapter 10). However, special attention is given to the following:

Measurement: Vital sign measurement gives important clues to the child's status. Blood pressure is measured in all four extremities, with pressure in the arm and leg on one side being measured simultaneously, and compared to the norms for the child's age (see Appendix B). The *pulse pressure,* or the difference between the systolic and diastolic pressures (normally 20–50 mm Hg), can be elevated or decreased with certain cardiac dysfunction.

Inspection: Assessment of skin color, particularly any degree of cyanosis, is important. Cyanosis in children with

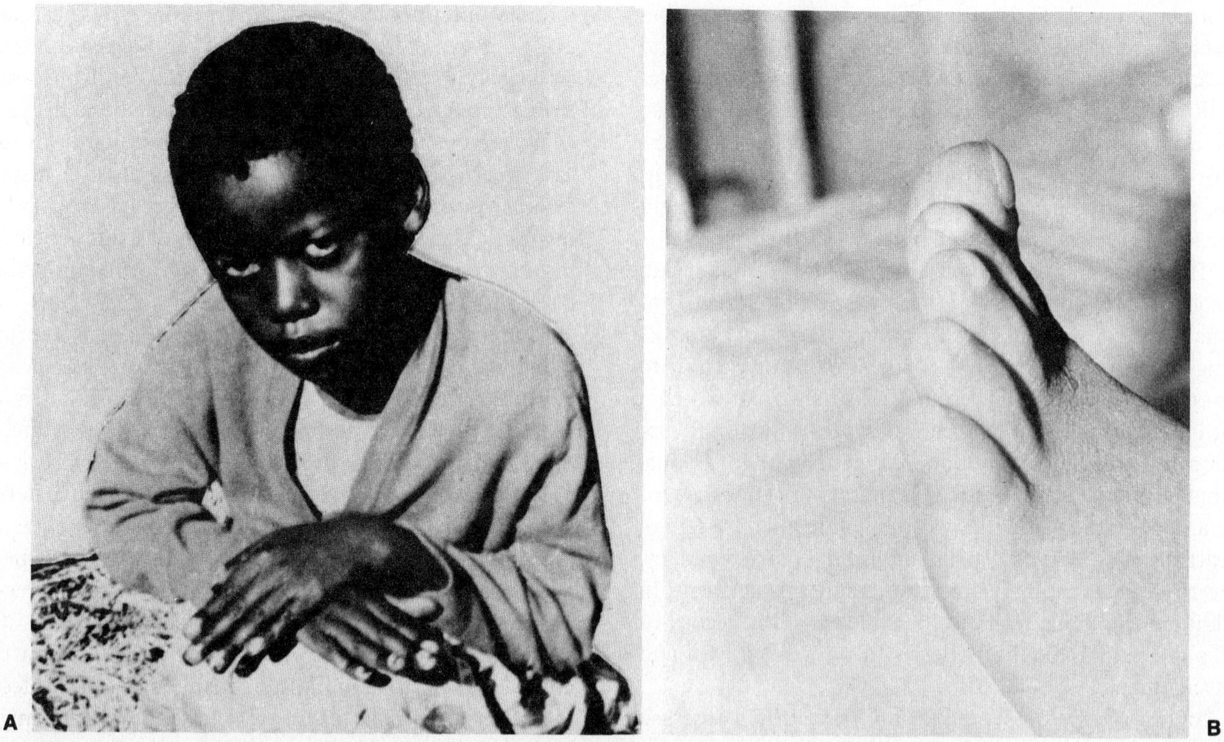

A. This child had a severe cyanotic cardiac defect. Note the crouched posture and the swelling fingertips into clublike configuration. ***B.*** *Note clubbing of the toes. (From Purtilo DT:* A Survey of Human Diseases. *Addison-Wesley, 1978, p. 68.)*

TABLE 23-1 Abnormal Pulse Patterns

Pulse	Characteristics
Thready pulse	Weak, difficult to palpate, seems to appear and disappear
Water-hammer (Corrigan's) pulse	Very forceful and jerky, associated with wide pulse pressure
Pulsus alternans	Alterations of weak and strong beats without changes in cycle length
Paradoxical pulse	Force weaker with inspiration and stronger with expiration
Sinus arrhythmia pulse	Rate increases with inspiration and decreases with expiration
Bigeminal pulse	Beats occur in pairs because of premature beats

dark skin is most evident in the mucous membranes of the mouth, which might have a violet hue. The extent of any cyanosis, the effect of activity on skin color, and how color reacts to oxygen administration (if ordered) is noted. The child's posture, the extent of any edema, and any clubbing (widened, thickened fingertips or tips of the toes) due to chronic hypoxia is described.

Palpation: Peripheral pulses are palpated and any abnormal pulse is recorded (see Table 23-1). Digits are palpated for capillary refill to assess tissue perfusion. Because hepatomegaly (enlarged liver) is one of the cardinal signs of congestive heart failure, it is important to assess liver size in a child with cardiac problems.

Auscultation: The heart is auscultated with a stethoscope. Murmurs can occur at various points in the cardiac cycle and are caused by the turbulence of blood as it passes between cardiac chambers or into major vessels. Murmurs are classified as *innocent* (functional, benign), meaning that there is no cardiac pathology, or as *organic,* meaning that there is cardiac pathology. (Murmurs are described in Tables 23-2 and 23-3).

TABLE 23-2 Six Criteria Describing Cardiac Murmurs

Criterion	Description
1. Timing in the cardiac cycle	Murmurs can occur in systole (between S_1 and S_2) or during diastole (between S_2 and S_1). The timing can be broken down more specifically within systole or diastole. For example, a systolic murmur can be described as early systolic, midsystolic, late systolic, or holosystolic (pansystolic, or occurring throughout systole). Similar descriptions are used for diastolic murmurs. A continuous murmur is one heard throughout systole and diastole
2. Frequency	Frequency refers to the sound of the murmur, which may be high-pitched, low-pitched, or medium-pitched
3. Location	The anatomic location is noted where the murmur is heard best (for example, the left sternal border in the fourth intercostal space)
4. Radiation	Radiation indicates where, besides the location, the murmur is heard
5. Intensity	The intensity, or loudness, of murmurs is graded on a scale from I to VI, with I being the softest and VI the loudest (see Table 23-5). Intensity may have variations. Crescendo murmurs begin softly but become louder. Decrescendo murmurs begin loudly and become softer. Crescendo-decrescendo murmurs start softly, become louder, and then become soft again
6. Effect of respiration and position	The nurse notes whether the murmur increases, decreases, or remains the same during inspiration, expiration, and position changes

TABLE 23-3 Scale of Intensity of Heart Murmurs

Murmur	Characteristics
Grade I	Faint, requires careful listening
Grade II	Quiet but readily heard
Grade III	Moderately loud, no thrill
Grade IV	Loud, usually associated with thrill
Grade V	Very loud, thrill present, can be heard with only partial contact of stethoscope and chest
Grade VI	Loud, thrill present, can be heard with stethoscope off chest wall

Validating Diagnostic Tests

Children with heart disease are subjected to many laboratory studies. The experience might be new or familiar to the child, but either way, it frequently creates considerable anxiety. The procedures and equipment often are frightening, so preparation of the child for the procedure and support during and after the procedure are primary nursing responsibilities (see Chapter 20).

Blood tests Since one of the major functions of the cardiovascular system is to transport oxygen to the organs, blood studies to measure hemoglobin and hematocrit levels are basic information for assessing and managing children with cardiac defects. The body compensates for chronic hypoxia by producing increasing amounts of hemoglobin, thereby resulting in polycythemia.

Children with fluid retention might have low serum electrolyte levels because of a "dilutional" effect. Although the initial serum results, particularly of sodium, might be low, the actual levels are normal. Once diuretic therapy is given, the results return to normal. Long-term diuretic therapy might be manifested by reduced serum potassium and chloride.

The nurse observes for bleeding or bruising after blood is withdrawn. If an arterial sample is obtained, the nurse applies direct pressure to the site for at least 5 minutes and longer if bleeding persists. To prevent the trauma of repeated tests, the nurse handles specimens carefully and exactly according to instructions (for example, protected from exposure to air, packed in ice). If blood gases (Po_2, Pco_2, pH, and O_2) are to be measured from a capillary sample, the nurse applies a warm compress to the site for 10 minutes before collecting the sample. This procedure increases the reliability of results. Providing a syringe and a doll and letting the child perform tests on the doll might help the child to work through the experience. Using play in this way also gives the nurse an opportunity to assess the child's perception of the event.

Cardiographic studies Cardiographic studies are painless, but the equipment might be frightening to the child. The nurse informs the child that the test will show the

ASSESSMENT GUIDE The Child with a Cardiovascular Problem

Assessment questions	Supporting data
Does the parent (or the child) report that the child is excessively fatigued?	Poor infant feeding; weak cry; exercise intolerance with frequent rest periods for the older child; dyspnea; squatting posture during physical exertion.
Does the child's skin appear mottled, pale, or cyanotic?	Skin changes on mild exertion, during exercise, during stress, or constantly; diaphoresis (sweating); edema (often a late sign of congestive heart failure), usually periorbital or sacral but might occur in extremities; poor tissue perfusion of fingers or toes; bruising
Has the child experienced repeated respiratory infections, difficulty breathing, or cough?	Tachypnea; hacking or congested cough; altered breath sounds; dyspnea; signs of respiratory distress (see Chapter 22)
Has there been a history of maternal infection during pregnancy with this child (eg, rubella, cytomegalovirus); maternal diabetes, alcoholism, poor nutrition, medications related to cardiac defects (eg, hormones, anticonvulsants) or radiation? Has the child experienced any illness such as scarlet fever, streptococcal pharyngitis, or Kawasaki disease (see Chapter 25); does the child have a genetic defect (eg, Down's syndrome), or are there any genetic disorders or congenital heart disease in any blood relative?	Alterations in heart rate (tachycardia); alterations in cardiac rhythm—arrhythmias, abnormal pulse pattern (Table 23-1); alteration in cardiac sounds—displacement of apical beat and/or point of maximal impulse, palpable thrill or heave, murmur (Table 23-2), click, snap, friction rub, gallop rhythm, fixed split of S_2; alterations in blood pressure—lower blood pressure in legs than arms or difference in pressure between arms, hypertension; decreased peripheral pulses, widened pulse pressure; delayed capillary refill; coolness, pallor, or mottling of extremities; clubbing of fingers and toes; polycythemia; distention of jugular veins; precordial bulge
Does the child have a history of feeding difficulties, poor weight gain, or decreased growth in relation to norms?	Anorexia; nausea, vomiting, diarrhea; abdominal pain and tenderness on palpation; hepatomegaly (liver enlargement); ascites (fluid in the abdominal cavity); poor muscle development with thin extremities

Additional data: Changes in urine output with alterations in urine specific gravity; fainting; anxiety, restlessness, alterations in level of consciousness, seizures.

doctors and nurses how the heart is working. Older children might be interested in more details regarding the specific test. The nurse reminds the child that it is very important that the child remain still and quiet during procedures. (Cardiographic studies are summarized in Table 23-4.)

Electrocardiogram The *electrocardiogram* (ECG) is a measurement of the electrical activity of the heart. It is used to detect cardiac rhythm and cardiac chamber thickness (hypertrophy). The normal electrocardiogram consists of a P-wave; a P-Q interval; Q-, R-, and S-waves; an S-T interval; and a T-wave. The P-wave reflects electrical activation of the left and right atria (Fig. 23-1). The P-Q interval reflects a pause during which the electrical impulse travels from the atria to the ventricles through the atrioventricular junction and bundle of His. The QRS deflection indicates ventricular electrical activity. The S-T interval reflects the delay between depolarization and repolarization. The T-wave results from ventricular repolarization.

Because electrical activity begins in the sinus node and progresses through the atria and then the ventricles, the normal electrocardiogram is characterized by a P-wave followed by a QRS complex and then a T-wave. The appearance of the P-wave and QRS complex is affected by the thickness of the respective chambers and by the exact route by which myocardial depolarization occurs. Thus the electrocardiogram is useful for detecting enlargement of cardiac chambers and determining whether the sequence of electrical conduction through the heart is normal. Interpretation of electrocardiograms is complex and requires special

TABLE 23-4 Cardiographic Studies

Study	Purpose	Procedure	Nursing management
Electrocardiogram (ECG)	Measure electrical activity of heart in one dimension (plus time) to detect arrhythmias, cardiomegaly, myocardial hypertrophy	Electrodes attached to arms, legs, chest. Electrical activity recorded on graph	Explain procedure to the child. Instruct child to remain still during procedure. Allow child to "play ECG" with doll. Clean off electrode jelly after procedure
Vectorcardiogram	Measure electrical activity of heart in three dimensions (plus time) to detect changes relative to altered conduction (arrhythmias, cardiomegaly)	Same as for ECG	Same as for ECG
Phonocardiogram	Obtain visual image of heart sounds and, in combination with ECG, timing of cardiac events	Microphone or transducer moved over chest. Pattern of heart sounds recorded on strip-chart graph	Explain procedure to child. Instruct child to remain still and quiet during procedure. Allow child to "play phonocardiogram" with doll. Practice procedure ahead of time
Echocardiogram	Visualize cardiac structures by recording sound waves bounced off of them	Same as for phonocardiogram	Same as for phonocardiogram
Radiography	See cardiac structures to detect abnormalities and distinguish cardiac from pulmonary disease. Assess volume of pulmonary blood flow. Detect (with barium) aberrant blood vessels around esophagus	Standard anteroposterior and lateral views taken of chest Barium esophagogram	Describe room and equipment to child. Explain procedure to child. Remain with child if appropriate (see Chapter 20). Instruct child to remain still while radiographs taken. Explain use of barium and need to drink special liquid, lie on table that will tilt, probability of white bowel movements due to barium
Radioisotope scanning	Visualize anatomy and hemodynamics in cardiac structures. Measure left ventricular ejection and chamber volume	Isotope injected intravenously. Scanner detects and records isotope distribution on chart	Explain procedure and equipment to child. Prepare child for insertion of intravenous line
Cardiac catheterization	Measure oxygen saturation and pressures in cardiac chambers and major vessels. Measure direction and volume of blood flow. Assess anatomy of cardiac structures. Assess electrophysiologic function of the heart	Cardiac catheter introduced into femoral or brachial vessel and advanced to the heart Catheter guided into cardiac chambers and major vessels (visualized by fluoroscopy). Pressure and oxygen saturation measured at various points. Radiopaque dye injected into catheter. Blood flow visualized by fluoroscopy; radiographs taken at selected times. Balloon septostomy may be done during procedure	Obtain history and perform physical assessment prior to procedure. Explain procedure to child and parent. Obtain baseline vital signs. Document pulses distal to catheter site. Keep child NPO 4–6 hours prior to procedure. Withhold digoxin, as ordered. After procedure, monitor for signs of complications (arrhythmias, hemorrhage, infection, impaired circulation, adverse reaction to dye or medication, dehydration). Encourage fluids once fully awake (about 1–2 hours after procedure). Keep involved extremity straight and relatively immobile for approximately 6 hours. Prepare the child and family for discharge, if appropriate

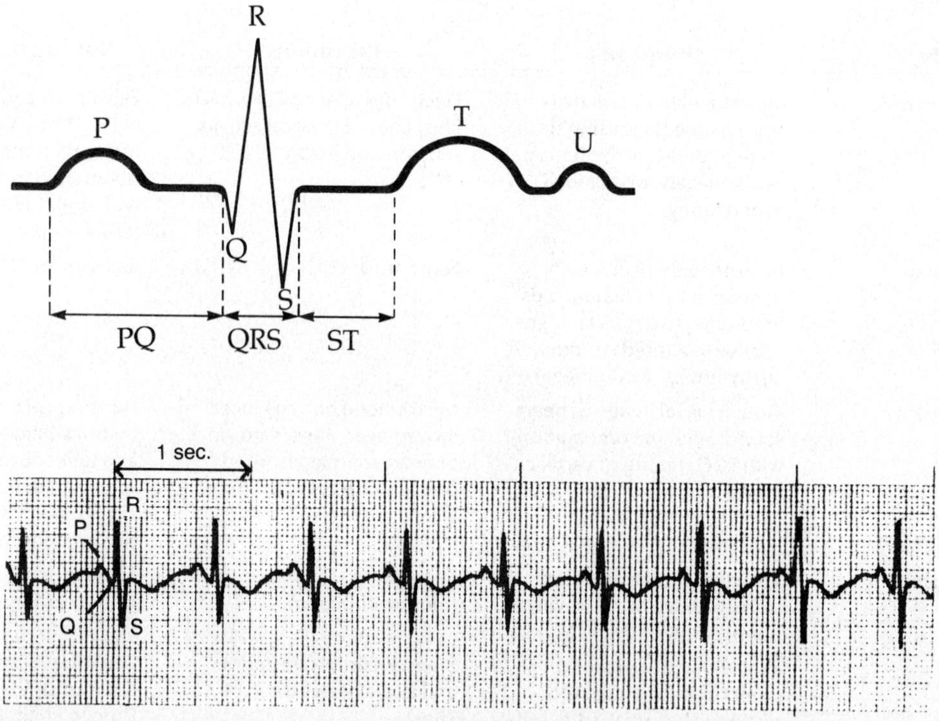

FIGURE 23-1
Normal electrocardiogram.

training and experience. (Normal electrocardiographic findings are in Table 23-5; a few common arrhythmias are presented in Fig. 23-2.)

Vectorcardiogram Because the heart is a three-dimensional structure, its electrical activation is also three-dimensional. Unlike the electrocardiogram, which reflects electrical activity in only one physical plane (plus time), the *vectorcardiogram* reflects electrical activation of the heart in three dimensions (plus time). The vectorcardiogram can reflect cardiac chamber enlargement when the electrocardiographic assessment is indefinite.

Phonocardiogram The *phonocardiogram* (Fig. 23-3) is recorded using a microphone placed on the child's chest. The heart sounds are recorded on a strip-chart recorder. Combined with a simultaneously obtained electrocardiogram and carotid pulse tracing, a phonocardiogram can measure time intervals between important cardiac events.

Echocardiogram *Echocardiography* is a technique of visualizing cardiac anatomy by recording sound waves reflected from cardiac structures. Sound is beamed through

TABLE 23-5 Normal Electrocardiographic Findings

Measurement	Norm
Rate	The number of beats per minute depends on oxygen needs and electrophysiologic function. The normal range varies with age
Regularity	The interval between beats (R–R interval) should be consistent
Association between P-wave and QRS complex	The P-wave should precede each QRS complex, and the P–R interval should be consistent
Configuration of P-wave, QRS complex, and T-wave	The configuration should be consistent for each

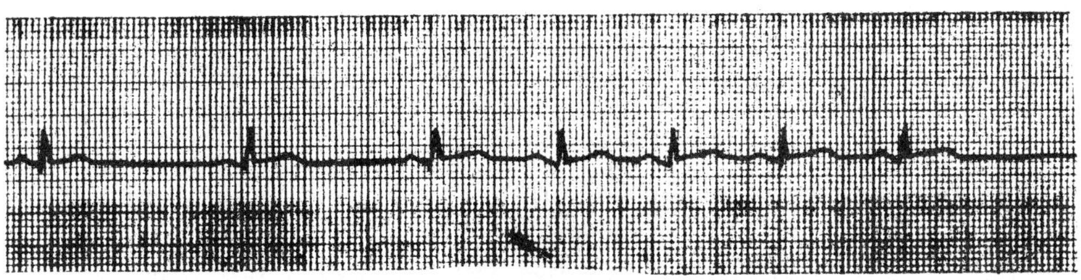

Sinus arrythmic

Originates in SA node
Rhythm is irregular and is influenced by respirations and vagal tone
P–R tone interval is normal
P-waves precede each QRS
QRS complex and T-waves are normal

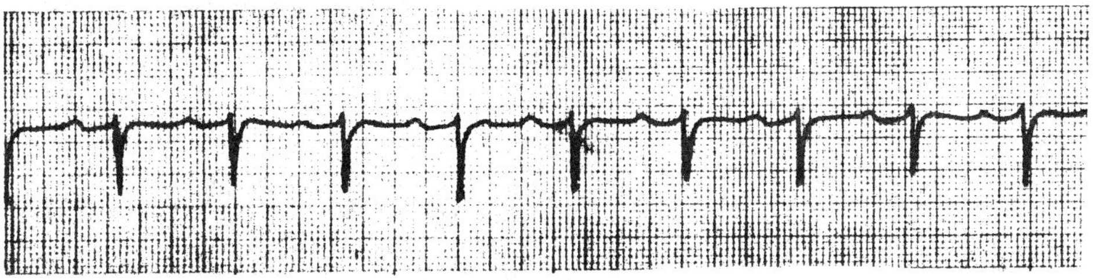

First-degree heart block

Conduction through AV node is delayed
Rate is normal
Rhythm is regular
P-waves precede each QRS
P–R interval is long (>0.2 seconds)
QRS is normal

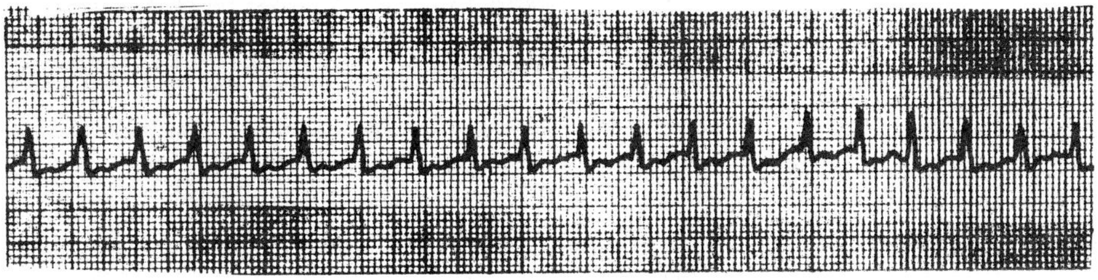

Paroxysmal atrial tachycardia (PAT)

Originates in ectopic focus in atria
Rate is rapid (160–240)
Rhythm is regular
P-waves precede each QRS
P–R interval may be shortened
QRS complex is normal

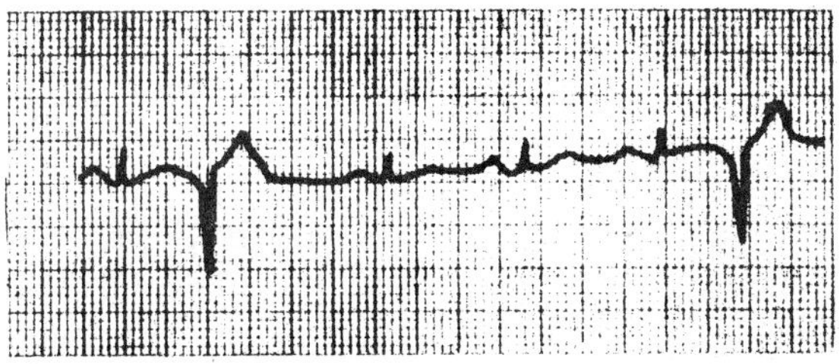

Premature ventricular contraction (PVC)
(Unifocal)

Impulse originates in ventricle prematurely and is followed by compensatory pause
Rate is normal
Rhythm is irregular
P-wave may be obscured by QRS of the PVC
QRS complex is wide and bizarre, originating from same focus in ventricle;
QRS shape is consistent (unifocal)

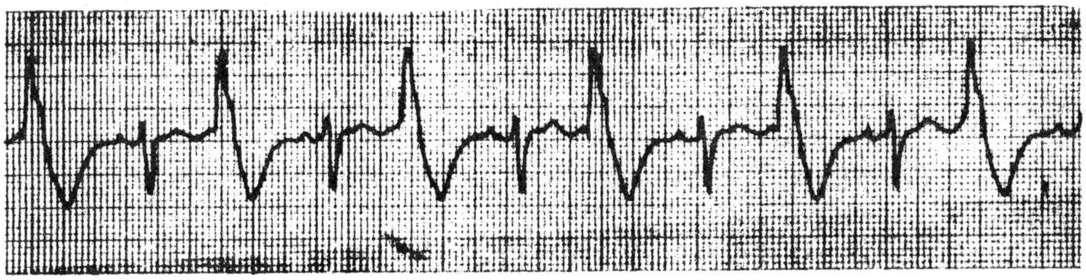

PVC is alternated with normal sinus beat

FIGURE 23-2

Abnormal electrocardiograms.

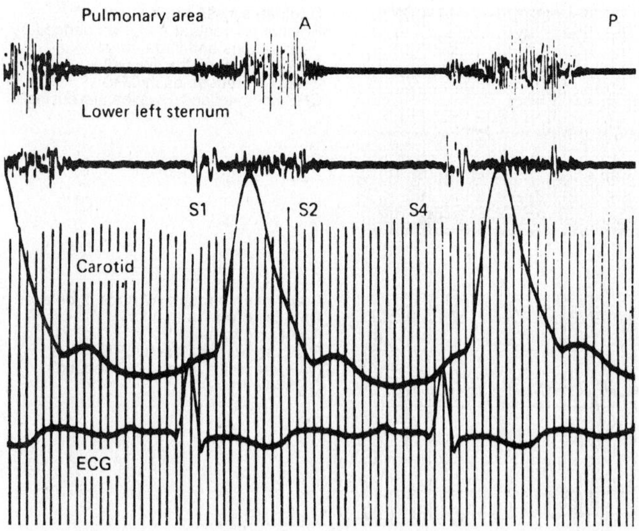

FIGURE 23-3
Phonocardiogram.

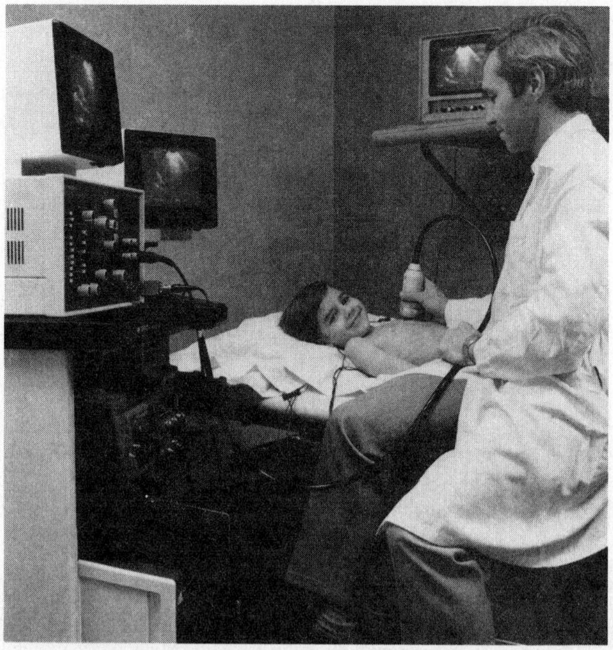

Echocardiography. (Courtesy of the Mayo Clinic, Rochester, Minnesota.)

the heart, and sound beams reflected from cardiac structures are recorded. There are two basic types of echocardiography: (1) M-mode and (2) two-dimensional (sector) echocardiography. M-mode echocardiography records only a very narrow beam of sound activity, which limits the structures that can be visualized. Two-dimensional (sector) echocardiography, as the term implies, allows the clinician to visualize cardiac structures in two dimensions (plus time). This technique provides much better definition of intracardiac structures than M-mode echocardiography.

Radioactive tracers *Radioactive tracers* use radioisotope techniques to define intracardiac anatomy, including shunts and anatomic details, and cardiac function such as hemodynamic measurements. Left ventricular chamber volume can be determined relatively easily and reproducibly by using these techniques. In addition, pulmonary blood flow can be mapped and alterations detected.

Cardiac catheterization *Cardiac catheterization* is an invasive procedure. A small catheter is usually introduced percutaneously into the large vessels (usually the femoral vein and artery) and advanced to the heart. The procedure is done in a room equipped for fluoroscopic visualization. A radiopaque contrast material injected through the catheter aids in fluoroscopic visualization of cardiac structure and direction of blood flow. The frequency of cardiac catheterization has diminished since echocardiographic techniques and information from such studies have improved.

Nursing Management for Procedures and Treatments

Cardiographic Studies

For all cardiographic procedures, practicing with the equipment ahead of time helps to diminish the child's fear during the procedure. For example, the child undergoing electrocardiogram needs to be given a chance to "play ECG" with a doll. Preparation for a phonocardiogram and echocardiogram is similar to preparation for an electrocardiogram, but in addition, a microphone or transducer is moved over the chest. It is important that the child hold still. Practicing holding still and using a "pretend transducer" ahead of time might alleviate anxiety and enhance cooperation.

Cardiac Catheterization

An increased number of cardiac catheterizations are now done on an outpatient basis. The child has the preprocedure examination and blood studies done the day prior to the exam. The nurse gives the parents and the child both oral and written instructions about the procedure to follow the evening and morning before the cardiac cathe-

PROCEDURE *Electrocardiogram*

- Explain to the child and parent that the purpose of the electrocardiogram is to record the activity of the heart in picture form. This can be compared to the idea of a television recording a picture of some activity.
- The child might be taken to a special room for the test.
- The child will be asked to lie on the back while electrodes are being applied. Assure the child that the test will not hurt.
- Show the child an electrode and allow the child to handle it in order to decrease anxiety.
- The electrodes will be placed in various locations on the body depending upon the reading desired. The arms, legs, and chest are areas frequently used. Conductor gel will be used under each electrode. The gel will feel cold to the child.
- During the time the tracing is taken, the child will hear a soft whirring machine sound. The child should be encouraged to remain quiet during the test and a parent may remain with the child for reassurance and to decrease anxiety.
- The test usually takes less than a half hour.
- After the procedure the gel is removed with mild soap and water.

terization. The family is told to call with any questions. Some institutions have developed booklets explaining the procedure and including pictures to color or activities to complete as a preparation aid.

A history and physical examination should be completed before cardiac catheterization. The thoroughness of this exam depends on the timing of the last exam and on any significant symptoms or changes that might be present. The physical examination provides baseline data and allows recognition of changes that might occur as a result of the procedure. Any sign of infection (for example, fever, cough, nasal discharge, sore throat) is reported to the physician. Infection increases the risk of the procedure considerably and is a contraindication except in an emergency.

It is helpful to mark with ink the exact location of pulses distal to the proposed catheter-insertion site. If a femoral vessel is to be used, the posterior tibial and dorsal pedal pulses are marked. The quality and strength of the pulse also is documented, as this information makes the critical assessment of pulses after the procedure more accurate.

Usually, a complete blood count and urinalysis are done before the procedure. Clotting studies might also be indicated. To prevent aspiration, the child is generally kept NPO for 4 to 6 hours before the procedure. Digoxin is usually withheld before the procedure, although this should be clarified with the physician. The nurse also inquires about allergies to medications, especially reactions to medication or the radiopaque contrast material that might have occurred during previous catheterizations.

Cardiac catheterization is often a stressful and frightening procedure for children, and careful preparation therefore is essential. Family members might also fear the diagnosis and prognosis that will be revealed, and this adds to their anxiety (see procedure for cardiac catheterization).

Possible complications following cardiac catheterization include cardiac arrhythmias, hemorrhage (from catheter site or from cardiac perforation), infection, swelling and inflammation at the site, phlebitis, thrombus, adverse reactions to radiopaque contrast material (dye), and dehydration. Skilled nursing care is essential if these complications are to be recognized or avoided.

When checking vital signs, the nurse also carefully assesses circulation in the extremity used for the catheterization. Arterial spasm, thrombus formation, phlebitis, or excessive swelling at the site all can obstruct blood flow into the extremity. The nurse palpates pulses distal to the catheter site. The opposite extremity can be used for comparison. If the pulses are not easily palpable, a Doppler device can be used to locate them. A weak or absent pulse is reported to the physician immediately. The nurse also assesses temperature, color, and capillary refill of the affected extremity. Coolness, pallor, cyanosis, swelling, and delayed capillary refill might be further indications of compromised circulation and should be reported. Wrapping the unaffected leg in a warm pack causes vasodilatation in both legs and might increase blood flow to the affected extremity. The affected extremity is not warmed, as the application of heat would increase metabolic demands at a time when circulation is

PROCEDURE *Cardiac Catheterization*

- Assess the child's perception of cardiac function, symptoms, and reason for hospitalization. Explain that the test will help the doctor know how to make the heart work better. Explain that the child will not be able to eat or drink before the test.
- Describe the appearance of the room and allow the child to visit if hospital policy allows. The child will be brought to the room by stretcher.
- Explain that the parent will not be allowed in the room with the child but will be waiting in a specified location and will return right after the test.
- Explain what the child will see in the catheterization room—people in gowns and masks, X-ray equipment, and a special table that moves. Allow the child to handle masks and gowns to become familiar with the equipment. Explain the test by using a doll for demonstration.
- The child will receive a premedication, which will cause drowsiness. Explain about the premedication just prior to its administration to decrease the anxiety time.
- The child will be placed lying down on the table and electrocardiogram leads will be placed on the arms and legs. Because it is very important for the child to be still, restraints will be placed on the arms and legs. Practice applying restraints so the child will know how they feel.
- A cutaneous or rectal temperature probe will be used during the test. Demonstrate the probe to the child.
- Tell the child that the doctor will wash the arm or groin with a special soap that will feel cold. Then some medicine will be given through a small needle. The needle will hurt a little but there will be no more pain.
- The doctor will make a small incision and will thread a catheter through. The child will not feel pain but might feel pressure as the tube is advanced. Dye is inserted through the catheter. The child might feel hot for a short time. When explaining this to the child, do not use the word "dye" as it could be confused with "die."
- X-rays will be taken, and the child will hear the noise from the X-ray machine as well as a loud banging noise as films fall into a collecting box. The lights in the room might be dimmed during the X-rays, but the room will not be completely dark. Tell the child that people might leave the room during this time, but they will return quickly.
- Tell the child that it is all right to sleep during the test or to ask questions. The child might like to listen to stories or music during the procedure.
- At the completion of the test the catheter is removed and a bandage is placed on the site. The child will return to the hospital room and the nurse will check pulses, blood pressure, and the bandage. An hour or so after the test the child can have something to drink. The child will need to remain in bed for several hours depending on the physician's order.

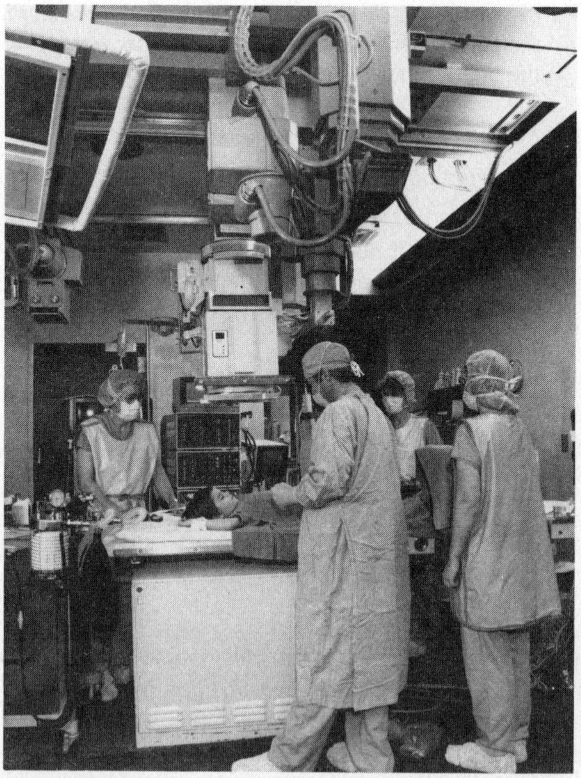

Cardiac catheterization laboratory. (Courtesy of the Mayo Clinic, Rochester, Minnesota.)

already compromised. If a thrombus is present, heparin therapy, surgery, or both might be needed.

The child usually is kept in bed for several hours after the procedure to reduce the risk of bleeding or trauma at the catheter site. A pressure dressing usually is in place. The nurse checks the site frequently for signs of bleeding, hematoma, or infection and protects the site from contamination, which can be difficult if the child with a femoral insertion wears diapers. Waterproof, clear plastic tape might be placed over the dressing to protect it from urine and feces, but the tape must not interfere with observation.

Dehydration might occur after cardiac catheterization. Not only is the child NPO before and during the procedure, but also, nausea and vomiting are common side effects of both the premedication and the contrast material, which might further limit intake and increase fluid loss. Additionally, the contrast material used is hyperosmotic and might cause hyperosmotic diuresis because large amounts of urine are needed to excrete the solute contained in the contrast material. Following catheterization, the nurse assesses the child's hydration status carefully. Intake, output, skin turgor, moistness of mucous membranes, and weight are monitored. Specific gravity of the urine is not useful, as abnormally high specific gravities are common because of the excretion of the contrast material. As soon as the child is fully awake, oral fluids are encouraged to maintain hydration and aid in the excretion of the contrast material. If the child is unable to tolerate oral fluids, intravenous therapy might be indicated.

Adverse reactions to the contrast material include elevated temperature, urticaria, wheezing, edema, dyspnea, headache, tremor, nausea, and vomiting. These are reported to the physician. Anaphylaxis, flushing, dizziness, and hypotension generally occur shortly after the dye is administered and are problems during but not after the procedure.

Children are often frightened after cardiac catheterization. They are awake but often groggy during the procedure. They hear comments by the staff that they might not understand. The sounds, sights, and sensations might be scary, and misperceptions are common. After the procedure, the nurse needs to provide opportunities or give suggestions to the parents about ways to assist the child to talk about the perceptions of the procedure. Therapeutic play in the presence of a familiar and trusted person therefore should be a routine postprocedure intervention (see Chapter 19).

Monitoring Devices

Cardiac monitor *Cardiac monitors* are often used for ongoing assessment of cardiac rhythm and rate. Monitors vary in type from those that simply measure heart rate to those that provide a continuous visual electrocardiographic display on an oscilloscope. If cardiac arrhythmias are an actual or potential problem, a monitor with continuous oscilloscope display and printout capabilities is most helpful. The printout provides a permanent record of the arrhythmia. It is essential that any electrical equipment be properly grounded.

Electrode pads are applied for a specific lead pattern. The electrodes must be applied carefully to ensure a clear tracing of cardiac rhythm. If the oscilloscope picture is unclear, the electrode pads and all connections should be rechecked. Upper and lower pulse limits should be set according to the child's age and condition. If the child's pulse exceeds the upper limit or drops below the lower limit, an alarm sounds. With some monitors, a printout is obtained automatically if the alarm is triggered. It is essential that the alarm be set at all times.

When an alarm sounds, the nurse quickly observes the rhythm tracing on the oscilloscope and assesses the child directly. Often, the alarm results from a mechanical problem, such as a loose electrode pad or loose wire, rather than an arrhythmia, but it is important to assess the child directly to make this determination. If an arrhythmia is present, a permanent tracing is obtained, and the nurse assesses the child's color, respiratory rate and effort, changes in sensorium, position, activity, precipitating factors, and anxiety. Depending on the child's condition and the nature of the arrhythmia, the physician might have to be notified.

The nurse explains the monitor's basic function and sounds to the child and family. Family members should hear the alarm sound before the alarm goes off unexpectedly. They should understand that the alarm does not necessarily mean that the child is in danger and that a nurse will always respond immediately if the alarm sounds.

Occasionally, anxious children or parents focus all concerns on the monitor and feel that they must personally observe the rate and rhythm. In some cases, this response represents a lack of trust in the staff. More often, however, it is an attempt by parents to alleviate a feeling of powerlessness by "doing something." The nurse who recognizes monitor watching as symptomatic of a deeper issue, such as lack of trust or a sense of powerlessness, can address that issue.

Sometimes a child or parent becomes somewhat dependent on the monitor. The continuous audible pulse provides a certain sense of reassurance, as does the prompt response of the staff to the alarm. Anxiety might result when the monitoring is discontinued, and the parent might fear that an arrhythmia will be missed. A thorough discussion of the rationale for discontinuation usually reduces such worries.

STANDARDS OF NURSING CARE *The Child Following a Cardiac Catheterization*

GUIDE FOR NURSING MANAGEMENT

Nursing diagnosis	Intervention	Rationale	Outcome
1. Potential for alterations in cardiac output: decreased (stressor: arrhythmia from interference with conduction of impulses from catheter irritation; septal perforation)	Monitor vital signs every 15 minutes until stable, then every 2–4 hours.	Close monitoring of vital signs will reveal any changes.	The child's cardiac rate and rhythm is similar to preprocedure range. The child's urine output is normal for the child's age and weight. The child's respiratory rate and effort is similar to that prior to procedure.
	Auscultate apical pulses to detect irregularities and observe for irregularities on the cardiac monitor. Report arrhythmias to physician.	Listening to the apical pulse for a full minute will make any altered rhythms evident—whether slow, fast, or irregular.	
	Observe for signs of congestive heart failure—audible breath sounds, edema, diaphoresis.	Congestive heart failure might follow arrhythmias.	
2. Potential for alteration in peripheral tissue perfusion (stressor: hemorrhage from site, arterial or venous clot obstruction interrupting blood flow)	Maintain pressure dressing over catheter site for 24 hours (or as ordered). Observe catheter site frequently for signs of bleeding.	A pressure dressing promotes hemostasis. Frequent monitoring is necessary to quickly identify any bleeding from the catheter entry site.	The child's peripheral pulses are palpable. The extremity is pink and warm, and the child does not complain of numbness or tingling. Capillary refill is adequate. The child's hematocrit remains at the preprocedure level.
	Minimize movement of affected extremity. Keep leg straight and flat for at least 6 hr postprocedure.	Minimal activity fosters clot formation and promotes hemostasis at the site.	
	Compare 6-hour postcatheterization hematocrit with the value of the precatheterization hematocrit to determine degree of possible blood loss. To detect weak or absent pulses, palpate pulses distal to the catheter site at the same frequency schedule as vital signs. Use the opposite extremity for comparison.	Internal hemorrhage or oozing is identified by the quality of the heart beat and a marked drop in hematocrit, also by weak vital signs, a thready pulse, and drop in blood pressure.	
	Monitor warmth, color, and capillary refill of the extremity.	Obstruction or hemorrhage will cause weak, distal pulses and diminished blood flow to the extremities, resulting in a cool, pale extremity with poor capillary refill.	
	If pulses are weak or not palpable, use Doppler or another similar device.	A Doppler device detects waves by ultrasound when the waves might not be able to be palpated.	
3. Potential for fluid volume deficit (stressor: nausea, vomiting, side effects of medications. Diuresis caused by opaque contrast material used during procedure)	Monitor intake and output hourly.	A fluid deficit is quickly noticed by an intake-output imbalance. The contrast material is a diuretic that can increase fluid loss.	The child retains fluids. The child's skin turgor is adequate and the child has moist mucous membranes. Urine output is appropriate for the child's age and weight.

STANDARDS OF NURSING CARE *The Child Following a Cardiac Catheterization (Continued)*

GUIDE FOR NURSING MANAGEMENT

Nursing diagnosis	Intervention	Rationale	Outcome
	Encourage child to drink fluids once fully awake. Start with clear liquids.	Gradual introduction of clear fluids decreases the likelihood of nausea and reduces the risk of aspiration from vomiting.	
	Observe for signs of dehydration (poor skin turgor, dry mucous membranes, absence of tears, sunken fontanelle). Observe and report vomiting or fluid refusal. Intravenous fluids might be required if oral intake is not adequate.	Early identification of dehydration allows for prompt correction with intravenous fluids.	
	Adjust intravenous infusion rate according to fluid intake for children with polycythemia, for whom adequate hydration is critical.	Maintaining fluid balance is more critical for children with polycythemia because of the increased viscosity of their blood, and because there is an increased risk for thrombus formation in these children if they are not well hydrated.	
4. Potential for infection (stressor: invasive procedure and break in skin)	Protect catheter site from contamination. For infants with a femoral catheter site, protect the pressure dressing from urine and stool with plastic tape. Change diapers often. Change dressing if contaminated with feces.	The femoral artery and vein are used for inserting the catheter. An open area exposed to urine and feces in the infant increases the risk of infection. Frequent changing and cleansing of contaminated areas are the best ways to prevent bacteria growth.	The child's catheter site heals without signs of infection (redness, warmth, purulent drainage, fever).
5. Potential for alteration in comfort (stressor: discomfort at catheter insertion site)	Observe for signs of pain at site (usually mild discomfort) and ask child to report pain. Administer analgesics. Provide comfort measures (rocking, holding, gentle touch, position change, diversion).	Discomfort should be mild. If severe or sharp pain is present, it might be a sign of a complication and needs to be reported immediately. Distraction is an effective reliever of mild discomfort.	The child states feelings of comfort. The child is able to be distracted easily and can obtain adequate rest.
6. Potential anxiety (stressor: misconception about procedure. Necessary separation from parents at time of procedure. Strange environment)	Identify fears and misperceptions.	Understanding why the procedure is needed and what exactly will happen at the time and exploring the room and the equipment help to reduce fear.	The child verbally expresses concerns or asks appropriate questions. The child is able to express fears through play.

(Continues)

STANDARDS OF NURSING CARE *The Child Following a Cardiac Catheterization (Continued)*

GUIDE FOR NURSING MANAGEMENT

Nursing diagnosis	Intervention	Rationale	Outcome
	Encourage the child to talk about the procedure.	Allowing the child to express concerns enables the staff to correct any errors or misunderstanding and to clarify and remove unwarranted fears. If children are supported and told that their concerns are legitimate, their confidence is bolstered and they are more likely to ask questions and ask for support.	
	Encourage therapeutic play.	Play is the way younger children put events, fears, and anxieties into perspective. Play allows them to be in control and to express fears in a nonthreatening way.	
7. Potential for knowledge deficit concerning home care (stressors: inadequate preparation, limited understanding of procedure)	Teach child and family how to care for catheter site at home: Allow older child to shower; give infant and young child a sponge bath for 3 days, then give tub bath. Change small bandage over catheterization site daily (or more frequently as needed) for 3 days. Observe for signs of inflammation or excessive tenderness; if these are present, report to physician.	Adequate discharge planning facilitates home care and reduces parental anxiety. Risks of complications are reduced when parents know what to do and what to watch for.	The parents can describe and demonstrate proper care of the catheter site. They can list signs of possible complications and know how to contact the physician.

Holter monitor A *Holter monitor,* which is worn by the child, provides a continuous electroradiographic recording for 12–24 hours. Sporadic arrhythmias that might not be detected during a regular electrocardiogram might be identified as the child proceeds with usual activities. Electrode leads are placed on the child's chest and arms and connected to the small recorder or transmitter, which is held in place by a harness the child wears.

Principles of Nursing Care

Acute Care Needs

Children with heart disease need careful, ongoing assessment. The condition of a child with serious heart disease can change rapidly, and the nurse therefore needs to recognize such changes quickly.

⊛ Potential alteration in cardiac output: decreased

The body's demand for oxygen directly affects cardiac workload. Therefore, a major nursing goal in caring for a child with cardiac disease is to minimize the oxygen needs of the body.

Providing adequate rest Because oxygen consumption is generally lowest when the body is at rest, the nurse organizes care so that the child's rest is disturbed as little as possible. Each intervention or procedure (bath, turning, vital signs) stresses the child and increases oxygen needs.

The nurse organizes care after careful assessment of the child's tolerance of procedures. Some children can tolerate several interventions or procedures at one time. This allows longer periods of uninterrupted rest. Other children show signs of distress (increased pulse and respiration, dyspnea, increased cyanosis) with even brief disruptions of rest. For these critically ill children, each activity (for example, turning, eating, voiding) is alternated with rest periods to allow time for recovery. Optional activities, such as complete baths and changes of linen, can be deferred until the child's condition improves. The nurse also schedules meals, naps, and procedures to coincide with the child's usual sleep pattern to further reduce stress and facilitate rest.

Interruption of rest periods should be avoided. The nurse might need to remind other members of the health care team of the child's need for undisturbed rest and often works with the team members to plan necessary activities accordingly.

If the child's rest is disturbed by irritability and restlessness not relieved by comfort measures, the physician might prescribe a sedative. Morphine sulfate is usually the drug of choice. The nurse rules out hypoxia as the cause of the child's restlessness and irritability before administering the sedative. Once the sedative is administered, it will mask these symptoms, so the nurse needs to be alert for other signs of hypoxia in the sedated child (see Chapter 22). The nurse also assesses respiratory rate, as respiratory depression is an adverse effect of sedation.

Anticipating the child's needs Anticipating the child's needs prevents unnecessary crying and frustration. The stress of crying increases oxygen demands and wastes limited energy. Although it is probably impossible to prevent crying entirely in infancy or early childhood, the nurse can reduce the frequency and intensity of crying episodes by careful attention to the child's needs for food, water, comfort, holding, and stimulation. For example, the nurse feeds an infant at the first sign of hunger cues (such as sucking on fists or restlessness). For older children, the nurse can place items they are likely to need within easy reach. This prevents exertion and frustration on the part of the child. The nurse also answers all call lights promptly. A prompt response is helpful in reducing the energy expenditure in an acutely ill child. The nurse tapers this approach as the child's condition improves.

Minimizing anxiety Anxiety stimulates the sympathetic nervous system and results in increased cardiac work. Although elimination of all anxiety is neither possible nor desirable, reduction of excessive and unnecessary anxiety is important in the care of the child with heart disease. The nurse needs to be alert for both verbal and nonverbal signs of anxiety.

The nurse needs to be sensitive to spoken and unspoken concerns. Questions that the child or the parents have need to be answered as clearly and honestly as possible. For questions that are best answered by the physician, the nurse helps the family formulate and present these questions.

Preventing hyperthermia and hypothermia Both hyperthermia and hypothermia increase the body's need for oxygen. If the child is in an insufficiently warm environment, metabolic rate increases to produce heat and maintain body temperature. Increased metabolism requires increased oxygen, and the heart must work harder to meet this demand. If the heart and lungs are unable to provide the additional oxygen, anaerobic metabolism with resultant metabolic acidosis might occur.

Infants are particularly susceptible to heat loss. Changes in temperature can be subtle and might occur undetected over an extended period. The nurse places young infants in isolettes, where they can be kept warm and can be closely observed. The nurse appropriately dresses older infants and children and keeps their rooms warm. The child's bed or play area should not be near cold external walls or windows. The infant's heat loss by evaporation can be minimized by uncovering only one body part at a time during the bath and drying it thoroughly. Wet linen is changed promptly.

Fever also increases metabolic rate and the need for oxygen. As a rule of thumb, the heart rate increases 10 beats per minute for each degree of temperature over 99. Therefore, fever can have a significant impact on a circulatory system that already is compromised. The nurse monitors the child's temperature on a regular basis and, in cases of fever, gives antipyretics, such as acetaminophen. Giving the child sponge baths with tepid water might be helpful, but it is important to avoid chilling.

Facilitating cardiac function

Decreasing excess circulating volume Reducing the workload of the heart involves eliminating excess sodium and fluid, which increase the circulating blood volume. Re-

TABLE 23-6 Diuretics Used in Congenital Heart Disease

Drug	Side effect	Nursing implication
Furosemide (Lasix) Potent, rapid-acting	Electrolyte imbalance (especially hypokalemia), dehydration, hypotension, nausea, vomiting, diarrhea, dermatitis, ototoxicity	Monitor blood pressure. Monitor fluid intake and output. Weigh child daily. Encourage foods high in potassium or give potassium supplements
Chlorothiazide sodium (Diuril) Inhibits sodium and potassium reabsorption in renal tubule	Nausea, weakness, dizziness, paresthesias, cramps, rash, hypokalemia, metabolic alkalosis, thrombocytopenia	Encourage foods high in potassium. Monitor fluid intake and output. Schedule doses to avoid nocturia. Inspect skin and mucous membranes for petechiae. Discontinue 48 hours before surgery
Spironolactone (Aldactone) Potassium-sparing, promotes sodium excretion Often used in conjunction with thiazides	Lethargy, headache, drowsiness, cramps, nausea, vomiting, hyperkalemia, rash, ataxia, impotence, hyponatremia	Monitor intake and output. Monitor for hyponatremia and hyperkalemia

ducing the heart's workload in this way is called *preload reduction.* This process most commonly is accomplished with diuretics. Intake of excessive sodium (salty foods) is avoided, and a low-sodium diet might be necessary. Restrictions on oral intake of fluid usually are not needed, except for severe heart failure. Dehydration must be avoided, especially in children with polycythemia.

Diuretics vary in their action, therapeutic effects, side effects, and adverse reactions. The nurse therefore needs to be familiar with specific types of diuretics to monitor their effects and the child's tolerance. Excessive fluid loss and electrolyte imbalances are possible consequences of diuretic therapy. Furosemide and the thiazides promote the excretion of potassium and potassium supplements often are indicated. Spironolactone, which spares potassium from excretion, can be used in conjunction with thiazide. Excessive potassium loss is a particularly serious problem in children who take digitalis, because hypokalemia enhances the effect of digitalis and might cause toxicity. (The most commonly used diuretics are summarized in Table 23-6.)

Minimizing resistance to cardiac outflow Reducing the work of the heart can also be accomplished by decreasing resistance in the systemic circulation, a process called *afterload reduction.* This is accomplished by administering vasodilators and antihypertensives. (Commonly used agents are summarized in Table 23-7.) These are potent medications, and the nurse is ever alert for serious side effects, especially hypotension. The nurse closely (every 30 minutes) monitors the blood pressure after administering the drug. Decreased respiratory rate and effort are the expected therapeutic effects from the medication.

Improving myocardial function Myocardial function is enhanced by digitalis, a cardiac glycoside that increases myocardial contractility, decreases the rate of contractions, slows conduction through the atrioventricular node, and promotes diuresis because of increased blood flow through the kidneys. Effective digitalis therapy results in an increase in cardiac output and a reduction in heart size, venous pressure, edema, and liver size (Meissner and Gever, 1980).

Two preparations, digoxin and digitoxin, are commonly used. Digoxin is used almost exclusively in children because its onset of action is more rapid than that of digitoxin and its rapid rate of excretion reduces the risk of toxicity. Digoxin can be given orally, intravenously, or intramuscularly. Oral preparations include a sweet-flavored elixir for infants and younger children and tablets for older children and adolescents.

Initiation of therapy is termed *digitalization.* Loading doses of the drug are given at 6- to 8-hour intervals to achieve therapeutic levels. After therapeutic levels have been reached, a maintenance dose is given every 12 hours (Table 23-8). Serum levels are checked, and the range of serum levels considered to be therapeutic is 1.7–2.0 mg/mL.

Digoxin is a potent medication with a relatively narrow therapeutic range. Fisch (1971) states that

> The margin of safety between the therapeutic and toxic and the toxic and lethal dose is relatively narrow. It has been estimated that

TABLE 23-7 Medications for Afterload Reduction: Vasodilators

Drug	Side effects	Nursing implications
Tolazoline hydrochloride (Priscoline)	Nausea, vomiting, gastric irritation, hypotension, hypertension, tachycardia, other cardiac arrhythmias, tingling	Give with meals or with milk to reduce gastric irritation. Check pulse and blood pressure regularly, ½–1½ hr after oral administration. Check pulse and blood pressure more frequently with IV administration, starting 15 min after dose is given. Caution child about postural hypotension and assist child as needed
Prazosin hydrochloride (Minipress)	Dizziness, headache, drowsiness, tachycardia, syncope, hypotension, vomiting, diarrhea, constipation, rash, urinary frequency, impotence	Monitor pulse and blood pressure carefully after administration (peak action 2–4 hr). Caution child to change positions slowly and avoid situations where injury could occur due to syncope. Assist child as needed
Sodium nitroprusside (Nipride)	Hypotension, mild decrease in cardiac output, nausea, retching, increase or decrease in pulse rate, restlessness, agitation, muscle twitching, rash	Give by IV route only. Use infusion pump to ensure precise control of rate. Monitor pulse and blood pressure vigilantly. Monitor intake and output

TABLE 23-8 Digoxin Dosages

Objective	Oral administration	Intravenous or intramuscular administration	Schedule
Digitalization (dose per 24 hr)	0.06–0.08 mg/kg	0.03–0.06 mg/kg	Initial dose: 50% of 24-hr total Second dose: 25% 6–8 hr later Third dose: 25% 6–8 hr after second dose
Maintenance (dose per 24 hr)	20%–25% of digitalization dose	10%–20% of digitalization dose	Divided equally into two doses: one dose given every 12 hr

Electrocardiograph is assessed before each dose is given. Ideally, cardiac monitor is in place during entire procedure.

when the desired therapeutic response is attained, 60 percent of the toxic dose has been administered; and when toxic reaction is manifested, approximately 50 percent of the lethal dose is ingested.

For this reason, the utmost care is required when calculating and preparing dosages. An error in decimal placement could result in administration of a lethal dose. Institutions often have special policies for safe administration of the drug.

Digitalis toxicity is a serious complication. The nurse observes carefully for signs of digitalis toxicity with all children on this drug. Toxicity can occur at any time during therapy, but the times it is most likely to occur are during digitalization, dosage adjustment, or episodes of hypokalemia.

Signs of digitalis toxicity vary, but changes in cardiac functioning usually are present. Cardiac manifestations include bradycardia, pulse deficit (apical pulse by auscultation greater than palpated radial pulse), and arrhythmias.

The nurse checks both apical and radial pulses for a full minute prior to administration of the drug. If the apical pulse is abnormally slow or if a pulse deficit is present, the drug is withheld, and the physician is notified. The apical rate requiring that the drug be withheld is not absolute but varies according to the child's age and apical rate prior to digitalization. If the pulse rate is significantly lower than previous rates or if there is a progressive downward trend over time, the dose is withheld pending specific orders from the physician. Usually, the child is on a cardiac monitor when therapy is initiated. A prolonged P-R interval (signaling first-degree heart block) and sinus bradycardia are both early signs of toxicity. Premature ventricular contractions, varying degrees of heart block, and ventricular tachycardia are other electrocardiographic changes associated with toxicity.

Anorexia, nausea, and vomiting are among the earliest manifestations of toxicity. Although vomiting for other reasons is not uncommon in children, especially infants, its occurrence should always raise suspicion of toxicity and be reported to the physician.

Neurologic manifestations of toxicity include headache, drowsiness, insomnia, dizziness, and confusion. Such visual disturbances as halos around objects, glittering spots, variations in color perception, and reading difficulty might occur. Young children have difficulty describing these symptoms; hence, they might go undetected. Older children usually are more reliable in their descriptions.

Hypokalemia (low serum potassium) enhances the effect of digitalis and increases the risk of toxicity. A dose that is correct in normal circumstances can cause toxicity in the presence of hypokalemia. Potassium depletion occurs as a result of the following:

1. Inadequate intake—administration of an intravenous fluid that does not contain added potassium, limited intake of nutrients
2. Excessive losses—diuretic therapy, diarrhea, vomiting, nasogastric suction without potassium replacement, hyperglycemic diuresis, corticosteroid therapy
3. Fluid shift—shift of intracellular fluid (K^+) to replace extracellular fluid (Na^+) loss, for example, metabolic alkalosis

If the child is receiving a potassium supplement at home, the nurse alerts the physician of this fact. Based on the child's clinical status and results of serum potassium levels, the physician decides whether or not to prescribe potassium. If the level is low, the physician is notified, and digoxin is withheld. Clinical signs of potassium depletion include muscle weakness, hyporeflexia, ileus, apathy, drowsiness, irritability, and fatigue. Electrocardiographic changes include prolonged Q-T interval, a widening and lowering of T-waves, and depression of the S-T segment.

❀ Potential activity intolerance

Because exercise tolerance is an important measurement in assessment of cardiac function, the nurse monitors the child's activity level to assess the physiologic and psychologic responses to activity or its limitation. Many children with heart disease do well at regulating their own activities. These children are sensitive to internal cues that indicate the need to rest. Such children usually do not need external restrictions on activity, but the nurse continues to monitor their response to activity and notes evidence of exercise intolerance.

Other children do need external controls to limit activity. In some types of heart disease, there are medical indications for restricted activity even though activity does not produce symptoms, and it might be hard for the child to understand the importance of rest if play activities cause no distress. Other children might persist in activity to the point of distress and beyond. They seem unable to regulate activity in response to internal cues. In an older child, persistent activity might be a form of denial or an effort to prove that "everything is OK."

Children who are unable to follow activity restrictions need a clear, age-appropriate explanation of why restrictions are necessary. They also need to be told exactly what their limits are, and these limits need to be enforced consistently. Allowing the child to express or "play out" frustration and anxiety related to activity restrictions is helpful. If the child seems to be using persistent activity as a form of denial, basic anxiety about the physical condition must be addressed. It is important to plan quiet activities with children to keep them occupied and stimulated while at rest. The nurse also must remember that the imposition of activity restrictions on a child who is normally active does not necessarily reduce cardiac workload. Sometimes the frustration of imposed bed rest creates more work for the heart than limited out-of-bed activity. Therefore, the nurse assesses each child individually and discusses appropriate activity limitations with the physician.

The nurse knows that the overall goal of activity restrictions is to reduce strain on the heart. If a particular restriction, such as confinement to bed, creates undue frustration and tension in the child, the restriction might actually increase the workload of the heart. The nurse therefore assesses each child individually and discusses appropriate activity limitations with the physician. The nurse then works with the parent to find ways of limiting activity while avoiding unnecessary frustration. One young child, for example, rejected the notion of staying in her crib, but she was content to play quietly in a high chair or playpen.

In assisting a child to adapt to restricted activity, the nurse first assesses the child's perception of the restrictions. Young children might feel that restriction is a form of punishment. Older children might feel that they are being "babied." Once the nurse understands the child's perception, it is possible to explain the rationale for restrictions in an honest and age-appropriate way and to correct any unrealistic expectations or worries the child might have.

For a small number of children, such as those with critical aortic stenosis, increased physical activity does not produce obvious symptoms but carries a risk of myocardial ischemia, arrhythmia, and death. It is often difficult for these children to understand why vigorous physical activity must be avoided when it does not seem to cause them any problems.

A second group of children whose activity must be limited includes those with heart failure and certain cardiac-related diseases, such as rheumatic fever. For some of these children, bed rest is ordered for an extended period of time. During the acute phase of the illness, the child feels ill and wants to rest. During the recovery phase, however, the child feels well enough for active play. Now the child has a difficult time understanding why such play continues to be contraindicated medically.

⊛ Potential impaired gas exchange

Alveolar gas exchange is often impaired in children with heart disease because of alterations in pulmonary blood flow, pulmonary congestion, or both. A major nursing goal is to facilitate optimal gas exchange.

Positioning Placing the child in a semi-Fowler's position prevents abdominal organs from exerting pressure on the diaphragm and allows greater expansion of the lungs. The nurse places an infant in an infant seat or car seat to maintain an upright position. If the infant is in an isolette, the nurse raises one end of the platform to create a 30- to 40-degree slant. A padded sandbag placed under the infant's buttocks and thighs helps to maintain the position and prevent the infant from sliding downward when the platform is slanted.

To avoid pressure on the chest wall, the nurse keeps the infant's clothing loose and nonrestrictive. The infant's arms are placed at the side and not over the chest.

Oxygen therapy Supplemental oxygen is used to improve tissue oxygenation. The oxygen is warmed to prevent chilling and is humidified to prevent drying of the mucous membranes. Oxygen concentration is monitored carefully. Supplemental oxygen is not always beneficial for the child with heart disease. If it is given for a trial period, the nurse carefully documents its effect on the child's color, vital signs, respiratory effort, and comfort.

Humidification Humidification without oxygen might help liquefy secretions. When using mist therapy, the nurse keeps clothing and bedding dry to prevent chilling.

Suctioning If there is pulmonary edema, the nurse might need to use suctioning to keep the airway clear. Suctioning is stressful for the child and causes discomfort, hypoxia, fatigue, and irritation to the mucosa. In addition, stimulation of the vagus nerve during suctioning can cause bradycardia. Before and after tracheal suctioning, the nurse provides the child with some additional oxygen, usually by mask. Careful auscultation of breath sounds before and after suctioning is done to assess the effectiveness of the procedure. Excessive suctioning is harmful and therefore is avoided. The nurse judges in each instance whether the child benefits sufficiently from the suctioning to make it worth the disadvantages.

Chest physiotherapy Chest physiotherapy might be helpful to the child with pulmonary complications of cardiac disease (see Chapter 22). The full procedure, which includes postural drainage, percussion, and vibration, is very exhausting. In children with heart disease, only a few positions usually are used per session, and postural drainage might not be included. The nurse auscultates the lungs and reads recent radiographic reports and then decides which areas of the lung to percuss. The nurse also carefully monitors the child's tolerance of the procedure and discusses signs of distress with the physician. The benefits of chest physiotherapy must be weighed against the stress it causes. Modifications, such as more frequent but shorter sessions, might be needed.

Bronchodilators Bronchodilators (mainly xanthines, such as aminophylline) are sometimes prescribed to improve ventilation of the lungs. The nurse monitors the effects of these powerful drugs on the cardiac, pulmonary, and central nervous systems. Cardiovascular effects of the xanthines include myocardial stimulation, tachycardia, hypotension, palpitations, and arrhythmias (extrasystoles). In addition, xanthines can increase the potential toxicity of digitalis preparations. For these reasons, bronchodilators are used cautiously and with careful monitoring in children with heart disease.

⊛ Potential fluid volume alterations

Proper fluid volume balance is of critical importance to the child with heart disease. Excess fluid causes additional work for the heart. Dehydration is a serious condition for all children, but it is especially serious for children with cyanotic heart disease. If the child also has polycythemia, dehydration further increases the viscosity of the blood and increases the risk of thrombus formation and stroke.

The nurse accurately measures and records all fluid intake and output for children hospitalized with cardiac disease. Parents and children are instructed in the importance of notifying the nurse or self-recording all intake and output.

The nurse carefully compares the intake and output at regular intervals and notes excessive or inadequate fluid intake. Disparity between fluid ingested and urine excreted is reported to the physician. Decreased urine output (in relation to intake) might indicate fluid retention. Increased urine output might be a positive response to diuretic therapy but, if excessive, can cause dehydration.

Weight is one of the most reliable indicators of fluid balance. All children hospitalized with heart disease are weighed at least daily. Increased weight might indicate fluid retention, worsening of congestive heart failure, and poor perfusion of the kidneys. Decreased weight might indicate inadequate intake or diuresis in response to therapy.

Other clinical indicators of fluid balance that the nurse assesses on a regular basis include the moistness of the mucous membranes, tension of the fontanelle, the presence of edema or ascites, and the presence or absence of tears in infants older than 6 weeks.

Fluid restrictions might be required in congestive heart failure. (Interventions related to oral fluid restriction are discussed in Chapter 20.) Intravenous fluids also must be administered carefully. The nurse uses an infusion pump or burette to prevent excess fluid administration, which might cause circulatory overload.

Of critical importance is not to introduce air emboli and particulate matter intravenously in a child with a right-to-left shunt. In a right-to-left shunt, a portion of the venous blood shunts directly to the left heart and systemic circulation without passing through the lungs. It is in the lungs where air emboli normally are absorbed and particulate matter is filtered. Therefore, in a right-to-left shunt, air emboli, clots, bacteria, and particulate matter might travel directly to the brain or other organ, causing infarction, infection, and tissue damage.

Potential for infection

Children with heart disease are at special risk for respiratory infections and bacterial endocarditis. Nursing goals related to preventing infection include avoiding exposure to and detecting early any signs of infections.

Respiratory infections Altered pulmonary blood flow and pulmonary congestion make the child with some forms of heart disease more susceptible to lower respiratory infections. Recurrent pneumonia is one of the common symptoms of congenital heart disease. Respiratory syncytial virus (RSV) is one of the more frequent causes of acute lower respiratory infections in infants. Research by MacDonald (1983) and associates compared the effect of RSV infection on infants with congenital heart disease to infants without heart disease. Results indicated that infants with congenital heart disease had significantly more severe disease than infants without heart disease and required intensive care and assisted ventilation more frequently.

When RSV infection is prevalent in the community, children with heart disease should not be admitted to the hospital for elective procedures. Hospital personnel need to be aware of the significant risks that respiratory infection presents to these children. Anyone, whether hospital personnel, visitor, or another patient, who has a respiratory infection must be careful not to expose children with heart disease to the infection. Clearly, children with heart disease cannot share rooms with children who have respiratory infections. Correct hand washing is essential, as contaminated hands are one of the major sources of contagion. If children with active respiratory infections are present, strict isolation procedures must be employed according to hospital policy.

The nurse needs to be alert for early signs and symptoms of respiratory infection in children with heart disease. Rhinorrhea, cough, fever, sore throat, and headache should be reported to the physician promptly so that appropriate evaluation and therapy can be initiated. When antibiotics are used for treatment of bacterial infection or prevention of secondary bacterial invasion, they are administered at equally divided intervals to ensure constant therapeutic serum levels.

Bacterial endocarditis Children with congenital heart disease and rheumatic heart disease are at risk for developing *bacterial endocarditis,* an infection of the valves and inner lining (endocardium) of the heart. Endocarditis usually occurs as a sequela to bacteremia, which might result from dental work; from any manipulation of the genitourinary tract (including catheterization) or gastrointestinal or respiratory tracts; from prolonged intravenous infusion; from cardiac catheterization and surgery; or from childbirth. It is also associated with infectious disease such as tonsillitis, pneumonia, and pyoderma.

Susceptible children generally are treated with prophylactic antibiotics before and after invasive procedures and during febrile illness. Parents must be taught about the importance of prophylaxis and the necessity of informing dentists and other health professionals of the child's increased risk status.

Signs and symptoms of bacterial endocarditis include unexplained fever, chills, lethargy, petechiae, splenomegaly, and congestive heart failure and are reported to the physician promptly. Early treatment is important if cardiac damage is to be minimized and complications (for example, emboli to various organs, brain abscess) prevented.

⊛ Potential knowledge deficit regarding management of hypoxic spells

Hypoxic spells, also called hypercyanotic episodes or "tet" spells, occur with some forms of cyanotic heart disease, most often tetralogy of Fallot or other defects causing right ventricular obstruction. Hypoxic spells usually result from an abrupt reduction in pulmonary blood flow. During the episode, the child becomes agitated, dyspneic, and limp and develops severe cyanosis. The child might rub the hands over the chest as if experiencing pain. The onset usually is sudden and unpredictable. Disappearance of a systolic murmur might be noted. Severe spells might progress to unconsciousness, seizure, and death.

Hypoxic spells require immediate treatment. The child is soothed and held in a side-lying, knee-chest position with the head and thorax slightly elevated. If the spell does not resolve, morphine sulfate (0.01–0.05 mg/kg subcutaneously) is administered, and oxygen might be given. If the child is known to have such episodes, it is helpful to have a syringe containing the correct dose of morphine available for immediate use. Increased frequency or severity of hypoxic spells is an indicator for surgical intervention.

Metabolic acidosis results if the spell does not resolve quickly. Intravenous phenylephrine hydrochloride (Neo-Synephrine) sometimes is used to increase systemic resistance and thereby to reduce the right-to-left shunt. Occasionally, an episode continues despite interventions, and emergency surgery is necessary.

The nurse teaches the parent to manage hypoxic spells, in case a spell occurs at home. The parent is taught to place the child in a knee-chest position and provide oxygen if it is available. The physician should be contacted if a spell does not resolve quickly, and the child should be taken to the hospital immediately. The most effective way for parents to learn management of hypoxic spells is to observe competent professionals calmly and skillfully manage a spell in the hospital. Instead of ushering the parent out of the room during a spell, the nurse can encourage the parent to observe and even participate in the child's care. After the episode, both parent and child should be given an opportunity to discuss the anxiety engendered by the spell and review steps in its emergency management.

⊛ Potential knowledge deficit regarding cardiac surgery

Parent preparation for cardiac surgery usually begins at the time of diagnosis. At that time the nature of the defect is described and the possibility of surgery often is introduced. Parents face the prospect of surgery with emotions that are different and sometimes conflicting. For some, the operation represents a resolution of the child's problem and a hope for a normal life. For others, surgery represents the threat of losing the child through death. Most parents feel a painful ambivalence—hope for improvement in the health of the child and fear of the loss of the child.

Parents must be prepared for both the preoperative and postoperative experiences the child will face. The nurse can use a diagram or doll to explain the incision. The nurse also describes or shows parents the equipment they will see, such as arterial and venous catheters, chest tubes, nasogastric tubes, pacemaker wires, urinary catheters, respirator, and electrocardiographic monitor. The nurse needs to warn parents that children are unable to speak while endotracheal tubes are in place. The nurse explains alarm systems so that parents will not become unduly frightened when an alarm sounds in their presence. Parents are also forewarned that blood in the chest tubes is normal. Unless the parents understand the reasons for such postoperative procedures as suctioning, turning, and chest physiotherapy, these procedures might be perceived as unnecessary or cruel.

The parents need special support at the time the child leaves them for the operating room. Although the parent might appear calm and composed, the fear of never seeing the child alive again is often just below the surface. Remaining with the parent for a time in the waiting area is therefore an appropriate intervention. The long wait during surgery can be agonizing. Parents should be informed that operating room schedules are never exact and that the surgery that is not over at the anticipated time does not mean problems have occurred. Parents tremendously appreciate periodic progress reports, however simple.

Despite careful preparation, a parent is often shocked to see the child postoperatively in the intensive care unit. The shock is less severe if the parent has visited the intensive care unit ahead of time and has been exposed to its myriad sights and sounds.

At each point in the preoperative discussion, the nurse emphasizes what the child will see, hear, and feel, as these sensations are of primary importance, particularly to the young child. Older children are more interested in the rationale for various procedures.

Many children benefit from seeing where their parents will wait during the surgery, visiting the intensive care unit, and meeting the nurses there. This is anxiety-producing, but the experience allows children to prepare themselves. It is not a desirable experience for all children, however, as the child who is very anxious might not be able to tolerate the stress of seeing the intensive care unit ahead of time.

Most children, however, benefit from an introduction to certain kinds of postoperative apparatus. These include:

1. *Endotracheal tube*. The nurse explains that the child will not be able to talk while the tube is in place but will be able to talk after the doctor takes it out, although the throat might be a little sore.
2. *Nasogastric tube*. The nurse explains that this tube helps the child not to feel like vomiting and therefore to be more comfortable right after surgery.
3. *Chest tube*. The nurse can connect the chest tube to a small saline bottle with red water in it to demonstrate the bloody drainage that is normal.
4. *Intravenous and intra-arterial catheters*. The nurse connects these to small saline-filled bottles to demonstrate how the child will get "drinks" of water, since the child will not be able to drink by mouth for a couple of days.
5. *Electrocardiographic leads and monitor*. The nurse reminds the child of having a "heart test" done and encourages the child to feel and put the pads on the doll.
6. *Urinary catheter*. The nurse explains that the child will not have to go to the bathroom because the catheter will collect the urine.

It is important to reassure the child that these apparatuses are not permanent and will be removed in the first few days after surgery.

Age-appropriate explanations are another vital aspect of preoperative preparation. The nurse tells the child that there will be pain and that medicine is available to relieve the pain. Usually, narcotics are given intravenously in the intensive care unit; however, if injections will be required, the child is informed. The nurse can explain that the little hurt of the needle will make the bigger hurt of the incision go away. The nurse explains postoperative procedures, such as coughing, deep breathing, and turning, which can be practiced.

The child is reassured that all the doctors and nurses understand that children feel like crying when they feel scared or if something hurts and that it is all right for the child to cry or tell them when something is wrong. The doctors and nurses then will try to help the child to feel better.

Using the doll, the nurse demonstrates placement and removal of the tubes. The nurse explains that after a time in the intensive care unit, the child will stay in a regular hospital room for a few days and then can go home. The doll should then be changed to street clothes to emphasize this important point.

Nutritional Needs

⊛ Alteration in nutrition: less than body requirements related to inadequate intake

Children with heart disease often have special nutritional needs. Growth retardation is common in children with congenital heart disease. Factors that play a role in growth failure include the following:

- Inadequate intake of nutrients related to fatigue
- Chronic hypoxia that affects the use of nutrients at the cellular level
- Hypermetabolism
- Malabsorption of nutrients
- Anorexia secondary to medications

Promoting adequate intake A major nursing goal is to provide adequate intake of nutrients and calories. Sucking requires a significant expenditure of energy, and infants with heart disease often become exhausted and dyspneic before they can consume an adequate volume of formula. Such infants are likely to suck and pant alternately through the feeding until they become fatigued and give up. Holding the infant in a semiupright knee-chest position helps to prevent fatigue and enables the infant to eat more. Using a soft nipple designed for premature infants reduces the work of sucking. The hole in the nipple might be enlarged slightly, although if the hole is too large, the infant might become overwhelmed by the volume of formula and might choke and aspirate some of it. The infant is allowed to pause and rest as needed and is not forced to eat when fatigued. The infant is held during feedings. If the infant is receiving oxygen, it must be continued during the feeding. Infants are fed at the first sign of hunger and are not allowed to tire themselves by crying. Other procedures are scheduled so that the child receives adequate rest prior to the feeding and is not disturbed after the feeding. Small feedings are offered frequently, such as every 2–3 hours around the clock. Smaller feedings minimize fatigue, and the small volume of food exerts less pressure on the diaphragm (Cloutier and Measel, 1982).

The nurse informs parents that infants with heart disease will not sleep through the night at the same age as normal children. The infant needs these additional months of night feedings in order to receive adequate intake to meet metabolic needs. The nurse helps the parents see the importance of sharing the nighttime feeding task and enlisting the help of others as needed. After feedings, the infant is placed in a semi-upright position (such as in an infant seat) to reduce the risk of vomiting and to facilitate respirations.

Breast-feeding might require more energy than bottle-feeding. Breast-feeding is not contraindicated if the infant is able to obtain enough milk without undue effort. If the infant does become fatigued and the mother remains committed to breast-feeding, breast milk can be expressed and fed by bottle or gavage. Some infants are placed on a schedule that alternates bottle and gavage feeding. If gavage or gastrostomy feedings are necessary, the infant should be provided with a pacifier during the feeding. In a few cases of severe heart disease, parenteral nutrition might be required (see Chapter 27).

High-calorie diets To provide as many calories as possible, special formulas containing 24–30 calories per ounce can be used. These formulas have additional carbohydrates, making them concentrated. Therefore the caloric increase must be introduced gradually, or diarrhea might result. The nurse offers water between feedings so that the child receives an adequate amount of free water to prevent dehydration.

Solid foods provide additional calories with limited expenditure of energy and often are introduced early for children with heart disease. Fluid intake remains important and the nurse ensures that the child continues to receive adequate fluid. Self-feeding and use of a cup should be encouraged at the usual ages as long as the child maintains an adequate intake. If the child's own intake is inadequate, the parent can let the child handle food and self-feed while continuing to feed the child.

Children should be offered a choice of high-calorie, nutritious foods at mealtimes and as snacks. While high-calorie, nutritious snacks, such as milkshakes, are encouraged, empty-calorie snacks are avoided because they require energy to ingest and digest but do not provide essential nutrients.

Iron supplementation It is important to prevent iron-deficiency anemia in children with cyanotic heart disease and polycythemia. Supplemental iron often is prescribed to prevent this condition. Research by Linderkamp (1979) indicates that viscosity of the blood increases in the presence of microcytosis associated with iron-deficiency anemia. The increased viscosity increases the risk of thrombus formation and cerebrovascular accident.

If an iron supplement is prescribed, the nurse teaches the parents the correct procedure for giving the medication to prevent staining of the teeth. The nurse also emphasizes the importance of preventing accidental overdose.

Sodium restriction A low-sodium diet might be advisable for some children with heart disease, especially for those with congestive heart failure. Sodium restriction is usually accomplished by never adding table salt to the food and by avoiding heavily salted foods (potato chips, bacon, pickles). Low-sodium milk formulas are available. Infants often accept these well, but older children might find them unpalatable. Breast milk is low in sodium and is acceptable for infants on low-sodium diets.

A nutritionist can provide helpful information for planning the nutritional needs of a child on a sodium-restricted diet. Both the parents and the child need to understand the importance of minimizing the intake of salt and how to accomplish this on a day-to-day basis. Parents need to know which foods are high or low in sodium, how to read labels for sodium content, how to modify recipes to reduce sodium, and how to order low-salt foods in a restaurant.

Developmental Needs

Most children with heart disease are intellectually and developmentally normal. Some children, however, particularly those with cyanotic heart disease, are at risk for developmental delays.

⊛ Altered growth and development related to effects of physical limitations

Chronic heart failure or chronic hypoxia limits strength and endurance, delaying the development of gross motor skills. Perceptual motor function and motor coordination are decreased in children with cyanotic heart disease.

Newburger and colleagues (1984) studied the effects of chronic hypoxemia on cognitive function. Their study indicated a correlation between cognitive impairment and increased age of repair in children with cyanotic heart disease. This lag was in part related to physical incapacity, and gains in IQ scores were seen after surgery when physical capacity and endurance increased.

Congenital heart defects might occur in association with other abnormalities. For example, 40% of children with Down's syndrome also have congenital heart defects (Scoggin and Patterson, 1982). Children with cyanotic heart disease are at risk for severe hypoxic episodes and cerebrovascular accidents. Either one of these risks might impair neurologic function.

Parental attitudes can affect the child's development. If a parent thinks the child is less capable than normal, this attitude is communicated to the child, who begins to feel inadequate in meeting developmental challenges. A parent who fears that increased motor activity will be harmful to the child does not encourage the child to try new skills.

Occasionally a parent's fears actually prohibit developmental progress.

Because independence is an important determinant of self-esteem, children need to be encouraged to assume as much independence as they are able. This often is difficult for children with cardiac disease. Parents find it easier and faster to do something for the child than to let the child spend the time and exert the effort to do it alone. This is particularly true if the child's efforts result in worsening existing symptoms. Often, a well-intentioned but misinformed parent prevents the child from doing things independently.

Altered growth and development related to environmental and stimulation deficiencies

Parents need help from the start to understand the hazards of overdependence. The parent who feels guilty, angry, or inadequate might do extra things for the child to compensate for these feelings. To counteract this natural tendency, the nurse helps the parent to focus on the child's capabilities rather than the child's limitations. The nurse also encourages the parent to identify personal adequacies as a parent. A parent who feels adequate most of the time is less likely to try to compensate for occasional feelings of inadequacy by doing too much for the child (Gottesfeld, 1979).

As children develop, parents should encourage them to assume increasing responsibility for their own care. Older children can be responsible for taking their own medication, observing appropriate limits, and observing dietary restrictions.

An infant or child with heart disease needs but might not receive the same type of developmental stimulation as a normal child. For example, children with heart disease might not have the physical capacity to explore the environment to the same extent as a normal child and might not receive the same type of encouragement from adults. Instead of being told to "Go on—try harder," the child with cardiac disease might be told "Don't try so hard—be careful."

The nurse works with the parent to develop strategies to help the child experience normal activities while preventing undue cardiac stress. For example, the normal infant crawls from room to room, but the infant with cardiac disease might need to be moved from room to room to experience new sights and sounds. A normal infant might be able to sit alone at 6 months of age. The 6-month-old infant with cardiac disease might need to be propped or held so that the world is seen from an upright position and the hands are free for manipulation of objects. A young child with heart disease might not have the stamina to walk alone but can experience the sensation of moving in an upright position if an adult provides support while the child moves the feet and legs. With a mobility aid, such as a walker, the child can move about easily with limited expenditure of energy. Parents need to bring stimulating experiences to their children with cardiac disease.

The child with heart disease might be physically small and might be passive rather than active. Because of these characteristics, parents often think that the child is younger and less capable than might actually be true. Nurses need to be alert for these assumptions and help parents provide appropriate activities that foster normal development.

Because the child with heart disease might have limited energy, it is important to avoid overstimulation and fatigue. A regular routine that includes play times and rest times is beneficial and aids in integrating the child's developmental activities into the family's day.

The nurse assesses the parent's understanding of the child's heart disease. Many people have limited knowledge of normal cardiac structure and function. Therefore, an explanation of the normal circulatory system often must precede a description of the child's problem if the parent is to understand the significance of the defeat, its symptoms and its treatment. Simple, two-dimensional drawings of cardiac structures are useful teaching tools.

The nurse also teaches the parent what the child's defect is *not*. The parent might be unnecessarily fearful that, for example, the child with heart disease will have a sudden heart attack and die, as adults with heart disease do. Whereas this is a risk for a small number of children with some defects, most parents can be reassured that the child is not at risk for a "heart attack." It is important to discuss the parent's fears and to help the parent to distinguish unrealistic fears from realistic concerns.

Discipline Discipline is a special issue for children with some forms of cardiac disease. If symptoms worsen when the child becomes upset or cries, the parent might go to extremes to appease the child and prevent such episodes. Although this meets the short-term goal of preventing hypoxemia and dyspnea, it is not consistent with the long-term goal of raising a well-adjusted child who can delay gratification. Reasonable efforts to meet the child's needs help to prevent unnecessary frustration, but parents cannot and should not try to prevent all crying. Most children with cardiac disease stop crying on their own when crying becomes too tiring. Unless specifically advised otherwise by the physician, the parent can assume that normal episodes of crying are not harmful to the child, even though symptoms might worsen. The parent needs to learn early to prevent manipulative behavior by the child (for example, "If you don't let me have a cookie, I'll cry and turn blue!"). The nurse encourages the parent to recognize the child's positive behaviors and ignore negative behaviors as much as possible. When the child learns that the parent is not upset by negative behaviors, the child will be less likely to use symptoms to manipulate the parent.

The parent also needs guidance and support in management of day-to-day issues in raising a special child. The child needs to develop an understanding of the disease and an increasing responsibility for self-care. The child is treated as much like siblings as possible with respect to household tasks, discipline, and responsibilities, although modifications might be necessary, depending on the child's physical status. A child with heart disease might not be able to do yard work but could be responsible for folding laundry and other less physically demanding jobs. Parents must understand the hazards of overprotection, overindulgence, and undue restrictions at home or at school. The cardiologist is responsible for determining what restrictions, if any, are needed for the child. The nurse works with the parents in applying these restrictions to particular situations. Unless contraindicated, the child should attend school regularly and participate in permitted activities with peers. Parents should consult with the doctor or nurse if they are uncertain whether an activity is allowed. It is better to check than to impose an unnecessary restriction on the child.

Emotional Needs

Children with congenital heart disease have an incidence of psychologic maladjustment similar to that of children with other chronic disease (see Chapter 14). Psychosocial problems might lead to emotional disability, which is more serious than the physical disability caused by the heart disease. Clearly, attention to the emotional needs of children and families is of paramount importance. Nurses and other health professionals need to promote realistic and appropriate parenting if the child is to develop as a socially competent and productive individual.

⊛ Potential alteration in family processes

Many children with heart defects, especially acyanotic defects, do not have obvious symptoms. It is often difficult for parents of these children to believe that an infant has a serious, perhaps life-threatening condition. A parent might "shop around" for other physicians who will reassure the parent that the infant is healthy. Heart disease often is not apparent at birth, and symptoms might not appear for several weeks. The parent typically is delighted and relieved initially to hear that the infant is normal, only to be told a few weeks later that the infant is ill. To be told that the infant is healthy and then to discover that the infant is ill is a particularly difficult adjustment for a parent. A parent often does not understand the reason for the time lapse between the birth of the child and the diagnosis. The parent might conclude that the physician either "missed" the diagnosis or tried to hide the truth. A loss of trust in health care providers might result.

The parent might experience feelings of anger because the child is not normal. This anger might be directed at themselves, the sick child, the spouse, the healthy siblings, God, or the professonal involved in the care of the child. Professionals must recognize the source of the anger and allow the parent time to deal with it. Reacting angrily to the parent's anger only intensifies the problem. Nurses help the parents to deal with these feelings. By discussing with the parents how vital their love and concern is to the child's care, the nurse redirects the parents' energy. While the technology of health care might be impressive, the child's confidence in the parent's love and protection is truly central to the child's well-being. Parents are encouraged to participate as fully as possible in their child's care. At the same time, the nurse acknowledges the parents' disappointment and anger concerning the reality of the diagnosis.

Caring for children with serious heart disease on a day-to-day basis can be demanding and stressful. Frequent feedings, special medications, and constant vigilance lead to tensions and exhaustion. Parents often feel inadequate in dealing with children's complex needs. The parent might see the child's symptoms (for example, poor feeding, irritability) as proof of parental failure. Activities such as feeding, which are ordinarily pleasurable, become ones of high anxiety when the child has heart problems.

⊛ Anxiety related to perceived threat to the child's health status

Anxiety and fear are common reactions when a parent learns of the child's heart disease. The term *heart* has metaphysical as well as biologic connotations. The heart has a special significance not associated with other organs. The diagnosis of heart disease is frightening, and the parent often is anxious about the child's survival. The symptom of cyanosis is especially anxiety-provoking, and it is very frightening for a parent to watch the child turn blue during feedings or other activities. Impending surgery also creates tremendous conflict and ambivalence in many parents. Although the parent realizes that surgery should improve the child's condition, the threat of death also is present. The parent faces the pain of deciding whether to let the child live with present impairments or to risk the loss of the child.

Anxiety is more likely if the child has had critical episodes during which the parents feared the child would not recover. Parental fears are often transferred to the child, who then feels vulnerable and fearful. Parents with exaggerated fears often have misperceptions about the cardiac disorder despite repeated explanations from professionals.

Anxious parents often hear explanations that are quite different from what a professional actually said. For example, one mother had repeatedly been told by the cardiologist that her son had no need for activity restrictions and should be treated like any other 14-year-old boy. At one clinic visit, the mother stated that she always had treated him absolutely normally—this said as she tucked in his shirt and bent to tie his shoe. Clearly, her anxiety influenced how she interpreted "normal" in the case of her son. Nurses help parents to distinguish realistic fears from unfounded anxiety.

When the child and family are unable to accept the fact of heart disease, cooperation with the therapeutic regimen is jeopardized. For example, a 7-month-old infant with chronic congestive heart failure related to a congenital defect was well-stabilized on digitalis. For no apparent reason, the child's condition deteriorated abruptly, and he needed emergency intervention. The mother later confided that the child seemed to be doing so well that she was sure his heart was better and that he no longer needed his medicine; she therefore did not give the digitalis. In this situation, the mother's anxiety led to her inability to accept the reality of the child's defect. Her denial of her son's diagnosis and need for treatment was related to her hope that the defect would go away; however, her behavior was life threatening.

⊛ Potential body image disturbance

Several factors determine the effect that the heart problem has on the child's body image. A major factor is the child's perception of the heart disease. This depends in part on the child's concept of the heart. Reif's (1972) studies of how children of different ages conceptualize the heart indicate that children betwen 4 and 6 years of age have a general idea of the heart's anatomic position. They characterize it as having a valentine shape and making tick-tock sounds. Children between 7 and 10 years of age realize the heart is not shaped like a valentine, and they recognize that the heart plays a vital role in body functions, although they are not generally sure what that role is. By 10–11 years of age, children have a basic understanding of how the heart works and why cardiac function is necessary to life.

Older children are more likely to have a realistic perception of their illness because of their better understanding of the circulatory system. Children under 8–10 years of age, particularly those in early and middle childhood, are likely to have misperceptions regarding the meaning and cause of their illness. For example, one 6-year-old believed her heart became "sick" because she "ran too much." Their inaccurate cause-and-effect reasoning might lead children to believe that their parents, siblings, or they themselves are responsible for the defect. Children might feel guilty or angry, depending on who they believe "caused" the disease.

Health Maintenance Needs

⊛ Potential for impaired home maintenance management

Observing for symptoms Once the parent understands the basics of the child's heart disease, the parent can better appreciate why certain signs and symptoms might occur. The nurse teaches the parent which signs and symptoms to watch for and what to do if these become evident. The specific symptoms that the nurse teaches depend on the nature of the child's disease. In general, the parent is instructed to observe and report fever, decreased intake, increased respiratory rate or pulse rate, difficult breathing (shortness of breath, congestion, grunting, retractions, cough), edema (swelling), increase in cyanosis, pallor, decreased urine output, and vomiting or diarrhea.

The child's hospital stay is an important opportunity to teach parents about monitoring the child at home. For example, during hospitalization, parents might practice counting respirations (and pulse if indicated) under the guidance of the nurse. Parents might practice how to use a thermometer safely and to read it accurately. The nurse also can evaluate parental awareness of symptoms. When a parent accurately assesses symptoms, the nurse can validate and reinforce the parent's judgment. Some parents miss important symptoms, whereas other parents overreact to minor findings. The nurse therefore identifies patterns of over- or underreaction prior to the child's discharge, as errors in judgment might have serious consequences for the child's health. If parents over- or underreact, the nurse gives corrective feedback. Underreaction to symptoms might be a form of denial (a maladaptive behavior in cases of chronic illness); overreaction might be a manifestation of anxiety. In either case, the underlying issues must be addressed.

Administering medications One of the major parental responsibilities is the administration of medications. The nurse carefully explains to the parents why the drugs are given, how they affect the body, what the side effects are, and what precautions are necessary. Parent education should begin when the medication is started. Attempting to do all of the teaching about medications just prior to discharge increases the risk of misunderstandings and mistakes.

Teaching can begin by having the parents observe the nurse measure and administer the medication. After the parents understand the procedure, the nurse supervises them as they measure the medication and give it to the child. The nurse offers suggestions that will make the task easier and enhance the parent's confidence. The child gets used to the parent's methods before going home, and if problems arise (vomiting, refusal) the parent can handle these with guidance from the nurse.

Some people have difficulty reading and using the dosage scales on syringes or droppers. Enlarged visual aids might be helpful during the learning period. Parents should be taught to place a liquid medication slowly in the side of the child's mouth about halfway back while the child's head is slightly elevated. If the medication is mixed with food, only a small amount of food should be used. If the child fails to finish the food, there is no way of knowing how much medication was taken. Parents also need to be aware of the risk of accidental overdose and the importance of safe storage of the drug. Written information on the drug container is valuable. Drugs vary considerably with respect to action, dosage, and side effects, and it is often difficult for parents to keep the drugs straight, especially if the child is taking several.

Digoxin In a survey of parents whose children received digoxin, it was found that frightening gaps in the parents' knowledge were present, particularly in regard to symptoms of digoxin toxicity. With a drug as potent and potentially dangerous as digoxin, it is essential that parents are given careful instruction regarding dosage, administration, signs of toxicity, and management of common problems.

Jackson (1979) notes that the following points should be included in teaching family members about digoxin:

1. Digoxin is a very effective but very potent medication. It enables the heart to pump more effectively with a slower and more regular rhythm.
2. The major danger is digoxin toxicity. It is important to recognize signs of toxicity as early as possible. Signs of toxicity include loss of appetite, vomiting, and slow or irregular pulse. If any signs of digoxin toxicity occur, the physician should be notified.
3. Digoxin should be given exactly as prescribed. It is dangerous to give more or less than prescribed.
4. It is important to give the medicine every 12 hours.
5. Digoxin is absorbed better if given 1 hour before or 2 hours after a meal.
6. If a dose is forgotten and 4 hours or less have elapsed since the dose was due, the dose may be given, and the next dose should be given at the regular time. If more than 4 hours have elapsed, it is best to skip the dose entirely. The subsequent dose should never be doubled or increased to make up for the forgotten dose.
7. If for any reason two doses are missed, the physician should be notified.
8. Most children like the taste of digoxin. If, however, the child spits out the medicine, the dose should *not* be repeated unless the parents are sure none of the medication was swallowed.
9. If the child vomits within 15 minutes of receiving the digoxin and it seems that all or most of the digoxin was lost, all or part of the dose may be repeated. If the child vomits more than 15 minutes after the dose, it should *not* be repeated, as part of the digoxin will already be in the bloodstream. The normal dose should be given at the next regular time. If the child vomits all or part of two doses of digoxin, the physician should be notified.
10. If the child becomes ill and has loss of appetite, vomiting, diarrhea, difficulty breathing, or a slow or irregular pulse, the physician should be notified.
11. Digoxin must be stored in a place that is safe from all children. Accidental overdose might be fatal.
12. If accidental overdose should occur, the child should be taken immediately to the nearest emergency room. Ipecac should be given before transport if the child is conscious. The medicine bottle should be brought along also.

Recommendations vary, depending on institutional policy and the physician's preference, about whether the parent should take the child's pulse before giving digoxin and at what point (pulse rate) the drug should be withheld.

Diuretics Diuretics are used frequently in children with heart disease. Instructions for parents vary according to the specific diuretic agent prescribed. When potassium-excreting diuretics are used, the parent must understand the risk of hypokalemia. If the child also is receiving digoxin, the parent should be aware that low potassium levels might precipitate digoxin toxicity. Signs of hypokalemia include anorexia, nausea, vomiting, numbness, confusion, irritability, and weakness. Parents should know which foods are high in potassium; these include bananas, oranges, grapefruit, prune juice, canned apricots, milk, carrots, and potatoes. If potassium supplements are ordered, the nurse instructs the parent in their use. Illnesses that result in decreased appetite, vomiting, or diarrhea increase the risk of hypokalemia. The parent therefore is encouraged to notify the physician if this occurs.

Doses should be scheduled so that diuresis does not occur at night in children who are toilet-trained. If diuretics are given in the late afternoon or evening, enuresis might occur. It might not be possible to avoid late-day administration for children with serious disease, however, as the priority is to maintain a steady serum level. Parents should understand that increased urine output is an expected effect. Decreased output, edema, and respiratory distress might indicate that the diuretic is ineffective and that the physician should be notified.

Skin and mucous membranes should be inspected daily for petechaie and other signs of bleeding if the child is receiving large doses or prolonged therapy with thiazide diuretics. Complete blood count, serum electrolytes, blood urea nitrogen, creatinine, uric acid, and blood sugar should be checked periodically for children receiving thiazide diuretics.

A potassium-sparing diuretic, such as spironolactone (Aldactone), may be used in conjunction with another diuretic such as one of the thiazides (Diuril). Because this drug prevents the excretion of potassium, it helps to counteract the potassium-losing effect of other diuretics, but hyperkalemia is a risk, particularly if this drug is used alone.

Preventing infection The nurse informs the parents that children with heart disease are at special risk for infection. Generally, parents must avoid exposing their children to persons who might have communicable diseases. This is not easy to do, since social contact is desirable for children, and infectious diseases are common in children. Siblings also bring illnesses home from school, and casual contacts at public places, such as stores and places of worship, might lead to infection. Commonsense precautions are indicated. Correct and frequent hand washing by everyone in the home is of primary importance. Isolating sick individuals from the child provides some protection. Use of common drinking glasses should be avoided. Infants should not be taken to crowded places where exposure cannot be controlled. If the child attends a day-care center or school, teachers must be told about the risk from infectious disease. The child might need to remain home in order to prevent exposure to illnesses "going around" at school.

Parents need not, however, be so frightened by the risk of infection that their children are never allowed to leave the house or play with other children. The goal is to strike a balance between avoiding unnecessary exposure and providing social contact. If signs of an infectious disease do occur, the physician should be notified.

Virtually all children with organic heart disease require prophylactic treatment with antibiotics to reduce the risk of endocarditis associated with dental work, minor surgery, and illnesses. The nurse therefore instructs parents to tell others involved in the care of their children about the presence of heart disease. For example, doctors, dentists, and emergency room personnel who evaluate and treat the child must be informed. Early symptoms of subacute bacterial endocarditis include fever, chills, and lethargy. These should be reported to the physician.

In addition to the special care related to the cardiac disease, the child needs routine health care. Regular assessments, immunization, recommended laboratory studies (urinalysis, hemoglobin), vision and hearing screening, developmental screening, and anticipatory guidance are especially important for the child with heart disease.

Regulating temperature Because both hyperthermia and hypothermia increase the child's (and especially the infant's) need for oxygen, the nurse discusses with the parent the need to prevent chilling or overheating in the child. Young infants are most susceptible to temperature variations in response to environmental conditions, and special precautions might be necessary. Diaphoresis, which might occur in infants with heart failure, can increase the risk of chilling.

The Child with Complications Related to Cardiac Dysfunction

Congestive Heart Failure

Congestive heart failure is a condition in which the heart is unable to supply blood to the body in sufficient quantities to meet the metabolic requirements of the organs. Congestive heart failure is a manifestation of an underlying disease rather than a disease in itself. It can be due to reduced myocardial function or to abnormally increased demands placed on the heart.

Compensatory mechanisms Prior to the development of congestive heart failure, compensatory mechanisms are activated by the body in an attempt to maintain cardiac output and appropriate blood pressure.

Sympathetic nervous system mechanism Decreased blood pressure stimulates vascular receptors and baroreceptors in the aorta and carotid arteries, which in turn trigger the sympathetic nervous system. Release of catecholamines increases the rate and force of myocardial contraction. Catecholamines also increase venous tone, so that blood is returned to the heart more effectively.

Decreased blood pressure also stimulates the renin-angiotension mechanism in the kidneys (see Chapter 28). The vasoconstrictive action of angiotensin causes decreased circulation to the skin, extremities, splanchnic bed (viscera), and kidneys. This action maximizes the blood flow to the heart, lungs, and brain. Pallor, cool extremities, and weak peripheral pulses might be present. The decreased renal blood flow stimulates the release of aldosterone, resulting in retention of sodium and water. The increased fluid, or *hypervolemia,* increases the workload of an already stressed myocardium.

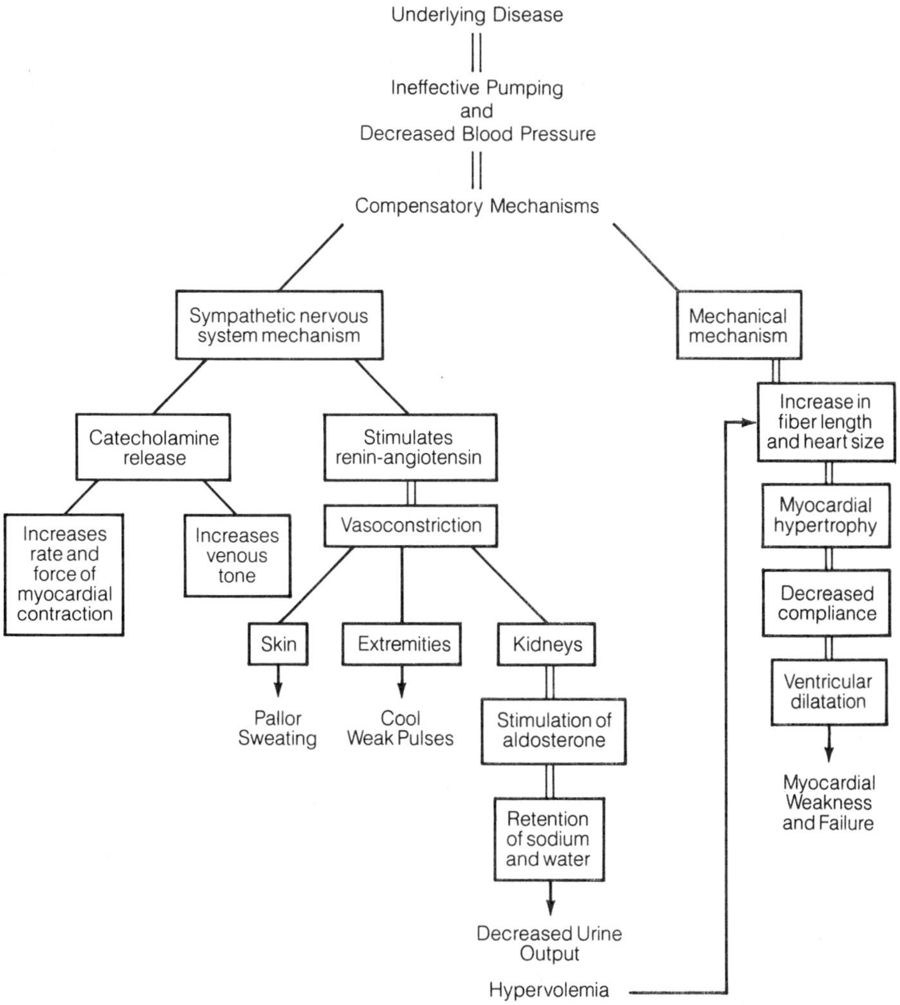

FIGURE 23-4
Mechanisms leading to congestive heart failure.

Mechanical mechanisms Poor peripheral perfusion and hypervolemia cause an increase in myocardial fiber length and heart size as the heart works harder to maintain cardiac output. The heart muscle thickens (myocardial hypertrophy) in an attempt to maintain cardiac output by increasing pressure in the ventricles. Myocardial hypertrophy is effective temporarily, but as muscle mass increases, compliance decreases, and greater filling pressure is required to achieve an adequate diastolic volume. Also, the increasing muscle mass might outgrow its blood supply, resulting in myocardial ischemia (decreased circulation).

Ventricular dilatation results as myocardial fibers stretch during diastole to accommodate increased ventricular volume. A mild-to-moderate stretch increases the force of the contraction, but beyond a certain point, contractility does not increase (Figure 23-4). Although compensatory mechanisms can help the child live longer, all mechanisms can increase cardiac work load causing eventual myocardial weakness and failure.

Types of congestive heart failure Congestive heart failure can be classified as left-sided or right-sided heart failure. Because each side depends on the effective function of the other, failure of one side usually results in reciprocal failure in the other side. In children, clinical right- and left-sided failure usually occur together.

Left-sided failure Because the left ventricle is unable to empty completely during systole, end-diastolic pressure and volume increase, and the left atrium is unable to expel blood into the left ventricle. Pressure in the left atrium rises, and blood returning from the pulmonary circulation is unable to enter the left atrium. Then, as blood backs up, pressure in the pulmonary veins increases. As the pressure buildup in the capillaries continues, fluid leaks from the capillaries to the interstitial spaces. When the amount of leaked fluid exceeds the capacity of the lymphatics to remove it, pulmonary edema results.

Right-sided failure When the pressure in the pulmonary vasculature is elevated, the right ventricle is unable to eject the blood completely into the pulmonary artery. The resultant increase in right ventricular end-diastolic pressure prevents emptying of the right atrium. Elevated atrial pressure inhibits the return of blood from the superior and inferior venae cavae. Elevation of pressures in the systemic venous circulation results in systemic congestion and edema.

Causes of congestive heart failure *Congestive heart failure* is a poor term because the signs and symptoms of congestive heart failure can occur when the heart is not truly "failing." In many instances, the heart meets increased demands and functions normally, perhaps supernormally. In addition to its inaccuracy, the term congestive heart failure is frightening to patients and families because *failure* implies cessation of function.

Causes of congestive heart failure can be classified as (a) increased volume, (b) obstruction to outflow, (c) ineffective myocardial function, (d) arrhythmias, or (e) excessive demand for cardiac output. In congestive heart failure due to increased volume, myocardial function is normal, but the heart is called on to pump an excessive volume of blood. Excessive volume might be due to hypervolemia, which could be caused by excessive fluid intake or retention. Fluid retention alone usually does not cause congestive heart failure, but it might complicate failure from other causes. In children, the demand for the heart to pump an increased volume is caused most often by congenital defects and altered hemodynamics. For example, in some defects a certain volume of blood ejected from the left ventricle returns directly to the heart without perfusing any organ. The heart must pump this recirculated blood in addition to the normal volume it ejects into the systemic circulation. Compensatory mechanisms that enable the heart to pump the increased total volume of blood include increased heart rate (tachycardia) and increased size of the pumping chambers (myocardial hypertrophy and dilatation). Despite the tachycardia, cardiomegaly, and diagnosis of congestive heart failure, the heart muscle is functioning normally.

Congestive heart failure due to obstruction to outflow might occur if the normal myocardium is expected to pump against increased resistance. Structural defects in the valves or major vessels might cause obstruction to outflow. Pulmonary disease and pulmonary arterial hypertension are two conditions that increase the resistance in the lungs and the work of the right ventricle. Congestive heart failure that occurs as a result of pulmonary pathology is termed *cor pulmonale*. Severe systemic hypertension also increases systemic resistance to outflow and can cause congestive heart failure.

Although congestive heart failure in children usually is due to abnormal stresses placed on the heart, sometimes it is due to a primary heart muscle disorder. Causes of primary myocardial dysfunction include rheumatic fever, infectious myocarditis, idiopathic congestive cardiomyopathy, and mucocutaneous lymph node syndrome (Kawasaki disease).

Congestive heart failure can accompany certain arrhythmias. Complete atrioventricular block, which results in an abnormally slow heart rate, or sustained primary tachycardia can lead to congestive heart failure. With tachycardia, there is insufficient time for ventricular filling, and cardiac output is therefore decreased.

Congestive heart failure due to excessive demand for cardiac output can occur with severe anemia. Because anemia reduces the oxygen-carrying capacity of the blood, the heart must pump more blood per minute to supply the tissues adequately. If the volume of blood required by the tissues is greater than the pumping capacity of the heart, congestive heart failure occurs.

Clinical manifestations Signs and symptoms of congestive heart failure are summarized in Table 23-9. Children with compensated congestive heart failure might not show any symptoms during daily activities. The presence of compensated failure can be demonstrated, however, by measuring the child's total working capacity using a bicycle ergometer or a treadmill. Patients with compensated congestive heart failure have reduced working capacity when the cardiovascular system is stressed.

As the degree of congestive heart failure increases, the cardiovascular system can no longer compensate adequately, and symptoms of cardiovascular insufficiency occur at rest or with minimal stress. Tachycardia, one of four cardinal signs of congestive heart failure, develops as the heart attempts to compensate for decreased efficiency with an increased rate. This compensatory mechanism has disadvantages. Tachycardia decreases diastolic filling time, which results in reduced ventricular filling and reduced coronary blood flow (coronary blood flow occurs during diastole). In addition, tachycardia increases the oxygen needs of the myocardium. Cardiomegaly due to hypertrophy and ventricular dilatation is a second cardinal sign of congestive heart failure.

Clinical manifestations related to pulmonary edema result from left-sided failure. Tachypnea is a third cardinal sign of congestive heart failure. Dyspnea, retractions, nasal flaring, expiratory grunt, cough, rales, rhonchi, and orthopnea are all manifestations of left-sided heart failure.

Edema from right-sided failure usually is not observed in infants. If present, it is most commonly seen in the periorbital and sacral areas. In older children, dependent edema in the legs and sacrum is observed. Pitting edema and ascites (fluid in the peritoneal cavity) also might be noted. Weight gain is an indication of fluid retention both in infants and in older children.

Hepatomegaly is a fourth cardinal sign of congestive heart failure and results from elevated pressure in the in-

TABLE 23-9 Signs and Symptoms of Congestive Heart Failure

Infants	Older children and adults
Tachycardia	Tachycardia
Tachypnea	Tachypnea
Hepatomegaly	Hepatomegaly
Cardiomegaly	Cardiomegaly
Gallop rhythm	Gallop rhythm
Oliguria	Oliguria
Diaphoresis	Diaphoresis
Rales, gasping, and grunting expirations are late signs	Rales
Poor feeding, slow growth pattern, fatigue	Exercise intolerance
Hypotonia, flaccidity	Dyspnea, shortness of breath; orthopnea, nocturnal dyspnea
Dyspnea, costal retractions (if severe), subcostal retractions	Edema, weight gain
Periorbital edema	Pallor, mottling of skin
Pallor and mottling of skin, transient duskiness	Dry, hacking cough
Persistent, hacking cough	Poor peripheral circulation, cold extremities
Poor peripheral circulation, cold extremities	Hypotension
Hypotension	

ferior vena cava. Elevation of pressure in the superior vena cava might result in distention of jugular veins.

Nursing management The nursing care of children with congestive heart failure is directed toward reducing the cardiac work load and enhancing cardiac output. Monitoring activity and promoting rest, careful recording of intake and output, and observing for signs of fluid retention are essential. Monitoring vital signs, limiting activities that cause stress, and administering prescribed medications such as digoxin and diuretics while noting their effects are important nursing interventions. The nurse carefully observes the child for subtle changes in appearance that might indicate fluid accumulation and for disposition changes that would indicate decreased activity tolerance or anxiety and restlessness from hypoxemia. Daily weights, measurement of abdominal girth, frequent position changes, dietary and environmental modifications to promote rest, and frequent vital signs and breath sounds are part of the nursing care for children with congestive heart failure.

Exercise tolerance test. (Courtesy of the Mayo Clinic, Rochester, Minnesota.)

The Child Undergoing Cardiac Surgery

Cardiac surgery is a stressful experience for both the child and the family, and the quality of nursing care in the perioperative period is a critical factor in the child's recovery. Although excellent physical care is of primary importance,

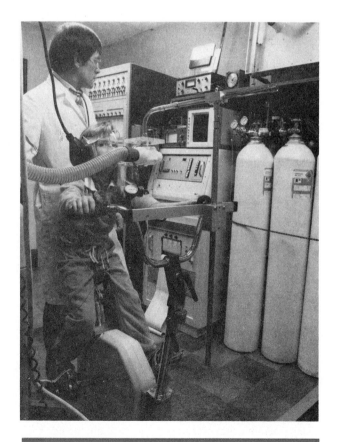

promotion of the child's psychologic adjustment is an integral part of nursing care.

Cardiac surgery may be done on an emergency basis or on an elective basis. *Closed-heart surgery* involves structures related to the heart but not the heart muscle itself and can be done without cardiopulmonary bypass. *Open-heart surgery* involves structures within the heart, necessitates an incision into the myocardium, and requires cardiopulmonary bypass. Palliative surgery provides a temporary or partial correction, whereas corrective surgery provides a permanent and total correction of the defect. Unfortunately, only palliative surgery is possible for some defects. Generally, the younger the child, the higher the surgical risk.

Preoperative management Preoperative assessment data include the following:

1. *Laboratory data.* Tests that are routinely done before surgery include chest radiographs, electrocardiogram, complete blood count, serum electrolytes, clotting studies, and urinalysis. Other studies, such as echocardiogram and cardiac catheterization, are done if necessary.
2. *Vital signs.* Temperature, pulse, respiration, and blood pressure are monitored prior to surgery.
3. *Sleep-wake patterns.* The nurse notes the child's usual pattern of sleep and activity. This information can be used postoperatively to plan periods of rest that coincide with the child's usual pattern. Stressful procedures can be scheduled during normal waking times when hydrocortisone secretion is likely to be highest.
4. *Height and weight.* These must be accurately measured and recorded, as they will be used in calculation of medication doses and fluid orders.
5. *Intake patterns.* Fluids and foods that the child particularly enjoys are documented. Information about the usual amount and times of intake can be used to plan progressive introduction of oral intake postoperatively. For example, a young child who is used to a bottle early in the morning might obtain some comfort by receiving a portion of the day's fluid allotment at that time.
6. *Elimination patterns.* The nurse needs to understand the words the child uses for bowel and bladder functions. Information on the usual pattern of urination and defecation will be useful in helping the child resume these functions as soon as possible after surgery.
7. *Signs of infection.* Any sign that might indicate the presence of an infection is reported to the physician. Surgery usually is contraindicated if infection is present.

Preoperative skin preparation, which might include bacteriocidal cleansing and shaving, is usually ordered, although this varies depending on the surgeon and the institution.

The nurse also needs to check all medication orders carefully. Generally, digitalis is withheld for 24 hours before surgery. Other medications might be initiated, discontinued, or modified. Any order that is unclear is reviewed and verified with the physician.

Intraoperative management Repair of intracardiac lesions requires the use of cardiopulmonary bypass. This is accomplished by use of a pump oxygenator with a high-efficiency heat exchanger. A cannula collects the venous blood at the right atrium and diverts it to the machine, where carbon dioxide is removed and oxygen is added. The oxygenated blood is returned to the circulation through a cannula that enters the ascending aorta and is circulated through the body, perfusing the organs and body tissues.

Hypothermia reduces the metabolic demands of the heart and other organs and usually is used in conjunction with cardiopulmonary bypass. The child's temperature is reduced to 20–30°C to compensate for reduced blood flow during bypass. For small children with complex intracardiac lesions, profound hypothermia might be required. The child initially is cooled to a core temperature of 28°C, is placed on cardiopulmonary bypass, and then is cooled rapidly to 15°C. At that point, bypass circulation is terminated. This provides a bloodless operative field and a motionless heart. After the lesion is repaired, bypass is resumed, and the child is rewarmed. Children are able to tolerate up to 60 minutes of profound hypothermia with total circulatory arrest.

During surgery there is constant monitoring of blood volume, arterial blood gases, blood pressure, and other indexes of cardiac output.

Postoperative management Care of the child who has had cardiac surgery is complex and challenging. After surgery, the child is transferred directly to the intensive care unit and remains there until stable, generally for 1–3 days. Although cardiovascular function is of primary concern, virtually every organ can be affected by cardiac surgery. Therefore, assessment must be constant and comprehensive. The nurse therefore makes astute observations so that subtle signs of potential problems are identified early and complications are prevented. The goals of nursing care in the early postoperative period include:

Preventing complications (Table 23-10)
Detecting potential problems early
Minimizing the psychologic trauma of the surgical and intensive care unit experiences

TABLE 23-10 Postoperative Complications of Cardiac Surgery

System	Complication
Cardiovascular	Decreased cardiac output Congestive heart failure Tamponade Arrhythmias Shock
Renal	Acute tubular necrosis
Respiratory	Atelectasis Pneumonia Pneumothorax Emboli
Neurologic	Emboli (air or particulate) Decreased cerebral blood flow
Infection	Wound Mediastinal Endocarditis Sepsis
Fluid and electrolyte	Hypervolemia/hypovolemia Acidosis Hypokalemia/hyperkalemia Hypocalcemia
Hematologic	Surgical bleeding Thrombocytopenia Disseminated intravascular coagulopathy Bypass-related coagulopathy Anemia

The details of care during the immediate postoperative period require special education and training in intensive care procedures and as such will not be specified.

Once stable, the child returns to the pediatric unit where the recovery process is monitored and preparation is made for discharge.

Managing convalescence Once the child is physiologically stable and is transferred out of intensive care and returns to the pediatric unit, the nurse plans interventions to help the child gradually resume normal activity and responsibilities and to prepare the family for discharge.

The nursing care for the child at this stage is similar to that of any child following major surgery. The nurse monitors cardiovascular status by auscultating heart sounds, palpating peripheral pulses, and measuring vital signs. The nurse also auscultates breath sounds, encourages deep breathing and coughing, provides chest physiotherapy, records intake and output, and notes the nutritional value of the child's food intake. The incisional sites are inspected daily for signs of infection as are lab value reports. As the child becomes more active, periods of activity are alternated with quiet times until the child regains strength.

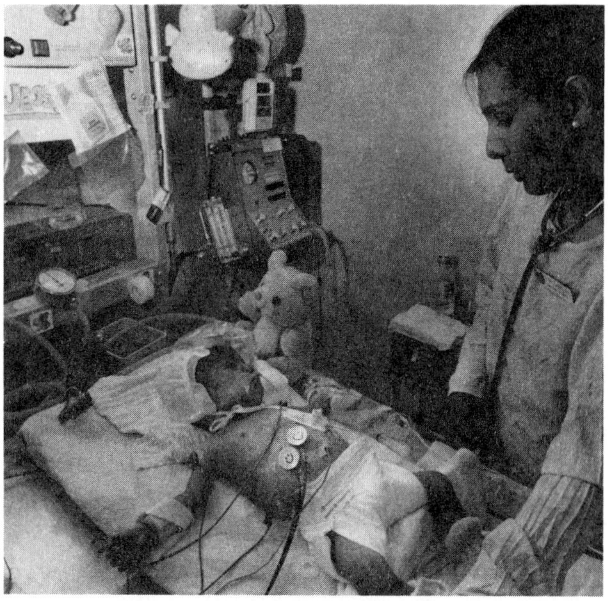

Child in intensive care unit after cardiac surgery.

All procedures are explained to the child before they are done, with an emphasis on what the child will feel. Explanations of the necessity of surgery and treatment in the intensive care unit should be repeated to dispel misperceptions. Therapeutic play is begun when the child is ready. If the child is hesitant to play, the nurse can play through some of the experiences the child has had.

Occasionally, a child exhibits angry or rejecting behavior toward a parent. This is very difficult for most parents to handle, although this behavior often is a positive comment on the parent-child relationship. The child might be angry that the parent has failed to provide protection and has allowed the surgery to occur. Children who are sure of their parents' love, however, know that the anger will be accepted and that their parents will continue to love them. Parents often need to have this behavior interpreted for them, and they might need help in understanding the importance of remaining with the child and providing consistent support.

The nurse assesses the child's readiness to relinquish the "sick role" and to assume more healthy behavior. The nurse also is alert for signs that the child is seeking secondary gain from symptoms or surgery. The nurse can promote the child's adjustment in this area by gradually expecting more independence and more self-care from the child.

Preparation for discharge A parent might need help in adjusting to the child's condition after surgery. The physician and nurse therefore address directly the importance of allowing the child appropriate independence, with its privileges and responsibilities. In preparation for discharge, the parents should learn to provide care in the hospital. They should have experience giving medications and performing treatments. The family needs instructions regarding medications, diet, activity restrictions, return to school, care of the incisions, and signs and symptoms to report. Follow-up appointments and the name and number of people to call with questions should also be provided.

Behavior disturbances in children after discharge are relatively common and include nightmares, sleep problems, overdependence, and separation anxiety. The nurse can discuss with parents how to handle these problems if they occur. Parents should encourage their children to continue to talk about the hospitalization and surgery. In play, a toy doctor or nurse kit is very helpful, as are pictures of the hospital and visits to the hospital. Although it is important to compliment children on how well the experience was handled and on how brave they were, praise should not be emphasized unduly. Rather, the child should be encouraged to seek gratification from normal, healthy experiences.

Congenital cardiac defects are discussed in Table 23-11.

The Child with Subacute Bacterial Endocarditis

Subacute bacterial endocarditis is an infectious disease that usually involves abnormal portions of endocardium or endothelium associated with a cardiac or vascular malformation. Subacute bacterial endocarditis can complicate even hemodynamically insignificant lesions, such as a small ventricular septal defect or a mitral valve prolapse. Endocarditis occurs most frequently in children with bicuspid aortic valve, patent ductus arteriosus, coarctation of the aorta, ventricular septal defects, tetralogy of Fallot, and aortic stenosis. The microorganism, commonly an alpha streptococcus, gains entry to the circulation through an interruption of the skin or mucous membranes. Because the alpha streptococcus is a natural inhabitant of the mouth, its entry into the vascular system can occur during dental manipulation. This is why subacute bacterial endocarditis prophylaxis is indicated for dental procedures.

Clinical manifestations The child with subacute bacterial endocarditis usually has an unexplained fever and an underlying cardiovascular malformation. Frequently, subacute bacterial endocarditis is associated with anemia, fatigue, splenomegaly, petechiae, splinter hemorrhages under the nails, and raw spots on palms and soles. Tender areas of inflammation might develop on the finger pads. The diagnosis of subacute bacterial endocarditis is confirmed by blood cultures.

Treatment Untreated subacute bacterial endocarditis is uniformly fatal. With antibiotic treatment, however, the infection can be eradicated. Treatment must be continued 3–6 weeks. Although curable, subacute bacterial endocarditis can cause further damage to infected heart structures while it lasts. If, for example, an abnormal aortic valve is infected, valve function can be diminished further by the infection. Antibiotic therapy might be less effective in the presence of prosthetic material, such as an artificial valve. Occasionally, the infection cannot be eradicated with antibiotics until the prosthetic material is removed.

The risk of developing subacute bacterial endocarditis can be reduced in susceptible children if antibiotics are administered before and after the skin or mucous membranes are violated, particularly during dental work. Penicillin is the drug of choice if the child is not already receiving penicillin and is not allergic to it.

Nursing management The nurse plays an important role in the prevention of subacute bacterial endocarditis by

- Reinforcing teaching about the importance of prophylaxis
- Teaching parents and children when and how antibiotics are to be administered
- Emphasizing the importance of oral health maintenance to reduce the chance of bacterial invasion
- Instructing parents to notify the physician if symptoms of subacute bacterial endocarditis occur

All those involved in the child's care (dentists, emergency room personnel, school nurse, and others) should be informed of the child's susceptibility.

Treatment of subacute bacterial endocarditis requires hopsitalization for a prolonged period. Children need careful preparation for intravenous therapy and blood cultures. The nurse discusses with the child the need for hospitalization and activity restrictions and helps the child cope with these aspects of care.

Intravenous antibiotics must be administered on schedule to maintain therapeutic serum levels. The nurse monitors carefully for side effects. Prolonged use of high doses of intravenous antibiotics can cause inflammation of the vein. The nurse also observes closely for signs of complications, namely, congestive heart failure and embolism.

(text continues on p. 761)

TABLE 23-11 Congenital Cardiac Defects

The child with an acyanotic cardiac defect

Patent ductus arteriosus

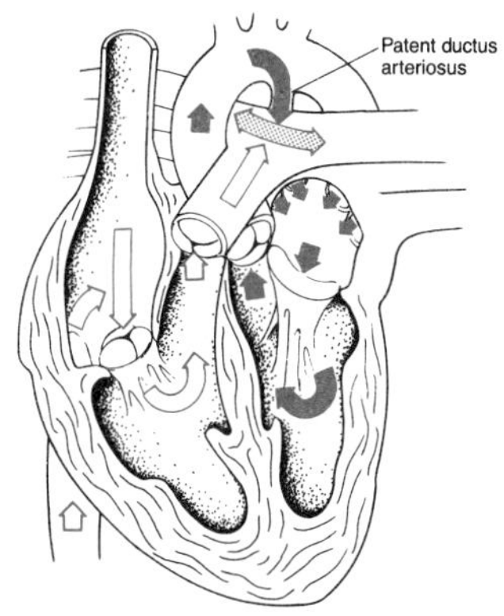

*Patent ductus arteriosus.**

Definition
Failure of the ductus arteriosus to close thus enabling oxygenated blood that has been ejected from the left ventricle to the aorta (high pressure) to flow into the pulmonary artery (lower pressure) and the pulmonary circulation. This altered flow creates increased volume in the lungs and left cardiac structures resulting in volume overload. Occurs in 1 of 2,000 live births and accounts for 10% of congenital heart disease.

Clinical manifestations
Machinery-hum murmur heard at the upper left sternal border across the back. If the volume of blood passing through the persistent patent ductus is large, it can result in left atrial and left ventricular enlargement, increased pulmonary pressure leading to pulmonary edema, and congestive heart failure. If the volume of blood is small, these effects are minimal.

Treatment
Surgical ligation (tying) of the vessel. This can be done relatively safely in patients of all ages. In premature infants, the ductus arteriosus sometimes can be closed using prostaglandin synthetase inhibitors, such as indomethacin, as an alternative to surgical ligation.

Nursing management
When indomethacin is used side effects may include oliguria, gastrointestinal bleeding, platelet dysfunction, and possibly bilirubinemia. Nursing care involves obtaining baseline values for blood urea nitrogen (BUN), serum creatinine, serum bilirubin, clotting function, and vital signs. The nurse monitors cardiovascular status to detect evidence of patent ductus arteriosus (heart murmur, wide pulse pressure, bounding pulses, congestive heart failure); urine output for blood and protein in the urine; BUN and serum creatinine levels; platelet count, prothrombin time, partial thromboplastin time; and observes for signs of gastrointestinal bleeding in stools and gastric aspirate.

If surgery is necessary, preoperatively the nurse reviews and provides the parents with a list of the early indicators of increased cardiac workload such as fatigue with previously tolerated exercise, increased pulse and respiratory rate, and evidence of puffiness around the eyes and weight gain, plus resources to serve as supports. Postoperatively the nurse promotes recovery by effectively managing the child's pain to prevent respiratory and skeletal complication. The time in intensive care is brief as the child is extubated shortly after surgery, gradually begins sips of water, and has the chest tube removed the following morning. Since the incision is on the left side of the chest, many nerve endings are involved, pain is intense, and the child resists movement. The nurse employs creative measures to have the child cough, deep breathe, turn, and ambulate with good posture. The child tends to guard the surgical site and lean toward the left when walking. If the child's posture is not corrected, a secondary scoliosis (curvature of the spine) might develop and if fluid accumulates in the lungs, respiratory complications might occur.

Coarctation of the aorta

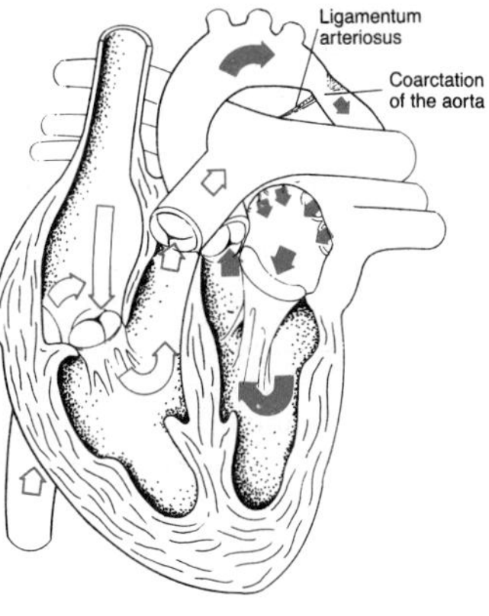

Coarctation of the aorta.

Definition
A shelflike projection of tissue into the lumen of the aorta usually just distal to the origin of the left subclavian artery resulting in a narrowing of the aorta. Occurs in 1 of 13,000 children. It causes increased systolic blood pressure proximal to the narrowed area and decreased systolic blood pressure distal to the narrowed area.

*Key to arrows in artwork throughout table appears in figure on p. 712.

(Continues)

TABLE 23-11 Congenital Cardiac Defects *(Continued)*

The child with an acyanotic cardiac defect

Coarctation of the aorta *(Continued)*

Clinical manifestations

The severity of manifestations depends on the degree of narrowing. Pulses are diminished and blood pressure is low in the lower extremities while pulses are normal-to-increased, blood pressure is high in the upper extremities. Lower extremities cool and are prone to muscle cramps during exercise. Possible complaints of headaches or dizziness, episodes of fainting, and nose bleeds secondary to hypertension. If severe, particularly in infants, symptoms of congestive heart failure might be present.

Treatment

Significant narrowing is treated by surgical removal of the aortic obstruction either by excising the shelflike membrane and patching the aorta or by cutting out the narrowed section of the aorta and sewing the two ends of the aorta back together. Children with congestive heart failure are treated with digitalis and diuretics prior to surgery. Coarctation repaired prior to one year of age can recur.

Nursing management

The nursing care needs of this child are similar to those of the child following correction of a patent ductus arteriosus since a left thoracic surgical incision is used. The nursing care focus is on pain management, pulmonary hygiene, and early ambulation with good posture.

Ventricular septal defect (VSD)

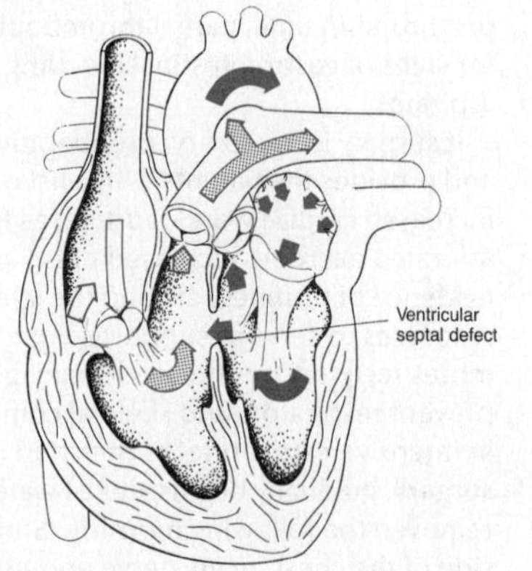

Ventricular septal defect.

Definition

An opening or openings in the septum between the two ventricles. Usually located in the upper membranous but sometimes in the lower muscular portion of the septum. Occurs in 1.5–2.5 of 1,000 live births and comprises 20% of all forms of congenital heart disease. During systole some of the oxygenated blood in the left ventricle (high pressure) is ejected through the opening into the right ventricle (low pressure) rather than into the aorta. This oxygenated blood plus the deoxygenated blood in the right ventricle is ejected into the pulmonary artery. Thus an increased (the larger the hole, the greater the increase) amount of blood enters the pulmonary circulation and returns to the left atrium and left ventricle. This might result in pulmonary edema and enlargement of the left heart. If the hole is large, pressure in the right ventricle and pulmonary arteries becomes elevated resulting eventually in obstructive pulmonary vascular disease.

Clinical manifestations

If the VSD is small, the child might be asymptomatic, the only sign being a characteristic murmur. If the VSD is large, symptoms of congestive heart failure and pulmonary edema appear within the first year of life. Severity of these symptoms depends on the size of the hole and whether or not any other cardiac defects are present.

Treatment

Small, hemodynamically insignificant defects require no specific treatment and most close spontaneously. For medium and large defects (defined as having 40%–65% of the pulmonary blood flow originating from the left-to-right shunt), symptoms of congestive heart failure are managed medically with digitalis and diuretics until surgical closure can be done or until spontaneous closure occurs. The surgery requires a midsternal incision and use of cardiopulmonary bypass. The hole is closed by either suturing it together or by sewing a patch (usually Dacron) over the hole. Complete repair is preferred, however, if the infant is a poor surgical risk, a palliative procedure, in which a small constricting band is placed around the pulmonary artery to reduce blood flow to the lungs, may be done. The procedure is known as pulmonary artery banding (PAB). The procedure is brief and does not require cardiopulmonary bypass.

Nursing management

Preoperative nursing care focuses on teaching the parents about the signs and symptoms of congestive heart failure, administration and side effects of medications, careful monitoring of the child's exercise tolerance, and monitoring of the child's eating patterns, growth, and general health status. The parents are told that worsening of any of these parameters necessitates medical and often surgical intervention. The nurse prepares and supports the parents and the child for any surgical and postoperative experiences. Postoperative care requires highly skilled nursing care, much of which is technical since the child's vital functions, such as respiration, heart rate, and blood pressure are monitored and at times controlled by external machines. In addition, the cardiac status is continuously monitored by intracardiac pressure monitoring devices.

TABLE 23-11

The child with an acyanotic cardiac defect

Ventricular septal defect (VSD) *(Continued)*

Once stable, the child returns to the regular unit. Nursing care during the remainder of the recovery phase is similar to that of any postoperative patient. When a midsternal incision is used, there are fewer complaints of pain since there are few nerve endings in that area. Generally it takes a few days for the body to recover and adjust to the change in blood flow. During this time, the child's vital signs, activity tolerance, eating, fluid balance, and respiratory status are monitored closely. The nurse discusses discharge care with the parents including activity, incision care, diet, medications, and some of the anticipated changes and abilities that the child will experience with improved exercise tolerance and energy. In addition, the nurse might discuss changes in role relationships as older children now are able to be more independent.

Atrial septal defect (ASD)

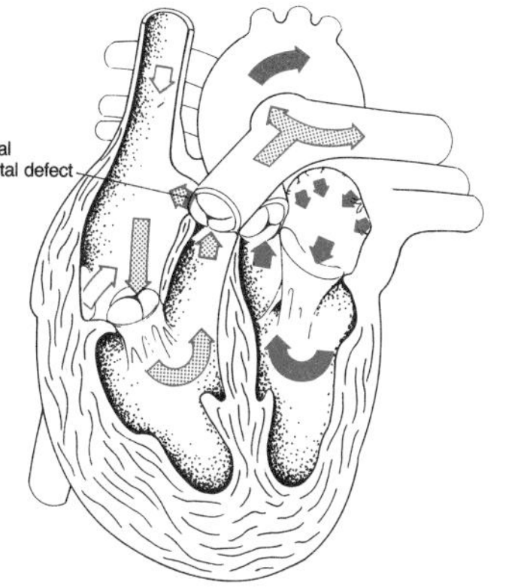

Artrial septal defect: ostium secundum.

Clinical manifestations
The child with an uncomplicated ASD usually is asymptomatic and diagnosed by the presence of a systolic ejection murmur heard at the left upper sternal border. Sometimes the child has some exercise intolerance. There is mild-to-moderate cardiomegaly and pulmonary vascular disease increases gradually over time.

Treatment
In boys, an ASD of significant size is repaired surgically otherwise complications such as congestive heart failure and atrial arrhythmias might develop during adulthood. In girls, all ASDs are repaired because of the increased risk of paradoxical emboli during pregnancy. The operation is performed when the child is about 4–6 years of age and requires cardiopulmonary bypass.

Definition
An abnormal hole in the atrial septum. The ostium primum defect is located low in the atrial septum and adjacent to the mitral valve annulus. The ostium secundum defect is located in the central portion of the atrial septum in the region of the fossa ovale. The secundum defect is the most common type accounting for 9%–10% of all congenital cardiac malformations. The ASD allows some of the oxygenated blood in the left atrium (high pressure) to flow into the right atrium (low pressure) thus increasing the volume of blood and work load of the right side of the heart and resulting in right sided enlargement. The increased volume of blood being pumped through the pulmonary circulation can result in mild or moderate pulmonary edema.

Nursing management
Because the majority of children with an ASD are asymptomatic, one of the nursing challenges is reinforcing and explaining the rationale for surgery when there are no current problems. Parents might verbalize concern that they are making the right choice to subject their child to open-heart surgery and will need time and support to accept the diagnosis and treatment plan. Therapeutic play both before and after surgery helps the child to work through why the "hurt" of surgery and separation was necessary when there were no symptoms of feeling ill. Fortunately, recovery is rapid and the child usually is discharged within a week.

Endocardial cushion defects

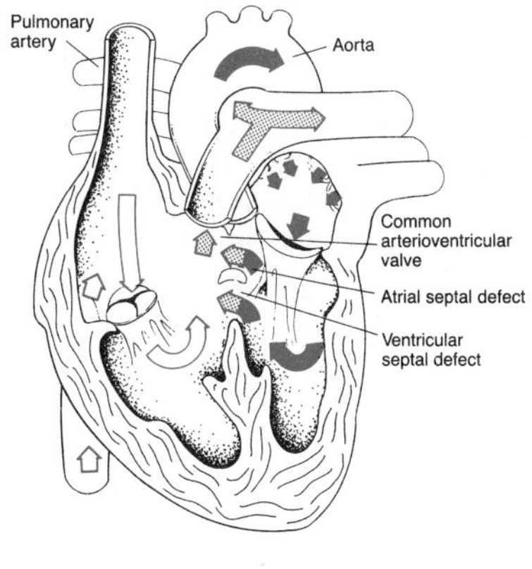

Complete atrioventricular canal.

Definition
Defects in the embryonic formation of the endocardial cushions (endocardium and valve leaflets) result in a spectrum of malformations, ranging from minor to major atrioventricular canal defects. Endocardial cushion defects are classified as a complete or an incomplete atrioventricular canal. An *incomplete atrioventricular canal* consists of an incomplete formation of the mitral valve and sometimes a prium (low) ASD. The ventricular

(Continues)

TABLE 23-11 Congenital Cardiac Defects *(Continued)*

The child with an acyanotic cardiac defect

Endocardial cushion defects *(Continued)*

septum is always intact. A *complete atrioventricular canal* consists of incomplete formation of the mitral valve and tricuspid valves, a prium ASD, and a high VSD. If the valvular defect is extensive, there may be one common atrioventricular valve instead of two separate atrioventricular valves, which when combined with the ASD and VSD allow for four-way communication among the left ventricle and left atrium and right ventricle and right atrium.

Clinical manifestations

In both types there is some degree of increased pulmonary blood flow and volume overload in the left and right ventricles. The incomplete form mimics the clinical picture of an ASD. If the mitral valve defect is significant, there will be regurgitation (upward movement) of blood from the left ventricle through the defects to the right atrium thereby increasing pulmonary blood flow. In complete atrioventricular canal, the combined left-to-right shunting and atrioventricular valve insufficiency result in elevated atrial pressures, increased pulmonary congestion and edema, congestive heart failure, and delayed growth. Endocardial cushion defects are the most common cardiac defects in children with Down's syndrome.

Treatment

The goal of treatment is to control pulmonary hypertension and prevent significant pulmonary vascular obstructive disease. The optimal treatment is surgical repair consisting of closure of the septal defects, and repair of the mitral and tricuspid valves. A midsternal incision is used as well as cardiopulmonary bypass. If the child is a poor surgical risk, a band may be placed on the pulmonary artery to decrease the blood flow to the lungs and to slow pulmonary changes. The congestive heart failure is managed with digitalis and diuretics.

Nursing management

The nurse teaches and supports the parents in the ongoing care of the child relative to medications, diet, activity, and general health status. These children are very susceptible to bacterial infections that invade the heart. They require antibiotic therapy before and after surgical correction. Following the intensive postoperative period, the nurse works closely with the family in planning the ongoing care of the child, remembering that many of these children have multiple needs after their cardiac problems are corrected.

Pulmonic stenosis (PS)

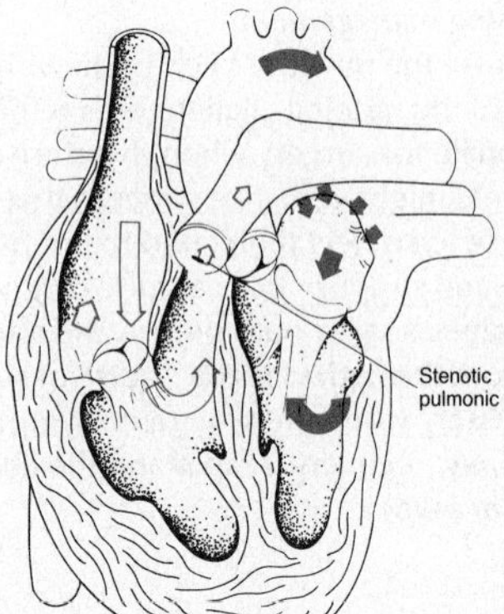

Pulmonic valve stenosis.

Definition

A stenosis (narrowing) at one or more sites in the outflow tract of the right side of the heart creating an abnormally small opening through which the right ventricle ejects blood to the pulmonary artery. The right ventricular systolic pressure becomes elevated abnormally in an effort to eject the normal amount of blood.

Clinical manifestations

If mild, the child is asymptomatic, and the lesion is detected by the cardiac murmur. If severe, there can be right ventricular failure and low cardiac output. If severe in newborns with a patent foramen ovale, there might be cyanosis as a result of right-to-left atrial shunting.

Treatment

Mild pulmonic valve stenosis requires no specific treatment. Severe stenosis requires valvotomy (opening of the valve).

Nursing management

Preoperatively the nurse provides teaching and support for the family and uses therapeutic play for the child to express and work through fears and concerns about the surgery and postoperative period. Usually the recovery period is short and without complications so discharge preparation must begin as soon as the child returns to the pediatric floor.

TABLE 23-11 *(Continued)*

The child with an acyanotic cardiac defect

Aortic stenosis (AS)

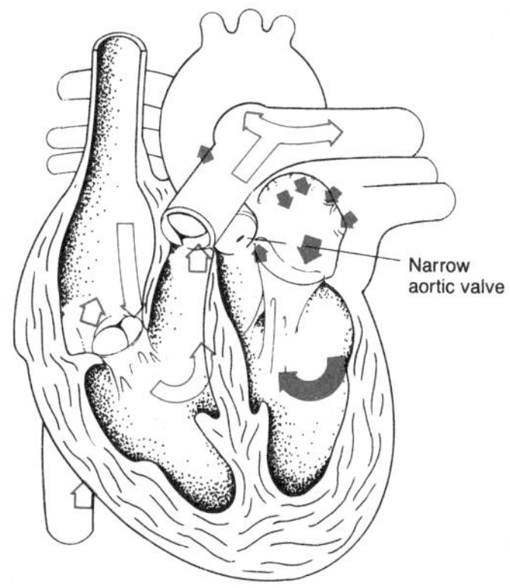

Aortic stenosis.

Definition

An abnormally small orifice (opening) in the aortic valve. Frequently the valve is malformed and the leaflets are thickened and relatively noncompliant. The left ventricle must generate abnormally high systolic pressure to pump a normal amount of blood resulting in left ventricular hypertrophy.

Clinical manifestations

In mild or moderately severe aortic stenosis, the child is asymptomatic and the lesion is detected through cardiac murmur. Severe aortic stenosis can be associated with syncope, reduced exercise tolerance, and fatigue. In infants, severe aortic stenosis can cause congestive heart failure.

Treatment

Mild aortic stenosis requires no treatment, but may be progressive so does require ongoing assessment. Moderate and severe aortic stenosis require operative relief by aortic valvotomy. Aortic valve replacement might be necessary in late childhood as aortic incompetence is a potential complication of valvotomy.

Nursing management

The nurse provides care similar to that described for the child with pulmonic valve stenosis.

The child with a cyanotic cardiac defect

Tetralogy of Fallot (TOF)

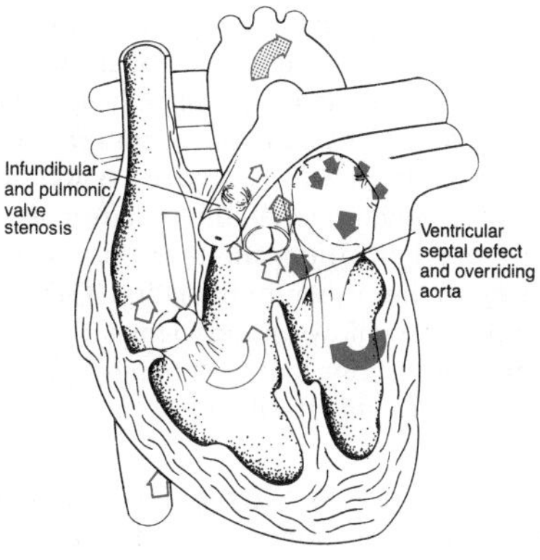

Tetralogy of Fallot.

Definition

A combination of four defects (1) a ventricular septal defect, (2) pulmonary stenosis, (3) an aorta that overrides the VSD, (4) right ventricular hypertrophy. The degree of right ventricular hypertrophy and the extent of shunting is related to the severity of pulmonary stenosis. If the stenosis is mild, there is little increase in the systolic pressure of the right ventricle. TOF comprises 10% of congenital cardiac malformations and is the most common cyanotic defect.

Clinical manifestations

The principal clinical manifestation is cyanosis, which varies in degree, depending on the severity of pulmonary stenosis. The infant with minimal pulmonary stenosis has mild right ventricular outflow obstruction and a left-to-right shunt and is not cyanotic. As the infant grows, however, the degree of stenosis increases and the direction of the shunt changes, resulting in cyanosis. If the infant's pulmonary stenosis is significant, there is a right-to-left shunt and cyanosis. The child with TOF might have hypoxic spells. These usually occur 1–2 hours after the child awakens but seldom occur prior to two months of age. These children might curl into a knee-chest position or squat after exertion. A squatting posture decreases pulmonary vascular resistance, increases pulmonary blood flow and improves

(Continues)

TABLE 23-11 Congenital Cardiac Defects *(Continued)*

The child with a cyanotic cardiac defect

Tetralogy of Fallot (TOF) *(Continued)*

oxygenation. Besides cyanosis, hypoxic spells, and frequent squatting, the child is underweight, has a systolic murmur with prominent ejection click, and polycythemia. Clubbing of the nailbeds might be present in the older infant and child. Polycythemia places the child at risk for central nervous system emboli, thromboses, and abscesses.

Treatment

Definitive treatment for TOF is surgical closure of the VSD and correction of the PS. The success of this procedure depends on the size and distribution of the pulmonary arteries and the size of the left ventricle. In small infants and children with markedly underdeveloped pulmonary arteries, total surgical correction might not be feasible. In these cases, a systemic-to-pulmonary arterial shunt might be created (Blalock-Taussig). Results are often unsatisfactory following the creation of a shunt and its later repair at the time of corrective surgery. Some cardiac centers have had good results with total corrective surgery during infancy by using deep hypothermia (core cooling) and limited cardiopulmonary bypass.

Nursing management

The infant with cyanotic heart disease is diagnosed at birth or shortly thereafter. The nurse supports the parents as they experience basic emotional responses to the birth of a defective infant (see Chapter 14). As the parents are ready, the nurse begins to prepare them to care for the infant at home prior to the surgery. With decreasing anxiety, the parents become more receptive to teaching and more involved in the care of their infant. Teaching is individualized to the needs of the family, but generally includes information on feeding techniques, on positioning for comfort and for maximizing cardiac output, on identifying signs and symptoms that need to be reported, on preventing chilling, and dressing the infant properly, and on managing hypoxic spells. The parents are given a written copy of the information as well as a phone number and the name of a contact person to call whenever they have a question or need reassurance.

Postoperatively, the greatest difference is that the child who was cyanotic is now "pink." After surgery, the child requires intensive monitoring for several days and once stable returns to the pediatric unit. Discharge teaching focuses on treating the infant as a normal child and helping the parents anticipate changes in the infant's feeding and activity tolerances.

Transposition of the great arteries (TGA)

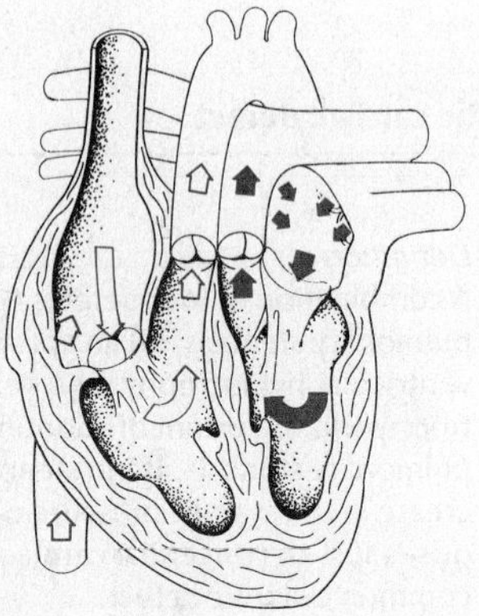

Transposition of the great arteries.

Definition

The aorta arises from the right ventricle and the pulmonary artery arises from the left ventricle thus creating two independent circulations. Oxygenated blood circulates through the pulmonary circulation to the left atrium and left ventricle and then returns to the pulmonary circulation via the pulmonary artery. Deoxygenated blood from the two vena cavae pass through the right side of the heart only to be recirculated through the systemic circulation via the aorta. This second most common cyanotic cardiac condition is incompatible with life.

Most infants with TGA have a patent foramen ovale that allows some oxygenated blood from the left atrium to shunt into the right atrium and then this mixed blood is pumped through the systemic circulation. Others might have a PDA or a VSD, which allows blood to mix. In general, the more abnormal communications that exist between the two circuits, the less cyanotic the infant will be.

Clinical manifestations

These neonates are cyanotic, generally large for gestational age, full-term, and otherwise healthy. There may be a family history of diabetes. Cyanosis and hypoxia increase as fetal structures begin to close after birth. Transposition of the great arteries causes an abnormal increase in pulmonary blood flow resulting in pulmonary edema and congestive heart failure. Like all children with cyanotic heart disease, these infants are at risk for polycythemia, with secondary complications of stroke, severe headache, and brain abscess.

Treatment

The neonate with TGA requires emergency treatment. Cardiac catheterization is done, and balloon atrial septostomy (Rashkind procedure) is performed to create a large opening in the atrial septum and increase interatrial mixing of oxygenated and deoxygenated blood. A neonate with TGA and a large VSD might require banding of the pulmonary artery to prevent pulmonary vascular obstructive disease secondary to pulmonary hypertension. As always, congestive heart failure is treated with digitalis and diuretics. Ultimately, surgical correction is performed to direct all the deoxygenated blood to the pulmonary circulation and the oxygenated blood to the systemic circulation.

TABLE 23-11 (Continued)

The child with a cyanotic cardiac defect

Transposition of the great arteries (TGA) *(Continued)*

Nursing management

The emergency nature of this defect and the need for immediate surgery adds to the parental stress and might prolong their emotional response to having a defective infant. The nurse caring for the infant helps to facilitate the attachment process by keeping the family, and especially the mother who might be at a different hospital, informed about the infant. A daily phone call to the mother and encouraging the father to take pictures to share with the mother is helpful. If a palliative procedure was done, discharge teaching is similar to that for the infant with TOF, however, this infant does not have hypoxic spells but might develop congestive heart failure.

If corrective surgery was done, nursing care following the intensive care period focuses on convalescence and is adapted to the developmental level of the child. Most medical centers prefer to do the surgery prior to the infant's first birthday.

Tricuspid atresia

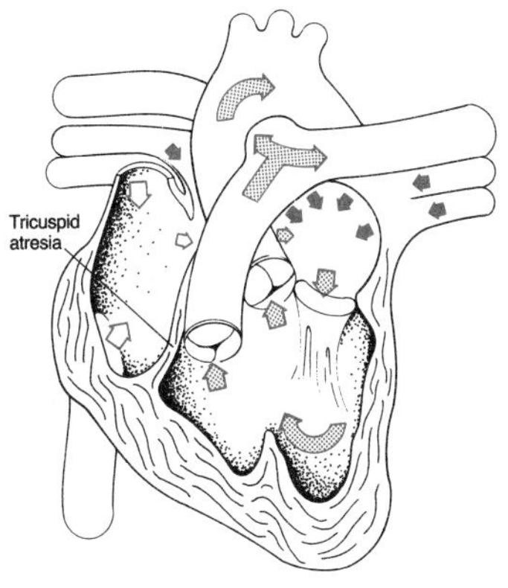

Tricuspid atresia.

Definition

In this condition, the triscupid valve did not develop and there is no communication between the right atrium and the right ventricle. Survival is not possible unless an interatrial communication or its physiologic equivalent is present. Usually, the right ventricle is hypoplastic (underdeveloped), and VSD and pulmonary stenosis may be present. The aorta and pulmonary artery might be normally related or transposed such that the aorta arises from the hypoplastic right ventricle and the pulmonary artery arises from the left ventricle. The relative amount of blood entering the pulmonary artery and the aorta depends on the position of the great arteries, the presence and severity of pulmonary stenosis, and the size of the intraventricular defect. In this cyanotic defect, the degree of cyanosis is inversely proportional to the volume of pulmonary blood flow. It accounts for 2% of congenital cardiac defects.

Clinical manifestations

In addition to cyanosis there is a harsh, blowing murmur heard at the left sternal border. The increased volume of blood pumped by the left ventricle eventually leads to left ventricular failure. If the interatrial communication is small, right atrial enlargement, significant hepatomegaly, and low cardiac output can occur. This infant tires easily, feeds poorly, has delayed growth and development, experiences dyspnea and tachypnea, and might have hypoxic spells. The older infant and child also has clubbing of the nailbeds.

Treatment

Because of left ventricular volume overload, these children benefit from digitalis therapy. Palliative operations include pulmonary artery banding for excessive pulmonary blood flow or a systemic-to-pulmonary artery shunt if pulmonary blood flow is deficient. For children with adequate left ventricular function and a relatively normal pulmonary vascular bed, a "physiologic" surgical repair is possible (Fontan procedure). This operation consists of closure of the interatrial communication, connection of the right atrium to the pulmonary artery by a synthetic conduit with valve, and isolation of the pulmonary artery from the ventricle (Fontan and Bandet, 1971). The chief negative result of this operation is that blood must flow into the pulmonary artery without benefit of a ventricular pump. Many children are markedly improved, but others have chronic fluid retention and reduced exercise tolerance.

Nursing management

The parents whose child has tricuspid atresia need time to adjust to the diagnosis. The nurse first helps the parents work through their grief and accept the diagnosis. Teaching and support for discharge then follow, including information about the administration of digitalis and diuretics, as these children are at high risk for congestive heart failure. Although surgery exists to help some of these children, not all are candidates, and complications are more frequent than in other conditions.

(Continues)

TABLE 23-11 Congenital Cardiac Defects *(Continued)*

The child with a cyanotic cardiac defect

Truncus arteriosus

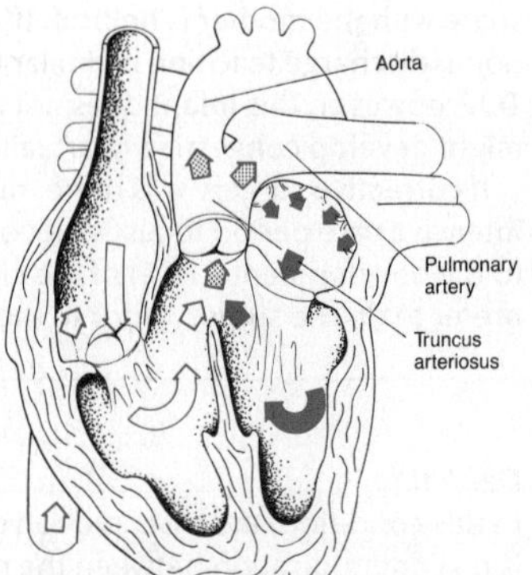

Truncus arteriosus.

Definition

One artery (the truncus), rather than two arteries (aorta and pulmonary artery), arises from the ventricles and then divides in one of three ways into the two arteries. The pulmonary artery might arise from the truncus as a single vessel that then divides into the left and right pulmonary arteries (truncus I). Alternatively, the right and left pulmonary arteries might arise as separate branches from the side (truncus II) or from the posterior aspect (truncus III). There always is a large intraventricular septal defect positioned below the origin of the truncus.

Clinical manifestations

Unless the pulmonary arteries are abnormally small, there is increased pulmonary blood flow at high pressure. This combination results in pulmonary edema and congestive heart failure plus potential early pulmonary vascular obstructive disease. If the pulmonary arteries are abnormally small, there is reduced pulmonary blood flow and cyanosis is present. Neonates with truncus arteriosus might appear normal, cyanotic, or have severe pulmonary edema at birth, depending on the size of the pulmonary arteries. As pulmonary vascular resistance declines after birth, congestive heart failure and pulmonary edema increase. Often the congestive heart failure and pulmonary edema are difficult to control even with digitalis and diuretics. If growth failure occurs despite optimum medical management, surgical intervention is necessary.

Treatment

Palliative banding of one or both pulmonary arteries might be done to reduce pulmonary blood flow. "Corrective" surgery consists of closing the VSD, removing the pulmonary arteries from the truncus arteriosus, and interposing a valve-containing conduit between the right ventricle and the distal pulmonary artery. This operation is performed before the child is 2 years of age, otherwise pulmonary vascular obstructive disease can occur. Because the lumen of the conduit usually is too small to accommodate the pulmonary blood flow of an adult, it must be replaced as the child grows.

Nursing management

As with the family whose child has tricuspid atresia, this family needs support, time, and repeated explanations. The focus of teaching is the identification and management of congestive heart failure. These children are monitored closely for changes in cardiac output and pulmonary vascular disease. The nurse works with the parents to find the balance between providing conscientious care and not being too overprotective.

NURSING CARE PLAN *Child with a Ventricular Septal Defect*

Assessment data: Matthew is an 8-month-old infant who was diagnosed as having a large ventricular septal defect at 2 weeks of age. He was hospitalized at that time with mild-to-moderate congestive heart failure (CHF). Diagnosis was confirmed by cardiac catheterization. He was stabilized on digoxin and discharged at 3½ weeks of age. He did well at home until 1 month ago, when he developed a cough and respiratory congestion. He became short of breath, pale, and diaphoretic while feeding and has not gained weight in the last 1½ months. Matthew was taking a 6–7 oz bottle of formula 4–5 times a day, but since becoming sick he has been taking 3–4 oz every 3–4 hours. He also eats strained baby food three times a day. He currently is being admitted to the hospital for evaluation of worsening CHF.

Matthew is the third child in the family, which consists of his mother, father, and two older sisters, ages 3 and 5. Matthew's mother, who plans to stay with him in the hospital, reports that he usually smiles and babbles but that for the last few days he has been "too sick." She says, "It would have been terrible if we had lost him before, but if anything happened now, I know we couldn't take it."

Nursing diagnosis	Intervention	Rationale
1. Alteration in cardiac output: Decreased related to presence of edema, easy fatigability, poor growth	Organize nursing care to provide periods of uninterrupted rest. Eliminate unnecessary interruptions in the acute phase of illness.	Oxygen needs are lowest when the child is at rest. Each episode of stress increases oxygen needs and therefore increases the work of an already stressed myocardium.
	Plan meals, rest, and procedures to coincide with the child's usual sleep-wake cycle.	Hydrocortisol secretion is likely to be highest at times the child is normally awake.
	Coordinate procedures with other members of the health care team to ensure uninterrupted rest.	Although nursing care might be well planned, interruptions by other team members might interrupt the child's rest and must be avoided.
	Attend to the child's needs promptly to reduce crying and frustration.	Crying increases oxygen needs and wastes limited energy.
	Avoid chilling by dressing the child appropriately for ambient temperature, keeping the child warm during the bath, and changing wet linen promptly. Report temperature elevations promptly.	Both hypothermia and hyperthermia increase metabolic rate and oxygen needs. With exposure to cold, metabolic rate might increase to maintain temperature in a normal range.
	Monitor vital signs every 30 min–1 hour during the acute phase. Monitor frequently cardiovascular status, including heart sounds, liver size, and peripheral perfusion.	Signs of improvement or deterioration might require prompt, appropriate action.
	Administer digoxin as ordered. Observe for toxic effects.	Digoxin is a highly toxic drug that must be given cautiously.
	Administer diuretics as ordered.	Diuretics are given to promote diuresis and reverse fluid retention.
	Monitor serum electrolyte values: prevent hypokalemia by administering the potassium supplement as ordered and encouraging foods high in potassium.	Digoxin toxicity is more likely to occur in the presence of hypokalemia.
	Monitor for signs of hypokalemia, particularly if the child is receiving a diuretic for CHF.	Some diuretics promote excretion of potassium.

(Continues)

NURSING CARE PLAN *Child with a Ventricular Septal Defect (Continued)*

Outcome: Matthew returns to previous tolerance of eating and activity, according to mother. Matthew stays awake for the entire feeding. Matthew takes his medications. Matthew demonstrates adequate cardiac output as pulse rate remains 95–135/min.

Nursing diagnosis	Intervention	Rationale
2. Ineffective airway clearance related to excessive secretions and decreased energy secondary to dyspnea, cough, and tachypnea	Monitor frequently respiratory rate, characteristics of respiration, and breath sounds.	Chanages in condition require prompt treatment.
	Position in semi-Fowler's and alternate use of infant seat with elevation of head of bed. Place sand bag under knees to maintain semi-Fcwler's position while allowing position changes.	Elevation prevents abdominal organs from pressing on the diaphragm and allows for greater expansion of lungs.
	Use knee-chest position for variety and relief of distress.	Without position changes, skin breakdown might occur.
	Dress the child in loose, nonrestrictive clothing.	Tight clothing limits thoracic expansion.
	Administer oxygen as ordered and monitor effect.	Supplemental oxygen improves tissue oxygenation and decreases cardiac workload.
	Provide humidification as ordered.	Humidity helps to liquefy respiratory secretions.
	Keep clothing and bedding dry.	
	Use a face mask instead of a tent for oxygen and mist, if feasible, to minimize the child's stress.	Face masks provide adequate oxygen and humidity levels in most situations and are less frightening and isolating than tents.
	Have suction available at the bedside in case the child is unable to cough up secretions.	Suctioning might be necessary to keep the airway clear.
	Provide chest physiotherapy as ordered. Monitor breath sounds before and after treatments. Concentrate on areas most in need of drainage. Modify the procedure if needed to reduce stress to the infant.	Postural drainage and percussion help to mobilize and remove secretions from the lungs. If the procedure increases the child's distress, modifications might be needed.

Outcome: Matthew demonstrates decreased respiratory distress (20–40/min). Matthew cooperates with being in the oxygen tent except for feedings. Matthew coughs productively in response to position changes and chest physiotherapy.

Nursing diagnosis	Intervention	Rationale
3. Alteration in fluid volume: Excess related to compromised regulatory mechanisms secondary to edema, fluid retention	Administer diuretics as ordered. Check serum electrolytes prior to giving furosemide (Lasix) and withhold if hypokalemia is present. Monitor for side effects, especially hypokalemia.	Diuretics promote the excretion of excess fluid, sodium chloride, and, with some drugs, potassium. Hypokalemia increases risk of digitalis toxicity.
	Weigh the child b.i.d. on the same scale.	Weight is one of the most sensitive indicators of fluid balance.
	Monitor intake and output. Check urine specific gravity of each voiding.	
	Assess hydration status frequently.	Diuretics can cause dehydration.
	Observe fluid restriction as ordered.	If fluid balance is fragile, a small increase in fluid might worsen congestive heart failure symptoms and fluid retention.
	Observe for signs of fluid retention—periorbital or sacral edema.	

Outcome: Matthew voids in amounts consistent with intake. Matthew shows no evidence of fluid retention (periorbital or sacral edema).

NURSING CARE PLAN *Child with a Ventricular Septal Defect* (Continued)

Nursing diagnosis	Intervention	Rationale
4. Activity intolerance related to imbalance between oxygen supply and demand secondary to dyspnea and irritability with mild activity	Monitor child's physiologic responses to nursing care activities, such as feeding, chest physiotherapy, and bathing.	Activity tolerance is an important parameter in the assessment of cardiac function. Decreased tolerance indicates decreased cardiac function.
	Modify procedures to decrease stress if necessary.	Modification might be needed to minimize oxygen needs and conserve energy.
	If confinement in bed or infant seat causes undue frustration, modify plan to include more holding, walking (portable oxygen), and quiet stimulation while in bed or infant seat.	Frustration of imposed inactivity might create more work for the heart than limited out-of-bed activity.
	Monitor tolerance of activity.	
Outcome: Matthew plays without distress. Matthew's mother states that he has increased attention span and interest in toys and food.		
5. Alteration in nutrition: Less than body requirements related to inability to take in adequate calories and increased metabolic demand for calories	Feed the infant in a semi-upright, knee-chest position.	This position prevents fatigue and minimizes abdominal pressure on the diaphragm.
	Use a soft nipple and enlarge the hole in the nipple if needed. Allow the infant to pause and rest as needed.	This allows the child to obtain more milk with less energy expenditure.
	Feed the infant at the first sign of hunger. Do not allow the infant to tire self by crying.	Crying wastes valuable energy needed for sucking.
	Provide adequate rest before and after feeding.	If fatigued, the infant will be unable to ingest and digest an adequate amount of formula.
	Provide frequent, small feedings, for example, 4–5 oz of 20-calorie/oz formula every 3 hours.	Smaller feedings minimize fatigue and exert less pressure on the diaphragm.
	Feed the infant cereal and strained foods at usual times and in a manner used at home.	Maintenance of homelike routine that the infant is familiar with will facilitate intake.
	Weigh the infant twice a day.	If adequate calories are consumed, slow, steady growth is reflected by weight gain.
	Increase caloric value of formula to 24–26 calorie/oz by adding polycose.	Polycose is carbohydrate that adds calories without increased effort of intake or volume of intake. This helps in growth and weight increase.
	Feed per nasal-gastric tube as a last resort if the infant is too exhausted to eat or if eating increases cardiac workload excessively.	This enables the infant to be nourished without stress or increased cardiac demand.
Outcome: Matthew gains weight and length steadily along designated percentile curve. Matthew ingests at least 700 calories per day. Matthew requires fewer rest periods during feeding.		
6. Altered growth and development related to effects of physical disability and inability to perform activities according to age-related norms	Provide quiet types of stimulation during the acute phase (for example, colorful mobile, small objects to hold and manipulate, peek-a-boo, music, soft toys to hold).	Quiet stimulation prevents boredom and frustration while maintaining the infant's interest in the environment and conserving energy.
	As Matthew's condition improves, provide for more vigorous activity (for example, blanket on floor for play, bouncing chair, sitting with pillow support). Change scenery and toys frequently throughout the day. Engage Matthew in verbal games.	The child might lack the energy and motor skills to obtain own stimulation, so stimulating experiences should be provided.

(Continues)

NURSING CARE PLAN *Child with a Ventricular Septal Defect* (Continued)

Nursing diagnosis	Intervention	Rationale
	Explore parents' feelings and perceptions about Matthew's development.	Parents might fear that the child is retarded or that delays are due to inadequate parenting.
	Point out areas of developmental success that parents might not recognize (for example, verbal, cognitive, social).	Parents might need help in seeing subtle but important signs of progress.
	Teach parents about Matthew's need for age-appropriate stimulation. Suggest toys and activities.	Parents might underestimate the infant's developmental level because of small size and gross motor delays.
	Assure parents that Matthew will limit his own activity and that they do not need to inhibit his activity except during acute periods.	Parents might inappropriately inhibit the child's physical activity to prevent "strain on the heart."

Outcome: Matthew does age-appropriate activities and skills according to the Denver Developmental Screening Test. Parents describe appropriate ways to promote Matthew's development.

Nursing diagnosis	Intervention	Rationale
7. Alteration in family processes related to hospitalization of child	Encourage the parents to participate actively in all phases of Matthew's care.	Presence of parents helps alleviate stress of strange environment for the infant.
	Arrange to have Matthew cared for by two or three primary nurses.	Care is less stressful for the infant if he develops relationship with familiar nurses.
	Ask the parents to bring familiar toys and objects from home. Allow siblings to visit frequently. Make the hospital routine as homelike as possible.	Familiar objects, people, and routines make the hospital seem less strange.
	Provide for periods of holding, rocking, and play by nurses, separate from procedures.	This promotes trust and prevents perception of nurses as people who only bring discomfort and stress.
	Acknowledge and respond to signs of stress and discomfort.	This promotes trust between infant and nurses.
	Arrange for siblings to visit for short time periods to maintain the family unit.	This helps to decrease the sense of anxiety for siblings and might help them understand why parents are not at home as much as usual.
	Encourage siblings to visit and take time to observe their reactions during visits.	It might be necessary to discuss siblings' reactions with parents.
	Assist parents to identify common fears and fantasies in siblings of the hospitalized child and how to deal with these.	Siblings frequently have many fears and fantasies, including guilt, fear for their own health, and jealousy. These are often expressed indirectly and are hard for parents to recognize.
	Encourage parents to spend time together each day. Provide care for Matthew during that time.	It is important for parents to maintain their own relationship during periods of stress.
	Determine parents' awareness of the needs of siblings at home.	Parents are often so focused on the needs of the sick child that they are unaware of the needs of siblings.

Outcome: Matthew's parents participate in his care. The family spends time together in the hospital. The parents discuss sibling reactions and needs with supportive personnel.

NURSING CARE PLAN *Child with a Ventricular Septal Defect* (Continued)

Nursing diagnosis	Intervention	Rationale
8. Parental anxiety related to uncertainty of future health status of son	Accept parents' expressions of anxiety and explain them to other staff members as needed.	Interpretation of parents' negative behavior to other staff members might prevent conflicts.
	Encourage the parents to ask questions and talk about feelings and fears.	Accurate information and expression of fears lessen anxiety.
	Encourage the parents to participate in Matthew's care and in decision making about his care.	Participation in care minimizes feelings of powerlessness and helplessness.
	Assist the parents in identifying methods of managing stress and anxiety that have been helpful before (time alone with spouse, walks, exercise, prayer).	Previous methods of coping might be helpful in current stressful situation.
	Assist the parents in obtaining support in the community (chaplain, parent support group, etc.).	Parents might be unaware of resources or might need help in contacting them.

Outcome: Parents express anxiety by asking questions. Parents identify and use previously helpful coping strategies. Parents discuss their needs with each other and with other family members.

The Child with Hypertension

Systemic arterial hypertension is much less common in children than in adults. Because blood pressure increases during childhood, blood pressure norms must be related to the patient's age or other indices, such as size or stage of maturation. For example, a blood pressure of 120/70 is normal for a 16-year-old boy but is abnormally elevated for a 4-year-old boy. (Normal blood pressure measurements are listed in Appendix B.)

Hypertension can be primary or secondary. Primary, or essential, hypertension has no known cause and is the most common form of hypertension in adults and probably in children. Numerous causes of secondary hypertension are known: the most common causes are renal disease and coarctation of the aorta. Renal diseases that can cause secondary hypertension include pyelonephritis, glomerulonephritis, hydronephrosis, and renal artery disease.

All children should have their blood pressure measured at some time during childhood and adolescence. Children with elevated blood pressure should be referred for appropriate evaluation and, if necessary, treatment. Treatment varies but generally consists of weight reduction (if needed), a low-sodium diet, diuretic therapy, and stress reduction.

Essential Concepts

- The heart is a muscular organ consisting of two atria (receiving chambers), two ventricles (pumping chambers), four valves (the tricuspid, pulmonic, mitral, and aortic valves), and an electrical conduction system (sinus and atrioventricular nodes and Purkinje fibers).
- Normally, there is no communication (opening) between the right heart, which receives deoxygenated blood from the systemic circulation and pumps it to the lungs, and the left heart, which receives oxygenated blood from the lungs and pumps it into the systemic circulation.

- Before birth, the fetal lungs are collapsed, and gas exchange takes place in the placenta; the blood bypasses the collapsed lungs by means of the ductus arteriosus and the foramen ovale.
- A shunt is an abnormal communication between the left and right sides of the heart.
- In a left-to-right shunt, the right ventricle pumps an increased volume of blood at increased pressure into the pulmonary arteries and lungs, causing dilatation and hypertrophy of the right ventricle, pulmonary edema, susceptibility to respiratory infection, tachypnea, and dyspnea.
- In a right-to-left shunt, deoxygenated blood flows into the aorta resulting in hypoxemia and cyanotic heart disease.
- An obstruction defect is a lesion or malformation in the heart valves or great vessels that impedes the forward flow of blood.
- Assessment history for the child with cardiovascular dysfunction includes data about exercise intolerance, cyanosis, diaphoresis, feeding difficulties, respiratory distress (particularly hypoxic episodes), growth and development, past health history, and family health history.
- Physical examination of the child with cardiovascular dysfunction includes measurement of vital signs, height, and weight; inspection of the skin for pallor or cyanosis, of the chest for convexity, and of the fingers and toes for clubbing; palpation of peripheral pulses, of the liver for signs of hepatomegaly; and auscultation of heart and breath sounds.
- Diagnostic tests used in assessment are hematologic and blood chemistry studies, cardiographic studies, and cardiac catheterization for which the child needs adequate preparation.
- Care of the child following cardiac catheterization involves assessment for complications, including arrhythmias, hemorrhage, infection, edema, thrombus formation, adverse reactions to contrast media, and dehydration following the procedure.
- In caring for the child with cardiac disease, the nurse can minimize cardiac workload by providing adequate rest, anticipating the child's needs, minimizing anxiety, preventing hyperthermia and hypothermia, eliminating excess sodium and fluid from the body, monitoring fluid balance, and administering drugs that reduce systemic resistance to cardiac outflow and enhance cardiac function.
- Children with heart disease are at risk for respiratory infections and bacterial endocarditis, an infection of the valves and inner lining (endocardium) of the heart.
- Hypoxic spells, which are usually due to an abrupt reduction of pulmonary blood flow, are managed by placing the child in a side-lying, knee-chest position; administering oxygen; administering morphine; and, if these measures fail, performing emergency surgery.
- Besides adequate intake, the nutritional needs of the child with cardiac disease might require high-calorie diets, low-sodium diets, and iron supplementation.
- The nurse helps parents to promote the child's normal growth and development by instructing them about the child's need for exercise, activity, stimuli, discipline, realistic limits on activity, and as much independence as possible.
- In caring for the health maintenance needs of children with cardiac disease, the nurse teaches parents to observe for symptoms, administer medications safely (especially digoxin), prevent infections, and regulate temperature.
- The nurse informs parents of children with organic heart disease about the need for prophylactic antibiotic administration at the time of any dental work, minor surgery, or illness, to reduce the risk of bacterial endocarditis.
- Congestive heart failure can be due to hypovolemia, obstruction to cardiac outflow, ineffective myocardial function, arrhythmias, or excessive demand for cardiac output; signs and symptoms include tachycardia, cardiomegaly, tachypnea, dyspnea, hepatomegaly, and weight gain from edema.
- The physiologic effects of most acyanotic defects have to do with volume overload in the right ventricle and pulmonary circulation, with resultant congestive heart failure and pulmonary edema.
- The cardinal signs of cyanotic cardiac defects are the signs of hypoxia, which include cyanosis, respiratory symptoms, poor growth, and exercise intolerance.
- In assessing the child with hypertension, it is important to remember that blood pressure increases during childhood and must be compared with norms for the child's age, size, and stage of maturation.

References

Castaneda R et al: Tetralogy of Fallot: Primary repair in infancy. Pages 63–69 in: *The Child with Congenital Heart Disease After Surgery.* Kidd BSL, Rowe RD (editors). Futura, 1976.

Cloutier J, Measel CP: Home care for the infant with congenital heart disease. *Am J Nurs* (Jan) 1982; 82:100–103.

Feldt RH (editor): *Atrioventricular Canal Defects.* Saunders, 1976.

Fisch C: Digitalis intoxication. *JAMA* (June) 1971; 216:1770–1773.

Fontan F, Bandet E: Surgical repair of tricuspid atresia. *Thorax* 1971; 26:240–248.

Gottesfeld IB: The family of the child with congenital heart disease. *Am J Matern-Child Nurse* (March/April) 1979; 101–104.

Huntington J: Care of the child with a disorder of the cardiovascular system. Pages 97–150 in: *Critical Care Nursing of Children and Adolescents.* Oakes AR (editor). Saunders, 1981.

Jackson PL: Digoxin therapy at home: Keeping the child safe. *Am J Matern-Child Nurs* (March/April) 1979; 105–110.

Krovetz LJ, Gessner IH, Schiebler GL: *Handbook of Pediatric Cardiology.* University Park Press, 1979.

Linderkamp P: Increased blood viscosity in patients with cyanotic congenital heart disease and iron deficiency. *J Pediatr* (Oct) 1979; 95(4):567–569.

MacDonald NE: Respiratory syncytial viral infection in infants with congenital heart disease. *N Engl J Med* (Aug) 1983; 307: 397–400.

Meissner JE, Gever LN: Reducing the risks of toxicity. *Nurs '80* (Sept) 1980; 29–38.

Moss AJ, Adams FH, Emmanouilides GC: *Heart Disease in Infants, Children and Adolescents.* Williams & Wilkins, 1977.

Newburger JW et al: Cognitive function and age at repair of transposition of the great arteries in children. *N Engl J Med* (June) 1984; 310:1495–1499.

Reif K: A heart makes you live: What children believe about their hearts. *Am J Nurs* (June) 1972; 72(6):1085.

Scoggin C, Patterson D: Down's syndrome as a model disease. *Arch Intern Med* 1982; 142:462–464.

Additional Readings

Agamalian B: Pediatric cardiac catheterization. *J Pediatr Nurs* 1986; 1(2):73–79.

Anderson DJ, Thibault J: Nursing management of the pediatric patient with Kawasaki's disease. *Issues Compr Pediatr Nurs* (Jan/Feb) 1981; 5(1):1–10.

Boll TJ, Dimino E, Mattsson AE: Parenting attitudes: The role of personality style and childhood long-term illness. *J Psychosom Res* 1978; 22(3):209–213.

Brantigan CO: Hemodynamic monitoring: Interpreting values. *Am J Nurs* (Jan) 1982; 82:86–89.

Broda D: Extending the role of the coronary care nurse. *Superv Nurse* (June) 1981; 12(6):48–50.

Caire JB, Erickson S: Reducing distress in pediatric patients undergoing cardiac catheterization. *CHC* 1986; 14(3):146–152.

Campbell C: Careers—Cardiothoracic nursing: Heart and soul. *Nurs Mirror* (Feb 10) 1982; 154(6):44.

Carnevale FA: Nursing the critically ill child. *Focus Crit Care* 1985; 12(5):10–13.

Cavanaugh AL, Mancini RE: Drug interactions and digitalis toxicity. *Am J Nurs* (Dec) 1980; 80:2170–2171.

Chelton SZ, Williams WH: Heart valve replacement in infants and children. *Crit Care Q* 1985; 8(3):29–37.

Click LA: Cardiac arrhythmias in infants and children. *Crit Care Q* 1985; 8(3):9–18.

Cohen MA: The use of prostaglandins and prostaglandin inhibitors in critically ill neonates. *Am J Matern-Child Nurs* (May/June) 1983; 8:194–199.

Dance D, Yates M: Nursing assessment and care of children with complications of congenital heart disease. *Heart Lung* 1985; 14(3):209–213.

Engle MA: Management of the child after cardiac surgery. *Pediatr Ann* (April) 1981; 10(4):53–60.

Fisk R: Management of the pediatric cardiovascular patient after surgery. *Crit Care Q* 1986; 9(2):75–82.

Foster SD: MCN pharmacopoeia. Indomethacin: Pharmacologic closure of the ductus arteriosus. *Am J Matern-Child Nurs* (May/June) 1982; 7:171–172.

Freis PC: Sounds of a healthy heart. *Issues Compr Pediatr Nurs* 1979; 3(7):1–4.

Gersony WM, Bierman FZ: Cardiac catheterizaton in the pediatric patient. *Pediatrics* (May) 1981; 67(5):738–740.

Hall RK: Oral and dental changes and management of children with cardiac disease. *J Int Assoc Dent Child* (June) 1980; 11(1): 19–28.

Hazinski MF: Critical care of the pediatric cardiovascular patient. *Nurs Clin North Am* (Dec) 1981; 16(4):671–697.

Johnson DL: Pediatric arrhythmias: A nursing approach. *Dimens Crit Care Nurs* (May/June) 1983; 2(3):147–157.

Kern LS, O'Brien P: The Fontan procedure. *Heart Lung* (Sept) 1985; 14(5):457–467.

Loeffel M: Developmental considerations of infants and children with congenital heart disease. *Heart Lung* (May) 1985; 14(3): 214–217.

Longo A: Teaching parents CPR. *Pediatr Nurs* (Nov/Dec) 1983; 9(6):445–447.

L'Orange C, Werner-McCullough M: Kawasaki disease: A new threat to children. *Am J Nurs* (April) 1983; 83(4):558–562.

Malinowski P et al: Transposition of the great arteries. *Crit Care Nurse* 1985; 5(3):35–48.

McElnea J: Spotlight on children. Childhood hypertension. *Nurs Times* (Sep 29–Oct 5) 1982; 78(39 Suppl):5–6.

McEvoy M: Functional heart murmurs. *Nurs Pract* (March/April) 1981; 6:34–36.

Miles MS, Carter MC: Coping strategies used by parents during their child's hospitalization in an intensive care unit. *CHC* (Summer) 1985; 14(1):14–21.

Nadas AS: Update on congenital heart disease. *Pediatr Clin North Am* (Feb) 1984; 31(1):153–164.

Ng L: Nursing aspects of the surgical treatment of idiopathic hypertrophic subaortic stenosis. *Heart Lung* (July/Aug) 1982; 11(4):364–375.

Norwood WI, Lang P, Hansen DD: Physiologic repair of aortic atresia-Hypoplastic left heart syndrome. *N Engl J Med* (Jan 6) 1983; 308(1):2326.

Page GG: Tetralogy of Fallot. *Heart Lung* (July) 1986; 15(4): 390–399.

Pasternack SB: Hypertension in children and adolescents. *Issues Compr Pediatr Nurs* (Dec) 1979; 3(7):23–57.

Pelletier L: Collecting information: A way to cope with cardiac surgery. *Matern-Child Nurs J* 1981; 10(3):143–154.

Phillips JM, Raviele AA: Diagnostic and therapeutic techniques in pediatric cardiology: Past, present, and future. *Crit Care Q* 1985; 8(3):1–7.

Pless IB: Chronic disease in children: Current controversies and technical advances. *Pediatr Clin North Am* (Feb) 1984; 31(1): 259–273.

Powers D: Nursing care study: Subacute bacterial endocarditis. *Nurs Times* (April 20–26) 1983; 79(16):50–53.

Pyles SH, Stern PN: Discovery of nursing gestalt in critical care nursing: The importance of the gray gorilla syndrome. *Image* (Spring) 1983; 15(2):51–57.

Rehm RS: Teaching cardiopulmonary resuscitation to parents. *Am J Matern-Child Nurs* (Nov/Dec) 1983; 8(6):411–414.

Reid TJ: Newborn cyanosis. *Am J Nurs* (Aug) 1982; 82: 1230–1234.

Rice V: Shock, a clinical syndrome. Part I: Definition, etiology, and pathophysiology. *Crit Care Nurse* (March/April) 1981; 1(3):44–50.

Rogers TR et al: Heart surgery in infants: A preliminary assessment of maternal adaptation. *Child Health Care* (Fall) 1984; 13(2):52.

Rushton CH: Preparing children and families for cardiac surgery: Nursing interventions. *Issues Compr Pediatr Nurs* (July/Aug) 1983; 6(4):235–248.

Ruttenberg H: Nonsurgical therapy of cardiac disorders. *Pediatr Consult* 1986; 5(2):1–12.

Sasso SC: MCN pharmacopoeia. Prostaglandin E_1 for infants with congenital heart disease. *Am J Matern-Child Nurs* (Jan/Feb) 1983; 8(1):29.

Saul L: Heart sounds and common murmurs. *Am J Nurs* (Dec) 1983; 83:1680–1689.

Scordo KA: Taming the cardiac monitor. Part 2. Understanding what the monitor's telling you. *Nurs '82* (Sept) 1982; 12(9): 61–67.

Slota MC: Cardiac pacemakers in children. *Crit Care Nurse* (Nov/Dec) 1981; 1(7):35–41.

Slota MC: Congestive heart failure. Part II: Medical and nursing management. *Crit Care Nurse* (Nov/Dec) 1982; 2(6):58–63.

Slota M: Pediatric cardiac catheterization: Complications and interventions. *Crit Care Nurse* (May/June) 1982; 2(3):22–26.

Stachura L: Care of the infant with ductus-dependent disease receiving prostaglandin E_1. *Issues Compr Pediatr Nurs* 1984; 7(4/5):203–215.

Stewart P: The young cardiac patient: Management considerations. *Pediatr Nurs* (Jan/Feb) 1980; 6(1):E–F.

Stroud ET: Acquired, chronic aortic insufficiency in the child. *Nurs Pract* (Nov/Dec) 1980; 80:26–27.

Utz SW, Grass S: Mitral valve prolapse: Self-care needs, nursing diagnoses, and interventions. *Heart Lung* (Jan) 1987; 16(1): 77–83.

Uzark K et al: Primary preventive health care in children with heart disease. *Pediatr Cardiol* (Oct/Dec) 1983; 4(4):259–263.

Van Breda A: Postoperative care of infants and children who require cardiac surgery. *Heart Lung* (May) 1985; 14(3): 205–208.

Vincent RN, Collins GF: Cardiac embryology and fetal cardiovascular physiology. *Crit Care Q* (Sept) 1986; 9(2):1–5.

Youssef M: Self control behaviors of school-age children who are hospitalized for cardiac diagnostic procedures. *Matern-Child Nurs J* (Winter) 1981; 10(4):219–284.

Chapter 24

Protection

Implications of Inflammation and Altered Skin Integrity

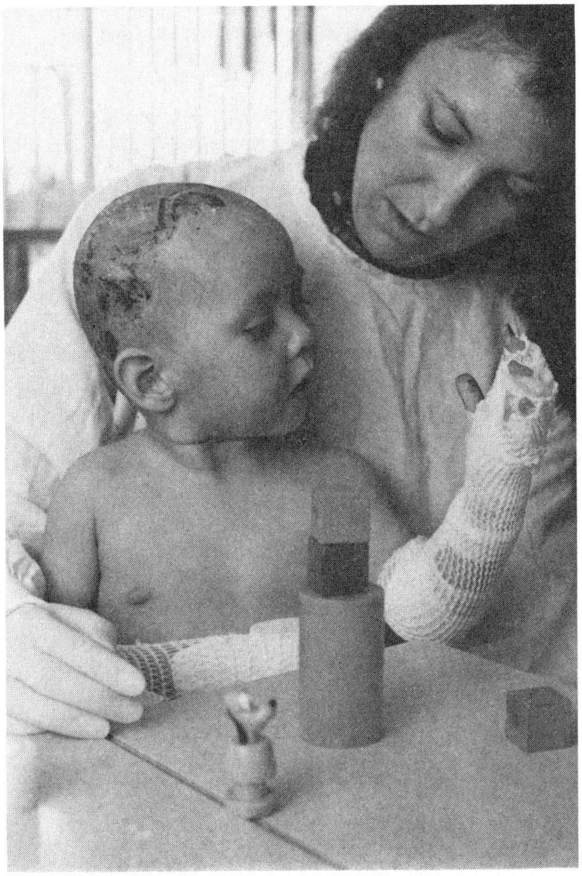

Chapter Contents

(Continues)

Cross Reference Box

To find these topics see the following chapters:

Congenital birthmarks	Chapter 18
Diaper dermatitis	Chapter 4
Milia	Chapter 4
Miliaria (prickly heat)	Chapter 4
Minor lacerations	Chapter 18
Monilia (thrush)	Chapter 18
Pediculosis	Chapter 18
Scabies	Chapter 18
Seborrheic dermatitis (cradle cap)	Chapter 4
Tinea capitis, corporis, pedis, and cruris	Chapter 18
Viral warts	Chapter 18

Objectives

- Describe the structure and function of the skin.
- Describe the history and physical examination required to evaluate the child with altered integument.
- Define the procedures and treatments involved in wound care and skin grafts.
- Explain acute care, nutritional support, and developmental needs of children with skin injuries.
- Explain the physiologic processes, medical treatments, and principles of nursing management for skin infection or inflammation.
- Outline the standard classification of burns according to the severity of injury and complicating factors.
- Describe the ways in which the medical and nursing management of the child with a burn respond to alterations in the body's systems.
- State the nurse's responsibilities in the care of specific areas after a burn.
- Describe the chronic-care measures for the child with a burn.
- Explain the physiologic processes, medical treatments, and principles of nursing management for the child with frostbite.
- Describe the nursing management for the child with severe surface injuries.

ESSENTIALS OF STRUCTURE AND FUNCTION
The Skin

Understanding the structure and function of the skin is necessary in order to assess properly the changes it undergoes. The skin begins to develop at about the eleventh week of gestation and undergoes developmental changes throughout the life span. Although the skin has similarities, there is considerable variability from individual to individual in terms of color, texture, pH, moisture, and temperature. These variations depend on the care of the skin, age, sex, and racial origin of the individual, and degree of exposure to the elements. The nature of skin varies in different parts of the body of the same individual and at different times during the life span. For example, the dermis is thinner in newborn infants than it is in adults, the amount of sebum and sweat is less, and the skin is less acidic, leaving infants more susceptible to skin alterations (Prugh, 1983).

The skin is structured to form an elastic and resistant covering for internal body structures. The internal fluid mechanism of the body is partially maintained by the skin and it prevents the excess loss of body fluids so long as the surface membrane is intact. When the surface is lost, such as in severe tissue injury or burns, large amounts of fluid, electrolytes, and proteins might be lost from the body. In fact, one of the more accurate indicators of hydration status in children is the quality of the skin.

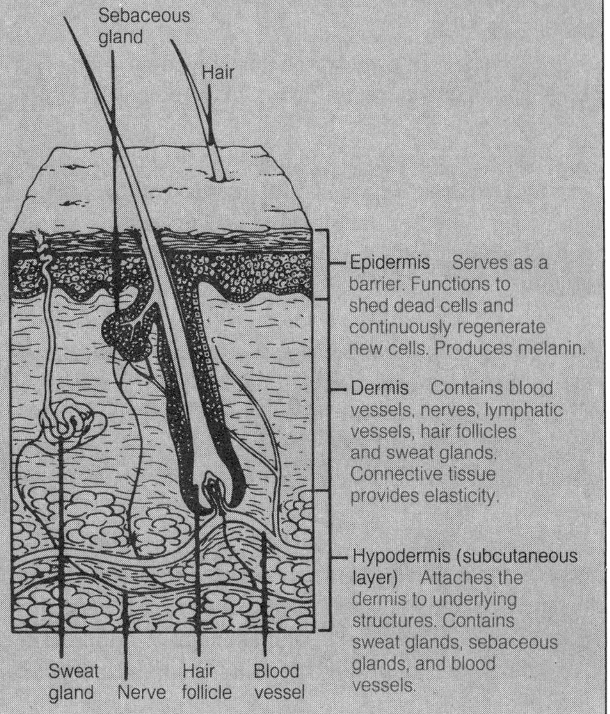

Structure and function of the skin.

Glossary

Apocrine glands Large sweat glands located in axillas, anal, genitocrural, and mammary areas.

Dermis The skin layer just under the epidermis. Location of blood vessels, nerves, lymphatics, hair follicles, glands, and connective tissue.

Eccrine glands Small sweat glands that help to control body temperature.

Epidermis The outer, thin surface of the skin. Covers the entire body and gives rise to nails, hair, sebaceous and sweat glands. Contains five layers, one of which is regenerative (see figure on skin structure).

Hypodermis Subcutaneous tissue containing sweat and sebaceous glands and blood vessels. Attaches the skin to underlying structures.

Melanin The principal pigment of the skin. Skin color varies depending on the activity of the melanin-producing cells. Other factors that affect skin color include the amount of blood in cutaneous capillaries as well as the degree of oxygenation of the blood. Other pigments such as carotene will affect skin color.

Sebaceous glands Glands that secrete sebum, a fatty acid. Sebum provides a protective coating thought to have some bacteriocidal effect. It helps maintain an acidic skin pH of between 4.5 and 6.5.

The skin is a complex, essential organ. It functions as both a physiologic and psychologic protector of the body. As a physiologic protector, it protects humans by inhibiting an excess loss of water and electrolytes, by providing an acid covering to protect the body from irritants and sources of infection, and serves as a thermoregulator by preventing loss of body heat.

As a psychologic protector the skin functions as an organ of perception and communication. In conjunction with the cerebral cortex, it is the vehicle for perceiving sensations of pain, temperature, touch, and pressure. Additionally, it reflects and expresses emotions and internal conflict through changes in color and temperature and through responses such as sweat production and secretion of sebum (fatty acids).

The appearance of the skin contributes to the development of the child's body image as part of self-esteem. As such, appearance contributes to the health and well-being of the child and plays a role in ego development. Consequently, the developing child's self-esteem is a significant concern for the nurse caring for a child with a skin alteration.

Nurses working with children, whether as inpatients or outpatients, are likely to encounter skin alterations because they are one of the most frequently seen health problems. Several premises about skin alterations have implications for nursing care. Skin alterations in children and youth might:

- be major or minor, congenital or acquired, acute or chronic, self-limiting or requiring treatment
- be associated with developmental level and consequently seen in some age groups and not in others
- be a manifestation of systemic disease
- have prodromal symptoms prior to the appearance of the skin alteration
- be caused by any number of agents or be autoimmune in origin
- have a different appearance in the child than in the adult
- be affected by interrelated factors such as nutritional status, age, pH, adequate blood supply, and psychosocial factors

Assessment of the Child with Altered Integument

History

It is essential to observe the child carefully and obtain an accurate history before planning nursing care. Important factors to consider include recent changes in lifestyle, skin alterations in family members, and particularly any known allergies. The initial interview elicits information regarding any trauma, recent infection, recent medications, or exposure to communicable disease.

Both child and parent can provide historical information. The nurse can structure the interview around the following:

1. *Description of associated symptoms*—Has there been any fever, stomachache, headache, dizziness, nausea, vomiting, runny nose, watery eyes, or cough? Any of these can be associated with communicable diseases or allergies. Fatigue, pain, itching, swelling, or redness are associated with inflammation and infection.
2. *Exposure to communicable disease or unusual substances*—A number of communicable diseases causing skin rashes are transmissible. The mode of transmission varies depending on the disease. Types of foods, beverages, and medications give clues to allergic responses. Changes in the child's environment, such as a new pet, and changes in habits, such as the use of a different type of soap, shampoo, or laundry products can be significant. Information about where the child plays might reveal contact with plant oils.
3. *Description of lesions*—The nurse asks when any rashes, lesions, or traumatic skin alterations first appeared and whether their appearance changed. If the lesions are larger, redder, or blistered, or have undergone some other changes, this is useful information. Whether any lesions have spread over the body and the direction of the spread are important facts also.
4. *Sensations from alterations*—The child is asked to describe how the skin feels. For example, does the child experience pain or itching? Is the skin hot, scaly, dry, oily, smooth, or rough? Have there been any secretions and what is their appearance?
5. *Treatments and results*—The nurse obtains information about the effectiveness of any treatments. The child's emotional response to any skin alteration is noted also, keeping in mind that a variety of adaptive and maladaptive responses might be evident.

Physical Examination

The nurse's eyes and hands are the most effective tools for examining the patient's skin. The description derived from inspection and palpation of lesions will be essential in helping to obtain solid baseline information about the child's dermatologic condition. Assessment of skin lesions is directed toward determining their type and size, their configuration, their distribution and location, and their texture and color.

Type and size of lesions Lesions are classified as either primary, secondary, or vascular. *Primary lesions* are those that arise in previously normal skin. *Secondary lesions* result from changes in the primary eruptions. *Vascular* lesions contain blood vessels. The most frequently seen childhood lesions are described in Table 24-1. The size of lesions is measured in centimeters (cm) if they are large enough to measure.

Configuration of lesions The configuration, or pattern a group of lesions assumes, can be important in assessing the dermatologic condition. Patterns fall into four major classifications:

Annular—lesions that have a ringlike pattern

Iris—lesions resembling a bull's eye

Linear—lesions that assume a straight line, often resembling a streak

Marbling—lesions that resemble swirls; sweeping brush-like patterns

Lesions also can be symmetric or asymmetric in shape.

Distribution and location of lesions The nurse records the areas of the body in which the lesions are found, whether the lesions are generalized or localized (for example, on the face, trunk, or extremities), and their distribution (clustered, coalesced, or discrete). Some areas of the body have a tendency to develop particular dermatologic conditions. For example, a localized, discrete rash is seldom caused by a systemic disease or reaction to a food or drug; however, a generalized rash, which often occurs abruptly in hospitalized patients, is frequently a reaction to a drug or some other allergen. The most common appearance of lesions caused by a drug reaction is *urticaria* (hives). These lesions can persist for as long as 1 week or more after the drug that caused the reaction has been discontinued or contact with the allergen has ceased. Occasionally, skin lesions will seem to disappear, only to reappear elsewhere, especially with bathing or exposure to cold or heat.

Texture and color of skin The nurse notes the consistency, texture, and color of the child's skin and any lesions. Moistness, smoothness, and dryness of the skin are considered in determining its texture and consistency. The nurse also considers the skin's color and degree of cleanliness. The skin's turgor can be checked easily by pinching it slightly (see Chapter 21).

The color of the lesions can range from yellow, pink, red, and bluish to gray, brown, and amber. Lesions also can be black or white. The color of the lesions is an important diagnostic guide. To assess color, the nurse considers not only the color of the lesions but also skin color in general. Nonglare daylight is considered the best for examining skin color and will help the nurse make an objective assessment. The nurse needs to be astute in making observations on darker-skinned persons because skin coloring can vary the appearance of lesions. The skin color of members of darker-skinned races often varies from black, yellow-brown, and reddish-brown to tones similar to those of whites. Comparing the unaffected skin with the affected skin is one way of observing color alterations. When assessing the color of the lesions, the nurse considers not only the present color but also color changes, the length of time the color has been present, and the sequence of the color change. The nurse also considers the effect of skin alterations on other body systems.

Validating Diagnostic Tests

Tests used to diagnose skin conditions are relatively benign and noninvasive. A simple explanation to the child that is appropriate for the child's developmental level will ensure cooperation and facilitate the procedure. Inspection of the skin and description of lesions are essential first steps in diagnosing a skin condition. Shining a flashlight sideways onto the lesion enables the nurse more easily to determine configuration. A magnifying lens is useful in helping to determine the topography of a lesion, as well as in locating parasites on the skin. Microscopic examination of a sample of infected skin is another direct means of diagnosing a skin condition.

To obtain a sample for direct microscopic examination, a scraping of the skin is necessary. Skin scraping for microscopic examination is done with a razor blade but is essentially painless. The child is encouraged to remain still and is told that the procedure feels like being scratched lightly.

A smear, culture, or biopsy might be obtained from skin lesions for further examination. Skin scrapings and wound cultures assist in determining causative organisms so that appropriate therapy can be instituted. Before specimens are taken, the skin lesion needs to be cleansed with a 70%

TABLE 24-1 Frequently Seen Childhood Skin Lesions

Primary lesion	Description
Macule 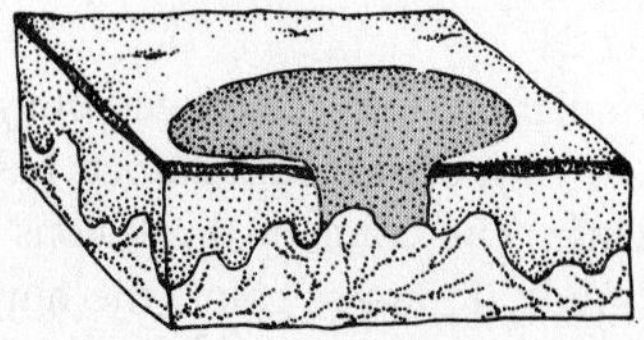	Flat, circumscribed, usually smaller than 1 cm; color differs from surrounding skin
Papule 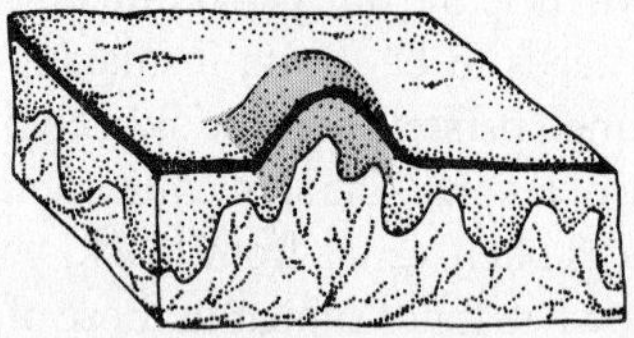	Raised, solid, sharply circumscribed, small (0.5 cm–1 cm in diameter), and colored in various shade of pink to red
Nodule	Small (1–2 cm), solid, in dermal layer of skin or subcutaneous tissue
Tumor	Solid, larger than 1–2 cm, soft or hard consistency, might lie deep in tissues
Wheal 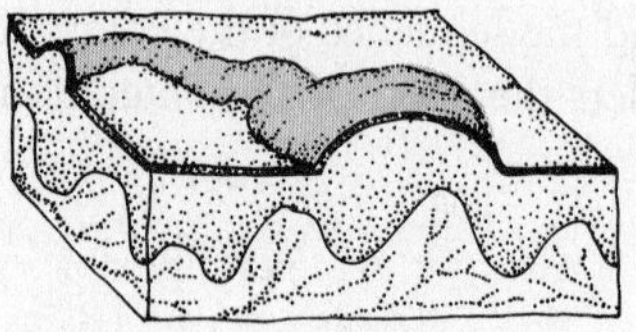	Circumscribed, flat-topped, relatively transient with irregularly shaped borders
Cyst	Nontender, fluid-filled mass, may be ganglion or tumor
Vesicle 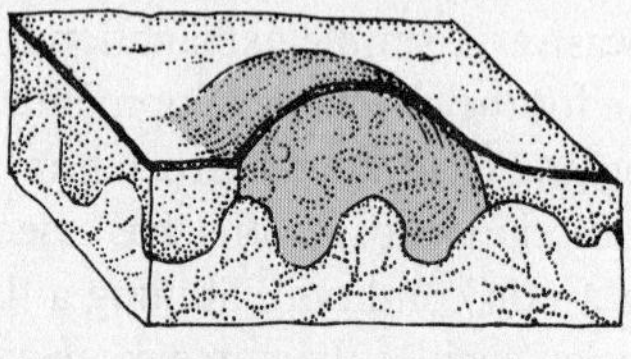	Small, less than 0.5–1 cm in diameter, circumscribed, elevated, fluid-filled
Bullae 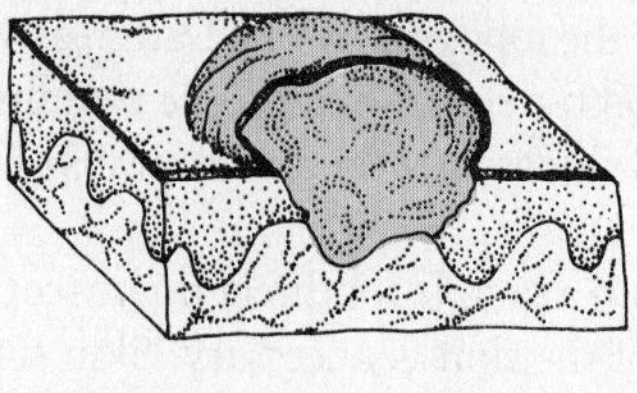	Larger than a 1-cm vesicle
Pustule	Vesicle that contains purulent exudate
Petechia	Circumscribed, sometimes elevated minute skin hemorrhage
Purpura	Circumscribed, elevated similar to petechia, but larger

TABLE 24-1 ***(Continued)***

Secondary lesion		Description
Scales	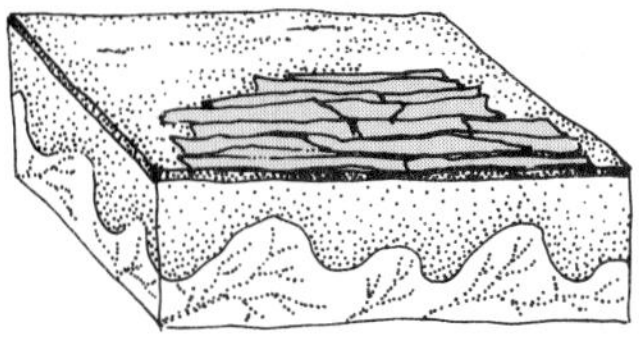	Thin flakes of exfoliated epidermis
Crusts	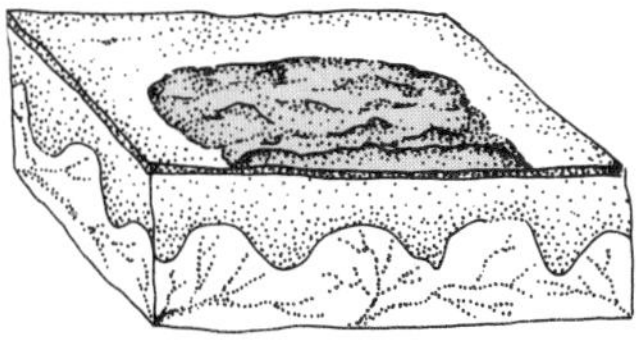	Dried serum, blood, or purulent exudate
Excoriation	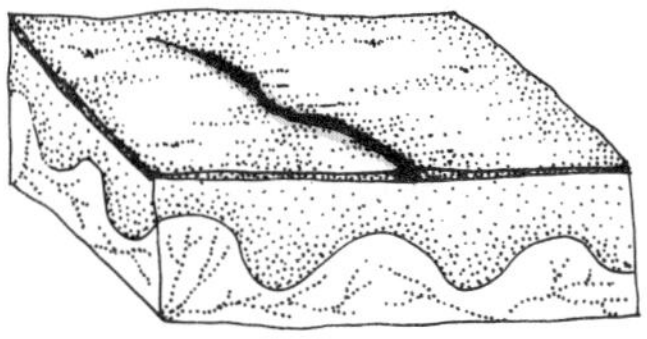	Mechanical removal of the epidermis, a scratch or scrape
Erosion		Moist, often-depressed lesion from loss of the superficial epidermis
Ulcer	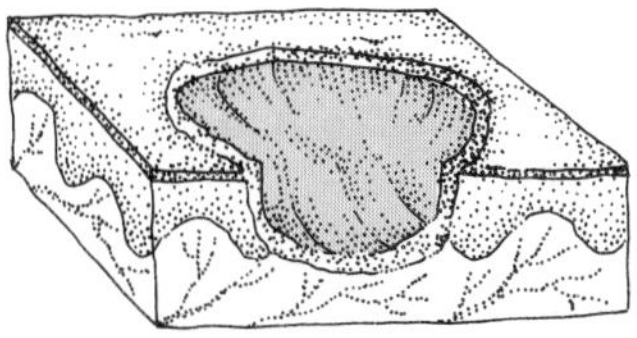	Deeper loss of skin surface often to dermis and subcutaneous layers
Fissure	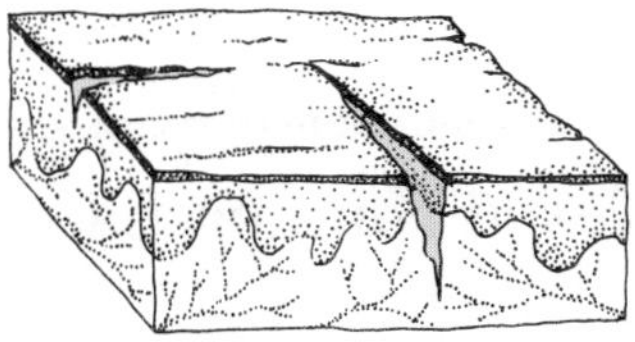	Deep, linear cleavage extending into the dermis
Lichenification		Thickened and roughened skin with increased visibility of skin furrows
Atrophy		Thinning of skin
Scar		Dense connective tissue resulting from destruction and healing of skin
Keloid		Hypertrophied scar
Striae		Pale, white, thin stripes, although purple during initial stretching

ASSESSMENT GUIDE *The Child with a Problem of the Integumentary System*

Assessment questions	Supporting data
Has the child experienced a thermal injury? **Note:** moderate or major burns or frostbite are medical emergencies and require immediate, emergency care	Tissue injury classified by depth (partial thickness or full thickness) and extent (percentage of body surface injured) (see discussion related to burns on p. 783 and frostbite on p. 796); thirst, restlessness, decreased blood pressure, increased pulse, and other signs of fluid volume deficit (see Chapter 21); dyspnea, retractions, nasal flaring and other signs of respiratory obstruction (see Chapter 22); nausea, vomiting, abdominal pain, decreased gastrointestinal motility; alteration in consciousness; generalized edema; numbness, tingling, pallor of fingers or toes
If the child has a rash, when did the rash first appear? How did the rash spread? Does it itch? Describe the lesions	Lesions (vary in appearance, extent, and location according to the cause)
Has the child been in contact with poison ivy, oak, or sumac, a new pet, new soap, shampoo or laundry products different foods, or medications?	Urticaria (hives); intense pruritis; draining lesions that crust; dry, thick, leathery skin, particularly in antecubital and popliteal creases as well as the back of the ears and neck; possible rhinitis, wheezing, itchy eyes; purpura, particularly on legs, thighs or buttocks
Has the child been recently exposed to any communicable condition or tick or flea bite?	Fever, sore throat, headache, nausea, vomiting, anorexia; enlarged lymph nodes; appearance of rash varies in location, onset, and type of lesions (see Chapter 18); white plaques on the tongue and mucous membranes
Has the child sustained a laceration, contusion, or abrasion, or does the child appear to have a skin infection?	Redness, edema; red streaks radiating from the affected part; fever, enlarged regional lymph nodes; honey colored or purulent drainage from any wound or lesion; decreased joint mobility coupled with rash on the face or over the joints

alcohol solution so that topical medication, if present, can be removed.

Complete blood counts and serum electrolyte levels are helpful to diagnose skin conditions as well as to monitor progress (such as in burn patients). Skin tests are useful in diagnosing allergic reactions (see Chapter 25). Other types of skin tests, such as the tine test for tuberculosis, test for exposure to an infectious organism. When preparing the child for any type of skin test, the nurse explains the purpose of the skin test and the procedure that will be used. The nurse notes on the record if the child is taking steroids or immunosuppressive drugs. The child and family are told that a positive skin test for an infectious disease does not always indicate an active infectious condition because the organism might be in an inactive, or dormant, state. Skin tests are not done on inflamed skin. In such a case it is likely that the test would aggravate the skin disorder and would also make it difficult to interpret the results accurately.

Other methods of diagnosing skin alterations include a diascope (glass pressed against a lesion) or a Wood's light. The Wood's light is a fluorescent light that reflects a particular color depending on the organism involved.

Principles of Nursing Care

Acute Care Needs

Impaired skin integrity related to irritants secondary to developmental factors

Skin care Keeping the skin clean and moist and free of irritants promotes healing, helps to prevent infections, and restores skin integrity. Skin irritants include urine, feces, and excessive perspiration, particularly in intertrigenous (skinfold) areas. In infants, friction from improperly placed diapers might irritate the skin. Diapers washed in certain types of soap and not rinsed sufficiently also might cause irritation. If cloth diapers are worn, a nonirritating soap should be used. The nurse might teach the parent how to diaper the infant so that rubbing does not occur. If too much moisture is a problem after cleaning the skin, exposing the area directly to sunlight or artificial light for short periods may help to keep the area dry.

The nurse is careful when cleaning the infant's or child's skin. Bland soap and water and a soft washcloth should be used, and vigorous rubbing is avoided. Because the intertrigenous areas are potential sources of irritation, care should be taken to cleanse them, particularly after every diaper change. After washing, the skin is patted dry.

Baths Baths often are helpful in minimizing the inflammatory process of skin lesions. When dryness and chapping are evident, the use of soap should be minimized. The use of bath oils is a simple way to manage dry, scaly skin. Bathing adds moisture to the skin, and the oil helps to retain the moisture. Mineral oil is an inexpensive substitute for bath oil. The disadvantage of mineral oil is that it lacks a surfactant to make it mix with water.

Oil baths such as Alpha Keri or Domol (1–2 tsp per tub of water) might alleviate drying as well as soothe the skin. Other cooling, antipruritic baths such as Aveeno (1 c per tub of water) or tar baths might help to minimize pruritus (itching). Adding baking soda to the bath water is an inexpensive method of relieving pruritus.

Shampoos Certain shampoos are used to treat skin conditions affecting the head. Available pediculocides (lice treatments) can be found in shampoo form, allowing for more effective treatment (see Chapter 18). The many varieties of dandruff shampoo presently on the market also can be used to treat and control seborrheic dermatitis in infants (cradle cap) (see Chapter 4). The major difficulty with the use of medicinal shampoos is that they must remain on the scalp for a certain amount of time (usually several minutes) to be effective. This might be difficult to achieve with young children. Shampooing the child's hair during the bath and allowing the child to play with bath toys while the shampoo remains on the child's head usually is successful. However, nurses need to caution parents that medicinal shampoos can irritate the eyes.

⊛ Impaired tissue integrity related to mechanical, chemical, or thermal irritants causing wounds or lesions

Wound care

Cleansing A variety of topical preparations are used to clean minor and severe wounds. The purpose of thorough cleansing is to reduce the development of inflammation and infection. Each preparation has its advantages and disadvantages and may be used according to institutional protocol. PHisoDerm and povidone-iodine solutions (Betadine) are commonly used wound-cleansing agents and are readily available for home use. Other solutions used for wound cleansing include Merthiolate (thimerosal) and hydrogen peroxide (Table 24-2).

It is important to remember that children are very concerned about the pain associated with wounds and might resist effective cleansing if they anticipate that the solution will cause additional pain. None of the previously mentioned solutions is painful when applied to wounds, although the effervescence of hydrogen peroxide can be irritating to some children.

Topical agents After thorough wound cleansing, application of a dressing and topical anti-infective agent inhibits bacterial growth in most wounds. The more common anti-infective ointments are presented in Table 24-3. Topical agents can be applied to the dressing or directly to the wound itself using sterile technique.

Anti-inflammatory steroidal lotions, creams, and ointments (eg, hydrocortisone) are used for certain rashes or lesions. They are used with caution to prevent systemic absorption of the steroid (see Chapter 25 for a discussion of steroids).

Other lotions, such as calamine or caladryl, are applied to the skin to control itching. Like the steroids, however, systemic absorption is a possibility when these are used on draining lesions. Benadryl toxicity has become a problem with the overusage of caladryl lotion.

Antifungal creams and ointments, such as Tinactin, need to be applied for at least two weeks for maximum effect against stubborn fungal infections. (See Chapter 18 for a discussion of fungal infections.)

Dressings Dressings serve a number of purposes. They keep the topical agent in contact with the wound or lesion and enable the patient to be ambulatory. They protect the wound from contamination, scratching fingers, bumps, and passing air currents, which might cause pain over exposed nerve endings.

Dry dressings Several different sizes and types of pads can be used to cover wounds. Plain sterile gauze pads come in sizes ranging from 2″ × 2″ to 4″ × 4″. Oversized thick gauze pads can be used on buttocks, back, chest, and abdominal wounds. Oval pads are made specifically for eye wounds. Nonstick Telfa pads are useful for abrasions, although they have limited absorbency. Band-Aids come in various shapes and sizes. Many are colorfully decorated to appeal to children.

Depending on the extent of the wounds or lesions, dressings may be secured with tape. Adhesive tape is used fre-

TABLE 24-2 Some Common Antiseptic and Cleansing Agents

Solution	Action	Nursing consideration
PHisoDerm	Mild topical antiseptic	Nonirritating; readily available for home use
Povidone-iodine (Betadine)	Antimicrobial; effective against gram-positive and gram-negative organisms, fungi, yeast, and viruses	Available for home use; nonirritating; not to be used on extensive wounds because of the possibility of systemic absorption
Thimerosal (Merthiolate)	Bacteriostatic; fungistatic; not as effective an antibacterial agent as others	Nonirritating; needs light-resistant container; used more as an antiseptic than cleansing agent; compatible with soaps
Hydrogen peroxide	Somewhat antibacterial; cleans wounds by release of oxygen (effervescent effect)	Nontoxic; can be used for oral wounds or lesions; must be stored in light-resistant container; should be rinsed from a wound with sterile saline when effervescent action stops
Aluminum acetate (Burow's)	Mild antiseptic, astringent	Relieves pruritis; do not use the solution if it contains a large amount of precipitate

TABLE 24-3 Topical Anti-Infective Agents

Preparation	Effect	Nursing consideration
Povidone-iodine (Betadine)	Antibacterial for gram-positive and gram-negative organisms; also effective against fungi, viruses, and protozoa	Nonirritating
Bacitracin	Antibiotic; effective against gram-positive and gram-negative bacteria, including streptococci and staphylococci	Should not be used on large surface wounds because of systemic absorption; particularly effective in treating impetigo of staphylococcal or streptococcal origin; nonirritating
Neosporin (polymyxcin B–bacitracin-neomycin)	The combination of antibiotics is more effective than any individual one against a broad spectrum of organisms	Nonirritating; also available in generic form—triple antibiotic ointment
Polymyxin B	Effective against gram-negative organisms; not effective against gram-positive organisms or fungi	Sensivity might cause irritation and burning; usually found in combination with bacitracin
Neomycin	Broad-spectrum antibiotic	Can be irritating to abrasions

quently; however, it can cause a contact dermatitis in susceptible children. Various forms of hypoallergenic tape are available. Tape will adhere to the skin better if tincture of benzoin is applied first. Benzoin serves a secondary purpose of protecting the skin from the irritation of the tape.

Dressing materials also include many kinds of gauze. Fine-mesh or wide-mesh gauze over wounds helps in debridement when the dressings are removed. Kerlix wrap works well on extremities, whereas Kling, or flexible, gauze wrap is needed for small fingers and toes. Stockingette, or tube gauze, also is useful for securing dressings to fingers and is particularly helpful for head dressings.

Removal of even minor dressings can be traumatic to a child. Some children like the tape removed quickly, whereas others prefer the slower method. The nurse inquires about children's preferences and also allows them to remove their own dressings if they so desire. If dressing changes are extensive and frequent, the use of gauze wrap to secure pads is preferable to tape. For major lacerations, particularly lacerations of the abdomen, the use of Montgomery straps reduces irritation from constant tape removal. See the section entitled "Burn Wound Dressings" later in this chapter for specific approaches to burn dressings.

Compresses Compresses, or moist dressings, are applied to relieve inflammation, to soften crusted lesions, or to promote comfort. Warm compresses often are used on open wounds or on areas of skin inflammation. Compresses are soaked and wrung gently in the prescribed solution (usually normal saline). The solution has been heated to the ordered temperature. Some institutions use prepackaged moist dressings that are heated under a special lamp. Compresses to open wounds require application using sterile technique. Once applied to the child, warm dressings are covered with plastic wrap and a towel to retain heat. Often a source of external heat such as a thermal pad is used to assist with heat retention. The nurse is careful to ensure an accurate temperature of hot packs to prevent burning of the skin (usually 40.5°C or 105°F).

Cool compresses relieve itching and irritated skin and often are used to treat dermatitis (skin inflammation). They are applied like hot compresses; however, they are not covered with plastic wrap. The compress is left open to the air to promote evaporation and skin cooling. When the compress is warm, it is removed, soaked again in the solution, and reapplied. Children might resist cool compresses, particularly if a large area is to be treated. The nurse ensures that the child remains warm throughout the procedure since evaporation on a small area can cause the child to feel a generalized cooling.

Wound closure Wounds will not heal until closure occurs, even though some granulation tissue (beginning healing) has formed. If wound edges are not closely approximated, if infection is present, or if there is poor blood supply to the injured area, the wound will not heal without leaving a large scar.

Adequate cleansing is required for all wounds to prevent infection. Suturing is required for some, depending upon the type, extent, and depth of the injury. The nurse assesses the type and depth of any laceration to determine whether suturing is required (see Chapter 18). In the event that the wound is not severe enough to need sutures, the nurse can use alternate methods to maintain proper closure. Butterfly-shaped bandages can either be bought or made out of adhesive tape. The advantage of this type of closure is that it provides proper tension on the edges of the laceration while leaving enough of the laceration exposed for more rapid healing. Steri-strip closures completely cover the laceration while providing tension for wound closure. They are particularly effective with jagged, uneven lacerations and may be used in place of sutures for this type of wound. When applying either butterfly or steri-strip closures, the nurse might first apply tincture of benzoin to skin areas that will come in contact with the tape but not over the wound itself. The major disadvantage with using both of these types of closures is that children tend to pick at the tape, thus destroying the tension and resulting in a larger scar.

Skin grafting Skin grafts are thin layers of integumentary tissue used to close wounds such as severe abrasions or extensive thermal injuries that cannot heal by any other method.

The functions of skin grafts include the following:

1. To cover a wound to prevent infection or to decrease fluid or heat loss from the wound
2. To improve joint mobility
3. To improve cosmetic appearance

Skin grafts can be permanent or temporary. There are three major types of grafts:

Autografts—permanent grafts taken from the child's own skin.

Allografts—temporary grafts taken from the skin of an individual of the same species. These include skin from human donors and cadavers and from chemically treated amniotic membranes. Allografts are used to cover wounds temporarily while donor sites heal. They prevent fluid and heat loss and serve as a natural barrier against infection. The body will begin to reject allografts after approximately 10 days.

Heterografts—temporary grafts taken from species other than human, usually pigs. They serve the same purpose as allografts and are removed after 10 days.

Most skin grafts are split-thickness in depth, including the epidermis and part of the dermis. They vary in thickness from 0.012 in. to 0.24 in. (Fig. 24-1).

The graft recipient site is prepared for grafting by hydrotherapy and *debridement* (the removal of dead skin) (see p. 789). Dead skin is removed by layers until a bleeding bed is reached. The bed must be free from debris and bacteria and must have a good blood supply to ensure that a graft will take.

The donor sites are selected from unaffected areas, excluding the face, joints, and the dorsa of the hands. Whenever possible, sites that usually can be covered by clothing, such as the buttocks and thighs, are chosen, since some discoloration can remain long after the site has healed.

From the time the child is admitted for grafting the

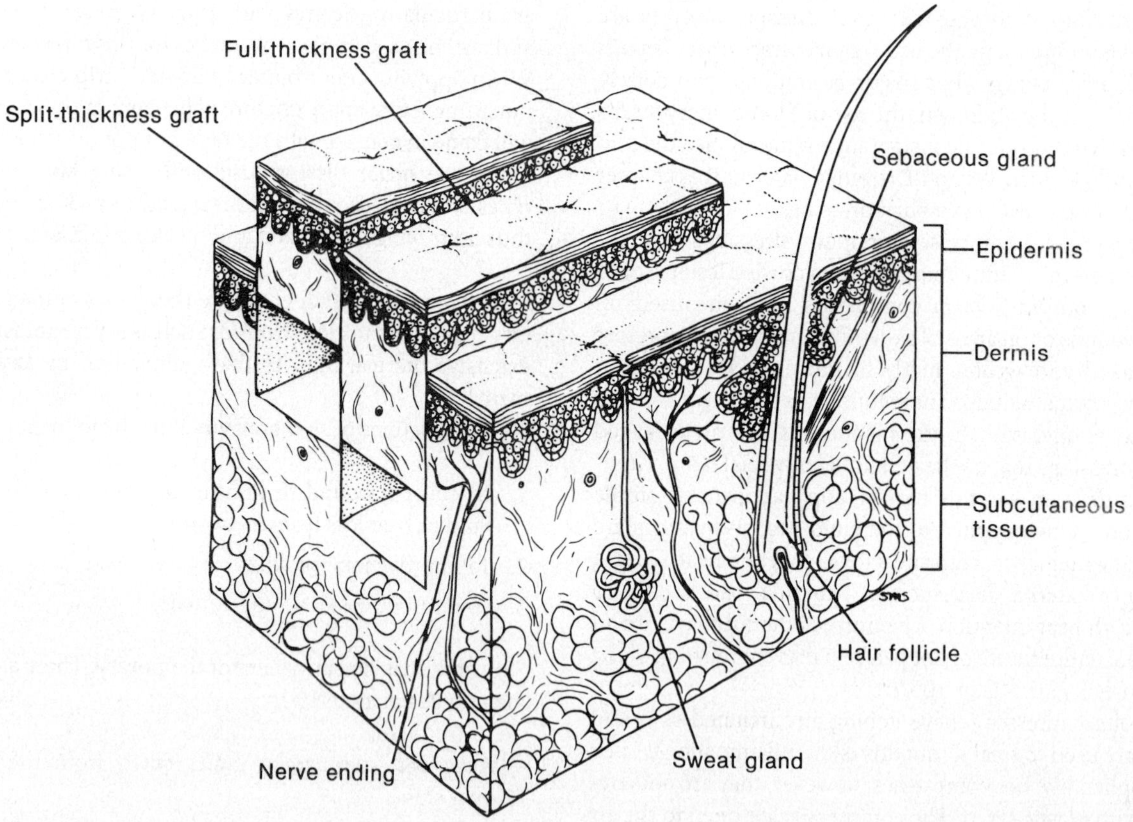

FIGURE 24-1
Two types of grafts are illustrated—the split-thickness graft, which includes all of the epidermis and part of the dermis, and the full-thickness graft, which includes all of the epidermis and dermis.

donor sites must be protected from infection and irritating topical agents that might be used to treat the wounds. Covering the donor sites with gauze impregnated with petroleum jelly protects the skin.

Once the graft is cropped (taken from the donor site), the goals are to prevent infection, promote healing, and ready the site quickly for recropping. Donor sites can be used after 10–14 days. If Scarlet Red fine-mesh gauze is used to promote healing of the site, the child needs to be informed preoperatively. The red color can be extremely frightening to the unprepared child. When the scalp is used for a donor site, parents and children need reassurance that the hair will grow back.

All donor sites are painful initially but will feel much more comfortable within a few days. As healing progresses, they begin to itch and must be protected from children's scratching and rubbing.

Nursing goals for skin grafting include preventing infection, supporting healing, and decreasing scarring. A primary nursing intervention is to maintain immobility of the grafted site. Immobilization is required until the circulation between the graft and the bed begins to be established (usually 3–4 days).

The nurse observes the site for signs of graft rejection and reports any sloughing or signs of circulatory compromise (such as pallor) or infection. Other nursing measures are related to the prescribed care of the site and might include dressing changes and specialized procedures such as rolling the graft to remove serous fluid pockets.

Maintaining immobility is a challenge to the nurse, particularly when working with children whose cognitive level does not permit understanding of the reasons for the immobility. The use of distraction and quiet play or story time assists the nurse to keep the child still (see Chapter 20 for a further discussion of immobility). Occasionally special splints might be needed to immobilize the graft site.

⊛ Potential alteration in comfort: itching

Pruritis (itching) is the most frequently seen reaction in skin conditions. Pruritis is either localized or generalized, depending on the skin condition and other factors. One feature of pruritis is its intermittent character, being more severe in the evening and during the night. Managing pruritis is one of the nurse's key responsibilities in caring for children with dermatologic conditions.

Bath oils, Aveeno (colloidal oatmeal), or baking soda baths can be used to relieve generalized itching. The use of play as distraction is an important nursing intervention. Children who are enjoying themselves tend to focus less on the pruritis.

Warm, irritating, and tight clothing is avoided. Cotton fabrics are preferred because of their breathability. Wool is contraindicated because the fibers can promote itching.

Depending on the severity of the condition, the physician might prescribe topical steroids, oral steroids, or antihistamines to relieve itching.

Potential for infection

Pruritis is one of the most common causes of secondary infection in children with skin alterations. Preventing secondary infections from scratching is important. The child's nails should be cut short and the hands kept meticulously clean. Children who are old enough should cut their own nails. It is essential to explain to the older child the importance of avoiding scratching and the precautions needed to prevent alterations in skin integrity.

Wearing cotton gloves at night is useful with school-age children and adolescents to prevent scratching during sleep. For young children elbow restraints or Duncan sleeves are helpful and for infants the hand covers on long-sleeved tee shirts aid in protecting them from scratching. The nurse or parent checks the child periodically to ensure that freedom of movement is not completely restricted if these means are used to prevent scratching.

With any type of compromised skin, infection is a possibility from breach of the body's first line of defense. Wound cleansing and applying topical anti-infectives can reduce the incidence of infection in many cases.

Puncture wounds, which close over quickly, and other dirty wounds are prime sites for rapid multiplicaton of the anaerobic organism *Clostridium tetani*. *C. tetani*, which is found in dirt and areas contaminated by animal excrement, can cause tetanus (lockjaw). Tetanus is fatal in 30%–70% of people who contract it (see Chapter 31). Children can receive puncture wounds from nails, pins, and wood splinters. Usually, penetration is superficial and the object can be removed easily. The small puncture wound does not bleed readily, so it should be squeezed gently to promote bleeding and to flush out the bacteria. This is especially important if the penetrating object is a rusty nail.

Since tetanus can occur as a result of even minor wounds and lacerations, the nurse obtains information about the child's primary immunization series of DPT (diphtheria, tetanus, and pertussis) (see Chapter 11). Since booster doses of tetanus toxoid (Td and DT) are given on a routine basis, information about the child's last tetanus booster is necessary. Tetanus prophylaxis is recommended for children with wounds (see Table 24-4).

TABLE 24-4 Tetanus Prophylaxis

Immunization history	Type of wound	Prophylaxis
Unknown, or less than three doses of DPT or DT	Clean, minor	Td*
	All others	Td and TIG**
Three or more doses	Clean, minor	Td only if last booster was longer than 10 years prior to injury
	All others	Td only if last booster was longer than 5 years prior to injury

*Give Td if the child is older than 7 years; give DT if the child is younger than 7 years and if pertussis vaccine is contraindicated.
**TIG, tetanus immunoglobulin.

SOURCE: *Morbidity and Mortality Weekly Reports* (Oct 4) 1985; 34/39:607–609.

Potential alteration in comfort: pain

Pain is associated with some integumentary alterations. The nurse assesses the child's perception of pain, its location, and its intensity through the use of an objective pain assessment tool (see Chapter 20). Pain is a means of protecting the body whenever physiologic or psychologic disturbances occur. Pain warns the individual that some type of trauma is occurring.

When the child is in pain, the nurse's primary responsibility is to reduce or eliminate it. The nurse minimizes or eliminates other discomforts because they might aggravate pain. Noxious stimuli that might intensify the child's reaction to pain should be removed if possible.

It is essential to make every effort to ensure that the child is comfortable and safe. If medications for pain are ordered, the nurse and child decide together when they are needed. The nurse can medicate the child prior to procedures such as baths or dressing changes that cause the child pain.

Cool compresses, such as Burow's solution, might relieve the pain from localized inflammation. Warm saline compresses also are effective to relieve pain related to certain conditions, such as suspected infection.

The nurse needs to make every effort to recognize factors that enhance comfort and relaxation without medication. The nurse provides reassurance and helpful diversions, eliminates stress and distractions that stimulate pain, and provides a climate that is conducive to rest and relaxation. The nurse needs to remember that individuals respond differently to pain because of their pain tolerance and cultural orientation to pain.

⊛ Potential fluid volume deficit

Cell production is impaired by dehydration; consequently, healing is slowed. Maintenance of the child's fluid and electrolyte balance is critical to the nurse caring for the child with a skin condition. Fever resulting in increased fluid loss might occur with some skin alterations. The relationship between intake and output and fluid and electrolyte balance is complex (see Chapter 21). Alterations in body temperature and maintenance of homeostasis depend to a large extent on the regulation of fluid balance. The nurse checks the child's temperature periodically to determine whether it is elevated. Antipyretic drugs can be used to lower the temperature, as well as mechanical means to cool the child (eg, sponging).

The nurse gives particular attention to weeping lesions or thermal injuries because fluid loss through these areas can be extensive. Careful monitoring of intake and output is essential for children with fluid alterations. Encouraging fluid to meet the child's daily fluid maintenance, with additional fluids if the child has extensive fluid loss, is a necessity. (See Chapter 21 for additional interventions for the child with a fluid and electrolyte imbalance.)

Nutritional Needs

⊛ Potential alteration in nutrition: less than body requirements

Wound healing is delayed by inadequate nutrition. Cell production is impaired by nutritional deficiencies, particularly vitamin C and protein deficiencies. For wound healing, the following nutritional needs must be met:

1. Sufficient protein and carbohydrate intake to prevent a negative nitrogen balance, hypoalbuminemia, and weight loss (50 to 120 calories/kg depending on the age of the child)
2. Increased daily intake of vitamins and minerals:
   a. Vitamin A—10,000–50,000 IU
   b. Vitamin B—0.5–1.0 mg/1000 dietary calories
   c. Vitamin B_2—0.25 mg/1000 dietary calories
   d. Vitamin B_6—2 mg
   e. Niacin—15–20 mg
   f. Vitamin B_{12}—400 mg
   g. Vitamin C—75–300 mg
   h. Vitamin D—400 mg
   i. Vitamin E—10–15 IU
   j. Traces of zinc, magnesium, calcium, and copper (Carpenito, 1983)

The nurse encourages the child with a skin condition to eat well-balanced meals. Adequate nutrition is essential to the healing process.

The child with extensive surface injuries requires significantly higher (up to 150%) caloric and protein intake because of protein loss and markedly increased metabolic needs (Rosequist and Shepp, 1985). These needs usually cannot be met with conventional IV solutions, so total parenteral nutrition is required (see Chapter 27).

Developmental Needs

⊛ Potential alterations in growth and development

Nurses need to continue to foster development leading to independence in self-care tasks for children with skin conditions, just as they would with any other child. Infants with skin conditions need to be talked to, held, and cuddled. They need freedom to move around and mobiles to watch. For the most part, skin lesions should not inhibit the infant's developmental needs. Appropriate nonallergenic toys should be offered to the infant. The nurse provides auditory, visual, and kinesthetic (movement) stimulation. Tactile stimulation is especially important since it occupies the infant's hands, thus decreasing scratching.

For children in early childhood, the nurse might need to ensure that the environment will promote healing rather than exacerbate the skin condition. Preschool children might be more sensitive to their lesions because other people notice them. Dramatic play might help these children decrease the frustrations or negative feelings associated with their skin conditions. Children of early childhood age should be encouraged to engage in age-appropriate activities.

By middle and late childhood, children can understand their skin conditions and follow through with self-care management when it is appropriately demonstrated to them. They might need help in accepting themselves if their peers, family, and other significant others have difficulty accepting them. The child's reaction to skin lesions cannot be predicted. Some children cope well, whereas others respond emotionally and behaviorally. Self-care and other activities, such as bathing and nail cleanliness, appropriate to their age and skin condition should be promoted in these children. Because these children are generally energetic and cooperative, the nurse might find it easy to help them understand the nature and care of their skin conditions.

The stresses on the adolescent's psychic energy are many and varied. A skin condition compounds the complexity of the adolescent's life. Helping adolescents feel good about themselves is crucial. Many adolescents with skin conditions have a significant degree of anxiety. The emotional reactions are manifested in a variety of ways, which include self-consciousness, withdrawal, and excessive attention to cleanliness.

Determining the child's and parent's level of knowledge and beliefs and fears about skin alterations helps the nurse in planning care.

The Child with Infection

Wounds become infected when treatment is inadequate or delayed or when they become contaminated in spite of precautions. Signs and symptoms of infection develop in the first 24–48 hours. Local manifestations of infection are pain, redness, warmth, swelling, drainage, and sometimes enlarged adjacent lymph nodes. General malaise and fever develop later if the infection progresses. When a sutured wound becomes infected, the physician might remove every other stitch to allow for drainage.

Warm saline soaks, frequent dressing changes, and topical antibiotics might be sufficient to treat the infection. However, in case of an abscess, needle aspiration of purulent material or incision and drainage of the wound under local anesthesia might be needed. Oral antibiotics, intramuscular long-acting penicillin, or intravenous antibiotics help to combat these infections.

An untreated wound infection can lead to invasive local infections and even to septicemia and death.

Cellulitis

Cellulitis is an invasive infection that occurs when organisms such as *Staphylococcus aureus, β-hemolytic streptococci,* and *Hemophilus influenzae* destroy tissue defenses. These microorganisms produce hyaluronidase, which destroys tissue barriers against the invasion and spread of bacteria.

Bacteria can enter through an open wound or at an intravenous site. Often, however, there is just a vague history of recent trauma with no break in the skin or history of injury.

The infected part of the body is red, swollen, warm, and painful. Red streaks from the wound might be present, and adjacent lymph nodes are enlarged and painful. The child's temperature usually is elevated.

Treatment includes immobilization and elevation of the infected part; warm, moist packs; fever control; and systemic antibiotics. Intravenous antibiotics such as oxacillin and dicloxacillin are given if the infection is serious. Treatment with oral antibiotics might be adequate to combat less severe cellulitis.

Nursing management includes application of warm compresses, maintenance of immobilization and elevation of infected part, and accurate IV antibiotic administration. Should the wound begin to drain, wound cultures are taken and wound and contact precautions followed. The nurse observes the child for signs of septicemia, including high fever, chills, and disorientation.

Impetigo Contagiosa

Impetigo is one of the most contagious skin conditions of childhood. Group A streptococci and *Staphylococcus aureus* are the most frequent causative organisms. Impetigo is the most common *pyoderma* (pus in the skin) infection in children. Predisposing factors are crowded living conditions, poor personal hygiene, and a hot, humid environment. Impetigo probably is spread by direct contact with an infected person. It can be spread by the child from its primary site to other sites on the child's body.

Clinical manifestations The lesions are discrete and coalesced. They begin as papules and progress to pustules, vesicles, and bullae surrounded by narrow areolas of erythema. Lesions tend to be seen primarily on the forearms and lower parts of the leg. Lesions also group around the mouth and nose. The vesicles and bullae rupture easily and release a thin, yellowish fluid. This serous discharge dries and forms a thick, soft, honey-colored crust. The bullous type of impetigo seems to be associated with group II staphylococci, whereas the vesicopustular form seems to be caused by group A β-hemolytic streptococci. It is sometimes hard to distinguish between impetigo and chickenpox.

Treatment Topical treatment might be indicated. Treatment is based on the age of the child and severity of the condition. Cleansing the lesion daily with soap and water or alcohol aids in removing the crusts. Lubricants are helpful in removing crusty scabs. Cleansing of the lesions is sometimes painful but is essential to prevent secondary infection.

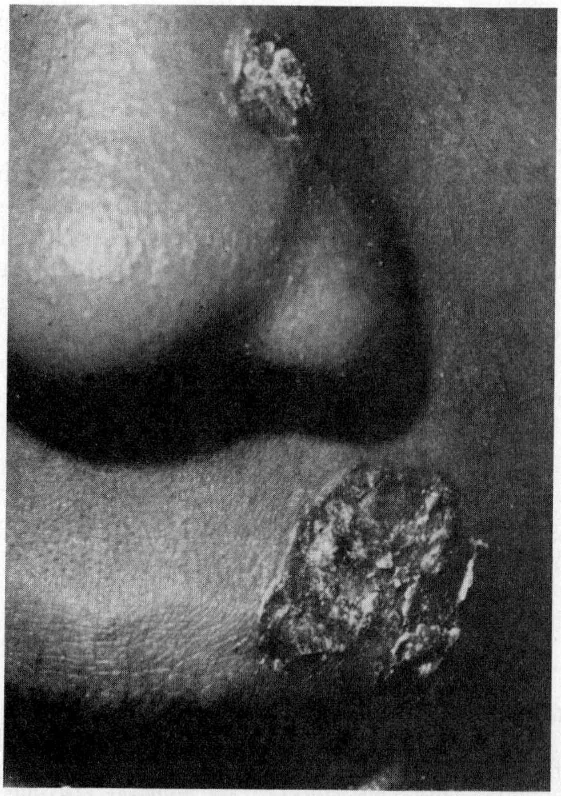

Impetigo (From Binnick SA: Skin Diseases: Diagnosis and Management in Clinical Practice. *Addison-Wesley, 1982.)*

If the child has a severe case of impetigo, systemic antibiotics might be required. The application of topical antibiotics (such as Neosporin ointment or Mycitracin ointment) might be helpful if the infection is extensive. In extensive conditions the treatment depends on the causative organism. If extensive disease is caused by group A β-hemolytic streptococci, penicillin, 25–40 mg/kg/day, usually divided into several doses for 7–10 days, or erythromycin, 40–50 mg/kg/day in divided doses, is given for 10 days. If the extensive infection is caused by staphylococci, cloxacillin, 50–100 mg/kg/day in divided doses for 7–10 days, or dicloxacillin, 25–50 mg/kg/day in divided doses for 7–10 days, is given. Intravenous antibiotic therapy might be essential for children with disseminated impetigo (involving internal organs).

Nursing management The nurse explains to the child and parent the importance of taking the medication as prescribed. They need to know that the prescribed antibiotic reduces the risk of complications and decreases the ability of the causative organism to spread to intimate contacts. Signs of side effects from the drug should be noted. The nurse observes children taking antibiotics for allergic reactions, which might include rashes. Children taking erythromycin should be observed for stomatitis and gastrointestinal disturbances. The nurse also notes resistance of the organism, particulary in cases where the antibiotic has been used for an extended period. Fever might be an early indicator of resistance.

If the impetigo is caused by β-hemolytic streptococci, the nurse follows the family to ensure that there are no symptoms that suggest the development of acute glomerulonephritis several weeks after the lesions have healed (see Chapters 25 and 28). Children under 6 years of age seem particularly susceptible to this complication. The parents should report any puffiness around the child's eyes or any sign of blood in the urine (urine might be cola colored).

The nurse avoids alarming the parents when telling them about the possibility of kidney complications; however, parents should be cautioned to be alert for signs of kidney involvement.

Handwashing after caring for a child with impetigo is important to prevent spread. The nurse also teaches the child good hygiene to prevent spread of the infection. The child with impetigo should have daily soap baths, and the child's washcloths and towels should not be interchanged with those of other individuals. The nurse encourages a balanced diet because proper nutrition aids in wound healing. Finally, the nurse helps the child and the family to cope with the condition.

The child's involvement in self-care might be helpful in coping with the condition. Having the child apply topical ointment to lesions when indicated is one way of involving the child. Allowing the child to cleanse the lesions encourages responsibility for self-care. The nurse demonstrates how to perform aspects of care, observes as the child performs the various aspects of care, and reinforces the procedure. Teaching the child that other people might get the condition if good hygiene is not practiced might help the child to begin to learn about the modes of transmission and also might encourage the child to assume responsibility for the prevention of health problems in other people.

Acne Vulgaris

Acne is the most common skin condition of adolescence. It affects 80%–90% of children in this age group. Acne is particularly distressing to teenagers because it undermines their self-confidence at an age when they already are struggling with their identity and feeling most insecure. As the androgen level rises in the adolescent, the sebaceous glands, which have not been as active before the adolescent years, become more active and produce more sebum. The sebum, along with oxidized fatty acids and accumulated dirt on the skin, form *comedones* (blackheads). The bacteria on the skin (*Corynebacterium acnes*) thrive in the retained secretions and form pustules. Papule formation also occurs. In addition to comedones, papules, and pustules, cysts and nodules also might occur. The lesions are located primarily on the face, back, and chest. Lesions also might be seen on the neck and arms.

Treatment The role of diet in the management of acne is highly controversial. Acne is influenced by many factors. Lifestyle, which includes diet and other factors such as physical and chemical exposures, might influence acne. It appears that exposure to environmental substances such as bromides, iodine, and chlorine can aggravate acne to a greater degree than any type of food (Epstein, 1983). A wholesome lifestyle should be encouraged that includes minimizing stress, getting adequate rest, and eating nourishing foods for a balanced diet.

Estrogens might be prescribed to aid in suppressing sebaceous gland activity. Oral tetracycline has been found effective in treating acne when a large number of pustules and cysts are present (Czernielewski and Skwarczynska-Banys, 1982). The side effects of tetracycline include phototoxicity and an inability to concentrate urine. Therefore, adolescents with renal problems should not be given the drug.

A corticosteroid such as prednisone might be used to reduce inflammation. Ultraviolet light also might be used to treat the condition. Topical preparations such as benzoyl peroxide or retinoic acid also might be useful in treating acne.

Cleanliness is particularly important. Keeping the face clean and following washing with a mild astringent is helpful. The goal is to maintain a mild peeling of the skin. Facial scrubs that contain abrasives should be used infrequently since they can increase skin irritation.

Nursing management The nurse discourages the use of greasy ointments and creams and cautions the adolescent not to pick at or squeeze the lesions. Squeezing might injure underlying tissue and cause scarring. Rubbing the skin too hard also should be avoided to prevent damage.

The nurse encourages the adolescent to keep the skin clean. Alcohol or other astringents might be useful in helping to cleanse and dry the skin, thus preventing the formation of comedones. Anti-acne soaps and lotions will aid in drying the skin. When the skin dries, the sebum is released more freely, so an initial increase in oiliness might be observed.

The nurse ensures that tetracycline, when ordered for adolescents, is taken with water and on an empty stomach. Tetracycline is not given with milk products because they interfere with its absorption. Tetracycline should be used with caution in adolescent girls who might become pregnant because the drug could damage the fetus. Certain preparations of retinoic acid (eg, Accutane) prescribed for oral use can cause fetal anomalies. These preparations are contraindicated for adolescents when there is any possibility of a pregnancy.

The psychologic aspects of the acne are important to the adolescent's developmental tasks and body image. Some authorities believe that stress exacerbates the condition. The rapidity of both physiologic and psychologic changes makes the adolescent extremely vulnerable to identity problems. A number of adolescents with cutaneous alterations are likely to experience anxiety and depression related to feelings about self and self-worth. Successful nursing management depends not only on treating the cutaneous alterations but also on helping adolescents cope with their feelings of frustration and self-consciousness and problems with self-esteem.

The Child with an Inflammation

Eczema (Atopic Dermatitis)

Eczema (atopic dermatitis) is a genetically determined condition. It can occur any time from birth to adulthood and the condition might be mild or severe, acute or chronic. Eczema is a disease of allergic origin that can be aggravated by stress. Common causes of the disease are food allergies, hair, feathers, certain fabrics, and environmental pollutants. It occurs more frequently in girls, most frequently in infants and children of early childhood age, and can be associated with asthma or rhinitis. There tends to be a familial pattern with the occurrence of this disease, and it is theorized that high levels of IgE production (see Chapter 25) in certain children are genetically controlled through multifactorial inheritance (Rocklin, 1984). Eczema occurs as a result of elevated levels of IgE specific for certain allergens, which elicit an inflammatory response in the skin. Eczema can occur as a single episode, resolving after the allergen is removed, or it can become chronic with remissions and exacerbations.

Clinical manifestations Eczema is characterized by very dry skin, severe pruritis, and erythematous papular and vesicular lesions. There is edema, oozing of serous drainage from the lesions, and crusting. Laboratory values reveal an increase in IgE levels and increased eosinophils. The onset of eczema can occur at different ages, and clinical manifestations vary accordingly:

Infants—Can start as early as 2 months of age and might last up to 2 years. Lesions appear first on the cheeks, forehead, and scalp. The lesions spread to other parts of the body, including the trunk and extensor surfaces of the extremities. Oozing and crusted lesions predominate.

Children—From 2 years to adolescence. The skin appears scaly. The distribution of crusted lesions is more predominant on trunk and extremities than on the face. The skin begins to thicken, particularly in creases, such as the popliteal and antecubital areas, and on the back of the ears and neck.

Adolescents—Skin continues to thicken and takes on a leathery appearance. Lesions occur on hands and feet with scaly skin elsewhere.

All forms of eczema cause intense pruritis; thus, the risk of secondary infection from scratching is high.

Treatment The management of dry and itchy skin is critical in the care of children with atopic dermatitis. Most children with eczema are managed at home but in severe and intractable cases, hospitalization might be indicated. Bathing is minimized although close attention is given to cleaning and drying the diaper area in infants. Mild soaps such as Dove or Neutrogena are used for bathing. Lubricants are applied over slightly moist skin rather than placed in the bath water. This seals in moisture and rehydrates, lubricates, and moistens the skin. Tepid, rather than hot, baths are given because they are less drying.

Topical steroid ointments, creams, or lotions such as hydrocortisone, triamsinolone (Kenalog, Aristocort), or betamethasone (Valisone) are often prescribed to reduce inflammation. Caution should be exercised when using topical steroids since systemic effects can result from absorption of steroids through open, draining skin lesions. Antihistamines such as diphenhydramine hydrochloride (Benadryl) or chlorpheniramine maleate (Chlortrimeton) are prescribed to reduce itching. These medications can cause drowsiness.

Nursing management Nursing goals are directed toward relieving pruritis and preventing secondary infection.

Since emotional stress can increase perspiration, which contributes to pruritis, sources of stress for the child should be reduced. In infants, the pruritis itself is stressful. Encouraging hand exploration and other normal developmental play activities provides distraction and occupies hands. Occasionally, a parent experiences increased stress in reaction to the child's appearance. Because this stress can be communicated to the infant, the nurse encourages stress reduction techniques for parents. The nurse also encourages the parent to cuddle the baby frequently to promote attachment. Older children whose eczema seems to be exaggerated by stress can benefit from the stress reduction exercises in Chapter 16.

The type of clothing worn is important. Wool near the skin is uncomfortable. Wool garments are undesirable because they irritate the skin. Soft cotton clothing is recommended. Sweaters of acrylic yarn provide warmth without the irritating qualities of wool. Clothes or toys that have potential allergenic properties should be avoided because children with atopic dermatitis are predisposed to other allergic conditions such as asthma.

Warm, wet compresses using Burow's solution might have a soothing, antipruritic and antiseptic action on the inflamed skin and are used frequently for oozing lesions. It is important to keep the child warm and to wet the compresses moderately. The child's fingernails should be cut to avoid developing a secondary infection from scratching. Mitts and/or elbow restraints to prevent scratching also have been suggested.

Eliminating the allergen, if the allergen can be identified, is helpful. Since the precipitating factor in infantile eczema might be food, it is recommended that the introduction of solid foods and citrus juices in infants be delayed until 5–6 months of age. This is particularly important for children who have a strong familial history of allergy (see Chapter 25).

Psoriasis

Psoriasis has an insidious onset and initially resembles atopic dermatitis. The plaques, however, are erythematous, and the scales are not greasy. Psoriasis is an inherited disorder with a complex genetic mechanism. The condition rarely occurs during infancy and early childhood but may be seen in children 5 years of age through adolescence. It is associated with decreased sweating.

Clinical manifestations The lesions begin as small, reddish, pinpoint papules surrounded by fine scales. The papules coalesce and form plaques. Sharply demarcated scales that are grayish or silvery white characterize the lesions. The lesions are located on the scalp, ears, forehead, and around the eyebrows, trunk, genitals, elbows, and knees. A sore throat usually precedes the eruption by 2 or 3 weeks.

Treatment The treatment of psoriasis is varied and depends on the stage of the condition. Treatment for 90% of the children with this condition requires topical therapy—corticosteroids, tar, or anthralin. Treatment must be vigorous and performed daily and is long term. In severe cases steroid cream and occlusive plastic wraps also might be necessary. When the soles of the feet are involved, the application of corticosteroid cream followed by the use of plastic wrap is an effective treatment.

Topical steroids are the mainstay of treatment for ordinary plaque psoriasis. According to Zackheim (1984), ointment bases provide greater activity than cream bases. The use of plastic occlusion enhances the effectiveness of either form. The most common complication of topical steroids is cutaneous atrophy. Intertrigenous areas and regions occluded for prolonged periods are particularly susceptible to cutaneous atrophy.

Systemic therapy will depend on the severity of the condition. Systemic treatment might include the use of antimetabolites such as methotrexate. Methotrexate helps to control or minimize psoriasis and psoriatic arthritis. Hepatotoxicity is a side effect of this drug. Exposure to psoralens and ultraviolet light (PUVA) might be effective in some cases of severe and extensive psoriasis. This treatment, however, might be carcinogenic and consequently is used cautiously. Etretinate, a new vitamin A derivative, is also effective in suppressing some severe forms of psoriasis.

Nursing management The nurse helps the family to adhere to the medical regimen and encourages patience because psoriasis is a difficult condition with which to cope. Progress is often slow. Helping children or adolescents cope with this condition is a challenge. Children of late childhood age and adolescents are particularly vulnerable in terms of having their psychosocial and developmental needs met. During the late childhood period, children are involved in many peer activities. Being selected for teams and participating in structured group activities are important aspects of the child's life. During the late childhood period, children also are learning to be thoughtful and considerate of others. Name calling might occur. Children with psoriasis are not very attractive because of the skin lesions. They might be viewed as being undesirable because of their appearance. Adolescents who are working on self-identity need support in coping because improvement is generally slow.

The Child with a Burn

Burns are a leading cause of accidental injury in children. Those who survive burn injuries endure pain, lengthy hospitalization, and disfiguring scars. The patterns of injuries are predictable by age group, coinciding with physical, cognitive, and emotional growth and development. At least 75% of childhood burns are preventable (see Chapter 12).

Children receive thermal burns from hot liquids, such as soup, coffee, tea, and boiling water; hot surfaces, such as radiators and irons; and contact with flames, as in match play, gasoline play, and house fires. Electrical burns occur when children bite into cords or extension plugs, or when they climb trees or telephone poles and play near high-tension wires. Electrical burns often are deep and disfiguring, damaging muscle and bone and often leading to limb amputation. Chemical burns occur most frequently among toddlers and are caused by handling and ingesting corrosive household cleaners. Overexposure to sunlight and high-dosage radiation also cause burns.

Burns are classified according to the percentage of total body surface area (TBSA) affected and according to the depth of damage to the skin and underlying structures.

Percentage of Injury

The rule of nines (Fig. 24-2A), useful in estimating burn size in children 10 years of age and older, is inaccurate for the younger child. The Lund and Browder chart (Fig. 24-2B) takes into account changing body proportions in the growing child. Fluid needs are calculated according to the percentage of injury and the child's body weight, so estimates must be accurate. Diagrams of the body are included in the burn chart. They can be color coded to denote areas of burn and varying depths.

Depth of Injury

Partial-thickness burns In partial-thickness (first- and second-degree) burns, the epidermis and part of the dermis are destroyed, leaving hair follicles and sweat glands intact (see Fig. 24-3). Some scalds and flash burns are superficial partial-thickness injuries (involving the epidermis), which heal in 1–10 days. Deep partial-thickness burns (involving the epidermis and part of the dermis) can take up to 6 weeks to heal and might eventually require skin grafting. If protected from injury and infections, partial-thickness burns heal by reepithelialization.

Typically, partial-thickness burns include sunburns, flash burns, and scalds. The shallower partial-thickness burn is reddened, dry, painful, and edematous. The deeper partial-thickness burn is reddened, painful, and edematous and is also moist and often blistered. Tissue blanches and refills with pressure, indicating intact capillaries.

Full-thickness burns Full-thickness, or third-degree, burns destroy the dermal layer down to and often including subcutaneous fat. Hair follicles, sweat glands, sebaceous glands, and nerves are destroyed (see Fig. 24-3). Some

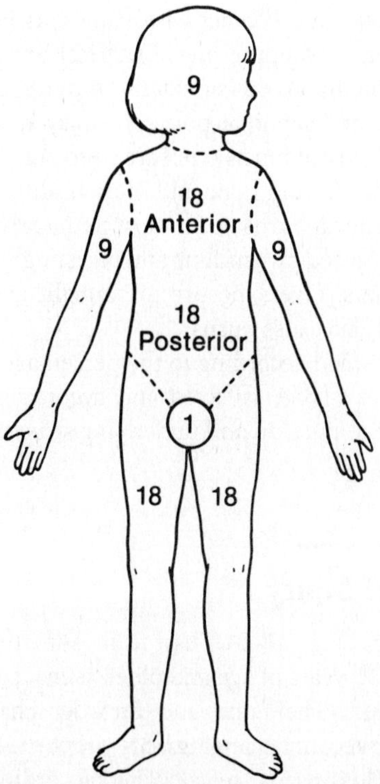

A

B

AREA	1 yr.	1–4 yrs.	5–9 yrs.	10–14 yrs.	15 yrs.	Adult	2°	3°
Head	19	17	13	11	9	7		
Neck	2	2	2	2	2	2		
Ant. Trunk	13	13	13	13	13	13		
Post. Trunk	13	13	13	13	13	13		
R. Buttock	2½	2½	2½	2½	2½	2½		
L. Buttock	2½	2½	2½	2½	2½	2½		
Genitalia	1	1	1	1	1	1		
R.U. Arm	4	4	4	4	4	4		
L.U. Arm	4	4	4	4	4	4		
R.L. Arm	3	3	3	3	3	3		
L.L. Arm	3	3	3	3	3	3		
R. Hand	2½	2½	2½	2½	2½	2½		
L. Hand	2½	2½	2½	2½	2½	2½		
R. Thigh	5½	6½	8	8½	9	9½		
L. Thigh	5½	6½	8	8½	9	9½		
R. Leg	5	5	5½	6	6½	7		
L. Leg	5	5	5½	6	6½	7		
R. Foot	3½	3½	3½	3½	3½	3½		
L. Foot	3½	3½	3½	3½	3½	3½		
TOTAL								

FIGURE 24-2
Two methods of determining the percentage of TBSA. ***A.*** *The rule of nines is used with children 10 years of age and older.* ***B.*** *The Lund and Browder method is used for children younger than 10 years. (From Artz CP and Moncrief JA:* The Treatment of Burns, *2nd ed. Saunders, 1969. Reprinted with permission.)*

clinicians classify burn injuries that damage underlying fat, muscle, and bone as fourth degree in depth. The full-thickness burn is pearly white, tan, brown, mahogany, or black in appearance. The tissue feels dry and leathery, does not blanch and refill, and is not painful. The burned tissue of a full-thickness injury is called *eschar.* Once dermis and dermal structures are destroyed, skin regeneration cannot take place. Skin grafting is necessary to close the full-thickness wound.

Classification of Burns

The American Burn Association has classified burns according to the severity of the injury and complicating factors (Artz et al., 1979). The small child with a burn of 10% or more, however, will require as much attention as the older child with a larger burn.

Minor burns include partial-thickness burns involving less than 15% of the TBSA and full-thickness burns involving less than 2% of the TBSA.

Moderate burns include partial-thickness burns involving 15%–30% of the TBSA and full-thickness burns involving less than 10% of the TBSA, except in small children and when the burns involve critical areas.

Major or critical burns include burns complicated by respiratory tract injury, partial-thickness burns involving 30% or more of the TBSA, and full-thickness burns involving 10% or more of the TBSA.

Burns of the face, hands, or feet are considered major because these are critical areas of function and appearance. Burns of the genitals are also in this category because this area harbors many bacteria.

Hospitalization is indicated for any children with moderate or major burns and sometimes children with minor burns involving 10% of the TBSA. Children under 2 years of age, unless the burn is very small and superficial, also should be hospitalized. Other burn categories in which children should be hospitalized include electrical burns; deep chemical burns; burns complicated by fractures or soft tissue injury; burns complicated by concurrent health problems such as obesity, diabetes mellitus, epilepsy, or renal disease; and burns in which child abuse or neglect is suspected (see Chapter 13).

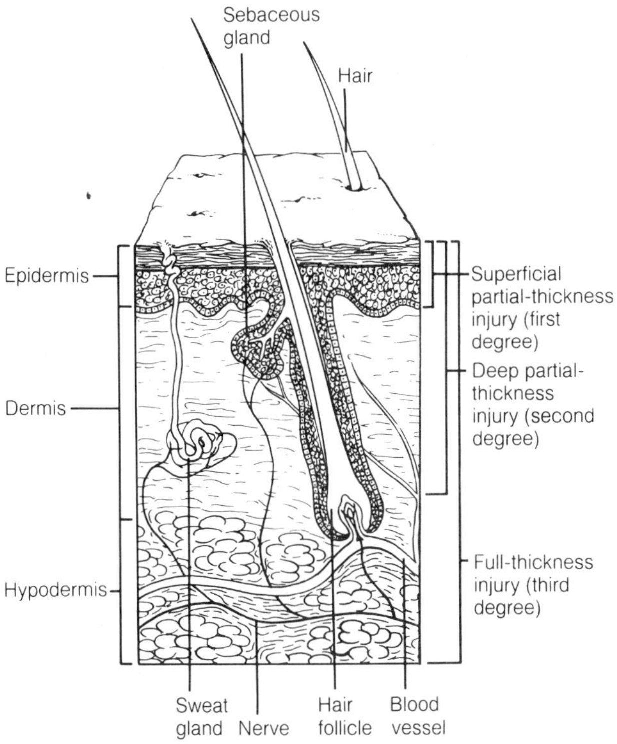

FIGURE 24-3
Depth of injury.

Medical and Nursing Management During the Emergent Phase

The *emergent phase* of care is the time needed to resolve immediate problems resulting from the burn injury. This phase usually lasts from 1 to 5 days depending on the severity of the burn.

Care at the scene of the injury The earliest part of the emergent phase is care at the scene of the injury. Stopping the burning process is the first step at the scene of injury. The longer the burning agent is in touch with the skin, the deeper the wound.

Methods for cooling burning tissue from flame, scalds, chemical, and electrical burns are illustrated in the First Aid Table (Table 12-6).

Electrical burns require specialized assessment. Because electrical current can take a variable course throughout the body, the nurse looks for current entrance and exit burns and suspects deep injury when electricity is the causative agent of a burn. On the surface where the electrical current entered and existed, there might only be a small-diameter burn that appears whitened, reddened, or charred. However, massive soft tissue, muscle, and bone damage might be present under the skin, and the area must be assessed carefully for circulation, sensation, and motion. In addition, electrical current is known to cause ventricular fibrillation and cardiac arrest. Cardiopulmonary resuscitation might be necessary at the scene.

Once the wound is cooled and clothing removed, the patient is at risk for rapid heat loss. Protective skin that helped to maintain body temperature has been lost or damaged. It is important to keep the child warm during transport to the hospital. Clean sheets and blankets are adequate, although many transporters still use sterile linen with burn victims. Rapid transport to an emergency room is crucial for the burned child because the hypovolemic shock that develops after burns can be life threatening. This is a time of crisis for the family as well as the child, and they too need careful attention.

Inhaling smoke in an enclosed space can lead to pulmonary edema and respiratory failure. Where there is smoke, there is carbon monoxide, which is the end product of the incomplete combustion of organic material. Carbon monoxide is readily absorbed from the lungs into the bloodstream and causes loss of consciousness at certain blood levels. Many burn victims are awake and alert at the scene, but those who have inhaled smoke containing carbon monoxide and other toxins often need cardiopulmonary resuscitation.

Stabilization and transfer The second phase of emergent care involves stabilization in the emergency room followed by transfer to the inpatient unit or burn center. Immediate nursing and medical management in the emergency room must focus on providing a secure airway and adequate ventilation and beginning fluid resuscitation. Wound care is not the first priority.

Severe burns cause alterations in all body systems. These are illustrated in Table 24-5 and provide the basis for medical and nursing management of the burned child.

Alterations in respiratory function

Upper airway obstruction Establishing and maintaining an open airway is of primary importance prior to transporting a burned child from the emergency room. The child needs nasotracheal intubation before edema, which develops rapidly, narrows the airway, and makes the procedure difficult. A tracheostomy is avoided unless oral or nasal tracheal intubation is impossible. An incision into burned neck tissue can result in extensive pulmonary infection.

Injury to bronchi and lungs Symptoms of smoke inhalation injury often are not immediately evident but appear 6–24 hours after the fire. Increasing respiratory distress

TABLE 24-5 Alterations Following Moderate to Critical Burns: Body System Manifestations

Respiratory system

Upper airway obstruction and respiratory distress caused by edema from inhalation of superheated air

Injury to lower airway from smoke inhalation

Carbon monoxide poisoning and hypoxia from end products of combustion

Atelectasis and respiratory failure from damage to lungs cause pneumonia

Pulmonary edema is possible in young children from too vigorous fluid replacement

Chest circumferential burns might limit chest wall excursions

Fluid and electrolytes

Fluid volume deficit from leakage of fluid from the body as well as from fluid shifts from vascular to interstitial compartment

Vasoconstriction in an attempt to preserve fluid volume and prevent hypovolemic shock

Appearance of edema from increased fluid in interstitial spaces

Alterations in fluid output

Alterations in hemoglobin and hematocrit

Initial increase in serum potassium from the tissue injury followed by excess excretion

Gastrointestinal system

Gastric dilatation and paralytic ileus

Thirst in response to hypovolemia

Stress ulcers from increased gastric acid production

Renal system

Reduced blood flow to kidneys

Potential for acute tubular necrosis from obstruction of renal tubules

Urinary tract infections from in-dwelling catheter

Kidney damage from nephrotoxic antibiotics

Neurologic system

Burn encephalopathy—seizures, delirium, and coma can occur

Metabolic system

Increased metabolic rate from the insult of an open wound

Release of catecholamines from burn stress leads to hypertension

Delayed growth and maturation from body's need to use energy for wound repair

Hematologic system

Initial elevation of hematocrit from fluid loss; decreased hematocrit with fluid replacement

Decreased platelet count yields coagulation disorders

and deteriorating blood gases indicate the child's need for ventilatory support. Administration of 100% oxygen should be started as soon as possible after the injury if carbon monoxide poisoning is a possibility.

Treatment often includes bronchodilators to reduce bronchospasm. Pulmonary cleansing using suctioning, percussion, clapping, postural drainage, and frequent position changes helps to prevent the atelectasis and pooling that leads to infection (see Chapter 22). Although pressure cannot be applied directly to burns, modified chest physical therapy and position changes are possible.

Children who survive severe smoke inhalation injuries and their complications might have permanent scarring of lung tissue, but the long-term effect on pulmonary function has not been documented.

Other pulmonary problems Infants and small children are susceptible to pulmonary edema if fluid resuscitation is too vigorous. They seem less and less able to tolerate the fluid loads required for the frequent skin grafting procedures. Careful monitoring of urine output and central venous pressure is essential in these patients.

When full-thickness burns encompass the circumference of the chest (circumferential), constricting eschar might limit chest wall excursions. The child's lungs become more and more difficult to ventilate. Escharotomies (incisions into eschar) relieve the pressure and allow for greater chest expansion.

Fluid volume replacement During the first 72 hours after a burn, fluid shifts dramatically from the vascular into the interstitial spaces. This rapid fluid shift, combined with the excessive loss of fluid through the burned skin, causes hypovolemia and signs of shock (thirst, restlessness, increased pulse, decreased blood pressure). In addition, because of the increased fluid in the interstitial space, the child appears greatly edematous.

The fluid that moves from the circulating volume to the interstitial spaces in burn shock consists of water, electrolytes, and albumin. Fluid resuscitation formulas are used as guidelines for treating burn shock. A formula specifying the amounts of replacement intravenous fluids is used in conjunction with close monitoring of vital signs, urine output, level of consciousness, and laboratory values. Fluid resuscitation formulas calculate the amount of water, crystalloid (Lactated Ringers) and colloid (albumin or fresh-frozen plasma) to be replaced.

Scrupulous monitoring of fluid replacement and fluid and electrolyte balance is essential. A urine output of 1 mL/kg bodyweight/h reflects proper hydration. An output of more than 1.5–2.0 mL/kg/h indicates fluid overload and needs to be reported.

Medical and Nursing Management During the Acute Phase

As capillary permeability returns to normal (beginning on the third to fifth day), reabsorption of edema fluid begins and diuresis (increased urine output) follows. This signals the beginning of the *acute phase*. Resuscitative fluid replacement drops significantly. Daily fluid and electrolyte needs, however, remain increased. Evaporative water loss through the burn wound is far in excess of that lost through normal skin and large amounts of sodium and plasma protein continue to leak through the open wound.

Because potassium is released from injured cells, serum potassium rises in the first 24–48 hours after burn injury. Once diuresis occurs, potassium is excreted causing serum levels to drop and necessitating replacement. The nurse closely monitors electrolyte values and the electrocardiograph monitor (ECG) for signs of hypokalemia (see Chapter 21).

Throughout the entire recovery process, fluid and electrolyte balance fluctuates with surgical procedures, sepsis, and evaporative losses. Careful monitoring is needed until the wound is closed.

Alterations in renal function The rapid reduction in circulating fluid volume that occurs after a burn reduces blood flow to the kidneys. In children with underlying kidney disease, extensive thermal injury, or electrical burn, an osmotic diuretic such as mannitol is given to prevent renal damage.

Urinary tract infections from ascending bacteria are common in the burn patient. The in-dwelling Foley catheter often sits in close proximity to the burn wound. Maintenance of a closed drainage system is a most important preventive nursing measure.

Alterations in gastrointestinal function Gastric dilatation and paralytic ileus often occur following a major burn, and digestion virtually ceases. The child is placed on NPO. A nasogastric tube is inserted and attached to suction in the emergency room to prevent vomiting and aspiration. Antacids are begun soon after admission to avert a Curling's or stress ulcer, a complication of burns in the past. This therapy continues while the stress of acute illness persists. Paralytic ileus will resolve and allow for oral intake 2–3 days after injury. The resumption of bowel sounds is one indicator that gastrointestinal function has returned.

Alterations in neurologic function Prolonged anoxia caused by smoke inhalation might leave the child in an unresponsive state for days after the burn injury. Most burned children, however, are awake and lucid on admission to the hospital and for a number of days afterward. For the child with a major burn, alterations in consciousness and activity, ranging from unresponsiveness to agitation and hallucinations, are common phenomena after the first week. The combination of sensory overload, sleep deprivation, and pain can account for profound withdrawal or combativeness seen in many children the second or third week of hospitalization. Some patients might need psychotropic drugs as part of a behavior management plan.

The nurse observes the child closely for signs of burn encephalopathy (neurologic dysfunction)—delirium seizures and coma.

Alterations in hematologic function Red blood cells are thought to have a shortened half-life in the burn patient. This, combined with blood loss from escharotomies, wound debridement, and surgery, results in anemia. A decrease in circulating platelets contribues to coagulation disorders. Frequent transfusions are necessary to maintain even low-normal hematocrits and hemoglobin levels throughout the acute-care phase.

Alterations in metabolism The body responds to the insult of a large, open burn wound by increasing the metabolic rate. Oxygen consumption increases as temperature, respiratory rate, and heart rate rise. At Shriners Burn Institute in Boston, children are placed in bacteria-controlled nursing units. These are plastic tentlike structures with laminar airflow. They protect the child from cross-infection and provide a warm, moist environment. The temperature inside the tent is kept at approximately 86°F with humidity at 85%. Those who recommend this type of environment believe that it reduces evaporative water and heat losses from the wound and unburned skin and in turn reduces the expenditure of calories (Burke et al., 1977).

Wound management During the acute phase of burn care, the burn team concentrates on preventing wound infection, closing the wound as quickly as possible, and managing the numerous complications that can occur as part of the burn illness.

Any break in the skin weakens one of the body's main defenses against the invasion of microorganisms. Closing the burn wound quickly and thus preventing infection is a high priority.

Wound care can begin as soon as an airway is established, vital signs are stable, and fluid resuscitation is well under way. Personnel performing wound care wear sterile gowns, gloves, masks, and caps to prevent contamination.

Initial cultures give baseline data about wound flora. This information might be helpful later on in establishing a time and possible source of contamination. Nurses and physicians collaborate to estimate and record the size and depth of the injury. Many burn centers keep photographic records of the patient's wounds from the time of admission.

Surgical soap solutions are used to clean the wound. Many burn specialists recommend leaving blisters intact as a natural sterile dressing. Dead skin from broken blisters can be debrided with sterile forceps and scissors.

Escharotomy Full-thickness burns that encompass the whole circumference of the extremities, fingers, toes, and chest need careful attention in the first hours after injury. Edema fluid accumulates rapidly under unyielding eschar and puts pressure on underlying blood vessels and nerves. Careful checks of circulation, sensation, and motion are necessary whenever there is a circumferential burn. Children's fingers and toes are very small and thin, and circulation is cut off quite easily. As circulation becomes impaired, hands and feet become cool, pale, or mottled; the child might complain of tingling or numbness. Capillary refill in nail beds is slow or absent, and pulses are difficult to palpate distal to the injury. When constricting eschar interferes with circulation or, in the case of the chest, lung expansion, the physician performs an *escharotomy* (incision into eschar) to relieve the pressure. After the escharotomy, it is important to continue checking circulation, sensation, and motion. Even with the extremities elevated, edema fluid continues to accumulate. It is helpful to leave a small window in the dressing where a pulse can be checked and to leave unburned fingers and toes exposed to check temperature and color. Often, the escharotomy incision must be deepened and extended in the first 24 hours to relieve increasing pressure.

Topical agents Several topical agents are used to treat burns. Each agent has its advantages and disadvantages. All work to protect wounds from the invasion and multiplication of microorganisms. They cannot be totally effective because bacteria become resistant to antimicrobial therapy with repeated exposure, and new agents are always being developed to counteract virulent strains of microorganisms. The three most frequently used topical agents are silver nitrate 0.5% solution, silver sulfadiazine cream 1% (Silvadene), and mafenide acetate 10% (Sulfa mylon). Other agents used include povidone-iodine (Betadine), cerium nitrate cream or solution, and nitrofurazone (Furicin).

Topical agents are applied using sterile technique, with a gloved finger or a tongue depressor. Previously applied agents are removed prior to new application to facilitate wound assessments. This removal is usually done during hydrotherapy.

A recent innovation in burn wound management is debridement using travase ointment. Travase is an enzyme that dissolves dead tissue and prepares the burn site for grafting. When using travase, the burn must be cleansed of all metal solutions (eg, silver nitrate). The ointment is applied and covered with moist dressings and reapplied three to four times daily.

Burn wound dressings Gaining proficiency in changing burn dressings requires time, practice, and attention to detail. During the first hours after a burn, while edema is increasing, the nurse wraps dressings loosely to prevent circulation from being impeded. To avoid interference with respiration, the nurse does not wrap the chest circumferentially in the emergent phase of care. Once the child feels better and is ambulatory, dressings must be secure but allow for maximum mobility. Fingers and toes should be wrapped separately so that surfaces do not adhere, forming weblike scar bands as they heal. Elasticized netting material can be used over dressings to keep them in place. This netting can be very useful for the toddler with a scald burn to the chest who is going back and forth to the playroom. Occasionally, infants and toddlers with silver nitrate dressings on their arms and hands will chew or suck on them. A protective drape over the area helps to prevent silver nitrate ingestion.

Adhesive tape cannot be used on facial burns. Endotracheal tubes can be secured with cloth tape tied around the tube and then around the head. When the ears are burned, gauze pads placed under each pinna prevent adherence to the scalp during healing. To prevent contamination of the wound, the nurse shaves surrounding hair, except for eyebrows. Liquid barrier drapes secured over thigh dressings help to prevent contamination with urine or feces. Splints that maintain joints in a position of function can be made on admission and remodeled to fit over dressings. Kerlix secures splints well.

Hydrotherapy and debridement The eschar of full-thickness burns is necrotic tissue, a perfect breeding ground for bacteria. Prompt removal of this eschar and preparation of a healthy bed to receive skin grafts are central to good wound care. Hydrotherapy involves showering the wound with water or soaking in a whirlpool, tub, or Hubbard tank once or twice a day for 20–30 minutes. This helps to soften and loosen eschar. Patients who are critically ill, whose body temperatures are abnormally low or high, and those with electrolyte imbalances cannot tolerate hydrotherapy. However, this form of wound care works well for less critically ill patients. Hydrotherapy helps to clean not only the wound but the entire body. It also helps to maintain range of motion. With the open wound, isotonic saline works best to prevent the loss of electrolytes and protect granulation tissue. A detergent is used to promote mild cleansing. The temperature of the solution should be 94–97°F.

Patients who undergo hydrotherapy find it painful and frightening, especially at first. The nurse administers pain medication at least 20 minutes prior to the procedure. As eschar softens, skilled nurses debride the wound with forceps and scissors. Although the task has to be completed, children need breaks to regroup their defenses. The experienced nurse learns how much is "enough" each day for each child, balancing the child's need for control and respite with the need to debride the wound and prepare recipient skin graft sites. Carefully planned teaching and behavior modification programs can help to provide the consistency and predictability needed by children who are enduring this daily suffering. Wounds often bleed during debridement. Pressure, sometimes cautery, and occasionally sutures are used to check this bleeding.

As the eschar separates and is debrided away, a bed of granulation tissue forms at the juncture of healthy and necrotic tissue. A healthy, uninfected granulation bed that is ready for grafting is red, flat, vascular, and low in bacteria count. Preparing the deep, full-thickness burn wound for grafting with hydrotherapy and debridement takes a number of weeks. Prompt surgical excision of eschar followed by placement of skin grafts is one treatment method preferred by some burn centers.

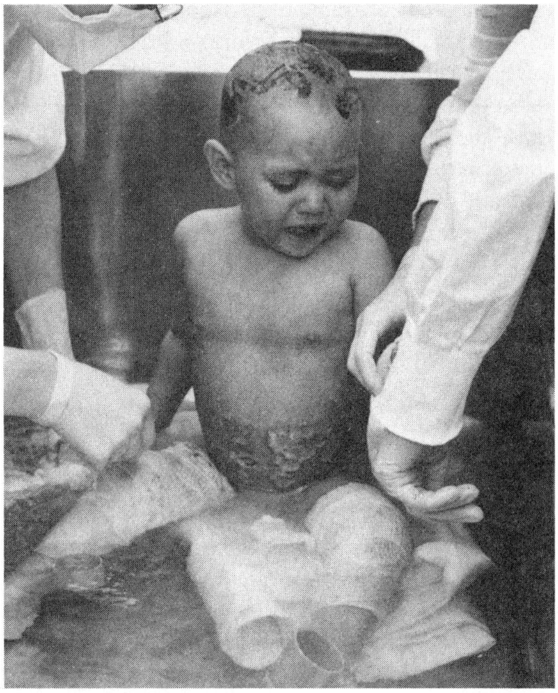

Hydrotherapy to remove dressings and eschar is extremely painful for the child and can be interrupted periodically to allow the child a respite from the procedure.

Preventing infection In spite of topical agents, early excision and grafting, careful hand washing, and aseptic technique for wound care, burn wounds can become infected. Contamination from the body's own flora and cross-contamination between patients are difficult to prevent.

The usual nursing measures to prevent the spread of infection between patients, such as hand washing, are even more important when caring for children with burns. Other measures might include environmental control with laminar airflow rooms and protective isolation (see Chapter 25).

Signs and symptoms of infection are the same for all kinds of skin wounds and include increased pain, swelling, redness in surrounding tissue, heat, and increased exudate that might be purulent or foul smelling. Skin grafts will literally disintegrate if placed on an infected recipient bed. Daily wound surface or biopsy cultures give data on predominant flora as well as an estimate of the amount of growth. Topical agents might be changed, grafting delayed or advanced, and frequency of dressing changes increased on the basis of the amount of exudate and type of organism growing on a particular wound.

Systemic sepsis can begin from a number of sites. The burn wound is an obvious site. Other sites include intravenous lines and their insertion sites, Foley catheters, and boggy, atelectatic lungs, where pneumonia organisms breed. Septicemia is a catastrophic illness for any patient. It often begins with subtle changes in the sensorium and decreased gastrointestinal motility but can quickly progress to circulatory collapse, coagulopathies, and even death. Intravenous antibiotic therapy often is begun with the first symptoms, and life supports are initiated to treat shock and respiratory failure. Children do survive sepsis with expert medical and nursing care, but treatment can be difficult because the causative organisms become resistant to antibiotics. There is a race against the clock to cover the burn wound and thus restore an important defense against infection before virulent organisms do irreparable damage.

Medical and Nursing Management During the Rehabilitative Phase

Nutritional management The most expert and vigilant wound care will be fruitless if the patient's nutritional needs are neglected. Caloric requirements increase significantly after burn injury in response to the accelerated metabolic state. Energy stores dwindle rapidly, and catabolism persists if body stores are not replenished and maintained. Protein is lost through the burn wound, along with heat, water, and electrolytes.

Immediately after a significant injury, the child receives no food or fluid by mouth for 24–48 hours because of decreased gastrointestinal motility. Once peristalsis returns, the nurse can begin feeding the child by mouth or nasogastric tube.

Whether to eat or not can become a control issue with incapacitated children, but even the cooperative child with an adequate appetite has difficulty taking in the amount of calories needed for wound healing. When there is a major burn, tube feedings and hyperalimentation will be needed to provide the necessary nutrients (see Chapter 27).

From the first day of injury onward, nurses need to pay careful attention to the nutritional needs of the burned child. Consulting with a nutritionist and the parent can help the nurse to design a meal plan that will provide the child with maximum calories. The occupational therapist can be called on to fashion adaptive devices to make self-feeding possible. The child should be given as many choices as possible, have food from home brought in if appropriate, and have mealtimes scheduled far apart from dressing changes.

Body weight measured twice a week helps the nurse to evaluate the effectiveness of the nutritional plan. The daily calorie count is an assessment procedure the child can participate in.

The proper mix of fats, proteins, and carbohydrates will vary for each child depending on the size and depth of the injury. The nurse might consult with hospital nutritionists to plan the pattern of meals and snacks that will meet the calculated daily requirements for the child.

Pain management Pain is one of the first words that comes to mind when burns are mentioned, but little has been written on pain management specific to burns. Having a burn means having pain that recurs and often intensifies. Repeated, painful treatments are also a necessary part of the recovery process.

Nurses speak of how difficult it is to carry out procedures such as hydrotherapy, debridement, and dressing changes day after day. It can be especially difficult to care for children who are too young to understand the reasons for all the pain. Balancing pain control with a number of other nursing goals is challenging. In the emergent phase of care, intravenous narcotics are effective in relieving pain. Morphine sulfate is used commonly. A small amount of morphine can be given intravenously and repeated as needed if the patient's vital signs remain stable. Tranquilizers given along with the narcotics help to decrease the patient's anxiety.

Intramuscular injections are avoided. Because of rapidly accumulating edema throughout the body, medications pool and are absorbed erratically from the intramuscular site. Unburned skin sites must be preserved for donor grafts, and any unnecessary breaks in the skin are portals of entry for infectious organisms.

A variety of different types of oral or intravenous analgesics will be needed throughout the course of hospitalization for hydrotherapy, debridement, and dressing changes. Children might become dependent on narcotics, requiring a gradual tapering of the drugs later on. They also might become tolerant of the drugs, needing larger doses for a period of time to provide adequate pain relief.

As regards pain control and burns, the nurse maintains a difficult balance. The child's pain must be reduced for procedures, but the child must remain alert enough for mealtimes to ensure proper caloric intake.

Touching and stroking, typically used by parents and nurses to express caring and give comfort, might be painful to the burned child. Parents need help to find ways to express their caring, to learn to hold their children in a nonpainful position, and to find unburned areas and areas not used for donor sites that they can touch and rub.

Even the most gentle and careful wound care can seem like an attack or assault to the child. A young child might interpret dressing changes as punishment in spite of reassurances and explanations. The response to injury from burns and hospitalization parallels the response of different age groups to illness and hospitalization.

For burn patients, anxiety and the intensity of the pain experience are closely linked. Whatever reduces the child's anxiety level will be helpful in the midst of painful procedures. Providing the child with some control during a painful procedure reduces the child's anxiety level. Giving the child choices such as which dressing to do first or how fast to remove the gauze allows the child a measure of control. Being predictable regarding the time and place for painful procedures also reduces anxiety.

Paying attention to each child's level of pain tolerance during a procedure is important in helping the child stay in control. Pausing to allow the child to take a deep breath, regroup, and get ready for the next few minutes of debridement helps the child master the situation because it is broken up into manageable parts.

Nurses experienced in burn care wonder about the long-term effects of so much pain and suffering on children. They comment, however, on the resilience and adaptability of children. Hospitalization and illness can be a difficult time for families but a time of growth and positive change as well. Providing opportunities for the child to express anger and hurt during painful procedures and during play, as well as helping the child to maintain control of and master the situations encountered, are part of nursing care (Bernstein and Robson, 1983).

Functional management

Contractures Burn wounds tend to heal in positions of flexion, resulting in decreased function, especially if the affected area is a joint. Joints need to be maintained in neutral positions or in extension and should be put through range of motion at least twice a day from the time of admission. However, after grafting is done, immobility is enforced for 5–10 days to allow the graft to take.

Since flexion contractures are a common problem, a positional and exercise routine is established in collaboration with the physical therapist. Splints are used when burns affect skin over joints. They are constructed so that they can fit over dressings and be secured with Velcro® fasteners or wrapped with Kerlix gauze. Splints are altered as edema subsides and the child's condition improves. The depth of the burn and the severity of scarring will determine how much time a splint must be worn.

Scars Scar formation is a major problem as burn wounds heal and for many months following healing. Scar tissue can impinge on joint function and distort the child's appearance. When the inflammatory process is intense and prolonged, as it is with deep partial-thickness and full-thickness burns, hypertrophic scars form. These scars are reddened, raised, firm, and almost woody in appearance. Eventually, the scar will lose its red color, flatten out, and become more pliable. However, the nurse can do a great deal to prevent or decrease contractures and disfigurement.

Experience in burn centers shows that pressure evenly distributed over the healed wound helps to lessen hypertrophic scar formation. Pressure garments are commercially available that fit any part of the body. When the wound is almost healed, the patient can be measured for pressure garments. The nurse can use ace bandages over healed wounds while waiting for the pressure garments to be made and delivered. Continuous wearing of pressure garments seems to work best for reducing scars. The nurse instructs the family on the care of the elasticized pressure garments and skin care for healed wounds.

Skin care after healing Families and patients might be reluctant to touch, wash, and care for healed wounds. The goal of any discharge teaching is to ensure that patients are comfortable caring for themselves or that their families are comfortable with the care before discharge. The nurse can give them written guidelines and the name of someone they can call with questions.

Emotional needs The first hours and days after a child has been burned are times of repeated crises. For weeks after a major burn injury, the main issue is survival while the wound remains open and the threat of sepsis persists. Children with less serious burns are still caught up with the crises of sudden hospitalization, painful treatments, and surgery. Questions and worries about loss of function, scarring, and disfigurement usually do not appear until the wounds begin to heal.

With an accident and something as painful and visible as a burn, the guilt that parents often feel when their children are hospitalized seems doubly intense. Often, the injury occurs because of carelessness or a momentary lapse in parental attention. The guilt is something parents, caregivers, siblings, and victims themselves carry for years to come.

Often, significant losses have occurred in a house fire. Other family members, an entire home, personal possessions, or a pet might have been lost. Parents and other family members of a child with major burns face weeks and months of crises and adjustments.

The nurse learns to listen and offer opportunities for parents and children to express their feelings of guilt, anger, fear, and frustration. Each trip to the operating room might provoke a recurrence of the feelings they experienced when the accident first happened. Parents' groups, siblings' groups, and individual counseling are ways families and burn victims can obtain support and learn to cope.

Infancy and early childhood are particularly vulnerable times for children with burns, who are unable to understand the need for painful treatments. Infants who see only the masked faces of parents and staff for days on end are missing an important part of the usual stimulation and cues about the world around them. Young children should be allowed to see full faces, especially those of their parents

Discharge Instructions for Burn Patients

For healed superficial burns and donor sites

Cleanse daily with mild soap and water. If possible, take a bath or shower and wash the entire skin with a washcloth

Use a nonperfumed lubricating cream or ointment, such as petroleum jelly, on the wound after the bath

Protect the wound from the sun. Cover healed areas with light, loose clothing. Wear a hat with a brim and apply a sunscreen to areas that are difficult to cover in warm weather such as the face, hands, and feet

Feel free to swim in any water—salt, fresh, or pool. Water is a great place for exercise, too. Remember to reapply sunscreen each time you get out of the water

For healed deep burns

Follow the instructions for healed superficial burns

Liberally apply lubricating cream. Because the burn has destroyed oil-producing glands, cream needs to be applied at least two or three times a day. Check the skin for dryness and flaking, a sign that more lubricating cream is required

Once a day, clean the pockets and crevices of scars with cotton-tipped applicators

Use medication as prescribed to reduce itching, which is one of the biggest complaints with burn scars

Use pain medication as prescribed. Sometimes, scars are painful, possibly as a result of nerve regeneration. In most cases no medication will be needed after discharge

Often, blisters on scar tissue break, leaving abrasion-like wounds. Apply mercurochrome or recommended cream or ointment to those superficial areas of breakdown

Clean any open areas, including areas where a blister breaks, with soap and water. Then apply mercurochrome and cover the area with a gauze bandage before applying the pressure garments. If necessary, use nonirritating paper tape to secure gauze pads

If an infection appears to be developing, or if you have any questions about the condition of your skin, wearing and fit of pressure garments, or any other problems, call ____________________

SOURCE: Surveyer JA, Clougherty DM: Burn scars: Fighting the effects.

and significant caregivers. Because small children cannot voice their needs and hurts, nurses need to remember that they still require analgesics before painful dressing changes and other procedures.

The nurse is careful to protect the burned child from contact with contaminated objects. Familiar blankets, cuddly toys, and plastic toys can be sterilized and provide comfort and entertainment.

In middle and late childhood children also need the comfort of the familiar. Playtime is doubly important when so much of the child's day is unpleasant and full of pain. Even when extremities, hands, and feet are burned and bandaged, children can play with their eyes and imaginations.

Sleep disturbances and nightmares about the accident are common after burn injuries and usually decrease with time and healing. The nurse helps children cope with disturbing dreams by listening, reinforcing reality, and acknowledging the connection between the dreams and the frightening experience they have been through. It is also important to adhere to bedtime routines and provide for periods of undisturbed sleep. For some children, nighttime sedation is necessary.

Living with disfigurement Children of all ages and their families need to cope with the visible and long-lasting effects of burns. Scarring and functional limitations are two major adjustment problems.

Children can develop a positive self-concept, regardless of scarring or functional limitations, with support from families and friends. Focusing on gains and potential rather than sickness and limitations is helpful to the child at any developmental level.

Because children with burns might be not only visibly scarred, but functionally limited, they often are stared at, teased by other children, or avoided. Role playing can help the child to cope positively with situations that might be encountered. Consultation and collaboration between the family, burn team, the school, and the child's friends will help to prepare for the child's return home and to school.

The return home can be both happy and difficult for families. The initial sense of elation might be followed by a let-down, lonely feeling once the realities of daily life become obvious. Follow-up care by the health team is essential to ease the transition. Peer support can increase the child's sense of control and self-concept. Resources for caring for patients in the acute phase of burn care are available throughout the country, but ongoing services are needed for children who have suffered major burn injuries if they are to develop optimally and lead fulfilling lives.

(*text continues on p. 796*)

STANDARDS OF NURSING CARE *The Child with a Major Burn*

RISKS

Assessed Risk	Nursing Action
Nausea, vomiting, and abdominal distention from decreased gastrointestinal motility	Listen for bowel sounds once every eight hours. Maintain the child on nothing-by-mouth status (NPO) until bowel sounds return. Insert nasogastric tube as ordered and attach to low suction. Observe and record amount and characteristics of drainage. Administer antacid or cimetidine as ordered.
Fluid volume deficit from leakage of fluid from the burn	Monitor the child's vital signs frequently and observe for alterations indicating impending shock (decreased blood pressure, increased pulse, restlessness). Administer intravenous fluids to obtain a urine output of at least one mL/kg/h. Insert a Foley catheter for accurate monitoring of output. Determine the child's weight and weigh daily. Monitor any changes in level of consciousness. Monitor laboratory studies—hematocrit, hemoglobin, electrolytes, blood gases, and other blood chemistries.
Respiratory distress from edema, smoke and heat inhalation, and decreased chest excursion from circumferential burns	Observe the child closely for signs of respiratory distress—labored breathing, retractions, increased respirations, decreased breath sounds, increased pulse. Monitor blood gases for alterations. Position the child with the head of the bed elevated to promote effective chest expansion. Observe the nose and mouth for evidence of soot; the eybrows, eyelashes, and nasal hairs for singing; and the voice for hoarseness. Administer 100% humidified oxygen if ordered. Assist with ventilation, intubation, or chest escharotomy as needed.

GUIDE FOR NURSING MANAGEMENT

Nursing diagnosis	Intervention	Rationale	Outcome
1. Potential alteration in body temperature (stressor: trauma to and removal of skin, increased metabolic rate in response to trauma)	Monitor the child's body temperature every hour. Use a continuous probe if temperature is unstable.	The child's thermoregulatory mechanism is drastically altered with severe tissue injury.	The child's body temperature will remain within normal limits. The child will not complain of being cold.
	Maintain room draft-free with temperature and humidity at increased levels (room temperature to 80–90°F and humidity to 80%–90%) or use warming lamps as needed to maintain child's body temperature.	Increasing the room temperature and humidity decreases evaporative fluid and heat loss.	
	Undress and redress one wound at a time.	This avoids unnecessary exposure.	
	Use bed cradle when treating wounds by the open method.	A covered bed cradle will retain warmth even though the sheet doesn't touch the child.	
2. Alteration in comfort: pain related to the injury and exposed nerve endings	Observe child for verbal and nonverbal signs of pain.	Child might not verbalize pain but might be restless or use facial grimacing.	The child can tolerate wound care and other treatments without an abnormal amount of pain. The child is able to obtain rest.
	Use comfort measures as possible.	Touching or stroking unburned skin provides essential contact.	
	Administer intravenous or oral medications as ordered, particularly prior to wound care and dressing changes.	Morphine sulphate might be required initially for pain relief because of the severity of the pain. Pain meds prior to treatments help to reduce pain sensations.	
	Encourage parent's participation in giving comfort.	The child might accept comforting by the parent more easily.	

(Continues)

STANDARDS OF NURSING CARE *The Child with a Major Burn (Continued)*

GUIDE FOR NURSING MANAGEMENT

Nursing diagnosis	Intervention	Rationale	Outcome
3. Anxiety related to unknown outcome secondary to the severity of the burn and the goals of treatments	Allow the child and family verbally or nonverbally to express their feelings.	Ventilating feelings of anxiety allows for obtaining a realistic peception of the event and can avoid crisis.	The child and family will state that they are less anxious. The child can identify and use techniques that reduce anxiety.
	Reassure the child and family that everything possible is being done to help the child's recovery.	Reassurance can be calming.	
	Provide a quiet, private location where family members can talk or cry.	Respecting the feelings of others while encouraging expression of feelings reduces unmanageable anxiety.	
	Provide quiet diversionary activities according to the child's age and physical limitations.	Diversion can reduce anxiety by taking the child's mind off problems temporarily.	
	Encourage relaxation techniques such as slow, deep breathing; conscious muscle relaxing; imagery.	Conscious relaxation can reduce anxiety.	
4. Potential infection (stressor: tissue destruction and increased environmental exposure to pathogenic organisms)	Provide tetanus prophylaxis as ordered.	Compromised skin defense can allow the growth of anaerobic organisms.	The wound appears clean and free from purulent drainage. The child's temperature remains within normal limits. Wound cultures are negative for pathogenic organisms.
	Apply topical agents and dressings as ordered.	Topical agents keep the burn covered, and their antimicrobial action assists with infection prevention.	
	Administer penicillin prophylaxis if ordered.	Systemic antibiotics are often prescribed to prevent infection.	
	Use careful aseptic technique throughout all wound care. Dress wounds on each body part separately using new equipment and gloves for each dressing.	These are measures to prevent infection by limiting exposure to organisms.	
	Observe the wound at each dressing change for wound redness, swelling, and increasing pain.	Increased drainage or signs of purulence as well as pain, redness, and edema indicate infection.	
	Obtain baseline wound cultures.	Baseline data assists with monitoring progress.	
	Compare progress of wound healing with baseline wound photographs.	Photographs provide a visual record for monitoring healing.	
	Cleanse wound with antiseptic except around eyes; use normal saline in eye area. Debride dead skin as ordered.	Cleansing and debridement help reveal healing tissue and limit growth of anaerobic organisms.	
	Be informed concerning ophthalmology; consult for patients with facial burns and apply ophthalmic ointments as ordered.	Facial burns might indicate eye injury.	
	Check circulation, sensations, and motion below areas of burns of extremities.	Careful monitoring will detect circulatory compromise from edema or eschar.	
	Assist with escharotomies as needed. Pack incisions with gauze to control bleeding.	Dead tissue is incised to reduce circulatory compromise.	

STANDARDS OF NURSING CARE *The Child with a Major Burn (Continued)*

GUIDE FOR NURSING MANAGEMENT

Nursing diagnosis	Intervention	Rationale	Outcome
	Shave hair from areas close to wound (except for eyebrows).	Hair can carry organisms.	
	Monitor vital signs and report a rectal temperature of 101°F or 38.3°C or more to the physician.	An increased temperature can indicate infection.	
	Use fluid barrier drapes over the dressing; change dressing immediately if contaminated.	Fluid barrier drapes prevent contamination from urine or feces.	
	Obtain urine, stool, and wound cultures twice a week.	Frequent routine cultures monitor infectious processes.	
	Use infection control measures according to hospital policy.	Protective isolation and strict hand washing reduce the chance of infection.	
	Instruct the family in protective techniques.	Families need to be with the child to learn and practice proper technique.	
5. Knowledge deficit related to activity limitations secondary to graft care	Observe the graft frequently for a healthy pink color.	Alterations in the color of the graft might indicate rejection.	The graft will begin to take by the tenth postoperative day. The child can explain the necessity for and cooperate with the immobility.
	Monitor the graft site for the collection of serosanguineous fluid under the graft and at the edges.	Serosanguineous fluid under the graft impedes proper contact between the graft and the skin.	
	Restrain the extremities as needed when the child is awake. Restrain the extremities at all times when asleep.	Immobility is necessary for the graft to adhere.	
	Administer pain medication as indicated.	Pain medication relieves discomfort and reduces restlessness, which might interfere with healing.	
	Maintain flat position in bed or slightly elevated.	Bending at the waist will impede healing if the graft is to the chest or abdomen.	
	Teach the child and family the importance of immobility and other aspects of graft care.	Knowledge reduces anxiety.	
	Consult a child-life therapist and provide diversional activities.	Diversional activities keep the child occupied and divert the focus from the discomfort caused by the immobility.	
	Monitor the child for problems associated with prolonged immobility.	See Chapter 20.	
6. Potential for ineffective family coping (stressor: the child's hospitalization, feelings of guilt, possible preexisting family stress)	Assist the family with expressions of feelings of guilt or loss of control.	Verbalizing feelings allows the family to face reality and begin to cope realistically.	The family is able to identify strengths as well as behaviors that indicate maladaptive coping. The family is able to use appropriate resources for support.
	Encourage the family to participate as much as possible in the child's care.	Participation in care increases feelings of control.	
	Assist the family to identify coping strategies that have been successful for them previously.	Using successful coping strategies increases the chance for successful coping with a new situation.	

(Continues)

STANDARDS OF NURSING CARE *The Child with a Major Burn (Continued)*

GUIDE FOR NURSING MANAGEMENT

Nursing diagnosis	Intervention	Rationale	Outcome
	Observe for possibility of abuse when burns appear suspicious (eg, with bathtub immersion burns, the child's feet, ankles, and buttocks might be the only areas damaged) and refer to social service if necessary.	Burns, particularly when regularly shaped, might indicate object used during child abuse. Immersion burns have "glovelike" appearance.	
7. Potential for body image disturbance (stressor: guilt, scarring, loss of peer contact, absence from family)	Encourage frequent family visiting within the limits of the protective isolation; encourage peers to write or call; have family arrange for a tutor when the child is able to resume studies.	Family visiting allows the child to maintain contact and feel a part of what is happening at home. Maintaining contact with peers keeps the child in touch with school and extracurricular activities.	The child demonstrates an interest in appearance. The child maintains contact with family and friends. The child will express acceptance of self.
	Facilitate the child's and family's expressions of anger, guilt, or depression; refer to a mental health nurse if warranted.	Expression of anger or guilt is the first step toward accepting the injury and its consequences.	

The Child with Frostbite

Children are subject to a second type of thermal injury, *frostbite,* which results from exposure to cold rather than heat. Like burns, frostbite can be mild, moderate, or severe, depending on the extent of tissue injury. It is classified as frostnip, superficial frostbite, deep frostbite, or fourth-degree frostbite (Rolnick, Stair, and Silfen, 1980).

Frostnip—mild freezing of the epidermis; appears as a small, pale area and can be readily rewarmed by contact with warm clothing or a part of the body

Superficial frostbite—either partial- or full-thickness injury; partial-thickness symptoms are white, cold area on skin surface, severe pain, erythema, burning, and pruritis on rewarming; full-thickness symptoms similar to partial-thickness symptoms, although erythema and blisters present 24–48 hours after rewarming; blisters replaced by eschar, which sloughs off leaving healthy tissue

Deep frostbite—affects underlying tissue; skin white or cyanotic, cold and hard to the touch, absence of sensation; extensive pain, edema, and blistering with rewarming; healing takes up to three months; pain during healing indicates more hopeful prognosis

Fourth-degree frostbite—same symptoms as deep frostbite but no pain on rewarming; gangrenous areas separate after approximately four months; surgical amputation might be needed

Several factors contribute to the occurrence of frostbite; the major one is hypothermia. *Hypothermia* occurs when body temperatures drop below 95°F. At that point the individual begins shivering. Shivering produces heat and is the body's attempt to compensate for the cold. When core body temperatures drop to below 90°F, the child is considered to be experiencing severe hypothermia. Severe hypothermia is detrimental to all body systems and, if untreated, can cause death.

Peripheral vasoconstriction in response to the cold increases the blood flow to the heart. Reduced tissue oxygenation combined with restricted blood flow from tight clothing (for example, boots and gloves) can result in tissue freezing and frostbite. Rewarming the frostbitten area without damaging the tissue further is a nursing and medical challenge. When a child is experiencing frostbite, initial assessment should focus on determining the presence and extent of hypothermia. Mild hypothermia can be treated by moving the child to a warm environment, removing wet clothing, and wrapping the child loosely in blankets. Shivering and environmental warmth might correct the problem. Children with severe hypothermia should be hospitalized and might be treated with fluid volume replacement and warming blankets or other warming techniques. Severe hypothermia must be corrected before attention can be given to frostbitten areas.

The frostbitten tissue should be rewarmed by immersion in warm, agitating water (temperature of 100 to 105°F or 37.8 to 40.5°C). The child should receive medication for pain. All frostbitten areas should be handled gently to minimize additional trauma.

The care of the hospitalized child after rewarming is similar to the care of the child with burns and includes protective isolation, hydrotherapy and debridement, and physical therapy. Unlike nursing care for burns, dressings are seldom used. The nurse elevates the child's extremities and uses a bed cradle to reduce pain from the pressure of bed clothing. The child's diet should be high in protein and calories to promote healing. Antibiotic administration or tetanus prophylaxis might be indicated.

Unless the frostbite is fourth degree, the child can be expected to experience pain and can be medicated accordingly. Psychologic alterations caused by severe pain, isolation, and the shock of tissue necrosis are common (Boswick et al., 1983). Signs of depression require understanding and encouragement from the nurse.

Amputation and/or skin grafting might be required after months of healing. Concurrent alterations in body image demand sympathetic and therapeutic nursing care. The long-term effects of frostbite might include scarring, infection, graft rejection, skin sensitivity to cold, and growth retardation in children whose epiphyses are involved.

Teaching the principles of frostbite prevention is a nursing responsibility. Children should be advised to wear appropriate clothing when going out in the cold. Wearing many layers of clothing is preferable to wearing one layer of heavy clothing because air is trapped between layers and acts as an insulator. Hats should always be worn because a large amount of body heat can be lost through the head. Mittens are preferable to gloves because the finger contact allows for more warmth. Tight-fitting boots should be avoided. Children should be advised to come in when their clothing is wet.

Frostbite damage can be more severe if the affected area is rewarmed and then refrozen. If it appears that a continuous source of warmth will soon be available, it is better to wait before attempting a rewarming procedure (Bangs, 1982).

The Child with Severe Surface Injuries

Child victims of automobile or motorcycle accidents are subject to severe contusions (bruises), abrasions (scrapes), and lacerations, along with associated injuries such as fractures, head trauma, and internal organ injury. After initial assessment and management of life-threatening problems, the nurse gives attention to surface injuries. The child's appearance, particularly if injuries are extensive, might daunt even the strongest of nurses.

First priority after stabilization is cleansing of the wounds to prevent infection and the administration of tetanus prophylaxis, if indicated. This becomes a difficult task because in all probability the wounds will be heavily contaminated with dirt and other matter. Miller (1980) recommended the following steps for effective cleansing of contaminated wounds:

1. Soak or scrub abraded and lacerated areas with povidone-iodine for 10 minutes.
2. Follow with sterile water or saline irrigation.
3. Remove contaminated particles with sterile applicator sticks or a small sterile hemostat after anesthetizing the area.
4. Cover with a dry sterile dressing over a topical anti-infective agent.
5. Recommend suturing if necessary.
6. Observe and assess for signs of infection.

Depending on the associated injuries, the child might or might not be able to be sedated for wound cleansing. In all likelihood sedation will be contraindicated because of potential head injury. The nurse explains the procedure to the child and reassures the child that the local anesthetic will limit the pain.

The child with severely denuded skin from extensive abrasions requires careful nursing management. Because fluid seeps through the wounds, nursing care is similar to that for burns, with particular attention to maintaining the fluid and electrolyte balance. Rehabilitative problems of preventing contractures, reducing scar formation, and preventing emotional and social problems are important nursing considerations.

NURSING CARE PLAN *The Child with Severe Surface Injuries*

Assessment data: Paul, a 14-year-old, is admitted to the Pediatric Unit after having been thrown from an automobile during a collision. He is awake, but drowsy, and complaining of a severe headache. His vital signs are presently stable. He sustained severe abrasions to his face, chest, and anterior surfaces of his arms and legs.

Nursing diagnosis	Intervention	Rationale
1. Potential for ineffective airway clearance (stressor: obstruction from trauma-related edema and possible altered level of consciousness)	Observe Paul for signs of respiratory distress—poor color, dyspnea, retractions. Know results of blood gases.	Signs of respiratory distress might indicate impending obstruction. Blood gases indicate the state of oxygenation.
	Position Paul with head slightly elevated.	Head elevation facilitates respirations and aids in preventing cerebral edema.
	Assist with endotracheal intubation and ventilation as needed.	Endotracheal intubation maintains the child's airway.
	Monitor Paul's level of consciousness.	Tendency for increase in secretion accumulation when semi- or unconscious.

Outcome: Paul will be free from respiratory distress.

Nursing diagnosis	Intervention	Rationale
2. Potential ineffective breathing pattern (stressor: pain)	Observe Paul for changes in respiratory status, particularly shallow respirations and decreased breath sounds.	Shallow respirations and decreased breath sounds indicate compromised breathing.
	Be knowledgeable of baseline radiograph report.	A baseline radiograph assists with monitoring lung changes.
	Have Paul breathe deeply and turn every hour as injuries allow; breaths should be slow and easy.	Deep breathing and turning promote lung expansion and prevent pooling of secretions. Slow breaths are less painful.

Outcome: Paul will be able to take deep, slow breaths to increase effectiveness of breathing pattern. Paul's blood gases will be within normal limits and he will be free from respiratory distress.

Nursing diagnosis	Intervention	Rationale
3. Potential fluid volume deficit (stressor: plasma and blood loss from multiple severe abrasions and possible internal trauma)	Monitor vital signs for decreased blood pressure and increased pulse. Observe Paul's skin color and turgor and any changes in sensorium.	Altered vital signs might indicate impending shock.
	Assist in establishing large needle bore intravenous lines.	Large needles are preferred for transfusions.
	Monitor IV fluid rate. Insert a Foley catheter as ordered and monitor Paul's urine output. Check urine specific gravity every 4 hours.	Adequate specific gravity (1.010–1.030) and urine output (1–2 mL/kg/h) is indicative of fluid balance; blood in the urine might indicate renal system problems.
	Obtain a baseline weight and monitor weight daily.	Weight can provide data regarding fluid balance.
	Monitor laboratory studies of electrolytes and hemoglobin and hematocrit.	Electrolytes are lost with fluid shifts; decreased hemoglobin and hematocrit might indicate internal bleeding.
	If ordered, insert a nasogastric tube and monitor drainage.	Bloody drainage might indicate internal hemorrhage; Paul remains NPO until gastrointestinal function returns and there are no complications from his injuries.
	Keep NPO while nasogastric tube is in place. Auscultate for presence of bowel sounds.	

NURSING CARE PLAN *The Child with Severe Surface Injuries* (Continued)

Nursing diagnosis	Intervention	Rationale
Outcome: Paul appears to be well hydrated with good skin turgor and urinary output appropriate for age and weight. Urine specific gravity and serum electrolytes are within normal limits.		
4. Sensory-perceptual alterations related to strange environment and possible sequelae to neurologic trauma	Perform neurologic checks every 15 minutes (see Chapter 31).	Careful monitoring ensures rapid treatment of complications.
	Institute seizure precautions (see Chapter 31).	Seizures are possible with a head injury.
	Provide a calm, restful atmosphere.	This promotes relaxation and rest.
	Observe for clear fluid drainage from nose or ears.	This could be cerebrospinal fluid leakage from a skull fracture.
	Talk with Paul frequently as to where he is and what happened.	This helps to determine level of consciousness and provides reality orientation.
	Provide stable environment.	
Outcome: Paul responds appropriately to environmental stimuli. Paul appears more alert and interested in his surroundings.		
5. Potential for infection (stressor: impaired skin integrity, dirty wound)	Clean the abrasions with povidone-iodine for 10 minutes.	Povidone-iodine is an antimicrobial agent.
	Irrigate abrasions with saline.	This helps loosen embedded dirt.
	Apply antimicrobial topical agent and dry sterile dressing.	The dressing keeps the agent in contact with the wound and prevents wound contamination.
	Observe for signs of infection—increased body temperature, redness at the wound site, signs of purulent drainage.	Infection needs to be treated promptly.
	Administer antibiotics if ordered.	Systemic antibiotics can prevent infection.
	Obtain baseline wound cultures.	Assists with monitoring wound status.
	Change dressings immediately if contaminated with urine or feces.	Urine and feces contaminate the wound and lead to wound infection.
	Administer tetanus prophylaxis as ordered.	This prevents the development of tetanus from dirty wounds.
Outcome: Paul's abrasions appear clean and free from debris. Wound cultures remain negative.		
6. Alteration in comfort: pain, related to injuries	Give soothing rubs to unabraded back.	Rubbing promotes comfort.
	Provide diversion—quiet music or television, or talking quietly to Paul.	Pain medication is contraindicated with head injury; distraction helps reduce pain.
	Encourage short visits from peers.	
	Ensure adequate rest and freedom from interruption as much as possible.	Organized nursing care reduces stimulation and therefore discomfort.
Outcome: Paul appears comfortable as evidenced by calm facial expression and the ability to relax. Paul can verbalize feelings of pain and request assistance.		
7. Knowledge deficit related to inadequate understanding of seat-belt safety	Teach Paul about automobile dangers; explain about propulsion forces during an accident; encourage future seat-belt use.	Seat belts restrain a person from forceful forward propulsion during an automobile accident.
Outcome: Paul will list reasons for using an automobile seat belt.		

Essential Concepts

- The major function of the skin, a complex essential organ, is to protect the tissues it encloses against external environmental factors.
- In addition to being a protector, the skin acts as a sensor and thermoregulator and aids in secretion, excretion, and absorption.
- The history, which is essential for any treatment of a skin injury, includes changes in lifestyle, family members' skin alterations, known allergies, exposure to substances or ill persons, length of time lesions have been present, and a thorough description of any lesions.
- The nurse assesses lesions for type and size, configuration, distribution, location, texture, and color.
- Four elements of skin and wound care are cleansing, administering topical anti-infective agents, applying dressings and compresses, and providing for wound closure.
- Interventions to meet the acute care needs of the child with an integumentary condition are directed toward restoring altered skin integrity, managing itching and pain, preventing infection, and preventing a fluid volume deficit.
- Because nutrition is essential to the healing process, the nurse encourages the child with a skin condition to eat well-balanced meals. Children with extensive wounds might need up to one and one half times the usual requirements for protein and calories.
- When caring for children with skin conditions, nurses foster development leading to independence in self-care tasks.
- Infections of the integumentary system include cellulitis, impetigo, and acne vulgaris.
- The child with a skin inflammation might experience atopic dermatitis (eczema) or psoriasis.
- Nursing management of the child with a thermal or severe surface injury includes preventing respiratory distress, providing for fluid and nutritional needs, preventing wound infection, preventing complications related to other body systems, and helping the child develop a positive self-concept.

References

Artz CP, Moncrief JA, Pruitt BA: *Burns: A Team Approach.* Saunders, 1979.

Bangs C: Caught in the cold. *Emerg Med* 1982; 14:29–39.

Bernstein NR, Robson MC (editors): *Comprehensive Approaches to the Burned Person.* Medical Examination, 1983.

Boswick JA et al: Helping the frostbitten patient. *Patient Care* 1983; 17:90–115.

Burke JF et al: The contribution of a bacterially isolated environment to the prevention of infection in seriously burned patients. *Ann Surg* 1977; 186:377–387.

Czernielewski A, Skwarczynska-Banys E: Oral treatment of acne vulgaris and oil acne with tetracycline. *Dermatologist* 1982; 165:62–65.

Epstein E: *Common Skin Disorders: A Physician's Illustrated Manual With Patient Instruction Sheets.* Medical Economics, 1983.

Miller M: Cycle trauma. *Nurs '80* (July) 1980; 10(7):26–31.

Morbidity and Mortality Weekly Reports (October 4) 1985; 34(39): 607–609.

Nurses' Drug Alert: Tetanus prophylaxis. *Am J Nurs* (April) 1984; 84:493–494.

Prugh DG: *The Psychosocial Aspects of Pediatrics.* Lea & Febiger, 1983.

Rocklin R: Immunologic diseases—a conference at Children's Hospital Medical Center, Boston, March 20, 1984.

Rolnick M, Stair T, Silfen E: Frostbite—easily prevented, responsive to treatment. *Consultant* (Dec) 1980; 20:133–141.

Rosequist CR, Shepp PH: The nutrition factor. *Am J Nurs* (Jan) 1985; 85(1):45.

Zackheim H: Treatment of psoriasis: Use of corticosteroids. In: *Controversies in Dermatology.* Epstein E (editor). Saunders, 1984.

Additional Readings

Carpenito LJ: *Nursing Diagnosis: Application to Clinical Practice.* Lippincott, 1983.

Fleming J: Common dermatologic conditions in children. *MCN* (Sept/Oct) 1981; 6(5):347.

Frankenburg W, Thornton S, Chors M: *Pediatric Development Diagnosis.* Thieme-Stratton, 1982.

Goldsmith LA (editor): *Biochemistry and Physiology of the Skin.* Oxford University Press, 1983.

Hurwitz S: *Clinical Pediatric Dermatology*. Saunders, 1981.

Jackson S: Dealing with burns. *RN* (Oct) 1984; 47(10): 35–39.

Johnson C, Cain V: Burn care: The rehabilitation guide. *Am J Nurs* (Jan) 1985; 85(1): 48–50.

Kavanagh C: A new approach to dressing change in the severely burned child and its effect on burn-related psychopathology. *Heart Lung* 1983; 12(6): 612–619.

Kavanagh C: Psychological intervention with the severely burned child: Report of an experimental comparison of two approaches and their effects on psychological sequelae. *Am Acad Psychiatry* 1983; 22: 145–156.

Kavanagh C, Freeman R: Should children participate in burn care? *Am J Nurs* (May) 1984; 84: 601.

Laude TA, Russo R: *Dermatologic Disorders in Black Children and Adolescents*. Medical Examination, 1983.

LaVoy K: Dealing with hypothermia and frostbite. *RN* (Jan) 1985; 48(1): 53–56.

Neuberger GB, Reckling JB: A new look at wound care. *Nurs '85* (Feb) 1985; 15(2): 34–41.

Neuberger GB, Reckling JB: Wound care: What's clear, what's not. *Nurs '87* (Feb) 1987; 17(2): 34–37.

Nurs '85 (June) 1985; 15(6): 53–57.

Robertson K, Cross P, Terry J: Burn care the crucial first days. *Am J Nurs* (Jan) 1985; 85(1): 30–43.

Sebilia A: When was your last tetanus shot? *RN* (Aug) 1984; 47: 18–24.

Surveyor J: Smoke inhalation injuries. *Heart Lung* 1980; 9: 825–832.

Chapter 25

Defense

Implications of Impaired Immunity

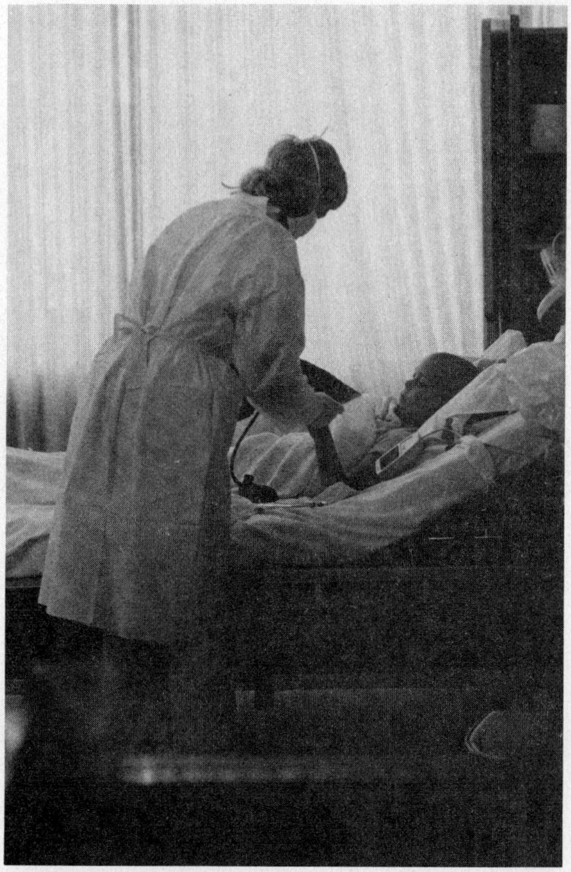

Chapter Contents

The Child with an Immune Deficiency

Acquired Immunodeficiency Syndrome
Humoral Deficiency—Agammaglobulinemia
Mixed Immune Deficiency—Wiskott-Aldrich Syndrome
Severe Combined Immunodeficiency Disease

The Child with an Autoimmune Disease

Acute Rheumatic Fever
Juvenile Rheumatoid Arthritis
Systemic Lupus Erythematosus
Acute Glomerulonephritis

The Child with an Immune Complex Disease

Mucocutaneous Lymph Node Syndrome—Kawasaki Disease
Shönlein-Henoch Purpura

The Child with an Allergic Reaction

Localized Allergic Reactions
Systemic Allergic Reactions

The Child with a Specific Allergic Reaction

Anaphylaxis
Food Allergy
Contact Dermatitis
Allergy to Bites and Stings

To find these topics, see the following chapters:

Acute glomerulonephritis	Chapter 28
Allergic rhinitis	Chapter 18
Asthma	Chapter 22
Cancer	Chapter 33
Diabetes	Chapter 29
Eczema	Chapter 24
Scarlet fever	Chapter 18
Streptococcal pharyngitis	Chapter 22

Objectives

- Define the body's nonspecific and specific defenses.
- Describe the disease processes associated with altered immune system function.
- Describe the assessment process related to immune system dysfunction.
- Describe the essential acute-care, developmental, emotional, nutritional, and health maintenance needs of children with immune dysfunction.
- Explain the physiologic processes, common medical treatments, and principles of nursing management for immune deficiencies.
- List the principal autoimmune and immune complex diseases.
- Describe the usual manifestations of hypersensitivity reactions.
- List the common irritants that cause allergic reactions.
- Describe the assessment process specific to allergic reactions.
- List the signs and symptoms for specific allergic manifestations.

ESSENTIALS OF STRUCTURE AND FUNCTION
The Immune System

Glossary

Antibody Protein formed by plasma cells. Antibodies attach to antigens to facilitate antigen destruction (antibody-antigen complex, or immune complex). Each antibody is specific to the antigen it destroys. Antibodies are known also as immunoglobulins (see table describing characteristics of immunoglobulins).

Antigen Substance such as an organism, toxin, or tissue that the body recognizes as foreign and attempts to neutralize or destroy through an immune response (see figure showing the antigen-antibody complex).

Autoantibody Antibody (immunoglobulin) formed in response to the body's own tissue (termed self-antigens).

Autoimmunity Reaction in which the body produces autoantibodies in response to its own antigens, thereby destroying normal tissue.

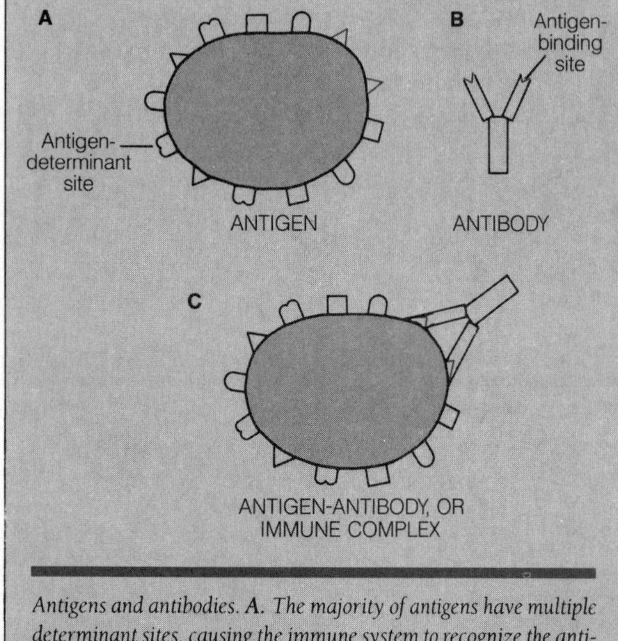

*Antigens and antibodies. **A.** The majority of antigens have multiple determinant sites, causing the immune system to recognize the antigens as foreign bodies. **B.** Each antibody protein has combining sites that makes it specific for a particular antigen. **C.** The lock-and-key combination of antigen and antibody is known as the immune complex.*

Immunoglobulins

Class	Normal serum levels	Associated characteristics
IgG	0.8–1.6 g/dL	Most common antibody found in blood and body tissues. Can cross the placenta into fetal circulation, thus giving the newborn the ability to resist infection. Coats microorganisms, allowing for faster recognition and elimination by phagocytes. When combined with an antigen, can activate the complement system, which helps destroy foreign substances and mediates the inflammatory response
IgM	0.06–0.2 g/dL	First antibody produced in an immune response. Present mainly in the blood and too large to cross the placenta. Effective against microorganisms because of its multiple antigen-binding sites. Can activate the complement system
IgA	0.15–0.4 g/dL	Found in body secretions such as saliva, tears, and sweat. Is present on mucosal surfaces of the gastrointestinal and respiratory tracts, where it protects mucosal surfaces from antigen invasion. Is passed to the infant via breast milk, thus conferring immunity to certain diseases
IgE	Trace	Serves a protective function on mucosal surfaces. Attaches to the surfaces of certain cells, causing them to release chemical substances, such as histamine, which can result in an allergic response
IgD	Trace	Present in only trace amounts in the blood. Functions are generally unknown

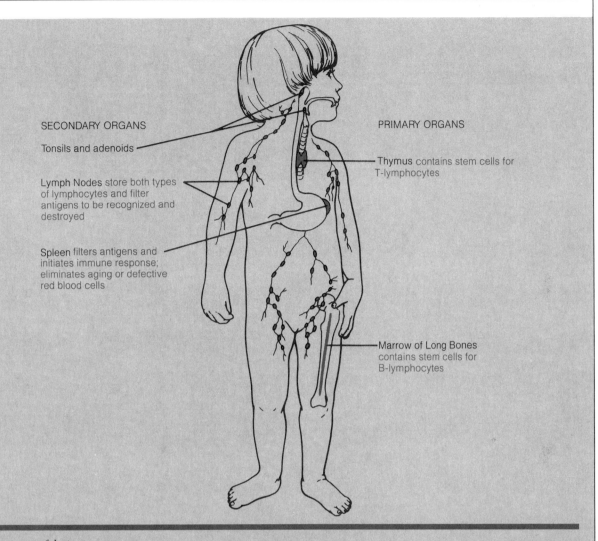

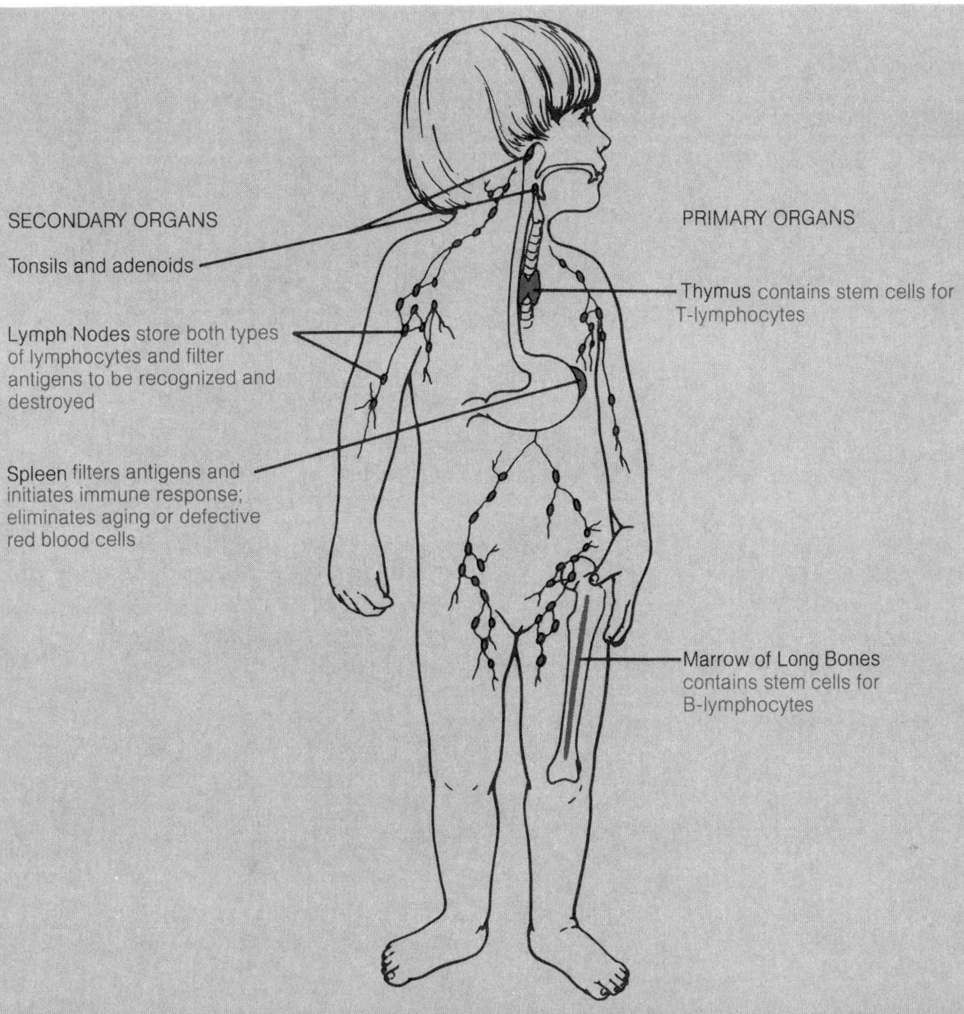
SECONDARY ORGANS
Tonsils and adenoids
Lymph Nodes store both types of lymphocytes and filter antigens to be recognized and destroyed
Spleen filters antigens and initiates immune response; eliminates aging or defective red blood cells
PRIMARY ORGANS
Thymus contains stem cells for T-lymphocytes
Marrow of Long Bones contains stem cells for B-lymphocytes

Major organs of the immune system.

Cellular response Immune response that defends against viruses, protozoa, fungi, tumor cells, and other tissue the body recognizes as foreign (grafts). Cellular responses include delayed hypersensitivity reactions.

Complement Series of nine proteins and enzymes that assist with immune system response to an antigen.

Humoral response Immune response that defends against bacteria and some viruses. B-lymphocytes (B cells) mature into plasma cells, which produce specific antibodies in response to the presence of an antigen.

Immune system Network that consists of primary and secondary organs that activate a response to a foreign agent. Cellular components include lymphocytes, which react in specific ways to destroy foreign substances, and phagocytes, such as macrophages, neutrophils, basophils, and eosinophils, which engulf and destroy foreign substances and release chemicals that enhance an immune response (see figure showing immune system organs).

Immunity Protection against disease. Immunity can be natural or artificial, passive or active. Passive immunity is short-lived because it does not require active participation of the immune system. Examples include:

natural passive immunity—IgG protection to an infant passed through the placenta

natural active immunity—immunity gained from the communicable diseases of childhood

artificial passive immunity—gamma globulin administration to temporarily protect a child from a disease such as hepatitis

artificial active immunity—childhood immunizations (see Chapter 11).

(Continues)

ESSENTIALS OF STRUCTURE AND FUNCTION *(Continued)*

The Immune System

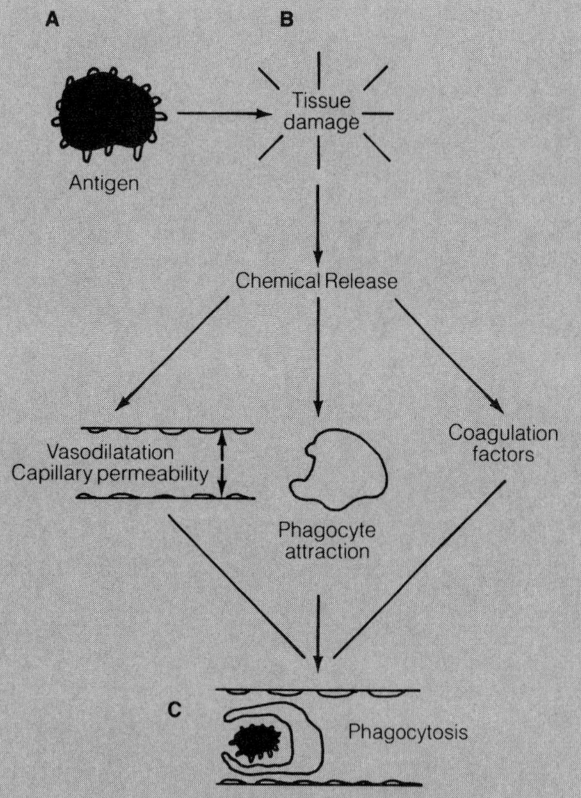

*Inflammatory response. **A.** Antigen entry causes tissue damage at the site. **B.** Damaged tissue releases chemicals that cause (1) vasodilatation and increased capillary permeability at the site, (2) attraction of phagocytes, and (3) release of coagulation factors to seal off the site and prevent spread of the antigen. C. Phagocytes engulf antigens and die. Further tissue damage releases toxins, causing fever and pain. Accumulation of byproducts is removed and cleared by the regional lymph nodes. Antigen is destroyed and the process subsides.*

Nonspecific immune response (inflammation) Response that occurs when an antigen has penetrated the first lines of defense. The antigen entry stimulates a release of chemical substances that cause vasodilatation, increased capillary permeability, and migration of phagocytes to the site. The action of the response can, but does not always, produce fever, pain, and purulence (pus) at the site. Because of the increased number of phagocytes needed in an inflammatory response, the bone marrow produces a high number of new leukocytes, causing an increase in the number of circulating white blood cells (leukocytosis). Prodromal symptoms of communicable diseases are an example of the nonspecific immune response (see figure showing inflammatory response).

Specific immune response Final line of body defenses, which responds specifically to antigens. The specific response not only destroys the antigen but also develops a memory that will reactivate the response if the antigen invades again. The two classifications of specific immune response are *humoral response* and *cellular response*. Each is specific against a particular type of antigen. The cellular response cooperates with and enhances the humoral response.

T cell (T-lymphocyte) Mediator of the cellular response.

Titer Measurement of the amount of circulating antibody in the blood.

The human body has a network of defenses to keep it intact and free from disease. Intact skin and mucous membranes are the body's first defenses against invasion by pathogens. Acid secretions, such as those produced in the gastrointestinal tract, also help to protect the body. When the first line of defense is crossed, the body activates its immune system to attempt to rid itself of the foreign agent and preserve health.

The major functions of the immune system are threefold: (1) to defend the body against invasion by such pathogenic agents as bacteria, viruses, parasites, and toxins, (2) to provide a surveillance system that identifies and controls rapid multiplication of abnormal cells (cancer), and (3) to clear adequately from the body the by-products of its own responses. The immune system is able to carry out its functions because of mechanisms that enable it to recognize agents foreign to the body and to ignore that which is part of the body. These mechanisms also maintain a "long-term memory" of foreign substances and react specifically against an infinite variety of pathogens. The actions of a properly functioning immune system are continuously effective, barring any trauma or insult to the system itself that alters the immune response.

Problems resulting from alterations of the immune system can affect persons at any point in the life cycle. Many of these diseases affect children younger than age 20. Immune system diseases can be physically debilitating as well as emotionally overwhelming, and they provide a challenge for effective nursing care. Conditions that affect the system can be grouped into the following four major categories: (a) immune deficiency diseases, (b) autoimmune diseases, (c) allergic manifestations, and (d) cancer. (Cancer is discussed in detail in Chapter 33.)

Assessment of the Child with Immune System Dysfunction

Immune system function can be altered in a variety of ways. Prolonged stress can result in diminished immune system function and increased susceptibility to disease. More severe problems resulting from immune system dysfunction are classified according to the specific function affected. For example, a child will have an increased susceptibility to infection if there is a problem with the efficiency of the cellular or humoral responses. Defects in immune surveillance can result in tumor development. Ineffective clearing of antigen-antibody complexes can precipitate an autoimmune reaction. Hyperactive immune system function causes allergy. (Table 25-1 lists specific immune system dysfunctions that the nurse needs to consider when assessing the child.)

History

A child with a suspected immune system disorder can exhibit symptoms that are often bewildering as well as frightening. Because many of these disorders mimic one another, a careful history is essential.

In addition to the routine information about the child, the nurse first obtains a description of the course of the disease up to the time of the interview. Relevant data include the age of the child, occurrence and pattern of fever or rash, and a description of colds or infections experienced during the past year. Particularly important when inquiring about recent infections is to document any history of a sore throat,

TABLE 25-1 Classification of Immune System Dysfunction

Classification	Definition	Example
Immune deficiency diseases	These result from an interruption in the cellular or humoral response, or both. Diminished production of antibodies or of T-lymphocytes causes decreased resistance to infection and the body's ability to recognize and eliminate tumor cells	*Humoral:* Agammaglobulinemia; hypogammaglobulinemia *Cellular:* Acquired immune deficiency disease (AIDS) *Combination:* Wiskott-Aldrich syndrome; severe combined immunodeficiency disease (SCID)
Autoimmune	The body's ability to distinguish self from non-self is impaired. The body begins to attack its own healthy tissue. Precipitating factors often are unclear	Acute rheumatic fever (ARF); juvenile rheumatoid arthritis (JRA); systemic lupus erythematosus (SLE); erythema multiforme, juvenile diabetes (see Chapter 29)
Immune complex diseases	Incomplete clearing of immune complexes by the lymphatic system allows them to remain in circulation. They become caught in small blood vessels of various body systems and initiate an inflammatory response	Acute glomerulonephritis (AGN); Shönlein-Henoch purpura; mucocutaneous lymph node syndrome—Kawasaki disease
Allergy	A hyperactive immune response to certain antigens (allergens). IgE production in response to the allergen causes cells to rupture and release chemicals having adverse effects on various body systems	Asthma; eczema; contact dermatitis; anaphylaxis

ALLERGY SURVEY SHEET

Name ______ Age ____ Sex ____ Date ______

Chief complaint

Present illness

Associated allergic symptoms

Eyes:	Pruritis ____	Burning ____	Tearing ____
	Swelling ____	Dark circles ____	Discharge ____
Ears:	Pruritis ____	Fullness ____	Popping ____
	Frequent infections ____		
Nose:	Sneezing ____	Rhinorrhea ____	Obstruction ____
	Pruritis ____	Mouth breathing ____	
	Prurulent discharge ____		
Throat:	Soreness ____	Postnasal discharge ____	Mucus in A.M. ____
	Itchy throat ____		
Chest:	Sputum ____	Dyspnea ____	Wheezing ____
	Color ____	Rest ____	
	Amount ____	Exertion ____	
Skin:	Dermatitis ____	Eczema ____	Urticaria ____

Family allergies

Previous allergic treatment or testing

Skin testing

		Improved	Unimproved
Drugs taken	Antihistamines	____	____
	Bronchodilators	____	____
	Nose drops	____	____
	Hyposensitization	____	____
	Antibiotics	____	____
	Steroids	____	____

Physical agents and habits. Is the child bothered by

Cigarette smoke ____	Heat ____	Air conditioner ____
Cold ____	Muggy weather ____	Weather changes ____
Perfume ____	Paints ____	Insecticides ____
Cosmetics ____	Chemicals ____	Hairspray ____
Pollens ____	Clothing ____	Sun ____
Animals/feathers ____	Dust ____	Adhesive tape ____

Food agents. Describe reaction to

Formula ____	Cereals ____	Fruits ____
Vegetables ____	Meats ____	Juices ____
Cheese ____	Milk ____	Eggs ____
Soda ____	Fish ____	Nuts ____
Citrus ____		

In infants: How and when were foods introduced?

FIGURE 25-1

Allergy survey sheet. This survey should be filled out by the nurse, not the parent, because questions might need clarification or information might need expansion. (Adapted from Patterson R: Allergic Diseases—Diagnosis and Management. *Lippincott, 1980 pp. 78–79.)*

Where symptoms occur

Place of residence at onset
Place of residence since onset
Symptoms better indoors or out
Effect of school
Effect of staying elsewhere nearby
Effect of hospitalization
Do symptoms occur around

Old leaves ______	Hay ______	Lakeside ______
Barns ______	Summer homes ______	Damp basement ______
Dry attic ______	Lawn mowing ______	Animals ______
Other ______		

Home: City ______ Rural ______
House ______ Age ______
Apartment ______ Basement ______ damp ______ dry ______
Heating system ______
Pets ______ dog ______ cat ______ hamster ______ bird ______

Bedroom: Type	Age	Living: Type	Age
Pillow ______	______	Rug ______	______
Mattress ______	______	Furniture ______	______
Blankets ______	______	Curtains ______	______
Furniture ______	______	Stuffed animals ______	______
		Security blanket ______	______

Are symptoms worse anywhere else in home?

When symptoms occur

Time and circmstances of first episode
Prior health
Course of illness over time
Time of year Perennial ______
Seasonal ______
Seasonally exacerbated ______
Time of week (weekends vs weekdays)
Time of day or night
After insect stings

What does child or family think makes the child worse?

Is the child ever free of symptoms?

Other comments

FIGURE 25-1
(Continued)

especially in conjunction with a fever. The nurse also notes any recent history of "flu" symptoms and any injuries.

Since some of the immune system diseases can be triggered by exposure to a drug or toxic chemical, it is essential for the nurse to determine what medications, if any, the child had received prior to onset of symptoms. Particularly important is a history of the child's taking antibiotics or sulfa. Also, the nurse notes any unusual environmental factors, particularly exposure to toxic chemicals.

A history of joint pain necessitates questions directed toward the pattern of the pain—for example, the time of day it occurs, the joints involved, and the transiency of the pain. It is important also to note any recent disappearance of joint pain. The immune system disorders that affect joint function differ according to the number and location of joints involved.

The nurse documents any allergic or hypersensitivity reactions. A history of persistent rhinitis, headaches, or respiratory congestion can indicate an allergic manifestation of which the child's family might be unaware. The nurse records any allergy desensitization regimen. An allergy survey (Figure 25-1) can be taken in the hospital, or a home assessment can be performed by a visiting nurse.

The nurse notes whether the child is appropriately im-

ASSESSMENT GUIDE *The Child with an Immune System Dysfunction*

Assessment questions	Supporting data
Has the child experienced repeated and frequent illnesses?	Thin appearance, failure-to-thrive; thin, lifeless hair; persistent bacterial (eg, *Staphylococcus, Streptococcus, Hemophilus influenzae*), viral, fungal (eg, monilia), or parasitic infections; enlarged lymph nodes; prolonged diarrhea; alterations in lymphocytes (see Table 25-2); fatigue
Does the parent or child report that the child has had a recent sore throat or scarlet fever?	Fever; joint inflammation and pain; chorea (muscle twitching); cardiac irregularities (eg, murmurs, friction rub, tachycardia, abnormal ECG); elevated white blood cell count, erythrocyte sedimentation rate, and anti-streptolysin titer; subcutaneous nodules; red lines on the skin
Impetigo?	Decreased urine output with cola colored urine; hematuria, proteinuria; elevated blood pressure; edema, especially periorbital; elevated antistreptolysin titer and blood chemistries
Is the child manifesting any limitation or pain in one or more joints? Document that pattern and type of pain and the joints involved.	Joint edema and effusion; limited joint range of motion; fever; rashes; fatigue
Has the child recently been exposed to any new medication, infection, foods, or been under increased stress? Do any family members have a history of immune system alterations, including allergies? Are immunizations up to date?	Skin alterations possibly including urticaria, weeping lesions, butterfly-shaped rash on the face, generalized rash, purpura, or hair loss; fever; respiratory alterations (eg, dyspnea, wheezing, cough, congestion, signs of respiratory distress); nausea, vomiting, or signs of gastrointestinal obstruction; alteration in urine values

Additional data: Cherry red tongue and pharyngeal area; Raynaud's phenomenon (vasospasm in fingers and toes); desquamation (skin peeling) of the palms and soles; corneal ulceration, conjunctivitis, iridocyclitis (inflammation of the iris and ciliary body of the eye); irritability, seizures, and other neurologic alterations; residual cardiac damage

munized and also records any reactions to immunizations. For instance, certain vaccines, such as the MMR (see Chapter 11), can cause a reaction in a child allergic to eggs or feathers.

Finally, since some immune disorders have a hereditary pattern, it might be necessary for parents to check the family records or talk to relatives about family incidence. Often, however, no known hereditary pattern will be evident.

Validating Diagnostic Tests

Much of the laboratory work performed for diagnostic workup of immune diseases involves serologic studies (Table 25-2). Remembering that children of various age groups are affected differently by venipunctures, the nurse explains the procedure to the child as carefully as possible to minimize traumatic effects.

Principles of Nursing Care

Although immune system disorders differ widely as to etiologies and symptoms, they have some features in common. For this reason, much of the nursing care of children with these problems can be applied to a variety of situations. Immune disorders can, however, affect more than one body system. In such instances, nursing interventions are similar to those for children with specific system disorders.

Acute Care Needs

Potential for infection

Some alterations in the immune system can result in severe, overwhelming infections for the child, related to abnormal

TABLE 25-2 Studies for Immune System Dysfunction

Test	Normal values		Alteration/clinical significance
White blood cell count (WBC) Number of WBC in 1 μL (mm^3) of blood		(× 1000 cells/μL)	*Increased:* Stimulation of bone marrow by invading organisms, bacteria
	Newborn	9.0–30.0	*Decreased:* Bone marrow depression from viruses or toxic chemicals
	Neonate (1 mo)	5.0–19.5	
	Infant (1–3 yr)	6.0–17.5	
	Child (4–13 yr)	4.5–15.5	
	Adult	4.5–11.0	
Differential white count*		(%)	*Increased:* Infection
Neutrophils	Newborn	32–62	*Decreased:* Viral or protozoan infections along with increased immature neutrophils during very severe infection indicates body's lessening ability to fight infection
	Infant (1 yr)	23	
	Child (10 yr)	31–61	
	Adult	54–75	
Basophils	Newborn	0.5–1.0	*Increased:* Hemolytic anemias, Hodgkin's disease, infections (particularly during phase of recovery)
	Infant (1 yr)	0.4	*Decreased:* Acute allergic reactions, anaphylaxis, stress
	Child (10 yr)	0.5	
	Adult	0–1	
Eosinophils	Newborn	2–2.5	*Increased:* Various allergic conditions, parasitic infestations, Hodgkin's disease, sickle cell anemia, postsplenectomy
	Infant (1 yr)	2.6	*Decreased:* Stress (burns, trauma, surgery, excess exercise)
	Child (10 yr)	2–2.5	
	Adult	1–4	
Lymphocytes	Newborn	26–36	*Increased:* Infections (acute and chronic, bacterial and viral), lymphocytic leukemia, non-Hodgkin's lymphomas, during antibody formation with young children
	Infant (1 yr)	61	*Decreased:* Stress responses to trauma or burns, Hodgkin's disease, immunoglobulin deficiencies, leukemias (chronic granulocytic or monocytic)
	Child (10 yr)	28–48	
	Adult	25–40	
Monocytes	Newborn	5–6	*Increased:* Infections including bacterial, viral, rickettsial; subacute bacterial endocarditis, malignant tumors, Hodgkin's disease, non-Hodgkin's lymphomas
	Infant (1 yr)	5	
	Child (10 yr)	4–4.5	
	Adult	2–8	
Serum immunoglobulins (see Essentials of Structure and Function)			*Increased:* Increase in IgE implicates an ongoing allergic response *Decreased:* Increased susceptibility to infection
Rheumatoid factor (RF)	0		*Increased:* Present in many autoimmune diseases, especially juvenile rheumatoid arthritis
Antinuclear antibodies (ANA) (antibodies to cell nuclear components [i.e., anti-DNA and anti-RNA antibodies])	0		*Increased:* Autoimmune diseases such as systemic lupus erythematosus and juvenile rheumatoid arthritis
Antistreptolysin titer (ASO)	150 μ/mL		*Increased:* Indicative of recent or current streptococcal infection, acute rheumatic fever, acute glomerulonephritis
Complement tests (measures individual components of the complement cascade)	Negative		*Increased:* Inflammation *Decreased:* Decreased C_2 implicates systemic lupus erythematosus
Erythrocyte sedimentation rate (ESR) (measures the rate at which erythrocytes precipitate out of solution)	12 mL/h		*Increased:* Inflammatory diseases, acute rheumatic fever, acute glomerulonephritis, Kawasaki disease

(Continues)

TABLE 25-2 Studies for Immune System Dysfunction *(Continued)*

Test	Normal values	Alteration/clinical significance
LE cell	0	Present in children with systemic lupus erythematosus and some other autoimmune diseases
Allergy skin tests (introduction of an allergen by skin prick, scratch, or intradermal method)	No reaction	Presence of wheals (immediate hypersensitivity) indicates reaction to a specific allergen
Intradermal skin tests (PPD, Mantoux) (tests function of cellular response)	Presence of a wheal after 48 hours	*Reaction:* Indicates actively functioning cellular response *No Reaction:* Can indicate diminished T-cell activity
Radioallergosorbant tests (RAST) (in vitro allergen/antibody combination)	Negative	Positive result indicates allergy to the allergen being tested

*Percentage of various types of WBC seen on examination of a slide of peripheral blood.

lymphocyte number and function. Protecting the child from infection is a primary nursing responsibility. Children with immune deficiencies need scrupulous protection from infection while in the hospital. The nursing goal is to protect the child from exposure to as many pathogens as possible.

Because the effectiveness of traditional protective isolation has been questioned (Jackson and McPherson, 1986), a *laminar airflow system* is the preferred method of providing a germ-free environment for those children who require it. A laminar airflow unit consists of a fan blowing air at a constant speed through two filters into the child's room. The filters remove not only dust particles but also extremely small contaminants, resulting in almost 100% sterile air. This unit might be in a room or a series of rooms joined by a separate corridor. Access to the rooms is limited and everything is decontaminated prior to entry. Every item entering the room must be heat sterilized or disinfected. This requirement includes such items as equipment, food, medications, toys, and linens.

Protection for most children is accomplished by placing the child in a single room, observing strict handwashing prior to entry, and making sure all who enter the room are free from infection. In hospital settings without access to a laminar airflow system, protective isolation might still be in use. The child is placed in a private room with the doors to the corridors closed at all times. Entry to and exit from the room is through a clean anteroom large enough to allow for dressing in the appropriate sterile clothing.

Care for a child in any type of protective environment presents a nursing challenge. The balance between adequately meeting the child's social and emotional needs without jeopardizing the physical needs is a delicate one requiring creative nursing approaches.

⊛ Potential for impaired physical mobility

Preventing joint contractures Some of the immune system diseases cause pain and partial limitation in one or more joints. Nursing care then must be directed toward prevention of joint contractures.

A physical therapy program usually is established for the child. This program might encompass not only exercises to maintain mobility but also other treatments such as whirlpool, heat application, and instructions for promoting self-care activities. It is imperative that the nurse and physical therapist communicate carefully for a coordinated, consistent approach. A timetable for exercises needs to be posted in such a way that nurses on all shifts can continue the therapy.

The nurse performs range-of-motion exercises of both affected and unaffected joints. The child should perform active exercises when possible, and the nurse encourages this by using play to promote activity. The use of nerf balls, trapezes, modeling clay, and any other tools for facilitating joint activity is beneficial. Games between similarly affected children not only promote physical health but also answer a need for social contacts among peers. The nurse emphasizes the importance of continuing the exercise regimen at home.

Preventing hazards of immobility In addition to joint contractures, some immune system disorders can cause severe complications to the heart and kidney if measures are

STANDARDS OF NURSING CARE *The Child in a Protective Environment*

GUIDE FOR NURSING MANAGEMENT

Nursing diagnosis	Interventions	Rationale	Outcome
1. Potential for infection (stressor: altered body defense systems)	Place child in a single room if no laminar airflow unit is available; others need to be free of active infection before entering.	Removing the child from other hospitalized children and contact with anyone who is infected reduces the chances the child will contract an infection.	The child will not exhibit any signs of infection—fever, respiratory distress, enlarged lymph nodes, or specific symptoms related to infection in body systems.
	If the child is on protective isolation or in a laminar airflow room, sterilize or disinfect all items to enter the room. Use sterile gown, mask, and gloves when entering the room. Remove all contaminated items such as caps, scissors, and watch before entry. Possible use of head and shoe covers. Consult with dietary department about sterilizing food, containers, and utensils.	Sterilization reduces the spread of organisms to an immunologically depressed child.	
	Coordinate nursing care so as not to have to leave the room.	Reducing the number of entries to the room reduces the chances the child will contract an infection.	
2. Sensory deprivation related to environmental and social isolation	Talk to the child when providing care. Orient young children frequently as to time and events. Play verbal games. Use the child's name frequently.	Verbal stimuli reduce sensory deprivation. Orienting the child prevents confusion resulting from loss of time sense.	The child is alert, responsive, and not withdrawn. The child is free from disorientation, depression, or extreme irritability.
	Provide tactile stimulation in the form of comfort measures. Cuddle all babies as often as possible.	Tactile stimulation conveys security to the child and reduces problems resulting from isolation.	
	Provide visual stimulation in the form of disinfected mobiles, crib toys, and other age-appropriate toys to enliven the environment. Provide a colorful plastic calendar for older children to maintain time orientation.	Visual stimulation promotes normal development while reducing sensory deprivation.	
	Enter room regularly and plan with the child times to be in the room so child can anticipate arrival.	Anticipation combined with orientation helps reduce the effects of isolation.	

STANDARDS OF NURSING CARE *The Child in a Protective Environment (Continued)*

GUIDE FOR NURSING MANAGEMENT

Nursing diagnosis	Interventions	Rationale	Outcome
3. Fear related to inability to recognize caregivers and loss of familiar surroundings	Explain to the child the purposes of isolation if the cognitive level is appropriate. Identify self when entering the room. Reassure infants with a calm, soothing voice and plenty of cuddling. Use primary nursing whenever possible. Provide the child with familiar comfort items such as a blanket or stuffed animal.	Assisting the child with identification and with making the environment more comfortable and familiar increases security and control and decreases fear.	The child exhibits a trusting attitude toward caregivers, including calling the nurse by name, decreased restlessness, and increased cooperation with care. The child will cry less frequently.
4. Social isolation related to separation from family and familiar environment	Encourage frequent visits from parents. Teach parents how to enter the room and include parents in child's care whenever possible. Encourage the parents to increase verbal contact with the child.	Including the family in the child's care, after appropriate instruction in precaution technique, helps maintain the family structure and assists the child to cope with the separation imposed by the isolation.	The child will express an interest in family events. If old enough, the child will ask about peers and activities going on at school.
	Talk about the family to the child when the family is absent. Discuss what the family members might be doing at home. Support the child when the parents leave. Encourage the parents to bring familiar, sterilizable objects from home	Verbal reminders of the family help the child maintain contact and keep up with current family events, thus reducing the effects of social isolation.	

not taken to prevent their occurrence. For this reason, complete bed rest or severely limited activity might be required until the danger of complications recedes. Complete bed rest, however, also can be hazardous. Therefore, the nurse addresses the problems of the hazards of immobility, which can affect body systems, and takes regular measures to prevent them (see Chapter 20).

Potential impairment of skin integrity

Children with immune diseases often exhibit peculiar skin manifestations. For example, the child with lupus erythematosis might demonstrate a classic butterfly-shaped rash on the face. Lesions seen in children with immune dysfunction can include bullae, dry scales, and purpura, among others.

The lesion differs according to the specific dysfunction. Because of these inherent skin sensitivities, the nurse needs to be more vigorous than usual with efforts to prevent skin breakdown during periods of immobility. Care of skin lesions depends on the type of lesions involved.

Alteration in comfort: pain related to inflammation

Because the inflammatory process causes local pain, pain relief is a nursing priority. Heat applications, if ordered, can relieve painful joints and inflamed areas. Certain medications might be ordered to reduce inflammation and provide relief from pain (Table 25-3). (Distraction and other nonmedicinal pain relief measures are described in Chapter 20.)

TABLE 25-3 Medications Used for Immune System Dysfunction

Medication	Effect	Nursing implications
Salicylates (eg, aspirin, Empirin, Anacin)	Anti-inflammatory analgesic	Salicylates are given in doses high enough to relieve symptoms but below blood level of 25 mg/100 mL. Observe for signs of toxicity—headache, tinnitus, dizziness, and confusion. Monitor serum salicylate level. Give with meals or antacids to prevent gastric irritation. Salicylates can increase bleeding tendencies and epistaxis is not unusual
Corticosteroids	Topical—anti-inflammatory	Topical steroids can be applied in a cream or lotion base. Observe for systemic effects related to overabsorption through the skin (see systemic anti-inflammatory)
	Systemic—anti-inflammatory	Give with meals or milk to prevent gastric irritation and internal bleeding. Monitor blood pressure. Observe child for side effects—moon face, fluid retention, decreased urinary output. Taper the dose down when removing the child from the medication to prevent adrenal cortex dysfunction. Protect the child from sources of infection, since symptoms of infection are masked by the medication
Antihistamines (eg, Benadryl, chlorpheneramine, brompheneramine)	Blocks the adverse effects of histamine	Observe the child for drowsiness or excitability. Assure the child's safety—bed rails elevated and close supervision when ambulatory

Nutritional Needs

⊛ Potential alteration in nutrition: less than body requirements

Inadequate nutritional status is a major contributor to dysfunction of the immune system (National Dairy Council, 1985). Deficiencies in protein, particularly, can decrease the body's ability to fight infection. Because infection or fever increase the metabolic rate, the child with an infection might not receive enough nutrients to combat the infection and protect against further infection.

Generally speaking, children with immune system disorders should maintain their usual diet if that diet contains adequate nutrients for growth and development. Increased protein consumption might be advised at times when the child's metabolic rate might be increased.

Children with food allergies have unique dietary problems. Because food is a common source of allergens, it might be necessary for the nurse to assist the child and family with identification of allergens and with dietary management.

Breast milk is considered to be allergen-free. If the mother is unable or unwilling to breast-feed her infant, hypoallergenic formulas might be advised for children with a familial allergic history or known allergy to formula. Hypoallergenic formulas include soybean preparations such as Isomil or Prosobee. In extreme cases, meat-based formula might be recommended to fulfill nutritional requirements.

The child might be older, however, before a food allergy is evident. Pinpointing the foods responsible is time consuming and requires much patience and strict adherence to a prescribed dietary regimen.

The physician might prescribe an *elimination diet*. Elimination diets are used to pinpoint a specific food allergen. The child or parent keeps a diet record for an established time period, noting any reactions. After that, suspected allergens are eliminated one at a time from the diet, each for a period of several days. If reactions subside, that food is implicated as an allergen. Elimination diets often are followed by *food challenges*. The allergen is reintroduced to confirm the allergic response.

Elimination diets are often done at home. The nurse is then responsible for making certain both child and family understand what is expected. The child's cooperation should be enlisted whenever possible. Because there are so many sources outside the home where the child has access to food, the child's active participation is essential for a successful test.

Once specific allergens have been identified, the general treatment is avoidance. All foods containing the allergen should be eliminated from the diet. Parents need to become label watchers. So many foods are combined with others, either as preservatives, flavoring, or coloring, that the parent should avoid some packaged foods. Food preparation then can place an added burden on the parent who prepares the foods. Children need to be taught which foods to avoid, including hidden ingredients in common foods. A dietary consultant can assist the parent to adapt to specific diet constraints while providing adequate nutrients for growth. Children need to be supported in the adjustment to a new dietary regimen. Older children tend to cooperate with dietary restrictions since they know they might experience reactions if they don't.

Developmental Needs

Potential for altered growth and development

Some children with immune system disorders require hospitalization only during a short, acute phase of a self-limiting disease. Others can expect long hospital stays or repeated hospitalizations.

Promoting normal development Children with immune system disorders, like other hospitalized children, need to continue their normal developmental progress within the hospital setting. Those children in the hospital who are acutely ill will have most of their developmental needs met secondarily to physical needs. Children hospitalized on a longer-term basis and those who are repeat admissions have unique developmental problems because of interruption in normal routine. (Chapter 14 discusses nursing care of the child with a chronic condition.)

Providing appropriate toys and games and encouraging the child to participate in care and in decision making helps promote normal development. Allowing the older child to telephone friends to maintain peer relationships is helpful. If visiting is impractical, as it might be for the isolated child, some effort should be made for the child to receive letters or tapes from friends. Children should be allowed to make some decisions about their care and to have some control over their environment.

Promoting independence The development of independence and responsibility for oneself is a process spanning several developmental stages. Children are normally encouraged to assert themselves and to assume responsibility for self-care while adhering to limits set by the parents. Unfortunately, it is easy to shelter a child suffering from a chronic illness whether out of guilt or from a sense of overprotectiveness. To a child with a chronic allergic disease, limiting independence and responsibility, regardless of age, can be destructive. The feelings evoked in the child not only retard normal development but also cause anger and frustration, both of which are detrimental to disease control.

A principal nursing intervention in the care of a child with an allergic problem is to encourage the parents to let go and treat the child as normally as possible. This requires great effort on the part of parents, because in actuality they must maintain control until the child is old enough to assume responsibility for self-medication. Interventions toward this goal need to be initiated on first contact with the family and reinforced consistently thereafter.

Children at an early age recognize overprotection and fast learn to manipulate parents accordingly. The nurse can assist parents to break the cycle by encouraging them to be firm and to recognize and limit manipulative behavior. Parents need support to break the cycle, but the results are worth the effort.

Emotional Needs

Anxiety related to uncertain health status

Both children who suffer from immune system disorders and their families can experience anxiety related to the severity of the disease, to the sometimes uncertain prognosis, or to the treatment and care provided. Nurses first need to support the child and family during the acute, somewhat frightening phase of illness. If the disease is self-limiting, the nurse needs to give reassurances that, as ill as the child might appear, with precautions, the child might recover with no permanent aftereffects. Because some of these conditions affect vital body organs such as the kidney and the heart, reassurance might be difficult. The nurse can help the family express fears and view the condition realistically. The reassurance, combined with nursing efforts to prevent complications, presents a nursing care challenge.

Children with immune deficiency disorders might be in more of a life-threatening situation than those with other kinds of illnesses. A normally simple infectious process could be fatal. Parents, and the child if capable of understanding, need vigorous support. They need encouragement to develop a positive attitude for living as well as needing help with the adjustment to the possibility of death. The nurse intervenes to facilitate the anticipatory grieving process where applicable.

Potential for ineffective individual coping

Stress, particularly when prolonged, weakens the immune system's ability to fight infection and can exacerbate symptoms of immune system dysfunction. Many diseases have an emotional, psychologic component. Whether the disease triggers the emotional problem or whether the emotional problem triggers the disease is often uncertain. Causes of stress are both internal and external. In additional to the feelings of stress from within, due to handling the adjustment to acute or chronic disease, the child is affected by external stress in the environment. The nurse attempts therefore to reduce internal and external sources of stress.

Techniques to reduce stress can be as simple as counting to ten or as complicated as meditation. Usually, the relatively simple technique of slow, deep breathing combined with complete muscle relaxation will ease feelings of stress. Children should be encouraged to practice relaxation for several minutes daily. (Relaxation techniques are described in Chapter 16.)

⊛ Potential for ineffective family coping

Parents too might respond adversely to the stress of the child's illness and hospitalization. Interventions then consist of assisting the parents to recognize and cope with the causes of stress. This assistance might include referrals to a social service agency for assistance with the financial burden. Coping with stress might involve encouraging the parents to take time off for themselves or for special attention to other children in the family.

Relaxation techniques should be taught to both parents and child. If parents are able to control their feelings of stress while the child is ill, the child will be calmer and complications might be avoided.

⊛ Potential alteration in self-concept

Some body changes can result from immune system disease. Some, like the effects of steroids, are temporary, whereas others such as joint limitation might be more permanent. The skin manifestations associated with some immune system diseases, particularly allergies, can be detrimental to body image.

In addition to the support ordinarily given for an alteration in body image, the nurse needs to teach the child and parents to cope with teasing. In some instances, these skills might involve having the child teach peers about the illness; they might involve teaching the child a quick comeback; or they might involve suggesting methods of minimizing the appearance change. The more comfortable children feel with their peers, the more responsive they'll be with any restrictions imposed by the disease.

Parents also need to be taught to assist the child to cope with the inevitable uncomfortable situation. The nurse can present some common situations to parent and child, although these depend on the child's age level. Discussing how each would handle the situation will allow the nurse to intervene. Above all, good communication between parents and child is essential for optimum emotional health.

Health Maintenance Needs

⊛ Potential knowledge deficit regarding home management

When preparing a child with an immune system disorder for discharge, the nurse acquaints the family with plans for follow-up care. Disease complications might not appear for several months to years after recovery. The child and family should be alerted to symptoms of complications or of disease exacerbation. Regular examinations probably will be required.

Some children might be discharged with joint limitation, necessitating regular physical therapy. The therapist demonstrates and explains any home care therapy regimen including range-of-motion exercises and prevention of joint contractures. The nurse assists the parents to plan for this at home. If the child is to return to school, therapy might be needed during the school day. The nurse then communicates with the school nurse, both orally and in writing, about exactly what needs to be done to maintain continuity of care.

The Child with an Immune Deficiency

Children who have deficiencies in cellular immunity exhibit signs of repeated infections from viruses, fungi, and parasites. Because of diminished T-cell activity, discrimination between "self" and "nonself" is impaired, resulting in an increased potential for developing malignancies.

Acquired Immunodeficiency Syndrome

Acquired immunodeficiency syndrome (AIDS) is a fatal immune disorder that primarily affects the cellular immune response. Cells that normally help the immune response are ineffective in children with AIDS. Thus, the cellular defense is turned off far more frequently, allowing the child to be overrun by infections not usually seen (these are termed *opportunistic infections*). Opportunistic infections include severe manifestations of herpes, cytomegalovirus, fungal infections, and protozoan pneumonias (*Pneumocystis carinii*). A rare type of skin cancer, Kaposi's sarcoma, is seen in adults with AIDS, but seen infrequently in children (Thompson and Gietz, 1985).

Although a relatively rare disease that mainly affects members of certain high-risk groups, AIDS has increased dramatically between its recognition in 1979 and the present. The groups most prone to developing AIDS include male homosexuals, addicts of intravenous drugs such as heroin, hemophiliacs or others receiving transfusions, Haitian people living in the United States, sexual partners of those infected with the virus, and infants and children of people in these high-risk groups.

Clinical manifestations Infants and children with AIDS have clinical manifestations similar to those of adults. The child might exhibit failure to thrive, persistent monilial infections, prolonged diarrhea, lymph node enlargement, repeated otitis media, and other infections. Usually, the child is connected in some way to a high-risk group.

Recently, infants have been identified that have most likely been exposed to an AIDS infection prenatally. These infants demonstrate similar clinical features that resemble, but are different from, children with fetal alcohol syndrome. These features include small for gestational age, microcephaly with a prominent forehead, altered facial features, blue sclerae, and repeated infections during early infancy.

Diagnostic evaluation Laboratory studies might reveal excess gamma globulin levels and excessive suppressor T cells in relation to helper T cells. The cause of AIDS is linked to a virus—human T-cell lymphotropic virus-III (HTLV-III), also called human immune virus (HIV). Antibodies to AIDS-related virus have been discovered in the serum of children with suspected AIDS.

The mechanism of AIDS transmission to infants has not yet been established, although it is believed to be transmitted during pregnancy or delivery from the infected mother. Older children have contracted AIDS through contaminated blood transfusions, although the incidence of this is decreasing because most blood is now tested for the presence of AIDS antibodies. AIDS also can be transmitted to children by sexual abuse from an infected person. Interpersonal contacts in school or day care are not known to be a source of transmission of the virus.

Treatment Treatment for AIDS is directed toward managing the opportunistic infections. Research continues into discovering a cure, a vaccine, or a medication that will prevent the virus from reproducing.

Nursing management Nursing care for children with AIDS is supportive and similar to that for any child with an immune deficiency. Protection from infection is of primary importance. Hospitalized AIDS patients usually are on blood, needle, enteric, urine, and secretion precautions. Strict handwashing is required and gloves should be worn when handling any of these sources of possible transmission of the disorder. Gowns are worn if the child is bleeding heavily. Masks are necessary only when the child is coughing productively. A private room is not necessary unless the child is coughing or bleeding excessively or has draining wounds.

Children with AIDS can be managed successfully at home if they do not have a serious infection requiring hospitalization. The nurse supports the parent and child to help them cope with the implications of the diagnosis and to provide the optimal quality of life for the child. (See Chapters 14 and 17 for nursing care of the child with a chronic condition and for care of the child who is dying.)

Unfortunately, the wide publicity surrounding AIDS has led to many misconceptions about its transmission. Children have been barred unnecessarily from schools and public places, to their emotional and developmental detriment. Nurses can be advocates for these children and should attempt to reduce fear of the disease by providing appropriate information to the community.

Humoral Deficiency—Agammaglobulinemia

One of the primary manifestations of a deficiency in humoral immunity is *agammaglobulinemia,* or complete deficiency of immunoglobulin. This disease can be inherited or acquired. The disease is seen mainly in young boys, although symptoms usually don't appear until 9 months to 2 years of age, probably because of the lingering effect of maternal antibodies.

Some children experience *hypogammaglobulinemia,* which is a much milder form of immune deficiency resulting from a decrease rather than an absence of immunoglobulins. These children typically manifest frequent, recurrent infections, particularly when they reach school age, and are exposed to pathogens in school. Treatment might involve gamma globulin injections to boost immune system function.

Clinical manifestations The child demonstrates high susceptibility to bacterial infections, particularly to common bacteria—*Staphylococcus, Streptococcus,* and *Hemophilus influenzae*. Children often appear thin and ill-looking. Their hair appears lifeless and dull. Unless the disease is recognized early, death can occur from infection. When recognized, this disease can be successfully treated.

Diagnostic evaluation Children who have repeated bouts with pneumonia or skin infections should be tested for agammaglobulinemia. Laboratory results will demonstrate low or nearly absent levels of IgG. Examination of lymph nodes or bone marrow will reveal a deficiency of plasma cells. Levels of T-lymphocytes are normal.

Treatment Antibiotics are administered to treat infections, and injections of gamma globulin are given on a monthly basis.

Nursing management The nurse teaches the parents about preventing infections. Cleanliness, avoiding crowds, and prompt treatment for the earliest signs of infection should be emphasized.

Careful administration of gamma globulin is essential. Injections are given intramuscularly and, depending on the size of the child, might need to be given in divided doses. The nurse and parents can give extra support to the child at the time of injections, since they can be a frightening as well as a painful experience.

Often, prophylactic chest physical therapy is ordered to prevent pneumonia. The nurse demonstrates this procedure to the parents and asks for return demonstrations until the parents appear to be competent. On hospital discharge, a visiting nurse referral would be helpful in most instances. The nurse can assist parents with preventive measures as well as reinforce the chest therapy technique.

Mixed Immune Deficiency—Wiskott-Aldrich Syndrome

Young boys are most commonly affected by *Wiskott-Aldrich syndrome,* a sex-linked recessive disease. The syndrome is classified as a mixed immune deficiency disease since it affects both the cellular system and the humoral system. The body cannot produce antibodies, and there appears to be an associated loss of cellular immunity. The immune system appears to function normally, initially, and symptoms do not appear until about 1 year of age. This disease is usually fatal with death occurring before age 6 as a result of hemorrhage or overwhelming infection. These children also are susceptible to malignancy.

Clinical manifestations Along with repeated infections and eczema, which indicate alteration in immune system function, the child has an associated thrombocytopenia. Bleeding is the most common clinical sign that brings the child for diagnosis. Infections can be bacterial or viral in origin.

Diagnostic evaluation Serum IgG levels are normal, but IgM is greatly reduced. There is also a decrease in T-lymphocytes. Blood work reveals decreased and abnormal platelets, although this can be corrected by platelet transfusions.

Treatment Topical steroids are applied to eczematous skin, and antibiotics are administered prophylactically for infections. Platelet transfusions are successful in temporarily correcting the thrombocytopenia. Gamma globulin is given to provide increased resistance to infection. No one treatment is known to cure or completely correct the disease. Recently, bone marrow transplantation has been attempted and has been successful in curing the disease (Nuscher et al., 1984). With early treatment, the prognosis for these children is optimistic.

Nursing management Interventions are directed toward prevention of infection. Parents are taught to apply topical steroids and to observe the child for adverse effects. The nurse carefully monitors transfusions, particularly observing for reactions. The parents are encouraged to protect the child from bruising, while still allowing development to proceed as normally as possible. Guidance is similar to that given to parents whose children have hemophilia. For example, the use of padded clothing and protective helmets is helpful when the child is learning to stand or walk (see Chapter 26). Because this disease is sometimes fatal, the nurse intervenes to facilitate the grieving process (see Chapter 17).

Severe Combined Immunodeficiency Disease

Rarely, children demonstrate a severe congenital combined humoral and cellular deficiency called *severe combined immunodeficiency disease* (SCID). Lymphoid tissue in these children is incompetent and is lacking both classes of lymphocytes. Children with SCID are unable to combat any antigens and must live in an antigen-free environment, such as a laminar airflow room, or in a "bubble" in order to survive. Recent success with bone marrow transplantation promises hope for these children.

The Child with an Autoimmune Disease

Acute Rheumatic Fever

Acute rheumatic fever (ARF) is an autoimmune disease that occurs as a result of invasion by group A β-hemolytic streptococci. ARF is not a contagious disease, although the precipitating factors—streptococcal pharyngitis or scarlet fever—are contagious. The risk for ARF increases if streptococcal infections are not treated properly.

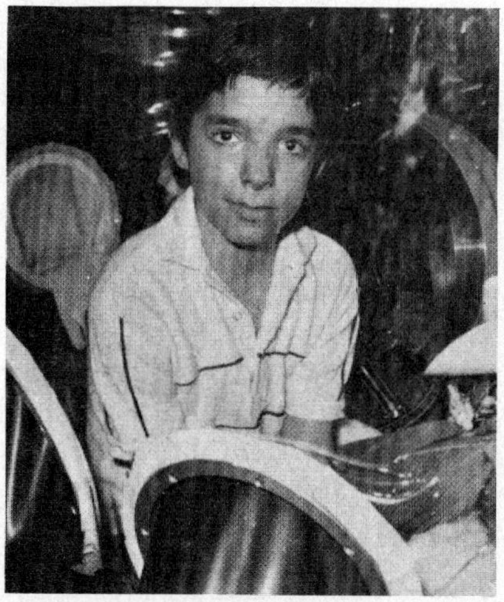

A child with SCID in an antigen-free bubble. (Courtesy Baylor College of Medicine; from Jenkins J: Human Genetics. *Addison-Wesley, 1983.)*

The exact etiology of this disease is still theoretic, but the generally accepted theory is that the streptococcal organism triggers the body to turn against its own connective tissue. This causes inflammatory responses in the myocardium and connective tissue portions of the heart (carditis), joints, and eyes.

ARF can affect children of all ages, but it primarily affects children in middle to late childhood. Close contact in a classroom can enhance the transmission of streptococcal diseases, as can any overcrowded living conditions. ARF is a self-limiting disease, usually resolving in 3 weeks.

The incidence of streptococcal-related immune disease has decreased dramatically since the discovery and widespread use of penicillin. Recently, however, the incidence of ARF has increased in some areas of the United States. Although the reason for this is not known, it is suspected that the increase is due to a combination of three factors (Centers for Disease Control, 1987).

1. Increased genetic predisposition.
2. An increasing number of rheumatologic strains of streptococci.
3. Changes in the incidence, detection, and treatment of streptococcal infections.

Clinical manifestations Acute onset of arthralgia (joint pain) often occurs first in one or more joints, and usually occurs in major joints. Arthralgia is transient and does not produce contractures. Subtle onset of chorea (involuntary muscular twitchings of trunk and limbs) might be the first manifestation in older children. Carditis, as detected by murmurs and ECG changes, is seen more frequently in young children. The onset of carditis might be acute, with chest pain and dyspnea, or be subtle.

Diagnostic evaluation Additional signs and symptoms associated with ARF are required for making a positive diagnosis of the disease. These include some combination of the following (known as the revised Jones' criteria):

- Major criteria
  Polyarthritis (joint inflammation in more than one joint)
  Carditis (inflammation of myocardium and valves)
  Erythema marginatum (wavy red lines on the skin outlining areas of normal skin)
  Chorea (involuntary twitching)
  Subcutaneous nodules (small movable knotlike areas just beneath the skin at the joints)
- Minor criteria
  Fever
  Arthralgia
  Alteration in electrocardiogram
  Previous history of ARF
  Leukocytosis
  Elevated erythrocyte sedimentation rate
  Positive C-reactive protein

For a positive diagnosis of ARF, two major criteria or one major and two minor criteria plus a history of a recent streptococcal infection (positive throat culture, scarlet fever, elevated antistreptolysin titer) must be present. A highly elevated erythrocyte sedimentation rate (ESR) is secondary to the inflammatory autoimmune reaction.

Treatment Treatment of ARF is directed toward preventing cardiac complications. Aspirin is prescribed for its anti-inflammatory properties and for pain. Prednisone also is given if carditis is present. Complete bed rest is maintained until the ESR drops to within normal limits. A throat culture is performed, and if it is positive, the child is treated with antibiotics.

Once a child has been diagnosed as having rheumatic fever, prophylactic penicillin is administered to prevent future occurrences. Penicillin prophylaxis continues until the child is 20 or for five years after the disease, whichever is longer. It can be taken again at any other time that exposure to streptococcal infection is likely (such as during dental work). Penicillin is not effective in treating the cardiac problems; its use is to prevent recurrence by preventing streptococcal infection.

Nursing management Maintenance of bed rest to prevent cardiac complications is a major intervention for a child with ARF. Damage to cardiac connective tissue can lead to mitral valve disease in later life. Because movement is strictly limited, the nurse needs to use ingenuity to present diversionary activities that are interesting, age appropriate, and quiet. School work should be continued, and the child should maintain contacts with family and peers. For some children, strict bed rest is extremely anxiety provoking, placing undue stress on the heart. Occasionally, limited activity will be allowed to minimize anxiety. Nursing interventions are directed toward preventing the hazards of immobility.

Because ARF can result in cardiac damage, parents and children might have undue anxiety. Contact between the nurse and family should encourage verbal expressions of concern. With prompt treatment and proper rest, complications can be minimized.

Juvenile Rheumatoid Arthritis

Juvenile rheumatoid arthritis (JRA) is a relatively common long-term autoimmune disease of the connective tissue. The course of JRA consists of spontaneous exacerbations and remissions. Antigen-antibody complexes lodged in the joints cause joint inflammation. This eventually can lead to joint limitation and subsequent bone destruction. In some cases, circulating antigen-antibody complexes can cause tissue injury in other body systems that contain connective tissue.

JRA can affect children of all ages and affects girls approximately five times as often as boys. It affects children differently, but disease patterns usually have the following three courses:

1. *Monoarticular (pauciarticular)*—30%–40% of cases. Fewer than four joints are affected. Girls tend to develop iridocyclitis (inflammation of the iris and ciliary body). Arthritic symptoms are generally mild with joint stiffness in the morning lessening during the day. Boys demonstrate arthritis in lower extremities. They can develop spondylitis.
2. *Polyarticular*—40%–50% of cases. Greater than four joints are affected. The presence of the rheumatoid factor for IgM indicates a poorer prognosis in this type. Disability can be mild to severe.
3. *Systemic*—20% of cases. Begins with high fever, rash on trunk and extremities, anorexia, and weight loss. Joint involvement occurs later in the disease process. Additionally, there might be carditis, pleurisy, pneumonia severe anemia, and enlargement of the liver. Disability ranges from mild to severe.

The joints usually affected are the knees, wrists, ankles, elbow, and neck. Joint stiffness is worse in the morning or after sitting for a period of time (a condition called the *gel phenomenon*). The prognosis is variable and seems to be worse with an increased level of rheumatoid factor. Many children experience spontaneous remissions within 1–2 years. Others, approximately 30%, continue to have the disease, creating permanent disabilities. Children with these disabilities often have retarded physical growth because of destruction of bone epiphyses.

Clinical manifestations The symptoms of JRA depend somewhat on the number of joints involved and the disease progression. For a suspected diagnosis of JRA, joint limitation, swelling, and pain should be of six weeks duration (Rennebohm and Correll, 1984). Some children initially experience high fever with transitory rash, whereas others complain of vague symptoms including malaise, low-grade fever, irritability, anorexia, and joint pain.

Diagnostic evaluation Hematologic tests are performed to establish the diagnosis. Serum usually reveals leukocytosis and positive antinuclear antibodies. Many children demonstrate an elevated ESR and ASO titer, which can occasionally confuse the diagnosis with ARF. Rheumatoid factor is present in most cases, but it is not specific for rheumatoid arthritis, as positive results are associated with most polyarticular disease.

Radiographs of the joints reveal joint effusion and possible degeneration. Approximately one child in ten will develop iridocyclitis. This is diagnosed by slit-lamp eye examination.

Treatment Treatment of JRA is directed toward pain relief, reduction of inflammation, and prevention of joint contractures. Nonsteroidal anti-inflammatory agents such as tolmetin sodium (Tolectin), indomethacin (Indocin), and naproxen (Naprosyn) might be prescribed, depending on the child's age. Aspirin, however, is used most frequently. Aspirin is given in doses of 80 mg/kg/day. This is high enough to decrease inflammation and to provide analgesic effect, but low enough to avoid toxicity. Salicylate levels are monitored to maintain blood levels of 20–30 mg/dL.

Gold salts sometimes are given, although their therapeutic value in children is questionable. They are given in weekly injections over a period of several months before their therapeutic effects become evident.

Corticosteroids are not ordinarily prescribed because of their serious side effects and also because of their tendency to mask other infections. Corticosteroids, however, are prescribed because of carditis or because other treatment has failed and a massive effort is needed to reduce the inflammatory process.

In addition to drug therapy, a regular program of physical therapy and exercise is ordered. This can include exercise of the joints and applications of heat in various forms, including wax treatments, hot packs, and whirlpool. In some cases immobility of an affected joint is desired. Immobility can be accomplished with either traction or a splint, depending on the joint involved.

Because of the long-term nature of the disease, the family can experience an overwhelming financial burden. If this happens, they might become more susceptible to claims of miraculous cures. Quackery has become a thriving business that directs itself to making money for so-called cures of arthritis. It is the health team's responsibility, and a necessary part of the treatment scheme, to be educated and to educate patients and parents to avoid quick cures. Pamphlets published by the US Government Printing Office and the Arthritis Foundation give objective views about legitimate treatments and list those treatments that are questionable.

Nursing management Nursing care of the child with JRA is multifaceted and challenging. It provides nurses with the opportunity for giving holistic care while excelling as team coordinators. Children might be hospitalized during the diagnostic period or during acute flare-ups. Usually, stress for the child is minimal if the child can be at home participating in as many activities as possible.

Since this condition can result in repeated hospitalizations for the child, continuity of care is vitally important. The principle nursing goal is to prevent complications without restricting the child's normal development. Additionally, the nurse needs to encourage the parent to strike a healthy balance between protection and overprotection. The child's independence and full participation in the therapy is essential for the most positive results.

While the child is hospitalized, interventions are directed toward preventing joint contractures, alleviating pain, and providing emotional support. Teaching parents and children about the expected course of the disease reduces anxiety and stress, which can exacerbate the condition.

Preventing joint contractures A program of exercises will be provided for the child with arthritis. The strenuousness of the exercise regimen increases as the child's condition improves. Both passive and active range-of-motion exercises alleviate morning stiffness. Performance of activities of daily living increases joint mobility. As the child improves and pain decreases, the child can and should exercise daily with enjoyable activities appropriate for developmental level. Activities such as swimming, bicycling, and dancing promote mobility without undue strain on affected joints. Contact sports are avoided.

Occasionally, splinting might be necessary to keep affected joints in proper alignment. Parent and child are taught the proper application of the splint.

Relieving pain Swollen, arthritic joints can be extremely painful. In addition to pharmacologic pain relief, other measures can be taken. Proper positioning in bed promotes comfort and minimizes joint stiffness. The child lies flat in a supine position, or prone. A bed cradle can be used to take the weight of the sheets off the painful joints. Slow, gentle movements are less painful than abrupt movements.

Applications of heat can relieve joint pain. Heat application can be in the form of warm showers or baths, hot moist packs or hydrocollator packs, whirlpool, or warm paraffin application. Occasionally, application of cold is more effective.

Providing emotional support Nurses identify and work with any recognized emotional problems but, more importantly, assist parents to recognize problems and intervene. Parents often have difficulty letting go and encouraging the child to perform at an appropriate developmental level. The concern is that the child will become overtired and precipitate an exacerbation. The opposite extreme, however, is an overprotectiveness that stifles normal development. The nurse then works with parents and children and teaches them to recognize fatigue and limit activity accordingly. The child should be encouraged to exercise moderately. Attention is focused on adequate rest and good nutritional habits. Relief from stress is important to the child's well-being; the nurse therefore teaches stress reduction measures to the child and family.

Discharge preparation When preparing for the child's discharge, the nurse refers the child to a visiting nurse for continuity of care in the home. Parents are taught heat application and physical therapy routines. The Visiting Nurse Association (VNA) might be able to help obtain any needed equipment.

Parents are encouraged to explain to the school teacher what can realistically be expected from the child. The disease has an unpredictable course, and severity of symptoms can vary from day to day. Flexibility is required from all concerned.

The Arthritis Foundation has local chapters in every state and is available as a resource to the public. Parents should be encouraged to contact the Foundation for further information about the disease and its implications for home care.

NURSING CARE PLAN *Child with Juvenile Rheumatoid Arthritis*

Assessment data: Nancy is a 13-year-old girl admitted to the hospital with pain, swelling, and joint limitation to both knees and her right ankle. She has complained of stiffness of her legs in the morning for seven weeks, and she walks with a mild limp that improves during the day. Her serum studies reveal mild leukocytosis, presence of ANA and rheumatoid factor, and a markedly elevated ESR. She is diagnosed as having juvenile rheumatoid arthritis, and a physical therapy evaluation has been ordered. Nancy is due to start a new school in a few weeks, and her parents are concerned that she might have problems if she is not there initially. Her physician will discharge her as soon as she and her parents understand her medical regimen.

Nursing diagnosis	Intervention	Rationale
1. Impaired physical mobility related to pain and stiffness in the joints	Plan a daily program of rest, exercise, and proper positioning.	Moderate exercise is essential for maintaining joint mobility.
	Teach range-of-motion exercises and muscle-strengthening exercises.	Gentle range-of-motion and muscle-strengthening exercises assist with relieving morning stiffness.
	Combine play and exercise with the use of balloons, balls, clay, riding a bicycle, swimming, and dancing.	Making exercise enjoyable will encourage the child to adhere to the daily routine.
	Discuss with Nancy how to monitor participation in any strenuous sport by balancing activity with symptoms.	Avoiding heavy exercise and contact sports is necessary to prevent undue strain on joints.
	Discuss with Nancy and parent the need to pace physical activity with rest and to heed warning signals of fatigue and pain.	Overuse of joints can lead to an exacerbation.
	Warn Nancy and family that sitting or reclining in one position for any extended length of time tends to weaken muscles and stiffen joints.	Maintaining one position for a length of time leads to the "gel phenomenon," or increased muscular stiffness and pain. Adequate rest is essential to prevent or reduce stress.

Outcome: Nancy and her family can describe and demonstrate her daily exercises. Nancy will not experience any permanent effects of limited mobility. Nancy can assess and respond to her own tolerance for activity.

Nursing diagnosis	Intervention	Rationale
2. Alteration in comfort: pain related to joint inflammation and swelling	Discuss use of heat to reduce morning stiffness and relax muscles; suggest taking a warm bath for 20 minutes in the morning; discuss the use of hot packs to relieve discomfort of an isolated joint and remind family of safety precautions.	Heat reduces morning stiffness by relaxing the muscles. The water should not be hot enough to burn.
	Explain to Nancy and family that a splint might be used during times of severe inflammatory response and pain to rest the joint. Remind them that the splint should maintain the joint in a position of function and be comfortable.	Nighttime splints prevent contractures and promote joint function.

(Continues)

NURSING CARE PLAN *Child with Juvenile Rheumatoid Arthritis (Continued)*

Nursing diagnosis	Intervention	Rationale
	Review with Nancy and family the medication regimen of aspirin and its beneficial anti-inflammatory effects.	Aspirin is an anti-inflammatory and analgesic agent that reduces pain and joint inflammation.
	Monitor serum salicylate levels.	The serum salicylate level is carefully controlled to be effectively high, but not high enough to be toxic.
	Observe for and teach Nancy and her family signs and symptoms of aspirin toxicity—headache, dizziness, tinnitus, and confusion.	These are signs of salicylate toxicity.
	Give aspirin with meals or directly after meals.	This reduces gastric irritation.
	Observe carefully for any signs of external hemorrhage, epistaxis, or internal bleeding—decreased blood pressure, increased pulse, restlessness; discontinue aspirin with physician approval at least 48 hours prior to a surgical procedure.	Aspirin prolongs the bleeding time and can cause internal bleeding if given in high doses.

Outcome: Nancy will experience and verbalize relief from pain and joint stiffness. Nancy and her family will describe and demonstrate pain relief measures.

Nursing diagnosis	Intervention	Rationale
3. Potential for ineffective individual coping (stressors: starting a new school, inability to "keep-up" with peers)	Contact the school nurse regarding the physical aspects of the classrooms and how the schedule might be adapted for Nancy to avoid fatigue.	Knowing what to expect in a new situation reduces stress.
	Encourage Nancy to join school and extracurricular activities as a way of keeping involved and meeting new friends.	Joining clubs and school activities promotes normal adolescent development and helps the adolescent cope with meeting peers.
	Encourage Nancy to be independent and to assume responsibility for her care.	Development of independence is a normal task for the adolescent.
	Teach stress relaxation exercises and encourage her to use them at the first indication of stress or anxiety.	Stress can exacerbate the disease by further altering immune function.
	Assist Nancy to express her feelings, fears, and frustrations about the disease and its limitations.	Expression of feelings helps bring things into perspective and reduces fear and anxiety.
	Introduce Nancy to other children who are coping well with the condition; encourage them to share successful coping strategies.	Peer support is important to the adolescent.

Outcome: Nancy will deal appropriately with stressful situations using effective coping strategies. Nancy will describe and demonstrate relaxation techniques to be used to cope with stress. Nancy will adjust easily to her new school.

Nursing diagnosis	Intervention	Rationale
4. Potential for ineffective family coping (stressors: unfamiliarity with the disease process and its prognosis)	Teach the family about Nancy's condition and its probable course; remind them to keep physician appointments and to be aware of any changes in her condition.	Knowledge reduces fear and anxiety and allows the family to be in better control. Follow-up visits are essential to detect changes in condition (such as iridocyclitis) that might not appear for several months.

NURSING CARE PLAN *Child with Juvenile Rheumatoid Arthritis (Continued)*

Nursing diagnosis	Intervention	Rationale
	Discuss with family Nancy's needs to be independent and to engage in the usual age-related activities.	Promoting the child's independence is essential for effective adherence to the medical regimen.
	Encourage family members to verbalize their feelings, anger, frustration, and fears about Nancy and resultant family dynamics.	Verbalizing fears helps to maintain a realistic perspective on the problem and reduces anxiety.
	Suggest support groups for parents that provide education, discussion, referrals for specialized care and financial aid as needed.	Available resources can assist the family to cope with the long-term nature of the child's condition—emotionally and financially.

Outcome: Nancy's family will cope effectively with the chronic nature of Nancy's condition. Nancy's parents can demonstrate effective coping strategies (eg, verbalizing feelings, obtaining appropriate information, contacting a support group).

Systemic Lupus Erythematosus

Systemic lupus erythematosus (SLE) is a complex condition that generally affects women of childbearing age, although the disease is seen frequently in younger girls. Lupus disease is not rare, and 20% of cases affect girls over age 8 (Behrman and Vaughan, 1983). The disease rarely affects boys, the female-to-male ratio being approximately 5 to 1. Less than 30 years ago, SLE was considered to be a fatal disease. Now, with improved approaches, approximately 90% of those affected can achieve a remission of 10 years or longer, although the disease might not be curable.

Lupus affects nearly all body systems and thus is a complex immune system disease. The cause is unknown although several precipitating factors are acknowledged. Disease onset can be triggered by exposure to ultraviolet light, drugs, pregnancy, or stress.

The immune mechanisms are unclear. The triggering event might cause cells to rupture and release their nuclear content, which then becomes antigenic. Autoantibody-antigen complexes lodge in multiple body tissues—skin, joints, heart, lungs, kidneys, brain, and circulatory vessels—and produce on-site inflammatory reactions. Because of an increased incidence in families, theories suggest that a genetic influence might be involved.

The prognosis of patients with SLE is good and is improving as more research is conducted to determine the nature of the disease. The prognosis is, however, related to the involvement of vital organs, particularly the kidneys. Depending upon the location of antigen-antibody complexes in the kidneys, they can be more or less responsive to therapy. Fatalities are due to renal failure.

Clinical manifestations Initial clinical manifestations include fatigue, weight loss, fever, alopecia (hair loss), and joint tenderness. These symptoms might be accompanied by mental or emotional alterations, including headaches and seizures. Erythematous rashes appear. A classic symptom is the butterfly rash that affects both cheeks and the nasal bridge. The symptoms usually seem worse after exposure to the sun. A small percentage of patients experience ongoing Raynaud's phenomenon, which is peripheral vasospasm causing pallor and numbness in fingers and toes in response to exposure to cold or emotional stress.

Later, more severe symptoms related to the body systems affected appear. As the disease progresses, increased systemic involvement might occur. Proteinuria (protein in the urine) is one of the first signs of antigen-antibody complexes in the kidney. Complexes in the lungs cause pleurisy, and cardiac inflammation is detected by ECG or murmurs. Anemia, leukopenia (decreased leukocytes), and a decrease in platelets might occur.

Diagnostic evaluation Because of its similarity to many of the other immune system disorders, the disease can be difficult to diagnose. Laboratory studies can indicate a positive LE cell, decreased complement levels (particularly C_2), positive C-reactive protein, and positive test for syphilis. Any or all of these can be present in other immune system

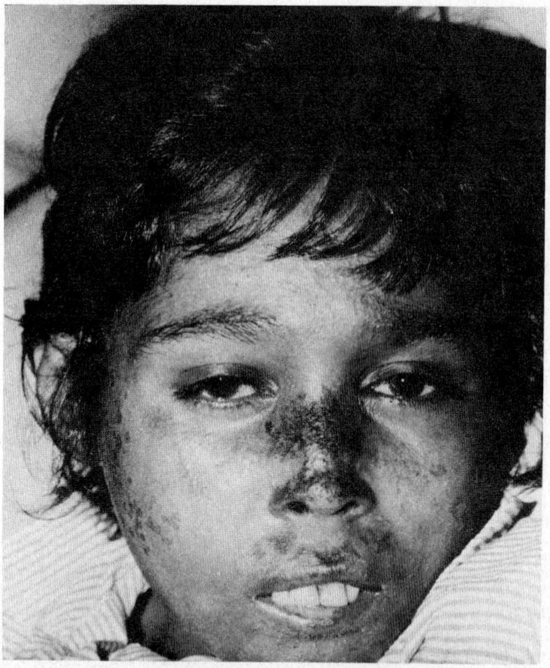

A young girl with a butterfly shaped rash of lupus erythematosis. (From Purtilo DT: A Survey of Human Diseases. *Addison-Wesley, 1978.)*

disorders. The definitive test for a positive diagnosis of SLE is the presence of ANA (antinuclear antibodies) and, more specifically, the anti-DNA antibodies.

Treatment Because disease exacerbation tends to increase during times of sun exposure or stress, treatment is initially directed toward avoiding trigger mechanisms. Girls are encouraged to avoid the sun totally or to apply an effective, high-factor sunscreen during exposure to direct or indirect sunlight. The holistic approach encourages plenty of rest, good nutritional habits, and a positive outlook on life. Infections are treated vigorously.

If arthritis occurs, salicylates are ordered both as anti-inflammatory agents and as pain relievers. The dosage is regulated so that serum levels are maintained at the upper limit of the therapeutic range. Other medications frequently used to treat SLE are antimalarial agents, such as chloroquine, and corticosteroids. Chloroquine is often given in conjunction with steroids to enhance effectiveness and to allow for a reduced steroid dosage. Anticancer drugs, such as methotrexate and nitrogen mustard, have been tried with some success. Their severe side effects can, however, prohibit their use on a general basis.

Careful monitoring of levels of complement, anti-DNA antibody, and antigen-antibody complexes can prevent serious complications by ensuring prompt treatment. Stress can exacerbate the condition. A referral for mental health and emotional counseling is indicated for obvious problems.

Nursing management Nursing care is directed toward maintaining open lines of communication among nurse, client, and family. The nurse follows principles of care for any child with a long-term condition (see Chapter 14). Because stress can adversely affect the child, stress reduction techniques are taught. Promoting adequate rest and proper nutrition is essential.

Because many patients are adolescents, appearance is a major concern. Alopecia can be distressing. The nurse might encourage using a wig and other aids to improve or maintain appearance. Nurses also promote independence and self-care. Medication schedules are planned to coordinate as much as possible with the patient's lifestyle. Adolescents can administer their own medicines and should be taught to recognize undesirable side effects. Some parental control is needed, however, because adolescents might skip doses in the normal spirit of rebellion.

If Raynaud's phenomenon presents a problem, measures to prevent its occurrence should be discussed. When the child expects to be exposed to the cold, layered clothing is the dress of choice. The air space between layers insulates. Mittens are preferable to gloves, and wide-toed boots allow for freedom of toe movement. Mylar or silk gloves and sock liners help retain warmth.

Raynaud's phenomenon occurs in summer as well as in winter, so the child should avoid swimming in cold water. Something as simple as holding an ice cream cone can trigger vasospasm. Simple measures such as wrapping the cone or ice cream stick with paper napkins will alleviate the problem.

If the child cannot participate in normal activities, the nurse attempts to discover areas in which the child can excel while not overextending. Excellence in some areas will foster improved self-image and a more positive outlook on life.

The Lupus Erythematosus Foundation has chapters in many cities and states. It is a helpful resource as it offers support to clients and families and disseminates information to the public for increased public awareness.

Acute Glomerulonephritis

Acute glomerulonephritis (AGN), like ARF, is an autoimmune disease occurring in response to a previous streptococcal invasion. It does resemble an antigen-antibody complex disease, however, since the inflammatory response in the kidneys is related to incomplete clearing of complexes. Unlike ARF, AGN does not necessitate an upper respiratory infection, since the disease can occur as a result of organisms entering through the skin, as in streptococcal impetigo. AGN mainly affects young boys and can occur as close as 3 days after development of an untreated streptococcal infection.

Theories about causes of AGN differ, but researchers generally suspect that antigen-antibody complexes lodge in the Bowman's capsule of the kidney, leading to inflamma- and obstruction. This process causes decreased glomerular filtration. Consequently, less sodium and water are passed to the tubules for reabsorption and excretion. The kidneys enlarge, and sodium and water are retained, leading to edema. Because of the fluid overload, the child can develop congestive heart failure. The kidneys can eventually shut down if the disease is not treated.

Along with the edema, the child can experience hematuria, hypertension, and decreased urinary output. Laboratory tests reveal a high ASO titer, leukocytosis, anemia, increased blood urea nitrogen (BUN), and decreased creatinine. Urinalysis yields increased blood, leukocytes, protein, and cells (see Chapter 28 for treatment and nursing care).

The Child with an Immune Complex Disease

Mucocutaneous Lymph Node Syndrome—Kawasaki Disease

Kawasaki disease affects children of both sexes, although boys predominate. Average age of onset is 4 years. The disease is not contagious and its precipitating factor is unknown. An increase in the ESR and circulating immunoglobulin levels, along with a markedly elevated white blood count ($15-40 \times 10^3$) and an elevated platelet count (above 500,000), points to an inflammatory response of an immune complex disease.

Kawasaki disease affects multiple body systems, predominantly the skin, mucous membranes of the respiratory tract, lymph nodes, and heart. Fatality rate is low, with death being the result of cardiac difficulties, particularly aneurysms. The risk of fatality is greater in boys under 1 year of age.

The syndrome is self-limiting and usually resolves after 3 to 4 weeks. A small percentage of children are left with residual cardiac damage that might not appear until years after the disease onset.

Clinical manifestations Because the symptoms mimic other diseases, criteria have been established for diagnosis. The occurrence of fever plus four of the other five criteria are necessary for positive diagnosis.

Diagnostic criteria for Kawasaki disease are:

1. Fever lasting five or more days
2. Bilateral conjunctival congestion
3. Alterations in the mucous membranes of the mouth and upper respiratory tract such as red, dry, fissured lips, bright red "strawberry" tongue, and inflamed and infected pharyngeal area
4. Edema and erythema of the extremities, peeling of the palms of the hands and soles of the feet, desquamation beginning at the fingertips and tips of the toes
5. Varied type rash on trunk and extremities
6. Cervical lymph node enlargement

Kawasaki disease begins with a high fever, followed by generalized rash, nonpurulent conjunctivitis (inflamed conjunctiva), oral and peripheral changes, and enlarged lymph nodes. Children with the disease are extremely irritable, reminiscent of increased central nervous system pressure. They appear acutely ill. As the disease progresses, they might experience symptoms of arthritis. Cardiac changes appear on ECG.

Diagnostic evaluation Blood work reveals a highly elevated white blood count ($15-40 \times 10^3$). The platelet count is increased above 500,000 after the second week. The increase in platelets causes obstruction of the capillaries in the fingers and toes, resulting in peripheral stasis and necrosis. The ESR is usually elevated, as are immunoglobulins in some cases. Blood tests are negative for ANA and LE cell. ECG monitoring is performed regularly and usually indicated cardiac changes during the acute stage. Desquamation (peeling) of the skin on the fingers, palms, and plantar surfaces occurs during the second week. The ECG usually will revert to normal on disease resolution.

Treatment Treatment is symptomatic. There is no known drug that will enhance recovery or prevent complications. High doses of aspirin are given for anti-inflammatory and analgesic effect and to reduce platelet obstruction of the capillaries. Whether or not aspirin can prevent the occurrence of cardiac sequelae is unclear.

Nursing management Interventions during the acute phase of the disease are directed toward maintaining comfort. Fever control and the promotion of adequate hydration are essential. The nurse gives mouth care to children with oral lesions. Environmental stimuli are reduced to minimize irritability. Supportive care to parents is essential, particularly since the child appears so acutely ill and is at risk for cardiac complications. The nurse observes for changes

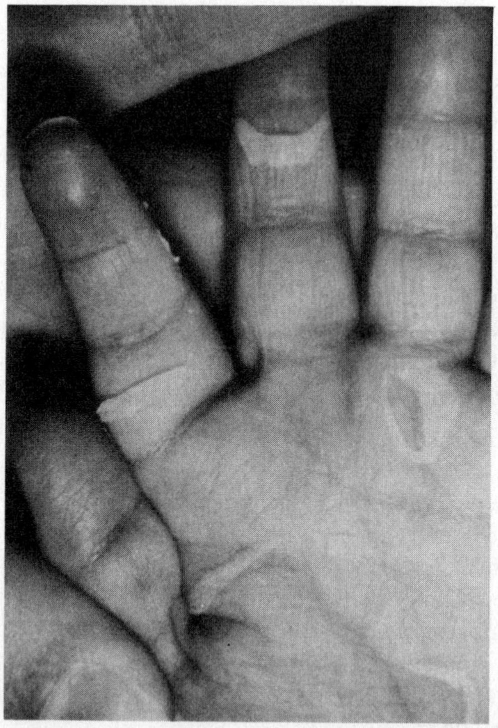

Desquammation of the fingers in a child with Kawasaki disease. (From Pickering L, Dupont H: Infectious Diseases of Children and Adults: A Step-by-Step Guide to Diagnosis and Treatment. *Addison-Wesley, 1986.)*

in vital signs and reports the occurrence of tachycardia or arrhythmias to the physician.

Parents are allowed to express their concerns but can be assured of the child's spontaneous recovery. Discharge preparation emphasizes the need for regular cardiac testing for early recognition of cardiac complications.

Shönlein-Henoch Purpura

Shönlein-Henoch (SH) purpura is a disease that can be precipitated by exposure to medications, infection, or insect bites. It is a relatively common condition affecting children 2–8 years old, with boys being affected twice as often as girls (Behrman and Vaughan, 1983). The immune insult causes an increase in circulatory immune complexes of IgG, which effuse into skin, mucous membranes, joints, and other body systems (*Nursing Mirror*, 1983).

SH purpura is a self-limiting disease that usually resolves in approximately 6 weeks. Full recovery is expected, although the child might experience sudden gastrointestinal complications, intussusception being the most common (see Chapter 27). Occasionally, acute or chronic renal problems develop that mimic glomerulonephritis.

Clinical manifestations The onset of SH purpura can be sudden or gradual. The child might complain of abdominal cramping or nausea. Arthritislike symptoms affect various joints, usually of the lower extremities. Purpuric lesions most often appear on the buttocks and legs, although they can also appear elsewhere. Over the course of the disease the lesions change color from pink to purple, then fade to yellowish brown before disappearing. The child might be febrile.

Diagnostic evaluation Blood studies reveal leukocytosis, elevated ESR, and elevated IgA concentrations. Bleeding and clotting times generally are normal, as are platelet counts. Unless internal bleeding occurs from gastrointestinal or renal complications, hematocrit and hemoglobin also will be within normal range. Urinalysis will demonstrate increased leukocytes and erythrocytes if there is kidney involvement. The stool should be examined for presence of occult blood.

Treatment Treatment is symptomatic. Salicylates are prescribed for pain. The child is observed for gastrointestinal complications and signs of nephritis (inflammation of the renal nephron). Renal involvement usually resolves but might recur later in life as chronic renal disease. Rarely, the child might exhibit signs of central nervous system involvement. Treatment with steroids seems to alleviate this condition.

Nursing management Primary nursing interventions include observation for internal organ involvement. Vital signs, particularly blood pressure, should be performed on a regular basis to detect indications of internal bleeding. The nurse keeps accurate records of intake and output and observes or tests urine and stools for presence of frank or occult blood. A markedly decreased urine output might be indicative of impending renal failure. A careful description of pain will assist the physician to diagnose problems.

If the child experiences any transient arthritis, the nurse emphasizes to the child and parents that this is temporary and will resolve itself. Diversionary activities include range-of-motion activities to exercise joints. If the child is confined to bed, the nurse takes precautions to prevent complications from immobility.

Discharge preparation includes instructions to parents for recognizing signs of renal difficulty. The nurse cautions parents that kidney problems might not appear for many years and that, when old enough, the child should be advised of symptoms. If a drug has been implicated as a possible cause, it should be avoided in the future. Any sign of frank blood in the urine or stool should be immediately reported to the physician. Parents should be encouraged to keep follow-up appointments.

The Child with an Allergic Reaction

An *allergic* reaction is a result of a hyperactive immune system response. *Immediate hypersensitivity* reactions are caused by IgE response to an allergen. The IgE binds to cells causing them to rupture and release chemicals that might have adverse effects on the body, including such symptoms as respiratory distress, skin manifestations, and vascular hypotension and shock. *Delayed hypersensitivity* is caused by a T-cell response to certain allergens, a reaction that occurs usually 48 hours after exposure to the allergen.

Allergic reactions can be local or generalized and they can be immediate or delayed. Initial contact with an allergen does not usually evoke a hypersensitivity response and histamine release. Subsequent exposures, however, will activate histamine release.

Localized Allergic Reactions

Integument Allergic skin manifestations include a variety of rashes, most common of which are eczema, urticaria (hives), and lesions from contact allergens. Pruritis (itching) from any of these can be severe and can cause the child extreme discomfort.

An eczematous rash initially might be dry and red, followed by scaling. If the eczema becomes chronic, skin thickening can occur, causing a leathery appearance. Itching is constant and can be exacerbated by dryness. (Eczema is discussed in Chapter 24.)

Urticaria is caused by the release of histamine. Capillaries in the skin dilate and allow exudation of fluid, causing raised, plaquelike wheals that can be intensely itchy. Hives can differ in size from pinpoint to extremely large. Hives are transitory in nature, appearing, disappearing, and reappearing in various body locations. They can be acute or chronic and are caused by a wide variety of environmental factors, including pressure, heat, cold, food, drugs, and stress. Often, there is no observable cause, and the urticaria resolves spontaneously. Antihistamines are given to reduce the pruritis by decreasing the histamine action.

Contact dermatitis most frequently consists of erythema followed by the appearance of vesicles that, on rupture, form yellowish crusts. Severe cases can involve constant weeping of fluid with subsequent loss of the surface skin layer. Pruritis can be intense.

Allergic skin manifestations can occur singly or in combination with one another, depending on the irritant and the magnitude of the response. Urticaria is also a symptom in systemic allergic responses.

Mucous membranes Allergens can affect the mucous membranes of the eyes and the upper respiratory tract. The membranes become red, edematous, and itchy, with an increase in clear mucous discharge. Rhinitis and conjunctivitis are common examples of eye and upper respiratory allergic manifestations. They often occur together as a result of seasonal pollen and are referred to as hay fever. Frequent sneezing is an initial symptom, followed by itchiness and rhinorrhea. Some children have dark circles under their eyes that do not disappear. This might be an indication that the child is suffering from an inhalant allergy. Edema of nasal passages can cause a sinus headache.

Systemic Allergic Reactions

Gastrointestinal system Histamine causes spasm of the smooth muscles, resulting in gastrointestinal symptoms on contact with an allergen—usually food. Symptoms include abdominal cramping, nausea, vomiting, and diarrhea. In infants, colic is the predominant manifestation.

Respiratory system Lower respiratory tract allergies are complicated by histamine's effect on smooth muscles. Smooth muscle spasm of the bronchioles can cause bronchospasm. Bronchospasm leads to air trapping in the lungs, with a resulting disturbance in oxygenation (asthma). Asthma can be precipitated by a number of irritants, including pollens, molds and mildews, dust, animal dander, foods, environmental temperature changes, and stress. (Asthma is discussed in Chapter 22.)

Vascular system Vasodilatation in the brain can cause migraine headaches. These headaches are severe and are often accompanied by nausea, vomiting, and light sensitivity. Foods have been implicated as precipitating factors, particularly those containing amines such as chocolate, cheese, alcohol, and citrus fruits. Avoidance of a known precipitator will reduce the attacks. Ergotamine, a drug that promotes vasoconstriction, has been effective when given at the onset of an attack of migraine.

Anaphylaxis *Anaphylaxis* is a systemic allergic response to an excessive release of histamine. The response can occur

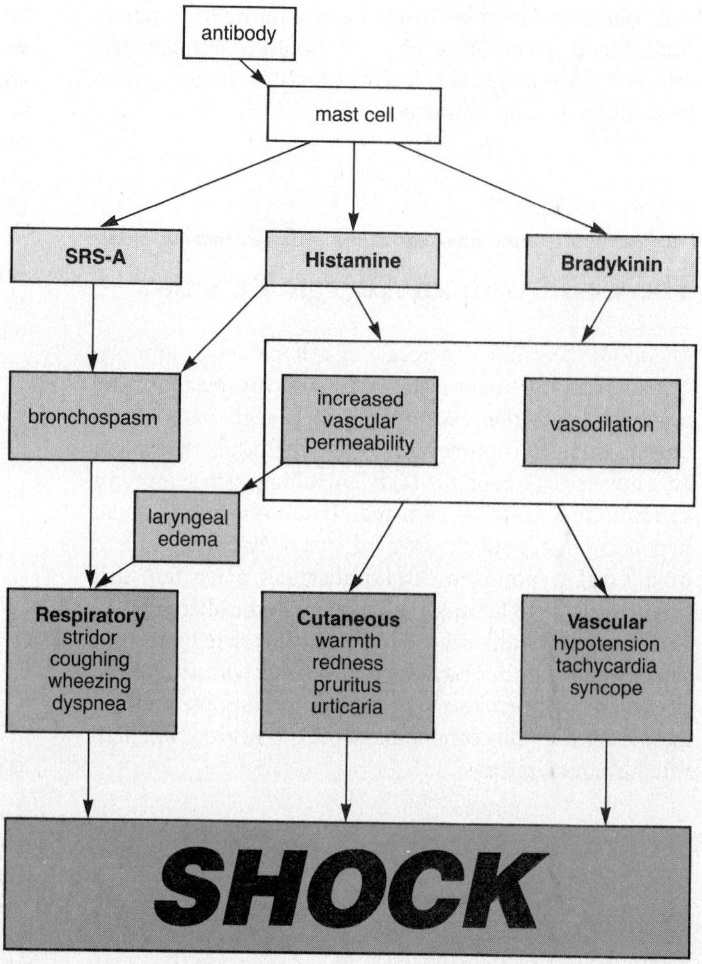

FIGURE 25-2

Mechanisms of anaphylaxis. Anaphylaxis is initiated by antigens interacting with antibodies on the surfaces of mast cells and basophils, which then release certain chemical mediators, such as SRS-A, histamine, and bradykinin. These mediators have profound effects on the pulmonary and vascular systems, resulting in bronchospasm, increased vascular permeability, and laryngeal edema. These physiologic changes in turn produce a variety of respiratory, cutaneous, and vascular signs and symptoms that can be precursors to shock. (From Harmon A, Harmon D: Anaphylaxis—sudden death anytime. Nurs 80 *[Oct 1980; 8:43]. Copyright © 1984, Springhouse Corporation. All rights reserved.)*

suddenly after exposure to an allergen that has not previously evoked a reaction. In addition to histamine, two other chemical mediators affect the magnitude of the response—SRS-A and bradykinin (see Fig. 25-2). Because these do not respond to the administration of antihistamines, the reaction can be severe and life-threatening.

The most common precipitating factors for anaphylaxis are insect stings, penicillin and penicillinlike drugs (particularly when administered intravenously), and foods.

The Child with a Specific Allergic Reaction

Anaphylaxis

Anaphylactic reactions can occur both in and out of the hospital. They are life-threatening, and medical and nursing interventions must be immediate. Initial symptoms of impending anaphylaxis include sneezing, generalized urticaria, weakness, and restlessness. These symptoms might be followed by laryngeal spasms and edema, gastrointestinal symptoms, dyspnea, and signs of circulatory collapse. If the condition is untreated, death occurs from blocked airway and vascular shutdown. Anaphylaxis can occur from seconds to approximately 30 minutes after exposure to an allergen.

Anaphylactic reactions most often occur as the result of an insect sting but can follow administration of certain medications or desensitization injections. Supportive therapy must be administered immediately to prevent shock.

Emergency treatment In case of an insect sting, a tourniquet should be applied just proximal to the sting site, if possible. The tourniquet should be tight, but not tight enough to cut off the circulation to the limb. Immediately afterward, the child should receive 0.1–0.5 mL of 1:1000 aqueous epinephrine subcutaneously, depending on body weight (0.01 mL/kg of body weight). The injection is repeated at 20-minute intervals until help is obtained. The child also is treated for shock by being kept warm and lying flat or with feet slightly elevated. If the child is conscious, nonalcoholic liquids are administered slowly.

In a controlled setting such as a physician's office or hospital, the epinephrine should be followed by diphenhydramine (Benadryl) given intravenously or intramuscularly. An IV is started to maintain a line for fluid replacement in case of shock. The nurse maintains an adequate airway and keeps a tracheostomy kit and a laryngoscope available at the bedside. The nurse monitors vital signs frequently, especially blood pressure, and observes for signs of shock. Should the child appear to have signs of impending circulatory collapse, extra fluids and plasma expanders are given intravenously.

Epinephrine is a drug that causes vasoconstriction. Its effect is rapid but lasts for only a short time. It is given to prevent circulatory collapse and effects this by causing vasoconstriction and resulting increase in cardiac output. Children receiving this drug experience tachycardia and possible heart palpitations. For this reason, the child might be extremely frightened and experience a high degree of anxiety. The nurse can reassure the child that these effects are normal and will eventually disappear.

Desensitization Under some circumstances, allergen desensitization might be indicated. Desensitization might be seasonal or year-round depending on the allergens involved. The procedure involves injecting minute amounts of the allergen subcutaneously to trick the immune system into accepting the allergen. The underlying principle is that by introducing allergens in extremely small quantities the immune system will develop tolerance to it.

Injections are usually given weekly, with gradually increasing allergen concentrations until tolerance is reached. Monthly maintenance doses are then administered. If the child develops a local or systemic reaction, the schedule reverts to the previous concentration that did not produce a reaction. If the procedure provides allergy relief, it is usually discontinued after 2 years.

The child and family need to know about the injections, and they need to understand that the child must remain in the physician's office for at least 20 minutes after each injection to be observed for reactions. The nurse in the office is always alert for signs of anaphylaxis, and epinephrine should be available at all times. Children should wear medic-alert tags if anaphylaxis is a possibility.

Food Allergy

Any food can be allergenic to a specific individual. Frequently seen food irritants include milk, wheat, eggs, citrus fruits, chocolate, nuts, and shellfish. Certain preservatives can induce an allergic response. For infants, all common food allergens are best withheld from the diet until after 6 months of age. Since cow's milk is a common irritant, mothers who have a known allergic history or a familial history of allergies should breast-feed exclusively for at least 6 months before adding foods or milk products. Foods should be added to the baby's diet one at a time and spaced several days apart to observe for an allergic response.

Food allergies take many forms, including rashes, irritation of the gastrointestinal tract, respiratory manifestations, and irritation of the neurologic system (headache, irritability).

Known food allergens such as orange juice and tomatoes might be mixed into commercial baby food preparations either to flavor or to preserve. Parents should be taught to read labels prior to giving their children commercial baby food.

Aside from a milk-free diet, frequently seen special diets might be gluten-free, wheat-free, egg-free, or a combination of all. The dietitian will have resources to recommend for meal planning and books containing recipes. To minimize the "difference" for a child, as much dietary planning as possible should include foods children generally enjoy. Many recipes can be adapted to fit dietary restrictions. For instance, some recipes can be made without eggs by increasing the amount of baking powder and soda used and by adding other spices and flavorings. If recipes call for small amounts of milk, substitute water or juice or soybean baby formulas (White and Owsley, 1983). Many other grain flours which might actually add to the flavor can be substituted for wheat flour in recipes.

Contact Dermatitis

Contact dermatitis is a delayed hypersensitivity reaction that usually doesn't appear until 12–48 hours after exposure to the allergen. It is usually a localized reaction but can be systemic, as seen in contact with plant irritants. Generally, allergens implicated in contact dermatitis are detergents, clothing, cosmetics, and such plants as poison ivy, oak, and sumac. Irritants such as permanents and hair-coloring kits and sunscreens containing para-aminobenzoic acid (PABA) also are implicated.

The immune response to a contact allergen can diminish over the years as long as contact is avoided. Subsequent accidental contact might yield a milder response.

Clinical manifestations The weeping and crusting rash seen in contact dermatitis can be severe and can result in sloughing of the surface skin layer. Poison plant irritants such as ivy, oak, and sumac also can cause severe systemic reactions. The episode usually begins with mild erythema and fluid-filled vesicles at contact sites. Eventually all exposed body areas might become involved. As the reaction continues, the child might exhibit generalized erythema, edema, urticaria, and fluid seepage. Itching is intense. Particularly if the oil has been carried by smoke, the face can be extensively involved, causing periorbital edema. The child might be unable to open the eyes and will be excessively uncomfortable.

Treatment Treatment for mild cases of contact dermatitis involves the administration of antihistamines to control itching and the histaminic release. Additionally, topical drying lotions such as calamine are recommended. Corn starch or baking soda baths might relieve pruritis.

Some over-the-counter preparations of 1/2% hydrocortisone cream can be used for the treatment of contact dermatitis. Pharmacists discourage their use with open skin, however, because of the danger of absorbing the steroid.

Severe and systemic manifestations of dermatitis can be treated with an adrenocortical steroid (glucocorticoid). An initial injection of prednisolone will be followed by oral medication in a tapered-dose schedule, taking approximately 6–7 days to complete. For weeping skin, Burow's compresses are recommended several times a day, although the solution should not be used on the eyes. Again, the child is advised to avoid the allergen.

Nursing management Nursing management for mild cases is similar to that for eczema (see Chapter 24). Children with severe manifestations should be observed for alterations in fluid balance as well as for an impending anaphylaxis. Antihistamines are given for itching. The nurse observes for side effects of steroid administration. Supportive measures are required if the child has severe manifestations. Reassurance should be given that the reaction is self-limiting and usually disappears within 2 weeks. Children treated by systemic steroids demonstrate marked improvement within 48 hours.

Allergy to Bites and Stings

Reactions to stinging insects range from mild to severe depending on the allergic tendency of the child and the frequency of prior exposure. Reactions can become progressively more severe with each sting. Insects most often implicated in allergic reactions are those of the hymenoptera class—bees, yellow jackets, wasps, and hornets. Bees leave a stinger, the rest bite.

Symptoms of allergic sting reactions can range from mild to severe. Normal response to a sting includes erythema, the presence of a small wheal, and itching. The reaction subsides in a matter of hours. A more severe reaction includes localized swelling and erythema extending out from the sting site. Systemic reactions might include anaphylactic shock. Some children also might experience a delayed toxic reaction.

The pain from stings can be relieved with applications of meat tenderizer in paste form. Unless the stinger is removed carefully, the toxin can remain active at the site, increasing the severity of the reaction. The stinger is removed by scraping it out horizontally. Removing a stinger with tweezers can be harmful because the pressure might force the venom from the sac into the child's skin. The nurse observes the child for manifestations of systemic reaction and institutes measures to treat anaphylaxis if necessary.

The nurse teaches the child and the family measures to decrease exposure to stinging insects. Shoes or sneakers should be worn when the child is outdoors. If hiking, long pants and long sleeves are advisable, and the child should avoid bright-colored clothing and perfumes or scented cosmetics.

Sting kits are produced by a variety of manufacturers, and all include a tourniquet, injectible epinephrine, and an antihistamine or sublingual isoproterenol hydrochloride (Isuprel). A child who has had a systemic reaction to an insect sting should have a kit available when outdoors and should be taught to use the kit appropriately.

Essential Concepts

- The human body has a network of defenses to keep it intact and free from disease.
- The major functions of the immune system are to defend the body against invasion by pathogenic agents such as bacteria, viruses, parasites, and toxins.
- Alterations in immune system function include immune deficiency diseases, autoimmune diseases, antigen-antibody complex diseases, allergy, and cancer.
- Immune deficiency diseases affect both cellular and humoral response, causing decreased resistance to infection and malignancy.
- Autoimmune diseases involve a lack of recognition of "self," and overproduction of antibodies destructive to normal tissue.
- Immune complex diseases result from trapping complexes in body systems and subsequent inflammatory response.

- Allergy is a hyperactive immune response to an allergen that causes hypersensitivity reaction in various body systems.
- Assessment of the child with an immune system dysfunction includes history, physical examination, and laboratory studies.
- Acute-care needs of the child with immune system dysfunction include administering pain relief, preventing the hazards of immobility, maintaining intact integument, and protecting from infection.
- Medications common to children with immune system disorders include salicylates, antihistamines, and corticosteroids.
- Children with immune system disorders might need a diet with increased protein or a special allergy diet.
- Emotional needs include adjustment to chronic disease, reduction of stress, promotion of independence, and adjustment to the life-threatening nature of some conditions.
- Some complications of immune system disorders do not manifest themselves until years later, and parents are encouraged to provide regular medical care.
- Immune deficiency diseases include AIDS, agammaglobulinemia, and Wiskott-Aldrich syndrome.
- Autoimmune diseases include acute rheumatic fever, juvenile rheumatoid arthritis, systemic lupus erythematosus, and acute glomerulonephritis.
- Immune complex diseases include Kawasaki disease and HS purpura.
- Allergic reactions can be local or generalized, immediate or delayed.
- Local reactions affect skin and mucous membranes. Systemic reactions affect most other body systems.
- Anaphylaxis is a sudden occurrence of vascular collapse due to a massive release of histamine.
- Allergic irritants include environment, food, insects, and medications.
- Common food allergies are to milk, eggs, and wheat, and dietary modifications might be made for each.
- Stress reduction and relaxation techniques can alleviate and prevent the allergic response.
- Specific allergic manifestations in children include anaphylaxis, food allergies, contact dermatitis, sting allergy, eczema, and asthma.

References

Behrman RE, Vaughan BC: *Nelson Textbook of Pediatrics*. 12th ed. Saunders, 1983.

Center for Disease Control: Acute rheumatic fever—Utah. *MMWR* (March 6) 1987; 36(8): 108–115.

Jackson MM, McPherson DC: Infection control: Keeping current. *Nurse Educator* (Jul/Aug) 1986; 11(4): 38–40.

National Dairy Council: Nutrition and the immune response. *Dairy Council Digest* (Mar/Apr) 1985; 56(2): 7–12.

Nursing Mirror, May 25, 1983 (inside back cover).

Nuscher R et al.: Bone marrow transplantation. *Am J Nurs* (Jun) 1984; 84(6): 764–772.

Rennebohm R, Correll J: Comprehensive management of juvenile rheumatoid arthritis. *Nurs Clin North Am* (Dec) 1984; 19(4): 647–662.

Thompson SW, Gietz KR: Acquired immune deficiency syndrome in children. *Pediatr Nurs* (Jul/Aug) 1985; 11(4): 278–280.

White J, Owsley V: Helping families to cope with milk, wheat, and soy allergies. *Matern-Child Nurs* (Nov/Dec) 1983; 8(6): 423–428.

Additional Readings

Abeles M et al.: Systemic lupus erythematosus in the younger patient: Survival studies. *J Rheumatol* (Jul/Aug) 1980; 7: 515–522.

Ammann A et al: Antibodies to AIDS-associated retrovirus distinguish between pediatric primary and acquired immunodeficiency diseases. *JAMA* (June 7) 1985; 253(21): 3116–3118.

Banwell B: Exercise and mobility in arthritis. *Nurs Clin North Am* (Dec) 1984; 19(4): 605–616.

Bennett JA: AIDS epidemiology update. *Am J Nurs* (Sept) 1985; 85(9): 968–972.

Bennett JA: HTLV III AIDS link. *Am J Nurs* (Oct) 1985; 85(10): 1086–1089.

Boland MG, Klug RM: AIDS: The implications for home care. *Matern Child Nurs* (Nov/Dec) 1986; 11(6): 404–411.

Buckley R: Immunodeficiency diseases. In: *Textbook of Rheumatology*. Kelley W et al. (editors). Saunders, 1981.

Campbell VG: Cover gowns for newborns infection control. *Matern Child Nurs* (Jan/Feb) 1987; 12(1):54.

Chipps B et al.: Diagnosis and treatment of anaphylactic reactions to hymenoptera stings in children. *J Pediatr* (Aug) 1980; 97:177–184.

Decker MD, Schaffner W: Risk of AIDS to health care workers. *JAMA* 1986; 256(3):3264–3265.

Groenwald S: Physiology of the immune system. *Heart Lung* 1980; 9:645–650.

Harmon A, Harmon D: Anaphylaxis—sudden death anytime. *Nurs '80* (Oct) 1980; 10:40–43.

Hood L et al.: *Immunology,* 2nd ed. Benjamin Cummings, 1984.

Hughes RB, Barley FK: AIDS from a school health perspective. *Pediatr Nurs* (May/June) 1987; 13(3):155–156.

Infection control guidelines. *Am J Nurs* (Feb) 1986; 86(2):12.

Kemp D: Development of the immune system. *Crit Care Q* 1986; 9(1):1–6.

Klug RM: Children with AIDS. *Am J Nurs* (Oct) 1986; 86(10):1126–1132.

Levine C (ed): AIDS: Public health and civil liberties. *Hastings Center Report* (Dec) 1986; 1–36.

Lewis E, Roberts J: Is autoimmunity a common denominator in immune complex diseases? *Lancet* (Jan 26) 1980; 1:178–180.

Lifson AR et al.: National surveillance of AIDS in health care workers. *JAMA* 1986; 256(3):3231–3234.

Lind M: The immunologic assessment: A nursing focus. *Heart Lung* 1980; 9(4):658–661.

Lindgren P: The laminar airflow room. *Nurs Clin North Am* (Sept) 1983; 18(3):553–561.

L'Orange C, Werner-McCullough M: Kawasaki disease: New threat to children. *Am J Nurs* (Apr) 1983; 83(4):558–562.

Lynch M, Gray J: Kawasaki disease. *Pediatr Nurs* (Mar/Apr) 1982; 8:96–101.

Medicus L: Kawasaki disease: What is this puzzling childhood illness? *Heart Lung* 1987; 16(1):55–59.

The new immunology: Helping the body heal itself. *Am J Nurs* (April) 1987; 87(4):455–473.

Neuberger G: The role of the nurse with arthritis patients on drug therapy. *Nurs Clin North Am* (Dec) 1984; 19(4):593–603.

Parker C: Food allergies. *Am J Nurs* (Feb) 1980; 80(2):262–265.

Patterson R: *Allergic Diseases—Diagnosis and Management.* Lippincott, 1980.

Pickering LK, DuPont HL: *Infectious Diseases of Children and Adults.* Addison-Wesley, 1986.

Schulman I: Idiopathic (immune) thrombocytopenic purpura in children: Pathogenesis and treatment. *Pediatr Rev* (Dec) 1983; 5(6):173–178.

Sherlock M et al.: Caring for the AIDS patient fearlessly. *Nurs 83* (Sept) 1983; 13(9):50–55.

Smith S: Physiology of the immune system. *Crit Care Q* 1986; 9(1):7–13.

Steinberg A: Management of SLE. In: *Textbook of Rheumatology.* Kelley W et al (editors). Saunders, 1981.

Taylor DL: Immune response. *Nurs 84* (May) 1984; 14:52–54.

Taylor DL: Anaphylaxis. *Nurs 84* (Jun) 1984; 14:44–45.

Thomas PA et al: Unexplained immunodeficiency in children. *JAMA* (Aug 3) 1984; 252:639–644.

Tortora GJ, Funke BR, Case CL: Specific defenses of the host: Immunology. Pages 396–433 in: Tortora GJ, Funke BR, Case CL.: *Microbiology: An Introduction.* Benjamin/Cummings, 1982.

Treating pateints with AIDS. *Health Affairs* 1984; 16: 16–18.

US Department of Health and Human Services: *Understanding the Immune System.* NIH 84–529, 1983.

US Task Force on Immunity and Disease: *Immunology.* US Department of Health and Human Services; NIH 80–940, 1980.

Vick R: *Contemporary Medical Physiology.* Addison-Wesley, 1984.

Chapter 26

Hematologic Composition

Implications of Altered Blood Elements

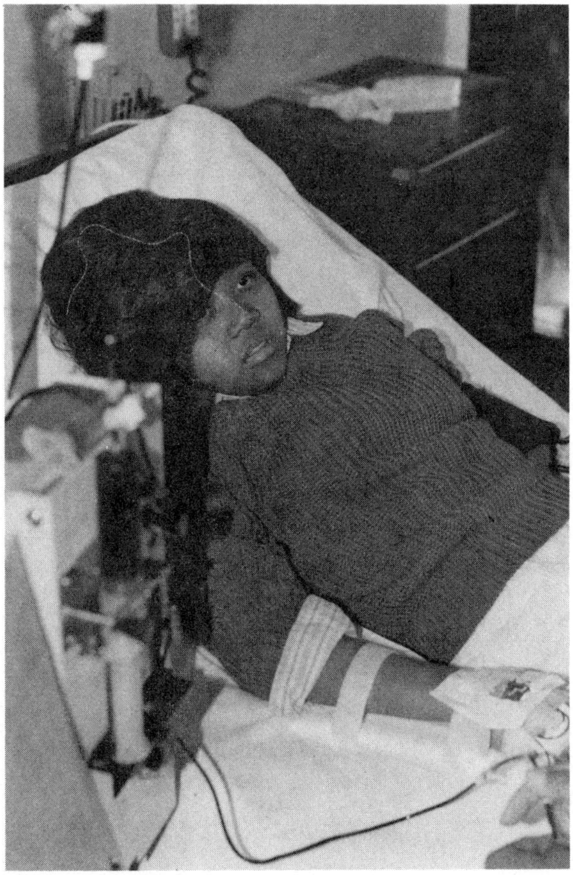

Chapter Contents

(Continues)

Cross Reference Box

To find these topics, see the following chapters:

Autoimmune disorders	Chapter 25
Epistaxis	Chapter 18
Hemorrhage	Chapter 12
Leukemia	Chapter 33

Objectives

- Describe the chief function of blood elements.
- Identify the laboratory tests (hematologic studies) used in the diagnosis of (1) anemias, (2) sickle cell disease and trait, and (3) clotting disturbances.
- List the topics most relevant to the history of a child with a hematopoietic disorder.
- Describe by body system the signs and symptoms that might be found in the physical examination of a child with (1) an anemic disorder and (2) a clotting disturbance.
- Describe the nurse's responsibilities regarding preparation for diagnostic tests, administration of blood transfusions, and bone marrow aspiration.
- Describe the principles of nursing care related to infection control and nutrition for the child with hematopoietic dysfunction.
- Compare and contrast the treatment and nursing management of children with red blood cell disorders (the anemias) and platelet disorders (clotting disturbances).

ESSENTIALS OF STRUCTURE AND FUNCTION

The Hematopoietic System

Blood consists of two components. The first component is the liquid, or plasma, portion, which contains proteins, carbohydrates, lipids, electrolytes, pigments, clotting factors, immunoglobulins, and many other substances. The second component is the cellular portion, which includes erythrocytes, leukocytes, and thrombocytes. All of these are descended from identical precursor cells (stem cells) in the bone marrow, which evolve and differentiate.

Glossary

Erythrocytes Red blood cells, which are circular and biconcave in shape, are used primarily by the body to transport oxygen and carbon dioxide. They give blood its color. Erythrocytes are produced in the marrow of short, flat bones and in the spleen and liver of the fetus and neonate (see figure showing erythrocyte formation).

Fetal hemoglobin (HbF) Has the ability to carry a larger amount of oxygen than HbA. Cells containing HbF are replaced by those containing HbA beginning shortly after birth.

Fibrinogen A protein dissolved in plasma that is converted to a threadlike filament (fibrin) necessary for clot formation. The conversion from fibrinogen to fibrin is prompted by actions of thrombin via blood coagulation factors (see figure showing hemostasis, coagulation).

Hematocrit Concentration of erythrocytes in a measured sample of blood. The level of hematocrit assists with determining the oxygen-carrying capacity of the blood.

Hemoglobin (HbA) Molecules located in each erythrocyte that combine with oxygen and carbon dioxide for transport to and from body tissues. The hemoglobin molecule contains protein structures and four nonprotein structures (hemes), each containing an iron atom (Fe^{2+}) as part of its structure. Each Fe^{2+} combines with one molecule of oxygen. For effective oxygen transport the body needs sufficient iron.

Leukocytes Nucleated cells whose primary function is to protect the body against infection.

Plasma Comprised of water (90%), dissolved proteins [albumin, fibrinogen (needed for clotting), immunoglobulins (antibodies)], electrolytes, hormones, gases (O_2 and CO_2), and metabolized products of digestion.

Thrombocytes (Platelets) Tiny nonnucleated elements of blood that assist with blood clotting (coagulation). Platelets trigger the release of coagulation factors (numbered I to XIII) that produce thrombin.

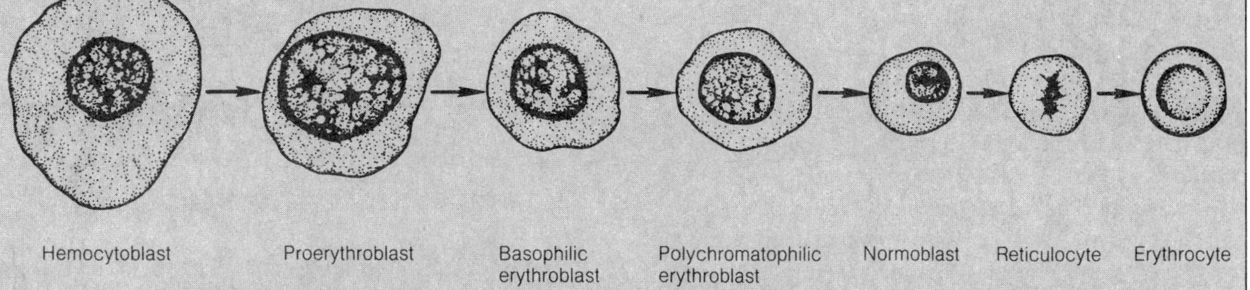

The process of erythrocyte formation is called erythropoiesis. Precursor cells become more mature as their concentration of hemoglobin increases. An inadequate supply of oxygen to the body stimulates kidney release of erythropoietin, a substance that stimulates erythrocyte production. Increased oxygen in the blood results in decreased erythropoietin and decreased erythrocyte production. (From Spence AP, Mason EB: Human Anatomy and Physiology, *3rd ed. Addison-Wesley, 1984.)*

(Continues)

ESSENTIALS OF STRUCTURE AND FUNCTION *(Continued)*
The Hematopoietic System

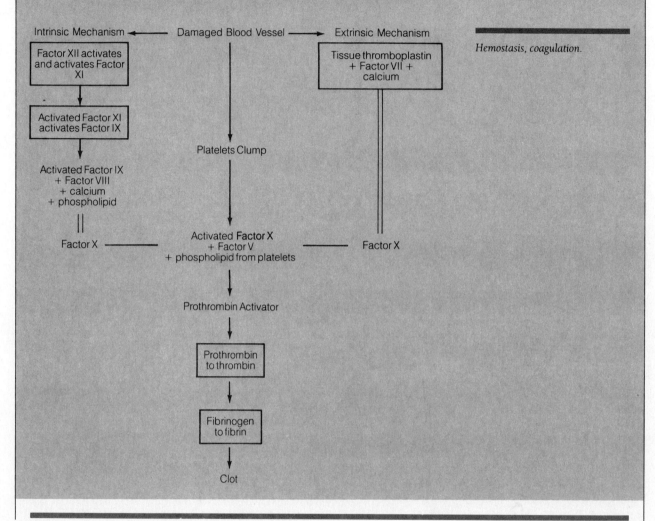

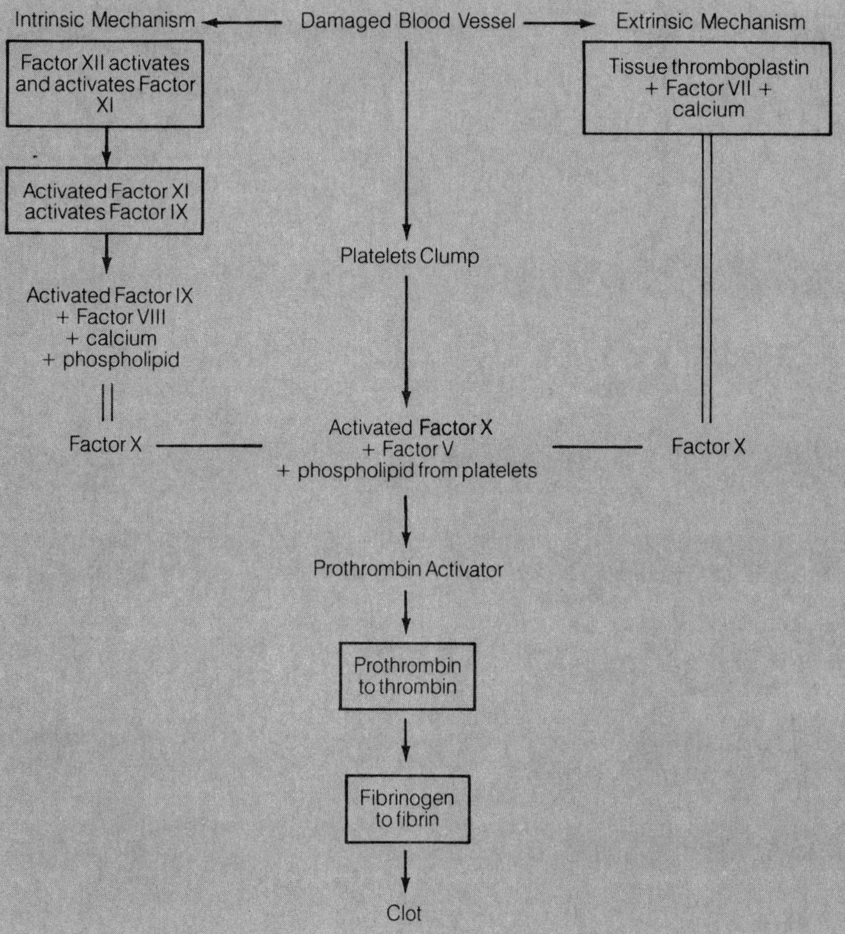

Hemostasis, coagulation.

Disorders associated with alterations of blood elements affect the function of erythrocytes (red blood cells), thrombocytes (platelets), leukocytes (white blood cells), or plasma. (Alterations in leukocytes are discussed in Chapter 25.) Alterations affecting erythrocytes reduce the oxygen-carrying capacity of the blood, causing anemia and its associated manifestations in the child. Alterations in thrombocytes can result in bleeding, either through a decrease in circulating platelets or through diminished platelet adhesiveness. A decrease in plasma levels of clotting factors also can result in prolonged bleeding. Regardless of the disease, children affected by disorders of hematologic composition require comprehensive nursing care that focuses on preventing complications and maintaining an optimal level of health.

Assessment of the Child with Hematopoietic Dysfunction

In assessing the child with *hematopoietic dysfunction* (alteration in the formation of blood cells), the nurse seeks data relevant to the suspected or diagnosed disorder. In anemia, for example, the nurse assesses the clinical manifestations of hypoxia (low tissue oxygenation). In clotting disorders, such as hemophilia, the nurse assesses the causes and effects of bleeding episodes. Assessment of the child with white blood cell disorders is described in Chapters 25 and 33.

ASSESSMENT GUIDE *The Child with a Problem Affecting Hematologic Function*

Assessment questions	Supporting data
Does the child appear pale, lethargic, fatigued, dizzy, or irritable? Does the child complain of numbness or tingling in the fingers and toes?	Decreased exercise tolerance; pale, possibly jaundiced skin; tachypnea, dyspnea, and increased respiratory effort (secondary to hypoxia); tachycardia, cardiomegaly, eventual congestive heart failure; edema (particularly of the hands and feet); decreased hemoglobin and hematocrit, altered erythrocyte indices, elevated bilirubin (see Table 26-1)
Is there a family history of anemia?	Positive sickle cell slide prep, abnormal bone marrow, presence of target cells
Does the child exhibit any signs of bruising, bleeding, or excessive skin discolorations? Is there a family history of clotting disorders?	Epistaxis (nosebleeds); petechiae (resemble flea bites), ecchymoses, hematomas, purpura; signs of circulatory collapse (decreased blood pressure, increased pulse, pallor, thirst); prolonged bleeding after surgery or trauma; occult blood in stool or urine; joint pain, swelling, and limitation; altered platelet count, coagulation factor levels, clotting times, and fibrinogen level (see Table 26-1)

Additional data: Exposure to drugs, radiation, chemicals; history of severe systemic disease such as leukemia or lupus erythematosus; protruding abdomen with splenomegaly; delayed growth

History

A comprehensive history of the child and family is essential to determine nursing diagnoses and interventions for children with hematopoietic alterations. Special emphasis is given to (1) a familial history of hereditary diseases; (2) adequacy of the child's diet, including dietary patterns; (3) history of chronic or recurring infections; (4) possible exposure to insecticides or any other toxic agents; and (5) physical activity and exercise tolerance. The family's cultural background and socioeconomic level also are noted since some blood disorders are linked to heredity, race, or place of birth.

Physical Examination

The child with anemia *Anemia* (deficiency in erythrocytes, hemoglobin, or both) alters the oxygen-carrying capacity of the blood. Anemia can be caused by excessive destruction or loss of erythrocytes, nutritional alterations, or genetic malformations of red blood cells. Many of the symptoms associated with anemia are related to the decrease in tissue oxygenation that it causes.

Anemias are classified according to the size of the red blood cells and their color or to the relative amount of hemoglobin. Anemias might be *microcytic* (undersized erythrocytes), *macrocytic* (oversized erythrocytes), or *normocytic* (normal in size). Anemias also might be *hypochromic* (decreased color) or *normochromic*.

Anemia results in a wide range of symptoms, depending on its severity and duration. Regardless of the cause of the anemia, the symptoms are similar. Typically, the child's skin looks waxy and pale. Hemoglobin and hematocrit levels are decreased as are the total red blood cells and reticulocytes. Erythrocyte indices (MCV, MCH, and MCHC in Table 26-1), which determine the volume and hemoglobin content of red blood cells, are altered, depending on the cause of the anemia. If the liver cannot keep up with the processing of by-products of erythrocyte destruction, bilirubin levels in the blood rise, giving the skin a yellow cast. When examining skin color in patients with dark skin, the nurse looks for pallor of the palms of the hands, mucous membranes, and conjuctivas and for yellow scleras (icteric scleras).

Anemic hypoxia affects the cardiovascular and respiratory systems. Decreased tissue oxygenation stimulates an increase in respiratory and heart rates in an attempt to increase the supply of oxygen to the tissues. Eventually, *cardiomegaly* (enlargement of the heart) and *dyspnea* (difficult or labored breathing) occur. If abnormally high heart and respiratory rates continue, congestive heart failure can develop because the efficiency of the heart muscle decreases when the fibers are stretched. Most children with anemia experience weakness and become fatigued easily. Anemic

TABLE 26-1 Normal Values, Alterations, and Clinical Significance of Hematologic Tests

Test	Normal values*		Alteration/clinical significance
Red blood cell count (RBC)	 Newborn (1–3 da) Neonate (1–4 wk) Infant (1–18 mo) Child (2–12 yr) Adolescent Male Female	*(M/μL)* 4.0–6.6 3.0–6.3 2.7–5.4 3.9–5.3 4.5–5.3 4.1–5.1	*Increased:* Anoxia, hemoconcentration, strong emotions can cause a temporary increase *Decreased:* Chronic infections; see hemoglobin and hematocrit alterations
Mean corpuscular volume (MCV) Average or mean volume of a single RBC; $MCV = \frac{Hct}{RBC}$	 Newborn (1–3 da) Infant (0.5–2 yr) Child (6–12 yr) Adolescent Male Female	*(μm^3)* 95–121 70–86 77–95 78–98 78–102	*Increased:* Macrocytic anemias including acute blood loss, hemolytic anemia, Down's syndrome *Decreased:* Microcytic anemias including iron deficiency anemia, thalassemia
Mean corpuscular hemoglobin (MCH) Average or mean quantity, by weight, of Hgb in a single RBC; $MCH = \frac{Hgb}{RBC}$	 Newborn (1–3 da) Neonate (1–4 wk) Infant (2–24 mo) Child (2–12 yr) Adolescent	*(pg/cell)* 31–37 28–40 23–35 24–33 25–35	*Increased* and *decreased:* See MCV alterations
Mean corpuscular hemoglobin concentration (MCHC) Average concentration of Hgb in a single RBC: $MCHC = \frac{Hgb}{Hct}$	 Newborn (1–3 da) Neonate (1–2 wk) Infant (1–24 mo) Child/Adolescent	*(% HB/cell)* 29–37 28–38 29–37 31–37	*Increased:* Severe and prolonged dehydration *Decreased:* Microcytic, hypochromic anemias (with decreased MCV) including iron deficiency, thalassemia, overhydration
Hemoglobin (Hgb)	 Newborn (1–3 da) Infant (2 mo) Child (6–12 yr) Adolescent Male Female	*(g/dL)* 14.5–22.5 9.0–14.0 11.5–15.5 13.0–16.0 12.0–16.0	*Increased:* Extracellular fluid volume deficit (signs of isotonic dehydration include acute weight loss, thirst, fatigue, dry mucous membranes, poor skin turgor, dry skin, absence of tears, sunken and soft eyeball, oliguria, anuria, longitudinal furrows on tongue) Transient exposure to high altitude *Decreased:* Anemia (signs include weakness, tachycardia, dizziness, dyspnea, cardiac failure, coma) Extracellular fluid volume excess (signs of isotonic overhydration include acute weight gain; no thirst; increase in pulse and blood pressure; polyuria; periorbital edema; signs of congestive heart failure—diaphoresis; signs of pulmonary edema—rales, dyspnea, cough; signs of cerebral edema—bulging, tense fontanelle in infant, convulsions, coma)

TABLE 26-1 (Continued)

Test	Normal values*		Alteration/clinical significance
Hematocrit (Hct)		(%)	*Increased:* Hemoconcentration (eg, from shock, surgery, severe burns, vomiting or diarrhea) *Decreased:* Anemia, hemodilution, leukemia
	Newborn (1–3 da)	44–75	
	Infant (2 mo)	28–42	
	Child (6–12 yr)	35–45	
	Adolescent		
	Male	37–49	
	Female	36–46	
Reticulocyte count The number of immature red blood cells		(%)	*Increased:* Sickle cell anemia, thalassemia major, chronic hemorrhage *Decreased:* Untreated iron deficiency and megaloblastic anemia, aplastic anemia
	Newborn (1 da)	3.2±1.4	
	Neonate (1–4 wk)	0.6±0.3	
	Infant (5–12 mo)	0.3–2.2	
	Adults	0.5–1.5	
Platelet count Number of platelets in 1 μL (mm^3) of blood	Newborn	84,000–478,000	*Increased:* Acute blood loss, iron deficiency anemia, trauma (surgery, fractures), altitudes, excitement, splenectomy *Decreased:* Acute lymphocytic leukemia, severe burns, septicemia, aplastic anemia, bone marrow depressant medications, incompatible blood transfusion
	Thereafter	150,000–400,000	
Bleeding time Amount of time it takes for bleeding from small superficial wound to stop	Newborn	1–8 min	*Increased:* Aspirin intake, coagulation disorders, acute leukemia, infectious mononucleosis, hypothyroidism
	Thereafter	1–6 min	
Whole blood clotting time Amount of time it takes for blood to clot in a glass tube	All ages	5–8 min	*Increased:* Clotting factor deficiencies, anticoagulant medications, leukemia, pneumonia, vitamin K deficiency
Prothrombin time (PT) Amount of time it takes for blood to clot after thromboplastin and calcium chloride are added to blood plasma. Detects deficiencies of Factors V, VII, and X, fibrinogen, and prothrombin	Newborn	< 17 s	*Increased:* Clotting factor deficiencies, vitamin K deficiency, anticoagulant medications, antibiotic therapy, coagulation disorders *Decreased:* Barbiturates, digitalis, and diuretic therapy, pulmonary embolism, oral contraceptives
	Thereafter	11–15 s	
Partial prothrombin time (PTT) A clotting test that measures activity of thromboplastin. Detects various factor deficiencies	Newborn	< 90 s	*Increased:* Anticoagulant therapy, deficiencies of clotting factors and vitamin K *Decreased:* Extensive cancer, after acute hemorrhage
	Thereafter		
	Nonactivated	60–85 s	
	Activated	25–35 s	
Thromboplastin generation time (TGT) Measures the blood's ability to generate thromboplastin. Distinguishes between Factor VIII and IX deficiencies	Newborn	8–20 s	*Increased:* Platelet deficiency, clotting factor deficiencies, anticoagulant medications
	Thereafter	8–16 s	
Fibrinogen level Measures fibrinogen levels in the blood	Newborn	125–300 mg/dL	*Increased:* Inflammatory conditions, pneumonia *Decreased:* Acute leukemia, severe hemorrhage or burns, severe liver damage
	Thereafter	200–400 mg/dL	

*Normal values can vary depending on laboratory method used.

hypoxia might cause dizziness, headache, irritability, decreased temperature tolerance, and tingling of the fingers and toes.

As red blood cells die and are removed by the spleen, the spleen enlarges, causing the child's abdomen to protrude. As the spleen invades the abdominal cavity, it pushes against other organs and against the diaphragm, resulting in further respiratory difficulties. Gastrointestinal symptoms of splenic enlargement include *anorexia* (loss of appetite), indigestion, pain, and frequently recurring diarrhea or constipation.

The child with clotting disturbances Disturbances of coagulation can be caused by a decrease in circulating platelets (thrombocytopenia) or by altered levels of clotting factors. Discolorations of the skin are characteristic signs of an alteration in the normal clotting mechanism. The nurse observes the skin for *petechiae* (small, purplish hemorrhagic spots that resemble flea bites); *ecchymoses* (bruises); and *hematomas* (tumors or swollen areas that contain blood).

If the child is bleeding at the time of the physical examination, blood pressure, heart rate, and respiratory status are monitored closely as are platelet levels. Prompt treatment is necessary during active bleeding episodes to avoid hypovolemic shock and other destructive results of frequent bleeding episodes.

The nurse observes the range of motion of all extremities. Loss of joint mobility might result from bleeding into joints and muscles or from disuse due to fatigue (as in anemia). The nurse notes how well the child is able to move each joint through its full range of motion and determines the need for assessment by a physical therapist.

Nursing Management for Procedures and Treatments

Preparation for Diagnostic Tests

The child undergoing diagnosis and treatment for specific diseases endures a multitude of tests and procedures. Evaluation of erythrocyte indices and other blood values often requires multiple venipunctures or finger sticks. The nurse explains all procedures completely to the child beforehand at the child's level of understanding. It is essential that the nurse or someone not involved in carrying out the procedure be with the child to provide emotional support. Holding the young child during and after the procedure increases comfort and security. The nurse might only need to hold the older child's hand to give emotional support. Infants and younger children might need to be properly restrained. Older children should participate in procedures if possible. This helps them to feel involved in their own care. Allowing the child to handle the equipment to be used in the procedure also decreases fear and anxiety.

Administration of Blood and Blood Products

Typing and cross-matching Medical therapy for hematopoietic dysfunction might include transfusions of whole blood or blood products to replace deficient blood components. No transfusion is without risk. The nurse caring for a child receiving a transfusion needs to be alert for the signs and symptoms of a reaction. Table 26-2 summarizes three of the major transfusion reactions.

Prior to giving a transfusion, the patient's blood and the donor's blood are typed and cross-matched as to group (A, B, AB, or O) and Rh factor (positive or negative). Blood-typing and cross-matching decrease the risk that the patient's and the donor's blood might be incompatible. Typing for HLA (histocompatibility locus antigen, which is present in lymphocytes) also might be done, especially if the patient requires repeated transfusions.

If blood is mismatched (a different blood group between donor and recipient or a different Rh factor), red blood cells clump together (agglutinate) and might occlude the blood vessels. Eventually, *hemolysis,* the destruction of red blood cells, decreases blood volume and causes the patient to go into shock. The patient then requires treatment to replace blood volume and avoid kidney shutdown.

Nursing considerations The nurse who is administering transfusions has many responsibilities besides watching for signs and symptoms of a reaction. Blood decomposes if it is exposed to room temperature for more than 4 hours, so the nurse stores it in a blood-storage refrigerator until it is needed. Intravenous medications are not routinely administered during the transfusion. If it is necessary to give a medication, the nurse stops the transfusion, flushes the intravenous line with normal saline, administers the medication, flushes the line again with normal saline, and then resumes the transfusion. If microaggregate filters are used, they must be changed every 2–4 hours according to directions.

Bone Marrow Aspiration

Bone marrow aspiration might be done to establish a diagnosis and is necessary when aplastic anemia (anemia from bone marrow failure) or leukemia (cancer of the blood-forming tissue) is suspected. In most red blood cell dysfunctions, only the initial aspiration is necessary. In the

TABLE 26-2 Transfusion Reactions and Nursing Interventions

Reaction	Cause	Symptom	Nursing intervention
Allergic (hypersensitivity)	Introduction of donor's allergens into recipient's blood (recipient allergic to the allergen)	Flushing Urticaria Wheezing Laryngeal edema Tightness in chest	Assess the patient for allergies Administer antihistamines or steroids prior to the infusion, as ordered Infuse blood slowly If reaction occurs (1) stop infusion and (2) have epinephrine available to treat respiratory distress or anaphylaxis
Hemolytic (incompatible)	Mixing of incompatible blood or blood-typing error	Reactions might occur within 10 minutes of transfusion Fever Headache Sharp lumbar (flank) pain Shaking Chills Nausea/vomiting Red or black urine (hemoglobinuria) Symptoms of impending shock	Type and cross-match blood prior to the transfusion Make a positive identification of the patient and blood to be transfused; verify with another nurse or physician Start the infusion slowly for 15–20 minutes or the first 50 mL of blood Monitor the patient closely—stay with the patient for the first 15 minutes If a reaction occurs (1) stop the infusion of blood and keep the intravenous line open at a keep-open rate; (2) return blood to the blood bank to cross-match again; (3) monitor the patient's vital signs every 5–15 minutes; (4) monitor the patient's urinary output hourly and insert a Foley catheter; obtain urine specimen and send to the lab; (5) watch for signs of intravascular coagulation; and (6) treat for shock using supportive medical therapies
Pyrogenic (febrile)	Introduction of foreign material into the patient's blood, which produces an antigen-antibody reaction	Chills Fever Headache Nausea/vomiting	Use aseptic technique in administration Monitor the patient's vital signs at least every 30 minutes to 1 hour during infusion Give antihistamines if ordered prior to infusion to alleviate a potential reaction, although effectiveness is questionable If reaction occurs (1) stop infusion and (2) report data to physician for evaluation

child with aplastic anemia or leukemia, repeated aspirations will be done.

The iliac crest is the most common aspiration site because it is a large marrow cavity in children. The sternum can be used in older children but should be avoided in young children because it is a fragile bone that is not fused, and vital organs are in close proximity to it.

Bone Marrow Transplantation

Bone marrow transplantation is becoming a frequently used treatment for patients with leukemia (see Chapter 33) and for aplastic anemia. Prior to bone marrow transplantation, total body irradiation and drugs are given to induce a deliberate suppression of the immune system. This process destroys any lymphocytes that might cause rejection of the transplant (see Chapter 25). As a result of this immunosuppression, all blood cell production ceases and the child becomes susceptible to overwhelming infections because of the absence of white blood cells.

The nurse assesses the child's and the family's understanding of the procedure and offers explanations, as needed. The child is cared for in a pathogen-free environment to prevent infection. Strict aseptic technique must be maintained before and after transplantation and the child needs to be protected from infection after discharge.

PROCEDURE *Administering Blood Transfusions*

- Explain to the child the purpose of the transfusion, that it is necessary to replace some of the blood that has been lost or to replace some of the substance in the blood that helps the child to be active and energetic.
- Obtain vital signs prior to the transfusion so there can be a basis for comparison during the transfusion.
- If ordered, administer medication 30 minutes prior to the transfusion to prevent an allergic reaction. Tell the child that this is necessary to make sure that the new blood will be able to work properly.
- Check the child's identification bracelet with another qualified health team member, as well as the child's blood type and match number and the type and match number of the donor blood. These are found on the unit of blood and on the blood verification slip from the blood bank. Check the expiration date on the blood.
- Flush the IV line with normal saline prior to administration since any solution containing dextrose can destroy the new cells. Set up the unit of blood with a blood filter (preferably microaggregate), which will filter out any particles, even as small as 20 to 40 microns.
- Tell the child that the transfusion will not hurt and should feel the same as the intravenous infusion. The blood infusion might feel cold. If the blood is warmed, a blood warmer, which heats the blood to between 32°C and 37°C, should be used.
- Attach the blood to the Y tubing of the IV and set at the prescribed drip rate. Use IV pump if indicated. Check the pump to be certain it is compatible with blood administration because compression of the tubing in some pumps can crush the blood cells.
- Stay with and observe the child for at least 15–20 minutes for a reaction. Take vital signs every 5–15 minutes for the first 30 minutes then every 30 minutes to an hour thereafter. Reassure the child. Use play as distraction if the child seems anxious.
- At the completion of the transfusion, the IV line is flushed with normal saline. Retake vital signs and resume or remove IV fluid as ordered.
- If there is any sign of a reaction, the transfusion is stopped and the physician notified. Hospital policy is followed regarding keeping the IV line open with normal saline and what to do with the discontinued blood.

Note: Small amounts of normal saline (1.0 mL) can be used for a flush to prevent fluid overload (Landier, Barrell, Styffe, 1987).

Principles of Nursing Care

Acute Care Needs

Activity intolerance related to imbalance between oxygen supply and demand

Because the oxygen-carrying capacity of the blood is decreased in the child with anemia, fatigue is a frequently seen symptom. Decreasing the oxygen needs of the child's body by conserving energy helps to prevent hypoxia. The nurse can accomplish this by providing a restful environment for the child and by helping the child to avoid stressful activities. Generally, the anemic child does not feel well and is fatigued easily, so it is fairly easy to limit the child's activities. Nursing activities and medical therapies are scheduled to maintain optimum rest. Disturbing noises are avoided, and regular nap or rest periods are scheduled. Procedures and stressful situations are avoided prior to meals so that the child is rested enough to eat a well-balanced diet.

Promoting effective respiratory function enhances oxygenation and decreases fatigue. The nurse helps the child to maintain an upright position, which decreases pressure on the diaphragm and allows greater lung expansion. An infant seat can be used to keep an infant upright. The nurse also promotes good hydration to liquefy secretions. Mobility and position changes prevent pooling of secretions and improve the oxygenation of blood in the lungs.

Potential for injury

Disturbances in coagulation result in hemorrhage of varying severity, particularly in response to trauma. The child

PROCEDURE *Bone Marrow Aspiration*

- Prepare child and parent for the procedure. Because bone marrow aspirations are done to rule out serious disease, the child and parent will be particularly in need of much reassurance and support. The child can be told that because it is necessary for the doctor to examine blood cells that haven't got into the bloodstream yet, the blood cells need to be taken directly from where they are made.
- Describe the position the child will be in during the procedure—on the abdomen with the hips elevated. Have the child practice being in the position. A folded blanket under the hips can elevate the hips and expose the posterior iliac crest.
- Explain how the hip will be washed with a special solution (povidone-iodine). This will feel cold to the child.
- After the hip is washed, the child will feel a temporary burning or stinging in the area from the subcutaneous injection of a local anesthetic. It often is better to tell a young child about the anesthetic just prior to the injection.
- When the local anesthetic has taken effect, the aspiration needle is inserted by the physician with a slight twisting motion until it is through the cortex of the bone and into the marrow. Tell the child there might be a feeling of pressure or a "pop" as the needle enters the marrow.

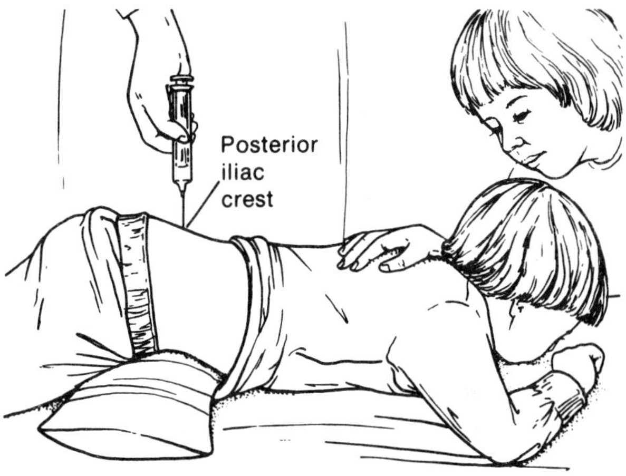

- As the marrow is aspirated by suction, the child might feel a sharp pain. The syringe is detached from the needle and the marrow is transferred to a glass slide. If white bone marrow spicules are seen, the specimen is adequate and the child can be reassured that the procedure is nearly over. If the specimen is not adequate, the suction is repeated.
- The needle is withdrawn and a pressure dressing is placed on the site. The child is comforted throughout the procedure and is encouraged to resume quiet play initially and then return to a normal activity level.

needs to be protected from any type of injury that could result in internal or frank bleeding. In the hospital the bedrails are raised and the bed is placed in the low position to prevent accidental falls. Bedrails are padded or bumper pads are used to prevent injury during sleep. The nurse alerts all health team members to the special need to protect the child from injury. It might be necessary for the nurse to supervise play and monitor the selection of toys. The child's nails are cut short to prevent scratching of the skin. Adolescents who need to shave are advised to use an electric razor rather than a straight-edge razor. Intramuscular injections are avoided. If they are required, the nurse applies prolonged pressure to the site. Mucous membranes in patients with clotting disturbances are prone to bleeding, so good oral care is necessary. Using a soft toothbrush and brushing carefully provides good hygiene while preventing injury.

Hypoxia that is associated with anemia can cause dizziness. The child who is dizzy might need assistance with position changes and with ambulation to prevent falls. The child is encouraged to move slowly and to sit or lie down if feeling dizzy.

Potential for infection

Patients with anemia might have a decreased resistance to infection either because of decreased tissue oxygenation or because of reduced production of infection-fighting white blood cells.

The best way to prevent infection is to protect the child from exposure to it. When hospitalized, the child should be in a private room or have a noninfectious roommate. No one with an active infection should come in contact with the child. This not only includes family and friends but also members of the health care team.

Oral hygiene and skin care can prevent skin breakdown and eventual infection. The nurse observes the child continually so that if signs of infection occur (unexplained fever, redness, swelling, and purulence at a local site), cultures can be obtained and antibiotics started promptly.

Outside the hospital environment, the child needs to avoid sources of infection. The child usually is allowed to return to school because developmental and social needs also need to be met. The family needs to be alert for signs and symptoms of infection so that immediate medical intervention can be initiated if an infection occurs. Routine immunizations and health care examinations should be maintained.

Nutritional Needs

⊛ Potential alteration in nutrition: less than body requirements

A continuous supply of fluid and nutrients is needed to maintain and nourish all the cells in the body. Attempts are made to meet the fluid requirement during the child's waking hours so that rest is not interrupted. Foods that are liquid at room temperature, such as ice cream, flavored gelatin, or Popsicles, can be used as fluid sources. The nurse offers fluids that the child likes, particularly if they are high in nutrient value, such as eggnog.

Some nutritional anemias, such as iron deficiency anemia, might even be avoided with a nutritious diet rich in iron and vitamins. The nurse teaches the parent to include foods high in iron such as red meat, fish, poultry, eggs, green leafy vegetables, potatoes, dried fruit, beans, and enriched bread and cereal in the child's diet.

Young children tend to resist foods high in iron and creativity is needed to provide an iron-rich diet. Raisins are popular with children but are used with caution for children in infancy and early childhood. Adding an egg to a milkshake provides extra iron. Children often will eat vegetables such as spinach or broccoli raw, in a salad or as finger food. Molasses cookies with raisins are a good source of iron and appeal to children.

Multivitamins might be prescribed along with the well-balanced diet. Vitamin C often is recommended because it enhances absorption of iron, or iron supplements can be given with citrus juice. Poor eating habits or inadequate absorption might cause folic acid and vitamin B_{12} deficiencies. These vitamins play a role in the formation of red blood cells; therefore, a deficiency in either or both of these substances can cause anemia. The child's diet should include foods rich in the deficient vitamin, and oral supplements might be needed to replenish the body's stores.

Infants over 6 months of age should be limited to 1 quart or liter of milk per day so that they will become hungry enough to eat solid foods rich in iron. New, unfamiliar foods should be offered one at a time so that the child can change food preferences and eating preferences gradually.

Older children, particularly adolescent girls, are also at risk of developing iron deficiency anemia as a result of fad or starvation diets, which are usually low in iron. These girls need to be encouraged to increase their iron intake with foods they might enjoy, such as dried fruits. The nurse explains the danger of starvation diets and provides diet teaching that encourages proper nutrition while maintaining a steady weight loss.

Whenever dietary restrictions are necessary, the nurse provides diet counseling for the child and family. They should be taught why dietary changes and good nutrition are essential.

Developmental Needs

⊛ Potential for altered growth and development

Children affected by disorders of the hematopoietic system often manifest the struggle between dependence and independence. Throughout their lives, many of them are dependent on others for assistance, for instance during transfusions, sickle cell crises, or other consequences of their disease. Since the developing child derives emotional satisfaction from self-care and acquiring independence, every effort should be made to encourage the child's active participation in care. As the child matures, increasing responsibility can be given in regard to diet, exercise tolerance, and safety. Parents are encouraged to allow the child freedom to explore while setting reasonable limits for safety. Parental overprotectiveness is a trap to be avoided so as not to stifle the child's emotional development.

Emotional Needs

⊛ Potential alteration in self-concept/self-esteem

Children with disorders of the hematopoietic system might have activity restrictions because certain activities increase their risk for complications from trauma or because chronic fatigue limits their energy expenditure. Activity restriction might make these children seem different from their peers, thus undermining their self-esteem and decreasing the satisfaction usually gained from social contact. Non-contact, but competitive, sports can provide team participation and a network of social interactions. The child's interest also can be directed toward extracurricular activities or clubs that do not require excessive use of energy. The child needs to be allowed to express any feelings regarding low self-esteem, and the nurse encourages parents to facilitate this process and to emphasize the child's strengths and realistic activity alternatives.

The Neonate with Hyperbilirubinemia

Hyperbilirubinemia (excess serum bilirubin) is a frequently seen problem in neonates. It can be caused by various conditions, including gastrointestinal dysfunctions such as biliary atresias or hepatitis (see Chapter 27), sepsis, and hemolysis (destruction) of erythrocytes.

Jaundice

Hyperbilirubinemia is characterized by *jaundice* (yellowish color of the skin), which is caused by an excess of bilirubin in the blood. *Bilirubin,* a product of hemoglobin breakdown, usually binds to albumin in the blood and is carried to the liver. In the liver it becomes attached to glucuronic acid (becomes conjugated) and is excreted in bile. Conjugated bilirubin is called direct bilirubin, and free, unconjugated bilirubin is referred to as indirect bilirubin. The normal serum direct bilirubin level is 0.1—0.4 mg/dL and the indirect bilirubin level is 0.2–1 mg/dL. Jaundice can become apparent with bilirubin levels greater than 2 mg/dL.

A variety of factors cause the breakdown of red blood cells in neonates, thus increasing the formation of bilirubin. Fetal erythrocytes have a shorter life span than those of an infant or older child (average 70 days as compared to 120); thus the fetus is constantly producing new cells and breaking down old ones. Because of the low arterial oxygen level experienced in the uterus, fetuses require more red blood cells than do infants. After birth, the breakdown of the excess numbers of fetal erythrocytes might be more than the infant's immature liver can handle effectively, resulting in a buildup of free bilirubin. This condition is known as *physiologic jaundice* (see Table 26-3).

Another cause of red blood cell breakdown is hemolysis, the destruction of both mature and immature red blood cells. Hemolysis usually is caused by blood group incompatibility between the mother and the fetus. When incompatibility is present, maternal antibodies cross the placenta and destroy fetal red blood cells.

Markedly excessive indirect bilirubin easily enters tissues with high lipid content and interferes with the metabolism of the cells. It also can cross the blood-brain barrier causing *kernicterus,* deposits of bilirubin in the brain. Kernicterus can lead to permanent brain damage.

Erythroblastosis Fetalis—Rh Incompatibility

Rh incompatibility is a major cause of hyperbilirubinemia. This occurs when an Rh-negative mother is pregnant with an Rh-positive child. During the first pregnancy or exposure to Rh-positive blood by transfusion, the Rh-negative woman develops anti-Rh-positive antibodies. This occurs because a minute amount of Rh-positive antigen has passed into her bloodstream from her fetus through the placenta. The mother is considered to be sensitized. During subsequent pregnancies with Rh-positive fetuses, the anti-Rh-positive antibodies cross the placenta and destroy the red blood cells of the fetus (Figure 26-1). The excess bilirubin from the hemolysis can cause kernicterus, severe anemia, brain damage, and death (Table 26-3).

Erythroblastosis fetalis can be suspected in any pregnancy where the mother is Rh-negative and the father is Rh-positive. Certain tests performed prenatally can assist in the evaluation of the fetus.

Amniocentesis indicates the presence of bilirubin in the amniotic fluid in fetuses with Rh incompatibility. Unfortunately, the amniocentesis itself has the risk of sensitizing the mother. Antibody measurements can be conducted on the mother. The indirect Coombs' test detects serum antibodies and can indicate previous exposure to Rh-positive antigen. Increasingly positive Coombs' tests in a pregnant woman might indicate the fetus is experiencing hemolytic difficulties that require immediate treatment in the form of intrauterine exchange transfusions.

Postnatally, a direct Coombs' test might be performed on umbilical cord blood to determine whether there are antibodies coating the infant's red cells. A strongly positive direct Coombs' test usually indicates Rh incompatibility.

Hydrops fetalis is an extremely severe case of hemolysis. In addition to the usual symptoms of erythroblastosis fetalis, the infant with hydrops fetalis has such a severe deficiency of protein in the blood that edema, a distended abdomen, and respiratory distress result. Few of these infants survive.

Rh incompatibility can now be prevented with injections of Rh_o (D) immune globulin (RhoGAM) within three days after each Rh-positive delivery or abortion. RhoGAM prevents the development of anti-Rh-positive antibodies. The effectiveness of RhoGAM can be increased if it is given once

TABLE 26-3 Neonatal Hyperbilirubinemia

	Cause	Clinical manifestation	Treatment
Physiologic jaundice	The liver is unable to handle increased breakdown of fetal erythrocytes	Jaundice, elevated total bilirubin; appears 24–72 hours after birth and lasts 3–7 days	Aimed at reducing bilirubin level; phototherapy if bilirubin level is increasing steadily; neutral thermal environment and adequate fluid intake
Rh incompatibility (erythroblastosis fetalis)	The condition occurs when a previously sensitized Rh-negative mother carries an Rh-positive fetus. Maternal antibodies cross the placenta and destroy fetal red cells	Jaundice appears within the first 24 hours after birth; elevated indirect and total bilirubin; strongly positive direct Coombs' test; anemia, enlarged liver; kernicterus (vomiting, hypoactive reflexes, increased muscle tone, apnea, cyanosis, seizures) if bilirubin >20mg/dL; condition worsens with subsequent pregnancies	Intrauterine exchange transfusions considered if amniotic fluid reveals increasing bilirubin or if maternal indirect Coombs' test is strongly positive; phototherapy; exchange transfusions; prevention by administration of RhoGAM (Rh_o D immune globulin) to the mother after every Rh-positive delivery or abortion and indirect Coombs' test during pregnancy
ABO incompatibility	The condition occurs most frequently when a group O mother carries a group A or B fetus. Naturally occurring antibodies cross the placenta and cause hemolysis of the fetal erythrocytes	Jaundice appears in the first 24 hours; elevated bilirubin; weakly positive direct Coombs' test; anemia; much less severe than Rh incompatibility and does not get worse with subsequent pregnancies	Phototherapy if bilirubin level is increasing or if infant is anemic
Breast milk jaundice	A chemical in the breast milk interferes with the liver's ability to conjugate bilirubin	Jaundice appears during the second week of life	Temporarily discontinue breast-feeding for 2–4 days until bilirubin levels fall

at 28 weeks of pregnancy and again after delivery. Once the woman has been sensitized, however, RhoGAM is ineffective.

ABO Incompatibility

ABO hemolytic disease is usually a mild and self-limiting condition that occurs most frequently when the mother is blood group O and the fetus is group A or B. Unlike anti-Rh-positive antibodies, which require prior sensitization before they cause fetal hemolysis, antibodies to group A or B seem to be naturally occurring in the person with group O blood. The infant with an ABO incompatibility will demonstrate a weakly positive direct Coombs' test in addition to other signs of hemolysis (see Table 26-3). Infants of subsequent pregnancies do not suffer more severely than the first infant with ABO incompatibility.

Nursing Management of the Neonate with Hyperbilirubinemia

Nursing goals in the care of the neonate with hyperbilirubinemia include early identification and the prevention of kernicterus and treatment-related complications. The initial interventions for infants with neonatal hyperbilirubinemia are supportive: closely observing vital signs and neurologic behavior, providing a neutral thermal environment, and providing adequate nutrition and fluids.

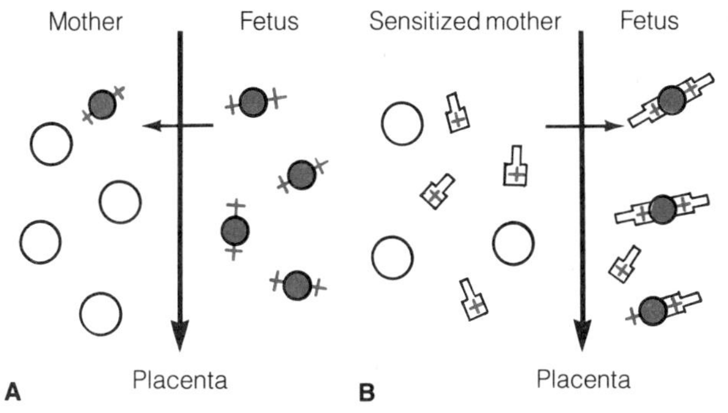

FIGURE 26-1

Erythroblastosis fetalis. ***A.*** *First pregnancy—mother becomes sensitized.* ***B.*** *Second pregnancy—antibodies attack and destroy fetal red blood cells.*

Adequate fluid intake is important because dehydration might worsen jaundice.

The nurse also monitors the serum bilirubin levels of all infants with jaundice until a definite decline is evident. If an infant's serum bilirubin level increases quickly soon after delivery, or if jaundice appears in the first 24 hours of life, attempts are made to lower the bilirubin level.

Phototherapy Phototherapy is begun when the bilirubin level is between 10 mg/dL and 15 mg/dL. Phototherapy is a treatment that exposes the infant to fluorescent lights, or lights in the blue spectrum. Phototherapy changes the indirect bilirubin into a water-soluble form that is able to be excreted in the bile and urine. Phototherapy provides radiant heat as well as light so that incubator and isolette temperatures are adjusted to maintain a neutral thermal environment (an environment that maintains the infant's core temperature between 36.5°C and 37.5°C). The nurse monitors the neonate's temperature frequently to detect alterations.

The neonate is covered minimally, mainly to protect the genital area and buttocks from the intense light. Most of the body is exposed to the light. A row of fluorescent light tubes is placed 18 inches above the neonate. The neonate is turned frequently (every 2 hours) for maximum exposure. Prior to instituting the phototherapy, the nurse gently, but securely, covers the infant's closed eyes with a mask to prevent retinal damage from the light source. The mask is removed at least once a shift to check for eye irritation or the development of conjunctivitis. The mask can be removed at other times to provide social or emotional stimulation.

Phototherapy increases insensible water loss, so fluid intake is increased. While the infant is receiving phototherapy, the nurse monitors bilirubin levels every 12 hours to determine the success of the treatment.

Phototherapy can cause dehydration, temperature instability, and metabolic imbalances. Occasionally, the skin turns a bronze color, or "flea bite" dermatitis occurs. The eye patches can scratch the infant's cornea if placed over open eyes. They occasionally slip down, blocking the nose and causing apnea (Stavis and Krauss, 1980). Therefore an infant receiving phototherapy isn't left alone in a nursery and ideally should be placed on an apnea monitor.

Loose green stools occur because the treatment increases bowel motility and decreases the activity of the enzyme that aids the digestion of lactose (Donlen and Budd, 1983). This can contribute to dehydration. Changing to a lactose-free formula helps to prevent this problem.

Phototherapy interrupts the attachment process because infants are separated from their parents and their eyes are patched so they cannot interact visually. Encouraging the parents to touch the infant frequently and to provide auditory stimulation in the form of soothing talk or soft music helps provide for the infant's emotional needs. The infant can still breast-feed and this is encouraged. Water supplements are necessary frequently, however, to keep the child adequately hydrated.

Exchange transfusions Exchange transfusions are used to lower indirect bilirubin levels and prevent brain damage in infants with severe hyperbilirubinemia—that is, cases occurring prior to 24 hours of age, hyperbilirubinemia with anemia, and indirect bilirubin levels in excess of 20 mg/dL. An exchange transfusion is performed by withdrawing a small amount of the infant's blood and infusing the same amount of warmed, fresh, or partially packed blood through an umbilical vein catheter. The neonate is typed and cross-matched prior to the transfusion and is given blood free of the offending antigens (eg, for Rh incompatibility, O negative blood is given since it contains no antigens, neither Rh nor blood group) (Ladewig et al., 1986).

The infant is kept NPO prior to and during the transfusion. The nurse closely monitors vital signs during the procedure, particularly the heart rate and ECG, since this procedure can cause arrhythmias. Electrolytes, especially calcium and sodium bicarbonate, are given to counteract metabolic imbalances present in the transfused blood. Heart failure can occur because of either fluid overload or rapid loss of blood volume. Hypothermia is possible if the blood is not adequately warmed. Bilirubin levels are closely monitored after the treatment to evaluate its success.

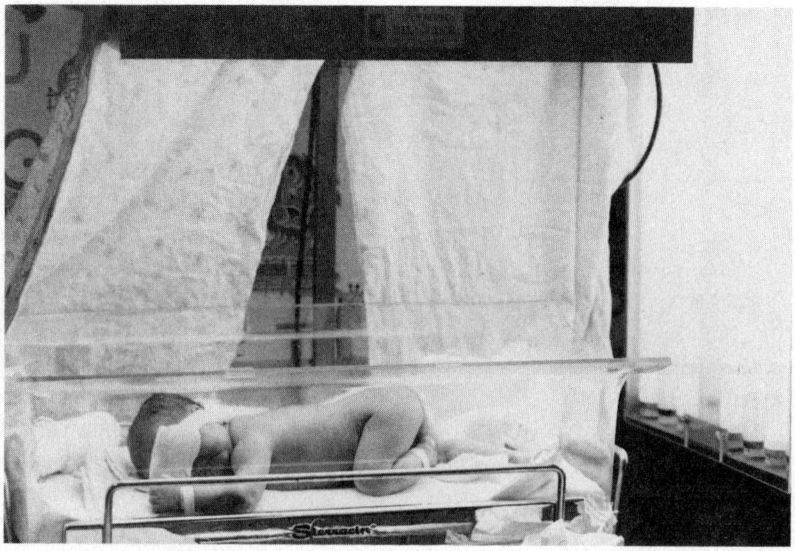

Phototherapy. (From Ladewig PA, London ML, Olds SB: Essentials of Maternal-Newborn Nursing. *Addison-Wesley, 1986.)*

The Child with Anemia

Iron Deficiency Anemia

Iron deficiency anemia is caused by an inadequate supply, intake, or absorption of iron. Iron is essential for the oxygen-carrying capacity of hemoglobin. Lack of iron results in smaller red blood cells and, in turn, decreased hemoglobin synthesis. Adequate daily ingestion of iron and iron released from disintegrating red blood cells supply iron for red blood cell production (*erythropoiesis*). Iron is absorbed primarily in the duodenum. When iron intake is inadequate, the body uses stored iron. When the stored iron is depleted, symptoms of anemia develop.

Iron deficiency is the most common cause of anemia in children. Infants between the ages of 6 and 24 months are prone to iron deficiency because their stores of maternal iron are depleted, and they become dependent on external sources. Unless iron is supplied in the diet the infant will become anemic. Other possible causes of iron deficiency anemia are (1) inadequate dietary intake of iron, such as might occur in bottle-fed infants who do not receive supplemental iron; (2) malabsorption of iron, such as occurs in chronic diarrhea, malabsorption syndromes, or gastrectomy; (3) blood loss caused by gastrointestinal bleeding, heavy menstruation, or hemorrhage; (4) excessive demands caused by periods of stress or rapid growth; and (5) intravascular hemolysis, resulting in hemoglobinuria.

Clinical manifestations Clinical findings of pallor, fatigue, and irritability, combined with a history of an iron-deficient diet, suggest iron deficiency anemia. When the hemoglobin drops below 6 g/dL, such symptoms as irritability, inability to concentrate, anorexia, and decreased activity are present. These are followed by cardiac irregularities and enlargement of the heart. Because iron deficiency anemia occurs gradually, most patients do not seek medical attention until it has progressed to an advanced stage.

Diagnostic evaluation The actual medical diagnosis is made following laboratory tests. The red blood cell count might be normal or slightly reduced. Hemoglobin is below the normal range for the child's age and usually below 10 g/dL. The hematocrit is below normal. The decreased red blood cell (erythrocyte) indices are important in diagnosis because they demonstrate the decrease in size and concentration of hemoglobin in a single red blood cell. The reticulocyte (immature red cell) count usually is low because the decreased availability of iron for synthesizing hemoglobin results in depressed production of red cells.

Treatment Treatment for iron deficiency anemia involves correction of any underlying problems (eg, hemorrhage or malabsorption), iron replacement therapy, and diet counseling. An oral preparation of ferrous sulfate or a combination of iron and ascorbic acid is given. Ascorbic acid given with the iron enhances its absorption. If the patient is uncooperative or if the gastrointestinal tract cannot absorb iron, the iron is administered parenterally.

Blood transfusions are rarely necessary in the management of iron deficiency anemia unless the deficiency has been caused by severe bleeding. If the anemia is profound or if infecton is present, transfusions of packed red blood cells might be prescribed.

Nursing management

Prevention Nutritional causes of iron deficiency anemia can be prevented. Regular monitoring of food intake and routine hemoglobin testing in children promotes the early identification and possible prevention of anemia. Any family history of anemia and special dietary practices, such as vegetarianism, need to be determined. The child's growth parameters are measured on a regular basis. Any change in growth or eating habits and unusual behavior (for example, pica) could be symptomatic of iron deficiency.

Infants require 8 mg/day of iron; this is best obtained from breast milk, from iron-fortified formula, from iron-fortified dry infant cereals, and from strained meats. Some mothers still use unaltered cow's milk to feed young infants. Whole milk does not provide the necessary quantity of iron. Unless the infant obtains iron from other sources, anemia is a great risk. Unfortunately, these infants appear to be thriving, and many of them grow fat on large quantities of whole milk. It is necessary for nurses to explain to parents that although the infant appears to be thriving, the diet is not supplying what the infant needs to stay healthy. This infant usually has a pale, pasty complexion.

The young child's iron requirement is 10–15 mg per day. For the finicky eater in early childhood this is extremely difficult. Often, children this age eat poorly, and it is a struggle for parents to ensure adequate amounts of iron. Nurses can recommend the use of cooked cereals like Cream of Wheat or oatmeal and the use of brown sugar or molasses instead of refined sugars. Bran muffins containing molasses and raisins are a good source of iron and they appeal to children of this age. Some mothers just mix molasses with milk as a flavoring.

Older children and adolescents are encouraged to avoid foods with empty calories. Nutritious snacks such as nuts and raisins or peanut butter crackers can be provided.

Interventions Nursing management of the child with iron deficiency anemia focuses on proper nutrition and cooperation with the medical regimen. The nurse informs the child and family that both dietary changes and supplemental iron therapy are needed to cure iron deficiency anemia.

The nurse teaches the child and family about the side effects of iron therapy, which include nausea, vomiting, and diarrhea or constipation. These symptoms might indicate a need to change the dosage. If the child is taking an oral iron preparation, it should not be consumed with milk or antacids beause they interfere with iron absorption. If a liquid iron preparation is being used, the child should drink it from a straw to prevent staining the teeth. Children who have not had ascorbic acid prescribed with the iron should take iron with a high vitamin C content juice. The nurse also warns the patient and family that the patient's stools will become black.

If intramuscular injections of Imferon are prescribed, the Z-track injection method is used to prevent the accidental deposition of iron in the skin. Deposition of iron in the skin could lead to a change in skin color or to scarring.

Dietary modifications are necessary indefinitely to keep the anemia from recurring, and oral iron supplements are taken until the prescription runs out. After the anemia subsides, the nurse encourages the parent to seek routine medical examinations for the child. Hemoglobin levels should be checked every 6 months to detect recurrences.

Aplastic Anemia

Aplastic anemia is a rare disease that affects approximately 5000 people a year in the United States (Goldstein, 1980). The mortality rate is high with 50%–60% of deaths occurring in the first 6 months after diagnosis (Hutchison, 1983). In aplastic anemia the formation of red blood cells, white blood cells, and platelets is depressed, resulting in profound anemia, leukopenia, and thrombocytopenia. Aplastic anemia is caused by injury, destruction, or low population of stem cells in the bone marrow. The disease can be primary (congenital) or secondary (acquired).

Approximately one-half of the aplastic anemias have an acquired or secondary cause. The most common causes of acquired aplastic anemia are (1) indiscriminate use of drugs such as chloramphenicol (an antibiotic); (2) irradiation; (3) toxic agents such as household dyes, paint removers, insecticides, and compounds with benzene; (4) severe diseases such as hepatitis or sepsis; and (5) immunologic deficiencies such as in leukemia. Approximately 50% are ideopathic, that is, having no known cause.

Clinical manifestations The symptoms of aplastic anemia result from the depressed blood elements. Progressive weakness, fatigue, tachycardia, tachypnea, and pallor are related to anemia resulting from the depression of erythrocytes. Ecchymosis, petechiae, and hemorrhage might result from thrombocyte depression. Leukopenia contributes to the occurrence of infection.

Diagnostic evaluation Peripheral blood studies reveal depression in blood elements. Hemoglobin is often below 8 mg/dL, leukocytes below $4000/mm^3$, and there are less than $100,000/mm^3$ of platelets.

Accurate diagnosis is by bone marrow aspiration and bone biopsy. The normally red marrow is yellow and fatty in patients with aplastic anemia. The marrow is lacking cells (hypoplastic).

Treatment The treatment protocol for aplastic anemia depends on the severity and prognosis of the disease in the affected child. Bone marrow transplantation is considered for children with a poor prognosis, that is, high risk of mortality within the first 3 months of diagnosis, if there is a compatible donor (Goldstein, 1980). If bone marrow transplantation is to be successful, it should be performed prior to the child receiving any blood transfusions or the transfusions can be of irradiated blood products. Minor antigens in donor blood can contribute to a transplant rejection. Bone marrow transplantation has been successful in almost 80% of patients who have not received prior blood transfusions (Hutchison, 1983).

Androgenic steroids (such as testosterone), both with and without corticosteroids (which enhance the effects of testosterone), are somewhat effective in instances where transplantation is out of the question. It is unknown exactly how androgens stimulate erythropoiesis. Response to treatment with androgens is slow (sometimes 3–10 months), and the child is provided with supportive therapy until there is a positive response. Supportive therapy includes blood component transfusions and aggressive antibiotic administration.

The possibility exists that aplastic anemia might be an autoimmune response against the marrow. Trials with globulins designed to suppress the autoimmune process have been somewhat successful.

Nursing management Nursing care for patients with aplastic anemia focuses on (1) preventing complications of infection and bleeding; (2) preparing the child and family for diagnostic and therapeutic procedures; (3) giving emotional support to the child and family during terminal illness; and (4) giving nursing care related to the therapy. Interventions are similar to those given to a child with leukemia (see Chapter 33).

Infection control The nurse protects the child from infection, giving special attention to the care of the skin and mucous membranes. Children with aplastic anemia are often placed in laminar airflow rooms or in strict protective isolation. Anyone entering the room abides by strict handwashing technique and wears sterile protective clothing.

In conjunction with protective isolation, the child is given at least daily baths with antibacterial agents (such as povidone-iodine solution) to keep the skin as free from pathogens as possible (Hutchison, 1983). Occasionally, oral antibiotics are administered to sterilize the gastrointestinal tract. Children are encouraged to adhere to strict handwashing.

The nurse monitors the child for signs of infection, particularly fever, and reports any immediately. Cultures of throat, urine, stool, and blood might be required to pinpoint the source of infection. Fever control is instituted as ordered. Aspirin is not used because it prolongs bleeding time.

The long-term psychologic effects of maintaining the child in a sterile environment have not yet been determined. The nurse provides as much verbal, visual, and tactile stimulation as possible (see Chapter 25).

Interventions for bleeding The decreased number of platelets in the blood makes the child susceptible to bleeding. The nurse protects the child from injury and carefully assesses the skin, urine, and stool for blood. Bleeding problems must be detected early so that prompt treatment can be initiated. Platelet transfusions are administered when the platelet count falls below $10,000/mm^3$–$15,000\ mm^3$ (Goldstein, 1980). Intramuscular injections are avoided for children with platelet counts below $50,000/mm^3$ (Hutchison, 1983).

The nurse gives frequent mouth care to provide comfort from bleeding mucous membranes and to prevent infection in the oral cavity. The use of a soft or sponge toothbrush or frequent rinses with a solution of salt and baking soda in water removes dried blood. Local pain control can be achieved through the use of lidocaine (viscous zylocaine), or Orabase ointment. Often, providing the child with Popsicles is all that is necessary.

The nurse is alert for signs of internal bleeding or intracranial hemorrhage. Frequent monitoring of vital signs and prompt reporting of alterations will limit the consequences of internal bleeding.

Emotional support The side effects of drug treatment can result in changes in the child's body image. For example, testosterone can cause deepening of the voice or hirsutism (abnormal hair growth), while corticosteroids might cause moon-shaped face. These changes might be difficult for the child to understand and accept. It is important for the nurse to approach the child in a positive manner and inform the child and family about the possible side effects before they develop.

If the child does not require hospital care, the nurse encourages the parent to make the child's life at home as

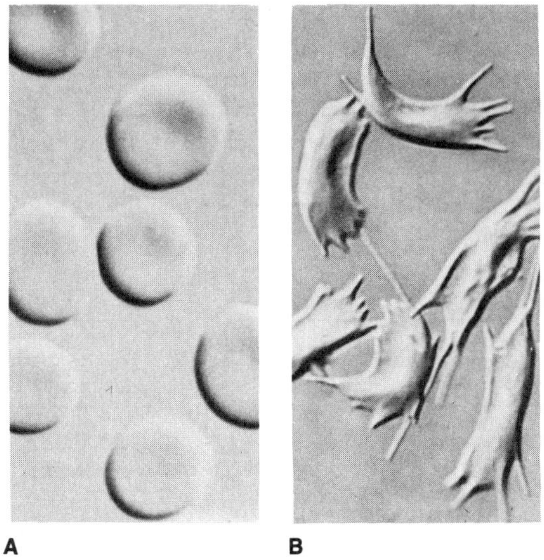

A. Normal red blood cells. *B.* Sickled cells. (From Jenkins J: Human Genetics. Addison-Wesley, 1983.)

TABLE 26-4 Comparison of Normal and Sickled Red Blood Cells

Characteristics	Normal cells	Sickled cells
Shape of RBC	Round	Crescent, or sickle
Life span of RBC	120 days	30–40 days
Oxygen-carrying capacity of Hgb	Normal	Decreased
Hgb per milliliter	12–14 g	6–9 g
Type of Hgb	Hgb A	Hgb S
Destruction rate of RBC	Normal	Greatly increased

normal as possible. Nursing care for the dying child is discussed in Chapter 17.

Sickle Cell Disease

Sickle cell disease is a frequently seen disease of genetic origin found predominately in blacks. Sickle cell disease is associated with the presence of hemoglobin S (Hgb S). Hgb S is an abnormal hemoglobin, which differs from normal adult hemoglobin (Hgb A) by having an altered amino acid component of its molecule. This alteration causes the normally round erythrocytes to become sickle, or crescent, shaped when the oxygenation of the blood is decreased (such as during physical exertion, dehydration, cold, or stress) (see Table 26-4).

The child with sickle cell disease inherits the homozygous gene (Hgb SS) via autosomal recessive inheritance pattern. All the child's hemoglobin will be abnormal in structure and the child will manifest signs of the disease. The sickle cell trait is heterozygous (Hgb SA). The child will have some normal hemoglobin and some Hgb S (25%–40%). The child will not exhibit symptoms except in conditions of high altitudes or in situations where oxygen levels are low, such as during extreme physical stress, surgery, or pregnancy.

Parents with sickle cell disease or trait can pass the condition on to their children. Approximately 1 out of every 10 black Americans has sickle cell disease or trait (Jenkins, 1983). Figure 26-2 illustrates the genetic transfer of sickle cell disease and trait.

Clinical manifestations In the child with sickle cell disease, Hgb S is present from the time of conception, but significant amounts of fetal hemoglobin tend to inhibit sickling and anemia until the infant is about 6 months of age. After 6 months of age, red blood cells with Hgb S begin to outnumber cells with normal hemoglobin, and signs of a progressive, lifelong anemia begin to develop (Johnson, 1985). The course of the condition is marked by physiologic crises. Complications of sickle cell disease can be recognized, predicted, and treated, but they cannot be prevented totally.

Frequently, the first signs of sickle cell disease are lack of appetite, irritability, and an increased susceptibility to infection. The child might be small for age and gain weight poorly. The mucous membranes are pale, and scleral icterus is evident. In the older child the trunk usually is short, the extremities long, the hips and shoulders narrow, and the hands and feet slender. Changes in the bone might be found radiographically as early as 6 months of age. Sexual maturation might be delayed or absent. The spleen might be palpable during the first decade of life. Later, the liver might be palpable, and cardiac complications can develop.

Associated manifestations of sickle cell disease include frequent severe infections, chronic leg ulcers, priapism (continual erection of the penis), decreased urine concentration with associated enuresis, hematuria, problems during pregnancy, and bone weakness. Patients with sickle

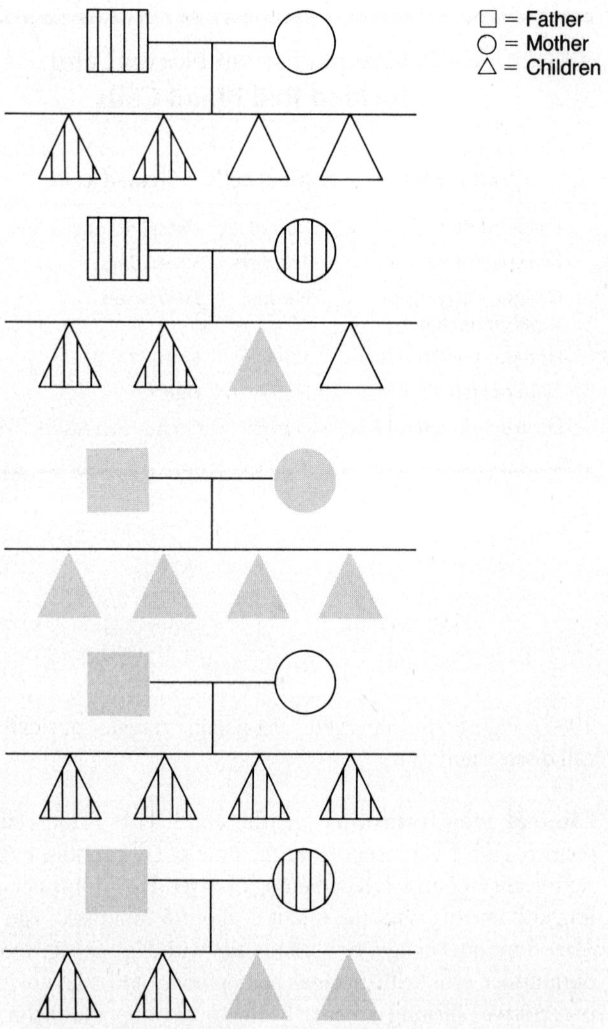

FIGURE 26-2
Genetic transfer of sickle cell disease. ***Solid*** *= sickle cell disease;* ***striped*** *= sickle cell trait;* ***open*** *= normal.*

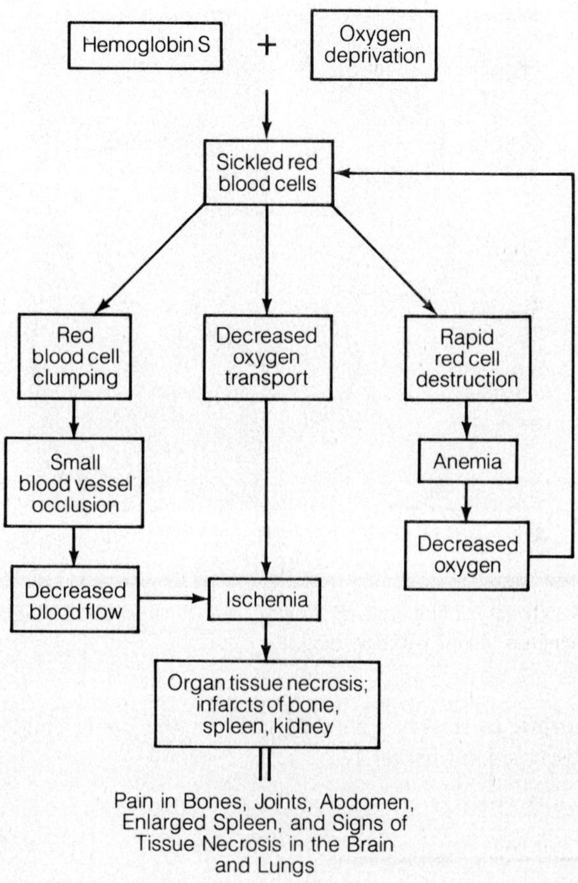

FIGURE 26-3
The sickling process and its physiologic effects.

cell disease also might have a lowered resistance to pneumococcal and salmonella microorganisms.

For variable periods, a child with sickle cell disease might have no complaints other than chronic anemia. Then, with the occurrence of a common childhood illness, such as tonsillitis or an upper respiratory infection, or for no apparent reason, the child becomes acutely ill. This sudden change in health is termed *sickle cell crisis.* Crisis occurs when physiologic stress reduces hydration or deprives the Hgb S of oxygen. Once it begins, the sickling process is self-sustaining because its anoxic effects cause further sickling. The sickling process and its physiologic effects are shown in Figure 26-3.

Sickle cell crises can be of the vaso-occlusive (thrombocytic), sequestration, or aplastic type (Table 26-5). Vaso-occlusive (thrombocytic) crisis, sometimes called "painful crisis," is the most common. In addition to the manifestations in Table 26-5, vaso-occlusive crisis can result in a group of skeletal problems known as hand-foot syndrome, seen in children 6 months to 2 years of age. The occlusion involves the short bones of the hands and feet. Painful swelling occurs in the hands and feet, with a decrease in the range of motion of the extremities involved. These symptoms are frequently confused with those of rheumatic fever or osteomyelitis.

The prognosis of sickle cell anemia is affected significantly by the quality of medical care and nursing management and the child's and family's response to the lifelong disease. The cause of mortality during the first years of life is usually from overwhelming sepsis and sequestration crisis.

TABLE 26-5 Types of Sickle Cell Crises

Pathophysiology	Clinical manifestation
Vaso-occlusive	
Red blood cell clumping blocks small blood vessels, resulting in tissue death. The crisis can last from four days to several weeks	Pain, distal ischemia (deficiency of blood); infarction (tissue death) in bones and joints, leading to swelling and pain; in the spleen, leading to abdominal rigidity, distention, pain, and fever, with eventual fibrosis and scarring; in the brain, causing stroke, hemiplegia, and death; and in the lungs, causing respiratory distress
Sequestration	
Sickling causes sudden pooling of blood in the spleen and liver. Prompt treatment can reverse the crisis	Enlargement of the spleen, liver failure and necrosis; circulatory failure causes signs of impending shock (extreme pallor, decreased blood pressure, rapid pulse)
Aplastic	
Bone marrow failure and increased destruction of red blood cells causes erythrocyte production shutdown lasting 10–14 days. Profound anemia results. This crisis usually ends spontaneously	Weakness, listlessness, tachycardia, tachypnea

As the child grows older, sickle cell crises occur less frequently.

Diagnostic evaluation All black persons should be screened for the presence of Hgb S, which is detected by blood tests such as the Sickledex test. If a sickling test is positive, the patient is tested further for the presence of active disease by hemoglobin electrophoresis, which determines whether the child has the trait or active disease. Hematology of the child with active disease reveals decreased hemoglobin and increased reticulocyte count.

Persons living in climates where malaria is prevalent have an advantage if they are carrying the sickle cell trait because the malarial parasite is incapable of invading the cells carrying Hgb S (Jenkins, 1983). Because many black Americans are descendants of equatorial Africans, it might be assumed that the presence of the sickle trait in black Americans has evolved from their protective mechanism against malaria. Under ordinary circumstances persons with sickle cell trait never develop or require treatment for sickle cell disease.

Treatment Therapy consists of treating the crisis symptoms and giving supportive care. Treatments and their objectives are as follows:

1. *Hydration*. Fluids are given orally or intravenously to produce hemodilution (an increase in the fluid volume of the blood), which helps to prevent sickling, pain, and thrombosis.
2. *Electrolyte replacement*. This counters the acidosis caused by hypoxia.
3. *Analgesic administration*. Acetaminophen is given for mild pain. Meperidine and morphine are reserved for extreme pain. Aspirin (in large doses) is avoided because it can worsen metabolic acidosis and can cause bleeding.
4. *Bedrest*. This conserves the child's energy.
5. *Antibiotic administration*. Antibiotics are used to treat or prevent infections. All patients over 2 years of age are given Pneumovax pneumococcal vaccine and can be given protection from *Hemophilus influenzae* type B to prevent meningitis.
6. *Oxygen therapy*. Reduced pulmonary oxygenation due to infiltrates and infarcts can lead to hypoxia. Oxygen therapy is reserved for children experiencing severe hypoxemia (low serum oxygen).
7. *Transfusion*. Packed red blood cells are administered to treat the anemia and reduce the number of circulating sickle cells. Exchange transfusions are reserved for life-threatening situations and are not employed routinely in painful crisis.

In children with splenic sequestration crisis, *hypovolemia* (reduced blood volume) is corrected promptly with volume expanders, and whole blood transfusions are required. Splenectomy is considered if the child has one or more severe crises because the spleen is one of the major sites of sickling, sequestration, and destruction of red blood cells.

Priapism is an occasional and painful effect of sickling. The usual treatment for priapism includes hypotonic fluids and warm baths. The erection needs to be relieved within several hours because of the danger of ischemia to the penile tissue. It might be necessary to aspirate the corpora cavernosa to relieve the erection.

Nursing management Helping the child and family adjust to a lifelong disease and preventing the sickling process are the two key factors in nursing management for the child with sickle cell disease. The nurse explains the disease and its effects to the child and family and informs and guides them in periods of crisis. Genetic counseling is strongly encouraged (see Chapter 15).

Preventing hypoxia Tissue hypoxia can initiate the sickling process, so it is essential that the child avoid factors that increase cellular requirements for oxygen. The nurse helps to avert hypoxia by the following:

1. Teaching the child to refrain from strenuous physical activities, such as contact sports, encouraging the child to participate in activities that are tolerated, and teaching the child to set realistic limits independently.
2. Teaching the child to avoid environments that are low in oxygen concentration such as high altitudes, unpressurized airplanes, and deep-sea diving.
3. Helping the child to minimize and deal with emotional and physical stress. This includes recommending stress reduction exercises (see Chapter 11) and encouraging parents to see that the child is protected from chilling and dehydration.
4. Protecting the child from known sources of infection and ensuring prompt treatment of any current infection.
5. Encouraging the child to drink one and one-half to two times the usual fluid requirements to facilitate hemodilution. The nurse informs the parents of the approximate number of ounces of fluid required daily. Less obvious sources of fluids such as ice creams and gelatins can be encouraged if the child is resistant to drinking large volumes.

Management of crises During a sickle cell crisis, intravenous fluid therapy might be combined with oral hydration because the child is less likely to eat and drink. The nurse carefully regulates the fluid intake and monitors the fluid and electrolyte balance. Accurate measurements of intake and output, of specific gravity of the urine, and of the child's daily weight enable the nurse to assess and manage hydration.

Because the child's anxiety during a crisis can increase the perception of pain, it is helpful for the nurse to use an objective pain assessment tool (see Chapter 20) to assess pain. Pain during a crisis can be managed with analgesics. Pain also is managed with comfort measures such as repositioning the child, immobilizing or elevating the painful part, or applying heat. Cold is not applied because it causes vasoconstriction, which extends the sickling process. Diversional activities usually are effective in taking the child's mind off the pain.

The nurse monitors the child's respiratory status so that proper interventions can be initiated in the event of respiratory distress. If oxygen is required, the nurse administers it by tent, mask, or nasal cannula, as appropriate for the child.

The child usually is fatigued and weakened during a sickle cell crisis, so it is fairly easy to provide bed rest. The nurse arranges nursing care, medical tests, and therapy so that the child receives maximum rest. Rest periods are scheduled prior to mealtimes so that the child will have the energy to eat. Play activities, which should not be strenuous, are essential for the child's development. The nurse also might be responsible for coordinating the daily visits of an occupational therapist.

Management of complications The child's neurologic status is closely monitored with frequent vital signs and neurologic checks (see Chapter 31). Alterations in consciousness, hemiplegia, or other adverse neurologic changes are reported immediately.

Vascular collapse and shock might occur as a result of a sickle cell crisis. The nurse observes the child for signs of shock: vital signs, blood pressure, and level of consciousness are closely monitored. Changes are reported to the physician immediately so that prompt treatment can be initiated. The nurse assists with blood transfusions as required.

Enuresis (bed-wetting) is caused by the increased fluid load and can be considered an effect of treatment. The nurse explains to the child and family that enuresis might occur. The nurse, or the parent if the child is at home, encourages the child to void before bedtime. However, the child is not awakened during the night because interruptions in the child's normal sleep patterns alter the child's ability to conserve energy.

Providing emotional support The nurse explains to the child and family the rationale and necessity for all treatments and diagnostic tests. It is essential for the nurse to be supportive during crises. Often families are anxious and fearful, and they should be given opportunities to express their fears.

The child and family can be helped to explore ways of adjusting to the limitations of a chronic illness (see Chapter 14). The nurse encourages the family to allow the child independence and freedom to develop normally within the constraints of the physical limitations imposed by the disease.

Parents might express guilt at having transmitted the disease to the child. They might need referral to counseling services or for genetic counseling.

Home management Because children with sickle cell anemia are susceptible to infection, and infection can precipitate a sickle cell crisis, well-balanced meals, protection from sources of infection, frequent medical supervision, and adequate rest are necessary. The parent is encouraged

STANDARDS OF NURSING CARE *The Child with Sickle Cell Disease*

RISKS

Assessed risk	Nursing action
Hypovolemia and shock during sickle crisis	Observe for signs of shock (restlessness, decreased blood pressure, increased pulse, pallor). Take vital signs hourly during crisis. Administer transfusions as ordered. Provide routine shock therapy (position flat, elevated legs, warmth, fluid volume restoration, vital signs, and monitoring level of consciousness).

GUIDE TO NURSING MANAGEMENT

Nursing diagnosis	Intervention	Rationale	Outcome
1. Alteration in comfort: pain related to physiologic tissue death, edema and limited motion secondary to vascular occlusion of sickling process	Determine the location of pain (joints, bones, abdomen) and note degree of warmth of affected extremity.	Noting the painful areas of the body, assist others to intervene appropriately and evaluate the child's progress. Promote continuity of approach.	The child's pain decreases and tolerance increases. The child states relief from pain.
	Administer nonaspirin analgesics as ordered.	Analgesics reduce pain; aspirin can exacerbate metabolic acidosis and hypoxia.	
	Reposition; immobilize or elevate the painful area.	Positioning and immobilization can relieve pain.	
	Apply heat.	Heat relieves pain without causing further vasoconstriction and occlusion.	
	Use diversional activities and teach relaxation exercises.	Diversional activities and relaxation exercises can take the child's focus away from the pain.	
2. Potential for impaired gas exchange (stressor: activities that increase cellular requirements for oxygen, growth spurt stress, high altitudes)	Monitor for signs of respiratory distress including cyanosis, alteration in blood gases, and difficulty breathing.	Hypoxia can alter respiratory patterns and effectiveness and can cause respiratory distress.	The child is free from respiratory distress (eg, no cyanosis, retractions or alterations in vital signs or blood gases). The child is well hydrated.
	Elevate the head of the bed.	Elevating the head of the bed facilitates adequate respirations.	
	Maintain a calm atmosphere.	A calm atmosphere decreases anxiety.	
	Observe for signs of fluid deficit and carefully monitor intake and output.	Maintenance of fluid volume is essential to maintain hemodilution and prevent sickling.	
	Maintain ordered intravenous fluid rate.	IV fluids assist in fluid volume maintenance.	
	Encourage the child to drink fluids (choose fluids the child likes) one and one-half times the fluid requirement for age and weight.	Drinking large amounts of fluids assists with hemodilution; creativity is needed to maintain large fluid intake and fluids that the child likes should be determined and encouraged.	

(Continues)

STANDARDS OF NURSING CARE *The Child with Sickle Cell Disease (Continued)*

GUIDE TO NURSING MANAGEMENT

Nursing diagnosis	Intervention	Rationale	Outcome
3. Potential infection (stressor: lowered resistance, decreased hemoglobin, chronic disease)	Observe for signs of infection: increased temperature, irritability or lethargy, decreased appetite, redness or swelling of tissue, pain.	Signs of infection need to be reported immediately so appropriate treatment can be initiated.	The child remains free from signs of infection.
	Protect child from known sources of infection.	This reduces the risk of contracting an infection.	
	Administer antibiotics as ordered.	Antibiotics are used to treat infection or to protect against infection in high risk situations.	
4. Activity intolerance related to imbalance between oxygen supply and demand	Organize nursing care to provide optimum rest by providing bed rest and scheduling rest periods as needed.	Organized nursing care allows for maximum rest.	The child appears well rested and free from fatigue. The child paces activities well.
	Encourage age-appropriate nonstrenuous activities.	Quiet activities divert the child while promoting rest.	
5. Knowledge deficit related to home management of the child with sickle cell disease	Teach the parents about the precipitators of a sickle crisis—dehydration, decreased oxygen, chilling, stress, strenuous physical activity.	Parents need to know precipitating factors in order to teach the child to avoid them.	The parents can explain the factors that precipitate a crisis and how to avoid them. The parents appear confident in their ability to care for the child and promote the child's optimal development.
	Encourage parents to protect the child from sources of infection and to obtain all routine immunizations, including protection against pneumococcal pneumonia and *Hemophilus influenzae* type B.	Infection can precipitate a crisis.	
	Emphasize the importance of increased fluid intake. Fluid intake should be one and one-half to two times maintenance fluid requirements daily.	More than maintenance fluid promotes hemodilution and reduces the risk for sickling.	
	Encourage parents to teach the child how to handle emotional and physical stress; include demonstration of stress reduction exercises.	Stress can precipitate a crisis; active coping with stress encourages self-care and independence.	
	Assist parents to express their concerns and anxieties about caring for a child with chronic concerns; refer for genetic counseling.	Allowing parents to express concerns helps them cope with the child's disease and its effects on the family.	
	Emphasize that the child can be encouraged to develop independence and responsibility for self-care.	Encouraging independence is important for the child's optimal development.	

to observe and report to the physician any signs of pain, weakness, pallor, swelling, fever, or alterations in level of consciousness.

Routine health promotion is recommended. The child should carry identification or a Medic-Alert Tag listing the diagnosis and, if possible, other related information.

β-Thalassemia (Cooley's Anemia)

Thalassemia is the name given to a group of hereditary hemolytic anemias that are caused by a deficiency in the normal synthesis of hemoglobin polypeptide chains. Unlike sickle cell disease, where there is an alteration in an amino acid component of the chain, thalassemia involves a decreased synthesis of the chain. This results in decreased hemoglobin in each erythrocyte. Subcategories of thalassemia are named according to the polypeptide chain affected, that is, as alpha-, beta-, gamma-, or delta-thalassemia.

In β-thalassemia the basic defect is a deficiency in the synthesis of β-chain hemoglobin molecules, which results in defective hemoglobin formation. Stimulated by inadequate supplies of hemoglobin, the bone marrow becomes *hyperplastic* (overproductive), forming red blood cells that are fragile and easily destroyed. The body attempts to compensate for the decrease in hemoglobin by producing fetal hemoglobin, which does not contain β chains.

There are two forms of β-thalassemia: thalassemia minor, the heterozygous form, and thalassemia major, the homozygous form, also known as Cooley's anemia. If the patient inherits only one thalassemia gene (which combines with a normal gene), mild to moderate anemia develops, and the patient is classified as having the heterozygous trait, or thalassemia minor. If two thalassemia genes are inherited (homozygous), the patient is born with the severe, life-threatening form (thalassemia major).

Thalassemia major is an autosomal recessive disorder. People whose ancestors lived near the Mediterranean Sea or in the Mediterranean Desert have the highest incidence of the disease, but it also can occur as a result of spontaneous mutations.

Clinical manifestations Thalassemia major is suspected in patients who exhibit signs of severe anemia (lethargy, pallor, weakness, and anorexia), who have a Mediterranean background, and who have the classic appearance of patients with the disease (thickened cranial bones, flat nose, and malocclusions of the teeth). Thalassemia major causes severe, progressive, hemolytic anemia that begins in affected infants at about 6 months of age, when the protective effect of fetal hemoglobin diminishes. The child's spleen enlarges with the increase in red cell destruction, causing an enlarged abdomen.

As the bone marrow becomes hyperplastic in an attempt to replace the red cells, it expands the marrow cavities of the bones, causing skeletal changes. The head enlarges, and facial features change to resemble those characteristic of patients with Down's syndrome. Chronic anemia causes growth retardation, so children with β-thalassemia commonly have small bodies. Bone cartilage thins with age, making the child susceptible to spontaneous fractures.

The child's skin is a muddy-yellow, or bronze color. This change in skin color is due to jaundice caused by increased bilirubin, pallor from the anemia, and iron deposits from excessive hemoglobin breakdown.

Cardiac complications, such as cardiomegaly, heart failure, or arrhythmias, are associated with β-thalassemia. These, along with liver and gallbladder complications, are related to a condition called hemosiderosis. *Hemosiderosis* is an accumulation in body organs of the iron-containing substance hemosiderin which results from the rapid destruction of defective red blood cells. The frequent blood transfusions that are required to maintain hemoglobin levels replenish the supply of red blood cells which, when destroyed, add to excess iron deposits and result in cellular damage.

Children with thalassemia minor usually exhibit no symptoms. Occasionally, a mild anemia might be present.

Diagnostic evaluation Hematologic tests reveal hypochromic, abnormally small red blood cells that are distorted in shape. Numerous target cells (bull's eye appearance) and numerous nucleated red blood cells are seen. There is also a predominance of fetal hemoglobin and decreased amounts of normal adult hemoglobin. Erythrocyte indices are decreased and bilirubin levels are increased.

Treatment There is no cure for β-thalassemia. Therapy consists of maintaining adequate hemoglobin levels to prevent tissue hypoxia. Frequent blood transfusions are required, but unfortunately, they increase iron overload of and subsequent damage to body tissues.

If the spleen destroys the transfused red blood cells, increasing the need for transfusions, splenectomy might be necessary. The major complication of splenectomy is infection, so prophylactic antibiotics and pneumococcal and meningococcal vaccines are given. Research is in progress on the use of bone marrow transplantation, but its effectiveness as a treatment for β-thalassemia has not yet been confirmed. Iron-binding agents, such as desferrioxamine (Desferol), are administered to remove excess iron from the blood. This is an attempt to reduce hemosiderosis.

The prognosis of the disease depends on its severity. Children with thalassemia major seldom live to adulthood.

Children with thalassemia minor require no treatment and can have a normal life span.

Nursing management Nursing care for children with thalassemia major is supportive. As with any child with anemia, interventions are directed toward preventing and reducing hypoxia. Oxygen therapy might be required.

Red blood transfusions are required to combat the anemia. The nurse administers blood transfusions and observes the child for signs of transfusion reactions. Frequent monitoring of vital signs is necessary to detect cardiac irregularities. The nurse also observes the child for signs and symptoms of hepatitis and iron overload.

As children with thalassemia major grow older, they might have difficulty adjusting to the body changes caused by the disease. They look different from their peers and usually cannot keep up during physical activities. These children need opportunities to express their feelings and guidance in handling the problems that might arise.

As many procedures as possible are done on an outpatient basis. Home care treatments can be arranged if the family is comfortable with them. The nurse arranges contact with community agencies that can give the child and family additional support. Thalassemia major eventually results in death. The children and their families need much support in dealing with crisis periods and the eventual death of the child. See Chapter 17 for methods of helping children and families through the death and dying process.

Because parents might have questions regarding the possibility of future offspring having thalassemia, genetic counseling should be made available (see Chapter 15). Patients with thalassemia minor, which is asymptomatic, should be informed that they can transmit thalassemia major to their children if their spouse or partner also has either thalassemia minor or thalassemia major. They can transmit thalassemia minor even when their partner is free of the trait.

The Child with Coagulation Dysfunction

Hemophilia

Hemophilia is a lifelong, hereditary disorder that is characterized by a disturbance of blood-clotting factors, particularly Factor VIII or Factor IX. A deficiency in either of these factors can adversely affect the production of thrombin, necessary for blood clotting.

The disease almost always occurs in males, at a rate of approximately 1 in 10,000 (Sergis-Davenport et al., 1983). Hemophilia is transmitted by females in a sex-linked hereditary pattern. The gene that causes hemophilia is carried on the X chromosome. A woman is considered a carrier if she carries the abnormal gene on one of her two X chromosomes. She will not have the disease, because the other X chromosome is normal. A male has one X and one Y chromosome. Therefore, if a male inherits an X chromosome carrying the hemophilia gene, he will have the disease. The disease can appear after several generations of disease-free males, or it can occur spontaneously from genetic mutation (Fig. 26-4).

In classic hemophilia A (the most common type), the patient's plasma is deficient in Factor VIII (antihemolytic factor [AHF] or antihemolytic globulin [AHG]). Normal individuals have Factor VIII at levels that vary from 50% to 200%. The degree to which a patient is deficient in Factor VIII tends to be familial. Children with hemophilia can have Factor VIII levels of 20% to less than 1%. Relatives with hemophilia have similar factor levels and symptoms. Table 26-6 illustrates how the level of Factor VIII affects the hemophiliac.

The second most common type of hemophilia is hemophilia B, or Christmas disease. It is caused by a deficiency of Factor IX, the Christmas factor, also known as plasma thromboplastin component (PTC).

Clinical manifestations The clinical manifestations of hemophilia A and B are similar. Hemophilia is seldom diagnosed in infancy unless there is excessive bleeding from circumcision, the umbilical cord, or birth trauma. Usually, bleeding episodes do not occur until early childhood, when the child becomes more active. Hematomas develop from minor bumps and falls or after immunization. Hemophilia can cause prolonged bleeding anywhere in the body. The child might bleed from the gums or from the loss of deciduous teeth.

Hemarthrosis, the oozing of blood into a joint cavity, such as the knee, elbow, or ankle, can cause the joint to become swollen, tender, and painful. The child might complain of stiffness or aching in the joint. Impaired mobility might be evident. Hemarthroses can occur once or twice a week with some children (Sergis-Davenport et al., 1983). Repeated hemorrhage into a joint results in damage to the synovial membrane, degeneration of articular cartilage, and formation of subchondral cysts. Long-range consequences, such as contractures and severe crippling, might develop.

Internal bleeding might cause severe physical complications. For example, bleeding into the neck or pharynx can cause airway obstruction; bleeding into the eyes or ears can destroy vision or hearing; and bleeding into the spinal column can cause paralysis. Spontaneous *hematuria* (blood in the urine) might occur two to three times per year.

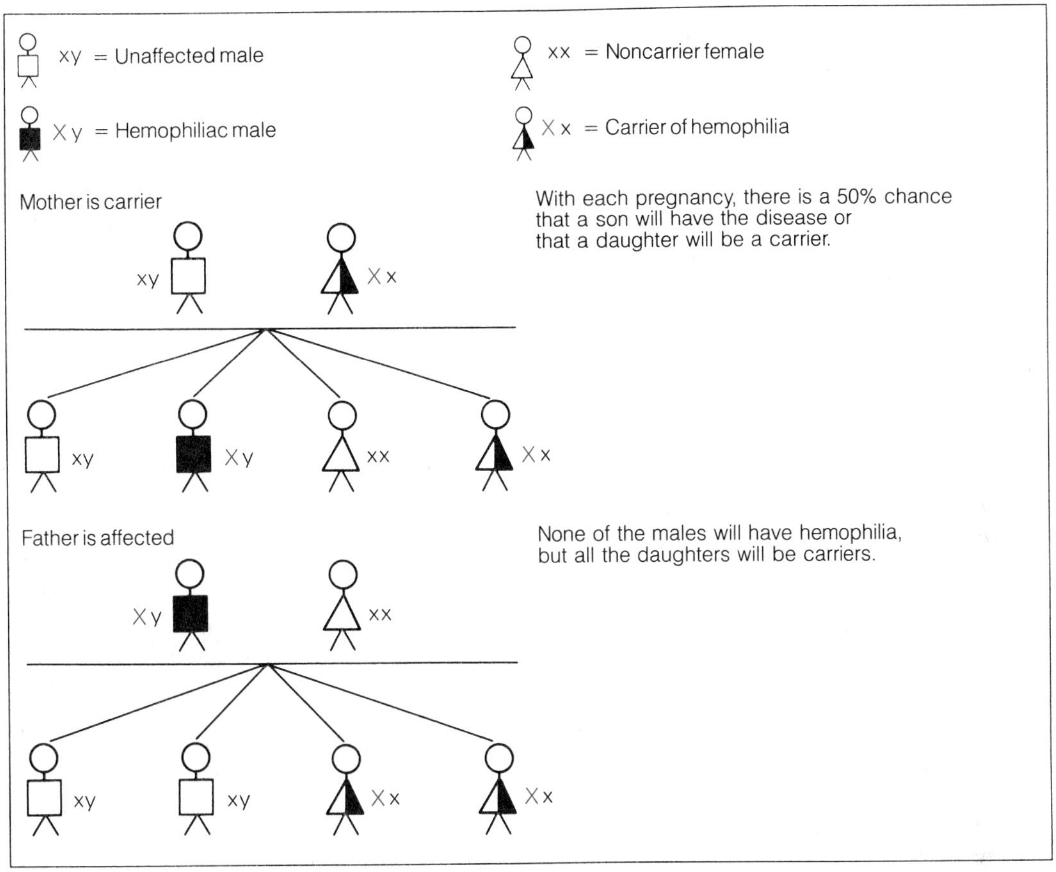

FIGURE 26-4
Examples of sex-linked hereditary patterns in hemophilia.

TABLE 26-6 Effects of Factor Deficiencies in Hemophilia A and B

Severity of hemophilia	Percentage of factor VIII or IX present	Characteristics
Mild	5–50	Bleeding only after severe insult
		Coagulation screening tests normal or low normal
Moderately severe	2–5	Infrequent spontaneous hemorrhages
		Significant hemorrhage after minor trauma
		Prolonged partial thromboplastin times
		Coagulation screening tests rarely passed
Severe	Less than 1	Frequent spontaneous hemorrhages throughout lifetime
		Coagulation screening tests always abnormal

Diagnostic evaluation Diagnosis usually is made on the basis of a prolonged bleeding episode following trauma or from a family history of hemophilia. Bleeding time is normal. Blood coagulation studies are done to determine which clotting factor is deficient. These tests include the prothrombin time (PT), partial thromboplastin time (PTT), thromboplastin generation test (TGT), and prothrombin consumption tests (see Table 26-1). There is usually a prolonged PT and PTT as well as increased TGT. Factor assays (eg, Factor VIII assay), which measure percentages of coagulation factors, assist in determining the percentage of deficient factor.

Treatment

Managing bleeding episodes Minor, external hemorrhage responds well to prolonged pressure and the application of cold. It is essential to stop the bleeding quickly to prevent damage to tissue, nerves, and joints. For more extensive bleeding episodes, the missing clotting factor is administered. Clotting factors can be administered prophylactically to reduce the numbers of bleeding episodes.

Three types of plasma products are available for the treatment of hemophilia A. Fresh-frozen plasma (FFP), obtained from fresh whole blood, is frozen and stored until needed. Once thawed, the plasma is administered promptly because Factor VIII deteriorates at room temperature. The amount of Factor VIII in the plasma depends on the donor's level of Factor VIII. Cross-matching for plasma administration is not necessary, although the child should be ABO compatible with the donor. FFP can be used for Factor IX deficiency also.

Cryoprecipitate of Factor VIII is prepared from fresh-frozen plasma. Like FFP, cryoprecipitate is obtained from plasma from a single donor. It is stored in the freezer until needed and must be used within 6 hours of thawing. There is no cryoprecipitate available for Factor IX deficiency. ABO and Rh compatability are preferred but not essential.

Lyophilized (freeze-dried) concentrates of Factor VIII are prepared by pharmaceutical companies from pools of plasma. Factor concentrate is stored in vials and refrigerated until needed. It is given, however, at room temperature. The dosage of factor concentrate is based on the amount required to achieve the desired level of the factor. Factor IX concentrates also are available.

The choice of product depends on several factors including risk, cost, and convenience. Cryoprecipitate has been used frequently for home treatment of hemophilia and has been preferred over concentrates because the risk of contracting hepatitis or acquired immune deficiency syndrome (AIDS) is decreased when there is a single donor. Heat treatment of concentrates greatly reduces the risk that the child will contract AIDS and somewhat decreases the risk of hepatitis.

Costs of the products vary from area to area, but because they are derived from whole blood, they are all extremely expensive. Blood donors usually are paid for the blood they give, and the cost increases as the product is refined. Heat-treated concentrates are more expensive than other products.

Accessibility, ease of handling, and storage are considered in selecting the product to be given. The concentrates are adaptable since they are stored in the refrigerator as opposed to the freezer. Both cryoprecipitate and concentrates are drawn up through a filtered syringe and administered IV by infusion set.

Because all of the substances used to treat hemophilia are blood products, the patient is at risk for serum hepatitis. Allergic reactions might occur from the infusion of fresh-frozen plasma but are rare with cryoprecipitate or the concentrates. Within the last few years hemophiliacs have been listed among the high-risk groups for contracting AIDS (see Chapter 25), although with the recent routine antibody screening of donated blood, the organism has been virtually eliminated from the blood supply.

Pain management Nonnarcotic, nonaspirin, or narcotic analgesics are prescribed to control pain, depending on its severity. Steroids have been used to decrease the inflammatory process in affected joints or to treat renal bleeds. Casts, traction, and joint aspiration might be necessary to preserve joint function. Surgical replacement of joints is considered in the event of total disability.

Nursing management

Control of bleeding The most important aspect of care for the child with hemophilia is control of active bleeding episodes. This is accomplished by administering the missing factor and taking nursing measures to stop the bleeding. External bleeding from a wound or mucous membrane can be controlled by applying pressure to allow clot formation and applying cold to promote vasoconstriction. The nurse instructs the parent to keep ice packs in the freezer for emergencies. Plastic bags of ice or a wet sponge placed in a plastic bag can be kept in the freezer, or commercially prepared cold packs can be obtained. Occasionally, topical hemostatics, such as Gelfoam, are applied to bleeding areas.

The parents are taught how to administer factor products. Pressure is applied to injection sites for at least five minutes after needle withdrawal. The parent is instructed to report immediately any abnormal pallor, weakness, restlessness, or other signs of internal hemorrhage. Severe headache, vomiting, and disorientation can indicate an intracranial bleed and should be reported immediately. Parents also report any signs of allergic or adverse reactions to the factor administration.

Management of joint hemorrhage and pain Joint hemorrhage and hemarthrosis occur most commonly in the knees, ankles, and elbows. When bleeding occurs, the child experiences discomfort and is unable to move the affected joint. Swelling occurs, and local skin temperature increases. The nurse, or the parent if the child is at home, administers the deficient factor and immobilizes the affected extremity during the acute bleeding episode. Immobilization controls pain and prevents further bleeding.

Pain from a joint hemorrhage is caused by pressure in the joint or muscle spasm. Cold packs alleviate the pain of acute hemorrhage. The joint is immobilized until active bleeding has ceased. Occasionally, splints are needed to maintain immobility and to provide comfort.

If pain persists, appropriate analgesics, such as acetaminophen, should be considered. Aspirin or any salicylate-containing compound is contraindicated because of its depressive effects on platelet function, which can last up to 10 days. The nurse cautions parents of patients with hemophilia to read the labels of all medications (such as cold tablets) for possible aspirin content. The parent can obtain a list of aspirin-containing drugs from the local pharmacy and, when in doubt, ask the pharmacist to select an appropriate over-the-counter analgesic.

Mild pain is treated with acetaminophen or propoxyphene compounds. For more severe pain, the physician might prescribe codeine, meperidine (Demerol), or morphine.

When active bleeding into a joint has stopped, exercise begins. Physical therapy promotes maximum function of the affected joints and maintains range of motion and tone of unaffected body parts. It might be necessary to continue the exercise program at home, in which case the nurse refers the patient to a visiting nurse or physical therapist for continuity of care.

Preventing injury The nurse teaches the families of children with hemophilia how to protect the child from injury without being overprotective. While the patient is in infancy, the parent should pad the crib and use nonbreakable feeding utensils. The home should have wall-to-wall carpeting to cushion falls. Toys should not have rough edges or sharp surfaces. Approved car seats should be used routinely. Routine health promotion is encouraged.

As the child becomes more active and begins to walk, play areas must be supervised. Knee and elbow pads and a helmet can help prevent injury while the child is mastering walking. The child should play on a fenced lawn rather than on a concrete yard or driveway.

The nurse informs the parent that because strong muscles help to protect the joints from bleeding, exercise should be encouraged. Swimming and quiet ball games are ideal for young children. Older children should not take part in contact sports, such as football, because of the obvious dangers. Snowskiing and tennis are not suitable because they place a great deal of strain on the knees and ankles, which could cause bleeding. Swimming, golf, and bowling are safe physical activities that can satisfy the child's competitive interests. It is generally felt that active hemophiliac children bleed less than sedentary hemophiliac children.

Discipline is important for the safety of young children with hemophilia. As young children, they must learn to obey safety rules, and, as early as possible, they must become responsible for their own safety. The nurse reminds parents that teaching their children self-discipline and instilling a sense of responsibility might well be the most important thing they can do to prevent injuries.

Routine health care needs Comprehensive management of the child with hemophilia should consist of a team approach that provides for the physical and psychologic needs of the child. The team should consist of the pediatrician, hematologist, orthopedist, dentist, social worker, physical therapist, psychologist, and nurse.

Hemophilia is a lifelong condition requiring continuity of care. All people who care for the hemophiliac child should be informed about the disorder and know what to do in the event of a bleeding episode. The parent is taught to handle minor wounds by adequate cleansing, application of pressure, and administration of factor if necessary. The dentist selected to care for the child needs to understand the disease and be aware of the need to administer the factor promptly when bleeding occurs. Factor VIII needs to be given prior to routine childhood immunizations. The child with hemophilia should wear medical identification jewelry and should be taught to recognize the earliest symptoms of bleeding so that prompt treatment can be instituted. A nutritional, but sensible, diet is important for children with hemophilia since excess weight can place excessive stress on muscles and joints that are prone to develop bleeding difficulties.

Emotional care Hemophilia is a chronic condition of childhood with acute episodes that might require hospitalization. The child with hemophilia is not an invalid and can progress developmentally within the safety and treatment guidelines of the disease. The National Hemophilia Foundation has more than 50 chapters across the country to help families of hemophiliacs with financial, psychologic, and medical care. The child's reaction to the disease or disability depends upon how well the family responds to the problems that arise. It is essential that the family members demonstrate a positive attitude toward the child with hemophilia to foster a safe environment and to increase the child's self-esteem.

Parents might have the guilt feelings associated with any genetically transmitted disease (see Chapter 15), and the family will encounter some of the problems associated with having a child with a chronic illness (see Chapter 14). Genetic counseling is made available to families with hemophilia to educate them about genetic transfer and to assist in coping with future pregnancies.

The child with hemophilia is encouraged to do as much as possible within the limitations of the disease. It is a natural tendency for parents to be overprotective in the hope of preventing situations that would precipitate a bleeding episode. Children who are not allowed to develop appropriately, however, can exhibit decreased self-esteem, increased manipulative behavior, and adverse emotional consequences. Educating the child about the disease and preparing the child to assume responsibility for actions and self-care can be the best prevention against injury, while allowing the child freedom to grow.

Idiopathic Thrombocytopenic Purpura

Idiopathic thrombocytopenic purpura, commonly known as ITP, is characterized by a reduction in the number of circulating platelets (thrombocytopenia), causing purpura, or bleeding into the tissues. In ITP the thrombocytopenia is caused by an antiplatelet antibody produced in the spleen (see Chapter 25 for discussion of the autoimmune response). The triggering agent seems to alter the surface of the platelets such that they become antigenic and are destroyed. Secondary causes of thrombocytopenia include systemic lupus erythematosus, past transfusions, drug sensitivities, hemolytic anemia, and a possible recent viral infection.

Clinical manifestations The platelet count in ITP is below 50,000/mm^3 and can plunge way below this level. The most common clinical signs of ITP are petechiae and areas of ecchymosis. Bleeding from mucous membranes in the mouth or nose, hematuria, bloody stools, and menorrhagia (excessive menstrual bleeding) are other manifestations of ITP.

Diagnostic evaluation Bone marrow examination is useful to rule out aplastic anemia or leukemia. A diagnosis of ITP is made if red and white blood cells in bone marrow are normal, the platelet count is decreased, and the bleeding time is prolonged.

There might be an elevation in IgG. Prothrombin time and partial thromboplastin time are normal. The tourniquet test, in which a blood pressure cuff is inflated to 100 mm Hg to test capillary fragility, is positive; that is, greater than 10–20 petechiae are present 5 minutes after the tourniquet release.

Treatment The treatment for ITP varies according to local protocol. The child's activity is limited and all contact with aspirin-containing drugs is eliminated. The administration of corticosteroids such as prednisone to suppress antibody response is controversial. Some physicians prescribe steroids for platelet counts less than 30,000 (Dubansky and Oski, 1986). Others use steroids only when there is high risk for marked bleeding, such as when the platelet count drops below 10,000.

Platelet transfusions generally are not beneficial since the antiplatelet antibody destroys the newly infused platelets. In recurrent or chronic ITP, a splenectomy is done to remove the major site of antiplatelet antibody production. Within 1–2 weeks after splenectomy platelet values are normal. Splenectomy frees 70%–90% of patients from the effects of ITP.

The prognosis for ITP is excellent. The majority of patients recover spontaneously within 6 months. In some instances the condition might become chronic.

Nursing management Families need a great deal of emotional support, especially during diagnostic procedures, because they might fear that their child has leukemia. Allowing parents to express their fears, while encouraging them to await the results of the bone marrow aspiration and other diagnostic tests, is helpful.

Acute care focuses on controlling bleeding and preventing hemorrhage (see the section on hemophilia). Pain is controlled with analgesics that do not contain aspirin. If steroids are prescribed, the nurse describes their side effects.

If splenectomy is indicated, the children and families need preoperative teaching (see Chapter 20). Because of the hazards of overwhelming infection after a splenectomy, patients are placed on prophylactic antibiotic therapy. The nurse instructs the child and family about preventing infections and seeking prompt medical attention if the child contracts any infectious disease.

Petechiae, purpura, and the side effects of steroid therapy change the physical appearance of the child. The nurse offers emotional support and reassures the child and family that recovery is likely to occur within 6 months, after which steroid therapy will end and the child's appearance will return to normal.

NURSING CARE PLAN *Child with Classic Hemophilia A*

Assessment data: Ryan is an 8-year-old boy with severe Factor VIII (less than 1%) deficiency. He was hospitalized for left elbow and proximal forearm soft tissue bleeding that occurred 2 days previously. He presently is being treated with a soft tissue splint and cryoprecipitate transfusion. Ryan is to wear the splint at all times, except during range-of-motion exercises four times a day. Ryan has had no other recent bleeding episodes. His last hemarthrosis occurred 8 months previously in the left elbow. All previous episodes have been stopped promptly with factor replacement therapy with no adverse effects.

Physical examination reveals a child of average height and below average weight. Resolving bruises are noted, primarily on lower extremities. Ryan complains of pain and stiffness of the left elbow upon movement. His fingers are warm and pink, with good capillary refill.

Ryan was diagnosed as having hemophilia when he was 9 months old. He lives at home with his parents and 5-year-old sister.

Nursing diagnosis	Intervention	Rationale
1. Alteration in comfort: pain related to bleeding into the joints and soft tissue	Observe Ryan for signs of pain.	Baseline data is useful in determining future needs for intervention.
	Position, support, and immobilize the affected joint; place a bed cradle over the joint.	Minimizing stress on the joint promotes comfort.
	Provide a restful, quiet, supportive environment.	A soothing environment relieves tension.
	Provide diversional activities and psychologic support.	Diversion focuses the child's attention on stimuli other than pain.
	Administer aspirin-free analgesics or narcotic analgesics, as ordered.	Aspirin-free, nonnarcotic analgesics reduce mild pain not relieved by comfort measures. Narcotic analgesics relieve severe pain. Aspirin prolongs clotting time.
	Explain to Ryan why he feels pain.	Information reduces fear.

Outcome: Ryan states he is free from pain. Ryan can identify measures that resulted in pain reduction.

Nursing diagnosis	Intervention	Rationale
2. Potential for injury (stressor: clotting dysfunction and developmental factors)	Instruct Ryan to avoid activities, such as contact sports, that increase the possibility of trauma.	These activities are potential sources of trauma.
	Encourage Ryan to participate in intellectual, creative, and physical activities (bike riding, swimming, bowling) that are not likely to cause trauma.	Strong muscles protect the joints from bleeding. Active children are less likely to bleed than sedentary children.
	Teach Ryan and family about good health habits, including adequate rest and nutrition.	These habits improve health status.
	Plan Ryan's physical education program with school personnel.	Awareness of the child's limitations helps school personnel to provide a safe and appropriate exercise program.
	Instruct Ryan's family that he must avoid all aspirin-containing drugs.	Aspirin and drugs containing aspirin interfere with platelet function, which could cause bleeding.

(Continues)

NURSING CARE PLAN *Child with Classic Hemophilia A (Continued)*

Nursing diagnosis	Intervention	Rationale
	Instruct Ryan and his family that he must wear the medical-alert tag and carry the medical-alert card at all times.	If bleeding should occur, prompt treatment can be given.
	Teach Ryan and his family to recognize the following signs of bleeding: blood in stools or urine, nosebleeds, tachycardia, faintness, confusion, and feeling of fullness in the affected area.	Recognizing the early signs of internal or external bleeding enables the child to obtain prompt treatment, which can minimize complications.
	Explain to Ryan and his family medical methods used to control bleeding: administration of blood factor; transfusion of whole blood or packed red blood cells when Hgb level falls.	Information about the medical regimen gives the family a better understanding of the child's need for care.
	Teach Ryan and his family emergency measures to control bleeding: application of pressure for 10–15 minutes, immobilization of the joint, elevation of the joint above the heart, and application of cold.	Prompt treatment with emergency measures minimizes bleeding by aiding in clot formation, decreasing blood flow to the extremity, and producing vasoconstriction.
	Instruct Ryan's family to seek medical assistance if bleeding is not stopped by usual measures.	It is essential to prevent complications of excessive bleeding.
	Protect Ryan from trauma in the hospital by padding bed rails, keeping bed in low position, assisting with ambulation and activities when necessary, rotating injection sites, and applying direct pressure over puncture sites.	These measures will minimize the risk of injury of bleeding.
	Establish routine good oral hygiene by referring Ryan to a dentist who is aware of Ryan's special needs and by teaching Ryan to use a soft toothbrush that has been soaked in water prior to brushing.	The dentist must be knowledgeable about hemophilia so that precautions can be taken when treating the child. Gentle cleaning of the teeth prevents mucosal bleeding.
	Teach Ryan and his family that special precautions should be taken during such procedures as dental work.	It might be necessary to give Factor VIII prior to some procedures to minimize the effects or bleeding.

Outcome: Ryan and his family can describe sources of injury and how to avoid them. They can demonstrate what to do when bleeding occurs. Ryan engages in safe activities.

Nursing diagnosis	Intervention	Rationale
3. Potential impaired physical mobility (stressor: edema and restricted movement from bleeding into joint, joint pain)	Maintain range of motion of unaffected joints and muscles by providing range-of-motion exercises while Ryan is on bed rest and by encouraging early ambulation and activity.	Exercise minimizes the loss of muscle tone, promotes circulation, and prevents contractures.
	Move the affected joint through passive range of motion, as ordered by the physician.	Passive range-of-motion exercises help prevent degeneration of the affected joint.
	Immobilize the joint during active bleeding.	Immobilization helps control bleeding into the joint and promotes absorption.
	Administer aspirin-free analgesics prior to range-of-motion exercises or physical therapy.	Reduction of pain enables the patient to better tolerate exercise and maximizes its effects.
	Encourage Ryan's family to participate in his exercise program.	Participation promotes the family's involvement in the child's care.

NURSING CARE PLAN *Child with Classic Hemophilia A (Continued)*

Nursing diagnosis	Intervention	Rationale
	Refer Ryan to a public health nurse and/or physical therapist for aid with his home care program.	Follow-up is needed to ensure that home care measures are being carried out.
	Provide a diet that is nutritious but does not allow for weight gain.	Obesity places additional pressure on weight-bearing joints.
	Encourage Ryan to participate in sports that maintain joint function but are not potential sources of injury.	Exercise helps maintain joint function.
	Educate Ryan and his family about the long-term consequences of hemarthrosis.	Education encourages prevention.

Outcome: Ryan and his family can identify measures to prevent joint contractures. The family assists Ryan to perform range-of-motion exercises.

Nursing diagnosis	Intervention	Rationale
4. Potential alteration in family process (stressors: imposed activity restrictions and home care demands)	Encourage Ryan and his family to discuss their feelings about hemophilia.	Knowledge about the effects motivates the child and family to follow the plan of care.
	Provide opportunities for Ryan's parents, especially his mother, to talk about the genetic component of the disease.	The child's mother might feel guilty that she passed this disorder on to her child.
	Find out how hemophilia has affected Ryan's parents' childrearing practices, for example, imposing discipline, setting limits, and fostering independence.	Parents need opportunities to learn which childrearing practices can best benefit a child with hemophilia.
	Foster Ryan's independence by allowing him to help make decisions about his care, focusing his attention on the things he can do, supporting his ego strengths, and fostering a positive self-image, encouraging him in self-care during hospitalization, and introducing him to other children with hemophilia who are adjusting well to the disease.	These measures promote self-esteem, a sense of control, a more positive attitude regarding the disease, and the opportunity to socialize with peers.
	Help Ryan and his family to identify factors that help them to cope well in crises, for example, previous coping patterns, the ability to seek out and use the help of others, and family stability.	Recognition of positive coping patterns prepares the child and family to use them during future crises.
	Encourage Ryan's family to join the National Hemophilia Foundation.	The famliy needs an opportunity to comunicate with other families having the same problems.
	Inform Ryan's family about possible sources of financial aid, such as the local chapter of the National Hemophilia Foundation and social service agencies.	Treatments for hemophilia can be very costly, and the family might need financial assistance.
	Encourage Ryan's parents to promote a sense of independence and responsibility as he grows older.	The child with hemophilia must learn to assume responsibility for self-care and should not be discouraged in this endeavor.
	Determine whether a home care program would be suitable for Ryan.	A home care program would allow the child with hemophilia and the family greater participation in treatment.

Outcome: Ryan and his family are able to discuss their feelings about the disease and its demands. They use available resources and can identify and use healthy coping strategies.

(Continues)

NURSING CARE PLAN *Child with Classic Hemophilia A (Continued)*

Nursing diagnosis	Intervention	Rationale
5. Potential knowledge deficit regarding home management (stressor: incomplete understanding of the disease, treatment, and complications)	Discuss with Ryan and his family the long-term effects of hemophilia.	Discussion increases cognitive knowledge.
	Explain to Ryan and his family all aspects of care and procedures involved in the treatment of hemophilia.	Knowing what to expect decreases fear of the unknown.
	Teach Ryan and his family the importance of preventive measures in the treatment of hemophilia.	Knowledge helps the child and family to understand and comply with preventive aspects of treatment.
	Discuss with Ryan's family the genetic components of hemophilia.	The family needs to know that subsequent offspring could have hemophilia.
	Refer Ryan's family to a genetic counselor.	A genetic counselor will be able to give the parents specific information about the genetic transmission of hemophilia in their own family.

Outcome: Ryan and his family can list the long-term health needs related to the disease. The family is aware of the implications of genetic transfer. The family can list potential complications.

Disseminated Intravascular Coagulation

Disseminated intravascular coagulation (DIC) is characterized by excessive coagulation followed by excessive bleeding. Massive fibrin formation occurs with the release of excess clotting factors following vascular injury. This causes the widespread development of thrombi (clots). Eventually, all the platelets and clotting factors are depleted, and the fibrinolytic (fibrin breakdown) mechanism is stimulated to dissolve the clots. This is followed by hemorrhage.

Disseminated intravascular coagulation is not a primary disease but rather is secondary to any number of acute pathologic processes. Common predisposing factors are respiratory distress syndrome, abruptio placentae, shock, acidosis, trauma, sepsis, and surgical procedures. It is unknown exactly how these acute conditions cause DIC.

Clinical manifestations Clinically, manifestations of DIC include (1) a tendency toward generalized bleeding; (2) ischemia of organs and tissue from vaso-occlusive thromboses; and (3) secondary anemia. Petechiae, ecchymoses, and hemorrhage, combined with evidence of thrombosis, are indicative of DIC. Thrombosis in a blood vessel serving the central nervous system causes changes in mental status. Thrombosis in a peripheral blood vessel might cause coolness and cyanosis of an extremity. Hematuria is a sign of renal system involvement.

Hematologic findings include decreased platelet and fibrinogen levels and prolonged prothrombin time (PT) and partial thromboplastin time (PTT).

Treatment Resolving the underlying disease process is the primary treatment for DIC. Heparin, an antagonist to thrombin, is given to inhibit further clot formation. When the platelet count rises and clinical findings suggest that DIC has ceased, heparin therapy is terminated. Replacement of platelets is seldom necessary, but platelets might be transfused after heparin therapy has begun. Whole blood or blood products can be given to replace the depleted clotting factor, but this treatment carries the risk of stimulating further clotting.

Nursing management Nursing care for children with DIC depends on the underlying cause of the condition. The nurse protects the child with DIC from any unnecessary bleeding episodes and is alert for signs and symptoms of vaso-occlusion and bleeding in the child who is at risk for DIC.

Essential Concepts

- Disorders associated with alterations of blood elements affect the function of erythrocytes (red blood cells), which carry oxygen; leukocytes (white blood cells), which protect the body from infection; and thrombocytes (platelets), which aid in coagulation and clotting.
- Assessment of the child with suspected or diagnosed hematopoietic dysfunction includes a complete history that focuses on familial hereditary diseases, nutrition, infection, possible exposure to toxic substances, and exercise tolerance.
- In the physical examination part of the assessment, the nurse gathers and assesses subjective and objective data relevant to the anemias or clotting disturbances.
- The child with anemia is likely to be pale, fatigued, and listless, and to have signs of hypoxia and splenic enlargement.
- The child with clotting disturbances is likely to have painful joints, skin discolorations, and other signs of internal or external hemorrhage.
- Diagnostic procedures and tests for blood disorders include hematologic studies and bone marrow aspiration, all of which are invasive or painful, necessitating careful preparation of the child and emotional support.
- Nursing responsibilities related to blood transfusions include explaining the procedure to the patient, verifying correct blood-typing and cross-matching between patient and donor, administering the transfusion, observing the patient for signs and symptoms of transfusion reaction, and beginning treatment if a transfusion reaction occurs.
- Interventions to meet the acute-care needs of the child with a hematopoietic dysfunction include promoting rest and good respiratory function to alleviate hypoxia and protecting the child from injury and infection.
- The nutritional needs of children with red blood cell disorders include a diet rich in iron and vitamins, particularly vitamin C.
- Meeting the developmental needs of the child with hematopoietic dysfunction involves encouraging the parent to promote the child's independence and self-care by giving the child increasing responsibility for diet, exercise tolerance, and safety.
- Interventions to meet the emotional needs of children with disorders of the hematopoietic system are directed toward encouraging development of a positive self-esteem.
- Dysfunctions of the hematopoietic system experienced by neonates include neonatal hyperbilirubinemia and ABO incompatibility.
- Hematopoietic alterations affecting red blood cell structure or function include iron deficiency anemia, aplastic anemia, sickle cell disease, and thalassemia.
- The child with a coagulation dysfunction might experience hemophilia, ideopathic thrombocytopenia, or disseminated intravascular coagulation.

References

Donlen JM, Budd RA: The low-birth-weight infant: A nursing perspective. In: *Neonatal and Pediatric Critical Care Nursing.* Stahler-Miller K (editor). Churchill Livingstone, 1983.

Dubansky AS, Oski FA: Controversies in the management of acute ITP: A survey of specialists. *Pediatrics* (Jan) 1986; 77(1): 49–52.

Goldstein M: The aplastic anemias. *Hosp Pract* (May) 1980; 15: 84–94.

Hutchison MM: Aplastic anemia: Care of the bone-marrow-failure patient. *Nurs Clin North Am* (Sept) 1983; 18(3): 543–551.

Jenkins J: *Human Genetics.* Benjamin/Cummings, 1983.

Johnson CS: Sickle cell anemia. *JAMA* (Oct 11) 1985; 254(14): 1958–1963.

Ladewig PA, London M, Olds S: *Essentials of Maternal-Newborn Nursing.* Addison-Wesley, 1986.

Landier WC, Barrell ML, Styffe EJ: How to administer blood components to children. *MCN* (May/June) 1987; 12(3): 178–184.

Sergis-Davenport E, Miller R, Comperts E: Overview of hemophilia. *Issues Compr Pediatr Nurs* (Sept/Dec 1983; 6(5–6): 317–328.

Stavis RL, Krauss AN: Complications of neonatal intensive care. *Clin Perinatol* (March) 1980; 7: 107–124.

Additional Readings

Buchanan GR: Disseminated intravascular coagulation. In: *A Practical Guide to Pediatric Intensive Care*. Levin B, Morris F (editors). Mosby, 1983.

Byrnes JJ: Thrombotic thrombocytopenic purpura. *Adv Intern Med* 1980; 26:131–157.

Clements MF, Blumenstein-Butler R, Meredith K: The development of a teaching model for patients with hemophilia and their families. *Issues Compr Pediatr Nurs* (June/Aug) 1984; 7(4–5): 213–217.

Dallman PR, Siimes MA, Stekel A: Iron deficiency in infants and childhood. *Am J Clin Nutr* (June) 1980; 33:86–118.

Dressler D: Understanding and treating hemophilia. *Nurs '80* (Aug) 1980; 10(8):72–73.

Gaddy Cohen D: ITP in children. *Issues Compr Pediatr Nurs* (Sept/Dec) 1983; 6(5–6):307–315.

Kneut C: Sickle cell anemia. *Issues Compr Pediatr Nurs* (Sept/Dec) 1980; 4:19–27.

Lanzkowsky P: *Pediatric Hematology—Oncology—a Treatise for the Clinician*. McGraw-Hill, 1980.

Lightsey AL Jr: Thrombocytopenia in children. *Pediatr Clin North Am* 1980; 27:293–308.

Masoorli ST, Piercy S: A lifesaving guide to blood products. *RN* (Sept) 1984; 32–37.

Moeller K, Swartzendruber EJ: Suppressing the risks of bone marrow suppression. *Nurs '87* (March) 1987; 17(3):52–54.

Nathan D, Oski F: *Hematology in Infancy and Childhood*. Vol II. 2nd ed. Saunders, 1981.

Nuscher R: Bone marrow transplantation. *Am J Nurs* (June) 1984; 84:764–772.

Peck NL: Action STAT: Blood transfusion reaction. *Nurs '87* (Jan) 1987; 17(1):33.

Reindorf CA: Sickle cell anemia. *Curr Concepts Pediatr Nurs* (Mar/Apr) 1980; 6(2):E to G.

Smith L: Reactions to blood transfusions. *Am J Nurs* (Sept) 1984; 84:1096–1101.

Chapter 27

Ingestion, Digestion, and Elimination

Implications of Inflammation and Obstruction

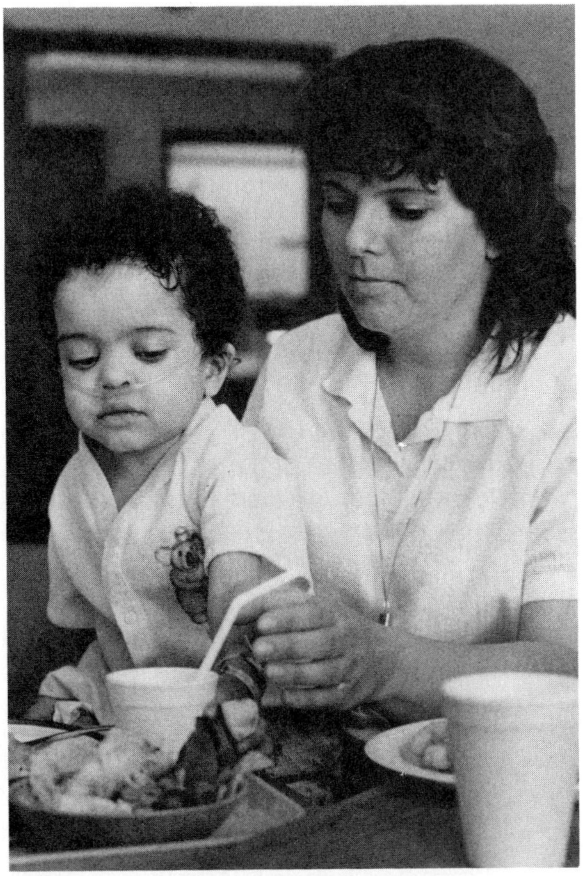

Chapter Contents

Alteration in nutrition: less than body requirements related to impaired use of food

Developmental Needs

Potential for altered growth and development

Emotional Needs

Potential alteration in parenting

Potential body image disturbance

Health Maintenance Needs

Potential for impaired home maintenance management

The Child with Problems Involving Ingestion

Cleft Lip and Cleft Palate
Esophageal Atresia and Tracheoesophageal Fistula

The Child with a Problem Affecting the Body's Use of Food

Phenylketonuria (PKU)
Gastroesophageal Reflux (Chalasia)
Celiac Disease
Short-Bowel Syndrome
Kwashiorkor

The Child with Existing or Potential Upper Gastrointestinal Obstruction

Pyloric Stenosis
Diaphragmatic Hernia

The Child with Existing or Potential Lower Gastrointestinal Obstruction

Intussusception
Umbilical Hernia, Gastroschisis, and Omphalocele
Congenital Inguinal Hernia and Hydrocele
Imperforate Anus
Hirschsprung's Disease (Aganglionic Megacolon)

The Child with a Problem of Inflammation

Appendicitis
Ulcerative Colitis and Regional Enteritis (Crohn's Disease)
Peptic Ulcer

Cross Reference Box

To find these topics, see the following chapters:

Abdominal pain	Chapter 18
Constipation	Chapter 18
Gastroenteritis	Chapters 18, 21
Foreign body ingestion	Chapter 18
Intestinal parasites	Chapter 18
Necrotizing enterocolitis	Chapter 34
Thrush	Chapter 18

The Child with a Problem Related to Interference with Metabolism of Nutrients

Hepatitis
Cirrhosis
Anomalies of the Biliary Tree

Objectives

- Describe the structure, function, and embryonic development of the gastrointestinal system.
- Describe the assessment criteria and diagnostic tests specific to assessment of the gastrointestinal system.
- Explain the principles of nursing care common to procedures and treatments involving the gastrointestinal tract.
- Define methods of feeding used for children with feeding problems.
- Explain the principles of nursing care for children undergoing abdominal surgery.
- Describe the essential developmental, emotional, and health maintenance needs of children with gastrointestinal dysfunction.
- Explain the physiologic processes, common medical treatments, and principles of nursing management for conditions hampering or preventing ingestion or digestion.
- Explain the physiologic processes, common medical treatments, and principles of nursing management for conditions interfering with the absorption or use of nutrients.
- Explain the physiologic processes, common medical treatments, and principles of nursing management for conditions characterizing inflammation of the digestive tract.
- Explain the physiologic processes, common medical treatments, and principles of nursing management for conditions affecting metabolism of nutrients.

ESSENTIALS OF STRUCTURE AND FUNCTION
The Gastrointestinal System

Embryonic Development of the Digestive Tract

The embryonic development of the gastrointestinal tract begins during the first 4 weeks of gestation. The embryonic tract begins as an internal tubelike structure (gut) that elongates and expands to form a continuous pathway extending from the mouth to the anus. The organs of the digestive system are formed from portions of the embryonic gut.

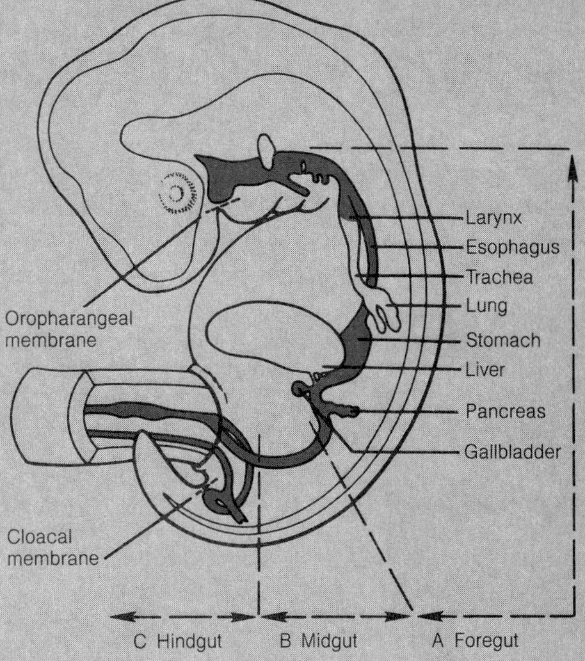

Primitive embryonic gut.

Glossary

Foregut The portion of the embryonic gastrointestinal tract that extends into the head and develops into the pharynx, esophagus, lower respiratory tract, stomach, portion of the duodenum, liver, pancreas, and biliary tree. The oropharyngeal membrane, which separates the foregut from the developing oral structures, disappears, thus providing an external opening through the mouth. (See figure showing embryonic gut.)

Hindgut Embryonic section of the tract that forms the final portion of the transverse colon, the descending colon, the sigmoid colon, the rectum, and the anal canal.

Abnormalities Associated with Abnormal Embryonic Development of the Gastrointestinal Tract

Abnormal process	Example
Failure to fuse Two surfaces that normally would join fail to unite, leaving the structure incomplete	Cleft lip and palate
Failure of or abnormal differentiation The mechanical separation of one structure into two fails to occur or there is a failure of separation by function	Duodenal stenosis from incomplete differentiation of stomach and duodenum
Atresia Abnormal closing of a structure that normally would remain open	Esophageal atresia, anorectal malformations, biliary atresia
Fistula An abnormal tubal connection from one surface to another that might be due to an incomplete separation or closure of a structure	Tracheoesophageal fistula, anorectal malformations with fistulas
Incomplete or abnormal misplacement Structures that normally move during development fail to do so	Volvulus from incomplete rotation of the gut

(Continues)

ESSENTIALS OF STRUCTURE AND FUNCTION *(Continued)*
The Gastrointestinal System

The cloacal membrane at the end of the hindgut separates the urogenital structures from the rectoanal structures. It degenerates, providing an external exit at the anus.

Midgut Embryonic gastrointestinal tract forming the small intestine, the cecum, the appendix, the ascending colon, and the initial portion of the transverse colon.

A number of processes affect the development of embryonic structures. Any interruption in the formation of these structures can cause abnormalities in their function. Many of these abnormalities are the direct result of developmental arrest: the structure fails to grow appropriately and maintains a primitive state (see table of abnormal development).

Physiology of the Digestive Tract

The digestive tract functions to ingest, digest, and absorb nutrients. Each portion of the gastrointestinal system is responsible for specific digestive functions. (See illustration of digestive tract.)

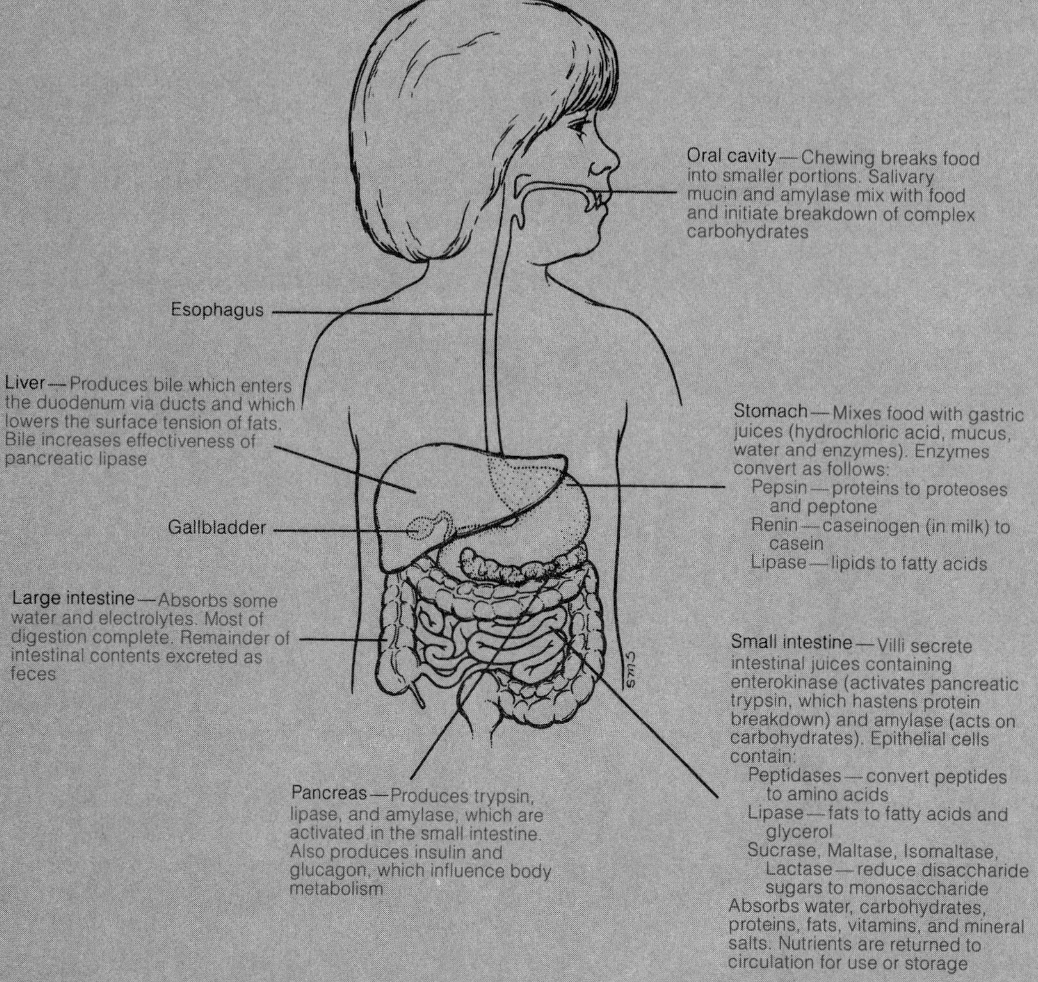

Oral cavity—Chewing breaks food into smaller portions. Salivary mucin and amylase mix with food and initiate breakdown of complex carbohydrates
Esophagus
Liver—Produces bile which enters the duodenum via ducts and which lowers the surface tension of fats. Bile increases effectiveness of pancreatic lipase
Gallbladder
Stomach—Mixes food with gastric juices (hydrochloric acid, mucus, water and enzymes). Enzymes convert as follows:
Pepsin—proteins to proteoses and peptone
Renin—caseinogen (in milk) to casein
Lipase—lipids to fatty acids
Large intestine—Absorbs some water and electrolytes. Most of digestion complete. Remainder of intestinal contents excreted as feces
Small intestine—Villi secrete intestinal juices containing enterokinase (activates pancreatic trypsin, which hastens protein breakdown) and amylase (acts on carbohydrates). Epithelial cells contain:
Peptidases—convert peptides to amino acids
Lipase—fats to fatty acids and glycerol
Sucrase, Maltase, Isomaltase, Lactase—reduce disaccharide sugars to monosaccharide
Absorbs water, carbohydrates, proteins, fats, vitamins, and mineral salts. Nutrients are returned to circulation for use or storage
Pancreas—Produces trypsin, lipase, and amylase, which are activated in the small intestine. Also produces insulin and glucagon, which influence body metabolism
SMS

The digestive tract functions to ingest, digest, and absorb nutrients. Food passes from the mouth through the esophagus, stomach, and intestines. Nutrients are absorbed into the circulation and wastes are excreted.

Disorders of the gastrointestinal system vary greatly in their impact on the lives of the affected child and family. Minor illnesses might cause inconvenience or disrupt the child's or family's life for only a brief period. Many disorders are life-threatening unless emergency treatment, often surgery, is instituted quickly.

Other gastrointestinal dysfunctions might be more chronic and can severely affect the child's growth and development. Any chronic disorder that disrupts the child's ability to eat and grow normally can have serious effects on the parent-child relationship. If the child fails to thrive, the parent might view this as a deliberate rejection of parental love and nurturance. Thus, nursing care of the child with a problem affecting the gastrointestinal tract involves promoting effective family coping as well as meeting the physical needs of the child.

Assessment of the Child with Digestive Dysfunction

A child suspected of having a gastrointestinal problem requires a complete physical assessment. In addition, the nurse pays particular attention to the functioning of the organs and to the processes of the gastrointestinal tract. (Tests used to diagnose gastrointestinal disorders are summarized in Tables 27-1 and 27-2.)

History

In addition to obtaining a standard history, the nurse questions parents of children with suspected gastrointestinal disorders about past events or behaviors that might point toward a diagnosis (eg, change in elimination or eating patterns). These questions are general but provide an overall view of the functioning of the child's intestinal tract.

A review of the child's prenatal history yields information that might aid in the diagnosis of a gastrointestinal disorder. This history includes the child's estimated gestation and birth weight. Any incidence of maternal polyhydramnios (excessive amniotic fluid) might indicate intestinal atresias or other defects of the intestinal tract. In addition, any family history of gastrointestinal anomalies can prove very important in establishing a working diagnosis.

Relevant data about the neonate include any observable anomalies such as protruding abdominal contents or facial defects. More subtle indicators of intestinal problems might include difficulty with initial feedings, episodes of aspiration, frequent vomiting or regurgitation, neonatal diarrhea, prolonged jaundice, gastric distension, respiratory distress, or failure to pass meconium.

The nurse questions the parents of an infant or child about any neonatal problems, growth patterns, weight gains or losses (particularly in relation to time involved), feeding history (breast- or bottle-feeding, vomiting, ability to suck), and the presnce of diarrhea or constipation. Any changes in elimination patterns or appearance and quantity of stools are noted. An in-depth dietary history is necessary for children with suspected food allergies or malabsorption syndromes.

A history of the current concern includes questions regarding the length of time that the child has experienced the problem and any outstanding gastrointestinal signs and symptoms. The qualities of the stools and vomitus are important in helping to reach a diagnosis. Therefore, the nurse asks the parent for or directly observes and records this information (see Assessment Guide).

The nurse also questions the parent and child about any abdominal discomfort, as the presence of pain requires more in-depth questioning. Frequency, intensity (severe, mild), nature (cramping, colicky), and location are assessed. The nurse questions the parent about the location of any pain occurring early in the course of the illness. (In appendicitis, for example, pain is frequently periumbilical before localizing in the right lower quadrant.) Timing of pain might also be significant and might, for example, occur before or after eating, defecating, or intense activity.

Changes in eating habits or abnormal eating patterns might indicate a gastrointestinal problem. For instance, children who have good appetites normally might exhibit sudden anorexia or nausea when eating. Adverse reactions to ingested foods (for example, diarrhea, abdominal distension) are important to note.

The nurse questions the parent closely regarding the onset of any jaundice, its duration, and any changes in its degree. Associated with the jaundice might be clay-colored stools and dark urine.

Validating Diagnostic Tests

Children with gastrointestinal disorders undergo a variety of diagnostic procedures. These might be invasive or noninvasive, and the child's need for preparation varies accordingly.

Noninvasive tests that might be used in the diagnosis of gastrointestinal disorders include flat-plate radiographs, stool tests, and barium swallow radiographs. Blood tests are frequently considered noninvasive, even though a venipuncture or fingerstick is necessary, and the child might perceive the test as threatening. Preparation for tests varies according to the developmental age and emotional needs of the child.

Invasive tests that might be used in the diagnosis of gastrointestinal disorders include barium enema, intestinal

TABLE 27-1 Diagnostic Tests Used in Gastroenterology

Test	Normal values *		Alteration/clinical significance
Serum chemistry			
Bilirubin Measures liver function	Total bilirubin Newborn Child Indirect bilirubin Direct bilirubin	mg/dL 1.0–12.0 0.2–0.8 0.2–0.8 0.1–0.4	*Increased:* Obstructive jaundice, hepatitis, cirrhosis, hemolytic jaundice, newborn hyperbilirubinemia
Ammonia Used as an indicator of hepatic protein metabolism	Values vary widely	40–110 mg/100 ml	*Increased:* Hepatocellular failure, Reye's syndrome
Alkaline phosphatase Index of liver and bone disease when matched with other clinical findings	Bodansky units/dL Children 5–14, adults 1.5–4.5 King-Armstrong units/dL Children 15–30, adults 4–13 Bessy-Lowery units/dL Children 3.4–9.0, adults 0.8–2.3		*Increased:* Obstructive jaundice, liver disease, metastatic bone disease, rickets, osteomalacia *Decreased:* Malnutrition, hypothyroidism, hypophosphatosia
Amylase	Children	45–200 dye U/dL	*Increased:* Pancreatic duct obstruction or inflammation, salivary gland inflammation *Decreased:* Hepatitis, cirrhosis, severe burns
Aminotransferases ALT (formerly SGOT) Presence of the enzyme directly related to number of dying cells and time lapse between injury to the tissue and test	Newborn (1–3 days) Infant (6 mo–1 yr) Child (1–5 yr) Older child (5 yr–adult)	IU/L 16–74 16–35 6–30 19–28	*Increased:* Cirrhosis, hepatitis, acute pancreatitis, acute renal disease, severe burns, hemolytic anemia, brain trauma, trauma to skeletal or cardiac muscle
AST (formerly SGPT) Test of enzyme level found mainly in liver. Evaluates liver function	Infant Children	IU/L below 54 1–30	*Increased:* Hepatocellular failure, cirrhosis, hepatitis, obstructive jaundice
Stool specimens			
pH	7–7.5		*Increased:* Base-protein breakdown *Decreased:* Acid-carbohydrate fermentation or disaccharide intolerance
Ova and parasites	0		*Increased:* Ameobae, *giardia*, helminths
Stool culture	No pathologic organisms		*Increased:* Certain forms of diarrhea
Stool electrolytes			*Decreased:* Sodium and chloride loss excessive in certain forms of diarrhea
Fecal fat	(One specimen or 72 hr collection.) On smear, fatty acid globules 1–4 μ in diameter		*Increased:* Idiopathic steatorrhea, ulcerative colitis, Crohn's disease, cystic fibrosis, malabsorptive syndromes, short-bowel syndrome, and other conditions
Trypsin	2+–4+ in children		*Decreased:* Some pancreatic diseases, might be absent in cystic fibrosis
Reducing substances	Negative		*Increased:* Disaccharidase deficiencies
Clinitest of liquid stool	Negative		*Increased:* Disaccharidase deficiencies

* Normal values might vary with laboratory method used.

TABLE 27-2 Other Gastroenterologic Studies

Test	Comments
^{131}I rose bengal	Hepatic retention of radioactive iodine is increased in obstructive jaundice. A diffuse nodular scan pattern indicates cirrhosis or hepatitis. A cystic scan pattern indicates choledochal cysts. Precautions must be taken because the isotope is excreted in the urine and stool of the child. All waste is considered radioactive, and no pregnant women are allowed to care for the child. A urinary catheter may be placed in young children to avoid contamination of linen with radioactive urine. Observe for allergy to iodine dye
Abdominal flat-plate and upright abdominal x-rays	Often used to diagnose or rule out pneumatosis intestinalis, free peritoneal air, organ displacement, subphrenic abscesses, intestinal obstructions
Upper-GI series	Used to diagnose esophageal abnormalities, gastric ulcers, bezoars
Small bowel follow through (SBFT)	Used to diagnose duodenal and jejunal ulcers, perforation, Crohn's disease, ileal stenosis or atresia, Meckel's diverticulum
Barium enema	Used to diagnose anal and rectal stenosis, rectal polyps, diverticulum, ulcerative colitis, Crohn's disease, Hirschsprung's disease, fistulas, intussusception
Intravenous cholangiography	Used to diagnose biliary tree anomalies (atresias, choledochal cysts, cholestasis)
Duodenal and jejunal biopsy or aspirate	Biopsies used for celiac disease, Crohn's disease, disaccharidase deficiencies. Aspirates used for pancreatic enzyme deficiencies, ova or helminths, *Giardia lamblia*
Rectal and colon biopsy	Used to diagnose Crohn's disease or ulcerative colitis, Hirschsprung's disease
Liver biopsy	Used to diagnose hepatitis, cirrhosis, other liver disease
Endoscopy	Fiberoptic examination for diagnosis of esophagitis, gastritis, ulcers, foreign bodies
Colonoscopy or proctosigmoidoscopy	Visualization of rectum and colon used to diagnose ulcerative colitis, Crohn's disease, anomalies, cause of bleeding, diverticulitis

ASSESSMENT GUIDE *The Child with a Gastrointestinal Problem*

Assessment questions	Supporting data
Does the child have any obvious abnormalities affecting the gastrointestinal system?	Presence of clefts of the lip or palate; alterations in the gag, suck, or swallow reflex; protruding abdominal contents; rectal or anal prolapse; closed anus; visible fistulas, fissures, or abscesses
Has the child experienced any alteration in feeding patterns or any growth delay?	Poor hydration status (see Chapter 21); nausea; vomiting: force (eg, projectile, regurgitative), color (eg, green = bile, clear = gastric, red = fresh blood, coffee ground = old blood), odor (fecal odor = obstruction), and time in relation to last meal; gastric distention and pain; visible peristalsis; failure-to-thrive; alteration in electrolytes and/or serum chemistries; occult blood in vomitus
Has the child experienced any alteration in elimination pattern?	Constipation; difficult defecation; abdominal pain and distention; absent or hyperactive bowel sounds; alteration in stool consistency, quality (eg, slimy, tarry, frothy, curdlike), color (eg, brown, black, green, yellow, white/clay, clear); occult blood, pus, reducing substances, or organisms in stools
Does the child appear to be in pain?	Anorexia, nausea, fever; changing pattern and location of pain (note and describe pain location and intensity)

Additional data: Cyanosis associated with feeding; copious oral or nasal secretions; respiratory distress after feedings or associated with abdominal pain and distention; history of food allergies or recent foreign travel; icteric (yellow) skin biopsy, endoscopy, colonoscopy, duodenal aspirates, and intravenous cholangiography (Table 27-2). Preparation for these need to be more extensive than for noninvasive tests because the child is more likely to fear the test and to fantasize about the experience. The child's concerns depend, however, on the child's developmental stage and previous experience with procedures or hospitalization. The nurse therefore plans according to the needs of the child and family. (Chapter 20 discusses principles of care for both invasive and noninvasive procedures.)

Nursing Management for Procedures and Treatments

Enemas

Many children require an enema or other bowel-cleansing routine prior to undergoing gastrointestinal procedures. Infants and young children require careful administration of enemas because of the small size of the rectal vault and the increased possibility of fluid and electrolyte imbalances associated with repeated enemas. The enema solution should be isotonic (usually normal saline). Plain tap water, which is hypotonic, or some hypertonic commercial enema solutions can cause rapid fluid shifts, leading to hypervolemia or hypovolemia and associated electrolyte imbalances. In small children, the usual procedure for "enemas until clear" might need to be modified to prevent these problems. The catheter used to administer the enema solution also should be flexible and well lubricated.

Suggested enema fluid volumes corresponding to age ranges are:

Age	*Volume*
18 months	50–200 mL
18 months–5 years	200–300 mL
5–12 years	300–500 mL
12 years and older	500–800 mL

Infants and young children who do not exhibit sphincter control need to be assisted in retaining the enema. The nurse firmly presses the buttocks together to prevent the immediate expulsion of the solution. Children who are still in diapers can be allowed to expel the solution into a diaper.

Medications

Laxatives such as mineral oil or magnesium hydroxide (milk of magnesia) might be prescribed to soften the stool and promote bowel emptying. Laxatives might cause cramping and discomfort. As with enema administration, the nurse observes the child for any alterations in fluid balance.

Other medications used prior to gastrointestinal procedures are antibiotics and anticholinergics. Kanamycin, neomycin, colistin, and other gut-specific antibiotics might be used to decrease the bacterial flora prior to surgery. Atropine, scopolamine, and other anticholinergic drugs might be administered in preoperative injections. These agents inhibit the production of saliva and mucus and would be particularly important for the child having surgery involving the oral cavity. The parent and child should be aware that anticholinergics can cause flushing and dryness of the mouth.

Dietary Modifications

The child undergoing gastrointestinal diagnostic tests might be placed on a restricted diet. The most common dietary change is to allow nothing by mouth (see Chapter 20 for the care of the child with NPO status). Other diet regimens might include clear liquids, full liquids, high- or low-fat diets, or exclusionary diets for certain disaccharides (sugars). Most hospitals maintain lists of foods that might be served for each type of diet. The nurse can often encourage cooperation with dietary restrictions by offering the child a choice of foods or by allowing substitutions whenever possible. If dietary restrictions are to be maintained for longer then 24 hours, the nurse might need to assess the child's intake for caloric and dietary sufficiency.

Gastric Decompression

Accumulation of gas and secretions in the gastrointestinal tract might require release through gastric decompression. Gastric decompression not only relieves pain from gas accumulation but also allows the gastrointestinal tract to rest until proper function returns. Gastric decompression is accomplished by the insertion of a nasogastric tube or by a gastrostomy (a procedure in which a tube is surgically placed and secured in the stomach through the abdominal wall).

Principles for nasogastric suction for children are similar to those for adults. The proper size tube is important (8, 10, 12, 14, depending on the size of the child). The nurse ensures that the tube is secured properly to prevent traction against the nares and ensuing pressure sores (see p. 890 for tube insertion in conjunction with procedure for gavage feedings).

The nurse prepares the child for insertion of the tube

PROCEDURE *Enema Administration*

- Explain the procedure to the child if the child is old enough to understand. Tell the child the purpose of the enema (eg, to help go to the bathroom, to help the doctor see if everything is all right with that part of the body). Assure the child that privacy will be respected.
- Have the child assume a left side-lying position with the upper leg bent and slightly forward. Keep the child covered except for the buttock area. Protect the bed with a plastic covering to prevent soiling. Have a bedpan readily available. The isotonic enema solution should be at body temperature and of an amount appropriate to the child's age and body size.
- Insert the lubricated tube no farther than 2–4 inches. Have the child take a deep breath while inserting the tube and insert very slowly and gently.
- Slowly insert the solution. Tell the child to take slow, deep breaths. If the child is unable to concentrate on breathing, have the child sing a song. The effect is the same and singing might distract the child. The child might feel the urge to defecate during the instillation. Encourage the child to retain the fluid as long as possible.
- If the child is undergoing a barium enema, the child's position might be changed in order to obtain the radiographs. The child will be asked to expel the barium in the radiology department.
- After an appropriate amount of retention time, ask the child to expel the enema. Describe and record the contents. Observe the child for any signs of fluid imbalance.

according to the child's developmental level. It is important to inform both child and family that nothing can be taken by mouth while the tube is in place. Involving the family in providing mouth care and providing a pacifier for the infant's sucking needs reduces the likelihood of inadvertent oral intake.

After insertion, the tube is connected to low suction. The tube should drain freely. Drainage should be clear to yellow-green. The presence of blood might indicate gastric wall irritation or trauma. Children undergoing prolonged gastric suctioning also are prone to mechanical irritation and development of gastric ulcers. Many physicians therefore prescribe prophylactic antacids in conjunction with intubation.

The nurse frequently checks the nasogastric tube for blockage. Signs of occlusion are absence of drainage or vomiting around the tube. In the case of suspected occlusion, irrigating the tube with saline might be necessary. If vomiting continues, it might be necessary to replace the tube.

Children who are receiving gastric decompression through gastrostomy ordinarily are not connected to suction. Instead, the open tube is placed to gravity drainage. As with nasogastric suction, a child with a gastrostomy for gastric decompression is NPO. Because gastrostomy is a surgical procedure, the usual preoperative preparation is followed.

The nurse records all gastric output (NG tube drainage, gastrostomy drainage, vomitus) in the intake and output record and reports any unusual color, odor, or substance. Large losses of fluid and electrolytes through gastric drainage might require additional intravenous fluid and electrolyte replacement. The nurse therefore observes for signs and symptoms of fluid and electrolyte imbalances in any child who is being decompressed (see Chapter 21).

Ostomy Care

Children undergo placement of ostomies for many reasons. Colostomies and ileostomies are most frequently performed because of congenital anomalies or because of bowel ischemia (decreased circulation to the area). Trauma or chronic inflammatory bowel disease might also necessitate ostomy placement.

The child who requires an ostomy requires age-appropriate patient teaching. The use of anatomically-correct dolls to demonstrate the procedure and the types of appliances the child might need postoperatively assists with high-quality preoperative teaching. Psychologic preparation of both child and parent is vital to their acceptance of the stoma as a condition allowing a normal life.

The nurse might be able to provide the parent and child with some measure of control during preoperative procedures by involving them in selection of the stoma site. This

STANDARDS OF NURSING CARE *The Child Undergoing Colostomy or Ileostomy*

RISKS

Assessed risk	Nursing action
Preoperative	
See risks from abdominal surgery	Perform necessary procedures related to gastric decompression, hydration status, respiratory function, prevention of infection, and hazards of immobility.
Postoperative	
Herniation of the stoma	Note the stoma size—stoma remains edematous for several days after surgery. Abnormal size after that might indicate herniation.
Circulatory compromise of the stoma	Note the stoma color—pale or livid color can indicate circulatory compromise.
Bleeding or infection of the stoma	Record and report any fresh bleeding or purulent drainage. Liquid stool is normal after bowel sounds return.

GUIDE FOR NURSING MANAGEMENT

Nursing diagnosis	Intervention	Rationale	Outcome
Preoperative			
1. Potential for infection (stressors: planned invasive procedure, presence of bacteria in bowel)	Administer oral or intravenous medications and saline or antibiotic enemas as required.	Antibiotics, particularly when applied directly to the bowel, decrease the risks of infection.	The child cooperates with the treatment. The child remains infection free.
	Maintain gastric suction or restricted diet if needed.	Both facilitate bowel cleansing by restricting passage of food through the tract.	
	Explain to child and family the need for the antibiotic enema and the procedure involved (see procedure box).	Explanations ensure cooperation. The longer the antibiotic remains in contact with the bowel, the more effective it is.	
2. Potential fluid volume deficit (stressors: NPO status, fluid loss through vomiting and/or diarrhea)	Determine need for intravenous fluids if child is NPO.	Children can be NPO for a while prior to surgery; this can lead to dehydration if fluids and electrolytes are not supplied.	The child appears adequately hydrated—intake is equal to that recommended for weight, voiding is frequent, skin turgor is good.
	Record intake and output, including emesis, enema return, and retained enema solution.	With any potential fluid volume shift, it is important to keep an accurate record of intake and output; retained enema solution is considered intake.	
3. Potential knowledge deficit concerning operative procedure and changes in body image (stressors: incomplete understanding, anxiety, cognitive level)	Teach a young child with concrete terms and drawings or ostomy doll showing ostomy at corresponding body part (urine collection bag can be used to illustrate appliance); describe all dressings and drains accurately (see Chapter 20).	Children should be prepared for surgery in an age-appropriate manner; the young child responds better to the use of concrete terms because of the child's cognitive level.	The child can explain ostomy surgery in language appropriate to developmental stage.

STANDARDS OF NURSING CARE *The Child Undergoing Colostomy or Ileostomy (Continued)*

GUIDE FOR NURSING MANAGEMENT

Nursing diagnosis	Intervention	Rationale	Outcome
	Begin teaching the older child several weeks before surgery, if possible, using drawings, dolls, or other models showing placement of ostomy and appliance; answer questions frankly and honestly; encourage child to express anxieties, ask questions, and perform self-care.	Older children might need a longer preparation time, particularly time to reflect on the procedure and to ask questions and express feelings.	
	Involve enterostomal therapist, if possible.	The enterostomal therapist is a person experienced in dealing with ostomies and with the reactions of patients and families.	
4. Potential parental knowledge deficit concerning the child's surgery and postoperative care (stressors: incomplete understanding of new information; anxiety)	Review need for ostomy; encourage questions; use doll or pictures to show stoma placement; explain future closure procedure if ostomy is temporary; begin explaining stoma care, familiarizing parent with basic equipment.	Parents need to be as adequately prepared as their children and also need time to express feelings and ask questions.	The parent can describe the need for and impact of the child's surgery and postoperative care.
Postoperative			
1. Impaired tissue integrity at the stoma site related to chemical irritants secondary to draining stool and ostomy appliance	Change dressings frequently, using Telfa; transverse, descending, or sigmoid colostomy might be left open to air.	Frequent dressing changes reduce the risk of infection; Telfa is less irritating to the stoma than gauze.	The stoma site will remain free from tissue breakdown. The site will be free from redness or excoriation.
	Apply occlusive ointment to skin around stoma site if ostomy has begun to drain and stoma appliance is not applied.	Occlusive ointment protects the skin around the stoma from excoriation by stools.	
	Apply ostomy bag if drainage is extensive or excoriating (which is common in ileostomy).	Ostomy bag protects the skin by containing stool rather than allowing it to remain on the skin.	
	Clean and dry skin thoroughly at stoma site before applying new appliance; use skin barrier (for example, karaya, Skin Prep, Stomadhesive) to protect skin from drainage. Cut the stoma pattern on the appliance 1/6 in. to 1/8 in. larger than the stoma.	Fecal material can be extremely excoriating; use of skin barriers as close to the stoma edge as possible minimizes the amount of the skin exposed to fecal material.	
	Observe for excoriation, weeping skin, maceration, infection, and ulceration at the stoma site.	Early intervention can prevent complications.	

(Continues)

STANDARDS OF NURSING CARE *The Child Undergoing Colostomy or Ileostomy (Continued)*

GUIDE FOR NURSING MANAGEMENT

Nursing diagnosis	Intervention	Rationale	Outcome
	Empty ostomy bag frequently.	The weight of the contents can pull on the skin. Increased traction on the ostomy appliance can cause it to separate from the skin, leaving the skin open to contact with fecal material.	
	Place a small amount of baking soda or mouthwash in the bag before reapplying.	These decrease odor (Adams and Selekof, 1986).	
2. Potential body image disturbance (stressors: change in appearance; ostomy appliance)	Allow both parent and child to express fears, perceptions, and psychologic distress; observe both parent and child for signs of extreme distress; for older child, encourage visit from another ostomate.	Another person with the same condition can be extremely supportive to a child.	Parent and child can express their fears and concerns about altered body image. The child expresses anger appropriately according to developmental level.
3. Potential knowledge deficit concerning stoma care (stressors: incomplete preparation or practice time)	Have parent and child observe nurse during stoma care and appliance change; explain all steps in these procedures.	Observation by parent and child is the first step in the learning process; it also encourages the child and parent to begin to accept the appearance of the stoma.	The child and family will demonstrate stoma care prior to discharge and will state feelings of confidence in their ability to perform care at home.
	Supervise parent and child as they perform ostomy care; verify that they are capable of performing care without assistance.	The child or parent needs to be competent in stoma care prior to discharge.	
	For older child, encourage as much self-care as possible.	Encouraging self-care encourages acceptance.	
4. Potential parental knowledge deficit concerning specific dietary needs (stressor: incomplete understanding of dietary alterations)	Explain any dietary restrictions or limitations (for example, limiting gas-causing foods such as cabbage or spices). Give the child applesauce or cranberry juice daily.	Gas-causing food might be uncomfortable for the child with an ostomy, particularly since there is an increase in odor. Applesauce and cranberry juice decrease gas (Adams and Selekof, 1986).	Parent and child can describe dietary needs and limitations.
	Explain need for increased fluid intake, especially following ileostomy.	Following an ileostomy, food isn't in the tract long enough for the body to completely reabsorb water, thus increased fluid is essential.	
5. Temporary activity intolerance related to potential injury to stoma and imposed limits	Explain all activity limitations, noting that child can resume all normal activities except contact sports once the site is healed.	Contact sports have the potential to damage the stoma.	Parent and child can give rationale for temporary activity limitations. The child will gradually return to normal activity without injury to the operative site.

STANDARDS OF NURSING CARE *The Child Undergoing Colostomy or Ileostomy (Continued)*

GUIDE FOR NURSING MANAGEMENT

Nursing diagnosis	Intervention	Rationale	Outcome
	Explain to the parent that a child who resumes normal activities begins accepting the ostomy.	Resumption of normal activity deemphasizes the ostomy, as children realize they do not have to greatly alter their lifestyles.	
6. Potential for impaired home maintenance management (stressors: inadequate home facilities, unavailability of resources, incomplete understanding of home management)	Provide parent with written instructions about care and return appointments.	Written instructions usually prevent forgetfulness.	Parent and child will explain the need for follow-up care. They are aware of community support systems.
	Provide a contact person (for example, public health nurse or enterostomal therapist) for questions that arise after discharge.	Knowing a person to contact after discharge gives the parent security in the knowledge that someone will be available to answer questions.	
	Provide parent and child any available helpful hints for ostomy care, as needed.	The more information that is provided, the easier it will be for parent and child to adapt; helpful hints usually are gained from experience and therefore are valuable pieces of information.	
	Inform parent about national organization of ostomates and any local community support groups that are available.	People in support groups usually are helpful in providing support and information to help the child and family adapt.	

is also a good opportunity for both parent and child to see and handle ostomy appliances, although several types of appliances might be tried before one is found to provide adequate skin protection, reasonable wearing time, comfort, and easy availability. The appliance will need to fit well while the child sits or bends, so selecting a site is best done when the child is awake and can participate as much as the child's developmental stage allows.

Ostomy care varies, depending on the placement site and on the location of the opening along the bowel. Ostomy supplies include a variety of protective agents and appliance sizes. Disposable rather than reusable appliances also have become more common now that the wide choice of disposable equipment allows for more efficient odor control and ease of application. When teaching a new ostomate and family, the nurse considers economic, physical, and psychologic needs. For example, parents with limited funds might prefer a reusable appliance. Parents might need to be informed that they are able to choose equipment other than the brand used by the hospital. Several companies supply pediatric ostomy appliances, and parents might wish to try several brands before making a choice. Ostomy bags can be made at home from sealable sandwich bags and stoma adhesive. Parents also need to be informed that a growing child is likely to need frequent readjustments of a permanent appliance and possible surgical revision of the stoma (see Standards of Nursing Care for the Child undergoing Colostomy or Ileostomy).

Principles of Nursing Care

Acute Care Needs

A child with a suspected gastrointestinal disorder requires close observation of functions related to the digestive tract. Nursing principles that are particularly important to these children include:

- intake and output records, stool records, emesis records (including nasogastric tube output)
- daily weight measurements
- infection control
- continued assessment for complications

All these needs can arise from the disease process (Table 27-3).

TABLE 27-3 Intake and Output Recording

Measurement	Data recorded
Intravenous fluids	Type of solution, rate of infusion, amount infused, blood products
Oral intake	Type and amount of oral liquids and solid intake if calorie count or dietary estimates are needed
Emesis, Levine tube/pump output	Quantity, quality, color, and presence of blood (if any)
Urine	Color, quantity, pH, and glucose (if needed)
Stool	Quantity, quality, consistency, color, texture, presence or absence of blood, pus, mucus, unusual odors, glucose, or reducing substances

⊛ Potential fluid volume deficit

Intake and output measurements The nurse closely monitors the child's hydration and electrolyte status (see Chapter 21). Intake and output records therefore are vitally important. Besides providing an indicator of fluid status, these records also help to identify changes in stool patterns, nutritional patterns, or recurring emesis.

Children with gastrointestinal problems frequently require fluid replacement by regular intravenous drip or by hyperalimentation (total parenteral nutrition). Fluid requirements are calculated on the basis of the child's age and weight. The degree of dehydration often determines the type of fluids and the speed at which fluids are delivered. Such conditions as diaphoresis (sweating) and certain metabolic and renal disorders require special considerations in fluid replacement therapy.

Children receiving hyperalimentation or constant-drip fluids might require infusion pumps for more accurate delivery of these fluids. For infants, infusion pumps for intravenous fluids are a safety measure and can prevent fluid overload or too rapid administration of intravenous fluids.

The nurse needs to consider amounts of liquid stool and urine as indicators of fluid status. Accurate measurement is important. Weighing infant diapers can give an accurate measure of output. All gastric output also is carefully measured. Gastric output is then considered when restoring fluids.

Weight measurements Children with gastrointestinal disorders causing fluid alterations, chronic or severe weight loss, or failure to thrive require frequent weight measurements. Although daily measurements are usually sufficient, certain children might need to be weighed more frequently. Those with severe fluid loss might need to be weighed as often as two to three times per day. Each child is weighed at the same time and on the same scale each day. Differences between scales can vary significantly enough to alter treatment regimens. Metabolic or bed scales might be needed for comatose children.

The child should be weighed in similar clothing each day. Infants are weighed without clothes or diapers, and older children remove excess clothing or slippers. Only clothing necessary for the child's sense of modesty should remain. The presence of an armboard or bulky bandage should also be noted in the weight records and the weight of the board recorded, if known.

⊛ Potential alteration in bowel elimination

Accurate monitoring of bowel elimination is essential in many problems affecting gastrointestinal function. A description of the color, quantity, consistency, and odor of the stool is important. The description allows the nurse to evaluate the results of the nursing or medical interventions. In addition, infants receiving total parenteral nutrition require continuous monitoring of all urine and stool output to indicate the response to the hyperalimentation. Children with severe constipation or encopresis (see Chapter 16) also require stool records to document and evaluate the condition.

⊛ Potential for infection

Because of the organisms involved, infection control is particularly important in gastrointestinal disorders. Diarrhea and hepatitis, for example, can be highly contagious.

Nurses need to be aware of routine infection control methods. To prevent cross-contamination between patients and to protect the nurse, hands are washed prior to entering a room, before caring for a patient, and before leaving the room. Parents, family members, and patients need to be reminded of the importance of hand washing, and nurses need to insist on cooperation. Some children with infectious dysfunctions of the gastrointestinal system might require special precautions such as enteric or wound and skin isolation procedures (see Chapter 20).

Potential knowledge deficit regarding gastrointestinal surgery
Children undergoing abdominal surgery require many of the same preoperative preparations as adults. For the child, age-appropriate explanations of the impending surgery also are important.

Because a large percentage of abdominal operations in children are emergency interventions, preoperative teaching often is extremely limited. The nurse attempts to explain to the child and family as much of what is taking place as possible, but the nurse also plans postoperative discussions with the child to minimize the effects of having been unprepared for surgery. The parent usually requires more intensive psychologic support if emergency surgery is necessary, so the nurse often needs to make a concerted effort to keep the parents informed of what is happening to the child (see Standards of Nursing Care: The Child Following Abdominal Surgery).

Complications related to gastrointestinal dysfunction Children with gastrointestinal problems might experience complications related to either the disease or the treatment. Nurses therefore need to observe children for changes that might indicate the onset of complications. Sepsis (blood infection) might occur as a severe consequence of some dysfunctions. Other complications include shock from hemorrhage or small or large bowel obstruction (Table 27-4).

Complications related to treatment can include stress ulcers, wound infections, and obstruction due to prolonged constipation or retained barium. Skin breakdown due to inappropriate positioning, insufficient perineal care, or ineffective ostomy care is an additional complication. Children receiving drip feedings or tube feedings are prone to fluid aspiration. Those children receiving hyperalimentation are observed for problems relating to fluid overload, hyperglycemia, or catheter contamination.

Nutritional Needs

Alteration in nutrition: less than body requirements related to impaired ability to eat
Children who cannot suck properly or who have had surgery requiring nasogastric tube placement lack sufficient oral intake. Nutritional deficit is a possibility.

Children who cannot maintain an adequate caloric intake require enternal or parenteral supplementation. Enteral alimentation (feeding) might include special formulas or diets and special techniques for providing these supplements (for example, continuous NG drip or gavage). Parenteral alimentation might include standard intravenous glucose and electrolyte solutions. (Table 27-5 lists standard and special infant formulas or supplements.) Children who are unable to take oral formulas by nipple might require tube feeding or special feeding nipples, cups, or spoons.

Enteral nutrition The two most common forms of tube feedings are gavage (through nasogastric tube) and gastrostomy feedings. Gavage feedings usually are temporary and are used when the child is unable to suck or swallow,

TABLE 27-4 Symptoms of Obstruction in the Small and Large Bowels

Symptom	Small bowel	Large bowel
Vomiting	Profuse, frequent, might or might not be bile-stained	Little or no vomiting Bile-stained
Dehydration	Occurs quickly	Little or none
Distension	Minimal	Occurs early, is often severe
Onset of symptoms	Rapid, acute	Slow, progressive
Pain	Severe, cramping, intermittent	Mild, steady rather than intermittent
Shock	Onset might be rapid because of massive loss of fluid into gut or because of sepsis	Less common unless colon ruptures
Stool	Stool and flatus remaining in colon might be passed initially	No stools

TABLE 27-5 Special Formulas and Formula Supplements

	Product	Manufacturer	Indications and comments
Electrolyte solutions	Pedialyte	Ross	Clear liquid diet for use in diarrhea and oral rehydration
	Lytren	Mead Johnson	Clear liquid diet for use in diarrhea and oral rehydration
Soy-based formulas	Neo-Mull-Soy	Syntex	Allergy to milk protein
	Prosobee	Mead Johnson	Allergy to milk protein
	Isomil	Ross	Allergy to milk protein
Elemental diets	Vivonex	Eaton	Dietary supplement or total diet
	Flexical	Mead Johnson	Contains soy and medium-chain triglycerides
Diets for malabsorptive conditions	Portagen	Mead Johnson	Used for short-bowel syndrome and fat malabsorption; fat is in form of medium-chain triglycerides and safflower oils
	Nutramigen	Mead Johnson	Enzymatic hydrolysate of casein frequently used in children with cystic fibrosis or any difficulty absorbing food proteins
	Pregestimil	Mead Johnson	Used for various malabsorption syndromes, contains medium-chain triglycerides
	CHO-Free	Syntex	Carbohydrate free (specific carbohydrates must be added as tolerated), often used in short-bowel syndrome
	Meat Base	Gerber	For allergy to milk protein and for children requiring a lower osmolality in formula
Low-phenylalanine formulas	Lofenalac	Mead Johnson	For children with phenylketonuria
	Albumaid XP	Ross	Used primarily for older children with phenylketonuria

STANDARDS OF NURSING CARE *The Child Following Abdominal Surgery*

RISKS

Assessed risk	Nursing action
Preoperative	
Bowel obstruction	Measure abdominal girth and monitor for distension, absence of bowel sounds, or acute pain. Report any of these to the physician.
Sepsis	Monitor and report changes in vital signs—tachycardia, tachypnea, hypotension, hypothermia.
Postoperative	
Routine postoperative risks—decreased cardiac output, ineffective breathing pattern, impaired physical mobility, and urinary retention	(See Chapter 20.)
Intestinal obstruction or paralytic ileus	Measure abdominal girth and monitor distension. Listen for return of bowel sounds. Monitor the pattern of pain. Maintain NPO with low suction to NG tube. Record characteristics of the first postoperative stool.
Sepsis	Monitor and report changes in vital signs as above.
Impaired wound healing	Observe and report unusual bleeding, purulence, redness, or edema. Change dressings as ordered using sterile technique.

STANDARDS OF NURSING CARE *The Child Following Abdominal Surgery (Continued)*

GUIDE FOR NURSING MANAGEMENT

Nursing diagnosis	Intervention	Rationale	Outcome
1. Potential knowledge deficit concerning preoperative procedures and operative events (stressors: inadequate understanding, cognitive level, emergency surgery)	Explain purpose of surgery in language that the child can understand. Use therapeutic play for young child and reinforce teaching that surgery is not a punishment but must be done to fix a problem.	Children understand better when explanations are geared to their cognitive level.	Child and parent are appropriately prepared for surgery and can explain what will be required postoperatively.
	Inform parent and child about preoperative procedures and reasons for them; include routine preoperative procedures such as blood tests, enemas, and injections with age-appropriate explanations.	Accurate information decreases anxiety.	
	Discuss specific postoperative preparation as indicated by the nature and severity of the problem.	Knowing what to expect ahead of time increases cooperation with the treatment regimen.	
2. Potential alteration in comfort: nausea and pain (stressors: presence of NG tube, incision)	Monitor vital signs.	Alteration in vital signs can indicate the child is in pain (increased pulse and blood pressure).	The child does not report any nausea. There is no vomiting around the tube. The child appears comfortable and relaxed.
	Maintain child NPO with NG tube.	NG tubes maintain an empty stomach to prevent postoperative nausea, vomiting, and strain on the suture line.	
	Check tube frequently for patency and proper functioning.	Frequent observation allows for earlier problem recognition.	
	Irrigate NG tube as ordered and whenever blockage is suspected.	Irrigation forces a mucus plug back into the stomach, thus clearing the tube; it also maintains patency of the tube lumen.	
	Connect NG tube to intermittent suction as ordered and monitor suction pressure.	Intermittent low suction is not irritating to the stomach and enhances effectiveness of the NG tube, thus decreasing gastric irritation.	
	Observe for blood in gastric drainage.	Blood in the tube is an early sign of gastric irritation or hemorrhage.	

(Continues)

STANDARDS OF NURSING CARE *The Child Following Abdominal Surgery (Continued)*

GUIDE FOR NURSING MANAGEMENT

Nursing diagnosis	Intervention	Rationale	Outcome
	Position NG tube to prevent tension on tape.	Tension on the NG tube increases discomfort and contributes to skin breakdown in the nares.	
	Encourage parent to hold infant or young child. Allow child to assume comfortable position unless otherwise indicated.	This decreases anxiety and consequently pain. Presence of and comfort from parent enhances child's coping.	
	Turn and reposition child every 2 hours.	Positional stiffness contributes to pain. Changes in position facilitate NG tube drainage.	
	Provide frequent mouth care with petroleum jelly to dry lips.	Dry lips increase discomfort.	
	Administer analgesics as needed. Record child's reaction to pain and need for medication.	Medication relieves pain and promotes rest.	
3. Potential alteration in fluid volume: deficit (stressors: fluid losses during surgery and via nasogastric tube, NPO status)	Maintain child NPO with NG suction until intestinal function returns. Replace gastric output with IV fluids if ordered.	Fluid replacement of gastric losses helps maintain fluid and electrolyte balance.	The child appears hydrated—good skin turgor, moist mucous membranes, adequate urinary output.
	Maintain intravenous fluids until oral fluid intake is adequate.	This prevents fluid deficit as a result of vomiting.	
	Record intake and output. Record first postoperative urine sample in order to verify kidney function.	Output is a valid indicator of the child's hydration status.	
	Monitor for signs of dehydration.		
	Record urine specific gravity a least once a shift.	Urine specific gravity, mucous membranes, and skin turgor are indicators of hydration status. Child's combined loss and increased need can exceed replacement; thus, need for close monitoring.	

STANDARDS OF NURSING CARE *The Child Following Abdominal Surgery (Continued)*

GUIDE FOR NURSING MANAGEMENT

Nursing diagnosis	Intervention	Rationale	Outcome
4. Potential knowledge deficit concerning postoperative condition and home care (stressors: incomplete understanding, new experience, anxiety, presence of other stressors in family)	Review any necessary wound care, dressing changes, and similar procedures.	Learning with the nurse's support decreases anxiety.	Child and parent are adequately prepared for discharge. Parent demonstrates all required procedures prior to discharge.
	Provide both written and oral instructions with return demonstrations.	Parent can review written instructions as a reinforcement for the oral instructions. Return demonstrations build confidence.	
	Inform parent about any supplies that might be needed on the child's return home; about diet, activity limitations, and return appointments; and about any possible complications (eg, increased temperature, nausea, vomiting) that should be reported.	The parent needs to be adequately prepared for situations to be encountered with home management.	
	Provide parent with a contact person in case questions arise (contact person might be public health nurse, primary care nurse, physician, or enterosomal therapist).	A contact person provides the parent with security and lessens reluctance to ask for assistance.	
	Remind parent that sleep problems and behavior problems, including regressive behaviors, are common reactions to hospitalization (see Chapter 19). Encourage parent to discuss hospitalization with the child and to seek help if child exhibits prolonged problems.	Often parents do not understand or know how to cope with the child's reactions to hospitalization. If informed that certain reactions are usual, their anxiety is decreased.	

when the child has respiratory or cardiac distress associated with nipple feedings, or when the child is unconscious. A gastrostomy tube might be indicated for children with anatomic anomalies of the oropharynx, esophagus, or cardiac sphincter of the stomach. Children who are dysphagic (cannot swallow) or who are severely mentally and physically disabled also might require gastrostomy placement.

Gavage feeding Gavage feeding involves intermittent placement of a feeding tube into the stomach through the nostril or mouth. The tube usually is removed after each feeding, and a new tube is placed for each successive feeding. Tubes left in place for several feedings require replacement every 24–72 hours. Older children, particularly those with chronic disabilities requiring long-term tube

PROCEDURE *Gavage Feeding*

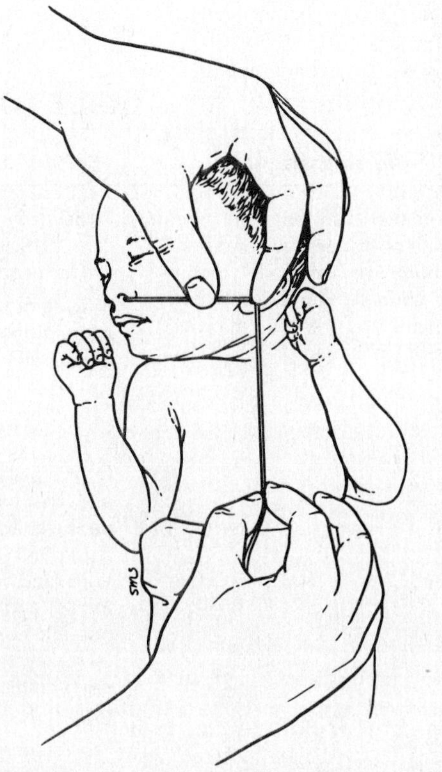

- Explain the procedure to the child if the child is old enough or aware enough to understand and cooperate. Tell the child that it will be necessary to swallow when directed, even though the child might not feel like doing so. Tell the child that after the tube is in, formula will be placed in the tube and go directly to the stomach. The tube is not removed after each feeding in older children in order to reduce the trauma of tube placement.
- Assemble needed materials: appropriately sized feeding tube (5–8 French for infants, 10–14 French for older children and thicker formulas), gavage feeding bag and tube setup, a 3–5 mL syringe, water or water-soluble lubricant, tape, stethoscope, and formula for feeding.
- After appropriate hand washing, swaddle wrap any child who is able to resist, or obtain assistance to hold child's arms and head. Position the child in a slightly right side-lying position or with chest elevated. Slight extension of the neck allows for easier viewing of the nares.
- Measure for the correct insertion length. Measure from mouth to earlobe for oral insertion (preferred with infants because they are nose breathers), or from tip of nose to earlobe for nasal insertion and then to a point midway between the distal xyphoid process and the umbilicus. Mark this length with a small piece of tape. Place a small piece of tape above the child's upper lip slightly below the nares.
- Lubricate the tube in the water or lubricant. Insert the tube with a firm, steady motion but do not force. Slight flexion of the neck facilitates correct tube placement during insertion. If difficulty is encountered, try the other nostril; pass to designated tape mark. The child might feel like gagging as the tube activates the gag reflex. Encourage the older child to swallow.
- Verify the proper position of the tube by aspirating stomach contents into attached small syringe. If no aspirate is visualized, inject 2–5 mL of air through the tube while listening with a stethoscope over the stomach (bubbling or gurgling indicates proper position), then withdraw the air.
- Wrap a strip of one-half-inch tape around the tube and secure it to the tape below the nares. Bring the tube to the side of the face and secure with tape again.
- Attach the gavage feeding bag and tubing setup to the tube. Pour room temperature formula into the holder and allow formula to flow by gravity (initial plunger pressure might be needed to begin flow). Regulate rate to approximate sucking rate. For more precise regulation of formula flow rate, attach tube to a gavage feeding infusion pump. Set flow rate so formula is infused within ordered time. The child will begin to experience a feeling of fullness. Allow infant to suck on pacifier during feeding to associate sucking with feeling full. A tube feeding should take as long as a normal bottle feeding (20–30 min).
- Flush the tube with sterile water or a small amount of air. Pinch the tube before removing to prevent leakage of formula. Gastric air is limited during gavage feedings. If an infant has been allowed a pacifier during feeding, it is very important to burp the infant well to prevent retention of swallowed air. Cuddling the infant during and after the feeding provides the association of security with the feeling of fullness. If the tube is to remain in place, the open end needs to be covered, usually with a gauze pad held in place with an elastic. Some NG tubes have a capping device attached to the tube. This device is put over the open end for covering.

PROCEDURE *Gastrostomy Feeding*

- Explain the procedure to the child if this is the first time the procedure is to be performed and if the child can understand. Tell the child that since the mouth and esophagus need a rest from food, the food needs to be placed directly into the stomach. This is done through the tube that the doctor already placed in the stomach.
- Assemble the needed materials—10–30 mL syringe, gavage feeding setup, infusion pump if rate needs to be precise, and prescribed room temperature formula.
- Attach syringe to gastrostomy and aspirate residue. The child might feel a slight tugging feeling. If amount of residue is large (5–10 mL for premature infants, 10–25 mL for newborn), replace residue and decrease present feeding by an equal amount. If residue continues or increases, report to physician.
- Pour formula into gavage feeding setup and regulate rate with thumb-screw. The child will experience a feeling of fullness in the stomach. Allow infants to suck on a pacifier while receiving formula so that the infant can make the connection between sucking and feeling full. Formula should flow easily. Feeding usually takes the same amount of time as a regular bottle feeding (20–30 min).
- When feeding is complete, clamp the tube. If gastric distension is observed, suspend the open end of the tube to allow for escape of trapped air.

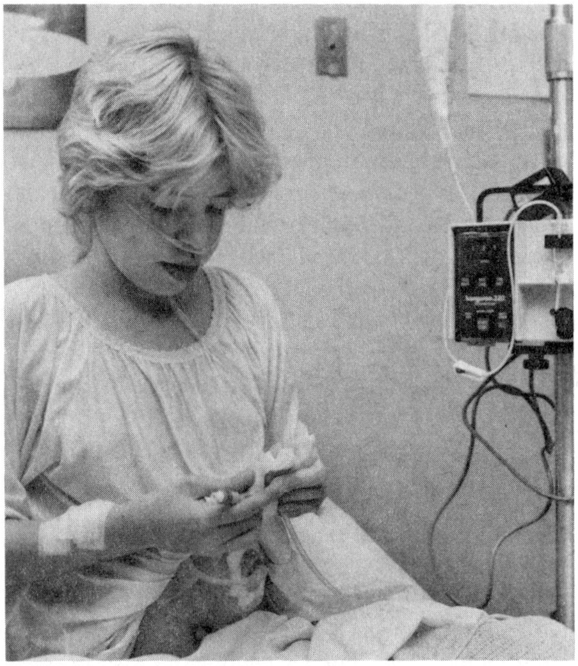

- Place the child in right side-lying or Fowler's position to promote gastric emptying. Cuddle infants as much as possible while keeping them in the position. This helps them associate pleasant feelings with food.

feedings, might only require tube changes every 3–7 days. Those requiring continuous drip feedings need frequent bottle changes to prevent bacterial contamination of formula that is at room temperature. Children receiving blender-prepared tube feedings might experience more problems with blockage of the tube than those receiving commercial formulas. One helpful measure is to color the formula of children on long-term tube feedings with food coloring. The color will distinguish the formula from mucus if there is a question of aspiration.

Gastrostomy feedings A *gastrostomy* involves operative placement of a tube through the abdominal wall and into the greater curvature of the stomach. To prevent the leakage of gastric contents into the abdominal cavity, the stomach is sutured to the peritoneal wall at the ostomy site. The tube is a large-lumen retention catheter; the large lumen facilitates holding the tube in place in the stomach. The site is kept clean and dry, and no dressing is required once healing has occurred. The nurse needs to prevent tension on the catheter, as this might cause bleeding or damage to the ostomy site.

Special feeding methods The child with neurologic or anatomic anomalies might require other feeding methods, which might include special nipples, spoons, or cups. Cleft palate nipples, lamb's nipples, or special cleft palate feeding systems (for example, Beniflex) might be required for children with cleft lips or palates. All of these methods allow the child to maintain adequate oral caloric intake.

⊛ Alteration in nutrition: less than body requirements related to impaired use of food

Children experiencing a change or disruption in gastrointestinal function require continued assessment of fluid and caloric intake. Fluid supplementation is important when the child cannot maintain oral fluid intake (for example, when the child is NPO) or when the child is losing large amounts of fluid and electrolytes (for example, in vomiting, diarrhea, or short-bowel syndrome). Adequate caloric intake is necessary to maintain normal growth and development. Caloric supplementation begins when nutritional deficit is a possibility as a result of calorie loss (diarrhea) or inability of the body to digest food. The goal of supplementation is to prevent negative nitrogen balance. For example, children with malabsorption syndromes or severely restricted diets require caloric supplementation in order to provide for normal growth.

Caloric requirements are calculated according to body weight, age, and physical activity.

Vitamin and mineral supplementation Children with increased metabolic needs or impaired gastrointestinal absorption might require vitamin and mineral supplementation. These supplements are given orally, intramuscularly, or intravenously. For example, children with steatorrhea (fatty stools), pancreatitis, or hepatic damage might require oral supplementation with water-soluble forms of the fat-soluble vitamins A, D, E, and K. Vitamin B_{12}, if indicated, might be given intramuscularly.

Children at general nutritional risk for other reasons might require supplementation of all vitamins and some minerals.

Parenteral nutrition When oral intake is restricted, inadequate, or impossible, parenteral nutritional supplementation might be necessary. Children requiring parenteral supplementation usually are malnourished as a result of a disease process or its treatment. Parenteral supplementation can consist of carbohydrates, protein, lipids, or any combination. In addition, certain vitamins, electrolytes, and trace minerals can be given intravenously if therapy is prolonged. *Total parenteral nutrition* (TPN), also referred to as *hyperalimentation,* is commonly used for conditions that prevent the absorption of nutrients from the bowel or for instances when the bowel requires complete rest.

The standard hyperalimentation fluid consists of a high concentration of glucose and amino acids. Glucose concentrations greater than 12% are irritating to peripheral vein walls and therefore usually are delivered through a central venous catheter. This catheter is placed through either the external jugular vein or the subclavian vein. If TPN is required on a long-term basis, a permanent catheter (for example, Broviac or Hickman) is tunneled into the vein through the chest wall.

An intravenous infusion pump carefully regulates the amount of solution to be administered. The pump also prevents blood backflow into the catheter tip from the increased pressure of the larger vein, thus preventing clot or embolus formation. An in-line micropore filter is used to prevent introduction of bacteria or air into the central circulation.

Complications Complications of hyperalimentation are related to the protein and glucose concentration, the rate of administration, the possibility of fat or air emboli, and infection related to contamination of the fluid, tubing, or insertion site. These complications can be life-threatening, and children undergoing TPN require close monitoring (Table 27-6).

Home hyperalimentation Home hyperalimentation is feasible for children who require long-term TPN. With home care, the adverse effects of prolonged hospitalization can be diminished. The cost of administration is minimized, and the family can function without dividing attention between home and hospital. (Assessment of the home environment and the feasibility of home care are discussed in Chapter 18.)

In addition to family resources and capabilities, the nurse asks whether the family's insurance company or another agency is willing to continue coverage once the child begins TPN at home. Many companies have agreed to extend coverage to home care once they have determined the 25%–35% possible savings.

Once the child and family are deemed candidates for home hyperalimentation, the nurse begins parent education. Parent and child teaching needs to be planned to minimize exposing the parent to a variety of contradictory or confusing techniques. Performing procedures in a consistent manner avoids confusion. Requesting that the community health nurse come in to the hospital to observe the parent demonstration ensures continuity of care.

The parent needs to learn the concepts, principles, and possible complications involved in the administration of TPN at home. Parents need both explanations and demonstrations of the necessary skills and should participate in their children's care at the hospital while supervised by the nurse.

With long-term hyperalimentation, the risk of physical complications increases. The hyperalimentation might interfere with normal growth. The child might be somewhat active, and the parent might find it necessary to enforce limits to prevent the child from dislodging the catheter.

Long-term hyperalimentation also has been associated with emotional difficulties. Emotional complications can include problems with body image, relationships, behavior

TABLE 27-6 Major Complications of Total Parental Nutrition

Complication	Prevention
Hyperglycemia (elevated blood sugar) or hypoglycemia (inadequate blood sugar)	Gradually increase the glucose content of the solution. Add insulin as directed for elevated serum and urine glucose. Maintain accurate rate of administration.
Emboli from air, lipids, or thrombus	Use an in-line micropore filter. Use an infusion pump. Change tubing quickly and remove air bubbles.
Infection	Use aseptic technique or follow institution policy for tubing or dressing changes.

disturbances, depression, and those associated with any chronic illness (see Chapter 14). The nurse evaluating the child receiving long-term TPN thus continually assesses the child and family for physical and psychologic complications of therapy.

Developmental Needs

⊛ Potential for altered growth and development

Children with gastrointestinal disorders might experience difficulty in meeting normal developmental needs. Prolonged gastrointestinal disorders frequently result in failure to grow and gain weight. Cognitive, musculoskeletal, and neurologic abnormalities resulting from chronic malnutrition or malabsorption can directly affect the child's ability to reach developmental milestones.

Developmental needs of infancy and early childhood, which include oral gratification, might be compromised by conditions affecting feeding or sucking. Frequent surgical repairs and special feeding methods also might prevent infants from receiving adequate oral stimulation. Malabsorption syndromes with resulting intestinal discomfort might lead children to refuse nipple feedings. Many children with failure to thrive develop alternative, inappropriate means of meeting oral needs, such as constant sucking of their hands, a specific pacifier, a piece of cloth or blanket, or their tongues.

Cuddling infants during feedings, regardless of the method, provides security that usually is associated with oral gratification. Giving a pacifier during tube or gastrostomy feedings provides oral gratification that is associated with stomach fullness.

Children undergoing long-term hyperalimentation or medical therapy also might experience restricted mobility and impaired motor development. Arm or leg restraints needed during intravenous therapy, together with the limitations of tubing length, might prevent the infant from learning to roll over, creep, crawl, or walk. Children with long-term malnutrition might not even have the muscle strength needed to elevate their heads or to sit without assistance. Older malnourished children might be unable to develop such motor skills as skipping or running.

The child needs to be encouraged to be as active as possible within limitations. Providing stimulating, but less active, forms of play promotes development. Combining infant exercise, passive range of motion exercises, and play can improve muscle tone, strength, and flexibility. Gross motor skills can be encouraged with careful parental supervision.

Emotional Needs

Families of children with acute or chronic gastrointestinal disorders experience a variety of reactions to the diagnosis, its implications, and the necessity for hospitalization. Nurses therefore need to involve families of ill children in planning and contributing to care.

⊛ Potential alteration in parenting

Parents of children born with congenital anomalies of the gastrointestinal tract need support while learning to cope with the implications of the defect. Parents of children with very obvious anomalies are at high risk for attachment problems because their expectations for a healthy, normal infant have been so quickly destroyed. The parent might be unwilling to look at the infant or provide anything but the most basic care. Infants who are separated from their parents immediately after birth or those who have dysfunctions that interfere with feeding also are at risk.

One of the major consequences of attachment problems is failure to thrive. Initial problems with attachment can be complicated if the infant has feeding difficulties because feeding promotes closeness between parent and child. Thus, the infant might exhibit failure to thrive from both organic as well as inorganic causes.

The nurse who recognizes that gastrointestinal dysfunction can interfere with attachment can do much to prevent complications. Emphasizing the infant's strong points, such as "Your baby seems to enjoy cuddling" or "What pretty eyes your baby has," encourages the parents to look beyond an obvious physical defect. Allowing the parent to participate in feeding also can promote attachment and increase the infant's feelings of security.

Potential body image disturbance
A child who has undergone a colostomy or ileostomy for any gastrointestinal dysfunction will be dealing with the effects of an altered body image. Regardless of the quality of the preoperative preparation, the child will undergo emotional responses to the physical change. The child might refuse to participate in care, touch, or even look at the stoma. The nurse helps the child verbalize feelings of anger and assists the child through the grief process.

Children with observable defects such as cleft lip and cleft palate might do well following repair while they are young. When they go to school, however, they might encounter adverse responses to their appearance or their ability to talk clearly. The nurse allows the child to verbalize feelings and assists the child through role play to handle uncomfortable questions or situations.

Health Maintenance Needs

Potential for impaired home maintenance management
Parents of children discharged from the hospital require specific information about home care. To prevent misunderstandings, the nurse provides both spoken and written instructions and a contact person or telephone contact in case the parent encounters difficulties.

Parents need instructions about medications, dietary restrictions, and feeding techniques. The nurse might identify commercially prepared formulas that are available at supermarkets and those that might be available or ordered from pharmacies. The nurse cautions the parent not to attempt to make home electrolyte solutions. These solutions can be dangerous and can adversely alter the child's electrolyte balance. If special formulas or diets are to be prepared at home, the parent requires teaching by the nurse or by a nutritionist.

Parents might need lists of acceptable foods or lists of specifically banned foods. A nutritionist might be able to provide recipe hints or guidelines to prevent a restrictive diet from becoming boring and repetitious.

The nurse explains any restrictions in activity with reference to the child's normal activities. The ultimate goal is for the child to return to optimal functioning as soon as possible.

The Child with Problems Involving Ingestion

Cleft Lip and Cleft Palate

Cleft lip and cleft palate are facial defects that result from failure of fusion of the primary or secondary palates during gestation. The primary palate is responsible for the development of the lip and anterior jaw. If closure is not completed by the seventh to eighth week of gestation, the infant is born with a *cleft lip*. Unilateral cleft lips usually are left-sided; bilateral cleft lips are more frequently associated with *cleft palates*. The cleft in the lip also varies in degree from a simple notch in the vermillion border of the lip to a separation that extends into the floor of the nose.

The hard and soft palates arise from the secondary palate. If the palatine processes fail to fuse before the twelfth week of gestation, a cleft of the hard or soft palate results. These clefts also vary in severity from a bifid uvula to a complete cleft of the hard and soft palates. They might be unilateral, bilateral, or midline. Cleft lip and cleft palate might occur separately or might be combined.

Clefts of the lip or palate are relatively common, occurring in about 1 in 1000 births in white Americans and less frequently in American blacks. Cleft palate alone occurs in about 1 of every 2500 births (Rudolph, 1982). Transmission of these defects appears to be multifactorial, and affected infants might have close relatives with the defect. Teratogens (environmental factors contributing to abnormal embryonic development) have been implicated in certain isolated occurrences. Cleft lip, either alone or in combination with cleft palate, is more common in males; cleft palate alone is more common in females. Clefts of the lip and palate often are seen with other chromosomal anomalies. Infants with either cleft lip or cleft palate therefore should be examined closely for other congenital anomalies, hearing defects, or mental impairment.

Clinical manifestations An examination of internal clefts should be done both visually and manually. Visual examination reveals obvious hard palate defects or more subtle defects such as soft palate irregularities or bifid uvula. Digital examination allows an assessment of the depth and degree of hard palate anomalies as well as assessment of the infant's sucking capabilities. Diagnosis includes classification of the type and severity of the defect as well as

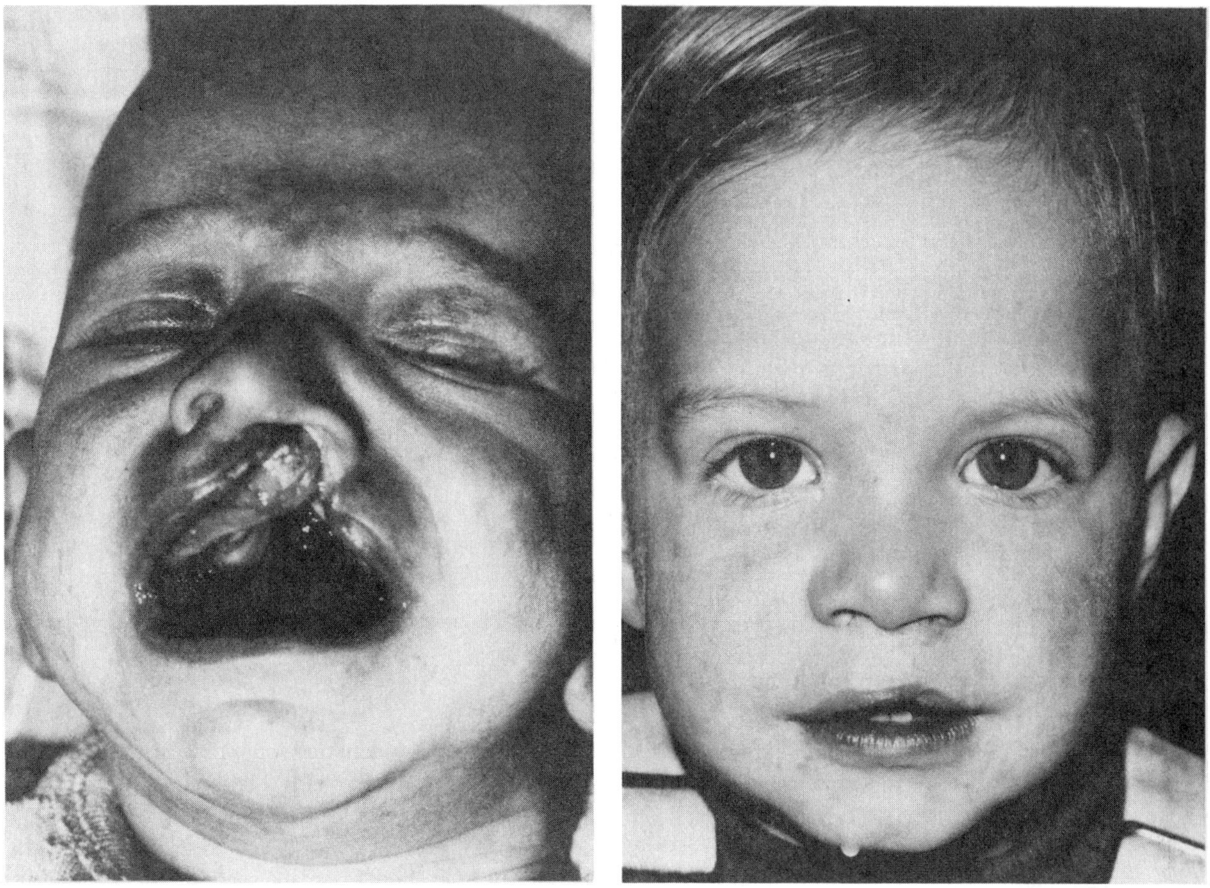

Child with a cleft lip and cleft palate, before and after repair. (Courtesy of David F. Sloan, MD.)

a thorough physical examination to rule out related birth defects.

The newborn with cleft palate might exhibit some immediate feeding difficulties. Fluids given to the infant can go through the open palate and out the nose. The infant sputters and coughs, and aspiration can be a complication. Newborns with cleft lip or cleft palate have difficulty creating the vacuum around the nipple that is needed for efficient sucking. As a result they become tired or frustrated before completing the feeding.

Treatment Initial medical management of the child with a cleft lip or cleft palate focuses on preventing aspiration of secretions and providing adequate nutrition. The child usually is unable to suck adequately on a standard nipple. Soft nipples with larger holes and longer spouts are used to provide formula while enhancing development of the muscles used for sucking, swallowing, and speech. Because the infant is unable to suck and swallow normally, secretions pool in the nasopharynx and might then be aspirated, so suctioning and careful feedings are important in the prevention of complications. Some mothers have been successful breast-feeding infants with cleft lip and cleft palate. Breast milk, if easily obtained, is preferable to formula because its antibodies provide some infection prevention. This immunity would be important to the infant with cleft palate who contracts frequent upper respiratory infections.

Surgical correction of a cleft lip Surgical correction of the lip defect usually is accomplished at 1 or 2 months of age or when the infant weighs at least 10 pounds, although surgery can be performed at any age. Repair at an early age can be more successful than that done when the child is older, more active, and better able to interfere with the healing process. Z-plasty, a type of closure consisting of a staggered incision line that minimizes retraction of the lip due to scar tissue, is the preferred procedure. It allows a natural-looking closure of the defect. After cleft lip surgery, a Logan bow (a metal wire arch) usually is attached to the cheeks with adhesive tape. This prevents tension on the upper lip and promotes healing with less chance of noticeable scarring.

Surgical correction of a cleft palate The timing for surgical correction of cleft palate is based on the severity of the defect. Correction usually is accomplished between 6 and 18 months of age but might continue in stages until the child is 4 or 5 years of age if the defect is severe. Early correction allows for development of more normal speech patterns. Delayed closure of large defects might require the use of prosthodontic appliances in addition to intensive speech therapy.

Long-term considerations are focused on promoting acceptable speech, preventing or correcting dental abnormalities, preventing and treating chronic ear infection, and providing psychologic support to the child. A hospital-based or community-based cleft palate team provides consistent long-term care for the child and family. The team consists of plastic surgeon, dentist, social worker, speech pathologist, otolaryngologist, orthodontist, nurse, psychologist, audiologist, and geneticist, among others. Speech therapy should begin early in life and might continue through adolescence. Orthodontia also is necessary throughout childhood to correct such problems as extra, malformed, or absent teeth. A myringotomy with tubes might be necessary to prevent recurring ear infections due to pooling of secretions in the nasopharyngeal area and improper drainge of the middle ear. The child might require counseling to cope with feelings relating to multiple surgeries, residual scarring, or noticeable speech defects.

Nursing management Immediate nursing care covers three essential areas: (a) maintaining a clear and adequate airway, (b) maintaining fluid and caloric intake, and (c) providing emotional support to the parents. Cleft lip is an immediately noticeable defect, and most parents are unaware of the advances in plastic surgery that now allow for a near normal appearance. Parents might require repeated reassurance from medical and nursing personnel. Before and after pictures of other children have been found to be effective in allaying parental fears (Colburn and Cherry, 1985). The nurse might also act as a role model by treating these infants like any others. Speaking to and cuddling these infants while feeding them allows parents to see that their children are indeed lovable human beings.

Nutrition: potential for fluid and calorie deficit Nutritional intake might be limited because the infant has trouble sealing the nipple well enough to create effective suction. The size of the defect might preclude breast-feeding, but mothers can express milk for bottle-feedings if they wish.

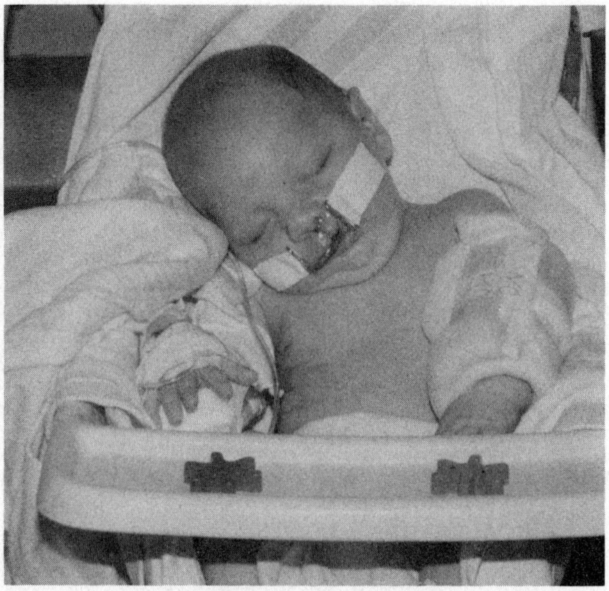

Child with a Logan bow. (Photograph by Judy Koenig.)

Special feeding systems and soft nipples with enlarged holes have been developed to aid in easier and safer nipple feedings. Some of these nipples are attached to soft plastic reservoirs that allow slow expression of the formula and limit the need for the child to create suction. Slower delivery of formula also prevents excess milk from escaping through the nose in infants who also have a cleft palate.

Infants should be held upright during feedings. This might be accomplished by holding the child's head while the child is in a seated position or by cradling the infant in the arm. A pillow propped between the nurse or parent's hand or arm and the chair arm can help hold the infant in a more upright position.

Because these infants do not "seal" the nipple well, they are prone to swallowing excessive amounts of air and require frequent burping. If the child with a cleft palate vomits, oropharynx and nasal passages require thorough bulb suctioning.

The nurse encourages parents to feed their infants as often as possible before discharge. Many nurses use these opportunities to teach any special feeding techniques and to assess parental knowledge and capabilities. The nurse often needs to reassure parents that it is normal for their infants to make loud noises while eating and that their infants might appear to choke more frequently than normal infants. With practice, the parent becomes familiar with the method and rate of feeding suited to the child.

Children who are incapable of nipple feeding might require tube or dropper feedings. Plastic medicine droppers might be used initially but are tedious and time consuming.

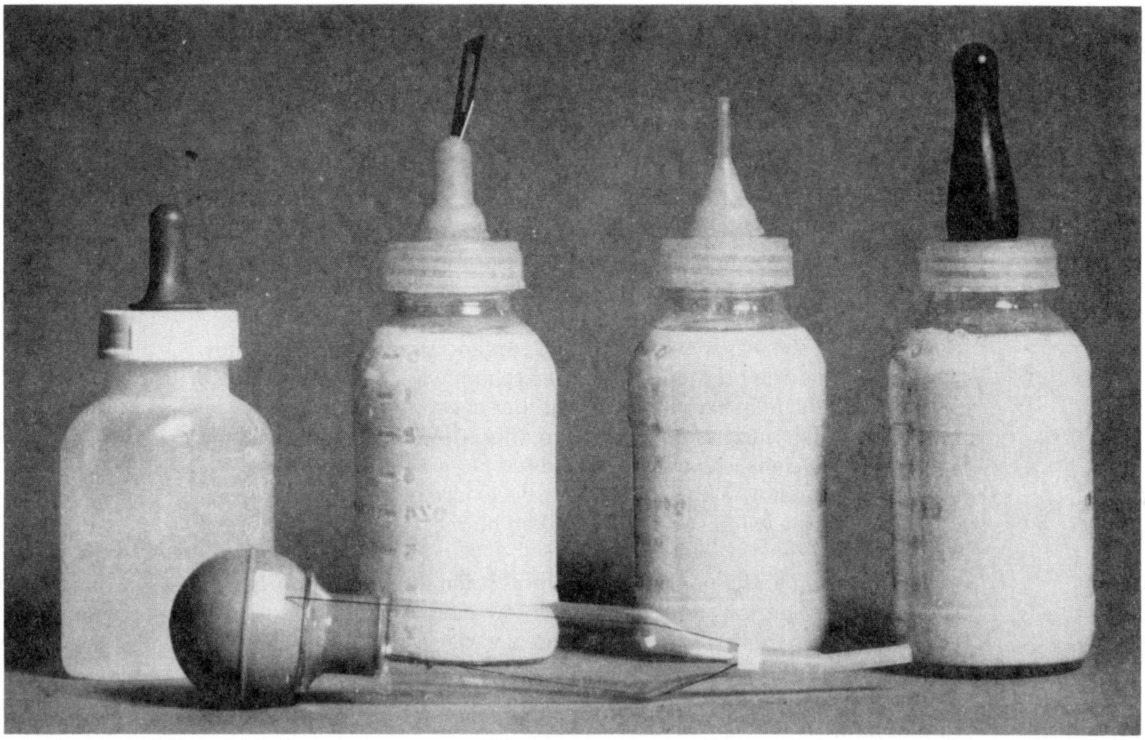

A variety of feeding methods are available for the infant with a cleft lip or palate.

Asepto or bulb syringe might then be used, or a homemade feeding system created. For this, a 12 or 14 French red rubber catheter is shortened, leaving the distal vents intact. A 10- or 20-mL Luer-lock syringe is then attached to the tubing. The result is a system that allows regulated delivery of very small amounts of formula. The flexible catheter can be placed so as to deposit formula at the center back or lateral back of the tongue. Occasionally a thin, flexible nipple can be used on the end of the Asepto syringe. Using the nipple allows more control over the amount of formula given. One of these methods is used after the initial surgery in order to avoid harming the suture line.

Preoperative preparation Immediate preoperative nursing care is directed toward instructing parents in the care of their children after surgery. The parent should be aware that the child will have both arms restrained in elbow restraints in order to prevent damage to the suture line. Children who will have cleft lip repairs are required to remain on their backs or sides and are not allowed to sleep in a prone position. Children with only palate closures can sleep in any position. The child is syringe-fed or cup-fed during the immediate postoperative period. Parental anxiety and the infant's reactions to changes in routine can be alleviated somewhat by practicing postoperative measures before surgery. Infants should be able to sleep comfortably in supine or side-lying positions. Occasional cup feedings at home might encourage more ready acceptance of this feeding method after successful cleft palate surgery.

Postoperative care Postoperative nursing care is focused on care of the surgical site. The nurse cleanses lip suture lines frequently according to hospital policy and following exactly the instructions of the plastic surgeon. Dilute hydrogen peroxide and cotton-tipped applicators are often used to remove all crusts or exudate. The nurse applies the cleaning solution with the applicator gently rolling, not rubbing, the tip to loosen crusts. Antibiotic ointment might be prescribed to prevent infection, maintain a supple incision line, and promote softening of any sanguineous crusts.

Feedings usually begin with clear liquids once the child is fully awake and are followed by full liquids as tolerated. Because of possible trauma to the incision line, children with lip repairs are fed by rubber-tipped syringe. Children with palate repairs are never tube-, syringe-, or fork-fed. Feeding by cup is preferable, although the side of a spoon to the lips might be acceptable. As with any surgery, vomiting

NURSING CARE PLAN *The Child with Cleft Lip and Cleft Palate*

Assessment data: Michael is a 2-month-old with a left-sided cleft lip and cleft palate. He was the product of an uneventful first pregnancy and weighed 7 lb 12 oz at birth. His parents were initially very upset that Michael was born with a defect. They received in-depth teaching and nursing support during his admission period and were able to speak to the pediatric plastic surgeon about repair options. They decided to wait until Michael weighed at least 10 lb. Their primary nurse encouraged them to feed Michael while she was there to offer support and suggestions, and they were able to decide on a feeding technique that was comfortable and provided adequate intake. Michael's mother chose to express breast milk for feedings and has not needed to offer formula supplementation. Michael now weighs well over 10 lb and has been admitted to the pediatric floor following his initial Z-plasty closure of his cleft lip. Repair of the cleft palate will be undertaken when he reaches 18–24 months of age.

On admission to the floor, the nurse notes that the Logan bow is intact over the surgical site; there is an intravenous line in his foot; and elbow restraints are in place. He is crying and flailing his arms. His parents state that they are very pleased with the repair but are somewhat hesitant to handle him so soon after surgery. They ask how to take care of him.

Nursing diagnosis	Intervention	Rationale
1. Potential impaired tissue integrity (stressors: developmental factors, easily disrupted surgical site, parental anxiety)	Maintain position of Logan bow.	Strips or Logan bow prevent lateral separation of suture lines.
	Maintain elbow restraints in place unless Michael is being directly supervised.	Elbow restraints prevent child from picking at surgical site yet leave hands free.
	Position Michael on his back or side only; an infant seat might be used.	Positioning prevents child from rubbing surgical site on bed linen.
	Perform lip and nostril care after feeding and as ordered. Use cotton-tipped swab and hydrogen peroxide diluted with normal saline (or water, as ordered). Apply antibiotic ointment or mesh gauze soaked in sterile water or saline to suture line as ordered.	Care for suture line, initially every hour, limits crusting, limits inflammation, and allows closer observation of site for infection.
	Allow no bottle or pacifier. Use nontraumatic feeding techniques (Asepto or bulb syringe, syringe with rubber tubing).	Sucking on nipple places undue pressure on site. Limiting trauma to site speeds healing and prevents scarring.
	Anticipate infant's needs.	Minimizing crying reduces tension on suture line.

Outcome: At discharge Michael's surgical site is clean and free from crusting. The suture line is intact and healing well.

NURSING CARE PLAN *The Child with Cleft Lip and Cleft Palate (Continued)*

Nursing diagnosis	Intervention	Rationale
2. Potential for ineffective airway clearance (stressors: edema at surgical site, increased thick secretions, nausea, and vomiting from anesthesia, vomiting from excess air swallowed during feeding)	Observe for respiratory distress.	Prompt intervention reduces the risk of complications.
	Reposition infant from side to back to side every 2 hours.	Frequent turning promotes more effective airway clearance.
	Burp after every ounce during feeding and elevate the head of the bed after feeding.	Asepto feedings allow the child to swallow air. If he vomits he might aspirate. Burping frequently and elevating the head of the bed decrease the risk of vomiting and aspiration.
	Explain rationale of the mist tent to parents. Keep infant and bed clothes dry.	A mist tent is used postoperatively to liquefy secretions and promote effective airway clearance.
	Clean nares gently with swabs and saline. Use suction equipment if acute respiratory obstruction occurs.	Patent airway ensures adequate respiration. Limiting suctioning limits trauma to site.

Outcome: Michael is free of respiratory distress.

Nursing diagnosis	Intervention	Rationale
3. Potential for alteration in nutrition: less than body requirements (stressors: difficult feeding, vomiting, fatigue from feeding)	Feed Michael slowly with frequent rests. Burp well.	Small, frequent feedings allow adequate time for the child to swallow completely, limit regurgitation, and prevent aspiration.
	Position on right side after meals or elevate the head of the bed.	Positioning aids gastric emptying and prevents aspiration.
	Allow rest after feeding.	Rest decreases the likelihood of regurgitation. Regurgitation can lead to decreased intake of nutrients.
	Progress slowly from NPO with IV status to oral fluid intake.	IV fluid ensures adequate hydration status during the immediate postoperative period. Slow progression of oral fluids limits vomiting.
	Progress from clear to full liquids until Michael is taking normal diet (breast milk).	Clear liquids are more easily tolerated in the initial postoperative period. Breast milk provides a balanced diet with sufficient calories and fluid plus a certain amount of disease protection.
	Feed in an upright position. Place dropper, special nipple, or rubber tubing of bulb syringe at the corner of the mouth and slowly drip in the liquid.	Feeding slowly and in an upright position prevents regurgitation.
	Feed Michael more frequently if feedings are not finished because he is fatigued.	Feeding by bulb syringe or dropper is much slower than by bottle, resulting in decreased intake and increased fatigue.
	Weigh q.o.d. and compare with previous weight for any increase or decrease.	Infant might lose weight after surgery; change in weight is a good indicator of adequacy of diet and nutritional status.

Outcome: Michael makes a successful transition from NPO with IV to adequate clear liquid intake within 12 hours of surgery. Michael's fluid and calorie needs are met as indicated by no weight loss.

(Continues)

NURSING CARE PLAN *The Child with Cleft Lip and Cleft Palate (Continued)*

Nursing diagnosis	Intervention	Rationale
4. Alteration in comfort: pain related to physical injury secondary to surgical incision	Observe Michael frequently for pain and discomfort. Offer comfort measures (holding, rocking, music, talking, position changes, toys). Medicate p.r.n. as ordered.	Distraction and comfort measures decrease anxiety and lessen sensation of pain. Frequent observations allow subtle signs of discomfort to be identified and interventions initiated before pain becomes severe.
	Use brightly colored mobiles and crib decorations to provide visual stimulation, and use music boxes or tape recorder for auditory stimulation.	These assist with maintaining the infant's interest and promote normal development.

Outcome: Michael appears comfortable and free of discomfort as evidenced by reduced crying, decreased restlessness, interest in playing, and ability to sleep.

Nursing diagnosis	Intervention	Rationale
5. Potential impairment of skin integrity (stressors: elbow restraints, limited movement of upper extremities)	Remove restraints one at a time when Michael is directly supervised. Remove restraints, give skin care, and perform range-of-motion exercises every 4 hours. Change positions every 2 hours.	Frequent position changes and release of restraints prevent harmful effects of limited mobility.
	Observe hands for signs of circulatory impairment (cold, pale, edematous).	Too tight restraints can interfere with circulation to the hands.

Outcome: Michael's arms and hands have good muscle tone and intact skin of good color and turgor.

Nursing diagnosis	Intervention	Rationale
6. Potential impaired home maintenance management (stressors: parental knowledge deficit, unfamiliarity with procedures)	Explain and demonstrate all facets of Michael's care to parents. Encourage parents to assume many caregiving tasks while the nurse is available for guidance and support. Begin home care instructions on return from surgery.	Adequate education, preparation, and support allow parents to reassume caregiving tasks with minimal fear that they might do something to harm the suture line and consequently Michael's appearance.
	Allow Michael's parents to discuss their feelings related to Michael's surgery and condition.	After initial surgery is over, parents begin to look forward to future surgery and care.
	Tell parents that the suture line probably will remain red for as long as a year following surgery.	Parents are less fearful when they know what to expect.
	Encourage parents to hold Michael frequently. Use this time to instruct parents in restraint care at home.	Demonstration of appropriate restraint care allows parents to practice this skill before discharge.
	Discuss infection prevention and feeding techniques since Michael is susceptible to otitis media.	Infants with cleft palate are susceptible to otitis media from increased susceptibility to upper respiratory infections.

Outcome: The parents express increased feelings of confidence in their ability to care for Michael. Michael's parents can demonstrate home care procedures—feeding, suture line care, and restraint care.

NURSING CARE PLAN *The Child with Cleft Lip and Cleft Palate (Continued)*

Nursing diagnosis	Intervention	Rationale
7. Parental anxiety related to perceived threat to son's health status secondary to concern about future surgery and therapy	Allow Michael's parents to discuss their concerns regarding need for continued follow-up, further surgery for cleft palate repair, and rehabilitative speech and dental therapy. Include parents in planning follow-up therapy for Michael.	Correction of cleft lip and cleft palate is long-term and requires considerable follow-up care. Parents who are able to discuss and plan for follow-up can understand that dental correction and clear speech are possible but will take coordinated effort over an extended period of time.
	Encourage parents to seek support from outside groups, particularly the Cleft Palate Association of America.	Contact with support group or other parents of children with cleft lip and cleft palate helps parents understand the long-term nature of care and helps them cope.

Outcome: Michael's parents express decreased anxiety and verbalize the reasons Michael will need follow-up care. Parents state that they have sufficient information and support to enable them to appropriately anticipate and plan for Michael's future health care needs.

can occur during the initial feedings, and parents should be aware that this is common. The infant who is cup-fed also requires frequent burping to prevent vomiting or abdominal discomfort.

Several types of restraints are available; the type used depends on the age of the child. Small infants might require elbow restraints only, whereas the older child might require elbow or wrist restraints. Children undergoing lip repairs might need vest or wrist restraints to prevent them from turning onto their abdomens. Restraints can be removed when the parent is holding or comforting the child but are best removed only one at a time. The nurse needs to caution the parent who removes restraints that the child's fingers should be kept away from the mouth. Extremely restless children might require diphenhydramine hydrochloride (Benadryl) or chloral hydrate sedation. Parents should know that their infants might be extremely restless, might appear uncomfortable, might cry more than usual, and might not be as easily comforted as before.

Children undergoing cleft palate repair have copious serosanguineous nasal discharge. Positioning the child can facilitate drainage of secretions and decrease risk of aspiration. Preoperative medications might cause oral secretions to be thick and sticky. A mist tent postoperatively helps alleviate this problem. Children with cleft palate repairs may lie prone. If oral suctioning is necessary to prevent aspiration, it is done with extreme caution, as gently as possible, and is directed toward the sides of the mouth and the lateral back side of the tongue. Following formula feedings with several sips of water helps prevent formation of sticky oral secretions. Adequate hydration also allows the production of adequate saliva.

Additional surgery might be necessary to revise lip scars, perform nasal realignment, or complete the palate repair later in early childhood. Referring the family to the American Cleft Palate Association might be indicated.

Esophageal Atresia and Tracheoesophageal Fistula

Esophageal atresia occurs when the cells of the embryonic foregut fail to develop, leaving a blind pouch. *Tracheoesophageal fistula* (TEF) arises when the foregut fails to differentiate into a totally separate esophagus and trachea. This results in an open fistula between the two structures. Although esophageal atresia or tracheoesophageal fistula might occur separately, the most common anomaly is a combination of both defects.

Esophageal atresia occurs in approximately 1 of every 3000–4000 live births. A high percentage of these infants are premature or of low birth weight (Rudolph, 1982). More than three-fourths of affected infants have defects consisting of a blind upper esophageal pouch with a fistula between the trachea and the lower esophagus (type C). (Figure 27-1 shows the five most common forms of TEF, along with their relative frequency of occurrence.) More than 25% of all infants with esophageal atresia or TEF have other congenital anomalies. Cardiovascular anomalies are most prevalent, but pulmonary, intestinal, genitourinary, and neurologic defects also can occur.

Clinical manifestations Infants with esophageal atresia or TEF might present a variety of symptoms, depending on the severity of the defect and the location of the fistula. They might develop cyanotic episodes and usually are unable to handle oral secretions. Copious oral and nasal secretions requiring frequent suctioning might be noted in the delivery room or nursery. The infant might cough or choke on secretions or become cyanotic because of laryngospasms. An attempt to pass a nasogastric tube indicates that the catheter cannot be passed into the stomach. All or any of these problems should lead to suspicion of esophageal atresia or TEF.

A history of maternal polyhydramnios also is common in infants with atresias. This is due to the inability of the infant to swallow and excrete amniotic fluid adequately in utero.

Less dramatic symptomatology might result in a missed diagnosis and further complications when the diagnosis becomes apparent with feeding. Feeding the infant with TEF type C causes regurgitation. The stomach might be enlarged with air that has passed into it through the fistula. Depending on the location of the defect, children with other types of TEF can aspirate during feeding.

Diagnostic evaluation Fluoroscopic studies and bronchoscopy are needed to determine the extent of the defect as well as the location of fistulas. If contrast material is used, it should be administered slowly and should be removed to prevent chemical pneumonitis. All contrast studies are dangerous because of potential aspiration or difficulty removing contrast medium and are only performed if safer tests are not effective.

Treatment Esophageal atresia is considered a surgical emergency. Initial care is directed toward preventing aspiration. Placement of a drainage tube through the nose and into the esophageal pouch allows frequent intermittent suctioning of pooled secretions (see Fig. 27-1C). Infants then remain in a high-Fowler's position to prevent reflux of gastric acid into the lungs through the fistula resulting in pneumonitis. For infants exhibiting gastric distension, a gastrostomy might be necessary to allow escape of trapped air.

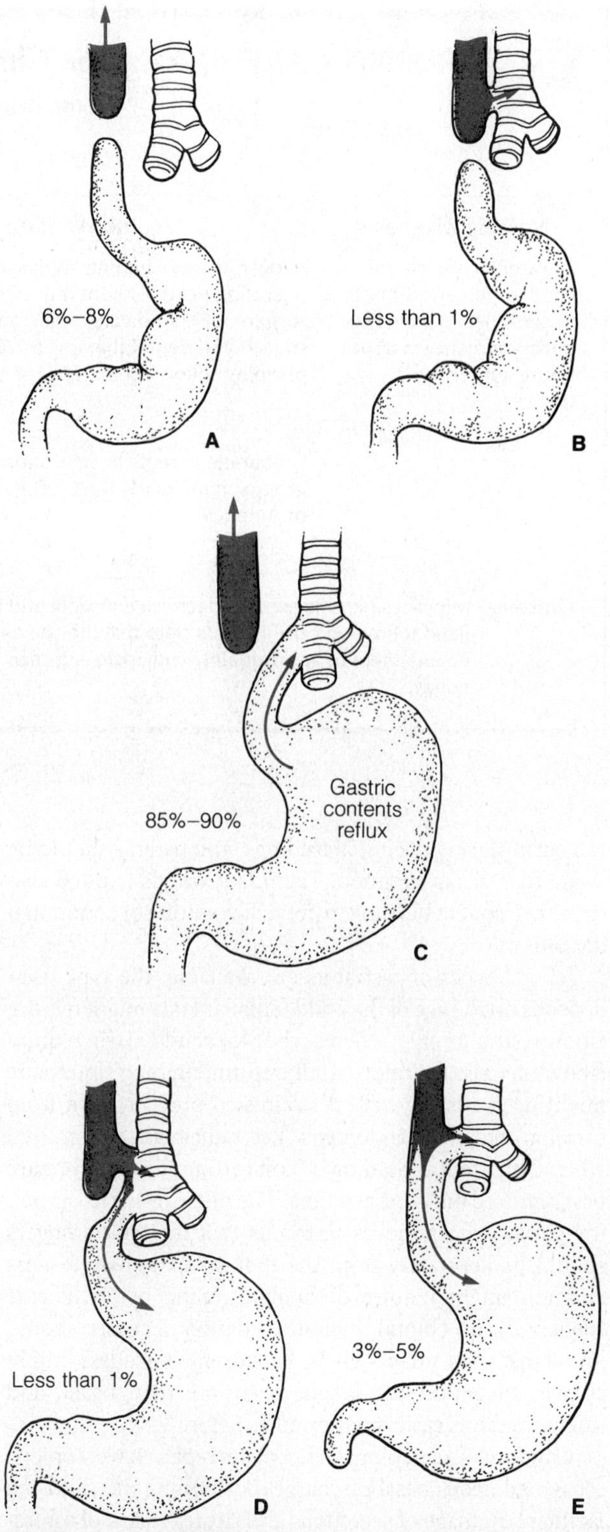

FIGURE 27-1

The five most frequently seen forms of tracheoesophageal fistulas and esophageal atresias, with their frequencies of occurrence. Arrows indicate what happens during infant feeding.

This also helps to prevent reflux of gastric acids into the trachea. Antibiotic therapy usually is instituted as a prophylactic measure in instances where aspiration pneumonia might have occurred.

Surgical repair is accomplished in single or multiple stages. In the single-stage procedure, all fistulas are closed, and an end-to-end anastomosis (joining) of the esophageal pouches is performed. If, however, the ends of the esophagus are separated by a wide margin or the child cannot tolerate extensive surgery, an alternative operation is performed. The fistulas are closed as before, but the proximal esophagus is brought to the outside of the neck (cervical esophagostomy). This ostomy usually is located at the left base of the neck and allows free drainage of swallowed secretions. A gastrostomy is necessary to provide feedings until a final reconstruction is done. When the esophageal pouches are widely separated an esophagoplasty is performed at 18–24 months of age. At that time, a segment of colon, previously cleansed with antibiotics, is removed and attached to both esophageal pouches to create a continuous esophageal passage. The newly constructed esophagus provides the same proximodistal peristalsis as a normal esophagus. The esophagostomy and gastrostomy are then closed.

The principal long-term complication of either type of surgery is esophageal stricture formation. Frequent dilatations often are necessary to prevent obstruction of the esophagus by scar tissue. Some surgeons perform dilatations at routine intervals as a preventive measure. Surgical revision of esophageal strictures might also be necessary. Colon transplants might become necessary for children who have frequent strictures and do not respond favorably to dilatations.

Nursing management The goals of preoperative nursing care for the infant with esophageal atresia or TEF are detection of the defect and prevention of aspiration. Nurses in the delivery room and newborn nurseries therefore suspect altered difficulty handling secretions. Although an infant might have other problems causing respiratory distress (for example, respiratory anomalies, brain damage, or cleft palate), the possibility of an atresia or fistula is much better discovered before feeding than afterward. Unfortunately, some infants are not diagnosed until after they have aspirated their first feeding. (This is why many institutions require the first feeding to be sterile water.)

Laryngospasm, a protective reflex to prevent aspiration, might cause the infant to become cyanotic. The nurse therefore suspects cyanotic infants with no known cardiac or respiratory anomalies of having anomalous formation of the esophagus and a possible connection between the esophagus and the trachea.

Because most infants have distal esophageotracheal fistula, affected infants should be placed in a head-up position in an isolette or radiant warmer (see Chapter 34). This position prevents reflux of damaging gastric secretions into the trachea. Suctioning of the esophageal pouch might be intermittent or continuous. Continuous suctioning prevents frequent blockage of the tube by mucus and prevents a sudden buildup of secretions. Low-pressure, continuous suctioning is therefore often preferred. The nurse also observes secretions for any evidence of fresh bleeding that might indicate an ulceration.

These infants are placed NPO, and a gastrostomy tube might be placed to gravity drainage to decompress the stomach. Gastrostomy feedings are *not* given before ligation (closing) of the fistula because of the possible reflux of stomach contents into the trachea. Infants receive intravenous fluid and electrolytes and might require hyperalimentation if surgery is postponed for more than 24–48 hours.

Postoperative care Immediate postoperative care includes care of the thoracotomy site (chest wall incision), chest tubes, and maintenance of ventilatory support when necessary. (See Chapter 23 for recommended care of the child who has undergone thoracic surgery.)

Infants who have undergone ligature of fistula or anastomosis of esophageal pouches are prone to pulmonary infections. The nurse therefore monitors the child closely for signs of atelectasis or pneumonia. Decreased breath sounds, increased respiratory rate, increased temperature, pallor, or cyanosis might indicate pulmonary infections or pneumothorax.

The infant usually returns with a gastrostomy, which serves several purposes. It allows initial gastric decompression after surgery, prevents mechanical irritation of the esophageal anastomosis site, and allows early reintroduction of feeding without harming the surgical sites. The gastrostomy tube is often left to gravity drainage to allow gastric decompression. When bowel sounds return, the gastrostomy tube might be elevated above the level of the stomach. This allows gastric secretions to pass through the pylorus yet allows escape of swallowed air through the open tube. Eventually the tube is clamped or plugged between feedings.

Infants who have undergone this type of surgery are susceptible to fluid and electrolyte imbalances and nutritional deficits. Loss of electrolytes through gastrostomy drainage during the first 48–72 hours might be significant. Many infants are placed on additional intravenous replacement therapy to prevent electrolyte disturbances. Accurate records of intake and output, including gastric drainage, are necessary.

The infant remains NPO until bowel sounds return and until there is no danger of disrupting the surgical site. Intravenous therapy provides hydration but often does not provide adequate calories. Infants who remain NPO for longer than 48–72 hours might require parenteral nutritional support. Infants who are gastrostomy-fed are given initial feedings of water or glucose and water. If these feedings are tolerated, the diet is advanced to include standard formulas that provide adequate calories for the infant's weight. Gastrostomy feedings are continued until the esophageal anastomosis has healed (10–14 days). Oral feedings then begin. Nursing care should include time to allow the child to learn to swallow.

Infants undergoing multiple-stage surgery return from surgery with a cervical esophagostomy. Because constant drainage of enzyme-rich saliva from the esophagostomy can cause excoriation of neck tissues, frequent, meticulous skin care is needed. A thin layer of an occlusive ointment is applied around the site. If excoriation is severe, a collection bag might be necessary, although this presents great difficulty because of the location of the esophagostomy and the nature of the secretions. A pacifier and "sham" feedings are encouraged to promote sucking and swallowing. Sham feedings consist of small amounts of liquids or pureed fruits, depending on the infant's age. Although the sham feedings are expelled through the esophagostomy, they allow the infant to experience varying taste and texture sensations. They assist the child with feeding after reconstruction is completed.

Needs of parents The nurse is concerned not only with the physical care of the infant but also with the emotional and educational needs of the family. Parents of children with congenital defects require intensive emotional support, but the emotional needs of parents are even greater when immediate surgery is needed for the infant to survive. Quiet, calm discussions about the infant's condition offer the parent a chance to ask questions and can help alleviate some of the stress. Ideally, these parents should receive as much preoperative information as possible and continued postoperative information and family advocacy.

Discharge preparation Parents of children undergoing multiple-stage surgery should be capable of caring for their children before discharge. The nurse provides both oral and written instructions along with actual demonstrations of gastrostomy feedings and esophagostomy care. The parent then returns the demonstration. If sham feedings are to be used, the parent should be aware of the frequency and amount of each feeding. Gastrostomy feeding supplies are often available through the hospital or might be provided by public health or Crippled Children's Services.

Nurses might need to encourage these parents to hold and cuddle their infants frequently. Because the normal attachment experienced during feeding has been disrupted, parents should understand that alternative contact is needed. Tube feeding while holding the infant is sometimes awkward, and the parent might feel more at ease with the young child lying down or in an infant seat during feedings. Parents should then make concerted efforts to cuddle after feeding or to provide frequent, close eye-to-eye contact throughout the day.

Infants who have the single-stage repair need to be observed for signs of stricture formation. The nurse explains and provides a written list of signs that indicate possible stricture formation and instructs the parent to contact the physician if any one of these signs occurs. Signs of stricture formation include choking or gagging on solid foods while tolerating pureed or liquid foods, refusing food and sometimes even liquids, dysphagia (inability to swallow), increased drooling, and frequent coughing and choking that appear to be related to swallowing.

The Child with a Problem Affecting the Body's Use of Food

Children are frequently admitted for a hospital workup because of failure to thrive, which is often used as a catchall admitting diagnosis for infants or young children who fail to grow and gain weight normally. Causes of failure to thrive in children might be inorganic (see Chapter 13) or organic. Organic causes of failure to thrive include a variety of disorders that interfere with the child's nutritional status. Specific organic causes include renal disturbance, gastrointestinal disorders, neurologic problems, cardiovascular anomalies, and general malnutrition or protein deficiencies. Only 10% of all cases of failure to thrive are found to have no organic cause.

Another general cause of failure to thrive is a mutation within the genetic codes of the cell that in turn leads to errors in body metabolism. These genetic defects are called *inborn errors of metabolism,* and they cause disturbances in the metabolism of amino acids, carbohydrates, lipids, minerals, vitamins, and other chemical processes. The clinical effects range from mild to severe. (Table 27-7 illustrates some of the inborn errors of metabolism that affect the gastrointestinal system.) Other alterations in the body's ability to absorb and use nutrients result from dysfunction affecting portions of the gastrointestinal tract and inadequate intake of appropriate nutrients.

Phenylketonuria

Phenylketonuria (PKU) is a condition that results from an interference with the body's metabolism of phenylalanine—an essential amino acid. Phenylalanine usually is converted

TABLE 27-7 Inborn Errors of Metabolism

Description	Clinical manifestation	Treatment	Nursing management
Lactose intolerance			
A deficiency or absence of lactase in the intestinal villi results in the body's inability to break down lactose. The excess lactose in the intestine is fermented by intestinal bacteria resulting in excessive amounts of lactic acid. Might affect up to 70% of American blacks but occurs in other people as well. Lactose intolerance also might be acquired from conditions resulting in decreased intestinal function	Abdominal cramps, distension and severe diarrhea. Stools are low in pH (below 6) and contain reducing substances	Lactose (milk product) free formula or diet	Test stools for pH and reducing substances (Clinitest tablets are used to test stools for presence of reducing substances). Give meticulous skin care to prevent excoriation from acidic stools. Give dietary teaching for lactose-free diet
Galactosemia			
Autosomal recessively inherited condition resulting in an absence of galactose-1-phosphate uridyl transferase, the enzyme required to convert galactose to glucose. Symptoms result from the buildup of improperly metabolized galactose. The condition can be fatal if not recognized early	Failure to thrive, enlarged liver, and cataracts. Child demonstrates progressive neurologic damage	Galactose-free formula or diet (no milk or other products containing galactose)	Give dietary teaching. Support child and family (see Chapters 15 and 17)

to tyrosine and proteins necessary for growth through an established metabolic pathway (Fig. 27-2A).

In PKU, the enzyme phenylalanine hydroxylase is missing, preventing the breakdown of phenylalanine for the body's use (Fig. 27-2B). Phenylalanine accumulates in the blood, and the acid by-products formed by abnormal metabolism accumulate in urine, sweat, cerebrospinal fluid, and other body tissues. Elevated serum phenylalanine causes severe neurologic damage with mental retardation. Because of associated interference with the production of tyrosine, and consequently melanin, the child with PKU usually is fair-haired and blue-eyed.

PKU is a relatively rare genetic disease that primarily affects Caucasians. It occurs as a result of an autosomal recessive inheritance pattern. Because the symptoms do not appear for approximately 6 months after birth, when the blood levels of phenylalanine are sufficiently high to cause damage, newborn screening for the disease is essential to avoid irreversible mental retardation.

Clinical manifestations Untreated infants develop a typical picture of moderate to severe mental retardation due to degeneration of the brain and defective myelination of the nerves. Eczema or seborrhea might be present, and there is a musty or mousy odor to the urine and sweat caused by the presence of phenylpyruvic acid. Infants might develop seizures, hyperactivity, a bizarre or schizoid personality, and marked behavior problems.

Diagnostic evaluation Phenylketonuria screening is mandatory in most states since the consequences of the disease are preventable. An initial serum phenylalanine (Guthrie) of above 4 mg/100 mL is diagnostic for PKU. For the measurement to be accurate, the infant must have ingested protein for at least 48 hours. Vomiting, NPO status, or early testing can lead to false-negative results, and many states require retesting of infants at 14–28 days of age. At that time a serum level of above 15 mg/100 mL is diagnostic.

Other tests are based on the presence of abnormal metabolic by-products that are present in the urine of affected infants, although it might take 2–4 weeks before the by-products are present in sufficient quantities for the test to be performed with any accuracy. Brain damage might already have occurred during this time. Experience has shown that children who begin dietary treatment within the first 2 to 3 weeks of life stand a greater chance of incurring no brain damage. For this reason, early blood tests are preferred.

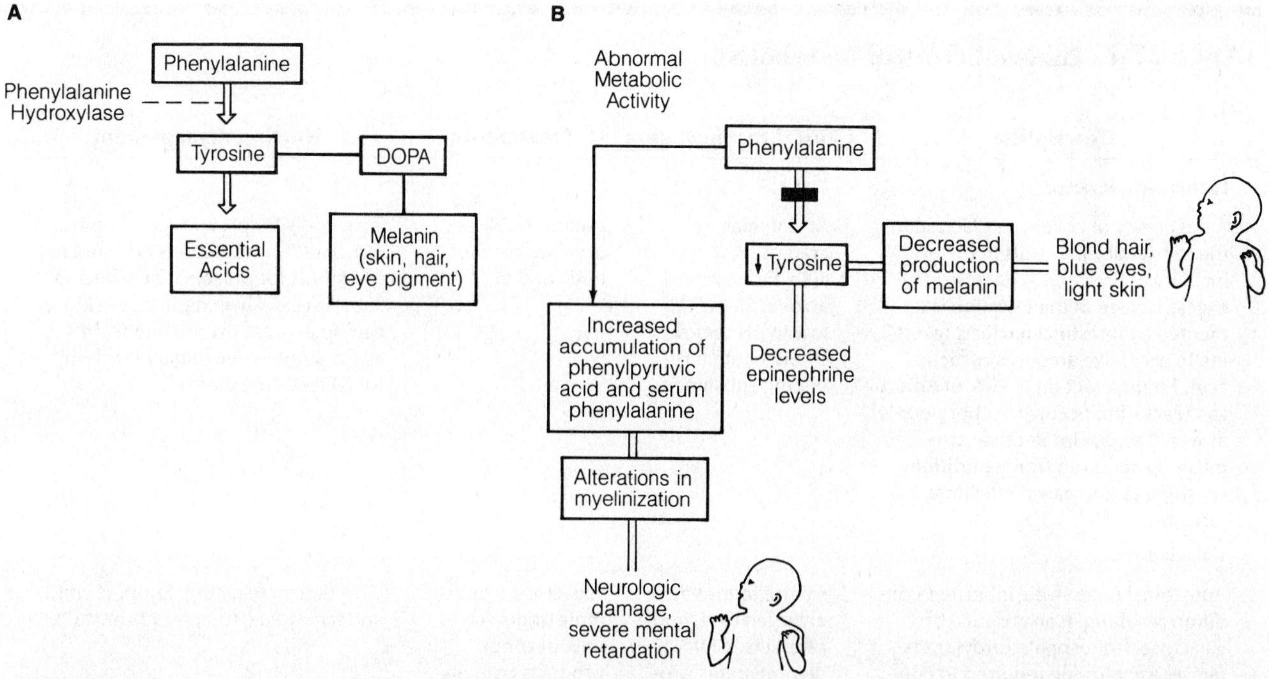

FIGURE 27-2
Pathophysiology of phenylketonuria.

Treatment Medical management is directed toward minimizing intake of dietary phenylalanine. Because phenylalanine is an essential amino acid, minimum intake of this substance is necessary, and because tyrosine is not being formed, an adequate amount of this amino acid is necessary also.

Infants are begun on a formula consisting of an enzymatic hydrolysate of casein (Lofenalac), which lowers the phenylalanine concentration from the normal 5% to approximately 0.4%. The diet is expanded to include low-phenylalanine foods as the child grows older. Foods such as fruits and juices, limited vegetables and grains, and pasta products are included. These foods supplement the phenylalanine-free formula. It is important to monitor serum levels of phenylalanine as an indicator of dietary control. Blood levels between 70 and 90 mg/kg for infants and 2 and 7 mg/kg for children appear to provide adequate growth without mental impairment.

Former protocol suggested that the diet be maintained until the child was at least 7–9 years old, at which time at least 90% of brain growth had occurred. Recent studies have recommended that the child continue the diet longer, possibly throughout life (Hayes et al., 1987). Because elevated levels of phenylalanine can cause congenital malformations in a fetus, any pregnant adolescent or woman with PKU needs to be on a phenylalanine-restricted diet.

Nursing management The long-term goals of nursing care are dietary education and emotional support. Because parents need first to become familiar with dietary requirements, nurses provide both oral and written information on phenylketonuria. Parents then face the importance of long-term dietary management and the problems it usually creates.

Special formulas are expensive. Children dislike the taste of these formulas, although the taste can be improved by flavoring with powdered drinks such as Kool-aid (Hayes et al., 1987). Low-phenylalanine foods (vegetables, fruit juices, limited cereals) can become restrictive and repetitive. Parents might encounter problems with dietary control when children become old enough to visit with friends or go to school. Peer pressure is difficult to handle and might cause the child to transgress on the diet.

Monitoring serum phenylalanine levels is an important part of follow-up care. Ideal serum phenylalanine levels are between 3 and 8 mg/100 mL. The nurse also observes the child for signs of phenylalanine deficiency. Metabolic acidosis and recurrence of skin rashes might indicate a deficiency. Height and weight growth patterns also can be adversely affected if intake of phenylalanine is cut too drastically.

Parents are given support in the management of the child with PKU. Discussing with them the child's possible resentment of the diet and methods of approach can prepare them to give the best possible support to the child. Parents are encouraged to obtain genetic counseling, and genetic counseling is recommended for the child at adulthood.

Gastroesophageal Reflux (Chalasia)

Gastroesophageal reflux (backflow) is a process that occurs when the cardiac valve at the distal end of the esophagus is relaxed or incompetent. This allows frequent reflux of gastric contents into the esophagus. A hiatal hernia might or might not be present.

Clinical manifestations Presenting symptoms might include a history of excessive vomiting during the first week or two of life. In severe cases, children who have been fed and then placed in a prone position in bed might regurgitate or vomit a large portion of their formula. Other problems encountered include esophagitis due to constant exposure to gastric acidity, aspiration pneumonia, weight loss, and esophageal hemorrhage. Reflux might trigger laryngospasm, manifested by choking, cyanosis, and periods of apnea.

Diagnostic evaluation The presence of reflux can be confirmed through a history of signs and symptoms or through the use of a barium esophagogram. The child swallows a bolus of barium and is then placed in a head-down position with the abdomen compressed. Radiographs indicate the presence of refluxed material that is not quickly cleared from the esophagus or repeated reflux of contrast material. Esophageal pH monitoring is another diagnostic test that aids in evaluating the presence of gastric acidity in the esophagus.

Treatment Medical management often is effective in handling reflux in infants but is less successful with older children. The routine approach includes careful and frequent burping followed by propping the infant in a semi-upright position (30–45 degrees) for an hour after each feeding. Recent research suggests that the child who is propped upright might experience more reflux episodes or that these episodes might last longer (Orenstein et al., 1983). Clinical implications of this research indicate that infants might experience less reflux and be less irritable if they are burped thoroughly during and after each feeding and then placed on their abdomens with the head of the bed elevated to a 30° angle for 2–3 hours. Placing the infant on a slant board helps to maintain this position. This routine is recommended until the disorder is outgrown, sometime between 4 and 6 months of age (Balistreri and Farrell, 1983). When infants are positioned upright to prevent severe reflux, however, they often remain upright for a full 24 hours throughout the day.

Formulas might be thickened with infant cereals to help prevent reflux. Antacids between feedings might be needed if esophagitis is present. More than half of these children respond well to therapy before reaching age 2.

If infants do not respond well to positional therapy or to thickened feedings, then surgery might be indicated to prevent the possible occurrence of aspiration pneumonia. The surgical procedures used create a mechanically competent cardiac sphincter and prevent further reflux.

Nursing management The goals of nursing care for the child with gastroesophageal reflux are to decrease the frequency of reflux, monitor the respiratory status if laryngospasms are frequent, maintain adequate nutrition, promote parent-infant bonding, and provide adequate infant stimulation if prolonged positional therapy is indicated.

Frequent small feedings of formula or formula with cereal, careful burping, and positioning during and after feeding are important nursing interventions. If a slant board is used, the nurse checks for adequate padding of the board and straddle bar and provides restraints that prevent the infant from slipping off the board. Minimal movement after feedings also helps decrease the incidence of vomiting.

If vomiting occurs, the character, frequency, amount, and time since the last feeding are documented. Accurate intake and output records are important. Infants who regurgitate large quantities of formula should be refed an amount equivalent to the lost formula.

If laryngospasms cause frequent periods of apnea, the infant might be placed on an apnea monitor (see Chapter 34). The nurse monitors the infant's respiratory status frequently.

Parents of infants with gastroesophageal reflux often feel inadequate in their parenting skills. They might, for example, have been told by well-meaning relatives that they are not feeding or burping their infants correctly. The frequent vomiting of feedings with resultant weight loss only contributes to parents' feelings of guilt. Because of this, parent-infant attachment might be impaired or delayed. An explanation of the physiologic cause of the infant's reflux helps parents realize that they are not to blame for their child's condition. Efforts to involve the parent in the child's feeding and physical care help facilitate attachment. The nurse encourages the parent to feed the child as often as possible during hospitalization so that the parent feels comfortable with the procedure on discharge.

Adequate stimulation becomes vitally important for infants confined to a slant board. Bright and colorful objects placed within reach, wrist rattles, and mobiles offer the infant a variety of stimulation. Talking to the infant with direct eye contact is important during feeding and diapering. Touching and stroking the infant provides tactile stimulation. Parents also can cuddle their infants upright on their shoulders, or with the child's head and chest higher than the stomach while held in the parent's arms. Care should be taken that the child is not held in such a way as to compress the abdomen.

If the child is discharged on an apnea monitor, the parents need to be instructed how to administer CPR should the alarm sound and the child has ceased breathing. Referral to a community health nurse for follow-up is essential for parent support.

Celiac Disease

Celiac disease is a malabsorption syndrome characterized by a permanent intolerance to gluten, a protein component found in wheat, rye, barley, and oats. The gluten-caused changes in the absorptive surface of the intestine greatly decrease the body's ability to use essential nutrients (Fig. 27-3). Celiac disease also has been called celiac sprue, nontropical sprue, or gluten-induced enteropathy. Although the etiology is not known, theories suggest an inborn error of metabolism or an impairment of immunologic function.

Clinical manifestations Biopsies of intestine show a flat mucosal surface, absence or atrophy of the villi, and the presence of deep crypts. Changes within the mucosa begin in the proximal small intestine and continue distally if the disease remains untreated. Initially, the reduced absorptive surface of the intestine causes a marked decrease in fat absorption, resulting in the production of large quantities of fatty, frothy, foul-smelling stools (steatorrhea). As the disease progresses, the absorption of proteins, carbohydrates, calcium, iron, and vitamins D, K, B_{12}, and B_9 (folic acid) is also impaired. These deficiencies can lead to hypoproteinemia (decrease in blood protein), osteoporosis (increased porosity of bone), osteomalacia (bone softening) from inadequate vitamin D, and hypoprothrombinemia (decreased blood prothrombin causing bleeding tendencies) from decreased vitamin K. Folic acid deficiency can contribute to anemia.

Symptoms of the disease can appear at any time after gluten-containing foods have been introduced into the diet. Although most of these children develop problems prior to age 2, symptoms can be delayed for many years. Early symptoms of the disease are subtle and include behavioral changes (such as apathy or irritability) as well as the physical symptoms of weight loss, abdominal distension, and diarrhea. Signs of progressive disease include colicky abdominal pain, vomiting, protuberant abdomen, subcutaneous fat loss, muscle wasting, and dependent edema of the lower extremities secondary to hypoproteinemia. Children are pale because of anemia, and bruising might develop secondary to inadequate vitamin K absorption. Late signs might include severe growth retardation osteoporosis and osteomalacia.

Diagnostic evaluation Diagnostic procedures include stool analysis of a 72-hour quantitative fecal fat level to determine the degree of steatorrhea. Assessment of serum protein, clotting factors, and electrolytes assists with the diagnosis. A sweat chloride test is frequently performed to rule out the possibility of cystic fibrosis. A duodenal and jejunal biopsy should be performed in order to ensure a definitive diagnosis.

Treatment Dietary management is the principal intervention in early or chronic celiac disease. The child is prescribed a gluten-free or gluten-restricted diet. Foods containing grains such as wheat, rye, oats, and barley are eliminated, and rice and corn are used as substitutes. Temporary parenteral hyperalimentation is necessary for children who are severely malnourished. Supplemental vitamins, calcium, and iron might be needed if malabsorption is severe.

Behavioral improvement is often noticed within the first few days of dietary treatment, with weight gain, increased appetite, and a decrease in frothy stools noticed several weeks later. Repair of diseased intestine proceeds proximally, and function might return to normal within months of beginning the new diet. The intolerance for gluten is permanent, and lack of adherence to a gluten-restricted diet can cause a relapse.

A severe crisis (celiac crisis) can develop when the child exhibits profuse, watery diarrhea and vomiting. The crisis causes severe dehydration and metabolic acidosis. Crises might be triggered by any intestinal infection, by fasting, or by ingestion of gluten-containing foods. Treatment is symptomatic and consists of gastric decompression and replacement of fluid and electrolytes.

Nursing management The long-term goal of nursing care is to provide dietary education and supervision. The nurse explains the disease and the rationale behind the gluten-free diet to the parent. A nutritionist is an excellent resource for nutrition education and dietary planning and is often able to provide special recipes for gluten-free foods.

Infants can be given standard infant formulas unless they are lactose intolerant. When cereal is introduced, rice cereal is permitted. The parent is encouraged to check labels on all baby foods for gluten content.

As the child grows, the nurse emphasizes the importance of screening the labels of all commercial foods for the presence of gluten or gluten-containing products. For example, such terms as *cereal fillers* or *hydrolyzed vegetable protein* indicate the presence of gluten. Many nutritionists can pro-

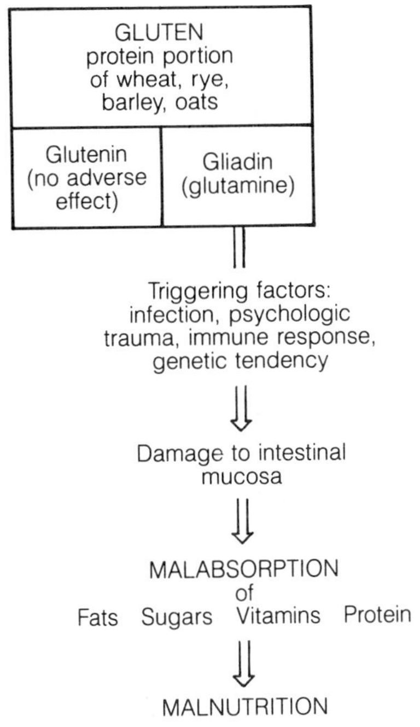

FIGURE 27-3
Pathophysiology of celiac disease.

vide a list of "safe" commercial foods as well as a list of ingredients that might indicate the presence of gluten in the product.

Initial dietary restrictions depend on the degree of inflammation present in the bowel. Children who exhibit lactose intolerance due to atrophy of the intestinal villi might be further restricted from milk-containing foods. Raw vegetables, gas-producing vegetables, raw fruits, and nuts might initially be restricted until inflammation subsides. Although most celiac patients can tolerate small amounts of gluten, the diet is continued for life. Older children and adolescents are often tempted to compromise their diets because the disease has been asymptomatic for long periods, and they feel "different" from other children because they are unable to eat spaghetti, hamburgers, hot dogs, or pizza. Because occasional dietary transgressions might not cause significant problems, transgressions only reinforce the child's view that the disease has been "cured." Research has shown, however, that a significant number of these people suffer relapse if dietary restrictions are not maintained.

Parental cooperation also might waver as the child continues to appear healthy on the restricted diet. Parents might need to be reminded of the child's appearance prior to dietary therapy and of the permanent growth retardation that is possible if dietary restrictions are not followed.

Boredom with a repetitive, bland diet can lead to dietary mismanagement. Children and parents should therefore learn to cook a variety of acceptable foods. The nurse might encourage older children and teenagers to discover foods or recipes that are acceptable and to begin developing a sense of responsibility toward their own dietary management.

Parents need to be aware of those factors that can lead to problems. Avoiding exposure to infections is important, and the development of diarrhea or vomiting warrants close observation if a crisis is to be prevented. Anticholinergics also have been implicated in the development of crises. Because these drugs are often prescribed as antihistaminics, mild sedatives, or preoperative medications, the parent or child needs to remind any physician or dentist of the child's intolerance before such drugs are prescribed.

Because the disease is chronic, many children of families develop emotional problems. The child's cooperation with dietary restrictions can change dramatically with age, and parents might find that normal childhood disciplinary problems are exacerbated by the restrictions required. See Chapter 14 for nursing care of a child with a chronic condition.

Short-Bowel Syndrome

One form of acquired malabsorption is frequently referred to as the *short-bowel syndrome*. This disorder usually occurs after massive resection of the small intestine performed to treat a number of gastrointestinal disorders. Although infants are capable of adapting to limited intestinal resection without problems, a resection of 25% or more of the small intestine can cause severe malabsorption.

The location of the resection is important in determining both the ultimate prognosis and the nature of the malabsorption. Malabsorption of such nutrients as iron, calcium, folic acid, bile salts, vitamin B_{12}, and other fat-soluble vitamins can occur. A decrease in the intestinal production of certain enzymes adversely affects the absorption of other needed nutrients. Fluid and electrolyte imbalances are common after major resections and might present a difficult management problem.

Treatment Treatment of infants with short-bowel syndrome is focused on maintaining nutritional status until normal intake is possible. Infants are frequently placed on long-term TPN and need adequate supplementation of trace elements and necessary vitamins until a normal diet can be resumed. Vitamin and mineral levels are measured to determine any deficiencies.

Infants begin oral feedings with small amounts of sterile water or isotonic electrolyte solutions. As the infant continues on the diet, isotonicity and osmolality of the formula can be adjusted according to the child's malabsorptive problem. Special hospital formulas are frequently used until the child's bowel can accommodate elemental diets or dilute standard formulas. (See Table 27-5 for special formulas.)

These infants are at high risk for many reasons. Hyperalimentation exposes them to systemic infections and certain nutrient deficiencies if they are not monitored closely. Frequent diarrhea can cause rapid dehydration, electrolyte imbalances, and excoriation of perineal skin due to nonabsorbed bile acids and enzymes. Circulating immunoglobulins might be decreased after massive resections, and frequent infections can cause major clinical setbacks.

With the advent of TPN, more of these infants are surviving than ever before, but physical, emotional, and social development might be affected because of prolonged hyperalimentation, chronic illness, and length of hospitalization. Many of these infants have remained on hyperalimentation for 6–12 months or longer.

Nursing management Nursing management is primarily symptomatic, and continued assessment of the child is important for planning care. Because of the prolonged hospitalization of these infants, the nurse takes care not to overlook signs or symptoms that require immediate attention.

Children on chronic hyperalimentation are monitored closely for signs and symptoms of complications. The nurse observes infants given oral feedings for signs of formula intolerance. A sudden change in stool frequency or character is the most common problem, but vomiting and gastric retention also might occur. These infants should be NPO with intravenous fluids until dietary changes can be tolerated.

Diarrhea is common in these infants. The nurse therefore monitors frequency, character, color, and volume of all stools. Tests for stool pH are also performed, and Clinitest can be used to identify any reducing substances in the stool and urine. Because stool and urine should be measured and tested separately, double diapering is the preferred collection method. This involves placing a folded diaper over the urinary meatus and another diaper over it in the usual way. Frequent applications of pediatric urine collectors can exacerbate already excoriated skin (Gantt and Thompson, 1985).

Strict intake and output records are important, whether the child is receiving hyperalimentation or oral feedings. Measurement of urine specific gravity is done to determine fluid status, and daily weight measurements are necessary.

Skin rashes or skin breakdown are common. Rashes might indicate trace element or vitamin deficiencies. Candidal rashes can cause severe skin breakdown in the perineal region, as can malabsorption of bile acids and enzymes. Antifungal creams are used to combat candidal infection, and exposure to air or warmth from a lamp might speed healing. The nurse needs to be aware of safety principles when using a gooseneck lamp to treat an excoriated buttock. The lamp is placed at least 18 inches from the infant, and a low-wattage bulb is used (45–60). The exposed area is checked at least every 5 minutes for reddening. This treatment is done for about 5 minutes 3 times a day. Active infants might need to be restrained during the treatment. Frequent skin care and thorough cleansings after each stool and voiding help prevent skin breakdown.

Although the many physical problems appear to be overwhelming, emotional concerns also are vitally important. Parents of these children have not only been faced with the necessity of immediate surgery for their infants but also have had to face long-term hospitalization and complex care regimens. Nurses need to encourage total family participation in the infant's care. Family dynamics are often strained because of prolonged hospitalization, and the extended family might play an important role in supporting the parents during these times. Support groups of affected parents and siblings might be informed by the nursing staff as an organized approach to aid these families, or families might develop individual support groups among themselves.

Family members should be encouraged to bring the infant mobiles or stuffed toys and should talk to and cuddle the infant whenever possible. This helps facilitate parental attachment and contributes to the infant's growth and development. Some parents feel that the infant clothes brought from home make their children more like individuals. The nurse therefore encourages all these activities.

Kwashiorkor

When the intake of protein is inadequate with respect to calories and other nutrients, the protein-energy deficiency is known as *kwashiorkor*. This disease affects mainly children from underdeveloped countries. Kwashiorkor can, however, result from certain chronic or acute conditions.

Clinical manifestations Symptoms of kwashiorkor include irritability and listlessness. Edema is typical, however, and can range from mild swelling of hands and feet to marked pritoneal fluid accumulations. Pigmentation in skin and hair is lost, and hair becomes brittle and sparse. A nondescript skin rash and fatty infiltrates of the liver are associated signs.

Nursing management Once the cause of the undernutrition is identified, interventions can be coordinated to provide an adequate and usable dietary intake. The addition of nutrients is gradual. The nurse plays a vital role in teaching and supporting the child and family during this transition to different dietary patterns.

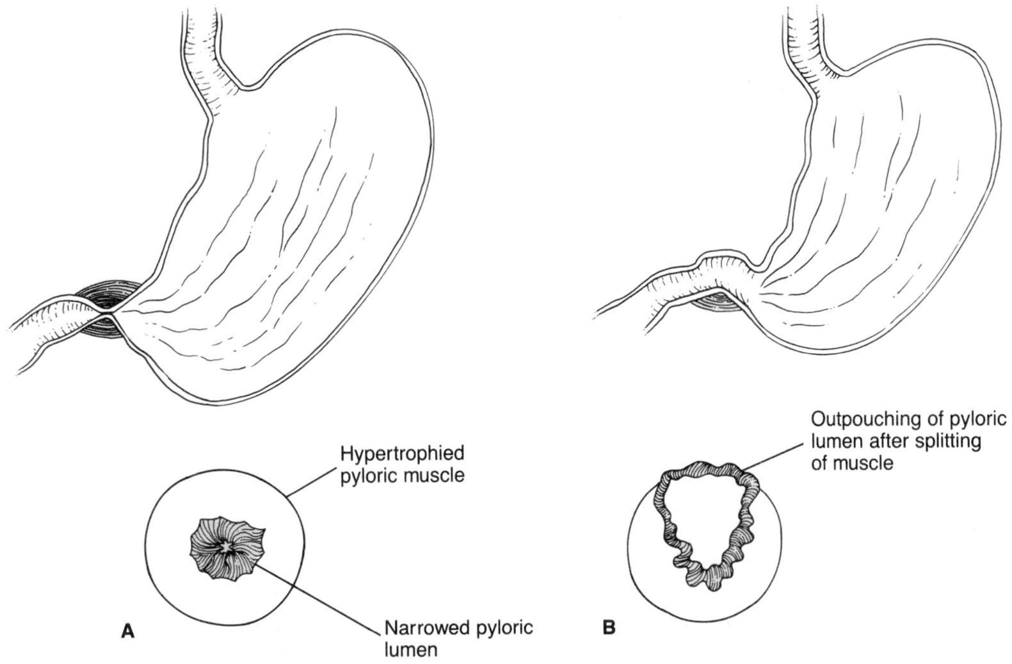

FIGURE 27-4
Pyloric stenosis. ***A.*** *Obstruction of pyloric lumen by hypertrophied muscle layers.* ***B.*** *Release of submucosal layer after pyloromyotomy.*

The Child with Existing or Potential Upper Gastrointestinal Obstruction

Pyloric Stenosis

Pyloric stenosis is the result of an increase in the amount of tissue and size of the circular muscle of the pylorus (Fig. 27-4). This causes narrowing, or stenosis, of the pylorus and effectively leads to an obstruction of the pyloric outlet.

Although the causative agent is unknown, heredity might play an important role. The disorder occurs more commonly in males (1:150) than females (1:750), and incidence is higher among first-born males.

Clinical manifestations Infants with pyloric stenosis have a variety of signs and symptoms. Because of the progressive nature of the obstruction, the infant might appear normal in the first week or two of life, but regurgitation or nonprojectile vomiting might begin in the second and third weeks. Projectile vomiting develops suddenly, becoming quite startling and forceful within 1–2 weeks of the initial onset. Projectile vomiting is sometimes forced 2 or 3 ft from the child. It might occur during or immediately after feeding or might be delayed for an hour or more. The emesis is not bile-stained but will contain gastric secretions, undigested formula, and, occasionally, flecks of blood. After vomiting, the infant appears voraciously hungry and usually takes another feeding immediately. Observation after feeding might show visible peristaltic waves moving from left to right toward the pylorus. Abdominal palpation might reveal a mass (approximately the size of an olive) in the epigastrium to the right of midline. This "olive" is present in an infant with a severely hypertrophic pylorus and is a classic indicator of pyloric stenosis.

Because of the incessant vomiting, the child will lose large quantities of chloride, sodium, and potassium and might present a clinical picture of failure to thrive and dehydration. Weight loss is common, and the infant can demonstrate loss of subcutaneous fat. Weight loss and dehydration are sometimes so rapid and severe that infants might present in critical condition with marked hypochloremic alkalosis.

Diagnostic evaluation Diagnostic studies include observation of the emesis pattern, palpation of the abdomen for presence of an "olive," and contrast studies. If contrast studies are necessary, the child is fed contrast material, and radiographs are taken to determine the obstruction. If pyloric stenosis is present, radiographs will show delayed or absent gastric emptying with the pylorus appearing as a narrow channel (commonly termed the "string sign").

Treatment Pyloromyotomy (dissection of the pylorus) is the standard surgical treatment for pyloric stenosis. Although nonsurgical treatment was once common, advantages of the present surgical procedure far outweigh the disadvantages of the slow and lengthy medical treatment.

Surgery usually is performed as soon as fluid and electrolyte imbalances have been corrected. It might be postponed for 2–3 days if the child is in severe imbalance.

Infants are NPO prior to surgery; gastric lavage is occasionally used to ensure that the stomach is totally empty at the time of surgery. Entry to the abdomen is through a small incision in the right upper quadrant. The muscle is split, thus enlarging the lumen.

The infant remains NPO for 4–6 hours after surgery. At that time, small feedings (approxmately 5 mL every hour) of glucose water or glucose and electrolyte solutions are begun. If these first feedings are retained, the volume of the feedings is increased. Dilute formula or breast milk is then introduced in small quantities. If tolerated, volume and concentration are increased until the child is tolerating full-strength feedings at 3- to 4-hour intervals.

Intravenous fluid administration continues until the child has shown the capability to retain adequate amounts of fluids by mouth, as these infants often experience some vomiting during the first 24 hours after surgery. If this occurs more than once, feedings might be withheld for several hours or might begin again with the first feeding of the regimen. Depending on the infant's ability to tolerate formula and retain feedings, a complete formula or breast milk diet might be reached within 24–36 hours. Many infants are discharged within 36–48 hours of surgery.

Nursing management Preoperative nursing care includes observation of the infant for signs and symptoms that facilitate the diagnosis of pyloric stenosis. Strict intake and output records are essential, and documentation should include not only the amount of emesis but also the character, quantity, and timing of emesis in relation to the last feeding. Frequent measurement of urine specific gravity is done to monitor the infant's state of hydration. Dehydrated infants require continued assessment for level of dehydration as well as for signs that might indicate an electrolyte imbalance (see Chapter 21). To prevent hyponatremia, vascular overload, or other complications, the nurse proceeds slowly with rehydration of severely dehydrated infants. Gastric lavage, if prescribed, is performed using isotonic saline irrigations in small amounts.

After surgery, care includes routine postoperative measures with continued observations for fluid and electrolyte imbalances. The operative site might be covered with collodion or with a small dressing. The nurse then keeps the site clean and dry to avoid infection and observes the infant for signs of inflammation.

The nurse also monitors the feeding regimen. Some hospitals have adopted standard postpyloromyotomy feeding schedules, although some surgeons prefer to individualize them.

Occasional emesis is common after surgery, so nurses need to inform parents that residual gastric irritation and individual reactions to anesthetics might cause intermittent vomiting during the initial 24–36 hours. Frequent or continued vomiting needs to be reported, and adjustments in the feeding schedule are made then. Infants can be placed in any position after surgery, but positioning in a right side-lying or Fowler's position promotes gastric emptying.

During preoperative and postoperative periods, the nurse encourages the parent to hold and cuddle the infant. Parental participation in feedings is also important when these are resumed postoperatively. Many of these parents might feel that the child's problem was a result of something they did or did not do. "Helpful" friends and relatives might have nurtured this sense of guilt. The nurse's explanation of the physical nature of the condition should therefore reassure parents that the problem does not reflect their parenting capabilities.

Diaphragmatic Hernia

Diaphragmatic hernias occur when the abdominal contents are displaced upward into the thoracic cavity through a defect in the diaphragm. The defect occurs most frequently in the posterolateral portion of the diaphragm; 85%–90% of hernias are found to be left-sided. This defect is the result of lack of fusion in the embryonic diaphragm and is rare, affecting 1 in 12,500 live births (Moynihan and Gerraughty, 1985).

Diaphragmatic hernia constitutes a medical-surgical emergency, and immediate surgery usually is necessary to prevent death. Mortality is related to age at onset of respiratory symptoms, with infants exhibiting symptoms during the first 48 hours of life having the poorest prognosis. The mortality rate for these infants is approximately 50%–65% (Moynihan and Gerraughty, 1985).

Clinical manifestations Infants present with a wide variety of symptoms depending on the location and severity of the defect. If the defect is small or herniation is limited, the infant might exhibit only mild respiratory distress.

These marginal hernias often are discovered later in life when the child develops frequent indigestion, hiatal hernia, or esophagitis due to the displacement of the stomach and distal esophagus. The most dramatic and most common clinical presentation occurs when most of the abdominal contents have been displaced into the thoracic cavity, leaving the child with a flattened (scaphoid) abdomen.

Hypoplasia (defective development) of the left lung is possible if herniation has been present during much of fetal life. The increased pressure within the thoracic cavity causes the mediastinum to shift toward the right, thereby impeding expansion of the right lung. These infants therefore experience acute respiratory distress with tachypnea, dyspnea, and cyanosis. Air swallowed during crying adds to gastrointestinal distension, thereby decreasing thoracic volume even more. Fatalities are usually the result of severe respiratory compromise, acid-base alterations, cardiovascular anomalies, or infection. Other factors such as prematurity or birth defects also contribute to the high mortality.

Diagnostic evaluation Confirmation of the diagnosis is reached through radiologic studies showing air-filled loops of bowel or a gastric bubble within the thoracic cavity. A diagnosis of diaphragmatic hernia is suspected if lung sounds are unilaterally absent or if the infant has a scaphoid abdomen.

Treatment Immediate respiratory support and resuscitation might be necessary while the infant is still in the delivery room. Emergency corrective surgery involves the return of all herniated contents to the abdominal cavity and closure of the diaphragmatic defect.

Nursing management The maternity or child health nurse is often the first to notice these infants' increasing respiratory distress and scaphoid abdomens. If a diaphragmatic hernia is suspected, the nurse places the infant with the head and chest above the abdomen. This position helps to reduce the intrathoracic pressure and allows downward displacement of the herniated abdominal contents. Placing the infant on the affected side assists with ventilation by relieving the pressure on the unaffected lung. An NG tube is passed and connected to intermittent suction, thereby preventing the infant from swallowing air, which only increases respiratory distress. Keeping the infant as quiet as possible prevents the swallowing of air that occurs normally during crying and minimizes stress to compromised cardiovascular and respiratory systems (Moynihan and Gerraughty, 1985).

Postoperative care is similar to that following most surgeries. Most infants require full mechanical respiratory support, however, and are cared for in the intensive care unit. In addition to providing respiratory support, the nurse attempts to keep the infant entirely free from stress to avoid raising the infant's pulmonary artery pressure. Parents often are not allowed to talk to or hold their infants for 3–5 days after surgery. Bonding difficulties resulting from the deemphasis on parental contact during the critical phase of care might be evident. The nurse encourages increased parental contact as soon as allowable.

The Child with Existing or Potential Lower Gastrointestinal Obstruction

Intussusception

Intussusception occurs when one portion of the intestine is telescoped into another (Fig. 27-5). Intussusception is the most common cause of intestinal obstruction in infants and young children. It is more frequently seen in males than females and might occur more frequently in patients with gastroenteritis, cystic fibrosis, or celiac disease. Identifiable causes for intussusceptions might be found in only 5% of the patients.

Intussusceptions are classified according to the involved segments of the intestine. Most are ileocolic and occur at the ileocecal valve. The terminal portion of the ileum telescopes into the cecum and colon, thereby obstructing the passage of intestinal contents.

Because of the constriction of the blood supply that occurs during the invagination, the involved bowel becomes edematous and fragile. This leads to bleeding within the intestines, and subsequent stools might contain red blood and mucus. These stools are described as "currant jelly" stools and occur in over half the affected children.

Clinical manifestations The classical presenting symptoms include severe paroxysmal abdominal pain in a previously healthy child. Children might scream and draw their knees upward during the spasms but appear to be comfortable between episodes and might even make attempts to play. Vomiting might occur, and the child might initially pass a normal stool. The longer the obstruction is present, however, the more lethargic and weak the child becomes. Continued obstruction leads to bile-stained emesis, currant-jelly stools, a shocklike syndrome with severe prostration, and eventual death.

Examination of the infant might show distension of the abdomen, tenderness, and some guarding of the affected site. A sausage-shaped mass might be felt in the right upper quadrant or in the epigastrium if the transverse colon is

FIGURE 27-5

Intussusception of the terminal ileum and ascending colon.

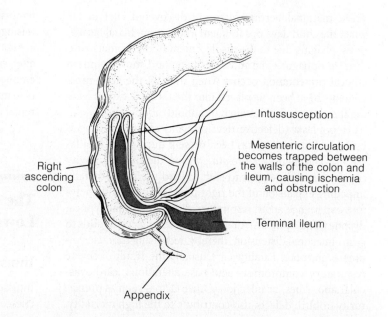

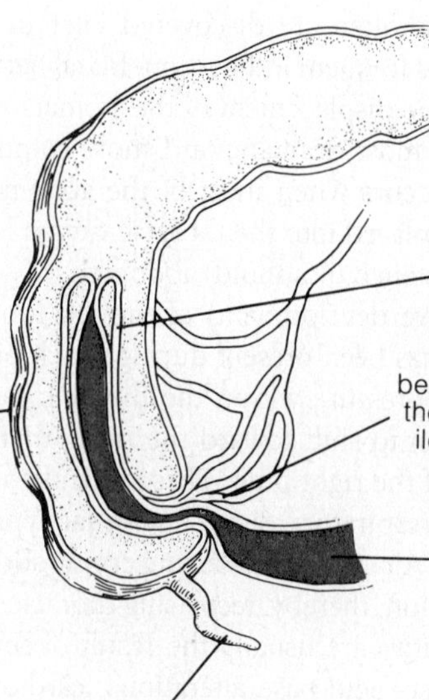
Intussusception
Mesenteric circulation becomes trapped between the walls of the colon and ileum, causing ischemia and obstruction
Right ascending colon
Terminal ileum
Appendix

involved. A rectal examination often reveals the presence of bloody mucus.

Diagnostic evaluation Diagnosis of intussusception is made with a combination of subjective and objective findings. The classic symptoms of intermittent intense abdominal pain, currant-jelly stools, and vomiting allow for an initial diagnosis. A barium enema might reveal the presence of an obstruction as well as the "coil-spring" appearance of barium within the intussusception itself.

Treatment If the diagnosis has been made within the initial 24 hours of obstruction or if there are no signs of shock or peritonitis, hydrostatic reduction by barium enema might be attempted. A Foley catheter is placed in the rectum and inflated. The buttocks are taped firmly together to prevent leakage of barium, and barium is then allowed to flow into the colon by gravity. Repeat or serial radiographs show free filling of the small intestine if the procedure has been successful. With early diagnosis, this procedure is successful in approximately 75% of cases.

If the procedure is not successful or if signs of sepsis or peritonitis exist, the child must undergo open surgical reduction of the intussusception. It might then be necessary to remove necrotic bowel to reestablish intestinal continuity.

Nursing management Documentation of severe intermittent abdominal pain, vomiting, or passage of currant-jelly stools helps to establish an early diagnosis. Attention is given to parent's interpretaions of the child's behavior. Because parents are more familiar with their children's reactions to pain or discomfort, they might provide an excellent history of the sudden onset of the obstruction.

For the child undergoing surgery, preoperative nursing care includes close monitoring of the child for signs of intestinal obstruction. Parental preparation includes not only a description of intussusception but also an explanation of reduction by hydrostatic pressure. If parents understand that hydrostatic reduction is not always successful, they can understand why surgery might then become necessary. Explanations should be accompanied by drawings or visual aids. A visual aid can be created by telescoping a section of Penrose drain. If the distal end is then clamped or tied and slowly filled with water, parents can see the principle of hydrostatic reduction in action.

Nasogastric suctioning and intravenous fluids are begun for any child for whom surgery might be necessary. Children exhibiting signs of shock or peritonitis might also require blood, plasma, and antibiotics prior to surgery. All stools are recorded with the presence or amount of fecal blood described. The passage of more than the initial normal stool might indicate spontaneous resolution of the obstruction.

The nurse observes children who have undergone hydrostatic reduction for passage of stool and barium, keeping in mind that a few children (less than 10%) who have undergone hydrostatic reduction have a recurrence of the intussusception and that this usually occurs within the first 36–48 hours of the initial reduction. Postoperative care of the child undergoing surgery for intussusception is similar to that for any child undergoing abdominal surgery.

Umbilical Hernia, Gastroschisis, and Omphalocele

An *umbilical hernia* is a protrusion of a portion of small intestine through an incompletely closed ring (umbilical ring) of muscle and fascia surrounding the umbilical cord. Umbilical hernias can be small (1–2 cm in diameter) or much larger. They occur more often in girls. These hernias usually are readily reduced by exerting gentle pressure with the fingers on the protrusion. Most eventually resolve spontaneously. Large umbilical hernias (greater than 2 cm) and those that persist into middle childhood usually are surgically repaired.

Gastroschisis is a rare congenital defect in the abdominal wall that allows evisceration (protrusion) of the abdominal contents. This defect is approximately 2–5 cm in diameter and is most often located to the right of an intact umbilicus. The degree of herniation varies and might include not only intestines but also other organs. Because there is no covering sac, the intestines are usually edematous, leathery, shortened, and malrotated. Malrotation is due to an incomplete rotation of the fetal intestine when reentering the abdominal cavity. In addition, the mesentery of the small intestine is not attached appropriately, and a *volvulus* (twisting of intestine) might occur (Fig 27-6). Edema, malrotation, or volvulus can cause obstruction.

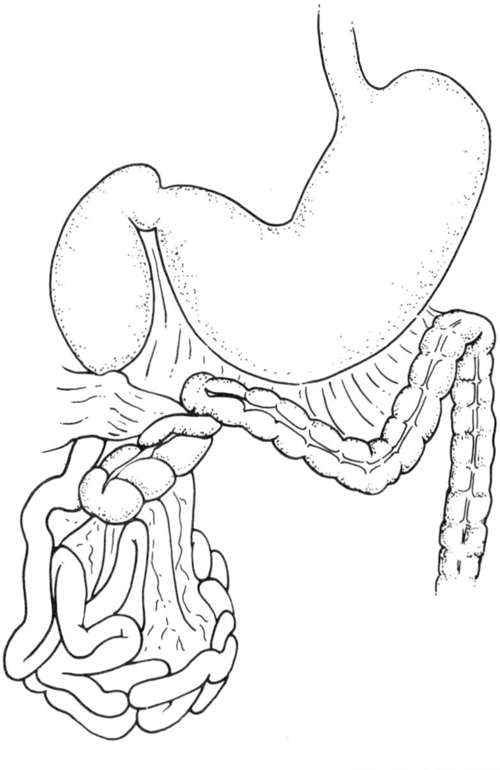

FIGURE 27-6
Malrotation and volvulus.

An *omphalocele* is an embryonic defect that occurs when the intestines fail to return to the abdominal cavity during the tenth week of gestation. Unlike gastroschisis, which does not affect the umbilicus, in omphalocele abdominal contents remain herniated into the umbilical cord. Because they are within the cord itself, they remain covered by the fetal amniotic membrane. The degree of herniation varies and might be slightly larger than an umbilical hernia to large enough to contain intestines and liver. Rupture of the sac might lead to further herniation, infection, or complete intestinal obstruction due to rotation of the intestines during rupture. Infants with omphalocele frequently have associated congenital anomalies.

Treatment Because of the extent of exposed bowel, infants with either gastroschisis or omphalocele might encounter complications involving massive heat and fluid losses, increased caloric requirements, intestinal obstruction, and infection of the site resulting in septicemia.

Initial treatment of the infant focuses on closure of the defect. If a large amount of the bowel has remained outside the abdominal cavity during fetal development, the cavity might be too small to allow primary closure of the defect without compromising intestinal circulation. In these cases, a prosthetic sac (or silo) of synthetic material (for example, Silastic) is placed over the protruding viscera, creating a pouch. The visceral contents are placed over the abdominal cavity to allow gradual return of contents into the cavity.

Once all contents have returned to the abdominal cavity, closure of skin and muscle layers can be completed. If gravity fails to return the intestines to the abdomen, additional surgery might be necessary.

Nursing management Preoperative assessment of the infant for signs of circulatory compromise, intestinal obstruction, and septicemia is an important nursing responsibility. Nasogastric suction is begun to prevent harmful distension of the bowel. The nurse needs to take great care to prevent infection when handling the exposed intestines in gastroschisis or the ruptured omphalic sac in omphalocele. The sac is kept moist with moist dressings covered with plastic wrap. The infant is placed in a supine position. Movement of the infant is minimized through use of restraints. The nurse keeps the infant warm. Support is given to the parents, and they are encouraged to verbalize their feelings about the infant's physical appearance. Postoperative nursing care is similar to that for any child undergoing abdominal surgery.

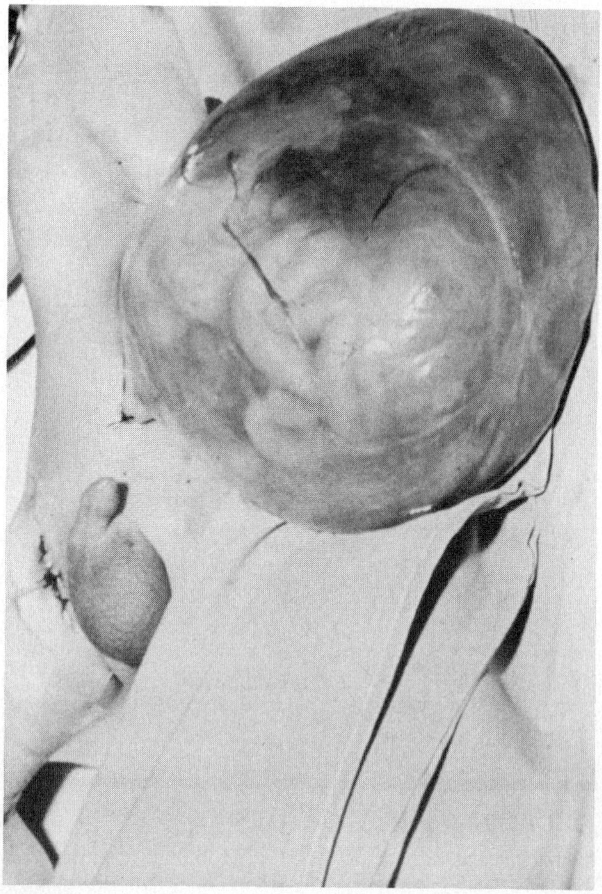

A

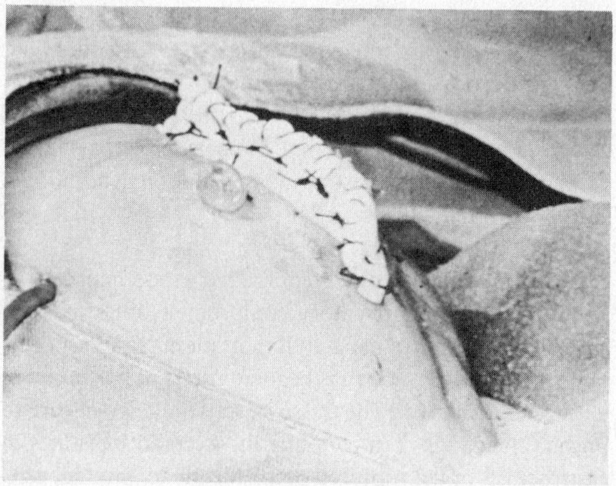

B

Infant with omphalocele. **A.** *An omphalocele sac is lying to the right of the abdomen.* **B.** *A silastic mesh bag covers the abdominal contents. Sutures in the bag decrease its size and move the abdominal organs back into the abdominal cavity. (Courtesy of Paul Winchester, MD.)*

Congenital Inguinal Hernia and Hydrocele

Inguinal hernias and hydroceles are due to defects in the closure of the lumen of the processus vaginalis during the eighth month of gestation. This pouch of peritoneum exits the inguinal canal at the external ring and precedes the testicle into the scrotum. Normally, the upper lumen atrophies, and the lower lumen (tunica vaginalis) encases the testicles. When the upper lumen fails to close, however, peritoneal fluid or intestines can be forced down the inguinal canal, through the external ring, and into the scrotum. Varying degrees of closure defects are possible. Large defects allow segments of small intestine to enter the canal, whereas small defects might only allow the entrance of peritoneal fluid. Presence of intestine within the canal indicates a hernia, while entrapment of fluid within the canal or scrotum describes a hydrocele (Fig 27-7).

Congenital inguinal hernias occur overwhelmingly in boys, but approximately 10% do occur in girls. The inguinal swelling is painless unless strangulation of intestines occurs, resulting in obstruction. The mass usually is reduced easily by gentle compression or might disappear when the infant is resting or feeding quietly. The defect becomes more noticeable during coughing, straining, or crying. In older children, hernias might appear more noticeable at the end of the day.

Strangulation (incarcerated hernia) occurs when the herniated loops of small bowel are trapped within the defect and cannot be reduced into the abdominal cavity. Symptoms of intestinal obstruction become evident, and the site might appear swollen, reddened, or warm. Gangrene of the intestine occurs if the hernia is left unreduced.

Treatment of choice for nonincarcerated hernias is the prompt surgical closure of the defect to prevent future incarceration. If incarceration has occurred, however, closed reduction might be attempted first. If successful, surgery might be delayed to allow healing of any damaged intestinal tissues. The infant awaiting surgery for incarcerated hernias is placed in a Trendelenburg's position to prevent further edema and damage of the affected intestine.

Most noncomplicated herniorrhaphies (repair of hernia) are now done on an outpatient basis. The wound frequently is covered with collodion or left open to the air to promote healing and allow thorough cleansing of the site. The nurse therefore informs parents of infants undergoing herniorrhaphies that these children require frequent diaper changes to prevent infection. Activity is not limited, and older children are encouraged to ambulate.

The nurse carefully observes children requiring surgical reduction of incarcerated hernias for signs and symptoms of peritonitis or complete bowel obstruction. Postoperative care for these children includes NG suctioning and intra-

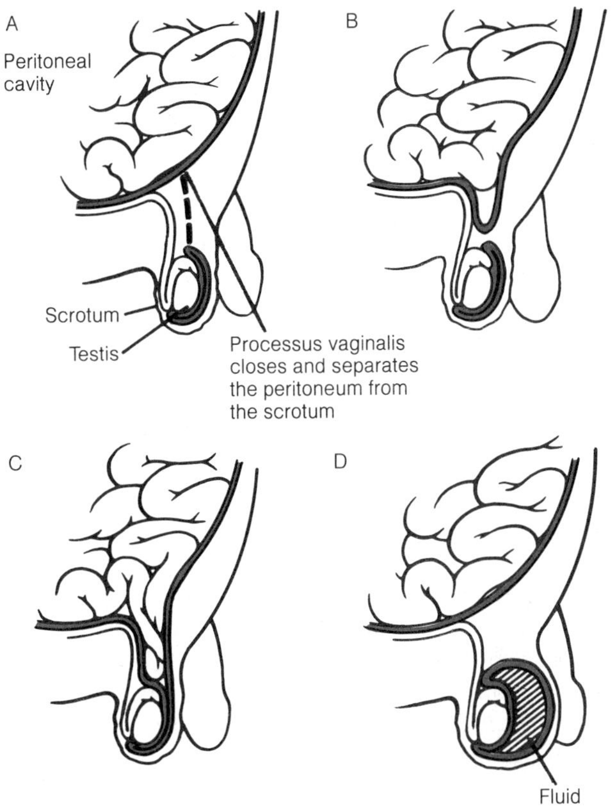

FIGURE 27-7

A. The processus vaginalis precedes the testis into the scrotum during fetal development, then fuses, separating the peritoneal cavity from the scrotum. B. Partially incomplete fusion of the processus vaginalis. C. Herniation of the intestine into the inguinal canal as a result of incomplete fusion. D. Noncommunicating hydrocele.

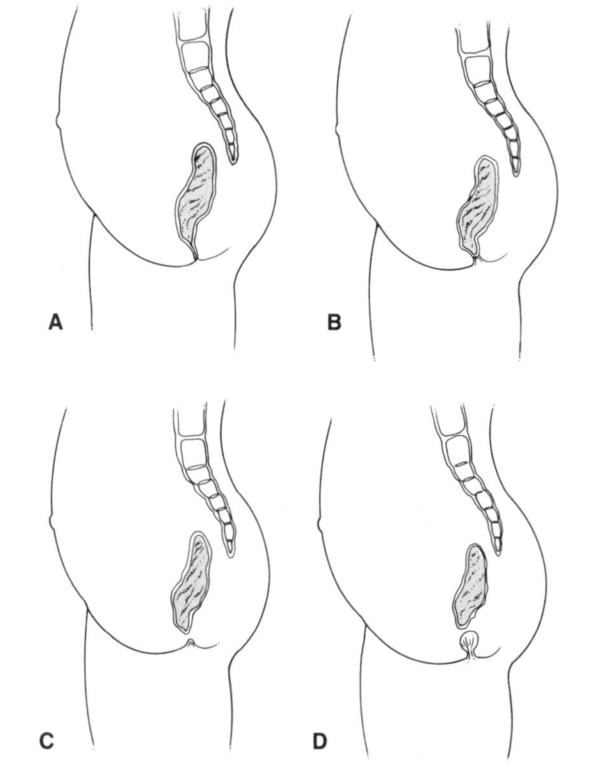

FIGURE 27-8

*Anorectal malformations. **A.** Anal stenosis. **B.** Membranous atresia. **C.** Anal agenesis. **D.** Rectal atresia.*

venous fluids, which are continued until normal bowel function returns.

A *hydrocele* also appears as an asymptomatic bulge in the inguinal and scrotal area, but, unlike the hernia, the hydrocele cannot be reduced, nor can it be produced by coughing or crying.

A *noncommunicating hydrocele* occurs when fluid is completely enclosed in the canal or scrotum. This fluid gradually reabsorbs and no treatment is necessary. When the lumen of the processus vaginalis remains open, a *communicating hydrocele* occurs. Fluid drains into the hydrocele from the peritoneum. Scrotal edema might appear greater at the end of the day because of gravity filling of the defect.

Surgery for repair of hydroceles involves closure of the connecting defect to prevent further collection of fluid within the scrotum. The continued presence of a hydrocele can predispose the child to traumatic hernias later in life.

Imperforate Anus

Imperforate anus is a term describing a group of anorectal malformations. Anomalies of this type occur in about 1 of every 5000 live births (Rudolph, 1982). The anus and rectum develop from the cloaca of the embryonic hindgut. Anything that impedes the development of the necessary rectal, anal, or urogenital structures results in an anorectal malformation. Anorectal malformations might affect genitourinary structures, most commonly by fistula.

Clinical manifestations In anal stenosis (Fig. 27-8A) the constricted anal opening might be noticed early in infancy during a digital exam or might only become apparent later, when the child encounters problems with chronic constipation, ribbonlike stools, and difficulty in toilet training. In anal membranous atresia (Fig. 27-8B), anal and rectal structures might appear normal except for the presence of a shiny, translucent membrane. Anal agenesis (Fig. 27-8C) accounts for 80% of all anorectal malformations. The rectum terminates in a blind pouch. Rectal atresia (Fig. 27-8D) occurs when the anal canal is appropriately developed but does not communicate with the rectum. The distance between the two structures might be significant, or they might be divided by only a membranous tissue. Fistulas connecting with the perineum, urethra, bladder, or vagina might be present in a large number of anorectal malformations.

Diagnostic evaluation Infants suspected of having anorectal malformations are evaluated in depth to determine the level of the defect and the presence or location of any fistula. Frequent abdominal radiographs are performed with the child in an inverted position. This allows air to fill the blind colonic pouch and permits clearer identification of the level of the defect. Another diagnostic tool is catheterization of any external fistulae, injection of contrast material, and subequent radiographs to provide a more exact classification of the defect.

Treatment Anal stenosis is most often managed with repeated manual dilatations of the anus. These dilatations are begun soon after birth and are continued by the parents once the child is discharged. To prevent accidental perforation parents need information regarding the proper technique of manual anal dilatation.

The type of surgical intervention is determined by the position of the defect. Low defects might be corrected by an abdominoperineal pull-through procedure with anoplasty or, in the case of anal membrane atresia, by anoplasty alone. High defects necessitate a temporary colostomy for at least 6–12 months. Surgery is then performed to correct any remaining fistulas and to position the bowel appropriately. Bowel control depends on location of the defect. When repaired, low defects usually allow the child to achieve continence without problems. The higher the defect, the less successful a bowel control regimen might be. Many children with high defects also have other pelvic anomalies, including vertebral defects and pelvic neurologic anomalies. Because of the anomalies, complete bowel continence might be extremely difficult or impossible to achieve. If innervation is affected, the child might lack the sensation of stool within the rectum and should be encouraged to defecate at the same time daily rather than waiting for the urge. A regimen of daily or every other day enemas or suppositories might be required if constipation is severe. If effective bowel control is not achieved before the child enters school or if chronic impaction is a problem, the child might be reassessed for placement of a permanent colostomy.

Nursing management The nurse is often the person who first identifies an anorectal malformation in a neonate, usually when attempting to take the initial rectal temperature. This is the reason the nurse never attempts to force a rectal thermometer when resistance is encountered. Other observations important in establishing a diagnosis are whether the child has passed meconium in the first 24 hours and whether meconium appears in an inappropriate place, such as the vagina or perineum.

Postoperative nursing care depends on the degree of surgery necessary to repair the defect. If an abdominoperineal pull-through is performed, nursing care includes prevention of infection at the surgical site, which might include either or both perineal and anal incisions. The site is kept very clean and observed for signs of infecton. The use of a gooseneck lamp or exposure to open air can promote healing of the site. When a colostomy is necessary, the nursing care plan incorporates postoperative colostomy care and instruction for the parents. Although these colostomies are present for only 6–12 months, appropriate care also needs to include prevention of skin breakdown or appliance leakage.

Information about bowel training becomes important in early childhood, and the nurse explains that children with anorectal malformations might encounter difficulty in toilet training. Parents are encouraged to use patience and persistence and should establish a daily routine when attempting bowel training.

Hirschsprung's Disease (Aganglionic Megacolon)

Hirschsprung's disease occurs when there is an absence of autonomic parasympathetic ganglion cells innervating a portion of the colon. Because of the absence of these ganglions, there is a lack of peristalsis and movement of feces within the affected segment. The section of colon proximal to the defect becomes greatly enlarged with entrapped feces and gas (Fig. 27-9).

The defect extends upward from the anus, and the severity of the condition is determined by the level at which active ganglia can be found. Approximately 90% of patients have an aganglionic segment that is limited to the rectosigmoid only. The rest vary upward to the hepatic flexure and in rare cases include the entire colon.

Clinical manifestations Lack of peristalsis results in constipation and signs of functional intestinal obstruction. Presenting symptoms vary from acute obstruction to chronic constipation, depending on the age of the child. Infants might fail to pass meconium or might have vomiting and abdominal distension. Emesis might be bile-stained and in severe cases might have the odor or texture of feces. Older infants might have histories of chronic constipation

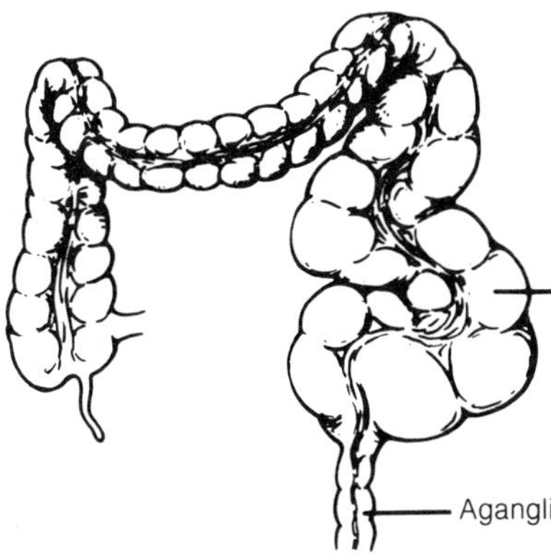

FIGURE 27-9
Aganglionic bowel as seen in Hirschsprung's disease.

alternating with diarrhea or histories of failure to thrive. Occasional bouts of constipation or diarrhea might develop into an enterocolitis with explosive diarrhea, fever, and severe dehydration. Fatalities can occur if enterocolitis is not treated immediately.

Older children exhibit increasing constipation and abdominal distension. Occasionally, a fecal mass might be present in the lower left quadrant, but the rectal vault is often empty of stool. These children often appear chronically malnourished, are often anemic, and exhibit malabsorptive hypoproteinemia (decrease in normal blood protein).

Diagnostic evaluation Diagnosis of aganglionic megacolon usually involves a rectal biopsy to determine whether ganglion cells are present. In small neonates, anorectal manometry might be preferred. This test attempts to mimic the presence of stool in the rectum by placing balloons between the internal and external sphincters. Children with megacolon exhibit abnormal contraction of the external sphincter without relaxation of the internal sphincter. Barium enemas might be used diagnostically, but their reliability for diagnosing aganglionic megacolon in neonates is questionable.

Treatment Treatment of Hirschsprung's disease in the older child might be limited to medical intervention with enemas, stool softeners, and low-residue diets. Such treatment is only palliative and successful if only a small portion of the colon is involved.

Surgical intervention is performed to remove the aganglionic bowel. Initially, a temporary loop or double-barrel colostomy is performed. A pull-through procedure involving removal of the aganglionic colon with reanastomosis of normal colon might be done with creation of the colostomy or later in a staged operation (colostomy followed by the pull-through, then colostomy closure). The timing of the colostomy closure is determined by the condition of the child and by the response to initial surgery. It is usually accomplished within 3–12 months. Only rarely is it necessary to maintain a permanent colostomy. In these instances, the extent of aganglionic colon is severe, and a permanent ileostomy might even be necessary.

Nursing management Preoperative nursing care focuses on observation and assessment of the infant. Once the diagnosis has been established and surgery is indicated, nursing care also involves preparing the child and parent for impending surgery. Physical care involves bowel preparation. In neonates with bowels that are still sterile, no preparation is needed. In older infants and children, preparation might begin several days prior to the surgery.

If low-residue or liquid diets are required at home before admission for surgery, parents need both oral and written instructions. If enemas are required at home, parents need instructions in preparing and performing an isotonic saline enema. The nurse then emphasizes the danger of tap water, soap, and commercial phosphate enemas. Isotonic saline solutions can be obtained without a prescription at pharmacies, or the parent can mix one teaspoon of noniodized table salt with one pint of lukewarm tap water. Return demonstrations by the parent are helpful in identifying needs for further instructions.

In addition to preparation through diet and enemas, systemic antibiotics might be given to reduce intestinal flora. Frequent oral administration of antibiotics might be used in conjunction with antibiotic enemas. Close monitoring of fluid status is necessary for children who are NPO and receiving repeated enemas. Small infants might require intravenous fluids if oral liquids are withheld for any length of time. Postoperative nursing care involves routine postabdominal surgery care as well as ostomy care.

The Child with a Problem of Inflammation

Appendicitis

Appendicitis occurs when the vermiform appendix becomes inflamed. This might be caused by a physical obstruction of the lumen by fecaliths (hardened feces) or by anatomic defects within the cecum itself. It is one of the most common diseases requiring abdominal surgery in childhood.

Although cases of appendicitis have been documented in infants under the age of 2, it occurs most frequently in later childhood and young adulthood.

Clinical manifestations The symptoms of appendicitis are diverse, and many cases therefore go unrecognized in children until rupture has occurred. The child might originally complain of a generalized periumbilical pain, with this pain later localizing in the right lower quandrant (a point halfway between the iliac crest and the umbilicus). Often there is rebound tenderness (the child complains of greater pain upon release of palpated pressure than while pressure is being applied). Fever and vomiting are usually present, and the child might complain of either diarrhea or constipation. Bowel sounds are decreased or absent. Children often remain lying on their sides with their legs drawn upward, a position they find the most comfortable. A normally active child might voluntarily remain quietly in bed.

Diagnostic evaluation A rectal exam is necessary to rule out other conditions and might be quite painful in a child with appendicitis. Laboratory tests usually reveal an elevated white blood cell count, although it is seldom higher than 20,000/mm^3. Abdominal radiographs reveal a fecalith or some other cause of obstruction, although these rarely confirm the diagnosis. Because the symptoms of urinary tract infection resemble those of appendicitis, a urinalysis is obtained to rule this out. In young children the symptoms mimic those of pneumonia and a radiograph is obtained to rule it out.

The child whose appendix ruptures might indicate a sudden lessening of pain, but if rupture has occurred with peritonitis following, the abdomen becomes more rigid, and the child exhibits obvious guarding of the abdomen. The fever might elevate dramatically, as might the white blood cell count.

Treatment An appendectomy (surgical removal of the vermiform appendix) is performed as soon as is feasible. The rationale is that it is much easier and safer to remove an intact appendix than it is to treat the resultant peritonitis if the appendix were to rupture. Children in shock or those exhibiting fluid or electrolyte imbalances are treated medically prior to surgery. Fluid replacements, NG suctioning, and antibiotics might be required initially to stabilize the child. Children with a suspected perforation should be positioned in a high-Fowler's position. This promotes pelvic pooling of any fecal leakage and might prevent the development of a subphrenic abscess.

Nursing management The goals of preoperative nursing care are to help establish a diagnosis and to prepare the child and parent for impending surgery. The first is accomplished through continued observation of the child's condition. Changes in behavior, location, or duration of pain; increase in vomiting; or any signs of shock or septicemia can become essential data when trying to diagnose appendicitis. Nurses functioning in a community or referral capacity need to remind parents that, because of the possibility of perforation, enemas, cathartics, or suppositories are contraindicated if appendicitis is suspected.

Preparation of the child and parents for imminent surgery involves interventions that are both physical and psychologic. Physically, the child usually requires rehydration or replacement of lost electrolytes. An NG tube might be placed and intermittent suctioning begun. Antibiotics might be required if a perforation is suspected.

The child is usually fearful and extremely anxious. This is often the child's first hospital stay, and the child might arrive with many preconceived notions of doctors, nurses, and hospitals. Children should receive concise, age-appropriate explanations of what will take place before surgery and after surgery (see Chapter 20). Postoperatively they will need to work out their reactions, preferably with the assistance of therapeutic play (see Chapter 19).

Psychologic support is important because of the emergency that appendicitis presents. Parents might express guilt for not having sought treatment earlier, or they might become hostile or anxious when surgery is not done immediately. They require patient and calm explanations of what is to be done and why. They need to be reassured that a well-hydrated, metabolically balanced child is a much safer surgical risk and that, for this reason, surgery might be postponed.

Postoperative nursing care of a child with simple appendectomy is basic care following any abdominal surgery. The hospital stay is usually only 2–5 days, and the child might resume normal activities quickly. Rough contact sports, abdominal muscle exercises, and heavy lifting are discouraged in the immediate postoperative period.

If a rupture of the appendix has occurred, Penrose drains are placed in the abscess site promoting healing from inside out and complete drainage of the abscess. The child should remain in a semi- or high-Fowler's position or can lie on the right side. Dressings usually are bulky in order to absorb copious drainage, which is extremely foul-smelling and irritating to abdominal skin. Frequent dressing changes are needed in order to prevent excoriation. These children might have to be placed on wound and skin precautions to prevent cross-contamination of other patients (see Table 20-5). Intravenous antibiotics are administered for 7–10 days and might be continued orally after discharge. The hospital stay varies from 1–3 weeks depending on the need for antibiotics. The surgical site is often allowed to granulate

TABLE 27-8 Ulcerative Colitis and Crohn's Disease (Regional Enteritis)

	Ulcerative colitis	Crohn's disease
Description	Extensive inflammation of the mucosa and submucosa of the colon and ranging throughout colon length. Occurs predominantly in adolescents. Familial tendency	Inflammatory condition affecting submucosa of the digestive tract. Most common in anus and terminal ileum. Affects segments of the digestive tract. Familial tendency. Incidence is higher than that of ulcerative colitis
Etiology	Unknown. Organic disease is exacerbated by emotional stress	Unknown
Clinical	Failure to thrive, abdominal pain, frequent liquid stools (10–20 times a day) containing pus and blood. Local tenderness on rectal examination. Leukocytosis, low grade fever, possibly arthritis. Normal barium enema. Microulcerations and pseudopolyps seen on rectosigmoidoscopy	Gradual onset of chronic fatigue, anorexia, occult bleeding. Generalized abdominal tenderness with possibly a right lower quadrant mass. Frequent diarrhea, fever, growth retardation, oral ulcerations, anal abscesses, and enlargement of regional lymph nodes. Fissures or fistulas seen by barium enema. Subclinical disease detected by biopsy
Treatment	Topical application of steroids via enema for mild disease. Systemic steroid and/or sulfasalazine therapy to achieve remission in moderate to severe cases. TPN for cases unresponsive to medication. Total colectomy with ileostomy for severe growth retardation, profuse hemorrhage, perforation, or malignancy	Same as for colitis—steroids, sulfasalazine, TPN. Surgery usually not effective in preventing recurrence
Nursing management	Long-term care (see Chapter 15). Teach stress reduction techniques (see Chapter 16). Diet therapy—high protein, high calorie, avoid foods causing pain or diarrhea. Small frequent snacks for children with anorexia. Care for oral ulcerations if present. Observe for medication side effects—give medications with milk and increase child's fluid intake. Preoperative preparation for ostomy if indicated	Similar to that for colitis. Frequent sitz baths to relieve perianal ulcerations and abscesses. Meticulous skin care
Prognosis	Increased risk of colonic cancer, greatly increased after ten years with the disease	Increased risk of cancer, although not so high as with ulcerative colitis

inward once drainage has ceased and the drain has been removed. Children might resume normal activities, but excessive activities as listed previously should be postponed.

Ulcerative Colitis and Regional Enteritis (Crohn's Disease)

Both ulcerative colitis and Crohn's disease are inflammatory conditions of the bowel. Although having similar clinical manifestations, they are dissimilar in many respects. (Table 27-8 compares the two diseases and their management.)

Peptic Ulcer

Peptic ulcer is a broad classification for any erosion of the mucosa of the stomach (gastric), pylorus, or duodenum. The causative agent of peptic ulcers is unknown, but hypersecretion of gastric acid and pepsin is considered a primary contributor to the development of these lesions. Another theory is that the protective mechanism of the stomach lining is in some way dysfunctional. Decreased mucus secretion, slow regeneration of damaged cells, and chronic irritation or inflammation might all be significant contributing causes.

The incidence of peptic ulcers in children varies widely from study to study. Boys are affected more often than girls, and children having close relatives with ulcer disease are also at greater risk. Young children might have either duodenal or gastric ulcers, while duodenal ulcers predominate in older children and adolescents.

Clinical manifestations Children vary dramatically in the clinical symptoms that develop. Adolescents tend to describe symptoms that are similar to the adult cycle of symptoms of pain-food/antacid-relief. They complain of a gnawing, burning pain in the epigastrium (heartburn), which develops several hours after meals. They might not experience vomiting or chronic abdominal pain. Young children, however, rarely have any standard group of symptoms. They complain of general intermittent abdominal pain, late night or early morning abdominal pain, preprandial (before meals) pain or postprandial pain, vomiting, or painless melena (black vomitus). The diagnosis of peptic ulcer therefore can be easily overlooked in a child exhibiting only intermittent abdominal pain.

Diagnostic evaluation Clinically, affected children might exhibit hematemesis, melena, or anemia. Endoscopy confirms the presence of an eroded site, and contrast studies (eg, upper GI series) might be necessary if a duodenal ulcer is suspected. Abdominal tenderness is noted during deep palpation of the epigastrium. Stools and emesis might be positive for occult blood.

Treatment Medical treatment of peptic ulcer is the first and safest choice. Dietary management limits foods that stimulate hyperacidity. Although bland diets and diets containing large amounts of milk and cream have been used in the past, they are less common now. Bland diets are difficult to maintain and might not offer the nutritional variety needed for growing children. Therefore, the diet is relatively free, but such items as tea, coffee, carbonated beverages, high-acid foods, and fried foods are restricted.

Frequent administration of antacids, as frequently as once an hour during the initial recovery period, is another component of treatment. Antacids containing magnesium hydroxide or magnesium trisilicate are preferred, although they might cause diarrhea and then need to be alternated with aluminum hydroxide antacids.

In addition to antacids, anticholinergic drugs or hydrogen ion blockers might be used. Preparations of propantheline bromide (Pro-Banthine), an effective anticholinergic, might be used to alleviate late night and early morning abdominal pain. Cimetidine (Tagamet), a hydrogen ion blocker, is one of the most commonly prescribed drugs in ulcer therapy.

Nursing management When the diagnosis of gastric or duodenal ulcer is confirmed in a child, the nurse formulates a coordinated plan of parent and child education to involve dietary and drug therapies as well as methods of stress reduction.

Because stress has been indicated as a possible contributor to hyperacidity, families usually need instruction in methods of reducing physical and emotional stress. Adequate sleep, small frequent meals, and regular exercise can aid in the reduction of physical stress, but disturbed family relationships might require counseling before emotional stress can be alleviated. Because children might use illness in a manipulative manner at home or school, difficulties with relationships in these environments also might require psychologic counseling.

The Child with a Problem Related to Interference with Metabolism of Nutrients

Hepatitis

Although *hepatitis* is technically any inflammation of the liver, the term has come to indicate the infectious process caused by specific viruses. The most commonly occurring viruses have been labeled hepatitis A and hepatitis B. They often produce the same clinical symptomatology, but their epidemiologic characteristics are distinctly different (Table 27-9). Other viruses can cause non-A or non-B hepatitis, and these should be considered until diagnostic tests can determine the causative virus. Exposure to hepatitis A confers immunity only for that type; exposure to hepatitis B confers immunity only for type B.

Two types of complications from hepatitis can produce chronic, progressive liver changes or even death. The first is *acute fulminating hepatitis* and is characterized by an extremely rapid onset with rapidly rising serum bilirubin. Encephalopathy (brain dysfunction), an increased tendency for hemorrhage, edema, and ascites (fluid in the peritoneal cavity) might develop rapidly into hepatic coma and death. The mortality rate exceeds 33%, with most deaths occurring within the first 1–2 weeks.

The second complication is *chronic active hepatitis* and is characterized by an insidious onset. It occurs more frequently in older girls.

Diagnostic evaluation Besides antibody tests, other tests can support the diagnosis of hepatitis. Pathologically, the functional liver cells are edematous or necrotic, with

TABLE 27-9 Hepatitis A and B

	Hepatitis A	Hepatitis B
Incubation	2–6 weeks from exposure to appearance of jaundice	2–5 months from exposure
Communicability	Oral-fecal contamination, food, water, fomites. Most communicable 2 weeks prior to jaundice. Can be transmitted parenterally	Parenterally through contaminated blood products or needles. Sexually transmitted. Frequently found in drug addicts. Communicable until B antigen disappears
Clinical manifestations	Acute onset of fever, malaise, gastric disturbances. Jaundice in 5–7 days with yellow sclera, dark urine, and clay-colored stools. Fatigue and mood swings	More insidious onset of fever, malaise, gastric disturbances, and jaundice. Arthralgia and dermatologic symptoms
Diagnosis	Presence of serum hepatitis A antibody	Presence of serum B surface antigen and B core antibody
Recovery	Icterus resolves after 4 weeks. Complete recovery in 1–3 months. Low mortality	Somewhat longer course. More serious disease with some fatalities
Precautions	Strict hand washing after using the toilet or handling contaminated diapers. Wash child's dishes in extremely hot, soapy water or in a dishwasher. Wash contaminated linens in hot, soapy water. Discard dressings or tampons in plastic sacks. No sharing any item in contact with saliva	Blood, needle, and body fluid precautions

infiltration by lymphocytes and macrophages. Cellular damage and edema can cause blockage of the biliary flow, which results in even more extensive damage. The damaged cells and blocked biliary flow are thought to cause the alterations noted in liver function tests. Elevations in aminotransferases (substances that indicate organ damage) such as ALT (formerly SGOT) and AST (formerly SGPT), alkaline phosphatase, and lactic dehydrogenase (LDH) levels indicate acute liver damage.

Obstruction of the biliary flow causes malabsorption of fat-soluble vitamin K and might result in a prolonged prothrombin time and bruising.

Treatment Treatment of uncomplicated hepatitis is palliative and directed toward management of symptoms: nausea, vomiting, anorexia, and easy fatigability. Hepatitis patients might find that low-fat foods are tolerated better than those with a high fat content. Foods that are high in carbohydrates are provided, and high-protein foods can be given unless there are indications of severe liver damage or impending liver failure. Frequent, small meals might appeal to the child more than larger quantities of food.

Nausea and vomiting can be triggered by high-fat foods or by odors such as tobacco smoke or cooking odors. Antiemetics are usually contraindicated because the damaged liver cannot metabolize them. If vomiting is severe, extremely small doses of antiemetics might be attempted. If vomiting is persistent it can lead to dehydration; then intravenous fluids might be necessary. All medications, especially those metabolized by or possibly toxic to the liver, should be limited.

Treatment of acute fulminant hepatitis is also symptomatic but focuses on the acute areas of encephalopathy, potential hemorrhage, ascites, negative nitrogen balance, and severe electrolyte imbalances.

There is no immunization available specifially for hepatitis A. Exposed persons might receive serum immune globulin (SIG) to prevent or to modify the course of the disease. Hepatitis B immune globulin can be given to those exposed to hepatitis B. A new hepatitis B vaccine is administered if serious exposure has occurred (Vargo, 1985).

Nursing management A large number of children with subclinical or uncomplicated hepatitis are cared for at home. (See Chapter 18 for guidelines to assess the feasibility of home care.) The goals for nursing care of these children are support measures and the prevention of further spread of the disease within the family.

Support measures include small, frequent meals or snacks that are high in carbohydrates and proteins but relatively low in fat. Parents must understand that their children have a physiologic reason for being anorexic and that they should not force these children to eat. The child's appetite might be better early in the morning, and the parent might find that a balanced breakfast is consumed more readily than lunch or dinner.

Parents need to understand that their children tire easily. These children frequently limit their own activities initially. Later in the illness, however, the child might begin feeling much more energetic and might wish to return to school or play, even though still quite jaundiced. Parents need to know that this is quite common and is a sign of beginning recovery. Children with hepatitis A are no longer considered infectious 7–10 days after the onset of jaundice and can therefore return to normal activities if they so desire. Children with hepatitis B are communicable until the antibody/antigen studies return to normal. Although the onset of fulminant hepatitis usually is severe and acute, cases have occurred in children with presumed benign hepatitis. The nurse therefore instructs parents to report immediately any signs or symptoms that might indicate severely impaired liver function. These include confusion, increasing lethargy, restlessness, sudden behavioral changes or inappropriate behavior, tremors of hands or feet, difficulty speaking, or unusual eye movement.

When caring for children with hepatitis at home, infection control measures are important (see Table 27-9). Care of the hospitalized child also includes (a) private room and private bath, if possible, (b) enteric isolation, including gowns and gloves for patient contact or linen changes (until hepatitis A is ruled out), and (c) blood, needle, and body fluid precautions for hepatitis B (see Table 20-5).

Cirrhosis

Cirrhosis is a widespread destructive and regenerative process involving the cells of the liver and caused by a variety of stressors (eg, hepatitis, biliary atresia, choledochal cysts, and drug or alcohol abuse). Cirrhosis in children also can be caused by cystic fibrosis, genetic metabolic syndromes, congenital viral infections, or chronic malnutrition.

Damage to the liver cells activates an overproduction of collagen at the sites of damage. This fibrous tissue adversely affects the structure and function of the liver.

Clinical manifestations Symptoms become evident only when destruction and scarring exceed cell regeneration. Initial mild symptoms include jaundice, failure-to-thrive, and pruritus (itching). Jaundice might vary in degree, might be present from soon after birth (in cases of children with biliary atresia or choledochal cysts), or might only become evident after a long-standing history of cirrhosis. Pruritus varies in intensity and can result in skin excoriation where the child scratches.

Children with severe liver damage might develop associated complications. Portal vein scarring results in a rise in portal vein pressure. This reduces the circulatory supply to the liver. The portal hypertension combined with decreased albumin levels causes ascites (leakage of serous fluid into the abdominal cavity and resulting enlargement of the abdomen). Consequently, respiratory distress might develop because of pressure on the diaphragm.

Varices (enlargement of veins) occur in associated organs, particularly the esophagus, in response to circulatory blockage in the liver. Blood-clotting factors, normally produced by the liver, are decreased, causing increased bleeding tendencies. Encephalopathy and coma are thought to result from the toxic effects of increasing serum ammonia levels due to progressive liver failure.

Diagnostic evaluation Altered liver function tests along with history of a hepatic insult help to establish a diagnosis. There might be a prolonged prothrombin time and a decrease in serum albumin. Upper GI series confirms the presence of esophageal varices. A liver scan indicates changes in liver size depending on the stage of the disease.

Treatment Medical treatment is symptomatic for most cirrhosis cases. Dietary management includes a high-carbohydrate, low-fat, moderate-protein diet. Water-soluble forms of fat-soluble vitamins A, D, E, and K are given. Vitamin B_{12} can be given by injection if necessary. If hepatic coma or encephalopathy is likely, a low-protein diet and avoidance of foods high in ammonia is recommended. Pruritis is very common and is frequently treated by giving cholestyramine (Questran) by mouth. This reduces itching by reducing the presence of bile salts but might result in further loss of essential vitamins.

More severe complications, such as portal hypertension or ascites, might be treated medically. These treatments, however, are rarely successful over long periods of time. Treatment of ascites includes a salt-restricted diet and the administration of diuretics. The administration of albumin temporarily corrects the deficit and helps to retain fluid within the vascular system. Ascitic fluid might also be removed by paracentesis (puncture of the abdominal cavity) if respiratory distress is severe.

Bleeding difficulties are helped by the administration of coagulation factors. Rupture of esophageal varices with resulting hemorrhage can be treated by compressing the bleeding varices with an inflated balloon on the end of a Sengstaken-Blakemore tube.

Nursing management Long-term goals of nursing care are physical and emotional support. Emotional problems are those common to children with a chronic or potentially fatal illness (see Chapters 14 and 17).

Mild pruritus can be managed by frequent cool soda baths, but this is seldom effective over a long period. Severe pruritus might require medication. Infants who scratch frequently require mittens to prevent excoriation of skin.

Because disturbance in blood clotting or the presence of esophageal varices can cause the child with cirrhosis to bleed severely, nurses need to observe for melenic stools or frank hematemesis. All blood tests should be performed during one venipuncture, if possible, and pressure should be applied on the site for a longer period than is normal. A pressure dressing might prevent severe bruising after venipuncture.

Children with edema should be discouraged from dangling their legs or wearing restrictive clothing. Scrotal edema might become quite severe, and a scrotal support might be necessary to prevent damage to the delicate skin. A salt-restricted diet might help, but only slightly.

Evidence of severe cirrhosis indicates a poor prognosis. Although liver transplantation is being researched and performed, its success in this situation still is marginal, and the availability of this procedure is limited. Nurses caring for children with end-stage hepatic failure therefore need to provide emotional support to the family and child.

Anomalies of the Biliary Tree

Biliary atresia and choledochal (common bile duct) cysts are the two most frequently occurring anatomic disorders of the biliary system. These might be two different manifestations of the same prenatal disease and constitute an acquired disease rather than a genetic anomaly. Biliary atresia might occur because of a failure in the development of the bile duct lumens, a defect that is classified as intrahepatic (within the liver) or extrahepatic (outside the liver). Intrahepatic atresia is very rare and might involve only the intrahepatic bile ducts or might also include defects in the production or synthesis of bile salts or bilirubin. Choledochal cysts occur at any place along the biliary tree. Theories about their origin vary, but the cause remains unknown.

Clinical manifestations Because biliary atresia is totally obstructive, signs and symptoms of liver damage become evident soon after birth. Early jaundice with elevated direct and indirect bilirubin levels is common, along with clay-colored stools and dark urine. Hepatosplenomegaly (enlargement of liver and spleen) is evident, and other complications develop by late infancy.

Choledochal cysts often are very thick walled and cause abdominal pain and jaundice. A mass usually is felt in the right upper quadrant. Liver enzymes and serum bilirubin levels are elevated. The cysts are thought to be present at birth, and early obstructive jaundice is often the initial clinical manifestation. The disease might progress to include symptoms of severe liver damage or hepatic failure.

Treatment Medical treatment of biliary atresia and choledochal cysts involves palliative treatment of complications. Liver function tests are monitored closely, and the child is observed for any signs of possible liver failure.

Surgical correction for external biliary atresia might involve reconstructing the biliary ducts with a portion of jejunum. This surgery is considered only marginally successful, and progressive liver disease is still quite common.

Present research and experimentation with total liver transplantation has been successful with some children and might be a greater success in the future. Children who survive the surgery appear to be healthy and have normal liver function. Results of longitudinal research, however, are not available yet.

Nursing management Nursing care of nonsurgical patients with biliary atresia or choledochal cysts is essentially the same as for children with cirrhosis or liver failure. Postoperative care of children undergoing surgical procedures is like that for any child undergoing abdominal surgery. Nurses need to be aware that surgery is rarely curative and that these children frequently are readmitted for complications of recurring liver damage or liver failure. The nurse might need to prepare the family for dealing with a chronic, potentially fatal disease (see Chapters 14 and 17).

Essential Concepts

- The gastrointestinal system functions to ingest, digest, and absorb nutrients. Digestion of food begins in the mouth and progresses through the esophagus to the stomach and intestines, where enzymes break down food substances for absorption.
- Assessment of the child with a suspected gastrointestinal disorder includes a complete history and physical assessment, together with relevant data about dietary history, gastrointestinal symptoms, and eating and bowel habits.

- Diagnostic tests for gastrointestinal disorders might require enemas, medications, or dietary modifications in preparation for the diagnostic test. Each of these procedures needs to be adapted to the age of the child and the developmental needs of both child and family.
- Gastric decompression for children requires choosing a tube of correct size, monitoring function and placement of the tube, observing drainage, and monitoring fluid and electrolyte status.
- Ostomy care involves extensive preoperative teaching for both child and family, which in turn involves selection of a stoma site and discussions about ostomy appliances and adaptations in daily living that allow normal functioning.
- Acute care needs for children with gastrointestinal disorders are directed toward counteracting fluid volume deficit, monitoring alterations in elimination, preventing infection and complications, and providing care for children undergoing gastrointestinal surgery.
- Nutritional needs for children with gastrointestinal disorders involve assessing caloric intake and counteracting a nutritional deficit by oral, nasogastric, or gavage feedings, or by hyperalimentation.
- The nurse prevents developmental delay by addressing needs of children with gastrointestinal disorders related to malnutrition, lack of oral gratification, or impaired mobility.
- Emotional needs of children with gastrointestinal dysfunction might require interventions directed toward strengthening a weak parent-infant attachment or promoting a healthy body image.
- Health maintenance for the child with a gastrointestinal disorder might involve ongoing medication, dietary modification, activity restrictions, and bowel-training regimens.
- Children with gastrointestinal dysfunction might experience problems related to ingestion, use of food, obstruction, inflammation, or the body's ability to metabolize nutrients.

References

Adams DA, Selekof JL: Children with ostomies: Comprehensive care planning. *Pediatr Nurs* (Nov/Dec) 1986; 12(6): 429–433.

Balistreri W, Farrell M: Gastroesophageal reflux in infants. *N Engl J Med* (Sept) 1983; 309: 790–792.

Colburn N, Cherry RS: Community-based team approach to the management of children with cleft palate. *CHC* (Winter) 1985; 13(3): 122–128.

Gantt L, Thompson C: Short gut syndrome in the infant. *Am J Nurs* (Nov) 1985; 85(11): 1263–1266.

Hayes JS et al: Managing PKU: An update. *MCN* (Mar/Apr) 1987; 12(2): 119–123.

Moynihan P, Gerraughty A: Diaphragmatic hernia: Low stress-higher survival. *Am J Nurs* (June) 1985; 85(6): 662–665.

Orenstein S et al: The infant seat as treatment of gastroesophageal reflux. *N Engl J Med* (Sept) 1983; 309: 760–763.

Rudolph AM (editor): *Pediatrics*. Appleton-Century-Crofts, 1982.

Vargo J: Viral hepatitis: How to protect patients—and yourself. *RN* (July) 1985; 47(7): 22–26.

Additional Readings

Atkins J, Oakley C: A nurse's guide to TPN. *RN* (June) 1986; 48(6): 20–24.

Barkin RM, Lilly JR: Biliary atresia and the Kasai operation: Continuing care. *J Pediatr* (June) 1980; 96(6): 1015–1019.

Bjeletich J. Hickman RO: The Hickman indwelling catheter. *Am J Nurs* (Jan) 1980; 80(1): 62–65.

Boarini J: The ostomy: What can go wrong. *Am J Nurs* (Dec) 1985; 85(12): 1358–1362.

Boyd CW: Postural therapy at home for infants with gastroesophageal reflux. *Pediatr Nurs* (Nov/Dec) 1982; 82(6): 395–398.

Burkle WS: What you should know about Tagamet: New drug therapy for peptic ulcers. *Nurs '80* (Apr) 1980; 10(4): 86–87.

Campbell DL: Congenital abdominal wall defects: Gastroschisis and omphalocele. *Neonatal Network* (Aug) 1982; 18–23.

Cargile N: Buying time when you face a bowel obstruction. *RN* (Aug) 1985; 48(8): 40–44.

Carr P: When the patient needs TPN at home. *RN* (June) 1986; 48(6): 25–27.

Chattriwalla Y et al: The use of cimetidine in the newborn. *Pediatrics* (Feb) 1980; 62(2): 301–302.

Colley R, Wilson J: Providing hyperalimentation for infants and children. *Nurs '79* (July) 1979; 9(7): 50–53.

Cupoli JM et al: Failure-to-thrive. *Curr Probls Pediatr* (Sept) 1980; 10(11): 1–16.

Dickinson R-J et al: Controlled trial of intravenous hyperalimentation and total bowel rest as an adjunct to the routine therapy of acute colitis. *Gastroenterol* (Dec) 1980; 79(6): 1199–1204.

Fox B, Stegall B: Take precautions now. *Nurs '85* (May) 1985; 15:48–49.

Gatch G: Gatroschisis and omphalocele. *Today's OR Nurse* (Jan) 1980; 1(1): 9–15.

Goldberg JH et al: A home program of long-term total parenteral nutrition in children. *J Pediatr* (Feb) 1979; 94(2): 325–328.

Hagenah GC, Harrigan J, Campbell MA: Inflammatory bowel disease induced remission. *Nurs Clin North Am* (March) 1984; 19(1): 27–35.

Hazle N: An infant who survived gastroschisis. *MCN* (Jan/Feb) 1981; 6(1): 35–40.

Hoas-Beckert B: Removing the mysteries of parenteral nutrition. *Pediatr Nurs* (Jan/Feb) 1987; 13(1): 37–41.

Hrabovsky EE et al: Advances in the management of gastroschisis. *Ann Surg* (Aug) 1980; 192(2): 244–248.

Kadner I-J: Inflammatory bowel disease. *Clin Symposia* 1982; 34(1): 3–32.

Kroner K: Are you prepared for your ulcerative colitis patient? *Nurs '80* (Apr) 1980; 10(4): 43–45.

Kurfiss-Daniels D: Positioning as treatment for infant gastroesophageal reflux. *Am J Nurs* (Oct) 1982; 82(10): 1535–1537.

Mabel DE et al: Practical problems in pediatric TPN—total parenteral nutrition. *Am J Intravenous Ther* (Oct/Nov) 1978; 5: 13–17.

Mayer T et al: Gastroschisis and omphalocele: An eight-year review. *Ann Surg* (Dec) 1980; 192(6): 783–787.

Morin CL et al: Continuous elemental enteral alimentation in children with Crohn's disease and growth failure. *Gastroenterol* (Dec) 1980; 79(6): 1205–1210.

Mowat AP: Viral hepatitis in infancy and childhood. *Clin Gastroenterol* (Jan) 1980; 9(1): 191–212.

Page-Goertz S, Stewart DR: Is the baby just spitting? Consideration of the gastrointestinal reflux. *Issues Compr Pediatr Nurs* (Apr) 1980; 4(2): 53–66.

Parfitt DM, Thompson VD: Pediatric home hyperalimentation—educating the family. *MCN* (May/June) 1980; 5(3): 196–202.

Perry SE et al: Gastrostomy and the neonate *Am J Nurs* (July) 1983; 83(7): 1030–1033.

Price SA, McCarty Wilson L: *Pathophysiology: Clinical Concepts of Disease Process.* 2nd edition. McGraw-Hill, 1982.

Sanchez CL: Nursing care of the infant and child with cleft lip and palate. *Point of View* (Jan) 1980; 17(1): 14–15.

Saxton D et al (editors): *The Addison-Wesley Manual of Nursing Practice.* Addison-Wesley, 1983.

Smith C: Assessing the liver. *Nurs '85* (July) 1985; 15:36–37.

Spenner D: When the baby is sick and the mother's concerns are ignored—pyloric stenosis. *Am J Nurs* (Dec) 1980; 80(12): 2222–2224.

Strauch B et al: Caring enough to give your patient control—Crohn's disease: Chronic, recurrent, and unpredictable. *Nurs '80* (Aug) 1980; 10(8): 54–59.

Tanner MS, Stocks RJ: *Neonatal Gastroenterology: Contemporary Issues,* Intercept, 1984.

Walker RM: Surgery for the child ostomate. *J Enterostomal Ther* (Jul/Aug) 1982; 9(4): 18–20.

Walsh M, Kliegman R: Necrotizing enterocolitis: The spectrum of disease. *Pediatr Basics* 1984; 40:4–7.

Weibley T et al: Gavage tube insertion in the premature infant. *MCN* (Jan/Feb) 1987; 12(1): 24–27.

Williams R: Congenital diaphragmatic hernia. *Heart Lung* (Nov/Dec) 1982; 11(6): 532–540.

Chapter 28

Genitourinary Transport

Implications of Inflammation, Obstruction, and Structural Abnormalities

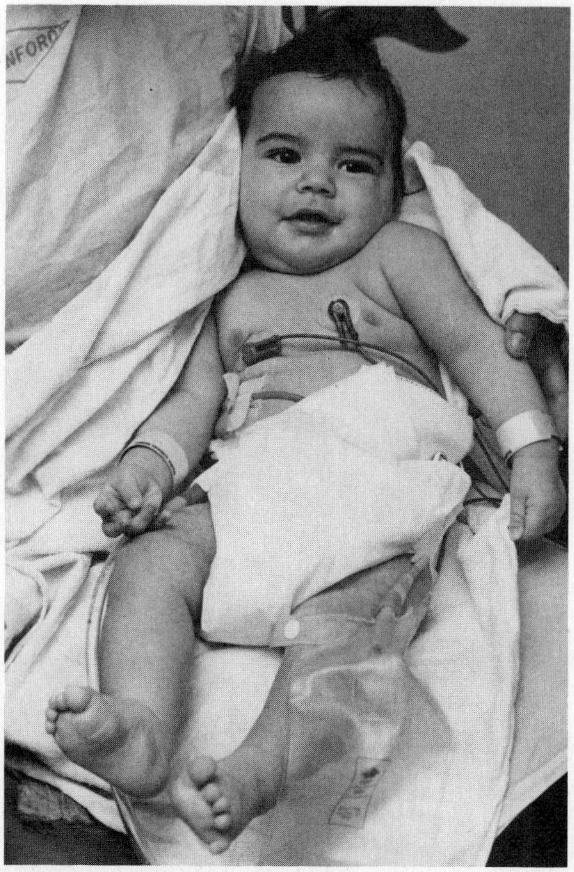

Chapter Contents

developmental or acquired imperfections secondary to deviations in structure and/or function of genitourinary system

Potential sexual dysfunction

Home Care and Health Maintenance Needs

Potential knowledge deficit concerning home management

The Child with a Problem of Infection

Acute Urinary Tract Infection
Toxic Shock Syndrome
Sexually Transmitted Diseases

The Child with a Structural Defect Involving the Genitourinary System

Hydronephrosis
Obstructive Anomalies of the Collecting System
Exstrophy of the Bladder
Reflux Anomalies of the Collecting System
Anomalies of the External Structures—Phimosis
Anomalies of the External Structures—Epispadias and Hypospadias
Cryptorchidism

The Child with a Problem with Filtration of Wastes

Acute Glomerulonephritis
Nephrosis—Nephrotic Syndrome
Acute Renal Failure—Acute Tubular Necrosis
Hemolytic Uremic Syndrome (HUS)

The Child with Chronic Renal Failure

The Child with Renal Trauma

Cross Reference Box

To find these topics, see the following chapters:

Enuresis	Chapter 16
Hydrocele	Chapter 27
Inguinal hernia	Chapter 27
Systemic lupus erythematosus	Chapter 25
Toilet training	Chapter 5
Wilms' tumor	Chapter 33
AIDS	Chapter 25

Objectives

- Describe the structure and function of the genitourinary system.
- List the criteria used in the assessment of a child with a genitourinary dysfunction.
- Describe principles of nursing care applicable to the child with a genitourinary condition.
- Explain the major treatment modalities and nursing management used for the child with problems related to genitourinary obstruction, infection, structural anomalies, and filtration of end products.
- Delineate nursing interventions to promote individual- or family-assisted self-care in a child with a long-term genitourinary dysfunction.
- Summarize the principles of preoperative and postoperative nursing care of the child undergoing genitourinary surgery.

ESSENTIALS OF STRUCTURE AND FUNCTION
The Genitourinary System

Glossary

Adrenal glands Located above each kidney. They produce hormones that assist with fluid and electrolyte regulation.

Bladder Muscular structure that collects urine for excretion. Bladder capacity increases with age from approximately 20 mL at birth to 700 mL in adulthood.

Kidney Organs (2) whose major functions are to maintain body homeostasis (acid-base and fluid electrolyte balance [Chapter 21]) and remove wastes from the body (see figure of urologic system). Kidneys are located in a position just above the waist in the flank.

Nephron The functional unit of the kidney, which regulates and maintains the volume and composition of body fluids and excretes soluble wastes. Components of the nephron include Bowman's capsule, tubules, loop of Henle, glomerulus, and associated venules and capillaries (see figure of nephron).

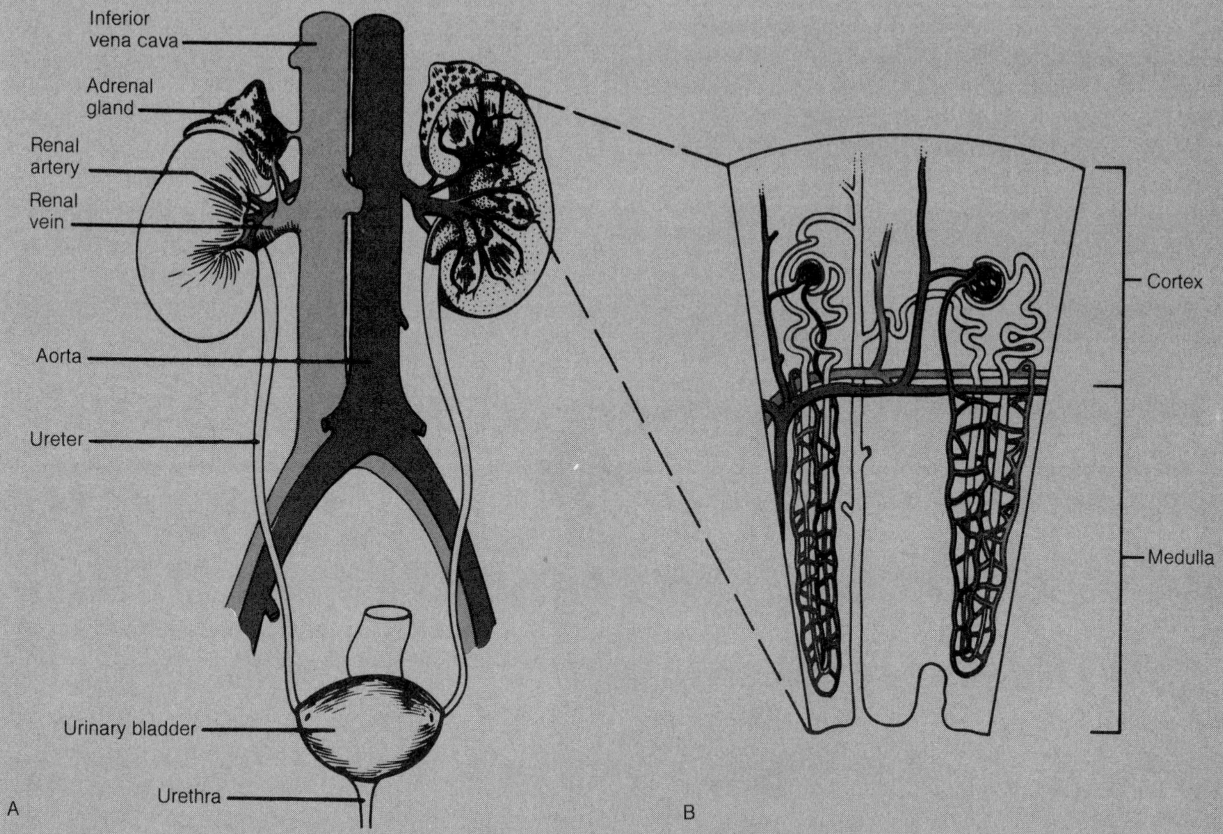

A. The urologic system. B. Nephrons in the renal cortex and medulla.

Ureters Long tubelike structures that transport urine from kidneys to bladder.

Urethra Tubelike structure that conveys urine from the bladder. The male urethra is approximately five times longer than the female urethra. The female urethra exits at the urinary meatus on the pelvic floor (Fig. 10-20). The male urethra transports both urine and semen and exits at the terminal meatus on the penile tip (Fig. 10-21).

Urine Hypertonic solution of fluid and waste products excreted by the body after essential nutrients and water are reabsorbed. Urine is acid, with a pH of 4.5–8.0. The acidification of urine is accomplished through the excretion of excess hydrogen and the retention of bicarbonate. The neutralization of ammonia is the major vehicle for hydrogen excretion.

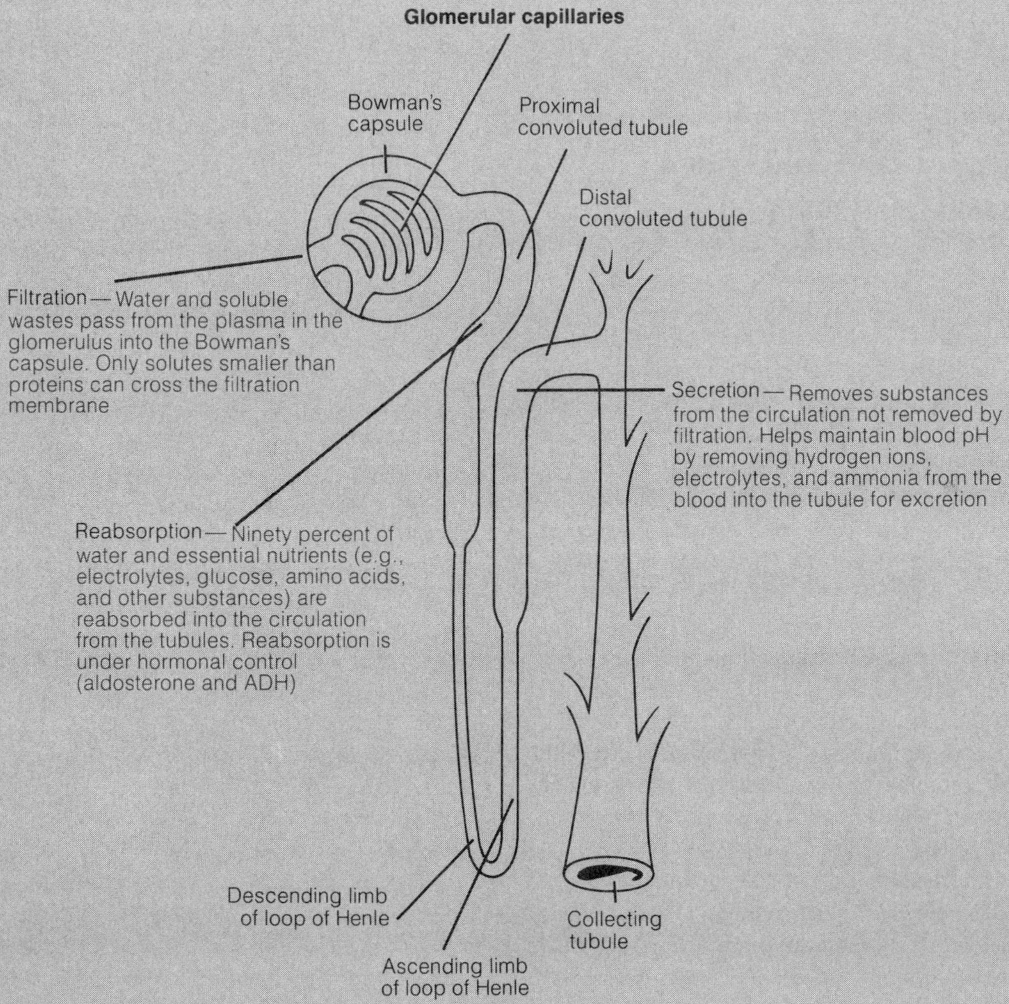

Nephron. Water and solutes (eg, electrolytes, glucose, ammonia) pass through the nephron and are reabsorbed into the circulation or excreted in the urine. Urine formation is regulated by three major hormones: Antidiuretic hormone (ADH) controls the rate of water reabsorption; aldosterone regulates sodium and potassium reabsorption; renin regulates blood pressure and thus the rate of filtration. (Adapted from Spence AP, Mason EB: Human Anatomy and Physiology, *3rd ed. Benjamin/Cummings, 1987.)*

The state of the genitourinary system contributes to the general good health and homeostasis of the child. Organs of the system interact and impact on other body systems to promote the constant composition and volume of body fluids through fluid regulation and elimination of wastes. Additionally, the system affects hormonal regulation, circulation, and reproductive function. Early diagnosis of pathology and appropriate interventions are critical for the optimal health of the child. Complex genitourinary dysfunction can lead to a state of chronic illness having serious effects on the child's growth and development.

Assessment of the Child with a Genitourinary Dysfunction

History

A detailed nursing assessment often begins with the prenatal history. Information regarding prenatal events such as maternal injuries, medications, or exposure to toxins might elicit helpful data. Relevant birth data include the presence of oligohydramnios (sparce amniotic fluid) or polyhydramnios (excessive amount of amniotic fluid) and the number of cord vessels, if known. Parental contact with any type of sexually transmitted disease also is important to note along with the treatment method employed.

Family history Because heredity affects the occurrence of some genitourinary diseases, a family history is essential. In addition to the usual information solicited in a nursing history, familial occurrences of hypospadias, polycystic kidney disease, or other genitourinary pathology might have bearing on the child's current problem.

Developmental history Essential to obtaining a history for the assessment of a child with a genitourinary problem is information about toilet training and normal urinary habits. Unusual delays in achieving urinary control can be significant, although if late control is usual for family members, this is less significant. Regression to wetting after control is attained can be related to psychologic factors, but persistent wetting requires medical attention. Generally, complete control is achieved by the end of early childhood. Close supervision by the child's primary medical care provider is necessary if urinary control is not achieved by the end of that stage.

Specific terms used by the child and family for urinary functions and organs should be recorded in the history. Embarrassment and difficulty verbalizing concerns are typical problems encountered with children and families affected by disorders of the genitourinary system. Future ease of communication with the child is enhanced if personal terms are used. Terms can vary widely according to cultural and intellectual background. They range from those that are anatomically and physiologically correct to those that are completely unrelated to the system. Some of the words might be seemingly appropriate to the child's culture but might be considered vulgar in other contexts. Use of terms will change as the child matures, and the older child, although embarrassed to use correct terminology, might fully understand it.

History of illness History of past infections; pain; undiagnosed fevers; and urine of unusual color, odor, or volume assist in the assessment of the child's genitourinary status. Recent changes in voiding patterns, alterations in the urinary stream, and changes in output are important additional factors to determine. Also, any history of vaginal or penile discharge or itching, or gastrointestinal complaints, can help determine if a problem exists. If sexually transmitted disease is suspected, children need to be asked about sexual contacts with possible carriers. Children can be assured that the information will remain confidential and be used only for purposes of informing contacts and health officials so that contacts can be treated.

If the child demonstrates a history of previous or repeated urinary tract infections, the nurse obtains information about the causative organism, if known; duration of the infection; and any successful treatment or medications. A history of previous surgical procedures or diagnostic studies helps the nurse clarify the integrity of the urinary system. Finally, before beginning the physical examination, it is important for the nurse to obtain a history of the presenting problem including precipitating factors, duration of symptoms, and home methods of treatment.

Physical Examination

Prior to conducting a physical examination, nurses carefully consider the approach to each child. Because genitourinary problems might involve a thorough examination of intimate body parts, children can be extremely threatened by the physical examination. Fear of the examination can alter other body responses—vital signs and abdominal reflexes. A calm, reassuring approach and verbal expressions of encouragement promote relaxation. Distraction techniques and use of play are particularly useful with the younger child. Explanations to the older child and reassurance that privacy will be respected ensure cooperation. The examination proceeds from the least to the most threatening system.

ASSESSMENT GUIDE *The Child with a Genitourinary Problem*

Assessment questions	Supporting data
Is the child experiencing any alteration in urinary elimination pattern? Describe the alteration	Decreased, forced, or intermittent urination; incontinence; abnormal placement of the meatus; alteration in the urinary stream; signs of fluid retention (see Chapter 21); edema; respiratory congestion; increased blood pressure; signs of dehydration (see Chapter 21); palpable kidneys; change in urine color and quality (eg, pale, cola color, cloudy, frothy); altered serum electrolytes and chemistries and urinalysis
	Increased frequency and urgency; pain (either lower abdominal or flank); fever, chills; positive urine, cervical, or urethral culture
Does the child have any observable abnormalities associated with the genitourinary tract?	Missing or abnormally placed meatus (might be associated with bending of the penis); open abdominal wall with protruding bladder contents; absent testes; inguinal bulge; scrotal edema; perineal inflammation, lesions, warts, or vaginal plaques
Has the child been exposed recently to any communicable disease?	Recent impetigo or streptococcal infection; elevated erythrocyte sedimentation rate or antistreptolysin titer (see Chapter 25); abnormal discharge; positive VDRL or gonococcal culture

Additional data: Abnormal position of ears (develop simultaneously with kidneys in the fetus); increased respiratory effort with edema; abdominal pain, nausea, vomiting, anorexia; short stature (usually in children with chronic renal insufficiency)

Privacy is most important during the assessment process. The child is properly draped at all times, and bedside curtains are closed. The child can decide whether parental presence is required.

Two aspects of the physical examination of the genital area are important. The first is that retraction of the testes occurs frequently during physical examination of a young boy and need not establish a diagnosis of undescended testicle. The nurse can observe for presence of the testes before proceeding with the scrotal examination. The second important aspect is that a vaginal examination usually is not necessary for the young girl. If the adolescent girl will be seen by a physician who will perform a vaginal examination, the nurse need not do so.

Validating Diagnostic Tests

A diagnostic workup for a child with a genitourinary problem can be quite complex. Some of the procedures involved are uncomfortable as well as embarrassing. The age and developmental level of the child is considered when doing pretest teaching since some children will react more strongly against tests involving the genitalia than will other children. Fears of mutilation, which are commonly seen in the early childhood period, can result in an extremely uncooperative child. Careful explanation and reassurance that no harm will occur as a result of the test might improve the situation. The presence of a familiar person or transition object during the procedure might help calm fears.

Noninvasive tests Routine blood and urine testing, including urinalysis, complete blood count (CBC), and serum values, assists in the assessment process. Normal values and the significance of abnormalities are summarized in Table 28-1. Despite advances in diagnostic technology, urinalysis remains the most important aspect of the initial evaluation of the genitourinary tract. If possible, a morning specimen is sent for analysis since the concentration and acidity changes as the day progresses. If possible, a clean-catch urine sample should be obtained.

Urine for culture and sensitivity (clean-catch urine) The nurse follows institutional procedure for procuring urine culture specimens. A midstream of clean-catch voided urine is collected from toilet-trained children after a thorough cleansing of the perineum. Girls are instructed to

TABLE 28-1 Alterations in Urine and Serum Values in Renal Disease

Test	Normal values*	Alteration/clinical significance
Urinalysis		
Color	Clear, amber	*Colored:* Some medications, that is, methylene blue, preparations of phenazophyridine hydrochloride (eg, Pyridium) *Dark yellow or orange:* Dehydration, fever *Red:* Blood
Turbidity	Clear	*Cloudy:* Sediment, possible bacteria
Specific gravity—ratio of density of urine to density of water	1.001–1.040; Usual child 1.003–1.010 Usual adult 1.015–1.025	*Increased:* Dehydration, nephrosis *Decreased:* Overhydration, inability to concentrate urine, glomerulonephritis, severe renal damage
pH	4.6–8.0, average 6.0	*Increased:* Persistent vomiting, alkalosis *Decreased:* Acidosis, nephritis
Protein	0	*Increased:* Present in renal diseases involving glomeruli and tubules, infections of kidneys, and other noninfectious processes
Glucose	0	*Increased:* Diabetes mellitus
Ketones	0	*Increased:* Acidosis
Cells	Few	*Increased:* Can indicate kidney, ureter, bladder pathology, depending on type
Erythrocytes (RBC)	0	*Increased:* Glomerulonephritis, trauma, pyelonephritis, tumors, contamination with menstrual flow
Leukocytes	Few	*Increased:* Urinary tract infection
Casts	0	*Increased:* Conditions of low pH, present in variety of kidney pathologies
Crystals	Some	*Increased:* Calculi
Serum		
Sodium	130–150 mEq/L	*Increased:* Sodium and water reabsorption and retention (edema) from decreased renal blood flow through glomerulus
Potassium	3.5–5.5 mEq/L	*Increased:* Renal failure, reabsorption of potassium and excretion of hydrogen ions
Chloride	95–108 mEq/L	*Increased:* Associated with some renal disorders
Phosphorus	2.3–4.1 mEq/L	*Increased:* Associated with kidney dysfunction, uremia, particularly tubular damage
Blood urea nitrogen	6–20 mg/dL	*Increased:* Inadequate excretion of urea due to obstruction or renal disease
Creatinine	0.6–1.5 mg/dL	*Increased:* Impaired renal function or urinary obstruction
Glucose	80–120 mg/dL	*Increased or stable:* Possibly indicative of diabetes mellitus
Hematocrit	Male: 37%–49% Female: 36–46%	*Decreased:* Response to bleeding in acute glomerulonephritis, trauma
Hemoglobin	Male: 13–16 g/dL Female: 12–16 g/dL	*Decreased:* Response to bleeding in acute glomerulonephritis, trauma

*Normal values might vary with the laboratory method used.

separate the labia and clean either side and the middle with three different wipes of a recommended cleaning solution. Cleaning proceeds from front to back to prevent contaminating the cleaned area. Boys are instructed to retract the foreskin gently and clean the tip of the penis. After cleaning either the labia or the penis, the child voids a small amount into the toilet, bedpan, or urinal and then a small amount into the sterile specimen receptacle. After being labeled correctly, the specimen is transported immediately to the laboratory. Any delay could result in multiplication of bacteria, leading to a false reading. If a delay is anticipated, the specimen is refrigerated. Nurses follow a similar cleaning procedure with untrained children. The cleaning is followed by the application of a sterile urine-collecting bag. The nurse observes the bag frequently to prevent contamination of the specimen from a loose bag.

Creatinine clearance test The creatinine clearance test (normal: male, 107–141 mL/min; female, 87–132 mL/min) measures glomerular filtration efficiency plus tubular excretion. A decrease in urine creatinine clearance indicates impaired renal function. Urine collected for 24 hours is required. A blood level for creatinine usually is done at some point during the 24-hour collection time and normally shows elevated creatinine if the clearance level is low. The container for a 24-hour collection is labeled with the time the collection is initiated, the child's name, and the name of the test. All urine samples are stored in the container. The collection begins after the child has voided and ends the following day with a final void just prior to completion time. A sign is placed on the child's bed and in the bathroom to save all voids. Older children and adolescents can share the responsibility for obtaining specimens if given adequate instruction and equipment.

Twenty-four-hour collection poses a problem for the untrained or incontinent child. Special collection bags with long polyethylene tubing are applied to the perineal area. The bag stays in place for the collection period and urine is emptied into the collection container via the tube.

Radiographic studies A simple flat plate of the abdomen allows visualization of the kidneys, ureters, and bladder (KUB). This radiograph is helpful when evaluating gross anatomic conditions (such as hydronephrosis).

Invasive procedures Adequate, honest preparation is most supportive to the child undergoing stressful procedures. When describing each test or procedure, the nurse carefully selects terms the child and family will understand.

Catheterization Bladder catheterization is a nursing intervention that the child with a genitourinary problem might face repeatedly. For young children this can be an unpleasant anxiety-provoking procedure. A successful initial experience facilitates subsequent catheterization. The purpose of the procedure is explained, and an estimate of the time the catheter is to remain in place is given. The use of dolls to demonstrate and explain the procedure is helpful, particularly with younger children.

The nurse explains to the child that there might be a feeling of pressure similar to the urge to urinate while the catheter is being inserted. The child should understand that, once inserted, the catheter presents no discomfort. Very young children might fear losing their insides through the tube, particularly if they see urine outflow. The sensitive nurse can anticipate this and give a realistic picture of what is happening.

Catheterization might be performed to empty the bladder prior to diagnostic tests, to obtain a sterile urine specimen, to measure residual volumes in the bladder, or to empty the bladder when the child is unable to void. The nurse needs to be familiar with the institution's procedure for bladder catheterization. Strict aseptic technique is essential as the urinary tract is most vulnerable to introduction of infection by catheterization.

Bladder tap Because a sterile urine specimen is difficult to obtain in infants, a bladder tap might be preferred. The technique requires a needle puncture of the skin and underlying bladder. The infant needs to be restrained during the procedure to prevent accidental trauma.

Pelvic examination A pelvic examination is performed to assess the structure of the reproductive organs or to obtain cervical specimens for examination or culture. The adolescent will need an explanation of the examination procedure and support during it. The nurse encourages the adolescent to breathe deeply and slowly to promote relaxation.

Cervical cultures might be required to diagnose gonorrhea or other sexually transmitted diseases (STD), such as *Candida, Chlamydia,* or *Trichomonas*. Serologic studies to support the diagnosis of a sexually transmitted disease include the Venereal Disease Research Laboratory (VDRL) slide test for syphilis and blood titers for herpes and AIDS antibodies.

Cystoscopy The cystoscopic examination is used to detect malformations of the bladder, ureters, and urethra. It is done under anesthesia for infants and children to ensure their cooperation. Cystoscopy allows visualization of the urethra and bladder by means of a lighted tubular lens. It allows visualization of ureteral orifices, removal of small calculi, and insertion of ureteral catheters if necessary.

PROCEDURE *Urinary Bladder Catheterization*

- Explain the procedure to the child using age appropriate concepts and familiar terminology. Tell the child the reason for the procedure and the estimated time the catheter will remain in (temporary or in-dwelling). Demonstrate the procedure on a doll and allow the child to see and touch catheters and drainage system.
- Have the child practice slow, deep breathing exercises and explain that the child will be asked to do this during the procedure. Tell the child that there will be a feeling of pressure when the catheter is being inserted and that the child might feel like urinating. Reassure the child that the feeling is normal and that the child shouldn't worry about having a urination accident.
- Gather catheter equipment together. Draw bedside curtains. Have the child lie supine with knees bent and totally relaxed. The child's legs are in a froglike position.
- After washing hands and putting on the gloves, clean the perineum as for a clean-catch urine. The area will feel cold.
- Ask the child to begin the breathing exercises as the lubricated catheter is being inserted. The child might feel some pressure. Use an appropriate size catheter. The lumen should be small enough for easy insertion but large enough to prevent leakage of urine (size #8 for infants and small children).
- Insert the catheter only until urine flow is observed. If the catheter is to be in-dwelling, insert slightly further and inflate the balloon carefully, then connect the catheter to the sterile drainage system. If catheterization is for purposes of relieving bladder distension or obtaining a sterile urine specimen, remove the catheter gently when the urine flow has ceased. In cases where the bladder is particularly distended, clamp the catheter at intervals to prevent a sudden rush of urine output.

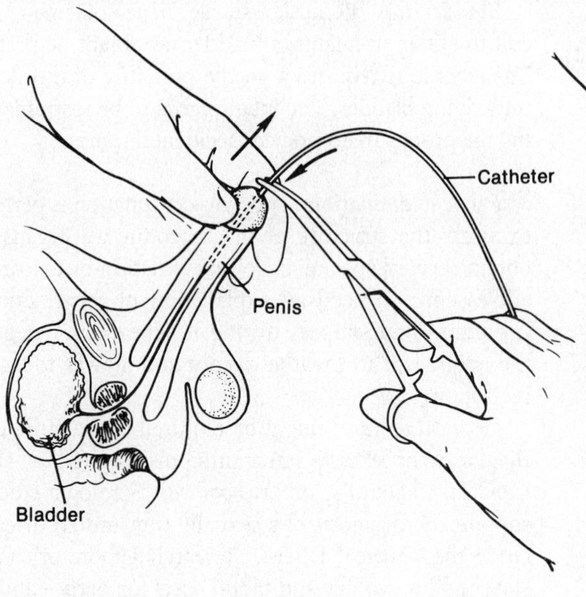

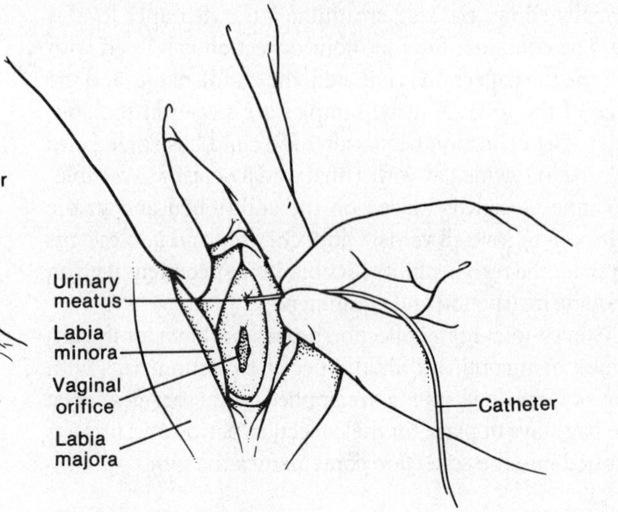

In addition to routine preoperative teaching, nursing preparation includes explaining the postoperative course. When voiding for the first time after a cystoscopy, the child might experience pain and burning. The child should be prepared for this discomfort and told that intake of extra fluid will alleviate the symptoms. The child is observed closely for postprocedural urinary retention and hematuria. If this is not the child's first experience, the retention might be intentional. Assurances can be given that with continued voids, discomfort lessens considerably. Often a warm sitz bath will relax the child, decrease bladder irritability, and encourage spontaneous voiding.

Radiographic studies Several invasive radiographic and urodynamic studies are used to assess the function and structure of the renal system. These include intravenous pyelogram (IVP), voiding cystourethrogram (VCUG examines urethra and bladder), renal angiography (visualizes renal circulation), and renal scan. Some of these studies require intravenous injections of a radiopaque contrast material. Whenever children are prepared to experience studies involving the use of a contrast material (radiopaque dye), the nurse is careful not to use the term dye as it is easily misinterpreted by children. The nurse explains how they will feel while the contrast material is being injected since it often causes a general feeling of warmth, particularly in the face. There might be a burning sensation at the injection site, radiating up the extremity. The child also might feel nauseous. Nurses can reassure the children that these symptoms will soon disappear. Young children can feel particularly apprehensive, and the presence of a parent or sympathetic nurse might ensure cooperation during the contrast material injection.

A nursing responsibility during radiographic studies is to obtain a history of any previous allergic response. In rare cases, the contrast material can precipitate an anaphylactic reaction, particularly in those children allergic to iodine and shellfish. Parents usually need to sign a special consent form for procedures such as an intravenous pyelogram because of this possibility, but they should be assured that the occurrence is rare. During the test, the child is observed for any local irritation or allergic response.

Principles of Nursing Care

Acute Care Needs

⊛ Alteration in urinary elimination pattern related to voiding pattern irregularities secondary to dysuria, hesitancy, urgency, retention

Children with genitourinary dysfunction will experience alterations in urinary pattern, depending on the cause of the dysfunction. For example, those children with obstructions can experience urinary retention, variations in the urinary flow, and incontinence. Children with urinary tract infections can have pain and urgency on urination. Children with renal dysfunction might experience marked decrease in urinary output followed by diuresis (excessive urination).

For children with any alteration in urinary elimination, the nurse carefully monitors the amount, color, and clarity of the urine. Providing privacy for urination is particularly important, since anxiety can alter the child's ability to relax the sphincter. Potty chairs or seats that fit on the toilet are more comfortable for the child who has been trained recently. Some young children are embarrassed to ask to go to the bathroom, so it is helpful for the nurse to inquire whether the child has to go. Any method that can assist the child, such as running water within the child's hearing, placing spirit of peppermint in the bedpan, or placing the child's fingers in warm water, is helpful.

Encouraging fluid intake in those children who can have unlimited fluids can improve the urinary output. Providing warm baths helps relieve bladder spasm. For children with urinary retention, bladder catheterization might be required.

Because normal voiding patterns can be interrupted following genitourinary surgery, the child is warned that this might happen. This can be particularly stressful for recently toilet-trained children, and parents should be cautioned to expect regressive behavior patterns.

⊛ Alteration in fluid volume: excess or deficit related to compromised regulatory mechanisms

Maintenance of fluid and electrolyte balance is of extreme importance in the management of the child with a genitourinary condition. The unique fluid management requirements of the child will be considered in prescribing intravenous fluid therapy and oral intake. The nurse then plays a major role by regulating the fluid intake according to the child's dysfunction and limits and by monitoring the child's intake and output carefully. Hourly checking and recording of intake and output is essential if the child is to remain adequately hydrated. A baseline urine output is 1 mL/kg of body weight/hour and slightly more for infants. Recommended fluid maintenance for children of various ages is given in Chapter 21.

Fluid restriction The child with impaired renal function immediately becomes involved in the complexities of fluid balance. Children with filtration problems (nephrosis, chronic renal failure) might be severely restricted to a few hundred milliliters a day. The child with severe genitourinary problems must deal with the frustrations of alternating severe restriction with no restriction.

Often, young children faced with the stress of restricted intake regress in response to feeling as if they have lost control of their bodies. The one control remaining is the refusal to eat or drink. This reaction is seen also in older children who perceive every other aspect of their lives to be beyond their control. A detailed assessment can be helpful in describing dietary likes and dislikes. Familiar foods and fluids offered by family members often are more acceptable to the young child. Control is assisted by offering children choices about types of food and fluid within their dietary limits.

When a child's fluid intake is severely restricted, it is essential that the nurse and parent be aware of exactly how much the child has consumed. This might include placing the total daily amount of allowed fluid in one container in the refrigerator. Fluids are removed from the container, and when the container is empty, no more fluid is allowed (Butler, 1985). A variety of fluids can be kept in several labeled containers and given until empty. Hard candies can be thirst quenching without added fluid.

Fluid encouragement Increased fluid intake is recommended in some urologic conditions and to increase the effectiveness of many urologic drugs. Children with urinary drainage devices (such as catheters and stents) need to be encouraged to drink large amounts of fluid. Fruit juices, particularly cranberry juice, are acceptable to children and are a convenient source of vitamin C.

Urine pH and specific gravity measurements assist the nurse in the assessment of the child's fluid needs. The goal of increasing or decreasing the type and amount of fluid is to maintain an optimal pH of 5.

Postoperative fluid needs Children recovering from genitourinary surgery present an additional challenge since their fluid needs correspond to their size and to the manipulation of their urinary tracts. Many children experience postoperative diuresis caused by urinary tract manipulation. This condition necessitates even more careful assessment of the child's fluid balance. The nurse needs to recognize quickly an intravenous infusion that is less than the prescribed volume or an inadequate oral intake and to correct the situation promptly to prevent dehydration.

Maintenance of fluid and electrolyte balance is a postoperative nursing challenge that can be facilitated during the preoperative period. Methods of drinking (bottle, cup) and the child's fluid preferences are included in the plan.

⊛ Potential for infection

Despite improved methods of preventing and treating infections, the genitourinary tract remains quite vulnerable. Predisposing factors such as structural abnormalities or stasis of urine and foreign bodies (such as catheters and stents) add additional risk.

There are several approaches the nurse can use to minimize infection. Good hand-washing procedure is essential when dealing with all patients. Thorough hand washing prior to and after contact with each patient will lessen incidence of cross-contamination. The use of aseptic technique when inserting catheters is a nursing measure that reduces the occurrence of infection.

The use of aseptic technique when in contact with the child's wound or intravenous site is essential. Any sign of infection (such as wound inflammation or intravenous-site phlebitis) is reported to the physician. Contaminated urine is contained and disposed of properly to prevent nosocomial (hospital-acquired) infection. Routine cultures of urine assist in the assessment of infection. Changes in the appearance of the child's urine (for example, sediment or odor) are indicative of infectious processes. Fever, flank pain, and urinary frequency also are common indicators of genitourinary inflammation.

⊛ Potential knowledge deficit concerning genitourinary surgery

Preoperative preparation for genitourinary surgery Often the preoperative preparation for the child facing genitourinary surgery begins shortly after admission to the nursing unit. A detailed assessment is important at this time so the nurse can plan an individualized teaching approach to the child and family. It is important that the nurse assess what the child and the parent understand about the anticipated surgical procedure.

The use of dolls to demonstrate the positions of tubes, dressings, and catheters can be particularly effective when teaching the child about genitourinary surgery. Familiarity with the postoperative equipment, such as catheters, drainage bags, mist tents, or other equipment, will reduce anxiety. The nurse gives a narrative description of the surgical experience, including what is to happen postoperatively and how the child will feel. If a recovering child with a similar surgical experience is available, the nurse encourages a sharing of experiences. Such a sharing experience would help the child having genital surgery to cope with any fears of castration or mutilation.

If immobility will be necessary in the postoperative period, the nurse prepares the child. Accurate information regarding the reason for immobility and the expected length of time involved will be helpful to the older child. The younger child might need reassurance that resuming appropriate physical activity is possible when the restriction is no longer necessary. A description of immobilizing devices such as restraints, testicular traction, bed cradles, and dressings will ease the postoperative course. The discussion of pain is as truthful as possible.

Postoperative care Any child experiencing genitourinary surgical procedures might expect to have one or more urinary drainage tubes, as well as the usual postoperative dressings, IVs, and routines. Postoperative nursing management is directed toward the areas of fluid and electrolyte balance, prevention of infection, relief of pain, prevention of injury, and management of other postoperative complications.

STANDARDS OF NURSING CARE *The Child Following Genitourinary Surgery*

RISKS

Assessed risk	Nursing action
Potential for routine postoperative complications—bleeding, pneumonia, urinary retention, infection	See Standards of Nursing Care—The Child Following Surgery in Chapter 20

GUIDE FOR NURSING MANAGEMENT

Nursing diagnosis	Intervention	Rationale	Outcome
1. Potential fluid volume deficit (stressors: postoperative diuresis, fluid loss during surgery)	Maintain the ordered intravenous rate.	Proper rate ensures adequate fluid replacement.	The child appears well hydrated. The child's urine output is within normal limits for age and body weight.
	Offer oral fluids when indicated according to the child's preference; monitor hydration status.	Oral fluids will gradually replace IV fluids to maintain adequate intake.	
	Measure output accurately every hour for 8 hours; measure output from each catheter and record separately.	Accurate output measurement assists with determining the child's hydration status.	
2. Alteration in comfort: pain related to physical trauma secondary to surgical incision	Observe for pain at incision site or bladder spasms.	Postoperative pain often focuses on the incision site. Catheterization can cause spasms.	The child appears relaxed. The child can participate in care. The child verbalizes relief from pain.
	Observe for restlessness, rigidity, or altered facial expression.	These are nonverbal signs of pain.	
	Check that catheters and stents are draining freely and hourly output is adequate.	Catheters or stents that become plugged by mucus shreds obstruct urine flow and can cause spasms.	
	Provide physical measures for pain relief—position change, back rub, releasing catheter tension, distraction.	Nonpharmacologic pain relief decreases the need for pain medication.	
	Administer prescribed medications.	Analgesics and antispasmodics relieve postoperative pain.	
3. Potential for injury (stressor: presence of urinary drainage tubes)	Tape catheters at exit site if ordered and to leg when possible; apply the tape so the catheter does not kink, twist, or rise against gravity.	Stabilization of catheters and stents prevents stress and trauma to the sites.	The catheters drain properly and remain straight and secure. The child shows no sign of trauma.
	Follow instructions for irrigation, instillation, and dressing changes.	Certain postoperative procedures are dictated by the individual institution.	

(Continues)

STANDARDS OF NURSING CARE *The Child Following Genitourinary Surgery (Continued)*

GUIDE FOR NURSING MANAGEMENT

Nursing diagnosis	Intervention	Rationale	Outcome
4. Potential for infection (stressors: invasive procedures, assault to primary defenses)	Maintain sterile drainage system.	Maintaining an intact system prevents the entry of organisms.	The child remains free of infection as evidenced by normal body temperature and negative urine culture.
	Follow routine care for urinary catheters.	Proper care of urinary drainage system reduces the risk of infection.	
	Monitor for fever, chills, flank pain, pain on urination, frequency, and bacteriuria. Obtain urine culture if fever present and when removing Foley catheter.	Bacterial count greater than 100,000 per mL indicates urinary tract infection.	
5. Potential for impaired physical mobility (stressor: imposed physical limitations following surgery)	Institute routine measures for preventing adverse effects of immobility (see Chapter 20).	Impaired mobility can cause muscle atrophy, constipation, urinary stasis, altered skin integrity, and respiratory compromise.	The child is free from signs of muscle atrophy, constipation, skin inflammation, and other hazards of immobility.

Nutritional Needs

Alteration in nutrition: less than or more than body requirements related to compromised use of nutrients secondary to loss or retention of protein and electrolytes

Diseases that adversely affect the kidneys can result in alterations in electrolytes (Na^+, K^+, and Ca^{2+}) and either increased loss of protein or inadequate excretion of protein wastes. Diseased kidneys have more difficulty excreting potassium and sodium, resulting in retention. Consequently, the increase in these electrolytes causes adverse effects on other body systems (see Chapter 21). The child might be placed on a sodium- or potassium-restricted diet. Foods that are fairly low in potassium are fruits such as apples and strawberries, whole grain foods, and vegetables.

Hypocalcemia is a risk in children with kidney damage, particularly from chronic renal disease. A deficit in the utilization of vitamin D results in decreased absorption of dietary calcium. Phosphorus retention inhibits absorption of calcium from the intestine. The resulting hypocalcemia triggers resorption (removal) of calcium from the bones. Resorption causes osteodystrophy (rickets-type bone dysfunction) and calcification of soft tissue. Active vitamin D and calcium supplements might be required to reduce this occurrence.

Limited protein intake might be recommended with certain conditions. Nursing management is directed toward maintaining weight while decreasing the protein portion of the diet. Of the total protein allowed in a limited protein diet, a major portion includes foods that promote growth (such as eggs, milk, meat, and whole grain).

The diet needs to consider the child's age, developmental level, and food preferences.

Developmental Needs

Potential altered growth and development

Facilitating adequate development Many children with genitourologic problems require frequent, often lengthy, hospitalizations, which might interrupt their developmental progress. Multiple surgical interventions often are necessary. It is not uncommon for these children to be forced to miss weeks or months of school. Whenever possible, attempts should be made to continue the child's education while still hospitalized. The parent is advised that although the child is ill, a routine as normal as possible should be encouraged. Tutors are available from the local school department for long periods of confinement either in the hospital or at home. Peers should be encouraged to visit.

Facilitating independence Problems of immobilization can frustrate a child's independence, resulting in potential disciplinary problems during hospitalization and later at home. As nurses plan for the child's care, they should anticipate the need for independence. Often even young children can assume responsibility for some part of their care. Self-care is encouraged during hospitalizaton and is incorporated into discharge planning.

Developmental considerations for adjustment Some genitourinary dysfunction can either prolong the achievement of continence in an untrained child or can cause a previously trained child to become temporarily incontinent. The nurse can encourage the parent to exercise patience, to use frequent praise, and to decrease expectations. (Toilet training is discussed in Chapter 5.)

The child experiencing urologic interventions is often physically incapacitated for varying lengths of time by the presence of urinary appliances. An infant learning to walk with the added burden of a bulky dressing is unaware of the situation. On the other hand, the preadolescent girl returning to school with a catheter draining into a leg bag must face a much more challenging adjustment.

Circumcision has entirely different implications for an infant than for an older boy. External appearance of the genitals is of different significance to children of various age levels. Nurses therefore consider the developmental stage when assessing impact of the disease.

Emotional Needs

⊛ Body image disturbance related to perceived developmental or acquired imperfections secondary to deviations in structure and/or function of genitourinary system

Alteration in body image is the major emotional adjustment of the child suffering from a disease of the genitourinary system. Infants and young children are not generally aware of body image in detail but are acutely aware of any gesture or motion that they perceive as threatening.

Children in early childhood are intensely aware of their body image. They might spend much time examining and exploring their bodies and those of their cooperative playmates. Children of this age with urologic problems often have their curiosity stimulated by the physical attention of professionals. The nurse therefore needs to be aware of this natural inquisitiveness.

For the child in middle and late childhood, the mere thought of "looking different" is anxiety-provoking. Because fads, styles, and group activities are important to children of this developmental level, being different as the result of a genitourologic procedure is a major stressor. Dietary restrictions, inability to participate in sports, and fear of embarrassment affect many of these children. Often the child perceives these problems as being as serious as the illness itself.

Although the goal is to increase the child's ability to "be like the other kids," the reality of the genitourinary problem makes this very difficult. Acceptance by family and peers is vital to the child. Unfortunately, the child's peers are often cruel without cognitive sense of the damage being done to the affected child. This is often a very difficult period for the parent and child. Expression of feelings by the use of play or art eases adjustment. The nurse allows parent and child to express fears, feelings, and frustrations as they begin this difficult adjustment. A parent should be comfortable with personal feelings about the situation before trying to assist the child.

The nurse attempts to reduce the stress the child might encounter when returning home. Often imaginative clothing designed to conceal drainage setups and creative approaches to difficult treatments evolve from discussion as concerned families and staff explore possibilities. For instance, a girl who must wear a urine-collecting appliance on her leg would profit from wearing loosely gathered knickers or slacks with banded bottoms, rather than conventional jeans. Manufacturers have produced pants similar to training pants for incontinent adults. Children who have problems with continence also benefit from this arrangement, possibly with the current fashionable underwear sewn over the training pant.

⊛ Potential sexual dysfunction

Any disturbance to the genitourinary tract is perceived as being of major significance during adolescence. Unfortunately, the response of adolescents experiencing stress can be negative. Sexual changes common to adolescence interfere with the adolescent's perception of illness and often intensify fantasies.

Fears of mutilation haunt many children with genitourinary problems. To minimize fears, interventions are explained with carefully chosen terms. Any manipulation of the penis or testes at this time gives rise to anxieties about future fertility or potency. Adolescent girls might be experiencing their first pelvic examination. Depending on what they have heard about the procedure, they also might fear loss of fertility, virginity, or harm to internal organs as a result of manipulation.

Occasionally, fertility can be compromised by repeated incidents of sexually transmitted diseases. The adolescent might be afraid to ask appropriate questions or to express fears. When working with adolescents, the nurse attempts to determine the amount of education the adolescent has received and works from the adolescent's knowledge base. The nurse emphasizes prevention as a way of minimizing adverse consequences. Nurses need to remember that since questions will surface again as decisions about marriage and family are made, it is helpful to provide a list of resources for subsequent reference.

Home Care and Health Maintenance Needs

⊛ Potential knowledge deficit concerning home management

Discharge preparation—catheterization Certain aspects of urinary tract conditions require special attention as the child prepares to go home. The physical care of urologic equipment at home requires understanding of simple aseptic technique and infection control. Procedures for dressings or irrigations and methods for emptying the bladder at home are taught early in the hospitalization so that all participants in care will have ample opportunity to learn and return the demonstration and gain confidence by repetition. For example, a young child discharged with home catheterization can eventually be taught to do the procedure alone. Meanwhile, both parents are taught catheterization technique, which in the home is simpler than with hospital equipment.

Unlike catheterization in the hospital, catheterization at home involves using a clean technique requiring no gloves, clean equipment (catheter and collection container), and thorough hand washing. After cleaning the area, an extra application of povidone-iodine preparation to the area is recommended before inserting the catheter. Expensive equipment is not required. Water-based diaper wipes can be used for cleaning with a clean plastic cup for collection. Catheters can be ordered through most medical supply stores.

To keep a routine check on urinary tract infections, home urine culture kits are available. They give results in 24 hours and, if positive, should be followed by a laboratory test for culture and sensitivity.

Older children and adolescents are encouraged to participate fully in their own care. There is no reason why self-catheterization cannot be performed at school, thus allowing for full school participation without being singled out as different. Although ureterostomies and ileal loop conduits are not frequently seen, children can be responsible for their own cleanliness and appliance changes. Prevention of skin breakdown is important, and the child should demonstrate competence in skin care.

Other discharge preparation Children with some genitourinary problems often are at risk because of the nature of the illness. Precautions necessary to protect the child's fragile renal function often include restrictions from vigorous play and from active sports. The nurse can suggest alternate activities that are suited to the child's personality and offer less physical risk. Sports, such as tennis or swimming, allow for both aerobic exercise and team participation and are enjoyed throughout the lifespan.

Because some genitourinary diseases require long-term care and frequent hospitalization, consideration is given to the effects on the child's schooling and peer relationships. To ease adjustment in school, the school nurse and teachers need to be aware of any special considerations such as special diets, self-catheterizaton, and need for extra time in the bathroom. Visiting nurse referrals are most beneficial for support and supervision after discharge from hospital care.

The Child with a Problem of Infection

Acute Urinary Tract Infection

Bacteriuria (the growth of bacteria in uncontaminated urine) indicates the presence of urinary tract infection even if no signs or symptoms of inflammation exist anywhere in the urinary tract. After respiratory infections, urinary tract infections (UTIs) are the most frequent type of childhood infection. The location in the urinary tract of the infection determines the clinical manifestations, which range from relatively mild asymptomatic infections in the lower tract to the more dangerous involvement of the kidney itself.

Except during the neonatal period, UTIs occur predominantly in girls and women. The incidence of urinary tract infection in boys is related to anomalies of the genitourinary system.

Urinary tract infections occur because of factors that allow bacterial entry into the urinary system. Major factors facilitating bacterial invasion in children include:

1. Anatomic factors such as the relatively shorter urethra in girls than in boys and the proximity of the urinary system to the anus and vagina. Some anomalies of the

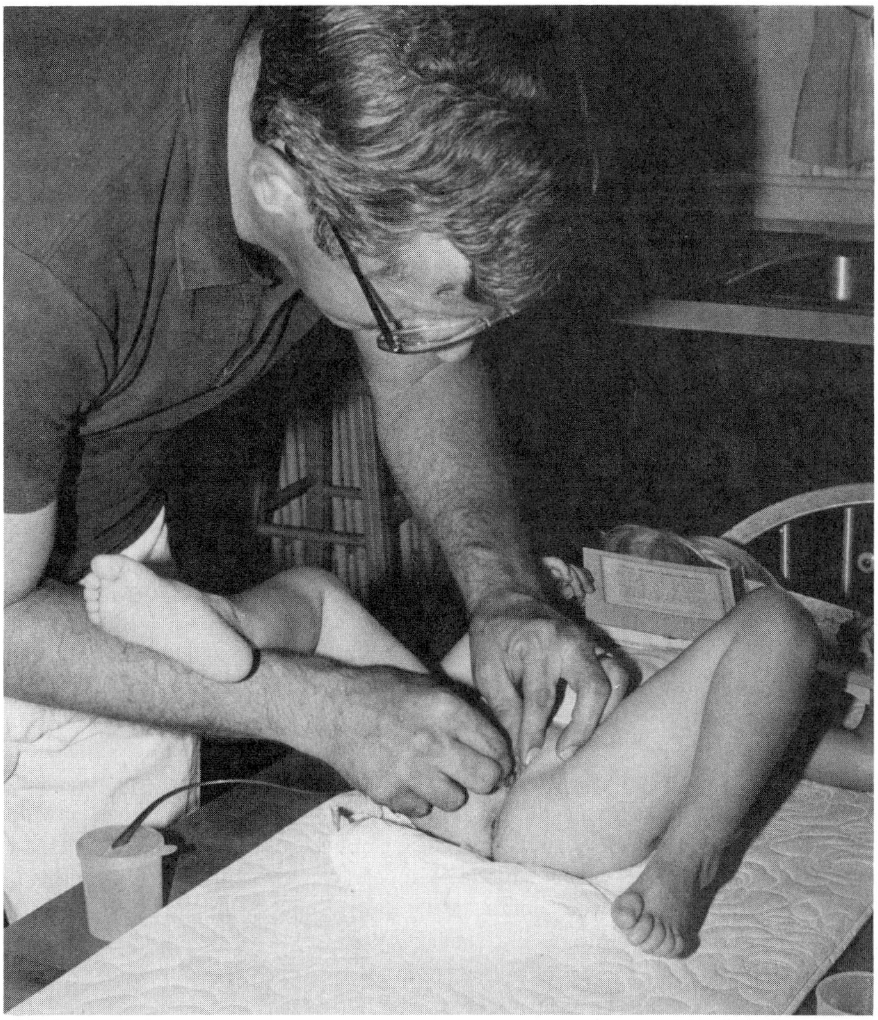

Catheterization at home requires clean technique. (Photograph by Judy Koenig.)

urinary tract such as vesicoureteral reflux or neurogenic bladder (bladder with inadequate innervation) can cause urinary tract infections

2. Incomplete bladder emptying due to structural anomalies or voluntary urinary retention
3. Irritants such as harsh soaps or detergents

Escherichia coli (gram-negative) is the most common infecting organism. Other causative bacteria include *Staphylococcus, saprophyticus, Klebsiella,* and *Proteus.*

Clinical manifestations Most UTIs are limited to the lower urinary tract and are related to *cystitis,* or inflammation of the bladder. Clinical signs and symptoms vary markedly and a significant number of children can have asymptomatic bacteriuria.

Infants and young children might exhibit gastrointestinal dysfunction and lower-abdominal pain. Poor feeding, irritability, and failure to thrive might be the only clues in infancy. Additional symptoms can include foul-smelling urine, urgency, frequency, dysuria (pain and burning on urination), dribbling, and recurrent enuresis (bed-wetting) in a previously trained child. Older children have the more classic picture of lower-tract infection: dysuria, frequency, urgency, and lower-abdominal pain.

Fever, chills, vomiting, and flank pain are signs of *acute pyelonephritis,* or upper urinary tract infection. Septicemia is a distinct possibility if the infection is not treated promptly.

Diagnostic evaluation Urine culture reveals significant bacterial growth. Bacterial counts of greater than 100,000 per mL are diagnostic of urinary tract infection. Counts of between 10,000 and 100,000 per mL are questionable and require further testing.

In addition to urine cultures, routine urinalysis is performed. Urinalysis might demonstrate pyuria (white blood cells in the urine) and possibly hematuria (bloody urine).

A first morning urine specimen is preferred for testing as it is more concentrated. If the specimen cannot be taken to the laboratory immediately, it is refrigerated since bacteria multiply rapidly at room temperature. If the specimen is obtained at home, the specimen container can be packed in ice for transport from home to the laboratory.

Additional urologic studies, such as IVP and VCUG, are performed on most boys with urinary tract infections because urinary tract infection in boys usually indicates underlying pathology of the urinary tract. In girls, such urologic studies generally are deferred until the second or third episode of urinary tract infection.

Treatment Treatment of a urinary tract infection includes eradicating the infection, recognizing and preventing relapses or reinfections, and correcting underlying abnormalities of the urinary tract.

To eradicate the current infection, an appropriate antimicrobial agent is selected. Drugs of choice are penicillin and sulfonamides such as sulfisoxazole (Gantrisin) or sulfamethoxazole-trimethoprim (Bactrim). More recently cefaclor (Ceclor) has been used to treat UTIs that are resistant to other antibiotics. Although effective, cefaclor is very expensive. A short course (2 to 3 days), or a large, single dose of antibiotic therapy can be effective treatment for an uncomplicated lower urinary tract infection.

Bacteria in the urine should disappear within 48 hours after antibiotics are started. A repeat urine culture is done at this time to determine if the chosen antibiotic is effective. One to two weeks following completion of the antibiotic therapy, another urine culture is obtained. Further cultures are obtained on a recommended schedule for several months to determine whether reinfection has occurred. If the child has repeated episodes of UTIs, a prophylactic regimen of low dose trimethoprim and sulfamethoxazole (Bactrim or Septra) might be prescribed.

Children with infections of the upper urinary tract are hospitalized for observation and for IV antibiotic therapy. Once acceptable blood antibiotic levels are reached and the child demonstrates no urinary tract abnormalities, the child can be discharged on oral antibiotic treatment. Treatment continues for 4 to 6 weeks.

Nursing management The nurse encourages the child to drink frequently in order to dilute the urine and flush the bladder. Although it is uncertain that acid urine can totally prevent urinary tract infections, acidic juices such as orange and cranberry appeal to children. They provide a good source of vitamin C while diluting the urine.

The child is taught to prevent urine retention by voiding frequently and completely emptying the bladder. Depending on the cause of the infection, the child might need home catheterization to prevent retention. Young children might need to be reminded more frequently to go to the bathroom in order to prevent unintentional retention. Warm sitz baths or a heating pad can be used to relieve lower abdominal pain.

If radiologic procedures such as IVPs or VCUGs are required, the nurse prepares the child and family for these intrusive procedures. It is important that the nurse ensure proper specimen collection when urine cultures are needed.

The child hospitalized for pyelonephritis can appear acutely ill. Management of high fever is an important nursing intervention. Intravenous therapy and provision for rest assist the child's recovery.

Parents and children are taught the possible causes and prevention of UTIs. Wearing clean, preferably cotton, underwear and wiping the perineal area from front to back until dry are emphasized. Children are encouraged to drink fluids and to void regularly. Harsh detergents or bubble baths are to be avoided since they serve as chemical irritants to the perineal and urethral areas. Sexually active adolescents should urinate both before and immediately after intercourse.

Home urine cultures might be recommended. The nurse ensures that the parent or child follows the recommended procedure. Home culture kits are available that provide evidence of any organisms on a culture plate in 24 hours. An accompanying color chart can help identify the organism as well as indicate a colony count. A dip-stick test, such as Microstix-Nitrate or N-Unistix, that determines the presence of bacteria in urine might be preferred.

The nurse emphasizes that the child must take all of the prescribed medication. Parents are given a schedule for follow-up cultures and doctor visits (see the Nursing Care Plan for the Infant with a Neurogenic Bladder).

Toxic Shock Syndrome

Toxic shock syndrome (TSS), which affects postpubescent young women, is a fulminating illness with sudden onset, severe multisystem involvement, and a relatively high fatality rate. The disease incidence is rare, but the greatest percentage of cases occur in young women or adolescents during their menstrual cycles. Incidence of TSS has been linked to tampon use, although the actual risk in tampon users is unknown.

Strong evidence suggests that the symptoms and effects of TSS are caused by toxins of phage group I *Staphylococcus aureus*. Theories suggest that tampons themselves do not carry the organism but do provide a medium for organism growth. *Staphylococcus aureus* can be cultured from the cervix or vagina of those affected.

NURSING CARE PLAN *Infant with a Neurogenic Bladder*

Assessment data: Marguerite is a 2½-month-old infant who has been hospitalized since birth while awaiting adoption. A product of a full-term pregnancy, she was delivered by cesarean section because of cephalopelvic disproportion. An ultrasound performed during labor revealed that she had an extremely large, full bladder. Observation and diagnostic workup during the neonatal period indicated a neurogenic bladder of unknown origin and uncertain prognosis for urinary control. Because of repeated urinary tract infections, the infant has been catheterized 4 times a day to remove residual urine from the bladder and has been placed on prophylactic trimethoprim and sulfamethoxazole (Bactrim). A couple has been found that is interested in adopting her, but is uncertain about being able to care for her bladder problem.

Nursing diagnosis	Intervention	Rationale
1. Reflex incontinence related to neurologic impairment secondary to uninhibited bladder contractions with incomplete emptying	At the 10:00 AM feeding time, remove Marguerite's diapers and observe for urination during or directly after feeding; be sure the infant is warm and loosely covered during feeding.	Most infants void during feeds.
	Record a description of the urine flow.	The description of urine flow can assist with determining pathology.
	Catheterize immediately after urination even if feeding is disrupted; measure and record the postvoid residual.	An accurate postvoid measurement monitors progress.
	Catheterize Marguerite again after feeding at 2, 6, and 10 PM.	Catheterization at regular intervals prevents urine retention and bladder distension.
	Observe Marguerite for bladder distension and irritability.	Bladder distension between catheterizations might indicate the need for more frequent catheterization.
	Observe and report alteration in bowel function.	A neurogenic bladder can be associated with nerve alteration in the bowel.
	Explain to the prospective parents that the infant's bladder dysfunction prevents her from fully emptying her bladder; describe how urine retention can favor organism growth and ascending infection of the urinary tract.	Understanding promotes compliance with a medical regimen.

Outcome: Marguerite's postvoid residuals decrease in amount. She does not demonstrate any bladder distension between catheterizations. The prospective parents can explain the physiologic basis for the treatment.

Nursing diagnosis	Intervention	Rationale
2. Potential for infection (stressors: urine retention, invasive procedure)	Catheterize q.i.d. using a size 8 straight catheter.	Regular removal of residual urine in the bladder reduces potential for organism growth.
	Demonstrate catheterization to prospective parents using clean technique.	Organism growth in the bladder is not appreciably increased with use of clean rather than sterile equipment; procedure is less complicated and more easily managed at home, thus resulting in better compliance.
	Encourage fluids—Enfamil 6 oz five times a day; give water between feedings as the infant will take; if the infant refuses water, diluted apple juice can be given.	Extra fluid dilutes urine and promotes more frequent voiding; juice might be more palatable and it increases urine acidity and possibly slows organism growth.

(Continues)

NURSING CARE PLAN *Infant with a Neurogenic Bladder* (Continued)

Nursing diagnosis	Intervention	Rationale
	Change diapers frequently.	Wet diapers provide a medium for organism growth and multiplication.
	Test urine for culture and sensitivity weekly.	Close monitoring of infection status is necessary to prevent complications from untreated UTI.
	Administer trimethoprim and sulfamethoxazole (Bactrim), ½ tsp twice a day, followed by sips of water.	Prophylactic administraton of antibiotic reduces incidence of UTI; Bactrim syrup is high in sucrose and should be rinsed from the mouth, even in an infant this young, to reduce incidence of damage to erupting teeth.
Outcome: Marguerite remains free from urinary tract infection as evidenced by negative weekly cultures, and absence of fever, irritability, anorexia, or changes in urinary output.		
3. Parental knowledge deficit related to incomplete understanding of home management secondary to inexperience and unfamiliarity with procedures	Clarify information regarding the infant's medical diagnosis and its impact on the prospective family.	Prospective parents need to know that the infant might never be toilet-trained, but eventually will be able to learn self-catheterization if necessary; infections need prompt treatment, and constant vigilance is essential.
	Allow time to answer prospective parents' questions.	This gives the nurse the opportunity to validate parents' understanding of the situation.
	Realistically explain the time commitment involved with the infant's care and problems they will encounter in addition to normal care.	Both prospective parents need to be involved in the infant's care—with both learning to catheterize. This allows greater freedom—one parent should not be tied down with care. Parents should explore resource people in their family or neighborhood who could catheterize the child when they need a vacation.
	Assess parental knowledge of well-child care.	Adoptive parents might have had little or no experience with infants.
	Explore with the prospective father any feelings he might have about catheterizing the infant.	Men and women both might have conflicting feelings about manipulating the genital area of opposite-sex children; allowing them to express their feelings provides a more realistic perspective.
	Teach both prospective parents how to catheterize the infant; observe return demonstration.	Parents must be confident and capable of assuming care before the infant can be discharged.
	Explain adaptations for home management: cleanliness and maintenance of catheters, use of home urine culture kits, how to obtain supplies, sterile urine collection for laboratory culture, positioning and restraint (if necessary) of infant.	The catheterization area at home should be preferably close to a bathroom for easy disposal; the infant should be catheterized on a flat surface at a comfortable height for the parent; no restraint is necessary while the infant is young, but this might need reconsideration when the infant is older and rolls over frequently; sterile urine lab culture kits should be provided for follow-up of a positive home urine culture; catheters should be washed with soap and water, dried with clean cloth and stored in a covered clean container—there is no need to sterilize.

NURSING CARE PLAN *Infant with a Neurogenic Bladder* (Continued)

Nursing diagnosis	Intervention	Rationale
	Teach measures for preventing urinary tract infections: wipe infant from front to back when cleaning perineal area, change diapers frequently, avoid leaving soap in the tub when giving baths, and encourage increased fluid intake.	These are measures that prevent urinary tract infection.

Outcome: Both prospective parents are interested in participating in Marguerite's care. Both can demonstrate skill with catheterizing. Both parents express confidence in caring for Marguerite. Both parents state they also feel confident and knowledgeable about well-child care.

Clinical manifestations The patient with TSS demonstrates a sudden onset of symptoms, usually around the time of menstruation. Nausea, severe vomiting, profuse liquid diarrhea, high fever (above 102°F), and severe abdominal pain might be the initial symptoms. These can be followed by signs of central nervous system alterations—severe headache, disorientation, irritability, and combativeness. On admission to the hospital, signs of fluid volume deficit with extensive peripheral edema, shock, and a diffuse erythematous rash are apparent. Involvement of the renal, hepatic, hematologic, respiratory, and integumentary systems also is likely. Desquamation of the hands and feet similar to that seen in scarlet fever occurs approximately a week after disease onset.

Diagnostic evaluation Laboratory values are altered according to the affected systems. There might be elevated levels of blood urea nitrogen, serum creatinine, bilirubin, and liver function studies. Altered bleeding and prothrombin times indicate hematologic involvement. Platelet levels become elevated after an initial thrombocytopenia. A highly elevated white count indicates infection.

Treatment Treatment for TSS is supportive. Massive fluid volume replacement with intravenous colloids is essential to reverse the effects of shock. Pulmonary therapy for lung involvement, heparin administration in conjunction with blood replacement for platelet and clotting alterations, and dialysis to restore fluid and electrolyte balance might be indicated. A course of antibiotic therapy can eradicate *Staphylococcus aureus* from vaginal secretions and possibly prevent recurrence of the disease. Although most patients recover, some might be left with residual damage to lungs or the peripheral vascular system.

Nursing management Intensive nursing observation is essential during the acute stage of TSS to recognize any deterioration in the patient's condition. Nursing care includes taking vital signs hourly, accurately recording intake and output, and monitoring for signs of impending renal failure or respiratory distress.

Toxic shock syndrome in adolescents, as in adult women, can be life threatening and requires critical-care nursing. The nurse is aware of family anxiety and should be available to answer questions. Information about the treatment should be provided and reassurance given when appropriate.

Discharge preparation includes teaching about perineal hygiene. Education regarding tampon use is an important nursing responsibility and a preventive measure. Those who have not had TSS can use tampons but should follow the following recommendations.

1. Alternate tampons with sanitary pads for light flow.
2. Change tampons frequently—every 1 to 8 hours for heavy to moderate flow.
3. Wash hands thoroughly prior to inserting the tampon.
4. Contact a physician immediately if sudden fever, vomiting, and diarrhea occur during the menstrual period, and immediately remove the tampon.

Patients who have had TSS should wait three months after the attack before resuming tampon use. For heavy menstrual flow, tampons can be used if changed every 1 to 4 hours. Tampons alternating with pads at night are recommended for moderate flow and pads only for light flow (Whettam, 1984).

Sexually Transmitted Diseases

Sexually transmitted diseases (STDs) are diseases transmitted primarily through sexual contact. These diseases can involve anal-genital, oral, ocular, and other body regions and are caused by a variety of bacteria, viruses, fungi, and other organisms.

The phenomenal increase in STDs since the 1960s has been attributed to many factors, such as increased sexual freedom without fear of pregnancy and a more permissive moral and social climate. Regardless of the reasons, STDs are occurring at significant levels in all strata of society.

Of primary concern is the extremely high incidence in people 15–24 years of age. The 15- to 19-year-olds in particular pose a difficult problem in that they might have restricted access to health care facilities and therefore might delay or avoid treatment. The nurse's role in teaching these adolescents and structuring health care environments receptive to their needs is essential (see Chapter 11).

It is mandatory to report many STDs to state health departments for identification and treatment of contacts and for compilation of health statistics. Nursing care of adolescents with STDs involves teaching effective methods for prevention. Promoting community awareness and responsible sex and health education is an additional nursing responsibility. Table 28-2 presents the most frequently seen STDs. Recently, chlamydial infections have become the most prevalent STD in the United States. Because they have not been reportable, their exact incidence is unknown.

The Child with a Structural Defect Involving the Genitourinary System

Hydronephrosis

Any partial or complete obstruction in the urinary tract can cause *hydronephrosis,* urine collection in the renal pelvis and calices. If the obstruction is uncorrected, intrarenal pressure rises, cyst formation is initiated, and circulation to the kidney is diminished. Eventually, there is atrophy of renal tissue leading to renal insufficiency.

Obstructions can occur anywhere in the urinary tract and can be congenital or acquired. They occur most frequently at the ureteral-pelvic junction (Fig. 28-1). Obstruction here occurs when abnormal muscle function within the ureter impairs the flow of urine from the kidney. Renal pelvic dilatation follows, and further mechanical obstruction occurs. Some other causes of obstruction include calculi (stones) and scar tissue or adhesions from inflammation.

Hydronephrosis can be unilateral or bilateral. The prognosis is directly related to the timing of diagnosis and intervention. If substantial irreparable damage is done to the renal tissue prior to intervention, chronic renal insufficiency persists.

Clinical manifestations There might be a decreased urine flow alternating with a sudden outrush as the rising renal pressure temporarily forces the obstruction aside. A history of repeated urinary tract infections with or without the upper-tract symptoms of flank pain, fever, and chills requires follow-up for hydronephrosis. In addition to flank pain, there can be abdominal pain or a sudden severe pain in the area of the kidney.

Young children might be completely asymptomatic except for a failure to thrive. Failure to thrive without any known or suspected cause indicates the need for a thorough series of urologic tests. Often the diseased kidneys are large enough to be easily palpable. Such tools as an IVP, ultrasound, and VCUG assist with locating the obstruction.

Preventive Teaching Guidelines for Reproductive Infections

Health teaching in the area of reproductive health is a primary responsibility of the nurse. Some guidelines for discussion include these:

Perineal hygiene should be practiced by both partners. Daily baths or showers with particular washing of the genital area might be helpful. Washing after intercourse might be advisable.

Both partners should urinate after sexual intercourse.

Adolescent girls should practice healthy urinary habits such as wiping from front to back, drinking fluids, and voiding regularly.

In order to avoid vaginal irritation, girls should wear cotton, loose-fitting underwear and should avoid bubble baths, hygiene sprays, and douching.

If using additional lubrication for intercourse, use contraceptive foams, creams, or jellies. These might provide some protection against sexually transmitted diseases. Petrolatum lubricants like Vaseline should be avoided as they tend to remain in the vagina and might promote infection.

Those who are sexually active with more than one partner should try to discriminate carefully and use condoms if at all possible.

TABLE 28-2 Sexually Transmitted Diseases

Disease	Causative organism	Epidemiology	Treatment	Nursing implication
Chlamydia trachomatis	*Chlamydia trachomatis* (tiny, viruslike bacteria) identified by culture and antigen tests; incidence over two million a year	Occurs in the sexually active; higher incidence in adolescents; risk increases with the number of sexual partners; can infect neonates of infected mothers with conjunctivitis, otitis, and pneumonia; symptoms of abdominal pain, vaginal discharge, proctitis, epididymitis	Three week course of tetracycline; erythromycin or sulfa for children and pregnant adolescents	Barrier contraception decreases risk, oral contraceptives increase risk; can cause sterility, ectopic pregnancies, and urethritis (in males)
Gonorrhea	*Neisseria gonorrhoeae* gram negative diplococcus; confirmed through cultures of infected sites—urethra, vagina, cervix, and rectum	Occurs in the sexually active; affects males and females equally, although symptoms are more acute in males; purulent discharge can be associated with urethritis, cervicitis, and symptoms of pelvic inflammatory disease; neonatal ophthalmia gonorrhea can cause blindness if not prevented	4.8 million units of procaine penicillin G IM or 3.5 G of oral ampicillin in a single dose; tetracycline if the organism is penicillin resistant	Incidence of fallopian tube adhesions and sterility is relatively high; gonorrhea in young children is suspect for child abuse; a systemic infection is possible with arthralgia, fever, chills, and skin lesions or rash; can be associated with syphilis
Herpes genitalis	*Herpes simplex* type II virus diagnosis based on clinical findings of lesions; titer for herpes antibody can be helpful	Transmitted by direct contact with lesions; virus can remain latent in the body causing recurrences; crossover between herpes II and herpes I (cold sores) is possible but not likely; symptoms include fever, malaise, burning sensation in area of erupting lesions; lesions are initially vesicular but quickly ulcerate	Spontaneous recovery in 3–6 weeks: recurrences can occur lasting 7–10 days and can be triggered by stress or illness; acetaminophen or aspirin for pain; sitz baths and heat lamp might promote drying of lesions	Genital herpes during pregnancy can cause spontaneous abortion (less than 20 weeks) or severe brain damage and congenital anomalies in infected neonates; cesarean delivery is preferred for women with active disease to prevent neonatal infection; increased risk of cervical cancer is associated with herpes
Syphilis	*Treponema pallidum* diagnosed by VDRL	Transmitted by sexual contact or congenitally; single chancre (ulceration) at exposure site resolves in 3–5 weeks (primary); secondary symptoms include symmetric rash and lymphadenopathy with flulike symptoms; tertiary stage can occur years after exposure and causes severe neurologic and cardiovascular disease	Penicillin; VDRL should be done at 3-month intervals for up to 2 years following treatment	Congenital syphilis is transmitted through the placenta after the 18th week of pregnancy; VDRLs are performed on pregnant women, usually at 7 months

(Continues)

TABLE 28-2 Sexually Transmitted Diseases *(Continued)*

Disease	Causative organism	Epidemiology	Treatment	Nursing implication
Vaginitis	Foreign bodies, nonspecific organisms, intestinal parasites, UTIs, *Candida albicans*, inadequate perineal hygiene	Common in females of all age groups; allergic vaginitis results from allergen or irritant in vagina such as vaginal sprays, douches, soaps, perfumes, powders; recent change in sexual partner can introduce new flora; intense itching might be associated with a thick white discharge *(Candida)*	Removal of allergen or foreign body; application of topical antifungal agents for 7–14 days to treat *Candida*—mycostatin is most commonly used; can be followed in 1–2 weeks by single dose of mycostatin-based vaginal suppository	Sitz baths might relieve itching and inflammation; *Candida* can be precipitated by antibiotic therapy and those antibiotics associated with it should be avoided; tampons should be removed frequently and attention sought if tampon becomes impossible to remove
Trichomonas vaginalis	Protozoa	Transmitted by sexual contact and possibly indirectly by bathing articles; highest incidence in females age 16–35 years (Noble, 1979); appearance of frothy, yellow-green foul-smelling discharge in copious amounts; severe itching and excoriation of vulva and perineum; asymptomatic in males	Metronidazole (Flagyl) to both partners after positive wet prep	Persons receiving metronidazole should not drink alcohol because of side effects of nausea and vomiting; not to be given during pregnancy

Treatment The goal of treatment is to preserve remaining renal function. The surgeon might excise the cause of obstruction (calculi, stricture) or reconstruct structural abnormalities (ectopic ureter, malformed ureter). Urinary diversion might be used as a temporary measure to decrease intrarenal pressure. It is accomplished by inserting a nephrostomy tube to drain the renal pelvis while awaiting surgery. If the routine surgical approaches to correct the obstruction are not feasible, nephrectomy might be considered.

Nursing management The child with hydronephrosis might be asymptomatic. If the nurse's physical assessment reveals mild discomfort, pain in the abdomen or flank, or diminished urine output, the nurse might suspect the presence of this condition. An accurate history from observant parents might indicate a gradual decrease in the number of voids if the child is still in diapers, but once the child is toilet-trained it becomes difficult for parents to provide this information.

Nursing care for the child with hydronephrosis is directed toward identifying and relieving the urinary stasis. Care is similar to that of any child undergoing genitourinary surgery. If the child is discharged with a nephrostomy, parents should be able to demonstrate tube and skin care and should be taught to prevent and recognize signs of infection. Long-term follow-up is essential.

Obstructive Anomalies of the Collecting System

Most anomalies of the urinary collecting system lead to restriction of urinary flow from the bladder. Although the causes might vary, treatment and nursing management are similar. The most frequent causes of flow restriction are urethral stricture (tightening or spasm of the urethral muscle) and posterior urethral valves (abnormal folds of mucosa at the male urethral opening).

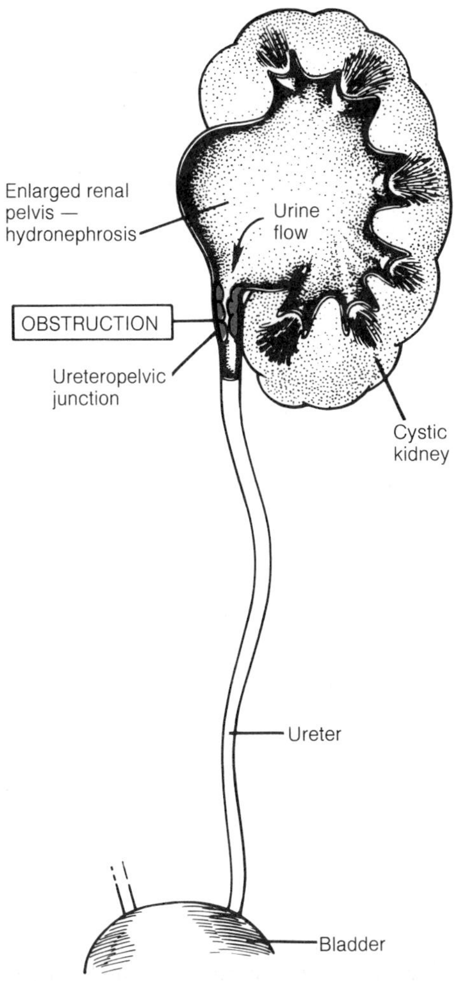

FIGURE 28-1

Obstruction at the utereropelvic junction impedes normal flow of urine from kidney to bladder. The collection of urine in the renal pelvis and calyces leads to hydronephrosis, cystic kidney, reduction of kidney circulation, and permanent kidney damage.

Treatment The usual intervention for mild stricture is urethral dilatation. Circumcision also might be indicated for boys. Catheterization can be necessary if the condition is acute or if dilatation is initially unsuccessful. Treatment for posterior urethral valves usually requires a long-term indwelling catheterization or surgical excision of the extraneous tissue.

Nursing management Assessment of voiding patterns and observation of the urinary stream is helpful in determining the extent of the flow obstruction. The plan of care is designed to assist in the restoration of urine flow and to prevent urinary stasis and the subsequent development of urinary tract infection. Close supervision of intake and output is essential along with observations of signs of retention (decreased output, bladder distension). If catheter drainage is to be used after the child's discharge, teaching begins as soon as possible. The child should become accustomed to the collecting device and clothing should be adapted to minimize the appearance of the device.

Exstrophy of the Bladder

Exstrophy of the bladder is a congenital malformation in which the lower portion of the abdominal wall and anterior wall of the bladder fail to fuse during fetal development. The bladder is visualized through the abdominal opening, revealing bladder mucosa and observable ureteral orifices. Hypospadias and epispadias (abnormal position of meatus on the penis) and other genital or bowel problems can be associated with this condition.

Because of the open bladder, there is constant drainage of urine. The fragility of the bladder mucosa as well as the direct access to the upper urinary tract through the open ureters predisposes the child to frequent infections.

The occurrence of bladder exstrophy is rare and is seen more frequently in boys. Children with exstrophy of the bladder are unlikely to attain normal urologic status. Simple closure is most often unsuccessful. Achieving continence without further diversion is unlikely.

Treatment Complete bladder turn-in might be attempted but is rarely successful. Its success usually depends on the amount of exposed bladder, and it involves more than one reconstructive procedure. Urinary diversion by ileal loop conduit is the treatment of choice. The surgeon takes a small portion of the ileum, sutures it to the ureters, which have been resected from the bladder, and to the skin, creating a stoma. Urine drains from the ureters, through the stoma, into a collecting appliance. Ileal conduit is favored over ureterostomies (both ureters brought to the skin) because it results in a single opening rather than bilateral openings. Reconstructive surgery is performed on the genitals to improve sexual function. Removal of the bladder might be included in the long-range plan.

Nursing management Exstrophy of the bladder is immediately noticeable at birth. During the newborn assessment, the nurse notes the size and extent of the defect, the condition of the mucosa, and the appearance of the surrounding skin (that is, color, amount, and turgor). Nursing interventions are directed toward preserving the integrity of the bladder mucosa, preventing an ascending infection, and maintaining fluid balance.

Frequent dressing or diaper changes will prevent skin breakdown and opportunity for infection. The dressing consists of a light petrolatum (Vaseline) gauze or a piece of cloth diaper covered with petrolatum. Petrolatum prevents adherence of the dressing to the fragile mucosa. Dressings are removed carefully to minimize bleeding.

The nurse supports the parents during their grieving process and their adjustment to their child's defect. Many questions and anxieties will surface, not only about urinary functions but also about appearance and the child's future reproductive capabilities.

Discharge teaching prior to reconstruction of the genitals includes proper dressing changes, infection control methods, and recognition of signs of infection or altered urinary function. Additional fluids will be needed in response to high temperature, infection, or hot weather. Home care should be adapted from that received during hospitalization. Every attempt should be made to provide a plan of care that is as uncomplicated as possible for the ease of the child and family. Parents are encouraged to promote the child's normal development while protecting the bladder from trauma. They need to be prepared to help their children deal with functional or cosmetic problems. Counseling might be advisable for families having difficulties in this area.

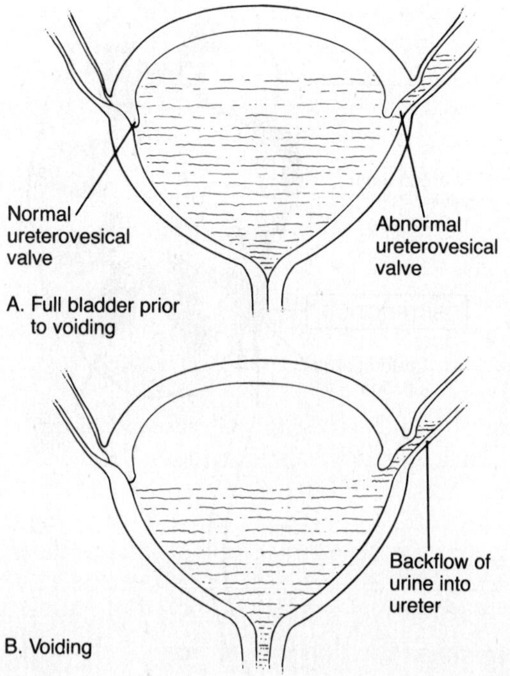

FIGURE 28-2
Vesicoureteral reflux.

Reflux Anomalies of the Collecting System

Reflux is a backflow of urine into either ureters or bladder, depending on location of the anomaly. Vesicoureteral reflux (Fig. 28-2) is the reflux of urine from the bladder into the ureters caused by defective implantation of the ureters. Urethrovesical reflux is a backflow of urine from the urethra into the bladder.

Both types of reflux cause persistent urinary tract infections and possible hydronephrosis. Abnormalities can be detected with IVP, VCUG, and cystoscopy. The prognosis for reflux is favorable with early detection.

Treatment Antibiotics are administered to treat the urinary tract infection. If the child does not respond to several months of medication, surgery might be recommended. Surgical reimplantation of the ureters in vesicoureteral reflux is the procedure of choice.

Nursing management Most ureteral reimplantation procedures involve the use of ureteral catheters or stents during the postoperative course. The stents are covered by sterile dressings and drain into a collecting apparatus. Initial gross hematuria is followed by gradual clearing as the postoperative period progresses. In addition to the stents, the child will have either a suprapubic or a straight catheter. Prior to discharge, all catheters are removed. The child is followed closely by a urologist after discharge.

Urethrovesical reflux can be minimized by attention to voiding patterns. The child is encouraged to void in a continuous stream and to empty the bladder completely. Nurses need to urge parents to observe for this. School teachers can be warned to allow the child sufficient time and opportunity for voiding during the school day.

Anomalies of the External Structures—Phimosis

Phimosis is a condition in which the prepuce is nonretractable from the glans penis. The foreskin contracts over the meatus, creating a diminished opening. Urine stream is obstructed and urination occurs only by force. The condition occurs mainly in uncircumcised boys.

A decreased urinary stream is the first sign. The pressure exerted on the area during urination causes inflammation of the foreskin with an infectious process leading to scarring and further adhesion of the foreskin to the glans.

Circumcision is the treatment of choice. This procedure involves excision of the foreskin to release the glans. Routine preoperative and postoperative nursing care is required. Older boys need careful explanation and demonstration of the surgical procedure. They need reassurance that the circumcision not only will relieve the problem but also will not destroy the function of the penis, although adjustment will have to be made to the alteration in its appearance. Postoperatively, the penis is covered with a petrolatum gauze. The site is tender for several days. The child is encouraged to void despite the burning that might be felt at the operative site.

Phimosis can be prevented easily with good nursing intervention. Neonatal circumcision usually prevents its occurrence, but circumcision is no longer recommended by the American Academy of Pediatrics as a routine procedure. Parents are taught to clean an uncircumcised penis properly. The foreskin need not be forcibly retracted for effective cleaning. Forcible retraction can cause inflammation leading to phimosis; thus the foreskin should be retracted gently and only to the point of resistance.

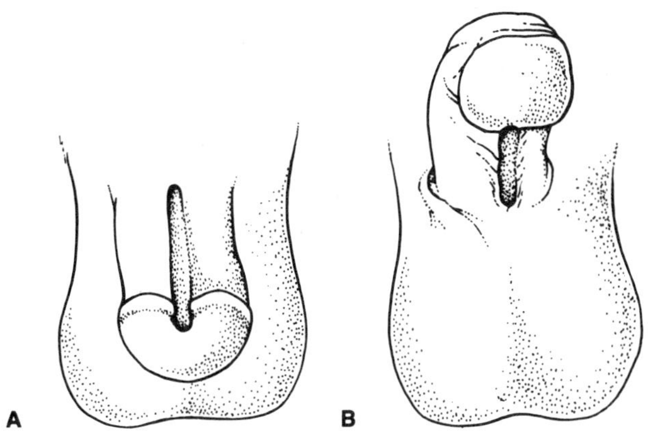

FIGURE 28-3

Anomalies of the penis. ***A.*** *Penile epispadias with dorsal chordee.* ***B.*** *Penile hypospadias with chordee.*

Anomalies of the External Structures—Epispadias and Hypospadias

Other anomalies of the penis include epispadias and hypospadias. Both of these conditions result in abnormal placement of the urinary meatus. Epispadias is rare, while hypospadias occurs more frequently and appears to have a familial tendency.

Clinical manifestations The urinary meatus in the child with hypospadias is located on the ventral surface of the penis on the shaft or near the glans. A less common site for the urethral opening is the scrotum or perineum. *Chordee,* a fibrous line of tissue causing a downward curve of the penis, is associated with this condition (Fig. 28-3). The extent of the chordee depends on the location of the meatus; that is, the farther back on the penis the location of the meatus, the greater the amount of chordee. The presence of a chordee can affect the child's future reproductive capabilities as well as his body image.

The urinary meatus in epispadias is on the dorsal surface of the penis. Epispadias also might be associated with abnormal fusion of the anterior abdominal wall, pubis, and bladder.

Treatment Urinary continence varies with the severity of the deformity. Urinary diversion often is necessary to achieve continence with epispadias. Management is the same as that for exstrophy of the bladder.

A satisfactory hypospadias repair straightens the penis; the child is then able to void while standing and ultimately will have the ability to inseminate directly. The single-stage repair usually is more successful than multistaged repairs, although it is not always feasible. In the one-stage repair, a skin graft or flap is used to extend the urethra to the tip of the penis. The chordee is released at the same time. If the urethra lies near the scrotum or in the perineum, a multistage repair is best The chordee is released initially. Subsequently, urethroplasty is performed in stages. A flap of penile skin is removed and an extended urethra is created with it. The meatus is then constructed as close to the tip of the glans as possible.

Nursing management Hypospadias or epispadias is discovered in the nursery by an alert nurse who discovers the abnormal meatus on assessment. Notation of any alteration in voiding is helpful to support the diagnosis. It is important for the nurse to assess the parent's understanding of the anomaly and the proposed plan for reconstruction.

Because reconstruction takes place during early childhood when fears of mutilation are prominent, the child's developmental, emotional, and psychologic needs are an important concern. Questions and fears might focus on genital manipulation and castration anxiety.

The child will have a modified catheter following corrective surgery for hypospadias. Dressing changes are specifically ordered by the surgeon, since considerable damage can be done if dressing changes are handled improperly. Frequently, the dressing is left untouched for several days as the skin graft flap heals.

It is beneficial to encourage diversional activities within the limits of extremity restraints, bed cradle, and prolonged immobilization after surgery. A normally active 2- to 5-year-old will present a particular nursing challenge. Encouraging imagination and using action toys can distract the child and make activity restrictions easier. The child and family should be well informed, prepared, and involved in the decisions about timing of admissions, or other aspects, whenever feasible.

Cryptorchidism

Cryptorchidism, or undescended testicle, is the failure of one or both of the testes to descend into the scrotum (usually during the seventh to ninth month of gestation). Failure to descend can be related to hormonal deficiency or mechanical problems such as a narrow inguinal canal, a short spermatic cord, or adhesions (Saxton et al., 1983). Because proper function of the testes depends on a temperature cooler than 98.6°F, failure to descend leads to decreased function and eventual atrophy of the gonad. Undescended testicles can be associated in some cases with an inguinal hernia on the involved side. True undescended testicles should not be confused with retraction of the testes in response to cold during examination (caused by spasm of the crimasteric muscle).

Treatment The testes descend spontaneously in many children during infancy. Orchidopexy is the preferred treatment for testes that do not descend spontaneously. The testis is surgically brought down into the scrotal sac and kept in position for several days by any number of different traction devices, such as a button on the outer scrotal surface or an elastic band attached to the thigh. The type of device is chosen by the surgeon. If the testis cannot be positioned correctly, the surgeon might remove it to minimize the risk of malignancy.

The prognosis varies with the timing of the repair. If cryptorchidism persists into adolescence, sterility can result. Risk of malignancy is elevated if atrophy occurs.

Nursing management In addition to routine preoperative preparation, the preoperative teaching includes a description of the tension device to be used. Postoperatively, the nurse checks the device for proper tautness. Bed rest is maintained until the tension suture is removed, usually in a few days. In conjunction with analgesics, ice packs often are indicated to relieve pain and to enable the child to tolerate keeping the leg extended. A bed cradle keeps pressure from bedclothing off the operative site.

The Child with a Problem with Filtration of Wastes

Acute Glomerulonephritis

Acute glomerulonephritis (AGN) is an immune complex disease that occurs in response to a previous invasion of group A beta-hemolytic streptococcus. The precipitating streptococcal infection usually affects the upper respiratory tract or skin (impetigo). Theories about causes of AGN differ, but the prevalent theory indicates that AGN might be an autoimmune response (see Chapter 25).

Autoimmune complexes lodge in the glomerulus and Bowman's capsule, leading to inflammation and obstruction. This process causes decreased glomerular filtration and tissue injury at the site. Consequently, less sodium and water are passed to the tubules for reabsorption and excretion. Because of the damage to the glomerular membrane, red blood cells and casts are excreted. The kidneys enlarge, and sodium and water are retained, leading to edema. Because of the increase in extracellular plasma volume, protein is excreted in the urine (Fig. 28-4).

The incidence of AGN varies with the environmental prevalence of streptococcal strains. The disease more frequently affects boys during early childhood. The prognosis for children with AGN is generally favorable, with the disease resolving spontaneously after a period of several weeks.

Clinical manifestations Hematuria and mild periorbital edema might be the first clinical manifestations. The urine can appear grossly bloody or be a dark brownish color (cola colored). As the disease progresses, the child might experience mild generalized edema (often evidenced only by weight gain), oliguria (decreased urine output), fever, anorexia, hypertension, and, rarely, central nervous system symptoms (headache, seizures). The child is at high risk for developing pulmonary edema or renal insufficiency. Occasionally there can be evidence of a transient nephrotic syndrome (see p. 956).

Diagnostic evaluation Urinalysis reveals white blood cells, red blood cells, protein, and cellular casts. There is an associated increase in urine specific gravity. Blood chemistries are elevated, especially blood urea nitrogen and serum creatinine. There also is an elevated erythrocyte sedimentation rate (ESR) and antistreptolysin titer (ASO) indicating exposure to streptococcal infection. Hemoglobin and hematocrit are decreased from hematuria.

Treatment Treatment necessitates hospitalization to monitor the disease progress and for recognition and prompt treatment of complications. Antibiotics are prescribed to treat any existing streptococcal infection. Careful and frequent monitoring of urinary output, weight, blood pressure, and blood chemistries helps to determine the fluid requirements. It is important to monitor carefully the fluid and electrolyte balance to reduce the risks of cardiac or renal failure. The child might be confined to bed, although some quiet activity is allowed. Children tend to mod-

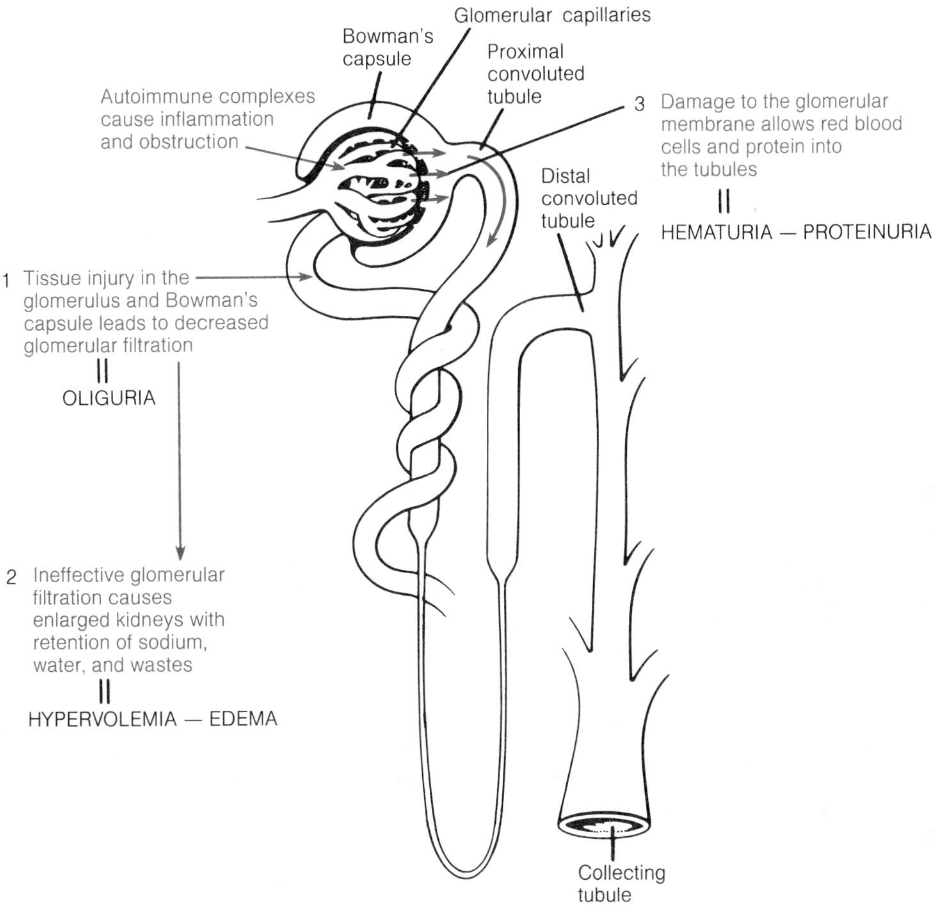
Glomerular capillaries
Bowman's capsule
Proximal convoluted tubule
Autoimmune complexes cause inflammation and obstruction
3 Damage to the glomerular membrane allows red blood cells and protein into the tubules
HEMATURIA — PROTEINURIA
Distal convoluted tubule
1 Tissue injury in the glomerulus and Bowman's capsule leads to decreased glomerular filtration
OLIGURIA
2 Ineffective glomerular filtration causes enlarged kidneys with retention of sodium, water, and wastes
HYPERVOLEMIA — EDEMA
Collecting tubule

FIGURE 28-4

Alterations in acute glomerulonephritis. (Adapted from Spence AP, Mason EB: Human Anatomy and Physiology, *3rd ed. Benjamin/Cummings, 1987).*

ify their activities according to their own tolerance. Children manifesting moderate hypertension might need antihypertensives.

If renal insufficiency is present, the child's fluid intake is generally restricted. Peritoneal dialysis can be used in cases of severe renal or cardiopulmonary problems.

Increased caloric intake is necessary to decrease tissue breakdown. If renal insufficiency is demonstrated, a low-potassium diet is recommended. Other dietary restrictions, such as low-protein or low-salt diets, vary but are generally unnecessary. Sensible limitation of protein and sodium, however, is desirable. Diuresis usually begins after several days and indicates a resolving disease process.

Nursing management The nurse assesses the family's awareness of the precipitating streptococcal infection. Physical examination identifies any clinical manifestations such as edema, weight gain, hematuria, and elevated blood pressure.

The goal of nursing management is to preserve renal integrity and prevent complications. Strict monitoring of intake and output is essential, as is daily weight measurement. Vital signs, serum electrolyte values, and urine examination results all are good indicators of the status of renal function. The child is observed for signs of renal deterioration such as diminished output or a change in laboratory values. Additionally, anxiety relief measures and quiet diversional therapy assist in the child's acceptance of the disease.

Discharge preparation includes encouraging follow-up blood pressures to confirm renal integrity. Parents might need to strip-test the urine for blood, although hematuria can be present to some degree for several weeks after other symptoms have disappeared.

Prevention of infection is important during this recovery period, since any infectious process will create excess strain on the kidneys. Although recurrences are rare, they are possible. Oral antibiotics are prescribed if there is a question of a repeat infection.

Acute glomerulonephritis is usually a self-limiting disease, resolving in approximately 14 days. Although further renal difficulties are uncommon, the child and family need to be alert to signs of renal complications. Long-term follow-up to assess renal status is necessary.

Nephrosis—Nephrotic Syndrome

Nephrosis is a syndrome, a group of conditions, characterized by proteinuria, hypoproteinemia (decreased serum protein), hyperlipemia (increased serum lipids), edema, ascites, and decreased urine output. Although its etiology is obscure, it is felt to be the result of an alteration of the glomerular membrane making it permeable to plasma proteins (especially albumin).

Plasma proteins enter the tubule and are excreted in the urine (causing proteinuria). The protein shift causes fluid from the plasma to seep into the interstitial spaces, resulting in lower circulating plasma volume (hypovolemia) and interstitial edema.

Hypovolemia activates the production of renin and angiotensin to stimulate adrenal secretion of aldosterone. Aldosterone in turn increases the reabsorption of sodium and water in the distal tubule. Additionally, lowered osmotic pressure of the blood triggers the production of ADH, thus further increasing the reabsorption of water. The generalized movement of water through the interstitial spaces adds to the edema (Fig. 28-5). The increase in blood lipids, especially cholesterol, might be due to metabolic error or might be an increase in production secondary to lowered serum albumin.

The course of the disease consists of exacerbations and remissions over a period of weeks to years. Treatment effectively shortens exacerbations. The disease can occur secondarily to other disease entities such as glomerulonephritis, lupus erythematosus, diabetes mellitus, and allergic responses. In the large majority of children with nephrosis, however, the cause is unknown. The prognosis is somewhat unpredictable since the disease can recur, although increased renal damage does not always occur.

Clinical manifestations Insidious or acute generalized edema usually is the first sign of nephrosis. Edema can be periorbital but is worse in the scrotum and abdomen (where it results in ascites). Affected children have such severe generalized edema that they experience dramatic weight gain. In addition to having edema, the child is pale, fatigued, and anorexic. Gastrointestinal symptoms can be present, and the ascitic abdomen demonstrates visible networks of blood vessels.

Urinary output is decreased. The urine might be dark and frothy from increased fat excretion and has an elevated specific gravity.

Children with nephrosis often experience respiratory distress from the fluid overload. They can demonstrate an increased susceptibility to infection, which is probably secondary to the decrease in plasma protein. Exacerbations of edema often occur after a recent infection. Malnutrition and muscle wasting can occur as a result of protein depletion but might not be noticed until the edema disappears.

Diagnostic evaluation Urinalysis reveals elevated protein excretion, as much as 30–40 g of plasma protein per day (Vick, 1984). Serum levels of blood urea nitrogen and creatinine usually are normal unless there is associated renal disease. The longer the edema lasts, the greater the chance of permanent renal damage. Blood cholesterol levels are increased because of the increase in circulating blood lipids. The ESR is elevated.

Treatment Treatment is directed toward decreasing the excretion of urinary protein and controlling edema. Additional goals include infection prevention, restoration of metabolic balance, prevention of renal damage, and correction of malnutrition.

Corticosteroids are prescribed to resolve the edema quickly. The child is maintained on steroids up to 12 months at the physician's discretion. Other pharmacologic therapy includes antibiotics for bacterial infections and thiazide diuretics during the edematous stage. Immunosuppressive drugs might be prescribed alone or in conjunction with steroids for children who do not respond well to steroids alone. In some instances anticancer drugs such as cyclophosphamide (Cytoxan) are effective in initiating remission. Diuresis and decreasing proteinuria signal remission. To prevent or control malnutrition, a diet high in protein is desirable. Salt is avoided and fluids limited.

Nursing management The nursing care for the child with nephrosis is similar to care for the child with glomerulonephritis, for much of the emphasis is on supportive measures. Although the prognosis for children with nephrosis is generally favorable, the course might be chronic.

The classical physical appearance of the child with nephrosis is one of lethargy, edema, pallor, and fatigue. Nursing management of these children therefore emphasizes rest and comfort measures with conservation of energy.

An accurate intake and output record, along with careful and frequent weight monitoring, assists the nurse to assess disease progress. Frequent urine checks for the presence of protein are essential. Measurements of abdominal girth correlate with the relative amount of edema. Significant changes in condition are reported to the physician.

The child with nephrosis requires scrupulous skin care because a break in skin integrity can easily cause infection. Frequent position changes are essential. Untrained children need meticulous perineal care because urine acidity predisposes the skin to breakdown. Diapers, whether worn or used as pads, are changed as soon as they are wet. Some of the newer plastic disposable diapers have extra layers to keep moisture from contacting the perineal area. Because of severe scrotal edema, pressure from a diaper might be extremely uncomfortable. In such cases, alternatives can be explored that allow for containing urine without the constriction. The skin around the scrotum should be gently cleaned and allowed to dry thoroughly to minimize skin breakdown. In some circumstances a scrotal support is necessary.

Diversional activities and schoolwork can be encouraged while the child remains in bed. If the course of the illness becomes prolonged, more creative approaches to deal with the problems of long-term immobility are required.

Because steroid therapy is indicated in the management of the child with nephrosis, the child is monitored for drug side effects. Unfortunately, many of the side effects of steroid therapy are unpleasant and make the child more uncomfortable. (See Chapter 25 for discussion of nuring care of the child receiving steroid therapy.) It is beneficial to the child and family to know that the side effects of steroid therapy will subside when the therapy is discontinued. Masked infection can be best detected by regular monitoring of the child's vital signs with close supervision of the child's temperature.

Dietary recommendations present a nursing challenge since it is difficult to encourage an anorexic child to eat the amount of protein required to prevent malnutrition and negative nitrogen balance. Small frequent feedings might be more palatable than larger meals; for example, baked custard can easily conceal an additional egg for extra protein.

Discharge preparation includes information about medications and their effects and about dietary maintenance. The parent might wish to speak to a dietitian to learn about incorporating the high amount of protein required into a palatable menu. Urine monitoring for protein is essential, although the testing method will vary. It is important to emphasize protection from infection, while encouraging normal activities.

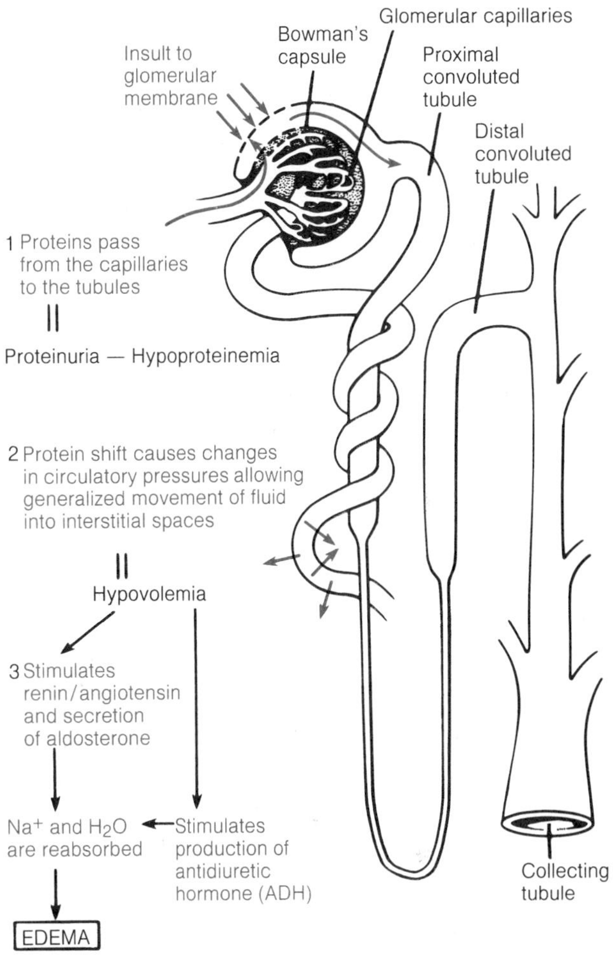

FIGURE 28-5

Alterations in nephrotic syndrome. (Adapted from Spence AP, Mason EB: Human Anatomy and Physiology, *3rd ed. Benjamin/Cummings, 1987).*

Acute Renal Failure—Acute Tubular Necrosis

Acute renal failure is caused by insult and damage to the renal tissue with resulting abnormalities in kidney function. The major clinical manifestations in acute renal failure are *azotemia,* or accumulation of nitrogenous wastes in the blood, and *oliguria,* urine output of less than 0.1 mL/kg/hr. Acute renal failure can be the result of prerenal factors, postrenal factors, or intrarenal factors. *Prerenal factors* include any problems affecting fluid volume of the circulation before it reaches the kidneys, such as loss of fluid and electrolytes from burns, diarrhea, and hemorrhage, or conditions such as congestive heart failure that decrease cardiac output. *Postrenal factors* include conditions that obstruct the renal system distal to the kidney tubules.

Approximately 75% of all cases of renal failure occur from *intrarenal factors* (Mars and Treloar, 1984), leading to acute tubular necrosis (ATN). Injury (either ischemic or nephrotoxic) to the renal tubules occurs when perfusion to the kidneys is reduced or from nephron damage by inflammation or by toxic agents. Injury causes tissue death (necrosis) with decreased blood flow through the glomeruli. This results in a decrease in the glomerular filtration rate with retention of wastes in the blood. Widespread necrotic patches in the renal tubules then occur, further reducing tubule effectiveness. Contributing factors to the occurrence of acute tubular necrosis in children include prerenal factors that remain uncorrected, infection, hypovolemia with shock, trauma and toxic drugs (particularly aminoglycosides), or chemical exposure.

Clinical manifestations Presenting symptoms in the child with acute renal failure include sudden oliguria and azotemia. Fluid retention and electrolyte imbalances—particularly hyperkalemia—gastrointestinal disturbances, anemia, and increased susceptibility to infection from a depressed immune system are associated symptoms. Some symptoms might be masked by clinical manifestations of underlying diseases.

There are three distinct recovery phases. The *oliguric phase* begins with a marked decrease in urinary output over a 24- to 48-hour period and lasts for approximately 7–14 days. The child's blood urea nitrogen and serum creatinine levels increase. If the cause of the acute renal failure is not hypovolemia, hypervolemia (fluid overload) is a common clinical manifestation. Excess fluid places a strain on the heart and can cause congestive heart failure. Hyperkalemia can cause cardiac irregularities, and the child might experience metabolic acidosis. Because of the decrease in the kidney's production of erythropoietin, a substance that stimulates bone marrow production of red blood cells, the child can experience anemia. Children with acute renal failure can have a decrease in T-lymphocyte production, which makes them more susceptible to infection.

The second phase of acute renal failure, the *diuretic phase,* is marked by a sudden increase in urinary output followed by 4–7 days of further, more gradual diuresis. The BUN continues to rise. Late in this phase the large amount of urine excretion is associated with excessive loss of sodium and potassium, resulting in electrolyte imbalance, the major complication of this phase. A decrease in the BUN signals beginning resolution.

The *recovery phase* lasts 2–3 months or for as long as a year. Tubular function returns, and all laboratory values return to normal. Some children are left with residual kidney damage, and complete recovery depends on resolution of the problem that originally triggered the acute renal failure.

Treatment Treatment of a child with acute renal failure depends on the underlying cause and contributing diseases. Interventions are directed toward restoring and maintaining fluid and electrolyte balance, removing obstructions, managing hypertension, and treating infection. The goal is to prevent permanent renal damage. Specific treatment measures include fluid restriction (unless the cause is hypovolemia), surgical removal of any obstructions, and dialysis to remove nitrogenous wastes and to correct electrolyte and acid-base imbalances until the kidneys can resume proper function. The administration of Kayexalate, a resin that exchanges sodium ions for potassium ions in the gastrointestinal tract, might be ordered if signs of hyperkalemia appear.

A diet high in carbohydrate and low in protein might be required, since the kidneys' ability to manage waste products of protein metabolism is impaired. Antibiotics are prescribed for infection. Aminoglycosides and other antibiotics that are nephrotoxic are avoided. Blood transfusions are ordered for internal bleeding or severe anemia (Hgb < 6 g/100 mL).

Nursing management Nursing interventions are directed toward monitoring and regulating fluid status, recognizing and reducing the effects of electrolyte and acid-base imbalances, preventing infection, providing adequate nutrition, and providing anxiety relief to child and family. Most children with acute renal failure are cared for in critical care units until the recovery phase because of the intensive monitoring they require.

Dialysis Some children with acute renal failure require dialysis to restore homeostasis and correct electrolyte and acid–base imbalances. *Dialysis* is an artificial, mechanical process for removing body wastes and maintaining fluid and electrolyte balance. Indications for treatment by dialysis are

Unresponsive hyperkalemia

Severe metabolic acidosis

Hypervolemia

Severe uremia

Blood urea nitrogen > 150 mg/100 mL

Congestive heart failure

Serum creatinine > 10–15 mg/dL (Reilly, 1983)

The underlying principle of dialysis involves the transport of water and other substances through an artificial or natural semipermeable membrane by the mechanisms of

STANDARDS OF NURSING CARE *The Child with Acute Renal Failure*

RISKS

Assessed risk	Nursing action
Electrolyte imbalance resulting from renal tubular damage	Monitor the ECG and observe for prolonged P-R interval and tall, peaked T-waves. Observe for other signs of hyperkalemia—muscle weakness, numbness and tingling, decreased blood pressure. Monitor electrolyte values (therapy begins when potassium is 5.5—6.0 mEq/L). Restrict dietary potassium. Monitor BUN and creatinine for changes over the course of the disease process. Monitor sodium levels carefully during the diuretic phase. Provide appropriate interventions if a child is being dialized.
Renal shutdown and uremia	Report any signs of deterioration in the child's condition immediately. Signs of impending renal shutdown include anxiety, irritability, seizures, hallucinations, anorexia, nausea, vomiting.

GUIDE FOR NURSING MANAGEMENT

Nursing diagnosis	Intervention	Rationale	Outcome
1. Alteration in fluid volume: excess related to compromised regulatory mechanisms secondary to altered electrolytes, azotemia, and oliguria	Accurately observe and record intake and output; measure urine pH and specific gravity every hour.	Accurate measurement of output is essential in determining the child's fluid status. Normal output is 1 mL/kg/hour. pH and specific gravity provide information about the concentration capabilities of the kidney.	The child's urine pH and specific gravity approach normal limits. The child loses 0.5%–1% body weight daily (Reilly, 1983). The child's urine output increases.
	Weigh frequently—daily or q8h during peritoneal dialysis. Measures need to be extremely accurate, so the same scale and clothing should be used; weigh child being dialized when the child is empty of dialysate.	Accurate weight measurements help determine fluid status.	
	Observe for signs of congestive heart failure and pulmonary edema.	Fluid overload can cause increased cardiac workload with resulting cardiac dysfunction.	
	Take frequent vital signs, particularly blood pressure, as often as every 15 minutes during periods of acute hypertension.	Frequent monitoring of vital signs allows the nurse to recognize complications quickly.	
2. Potential for infection (stressor: invasive procedures)	Administer antibiotics if prescribed.	Antibiotics are used to treat infection. All antibiotics with toxic effects to the kidneys must be avoided or used minimally and with great caution.	The child is free of infection as evidenced by absence of fever, pain, and irritability. Cultures are negative.
	Use strict aseptic technique for dressing changes and catheter care; wash hands frequently.	Aseptic technique decreases the risk of infection.	
	Obtain cultures if signs of infection appear.	Cultures of skin, catheters, urine, or blood help to determine the focus of infection.	

(Continues)

STANDARDS OF NURSING CARE *The Child with Acute Renal Failure (Continued)*

GUIDE FOR NURSING MANAGEMENT

Nursing diagnosis	Intervention	Rationale	Outcome
3. Potential activity intolerance (stressors: internal bleeding and subsequent anemia)	Monitor blood pressure; examine stool for occult blood, and observe for other signs of internal bleeding; administer transfusion if ordered.	Internal bleeding needs to be recognized immediately for treatment to be instituted.	The child appears to rest comfortably and pace activities appropriately.
	Conserve child's energy with organized nursing care; allow for maximum rest.	Well organized nursing care conserves the child's energy by allowing for maximum rest.	
4. Alteration in nutrition: less than body requirements related to hypermetabolic state secondary to imbalance between body's need for and ability to handle proteins	Provide a high calorie diet with protein of high biologic value.	Carbohydrates, proteins, and fats are rapidly metabolized. Protein intake is restricted because of the kidneys' inability to handle protein breakdown. Proteins with high biologic value provide optimum protein for growth with decreased consumption.	The child does not exhibit any signs of muscle wasting, severe weight loss, or malnutrition. The child eats the prescribed high calorie diet.
	Suggest total parenteral nutrition if child is experiencing anorexia, nausea, or vomiting.	It is important to maintain nutritional level if child is unable to eat. Parenteral nutrition can provide an appropriate level of nutrients.	
5. Anxiety of child and family related to perceived threat to health status secondary to uncertainty of the treatments and seriousness of the renal dysfunction	Give frequent explanations of procedures; allow for ventilation of feelings and give reassurance when appropriate; provide for child's developmental needs whenever possible.	Explanations and allowing the child and family to verbalize fears decrease anxiety.	The child and family express a decrease in anxiety level. The family states the nursing staff is available for questions.
	Teach family signs and symptoms of recurring kidney problems; encourage family to follow recommendations of physician for follow-up care.	Teaching the family allows for greater control and participation in care as well as rapid recognition of complications.	The parents can describe the signs and symptoms of recurring kidney problems and know when to contact the physician.

diffusion, osmosis, and hydrostatic pressure (see Chapter 21). Removal of wastes is accomplished by introducing a dialysate consisting of fluid, electrolytes, and glucose to one side of the membrane while the other side contacts the child's blood. The concentration of solutes in the dialysate pulls water, nitrogenous wastes, and potassium from the circulation, while maintaining or correcting serum concentrations of sodium, chloride, and certain other electrolytes. The composition of the dialysate determines the substances that are to be removed from or replaced into the circulation.

There are two major types of dialysis that are used to treat acute renal failure in children—peritoneal dialysis and hemodialysis. In *hemodialysis,* the semipermeable membrane is a sheet of treated cellophane located in a dialysis machine. Blood leaves the body through a cannula that has been inserted into a large vein, such as the femoral vein, or through an arteriovenous shunt or fistula. The blood circulates through the dialysis machine where it contacts the membrane and dialysis occurs. The blood then is pumped back into the body. Hemodialysis in children is an extremely delicate metabolic process. The nursing management of the child undergoing hemodialysis demands an understanding of the biochemical, metabolic, and technical intricacies of the artificial kidney. The nurse functioning in a hemodialysis unit therefore receives extensive orientation and education according to institution protocol.

Peritoneal dialysis is the physical movement of solutes through the semipermeable membrane of the peritoneum, where it comes in contact with the vascular supply of the area. Peritoneal dialysis can be accomplished manually via gravity (Fig. 28-6) or by machine. A catheter is sutured into the peritoneal cavity below the umbilicus. The dialysate is administered through the catheter, allowed to remain in the peritoneum where dialysis occurs, then removed or allowed to drain out.

Nursing interventions start with reassurance and support for the child and family before dialysis begins. A predialysis weight is essential, and children should empty their bladders before the procedure begins, if possible.

While the dialysis procedure is in progress, it is important that the nurse watch for any evidence of blood or purulence in the dialysate fluid. The nurse also maintains and records an accurate measurement of the intake and output of dialysate. The child's vital signs are generally taken every 15 minutes to hourly, when stable. Any major changes should be assessed and reported to the physician, particularly complaints of abdominal pain, sudden onset of profuse watery diarrhea, signs of respiratory distress, and any increase or decrease in blood pressure.

The child's weight and serum electrolytes as well as hemoglobin and hematocrit are monitored closely. If the child voids, the nurse measures the urine specimen for glucose, specific gravity, and presence of blood. The child is observed for signs of hyperglycemia, hypotension, or hypertension. Risks of peritoneal dialysis include infection, perforation of the bowel, and pulmonary edema. With the child lying flat during peritoneal dialysis, nursing interventions need to be directed toward comfort measures and providing distraction.

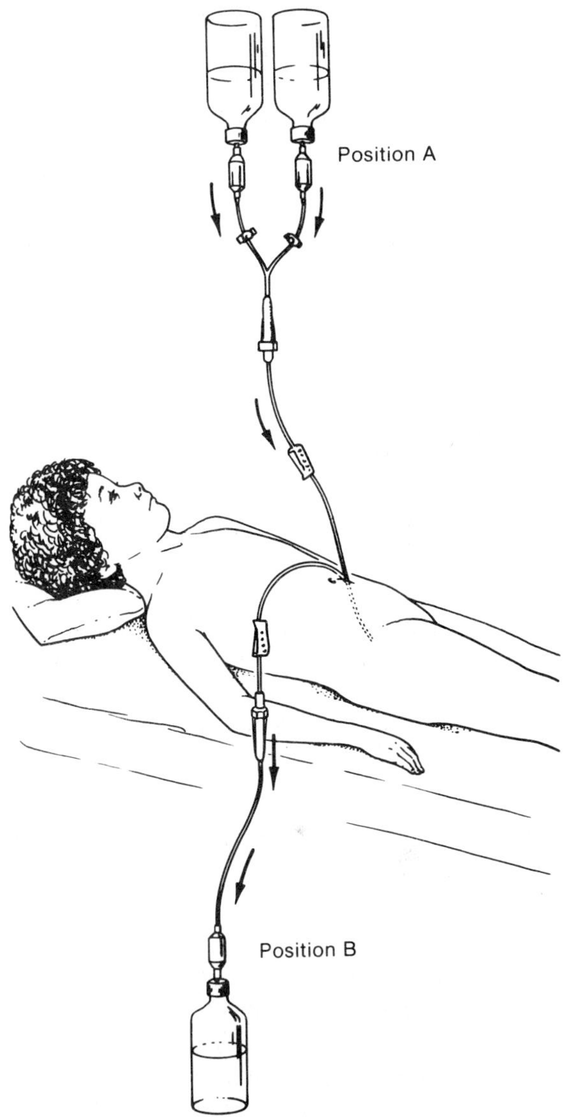

FIGURE 28-6
Manual peritoneal dialysis.

Hemolytic Uremic Syndrome

Hemolytic uremic syndrome (HUS) occurs mainly in children ages 2 months to 8 years. Although relatively rare, it is the most frequent cause of acute renal failure in children.

The etiology of HUS is not presently known, but both infectious agents (viruses and bacteria) and an immunologic response have been suspected. Damage occurs to the endothelial lining of the blood vessels, causing fibrin and platelet clot depositions and thrombocytopenia (decreased circulating platelets). The occlusion of the vessels, which occurs as a result of the deposition, fractures the red blood cells as they pass through the vessels. The damaged cells are quickly destroyed by the liver and spleen, resulting in hemolytic anemia. Because of the damage and occlusion of the vessels forming the glomeruli, acute renal failure develops. Approximately 80%–90% of children with HUS recover completely. Some are left with hypertension (Reilly, 1983).

Clinical manifestations HUS develops in two stages. During the prodromal stage (1–7 days), the child develops abdominal pain with nausea, vomiting, and diarrhea. There might be pallor, fever, irritability, signs of an upper respiratory infection, lymphadenopathy (enlarged lymph glands), skin rash, and edema. The prodromal phase is followed by an acute phase. Symptoms of the acute phase include severe gastroenteritis with bloody diarrhea, hemolytic anemia, hypertension, acute renal failure, and neurologic manifestations that range from irritability to seizures.

Diagnostic evaluation Laboratory studies reveal hemolytic anemia with decreased hemoglobin and hematocrit, thrombocytopenia (less than 140,000/mm^3), increased white blood cell count, BUN greater than 40 mg/100 mL, and increased creatinine. The child will experience hypertension and oliguria (Reilly, 1983).

Treatment The goal of treatment is to correct the hematologic alterations, improve the renal status, and manage the neurologic alterations. The child is placed on kidney dialysis. Aspirin might be given for its inhibitory effect on platelet function. The child is placed on seizure precautions (see Chapter 31).

Nursing management The nursing management of the child with HUS is similar to management of a child with acute renal failure. The nurse protects the child from injury during seizures and performs frequent neurologic checks.

The Child with Chronic Renal Failure

Chronic renal failure occurs as a result of progressive nephron destruction and diminished function of the kidneys over a prolonged period of time. It is said to exist when the kidneys are no longer capable of balancing the composition of body fluids. Symptoms of chronic renal failure are similar to those of acute failure. Elevated creatinine and blood urea nitrogen levels are caused by retention of nitrogenous wastes. Acid-base balance is impaired by the kidneys' inability to reabsorb bicarbonate. Anemia is the result of diminished or absent renal erythropoietin function, impaired release of stored iron, and iron deficiencies. Because the disease is insidious in onset, the body develops a tolerance to adverse effects of imbalance until kidney damage is severe.

Chronic renal failure can be caused by glomerulonephritis, diabetes mellitus, kidney infections, immune system disorders (particularly autoimmune disorders), or any other disorder resulting in kidney damage.

Chronic renal failure is divided into three stages. The first stage presents a decreased renal reserve with slightly impaired function, but blood chemistries are not affected. In the second stage, renal insufficiency is noted, and the glomerular filtration rate is less than 50% of normal. At this point, blood chemistries are affected with slight elevations of blood urea nitrogen and serum creatinine. In the third stage of chronic renal failure, known as end-stage renal disease, the child suffers from azotemia and *uremia* (azotemia plus clinical symptoms related to accumulation of nitrogenous wastes). Renal function is minimal or absent, and blood chemistries are abnormal.

Clinical manifestations The accumulation of nitrogenous wastes in uremia, along with the associated fluid and electrolyte and acid-base imbalances, adversely affects every body system. The child displays weakness, apathy, anorexia, severe bleeding tendencies with anemia, yellow skin, delayed wound healing, respiratory distress, and signs of metabolic acidosis. Signs of hyperkalemia occur when the kidneys no longer are able to handle potassium because of delayed excretion time. Edema is caused by the retention of sodium and fluid from the decreased glomerular filtration rate and continued reabsorption of sodium.

Over the long term, the child experiences alterations in the skeletal system with related growth delay. *Renal osteodystrophy* is a collective term for a variety of bone anomalies that result from the imbalance of calcium and phosphorus. Osteodystrophy is caused by the kidneys' inability to excrete phosphorus and decreased ability to synthesize the active form of vitamin D for calcium utilization. Because calcium is not absorbed from the intestine or utilized, bone resorption occurs, resulting in bone demineralization. The continued high level of serum phosphorus and the chronically depleted calcium causes secondary hyperparathyroidism (see Chapter 29). The excessive secretion of parathyroid hormone causes further demineralization. As a result of these bone changes, the child might experience spontaneous fractures.

The child with chronic renal failure manifests skin alterations. The skin becomes dry and itchy, probably due to hyperparathyroidism. In advanced disease, urea is excreted through the sweat and crystallizes on the skin. This is known as *uremic frost* and is a sign of end-stage renal disease.

If chronic renal failure goes untreated, neurologic manifestations appear. The child will experience coma and death.

Treatment The treatment for chronic renal failure is complex. The goal of conservative management of chronic renal failure is maintenance of metabolic homeostasis, which is achieved by maintaining a delicate balance between nutritional and pharmacologic alterations. As chronic renal failure progresses, biochemical manipulations become necessary, and a dialysis program is initiated.

Dietary management The purpose of strict dietary management in the child with chronic renal failure is to prolong life and postpone as long as possible the need for dialysis. The diet is carefully balanced to provide adequate nutrition for growth while working within the renal limitations. Generally, the diet provides adequate calories while somewhat restricting protein. Electrolytes are closely monitored and dietary intake is regulated according to the child's status.

The child receives 42–91 kcal/kg/day (infants 100–120 kcal/kg/day) (Lopes, 1983). Included in the caloric count is the recommended daily allowance for protein. The major portion of the protein is food with high biologic value such as eggs, milk, meats, and whole grains. Protein might be restricted if the child should start dialysis. Fluid intake is based on the child's fluid output (eg, if output is normal, fluids are not restricted; if the child is oliguric, severe restriction might apply).

If serum potassium levels are elevated, potassium is restricted. Because potassium is present in most fruits, restriction can cause constipation. A diet high in whole grains, vegetables, and low potassium fruits such as apples and strawberries can prevent this problem. Sodium is restricted if the child is hypertensive or demonstrates signs of edema or congestive heart failure.

Phosphorus intake is restricted. Breast milk is lower in phosphorus than cow's milk, so bottle-fed infants might require special formulas to reduce phosphorus intake. Administration of aluminum hydroxide gel interferes with dietary absorption of phosphorus and thus lowers the serum level.

Once the serum phosphorus is decreased, calcium supplements along with the active form of vitamin D (D-25-OH-D3) are prescribed to prevent hypocalcemia and osteodystrophy (Lopes, 1983). Vitamin D in inactive form assists with the absorption and use of calcium. Other vitamins and iron supplementation are recommended.

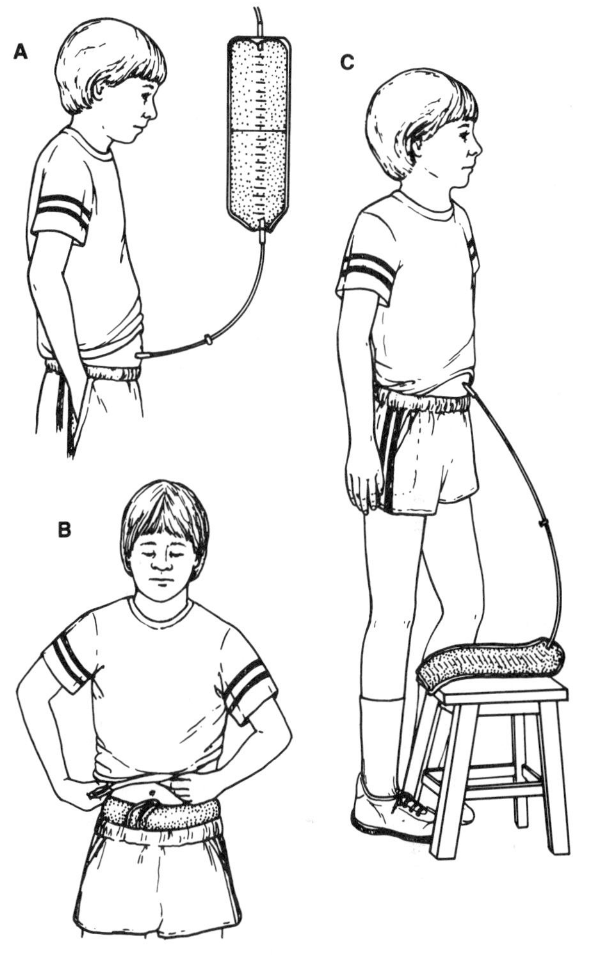

FIGURE 28-7

*Child undergoing continuous ambulatory peritoneal dialysis. **A.** Tenckhoff tube is surgically implanted in abdomen, below umbilicus. Dialysate bag is aseptically attached to tube, and fluid is allowed to flow into peritoneal cavity. **B.** Dialysate remains in peritoneal cavity about 4–6 hours. Bag may be rolled up and tucked under clothing, allowing child to pursue normal activities during dialysis. **C.** Fluid is drained out of peritoneal cavity by unrolling the bag and suspending it below the pelvis, allowing gravity to drain fluid into the bag. After drainage, child aseptically attaches a new bag of dialysate and refills the peritoneal cavity. Procedure is repeated 4–6 times per day.*

Management with dialysis When a decision is made to begin dialysis, a variety of factors are considered. Hemodialysis, although quickly effective, is done usually at a dialysis center, which requires the child to remain in the center for approximately 3–4 hours several days a week. Continuous ambulatory peritoneal dialysis is a relatively new alternative to hemodialysis for ambulatory patients. Its major advantages are the freedom of movement that it allows the child and the capability for management.

A catheter is surgically implanted into the abdomen for instillation of the dialysate. The procedure then involves attaching a bag of dialysate to the catheter, infusing the dialysate for 10–15 minutes, rolling the bag, and securing the bag and catheter to the abdomen. The child is then allowed normal activity for 4–6 hours (8–10 hours at night). After the allotted time, the dialysate is drained from the abdomen by hanging the bag lower than the pelvis. A fresh bag of dialysate is then attached and the process repeated. The cycle is performed three to five times a day, depending on the child's needs (Fig. 28-7). Because the catheter admits direct access to the peritoneum, the child and family must use strict aseptic technique whenever the catheter is manipulated. In addition, a thorough understanding of the procedure needs to be followed by repeated return demonstrations, so that the child and family can gain confidence. Use of a newly developed CAPD doll assists parents and children to visualize the procedure and to practice prior to performing the procedure on the child (Kennedy, 1985).

Renal transplantation Renal transplantation is becoming a viable alternative to lifelong dialysis for many children. The multidisciplinary approach necessary for renal transplantation can be exhausting. Consultations with specialists in orthopedics or internal medicine usually are requested, along with last-minute reviews of the child's status by infectious disease and hematology groups.

Nursing management The nursing management of the child with chronic renal failure is complex and challenging. An effective plan for management of these children demands not only understanding the highly complex physiologic disturbances, but, equally important, an awareness of and sensitivity in dealing with the overwhelming impact that this chronic illness has on the children and their families.

Coordinating care Nursing management is directed toward correcting metabolic imbalances, recognizing and managing neurologic complications, restricting fluids, and providing a diet high in calories but with restrictions of sodium, potassium, or protein. Unlike many other chronic states, end-stage renal disease challenges the medical and nursing professions to join their collective talents in an attempt to minimize the suffering of the children and families involved. A total team effort, communication, and support are demanded by this progressively destructive disease.

To facilitate a consistent approach to the care of a child with chronic renal failure, the nurse often assumes responsibility for coordinating efforts and activities of other health professionals, particularly regarding dialysis and dietary restriction. Because this is a progressively destructive disease, a long-range plan is developed as soon as feasible, and this information is shared with all involved. Family participation is crucial for the successful implementation of any plan, and parental input is essential.

Dialysis quickly becomes a major part of the life of the child and family. The impact is such that many previous priorities now require reassessment. Often the child and family must travel a considerable distance to reach the dialysis unit. Although dialysis units for adults are numerous, units dedicated to the treatment of pediatric renal failure are relatively few. Dialysis centers designed to treat adults often are not appropriate for the treatment of children.

Discharge preparation Home care of the child with renal failure often is a continuation of the care designed to meet the child's needs in the hospital setting. Parental involvement in the early days of the hospitalization will facilitate discharge teaching. Optimally, two members of the family should be taught to take the child's blood pressure. Often older children can learn to take their own blood pressure with little or no assistance. Return demonstration by all learners is essential before discharge, and the child and family should be comfortable with the demands and feasibility of care prior to discharge.

Rebellion against fluid and dietary restrictions and anger and resentment toward the restrictions of dialysis is not uncommon in children with renal failure. Encouragement of normal activities within the medical restrictions can increase the child's self-esteem. Nurses need to be aware of the implications of long-term illness (see Chapter 14) to care most effectively for children with chronic renal failure.

Parent and peer support groups can be extremely helpful with childhood catastrophic illnesses. The parents of children with chronic renal failure are no exception, and referral to such a group should be made whenever the resource is available. The traditional support systems such as psychiatry, psychology, social service, and the clergy are also important as the child and family deal with the illness.

Fear, anxiety, and expectations are all brought precipitously to the surface when the child and family prepare for transplantation. The nurse joins other health professionals as they strive to reassure and support the child and family during this stressful period. Children and families might experience emotional difficulties adjusting to a kidney transplant. The child will gain weight and appear healthier after transplantation, requiring a complete adjustment to a new body image and increased activity levels. Protective parents will need assistance to allow their child to become independent and live a more normal life. Children sometimes have difficulty accepting the transplant as part of themselves, and until they do so, they might be fearful and experience adjustment problems. The nurse can encourage the child to participate in normal activities for the child's developmental age (only contact sports are to be avoided). The child and family are encouraged to express feelings they might have about the transplant and its effects. Peer and group support can be recommended.

The Child with Renal Trauma

By far the most common cause of renal trauma in children is injury from automobiles. Motorcycle accidents and sports injuries with trauma to the genitourinary tract also are implicated in adolescents. Genitourinary trauma can cause blunt or penetrating injuries and should be suspected whenever there is injury to the flank, chest, abdomen, or pelvic area. Fractures of the ribs or pelvis indicate the need for follow-up for renal injury.

Because the kidney is protected by muscles, most renal trauma in adults results in minor injuries. In children, however, injuries can be more extensive because of less developed musculature and decreased body fat.

Assessment for genitourinary trauma includes inspecting the child for obvious contusions, abrasions, skin discolorations, and palpable masses. Gross or microscopic hematuria is present in children with renal damage and, depending on the extent of the injury, hemorrhage is a constant danger. The child might complain of pain in the flank, abdomen, or lower rib area. Radiographic examination might or might not reveal abnormalities. A sudden decrease in urinary output along with elevations in blood urea nitrogen and serum creatinine levels can indicate impending renal failure, particularly if the child is hypovolemic from hemorrhage.

Treatment for renal injury is conservative in most cases. If physical examination and radiographic studies are normal and the child demonstrates only microscopic hematuria, discharge with home observation might be indicated (Kearney and Finn, 1981). Children with abnormal findings usually are observed in the hospital to recognize quickly any deterioration in renal status. Nephrectomy might be performed if conservative treatment is unsuccessful (Cook, 1983). Trauma to the ureters, urethra, or genitals usually is handled surgically.

Accurate observation of the child with genitourinary injury is essential to effective nursing management. Frequent monitoring and recording of intake and output, vital signs, serum electrolytes, hemoglobin and hematocrit, and presence of hematuria gives clues to the child's renal status. The nurse measures abdominal girth daily to assess the size of any mass. Urinary catheter guidelines should be followed if the child has been catheterized. Quiet diversional activities occupy the child who is confined to bed. Discharge preparation needs to include information regarding signs of hemorrhage or renal damage, since complications can occur for up to 2 years after the injury (Cook, 1983).

Essential Concepts

- The state of the genitourinary system contributes to the general good health and homeostasis of the child.
- Concerns related to the system include maintenance of health and homeostasis, adjustments related to altered body image, and fears of mutilation or of sexual and reproductive deficits.
- Function of the renal system is concerned with regulation and maintenance of the composition and volume of body fluids and the excretion of soluble wastes.
- Assessment of the child with a genitourinary dysfunction includes data gathering and assessment of all body systems, since alteration in the genitourinary system can have adverse effects on the whole body.
- Some diagnostic tests for genitourinary function are embarrassing and invasive, and the child's privacy should be strictly respected.
- Urinary catheterization is performed to empty the bladder prior to diagnostic tests, to obtain a sterile specimen, to measure residual volumes in the bladder, or to empty the bladder when the child is unable to void.
- Acute nursing care involves managing alterations in urinary elimination patterns, monitoring and managing the often critical fluid and electrolyte balance, preventing infection, and providing preoperative preparation and postoperative management if indicated.
- The nutritional needs of children with renal dysfunction are related to the kidneys' inability to process wastes and might include restrictions or additions of protein, restrictions of potassium, sodium, or phosphorus, and additions of calcium and vitamins, depending on the dysfunction involved.
- Meeting the developmental needs of children with genitourinary dysfunction includes interventions directed toward facilitating adequate development in light of repeated hospitalizations and promoting the child's independence and self-care.
- Interventions to meet the emotional needs of children with genitourinary dysfunction include attention to problems resulting from lifestyle restrictions, alterations in body image, and questions regarding sexual and reproductive function.
- Special home care problems might include home catheterization or dialysis.
- Nursing interventions for the child with a genitourinary infection are directed toward careful assessment and supportive care during acute episodes and toward preventive education and counseling.
- Structural defects affecting the genitourinary system

include hydronephrosis, exstrophy of the bladder, obstructive anomalies of the collecting system, reflux anomalies of the collecting system, and anomalies of external structures such as phimosis, hypospadias, epispadias, and cryptorchidism.

- Acute glomerulonephritis and nephrosis are two renal dysfunctions that affect the filtration of wastes.
- Assessment and nursing management of these dysfunctions address imbalances of fluid and electrolytes.
- Acute and chronic renal failure have devastating effects on multiple body systems in the affected child and require meticulous assessment and critical-care management.
- Kidney dialysis can be used to treat renal failure by allowing the body to excrete wastes and correct fluid and electrolyte imbalance.
- Renal transplantation can allow the child recovery from end-stage renal disease, but transplantation is not without the potential for severe complications.
- Care of the child who has sustained genitourinary trauma requires accurate observation to recognize quickly signs of deteriorating renal function.

References

Butler B: Nutritional cornucopia. *J Nephrol Nurs* (Jan/Feb) 1985; 2(1):36–37.

Cook L: Renal trauma. *RN* (Feb) 1983; 46:58–63.

Kearney G, Finn D: Trauma to the genitourinary tract. *Emerg Med* (Aug) 1981; 13:69–79.

Kennedy J: The development of CAPD dialysis dolls. *J Nephrol Nurs* (Sept/Oct) 1985; 2(5):231–235.

Lopes G: A dietary approach to chronic renal failure. *Issues Compr Pediatr Nurs* 1983; 6:23–62.

Mars DR, Treloar D: Acute tubular necrosis—pathophysiology and treatment. *Heart Lung* (March) 1984; 13(2):194–200.

Noble RC: *Sexually Transmitted Diseases*. Medical Examination, 1979.

Reilly M: The renal system. Pages 387–408 in: *Pediatric Critical Care*. Bloedel-Smith J (editor). Wiley, 1983.

Saxton D et al: *The Addison-Wesley Manual of Nursing Practice*. Addison-Wesley, 1983.

Vick R: *Contemporary Medical Physiology*. Addison-Wesley, 1984.

Whettam J: Update on toxic shock: How to spot it and treat it. *RN* (Feb) 1984; 47(2):55–60.

Additional Readings

Bassing S: Saving the baby when mom has herpes. *RN* (Oct) 1985; 48(10):35–37.

Brown L: Toxic shock syndrome. *Am J Matern-Child Nurs* (Jan/Feb) 1981; 6:57–59.

Behrman RE, Vaughan VC: *Nelson Textbook of Pediatrics*, 12th ed. Saunders, 1983.

Brundage D: *Nursing Management of Renal Problems*. Mosby, 1980.

Ceccarelli CM: Hemodialytic therapy for the patient with chronic renal failure. *Nurs Clin North Am* (Sept) 1981; 16(3):531–549.

Centers for Disease Control: *Morbidity and Mortality Weekly Report* (Aug 17) 1984; 33:461–463.

Centers for Disease Control: *Morbidity and Mortality Weekly Report* (Sept 27) 1985; 34(38):590–595.

Chlamydia trachomatis infections: Centers for Disease Control: *Morbidity and Mortality Weekly Report* (Aug 23) 1985; 34(33): 535–735.

Coleman EA: When the kidneys fail. *RN* (July) 1986:28–34.

Gralton KS: Renal, endocrine, and metabolic crises. Pages 376–386 in: *Pediatric Critical Care Nursing*. Vestal K (editor). Wiley, 1981.

Hekelman F, Ostendorp C: Nursing approaches to conservative management of renal disease. *Nurs Clin North Am* (Sept) 1975; 10:431–448.

Hoarsley J, Crane J, Reynolds M: *Clean Intermittent Catheterization*. Harcourt Brace Jovanovich, 1982.

Hollander LA: Renal transplantation in school age children: Beyond physiologic care. *ANNA* (Aug) 1985; 12(4):252–254.

Larson E: Intransigent genital infection? Suspect chlamydia. *RN* (Jan) 1984; 47(1):42–43.

Lewis SM: Pathophysiology of chronic renal failure. *Nurs Clin North Am* (Sept) 1981; 16(3):501–513.

Murphy LM et al: Renal disease: Nutritional implications. *Nurs Clin North Am* (March) 1983; 18:57–70.

Pickering LK, DuPont H: *Infectious Diseases of Children and Adults*. Addison-Wesley, 1986.

Pope T: Toxic shock syndrome. *Nurs Pract* (Sept/Oct) 1981; 6: 31–32.

Quinlan MW: UTI: Helping your patients control it once and for all. *RN* (March) 1984; 47(3):42–43.

Rodrigues RD, Hunter RD: Nutritional intervention in the treatment of chronic renal failure. *Nurs Clin North Am* (Sept) 1981; 16:573–585.

Sorrels AJ: Peritoneal dialysis: A rediscovery. *Nurs Clin North Am* (Sept) 1981; 16(3):515–528.

Topor M: Chronic renal disease in children. *Nurs Clin North Am* (Sept) 1981; 16:587–597.

Wroblewski S: Toxic shock syndrome. *Am J Nurs* (Jan) 1981; 81:82–85.

Chapter 29

Metabolism

Implications of Altered Hormonal Regulation

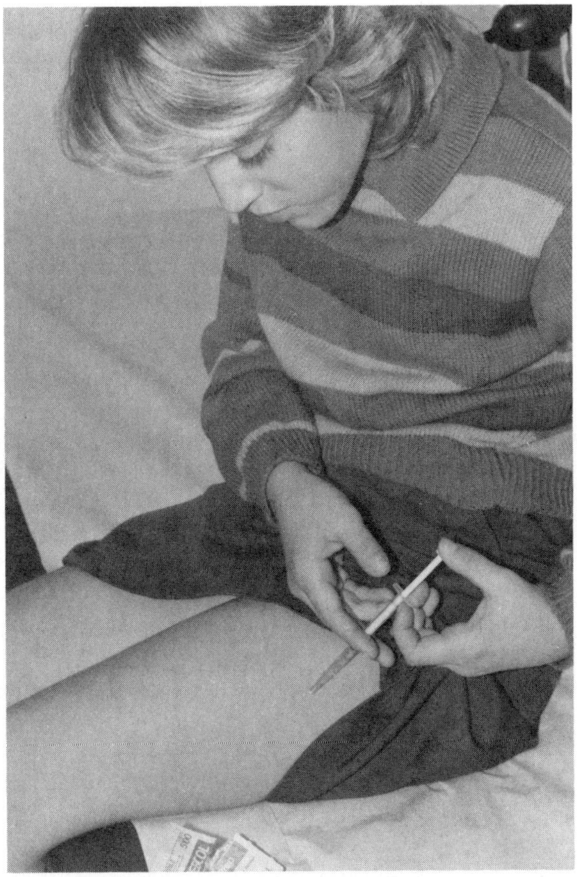

Chapter Contents

(Continues)

Potential knowledge deficit concerning home care management

The Child with Altered Secretion of Insulin

Diabetes Mellitus

The Child with Inappropriate Secretion from the Anterior Lobe of the Pituitary Gland

Growth Hormone
Growth Hormone Hypersecretion—Pituitary Gigantism
Growth Hormone Hyposecretion—Hypopituitarism
Gonadotropin Hypersecretion—Precocious Puberty
Adrenocorticotropin Hypersecretion—Cushing's Disease

The Child with Inappropriate Secretion from the Posterior Pituitary Gland

Posterior Lobe Hypofunction—Diabetes Insipidus

The Child with Inappropriate Secretion from the Adrenal Glands

Excessive Cortisol Secretion
Excessive Adrenal Sex Steroid Secretion—Adrenal Hyperplasia (Adrenogenital Syndrome)
Adrenal Cortex Hypofunction—Addison's Disease
Adrenal Medulla Hyperfunction—Pheochromocytoma

The Child with Inappropriate Secretion from the Thyroid Gland

Hyperfunction (Hyperthyroidism)
Hypofunction (Hypothyroidism)

The Child with Inappropriate Secretion from the Parathyroid Glands

Hyperfunction (Hypercalcemia)
Hypofunction (Hypocalcemia)

The Child with Inappropriate Secretion from the Gonads

Hyperfunction—Excessive Estrogen or Testosterone Production
Ovarian or Testicular Hypofunction—Delayed Sexual Maturation

Objectives

- Describe the assessment criteria for and physical examination of the child with endocrine dysfunction.
- Define the nurse's role in the procedures and treatments that involve the endocrine system.
- Outline the acute care, nutritional, developmental, emotional, and health maintenance needs of the child with endocrine dysfunction and the family.
- Explain the clinical manifestations, diagnostic evaluation, treatment, and nursing management for the child with diabetes mellitus.
- Describe the administration, measurement, dose adjustment, and storage of insulin.
- Explain the physiologic processes, treatments, and principles of nursing management for conditions involving inappropriate hormonal secretions from the pituitary gland.
- Explain the physiologic processes, treatments, and principles of nursing management for conditions involving inappropriate secretions from the adrenal glands.
- Explain the physiologic processes, treatments, and principles of nursing management for conditions involving inappropriate secretions from the thyroid gland.
- Explain the physiologic processes, treatments, and principles of nursing management for conditions involving inappropriate secretions from the parathyroid glands.
- Describe the physiologic processes, treatments, and principles of nursing management for children with hyperfunction of the ovaries or testes.
- Describe the physiologic processes, treatments, and principles of nursing management for children with delayed sexual maturity.

ESSENTIALS OF STRUCTURE AND FUNCTION
The Endocrine System

The neuroendocrine system, composed of the endocrine system and the nervous system, functions to achieve and maintain internal homeostasis. The endocrine system functions by circulating very small amounts of specific chemicals (hormones). The nervous system functions by sending nerve impulses throughout the body. Together, these systems regulate homeostasis, metabolism, growth, and reproduction.

Endocrine glands synthesize hormones that are proteins or compounds made from proteins or steroids. The endocrine glands are ductless; that is, they secrete the hormones directly into the bloodstream. Hormones circulate widely throughout the body but are highly specific in their action on organs (target organs). Hormones serve as messengers, providing communication between endocrine glands and target organs.

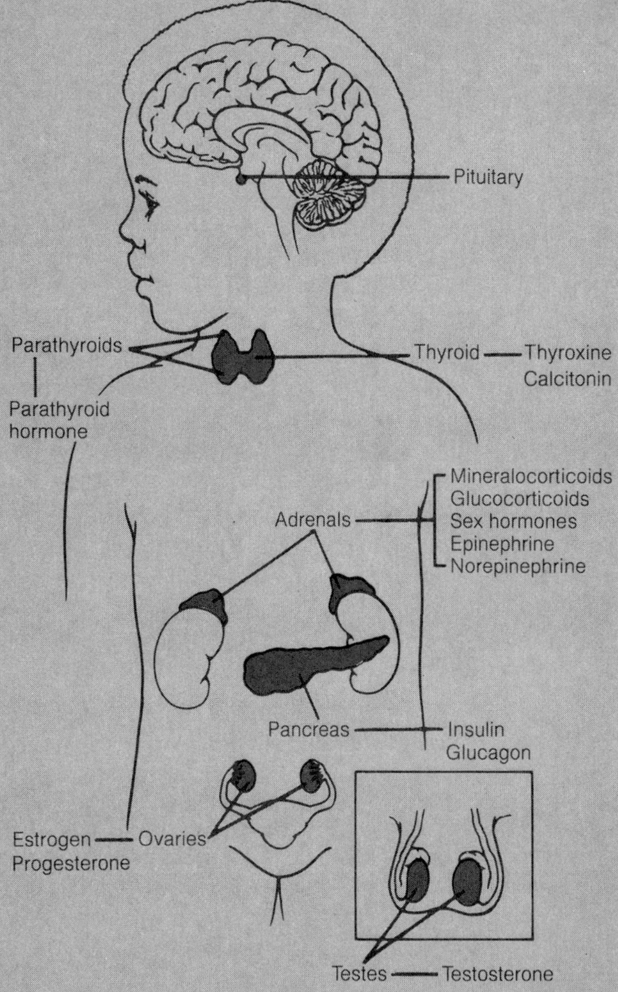

Endocrine system with hormones.

Glossary

Adrenal cortex The outer covering of the adrenal glands located on the top of each kidney. The cortex produces the corticosteroids, which include mineralocorticoids (eg, aldosterone), glucocorticoids, and sex hormones. Mineralocorticoids affect the mineral levels in the blood, particularly salt, by acting on the kidney tubules (see Chapter 28). Glucocorticoids promote metabolism, decrease inflammation, and increase blood sugar levels in response to long-term stress. Sex hormones (androgens and estrogens) are produced in small amounts.

Adrenal medulla The interior of the adrenal glands. The medulla synthesizes epinephrine and norepinephrine, which act on the sympathetic nervous system to produce the "fight or flight" mechanism.

Ovaries Paired almond-shaped glands located in the pelvic cavity. Ovaries produce estrogens and progesterones that initiate the development of secondary sex characteristics and support pregnancy and lactation.

Pancreatic islets of Langerhans Produce insulin and glucagon, which regulate blood sugar. Insulin facilitates the transport of glucose from the blood into cells to be used for energy. Glucagon increases blood glucose level by its action on the liver to release stored glucose.

Parathyroid glands Four glands adjacent to or embedded within the thyroid. They secrete parathyroid hormone, which is the primary regulator of blood calcium.

Pituitary gland Small gland located below the hypothalamus in the brain (see figure showing endocrine

(Continues)

ESSENTIALS OF STRUCTURE AND FUNCTION *(Continued)*

The Endocrine System

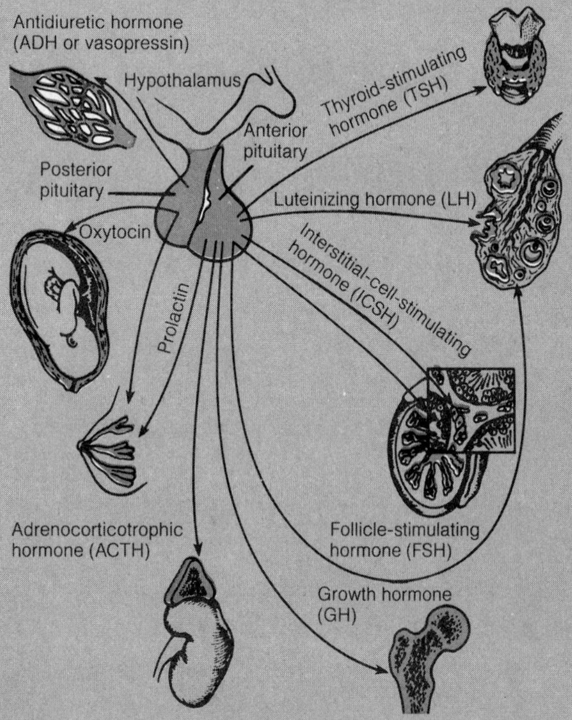

Functions of the pituitary gland: secretion of releasing hormones. (From Spence AP: Basic Human Anatomy. *1st ed. Benjamin/Cummings, 1982; p. 485.)*

system). The gland is divided into anterior and posterior lobes. Each secretes or stores and releases hormones with specific effects on the body (see table; figure showing pituitary function). Because of its location in the midbrain, it is susceptible to any disease, damage, or malformation affecting that portion of the brain.

Testes Paired oval structures suspended in the scrotum. The testes produce testosterone, which initiates puberty in boys and which promotes continuous production of sperm.

Thyroid gland Attached to the anterior and lateral aspects of the trachea. Synthesizes the metabolic hormone thyroxine with the help of iodine. Calcitonin, a hormone that decreases blood calcium levels, also is produced by the thyroid glands.

Hormones of the Pituitary Gland

Hormone	Effect
Anterior pituitary	
Somatotropin (growth hormone)	Converted by the liver to somatomedin, which promotes somatic growth and maintains blood glucose level
Follicle-stimulating hormone (FSH)	Stimulates seminiferous tubules to produce sperm in males; stimulates the secretion of estrogen and progesterone in females
Luteinizing hormone (LH)	Stimulates ovulation in females; stimulates secretion of testosterone in males; also called ICSH (interstitial cell-stimulating hormone in males)
Luteinizing-releasing hormone (LRH)	Stimulates the release of FSH and LH by the pituitary gland
Adrenocorticotropic hormone (ACTH)	Stimulates the adrenal cortex to convert cholesterol into adrenal steroids
Prolactin	Maintains milk production after childbirth
Thyroid-stimulating hormone (TSH)	Stimulates the thyroid gland to synthesize and release thyroxine
Posterior pituitary	
Antidiuretic hormone (ADH, also called vasopressin)	Stimulates distal loop of kidney to reabsorb water and sodium
Oxytocin	Stimulates uterine contractions and the "let down reflex" in breast-feeding women

The hypothalamus controls pituitary function by secreting small peptides that reach the anterior pituitary gland. By acting with the pituitary gland, the hypothalamus is involved with regulating appetite, sugar and fat metabolism, body temperature, maintenance of water balance, and secretion of inhibiting hormones such as somatostatin, which inhibits release of growth hormone.

Hormonal imbalances that develop during gestation, childhood, or adolescence have pronounced effects on children's physical health, growth, pubertal development, and body image. Parents' perceptions of and expectations for children with hormonal dysfunctions might be affected by the serious nature of the problems and the demands placed on the families by the management of the disorders.

The most frequently seen hormonal problem in children is diabetes mellitus. Other common hormonal problems of childhood are hypothyroidism, congenital adrenal hyperplasia, short stature, and precocious puberty. Nursing care of children with hormonal dysfunction is based on a recognition of the age and developmental level of the child; cultural, ethnic, and religious factors; socioeconomic status of the family; meaning of the illness to the child and family; structure of the family and roles of the family members; and an assessment of family strengths.

Assessment of the Child with Endocrine Dysfunction

The endocrine system regulates metabolism, growth, pubertal development, reproduction, fluid and electrolyte balance, and response to stress. In obtaining the history associated with the endocrine system, the nurse is sensitive to the important effects that endocrine function and dysfunction have on the child and family.

History

The prenatal history might reveal maternal endocrine dysfunction, which can affect fetal development. For example, maternal hyperthyroidism can cause either neonatal hyperthyroidism or congenital hypothyroidism. Diabetes during pregnancy is associated with a number of possible problems, including small-for-gestation infants, as well as hypoglycemia, respiratory distress, and congenital anomalies of the cardiac, musculoskeletal, renal, and gastrointestinal systems. Because the mother might feel guilty about possibly causing her offspring to have health problems, the nurse needs to phrase questions tactfully to minimize further emotional trauma.

Because some endocrine disorders are of genetic origin, a family history is essential. Many endocrine problems are thought to be inherited by X-linked or autosomal modes of transmission. The family history needs to include all blood relatives in the child's extended family.

Obtaining a history of the child's growth and attainment of developmental milestones is important because endocrine dysfunctions can alter growth and neurologic development. The nurse assesses the child's growth record, plotting the heights, weights, and head circumference measurements on standard growth charts (Appendix A). The average child should grow and gain weight at rates similar to those listed in Table 29-1. Some endocrine disorders can produce changes in the child's daily habits that can affect behavior. The nurse therefore asks about changes in school performance, constipation or diarrhea, heat or cold intolerance, changes in appetite or food preferences, and changes in sleeping habits. During the history-taking session, the nurse observes the child's behavior and requests for food, drink, and trips to the bathroom.

Physical Examination

Careful growth measurement is important for accuracy. The nurse double-checks the current measurements if they seem in doubt and records any marked deviation from previous measurements.

In assessing the child's general appearance, the nurse observes the child's body proportions to determine whether the limbs appear to be proportional to the trunk, that is, whether the arms and legs appear too long or too short. Changes in the ratio of upper and lower skeletal segments occur throughout childhood until they approach the adult

TABLE 29-1 Average Height and Weight Gain Per Year of Life

Age	Linear growth per year	Weight gain per year
0–12 months	10 in. (25 cm)	13–18 lb (6–8 kg)
13–24 months	5 in. (12.5 cm)	5–8 lb (2.5 kg)
25–36 months	4 in. (10 cm)	4–6 lb (2 kg)
37–48 months	3 in. (8 cm)	3–5 lb (1–2 kg)
4 years to puberty	2.0–2.5 in. (5.0–6.5 cm)	4–6 lb (2–3 kg)

ASSESSMENT GUIDE *The Child with Altered Hormonal Regulation*

Assessment questions	Supporting data
Does the child appear to have any abnormalities in appearance?	
Growth	Excessively tall stature; elongation of the mandible with malocclusion of the teeth; alteration in sexual maturation
	Subnormal growth rate; infantile features, hypoglycemia; deficiency in LH and FSH, excessive TSH
	Facial rounding with growth failure, muscle wasting and fatigue; skin striae and bruising; increased blood pressure
Sexual characteristics	Very early development of secondary sex characteristics (eg, breasts, pubic hair, menstruation, penile elongation); may be associated with short stature and early skeletal maturation
	Ambiguous genitalia in infants; rapid growth with early epiphyseal closure resulting in short stature; alterations in sodium and water balance resulting in hypovolemia and dehydration
	Delayed sexual maturation in girls associated with webbing of the neck and low hairline; elevated blood pressure; additional anomalies (eg, abnormal kidneys, coarctation of the aorta, pulmonary stenosis)
	Delayed sexual maturation in boys associated with breast enlargement
Has the child exhibited any fluid and electrolyte alteration?	Polyuria, excessive thirst, bedwetting; increase in appetite without substantial weight gain; fruity odor to breath associated with alterations in level of consciousness; glucose in the urine, alterations in serum electrolytes
	Polyuria, excessive thirst; decreased appetite with weight loss; dehydration; decreased urine specific gravity
Has the child experienced any alteration in activity level?	
Increased	Nervousness, irritability, weight loss with increased appetite; thyroid enlargement (might be associated with protruding eyes); hypertension and growth acceleration; heat intolerance; elevated thyroid hormone levels
Decreased	Significant slowing of linear growth; constipation; dry, thickened skin; coarse hair with possible excessive hair loss; cold intolerance; increased requirements for sleep; low thyroxine level, high TSH
Does the child have a family history of endocrine disorders?	

Additional data: Nausea, vomiting, abdominal cramping; changes in skin pigmentation; tetany; salt craving

ratio of 1:1. Assessment of arm span is accomplished by measuring the distance between the fingertips with the arms extended straight out from the shoulders. The nurse also observes the child's facial features for any of the following findings associated with endocrine dysfunction: flattened nasal bridge, small jaw and crowded teeth, bowing of the frontal bones of the skull, and the presence of a high, arched palate.

The eye examination includes checking for exophthalmos (bulging eyes) as well as assessing for visual acuity and visual fields. Ophthalmoscopic examination might reveal displaced lenses, cataracts, and retinal hemorrhages.

The amount of testosterone to which the fetus is exposed during development affects the appearance of the newborn's external genitals. Insufficient testosterone alters the male genitals and excessive testosterone alters the female genitals, resulting in abnormalities or ambiguous genitals. The female infant's external genitals are examined for enlargement of the clitoris, fusion of the labia, and hyperpigmentation (increased color) of the tissue. The male infant's external genitals are examined for the presence of testes in the scrotum, hyperpigmentation, hypospadias, and abnormal length or diameter of the penis. The length of the penis is measured by using a short, stiff ruler that is pressed gently into the symphysis pubis as the penile length is noted.

When assessing the sexual development of the adolescent or older child, the nurse evaluates whether the parent should stay or leave the room. The nurse provides the patient with a gown and cover sheet and requests that all clothing be removed. Examination of breast development and axillary hair can be accomplished while assessing the heart and lungs, and pubic hair can be assessed when evaluating femoral pulses.

Secondary sexual characteristics (pubic and axillary hair in both sexes, facial hair in males, and breast development in females) are the external markers that distinguish the sexes from each other but play no direct role in reproduction. Children with certain endocrine dysfunctions develop secondary sexual characteristics earlier or later than normal. Secondary sexual development is described and illustrated in Chapter 8 (see Figs. 8-1, 8-2, and 8-3).

Endocrine disorders might affect skin texture, temperature, turgor, and pigmentation. The nurse observes the skin for the following characteristics: thickness, coarseness, doughy feel, dryness, sallow color, moistness, warmth, hyperpigmentation of scars and skin folds, flushing, pigmented nevi (moles), and striae (lines).

The child's respiratory status is assessed, noting the character and rate of respirations. The child's breath is assessed for the presence of a fruity odor (a sign of ketoacidosis) by requesting the child to repeat a sentence.

Because thyroid disorders affect the child's neurologic status, the nurse performs a thorough neurologic examination. Deep tendon reflexes are assessed for sluggishness, briskness, and speed of return; the tongue for twitching; the hands for tremors; and the eyelids for lag. The child's level of consciousness, orientation, balance, and coordination also are described.

The nurse assesses blood pressure, pulse, and status of peripheral circulation because these parameters are affected by some endocrine dysfunctions. Any increase in muscle mass and muscle strength is noted because adrenal disorders can affect muscle tone.

While making objective observations during the physical examination, the nurse converses with the child and family, thereby obtaining additional subjective data. These data are then validated by the use of diagnostic laboratory and radiologic tests, when appropriate.

Nursing Management for Procedures and Treatments

Preparation for Diagnostic Tests

Children with suspected endocrine dysfunction undergo fairly extensive and sometimes invasive diagnostic workups. The nurse's role in the diagnostic workup might consist of coordinating the various procedures and explaining them to children and parents. Teaching children and parents how to collect urine specimens, providing emotional support to children during procedures, and ultimately teaching children and parents how to administer medications required for management of the endocrine dysfunction are important nursing actions.

Serum electrolyte values are helpful in assessing the child with an endocrine imbalance. For example, the serum calcium level might be decreased in a child who has a dysfunction of the parathyroid gland preventing secretion of parathyroid hormone (see Chapter 21 for serum electrolyte values).

Hematocrit and hemoglobin values can be altered in children with endocrine dysfunction. The measurement of glycosolated hemoglobin (HbA1c) gives an accurate picture of how the body has metabolized glucose during the previous 2–3 months (norm: 2.2%–4.8% of total hemoglobin).

Urine studies usually involve a 24-hour urine collection. These studies are summarized in Table 29-2. Other studies performed to evaluate endocrine function are found in Table 29-3.

For their own comfort and to assist the child in dealing with the new situation, parents need to be included in the preparation for diagnostic testing. The nurse is generous with time estimates because children and parents will become apprehensive in the face of unexpected delays. The nurse explains clearly what meals are omitted before certain procedures.

Care of a Child Receiving Steroid Therapy

Children with adrenal disorders take replacement (physiologic) amounts of cortisone because their adrenals do not produce sufficient glucocorticoids. Taking replacement doses (those needed to provide deficient steroids) does not place the child at risk for complications (infections, hypertension, gastrointestinal bleeding) that might occur when larger (pharmacologic) doses of steroids are used to treat renal disease, asthma, juvenile rheumatoid arthritis, and cancer (see Chapter 25). The most important aspect of

TABLE 29-2 Urine and Serum Studies for Evaluation of Endocrine Dysfunction

Test	Normal values*		Alteration/clinical significance
Urine			
	(mg/24 hours)		
17-ketosteroids	Infant (less than 1 yr)	under 1	*Increased:* Enzymatic deficiency, Cushing's syndrome, adrenogenital syndrome
Test of adrenal cortex function	Child (5–8 yr)	under 3	*Decreased:* Addison's disease
	Child (9–12)	approx. 3	
	Adult male	8–25	
	Adult female	5–15	
	(mg/M/24 hrs)		
17-hydroxycorticosteriods	Children to 16 yrs	3.1–10.0	*Increased:* Cushing's syndrome, stress
Test of adrenal cortex function			*Decreased:* Adrenocortico insufficiency, anterior pituitary hypofunction, severe anemia, starvation
Urinary-free cortisol	20–100 μg/24 hr		*Increased:* Cushing's syndrome
Test of adrenal cortex function			*Decreased:* Addison's disease, enzyme deficiency
Urinary calcium	10 mg/dL		*Increased:* Hyperparathyroidism
			Decreased: Hypoparathyroidism
Urinary sodium	40–180 mEq/24 hr		*Increased:* Enzymatic deficiencies, Addison's disease
Urinary vanillymandelic acid (VMA)	(24-hr specimen mg/g creatinine)		*Increased:* Tumors of the adrenal gland, neuroblastomas and other tumors arising in sympathetic or adrenal medullary tissue
	Infant (1–12 mo)	1.40–15.0	
	Child (5–10 yr)	0.5–6.0	
	Child (10–15 yr)	0.25–3.25	
Urine glucose	0		*Increased:* Diabetes mellitus, Cushing's syndrome
Urine for ketones	0		*Increased:* Diabetic ketoacidosis, metabolic acidosis
Serum			
Thyroid functions:			
Thyroxine (T_4) (Murphy-Pattec)	6.0–11.8 μg/dL		*Increased:* Hyperthyroidism, thyroiditis, thyrotoxicosis
Triiodothyronine (T_3UR) uptake ratio	25%–35% uptake		*Decreased:* Cretinism, goiter, hypothyroidism, myxedema
Free thyroxine (T_7)	1.3–4.4 index		
Thyroid-stimulating hormone (TSH)	Up to 0.2 mV/mL		
Glucose tolerance test	Fasting: 65–110 mg/dL 30 min: <155 mg/dL 60 min: <165 mg/dL 120 min: <120 mg/dL 180 min: fasting level or less		*Increased:* at 2 hours suggests diabetes mellitus; curves can be abnormal in Cushing's syndrome *Decreased:* after 2 hours suggests hypoglycemia

*Normal values may vary with laboratory method used.

steroid therapy for children with adrenal disease is ensuring regular (two to three times a day) administration of the medication. Without this daily steroid replacement, the children are in a state of adrenal insufficiency and at risk for developing adrenal crisis (hypotension, low blood sugar, and shock) should a significant stress (trauma, illness) occur.

The nurse explains to the child and family the importance of administering the medication every day at the appropriate time and works out an appropriate reminder system with them. The family is taught to watch for signs and symptoms of adrenal insufficiency (shocklike symptoms such as increased pulse and respiratory effort, decreased blood pressure, cold clammy skin, and cyanosis) and how

TABLE 29-3 Evaluation of Endocrine Function: Diagnostic Tests

Procedure	Purpose	Invasive	Preparation of patient
Thyroid scan (Image)	Assess size and character of the thyroid gland	Yes	If the scan is to determine the presence of thyroid cancer, the patient must stop taking thyroxine for 4–6 weeks and tri-iodothyronine 10–14 days prior to the scan
Pelvic/abdominal ultrasound	Assess ovaries and adrenal glands for size, masses, cysts	No	Encourage oral fluids to fill the bladder prior to the sonogram
Bone age radiograph of hand and wrist	Assess skeletal maturation	No	Might require a hemiskeletal survey for a very young child
CT scan of head	Examine head for masses near pituitary gland	Yes	Sedation might be required. Child who needs sedation might be allowed nothing by mouth prior to the scan
Luteinizing releasing hormone (LRH, or luteinizing hormone releasing hormone, LHRH) stimulation test	Evaluate pituitary gland's ability to release luteinizing hormone (LH) and follicle-stimulating hormone (FSH)	Yes	Patient might be allowed nothing by mouth several hours prior to the test
Thyrotropin-releasing hormone (TRH) stimulation test	Exaluate pituitary TSH reserve	Yes	The test is performed in the morning after an overnight fast. Blood pressure and pulse are monitored. Thyroxine is stopped for 14–28 days prior to the test
Adrenocorticotropic hormone (ACTH) stimulation test	Evaluate ability of adrenal cortex to synthesize adrenocortical hormones	Yes	Nothing by mouth allowed for 12 hours prior to the test
Human chorionic gonadotropin (HCG) test	Assess ability of testes to secrete testosterone	Yes	Serum testosterone level is measured before and after a series of HCG injections
Metyrapone test	Assess ACTH and cortisol production	No	Baseline 24-hour urine specimens are collected for 1–2 days, then metyrapone is given every 4 hours for six doses, after which urine specimens are collected for 24 hours. The patient cannot be taking diphenylhydantoin (Dilantin). If the patient is on cortisone, this medication must be stopped, which places the patient at risk for adrenal insufficiency
Dexamethasone suppression test	Study cortisol suppression in Cushing's syndrome	Yes	Dexamethasone is given every 6 hours for 2 days, then the serum cortisol level is measured, and urine is collected. The patient might develop adrenal insufficiency during this test

to obtain emergency treatment for it. The nurse also reminds the family that the steroid dose must be continued and increased during illnesses characterized by fever or anorexia. The family is cautioned against allowing any medical personnel to discontinue the steroids during an illness. To do so could lead to death from adrenal insufficiency.

Principles of Nursing Care

Acute Care Needs

Acute nursing care of the child with endocrine dysfunction involves prompt, skilled observation and intervention.

❀ Potential fluid volume deficit

Children with some disorders of the endocrine system experience diuresis with associated fluid imbalances. The nurse carefully monitors intake and output and intravenous fluid replacement. The urine is checked on a regular basis for specific gravity, and in the case of a child with suspected diabetes mellitus, for sugar and ketones. The nurse ensures adequate oral intake, taking into consideration the child's fluid likes and dislikes. Monitoring for signs of dehydration is essential (see Chapter 21 for nursing management of children with fluid imbalances).

Fluid imbalances can contribute to electrolyte imbalances. Also, children with endocrine dysfunction might present with or develop electrolyte abnormalities during treatment. A potassium deficit is suspected if the child complains of muscle weakness and has a weak pulse, absent reflexes, hypotension, or arrhythmias; this problem is recognized and treated promptly to prevent death.

The nurse also is alert for irritability, diarrhea, and oliguria, which are signs of hyperkalemia. Because excessive potassium levels slow or prevent the transmission of stimuli through the cardiac muscles, the child can experience intraventricular conduction disturbances.

Children who are hypocalcemic report a tingling sensation in the fingers and around the mouth, muscle cramps in the abdomen, and carpopedal (hand and foot) spasms or have convulsions. The child who is hypercalcemic has flaccid muscles, reports flank or deep thigh pain, has nausea and vomiting, or is stuporous.

The child with hyponatremia might appear very apprehensive, complain of abdominal cramps and have diarrhea; be hypotensive with a rapid, thready pulse; have cold, clammy skin; be cyanotic; and have seizures. With hypernatremia, the child might be agitated and appear flushed and have dry, sticky mucous membranes; a firm, rubbery turgor to the skin; and very little urine output.

In addition to the previously mentioned electrolyte abnormalities, children with endocrine dysfunction also might develop hypoglycemia, respiratory distress, and acidosis—all potentially fatal conditions that require intensive nursing care. (See Chapter 21 for nursing management of a child with an alteration in electrolytes.)

❀ Potential sleep-pattern disturbance

The child who is awakened at night because of frequent trips to the bathroom (nocturnal diuresis) can be irritable and fatigued. Children with accelerated metabolism also might not be able to sleep at night. Because fatigue is not conducive to recovery, the nurse ensures regular, adequate periods of rest during the day. These rest periods are recorded on the nursing care plan for all to follow. It is helpful if the child is encouraged to void prior to every rest period. Reducing the environmental stimuli, such as closing shades and doors and turning off any unnecessary machinery, can create an atmosphere for rest.

❀ Potential for injury

Endocrine dysfunction complicates the nursing care of the child undergoing surgery. The stress of surgery frequently changes the child's hormonal requirements leading to body injury if hormone replacement is not properly managed. When the nurse plans preoperative and postoperative care of the child with an endocrine dysfunction, the assessment must include (1) when the child received the most recent dose of hormone (insulin, hydrocortisone, vasopressin, propylthiouracil); (2) how long the child will be unable to eat and take oral medication; (3) the current measurements of blood pressure, pulse, blood glucose level, and serum electrolyte levels; and (4) the plans for the administration of hormones during surgery and recovery.

❀ Potential hypothermia

Children with some endocrine disorders feel cold most of the time due to a decreased metabolic rate. The nurse monitors the environmental temperature and ensures that the child is properly covered at all times. It might be helpful if the parent brings warm, winter-weight pajamas from home if the child is cold consistently.

Nutritional Needs

❀ Potential alteration in nutrition: more than body requirements

Certain endocrine disorders alter children's appetites, fluid requirements, and appetite control. Some dysfunctions increase the child's appetite and others cause the child to be thirsty and require an increased fluid intake.

Other endocrine disorders cause unusual or uncontrollable cravings. For example, one 11-year-old boy presented with complaints of weakness and nausea. Assessment of his food intake revealed a preference for salty foods, such as pretzels and dill pickles; he even reported drinking the liquid from the pickle jars. On physical examination, the nurse noted that the child had hyperpigmentation in his skin creases. Diagnostic testing confirmed that the salt craving was due to adrenal cortex hypofunction (Addison's disease).

A 24-hour dietary recall or a written 3-day dietary history provides nutritional assessment and aids planning and teaching in endocrine-related disorders. Children with diabetes require some dietary modifications to avoid hypoglycemia (low blood sugar) and hyperglycemia (high blood sugar). These special needs will be addressed in the section on the management of diabetes in children.

Developmental Needs

⊛ Potential altered growth and development

Identifying learning disabilities Several endocrine disorders might cause neurologic impairment and learning difficulties in children who develop these problems during infancy and the early childhood years when the brain is still developing. Congenital hypothyroidism, if not recognized within 1 or 2 months after birth, can cause serious mental retardation (cretinism). Severe or frequent hypoglycemia in young children has been associated with varying degrees of mental retardation and developmental delays. Girls with Turner's syndrome, a chromosome defect, frequently have difficulty with problems involving spatial relationships, so the nurse might consider an endocrine dysfunction when a short, prepubertal girl reports that she has problems in geometry but does well in other subjects at school.

Promoting independence and self-care Chronic health disorders might cause school absences, lack of participation in peer group activities, and an overprotective-dependent relationship between parents and chlidren. All of these factors can interfere with the child's development. Most endocrine disorders have few visible stigmas. This is a mixed blessing for the child, being positive in that the disorder is not visibly disabling, but negative in that some people might not believe that the child has serious health problems that can legitimately interfere with activities and responsibilities.

The nurse assists the child in meeting the need for independence through education and role playing and by providing support through listening. Contacting school personnel to alert them to the problem assists with a consistent approach to child and family. For example, one 13-year-old girl who had recently moved to another state elected not to tell her new classmates that she had diabetes for fear of being ostracized, yet she hesitated to join in activities with her new acquaintances because she feared having an insulin reaction (hypoglycemia). The nurse worked with this young adolescent for 6 months, teaching her to manage her diabetes with the goal of gaining self-confidence in meeting new people and interacting in new situations. They practiced role playing in telling new friends about the diabetes. The nurse realized the goal was achieved when this adolescent called one night from a slumber party with her new friends requesting advice on what to eat for a midnight snack following a vigorous game of volleyball.

Emotional Needs

⊛ Potential ineffective family coping: compromised

The child's ability to deal with a chronic endocrine dysfunction depends to a great extent on several variables: cultural influences, the child's age and developmental level, the family's perception of the health problem, and strengths of the family. (These variables are discussed in Chapter 14 in relation to chronic conditions in children.)

The child's cultural background contributes to the ways in which the endocrine disorder is perceived. The nurse adapts the method of and approach to teaching children and families to their unique cultural features.

The age at which children develop endocrine disorders can affect how they and their families perceive the seriousness of the disorder. Parents of infants and young children with diabetes mellitus might be so overprotective that they feel they cannot leave their children with babysitters and are reluctant to let their children enter school at the appropriate age. Family counseling might be indicated for families using maladaptive coping strategies.

⊛ Potential self-esteem disturbance

Children and families perceive health problems in different ways. Some of the variance in perceptions depends on how seriously ill the child is when the disorder is diagnosed or how physically abnormal the child looks because of the disorder. Parents of newborn girls with congenital adrenal hyperplasia generally are quite distraught initially because of the obvious virilization of the external genitals. These families often continue to be very apprehensive and somewhat overprotective about their daughters because the children can develop adrenal insufficiency quickly with intercurrent illnesses. These girls frequently view themselves negatively and have low expectations of their ability to handle situations. Newborn boys with this condition generally are not diagnosed until they are 10–14 days of age, at which time they usually are quite ill; in fact, some newborn boys nearly die before the diagnosis is made and treatment initiated.

Girls with Turner's syndrome and their families cope with the emotional burden of infertility and short stature. Children who develop Cushing's syndrome (adrenal cortex hyperfunction) have altered body images, emotional lability, and limitation of activity, to which they must adjust until the symptoms are relieved. Children with deficiencies in growth hormone frequently are treated as younger children, and parents, peers, and schoolteachers either limit their participation in activities or have unrealistic expectations of their physical capabilities.

The nurse assesses the child and family's strengths and builds on them. Parental support is the key to both good management of any health disorder and the child's development of positive self-esteem. The nurse provides support, objective observations, and information concerning child development as it relates to the child's needs for parental support with a given task. Parents who can develop realistic and responsible attitudes toward their children's health problems incorporate the children's health needs into the family's lifestyle and prevent the child from feeling different. This acceptance by the family helps the child become secure and develop a positive sense of self-esteem.

Health Maintenance Needs

Most endocrine disorders are chronic in nature and need to be evaluated regularly by a health care team. The nurse has the opportunity to build rapport with the child and family and provide ongoing education in the areas of health maintenance, parenting, and child development. This can be a distinct advantage over the acute-care setting, in which the nurse has less time for teaching such topics.

⊛ Potential knowledge deficit concerning home care management

The nurse assesses the family's beliefs about health maintenance and makes plans for ongoing education accordingly. Families who use health care facilities only for acute, episodic care might have difficulty comprehending the need for regular well-child checkups. For example, one mother commented when reminded about her daughter's appointment at the diabetes clinic that she had not planned to keep the appointment because her daughter was not sick that day.

Children over 6 years of age and their parents need to learn the basic survival skills associated with their endocrine disorder at the time of diagnosis. They need to demonstrate basic knowledge of the problem as well as competence and comfort in assuming the responsibility for managing the child's home care before the child is discharged. Survival skills include (1) understanding the action of the medication or medications to be administered; (2) knowing how to administer the medication and how to prevent, recognize, and treat any side effects of the medication; (3) knowing how to contact the health care team for follow-up and emergency care; and (4) being able to explain the child's health problem to family, friends, and school personnel. With time, the family will acquire a more thorough understanding of the disorder and its treatment as a result of practical experience, self-education, and continued teaching by health professionals.

The nurse does not attempt to teach the child and family everything at the initial contact because most people learn poorly under stressful conditions. The nurse identifies and concentrates on the basic skills and knowledge needed immediately by the family and teaches these facts slowly and patiently. Children with endocrine disorders have the same basic requirements for rest and stimulation as other normal, healthy children, although extra rest might be required by some children with endocrine dysfunction.

The family often finds a visiting or public health nurse helpful during the first few days or weeks at home to provide assistance in setting up home care. In many settings the nurse initiates the visiting nurse referral as part of the discharge planning. The nurse also can refer the family to community lay organizations such as Little People of America or the American Diabetes Association.

Frequently, a parent of another child with the same endocrine disorder can offer practical guidance to the parent of a newly diagnosed child on how to cope with everyday situations, where to obtain supplies, and the emotional stages experienced by children with chronic illnesses and their parents. The nurse might wish to be present during such a parent visit to gain personal insight into the reality of dealing with chronic illnesses in children.

At regular return visits, the nurse continues to provide anticipatory guidance and divides long-term goals (such as, "Johnny will be giving all his own shots by next summer") into smaller, more tangible steps (such as, "by the end of the month, Johnny will be selecting the sites for injections and mixing the insulins"). It is often advisable to schedule checkups just prior to potentially stressful events, such as the beginning of the new school term or vacation or anticipated developmental changes such as the onset of puberty.

Children also need anticipatory guidance. The nurse rehearses with children situations they will encounter such as, "What will you do about taking your afternoon dose of medicine when you go to play at a friend's house after school?" or "What do you want your friends to know about your condition?"

The Child with Altered Secretion of Insulin

Diabetes Mellitus

Diabetes mellitus is a disorder of carbohydrate metabolism that affects 1 out of every 500–800 children under 21 years of age. As such, diabetes mellitus is a frequently seen health disorder of children and adolescents. For carbohydrates to be metabolized correctly, insulin must be released in adequate quantities from the pancreas when the blood glucose level is rising. Any disruption in the release or effectiveness of insulin can lead to hyperglycemia (increased blood sugar). The release of insulin can be disrupted when there is damage to the insulin-producing cells in the pancreas.

Genetic factors Diabetes mellitus is classified as either *Type I* (juvenile-onset, insulin-dependent) or *Type II* (mature-onset, usually noninsulin-dependent). Type II diabetes is seen primarily in adults; however, certain adolescents can develop mature-onset diabetes of youth (MODY). These adolescents usually have a family incidence of mature-onset diabetes and develop symptoms similar to that of Type II diabetes.

Most children with diabetes have the Type I disorder. Recent research has demonstrated a genetic difference in the two types of diabetes; that is, a young child's diabetes probably is unrelated to the fact that an elderly relative has Type II diabetes.

Type I diabetes is associated with an increase in certain histocompatibility antigens (HLA). The HLA system is located on chromosome six and plays a central role in the immune response (see Chapter 25). The risk of acquiring diabetes appears to increase in children who inherit certain of these histocompatibility antigens. Children who have a sibling or a parent with diabetes have an increased risk for developing it. HLA typing (identification of the histocompatibility antigen) of families in which diabetes exists might predict more precisely the risk for diabetes. However, since no preventive therapy is available to at-risk siblings, HLA typing presently is used mainly for research purposes. Siblings might have periodic blood glucose testing, glucose tolerance tests, islet-cell antibodies tests, or glycohemoglobin measurements in an attempt to detect the disorder in its early stages.

Autoimmune factors Type I diabetes might or might not be associated with high levels of islet-cell antibodies at the time of diagnosis. Islet-cell antibodies are antibodies that damage the cells in the pancreas that produce insulin. Children who have islet-cell antibodies are at risk for developing thyroiditis and adrenal hypofunction as well as diabetes, whereas children without islet-cell antibodies do not appear to be at increased risk for the other autoimmune endocrine disorders (Guthrie and Guthrie, 1983).

The histocompatibility complex (HLA) is thought to direct the body's response to various antigens, including viral infections. Some investigators believe that children develop diabetes in response to the combination of having a genetic predisposition and HLA-directed response to viral infections, which culminates in the destruction of pancreatic beta cells. A virus similar to the Coxsackie B4 virus is one virus that has been implicated in the development of diabetes.

Environmental factors Certain environmental factors can contribute to the development of diabetes. Toxic chemicals, for example, can destroy beta cells.

Clinical manifestations The onset of diabetes mellitus in children and adolescents generally is fairly rapid, with the signs and symptoms appearing over a course of days to weeks. The classic symptoms of diabetes mellitus are polyuria (excessive urination), polydipsia (excessive thirst), polyphagia (excessive food intake), and weight loss (see Fig. 29-1). The parent might be particularly aware of nighttime bed-wetting or excessive thirst.

Polyuria is caused by the spillage of glucose into the urine when the renal threshold for the maximal reabsorption of glucose (160–200 mg/dL in most children) is exceeded. A resultant water loss occurs because of osmotic diuresis. Dehydration and an increase in serum osmolality result, which triggers compensatory polydipsia. Water losses can lead to intravascular volume depletion, decreased perfusion to the kidneys, and decreased glucose clearance by the kidneys, leading ultimately to an increased plasma glucose level.

Alteration in metabolism of fats—ketoacidosis In insulin deficiency, carbohydrates cannot be metabolized properly for energy. Lack of insulin triggers the process of *catabolism,* in which fat and protein are used for energy. This state of starvation signals the hypothalamus that body stores are being used, and the appetite will then increase (polyphagia), unless significant nausea is present. Despite the increased food intake, catabolism causes weight loss.

As fat is used for energy, the level of free fatty acids in the blood increases. The liver converts free fatty acids to the ketone bodies beta-hydroxybutyrate, acetoacetic acid, and acetone. The rate of ketone formation exceeds the capacity for peripheral use, leading to an accumulation of ketoacids and metabolic acidosis. Compensatory deep, rapid breathing (Kussmaul respirations) develops in an attempt to excrete excess carbon dioxide. The presence of acetone is responsible for the fruity breath sometimes observed in children with ketoacidosis.

Diabetic ketoacidosis is defined by a glucose level of over 300 mg/dL, a venous pH less than 7.4, a bicarbonate level less than 15 mEq/dL, glucosuria (presence of glucose in the urine), and ketonuria. The child's level of consciousness is affected by the progressive dehydration, acidosis, hyperosmolality, and diminished cerebral oxygen utilization. If not corrected promptly, diabetic ketoacidosis can lead to progressively worsening coma and death.

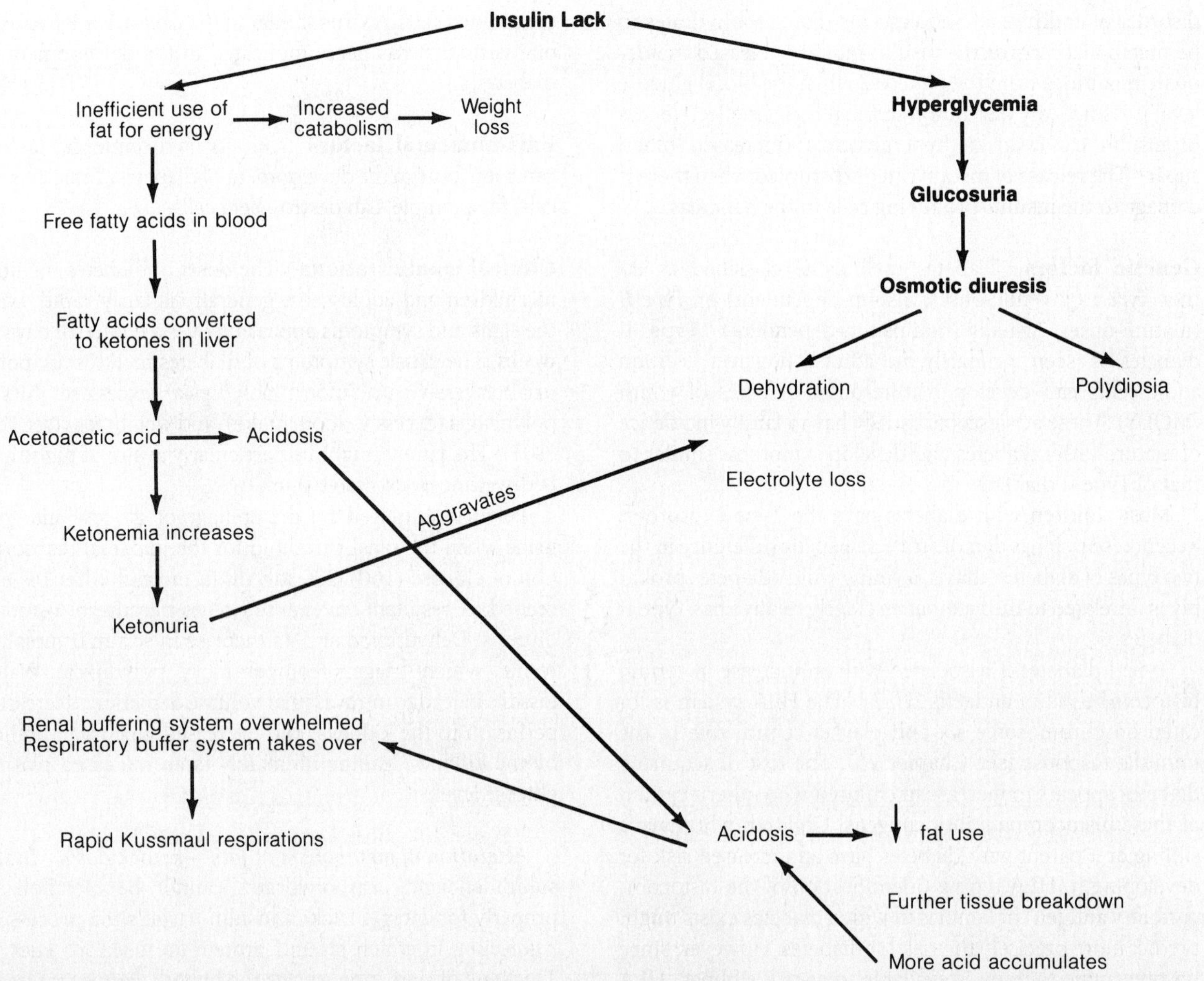

FIGURE 29-1

The body's response to lack of insulin.

Diagnostic evaluation Children of all ages can develop diabetes, even very young children. Often, infants and young children are very ill and in ketoacidosis when diagnosed. Health care providers and parents do not think of very young children as having diabetes and attribute their symptoms initially to gastroenteritis. A quick check of a urine specimen for glucose and the discovery of glucosuria leads to the diagnosis of diabetes in the young child.

A reliable index of long-term glucose control can be obtained from a blood test that determines the glucose concentration in the erythrocytes. Hemoglobin A_{1c}, or glycosylated hemoglobin, is hemoglobin to which glucose has been nonenzymatically coupled. Because the reaction is slow and continues irreversibly throughout the 120-day life span of the red blood cell, the results can accurately reflect glucose metabolism over the preceding 2–3 months. This test is not subject to variations in diet, exercise, stress, or time of day as are urine test results.

Other serum tests used to diagnose diabetes mellitus include a fasting blood sugar test (usually greater than 130 mg/dL) and a glucose tolerance test (elevated blood glucose greater than 200 mg/dL 2 hours after glucose administration). Urinalysis might reveal glucosuria and ketonuria. During diabetic ketoacidosis, arterial pH, serum CO_2, and electrolyte studies are obtained.

Treatment

Insulin Prior to the discovery of insulin in the 1920s, few people with diabetes survived more than a few years after diagnosis. Insulin functions in a somewhat poorly defined manner. It is known that insulin binds to insulin receptors on cell surfaces, allowing glucose to be taken up

TABLE 29-4 Types of Insulin and Their Actions

Name and classification	Onset of action	Peak action	Duration of action	Time of administration	Time when hypoglycemic reactions can occur
Rapid acting					
Crystalline zinc (CZ)	Within 1 hour	2–4 hours	5–8 hours	Before meals and when needed	Between meals
Regular	Within 1 hour	2–4 hours	5–8 hours	↓	Between meals
Semilente	Within 1 hour	6–10 hours	12–16 hours	Before breakfast	Around lunch
Intermediate acting					
Globin zinc*	Within 2–4 hours (faster as dose increases)	6–10 hours	18–24 hours (longer as dose increases)	Before breakfast	Around dinner time or before bedtime
Lente	Within 2–4 hours	8–12 hours	28–32 hours	↓	↓
Neutral protamine hasedorn (NPH) (isophane insulin)*	Within 2–4 hours	8–12 hours	28–30 hours	↓	↓
Slow acting					
Protamine zinc (PZ or ZP1)*	4–6 hours	16–24 hours	24–36 hours or more	Before breakfast	During night or early morning
Ultralente	8 hours	16–24 hours	36 hours or more	↓	↓

*These insulins have a modifying protein added (protamine or globulin).

by the cell. Factors such as obesity and hypercortisolism inhibit the action of insulin, whereas exercise promotes the action of insulin.

Insulin is measured in units. Insulin solutions and syringes are manufactured with 100 units of insulin per milliliter (U-100). Insulin syringes are calibrated so that each marking equals one unit. Insulin can be rapid, intermediate, or slow acting (see Table 29-4).

The amount and type of insulin prescribed depends on a careful consideration of the child's blood glucose level, diet, and amount of regular exercise. Blood glucose levels in normal children increase approximately one half-hour after eating and return to normal approximately 2 hours after a meal. In the diabetic child, the blood glucose level remains elevated much longer and needs the insulin to bring it down to within normal limits. Combinations of insulin are given so that peak action occurs approximately at the time the child's blood glucose level would be highest. For example, a short-acting and intermediate-acting insulin might be given before breakfast. The regular insulin would peak mid-morning, while the intermediate would peak late afternoon or early evening (see Fig. 29-2). Depending on the child's blood glucose level, insulin might be given again in the evening. Snacks often are given at mid-afternoon and bedtime to prevent hypoglycemic reactions at peak insulin time.

Nutritional management The child is placed on a diet program that is individualized according to insulin requirements and exercise levels. Depending on the center treating the child, the diet can be strictly enforced or altered depending on the changing needs of the child. Avoidance of refined and simple sugars and limitation of certain fats

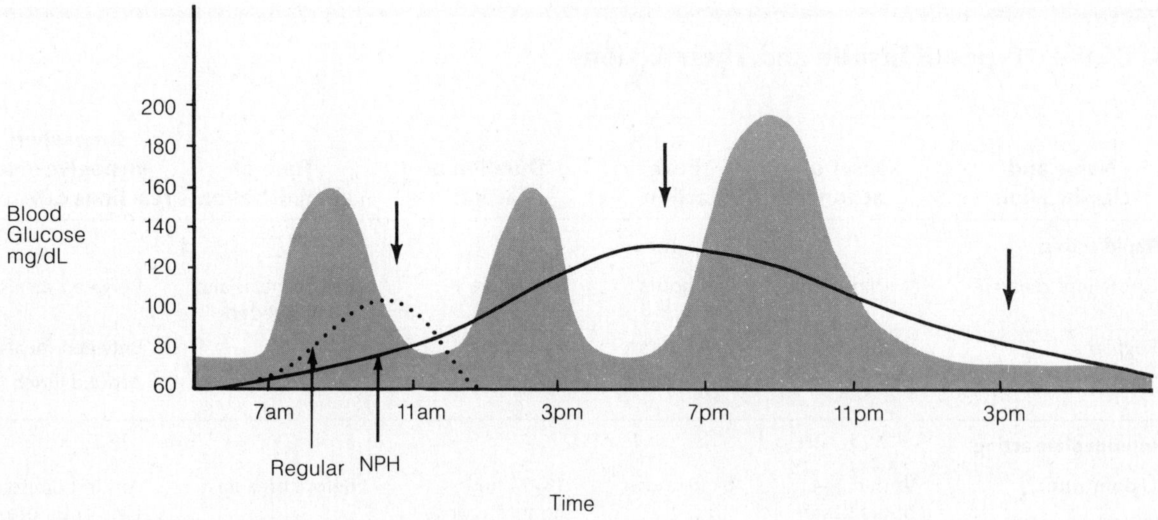

FIGURE 29-2

Blood sugar peaks when the child is receiving three meals. Effects of regular and NPH insulin given in one morning injection. Arrows indicate times most at risk for hypoglycemia.

usually are included in any diet plan. Because of the growth needs of children, the diet includes adequate milk and calories for the child's desired weight. Some diet plans use the American Diabetes Association food-exchange lists for structuring the diet.

Diabetic ketoacidosis When glucose control is not maintained or stress or illness cause blood glucose levels to rise, ketoacidosis (diabetic coma) results. The nurse performs careful assessment of the level of consciousness; of the state of hydration, including skin turgor, mucous membranes, neck veins, and blood pressure; and of cardiac status. A thorough but brief history of the events leading to ketoacidosis is taken. Treatment is planned to monitor the child's rehydration and return to metabolic normality and to prevent the complications of ketoacidosis (hypoglycemia, hypokalemia, and cerebral edema). Children in ketoacidosis have deficits in their water, sodium, potassium, and chloride chemistry. The degree of deficit depends on the length of time in ketoacidosis and the child's ability to maintain adequate fluid and electrolyte intake.

Bicarbonate replacement is used cautiously and sparingly to prevent cardiac arrhythmias and worsening acidosis. Bicarbonate usually is given when the arterial pH drops below 7.1. Metabolic acidosis generally is self-limiting with adequate rehydration and insulin therapy.

Insulin is given initially by IV bolus. Subsequently, IV fluid volume replacement along with continuous regular insulin drip helps reverse hyperglycemia. Initially a hypotonic IV solution is used. Dextrose is added to the IV solution when the blood sugar reaches 200–300 mg/dL to prevent hypoglycemia. Potassium and phosphate replacement might be required.

Nursing management

Care for the child in ketoacidosis Most of the hospitalizations for diabetic children are related to episodes of ketoacidosis either at the time of diagnosis or during acute illnesses that alter blood glucose control. Nursing care of the child in ketoacidosis involves intensive measures. Nursing interventions include hourly recording of the child's total fluid intake and urine output. If the child cannot void, a urinary catheter might be needed, although catheterization is not desirable because of the possibility of inducing a urinary tract infection and the rapid growth of bacteria in the high-sugar environment. The goal of fluid therapy should be a gradual decline in osmolality. However, a more rapid fluid administration might be required with a severely dehydrated child.

Because potassium deficit generally is the most pronounced electrolyte imbalance in ketoacidosis, the child's cardiac cycle is monitored. The nurse checks the cardiac monitor for signs of hypokalemia (prolonged Q-T interval, low T waves, presence of U-V waves, and depressed S-T segments) and, in rare cases, hyperkalemia (widened QRS complex and high-peaked T waves). Serum electrolytes as well as arterial blood gases are monitored closely.

Vital signs are monitored every one-half to one hour. Alteration in respirations, particularly the appearance of Kussmaul respirations, is significant and is reported immediately. The nurse monitors the child closely for signs of hypovolemic shock (see Chapter 21).

Several methods exist for administering insulin during ketoacidosis, such as intramuscular, intravenous, or some combination of these routes. Regular insulin is the only insulin that can be given intravenously. Insulin has a tendency to cling to the sides of the glass and plastic tubing used for intravenous administration. Priming the infusion set by running 50 mL of the insulin-prepared solution through the tubing and connectors before attaching it to the child helps to prevent this loss of insulin that would otherwise occur during the first few hours. The intravenous fluid is administered by a mechanical infusion pump to ensure a steady, safe flow.

Blood sugar levels are monitored every 1–2 hours. The goal is a gradual decline in the blood glucose level over several hours. Urine is tested for the presence of glucose or ketones.

In addition to the direct care outlined in the previous paragraphs, the nurse offers support to the child's parents and keeps them informed about all aspects of the treatment plan. After the child is stabilized, the family continues to adjust to the changes that will be occurring in their lives and continues to need support, teaching, and encouragement.

Insulin therapy Parents and most children over 12 years of age learn to administer insulin at the time of diagnosis. Some children younger than age 12 years also can be taught injection technique. Some health care teams insist that the child not leave the hospital until each parent has given the child at least one injection.

Learning to inject insulin is difficult for children and families. Accepting the fact that the child needs the injection is the first hurdle. The child and family are allowed to express their feelings of anger and frustration in a supportive environment. Children frequently ask why they must have insulin injections and secretly hope that they will eventually not need injections. They also might feel guilty and view the insulin injections as punishment for having diabetes. The nurse kindly but firmly explains the course of the disease so that children's and parents' expectations are realistic.

Teaching sessions for children and families are planned to be short so as not to be overwhelming. Using visual aids, role playing, and allowing child and family to handle equipment freely is essential. The nurse teaching families to inject insulin makes certain the family (1) knows the correct insulin to use; (2) knows how to draw up the insulin doses correctly; (3) has a plan for the rotation of injection sites; (4) can give the injection comfortably; and (5) has a place to record the insulin dose and site used. Figure 29-3 demonstrates one plan for the rotation of injection sites. Site rotation occurs both among areas of the body and within specific areas. Most children do not use the abdominal sites until adolescence. Even then, the abdomen often is a difficult area to use psychologically. For very young children, the buttocks often are the easiest site to use.

The nurse teaches and practices consistency in the order of drawing and mixing insulin preparations in a syringe. Most practitioners recommend drawing the short-acting (Regular) insulin into the syringe before the longer-acting insulin to prevent contamination of the short-acting insulin by the longer-acting preparation.

Insulin does not require refrigeration as long as it is not exposed to temperatures under 32°F or over 90°F. Extra, unopened bottles of insulin may be stored under refrigeration to prolong their shelf-life. The advantages of using nonrefrigerated insulin are that (1) insulin injections hurt less when the insulin is at room temperature; (2) there might be less tissue damage from insulin at room temperature than from chilled insulin; and (3) insulin suspensions (NPH and Lente) settle less out of suspension at room temperature than when refrigerated.

Insulin dose adjustment is a skill that many children with diabetes and their parents have learned in conjunction with regular home blood glucose monitoring. Table 29-5 presents guidelines for self-management and insulin adjustment based on premeal blood glucose levels. The nurse explores with the family the safest and most cost-effective methods for home insulin use.

Insulin pumps, which administer insulin in response to changing blood sugars, are available in portable form. The portable pumps are not widely accepted by children and adolescents because of the "hassles" associated with the visibility of the pump and the presence of the subcutaneous needle, which is part of the pumped insulin system. If the child and parent choose to use an insulin pump, the nurse teaches the child and family about the operation and care of the pump according to protocol for the particular system used.

Glucose monitoring Home blood glucose monitoring is the preferred method for careful assessment of the child's status. The child uses a lancet or Monoject type lancet to obtain the blood sample. Readings can be obtained by using a reagent strip (changes color with the amount of glucose in the blood) such as Chemstrip bG or Dextrostix, or a more accurate reading can be obtained by use of a meter. The recommended schedule for blood glucose monitoring is four times a day—before each meal and the bedtime snack. Additional readings might be necessary if the child's exercise level is increased or if hypoglycemia is a frequent occurrence.

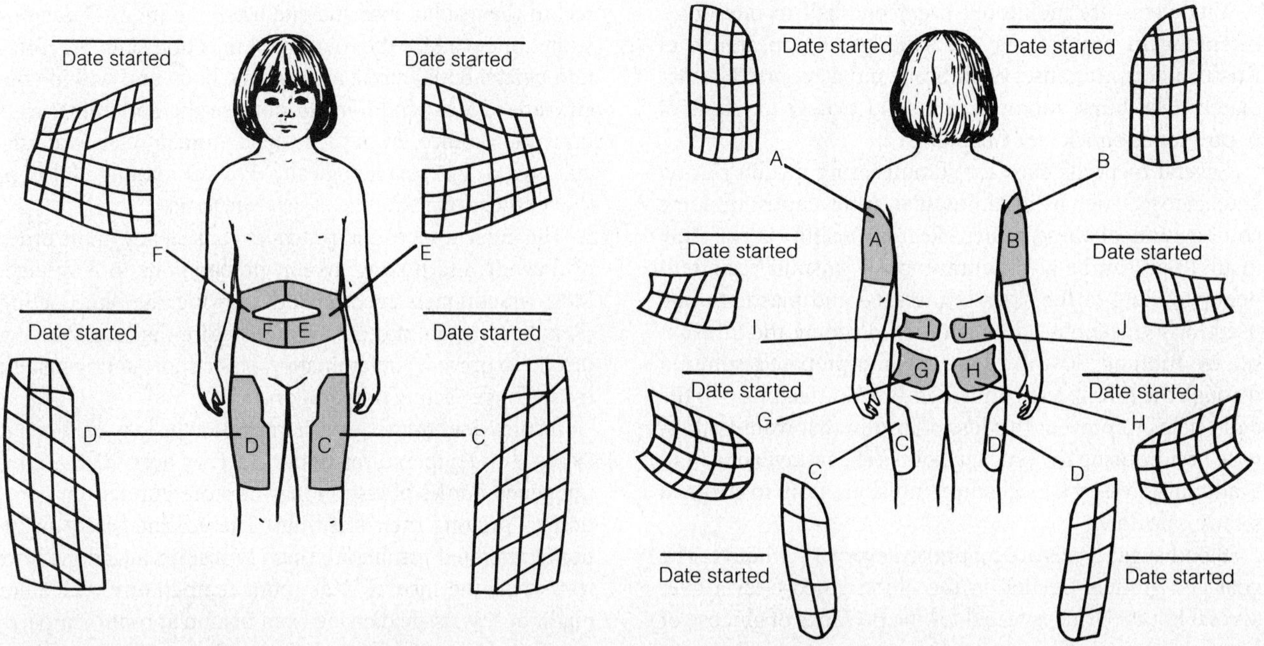

FIGURE 29-3

Sites for the rotation of insulin injections; rotation occurs within and among body areas

TABLE 29-5 Guidelines for the Self-Management of Diabetes

Actions to take	Before breakfast	Before lunch	Late afternoon	Before-bedtime snack	During the night
If blood glucose level is	**Too low**	**Too high**	**Too low**	**Too high**	**Too high**
First	Increase the protein in the bedtime snack	Omit the midmorning snack	Increase the carbohydrate in the midafternoon snack	Increase the evening short-acting insulin	Add or increase the long-acting insulin before the evening meal
Second	Reduce the evening long-acting insulin	Increase the morning short-acting insulin	Decrease the morning long-acting insulin	Add exercise after the evening meal	Check the blood glucose level at 3:00–4:00 AM
Third	Check the blood glucose level at 3:00–4:00 AM	Add exercise in the morning		Decrease the carbohydrate in the evening meal	Add exercise in the evening

Prior to the advent of home blood glucose testing, children with diabetes relied on the assessment of urine glucose spillage to evaluate insulin therapy. Urine glucose monitoring was somewhat inefficient because the lag time between the blood glucose increase and urine spillage of glucose can vary between 20 minutes and 2 hours. Relying solely on urine testing for self-assessment is less safe and less accurate. Urine testing is done, however, when the blood glucose level is greater than 240 mg/dL. It is necessary to monitor urine spillage and the presence of ketones to prevent ketoacidosis. Urine testing can be done with reagent strips. However, more accurate results are obtained by

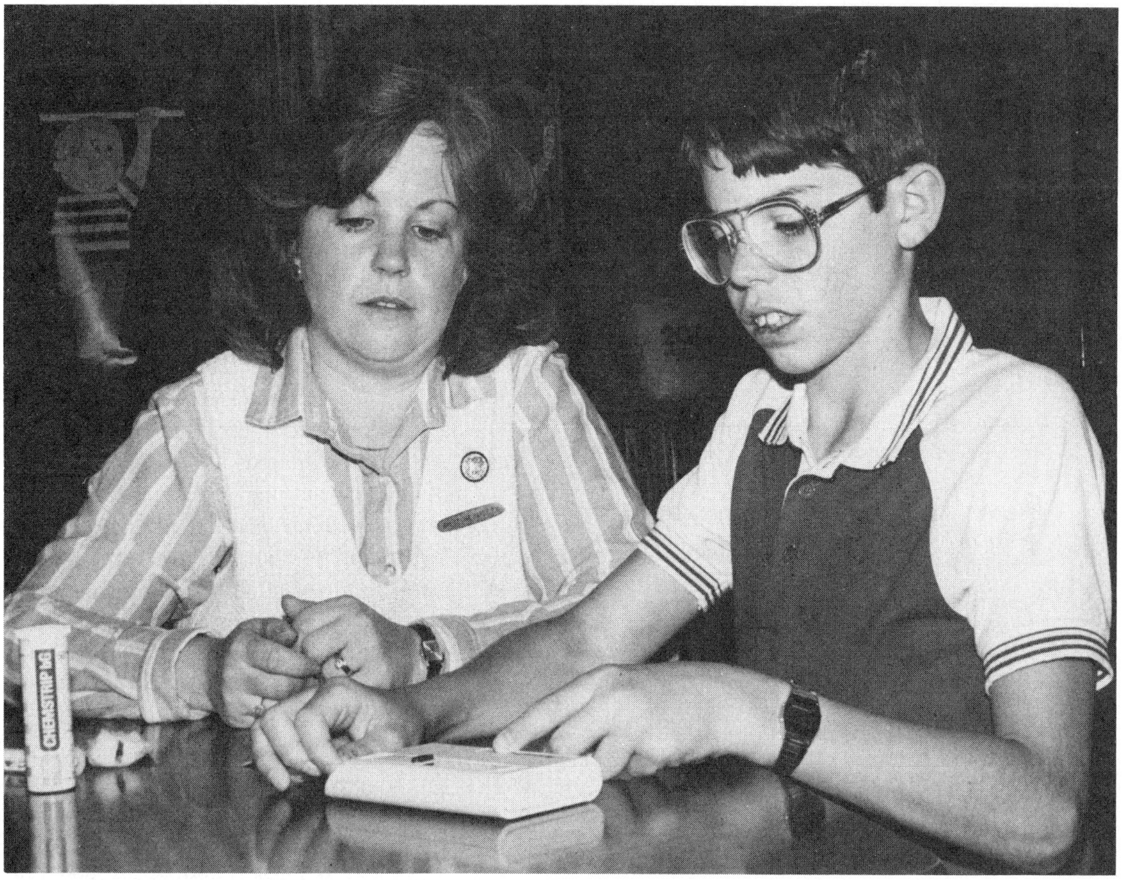

The child with diabetes monitors blood glucose through use of a reagant strip or glucose meter. (Photograph by Judy Koenig.)

using Clinitest and Acetest tablets. Clinitest tablets induce a chemical reaction when added to urine and water. The color change from the reaction (from dark blue to bright orange) indicates the approximate amount of glucose in the urine. Clinitest tablets require either two or five drops of urine. The two drop method is considered to be more accurate. Acetest tablets turn purple in response to a drop of urine containing ketone bodies. The child and parent are taught to use the double-void method and to test the second voided specimen. The nurse teaches the child and family to do urine testing and gives them guidelines for when the testing is to be done and the course of action to be taken should the child test positive.

Diet regulation All growing children require a balanced diet to provide adequate calories and nutrients, and children with diabetes are no exception. Regardless of the philosophy of the health care team toward dietary management, the goal is to provide a balance of nutrients aimed at sustaining growth and minimizing both hypoglycemia and hyperglycemia. The caloric level recommended for most children is based on age and weight.

Two approaches to teaching children about food management are the exchange lists and the free diet. Both systems restrict the types and amounts of simple sugars that are allowed. The *exchange lists* (Table 29-6) use six food groups to provide a framework for both qualitative and quantitative control of the diet. The *free diet,* a qualitative approach, strives to avoid a rigid structuring of food patterns. It does not define specific types and amounts of food. The rationale for the free diet stems from the concern that calorically controlled diets do not provide the necessary allowances for normal growth and development, and the strict monitoring of food intake has the potential for emotional harm (Heins, 1983). Children and their families also benefit from information about fast-food restaurants so that the child might eat with peers.

Self-testing Whether control is measured using blood or urine testing, the child and family need to learn the

TABLE 29-6 Exchange Lists for the Diabetic Diet

Exchange	Composition
Milk	Includes nonfat, low-fat, and whole milk. One exchange of milk contains 12 g of carbohydrate, 8 g of protein, a trace of fat, and 80 calories
Vegetable	One exchange of vegetables contains about 5 g of carbohydrate, 2 g of protein, and 25 calories
Fruit	One exchange of fruit contains 10 g of carbohydrate and 40 calories
Bread	Includes bread, cereal, and starchy vegetables. One exchange of bread contains 15 g of carbohydrate, 2 g of protein, and 70 calories
Meat	Lean meat: one exchange of lean meat (1 oz) contains 7 g of protein, 3 g of fat, and 55 calories
	Medium-fat meat: for each exchange of medium-fat meat, omit one-half fat exchange
	High-fat meat: for each exchange of high-fat meat, omit one fat exchange
	Fat: One exchange of fat contains 5 g of fat and 45 calories

proper technique, when to do the testing, how to record the results, and how to interpret the test results. Generally, the more often testing is performed, the more information is available on which to make decisions about diabetes management. Most children test in the morning before insulin and breakfast, in the late afternoon before insulin and dinner, and prior to the bedtime snack. Occasionally, tests are performed before lunch and during the night (2:00–4:00 AM). Some children also test before and after exercise to determine any necessary adjustments in insulin or food intake.

Timed collections of urine specimens can help to assess the total glucose spilled into the urine during specific times of the day or night. The child must begin and end a collection period with an empty bladder. All urine is then saved and measured at the end of the collection period. The urine is tested for glucose, and the amount of glucose spilled is calculated by multiplying the volume of the urine collected (in milliliters) by the grams per deciliter present in the tested collection. For example, urine collected from breakfast until lunch measured 300 mL and tested at 5 g/dL; therefore, 15 g of sugar were spilled. This information indicates a need to increase the morning Regular insulin.

Exercise planning When helping a diabetic child plan an exercise program, the nurse assesses the child's previous activity level and uses it as a guide for planning the type, intensity, duration, and frequency of exercise. The nurse then helps the child to establish short-term goals and identify bodily responses to exercise and the relationship of exercise, diet, and insulin. Exercise patterns in school are considered as well as exercise patterns after school and on weekends. The nurse might want to consult with the school regarding the amount of exercise and the times for recess and gym classes.

Exercise, although it requires additional glucose, is beneficial to the child with diabetes. In additon to the usual beneficial effects of exercise, the metabolic effects of frequent exercise are numerous. These include the reduction of insulin requirements, increased storage and utilization of glucose, and less extreme fluctuations in the diabetic's blood glucose level over a 24-hour period.

Although children with diabetes are encouraged to exercise, exercise is not without potential problems. Children and adolescents with diabetes might experience hypoglycemia during or after exercise because muscle and liver glycogen become depleted and the continued presence of injected insulin suppresses the hepatic output of glucose. Body tissues become more sensitive to insulin with exercise because of the increased affinity of the insulin-binding receptors. The nurse and the diabetic can rehearse exercise situations and plan changes in food intake or insulin dosage to prevent the occurrence of hypoglycemia.

The opposite problem (hyperglycemia and ketonuria) also might occur when a person with diabetes exercises. This is caused by the fact that production of glucose in the liver lags behind muscle use. Thus the liver produces the glucose after the muscles have stopped working, causing an "overshoot" of glucose. Based on this knowledge, the current recommendation is to exercise if the blood glucose level is under 200 mg/dL and there are no ketones present in the urine.

Skin care Parents often have questions about skin care (use of topical ointments, care of blisters, permitting children to go without shoes) because of the skin and circulatory problems older individuals with diabetes experience. Children with well-controlled diabetes have good white blood cell function and patent blood vessels so that the healing of skin injuries is generally uncomplicated. The nurse advises children and families to file toenails straight across and even with the end of the toe; to wear comfortable shoes; to care for blisters, cuts, or abrasions by cleansing with soap and water; and to go without shoes only where there is no danger of injuring the feet.

Adolescents and enuretic or pretoilet-trained young children with diabetes are susceptible to vaginal and perineal

Fast-Food Exchanges for Children with Diabetes

	Serving size	Calories (1 serving)	Carb. (g)	Pro. (g)	Fat (g)	Sodium (mg)	Exchanges (1 serving)
Kentucky Fried Chicken (edible portion of Original Recipe Chicken)							
Wing	1(56g)	181	6	12	12	387	½ Starch, 1½ Med.-Fat Meat, 1 Fat
Drumstick	1(58g)	147	4	14	9	269	2 Med.-Fat Meat
Side Breast	1(95g)	27	10	2	17	65	½ Starch, 2 Med.-Fat Meat
Thigh	1(96g)	278	8	18	18	517	½ Starch, 2 Med.-Fat Meat, 2 Fat
Center Breast	1(107g)	57	8	26	14	532	½ Starch, 3 Med.-Fat Meat
Cole Slaw	1(79g)	103	12	1	6	171	2 Vegetable or 1 Starch, 1 Fat
McDonald's							
Hamburger	1(100g)	263	28	12	11	506	2 Starch, 1 Med.-Fat Meat, 1 Fat
Quarter Pounder	1(160g)	427	29	25	23	718	2 Starch, 3 Med.-Fat Meat, 1 Fat
French Fries (Regular)	1(68g)	220	26	3	12	109	2 Starch, 2 Fat
Chicken McNuggets	1(109g)	323	15	19	20	512	1 Starch, 2 Med.-Fat Meat, 2 Fat
Egg McMuffin	1(138g)	340	31	19	16	885	2 Starch, 2 Med.-Fat Meat, 1 Fat
Shakey's							
Thin Cheese 13″ Pizza	1/10	140	18	9	5	315	1 Starch, 1 Med.-Fat Meat
Thin Pepperoni 13″ Pizza	1/10	183	11	17	8	455	1 Starch, 2 Med.-Fat Meat
Thin Onion, Green Pepper, Olive, Mushroom 13″ Pizza	1/10	171	21	10	5	395	1 Starch, 1 Med.-Fat Meat, 1 Vegetable
Thick Pepperoni 13″ Pizza	1/10	232	19	19	8	494	1 Starch, 2 Med.-Fat Meat
Taco Bell							
Beef Burrito	1	466	37	30	21	327	2½ Starch, 3 Med.-Fat Meat, 1 Fat
Beef Tostada	1	291	21	19	15	138	1½ Starch, 2 Med.-Fat Meat, 1 Fat
Taco	1	186	14	15	8	79	1 Starch, 2 Lean-Fat Meat
Tostada	1	179	25	9	6	101	1½ Starch, 1 Med.-Fat Meat

Excerpted from Franz M: Fast Food Facts, 1987, with permission of the author and publisher, Diabetes Centers, Inc., PO Box 739, Woyzata, MN 55391.

fungal infections. These infections can be minimized by maintaining good blood glucose control, keeping the perineal area as dry as possible, practicing good hygiene, and allowing air to reach the perineum by avoiding nylon underwear and tight-fitting garments.

Hypoglycemia Hypoglycemia needs to be treated promptly whenever it is suspected. Severe hypoglycemia leads to seizures, possible brain damage, and death.

Hypoglycemia sometimes is difficult to differentiate from hyperglycemia. Parents and school personnel can be given a

Parent Checklist

	Hypoglycemia	Hyperglycemia
Does the child appear to be	□ irritable, tired, headachy, dizzy, hungry, shaky, vomiting?	□ weak, thirsty, nauseous, breathing rapidly or deeply, going to the bathroom frequently?
Is the child's skin	□ pale and clammy?	□ flushed and dry?
Did the symptoms appear	□ suddenly?	□ gradually?
Has the child skipped a meal or suddenly increased exercise?	□ yes	□ no
Has the child experienced any recent stressful event or infection?	□ no	□ yes
Has the child's blood glucose been	□ lower than usual?	□ higher than usual?
Does the urine show any glucose or acetone?	□ no	□ yes
Does the child have a fruity breath?	□ no	□ yes

simple checklist to remind them of the symptoms while they are still learning about diabetes. Children over 5 years of age and parents, siblings, babysitters, athletic coaches, and school personnel should be familiar with the signs of hypoglycemia and know how to treat the condition when it occurs. Most children with diabetes experience mild hypoglycemia at least once a month because of the difficulty of balancing food, exercise, and insulin dosage.

Mild hypoglycemia can be managed with an oral feeding of a rapidly acting sugar (see Table 29-7). Generally, 10 g of carbohydrate (40 calories) is sufficient to bring the blood glucose level back to normal, although the symptoms of shakiness and headache might persist for hours after the blood glucose level has been normalized. The immediate treatment is followed with a meal or snack. If the child is in the hospital or clinic when hypoglycemia is suspected, the nurse performs a blood glucose test to determine the blood glucose level prior to initiating treatment. Each child's tolerance of a low blood glucose level is different, and knowing the level at which symptoms occur assists in regulating daily diet, insulin, and activity and in planning for special events for that child.

When the blood glucose has fallen to a very low level, the child might be semiconscious, combative, or unable to swallow and thus unable to take an oral feeding. Glucose pastes or gels can be squeezed into the pouches of the child's cheeks and the cheeks and neck massaged to speed up absorption of the glucose through the mucous membranes.

If the child does not respond to this treatment in 5–10 minutes, glucagon can be given as an intramuscular injection. Glucagon is a hormone made by the alpha cells of the pancreas, and when injected, it raises the blood glucose level by releasing glucose from glycogen stores in the liver and muscles. The dose of glucagon is 0.5–1.0 mg.

The child generally will awaken within 10–15 minutes, and a snack or meal is then taken to sustain the blood glucose level. The rapid rise in glucose following the administration of glucagon might cause nausea and vomiting, and the blood glucose level might remain elevated for as long as 24 hours after the episode of hypoglycemia. With severe hypoglycemia, the child might lose consciousness and/or exhibit seizure activity. If this occurs at home, the parents can give glucagon; however, the child also might require intravenous glucose to correct the problem.

Caution is taken with the concentration of glucose used to correct hypoglycemia and the rate at which it is administered. If the child remains in a postseizure state following severe hypoglycemia, continuous slow-drip intravenous glucose might be required for several hours to maintain blood glucose levels until the child is able to eat.

Because hypoglycemia can occur at any time, the nurse advises the child to wear a medical identification necklace or bracelet. Adolescents also need to mark their drivers' licenses and carry food in the car when driving. Most children keep snacks in their desks, school lockers, purses, or bookbags. After an episode of hypoglycemia has occurred and been successfully treated, parents, children, and health professionals need to discuss the cause of the hypoglycemia and take steps to prevent its recurrence.

Strategies for special problems Three special problems faced by the diabetic child are illness, growth spurts,

TABLE 29-7 Management of Hypoglycemia

Symptoms: Cerebral	Symptoms: Adrenal	Management	
Dizziness, headache, nausea, drowsiness, irritability, poor coordination, personality change	Shakiness, trembling, sweating, pallor, dilatation of pupils causing blurred vision	Give a snack of 10 g fast-acting sugar followed by a meal or snack	
		2 tbsp raisins	6–7 Lifesavers
		1 fruit roll-up	½ cup fruit juice
		½ can regular soda	5 sugar cubes
		⅓ bottle of Glutose	

SOURCE: Balik B, Haig B, Moynihan P: Diabetes and the school-aged child. *Am Matern-Child Nurs* (Sept/Oct) 1986; 11(5): 324–330.

and puberty. The nurse can offer strategies for coping with each of these problems.

Illness When a child with diabetes becomes ill, the family might encounter blood glucose levels that are above or below the child's usual level. In addition, ketones often develop. Illness is one of the most frequent causes of diabetic ketoacidosis.

The usual diet might be unpalatable, and the insulin dose might need to be adjusted. Frequent testing of blood and urine is needed to determine how well the diabetes is being controlled. The parent also is taught to be aware of the child's state of hydration because potassium imbalance is a special concern with dehydration.

Parents often question the use of over-the-counter medications (cough suppressants, cold remedies, and so on). These drugs are used with care because many contain concentrated sugar.

Health care professionals provide emotional support for the child and family during the illness and help them to make any needed insulin adjustments. On sick days, the meal plan emphasizes easily digested carbohydrates. If food intake is problematic (because of anorexia, vomiting, or nausea), insulin can be given in small, frequent doses to avoid potential hypoglycemia.

Most illnesses can be managed at home with careful monitoring by the parent in consultation with the health care team. If repeated vomiting occurs, the child will require emergency room evaluation and treatment with intravenous fluids. The nurse might encounter a parent who is very fatigued and discouraged because the child's condition did not improve despite all the efforts of home care. The nurse needs to recognize and praise the parent's efforts, while reassuring the parent that occasionally medical intervention is needed to restore balance. After the child's condition is stable, it is mutually beneficial for the nurse to spend time with the parent and review the events preceding the emergency treatment. This discussion will facilitate planning for management of the diabetes during future illnesses.

Growth All children require insulin to promote growth; the amount of insulin needed increases with growth. Children with diabetes, therefore, require periodic (three to four times per year) medical evaluations of their insulin requirements.

Additional calories are required during a time of increased growth whether the child is a diabetic or a nondiabetic. Sporadic growth spurts, a characteristic of children, are accompanied by a marked change in appetite and demand for additional food. Parents describe these periods as a time when their children consume enormous quantities of food during a week and then return to their usual eating patterns. The following week these parents often note an increase in their child's weight, height, or both.

When the nondiabetic child goes through a growth spurt, the pancreas is able to produce additional insulin to facilitate the metabolic process of carbohydrates and provide a supply of glucose required for cells' energy expenditure. The diabetic child is unable to tolerate the extra carbohydrates consumed. When additional insulin is not available to use the increased glucose produced and to convert it to energy, the kidneys waste it. Thus, when the child who has diabetes eats additional food to satisfy hunger, blood sugar levels increase and the child might experience signs of hyperglycemia.

The nurse advises parents concerning growth spurts and encourages them to provide additional, nutritionally adequate, well-balanced proportions of proteins, carbohydrates, and fats for their growing children. Insulin is then adjusted so glucose is available for cell energy and growth. For optimal growth, the child requires flexibility in diet and insulin requirements to allow for these sporadic episodes of increased need. Parents who are prepared for these episodes can make the necessary adjustments and prevent potential conflict between hunger and glucose control. Understanding their children's unique needs within normal growth and development will help parents enhance their children's sense of self-esteem rather than foster a sense of failure whenever glucose spillage occurs.

Puberty If the diabetes is adequately controlled, most children will enter and progress through puberty at the expected times (10–14 years of age for females and 11–16 years of age for males). Menstrual periods might be associated with hyperglycemia and ketonuria because of estrogen and progesterone changes. The dosage of insulin might need to be adjusted during this time.

The developmental tasks of adolescence might interfere with good glucose control and cause friction between the parent and adolescent. The nurse can intercede, acting as an interested third party when the parents or adolescents need to talk about their frustrations. As the child enters adolescence, the nurse reviews the treatment plan with the child. Alterations can be made at this time to accommodate as much as possible the adolescent's changing food and exercise preferences. Role playing is particularly helpful for teaching the adolescent how to handle complicated social situations where it is important for the adolescent to appear to be like peers. Smoking and drinking alcohol are to be discouraged strongly. Camps or peer support groups can be helpful to adolescents who are diabetic.

Prevention of complications Approximately 50% of individuals with diabetes develop microvascular disease of the retina (retinopathy) and kidney. Macrovascular disease (coronary artery disease and poor peripheral circulation) and neuropathy also can be complications. The debate regarding the cause of this process has raged for years. Some authorities feel that the vascular complications are related directly to hyperglycemia (and that careful glucose control might prevent or minimize the problems). Other experts feel that there might be various subtypes of diabetes, with some people being more susceptible to the development of complications.

Previously, no methods were available to control the blood glucose perfectly by the physiologic delivery of insulin; therefore, the question was unanswerable. With the advent of home blood glucose monitoring and portable insulin pumps, the questions might be resolved. However, because most individuals do not develop complications until at least 15 years after diagnosis, a generation of children using these latest management tools will have to be studied around the turn of the twenty-first century to assess the impact of improved control on the development of complications. The nurse observes each child on a regular basis for the early development of complications.

Coping and acceptance strategies Because their age, cognitive and development levels, and life experiences differ, children and adults (parents and health professionals) have different concerns about diabetes. It is unwise, impractical, and unsuccessful to use scare tactics (threats of possible vascular disease) to convince children to test more often, remember their injections, or eat appropriately.

Young children also have a difficult time accepting the fact that their parents have to hurt them purposefully to help them. Children at this level of moral development believe that the hurt is punishment for wrongdoing. The nurse and parent need to provide careful explanations for the child using age-appropriate terms and make a clear distinction between treating the disease and disciplining the child.

Children with diabetes might have difficulty understanding why they have to be different from their peers (see the discussion of chronic illness in Chapter 14). They are reminded constantly about the consequences of their disease because they have to eat certain foods according to a schedule, interrupt play for a snack or premeal testing and insulin, forego spontaneous trips for ice cream treats, and abstain from or limit their intake of sweets at birthday and school parties.

The daily insulin injections are not only bothersome but also the source of fearful fantasies. Many children have latent fears of self-injury or body mutilation related to the daily insulin injections.

In late adolescence individuals develop the ability for abstract thinking and can begin to perceive life with a career or job, family and home, or travel and adventure at 30 or 40 years of age and what it might be like. However, peer activities of the present are judged to be more important than tasks to ensure optimal glucose control. Adolescents might react to information about potential vascular complications in any one of several ways. They might become depressed, feeling as if a "big cloud" were hanging over them and that they are doomed no matter how hard they try to control the diabetes. The depression might be manifested in behavior such as total denial of the diabetes, refusal to take injections, inappropriate eating, and a general disregard for all preventive measures or early warning signs. Another adolescent might develop an all-consuming concern about the future and feel that "if only I work hard enough to keep my blood glucose normal, this won't happen to me." This person might be quite compulsive about glucose testing and elect to use an insulin pump or take multiple insulin injections every day in search of normoglycemia and be angry and frustrated when these hoped-for results are not achieved.

Parents also deal with concerns about diabetes in a variety of ways. They might attend compulsively to every facet of the child's diabetes management, or they might expect the child to assume total responsibility for the management (denial). Parents of young children might feel guilty about inflicting the pain of injections and blood testing. Parents of

NURSING CARE PLAN *The Child with Diabetes Mellitus*

Assessment data: Teri, an 8-year-old black girl, was diagnosed recently with type I diabetes mellitus. She presented with a 2-week history of vaginitis, polydipsia, polyuria, and weight loss. Teri lives with her single mother, 6-year-old brother, and 4-year-old sister in an apartment in a low-income neighborhood near the hospital.

Nursing diagnosis	Intervention	Rationale
1. Knowledge deficit concerning insulin therapy related to unfamiliarity with injection procedure and relation of insulin to the disease process	Disucss learning style preferences with Teri and her mother before teaching initial procedure, and plan the approach accordingly; keep teaching sessions short—no longer than 20 minutes.	Some people prefer oral communication, audiovisual materials, and demonstration/practice to reading educational materials. Learning occurs most easily when individual preferences are respected. Short teaching sessions decrease anxiety and allow the child and parent to absorb the information.
	Explain how the body repsonds to too much sugar (hyperglycemia), and provide the family with a list of related signs and symptons.	Knowing how the body responds to sugar leads into the discussion of what happens when insulin is not available to metabolize sugars.
	Explain the function and need for insulin as well as the types of insulin and their onset, peak, and duration.	Knowledge about insulin and its necessity for proper glucose usage is important to understanding and accepting the need for daily (and usually twice daily) insulin injections.
	Demonstrate the technique of drawing up insulin into a syringe and have the parent return the demonstration; Teri is receiving 5U Regular and 7U NPH insulin one-half hour before breakfast.	Demonstration and practice at the person's own pace enhance learning.
	Explain the method of giving the injection; have the parent practice on a doll before giving the injection to the child.	Practice on an inanimate object allows one to feel comfortable with the technique before needing to use it on a child.
	Explain site rotation and demonstrate use of the site rotation chart.	Use of the chart reinforces rotation of sites as a concrete guide available and lessens potential for subcutaneous tissue damage.
	Discuss care and storage of insulin and supplies.	Proper care of supplies is important to ensure sterility of equipment and safety.
	Explain how the body responds to too much insulin (hypoglycemia), and provide the family with a list of related signs and symptoms; give the family a list of fast-acting sugars to be given for hypoglycemic episodes; demonstrate the use of glucagon.	Prompt management of hypoglycemic episodes is essential. The child can learn to recognize her own symptoms and deal with them. Glucagon can be administered if the child is unable to eat or is unconscious.

Outcome: Teri's mother can confidently explain the action and purposes of insulin and can demonstrate appropriate injection technique. Teri and her mother can describe the signs of hypoglycemia and can list foods that can be given to counteract the hypoglycemia.

2. Knowledge deficit concerning dietary management of diabetes related to incomplete understanding of the disease process	Review and reinforce dietary teaching done by the nutritionist; discuss the role of diet in controlling blood glucose levels; discuss the specifics of Teri's diet and have Teri and her mother answer questions about kinds of food, amounts of food, and times of eating; emphasize the importance of not skipping a meal or snack.	A balanced diet consisting of proteins, carbohydrates, and fats is essential for growth and health. Consistent amount and pattern of food intake is necessary to maintain proper balance of insulin and sugar.

(Continues)

NURSING CARE PLAN *The Child with Diabetes Mellitus (Continued)*

Nursing diagnosis	Intervention	Rationale
	Have Teri and her mother plan a week's menu of meals and snacks.	Actual meal planning defines options and reinforces dietary teaching.
	Explain the effects of physical activity on the balance of sugar and insulin; discuss how to adjust insulin and food requirements for times of increased or decreased activity.	Insulin dosage and diet are prescribed for normal activity. When activity level is increased, more food or less insulin is needed; when activity level is decreased, less food or more insulin is needed.
	Discuss with Teri and her mother how to adjust diet and insulin during times of illness or emotional stress.	Illness and stress can increase blood sugar, necessitating alterations in diet and insulin.
	Encourage Teri's mother to contact the health care provider during times of stress; give her a phone number of who she can contact.	Failure to contact the health provider might result in inappropriate management and hospitalization.

Outcome: Teri and her mother can answer questions about her diet and about the effect of too much or too little food. Teri and her mother are able to identify times of stress and have learned how to adjust insulin and diet to maintain good control of diabetes.

Nursing diagnosis	Intervention	Rationale
3. Knowledge deficit concerning methods for glucose monitoring related to unfamiliarity with the procedures and meaning of test results.	Explain how blood glucose results relate to diabetic control and the insulin, diet, exercise interrelationship.	Control of diabetes depends on how much the child and parent know about it; the separate parts of management need to be explained as being interrelated to provide better comprehension of the condition and the importance of each phase of management.
	Teach Teri and her mother how to do blood glucose testing using reagent strips and urine glucose and ketone testing using Clinitest and Acetest tablets.	Blood glucose testing provides a more accurate picture of diabetic control. Urine should be tested when blood glucose rises above 240 mg/dL to monitor any ketoacidosis.
	Provide a chart and demonstrate how to record results.	Written results reduce the risk of forgetting and subsequent inappropriate management.

Outcome: Teri and her mother can demonstrate both blood and urine glucose testing and can correctly interpret and act on test results.

Nursing diagnosis	Intervention	Rationale
4. Impaired skin integrity related to altered metabolic state secondary to increased blood glucose	Teach Teri proper perineal care, including keeping the area as dry as possible, avoiding powders, and avoiding the use of nylon underclothing.	Moist areas support the growth of fungal organisms, which can then become clinically observable. Children with diabetes are more prone to developing vaginitis because of a carbohydrate-rich environment that supports organism growth.
	Teach Teri and her mother the importance of good skin care, prompt care of lacerations, and properly fitting shoes.	Long-term complications of improperly managed diabetes include circulatory compromise with delayed healing.

Outcome: Teri practices appropriate perineal hygiene to prevent a recurrence of vaginal infections. Teri and her mother can describe the potential long-term consequences of elevated blood glucose to the skin and institute appropriate measures to prevent infection and skin breakdown.

Nursing diagnosis	Intervention	Rationale
5. Potential alteration in health maintenance (stressors: change in routine at school, peer pressures, or possible financial difficulties)	Contact the school nurse and send her a written plan of care, including insulin dosage, snack schedules, schedule for glucose monitoring, and measures to be used for hypoglycemic episodes; provide the school nurse with a telephone number for questions.	Networking and collaboration with other health professionals increase the contact and coverage for the child and family. Persons interacting in the home and school environment might be better able to assess the child's and family's reaction to illness.

NURSING CARE PLAN *The Child with Diabetes Mellitus (Continued)*

Nursing diagnosis	Intervention	Rationale
	Encourage Teri to visit the nurse to go over the plan with her and to familiarize herself with the school facilities.	If the child is comfortable in the environment, she will be more likely to use resources appropriately.
	Refer Teri to the community health nurse for initial follow-up visits.	Follow-up is essential to be sure the family is carrying out the treatment plan in the home and not experiencing any difficulties.
	Encourage Teri and her family to attend lay diabetes meetings and explore any potential problems such as transportation; refer Teri to a scholarship program for summer diabetes camp.	The family might not be aware of the available resources for social support or how to contact other children and families who are dealing with diabetes also.
	Explore with the family and the social worker effective but least expensive diabetic equipment.	Use of bottled alcohol and cotton balls is less expensive than prepackaged alcohol swabs; a glass syringe with disposable needles is less expensive than disposable syringes; however, the family must be competent with sterilizing the syringe.
Outcome: Teri and her mother plan to use appropriate community resources to assist them with diabetic management. Teri can identify the appropriate people from whom to obtain assistance in school.		
6. Potential self-esteem disturbance (stressors: daily insulin injections, glucose monitoring, feeling "different," and uncertainty managing new diet and activity regimen)	Encourage Teri to participate in her usual activities with peers and family; incorporate the treatment plan into her routine as much as possible.	Preventing the child from feeling "different" can prevent self-esteem disturbance.
	Counsel the mother to be alert for any signs of rebellion or noncompliance with the treatment plan and to request reevaluation if this becomes evident.	Rebellion is usual during adolescent years and requires a reevaluation of the plan in order to answer the child's new physical and emotional needs.
Outcome: Teri demonstrates acceptance of her limitations and begins to acquire self-management skills. Teri's mother can describe signs of rebellion and will initiate reevaluation should such occur.		

older children might have mixed feelings of apprehension and relief as the children take over management tasks and become more independent. Parents of adolescents often have difficulty sorting out normal adolescent behaviors from problems related to diabetes.

Nurses and other professionals help children and parents set short-term and long-term goals for diabetes management by teaching them the concepts and skills needed to reach the goals, helping them to break down large goals into easily achieved smaller steps, and readily providing reinforcement and support (Table 29-8). The nurse can negotiate behavioral contracts with children and parents and thus achieve shared responsibility for the diabetes management.

Nurses need to be alert to the types of parenting known to place the child at risk for problems in adjusting to diabetes. The overprotective parent can place the child at risk for problems as can an overpermissive parent. The goal is to have parents be supportive and caring while allowing the child independence according to the child's developmental level and readiness to take control. Families with a diabetic child mourn their loss of flexibility and mourn the loss of a "healthy child." They might resent the work involved on a daily basis, have difficulty sharing the work of managing the diabetes, and encounter financial hardships associated with hospitalizations, supplies, and physicians' fees. The nurse helps the family to assess its strengths and to have realistic expectations of the child's ability for self-management.

Lay groups composed of the families and individuals with diabetes can be important resources for children and parents. Common concerns, fears, and problems as well as

TABLE 29-8 Guidelines for Diabetes Management Goals According to Age-Appropriate Steps

Age	Diet	Insulin	Testing
4–5 years	Helps pick foods based on likes and dislikes	Helps pick injection sites; pinches up skin; wipes skin	Collects blood or urine; watches parent do testing; colors test results on records
6–7 years	Can tell if food has no sugar, some sugar, or lots of sugar	Pushes plunger in after parent gives shot	Performs blood or urine test; records results; might need reminding; will need supervision
8–9 years	Selects foods based on exchanges	Gives own shots (at least once a day)	Does own blood test
10–13 years	Knows diet plan	Rotates sites; measures insulin	Looks for patterns in test results
14+ years	Plans meals and snacks	Mixes two insulins in one syringe (if needed)	Suggests insulin changes based on test patterns

SOURCE: *My Child Has Diabetes: A Book of Questions and Feelings.* Becton Dickinson Consumer Products, 1985, p. 7. Reprinted by permission.

possible solutions are shared and discussed. Social group activities such as fundraising to support research offer both hope and an opportunity for action. Diabetes camps are another resource and one viewed by many parents and professionals as the most important learning experience for children. In camp, skills are learned in an atmosphere of mutual support and peer acceptance while physical activity and wellness are stressed and experienced.

Diabetes is a challenging condition to manage. The nurse, working in a team with the physician, dietitian, psychologist, social worker, and other significant people, can offer vital support and education to the children and families who must live with this disorder.

The Child with Inappropriate Secretion from the Anterior Lobe of the Pituitary Gland

Growth Hormone

The final height of an individual is reached when the bone epiphyses (the lengthening part of bone) close and their cartilage is replaced by bone. Once the epiphyses have ossified, very little linear growth occurs. The anterior lobe of the pituitary gland secretes *somatotropin,* or *growth hormone.* Growth hormone affects all aspects of growth including linear, or skeletal growth, as well as protein, fat, and carbohydrate metabolism.

Growth Hormone Hypersecretion—Pituitary Gigantism

Growth hormone excess is rare in children. When it occurs in childhood, a tumor often is present in the hypothalamic-pituitary unit. These tumors increase the secretion of the growth hormone. If this process occurs prior to epiphyseal closure, linear growth might be considerable (7–8 feet in height). If excessive growth hormone secretion develops after epiphyseal closure, further linear growth does not occur, and the child does not achieve abnormally tall stature. The excessive growth hormone levels, however, do promote acromegaly (elongation of the mandible), causing malocclusion of the jaws and teeth; bony overgrowth of joints in the extremities, causing disabling arthritis; and an increased quantity of soft tissue at the heels, increasing shoe size.

A child with excessive growth hormone secretion frequently will have associated symptoms related to the effect of the tumor on other pituitary hormones or body structures. Alterations in FSH (follicle-stimulating hormone), LH (luteinizing hormone), and ACTH (adrenocorticotropic hormone) levels can cause delayed sexual development. Growth hormone stimulates release of glucagon by the liver, causing rising blood glucose. Pressure from a pituitary tumor can cause optic nerve deficit, resulting in visual impairment. Heart enlargement with hypertension and generalized visceral enlargement occur with excessive stimulation.

Treatment Treatment of growth hormone excess includes reduction or removal of the pituitary tumor. This is accomplished by surgical removal or by such techniques as cryosurgery or radiation. (See Chapter 31 for care of the child following neurologic surgery.) Replacement hormones usually are ordered after tumor removal. These might include androgens, estrogens or progesterones, and thyroid hormone.

Nursing management Nursing management includes screening young children for excessive growth. The child's height is plotted on growth curves at each visit. A sharply elevated growth curve is cause for concern and referral for evaluation is indicated.

Additionally, nursing management is directed toward providing preoperative and postoperative care, assisting the child to develop a positive body image, and monitoring for alterations in blood glucose and fluid balance.

Another disorder associated with tall stature, which needs to be differentiated from growth hormone excess, is cerebral gigantism. In this condition, growth hormone levels are normal, as are other endocrine functions. Children with this disorder have prominent foreheads and other cranial abnormalities, mental retardation, and advanced skeletal maturation. The cause of this condition is attributed to a cerebral defect rather than pituitary dysfunction.

Growth Hormone Hyposecretion—Hypopituitarism

In addition to its systemic growth-promoting effects, growth hormone also plays a role in glucose balance. It prevents hypoglycemia by decreasing glucose uptake by muscles and by stimulating glucagon secretion. As a result, growth hormone deficiency is suspected in a child who is growing at a subnormal rate (less than 1.5 in./yr) and who has hypoglycemia. Usually there is a history of an insult to the area of the pituitary gland (brain tumor, cranial irradiation, hydrocephalus, or encephalitis) or other associated pituitary deficiencies such as diabetes insipidus, ACTH deficiency, thyrotropin deficiency, or gonadotropin deficiency.

Clinical manifestations Children with growth hormone deficiency are short, although weight will be within normal range. They also have small, infantile features; crowding of the teeth; and chubby cheeks. There might be a high arched palate and a single central incisor. Deficiency of ACTH leaves the child with adrenal insufficiency (discussed in the section on adrenal gland hypofunction). Deficiency of LH and FSH will make pubertal development impossible without the administration of estrogen or testosterone. However, there is no effect on fertility unless there is a deficiency of gonadotropins. Thyroid-stimulating hormone (TSH) deficiency causes secondary hypothyroidism, which is treated with thyroxine replacement (see the section entitled The Child with Inappropriate Secretion from the Thyroid Gland). Usually, the child will have normal intelligence.

Some children have deficiencies in several or all of the anterior *and* posterior pituitary-stimulating hormones. This condition is known as *panhypopituitarism.* Many of these children have congenital anomalies of the midbrain that do not permit the proper development of the hypothalamus and pituitary glands. If the posterior pituitary lobe is also affected by the process that causes anterior pituitary hypofunction, the clinical manifestations will be related to deficiencies in posterior pituitary hormones as well.

Diagnostic evaluation Wrist radiographs evaluate bone age by examining epiphyseal activity. Serum hormonal levels reveal diminished levels of ACTH, LH, FSH, and growth hormone. A CAT scan might be performed to determine the presence of a tumor or lesion. The fasting blood sugar is decreased.

Treatment To document growth hormone deficiency, the health care team generally observes the child's growth rate for 6–12 months and then selects validating endocrine studies to determine growth hormone deficit. Treatment of growth hormone deficiency historically involved injections of human growth hormone. However, human growth hormone has been unavailable since 1985 because of the occurrence of a rare central nervous system disorder in some children who had received the hormone. The synthetic hormone Protropin is prescribed when there is a proven deficiency of growth hormone. It has demonstrated ability to increase the growth rates substantially without the adverse effects of the human growth hormone (Parks and Fischer, 1986).

In addition to administering synthetic growth hormone, replacing other deficient hormones is indicated. Any tumor is surgically removed or destroyed.

Nursing management The nurse's role during diagnostic testing is to explain the tests to the child and family and to ensure the timely collection and proper handling of blood specimens (correct tubes, labels, and icing of specimens) for endocrine studies. The nurse keeps the child NPO, observes for signs of hypoglycemia during the tests, and gives the child a snack following test completion.

Nursing care might involve referring the child for evaluation, assisting in the testing procedures, teaching parents to give the synthetic growth hormone injections, counseling the child about self-image, and assessing the growth response to therapy. If the child is prone to hypoglycemia, the nurse assists the parents in recognizing symptoms and having glucose pastes or gels on hand to give orally if severe hypoglycemia occurs.

Many children are quite short or grow very slowly but are not deficient in the growth hormone. In fact, it is more common to encounter this type of child than a child with a documented growth hormone deficiency. Some children are small in stature for genetic reasons. The parents might seek evaluation of their children's growth in the hope that their children will be spared the trauma they themselves might have experienced because of small stature. Nursing care for children and their families consists of counseling about appropriate clothing, physical activities, and the importance of tailoring expectations to the child's age rather than stature.

Another large group of children with small stature have constitutional delay of growth. These children generally grow at a normal rate, but they are at or below the fifth percentile for their age. Although most of these children eventually attain an average adult height, their entrance into puberty generally is delayed by 1–2 years as compared with their age-mates. Nursing care of children with constitutional delay of growth and puberty is similar to that for children with genetic short stature, except that the constitutionally delayed children generally can be reassured that they will attain average size by the time they are through growing.

Gonadotropin Hypersecretion—Precocious Puberty

One of the factors involved in the onset of puberty is the increased secretion of the gonadotropin hormones (LH and FSH). The onset of puberty is considered *precocious* (early) in girls younger than 9 years of age and in boys younger than 10 years of age. In girls, this process of early pubertal development is most frequently idiopathic, whereas in boys, intracranial tumors more often stimulate the early pubertal development.

Clinical manifestations Girls with precocious puberty generally present with premature *thelarche* (breast development), which is sometimes unilateral but frequently is bilateral. Pubic hair might or might not be present along with the early breast development. Examination of the vagina might reveal evidence of increased estrogen secretion; that is, the vaginal mucosa thins and becomes reddened. Menstruation might occur.

Boys with precocious puberty generally present with pubic hair. They also might have accelerated linear growth, increased muscle mass, testicular enlargement, and penile growth.

Diagnostic evaluation When a child develops precocious puberty, the history and examination focus on discovering the cause of the early pubertal development. Possible etiologies for precocious development of secondary sexual characteristics include an intracranial mass (central precocious puberty), an adrenal mass or enzyme defect causing excessive secretion of adrenal testosterone, or an ovarian cyst or tumor secreting excessive estrogens.

To assess the possibility that the pubertal development is caused by an intracranial mass, the nurse carefully checks the child's neurologic status. The child is questioned about the presence of any headaches or visual disturbances. An ophthalmologic examination is done to assess the child's visual fields and determine whether any papilledema exists. A CT scan of the child's head might be done to examine the hypothalamic-pituitary region for evidence of a mass. Pituitary gonadotropins are measured and might be elevated above normal.

Treatment and nursing management The child who is discovered to have an intracranial lesion is referred to a neurosurgeon, who assesses the feasibility and necessity of surgically removing the mass. Nursing care throughout this initial assessment phase includes obtaining a careful history of the pubertal development, coordinating the diagnostic evaluation, and supporting the child and parent through radiologic and laboratory procedures. Explaining puberty to the child and being present for support and teaching when the method of treatment is discussed is essential. (Additional nursing interventions are discussed in the section on the child with alterations in ovarian or testicular function.)

Adrenocorticotropin Hypersecretion—Cushing's Disease

Cushing's disease (ACTH hypersecretion) is rare in children. When present, it usually is caused by an intracranial mass in the hypothalamic-pituitary unit. Chronic ACTH oversecretion stimulates the adrenal cortex to produce excessive amounts of cortisol (glucocorticoid), which leads to the development of Cushing's syndrome (hypercortisolism). (The features of hypercortisolism are discussed in the section on adrenal gland hyperfunction.) Children with Cushing's disease generally undergo surgical removal of the intracranial tumor and/or have cranial irradiation. Before, during, and after surgery, these patients require stress (increased) dosages of steroid hormones (cortisone derivatives). Nursing care of these children includes a careful history of the progression of the symptoms, with close attention to symptoms of intracranial pressure from the mass, and support during the diagnostic procedures and surgery.

The Child with Inappropriate Secretion from the Posterior Pituitary Gland

Posterior Lobe Hypofunction—Diabetes Insipidus

To conserve the water needed for cellular function and the maintenance of blood volume, the hypothalamus produces antidiuretic hormone (ADH), or vasopressin, which is stored and released from the posterior pituitary gland. The distal renal tubules respond to ADH stimulation by conserving water.

Children with symptoms of polydipsia, polyuria, preference for ice water, the need to drink water during the night, decreased appetite, and weight loss are evaluated initially for the presence of diabetes mellitus. When no elevation in blood glucose or glucosuria is documented, these thirsty children often are discovered to have the "other" kind of diabetes—*diabetes insipidus*.

Diabetes insipidus can occur for several reasons. Central diabetes insipidus is caused by a lack of ADH. Nephrogenic diabetes insipidus is caused by renal unresponsiveness to ADH and is an X-linked recessive genetic defect. Nephrogenic diabetes insipidus does not respond to administration of vasopressin (ADH).

Central diabetes insipidus (ADH deficiency) can be caused by incomplete formation of the pituitary gland. It might occur following brain surgery or other central nervous system insult and be temporary in nature. Diabetes insipidus occasionally might be the presenting complaint when a child has developed an intracranial lesion.

Clinical manifestations The presenting clinical picture for central diabetes insipidus includes polydipsia, polyuria, failure to thrive or weight loss, irritability, fever, dehydration, or even hypovolemic shock. The child's 24-hour fluid intake and output are increased, and the urine specific gravity is very low. The serum osmolality is high, the serum sodium level is elevated, and the serum vasopressin level is low. With central diabetes insipidus, the polyuria, thirst, and other abnormalities will resolve with vasopressin therapy.

Diagnostic evaluation The diagnosis is made by a water deprivation test, which is a potentially dangerous test that should be done with the child in the hospital. Although the water intake is restricted, the volume of urine remains high. The nurse and physician carefully monitor the child's blood pressure, pulse, urine specific gravity, weight, urine output, serum osmolality, and clinical status. It is critical that the child is not allowed to become severely dehydrated during the test.

Treatment Treatment of acute dehydration caused by diabetes insipidus includes the administration of free water to correct the fluid deficit and use of an intravenous drip of aqueous vasopressin. Excessive vasopressin causes hypertension, hyponatremia, and water intoxication so the drug dose is calculated carefully to reduce risks.

Chronic management of central diabetes insipidus requires the administration of vasopressin, given either as an intramuscular preparation of Pitressin Tannate in Oil or as an intranasal spray of DDAVP (desmopressin acetate). The injectable Pitressin is given every 1–2 days but is difficult to mix and painful to receive. The DDAVP nasal spray is used every 12–24 hours.

Nursing management The nurse refers the child who has polydipsia and polyuria for evaluation. The nurse observes the child during the water deprivation test and teaches the child and family how to administer the vasopressin. Other interventions are directed toward supporting the family and the child with a chronic condition.

The Child with Inappropriate Secretion from the Adrenal Glands

Excessive Cortisol Secretion

The adrenal cortex might synthesize and secrete excessive amounts of cortisol for several reasons. Cushing's disease (excessive ACTH secretion) will stimulate the adrenal glands to secrete large amounts of cortisol. The adrenal cortex also is capable of functioning autonomously (independent of pituitary ACTH regulation) in the presence of adrenal tumors. The resulting disorder is Cushing's syndrome. Hypercortisolism also might result from steroid therapy for treatment of asthma, renal disease, or as part of chemotherapy for cancer.

Clinical manifestations Children with Cushing's syndrome have facial rounding, growth failure, truncal obesity, thinning of the extremities, muscle wasting, weakness, and fatigue. Skin changes show thinning with purplish-red striae and bruising caused by increased capillary fragility. The child might exhibit personality changes (becoming labile), buffalo hump on the back, hypertension, hyperglycemia, osteoporosis, and occasionally acne and other evidence of virilization (masculinization).

STANDARDS OF NURSING CARE *The Child with Diabetes Insipidus*

Assessed risk	Nursing action
Fluid volume deficit	Monitor the blood glucose level, glycosolated hemoglobin, and serum electrolytes. Test urine for sugar and acetone and measure specific gravity. Observe and record the child's intake and output. Observe skin color and turgor and moistness of mucous membranes. Encourage small, frequent amounts of fluids if the child is conscious and able to retain oral intake. Monitor the EKG for signs of hypokalemia.
Impaired gas exchange	Assess the level of consciousness. Monitor blood gas values. Note and report any changes in respirations such as Kussmaul respirations. Note any fruity odor to the child's breath.

GUIDE FOR NURSING MANAGEMENT

Nursing diagnosis	Intervention	Rationale	Outcome
1. Potential alteration in fluid volume: deficit (stressors: excessive urinary output, inability to conserve water)	Observe child closely for signs of dehydration. Monitor IV vasopressin administration carefully. Report immediately any signs of hypertension, hyponatremia, or water intoxication.	Early signs of dehydration, when detected, allow for early intervention.	The child appears well hydrated with urine output appropriate for age, skin turgor is good, and serum electrolytes are normal.
2. Parental knowledge deficit concerning administration of vasopressin related to unfamiliarity with procedure and action of medication	Demonstrate the administration of nasal vasopressin; have parents return the demonstration using saline until comfortable with the technique.	Vasopressin needs to be carefully administered. There is risk for error if the return demonstration is performed with the drug.	Parents can demonstrate how to administer vasopressin correctly and can recognize the signs of underdosage or overdosage.
	Inform the parents about the signs of incorrect dosage.	Pallor, abdominal cramps, and nausea can be signs of overdosage. Return of symptoms can indicate the dose is not sufficient.	
3. Potential for ineffective individual and family coping (stressors: alterations in lifestyle to accommodate disease limitations, anxiety)	Encourage the child and parents to talk about their feelings; facilitate expression of anger, guilt, and fear.	Expression of feelings allows the child and family to confront the implications of the disease and helps them cope.	The family is able to express feelings verbally about the child's illness; the child appears to be coping adequately.
	Discuss lifestyle adaptations and how to monitor child's hydration status and diet.	Including the treatment plan as much as possible in the child's lifestyle assists with coping.	

Diagnostic evaluation Evaluation of the child with suspected hypercortisolism includes examination of the blood and urine cortisol and ACTH levels, special suppression tests (metyrapone and dexamethasone), ultrasonography of the abdomen, CT scans of the head, and skeletal radiographs to look for evidence of osteoporosis.

Nursing management The nurse's responsibilities during this extensive diagnostic workup include instructing the child and parents about the procedure for 24-hour urine collection, providing support to an emotionally labile child, carefully timing the administration of medications and drawing of blood for the special diagnostic tests, and giving skilled nursing care to the child who requires surgery for the removal of tumors.

Excessive Adrenal Sex Steroid Secretion—Adrenal Hyperplasia (Adrenogenital Syndrome)

Adrenal androgens increase linear growth, stimulate growth of pubic and axillary hair, and increase the maturation of the epiphyses (growth centers) of the bones. The adrenal androgens are androstenedione, dehydroepiandrosterone (DHEA), and DHEA-sulfate. These hormones are excreted in the urine as 17-ketosteroids.

Excessive production of adrenal sex steroids might be caused by the presence of tumors or enzyme deficiencies. The child with a virilizing adrenal tumor might present with clitoromegaly (enlargement of the clitoris) in girls or penile enlargement (with concomitantly small testicles) in boys. Other signs include pubic and axillary hair growth, increased linear growth rate, increased muscle development, and acne. Urine and blood measurements of adrenal androgens are elevated in the presence of adrenal tumors.

The treatment is adrenalectomy (removal of the adrenal gland), followed by irradiation and/or chemotherapy if the tumor is malignant. Male virility is unaffected by adrenalectomy because most testosterone is produced by the testes.

Enzyme deficiencies in the metabolic pathways of cortisol and aldosterone bring about excessive formation of adrenal sex steroids. If the adrenal cortex is unable to synthesize cortisol and aldosterone, the message is given to the pituitary gland to release more ACTH for adrenal stimulation. This causes the adrenal gland to enlarge (adrenal hyperplasia). Because the adrenal gland is not able to respond to the ACTH, all the precursors of aldosterone and cortisol accumulate and are shunted along the pathway to the production of adrenal androgens. Thus, the adrenal gland secretes large amounts of testosterone and some estrogen.

The enzyme deficiency that causes congenital adrenal hyperplasia (deficiency of 21-hydroxylase) is the most common cause of ambiguous genitals observed in the neonatal period. Congenital adrenal hyperplasia is an autosomal recessive disorder.

Cinical manifestations Excessive androgen production in utero has little effect on the male fetus, other than possibly causing the penis to be slightly larger than average and causing some pigmentation of the scrotum. However, when the female fetus is exposed to excessive adrenal androgens, the external genitals become virilized (the internal sex structures are unaffected). The clitoris enlarges, and the labia partially or completely fuse to form what might appear

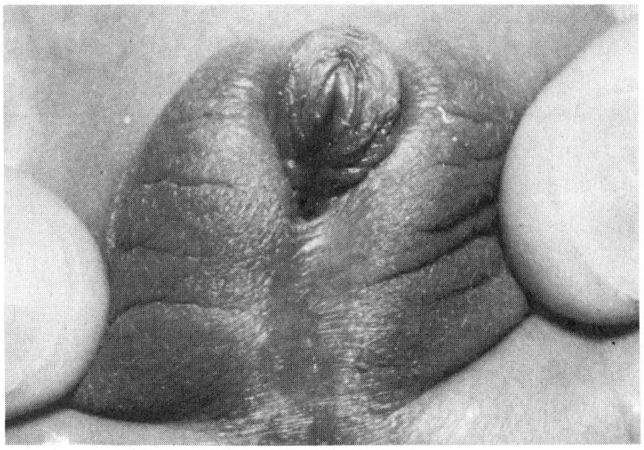

Partially masculinized external genitals of a child with congenital adrenal hyperplasia caused by adrenally produced androgen. (From Smith DW: Growth and Its Disorders: Basics and Standards, Approach and Classifications, Growth Deficiency Disorders, Growth Excess Disorders, Obesity. *Saunders, 1977, p. 132. Reprinted by permission.)*

to be a scrotum; however, there are no testicles present in the "scrotum."

Diagnostic evaluation The female child with this adrenal disorder will have a normal female karyotype (XX). There will be elevated levels of urinary 17-ketosteroids. Pelvic ultrasonography will identify internal reproductive organs.

The inability of the adrenal gland to produce aldosterone can result in sodium and water depletion with hypovolemia and dehydration in some children. Serum electrolytes might reveal depleted sodium and elevated potassium levels. Affected infants demonstrate failure to thrive with vomiting.

Treatment and nursing management Treatment of this disorder is surgical correction of the female's external virilization. Corticosteroids are given to reduce the pituitary stimulation of ACTH.

The nurse supports the parents of an infant with ambiguous gentials. Parents are extremely confused by the infant's appearance and might have difficulty accepting the fact that the infant is a girl. Depending on parents' expectations and emotional responses to their infant's appearance, there might be initial difficulties with attachment.

The nurse supports the parents by emphasizing the general health of the infant and encouraging the parents to hold the infant as much as possible. Although they might find accepting the infant as female difficult, the nurse encourages acceptance. The nurse uses neuter terms (baby, infant) when referring to the infant and suggests a delay in naming the infant and announcing the birth until the sex is confirmed. Explaining the physiology of adrenal androgens is helpful for parent understanding.

The infant is monitored closely for excessive sodium loss and for signs of dehydration. Genetic counseling might be indicated.

Adrenal Cortex Hypofunction—Addison's Disease

Glucocorticoid (cortisol) insufficiency can be caused by congenital absence of enzymes in the cortisol production pathway (adrenal hyperplasia), ACTH deficiency, or destruction of the adrenal cortex by infectious organisms (Waterhouse-Friderichsen syndrome). An autoimmune destruction of the adrenal cortex can lead to chronic adrenocortical insufficiency, or *Addison's disease*. Addison's disease is relatively rare and occurs usually in older children.

Clinical manifestations Glucocorticoid deficiency can be accompanied by mineralocorticoid (aldosterone) deficiency in many of the children affected. The child with mineralocorticoid deficiency exhibits salt craving, dehydration, and poor weight gain.

Children with adrenal cortex hypofunction develop muscular weakness and fatigue. They might be irritable, exhibit weight loss, and complain of nausea, vomiting, and diarrhea. Often, the child's skin pigmentation changes, which includes darkening of pigmented areas such as the nipples, scars, or hair.

An adrenal crisis (Addisonian crisis) can occur in response to illness or stress. This is an acute situation that requires rapid intervention. The child complains of nausea, vomiting, and abdominal cramping. There might be fever, hypotension, and cyanosis, with eventual hypovolemic shock and coma.

Diagnostic evaluation Evaluation for glucocorticoid insufficiency generally includes a morning serum cortisol level measurement, which will be low; a 24-hour urine specimen measurement for free cortisol, which also will be low; serum sodium and potassium level determinations; and a blood urea nitrogen (BUN) measurement. An ACTH stimulation test might be used to demonstrate adrenal unresponsiveness to ACTH.

Treatment Treatment for the child in adrenal crisis is directed toward stabilizing the child's fluid and electrolyte balance and administering cortisone replacement. Parenteral corticosteroids and intravenous fluid replacement are initiated and continued until the child is stable. The child might be placed on a cardiac monitor to detect potassium alterations and to monitor cardiac status. Oxygen is given for respiratory distress or cyanosis.

Long-term treatment includes oral corticosteroid replacement therapy. Treatment for mineralocorticoid deficiency is replacement therapy with 9-alpha-fluorocortisol or desoxycorticosterone acetate (DOCA). Carefully regulated amounts of salt might be added to the formula of the infant with mineralocorticoid deficiency. These bottles must be marked clearly because salt potentially is lethal for healthy infants.

Nursing management The nursing management of acute adrenal crisis involves monitoring blood pressure and serum electrolyte values, keeping an accurate record of the child's fluid intake and urine output, and assisting with the recovery process from dehydration and shock. Since the crisis can be caused by stress, illness, or cortisone withdrawal, the nurse obtains a history of the precipitating factor.

The nurse teaches the child and family about the administration of replacement hormones. The family needs to know the signs and symptoms of acute adrenal insufficiency and understand the need to increase the dose of glucocorticoid during stress or illness or when the child refuses to eat the normal diet. The family also needs to be aware of the signs and symptoms of excessive hydrocortisone therapy, namely, hypercortisolism (Cushing's syndrome).

One side effect of therapy for mineralocorticoid deficiency is hypertension, so the nurse monitors the child's blood pressure at follow-up appointments. Children with enzymatic deficiencies need close follow-up during their growing years so that dosages can be adjusted to allow for normal growth.

Adrenal Medulla Hyperfunction—Pheochromocytoma

Chromaffin tissue cells (found in the adrenal glands) synthesize, store, and secrete catecholamines (epinephrine and norepinephrine). *Pheochromocytomas* are tumors that arise in chromaffin tissues. This type of tumor is relatively rare in children but is twice as common in boys as in girls.

Children with pheochromocytoma, or adrenal medulla hyperfunction, experience hypertension, headaches, sweating, nausea and vomiting, weight loss, and visual disturbances, all related to excessive catecholamine production by the adrenal medulla. Evaluation of the child with suspected adrenal medulla hyperfunction includes studies of urinary and blood catecholamines and their metabolites. Treatment is surgical removal of the tumor. Prior to surgery, the excessive catecholamines need to be blocked by alpha-

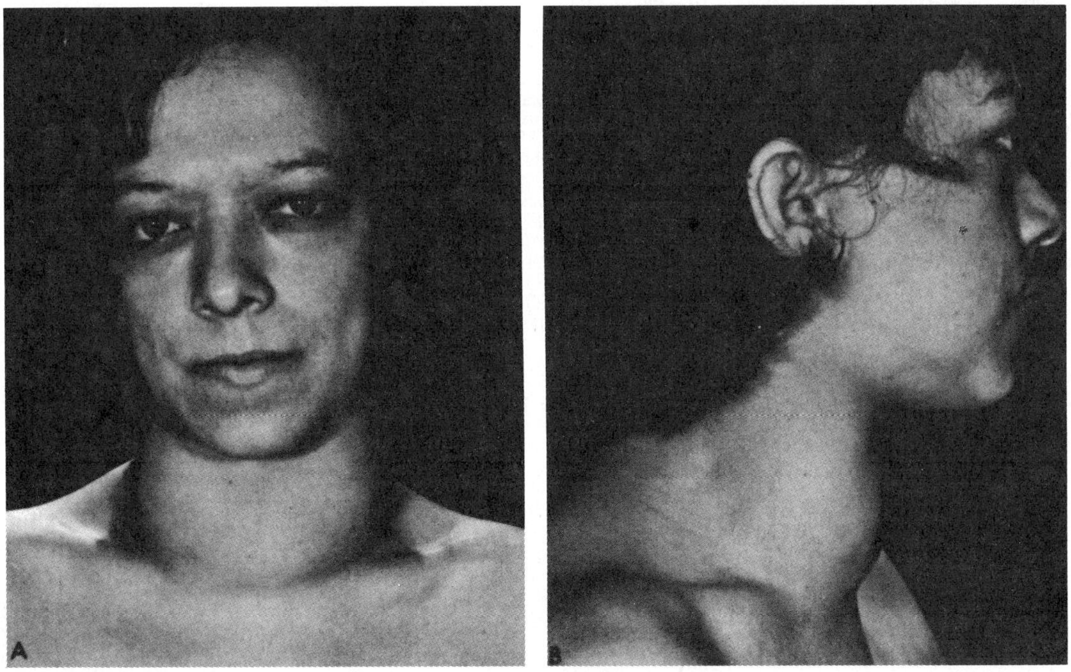

Hyperthyroidism. Note the sulcus between the thyroid and the lateral aspect of the neck, as well as the dilated veins overlying the thyroid gland. The only ocular abnormality was slight widening of the right palpebral fissure, without true exophthalmos. (From Williams RH: Textbook of Endocrinology. *6th ed. Saunders, 1981, p. 188. Reprinted by permission.)*

adrenergic agents. The side effects of these medications include hypotension, gastrointestinal irritation, and nasal congestion. The child might require glucocorticoids prior to surgery if a bilateral adrenalectomy is anticipated. Postoperatively, urinary catecholamines are measured to assess the effectiveness of the surgery.

The Child with Inappropriate Secretion from the Thyroid Gland

Hyperfunction (Hyperthyroidism)

Excessive production of thyroid hormones (T_3 and T_4) appears to be caused by an autoimmune process and is more frequently seen in girls than in boys. Since thyroid hormones regulate body metabolism, excessive production accelerates the metabolic process.

Clinical manifestations The child with hyperthyroidism presents with symptoms reflective of accelerated metabolism. These include weakness, tachycardia, irritability, nervousness, mood swings, weight loss with polyphagia, hypertension, and growth acceleration. The child might not be able to sleep at night. Tremors of the hands cause poor handwriting. The child might have firm thyroid enlargement (goiter), exophthalmos (protruding eyes), and a staring facial expression. Diarrhea and thin, velvety, moist skin with heat intolerance are frequently seen. The child with hyperthyroidism generally feels miserable.

Diagnostic evaluation Laboratory findings will include elevated thyroid hormone levels and suppressed TSH level. CT scans of the thyroid generally will demonstrate diffuse enlargement of the gland. In addition, the 24-hour uptake of the radioactive isotope of iodine (^{131}I) will be elevated.

Treatment Treatment goals are normalization of the thyroxine levels, reduction in the size of the thyroid gland, resolution of the exophthalmos, and resolution of the symptoms. Some of these improvements might not be evident for many months. The treatment of hyperthyroidism might involve surgical removal of the thyroid gland, reduction of the thyroid tissue using radioactive iodine, or conservative medical management using medication.

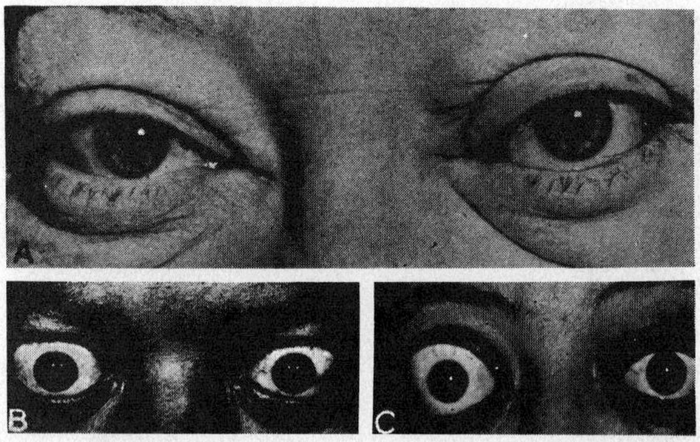

Exophthalmos. ***A.*** *Palpebral edema. Swelling of the eyelids masks the protruding eyeballs.* ***B.*** *Marked widening of palpebral fissures; slight palpebral swelling.* ***C.*** *Unequal degrees of ophthalmopathy. (From Williams RH:* Textbook of Endocrinology. *6th ed. Saunders, 1981, p. 190. Reprinted by permission.)*

With medical management, agents are used to block thyroid hormone synthesis, allowing the thyroid gland to "rest." These medications, which in effect block the action of TSH, are propylthiouracil (PTU) and methimazole. They must be taken every 8 hours for maximal effect. Methimazole and PTU have potentially serious side effects, including leukopenia, agranulocytosis (granulocyte suppression), rashes, arthritis, and hemolytic anemia. Complete blood counts are obtained routinely in children taking these medications. Whenever such a child has an infection, mouth sore, or unexplained fever, the medications are stopped, and a blood count is obtained. If a child develops these serious side effects of medical therapy, other corrective measures are considered.

Regardless of the course of treatment chosen (irradiation, surgery, or medical management), the child eventually will have subnormal thyroid hormone levels and require daily thyroid hormone replacement. Synthetic thyroxine is the usual form of medication given. There are virtually no side effects of this thyroxine preparation, which is chemically identical to human thyroxine.

Nursing management Nursing management of the child with hyperthyroidism might include referral for definitive diagnosis. The severely symptomatic child might require hospitalization for the treatment of tachycardia, hyperthermia, and exhaustion. The nurse designs a supportive, flexible care plan for the child, who literally might be unable to sit down or sleep. Exophthalmos might prevent the eyelids from closing completely in sleep; the child and parent need to learn how to instill artificial tears at bedtime and understand the importance of this medication in preventing corneal ulceration. The nurse also instructs the parent and child about the action of all medications prescribed, the importance of adhering to the medication routine, and how to observe for side effects of the medications. If surgery is elected, the nurse plans and provides appropriate care before, during, and following surgery.

The child with hyperthyroidism is usually quite uncomfortable, nervous, and moody. After the onset of symptoms and prior to treatment, school performance and peer relationships generally suffer. The parents often become frustrated with the child's behavior and their attempts to deal with it. The nurse might need to contact the child's school to explain the hyperthyroidism with regard to recent behavior and performance problems. The parent will need support in dealing with the child's behavior until the thyroxine level returns to normal.

Hypofunction (Hypothyroidism)

Hypothyroidism can be congenital or acquired. One neonate out of every 4000 live births has congenital hypothyroidism (La Franchi, 1982). Congenital hypothyroidism might be caused by nondevelopment or abnormal location of the thyroid gland during fetal life, TRH or TSH deficiency, enzymatic defects within the thyroid gland, or the transplacental passage of antithyroid medications.

Clinical manifestations Many states now require that neonates be screened for congenital hypothyroidism. This simple test can be done at the same time phenylketonuria (PKU), sickle cell, and other screening tests are performed. The neonate with hypothyroidism generally has a low thyroxine level and an elevated TSH level and might or might not have signs and symptoms of hypothyroidism. The symptomatic infant might have temperature regulation problems; sluggish reflexes; a large, protruding tongue; constipation or decreased stools; an umbilical hernia; a flattened nasal bridge; or mottling of the skin.

Mental retardation might occur if the infant is not treated promptly with thyroxine (within 3 weeks after birth). If the infant is not diagnosed until symptoms are evident, some intellectual impairment might have occurred already.

Children might acquire hypothyroidism from enzymatic defects or from a trauma to the hypothalamic-pituitary area that causes a TSH or TRH deficiency. Hypothyroidism might follow surgical removal of the thyroid tissue or might result from an autoimmune process that damages the thyroid.

Acquired hypothyroidism frequently is discovered when the child experiences a significant slowing in linear growth.

The child with acquired hypothyroidism might have cold intolerance; constipation; lack of interest in normal peer activities; dry, thickened skin; coarse hair; and increased sleep requirements. School performance and behavior might be ideal because the child has just enough energy to do schoolwork and is not easily distracted by the desire to participate in other activities.

Diagnostic evaluation Laboratory evaluation generally will demonstrate a low thyroxine level, a low level of free thyroxine, and a high TSH level. A TRH stimulation test might be performed if there is a question of pituitary dysfunction.

Treatment Treatment of congenital hypothyroidism consists of giving thyroxine daily. This pill can be crushed and given to the infant in a small amount of strained fruit. Treatment with thyroxine will be required throughout the infant's life. The amount of medication is adjusted for growth during childhood and adolescence. Follow-up consists of periodic assessment of the child's growth, weight gain, and attainment of developmental milestones. Intelligence testing prior to entering school might be indicated and helpful, particularly if the child was diagnosed after 2 months of age. Treatment of acquired hypothyroidism is identical to that for congenital hypothyroidism. The dosage of thyroxine is adjusted for growth during childhood and adolescence.

Nursing management Nursing management of the infant with congenital hypothyroidism includes supporting and counseling the parents (see Chapter 14). The nurse explains the function of thyroxine and the importance of administering the medication every day.

Encouraging the parent to provide stimulation is important for promoting development. At follow-up visits, the nurse might assess the infant's development using a standardized tool such as the Denver Developmental Screening Test (DDST). In states where neonates are not screened for congenital hypothyroidism, nurses carefully assess infants at well-child visits for symptoms of hypothyroidism.

Nursing management of the child with acquired hypothyroidism might involve referring a child who is growing poorly or who has other signs and symptoms of hypothyroidism. When thyroxine therapy is initiated, the nurse informs parents and teachers of the expected changes in the child's energy level and behavior. The child might appear to be hyperactive when compared with the previous hypothyroid demeanor. Nurses can help children and parents identify methods of remembering the daily medication.

The Child with Inappropriate Secretion from the Parathyroid Gland

Hyperfunction (Hypercalcemia)

Hyperfunction of the parathyroids, or *hypercalcemia,* is a serious medical condition. Hypercalcemia can be primary (caused by a tumor of the parathyroid) or secondary (caused by underlying disease, usually renal).

Hypercalcemia is defined as an abnormally elevated serum calcium level. Hypercalcemia can cause nephrocalcinosis (calcium in renal tubules), with hypertension and renal failure.

Signs and symptoms of hypercalcemia are polydipsia and polyuria, constipation, hypotonia (decreased muscle tone) and weakness, irritability, and listlessness. Laboratory evaluation will reveal normal or increased calcium levels, hypophosphatemia, an increased alkaline phosphate level, and an increased parathormone level. Radiographs might demonstrate bone demineralization.

Treatment Treatment of secondary hypercalcemia is accomplished by treatment of the underlying dysfunction (see Chapter 21). Acute treatment of severe primary hypercalcemia (serum calcium level greater than 15 mg/dL) consists of intravenous hydration and diuretic administration to promote calcium excretion. Supplemental potassium, phosphates, and magnesium salts restore electrolyte balance and promote reabsorption of calcium by bone. Calcitonin or mithramycin might be given to prevent bone resorption (release of calcium by bone into serum). Low dose corticosteriods might be prescribed. The child is placed on a low calcium diet.

After the hypercalcemic crisis is resolved, measures are taken to continue to decrease the serum calcium level, after which the parathyroids or parathyroid tumors are removed surgically.

Nursing management Nursing management of the child with hypercalcemia includes carefully monitoring fluid intake and output, monitoring serum electrolytes, collecting urine specimens to assess calcium excretion, and monitoring the child's cardiac status during acute treatment.

Hypofunction (Hypocalcemia)

Hypocalcemia is defined as an abnormally low serum calcium level. Hypocalcemia can be primary, that is, related to parathyroid dysfunction with decreased parathormone. Also, children develop secondary hypocalcemia with removal of the thyroid and associated parathyroid glands. Hypocalcemia can be a life-threatening condition because it can cause seizures and respiratory arrest.

Signs and symptoms of hypocalcemia are a tingling sensation of the hands and around the mouth; muscle cramps; muscle twitching; weakness; tetany and seizures; positive Chvostek's sign (seventh cranial nerve irritability); and positive Trousseau's sign (carpospasm when a blood pressure cuff is inflated). Some infants with hypocalcemia also might be lethargic, eat poorly, and vomit.

Premature infants who suffer birth asphyxia are likely to develop hypocalcemia in the first few days of life. Older children might develop hypoparathyroidism and hypocalcemia following thyroid surgery. Children with X-linked recessive or autosomal recessive hypoparathyroidism might have mild mental retardation, diarrhea, hyperreflexia, hypoplasia of dental enamel, brittle nails, and fragile hair, in addition to the other symptoms of hypocalcemia listed previously.

Treatment of acute, serious hypocalcemia includes the slow intravenous administration of calcium salts, with the nurse observing the cardiac monitor for bradycardia and the child's respiratory status closely because hypocalcemia can cause laryngeal stridor. A tracheotomy set needs to be at the child's bedside. The child with hypocalcemia might require the long-term administration of oral calcium gluconate, with the dosage adjusted to maintain a normal serum calcium level. Vitamin D supplements are given to enhance absorption of calcium. Parathyroid hormone replacements might be necessary. (See Chapter 21 for additional nursing measures for the child with hypocalcemia.)

The Child with Inappropriate Secretion from the Gonads

Hyperfunction—Excessive Estrogen or Testosterone Production

Excessive estrogen production in the young girl brings about early pubertal development (precocious puberty) and rapid bone maturation, with early closure of the epiphyseal growth centers and shortening of ultimate stature. Two causes of early puberty (gonadotropic hormone hyperfunction and adrenal tumors) have been discussed. The third source of early estrogen production is ovarian tumors and cysts. Ovarian cysts might require surgical removal but generally regress spontaneously. Regression of puberty occurs following surgical removal of tumors in young girls. If sufficient ovarian tissue remains, the child should enter puberty normally at the expected time. If all of the ovarian tissue is removed, estrogen and progesterone therapy will be required to complete secondary sexual development, and the child will be infertile.

Clinical manifestations Assessment of the child with precocious puberty (male or female) includes a careful history to obtain information regarding how long the parents have been aware of the signs of early puberty. The onset of the signs and whether the child's linear growth has accelerated are important to note. Occasionally a child with precocious puberty complains of headaches or visual disturbances (symptoms of an intracranial lesion), or the child has access to estrogens or androgens (oral contraceptives, estrogen-containing hand creams, or farm animal feed that is supplemented with androgens or estrogens).

During the physical examination, the nurse observes the amount of breast development, evidence of pubic hair, amount of axillary hair, presence of body odor, and evidence of estrogen effect on the vaginal mucosa in girls (or enlargement of the testicles and increase in penile length in boys). The child's pubertal development is compared with the Tanner standards (see Figs. 8-2 and 8-3). The nurse also assesses the child for impaired visual fields or evidence of papilledema.

Diagnostic evaluation Radiologic studies generally are ordered to assess the child's bone maturation and determine whether the skeletal maturation is advanced for the child's chronologic age. Pelvic and abdominal sonograms might be used to look for ovarian cysts or masses and adrenal hypertrophy or masses. A CT scan of the head might be ordered to look for intracranial masses, which could be the cause of the early pubertal development.

Laboratory assessment includes blood tests for the levels of LH, FSH, estradiol (estrogen), and testosterone. The levels of FSH, LH, and estradiol are very low in children between 1 month of age and puberty; however, the levels might be in the pubertal range in a child with precocious puberty. The level of testosterone is normally low in children between 1 month of age and puberty but might be elevated to the male pubertal range in a child with precocious puberty. If the testosterone level is elevated in a female, adrenal dysfunction is suspected.

The level of plasma 17-hydroxyprogesterone might be measured. This substance is a precursor of cortisol, and if elevated might suggest the presence of an enzyme deficiency in the adrenal cortex, which can cause the overproduction of testosterone. The level of urinary 17-ketosteroids, a byproduct of adrenal steroid production, is

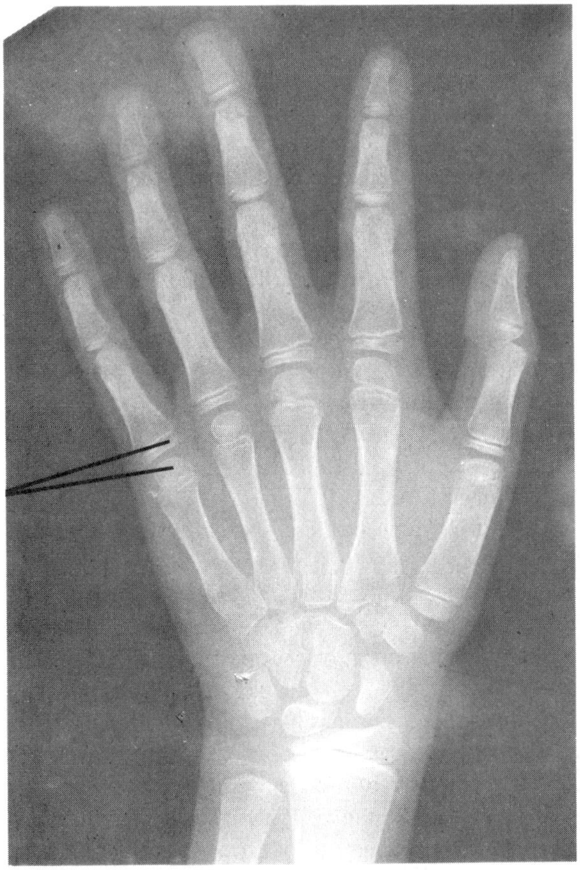

A

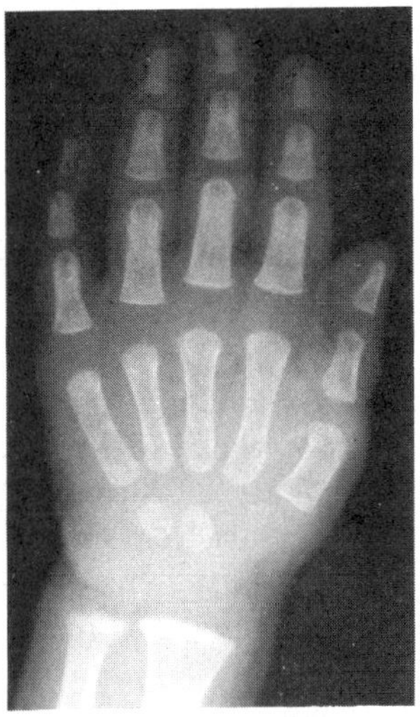

B

Radiographs of the right hand of **A**. *a 7-year-old child and* **B**. *an 18-month-old child. The spaces between the bones are the cartilage epiphyses of the various bones. In the 7-year-old, the epiphyses have ossified earlier than usual, leaving thin epiphyseal plates. (From Spence AP, Mason EB:* Human Anatomy and Physiology, *3rd ed. Benjamin/Cummings, 1987, with permission.)*

measured to evaluate the possibility that an adrenal tumor is the cause of the precocious puberty.

Treatment At present, there is no ideal therapy for children with precocious puberty. Medroxyprogesterone has been the most widely used agent to treat this problem. It arrests the progresson of secondary sexual characteristics by blocking the pituitary release of LH and FSH. Because precocious puberty is usually a process that waxes and wanes, many parents and physicians elect not to treat children with any medication but rather to observe the course of development and give the child guidance. Most parents agree with this philosophy of no treatment and ask for suggestions on how to deal with a large-for-age child in terms of peer relationships and parental expectations. The child with precocious puberty has to deal with peer reactions to early breast development, menses, pubic hair, penile growth, and the emotional changes that accompany puberty.

Nursing management Nursing intervention includes implementing diagnostic procedures and counseling parents and children. The nurse emphasizes that these pubertal developments are normal but are occurring at an early age.

Ovarian or Testicular Hypofunction—Delayed Sexual Maturation

Sexual maturation usually begins prior to 15 years of age in girls and before 16 years of age in boys; most girls have breast budding by 12 years of age, and most boys will have beginning testicular enlargement by 14 years of age. If a child shows no signs of pubertal development by 14 years of age, the cause for the delay should be assessed.

Children with a history of insult to the hypothalamic-pituitary region might not have the ability to release LH and FSH and have hypogonadotropic delay of puberty. This problem is not very common in general pediatric practice but might be present in children with other pituitary gland dysfunction or following central nervous system irradiation. A more common cause of delayed pubertal development is constitutional delay of growth (see the section on anterior lobe hypofunction). Puberty might be delayed in the girl because of ovarian deterioration.

The most common cause of ovarian dysfunction is *Turner's syndrome,* a chromosomal abnormality. The girl with Turner's syndrome most commonly has a 45XO karyotype rather than the normal 46XX female chromosome complement (see Chapter 15).

Clinical manifestations Turner's syndrome can be suspected at birth if the female infant has webbing of the neck and a low hairline, absent femoral pulses, puffy hands and feet, and a high, arched palate. If Turner's syndrome is diagnosed in infancy, no specific treatment is recommended until approximately 7 years of age or until the growth rate slows.

More often, Turner's syndrome is not diagnosed until the girl's linear growth rate decelerates in late childhood and/or she fails to have secondary sexual development in her adolescent years. She might have some of the stigmas associated with classic Turner's syndrome described previously along with hypertension and coarctation of the aorta.

Diagnostic evaluation Laboratory findings in the older girl with Turner's syndrome will include increased FSH and LH levels, decreased estrogen levels, delayed bone age, and the 45XO karyotype. Girls with Turner's syndrome might have single, rotated, or horseshoe-shaped kidneys. An intravenous pyelogram is needed to obtain this information. Girls with Turner's syndrome should be referred to a cardiologist for evaluation of hypertension because many girls with this condition have coarctation of the aorta or pulmonary stenosis.

Treatment If the child cannot release LH and FSH and has hypogonadotropic delay of puberty, regardless of whether the problem is with the hypothalamus (the hypothalamus cannot release LRH) or the pituitary (the pituitary cannot respond to LRH stimulation by releasing FSH and LH), the treatment is replacement therapy with estrogen and progesterone for girls and testosterone for boys.

When testicular function is questioned in a newborn male, a human chorionic gonadotropin (HCG) stimulation test is performed to determine the testosterone levels. In the newborn with a smaller than usual penis, a course of testosterone might be given and the penile response evaluated. Bilaterally undescended testicles (cryptorchidism) are associated more often with infertility than unilateral cryptorchidism. Young men with *anorchism* (congenital absence of the testes) will require testosterone therapy for secondary sexual development and usually elect to have prosthetic implants into the scrotum for cosmetic reasons.

Enzymatic deficiencies can cause incomplete masculinization of the external genitals and cause gynecomastia (breast enlargement) at puberty. Chromosomal abnormalities such as *Klinefelter's syndrome* (XXY karotype) prevent secondary sexual development. The therapy for many of these disorders is intramuscular injections of testosterone.

Most children do not require hormonal therapy for the treatment of delayed puberty caused by constitutional delay. Satisfactory coping with the delay can be achieved if the young adolescent is reassured of general good health and is given some estimate of when puberty will begin. However, adolescents who are significantly smaller than their peers might elect hormonal treatment to initiate the natural process of puberty. Males can be given a 3-month course of testosterone; size and pubertal development are assessed 1 month after the last testosterone injection. Generally, one to two courses of testosterone therapy are sufficient to launch a male into puberty.

Psychologically, adolescents might feel more assured of their sexual capacity if allowed to complete sexual maturation without further hormonal supplementation. Oral testosterone preparations are available but are less effective than the injectable forms and have been implicated in the development of hepatic dysfunction.

Girls might be given estrogen and progesterone to hasten secondary sexual development. Prolonged therapy is contraindicated because of the risks of estrogen therapy (blood clots, uterine cancer, hypertension, and migraine headaches) and the possibility of accelerating epiphyseal closure, resulting in ultimate short stature. Before recommending estrogen therapy, however, a family history pertaining to blood clots, cerebral vascular accidents, and migraine headaches is obtained and evaluated.

Understandably, parents are quite upset when the diagnosis of Turner's syndrome is made because these girls are infertile. The child who is under 12 years of age generally is told that she requires medication to promote linear growth. When she is old enough to be concerned about secondary sexual development and requires estrogen and progesterone therapy, the infertility problem is discussed. Current research with in vitro fertilization might allow females with Turner's syndrome to become pregnant at some point in the future. Emphasis is made that although the child will be sterile, her sexual function will not be diminished.

Treatment of Turner's syndrome involves the administration of an anabolic steroid or growth hormone to promote linear growth. Anabolic steroids might mature the skeleton more rapidly than the height advances, so periodic bone age radiographs are required. Estrogen therapy, daily or every other day, is initiated when the girl becomes uncomfortable with her lack of pubertal development. Progesterone is added later to stimulate menstruation.

Nursing management Nursing management of the child with delayed puberty might include referring the child for assessment, assisting in the initial assessment procedures, teaching the child and parent about testosterone or estrogen therapy, and counseling the child and parent about clothing appropriate for age and size.

Essential Concepts

- The endocrine system functions by circulating very small amounts of specific chemicals called hormones, which regulate metabolism, growth, puberty, and reproduction.
- Assessment of the child with possible endocrine dysfunction requires a complete history, including prenatal history and family history, and a physical examination, with special attention to appearance, vision, sexual development, and neurologic response.
- Because children with suspected endocrine disorders must undergo extensive diagnostic testing, the nurse coordinates the various procedures, teaches children and parents the correct methods, and offers emotional support to the family during testing.
- Acute care of children with endocrine dysfunctions might require prompt observation and intervention for children who present with fluid and electrolyte imbalance, alteration in their sleep/rest cycle, and alteration in body temperature, and who have the potential for injury from hormonal alterations during periods of stress.
- Interventions for children with nutritional alterations from endocrine disorders include planning for alterations in children's appetites, fluid requirements, and appetite control and, in some cases, food plan modifications to avoid hypoglycemia and hyperglycemia.
- Children with endocrine disorders might experience developmental delay from neurologic impairment and learning difficulties or from unresolved independence/dependence conflict.
- The child and family's ability to deal emotionally with a chronic endocrine disorder depends on the child's age and developmental level, seriousness of the condition, and impairment to the child's appearance or functioning that might alter the child's self-esteem.
- Because most endocrine disorders are of a chronic nature, children over 6 years of age and their parents need to learn basic survival skills at the time of discharge from the hospital, including undertanding the action of medications, knowing how to administer medications and prevent side effects, knowing how to contact the health care team, and knowing how to explain the disorder to family and friends.
- Alteration in pancreatic islet-cell function can lead to decreased or absent production of insulin and the occurrence of diabetes mellitus in children.
- Children with alterations in the anterior lobe of the pituitary gland can experience problems related to growth, sexual maturation, and excessive production of ACTH.
- For the child with posterior lobe hypofunction of the pituitary gland, or diabetes insipidus, nursing care involves observing the child during a water deprivation test and teaching the child and family to administer vasopressin or diuretics.
- Depending on the hormones affected, the child with inappropriate secretions from the adrenal cortex might experience Cushing's syndrome from excessive cortisol secretion, ambiguous genitalia from excessive sex steroid secretion, and severe alterations in fluid and electrolytes from insufficient secretion of aldosterone.
- Nursing management of a child with hyperthyroidism might include creating a supportive care program for the child who is very uncomfortable from increased metabolism, helping to allay the child's fears, instructing the parent about medications, and providing appropriate care if surgery is elected.
- For an infant with congenital hypothyroidism, the nurse supports and counsels the parent, explains the function of thyroxine and the importance of daily medication, and discusses infant stimulation.
- The nurse's role in caring for a child with inappropriate secretions from the parathyroid gland includes careful monitoring of fluid intake and urinary output, monitoring serum electrolytes, collecting urine specimens to assess calcium excretion, and observing the child's cardiac monitor during acute treatment.
- The child with excessive production of estrogen or progesterone from the gonads can exhibit precocious puberty, while the child with hypofunction of the ovaries or testes can experience delayed sexual maturation.

References

Guthrie D, Guthrie R: The disease process of diabetes mellitus. *Nurs Clin North Am* (Dec) 1983; 18(4): 617–630.

Heins JM: Dietary management in diabetes mellitus. *Nurs Clin North Am* (Dec) 1983; 18(4): 631–643.

La Franchi S: Hypothyroidism: Congenital and acquired. In: *Clinical Pediatrics and Adolescent Endocrinology*. Saunders, 1982.

Parks BR, Fischer RG: Growth hormone. *Pediatr Nurs* (July/Aug) 1986; 12(4): 302.

Additional Readings

Aurbach GS, Marx SJ, Spiegel AM: Parathyroid hormone, calcitonin and the calciferols. In: *Textbook of Endocrinology*. 6th ed. Williams RH (editor). Saunders, 1981.

Balik B, Haig B, Moynihan P: Diabetes and the school-aged child. *Am J Matern-Child Nurs* (Sept/Oct) 1986; 11(5): 324–330.

Bates S, Ahern JA: Tight control: What does it mean? *Am J Nurs* (Nov) 1986; 86(11): 1256–1257.

Burns EM: Diabetes mellitus and pregnancy. *Nurs Clin North Am* (Dec) 1983; 18(4): 673–685.

Cunningham LN, Barr P: Developing an endurance exercise program for the diabetic patient. *Diabetes Educ* 1982; 8(3): 11–13.

Etzwiler DD, Karam JH: Human insulin: How it looks now. *Diabetes Today Tomorrow* 1983; 3(1): 1.

Felig P: *Exercise and Diabetes*. Address at the Tenth Annual Meeting of the American Association of Diabetes Educators. San Antonio, TX, September, 1982.

Flavin K, Haire-Joshu D: The pharmacologic repertoire. *Am J Nurs* (Nov) 86; 86(11): 1244–1248.

Fow JM: Home blood glucose monitoring in children with insulin-dependent diabetes mellitus. *Pediatr Nurs* (Nov/Dec) 1983; 9: 439–442.

Haire-Joshu D, Flavin K, Clutter W: Contrasting type I and type II diabetes. *Am J Nurs* (Nov) 1986; 86(11): 1240–1243.

Hodges LC, Parker J: Concerns of parents with diabetic children. *Pediatr Nurs* (Jan/Feb) 1987; 13(1): 22–25.

Hoffman RG et al: Self-concept changes in diabetic adolescents. In: *Psychological Aspects of Diabetes in Children and Adolescents*. Laron Z, Galatzer A (editors). Karger, 1982.

Johnson S, Rosenbloom AL: Behavioral aspects of diabetes mellitus in childhood and adolescence. *Psychiatr Clin North Am* 1982; 5(2): 357.

Kaplan SA: *Clinical Pediatrics and Adolescent Endocrinology*. Saunders, 1982.

Lillo R, Masteller D: Outpatient management of children in diabetic ketoacidosis. *Pediatr Nurs* (Nov/Dec) 1982; 8: 383–385.

Loman D: Monitoring diabetic children's blood glucose levels at home. *Amer J Matern-Child Nurs* (May/June) 1984; 9: 192–196.

Moorman NH: Acute complications of hyperglycemia and hypoglycemia. *Nurs Clin North Am* (Dec) 1983; 18(4): 708–713.

Nemchik R: Diabetes today: A whole new world. *RN* (Oct) 1982; 45(10): 31–36.

Saucier CP: Self-concept and self-care management in school-age children with diabetes. *Pediatr Nurs* (Mar/Apr) 1984; 10: 135–138.

Saxton D et al. (editors): *The Addison-Wesley Manual of Nursing Practice*. Addison-Wesley, 1983.

Spies ME: Vascular complications associated with diabetes mellitus. *Nurs Clin North Am* (Dec) 1983; 18(4): 721–733.

Swearingen P: *Manual of Nursing Therapeutics*. Addison-Wesley, 1986.

White PC, New MI, Dubont B: Congenital adrenal hyperplasia. *N Engl J Med* (June 11) 1987; 316(24): 1519–1523.

Williams RH (editor): *Textbook of Endocrinology*. 6th ed. Saunders, 1981.

Chapter 30

Skeletal Integrity and Mobility

Implications of Inflammation and Structural Abnormalities

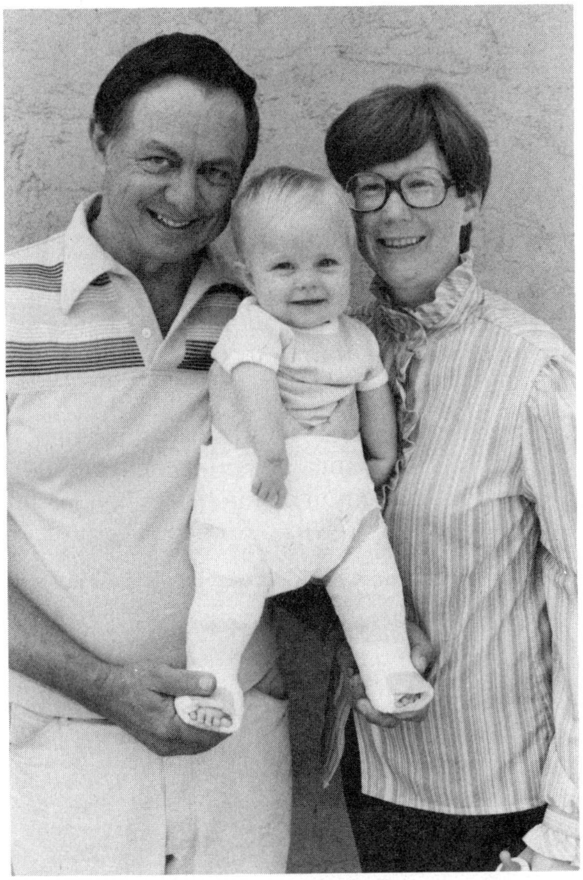

Chapter Contents

(Continues)

Objectives

- Describe the nursing assessment relative to a child with a skeletal dysfunction.
- Describe procedures and diagnostic tests the nurse uses to assess skeletal function.
- Describe nursing management related to treatment with casts, traction, braces, and frames.
- Identify nursing interventions used in preventing skin breakdown, controlling infection and complications, assessing and controlling neurologic and circulatory compromise, monitoring appliances and apparatus, and controlling pain.
- Describe preoperative and postoperative care of the child undergoing skeletal surgery.
- Identify the nutritional, developmental, emotional, and health maintenance needs specific to a child with a skeletal injury or disorder and the family.
- Explain why fractures heal more quickly in children than in adults.
- Describe emergency and definitive medical treatments and principles of nursing management for traumatic injury to bones and joints.
- Explain the physiologic processes, common medical treatments, and principles of nursing management for infections of bones and joints.
- Describe the chief abnormality, common medical treatments, and principles of nursing management of children with congenital and acquired skeletal dysfunctions.

ESSENTIALS OF STRUCTURE AND FUNCTION
The Musculoskeletal System

Because the skeletal structure of young children is somewhat cartilaginous, young children are less prone to severe fractures than adults. Their bones are better able to withstand the effects of severe stress. The thick periosteum and plentiful blood supply aid in healing, so children's bones heal faster than adults' bones with the same injury.

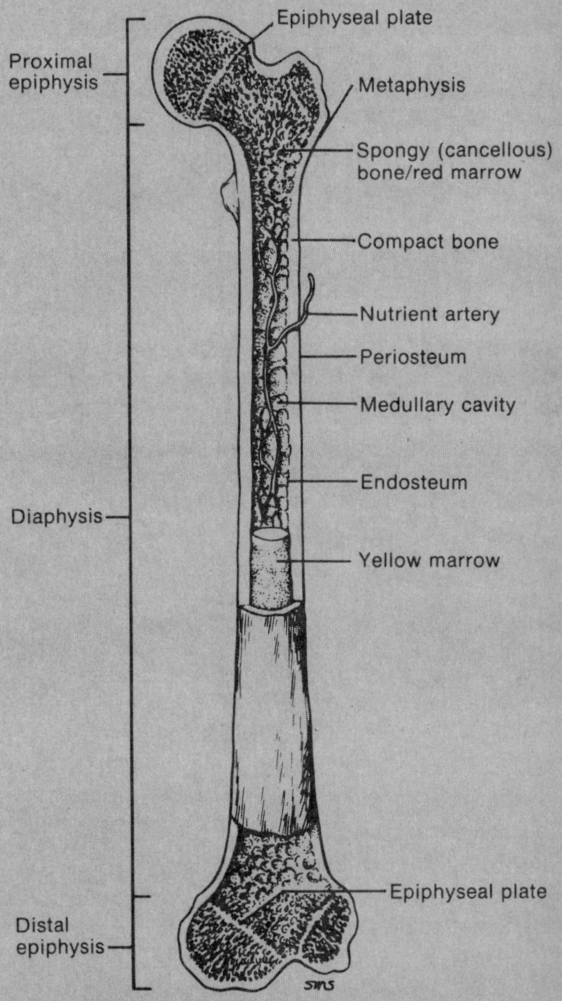

Parts of a long bone.

Glossary

Bones Protect the interior body organs. Long bones, which are found in the upper and lower extremities, carry the body's weight (see figure). Short bones are in areas where strength and compactness are needed. Flat bones are thin and provide structure. Bones increase in length until skeletal maturity, then only in breadth.

Diaphysis Bone shaft. The diaphysis is covered by compact bone and periosteum, a double layer of connective tissue. In children the periosteum is very thick and vascular. Bones are nourished by numerous blood vessels.

Epiphysis Growth end of long bones. The growth plate in the epiphysis is made of cartilage cells that develop and grow, causing the bone to increase in length. Injury to the growth plate can cause growth to be disrupted or to cease.

Joint A capsule enclosing articular (connecting) bone surfaces, ligaments, and muscles. The joint is lined with a synovial membrane, which secretes a viscous, clear fluid that nourishes the bone and lubricates the joint. The amount of joint movement is determined by the ligaments, muscles, and tendons on the adjoining bones.

Medullary cavity Interior of bones, which in young children is a site for blood cell production. By adolescence, the medullary cavity is a site for fat storage, with hematopoiesis occurring in the marrow of the cranium, sternum, ribs, vertebrae, and pelvis only.

Ossification The process of developing new bone. Osteoblasts produce new bone when activated. Hormones from the parathyroid and thyroid regulate the amount of calcium and phosphorus deposited in bone to give it strength. A diet that provides vitamin D, calcium, and phosphorus is essential for bone health.

Resorption The process by which old bone is dissolved. The destruction of old bone can release calcium into the circulation.

The skeletal system contributes to the body's form and function. It supports the soft tissues and enables movement. The bony skeleton of the body protects many organs: the skull protects the brain; the vertebrae protect the spinal cord; the rib cage protects the heart, lungs, liver, and spleen; and the pelvis protects the reproductive organs. The bones are also a reservoir for storing minerals, primarily calcium and phosphorus. Although these minerals are quite stable, they can be mobilized and circulated by the blood to meet the body's needs. Finally, the bones' red marrow is responsible, under normal circumstances, for the production of blood cells (see Chapter 26).

Nursing care of children with skeletal dysfunction often involves measures to offset the effects of immobility. The nursing care for the child with a skeletal disorder therefore is likely to involve teaching about adaptations needed for long-term care.

Assessment of the Child with a Skeletal Condition

History

A child with a problem involving the skeletal system seeks medical attention because of various signs and symptoms. Common complaints include deformity, a limp, pain, general or local weakness, and swelling and stiffness in joints. In obtaining a history, the nurse seeks to establish how the complaint, its characteristics, and its cause are related.

The history of the child's delivery can be significant. The child might have experienced trauma or injury at birth. Skeletal abnormalities might be noted at birth or during the initial neonatal assessment. For example, breech delivery is associated with an increased incidence of dislocated hip and torticollis, or wryneck (unilateral contracture of the sternocleidomastoid muscle).

A history of delayed or uneven achievement of developmental milestones occurs with certain skeletal conditions. If a child shows a clear preference for using one hand more than the other before the age of 2, for example, there might be a defect in the other hand; the dominant hand is not chosen prior to age two and frequently not before age four. Dislocated hip, if not diagnosed and treated in infancy, usually delays walking.

The nurse inquires about bone or joint disorders in other family members. Additional information about diseases, injuries, drugs, or exposures to toxins that have been linked to skeletal defects and disorders is helpful. For example, thalidomide, once believed to be an effective sedative and sleeping aid with few side effects, was found to cause serious skeletal defects (absence of or shortened limbs) when taken in early pregnancy.

It is important to know how a problem affects the child and family. Does the problem interfere with their lifestyle? Is the child's general health affected? Perhaps there are fears surrounding a problem or complaint. Exactly why was help sought?

Pain is associated with many orthopedic conditions in children. Remembering that many factors influence a child's perception of pain, the nurse can help interpret the complaint. For example, a young athlete might attempt to ignore or downplay pain in order to continue to engage in sports. Children in late childhood and adolescence likewise tend to minimize pain when around strangers so as to appear more grown up and strong. Occasionally, children magnify the amount of pain they feel as an attention-getting mechanism. The nurse encourages the parent to confirm the accuracy of statements the child makes about pain, if possible. For example, the child might complain differently at home than in the hospital. If pain is severe enough to prohibit activity, fear of pain or fear of loss of a function can greatly influence the child's description and expression of pain.

The nurse notes in the child's or parent's own words exactly how an injury happened. Injury is suspected if the child complains of sharp pain that worsens with activity and lessens with rest. Dull, boring pain that is constant, increases gradually, and awakens the child from sleep is likely to be due to infection or tumor growth. Table 30-1 lists conditions usually associated with sharp or dull pain.

Physical Examination

Physical examination for structural abnormalities includes inspection and assessing range of motion. The torso, hip, legs, and feet are primary inspection sites for determining skeletal dysfunction since many of the childhood skeletal abnormalities affect these areas.

The spine is inspected for curvatures such as *lordosis* (anterior curve), *kyphosis* (excessive posterior curve, humpback), or *scoliosis* (lateral curve). The child is observed from the back for a protruding hip, while standing, or an uneven thoracic area, while bending from the waist (Fig. 30-1). Instability or dislocation of the hip is evident from various signs, including uneven leg length, limited abduction, asymmetrical skin folds on the thighs, and a limp if the child is walking (see Chapter 10). Traumatic dislocation of the hip is not common in children. Its clinical appearance varies in relation to the position of the dislocation.

Leg length is assessed by comparing the levels of the knees and both sides of the pelvis and observing for functional curves of the spine. Although a degree of difference

TABLE 30-1 Pain in Presenting Orthopedic Conditions

Type of pain	Musculoskeletal condition
Sharp	Bone injury with muscle spasm
	Bone injury with periosteal tear
	Fracture
	Dislocation
	Slipped capital femoral epiphysis
	Fragment of bone in joint
	Joint strain
Dull	Tumor
	Osteomyelitis (bone infection)
	Muscle strain
	Sprain

between the length of the right and left legs is acceptable, any discrepancy greater than 1 cm might require referral. A significant leg length discrepancy, if untreated, can lead to degenerative problems in adult life. Gait is affected by leg length discrepancy, causing the head to bob excessively when the child walks. If weight bearing is painful, the child might assume a limp in response. A limp adopted in an attempt to reduce pain is called an *antalgic limp*.

The feet are examined for straightness and for adequate motion. Some children can exhibit mild turning in of the feet as a result of positioning in utero. These children will exhibit little resistance to passive range of motion. Children with severe foot deformities exhibit much resistance to muscle stretching.

Physical examination of the child with suspected musculoskeletal injury or fracture includes observation of signs of injury, such as contusions (bruises) or wounds. The nurse gently palpates the outline and shape of the bones, noting any abnormal prominence, malpositioning in relation to landmarks, or thickening. Any scars indicative of old injury or surgery are noted.

Examination of the child with suspected infection or tumor growth includes assessment of the skin. The nurse palpates the skin to determine its texture, turgor, and temperature and to detect lumps and swelling. Skin might be tender or reddened over an infected area. Warmth of the skin indicates increased vascularity (circulation) and can be an indication of infection. Warmth also might occur over a rapidly growing tumor. Cyanotic or cool skin is a possible indication of impaired vascularity. The nurse obtains baseline data about color, sensation, and motion of a body part to use in later assessments of innervation and vascularity.

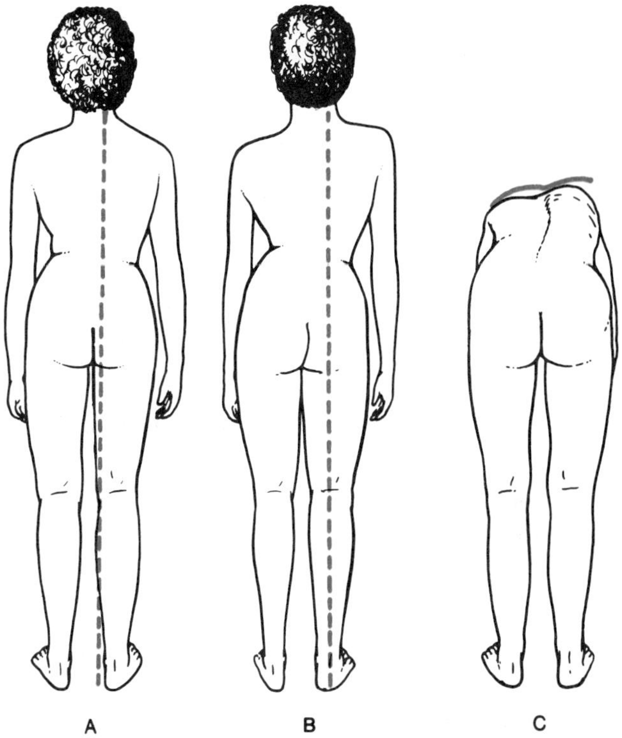

FIGURE 30-1
Lateral curvature of the spine. ***A.*** *Mild, compensated scoliosis.* ***B.*** *Severe, decompensated scoliosis.* ***C.*** *Rotation of the vertebrae and ribs; visible when the child bends over.*

Validating Diagnostic Tests

Radiographic studies In assessing a child with a condition involving the bone, radiographs are of primary value. They are used extensively for initial diagnosis. They evaluate treatment effectiveness and recovery. X-rays show bone density, breaks in the periosteum, irregularities, and areas of new bone formation.

Radiographs of joints can show narrowing of cartilage space, changes in joint surfaces, loose or foreign bodies, and peripheral new bone. Skeletal age can be determined by comparing a child's radiographs to the norm. Skeletal age has implications for treatment and expected outcome with various conditions.

Radiographs do not necessarily show pathologic changes in the young child. Occasionally special radiographic techniques such as computerized tomography (CT scan) or injection of radiopaque dye into a joint might be needed to establish a diagnosis. Radiographs are taken into consideration along with the history of the child's illness or accident and signs and symptoms.

ASSESSMENT GUIDE *The Child with a Skeletal Condition*

Assessment questions	Supporting data
Has the child experienced any recent trauma?	Tenderness, edema, pain at the site of injury; laceration, contusion, ecchymotic areas; feeling of numbness or tingling in an extremity distal to the injury; decreased sensation and movement in the affected body part
Is the child experiencing any pain or joint limitation? Describe the location, type (sharp, dull, boring, constant, intermittent, associated with weight bearing), and whether the pain increases or decreases with activity or rest	Redness and swelling associated with the painful area; purulent drainage; limp; guarding of an affected extremity; fever
Does the child appear to have any structural abnormality?	
Spine	Lack of symmetry of body parts; uneven scapulae, lateral curvature of the spine; one hip prominent; associated dyspnea; anterior or posterior curve
Hips	History of delayed walking; asymmetric gluteal or thigh folds; lurching or waddling gait
Legs	Uneven leg length; varus or valgus deformities of the knee ("bowlegs" or "knock-knees")
Feet	Equinus or calcaneus positions of foot and ankle. Forefoot turning in or out; resistant to passive range of motion

Additional data: Clear drainage from nose or ears indicating possible head injury; alteration in neurologic signs (see Chapter 31); signs of internal bleeding or hypovolemic shock (increased pulse, decreased blood pressure, restlessness, thirst, pallor)

Arthroscopy Arthroscopy is a technique for directly inspecting the interior of a joint, often the unstable knee joint, by means of a thin rod containing a camera and light source that is introduced through a cannula. It is frequently carried out while the child is under a general anesthetic but can be done with local anesthesia. The joint is distended with fluid for visualization. It is both a diagnostic and surgical tool. Corrective work such as shaving, cutting, or trimming sources of pain or irritation might be done during arthroscopy.

Laboratory tests Although history, physical examination, and radiographic studies usually are sufficient to identify a skeletal problem, laboratory tests might be used to diagnose and monitor a condition. For instance, in osteomyelitis (infection of the bone) the white blood cell count can be high. The white count is used to monitor the resolution of infection and evaluate the effectiveness of treatment. Hemoglobin or hematocrit values help assess blood loss after injury or surgery. Blood calcium levels can be used to monitor bone growth, bone healing, and the general health of the musculoskeletal system. They correlate with the resorption of calcium from bone. Blood calcium levels can be elevated during normal growth spurts or during bone healing.

Nursing Management for Procedures and Treatments

Internal Fixation and Fusion

Bony structures can be aligned in the most functional position following injury. In some circumstances it is impossible to achieve the best position for alignment without fixing the bones in position. Plates and screws sometimes are used to align bone and bone fragments after injury or as part of a surgical repair. Bone grafting, with or without metal instrumentation, might be used to fix the spine in an inflexible but more functional position (spinal fusion).

Following fixation or fusion, the child is immobilized and regains mobility gradually. The nursing care is similar to that for any child experiencing surgery and immobilization (see Chapter 20).

Casts

Types of casts A wide variety of casts is used to immobilize and position body parts (Fig. 30-2). The type of cast

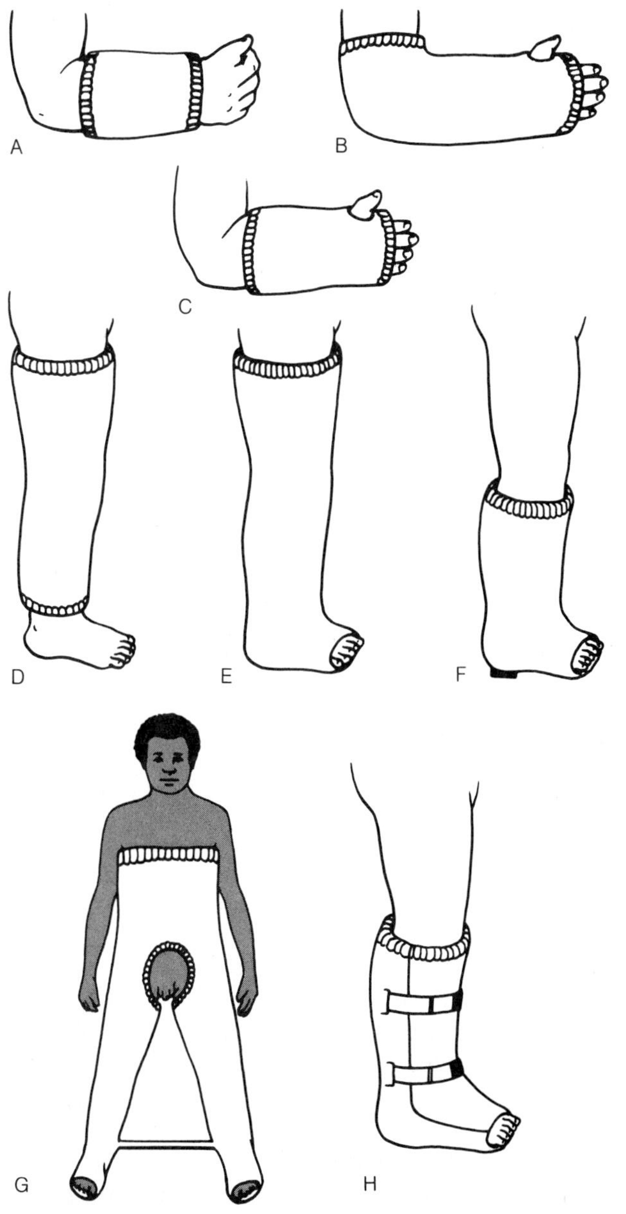

FIGURE 30-2
A. Cylinder cast, arm. B. Long arm cast. C. Short arm cast. D. Cylinder cast, leg. E. Long leg cast. F. Short leg walking cast. G. Hip spica cast. H. Bivalved cast.

used is determined by the site and extent of the injury or required correction.

Casts might remain on the child for the entire healing period or might be removed and reapplied periodically.

Casting material Casting material is of two basic types—plaster or synthetic. Synthetic casts can be fiberglass or polyurethane or a combination. Casting material comes in tape form and is applied, after being activated by water, heat, or light, in a similar fashion to any bandage. The cast is molded to the body and dries hard, leaving the casted portion in the required position.

Each casting material has its own advantages and disadvantages. Plaster casts tend to mold more easily, thus making them more useful for infants and young children. They also are less expensive. The major difficulty with plaster casting is that the cast must remain dry at all times, making it difficult to keep clean. The drying time is prolonged (usually longer than a day), and the chemical reaction caused by the interaction of water and calcium-laden cast tape can be uncomfortable for the child during drying.

Synthetic casts are lighter weight than plaster and allow for greater mobility. They dry quickly (often in less than 30 minutes). They are, however, more expensive than plaster and thus not suitable in situations where casts have to be replaced frequently. With permission, the child can get a synthetic cast wet. However, the cast must be thoroughly dried to prevent skin breakdown.

Cast application Stockinette or a nonabsorbent lining is applied to the area to be casted. Then rolls of wet plaster or synthetic material are wrapped around the body part to be immobilized. Because of the chemical reaction that takes place when rolls of plaster casting material become wet, the cast feels quite warm when it is first applied. As the chemical reaction ceases and the cast dries, water evaporates. The cast and the child then feel cold. The nurse needs to explain these sensations to the child to help the child feel less anxious and less frightened of the temperature changes.

Other nursing measures can increase the child's sense of control and comfort during a cast application. The nurse is aware of maintaining the child's privacy. Under certain circumstances (application of a body cast) the child might feel more comfortable if the stockinette is applied in the hospital room rather than in the open cast room. During cast application, the nurse needs constantly to be aware of the child's reaction so teaching can be reinforced and support given. The nurse might be asked to hold the injured area in position during casting. Humor can be used to lessen fears, decrease embarrassment, and promote the child's feelings of self-worth during casting.

Immediate cast care The edges of the cast need to be well padded and smooth to prevent skin irritation. If stockinette is used in a cast, it can be pulled out and over cotton padding and secured to the edge of the cast with a layer of cast material to provide a smooth surface against the skin. When the cast is dry, the nurse can add more padding by slitting the stockinette, inserting padding, and reattaching the stockinette to the outside of the cast with tape. If the

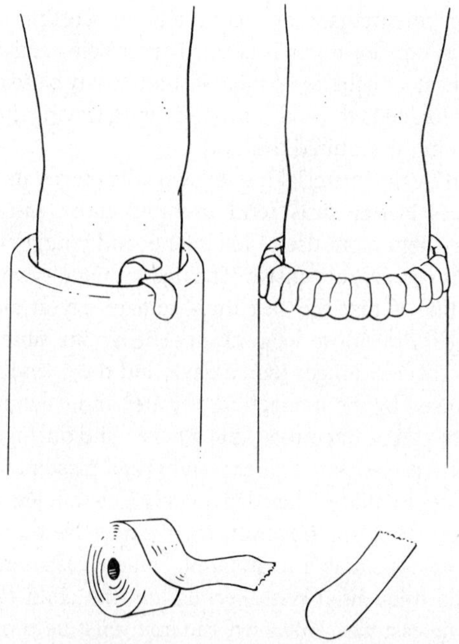

FIGURE 30-3
Petalling a cast. Tape edges are rounded to facilitate smooth application and prevent irritation and peeling from corners.

edges of a plaster cast are not smooth, one inch waterproof tape is cut and placed around the edge of the cast in the form of overlapping petals. "Petalling" is done when the cast is completely dry and can be redone if necessary (Fig. 30-3).

Synthetic casts are particularly rough and might have edges that need to be smoothed with a file when the cast is dry. This type of cast is petalled with moleskin to protect the skin from sharp edges.

Ongoing care of the child in a cast The nurse handles the child and the cast with care. While a plaster cast is drying, the child is turned every hour so the cast dries and hardens on both sides. While turning, the nurse handles the cast by the palms of the hands only, in order to prevent indentations. The cast is left uncovered for drying, although it is necessary to cover the child to provide warmth.

After the cast has dried, the nurse turns and repositions the child every 2–4 hours. More frequent repositioning is necessary if areas of the skin are subjected to pressure.

Edema is not an unusual occurrence in the child with a cast. Tissue injury from the skeletal trauma and vasoconstriction from the cast both contribute to edema. If the swelling is severe enough to compromise the circulation, muscle tissue death might occur. This is most likely in injuries of the wrist, ankle, or knee and is referred to as *compartment syndrome.* Tissue death can occur quickly, leaving the child with permanent muscle damage. In order to prevent or recognize potential compartment syndrome, the nurse monitors color, sensation, and motion in the body part distal to the cast. Pallor, numbness or tingling, pain, decreased pulse, or paralysis might indicate circulatory compromise. Initially, checks are made as frequently as every 30–60 minutes, since edema from the injury or surgery might exert pressure against the cast. After 24 hours, the nurse assesses color, sensation, and motion at least every 4 hours until cast removal. A casted extremity can be elevated on pillows to reduce edema.

Hemorrhage from skeletal injury or surgery is a potential complication. Often the cast will be stained with sanguineous drainage. A line is drawn around the stain and is marked with the time in order to assess whether active bleeding is occurring. A quickly spreading stain and other indications of bleeding are reported immedately.

Because visible signs of infection are difficult to observe in a child with a cast, the nurse feels the cast daily for "hot spots." These along with any foul odor, pain, drainage, or fever might indicate infection.

Safety is a most important nursing consideration. The nurse keeps small objects away from young children and tells older children never to put anything between their cast and skin. A child with a casted leg might be extremely off balance while standing or moving from bed to chair. Although children and adolescents might want to perform these tasks independently, the nurse's presence is required to ensure safety. Distraction is used to help keep children from becoming too active. If there appears to be a real potential for injury from excessive activity, the child can be restrained.

Protecting a cast from becoming soiled with food, urine, or feces can require a great deal of skill on the part of the nurse. The child's cast is covered with waterproof covering when the child eats or plays with materials that might soil the cast. Cleaning a soiled plaster cast is a problem. The cast can be cleaned with a slightly damp cloth and a mild powdered cleanser. Most synthetic casts can be cleaned with soap and water. Thorough drying is important. A blow dryer can be used on a cool setting to speed drying time. The dryer should not be used too close to the cast or child's skin because it can overheat the area. If the inside of a synthetic cast remains damp, the risk for skin breakdown and infection is increased.

Cast removal Removal of a cast by means of a cast saw can be very frightening for a child. As with cast application,

Special Considerations for a Child in a Hip Spica Cast

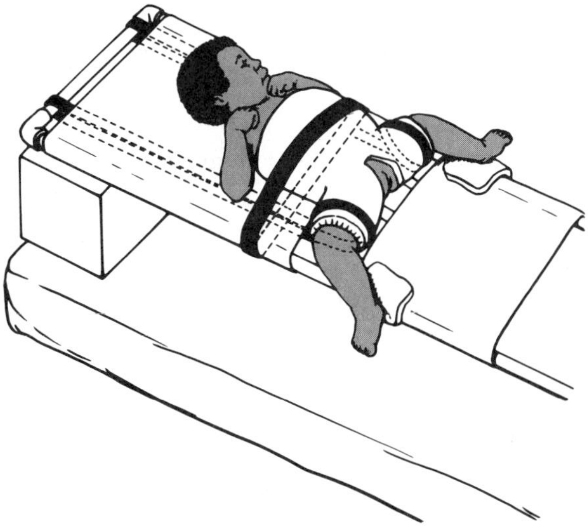

Turning—For cast drying and position changes, the child is turned frequently. The crossbar of a hip spica is not used to turn the child. Turning is accomplished by sliding the child to one side of the bed, then turning the child toward the opposite side. For the child's safety, the nurse informs the child exactly when the turn will occur (eg, on the count of three or when I say, "ready, set, go"). Depending on the child's age, weight, and ability to assist, two people might be required for turning.

Keeping clean—Plastic wrap is tucked under the edge of the cast near the perineal area and can be secured to a dry cast with tape. Plastic disposable diapers can be used for protection in an untrained child. The plastic protects the cast while the padding absorbs urine and stool. A sanitary pad can be used for additional absorption at night. The plastic and diapers are removed and replaced immediately if soiled. When a child in a spica cast or body cast uses a bedpan, the child's upper body needs to be slightly elevated so that urine and feces flow down into the bedpan and not up into the cast. The incontinent child in a spica cast can be elevated on a frame, such as the Bradford frame, which has an opening under which a bedpan is placed.

Promoting safety—The young child is restrained on the Bradford frame to prevent inadvertent falls. The nurse cautions the more active child against making sudden moves or turns without assistance. If safety is a concern, an older child can be restrained, although this is avoided if possible. The child is restrained if placed in a go-cart or low guerney. Some car seats can be adapted to accommodate the infant in a spica cast.

Providing for privacy—The child in a hip spica is covered at all times to maintain privacy. Hospital gowns are loose fitting and can accommodate the width of the cast. If the child wishes to wear underwear or nightwear from home, the seams can be slit and Velcro closures applied for easy removal of clothing.

Preventing muscle atrophy—Encourage the child to use actively all uncasted extremities. Use play as a mechanism for accomplishing this—Nerf® balls, clay, computer games, mobiles, etc (see Preventing Hazards of Immobility in Chapter 20).

Facilitating feeding—The infant in a spica cast is awkward to feed, but the nurse encourages the parent to hold and cuddle the infant during feeding whenever possible. The football hold, or holding the infant tightly against one side, can make breast-feeding easier. The infant takes from the breast on the same side. The parent supports the infant's head and the cast while burping. The slightly older infant or child can be fed solids while on the Bradford frame since the elevation of the frame is appropriate to prevent regurgitation. The nurse encourages the parent to cover the cast during feeding to prevent soiling. An assortment of large, colorful smocks can properly cover the child while making mealtime more interesting.

the child and family need preparation for the experience. The cast saw is noisy, and many children are afraid of being cut. Careful demonstration of the saw can lessen fears. The nurse demonstrates to child and parent how the saw stops when it touches skin. The child is assured that the cast saw will not cut the skin but that the vibrations might be felt, causing a sensation of warmth.

Before the cast is removed, the nurse describes to the child and parent how the skin under the cast will look. If a cast has been in place for a number of weeks, the skin will be flaky and brown because of the accumulation of dead skin. Application of an oil, such as baby oil, followed by gentle washing helps remove the dead skin. A casted extremity might appear slightly smaller than its counterpart from mild muscle atrophy. The body part will be stiff. Gentle coaching and exercise correct this problem.

STANDARDS OF NURSING CARE *The Child with a Cast*

GUIDE FOR NURSING MANAGEMENT

Nursing diagnosis	Intervention	Rationale	Outcome
1. Potential fear of cast application and removal (stressors: knowledge deficit, sound of cast saw)	Explain to child and parent procedures of cast application and sensations the child will experience (for example, warmth of wet cast); use a doll or real materials to demonstrate; allow the child to handle materials.	Knowledge of what is to occur reduces fear and allows the child and family a measure of control.	The child appears comfortable with the demonstrated procedures. The older child can verbalize understanding of the procedure and reduction of fear.
	Explain the procedure for cast removal; demonstrate use of a cast saw and how it vibrates rather than cuts.	Demonstration of the cast saw is crucial to the child's understanding that the saw will not cut the skin; the demonstration reduces the child's fear.	
2. Potential alteration in peripheral tissue perfusion (stressor: cast constriction)	Check color, sensation, and motion of skin distal to the cast every 30 minutes for the first few hours after application and every 1–4 hours thereafter and PRN.	The cast can constrict blood vessels and decrease circulation and reduce innervation to the casted area.	Circulation to the affected extremity appears adequate—skin is pink and warm, capillary refill is rapid; there is no numbness or tingling; fingers or toes move freely. Parent and child can describe signs of inadequate perfusion and can explain the importance of seeking immediate help if such signs occur.
	Mark and monitor the outline of any drainage stain on the cast. Record the time the cast is marked.	A rapid increase in the size of a drainage stain can indicate hemorrhage or draining infection.	
	Inquire about and observe for manifestations of pain on movement.	Pain, particularly after the third or fourth day; might indicate compartment syndrome.	
	Elevate casted extremity after cast application and if any swelling is evident.	Elevation improves venous return and reduces swelling.	
	Check the cast for tightness by slipping a finger under the edge and asking the child if the cast feels tight.	If slipping a finger under the edge of the cast is not possible, the cast is probably too tight and will lead to circulatory compromise.	
	Teach the child and parent all these measures and emphasize the importance of continuing cast checks after discharge; tell the parent to notify the physician if any signs of inadequate perfusion occur.	Knowledge increases compliance with the treatment regimen and allows for rapid identification of developing circulatory difficulties. Casts do not expand with growth and weight gain. Evidence of constriction appears several weeks after application.	
3. Potential alteration in comfort: pain (stressors: musculoskeletal injury, restriction of cast)	Administer analgesics as ordered and provide other measures to relieve pain (eg, distraction, imagery, relaxation, play, repositioning).	Relief of pain decreases anxiety and promotes the child's compliance with the treatment, as well as promoting muscle relaxation.	The child verbalizes relief from pain. The child is able to play and to sleep appropriately. The child appears more relaxed, less restless.

STANDARDS OF NURSING CARE *The Child with a Cast (Continued)*

GUIDE FOR NURSING MANAGEMENT

Nursing diagnosis	Intervention	Rationale	Outcome
	Use relaxation exercises during muscle spasms. Have the child take slow, deep breaths, or consciously attempt to relax each muscle group.	Concentrated relaxation can relieve muscle tenseness and thus muscle spasm.	
	Teach child and parent to identify and report sources of discomfort, such as muscle spasms, pressure sores, or skin irritation.	Accurate reporting of signs and symptoms can ensure rapid treatment of impending complications such as infection, tight cast, or skin irritation.	
4. Potential impaired skin integrity (stressors: pressure points or irritation from cast)	Handle a wet cast with the palms of the hands only.	Fingers can dent the cast and cause skin irritation under the dented areas.	Skin at or under cast edges is smooth and intact. There are no signs of indentation or irritation. Skin at bony prominences is smooth and nonirritated.
	Elevate the wet casted extremity on pillows without plastic covering.	Plastic covers can retain the heat from the chemical reaction of a plaster cast and cause burning of the skin. The cast dries more quickly if the moisture is not retained by plastic.	
	Remove any plaster flakes from the skin; smooth rough cast edges; when cast is completely dry, petal cast edges with water-repellent tape or moleskin.	Cast edges that are not smooth can irritate and break the skin.	
	Inspect skin under cast edges with a flashlight.	Routine inspection can spot irritation before the skin breaks down.	
	Instruct older child not to place objects between cast and skin; do not allow a young child to play with small toys that could be inserted under the cast.	Small objects under the cast place pressure on the skin causing irritation and breakdown.	
	Turn and reposition the child every 2 hours; rub bony prominences with lotion, but avoid using lotion or powder near cast edges. Follow protocol for skin care around cast edges.	Rubbing increases the circulation to pressure areas. Turning relieves pressure. Lotions and powder might cake and cause skin irritation. Moisture inside the cast provides a medium for organism growth.	
	Instruct child and family not to scratch skin under cast. Blow cool air between the cast and skin with a hair dryer set on cool to relieve itchiness.	Cool air relieves pruritis. The child might not be tempted to insert objects into the cast to scratch.	

(Continues)

STANDARDS OF NURSING CARE *The Child with a Cast (Continued)*

GUIDE FOR NURSING MANAGEMENT

Nursing diagnosis	Intervention	Rationale	Outcome
	Instruct child to report pain or discomfort under the cast; check the cast for musty odor; ask the child to report any warm areas that occur after the cast is dry.	Pain and musty odor might indicate infection.	
	Teach the parent how to carry out these measures at home; ensure that the parent knows when the physician should be contacted; instruct the parent not to let the child get dirt or sand under the cast.	Preventing skin irritation will reduce the risk of skin breakdown.	
5. Potential knowledge deficit of home care management of a child in a cast (stressors: anxiety, limited understanding, unfamiliarity with new procedures)	Teach the parent how to manage ambulation (for example, stair climbing); lift and move the child safely, using correct body mechanics. Instruct the parent in measures to prevent physical and developmental deficits or complications related to immobility (see Chapter 30).	Correct management increases safety for the child and family.	Parent can explain and demonstrate safe and appropriate home care.
	Teach parent and child how to keep child and cast clean with daily sponge baths of areas not covered by the cast, use of damp cloth and mild cleanser to wipe cast daily, and avoidance of lotions and powders around or under cast edges.	Adequate discharge preparation ensures adequate home care.	
	Instruct parent and child how to monitor elimination patterns, prevent constipation, keep cast sanitary and child's perineal area clean, and prevent or correct cast wetness if child is diapered or incontinent.	Giving the parent adequate information and demonstration increases their control.	
	Refer to a visiting nurse if appropriate.	A visiting nurse can accurately assess the home for factors contributing to successful home care; the nurse can provide the family with additional needed equipment or supplies.	

Traction

Traction is used to immobilize a body part, realign fracture fragments, and reduce muscle spasm, joint dislocation, or spinal curvature. A traction apparatus is a structure of weights and pulleys that exerts pull to maintain a body part in correct alignment for healing. A radiograph might be done while the child is in traction in order to monitor the placement of the bone fragments or to determine the need for alteration in the direction or amount of traction pull. There are two basic kinds of traction: skin traction and skeletal traction (Table 30-2).

Skin traction Skin traction is a noninvasive traction that achieves an external pull on a body part. Its advantages include ease of application and removal. It is especially useful for the child who does not need continuous traction. The effectiveness of skin traction is limited by the amount of pull that can be exerted on the skin.

Skin traction is applied by placing foam-rubber straps against the body part and then securing the straps with elastic bandages. Sometimes, the straps are adhesive-backed. If these are used, the nurse protects the child's skin by first applying tincture of benzoin to any skin area that will come in contact with the adhesive. Before applying skin traction, the nurse refers to the child's history to be sure that the child is not allergic to rubber or adhesive. If the child has a history of these allergies, an alternative method of treatment may be chosen. Sometimes wrapping the extremity in cotton batting prior to application of the straps provides a sufficient barrier to prevent an allergic response.

Unless contraindicated, the nurse removes the bandages securing skin traction at least once a shift to assess circulation and to provide skin care. The bandages are reapplied smoothly and securely. Adhesive-backed straps are not removed. Elastic bandages covering the adhesive straps can be removed for rewrapping; however, extreme caution is taken to be sure the adhesive straps are secure in order to prevent traction slippage or release. It is helpful to have assistance if elastic bandages are to be rewrapped. One person keeps the adhesive straps in place and the traction secure, while the other person reapplies the bandages.

The position of the traction weights is checked regularly, as are the ropes and pulleys. Weights swing freely except when the child might be out of the traction. The nurse does not change the prescribed amount of weight or remove the child without specific orders to do so.

Skeletal traction Skeletal traction is an invasive procedure that exerts traction by means of wires or pins inserted in the bone. Greater force can be exerted by skeletal traction, and it can be maintained longer than skin traction. The wire pins or tongs used for skeletal traction are inserted by the physician, usually under anesthesia. Skeletal traction is never removed for skin care.

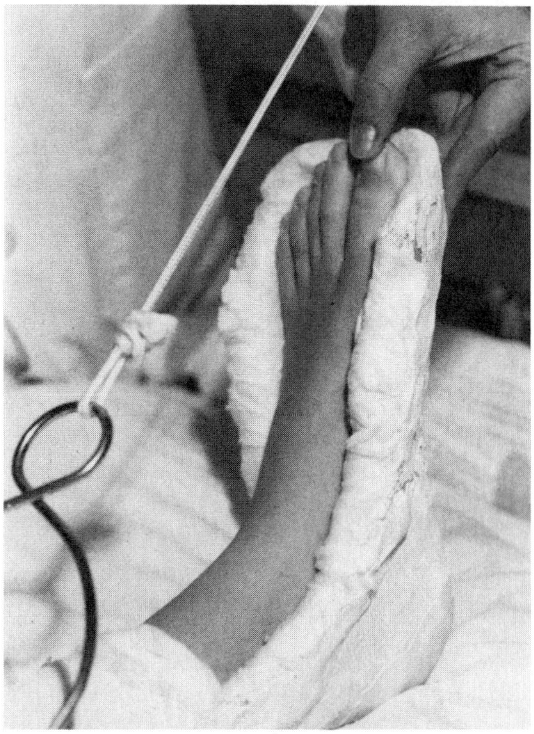

Assessing a child in skeletal traction. (From Swearingen PL: The Addison-Wesley Photo-Atlas of Nursing Procedures. *Addison-Wesley, 1984, p. 563.)*

As with skin traction, the nurse checks the circulation in the extremity. More frequent monitoring is necessary immediately after traction is applied or reapplied. The pin sites are monitored closely for signs of infection or "tenting" (new skin at pin insertion site attaching to the pin, creating triangle or tent configuration). If the child is in traction for a spinal condition, monitoring neurologic signs and symptoms is an important nursing measure.

If possible, the nurse prepares the child and family before traction is applied. Often, however, the child requires traction following an injury, and teaching and demonstrations must be done after traction is applied.

Besides pain, which can be present initially, immobility is perhaps the most difficult aspect of traction management for the child and the nurse. Because the success of traction depends on its correct maintenance, the nurse makes certain that the child and family understand the exact purpose of traction, how it works, and what they can do to help maintain it. Marking the bed or side rail with tape to indicate the child's correct position (for example, where head, shoulders, or feet should be) enables the child and family to participate in the child's proper positioning and traction

(text continues on p. 1025)

TABLE 30-2 The Child in Skin or Skeletal Traction

	Indications	Nursing considerations
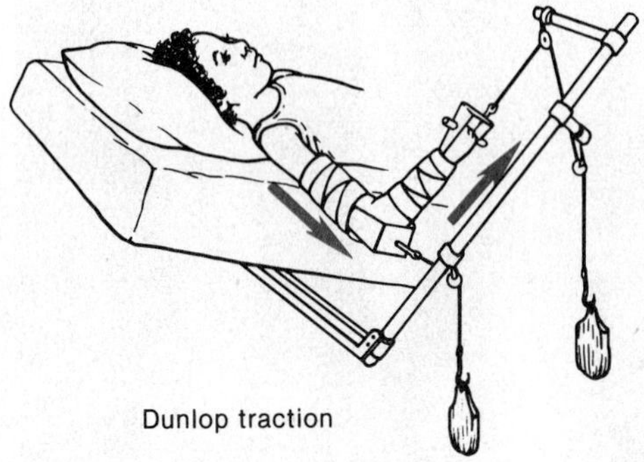 Dunlop traction	Supracondylar fracture of humerus (fractured elbow), postoperative immobilization, reduction of elbow contractures; can be skeletal traction also	Correct alignment is critical because of risk of arm contractures Pain that persists after immobilization might be a sign of circulatory or neurologic compromise
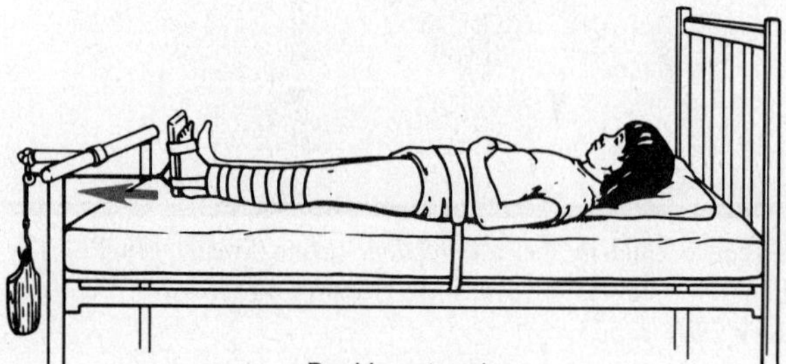 Buck's extension	Postoperative immobilization, reduction of hip or knee contractures	Pull of traction might cause child to slide toward foot of bed; traction is rendered ineffective if weights or ropes do not hang freely
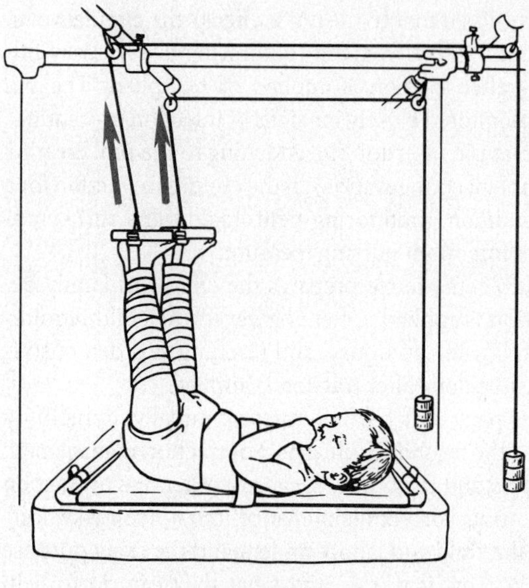 Bryant's traction	Reduction of fractured femur or congenitally dislocated hip in child less than 2 years of age and weighing less than 30 lb	Frequent assessment of circulation to legs, feet, and toes required because of risk of circulatory impairment due to low blood pressure in ankles, tight leg bandages, vasospasm from traction on blood vessels, or hyperextension of the knee Pain, particularly in the calf, is a sign of impending Volkman's ischemia Child's sacrum must be elevated enough so that nurse can slip hand between child's buttocks and bed or frame

TABLE 30-2 *(Continued)*

	Indications	Nursing considerations
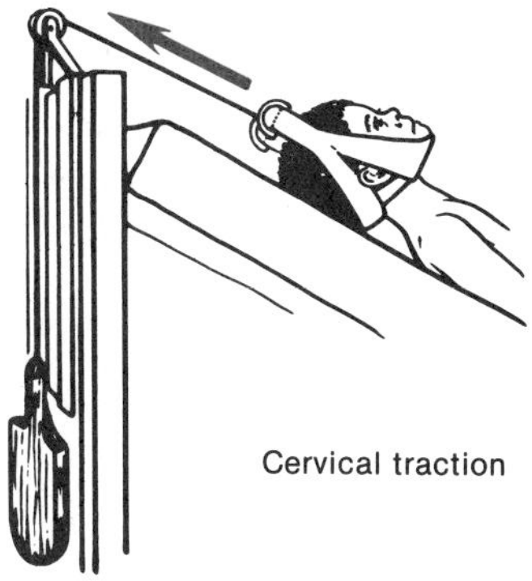 Cervical traction	Injury or disease of the cervical spine	Head of bed is elevated 15–20° Head must be kept straight
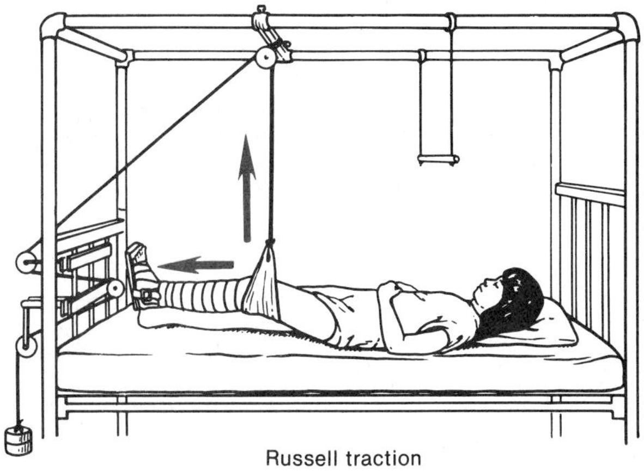 Russell traction	Postoperative immobilization of hip and knee, reduction of fractures of the femur	Sling position under knee is checked frequently Hip flexion must remain at correct angle Assess for compromised perineal nerve Child may need restraint to prevent slipping toward foot of bed
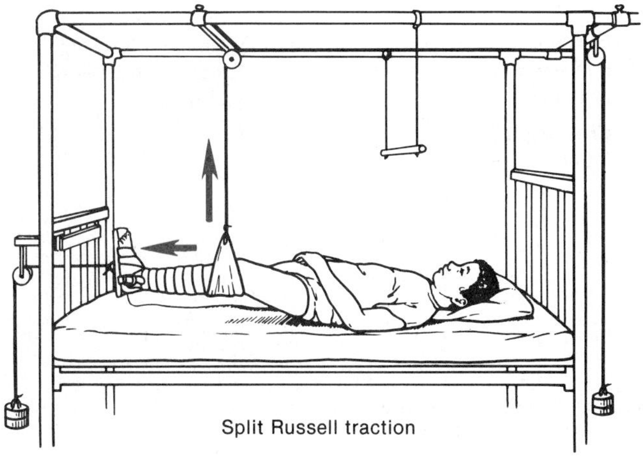 Split Russell traction	Postoperative immobilization, reduction of hip or knee contractures, dislocated hips	Considerations same as for Russell traction

(Continues)

TABLE 30-2 The Child in Skin or Skeletal Traction *(Continued)*

	Indications	Nursing considerations
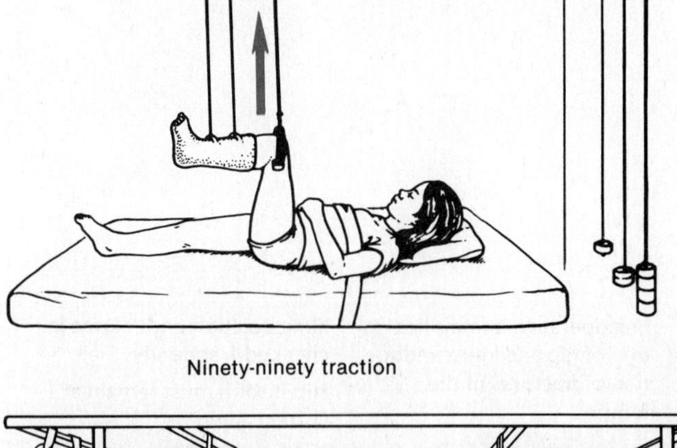 Ninety-ninety traction	Reduction of fractured femur	Alignment is monitored to ensure that child is positioned correctly for pull at a 90° angle Child is quite comfortable Care is simplified by height of traction apparatus above bed
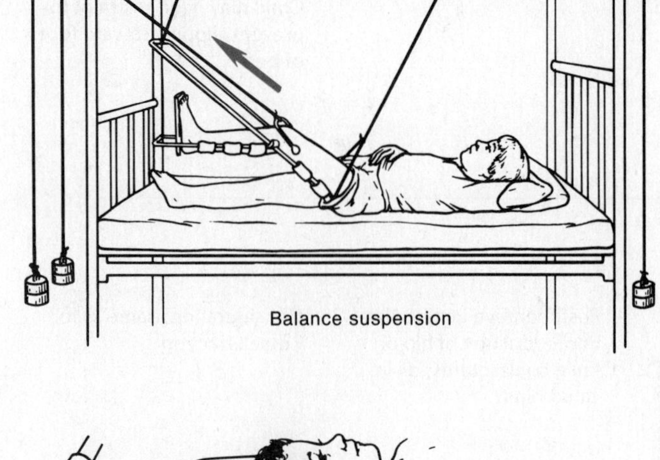 Balance suspension	Postoperative immobilization of hip or knee, musculoskeletal disease, fractured femur (with skeletal traction)	Involves care of Thomas splint with Pearson attachment Splint and attachments might have separate ropes and weights, allowing greater movement of the knee Child is relatively mobile Slight malalignment can be corrected by repositioning of the ring
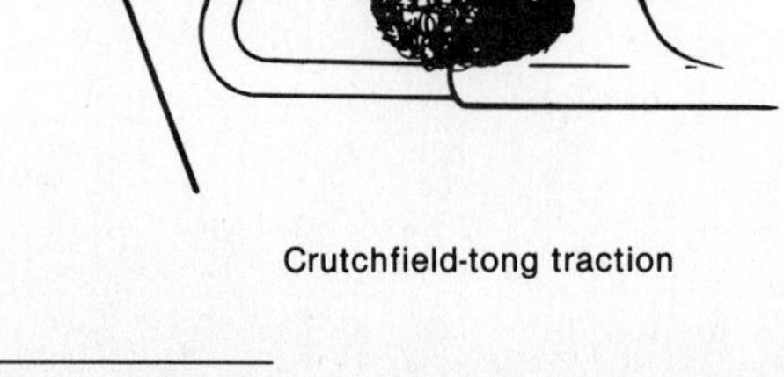 Crutchfield-tong traction	Pin sites are monitored for looseness of pins and signs of infection Child might be on a turning frame	Immobilization following spinal fusion, severe injury to cervical spine

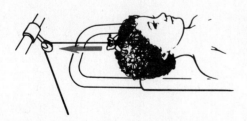

NOTE: Arrows indicate direction of pull exerted by traction. Straps or vest restraints and position of bed are sometimes used to keep the child positioned correctly and supplement countertraction exerted by the child's body weight.

maintenance. The child might also enjoy helping to see that ropes are centered in the pulleys and that weights hang freely. The child can use a trapeze hung from an over-bed frame to pull the body up in bed and help maintain proper body alignment.

If countertraction provided by the child's body weight is insufficient, traction can pull the child down in bed or to the side. A folded sheet used as a sling can help to maintain the correct position. Sometimes, elevating the foot or side of the bed on shock blocks suffices to counterbalance traction.

STANDARDS OF NURSING CARE *The Child in Traction*

RISKS

Assessed risk	Nursing action
Respiratory insufficiency, urinary retention, constipation, impaired skin integrity, or muscle atrophy from immobilization	Prevent hazards of immobility (see Chapter 20).

GUIDE FOR NURSING MANAGEMENT

Nursing diagnosis	Intervention	Rationale	Outcome
1. Potential fear concerning traction apparatus and restricted movement (stressors: traction equipment or frame, ropes, weights; play and self-care limitations)	Explain the purpose and function of traction to the child and family; use diagrams to illustrate the therapeutic pull of traction.	Knowledge assists with cooperation with the treatment. Knowledge decreases fear.	The child and family understand the purpose of traction and can explain how it works. They demonstrate confidence and lack of fear related to traction apparatus.
	Provide the child with a doll that is in traction; allow the child to manipulate a toy traction apparatus.	Visual and tactile images assist with learning and reduce fear of unfamiliar equipment.	
	Involve the child and family in maintaining traction and the child's correct position in bed.	Involving the child and family improves their understanding as well as encourages cooperation with the treatment.	
2. Potential alteration in peripheral tissue perfusion (stressors: constriction of elastic bandage, skeletal pin)	Monitor the extremity in skeletal traction every 30 minutes on the day of application; for skin traction monitor the extremity every 15 min for 30 min and then according to routine after each rewrap of the elastic bandage. Check for capillary refill, skin color and temperature (should be warm and pink), sensation, (no numbness or tingling), and motion. Check the peripheral pulse. Check the tightness of any elastic bandages. Immediately report any abnormal pain or signs of circulatory compromise for skeletal traction; for skin traction release and rewrap elastic bandage making it slightly looser.	Anytime the blood supply to a body part is impeded, there is decreased circulation, sensation, and motion. Careful monitoring translates into early intervention if blood supply is impeded.	Blood supply is not impeded as evidenced by good circulation, sensation, and motion checks.

(Continues)

GUIDE FOR NURSING MANAGEMENT

Nursing diagnosis	Intervention	Rationale	Outcome
3. Potential for injury (stressor: improper pull, inadequate restraints, presence of pin for skeletal traction)	Check traction apparatus to be sure that knots are secure and free from pulleys, weights are hanging freely (that is, not touching bed, floors, walls, etc), and ropes are centered in pulleys.	Alterations in the traction apparatus can adversely affect its function, causing further injury through incorrect pulling force.	The child remains in proper position relative to the traction. The child conforms to activity limitations that minimize injury risk.
	Check the child's position in bed and correct as necessary; mark head or foot of bed and side rails or sheets with tape to denote correct position of the child in relation to traction apparatus; do not elevate the head of the bed unless ordered.	Alteration in position can alter the effectiveness of the traction.	
	Use jacket restraints or elevate the bed on shock blocks as necessary.	These measures supplement the countertraction of the child's body weight. Because young children weigh so little, they get pulled toward the traction weights and alter the pull.	
	For skeletal traction, monitor pin site for infection or tenting; pad the pin ends.	Pin ends can scratch or injure an unaffected extremity. Pin entrance and exit sites are open wounds with potential for bacteria growth and infection. As the sites heal, the skin might adhere to pins creating additional injury when pins are removed.	
	For skin traction, check elastic bandages to be sure they are smoothly and securely wrapped.	Elastic bandages assist with the proper position of skin traction and prevent its sudden failure and subsequent injury.	
	Restrain child who is on a frame. Keep side rails elevated when no one is with the child.	An unrestrained, active child can easily fall out of bed and sustain an injury.	
4. Potential alteration in comfort: pain (stressors: muscle spasms, pull of traction)	Teach child to do relaxation exercises during muscle spasms; medicate if ordered; provide distraction; alter position.	Muscle spasms are particularly painful and get worse when the child is tense but lessen with deep breaths and distraction.	The child appears relaxed. The child can sleep and play.
5. Potential alteration in growth and development (stressor: long-term hospitalization)	Have the child help to plan a daily routine that alternates rest periods and active periods, time with others and time alone.	Including the child in planning promotes self-care, independence, and self-esteem.	The child demonstrates interest in self-care activities. The child is able to use age-appropriate toys and games. The child does not appear to be using regressive behaviors.
	Provide age-appropriate games and activities, particularly those involving physical activity, within the limits of the traction.	Age-appropriate activities help maintain developmental level.	

GUIDE FOR NURSING MANAGEMENT

Nursing diagnosis	Intervention	Rationale	Outcome
	Encourage the child to maintain contacts with peers and facilitate the child's making new friends in the hospital; assist the child in decorating the bed space.	Maintaining social contacts is important to the school-age child and adolescent and prevents isolation.	
	Encourage the child to keep up with schoolwork; provide opportunities for the chlid to do so.	Maintaining educational level prevents developmental delay.	
	Encourage exercise through use of play (for example, throwing foam balls, bean bags, or Velcro darts; kicking balls with unaffected leg; performing pull-ups on overhead trapeze).	Exercise prevents muscle atrophy and provides distraction.	
6. Potential for ineffective individual and family coping (stressors: fear, anger, guilt, lack of support)	Encourage the child and family to express fears, anger, and other negative feelings.	Verbalizing fears helps everyone to deal directly with them.	The family members appear relaxed with the child. Family members participate in the child's care and appear eager to assume the care at home. The family members can state what behavior they can expect from the child both in the hospital and at home.
	Offer toys appropriate to expressing aggression, setting limits when necessary.	Children who cannot verbalize fears can often act them out using imagination.	
	Provide information and reassurance as appropriate; refer to parent group for support or introduce child and family to someone who has had similar experience.	Reassurance reduces anxiety, and information provides a measure of control. Peer support from those with similar experience provides emotional strength and practical ideas.	
	Involve family members in child's care in the hospital and in discharge preparation.	Including family members in the child's care reduces the disruption in the family structure.	
	Encourage the family to continue home routines and family rituals.	Allowing the child's admission to disrupt the family as little as possible makes the child's return home an easier adjustment for all. Keeping as much as possible to home routine provides control, comfort with familiarity, and sense of stability.	
	Prepare the family for subsequent phases of treatment by explaining treatments and describing the child's expected reactions; explain the child's behavior to family members and prepare them to accept some developmental regression during the course of treatment.	The family copes more easily if it knows what to expect.	

Braces and Splints

Braces and splints are used to immobilize a body part in a position of function, to prevent weight bearing, to stabilize a joint, or to aid in the correction of a deformity. Braces allow the child's progress to be monitored on an outpatient basis, a distinct advantage over casting or inpatient traction.

The length of time a brace or splint is worn depends on its purpose. Braces used to correct deformities frequently are worn 23 hours a day, coming off only for bathing, skin care, and exercises. A brace or splint also might be removed for regular, prescribed periods, such as at night.

A brace is fitted to body curves so as not to create friction, skin irritation, or muscle misuse. The nurse assesses the child for circulatory or neurologic compromise and teaches parents to do so. Because braces and splints can exert pressure on the surrounding skin, regular skin care is required to prevent skin breakdown.

Braces are difficult and expensive to make and require special care if they are to remain functional and not irritate the skin. Leather portions are cleaned periodically with a leather cleaner or saddle soap. Plastic portions are wiped off with a mild soap-and-water solution daily. The screws are checked daily and tightened whenever necessary. Metal portions of the brace can be sharp or rough. These might require a protective covering of tape, plastic, or foam rubber to prevent damage to clothing.

Frames

Bradford frame Special frames facilitate care of the immobilized child. The Bradford frame is a rectangular lightweight metal frame covered with one long or two shorter pieces of water-repellent canvas separated near the center by 6–8 inches. The canvas is covered by blankets or other padding, then sheets or pillow cases are put over the padded canvas for comfort and cleanliness. The frame can be purchased, rented, or made by the family or facility needing it. The frame should be slightly larger than the child. It usually is placed so that its head and foot rest on two large wooden blocks that extend across the width of the bed. The head end of a Bradford frame is elevated for a child in a spica cast so that urine and feces drain down and away from the cast.

The blocks need to rest on a firm surface for stability. If the mattress is not sufficiently firm, a board of approximately the same size can be placed on top of the mattress. For safety and stability, the frame is secured at the corners to the bed frame or springs by four long, buckled straps. The child is secured to the frame by some form of restraint such as a vest or belt.

Stryker frame The Stryker frame is used for turning children who are immobile because of spinal injury or surgery. It consists of two canvas-covered frames that lock into a stand. The frame is longer and slightly wider than the child. A foot board can be positioned against the feet to maintain functional alignment when the child is supine. Armrests can be attached to the sides for comfort. Sheepskins, blankets, or Eggcrate® foam are placed on top of the canvas to protect skin from pressure.

The frame used when the child is supine consists of two pieces of canvas separated by a space to allow for positioning and use of the bedpan. The frame used for the prone position has one piece of canvas extending from the child's shoulders to the ankles and a small second piece of canvas to support the forehead. This allows the child to look down for reading or eating. A tablelike shelf is positioned under the upper portion of the frame to hold books, food, and supplies. Because the canvas ends at the child's ankle, it allows for functional positioning and full range of motion of the foot and ankle. The Stryker frame is narrow, so it is important that the child be restrained with a sheet or waist restraint and, if restless, restraints around the chest and thighs.

If possible, the nurse demonstrates the frame to the child prior to the treatment and allows the child to experience being turned. The nurse assures the child that turning is not dangerous. Once the child is immobilized on the frame, the nurse ensures that the stabilizer pin is secure and that restraints are kept fastened except during skin care.

The nurse enlists the help of trained personnel to turn the child. The child might feel more secure hugging the frame during turning. Before the child is turned, the unused half of the frame is applied and fastened securely to the lower half with safety belts so that the child is sandwiched between the two halves. The nurse then loosens the stabilizer pin, turns the frame smoothly and swiftly, and replaces the stabilizer pin immediately. The top half (formerly the bottom half) of the frame is removed, and the nurse repositions the child for comfort.

Principles of Nursing Care

Acute Care Needs

⊛ Potential impaired skin integrity

Casts, some traction apparatus, and braces can cause localized skin breakdown as they press or rub the skin. The nurse examines the edges of casts, traction equipment, splints, and braces for any rough areas. Measures such as

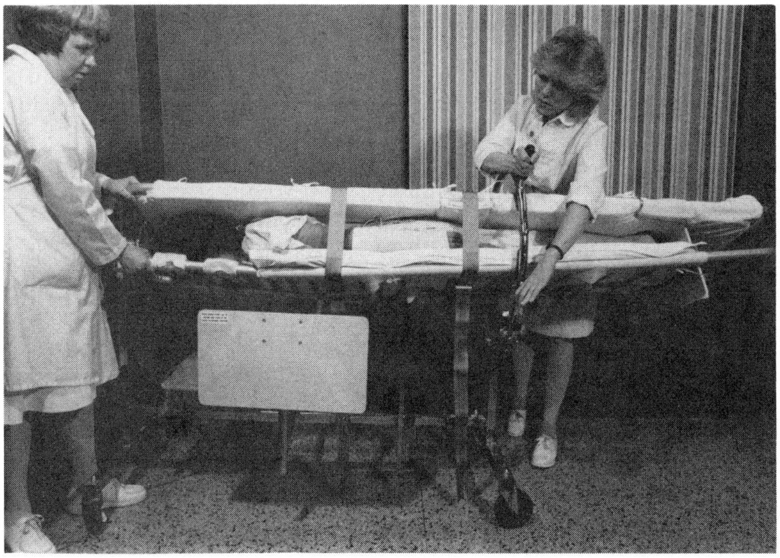

Stryker wedge turning frame. (From Swearingen PL: The Addison-Wesley Photo-Atlas of Nursing Procedures. *Addison-Wesley, 1984, p. 619.)*

petalling and padding can prevent excess friction that leads to impaired skin integrity. The nurse notes and reports any dents in a cast.

Alcohol or tincture of benzoin sometimes is used to toughen the skin at cast edges, under removable traction appliances, and over bony prominences that come in contact with removable appliances and apparatus. Toughening with alcohol is particularly useful for children who pull against a cast, brace, splint, or traction because of high activity level or neurologic impairment. The nurse uses alcohol with caution so the child does not inhale the irritating fumes.

It is important to prevent any extraneous material from getting between a cast and the child's skin. Parts of toys, food, and other small items are the usual culprits. The nurse covers the cast while the child is eating, keeps the bed clean and wrinkle-free, and keeps all small objects out of the child's reach.

Itching (pruritis) can prompt a child to insert an item under a cast. Relieving itching is an important nursing intervention to preserve skin integrity.

The nurse administers regular skin care to pressure areas. Skin care, provided to prevent irritation and breakdown, varies according to protocols but follows the general principles described in Chapter 20.

⊛ Potential for infection

Infectious microorganisms can enter the body at sites of skin breakdown or surgical incision and can cause skin infection, bone and tissue infection, or systemic infection. The keys to prevention of infection are correct skin care, preoperative skin preparation, and administration of antibiotics as ordered by the physician.

With skeletal traction, the site of pin or wire insertion is a potential focus of infection. There is controversy over whether the site should be cleansed daily or left alone following initial placement, and there is great variety among methods of pin care. Generally, the skin around the pin site is cleaned according to hospital policy to remove crusts and prevent the collecting of microorganisms at the site. Any skin tension, pulling, or tenting at the pin sites is reported immediately, since skin tension contributes to breakdown and infection.

Whether or not the nurse cleanses the pin site, several principles are involved in pin care. The nurse observes the site frequently for signs of infection, such as purulent drainage, crusting, swelling, and erythema that persist longer than 72 hours (Celeste, Folick, & Dumas, 1984). Any cleansing technique performed in the hospital should be sterile and performed gently so as not to introduce pathogens or traumatize the skin. A sterile gauze is often cut to fit around the pin. The nurse also assesses the site for any loosening or slipping of the pin.

The tips of the pins can be covered with gauze, rubber caps, or other protective material. This prevents puncture or scraping of the skin on other parts of the child's body.

⊛ Alteration in comfort: pain related to physical injury and biologic response secondary to circulatory compromise

The pain that results from skeletal manipulation can be extremely severe. Pain and swelling after surgery or a fracture can be expected to begin to diminish after approximately three days. If by the fourth day the pain has not diminished in intensity or has increased, the nurse suspects ischemia, or compartment syndrome. In addition to severe pain that appears to be muscle-related, other signs of ischemia include puffiness, pallor, and coolness of the extremity, paresthesias (numbness), paralysis, and absent pulse.

The nurse assesses for adequate circulation frequently but especially before medicating or explaining away pain related to a skeletal condition. To detect circulatory or neurologic compromise, the nurse assesses color, sensation, and motion in the body part distal to the cast or traction and reports any abnormality immediately. The nurse also attempts to decrease edema and increase circulation by elevating the edematous body part or loosening the elastic bandages of skin traction if neither intervention is contraindicated by the child's skeletal condition. If repositioning or elevation does not decrease the pain and signs of circulatory compromise, the physician is notified immediately.

Alteration in comfort: pain related to muscle spasms

Skeletal surgery involves much manipulation, pounding, and application of pressure. The child can experience painful spasms in muscles that have been stretched, pulled, and stabilized in new positions. With any sign or report of pain, the nurse first rules out ischemia as the cause. Traction can cause painful muscle spasms that require administration of muscle relaxants or analgesics. Constant pain, even if it is not severe, creates fatigue and restlessness and reduces energy needed for coping.

The child can be medicated for spasms, initially as frequently as every three hours. The nurse anticipates the pain if possible, since once the spasms have started, the child becomes more tense and the spasms increase. The nurse can use distraction, relaxation techniques, and play to deal with muscle spasm pain. These techniques seem to be more effective as the child's condition improves. Encouraging the child to breathe slowly and relax during the spasms can help. If the child is old enough to cooperate, use of imagery is helpful (eg, Imagine the pain is like a carousel. As the carousel slows, the pain goes away).

Impaired physical mobility related to imposed activity limitations

Immobility imposed by casts, traction, or a frame affects every system of the body (see Chapter 20). The nurse counteracts these effects by encouraging the child to move as much as possible, breathe deeply, participate in self-care, and perform prescribed exercises. The child benefits from activities and exercises that maintain muscle strength in noninvolved extremities. Turning, pulling up on an overhead trapeze, and lifting small weights strengthen muscles. The child can usually strengthen muscles of immobilized body parts by doing muscle-setting exercises, that is, by contracting and relaxing muscles without moving any joints.

Potential fluid volume deficit

Children who undergo skeletal surgery lose large amounts of blood because of the high vascularity of bone. This active loss of body fluids places the child at risk for hypovolemia. The nurse therefore reviews estimates of intraoperative blood loss and expects to see blood and fluid replacement after surgery.

Blood loss might not end with surgery, however, and the nurse is especially careful to monitor signs of bleeding at the operative site, vital signs, and laboratory values. If the operative site is casted postoperatively, the nurse observes the cast for serosanguineous staining and fresh bleeding. The nurse draws a circle around the initial serosanguineous stain and records the date and time. Additional circles are drawn to outline successive increases in staining. Because bone surgery results in postoperative blood loss, and bone oozes for a time following incision, some blood staining on the cast is normal. For some operations such staining can be considerable. Careful monitoring of fresh bleeding, vital signs, and hematocrit enable the nurse to detect signs of excessive blood loss.

Nutritional Needs

Alteration in nutrition: less than body requirements related to the child's inability to eat or anorexia

Eating independently is difficult for children who are partially immobilized by casts, traction, or frames. The nurse prepares and positions food on the tray so that it is easy to reach. Providing the child with finger foods, sandwiches, raw vegetables, and fruit helps maintain the child's independence and control over what is eaten. Straws inserted into covered cups of liquids promote self-feeding as well. The nurse might find it necessary to cut meat or other large pieces of food for the child or open dishes and packets of salad dressing, jelly, or seasonings.

Children who must remain flat in bed, especially in the supine position, require nursing ingenuity during mealtime. Those who can be turned have an easier time eating while lying on their side, with the tray placed on the bed beside them. For children who can be turned prone, such as those on a Stryker frame, the tray can be placed on a shelf underneath. Eating in these positions is fatiguing and often interferes with appetite. Intake is likely to improve if small meals and nutritious in-between-meal snacks are offered.

Independence and appropriate control over meals are crucial to the immobilized child since the need for nutrients is great and the child's opportunities to control the environment are few. The child is allowed to choose favorite foods from the menu and to choose the position for eating that is most comfortable. The nurse can inform the child that assistance is available but let the child decide when it's needed. The nurse assists the child to plan a diet high in fluids, protein, vitamins, minerals, and fiber to promote healing and combat the effects of immobility.

Developmental Needs

Potential altered growth and development

Treatment of skeletal conditions often requires long hospital stays with periods of home care after discharge. The child can be deprived of interactions and developmental opportunities normally supplied by school, family life, and peer association. Play, participation in self-care and hospital activities, opportunities to socialize, and encouragement with schoolwork all stimulate the child and promote normal growth and development. Maintaining contact with peers is particularly important and the child is encouraged to telephone or write letters to friends. Most hospital units allow peer visits.

Emotional Needs

The emotional needs of children with skeletal conditions are related to reactions to immobilization, casts and other appliances, and alterations in body image.

Ineffective individual coping related to situational crisis of immobilization

Some children find immobilization and restrictions difficult to accept, particularly since they feel well. Besides teaching and reteaching restrictions, the nurse might have to curb inappropriate behavior and set firm limits. Most children accept immobilizations and restrictions quite contentedly, perhaps because equipment, casts, or traction apparatus are concrete and constant reminders of the skeletal condition.

The child's apparent acceptance is sometimes superficial, however. Although the child might appear to adjust well initially, signs of maladjustment, such as anger, rebelliousness, frustration, and uncooperativeness, might manifest themselves later. These feelings diminish as the child begins to regain mobility. At this stage of treatment, many children make up for any setbacks they might have suffered in emotional development.

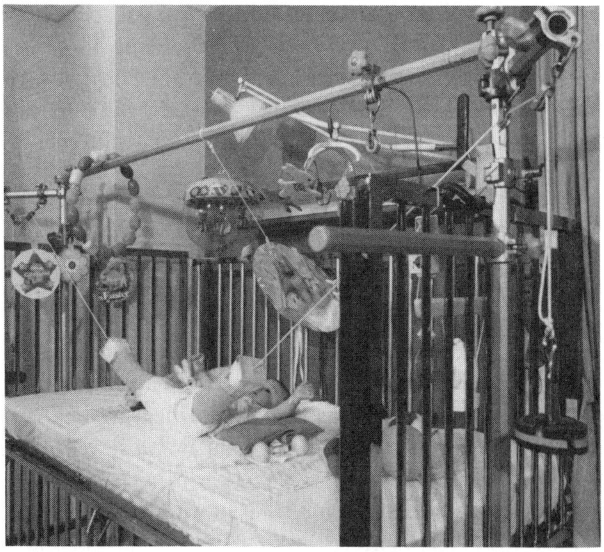

Meeting developmental needs of a child in Bryant's traction by providing visual stimuli, such as toys and mobiles. (From Swearingen PL: The Addison-Wesley Photo-Atlas of Nursing Procedures. *Addison-Wesley, 1984, p. 559.)*

The nurse, understanding that activity limitation is frustrating to any child, helps the child deal with the anger. Age-appropriate play activities such as pounding clay or other art materials helps the child release anger. Encouraging doll or puppet play or story-telling allows the child to appropriately act out hostility. Allowing the child as many choices in care provides the child with control and encourages self-care.

The child's emotional status throughout treatment depends on the suddenness of the condition's onset, severity of the condition, and length of treatment. The child who has survived an accident in which others have been injured or killed requires special nursing interventions and emotional support and might need referral for counseling.

Fear related to knowledge deficit concerning orthopedic apparatus

Casts, braces, splints, and traction devices often seem strange and frightening to the child. The nurse carefully explains and, if possible, demonstrates equipment before it is applied or used in the child's treatment. For example, the child with skeletal traction might wish to believe that a pin or wire does not pass through the bone. Though facts can frighten or alienate the child at first it is more helpful in the long run to tell the child the truth than to collaborate in deception. While explaining that the pin or wire does pass through the bone, the nurse reassures the child that the bone is not harmed. Use of dolls or puppets can help explain apparatus or allow the child to deal with feelings related to the apparatus.

Body image disturbance related to nonintegration of change in body function and appearance

The child might refuse to look at the traction apparatus, injury, or stained cast. These sights seem unattractive, and the child might fear that the traction pin will leave holes in the extremity, that the traction weight will make the extremity longer, or that a deformity is permanent. The child needs to express these feelings to someone who can sympathize with these concerns, take them seriously, and answer questions honestly. Some children cannot talk about their fears. For these children, another form of expression, such as doll play, the opportunity to handle equipment, and painting or drawing, are appropriate.

Children who are discharged with casts or braces are conscious of their appearance and might fear being teased, stared at, or questioned. Children with these fears need to practice responding to questions about their appearance so that they feel ready to relate to people outside the hospital. Role play is an effective method for helping children deal with uncomfortable questions. The nurse can suggest adaptations for clothing that are attractive and stylish while fitting over or around apparatus.

Health Maintenance Needs

Potential for impaired home maintenance management

Discharge preparation for the child who is hospitalized for a musculoskeletal condition includes teaching the parent assessment and protection of skin integrity; cast or brace care; turning; and use of crutches or other mobility devices. The nurse gives the parent instructions in writing. If the parent needs to adapt the home for the child's limitations or purchase or construct equipment, the nurse furnishes written instructions well before the child's discharge.

The nurse helps the family to plan alterations needed in the home to enable the immobilized child to participate in family life or get around using mobility aids. Environmental hazards, such as throw rugs, stairs, cords, and other obstacles, are safety hazards that are identified and minimized before the child returns home.

Crutch-walking is an important skill for the child to master prior to discharge. It is important to remind the child to stand up straight while using the crutches and not to lean on the crutch tops. The nurse checks for elbow flexion of about 30 degrees that indicates that the handgrip is at a correct level. The child is cautioned to be especially careful in wet weather that the crutch tips are dried prior to using them indoors, to prevent slipping. The nurse encourages the child to walk slowly and not to lend the crutches to others or use them inappropriately.

The nurse makes arrangements to ensure continuity of care. This might include scheduling follow-up appointments or referring the family to a community health nurse. In many states, the community health nurse, or public health nurse, assists families who need the help provided by Crippled Children's Services.

The Child with a Musculoskeletal Injury

Fractures

Types of fractures Children sustain fractures as a result of traumatic forces exerted on bone. Fractures can be sustained in almost any bone but are most frequently seen in the long bones of the legs and arms, the wrists, fingers, toes, and skull. Fractures can be *simple* or *closed,* that is, entirely below the skin surface, or *compound,* where one or both of the bone ends pierces the skin and leaves it open to organism entry. A *comminuted* fracture occurs when the bone is in multiple fragments. The break also is classified as complete or incomplete depending on the depth of injury. A spiral fracture affects the length rather than the width of the bone.

Children's bones, because of their greater flexibility, react to stress in different ways from those of the adult. They deform before breaking, and they might simply bend, buckle, or break incompletely.

A *buckle fracture,* also called a torus fracture, occurs most frequently in young children. The bone fails with compression forces, usually near the metaphysis. The fracture is seen as a raised or bulging area. In a *greenstick fracture,* forces cause a break through the periosteum and compact bone on one side, while merely bending the other side. Greenstick fractures are commonly seen in the forearm. Despite the flexibility of their bones, children are subject to other types of fractures in which the bone is broken completely.

Fractures that affect the epiphyseal, or growth, plate can

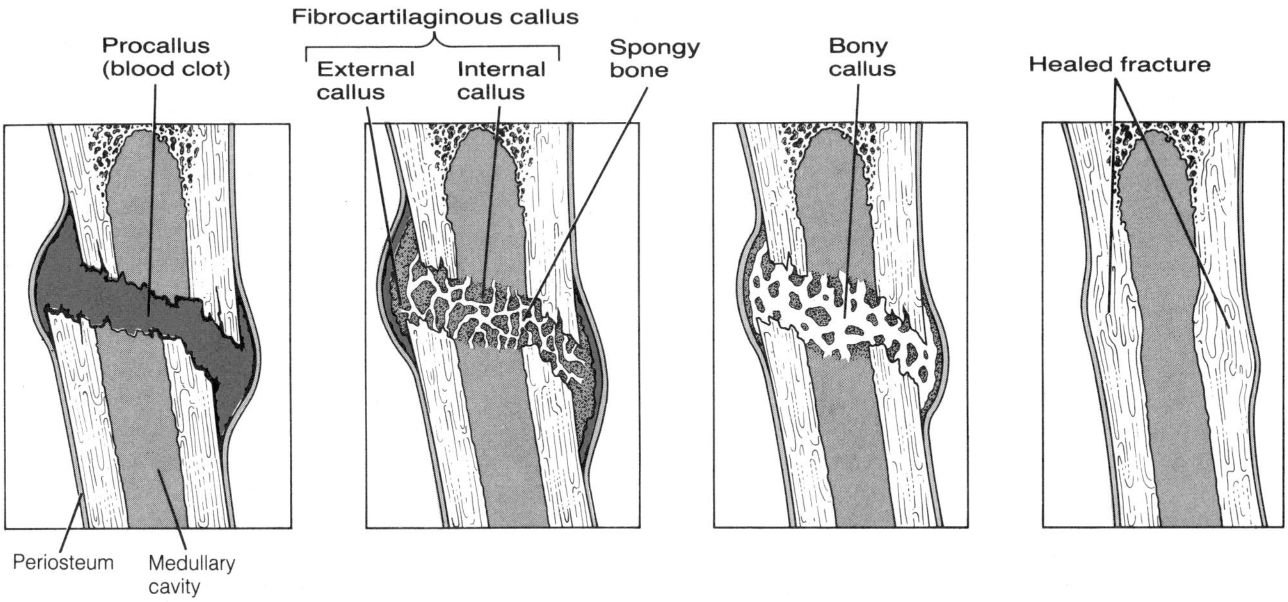

FIGURE 30-4

The process of bone healing. (From Spence AP, Mason EB: Human Anatomy and Physiology, *3rd ed. Benjamin/Cummings, 1987, with permission.)*

interrupt and alter growth. The impact of these fractures on growth depends on the area of the epiphyseal plate affected. For example, fractures that leave the germinal layer and blood supply of the epiphyseal plate relatively intact cause little growth retardation. On the other hand, fractures that destroy the germinal layer result in growth disturbance.

Injury that stimulates blood supply to the epiphysis and thus to the epiphyseal plate can lead to overgrowth of the affected bone. For this reason some fractures, particularly in the long bones, are set with some overriding of fracture fragments so that the healed bone will not be longer than the corresponding bone on the other side of the child's body.

Bone healing The factors affecting bone growth in children help explain differences between fractures in children and adults. Bones undergo much remolding as children grow. As the growing bone responds to the pulls of muscles and stresses for bearing weight, some natural realignment of fractured bone occurs. Fractures in young children and fractures that occur relatively close to the epiphyseal plate have more potential for this spontaneous correction. Spinal fractures and fractures in a plane other than the direction of joint movement do not realign spontaneously.

After a fracture has occurred and the bone fragments are in proper alignment, healing begins. The process of healing from the procallus stage to healed bone is illustrated in Figure 30-4. Fractures in children tend to heal more rapidly than those in adults. The blood supply to the bone is rich; the periosteum is thick; and the osteogenic activity is high. As age increases, the time involved in healing also increases. For example, a femoral shaft fracture in a neonate that would heal in 3 weeks heals in an 8-year-old in 8 weeks and in a 12-year-old in 12 weeks (Salter, 1983).

Clinical manifestations Signs and symptoms of fracture depend on the type of fracture present and whether it affects the diaphysis, epiphyseal plate, or epiphysis. Generally, a fracture causes sudden sharp pain at the time of the injury and tenderness at the site thereafter. Pain increases with movement and decreases somewhat with rest. The child usually cannot use the affected body part. Numbness and tingling in the extremity distal to the fracture site is a frequent occurrence.

There might be obvious deformity at the fracture site and abnormal positioning of the body part. Swelling varies, depending on the degree of soft-tissue damage and the displacement of bone fragments. There might be discoloration around the fracture site or frank bleeding from a wound communicating with a fracture. Bone fragments might be visible. Radiographs confirm the diagnosis.

Treatment Emergency treatment of fractures involves performing an initial assessment of bone injury and soft-tissue damage, preventing further injury, promoting comfort, and keeping the child NPO in case anesthesia or surgery is required. Any deformity is observed, and if only swelling is present, the area is gently palpated for the site of greatest tenderness. Color, sensation, motion, and pulses distal to the injury are monitored to detect neurologic or circulatory compromise. Splinting decreases both discomfort and the chance of further injury. A splint needs to immobilize the fracture site, including the joints above and below the injury. Outside the hospital or clinic, ingenuity might be needed to devise a splint using materials at hand (see Chapter 12 for first aid for skeletal injury). In the hospital, plaster might be molded to support the area or an aluminum splint applied.

The fracture is immobilized after it has been properly reduced or realigned. The fracture might be realigned by (a) closed reduction, or external manipulation of the body part; (b) open reduction, or surgery and internal fixation; or (c) traction. After alignment, the body part is placed in a splint or cast. For proper immobilization, the joint above and the joint below a fracture are included in the cast. Internal fixation devices (rods, pins, or wires) might remain in the bone unless they eventually irritate the skin, cause pain, or become superficial. Intermedullary rods (within the medullary cavity) frequently are permanent. Screws and plates used as internal fixation devices are removed after initial healing if they are thought to weaken the bone.

Radiographs are used to monitor alignment and healing. Increasing amounts of callus formation indicate progress. Radiographs might be taken as often as weekly while the child is in traction, preceding casting, and during the first few weeks following casting of fractures that are likely to lose alignment. Greenstick fractures can spring back to the position of injury, and other fractures can become displaced as swelling decreases and the cast becomes loose.

Follow-up assessment might be done every 3 months for the year following injury, particularly if leg length discrepancy is a risk. This allows for early identification of complications from the injury or fracture healing.

Nursing management A fracture usually occurs while the child is engaged in active play or sports or as a result of an accident. In either case, the child usually is frightened by what has happened. The child who is injured in athletic activity often worries about the return of full function. The accident victim might feel in some way responsible for the injury and possibly the injury or even death of another person. The teaching done during emergency treatment might be hurried. All these circumstances can cause the child to understand and remember little of what is said. The nurse therefore determines what information the child has retained, repeats teaching, and gives reassurances frequently to ensure the child's understanding of the injury and its treatment.

Nursing management might involve splint, cast, or traction care. Whatever treatment is used, the nurse monitors color, sensation, and motion in body parts distal to the fracture. Severe pain requires careful and thorough assessment because pain might indicate neurologic or circulatory compromise. Neurologic or vascular compromise necessitates immediate reporting to the physician for rapid intervention.

A major complication in the child with a fracture is fat embolism. Fat embolism occurs most frequently after fracture of a long bone such as the femur and can be life threatening. Fat globules from the fracture site are released into the systemic circulation and can lodge in lung capillaries, causing impaired gas exchange (Stevenson, 1985). The first 24–72 hours after the fracture are critical. If the child develops dyspnea or other signs of respiratory compromise, these should be reported immediately. The first sign of an embolism might be increasing blood pressure, so monitoring vital signs is essential. If any signs of embolism appear, the child is placed in a semi-Fowler position and oxygen is administered (Stevenson, 1985). Preventing the complications of immobility and watching for signs and symptoms of infection also are essential for any child with a fracture.

The parent is given written instructions about monitoring the child at home. Information includes how frequently to monitor circulation, what to look for, and how to maintain the cast. A follow-up appointment is written on the instructions.

Sprains, Strains, and Contusions

A *sprain* is a joint injury caused by pulling or tearing of a ligament. A *strain* is a muscle or tendon injury caused by stretching or overuse. A *contusion,* or bruise, is a skin and soft-tissue injury caused by a blow that does not break the skin. Although sprains, strains, and contusions make up most of the acute athletic injuries, epiphyseal injuries sometimes occur rather than sprains or strains in children.

Clinical manifestations Minor sprains cause tenderness at the point of injury and minimal swelling and loss of joint function but no abnormal movement of the joint. Moderate sprains cause swelling, local hemorrhage, moderate loss of function, and joint pain, particularly with activity or weight bearing. A severe sprain, in which the ligament is completely torn, usually causes less pain than a moderate sprain, but there is severe swelling, hemorrhage, and abnormal joint movement.

The signs of a strain's severity differ, depending on whether the injury affects the point of muscle origin or tendon insertion. Bleeding occurs with an injured muscle belly. Pain and soft-tissue swelling, rather than bleeding, characterize tendon injury. Relatively little pain occurs at the time of tendon or ligament injury, so complete tears of tendons or ligaments might at first be less obvious than muscle tears. For these reasons, strains or sprains involving the knee, Achilles tendon, finger, or shoulder can be difficult to diagnose unless the child reports that the disturbance in joint stability or function was preceded by a snapping, popping, or tearing noise.

Treatment Early treatment reduces recovery time. Ice, compression, elevation, and rest (ICER) are the emergency treatments for sprains, strains, and contusions. Twenty to 30 minutes of ice and compression applied immediately after the injury can reduce by half the time needed for recovery (Garrick, 1981). Except when surgical intervention is needed, ICER is continued for 24–36 hours. A complete tear is surgically repaired.

During healing, muscle tone is maintained with muscle-setting exercises. After the injury heals and pain is gone, the child works up slowly to preinjury activity levels.

Nursing management A nurse who witnesses an injury initiates first-aid treatment immediately. If ice is available, it is placed over the injury for at least 20 minutes. The area is wrapped so as to exert compression without interfering with circulation or innervation. While giving first aid, the nurse teaches the child and others who may be at the scene, including parents and coaches, the importance of applying ice and compression immediately to sprains, strains, or contusions.

During recovery, the nurse teaches the child muscle-setting exercises to maintain muscle tone and hasten the return to previous activity levels, or the child might be referred for physical therapy. The nurse cautions against returning to activities and sports too soon. Only when signs and symptoms have totally disappeared should the child resume strenuous activity. Children and even coaches sometimes try to rush the recovery period, thinking that activity can be resumed if it is not too painful. This could result in reinjury and an even longer recovery period.

Dislocations

Dislocation, or luxation, is displacement of the articular surfaces of a joint. Partial displacement is called subluxation. Dislocation of the femoral head occurs with severe trauma. Dislocation of the elbow and wrist are frequently seen in children. Posterior dislocation of the elbow usually results from a fall on the outstretched hand in which the radius and ulna are displaced posteriorly and upward. Dislocation of the wrist occurs commonly in young children who attempt to twist out of a parent's handclasp. Dislocation of the normal knee is not common.

Dislocation is very painful. Deformity at the joint might be obvious. There is often swelling, and joint motion is very painful and restricted.

Treatment for dislocation is closed, manual reduction or open, surgical reduction. Nursing management depends on treatment and the clinical situation. The child and parent need reassurance and support until the joint is reduced. Some children need preparation for general anesthesia and surgery. After reduction, the joint might be immobilized with a sling. After reduction, the nurse monitors the extremity for color, sensation, and motion to detect any neurologic or vascular compromise.

The parents are given a demonstration and written instructions on how to monitor circulatory status, how to apply the sling, and whom to contact if circulatory compromise occurs. The nurse informs the child and parent about any activity limitations and when to return for a follow-up examination.

The Child with a Structural Abnormality

Clubfoot (Talipes Equinovarus)

Clubfoot is a deformity in which portions of the foot and ankle are in various nonfunctional positions. The foot and ankle are in either the *equinus* (foot extended, toes lower than heel) or the *calcaneus* (foot flexed and heel lower than toes) position. The foot also can be in the *varus* (inverted, or turned in) or the *valgus* (everted, or turned out) position. Clubfoot can be unilateral or bilateral, flexible or rigid, mild or severe.

The deformity is almost always congenital. Its exact cause is unknown, though it does seem to have environmental and some inherited components. Incidence is highest in families who already have one child with a clubfoot. Incidence in the general population is 2 in 1000 (Salter, 1983). Clubfoot occurs more frequently in males than in females and can be associated with other congenital abnormalities such as spina bifida (see Chapter 31).

Clinical manifestations The most common deformity and the one that is usually called clubfoot is talipes equinovarus (Fig. 30-5). In *talipes equinovarus,* the foot twists inward and is in plantar flexion (pointed down). In severe forms, the foot has a clublike appearance.

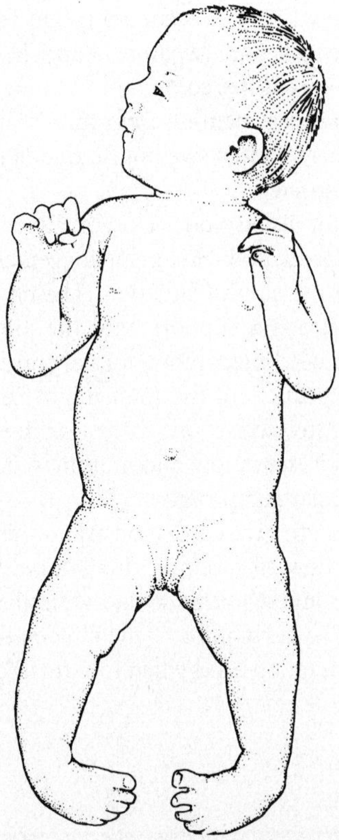

FIGURE 30-5

Talipes equinovarus (clubfoot). (From Saxton DF et al: The Addison-Wesley Manual of Nursing Practice. *Addison-Wesley, 1983, with permission.)*

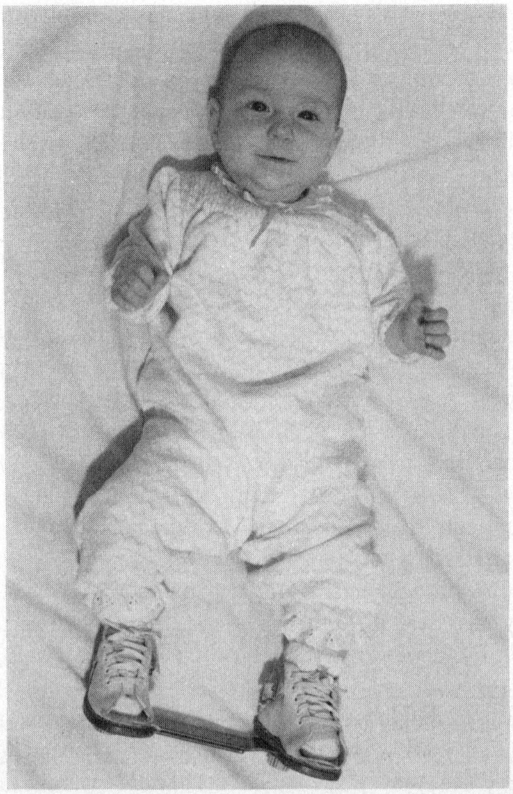

Denis-Browne splint. (From Swearingen PL: The Addison-Wesley Photo-Atlas of Nursing Procedures. *Addison-Wesley, 1984, p. 528.)*

Some children have a mild varus deformity of the forefoot (metatarsus adductus). The foot turns inward when the child lies, stands, or walks (pigeon-toed). This mild inversion differs from talipes equinovarus in that the foot is flexible, not rigid. The foot can be passively put through complete range of motion and readily corrects to a neutral position. Heel and leg size are normal. Mild, flexible clubfoot is possibly the result of intrauterine position, especially during the last month or so of gestation.

Talipes equinovarus is a rigid deformity. it can be so pronounced that the toes touch the inner side of the lower leg. The foot cannot be passively manipulated to a neutral position. The heel is small, and the leg becomes atrophied to some degree. There are soft tissue changes in the foot. Ligaments on the medial side of the foot and posterior aspect of the ankle are thickened and shortened. Muscles might be contracted.

Treatment Treatment for mild varus deformity includes stretching exercises and possibly special shoes. Passive stretching exercises might be prescribed alone or in combination with corrective shoes or splints. The parent is taught which exercises to do and how frequently to do them. Many choose to do these exercises during the infant's feedings. Feedings are quite equally spaced, and the parent is less likely to forget the exercises if they are part of another routine aspect of care.

Treatment for talipes equinovarus is initiated immediately after diagnosis. Because the infant's skeletal structure is more malleable, the earlier the treatment, the more favorable the results. If deformity is severe, treatment is often begun before the neonate is discharged.

Conservative treatment consists of manipulation of the foot away from the abnormal position and maintenance of the corrected position with adhesive strapping or a plaster cast. Serial restrapping or recasting follows at 1- to 2-week intervals. This routine accommodates the infant's growth and allows both repositioning and continual, gradual manipulation of the foot to an overcorrected position. An adhesive, nonirritating liquid, such as benzoin, can be applied to the skin before adhesive strapping or casting to prevent slippage and loss of correction. The cast might extend from toes to groin, with the knees flexed to control heel position and leg rotation. Exercises then are prescribed following the completion of casting or strapping to maintain the correction. The *Denis-Browne splint* is one of many treatment devices used in the correction of in-toeing and clubfoot. The feet fit into special shoes or padded forms, which are laced. The shoes or forms are fastened to an adjustable bar providing the appropriate degree of eversion, rotation, and dorsiflexion needed to achieve a mild degree of overcorrection.

When fully corrected, the foot is held in an overcorrected position by a cast, strap, or splint, such as a Denis-Browne splint, for several weeks. Then a bivalved cast or Denis-Browne splint is commonly worn at night to hold the foot in a slightly overcorrected position. During the day, the child wears special shoes constructed to maintain the desired corrected or overcorrected position.

Surgery and subsequent casting can continue well into adolescence. Treatment continues until walking and shoe wear show no residual or recurring deformity.

A rigid deformity might require surgical intervention. This often includes correcting soft-tissue deformities, for example, lengthening the heel cord and other tendons, dividing tight ligaments, and restoring bones to normal positions. In older children, bone wedges might be used to realign the bones of the foot. In infants and younger children, surgery usually is confined to the soft tissues so as not to interfere with bone growth. Following surgery, the foot is casted for several months.

Nursing management Following each application of straps or cast, the nurse monitors the infant's toes for color, sensation, and motion to ensure that the cast or strapping is not too tight. The nurse demonstrates cast care to the parents, particularly emphasizing aspects related to protecting the cast from soiling.

The nurse and parent provide stimulating activities to distract the infant who is casted. The parent is instructed to support the infant's normal development as much as possible.

If passive stretching exercises are part of the treatment, the nurse observes the parent's performance, explains the purpose and desired result of the exercises, and recommends appropriate times to do them (usually six times daily).

If surgery is required the nurse can help the parent to verbalize feelings of anxiety or guilt. The parent might need support during frequent visits to the doctor, clinic, or hospital, which can become time-consuming and difficult, depending on the family situation.

To increase success, treatment is initiated soon after diagnosis. This might compound parental stress because the parent also is adjusting to the distressing fact that the infant has a deformity. The nurse plays an important role in supporting the parent during initial decision making about treatment choices. By helping the parent to express concerns, providing answers to questions, and maintaining a positive and supportive attitude, the nurse helps the parent to establish coping behaviors necessary during the initial treatment and long follow-up required for the infant with clubfoot.

Congenital Dislocated Hip (Congenital Hip Dysplasia)

Congenital hip dysplasia is a condition in which one or both of the femoral heads is displaced from the acetabulum (hip socket) or acetabula. The cause is unknown, but the following factors seem to be relevant:

- Familial tendency
- Laxity of the hip joint capsule and associated ligaments
- Breech presentation at birth
- Postnatal positioning (eg, in baby carriers or swaddling that keep the hips adducted)

Dislocated hip is one of the most common congenital deformities in the Western world. It occurs in approximately 1.5 in 1000 live births, and it occurs in girls eight times more often than in boys. Both hips are affected in one-half of the cases (Salter, 1983). Deformity that develops in utero instead of after birth is more severe. Often, the hip is not dislocated at birth but merely shows a tendency to dislocate.

Congenital dislocated hip might be manifested as (a) an unstable hip in which the femoral head can be dislocated by manipulation (preluxation); (b) partial dislocation (subluxation) in which the femoral head has some contact with the acetabulum but is not in correct position; or (c) dislocation in which the femoral head has no contact with the acetabulum.

With dislocation, the femoral head fails to exert appropriate pressure against the acetabulum. This results both in delayed development of the femoral head and failure of the acetabulum to form correctly. As a result, the femoral head becomes small and flattened, and the acetabulum becomes shallow and eventually flat. The adductor muscles of the hip shorten and contract.

Clinical manifestations The child with dislocated hip might exhibit signs of shortening of the femur on the affected side. Either thigh or gluteal folds or both are increased on the affected side when the two legs are compared

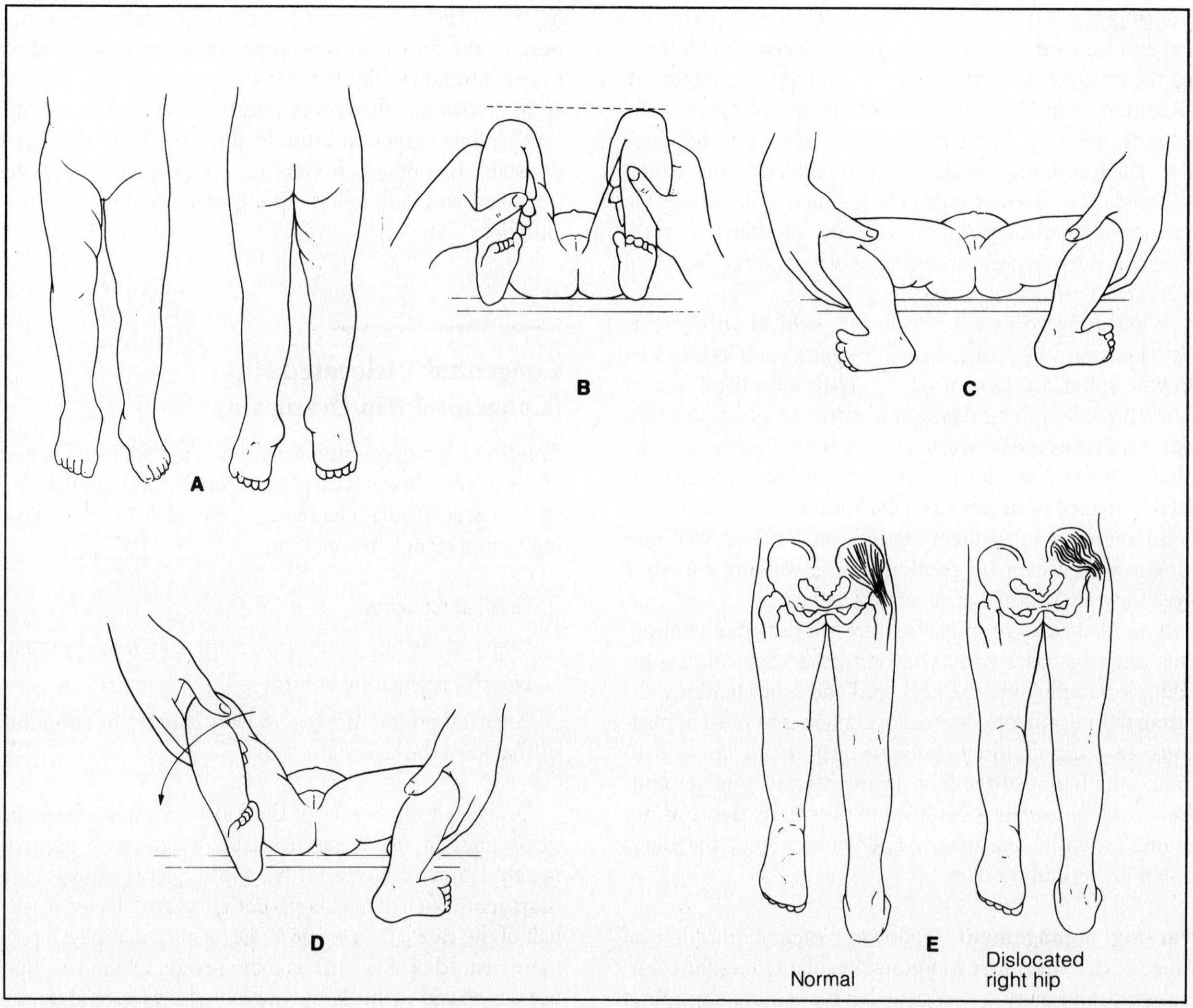

FIGURE 30-6

*Signs of unilateral dislocated hip in an infant. **A.** Unequal thigh folds. **B.** Galleazzi's sign. **C.** Normal abduction of the thighs. **D.** Limited adduction of the thighs. **E.** Trendelenburg's test.*

(Fig. 30-6A). If the infant is placed in the supine position and the hips flexed at 90° while the knees are bent, the level of the knee on the affected side will be lower than that of the other knee—positive Galeazzi's sign (Fig. 30-6B).

Abduction of the affected side is limited (Fig. 30-6 C & D). Sometimes, Galeazzi's sign or limitation of abduction are not apparent in the neonate, since there has not been enough time for muscle spasms and contractures to develop. After 4–6 weeks and some further shortening of adductor muscles, however, they become apparent.

Ortolani's click is a reliable sign of hip dislocation in the neonate (see Chapter 10).

The Trendelenburg test is used to assess hip dislocation in children who are old enough to stand and bear weight. When the child stands on the leg of the affected side, the opposite hip slants downward instead of remaining level (Fig. 30-6E). This is caused by the weakness of the hip abductor muscles. The downward slant of one hip is a positive sign of dislocation in the weight-bearing hip. If one hip is dislocated, the child walks with a characteristic limp known as the Trendelenburg gait. Dislocation of both hips causes a waddling gait and the child will have lordosis.

Diagnostic evaluation Detection often is the result of routine nursing assessment of the infant. Radiographic studies or sonography can confirm the diagnosis. If dislo-

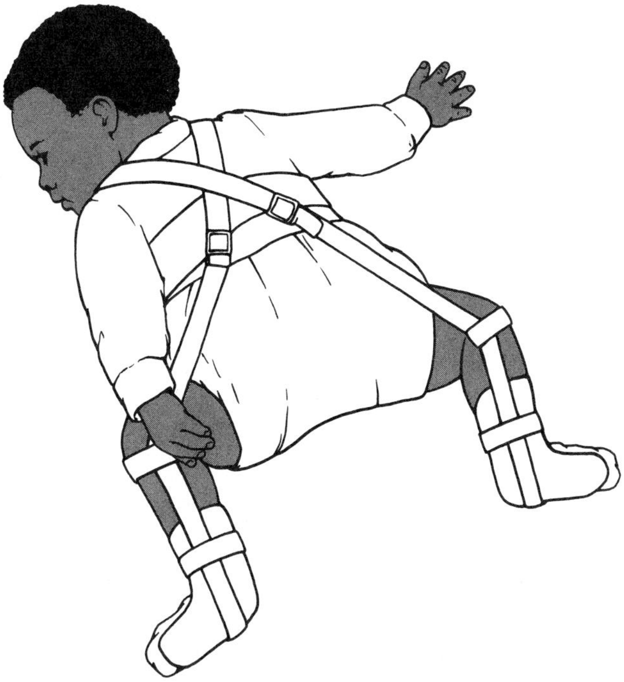

FIGURE 30-7

The child in a Pavlick harness for congenital dislocated hip.

cated hip is not diagnosed and treated in infancy, mastery of walking is frequently delayed.

Treatment Early detection and treatment is less complicated, more effective, and can prevent complications. Treatment varies with the severity of clinical manifestations and the age of the child. During the neonatal period, when the adductor muscles have not yet shortened or contracted, treatment consists of carefully positioning and maintaining the hip in abduction with the head of the femur in the acetabulum for several months, thus encouraging deepening of the acetabulum. This position is maintained by use of a splint such as the Frejka pillow or Pavlik harness or a hip cast. The Frejka pillow splint fits around the diaper area and between the thighs, so it is removed and reapplied with each diaper change. The Pavlik harness (Fig. 30-7) consists of straps passing from the shoulders and chest to the feet and lower legs. The harness often is readjusted to maintain the proper position of the head of the femur in the acetabulum.

If the dislocation is not treated until 2–3 months but before 12–18 months of age, traction for a number of weeks prior to casting generally facilitates proper positioning. Traction stretches the tightened muscles, allowing better placement of the head of the femur in the acetabulum. Closed reduction is then done with the child under general anesthesia, and a hip spica cast is applied to maintain the abducted position. The cast usually remains on for several months, being removed and reapplied as necessary to accommodate the child's growth.

Once contracture of the adductor muscles and accompanying displacement of the femoral head has occurred, usually after the child's first birthday, more extensive treatment is necessary. If soft tissue and muscle contractures are not severe, bilateral traction might serve to reposition the femoral head and achieve abduction. Closed reduction and casting follow. If the contractures are severe, traction followed by serial closed or open reduction might yield satisfactory results. While in traction and especially after cast application, the young child is often positioned on a Bradford frame.

During the course of treatment, periodic radiographs are taken to assess positioning of the head of the femur and depth of the acetabulum. If treatment is not begun until after the age of 18 months, increasing rigidity and changes in the femur and acetabulum will have progressed to a stage that is difficult to correct completely. Open reduction and such procedures as osteotomy (surgical incision into bone) and arthroplasty (surgical reformation of a joint) might be necessary. If congenital dislocated hip is untreated after the age of 7, treatment is very unsatisfactory.

Nursing management Nursing management for the child undergoing treatment for congenital hip dysplasia involves direct care and teaching related to splints and spica casts. The infant or child is growing and developing quickly, so nursing and home care are likely to require many adjustments during the months of treatment.

Parents of an infant in a Pavlik harness are cautioned not to remove the harness without expressed direction from the physician. The harness is the treatment of choice for most infants, but its effectiveness is directly related to parental compliance. The child can develop complications or achieve an unsuccessful reduction if directions are not followed.

The parent is taught to readjust the buckles if they become loose. Marking the straps with indelible ink to indicate the correct position will help the parent should the straps slip (Mulley, 1984). The parent sponge bathes the infant with careful attention to the skin under the straps. Diapers with elastic legs or plastic pants over cloth diapers can prevent soiling of the harness. The harness can be sponge cleaned on the child with mild soap and water (Mulley, 1984). The parent of a child in a hip spica cast needs to be given written directions for caring for the child (see the box Special Considerations for the Child in a Hip Spica earlier in this chapter).

Legg-Calvé-Perthes Disease (Coxa Plana)

Legg-Calvé-Perthes disease, a form of osteochondrosis also known as coxa plana, is a condition produced by avascularity (insufficient supply of blood vessels) in the femoral head. This self-limiting disease can produce a flattened femoral head, which has the potential for resulting in structural abnormality of the hip. It lasts from 2 to 8 years. The cause is unknown. Legg-Calvé-Perthes disease occurs in boys four times more often than in girls. Onset usually occurs when the child is between 4 and 8 years of age, but children as young as 3 and as old as 11 have presented with the disease. The disease can affect the entire capital (upper) epiphysis or only the anterior half or two-thirds.

Legg-Calvé-Perthes disease has several stages:

1. The incipient, or *synovitis,* stage can last from 1 to 3 weeks and is characterized by soft tissue changes with swelling of the synovial membrane and joint capsule. There might not be any noticeable clinical signs.
2. The second, or *avascular,* stage is often the first stage noted. It is characterized by interference with the blood supply to the head of the femur and death of osteocytes and bone marrow cells. The femoral head might be displaced laterally from the acetabulum. This stage lasts from several months to a year.
3. In the third stage, the *regenerative* stage, vascular and connective tissue invade the dead bone. The necrotic bone is absorbed and replaced by live though not yet calcified bone. The length of this stage varies depending on the extent of involvement.
4. In the fourth and final stage, ossification (formation of bone substance) occurs. Reossification takes about two years.

If there is a resulting discrepancy between the shape of the newly ossified femoral head and the acetabulum, degenerative changes will occur in adulthood.

Clinical manifestations Early manifestations of Legg-Calvé-Perthes disease are a limp and pain, which might be present for several months. The pain usually is referred to the knee, thigh, or groin. The child's complaints concerning the severity of pain vary, but severity usually increases with activity and decreases with rest. Symptoms might begin following an injury, but this is not generally the case. The child's limp is characterized by limited abduction and internal rotation of the hip. The combination of a history of pain, limp, and radiographic evidence of decreased bone cells in the affected femoral head lead to the diagnosis.

Prognosis varies and is related to several factors. First, the earlier the onset, the more favorable the prognosis. Younger children have more cartilage and less osseous bone and thus less risk of deformity. Second, prognosis is better if less than half of the femoral head is involved. Third, the earlier and more effectively the child is treated, the better the outcome.

Treatment The goal of treatment is to minimize or prevent damage and deformity to the femoral head and keep it in proper relationship with the acetabulum until healing occurs naturally. Some children are merely monitored for proper healing. For others, the femoral head is maintained in the acetabulum in a position of abduction through the use of casts, braces, or a special sling. Definitive treatment might or might not involve surgery.

An initial period of bed rest might be followed by application of Petrie casts or a brace which holds the femur in an abducted position so the head is well secured by the acetabulum. Weight bearing in this position is allowed because it minimizes focal areas of load thus decreasing distortion. If contractures are present as a result of the child's favoring the leg during the initial phases of disease, bilateral traction might be necessary to decrease muscle spasm and return full range of motion to the hip. The child sometimes wears a brace during the day, but traction or a bivalved cast might be used to maintain the proper position of the hip during the night.

Children under the age of 4 years are more likely to heal without deformity and therefore might be treated with traction until full range of motion is attained in the hip. After that, they might be ambulatory, without cast or brace, but are restricted from strenuous physical activity.

The child wears the brace or casts until the bone has reossified, which usually takes about 2 years. If only part of the femoral head is affected, the brace might be worn for less than a year.

Surgical intervention is needed if conservative methods of treatment do not keep the femoral head abducted adequately, if there is discrepancy between the reossified head of the femur and the acetabulum, or if conservative treatment is likely to be exceptionally long. Whatever surgical procedure is chosen, its goal is to ensure that the acetabulum covers the femoral head and keeps it abducted.

Nursing management Nursing management for a child with coxa plana is similar to that for any child in traction, casts, or brace. Once the femoral head has been positioned correctly, pain ceases. The child, being comfortable, also might be convinced that treatment is unnecessary. Because the child at the time of diagnosis is likely to associate disease and its accompanying restrictions with punishment, a major nursing goal is to ensure cooperation and understanding of treatment. The nurse can serve as a resource or refer the family to community agencies for additional teaching, answers to questions, reassurance, and support.

Children quickly adapt to wearing treatment devices and can achieve a surprising degree of activity. An active child who wears casts or a brace has the skin in these areas subjected to unusual pressure and stress. The nurse instructs the parent to pay particular attention to skin care in this area.

Some children undergo surgery to shorten the period of immobilization. Others do not choose surgery but need it even though their compliance with treatment was excellent. These children might have to work through feelings of discouragement and sometimes anger or guilt.

If the femoral head has residual damage (after healing), the hip does not function optimally. The nurse then assists the child to cope with repeated operations to fashion a congruous femoral head and acetabulum. These children sometimes experience degenerative changes or pain, necessitating corrective surgery for symptomatic relief at a later time.

Slipped Femoral Capital Epiphysis

Slipped femoral capital epiphysis is displacement of the head from the neck of the femur. Usually, the femoral neck moves upward and forward while the capital epiphysis (head) becomes displaced backward and downward. In the preslip phase, the growth plate widens, but the epiphysis is not displaced. Slippage is classified, according to the amount of displacement, as minimal (less than 1 cm), moderate (less than two-thirds the diameter of the femoral neck but greater than 1 cm), or severe (greater than two-thirds the diameter of the femoral neck). The slip can be acute or chronic.

The exact cause of slipped femoral capital epiphysis is unknown, but endocrine disturbance has been implicated. Slippage tends to occur in adolescents who are either large and obese or tall and thin. It might be related to excess growth hormone or decreased sex hormone. Occasionally, acute onset of symptoms follows trauma, but usually symptoms develop gradually.

Slipped femoral capital epiphysis usually occurs during periods of rapid growth in early adolescence (ages 13–16 in boys and 11–14 in girls). Boys are affected more frequently than girls, and a significant number of adolescents (around 30%) suffer slippage on both sides, one side after the other (Salter, 1983).

Clinical manifestations The adolescent with slipped femoral capital epiphysis complains of intermittent or constant pain and walks with a limp. The pain is described as being in the hip or groin area, the anteromedial aspect of the thigh, or the knee. Thigh or knee pain is generally referred from the hip. The adolescent tends to hold the leg in external rotation, and the range of motion of the hip is restricted (difficulty with internal rotation, abduction, and flexion). Lateral radiographs of the femoral neck confirm the diagnosis.

If the condition is untreated, further slippage can occur. The epiphysis eventually heals to the femoral neck, whether or not its position has been corrected. Hip abnormality and sometimes degenerative changes later result.

Treatment Preventing further slippage and damage to the epiphysis is the goal of treatment in the adolescent with slipped femoral capital epiphysis. From the time of diagnosis until after treatment, the adolescent does not bear weight on the affected side. Treatment varies according to the level of acuity and extent of the condition. If slippage is minimal, threaded wires are passed into the femoral neck and the epiphysis to stabilize the position and to promote epiphyseal closure. If slippage is more extensive, the positions of the femoral head and neck must be improved prior to internal fixation with pin or wires.

The adolescent who has experienced symptoms for less than 3 weeks might be placed in traction in order to return the epiphysis to a more normal position. The epiphysis then is fixed into position with pins. The adolescent ambulates with crutches until healing is complete.

With chronic slipped femoral capital epiphysis or with moderate to severe acute slippage, open correction (osteotomy) might be done. The epiphysis might or might not be pinned, depending on the surgical procedure. Both conservative and surgical methods have the risk of compromising blood supply to the femoral head with resultant deformity.

Prognosis depends on the degree of slippage and response to treatment. The earlier the condition is treated, the better the prognosis.

Nursing management Physical care for the adolescent being treated for slipped femoral capital epiphysis might include traction care and preoperative and postoperative nursing interventions. The nurse assesses the adolescent's progress and teaches the adolescent and the parent crutch walking safety and to observe for involvement of the opposite hip (limp, pain, restricted movement of the hip), because there is an increased risk that the second hip might become affected. Any pain and inadequate range of motion are reported immediately, since rapid initiation of therapy improves the prognosis.

Scoliosis

Scoliosis is lateral curvature of the spine. It involves both lateral deviation from the midline and rotation of a series of vertebrae. Scoliosis can be *functional,* in which temporary curvature is caused by posture or position changes, or *structural,* in which curvature is caused by changes in the bony structure of the spine, or the soft tissues surrounding the spine, or both.

In functional scoliosis, which is a postural habit, one long curve involves the thoraco-lumbar region of the spine. The child can voluntarily correct the curve, and the curve disappears when the child is lying down. The child with a pelvic tilt due to a leg length discrepancy, hip contracture, or other cause can have functional scoliosis. Functional curves do not become structural.

Structural scoliosis can be identified at any point in childhood or adolescence. If untreated, tissue changes and deformity can last throughout life. Structural scoliosis can be congenital or can be caused by such conditions as vertebral abnormalities, paralysis, or muscle disorders.

Idiopathic scoliosis, or scoliosis with no recognizable cause, is the most common form of structural scoliosis, occurring in 5 of 1000 persons in the population (Salter, 1983). By far the greatest number of children with idiopathic scoliosis have late-onset, adolescent, idiopathic scoliosis, usually occurring after age 10 and with a right thoracic curve. Girls are affected five to seven times more frequently than boys. Scoliosis tends to be familial, with incidence being much higher in families where another family member is affected than in the general population.

The deformity progresses during periods of growth and stabilizes when vertebral growth ceases. Slight increases (5°) in curvature can occur after childbirth and with aging.

Clinical manifestations The spine grows to maintain the body's balance. When a lateral curve develops, the spine and ribs rotate toward the convex portion of the curve. The abnormal forces pressing on the growing spine cause vertebrae to become wedge shaped. Muscles and ligaments are contracted and thickened on the concave side and thin and atrophied on the convex side of the curve. Occasionally, the body develops an associated compensatory curve to maintain posture and balance (Fig. 30-1A).

The rotation of the rib cage in the child with scoliosis can cause a visible hump, particularly when the child is bending forward (Fig. 30-1C). Forward rib rotation can lead to displacement of the sternum from the midline. The thoracic cavity becomes asymmetric and in severe cases can affect lung ventilation. With a curve of 50% or more, vital capacity can be affected, and a curve of 100% or more can cause rapid breathing or hypoxia.

Very severe scoliosis can be painful, but pain is not common in children. Back pain might, however, occur subsequent to degenerative changes.

Diagnostic evaluation Scoliosis might be identified during routine school or health screening. A parent might notice a discrepancy in the level of the child's hips or shoulders when the child is in a bathing suit or when trying to alter clothing. Radiographic examination confirms the diagnosis and classifies the curvature according to location, direction, angle, and the degree and direction of vertebral rotation. The age of the child at onset and the type and degree of curvature are major factors affecting the prognosis. The younger the child is at the onset of scoliosis, the more severe the deformity is likely to be. Generally, lumbar scoliosis has a much more favorable prognosis than thoracic scoliosis, which might progress to a sharp, unsightly curve.

Treatment For functional scoliosis, no treatment is necessary unless the curve is marked, in which case postural exercises or correction of hip deformity or leg length discrepancy might be done. Structural scoliosis—the most frequent type in adolescents—is treated as early as possible to prevent or lessen progression of the curve.

Structural scoliosis might be treated conservatively with exercises and frequent follow-up; with a brace or cast to stretch the spine, relax pressure on the vertebrae, and allow more normal growth; or with spinal fusion to stabilize the spine. Exercises improve posture and help to maintain flexibility of the spine. They might consist of general exercises, bending toward the outside of the curve and stretching the inside of the curve. Passive stretching exercises and back muscle-strengthening exercises sometimes are used, and the child is taught to breathe deeply to improve chest expansion. Occasionally, lateral electrospinal stimulation is used in the treatment of scoliosis. An electrical impulse is generated that stimulates muscle contraction, and thus muscle strengthening, and prevents worsening of the curvature.

For moderate or mild scoliosis, a brace or cast might be worn to provide pressure on the convex side of the curve or curves and to exert gentle straightening forces on the spine. A silastic brace, molded to the specific child, frequently is used. It is worn until growth is complete or until another form of treatment is started. The brace is used extensively if the child can be counted on to wear it full-time for as long as it is needed. To be as effective as possible, the brace must be worn for 23 hours a day. It is removed for hygiene and skin care only. A brace can be used to treat curves of less than 40°. It usually is worn for several years and the child is gradually weaned from it. Regular radiographs and follow-up during weaning ensure that the correction is maintained.

Spinal fusion stabilizes the spine and arrests progression of the curve. Spinal fusion is considered when the curve is physically or cosmetically severe, when a curve becomes progressively worse after conservative treatment, or for a backache that cannot be relieved. During posterior spinal fusion, the major curve is fused, preventing progression of the deformity.

Spinal fusion is accomplished by three methods: (1) Harrington rods, which are telescoping metal rods placed on the concave side of the curve to internally fixate the curve and provide safe straightening of the spine, (2) Dwyer instrumentation, which attaches a series of screws to the vertebrae then a cable is passed through and attached to the screws to provide straightening, and (3) Luque wires, which are thin flexible wires threaded through the vertebrae and wrapped around the fusion site and a verticle stable rod. Children with severe scoliosis might be placed in traction or a halo apparatus prior to surgery to begin stretching the spine and musculature in preparation for fusion.

Postoperatively, the spine is immobilized until the fusion is stable. The child is on bed rest until initial healing has begun. Any twisting or bending of the back is scrupulously avoided. The child might be on a turning frame, such as a Stryker frame. Because of the greater stability of instrumentation, the child with fixation devices such as Luque wires or Dwyer instrumentation is not on a frame but is log-rolled in bed. A child with Luque wires usually is out of bed early in the postoperative period.

After about 5 days to 2 weeks, most treatment plans involve removal of stitches and the application of a cast or brace. A silastic jacket-type brace is preferred and is increasingly being used. It enables the child to be much more mobile than the child who is casted.

Radiographs are taken to see if the desired correction has been maintained. If healing and position under the brace or cast are satisfactory, the child can be made ready for discharge and home care. Some children can be ambulatory after discharge, while others require bed rest at home. The child is scheduled for a medical evaluation about 3 months after surgery. The child usually is immobilized in the brace or cast for at least 3 months or until healing is complete, at around 6 months.

Nursing management Teaching is an ongoing nursing responsibility, especially for the child who is undergoing conservative treatment on an outpatient basis. The nurse teaches prescribed treatment routines, determines the child's and parent's understanding of these, and on return visits tries to obtain an honest record of the child's compliance. The nurse emphasizes to the parent and child that failing to follow the treatment could have adverse consequences. Because it is the child who must do the exercises or wear the brace, and because the child usually is at an age of growing independence, compliance with treatment is determined primarily by the child's motivation and understanding. The nurse gives the parent written information about types of exercise and an exercise schedule and supports the parent in emphasizing the importance of the treatment to the child. Scoliosis clinics might conduct or refer the child to peer support groups that can help maintain the child's compliance with the treatment regimen.

If the child is to wear a brace, the nurse assesses the child's acceptance of the brace and reinforces teaching about the need for cooperation. If lack of cooperation is identified early, the health care team can consider other approaches to treatment before the deformity has time to worsen. The nurse encourages the child to wear a light jersey under the brace and to check the brace regularly for loose parts.

Compliance is especially difficult for the child who views appearance or athletic participation as more important than a straight back. In teaching the child about activity restrictions, the nurse emphasizes that exercise and activity are very beneficial to the child wearing a brace. Strenuous gymnastics and contact sports are not appropriate, however, since they might endanger the safety of the child and others. Other exercises such as swimming and dancing are encouraged.

A child wearing a body cast or brace has many similar needs. Acceptance of altered appearance and care of the skin are areas of concern. Clothing needs to be attractive, large, loose fitting, and stylish. Emphasizing other aspects of appearance, such as an attractive hairstyle or makeup, can improve the adolescent's body image.

After cast application, the nurse assesses neurologic function, particularly in the hands, and reports immediately any altered sensations or signs of impairment.

If the child is to undergo spinal fusion, extensive preoperative preparation is necessary. The nurse ensures that the child is prepared for such experiences as being cared for in an intensive care unit and being immobilized on a turning frame or bed. The child and nurse practice the turning routine to be used postoperatively.

Postoperatively, the child is dependent, immobilized, and has experienced a large blood loss. The nurse therefore seeks to reduce the ill effects of these stressors. Assessment for complications such as decreased cardiac output, ineffective breathing pattern, and postoperative hemorrhage is important. The child usually returns with chest tubes. After manipulation of the vertebral column during surgery, altered neurologic function and paralysis are serious possible complications. The nurse carefully observes and documents color, sensation, and motion in all extremities and reports changes immediately. Prompt relief of stress on the nerves

(*test continues on p. 1048*)

NURSING CARE PLAN *The Adolescent Recovering from Spinal Fusion*

Assessment data: Carrie is a 13-year-old girl with a 70° curvature of the thoraco-lumbar spine who has undergone an anterior spinal fusion with Dwyer instrumentation. Donor bone for the fusion was taken from the excised rib. During surgery she received one unit of packed cells. Postoperatively, she spent the first 2 days in intensive care but was then transferred to the nursing unit to which she had been admitted preoperatively. Her chest tube was removed, her in-dwelling urinary catheter was removed, and she has voided independently. Bowel sounds have returned. She still has an IV but is tolerating oral fluids.

Assessed risk	Nursing action
Neurologic compromise from spinal manipulation	Check all extremities every 4 hours for adequate motion and sensation. Ask the child about any numbness or tingling. Check pedal and radial pulses and color and temperature of the feet and hands.
Postoperative hemorrhage	Change the dressings as ordered after removal of chest tubes. Monitor any amounts of frank blood on the dressings. Observe for decreasing hemoglobin and hematocrit levels
Postoperative urinary retention and paralytic ileus	See routine postoperative care, Chapter 20.
Complications of immobility—muscle atrophy, respiratory and elimination problems	See Standards of Nursing Care for the immobilized child, Chapter 20.

Nursing diagnosis	Intervention	Rationale
1. Alteration in comfort: pain related to physical injury secondary to surgical manipulation of ribs and spine	Medicate as ordered and observe response to medication.	Medication is administered to relieve severe pain and promote relaxation.
	Administer muscle relaxants as ordered.	Muscle spasms are frequently seen after spinal fusion.
	Identify Carrie's nonverbal indications of pain, such as increased restlessness, withdrawal, and anxiety; report these to all caregivers.	The child, particularly an adolescent, might not admit to pain. Subtle behavioral changes can indicate increasing pain.
	Reposition every 1–2 hours using log-rolling technique; three people are needed for turning—one on either side and one to support her head; KEEP SPINE STRAIGHT WHILE TURNING; place pillows at her back and between her knees.	Repositioning from back to side to side relieves pressure on the operative site and decreases pain. Unnecessary movement of the spine could contribute to injury.
	Remain with Carrie until the pain subsides; assist with diversionary measures (she likes music), and provide comfort measures.	Fear increases the perception of pain. Noninvasive pain relief measures can be very effective when combined with analgesics. Comfort measures improve feelings of well-being.
Outcome: Carrie expresses relief from pain. She is able to sleep and appears relaxed.		
2. Potential for ineffective breathing pattern (stressors: anesthesia, chest incision, pain, anxiety)	Monitor breath sounds, respiratory rate, depth of respirations, use of accessory muscles, color, temperature, and blood gases.	Early recognition of inadequate air exchange enables health team to prevent severe respiratory distress.
	Have Carrie turn side-to-side and breathe deeply at least every 2 hours. Use incentive spirometer or blow bottles.	Turning and deep breathing facilitate lung expansion and prevent pooling of secretions.

NURSING CARE PLAN *The Adolescent Recovering from Spinal Fusion (Continued)*

Nursing diagnosis	Intervention	Rationale
	Be sure that Carrie is comfortable prior to breathing exercises.	Pain can markedly decrease respiratory effort.
	Report any respiratory pain or related distress, decreased or absent breath sounds.	These could be signs of atelectasis or tension pneumothorax, a complication of anterior thoracotomy.

Outcome: Carrie remains free of respiratory distress and related problems as evidenced by adequate ventilation and absence of respiratory infection. Blood gases are within normal limits.

Nursing diagnosis	Intervention	Rationale
3. Potential alteration in cardiac output (stressors: operative blood loss, fluid loss, stress of surgery and anesthesia)	Observe dressing sites for serosanguineous staining and excessive blood.	Excessive bleeding could lead to hypovolemia and shock.
	Monitor fluid intake and output. Test urine specific gravity.	Urine output and specific gravity are excellent indicators of hydration. Decreased output with increased specific gravity can indicate dehydration.
	Monitor pulse and blood pressure and report changes to the physician.	Pulse and blood pressure changes occur relatively late in acute blood loss.
	Observe skin color, quality of tissue perfusion (capillary refill), hematocrit, hemoglobin, and warmth of extremities and monitor peripheral pulses.	Changes might indicate circulatory compromise.
	Provide a diet high in iron; Carrie likes eggs and raisins and all juices; administer ferrous sulphate as ordered.	Iron-containing foods help to correct anemia from operative blood loss by increasing the available iron for hemoglobin formation. Citrus juices enhance absorption of iron.

Outcome: Carrie appears hydrated. Her vital signs are stable and hemoglobin and hematocrit levels are increasing.

Nursing diagnosis	Intervention	Rationale
4. Potential impaired skin integrity (stressors: bed rest with pressure on bony prominences, mobility limitations)	Reposition and provide skin care every 2 hours.	Repositioning takes pressure off bony prominences and allows for adequate skin care.
	Use sheepskin or Eggcrate® foam pad on the mattress.	These promote more even distribution of weight and are more comfortable, thus preventing uneven pressure.
	Massage bony prominences and areas susceptible to pressure.	Massage promotes circulation to the area.

Outcome: Carrie's skin is smooth and intact without evidence of breakdown.

Nursing diagnosis	Intervention	Rationale
5. Potential alteration in nutrition: less than body requirements (stressors: anorexia, increased protein needed for healing)	Provide Carrie with a high-protein, low-calorie diet; include foods with roughage.	High protein is needed for healing. Calories are monitored so that the child's weight is appropriate for growth during the long period of relative immobility to follow. Roughage promotes bowel emptying.
	Offer small, frequent servings of well-liked foods, frequent snacks. (Carrie likes grilled cheese sandwiches.)	Small, frequent servings and favorite foods are most likely to be eaten. The child has poor appetite due to pain, dependence, and immobilization.

(Continues)

NURSING CARE PLAN *The Adolescent Recovering from Spinal Fusion (Continued)*

Nursing diagnosis	Intervention	Rationale
	Discuss the importance of adequate fluid intake and a balanced, high-protein diet.	The child should understand that adequate fluid intake is needed to prevent dehydration and hypovolemia; protein is necessary for healing.
	Ask Carrie's help in planning menus.	Feelings of control over treatment enhance cooperation.
	Arrange to have family, friends, or other patients join Carrie for meals.	The child is likely to eat better if mealtime is a pleasant and sociable event.
	Arrange for family or friends to bring Carrie's favorite foods from home.	Food from home can greatly stimulate appetite and make eating more appealing.

Outcome: Carrie will obtain the nutrients needed for proper healing and appropriate weight control. She will consume the calories recommended by the nutritionist.

Nursing diagnosis	Intervention	Rationale
6. Potential impaired social interaction (stressors: pain, limited physical mobility, or disturbance in self concept from surgery)	Organize Carrie's day and care according to her preferences and maintain a routine that allows for rest.	The child's maintaining some control over activities and routine is crucial to self-concept and cooperation.
	Place personal things, telephone, and call button nearby and encourage Carrie to use them.	The arrangement of the environment can greatly increase independence and promote positive sense of self.
	Plan activities according to position; move television, radio, craft materials, books within reach.	Diversions stimulate the child to maintain developmental level and to initiate activity according to the child's tolerance.
	Help Carrie to keep up with schoolwork. Have the parent bring schoolwork to the hospital, arrange for quiet study times, and determine whether a tutor is needed. Praise Carrie for tasks completed and help her to set attainable goals.	Keeping up with schoolwork is difficult but important to maintenance or increase in child's feelings of self-worth.
	Encourage Carrie to maintain contact with peers via the telephone and visits.	Maintaining contact with peers keeps the child interested in life outside the hospital, fosters self-esteem, and eases future reentry into normal life.
	Do passive and active range-of-motion exercises of the upper extremities at least four times a day.	Exercise maintains range of motion and some muscle strength and also reminds the child of eventual recovery and mobility.
	Plan with the surgeon and physiotherapist appropriate lower extremity activity, such as quadriceps-setting and knee and hip range-of-motion exercises and implement the plan.	Quadriceps exercises increase muscle strength and activity tolerance and promote adequate circulation to extremities.
	Plan for a gradual increase in activity as soon as the brace is applied.	Gradual activity increase reduces fatigue and promotes balance when the child is upright.

Outcome: Carrie's tolerance for activity increases so that she will have little adverse effect when adjusting to the brace. She maintains contact with peers and continues doing her crafts and playing games with others in the playroom.

NURSING CARE PLAN *The Adolescent Recovering from Spinal Fusion (Continued)*

Nursing diagnosis	Intervention	Rationale
7. Self-care deficit of hygiene, toileting, and dressing (level II) related to mobility restrictions from the surgical procedure	Arrange hygienic and grooming routines for times when pain is minimal (for example, following analgesic administration).	The child is more likely to participate if she is comfortable.
	Arrange grooming aids, food, and utensils for ease in self-feeding.	Participation in grooming and feeding fosters feelings of control and independence.
	Anticipate Carrie's needs for help during bathing, grooming, and toileting.	Having assistance readily available decreases the child's frustration, increases trust, and preserves dignity, while ensuring appropriate care.
	Encourage Carrie to verbalize feelings of embarrassment, frustration, or helplessness.	Expressing feelings helps child to cope with them.
	Assure Carrie that her helpless state is temporary and that results of treatment will be positive.	Reassurances remind child that dependence is temporary and help child to keep treatments in perspective.

Outcome: Carrie participates in her care as much as possible within her mobility limitations. She can discriminate between activities she can perform herself and activities with which she needs assistance.

Nursing diagnosis	Intervention	Rationale
8. Potential body image disturbance (stressors: temporary change in appearance and activities during time in brace	Encourage Carrie to discuss feelings of resentment and anger. Provide diversionary activity for tension release, such as latch-hook rug kits, painting, games.	Verbal and physical outlets help decrease the effects of dependence, immobility, and surgery that affect body image.
	Accept Carrie's need for periods of withdrawal and moodiness as she adjusts to change in body image and separation from peers and normal activities. Explain to the parent that these reactions are normal.	The child needs understanding and time alone to cope with physical and emotional aspects of treatment.
	Arrange to have former patients who have undergone the same procedure come to visit Carrie.	Talking to peers who have undergone spinal fusion helps the child cope with treatments, provides support and new friendships, and reassures the child that treatment will be "worth it."
	Prepare Carrie for the brace by having the brace fitter demonstrate it; discuss attractive and appropriate clothing that will fit over the brace; encourage her to stand straight when the brace is applied.	The better the child is prepared, the less difficult the adjustments.

Outcome: Carrie demonstrates interest in how she will look with the brace on. She is able to talk positively about her appearance and what she will look like at the end of the treatment. She cooperates with planning for appropriate clothing.

Nursing diagnosis	Intervention	Rationale
9. Potential mild impaired home maintenance management (stressor: anxiety, limited understanding)	Encourage Carrie's parents to participate in her care, particularly in activities of daily living that will require assistance when Carrie is discharged.	Preparation in the hospital ensures follow-through in the home.

(Continues)

NURSING CARE PLAN *The Adolescent Recovering from Spinal Fusion (Continued)*

Nursing diagnosis	Intervention	Rationale
	Teach Carrie and her parents how to apply and care for the brace with particular attention to skin care.	Adequate teaching and practice prevents complications and increases caregivers' confidence in their ability to manage.
	Inquire about the layout of the house and recommend modifications if necessary, with the addition of equipment such as a raised toilet seat and shower bars if needed.	Adaptations to the home might be required since Carrie will have difficulty sitting and will need to be somewhat inactive temporarily. Resources for adaptive equipment usually can be identified by the community health nurse.
	Explain Carrie's diet to the parents and encourage them to follow through.	Diet is important for continued healing.
	Describe Carrie's activity limitations—no prolonged sitting, no bending, no sports or activities that would stress the spine.	Appropriate activity is essential for adequate healing.

Outcome: Carrie's transition to home is well planned. Carrie's parents can demonstrate brace care and explain other aspects of her care. The parents have arranged to acquire any necessary adaptive devices.

can reverse neurologic compromise and prevent lifelong sequelae.

Immobility can cause gastrointestinal, urinary, and integumentary complications. A Foley catheter is used in initial postoperative management.

Postoperative back pain is at first severe, but after the first few days, it often is less severe than pain at the donor site or pain from flatulence. Pain is significant for the child who must be out of bed in the early postoperative period.

The nurse teaches the child who remains in bed to perform muscle-setting exercises and as much self-care as possible to combat weakness. The nurse involves the child in unit activities when the child feels well enough.

Getting up, when allowed, must be gradual to avoid dizziness and collapse. A child progressing directly from bed rest to sitting in a chair requires special attention and physical support from the nurse, because blood loss, bed rest, and pain all contribute to the potential for dizziness or fainting.

The child can be discharged after becoming ambulatory in the hospital, provided that radiographic examination shows that correction is being maintained and the fused area is not compromised. Before discharge, the nurse instructs the child to avoid strenuous activity until healing is complete. Sitting for long periods of time might be contraindicated. The child might need assistance with bathing and other activities of daily living. Encouraging the child to develop increased self-esteem is an important intervention. Although the child might be in a brace or cast for an extended period of time, attractive clothes, makeup, promotion of socialization with peers, and maintenance of a near normal routine assists with maintaining positive self-image.

Kyphosis and Lordosis

Kyphosis (hunchback) is an exaggerated posterior curvature of the spine, usually in the thoracic area. *Lordosis* is an exaggerated anterior curvature, usually affecting the lumbar spine. Deformity can be functional or structural. Functional, or postural, kyphosis or lordosis is caused by habitual slouching. Structural kyphosis, in which vertebrae become wedge shaped, can be congenital or acquired through spinal tuberculosis, myelomeningocele, tumors, or other structural damage to the spine.

Treatment and nursing management Treatment for mild kyphosis and lordosis requires postural exercises performed on a regular basis. Doing exercises and sleeping on a firm surface without a pillow are sometimes all that is needed to minimize deformity. If noncompliance with an exercise routine is a problem, muscle strengthening and postural recreational activity are encouraged. Swimming, aerobic or other dance, and gymnastics are examples of activities that assist the child to be aware of body position and posture. Exploring the reasons for poor posture is helpful, particularly with adolescent girls who might be slouching to hide breast development or because of low self-esteem. The nurse allows the child to express feelings, honestly discusses how the child can become more attractive with correct posture, and helps the child to feel more comfortable about body changes. The nurse also can teach the child how good posture benefits body mechanics and function.

Some children with severe deformities require braces or surgery for correction. In these cases, the nursing care is similar to the child with scoliosis.

Duchenne Muscular Dystrophy (Pseudohypertrophic Muscular Dystrophy)

Muscular dystrophy is the name of a group of genetically acquired diseases that cause gradual, progressive muscle wasting. Muscular dystrophy can affect children and adults depending on the type involved. The most frequently seen form of muscular dystrophy in children is Duchenne muscular dystrophy, or pseudohypertrophic muscular dystrophy.

Duchenne muscular dystrophy is a sex-linked inherited condition that affects primarily boys at a rate of 1 in 3000–4000 live male births. Symptoms appear when the child is between 2 and 4 years of age, with initial muscle weakness in the hips, shoulder, and spine. The progressive muscle wasting eventually affects all muscles of the body, including those of the respiratory and cardiovascular systems. Death occurs usually prior to 20 years of age from respiratory infection or heart failure.

Clinical manifestations Initial manifestations of Duchenne muscular dystrophy include an inability for the child to get up from a lying position and difficulty jumping. The child walks with a waddling gait from affected muscles in the hip girdle. As the condition progresses, the child has difficulty climbing stairs, getting up from a sitting position, and ambulating. The child might develop severe muscle contractures. If these are untreated, they totally limit ambulation and the child becomes confined to a wheelchair.

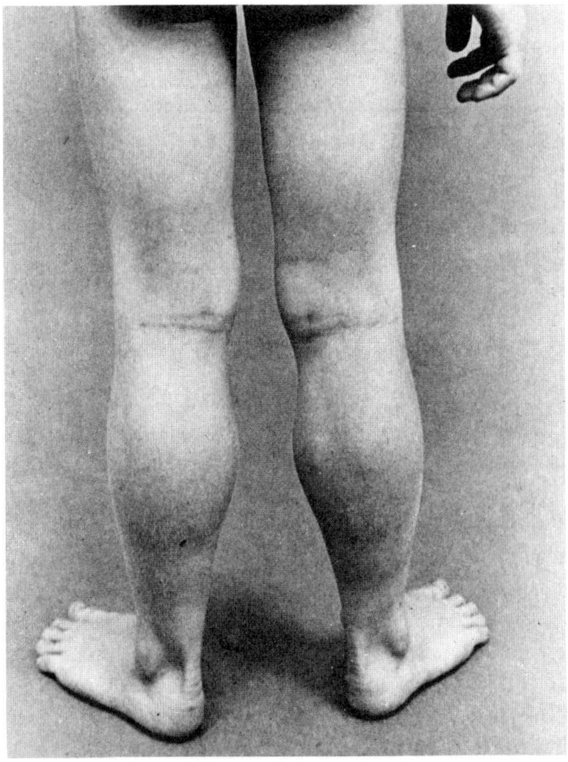

Pseudohypertrophy of calf muscles in muscular dystrophy. (From Purtilo DT: A Survey of Human Diseases. *Addison-Wesley, 1978, with permission.)*

A classic sign of Duchenne muscular dystrophy is pseudohypertrophy of the calf muscles. The calves appear large (hypertrophied), as if the child had strengthened them through athletics. In actuality, the enlargement is not due to increase in muscle size, but to muscle fibers being replaced by fibrous tissue and fat deposits.

Children with Duchenne muscular dystrophy can exhibit respiratory infections, particularly pneumonia, as the accessory muscles of respiration weaken. Some children have a seborrheic dermatitis. Scoliosis and shoulder disability can occur once the child is confined to a wheelchair.

Diagnostic evaluation Diagnosis of muscular dystrophy can be made through electromyogram (EMG), which is a procedure that can determine the motor potential of muscles. Muscle biopsy can demonstrate replacement of normal muscle fiber with fibrous tissue and fat.

One of the classic diagnostic signs of muscular dystrophy is an elevated CPK level. CPK (creatine phosphokinase) is an enzyme normally found in muscle tissue. When muscles waste, as they do in muscular dystrophy, the CPK is released into the circulation and can be detected by blood studies. Although symptoms of muscular dystrophy might not appear until the child is 2 years old, the elevated CPK is evident from birth. Boys with a family history of muscular dystrophy can have their CPK levels done to help determine whether they have the disease. By diagnosing the disease early, the child's independence can be prolonged because of early initiation of physical therapy, exercises, and social and psychologic counseling.

Treatment The goals of treatment for the child with muscular dystrophy are to facilitate ambulation and independence for as long as possible and to manage aggressively respiratory or cardiac difficulties. The child is placed on a regular exercise program of joint range of motion and stretching exercises. Stretching is particularly important to prevent contractures, which could limit ambulation. The child is encouraged to exercise according to developmental level as much as possible. Swimming is considered to be excellent exercise both for keeping limber and for allowing the child to participate in an athletic endeavor. Surgical release of contractures along with bracing is done to prolong ambulation.

When needed, assistive devices are used to facilitate activities of daily living. These might include bathtub rails, elevated toilet facilities, footboards to keep heel cords stretched, and clothing with Velcro-type fasteners that help the child dress and undress easily. The child's home can be modified so that the child can move about safely and easily. Rugs are removed, and the child's bedroom might be moved to the first floor. Rubber-soled shoes are advised to prevent slipping while walking.

Diaphragmatic breathing exercises might be recommended to keep the lungs inflated when respiratory muscles are weak. Percussion and postural drainage can be prescribed in combination with a positive pressure breathing apparatus (see Chapter 22) to assist with effective airway clearance. Antibiotics are given to children with pneumonia.

The parents are referred for genetic counseling. At present, the gene that codes for muscular dystrophy has not been positively identified, although scientists are quickly closing in on its location. Thus, the disease cannot be discovered by amniocentesis. Carriers have been identified through use of the CPK test. Like children with muscular dystrophy, carriers of the gene have elevated blood levels of CPK. Unfortunately, these levels tend to decrease as the girl becomes older so that by the time she reaches adulthood, the CPK level might not be detectable. This fact makes the CPK test for carriers only 70%–80% accurate.

Recently, a gene marker for muscular dystrophy has been discovered that can accurately predict whether a woman is a carrier of the muscular dystrophy gene. Blood samples from the woman and from other members of her family are required to trace the inheritance of the genetic marker. Identifying the marker in combination with the CPK test can predict whether a woman is a carrier of the gene with nearly 100% accuracy. (See Chapter 15 for a discussion of genetics and inheritance.)

Nursing management Nursing management is directed toward preventing contractures and encouraging independence and normal development. The nurse teaches the family the exercise regimen and encourages the child to exercise regularly. Prolonged bed rest of any kind is discouraged since it can accelerate the muscle weakening. If the child needs to be on bed rest for any reason, the nurse emphasizes to the parent that joint range-of-motion exercises need to be carried out frequently.

The nurse discusses safety in the home, particularly if the child is wearing braces to assist with ambulation. A home visit might be necessary to see if adaptation of the home environment is necessary. The nurse can talk with child and parent to plan for clothes that are in style, easy to put on and take off, and loose enough to cover any assistive devices.

The child who is wheelchair-bound will need to be placed on a low-calorie diet. Children confined to wheelchairs are at risk for becoming obese, thus placing additional strain on already compromised muscles. The nurse discusses any diet plan with the child and parent and tries to include in the diet foods the child likes. Fluids are encouraged to prevent urinary and renal difficulties caused by immobility.

Because muscular dystrophy is a fatal condition, the child and family will need much encouragement and support. The nurse encourages them to express their feelings and talk about any fears. (See Chapter 14 for the nursing care of the child with a chronic condition and Chapter 17 for care of the dying child.) Refer the family to the Muscular Dystrophy Association for psychologic and financial assistance.

The Child with Skeletal Inflammation

Infection of the Bone (Osteomyelitis)

Infection of the bone, or osteomyelitis, occurs 3–4 times more often in boys than in girls. Usually it originates from bacteria in the blood (hematogenous), but it can be an extension of a local infectious process or, as in a compound fracture, the invasion of microorganisms through an open wound (exogenous).

The metaphysis of the distal portion of the femur and the proximal portion of the tibia are the most frequent sites of osteomyelitis. In acute hematogenous osteomyelitis, factors in the medullary cavity can facilitate organism invasion (Fig. 30-8). Pus accumulates under the periosteum, causing elevation of the periosteum and compression of medullary circulation with resultant bone death. If the site of infection is near the epiphyseal plate, which it often is in children, new bone is developed in order to contain the infection. Eventually, the periosteum ruptures, causing release of purulent matter. The released purulence can infect the nearest joint. Occasionally, sinuses develop that allow purulence to infect the surrounding soft tissue or the skin. If the epiphyseal plate is heavily infected, there might be an adverse effect on the child's growth. Osteomyelitis can become chronic.

Clinical manifestations Signs and symptoms vary considerably with the severity, duration, and location of an infection, and with the age of the child. There might be a history of a recent upper respiratory, urinary tract, or other infection. Severe and constant pain is usual at the site of bone infection. The child might limp or fail to use an extremity. The area over the infection is tender to the touch. Once the periosteum ruptures and pressure exerted on the bone by pus is released, pain lessens. Pain usually is located over the metaphysis, as are local heat and swelling. Systemic signs of sepsis, including fever, vomiting, and even dehydration, might occur.

Diagnostic evaluation *Staphylococcus aureus* is the organism implicated in the majority of cases. *Hemophilus influenzae* and *Salmonella* also have been implicated. It is important to identify the organism prior to treatment in order to determine the most effective antibiotic. Blood cultures and aspiration cultures of affected bones or joints often reveal the causative organism.

The white blood cell count usually is elevated, though it can be normal, even in a severely ill child. The sedimentation rate is elevated. As the infection progresses, radiographs reveal local tissue density and then new bone formation and radiolucency in areas of abscess.

Treatment Treatment for acute hematogenous osteomyelitis is rigorous treatment with intravenous antibiotics. Antibiotics frequently are started as soon as blood studies are completed. Culture and sensitivity tests are done on local aspirates to identify the infectious microorganisms. Once identification is made, an appropriate antibiotic is given. Parenteral antibiotic therapy is continued for 4–6 weeks.

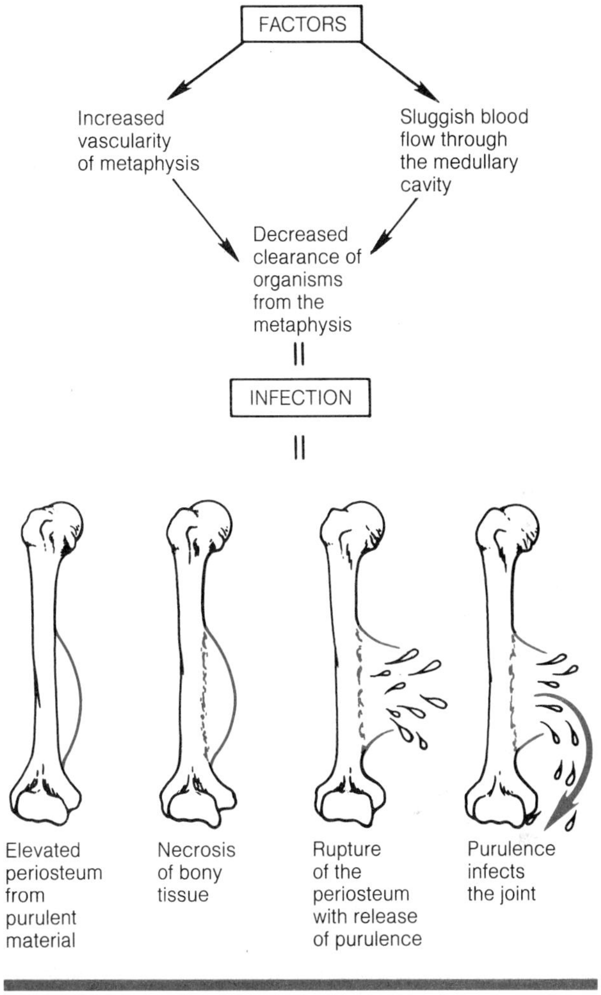

FIGURE 30-8
Pathophysiology of osteomyelitis.

Surgical treatment might be required to release the pressure of pus on the periosteum and to excise dead bone. If a correct diagnosis is not made promptly, the infection worsens, and the child is likely to undergo surgical drainage, to experience fever and pain, and to need long-term antibiotic therapy. Analgesics are prescribed for pain.

Nursing management Nursing care for the child with osteomyelitis centers around careful assessment of local and systemic signs and symptoms and provision of supportive care. Some children become very ill. The nurse ensures that blood for culture is obtained during temperature elevations. Treatment with intravenous antibiotics is prolonged, and the possibility of lengthy hospitalization stresses both the child and family (see Chapters 19 and 20). Wound and skin precautions are necessary for a child with a draining wound (see Chapter 20).

The affected limb requires immobilization during treatment, and this might be achieved through use of a cast or splint. Often a bivalved cast is preferred. The nurse provides appropriate cast care. The use of play and continuance of schoolwork helps distract the child while bed rest is required.

If the child is dehydrated from sepsis or vomiting, the nurse carefully monitors fluid intake and output. A diet high in calories, protein, and vitamin C is started as soon as possible to promote bone healing.

Maintaining long-term antibiotic therapy is difficult for the child and parent. More and more children with osteomyelitis are cared for at home with a heparin lock used to keep the vein open for antibiotic therapy. The parent is taught how to maintain the lock, mix and administer the antibiotic, and maintain safety by protecting the IV site from harm. Referral to a community health nurse for supervision of treatment is recommended.

Infection of the Joint (Suppurative or Septic Arthritis)

Infection of the joint, or septic arthritis, can originate from bacteria in the blood; direct extension of an infection, such as osteomyelitis; or direct inoculation from a wound. Infection causes the synovial membrane to produce increased amounts of synovial fluid and the joint to become distended. As infection progresses, pus accumulates in the joint. Destructive and degenerative changes occur, and the joint might eventually dislocate if the joint capsule becomes very distended.

The causative organisms include *Staphylococcus aureus*, group A beta-hemolytic streptococci, and *Hemophilus influenzae* (the most common cause in infants 6 months to 2 years of age). Therefore, a history of recent otitis media, streptococcal pharyngitis, impetigo, or invasive dental work might be given. With the general use of the *Hemophilus influenzae* type B vaccine in children under age two, the incidence in this age group can be expected to decrease.

Clinical manifestations The infected joint is painful, warm, and swollen and has extremely limited range of motion. The symptoms usually are acute. Extremities are moderately flexed due to muscle spasms. If the lower extremities are affected, the child limps or might refuse to walk. Ineffective or late treatment, especially when a major joint is affected, might cause a serious, lifelong disability.

Joint aspiration followed by culture of synovial fluid identifies the organism. The child's erythrocyte sedimentation rate is elevated. Tomography or bone scan can confirm the diagnosis.

Treatment The joint is immobilized. Traction might be applied to relieve muscle spasm, decrease pain, and separate joint surfaces. A splint can be used to immobilize the wrist or ankle. A 2–3 week course of systemic administration of antibiotics is prescribed to control the infection. If the infection is not controlled, the joint is surgically drained and irrigated with antibiotics. Eventually, range-of-motion exercises are started, but weight-bearing joints are protected from pressure until they again function normally. The child might need crutches temporarily. With early diagnosis and treatment, the prognosis for a return to normal joint function is good.

Nursing management Nursing management is similar to that for a child with osteomyelitis and involves caring for a child whose joint might be exquisitely painful or a child who is in traction. The needs of any immobilized child are addressed. As pain and swelling decrease, the nurse teaches the child and family about the importance of continuing to follow the prescribed treatment regimen. Compliance is necessary for a full recovery.

The Child with a Disease of the Bone

Osgood-Schlatter Disease

Osgood-Schlatter disease is tendonitis of the distal portion of the patellar tendon with secondary hypertrophic new bone formation (osteochondrosis) on the proximal tibial tubercle. There is tenderness of the patellar tendon and excessive enlargement of the proximal tibial tubercle. Osgood-Schlatter disease occurs primarily in adolescent boys who participate in sports. Symptoms usually follow a rapid growth spurt.

The disorder is caused by trauma or repeated stress in the area of the patellar tendon. Soft-tissue swelling and small, free bone particles anterior and superior to the tuberosity are visible on radiographs. The patella might be displaced anteriorly. If the condition has not already resolved, it will do so when the epiphysis closes and the tubercle fuses to the diaphysis. The bony prominence of the tibial tuberosity might be somewhat deformed, which can make kneeling uncomfortable. Rarely, the tubercle fuses early, eventually causing hyperextension of the knee. The patella might remain higher on the affected side, causing it to dislocate laterally or to contribute to degenerative arthritis.

Clinical manifestations The child experiences local pain in the anterior aspect of the knee, especially with running, jumping, squatting, use of stairs, and kneeling. Pain diminishes and might disappear with rest. There is excessive enlargement of the tibial tuberosity and thickening of the patellar tendon. No fluid is felt in the knee.

Treatment Treatment consists of restricting strenuous physical activities, such as sports, running, jumping, and long walks, for several months. This treatment is adequate in mild cases. In more severe cases, the knee is immobilized in a cylinder cast for several weeks. Strenuous exercise and sports are restricted for several months after cast removal. Anti-inflammatory agents injected into the affected tendon can provide symptomatic relief. Sometimes the tubercle is removed surgically.

Nursing management The nurse usually sees children with Osgood-Schlatter disease in an outpatient setting. One of the nurse's major goals is to convince the active child of the need for activity restrictions. The child needs to understand the importance of curtailing physical activity for what might seem like a very long time. The nurse can emphasize that time out will prevent complications and help the child or adolescent reach maximum athletic potential in the future.

Osteogenesis Imperfecta

Osteogenesis imperfecta is a condition that results in pathologic bone fractures. It is a connective tissue disorder primarily affecting the bone, causing fractures to occur in response to minor stressors. It usually is inherited as an autosomal dominant trait, although it can be inherited as an autosomal recessive trait.

Clinical manifestations Osteogenesis imperfecta congenita is a severe form of osteogenesis imperfecta that is evident at birth because of multiple fractures that have occurred in utero or during delivery. Children with this form are often stillborn or die soon after birth. They occasionally live through childhood, but they are bedridden. Osteogenesis imperfecta tarda is a less severe form of the disease. With this type, some children experience fractures in infancy (gravis form). The fractures heal at the usual rate, but bones are likely to refracture because of disuse atrophy following immobilization.

Some children have a very mild form of the condition, and medical attention is sought because of delayed walking or a fracture. Other children have multiple fractures and can be mistaken for battered children. The extremities might have angular deformities due to fractures. Children experiencing fractures early in life often have shortened stature due to deformities of the legs, overriding of fractures, compression, fractures of the spine, and kyphoscoliosis. There is usually little pain with the fractures of osteogenesis imperfecta because there is little soft-tissue trauma.

A classic sign of osteogenesis imperfecta is blue sclera. This sign, which is present in almost all children with the disease, is caused by thinness and translucency of the whites of the eyes (sclerae). The color varies from blue-white to deep sky blue.

The child's skin is thin, and the muscles have decreased tone. There might be subcutaneous hemorrhages, and any surgical scars are often wide. Ligaments are lax, and joints might have increased mobility.

The forehead is broad, and the shape of the head might be similar to a helmet. There is a deficiency of dentin, and teeth break easily, have poor resistance to caries, and hold fillings poorly. Deafness can result because of otosclerosis or pressure on the auditory nerve.

Treatment Treatment for osteogenesis imperfecta mainly consists of treating fractures. Proper alignment of fractures can decrease deformity, and intermedullary rods help correct angulation in some children. Immobility is discouraged to lessen disuse atrophy and thus the likelihood of refracture.

Nursing management Nursing management involves care of a chronically ill child with a deforming, debilitating, inherited condition (see Chapters 14 and 15). Nursing considerations vary from family to family because, among other reasons, the condition varies markedly in severity. Parents might be dealing with anger toward health professionals if the parents have been unjustly suspected of child abuse. The nurse allows for expression of feelings of anger or guilt.

Fragility of bones makes cautious handling of the child essential. Encouraging as much activity as possible during periods of immobilization can partially combat disuse atrophy.

Referral to the Osteogenesis Imperfecta Foundation can provide families with needed support and specialized services.

Essential Concepts

- The skeletal system, which is made up of bones, their joints, and attached muscles, ligaments, and tendons, supports and protects the body; enables movement; and contains marrow, which produces blood cells.
- Mechanical stress, trauma, circulation, nutrition, metabolism, and infection can affect bone growth and development both before and after birth.
- Diagnostic tests used in assessing skeletal conditions include radiographs, in which deformities or injuries can be seen; hematologic studies, which are used to assess and monitor infections related to surgery or injury; and serologic studies, which are used to detect congenital deficiencies of hormone secretion.
- Nursing care related to cast application and removal includes preparing the child and family by explaining the purpose of casting and describing the sensations caused by wet and drying casting materials; monitoring circulatory status and skin integrity; and, before removal, demonstrating use of the cast saw to lessen fears.
- In skin traction, pull is exerted on skin surrounding the body part; in skeletal traction, pull is exerted by means of wires or pins inserted in bone.
- Nursing care for the child in skin traction includes monitoring extremities for color, sensation, and motion; releasing traction, if permitted, to care for skin under bandages; helping the child to adapt to immobilization; and teaching the child and family the purpose of traction and ways in which they can help to maintain it.
- Skeletal traction requires the same measures as skin traction, except that the nurse does not release traction to provide skin care, but rather observes pin sites for signs of slippage or infection.
- Nursing care for the child with a brace includes maintaining skin integrity, ensuring that the brace fits correctly and comfortably, and teaching the child and parent about compliance with brace wearing and skin and brace maintenance at home.
- Nursing care for the child who is immobilized on a frame includes interventions to prevent physical and developmental complications of immobilization, to ensure that excreta do not remain in contact with the child's skin or soil the cast, to restrain the child to prevent falls or inappropriate movement, and to provide reassurance that being turned on a frame is not dangerous.
- Interventions to meet the acute-care needs of the child who is partially immobilized by a cast, traction, or brace include prevention of skin breakdown; control of infections and complications; controlling pain and muscle spasms; and preventing hazards of immobility.
- The nutritional needs of the child who has a skeletal condition or has undergone bone surgery include high-protein intake to promote healing, fluid intake above daily maintenance requirements, and a well-balanced diet containing adequate roughage to prevent constipation.
- Meeting the developmental needs of a child with skeletal dysfunction includes encouraging age-appropriate activities within limitations, promoting contact with family and peers, encouraging schoolwork, and preventing developmental delay.
- The emotional needs of the child with a skeletal condition relate to ineffective individual coping related to immobilization, anxiety about the orthopedic apparatus, and potential body image disturbance.
- Interventions to meet the health maintenance needs of a child with a skeletal condition frequently involve teaching about cooperation with the home treatment plan, ensuring that the home environment is safe for the partially immobilized child, arranging follow-up care, and referring the family to resources in the community.
- The child experiencing injury to the musculoskeletal system might experience a fracture, sprain, strain, contusion, or dislocation.
- Frequently seen structural abnormalities occurring in children with skeletal dysfunction include clubfoot, congenital dislocated hip, Legg-Calvé-Perthes disease, slipped femoral capital epiphysis, scoliosis and other spinal curves, and muscular dystrophy.
- The child with skeletal infection can experience infection in the bone (osteomyelitis) or joint (septic arthritis).
- Osgood-Schlatter disease and osteogenesis imperfecta are two bone diseases seen in children.

References

Celeste SM, Folick MA, Dumas KM: Identifying a standard for pin site care using the quality assurance approach. *Orthop Nurs* (July/Aug) 1984; 3:17–24.

Mulley D: Harnessing babies. *Am J Nurs* (Aug) 1984; 84:1006–1008.

Salter RB: *Textbook of Disorders and Injuries of the Musculoskeletal System,* 2nd ed. Williams & Wilkins, 1983.

Stevenson CK: Take no chances with fat embolism. *Nurs '85* (June) 1985; 15(6):58–63.

Additional Readings

A Comparison of plaster of paris and synthetic casts. *MCN* (May/June) 1986; 174–176.

Agee BL, Herman C: Cervical logrolling on a standard hospital bed. *Am J Nurs* (March) 1984; 84:315–318.

Allard JL, Dibble SL: Scoliosis surgery: A look at Luque rods. *Am J Nurs* (May) 1984; 84:609–611.

Behrman RE, Vaughan V: *Nelson Textbook of Pediatrics.* Saunders, 1983.

Benz J: The adolescent in a spica cast. *Orthop Nurs* (May/June) 1986; 5(3):22–23.

Brantley P, Cenella M: *The Nurse and Orthopedic Surgery.* The Orthopedic Nurses' Association, in cooperation with Howmedica, 1980.

Cuddy CM: Caring for the child in a spica cast: A parent's perspective. *Orthop Nurs* (May/June) 1986; 5(3):17–21.

Davis SE, Lewis SA: Managing scoliosis: Fashions for the body and mind. *Am J Matern-Child Nurs* (May/June) 1984; 9:186–187.

Derscheid G: Rehabilitation of common orthopedic problems. *Nurs Clin North Am* (Dec) 1981; 16:709–719.

Farrell J: *Illustrated Guide to Orthopedic Nursing,* 2nd ed. Lippincott, 1982.

Farrell J: Orthopedic pain: What does it mean? *Am J Nurs* (April) 1984; 84:466–469.

Francis EE: Lateral electrical surface stimulation treatment for scoliosis. *Pediatr Nurs* 1987; 13(3):157–160.

Garrick J: The sports medicine patient. *Nurs Clin North Am* (Dec) 1981; 16:759–767.

Gates SJ: Helping your patient on bedrest cope with perceptual/sensory deprivation. *Orthop Nurs* (March/April) 1984; 3:35–38.

Goldman L: The injured ankle. *Nurs Pract* (Oct) 1981:51–56.

Guerrein AT: Osteogenesis imperfecta: A disorder that breaks more than our hearts. *Am J Matern-Child Nurs* (Sept/Oct) 1982; 7:315–318.

Halladay J: Update on scoliosis. *Can Nurse* (Sept) 1984:44–45.

Hankin FM, Gragg AJ, Kaufer H: Bleeding beneath postoperative plaster casts. *Orthop Nurs* (Jan/Feb) 1983; 2:27–31.

Holland SH: Up-to-date home care of a baby in a hip spica cast. *Pediatr Nurs* (March/April) 1983; 9:114–115.

Ibrahim K: An overview of childhood fractures. *Pediatr Nurs* (Jan/Feb) 1984; 10:57–65.

Karn MA, Crawford AH: Postoperative nursing management of the patient following posterior spinal fusion. *Orthop Nurs* (March/April) 1984; 3:21–25.

Kelly DJ: The use of fiberglass as reinforcement with plaster casts. *Orthop Nurs* (Nov/Dec) 1983; 2:33–36.

King JP: Bones: How to grow new ones. *AORN J* (April) 1982; 35:968–975.

Kryschyshen PL, Fischer DA: External fixation for complicated fractures. *Am J Nurs* (Feb) 1980; 80:256–260.

Kylberg HK: Descriptions of growth disturbances in children with osteomyelitis at different ages. *Orthop Nurs* (Nov/Dec) 1983; 2:28–32.

Lentz M: Skeletal aspects of deconditioning secondary to immobilization. *Nurs Clin North Am* (Dec) 1981; 16:729–737.

McFarland MB: Encircling cast drainage: Is it valuable? *Orthop Nurs* (March/April) 1984; 3:41–43.

Mather LS: The secret to life in a spica. *Am J Nurs* 1987; 87(1):56–58.

Matsen FA III, Veith RG: Compartment syndromes in children. *J Ped Orthop* 1981; 1(1):33–41.

Milazzo V: An exercise class for patients in traction. *Am J Nurs* (Oct) 1981; 81:1842–1944.

Pashley J, Wahlstrom M: Polytrauma: The patient, the family, the nurse and the health team. *Nurs Clin North Am* (Dec) 1981; 16:721–727.

Ross DG: The knee. *Orthop Nurs* (Sept/Oct) 1983; 2:23–28.

Salmond SW: Trauma and fractures: Meeting your patient's nutritional needs. *Orthop Nurs* (July/Aug) 1984; 3:27–33.

Shesser LK: Car seat modification for children under treatment for congenital dislocated hips. *Orthop Nurs* 1985; 4(6):11–13.

Shesser LK, Kling T: Practical considerations in caring for a child in a hip spica cast: An evaluation using parental input. *Orthop Nurs* (May/June) 1986; 5(3):11–15.

Smith-Mather ML: The secret to life in a spica. *Am J Nurs* (Jan) 1987; 87(1):56–58.

Spickler LL: Knee injuries of the athlete. *Orthop Nurs* (Sept/Oct) 1983; 2:11–19.

Tachdjian M: *Pediatric Orthopedics.* Vols. I and II. Saunders, 1972.

Thomas PC: Nursing care of patients undergoing posterior fusion with segmental (Luque) spinal instrumentation. *Orthop Nurs* (May/June) 1983; 2:13–20.

Thomassen PF: Helping your scoliosis patient walk tall. *RN* (Feb) 1984; 47:34–37.

Thorne BP: A nurse helps prevent sports injuries. *Am J Matern-Child Nurs* (July/Aug) 1982; 7:236–240.

Tibbits CW: Adolescent idiopathic scoliosis. *Nurs Pract* (March/April) 1980:11–20.

Trigueiro M: Pin site care protocol. *Can Nurse* (Sept) 1983: 24–25.

Varni NA: Osteogenesis imperfecta: The basics. *Pediatr Nurs* (Jan/Feb) 1984; 10:29–33.

Villalon D, Smith MN: At home with traction. *Pediatr Nurs* (Jan/Feb) 1982; 8:15–16.

Waldvogel FA, Vasey H: Osteomyelitis: The past decade. *N Engl J Med* 1980; 303(7):360–370.

Wassell AC: Sports medicine: Acute and overuse injuries. *Orthop Nurs* (March/April) 1984; 3:29–33.

Wassel A: Nursing assessment of injuries to the lower extremity. *Nurs Clin North Am* (Dec) 1981; 16:739–748.

Williams PF: *Orthopaedic Management in Childhood.* Mosby, 1983.

Chapter 31

Innervation and Mobility

Implications of Altered Neurologic and Neuromuscular Function

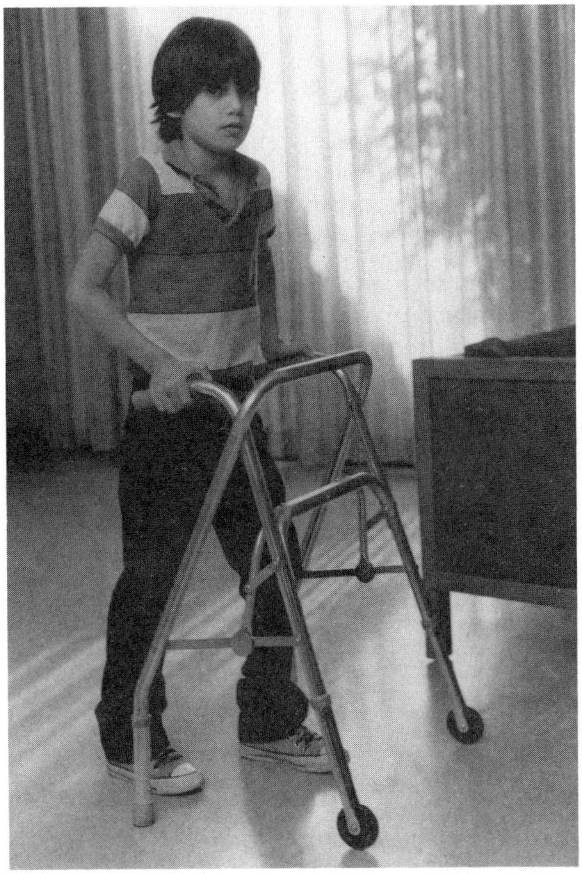

Chapter Contents

(Continues)

Cross Reference Box

To find these topics, see the following chapters:

Attention and activity disorders	Chapter 16
Learning disorders	Chapter 16
TORCH infections	Chapter 15

Objectives

- Describe the structure and function of the nervous system.
- Describe the assessment techniques specific to assessment of the nervous system.
- Explain the principles of nursing care common to procedures and treatments for neurologic dysfunction.
- Describe the acute-care needs specific to the child with increased intracranial pressure, the comatose child, and the child requiring neurosurgery.
- Relate the effects of long-term neurologic dysfunction to the developmental needs of children who are neurologically impaired.
- Describe the clinical manifestations, diagnostic methods, treatment, and principles of nursing management for the child with a seizure disorder.
- Describe the clinical manifestations, treatment, and principles of nursing management for each congenital malformation of the central nervous system.
- Explain the clinical manifestations, methods of diagnostic evaluation, treatment, and principles of nursing management for each infection of the central nervous system.
- Explain the clinical manifestations, treatment, and principles of nursing management for the child with a head or spinal cord injury and for the child with cerebral palsy.

ESSENTIALS OF STRUCTURE AND FUNCTION
The Neurologic System

The central nervous system and the peripheral nervous system interact with each other and with other body systems. They control functions as basic as breathing and blood circulation, muscle movement, and sensory perception, among others. In addition, they determine the higher level functions of cognition, speech, and the manipulation of ideas.

Glossary

Acetylcholine The primary neurotransmitter of the parasympathetic system.

Autonomic nervous system A division of the peripheral nervous system controlling involuntary, unconscious, neuronal functions through effects on smooth and cardiac muscle and glands of the body.

Central nervous system The brain, twelve cranial nerves, the spinal cord, and the origins of the nerves comprising the peripheral nervous system (see figures of brain and spinal cord section).

Cerebrospinal fluid Colorless fluid that circulates through the ventricles of the brain and the subarachnoid space and bathes the brain and spinal cord (see table, cerebrospinal fluid values and figure, cerebrospinal fluid circulation).

Extrapyramidal tract Motor pathways that do not cross in the medulla but are regulated by the cerebellum, midbrain, and brain stem to maintain muscle tone, posture, and refinement and coordination of movements.

Meninges Three-layered protective membrane (pia mater, arachnoid, dura mater) covering the brain and spinal cord and separated by the subdural and subarachnoid spaces (see figure, meningeal layers).

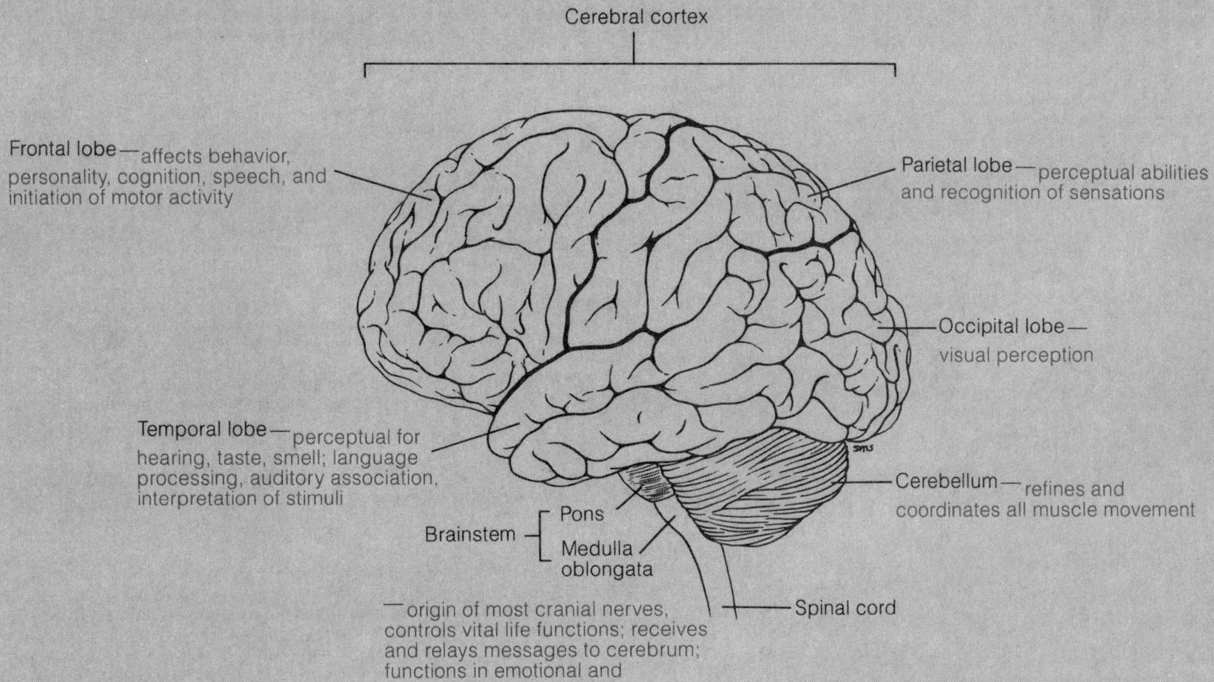
Cerebral cortex
Frontal lobe—affects behavior, personality, cognition, speech, and initiation of motor activity
Parietal lobe—perceptual abilities and recognition of sensations
Occipital lobe—visual perception
Temporal lobe—perceptual for hearing, taste, smell; language processing, auditory association, interpretation of stimuli
Cerebellum—refines and coordinates all muscle movement
Brainstem
Pons
Medulla oblongata
—origin of most cranial nerves, controls vital life functions; receives and relays messages to cerebrum; functions in emotional and instinctual responses
Spinal cord

Anatomic divisions of the brain with their physiologic functions.

(Continues)

The Neurologic System

Cerebrospinal Fluid Values

Characteristic	Normal value	Abnormal alteration
Color	Clear	Xanthochromic (yellowish) color is abnormal beyond the neonatal period; indicates hyperbilirubinemia or recent subarachnoid hemorrhage. Cloudy fluid indicates inflammatory purulence
Cell count	Neonate: < 15 leukocytes/mm^3 Child: 0–5 cells/mm^3 (all lymphocytes)	Elevated white blood cell count Bacterial meningitis: often $> 1000/mm^3$ (predominantly polymorphonuclear leukocytes) Viral meningitis: $< 500/mm^3$ (predominantly lymphocytes) Red blood cells indicate intracranial hemorrhage; might result from a bloody lumbar puncture
Protein	Neonates: 60–120 mg/dL Child: 15–45 mg/dL	Elevated in inflammatory diseases (meningitis, encephalitis), tumors, or degenerative conditions causing increased permeability of the blood-meningeal barrier
Glucose	One-half to two-thirds serum glucose level	Decreased in bacterial, tubercular, or fungal meningitis or meningeal tumor
Gram's stain	No organisms	Gram-positive or gram-negative organisms in bacterial meningitis

Neuronal tissue Grey (cortical) and white (subcortical) matter comprising the brain and spinal cord.

Neurotransmitter A chemical substance released by nerve cells that facilitates the passage of impulses along nerve pathways.

Norepinephrine The primary neurotransmitter of the sympathetic system.

Parasympathetic system A division of the autonomic nervous system with opposing physiologic effects to the sympathetic system (decreased heart rate, bronchial constriction, stimulation of gastrointestinal activity, and bladder emptying).

Peripheral nervous system Cranial and spinal nerves that connect to the brain and spinal cord and that carry sensory and motor nerve impulses to (efferent) and from (afferent) all areas of the body (see figure, nervous system components).

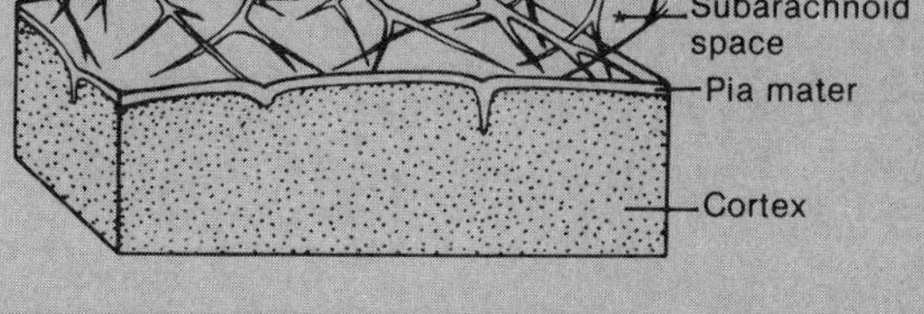

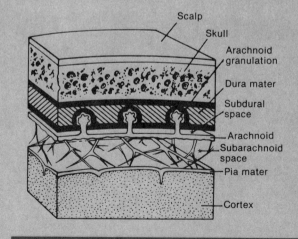

Meningeal layers covering the brain surface.

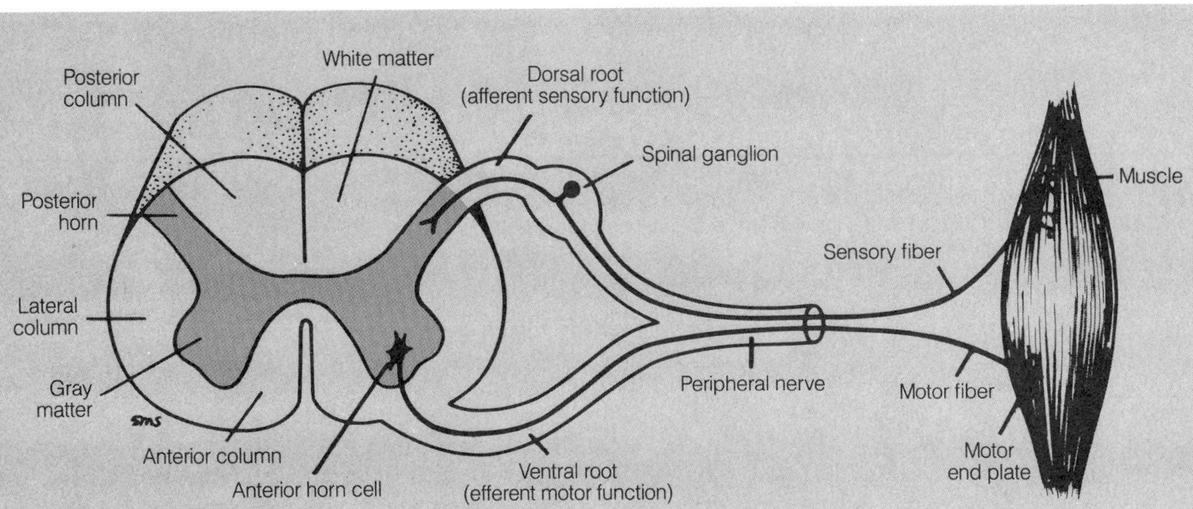

Cross-section of spinal cord with peripheral nerve innervation of muscle tissue.

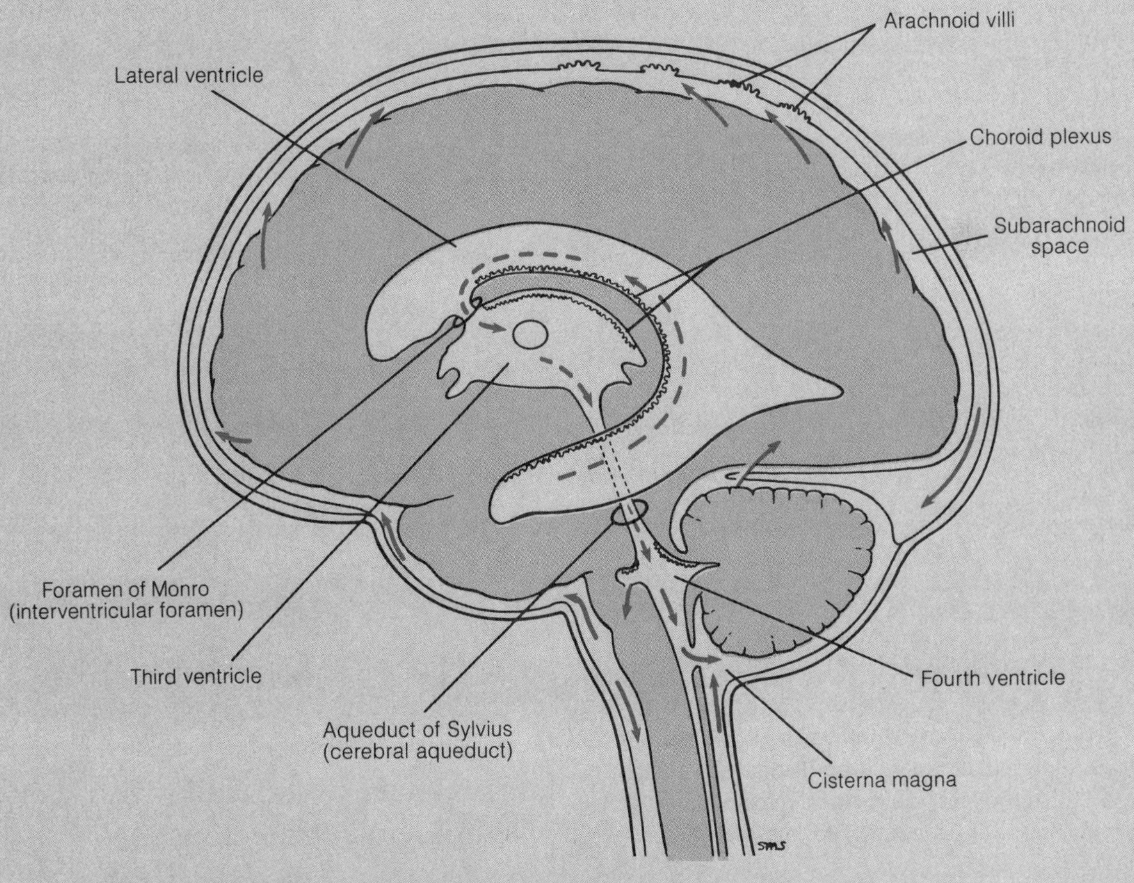

Cerebrospinal fluid circulation: CSF is formed continuously in the choroid plexus, enters the circulation, and is absorbed by the arachnoid villi. Any obstruction to its flow or abnormal CSF production increases the intracranial pressure.

(Continues)

ESSENTIALS OF STRUCTURE AND FUNCTION *(Continued)*
The Neurologic System

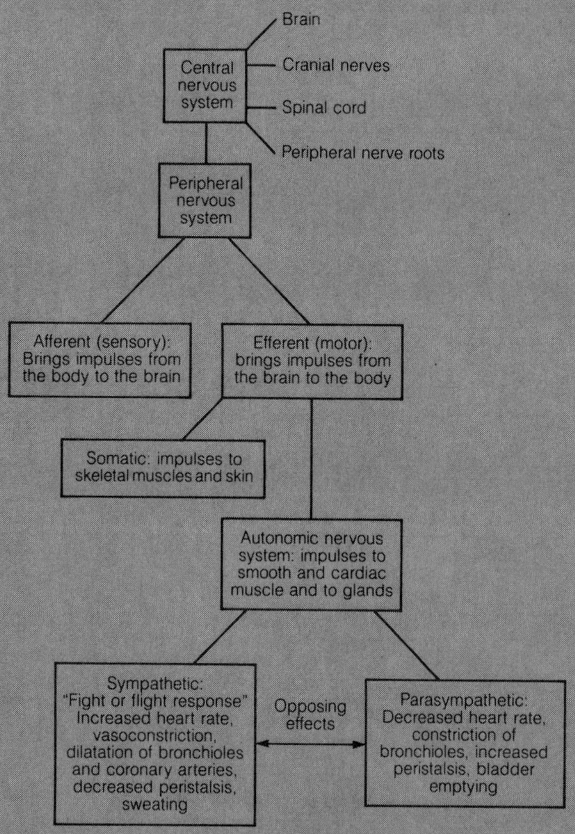
Brain
Central nervous system
Cranial nerves
Spinal cord
Peripheral nerve roots
Peripheral nervous system
Afferent (sensory): Brings impulses from the body to the brain
Efferent (motor): brings impulses from the brain to the body
Somatic: impulses to skeletal muscles and skin
Autonomic nervous system: impulses to smooth and cardiac muscle and to glands
Sympathetic: "Fight or flight response" Increased heart rate, vasoconstriction, dilatation of bronchioles and coronary arteries, decreased peristalsis, sweating
Opposing effects
Parasympathetic: Decreased heart rate, constriction of bronchioles, increased peristalsis, bladder emptying

Relationships between major nervous system functional components

Pyramidal tract Motor pathways that descend from a hemisphere of the cerebrum, cross to the opposite side in the medulla, and continue descending through the spinal cord to govern conscious muscle contraction on the opposite side of the body.

Sympathetic system A division of the autonomic nervous system, which mobilizes the body in response to pain, cold, strong emotion or other stresses and which results in the "fight or flight" response (increased heart rate, vasoconstriction, dilatation of coronary arteries and bronchioles, decreased gastrointestinal peristalsis, and sweating).

Muscle function depends on the integrity of each motor nerve and the skeletal muscle it activates (see cross-section of the spinal cord). Impulses originate in either the pyramidal or extrapyramidal tract and proceed along the peripheral nerve to the motor end plate. The release of the neurotransmitter acetylcholine at the motor end plate results in structural and chemical changes that cause muscle shortening, or contraction. The tracts function together to produce continuous, mild muscle contractions for tone, unconscious muscular activity, and voluntary movement.

The nervous system in the human being is extremely complex in both organization and function. It influences virtually all life processes and provides the individual with the primary means of perceiving and interacting with the environment.

Alterations of neurologic function in children can have significant effects on the child's growth and development. These range from subtle interferences associated with isolated perceptual weaknesses to the devastating multiple handicaps imposed by severe cerebral insult.

Assessment of the Child with Neurologic Dysfunction

Alterations in neurologic function might be readily observable or subtle. Because dysfunction of other body systems (metabolic, cardiovascular, and others) can accompany neurologic dysfunction, a thorough history is essential (see Chapter 9).

History

The maternal history of previous and subsequent pregnancies includes miscarriage, stillbirth, prematurity, congenital anomalies, or other conditions. The nurse then reviews the prenatal history for factors that might be associated with disorders of neurologic development. These include the use of medications, exposure to radiation, nutritional deficiency, alcohol or drug abuse, and maternal endocrine or metabolic disorders (such as hypothyroidism or diabetes). The nurse also reviews the pregnancy for any abnormalities.

The history of labor and delivery includes the length of labor, presence of fetal distress, presentation, type of delivery (vaginal or cesarean section), and umbilical cord prolapse or compression, all of which can be related to perinatal trauma. Birthweight is noted and considered in relation to gestational age. The nurse also notes the Apgar scores, presence of respiratory problems, and congenital anomalies apparent at birth. The neonatal history covers any difficulties such as seizures, jaundice, poor muscle tone, irritability, or feeding problems.

Physical Examination

The examination of the child with a neurologic problem includes a wide variety of assessments because virtually all life functions are regulated by the nervous system. Specific neurologic assessments include cerebral function, cranial nerves, cerebellar functions, motor and sensory systems, and reflexes. The nurse does not necessarily need to include all of these aspects in each evaluation but needs to be familiar with the complete neurologic assessment of children to provide knowledgeable management.

Cerebral function The child's overall cerebral function is assessed by the history, observation, and specific tests. The child's general behavior, level of consciousness, orientation, memory, intellectual performance, and integrative functions of language, sensory, and motor skills are evaluated. The most important aid in assessing cerebral function is a systematic developmental assessment using reliable tests and established norms.

The child's *level of activity* (for example, overactivity, lethargy), *mood* (irritability, apathy, lability), and *social responses* are important clues to neurologic function. *Behavioral characteristics* are assessed according to age. Some behaviors, such as tantrums and a limited attention span, are typical in younger children. Other deviations, including hyperirritability, indifference to environment, or delirium, are abnormal at any age.

Level of consciousness (LOC) is evaluated by the child's alertness, orientation, and ability to respond to verbal and physical stimuli. Lethargy, drowsiness, lack of orientation to familiar people or places, and decreased responsiveness indicate alterations in consciousness. The levels of altered consciousness can be defined as follows:

Stupor. The child is arousable for brief periods and can make simple verbal and motor responses. Stupor might alternate with periods of delirium, which is characterized by confusion and agitation.

Light coma. The child cannot be aroused and makes primitive and disorganized avoidance movements to painful stimuli.

Deep coma. The child does not respond to painful stimuli (eg, pressure on the fingertip at the nail bed or pinching pressure near the sternum) or responds with decerebrate posturing (rigid extension and pronation of the arms and extension of the legs).

Flaccid and apneic coma. The child's brain stem functions fail and respiratory effort stops. The child requires mechanical life supports and is considered to be brain dead.

These levels often are used to describe a child's alteration in consciousness. Because they are subject to the opinion of the nurse observer, however, they are not necessarily precise. Because of the importance of completely describing the child's activity and responses, a standardized assessment tool to measure and serially record the level of consciousness has been developed and is now in widespread use. This tool, called the Glasgow Coma Scale (GCS), measures eye opening and best verbal and motor response, assigning numeric values to specific observations. The total number of points can range from 3 to 14, with 7 or less considered coma. The tool allows for a rapid, objective evaluation that is easily recorded and is helpful in monitoring for any changes in status. (These measurements are illustrated in Table 31-1.) Level of consciousness in young children and infants is more difficult to assess. Activity level, motor responses, and recognition of familiar faces are helpful assessment criteria in young children.

Accurate assessment of intellect requires formal testing beyond the routine assessment. The nurse can, however, generally assess the child's cognitive abilities by observing the child's fund of general knowledge, performance of expected age-level tasks, and reasoning abilities (see Chapters 4–8). Immediate recall (short-term memory) and recall of previously learned material (long-term memory) is important to assess. Memory deficits can reflect language-

TABLE 31-1 Modified Glasgow Coma Scale

Number value	Eyes open	Best verbal response	Best motor response
5	Yes	*Infant:* Attends to noises and voices. Coos when viewing mother's face or in response to cooing by the nurse	*Infant:* Swipes at a bright object held within view. Spontaneous smile to tickling or other social stimulus. Purposeful reaching and grasping (over age 6 months)
		Early childhood: Able to identify mommy and daddy or other familiar people (eg, sibling, Big Bird, or other TV character). Might be able to associate time with meals or TV programs	*Early childhood:* Responds to "touch your nose," or "wiggle your toes"
		Middle childhood: Able to identify self by name and can name and describe friends. Can probably identify place but not necessarily time	*Middle childhood:* Obeys command to move body part
		Late childhood and adolescence: Oriented to familiar persons, place, and time	*Late childhood and adolescence:* Obeys command to move body part
4	Spontaneously	Able to respond verbally depending on age but is disoriented and confused	Purposefully tries to remove painful stimulus
3	To sounds and speech	Inappropriate verbal responses; uses words or phrases that make no sense	Arm flexion in response to pain (decorticate)
2	To pain	No intelligible verbalizations. Responds with incomprehensible sounds	Arm extension and internal rotation in response to pain (decerebrate)
1	None	None	None

processing disorders, visual memory problems, or more global cerebral dysfunction. Tests of memory need to be age appropriate. For instance, a 3-year-old might be expected to repeat three digits in a test of immediate recall.

Developmental screening includes screening for language processing, visual, motor and spatial relationships, and fine and gross motor skills. Delay in any of these areas might indicate an alteration in cerebral function.

Cranial nerve function Evaluation of the 12 pairs of cranial nerves can yield important information about underlying brain function and can help to localize specific deficits (Table 31-2). Examination of all the cranial nerves is difficult to obtain in young infants and children. The cranial nerves most frequently tested in the acute setting are the oculomotor (III), trochlear (IV), and abducens (VI) (tested together). Examining the pupils of the eyes for size, equality, and reaction to light is a part of a routine neurologic check. Neurologic checks are performed on a regular basis on any child with cranial trauma, seizures, or questioned cranial abnormality or inflammation. Information about other cranial nerve activity is gleaned more readily from careful observations of the child's activity and responses than from formal testing.

Cerebellar function The cerebellum coordinates and refines motor movements and maintains postural balance. Assessment is directed toward comparing the child's balance and coordination with expectations for age. A variety of tests can be used to determine cerebellar function, and the child's motor movements in play, dressing, and feeding also can be observed. (Tests for cerebellar function are described in Chapter 10.)

The nurse assesses balance by asking the child to stand with the feet together, arms outstretched, and eyes closed. A positive Romberg's sign is demonstrated when the child starts to fall during this test. The arms also are observed for excessive drift or abnormal hand movements.

Motor function The nurse assesses muscle tone by determining the resistance to passive range of motion of the trunk and extremities. Any of the following alterations in muscle tone might be present in a child with a neurologic dysfunction:

TABLE 31-2 Assessment of Cranial Nerves

Nerve	Assessment	Nursing implications
Olfactory (I)	Test child's ability to smell familiar odors (peppermint, peanut butter) with eyes closed	Impairment usually related to upper respiratory illness or allergic condition rather than neurologic dysfunction
Optic (II)	Measure visual acuity, visual fields. Fundoscopic exam (see Chapter 10)	Fundus of eye: optic disk edema (papilledema), retinal hemorrhage, and decreased venous pulsations indicate increased intracranial pressure. Environmental safety precautions and rehabilitation are required for the child with a visual field deficit (blindspot)
Oculomotor (III), trochlear (IV), and abducens (VI) (tested together)	Evaluate size, symmetry, and reaction to light. Test child's ability to move eyes to follow object in all directions (extraocular movements). Note nystagmus (rhythmic jerking of eyes)	Unequal pupils, decreased reaction to light, double vision, or paralysis of eye movement might indicate brain tumor, hemorrhage, inflammation, and increased intracranial pressure. Nystagmus can be associated with toxic reactions to drugs (especially phenytoin and phenobarbital)
Trigeminal (V)	Test facial sensation by child's ability to feel light touch. Assess motor function by strength and symmetry of jaw closure. Test corneal reflex—eyeblink to touching cornea with wisp of cotton	Assess the child's ability to chew and adapt feeding as necessary to avoid possible choking or aspiration. The absence of a corneal reflex requires the instillation of artificial tears (lubricant eye drops) to protect the cornea from abrasion
Facial (VII)	Note symmetry of facial expression and movement. Test facial muscle strength by having child close eyes tightly and press lips closed. Test child's ability to taste salt and sugar	Paralysis of the facial nerve (Bell's palsy) might be associated with otitis media and meningitis. Incomplete eye closure might require that a patch be worn to protect the cornea
Acoustic (VIII)	Assess hearing (see Chapter 32)	
Glossopharyngeal (IX), vagus (X)	Test child's ability to swallow. Assess gag reflex by stimulating pharynx with a tongue depressor or cotton-tipped applicator. Note a hoarse or stridorous vocal quality	Impairment can interfere with feedings so the nurse should attempt feeding techniques to reduce the risk of aspiration. Inability to swallow oral secretions requires positioning to facilitate drainage and oropharyngeal suctioning as needed
Accessory (XI)	Test movement and strength of the trapezius and sternocleidomastoid muscles by having child turn head to each side against resistance and elevate shoulders against resistance	Impairment interferes with head control. Measures are needed to provide head and neck support
Hypoglossal (XII)	Assess tongue movement by having child protrude tongue. Note symmetry, tremors, and ability to move tongue	Abnormal tongue movements are common in children with cerebral palsy. Impairment interferes with feeding and speech (refer to rehabilitation management, child with cerebral palsy)

Hypotonia reduced muscle tone. Infant may appear "floppy," lying in frog-leg position rather than in the normal flexed posture. When held suspended prone with the nurse supporting the chest, the infant makes no attempt to right the head and hangs in a dangling position

Flaccidity absence of normal resistance to passive movement of a body part

Hypertonia increased muscle tone. Abnormal muscle rigidity when the child is at rest

Spasticity prolonged muscular contraction and increased resistance of muscles to passive stretching

ASSESSMENT GUIDE *The Child with a Neurologic Dysfunction*

Assessment questions	Supporting data
Does the child have any observable structural or functional deformity?	
Head	Scleras visible above the iris (setting sun sign); head circumference above normal or increased growth outside normal curve
Spine	Presence of spinal dimple, hair tuft, or fluid sac; alterations in movement and muscle tone of the legs and feet including paralysis; lack of urinary and anal sphincter control, incomplete bladder emptying with frequent UTIs; decreased sensation below the level of the abnormality
General	Poor or absent gag, swallow, or sucking reflex; increased or decreased muscle size, strength, or tone (spasticity, abnormal movements or postures, paralysis); seizures
Has the child experienced any recent infection, or trauma to the head or spine?	Signs of increased intracranial pressure—bulging fotanelles (in infant); severe headache; vomiting (often projectile); leakage of clear fluid from the nose or ears; alterations in pupil size and response to light; diminished reflexes; positive Kernig's and Brudzinski's signs; inability to flex neck; alterations in level of consciousness
Does the child appear to have any alteration in level of consciousness? Is there a family history of seizures?	Seizures (describe type, pattern of frequency, progression, time, associated symptoms such as incontinence, cyanosis); abnormal posturing (decorticate, decerebrate); decreased level of response (by Glasgow Coma Scale)

Additional data: Petechial rash associated with signs of increased intracranial pressure; fever; abnormal CSF or EEG

Muscle strength is determined by observing the child's spontaneous activity in getting up from lying down or sitting, standing, and walking. The nurse notes symmetry, any weakness, and the degree of ease in movement. Strength also is assessed against resistance. Individual muscle groups are tested by having the child resist the nurse's movements.

The child's cooperation can be elicited by making a game of flexing or extending the head, trunk, and extremities against resistance. For example, the nurse might ask the child to keep the arm flexed while the nurse tries to extend it or keep the arms together while the nurse attempts to separate them. Active strength is assessed by having the child grasp the nurse's fingers and squeeze them. The nurse notes the presence and degree of weakness, paying particular attention to the equality of strength of the muscle groups of the two sides of the body.

Motor control and coordination can be assessed by developmental screening of age-appropriate motor tasks. The nurse assesses head control, sitting balance, standing, walking, and other age-expected motor milestones. The nurse observes the child manipulate toys, reach for objects, and perform bilateral hand activities to evaluate both fine motor control and hand preference. Dominance of one hand or the other normally does not develop before 18 months to 2 years of age. Preferential use of one hand before this age can indicate a weakness of the other hand. The nurse observes the child's gait for abnormalities of toe-walking, scissoring, unsteadiness, or asymmetric weakness or limp.

The nurse notes abnormal movements and postures with the child at rest and performing activities. Tremors on reaching, involuntary writhing movements of the extremities (*athetosis*), or irregular jerking movements (*chorea*) might be seen with motor dysfunction. These movements might become more pronounced as the child attempts motor control and diminish or disappear when the child is at rest and during sleep. Other abnormal movements might include tongue thrust, facial twitching or grimacing, and behaviors associated with various seizure activities.

Posturing can reflect alterations in muscle tone. Rigid arching of the back with neck extension is called *opisthotonos* and reflects hypertonic spinal extensors. This posture can reflect meningeal irritation or cerebral motor insult. Persistent tonic neck reflex posture at any age or elicited tonic neck posture after 6 months of age is atypical. The nurse notes any abnormal posturing of the extremities such as persistent arm flexion and fisting.

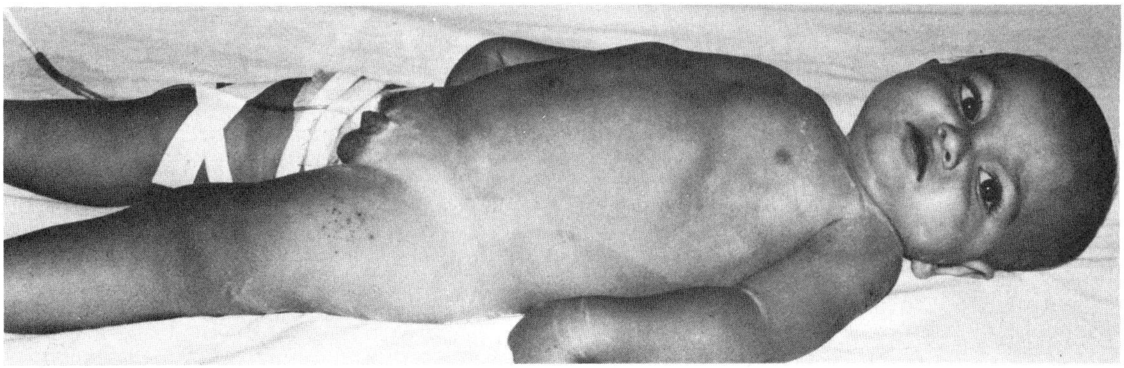

Decerebrate position. (From Purtilo DT: A Survey of Human Diseases. *Addison-Wesley, 1978, p. 427, with permission.)*

PROCEDURE *Electroencephalogram (EEG)*

- Prepare the child and parent for the procedure by giving a thorough explanation.
- Explain that the child will lie on the back to allow the technician to place the wires properly. The nurse or technician can handle the electrodes to show the child that they do not hurt.
- Describe how the electrode gel is placed on the child's head in multiple locations. The gel feels cool and damp and can be likened to toothpaste to increase the child's understanding.
- During the procedure the child will be encouraged to relax and remain still. The parent or trusted adult can remain with the child during the procedure to help the child relax. An activity such as storytelling or quiet singing promotes relaxation and helps the time pass quickly for an unsedated child.
- Explain that the child might be asked to breathe quickly at some point during the test.
- Electrodes are removed when the test is done. The older child might be interested to see the tracing and might understand the analogy to a television picking up a "picture" of the brain's activity. An EEG usually lasts no more than an hour.
- The child's hair is washed after the procedure to remove the gel or paste.

Characteristic postures are associated with severe brain insult and alterations of consciousness. In *decorticate* posturing the arms are held adducted with the elbows flexed and hands fisted over the chest, and the legs are extended. This posture usually reflects diffuse cerebral involvement. *Decerebrate* posturing consists of rigid extension, adduction, and internal rotation of the arms with the legs extended. This posturing indicates brain stem dysfunction.

Validating Diagnostic Tests

Radiographic and other neurodiagnostic studies (summarized in Table 31-3) are analyzed in conjunction with assessment data. These assist the nurse in completing the assessment.

Nursing Management for Procedures and Treatments

Preparation for Diagnostic Tests

The child with neurologic dysfunction might be functioning at a cognitive level below the chronologic age. The nurse therefore needs to perceive the child's level of understanding and any observable behavioral disorder to prepare the child accurately for diagnostic tests.

The *electroencephalogram* (EEG) is a frequently used noninvasive diagnostic test that requires the child to remain still and have electrodes applied to the scalp with a paste (see Table 31-3). The quality of the recording depends on the

TABLE 31-3 Radiographic and Other Neurodiagnostic Studies

Study	Organ	Procedure	Nursing management	Implication
Skull radiographs	Cranium	Single radiograph and various views of skull	Prepare for radiographic studies	Detects traumatic fractures and bony changes associated with congenital malformations, space-occupying lesions, and increased intracranial pressure
Computed tomographic (CT) scan	Internal structures of head	Intravenous injection of radiopaque dye (can be done with and without contrast). CT scanner takes multiple cross-sectional views of tissue density with data organized into composite pictures	Explain procedure and scanning equipment. Administer sedation	Determines size and position of ventricles, presence of masses, edema, and vascular changes
Cerebral angiography	Cerebral arteries and brain circulation	Sedation or general anesthesia. Injection of dye through femoral or carotid arteries. Radiographs	Explain procedure. Nothing by mouth according to protocol. Administer sedation. Posttest monitoring of vital signs and neurologic signs. Maintain immobility of injection site to reduce potential bleeding and edema—apply sandbag pressure as ordered. Check circulatory status in extremity distal to injection site for signs of obstruction	Detects blood vessel abnormalities, alterations of cerebral blood flow, and vascular tumors
Brain scan	Brain	Intravenous injection of isotope. Radioscanner detects presence of isotope and records the pattern on a chart	Explain procedure and equipment. Administer sedation if needed	Helps detect intracranial lesions such as tumors and abscesses
Myelography	Spinal cord	Lumbar puncture. Injection of dye into subarachnoid space. Radiographs of spine	Explain procedure and equipment. Administer sedation. Posttest monitoring of vital signs, neurologic signs for indications of adverse reaction	Determines trauma, mass, lesion, or other abnormality of the cord
Electroencephalogram (EEG)	Brain	Electrodes applied to head with conductive gel. Recordings taken during sleep, waking, hyperventilation, and stimulation with strobe light	Explain that electrodes do not hurt. Deprive child of sleep prior to test if ordered. Administer sedation if ordered. Allow trusted adult to remain with child during test. Wash hair after the procedure	Records electrical activity of the cerebral cortex. Identifies alterations in patterns due to seizures, trauma, or inflammation

TABLE 31-3 *(Continued)*

Study	Organ	Procedure	Nursing management	Implication
Subdural tap	Subdural space of cranium	Performed on infants and young children up to 2 years of age. Needle with stylet is inserted into the subdural space through the anterior fontanel or coronal suture. Stylet is withdrawn and fluid is allowed to flow out Amount of fluid withdrawn is limited to 15–30 mL from each side of the head. Stylet is replaced and the needle is withdrawn	Explain procedure to parents. Child is in the supine position with the head held firmly. Monitor child during the procedure for signs of shock or alteration in consciousness. After the test, maintain pressure dressing to the site, observe for fluid oozing from the site, and maintain child in an upright position or infant in infant seat	Detects and removes abnormal fluid collections in subdural space (effusion, hematoma). Collects fluid samples for laboratory analysis
Lumbar puncture	Cerebrospinal fluid system; lumbar spine	Needle with stylet is inserted into interspace between third and fourth lumbar vertebrae until the dural space is entered. Stylet is removed, and a three-way stopcock with a manometer is attached to measure CSF pressure. Cerebrospinal fluid samples are collected in numbered tubes. Stylet is replaced and needle is removed	Explain procedure. Position child on the side with spine curved. Hold child firmly with head flexed on chest and knees flexed on abdomen. Give child constant verbal support and reassurance throughout procedure. Monitor child's respiratory status during procedure. After the test monitor for headache, fever, or fluid leakage from puncture site. Assist with obtaining a blood sample to measure serum glucose. Have child lie flat after procedure to minimize spinal headache	Determines elevated CSF pressure. Collects CSF samples for culture, cell count, and protein and glucose measurements. Aids in diagnosis of meningitis, encephalitis, central nervous system hemorrhage, and increased intracranial pressure (ICP) (contraindicated in the presence of acutely increased ICP since it can cause cerebral herniation)
Electromyography (EMG)	Muscle	Needle electrodes are inserted into muscle to be tested. Electrical activity is recorded at rest and during muscle contraction	Explain procedure, discomfort, and need to hold still. Administer sedation if ordered. Ensure that child has an adult support figure during test. Tell older child that the test feels like "mosquito bites" and tingling	Measures electrical activity of muscle—differentiates nerve and muscle disorders
Nerve conduction studies	Peripheral nerves	Electrodes are taped to skin at points to be tested. Mild electric shock is applied as nerve stimulation. Velocity of transmission of nerve impluses is recorded	Same as for EMG	Measures velocity of nerve impulses along peripheral pathways. Detects nerve damage and demyelination

PROCEDURE *Lumbar Puncture*

- Prepare the child and parent for the procedure.
- Have the child practice the position if there is time before the procedure. The child assumes a side-lying position with knees tucked and chin flexed to the chest. The back is curved. The nurse or parent "hugs" the child to maintain the position. Infants can be positioned sitting with the back curved.
- Explain that the lower back (lumbar region) is washed first with a solution (povidone-iodine). This will feel cold to the child.
- Explain to the child that the doctor will have to administer an injection (local anesthetic) in the area of the back that was washed. The child will feel a stinging sensation that will last for less than a minute.
- After the anesthetic takes effect, the physician will insert a needle into the lumbar vertebral space. The child will feel pressure and possibly some shooting pain in the leg.
- Explain that the child will have to remain still for several minutes while the needle is in place. The physician will take CSF samples and measure the CS fluid pressure.
- When the needle is removed, light pressure and a Band-Aid are applied. A flat position for 4–6 hours after the procedure is recommended for children who have experienced headaches during previous lumbar puncture procedures.

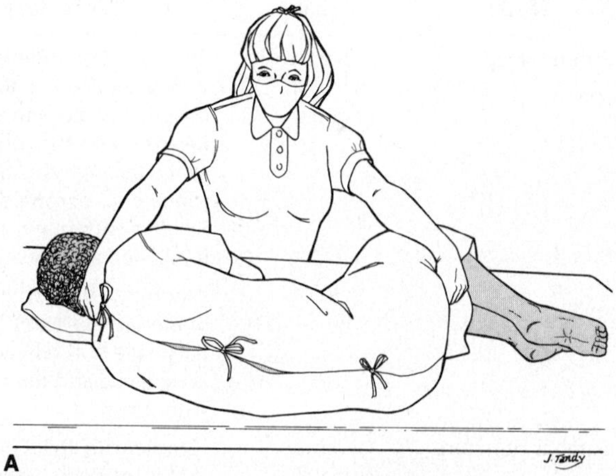

A

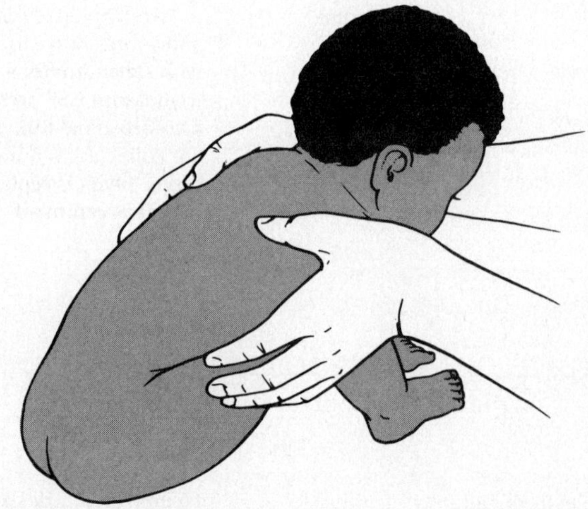

B

child remaining quiet and relaxed, which is more successful when the child is well prepared.

A lumbar puncture is performed to examine the cerebrospinal fluid (CSF) and measure its pressure (see Table 31-3). The nurse explains the procedure to the child in terms appropriate to the child's level of understanding, telling the child that this special test requires lying in a flexed position curled up like a ball. It is extremely important that the child know that a support figure will be present constantly to help hold the child still. Sedation is occasionally necessary. Because this procedure can seem very frightening to parents, the nurse describes the procedure to them and explains that there is relatively little danger to the child.

Radiographic studies include both single radiographs and more specialized procedures such as computed tomographic (CT) scans and angiography. Other procedures frequently used for diagnosis of neurologic dysfunction include subdural tap and electromyography (see Table 31-3). Any diagnostic test that requires a pretest sedative necessitates additional explanation to child and parent. The type and route of the sedative need to be described.

Habilitation and Rehabilitation Management

Care of the child with a neurologic deficit can involve habilitation. *Habilitation* often involves special management to improve deficit areas of function, help the child to de-

PROCEDURE *Computed Tomography (CT Scan)*

- Prepare the child and parent for the procedure. It is important to show the child a picture of the scanner and to explain that the child's head will lie inside the donut-shaped opening. Reassure the child that although the procedure will not hurt, the child's head will be strapped securely with a special type of hat or head band.
- Describe how the child will lie supine on the scanner table. The child's head will be immobilized. Because the room might be cold, the child can be told to ask for an extra blanket if needed.
- Explain that the child will be moved so that the child's head moves through the cylinder. The scanner looks like the front of a large washing machine. Depending upon institution policy, a reassuring adult might be allowed to remain in the room with the child. If not, the isolation might be frightening. The child is told that a nurse or the technician will talk throughout the procedure. A favorite blanket or animal, secured tightly so as not to interfere with the scan, might be comforting.
- During the procedure the child will hear a loud clicking or banging noise.

velop compensatory skills, and maximize the child's overall development.

Rehabilitation includes activities designed to restore a child to a previous level of function. Depending on the type of disorder, rehabilitative nursing measures include physical care, provision of adaptive equipment, developmental stimulation, and behavioral management.

The nurse is involved in the therapeutic management of neurologically handicapped children in acute-care settings, rehabilitation centers, and ambulatory and home-based programs. The nurse often coordinates multidisciplinary team efforts and acts as the family's liaison with various specialty services. Habilitation and rehabilitation programs for the child are planned and executed carefully by the child's therapeutic team. The plan is realistically based on a complete assessment of the child's physical, cognitive, social, affective, and environmental strengths and weaknesses. The plan also allows for the uncertain prognosis of some neurologic conditions.

Exercises The child with motor limitations often requires specific exercise programs to maintain joint mobility, strengthen muscle function, and increase endurance. Range-of-motion exercises are important for the child with paralysis, muscle weakness, or spasticity. Moving the child's extremities through their full flexion, extension, and rotation both helps to prevent joint contracture from disuse and improves circulation to the affected area. These exercises usually are carried out several times daily and can be incorporated into other care routines (bathing, dressing) and play activities.

Some exercises are directed toward strengthening specific muscle groups. For example, the paraplegic (paralyzed from the waist down) child might have an exercise program to strengthen the upper body and arms in preparation for walking with crutches and wheelchair mobility, which require considerable shoulder and arm strength. Push-ups and lifting weights in bed using a trapeze are additional muscle-strengthening modalities that can be used.

Young children can be moved through exercises passively. Active exercises are encouraged through the use of play, positioning, and stimulation. For example, placing a toy just out of reach and assisting the child to focus on the toy and to move toward it can promote desired motor movement. Mat exercises, balancing, and positioning promote development of head and trunk control. Water is an excellent medium for exercise. The child gains an appreciation of relaxation in water, while the resistance exerted by water during exercise can improve muscle tone. Older children can participate more fully in an exercise routine, particularly when incentives are used and praise is given for goal achievement.

The nurse encourages a positive attitude in child and family by incorporating exercises into meaningful activities. Using positive reinforcements such as achievement charts can help the child to remain engaged in what can otherwise be tiresome exercises.

Casts, splints, and braces Assistive devices are used to correct, maintain, and support body parts in a functional position when weakness, paralysis, or spasticity is present. Casts are used following orthopedic corrective surgery and as removable (bivalved) supports for intermittent use to maintain joint alignment and prevent contracture formation. (See Chapter 30 for care of the child in a cast.)

Like casts, splints maintain functional alignment of an affected body part. Handsplints are used frequently when a child's hand is weakened by hemiparesis, paralysis, or spasticity. The splint has a lightweight plastic posterior shell, and Velcro straps are used to hold the hand and wrist in

STANDARDS OF NURSING CARE *Rehabilitation for the Child with Impaired Neurologic Function*

GUIDE FOR NURSING MANAGEMENT

Nursing diagnosis	Intervention	Rationale	Outcome
1. Potential impaired physical mobility (stressors: poorly coordinated fine and/or gross motor movements; altered innervation of muscle groups)	Perform exercises as ordered.	Exercises maintain joint mobility and strengthen muscle function.	The child achieves maximum independent mobility. The child shows no evidence of joint contractures.
	Promote ambulation by applying any ordered assistive braces and by supervising and reinforcing the child's ambulation program. Provide a helmet if needed.	Braces support and stabilize the trunk and extremities for ambulation. A helmet can protect a child with impaired balance.	
	Alternate the child's position frequently (positions such as prone on wedge and legs elevated).	Frequent position changes prevent prolonged joint flexion and extension.	
	Position the child with supports to maintain correct alignment (abduction wedge between legs, footrests, and tray for elbow support, for example). Apply splints, braces, and bivalved casts as ordered.	Correct positioning reduces the risks of joint contractures.	
	Provide the nonambulatory child with a wheelchair, cart, or stroller. Ensure that the child in a wheelchair is adequately supported and is in good sitting alignment.	Exercise associated with wheelchair operation can prevent upper body contractures.	
	Teach the child independent mobility, transfers, and wheelchair operation.	These measures decrease the risk of injury.	
2. Potential impaired skin integrity (stressors: decreased ability to change position, altered nutritional status—excess or deficit)	Provide frequent skin care. Inspect the skin for pressure areas.	Frequent skin care and inspection can prevent skin breakdown. Friction areas can cause skin breakdown.	The child shows no evidence of pressure areas, decubitus ulcers, or abrasions.
	Provide sheepskin, Eggcrate® foam pad, alternating pressure mattress, flotation seat cushion, shoes without rough seams, and protective clothing.	These measures protect the skin and equalize pressure to the skin.	
3. Potential alteration in nutrition: less than body requirements (stressors: anorexia, difficulty with feeding or eating)	Position the child in optimal sitting alignment, especially when eating.	Sitting as high as possible facilitates passage of food.	The child's health status reflects adequate nutritional status. The child shows no evidence of feeding complications (airway obstruction or aspiration pneumonia).
	Adapt the consistency of the child's food to the child's ability to eat.	The child will take in more food if the food is of a consistency appropriate for the child's ability to eat and decreases risk of choking.	

STANDARDS OF NURSING CARE *Rehabilitation for the Child with Impaired Neurologic Function (Continued)*

GUIDE FOR NURSING MANAGEMENT

Nursing diagnosis	Intervention	Rationale	Outcome
	Provide special assistance as indicated (for example, manually closing the jaw or placing food between side teeth or at center of tongue).	Special feeding techniques can improve intake and lessen spilling.	
	Obtain adaptive feeding equipment for the child (see Chapter 14).	Adaptive equipment facilitates the child's independence in feeding.	
4. Potential altered urinary elimination pattern (stressors: incomplete or absent innervation to bladder; retention, dribbling)	Monitor urinary output. Perform alternate means of bladder emptying as ordered (Credé method and intermittent catheterization).	Adequate urinary output can prevent urinary tract infection.	The child voids in amounts appropriate for age, weight, and fluid intake.
	Ensure adequate fluid intake; include juices, especially cranberry.	Increasing fluids assists with flushing the genitourinary system and prevents urinary stasis.	
	Plan specified times during the day for voiding. Provide ostomy care for the child with ileal loop diversion.	Regular times for bladder emptying helps to prevent stasis and infection. See Chapter 28.	
5. Potential alteration in bowel elimination: constipation (stressors: incomplete or absent bowel innervation; inadequate intake)	Ensure adequate fluid intake, especially fruit juices.	Increased fluids assist with stool softening.	The child's bowel movements are regular and of soft consistency.
	Provide high fiber food such as fresh fruits, whole grain cereals, and bread.	Adequate fiber assists with regular bowel elimination.	
	Develop bowel program with regular toileting schedule, dietary adjustment, and use of suppositories.	Regular program encourages regular defecation and decreases the risk of constipation or stool incontinence.	
	Adapt toilet seat to provide support for trunk and extremities.	Bowel elimination is easier when the child is sitting upright.	
	Administer stool softeners as needed.	Stool softeners promote defecation and keep stool soft; child is less likely to become dependent on them.	
6. Potential impaired verbal communication (stressors: difficulty forming words or sentences; limited ability to verbalize thoughts)	Assist in developing alternative communication systems (gestures, sign language, communication board, typewriter, voice synthesizer, and so on). Exercise patience as the child attempts to communicate. Facilitate the use of the child's communication system by all who interact with the child.	Setting up a communication system that is understandable to all facilitates nursing care and promotes comfort for the child.	The child is able to communicate successfully.

(Continues)

STANDARDS OF NURSING CARE *Rehabilitation for the Child with Impaired Neurologic Function (Continued)*

GUIDE FOR NURSING MANAGEMENT

Nursing diagnosis	Intervention	Rationale	Outcome
7. Potential altered growth and development (stressors: uncoordinated fine and gross motor abilities)	Encourage mobility as a means of exploration.	Children learn by exploring.	The child achieves modified age-appropriate developmental tasks according to child's ability.
	Adapt play materials to enable the child to manipulate them. Provide stimulation appropriate to the child's developmental level.	Play encourages development.	
	Adapt self-care activities to facilitate independence (clothes with Velcro closures, elastic waist, shoes without laces, adapted feeding equipment, support bars in bathroom, and so on).	Achieving independence is a developmental task of childhood.	
	Praise and reinforce the child's attempts at mastery and independence.	Positive reinforcement is a form of encouragement.	
8. Potential self-esteem disturbance (stressors: feeling different, frustration with limitations)	Help the child and family to emphasize the child's strengths and abilities.	Focusing on the child's strengths increases self-esteem.	The child states an understanding of limits and demonstrates the ability to function within imposed limits. The child identifies personal qualities that indicate positive self-esteem.
	Set realistic rehabilitation goals.	Realistic goals prevent failure and decreased self-confidence.	
	Allow for the expression of frustrations, anger, sadness, and other emotional reactions.	Emotional expression that is accepted by the nurse reinforces the child's sense of self-worth.	
	Encourage opportunities for positive experiences with peers.	Positive acceptance by peers increases the child's acceptance of self.	
	Refer serious emotional disturbances of the child and family for appropriate intervention.	Professional counseling is needed for severe emotional disturbances to prevent adverse consequences.	
9. Potential knowledge deficit of home care (stressors: knowledge deficit, unfamiliarity with equipment or procedures)	Teach the child and family specific aspects of the child's rehabilitation (including all of the preceding interventions).	Adequate knowledge ensures optimal care.	The child and family demonstrate a knowledge of specific rehabilitation measures and health care maintenance. The family copes optimally with the impact of a disabled child. The child and family use resources as needed. The child successfully attends an appropriate educational program.
	Teach the elements of comprehensive child health and not just for the deficit areas.	Routine health care measures are important for any child with a chronic condition as they are for a well child.	
	Assist the family to prioritize the child's multiple needs; discuss ways that exercises and other therapeutic regimens can be incorporated into daily activities.	Prioritizing needs helps the family cope with the child's multiple problems.	

STANDARDS OF NURSING CARE *Rehabilitation for the Child with Impaired Neurologic Function (Continued)*

GUIDE FOR NURSING MANAGEMENT

Nursing diagnosis	Intervention	Rationale	Outcome
	Provide anticipatory guidance and support in helping the family to cope with the impact of the child's disability on siblings, family relationships, and lifestyle.	Assisting the family to express feelings about the child's disability increases family coping and acceptance of the child.	
	Refer the family to community agencies and organizations for children with special needs to provide: Counseling and support Health, educational, and therapy services Recreational opportunities Adapted equipment Advocacy	Referral to community agencies can increase information sources for the family.	
	Provide consultation and liaison for school placement.	Consultation facilitates the child's reentry into school.	

place. As with casts, the nurse moves the extremity gently to the desired position before applying the splint and checks for irritation and pressure sores. Resting splints are removed when the child is actively using the affected part. Assistive splints help to stabilize a joint or joints for functional use. Handsplints provide wrist and hand stability and can be fitted with attachments for eating utensils, pencils, typing pointer, and the like.

Braces of various types are used to stabilize a body part for functional use as well as to maintain alignment. Lower extremity and trunk orthoses (bracing devices) are used to control and support areas of neuromuscular weakness or imbalance for weight bearing, sitting, and ambulation. Below the knee, braces might be molded polypropylene shells that are worn inside the shoes to stabilize the foot and ankle. Other braces might assist motion with adjustable spring joints on vertical supports to aid plantar and dorsiflexion. The supports are attached directly to the shoe or to a molded insert by a band at the upper end around the calf.

More extensive lower extremity orthoses are used for hip and knee control and may be attached to body jackets for maximum support, such as for children with spinal cord lesions. Hip and knee joints on the braces have locking pins or slide bars to provide stability for standing but allow sitting with the joints unlocked. The inner surfaces of the brace that come in contact with the skin usually are padded with foam or soft leather to prevent pressure areas. Children should wear absorbent cotton undergarments and socks under braces to prevent skin irritation. The underwear worn beneath the braces must be close fitting and adjusted so that wrinkles do not create friction points. (See Chapter 30 for care of children in braces.)

Other equipment for the child with neuromuscular weakness or imbalance include prone standers, standing tables, chairs with added support and leg abduction wedges, overbed trapezes, and many other devices that are constructed to improve alignment and functional motor skills. The nurse ensures that the child's position is changed at regular intervals to prevent joint contractures and skin breakdown.

Mobilizing aids In addition to orthoses for stability, children with neuromuscular impairments often need assistive devices for mobility, either ambulatory instruments or wheeled apparatuses. Walkers, crutches, and canes provide added support for standing and walking, and the child's therapist teaches the proper use of these aids and gait technique. The nurse supervises and reinforces the child's ambulation, ensuring that safety measures (helmet, contact guarding) are used as needed to prevent injury from falls.

As the child becomes more ambulatory, an important aspect of the teaching program is learning how to fall without injury. Many children with neurologic impairments do not develop normal protective reflexes and need to be taught to balance, right, and break their fall should they trip or lose their balance. Different types of walkers and crutches give varying degrees of support and are chosen according to the child's strength and motor control. The child might begin ambulation with a rolling walker and progress to crutches as skill and strength develop.

Functional ambulation is possible for many neurologically disabled children, but for many of these children, ambulation might be slow-paced and require a tremendous energy expenditure. These children and others for whom weight-bearing ambulation is not possible benefit from mobility via wheelchairs, carts, and strollers adapted to their individual needs.

Adequate support is needed to maintain these children in correct alignment and provide stability for pushing themselves or engaging in activities with their upper extremities. Adaptations include footrests with straps, pelvic and trunk supports or safety belts, leg abduction wedges, headrests, and one-wheel driven or motorized chairs. The type of chair is selected to allow maximum mobility and independence while providing the necessary stabilization.

When positioning the child in a wheelchair, the nurse checks the fit and ensures that the child is adequately supported and in proper sitting alignment. Examples of improper fit include footrests that are too low or high, a seat that is too long and presses on the popliteal space, and a chair size that is too large, preventing the child from reaching the wheels and pushing independently.

The child with upper extremity strength is taught to propel, manipulate doors and ramps, and transfer to and from the chair independently. In all rehabilitative efforts, the goals are to increase the child's freedom and independence while providing adequate safeguards from accidents. The child's age and judgment ability are considered in allowing wheelchair access near such potentially dangerous areas as stoves, stairs, ramps, and so forth. The young child who is mobile on wheels is as capable as the nonimpaired youngster of exploring and being injured accidentally. The nurse teaches safety measures to parents of disabled children, particularly as previously immobile children learn new means of moving about.

Principles of Nursing Care

Acute Care Needs

Potential alteration in cerebral tissue perfusion

Increased intracranial pressure (ICP) can accompany a number of neurologic conditions and is particularly associated with craniocerebral trauma. Although the primary cause might differ, the physiologic principles of increased ICP in the various conditions are similar. (The mechanisms leading to increased ICP are shown in Figure 31-1.)

Normal ICP is a function of balance between the fixed volume of the rigid cranium and the volume of its contents—brain tissue, meninges, CSF (cerebrospinal fluid), and blood. For the pressure to remain constant once the fontanelles are closed, an increase in the volume of any one of these intracranial contents must be accompanied by a relative decrease in the volume of one or more of the other contents.

The neurologic system compensates for increased cranial volume by displacing more CSF to the spinal subarachnoid space. Additionally, CSF absorption is increased. In the infant the fontanelles widen to accommodate the increased volume. These compensatory mechanisms allow the brain to tolerate occasional temporary elevations in ICP. When the neurologic system is no longer able to reduce volume further, however, pressure inside the cranium rises. The child then experiences symptoms of increased intracranial pressure.

One cause of increased ICP is an increase in cerebral blood volume. The maintenance of cerebral blood volume is tied to the arterial carbon dioxide content. Thus, when the arterial CO_2 content is low, vasoconstriction results. When the arterial CO_2 content is elevated, such as in a hypoxic state, fever, or hypertension, the cerebral arteries dilate, increasing the intracranial volume.

An increase in ICP, whatever the cause, results in interference with the venous drainage. When this occurs, the pressure rises and impedes capillary circulation, thus reducing tissue perfusion. Decreased tissue perfusion in the brain leads to edema, tissue ischemia, further increased ICP, and eventually death.

The manifestations of increased ICP vary, depending on the age of the child, cause of the disorder, and rate (acute or chronic) at which the pressure develops. In infants the skull is able to expand as the volume of its contents expands. A tense, bulging fontanelle, separation of cranial sutures, and head enlargement are signs of increased ICP in infants and young children under 2 years of age. Because of the adaptive ability of the cranium, symptoms of disturbed brain func-

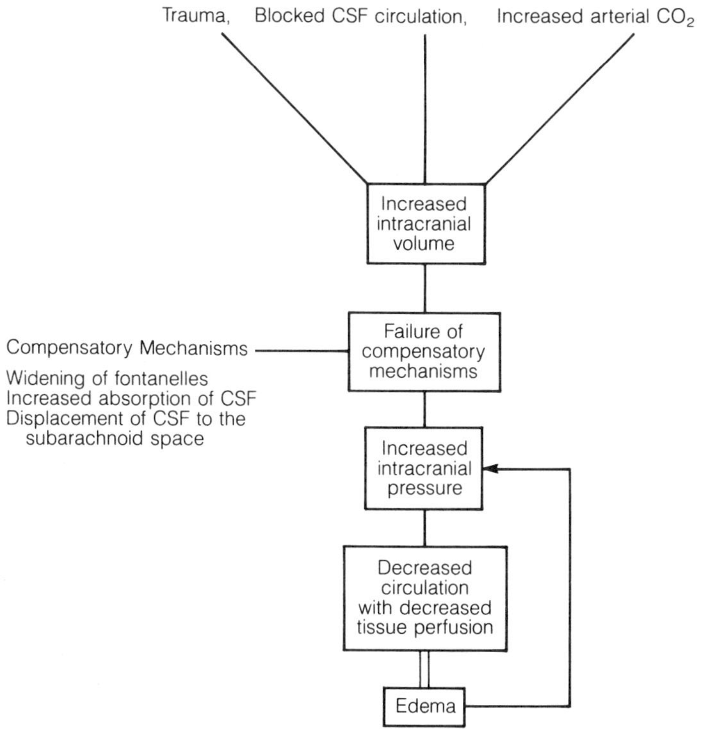

FIGURE 31-1

Mechanisms leading to increased ICP.

tion at this age might be minimal. Irritability, poor feeding, and delayed development might occur, but the more classic indicators of increased ICP often are not present.

Older children, whose compensatory mechanisms are limited, might develop headache, nausea, vomiting, alterations in behavior and consciousness, *diplopia* (double vision), and *papilledema* (optic disk swelling). As ICP increases, focal neurologic deficits of cranial nerve dysfunction (pupil reactivity changes, loss of oculomotor control), unilateral motor or sensory changes (hemiparesis), and seizures might develop. Advanced increased ICP causes the Cushing triad of slowed pulse, altered respiratory rate, and elevated systemic blood pressure. Progressive lethargy, stupor, and coma accompany untreated increased ICP.

A severe complication of increased ICP is the displacement of brain tissue (*herniation*) into an adjacent space. Herniation of cerebral tissue inferiorly across the *tentorium* (the barrier between the cerebrum and brain stem) can result in the compression of blood vessels, obstruction to the CSF flow, and injury to cerebral and brain stem structures. Cerebellar hernation also can occur, with displacement downward through the foramen magnum. Life-threatening deterioration of vital functions can result from brain stem compression secondary to herniation. Sudden increases in an already elevated ICP from fluid overload or hypercapnia (increased serum CO_2) can precipitate herniation as can a sudden reduction of CSF pressure from below (by way of a lumbar puncture).

The management of increased ICP is directed toward reducing intracranial volume and treating the underlying disorder. Osmotic diuretics (mannitol, glycerol) might be used initially to reduce acute brain edema. These agents remove tissue fluid rapidly when renal function is adequate. These agents usually are not continued on a long-term basis because a rebound elevation of ICP results from prolonged use. The child's electrolyte levels and urine output are monitored carefully.

Corticosteroids such as dexamethasone also are given to reduce brain swelling. Slower acting than the osmotic agents, steroids often are started concurrently with diuretics and become effective as the osmotic dehydrating action wears off. Corticosteroids are continued for longer periods than osmotic diuretics, depending on the child's condition. Antacid preparations are given orally or by nasogastric tube to prevent gastric irritation secondary to steroid administration. The nurse also observes the child for signs of gastric bleeding (hematemesis, positive stool guaiac).

Fluid restriction Fluid restriction can help to reduce increased ICP by decreasing the circulating blood volume. Fluid amounts below the usual maintenance requirements are ordered, and the child is monitored carefully to prevent fluid overload. The composition of the parenteral fluids administered is determined by the child's electrolyte and serum chemistries, but hypotonic solutions (such as .45% saline) are not used because they can further increase ICP.

The child's state of hydration is monitored continuously (see Chapter 21). Strict fluid restriction can potentially result in hypovolemic shock. The nurse therefore is alert for signs of this complication (increased pulse, decreased blood pressure, pallor, thirst, and alterations in levels of consciousness).

Temperature regulation Temperature regulation is an important aspect of management. Elevated body temperature increases cerebral blood flow and tissue oxygen requirements. It might be necessary to reduce the child's temperature by administering antipyretics or giving a sponge bath. The child's fluid intake is not increased to reduce fever because of the risk of overhydration.

In some children with severely increased ICP, hypothermia to subnormal body temperatures can be induced by the use of a cooling mattress or other devices. Intracranial pressure also can be relieved by barbiturate-induced coma (to reduce metabolic demands), removal of ventricular fluid, or decompressive craniectomy in selected cases, but these measures are reserved for the most severe forms of cerebral edema that do not respond to the traditional approaches.

Antibiotic administration Treatment of the underlying cause of the ICP includes antibiotic therapy for central nervous system infections, neurosurgical excision of accessible masses or lesions, or medical treatment of toxic or metabolic disorders. Conditions that obstruct the flow of CSF and result in hydrocephalus (increased CSF in brain ventricles) often are treated surgically with shunt procedures. In these procedures a pump is surgically placed to divert the CSF and reduce the ICP.

Nursing care of the child with increased ICP also includes continuous assessment of the child's state of consciousness, monitoring vital and neurologic signs, and employing measures to avoid increasing ICP. The child's level of consciousness is the most sensitive indicator of changes in ICP. Altered consciousness precedes other signs and symptoms of more advanced ICP elevations. The nurse is alert to subtle behavioral and cognitive changes in the child such as decreased responsiveness, confusion, or irritability. The child's condition might deteriorate rapidly, making serial assessments and early detection of changes vital to effective treatment.

Unless contraindicated (as in a question of spinal injury), the head of the child's bed is elevated 30–45° to improve fluid drainage from the brain. The child's head must be kept in neutral alignment. Neck flexion is avoided to prevent airway obstruction or impairment of venous return from the head. Stimulation and emotional agitation increase ICP, and nursing care is organized carefully and carried out gently to avoid unnecessary pressure increases from procedures and manipulations (such as tracheal suctioning or obtaining rectal temperatures). The nurse evaluates the need for restraints carefully because the child's combativeness will increase ICP. It is best to use the least amount of restraint possible and to apply protective coverings to infusion sites. The child's environment is kept as quiet as possible, and any avoidable stresses are removed. If more specialized measures are necessary to decrease the ICP, they are carried out in an intensive care setting.

❁ Potential sensory-perceptual alteration

Alterations in consciousness that result in sensory-perceptual changes can accompany a wide range of neurologic and systemic disorders in children. These include cerebral trauma, hemorrhage, infection, space-occupying lesions, or seizures. Coma is the most severe manifestation of sensory-perceptual impairment.

The comatose child's sensory perception is altered, and it might be difficult to determine how aware the child is of environmental stimuli. The nurse prevents sensory deprivation by providing meaningful stimulation for the child through touch, voice, and movement. The child's hearing might be intact, even though the child appears not to respond to auditory stimuli. Radio or television programs or tapes of familiar songs or stories that are selected carefully and geared to the child's developmental level can be played. The parent and those caring for the child are encouraged to talk to and avoid discussing the child or engaging in inappropriate conversation in the child's presence.

Nursing care for the comatose child The most important aspect of nursing management of the comatose child involves serial monitoring of neurologic status, including assessing vital signs, level of consciousness, and neurologic signs. The nurse particularly observes the child for changes indicative of improvement or deterioration in condition so that therapeutic interventions can be initiated if needed. The management of the comatose child with signs of increased ICP is the same as for any child with increased ICP.

Promoting effective airway clearance The nurse monitors the child's respiratory status and adequacy of ventilation continuously by assessing respiratory effort, auscultating breath sounds, and observing for fluctuations in arterial blood gases. Changing the child's position and performing chest percussion and postural drainage (unless contraindicated by increased ICP) help to mobilize secretions. The nurse suctions the child's secretions frequently to maintain clear respiratory passages.

The child might have an endotracheal or tracheostomy tube in place to ensure a patent airway and might require ventilator assistance. Respiratory care focuses on maintaining adequate arterial oxygenation and preventing complications from hypoxia, pneumonia, and atelectasis (see Chapter 22).

Monitoring fluid balance The nurse monitors the child's state of hydration by observing the serum electrolyte levels and urine volume and measuring specific gravity of the urine. The comatose child might develop water intoxication from inappropriate secretion of antidiuretic hormone (ADH) from the anterior pituitary gland. In this situation the child's urine output drops, the urine is concentrated, serum osmolarity decreases, and hyponatremia develops. This condition can cause elevations in ICP from overhydration and can result in death.

Inappropriate ADH secretion is treated by fluid restriction until the child's state of hydration becomes stable. Evaluation of urine output is accompanied by serum chemistries and osmolarity measurements to avoid incorrect fluid therapy.

Managing nutrition In cases of prolonged coma, the child's nutritional needs are met by nasogastric or gastrostomy tube feedings. The type, amount, and method of feeding might vary, but the nurse assesses the child's ability to tolerate feedings and prevents possible aspiration by positioning the child on the side with the head elevated. As the child's condition improves, oral feeding is begun with soft foods if adequate gag and swallow reflexes are present.

Preventing problems with elimination In the acute-care period, an in-dwelling catheter is used to measure urine output accurately. When the comatose child's condition stabilizes, the catheter is removed to reduce the incidence of bladder infection. Diapers or external collecting devices are used, and the nurse observes the child for bladder distension, changes in output, and frequency of voiding.

Stool softeners, bulk agents, or cathartics might be needed to prevent constipation. Loose stools often can be treated by dietary management. The perineum and buttocks of the comatose child who is incontinent must be cleaned thoroughly to prevent excoriation from soiling.

Preventing hazards of immobility Nursing measures also are directed toward preventing secondary effects of immobility involving the skin and circulatory and musculoskeletal systems. The use of a sheepskin or an alternating pressure air mattress, position changes, and skin care to stimulate circulation will prevent the formation of decubitus ulcers.

The nurse positions the child with the trunk and extremities in correct postural alignment and changes the child's positions from side to side and to semiprone at 2- to 4-hour intervals. The uppermost extremities are supported by pillows to prevent stress on the major joints (shoulder, elbow, hip, and knee). Antiembolism stockings can be used to improve venous return from the lower extremities. Passive range-of-motion exercises and intermittent splinting or casting to maintain functional position of the extremities can be used to help prevent contractures. Special boots can be worn to prevent foot drop.

The comatose child's corneal reflexes might be impaired, resulting in incomplete eye closure and subsequent drying and ulceration of the cornea. The nurse instills eye drops frequently because artificial tears might be needed to provide lubrication.

Neurosurgery—preoperative and postoperative care Children require neurosurgery for a number of pathologic conditions. In addition to routine preoperative and postoperative care, careful monitoring of neurologic status is essential. Complications from neurosurgery, such as increased ICP or infection in the form of meningitis, can have far-reaching consequences for the child's optimal development.

Nutritional Needs

⊛ Potential alteration in nutrition: less than body requirements

The child with a neurologic disorder might have feeding difficulties associated with impairment of the mechanisms necessary for normal eating and drinking. Feeding techniques are adapted for the child with cerebral palsy or any insult to the nervous system that interferes with motor control, coordination, and reflexes.

Impaired oromotor control can result in problems with sucking, lip closure, ability to move food in the mouth, and chewing. The child might exhibit abnormal reflex patterns such as tongue thrust or jaw clamping. Impaired swallow or gag reflexes can increase the risk of aspiration or airway obstruction.

Nursing management includes determining the child's feeding abilities carefully by obtaining a thorough history from the parent and observing the child while eating. Poor suck or food dribbling out of the mouth or being pushed out by tongue thrust are indicative of neuromuscular problems. The nurse gives the child a small amount of water and watches for any swallowing difficulties or choking. The nurse also observes the child's ability to use a bottle and nipple or cup and other eating utensils. Finally, the nurse evaluates the child's ability to self-feed.

Food, equipment, and techniques are adapted to compensate for a variety of feeding problems. Infants who suck and swallow poorly might need gavage feedings (see Chapter 27). Soft nipples or syringe-type feeders are helpful for some infants, as is thickening the formula slightly with a thickener such as baby cereal to aid swallowing.

Manual lip closure and jaw control are feeding techniques used with children with cerebral palsy. The nurse's

STANDARDS OF NURSING CARE *The Child Following Neurosurgery*

RISKS

Assessed risk	Nursing action
Postoperative complications such as hemorrhage, ineffective airway clearance, fluid loss, and neurologic dysfunction	See Chapter 20.
Increased intracranial pressure from surgical insult or shunt malfunction	Position the child with the head of the bed slightly elevated as ordered. Monitor the child for signs of increasing intracranial pressure such as increased blood pressure, headache, vomiting, irritability, and bulging fontanelles. Avoid overly vigorous chest physiotherapy or suctioning. Prevent factors that increase ICP by Maintaining optimal ventilation Monitoring intravenous fluid administration carefully to prevent overhydration Providing comfort and reassurance to decrease agitation Avoiding the use of restraints, which increase combativeness Reporting vomiting immediately and keeping the child on NPO status Using slow, gentle movements when positioning the child

GUIDE FOR NURSING MANAGEMENT

Nursing diagnosis	Intervention	Rationale	Outcome
1. Potential alteration in comfort: pain (stressors: incision, headache)	Observe for signs of pain at incision sites, headache, and neck pain.	Early recognition of pain allows for rapid pain relief.	The child appears comfortable and able to obtain rest. The child identifies pain relief measures that are effective.
	Differentiate postoperative pain from signs of meningeal irritation.	Meningeal irritation (headache combined with nausea, vomiting, neck rigidity, back arching, and alterations in vital signs) needs to be reported immediately.	
	Change the child's position, keeping weight off the operative site; apply cool compresses to the eyes and forehead; and darken the room.	These measures are effective nonpharmacologic pain relief measures.	
	Administer analgesics if not contraindicated by the child's neurologic status. If analgesics are permitted, select a medication with the least potential for central nervous system depression.	Because of the central nervous system insult during surgery, CNS depressants can adversely affect the child because they can increase the CNS depression caused by the surgery.	

STANDARDS OF NURSING CARE *The Child Following Neurosurgery (Continued)*

GUIDE FOR NURSING MANAGEMENT

Nursing diagnosis	Intervention	Rationale	Outcome
2. Potential for infection (stressors: break in primary defenses at surgical incision, invasive procedures, presence of shunt)	Use aseptic technique for dressing changes.	Aseptic technique decreases the risk of organism entry from the nurse.	The child remains free of any infection.
	Observe for erythema and drainage from incision sites; note the type of drainage; report immediately the drainage of clear fluid (cerebrospinal fluid), particularly if it tests positive for glucose by Dextrostix.	Clear drainage that is determined to be cerebrospinal fluid can indicate that there is an entry to the CNS for organisms.	
	Observe and report meningeal irritation.	Meningitis is an infection of the CNS.	
3. Potential injury (stressors: strain or tension on incision with movement; use of turning frame)	Position the child's head to lie on the nonoperative side unless ordered otherwise.	Keeping weight off the operative site decreases trauma and the risk of injury.	The child shows no evidence of trauma to operative areas such as pain, hemorrhage, neurologic complications, or separation of the suture line.
	If the operative site is occipital or cervical, do not rotate head when turning; use a log roll and move child's head and neck as one unit.	Keeping head and neck aligned prevents strain on the suture line.	
	Use a Stryker frame as ordered to immobilize the spine. Follow safety guidelines when turning the frame and child.	Ensure turning child as a unit to decrease strain on the suture line after spinal surgery.	
4. Potential body image disturbance (stressors: loss of hair, facial edema and bruising)	Prepare the child and family preoperatively for the child's postoperative appearance (shaved head, eye edema, bulky head dressing).	If the child and family are prepared, they won't be as upset after surgery.	The child and family demonstrate acceptance of the child's altered appearance.
	Provide a hat or scarf for the child. Suggest that the family obtain a wig until the child's hair grows in, if appropriate.	Providing cover to the operative site gives the child a more normal appearance while hair grows and decreases reaction to the change in appearance.	
	Support the child and family in coping with the emotional impact of altered body image.	Allowing the child and family to express their feelings helps them to cope.	
5. Potential knowledge deficit concerning home care (stressors: limited understanding of new procedures to learn)	Teach the child and family the signs of increased ICP, shunt malfunction, central nervous system infection, and wound infection.	Adequate teaching ensures early recognition of complications.	The child and family can describe the signs of complications. The child and family demonstrate knowledge of home care and importance of follow-up evaluations. The school-aged child continues schooling successfully.

(Continues)

STANDARDS OF NURSING CARE *The Child Following Neurosurgery (Continued)*

GUIDE FOR NURSING MANAGEMENT

Nursing diagnosis	Intervention	Rationale	Outcome
	Teach the family to pump the shunt, if indicated.	Pumping the shunt facilitates circulation of cerebrospinal fluid. Proper technique is important to prevent damage to the shunt.	
	Advise the child and family about any activity restrictions and the need for safety precautions such as a helmet.	The family will feel more confident if they know how to plan for their child's activity and safety.	
	Instruct the family about the medications to be given at home (such as anticonvulsants and antibiotics).	Accurate medication administration is important for optimal recovery.	
	Refer the family to community agencies for teaching and support as needed.	Community resources can provide additional information to families.	
	Give the family specific information regarding postoperative follow-up plans, particularly neurosurgical appointment and the school-aged child's reentry to school.	Parents need to understand all follow-up plans to ensure adequate health care for the child.	

hand is placed along the side of the child's jaw, and the index and middle fingers gently close the child's lips after food is put in the child's mouth. This is best accomplished by sitting beside or behind the child and using the other hand to feed the child. The child can either sit in the nurse's lap or upright alone with adequate support.

Actual feeding techniques can be adapted to the child's needs. A small Teflon-coated spoon is useful because it is easier for the child to get the food off the spoon, and it avoids trauma from biting down on a hard spoon. The nurse might have to place food partway back on the child's tongue or between the side teeth so that the child can manage it. Feeding programs to facilitate eating and improve the child's oromotor control are developed by a multidisciplinary team that includes the nurse, dietitian, and speech and occupational therapists. (See Chapter 14 for additional assistive feeding devices.)

The consistency and type of food might have to be adjusted for the child with neuromuscular impairment. Children with difficulties in chewing or swallowing need soft or semisoft food. The chronic feeding problems some children experience can lead to nutritional inadequacies and debilitation. High-protein, high-calorie dietary supplements can be added in forms that the child will tolerate (such as puddings or frappes).

Nasogastric or gastrostomy routes might be used to feed children with impaired consciousness. This form of feeding also might be necessary for severely disabled children who cannot handle food orally. The type of formula, procedure, and schedule will vary according to the child's needs and institutional protocols. (See Chapter 27 for principles of nasogastric or gastrostomy feedings.)

Potential alteration in nutrition: more than body requirements

The dietary needs of some children with neurologic dysfunction are related to obesity caused by excessive food intake and relative physical inactivity. Obesity can inhibit rehabilitative progress by making ambulation and mobility

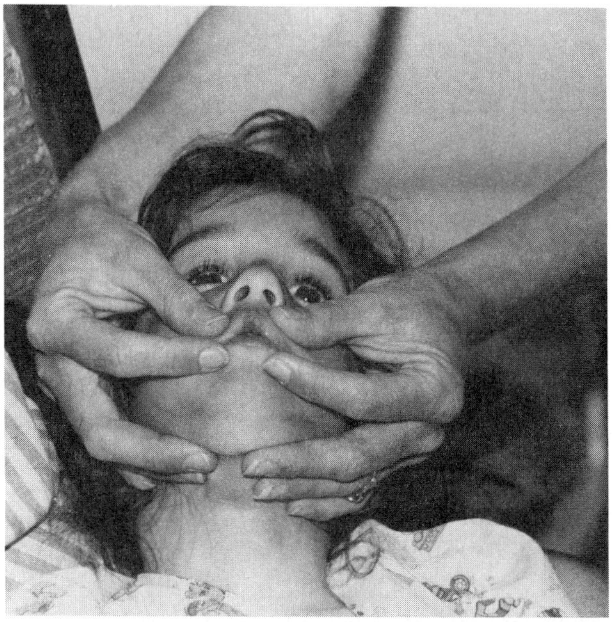

Manual lip closure and jaw control can be used as a feeding technique for children with cerebral palsy.

more difficult. In addition, excessive fatty deposits might increase the child's risk for skin breakdown. Because the child with motor impairment expends few calories, dietary management focuses on weight control while ensuring sufficient nutrients for health and growth.

The nurse is sensitive to the child's psychosocial as well as physical needs in developing a dietary plan. Disabled children and their families might have developed patterns of using food as a form of gratification to replace other pleasures precluded by the children's limitations. The nurse assesses the dynamics contributing to the child's weight problem and develops meaningful incentives to alter dysfunctional behavior patterns associated with food. Dietary planning to prevent obesity in disabled children is better than treating the disabled child who is already overweight.

Developmental Needs

The developmental needs of children with neurologic dysfunction are similar to those of all children, but because of their particular deficits, special interventions might be needed to help neurologically impaired children achieve success in developmental tasks. Cognitive, sensory, behavioral, or motor impairments can greatly affect the child's acquisition of skills, adjustment to the environment, and emotional well-being.

⊛ Potential altered growth and development

All infants and children need a variety of sensory and motor experiences to stimulate cognitive and psychosocial growth. The normal exploration of the environment and seeking of stimulation might be impossible for the child with motor, cognitive, or communication limitations caused by neurologic dysfunction.

The child can benefit from being exposed to age-appropriate stimuli and given the opportunity to build compensatory strengths such as wheelchair mobility to broaden the possibilities for exploring the environment. Adapting wheelchairs to provide trunk stability and free the child's hands for manipulation and stabilizing toys or books can increase the child's independence and opportunities for stimulation.

Early intervention programs with neurologically impaired children often place a great deal of emphasis on stimulation. When based on a thorough assessment of the child's capabilities and family strengths, individualized programs of sensorimotor stimulation might be recommended by a team with expertise in this field. The nurse is responsible for evaluating the appropriateness of stimulation programs for the child and family.

In their enthusiasm to stimulate the disabled child, however, health care professionals need to avoid overwhelming either the child or the family with time-consuming and exhausting programs. It is worthwhile working with parents to help them discover opportunities to provide sensorimotor stimulation for the children in their everyday care and recreation activities (such as during bath or mealtimes, while shopping, and so forth).

The educational needs of children with neurologic disorders range from the severely disabled child's need to learn self-help skills to the learning disabled child's need for compensatory reading instruction.

The neurologically impaired child might continue to require the special treatment of a hospital-based or private school, but these children are being included increasingly in public school programs. School nurses, in particular, face tremendous challenges in educating staff, providing direct health services, and promoting the neurologically impaired child's adjustment in the school setting. The school nurse can act as a liaison between the home, school, and medical care facility regarding the child's health needs. Duties can include monitoring seizures and medication administration, feeding programs, respiratory care, or specialized bowel or bladder programs. The nurse often is a consultant and resource person in coordinating the child's school program, incorporating data from health care assessments and family information both to facilitate the child's adaptation and to ensure communication between home, school, and health care agencies.

Children with neurologic impairments might be hospitalized repeatedly for medical management or surgical procedures. Their school programs can be interrupted frequently, interfering with their academic progress. Whenever possible and as much as possible, educational routines should be part of care for these hospitalized children (see Chapter 20). Collaboration with the family and school is also necessary in discharge planning to prepare for the child's reentry to school.

⊛ Potential impaired social interaction

The dysfunction in motor control, communication, or cognition that can accompany neurologic disorders might interfere with the child's ability to interact socially and to develop social skills. Difficulties can arise not only from the child's limitations but also from the reaction of other people to the child's differences. The child's opportunities for socialization outside the family might be limited by dysfunctional reactions to disabling conditions.

For example, others might be reluctant to socialize with a nonverbal child with cerebral palsy, a child with seizures who wears a helmet, or a child with musculoskeletal or some other deformity who appears "different." Dysfunctional reactions often are based on fear and a lack of understanding about the disabling condition. Those who do interact with neurologically impaired children tend to relate to them below their level of maturity, treating them as if they were mentally retarded, regardless of their actual cognitive level.

To meet the child's socialization needs, nursing care is based on an assessment of the child's psychosocial developmental level, interactional style, and any physical or emotional barriers to social encounters. During hospitalization, neurologically impaired children, surrounded by strangers and in unfamiliar environments, might feel even more isolated than they do in their daily lives. The nurse becomes familiar with any alternate communication system the child uses and ensures that this system is used consistently.

The nonverbal child who cannot communicate is particularly vulnerable to social isolation. Devices such as a communication board, mechanical communicator, or description of the child's gesture or signing system should be readily accessible and not put away in a drawer.

The nurse enhances the child's socialization by encouraging interaction with peers, role modeling, providing simple explanations and assistive cues such as "Jenny is a whiz at that game and would like to play it with you. She might have trouble moving the pieces, but I'll bet that you could help her with that." Children can accept individual differences more readily than some adults when adequately guided and can contribute significantly to the overall social adjustment of neurologically impaired children in the hospital, at school, or in the community.

The child whose neurologic dysfunction is manifested behaviorally might exhibit inappropriate social skills such as impulsivity, disinhibited responses, or negativism. Peer interaction is hampered by the child's behavior, and the child often is rejected by other children. Specific behavior management programs developed using a team approach that includes parents and others involved with the child can be helpful. Teaching children to share, take turns, and recognize other people's needs is undertaken in structured situations, and the goal is for the children to learn a particular social skill, generalize it to other situations, and derive satisfaction from the resulting appropriate interpersonal relationships.

Emotional Needs

⊛ Potential ineffective individual coping

The neurologically impaired child often is more dependent because of motor or developmental limitations. Physical dependency might stem from neuromuscular weakness and lack of motor control, with the child requiring assistance with such activities as eating or dressing. The neurologically impaired child might have the same needs for independence as nonimpaired children but has fewer opportunities to achieve independence. Neurologically impaired children often become frustrated by their limitations and necessary reliance on others.

Parents might have ambivalent feelings about encouraging independence. They fear for their children's safety, and at times they are gratified by their children's dependence. The nurse assesses the parent-child relationship and the child's abilities and counsels the family to help them to maximize the child's independence.

The child's independence can be enhanced by providing equipment that can be manipulated independently and by giving the child enough time to persevere in attempts to become more independent. Clothes with Velcro closures, built-up spoons or other adapted eating utensils, and stabilizing play materials such as books or games will enable the neurologically impaired child to perform aspects of self-care and learn and play without constant adult attendance.

Parents often find it easier to assume the care themselves than to let their children do as much as they can by themselves. The nurse helps the parents to see the value of fostering their children's independence to increase their self-image and future self-sufficiency. (The care of the child with a chronic condition is discussed in Chapter 14.)

In caring for the neurologically impaired child, the nurse provides a balance between allowing the child to perform as many tasks and make as many decisions as possible while preventing frustration and unnecessary failures. Letting children choose when treatments or exercises will be done, allowing them to select their own menus, and giving them the freedom to move in their wheelchairs are some ways to give children the control they might lack in other areas.

The Child with a Seizure Disorder

Seizures

Seizures are among the more common manifestations of neurologic dysfunction in childhood and are associated with a variety of acute and chronic conditions. A *seizure* is a sudden, transient alteration in brain function that is caused by the excessive, disorderly discharge of electrical impulses by neuronal tissue. Alterations of consciousness and motor, sensory, or autonomic function are clinical manifestations of seizure activity, which can occur as a single episode or recur intermittently. Different characteristic seizure patterns, such as convulsions, lapses of consciousness, and behavioral disturbances, reflect the type of abnormal electrical activity and area of brain involvement.

Incidence estimates of seizures among children vary depending on age and seizure type. Up to 6% of all children experience one or more seizures by adolescence, but the majority of seizures are single, nonrecurrent episodes associated with acute illness and fever (Conway-Rutkowski, 1982).

A seizure disorder, or *epilepsy,* is a condition in which the child experiences chronic recurrent seizures. Epilepsy affects a very small number of individuals. Seizures are more frequently seen in the first two years of life because of the immaturity of the nervous system.

Seizures are categorized according to etiology, clinical manifestations, and electroencephalographic pattern. Because seizures are not a specific disease entity but a symptom of an abnormality of brain function, a variety of factors might be responsible.

At different ages, certain causes are more common. In the neonatal period, the effects of perinatal insult by anoxia or hemorrhage and congenital brain defects are frequent causes of seizures. In later infancy and early childhood, febrile convulsions, seizures associated with central nervous system infections, and congenital malformations are common causes. Other causes of seizures might include seizures resulting from trauma, metabolic disorders, toxins, and space-occupying lesions such as tumors. Beginning at about 3 years of age and continuing throughout adolescence, the cause of recurrent seizures cannot be determined in most children, and the disorder is referred to as *idiopathic epilepsy.*

Clinical manifestations Seizures are classified as *generalized* (involving both brain hemispheres) or *partial* (involving a localized area of the cerebral cortex). (The types and descriptions of seizures observed in children are summarized in Table 31-4. Neonatal seizures are discussed in Chapter 34.)

Depending on the type of seizure, the child might experience an aura or warning sensation just before the onset of the attack. Abdominal pain, nausea, feeling "shaky," dizziness, sudden fear, and visual or auditory sensations are among the auras described by children and adolescents. Grand mal and psychomotor seizures frequently are preceded by an aura.

A seizure episode is usually self-limiting and by itself causes no acute injury. The sudden loss of consciousness and forceful muscle contractions that often accompany seizures, however, can result in injury from falls or striking objects. Children with atonic or myoclonic seizures can suffer severe trauma to the face and teeth from head drop attacks. Another secondary complication from seizures occurs during mealtime aspiration of food. The child also might aspirate excessive oral secretions produced during a generalized seizure.

After a grand mal or psychomotor seizure (the postictal phase), the child is often confused, drowsy, and might sleep for variable periods of time. Some children complain of headache and experience fatigue for a day or two after a gran mal seizure. In contrast, there is usually no postictal drowsiness following absence (petit mal) seizures or minor motor attacks, and the child immediately resumes previous activities.

Diagnostic evaluation One of the most important aspects in the diagnostic evaluation of seizures is a detailed history, which is obtained from both the parents and, if possible, the child. The purpose of the history is to determine whether the episodes represent seizure activity, the type of seizure, focus (if any), and possible causes for the disorder.

The practitioner evaluating the child is seldom present during a seizure and must obtain a detailed clinical description of the episode, including preceding events (illness, fever, injury, and so forth), any aura or warning, and an exact description of the seizure and the child's behavior during the postictal period. The sequence of events, responsiveness of the child, parts of the body involved, and duration of the seizure are helpful in defining the type of seizure. It is important to determine any localizing signs that might indicate a focal origin. The child's age at onset, frequency of seizures, and any factors that precipitate the attacks also are

TABLE 31-4 Types of Seizures

Type	Description
Generalized seizures Major motor (grand mal)	Might be preceded by an aura. Initial loss of consciousness. Tonic phase involves rigid extension of the body; eye deviation; apnea; cyanosis; increased salivation; and loss of bladder and bowel control. Clonic phase involves rhythmic jerking movements. Postictal phase involves confusion and sleep. Seizure lasts 2–5 minutes or longer. Variable frequency
Absence (petit mal)	Onset between 3 and 8 years of age. Brief (few seconds) staring spell. Loss of awareness, with or without minor muscle twitching (face and hands). No loss of postural tone. Several to hundreds of episodes every day
Minor motor—atonic	Onset between 3 and 8 years of age. Brief (few seconds) loss of muscle tone. Head drop; upper body drop; or full body drop. Frequency is variable—often daily or weekly episodes
Minor motor—myoclonic	Onset between 3 and 7 years of age. Brief (few seconds) muscle flexor spasm. Forceful head drop; arm extension; trunk flexion. Variable frequency—daily to weekly episodes
Infantile spasms	Onset between 3 and 9 months of age. Brief (momentary) flexion of neck, trunk, and legs ("jack-knife" seizures). Recurs in clusters of episodes—up to hundreds of times daily. Disappears after infancy; often replaced by other types of seizures in later childhood; usually accompanied by psychomotor impairment. Characteristic electroencephalographic pattern (hypsarrhythmia)
Partial seizures Focal	Localized motor or sensory disturbance, generally without impairment of consciousness. Often unilateral. Motor—twitching of face, hand, foot might progress to entire side of body (Jacksonian seizure) Sensory—tingling, numbness, or other altered sensation of affected body part Child might have weakness of the affected muscle group (Todd's paralysis) lasting hours to days following the seizure. The duration usually is several minutes. The frequency is variable
Psychomotor	Might be preceded by an aura. Widely varying manifestations. Behavioral and sensory alterations—most commonly staring; repetitive motor activity (automatisms) such as lip smacking, chewing, eye blinking, and fumbling with hands; confused state, mumbled speech; bizarre behavior (such as purposeless walking or running, undressing, aggression if restrained). Postictal fatigue and sleep. Duration is 5–10 minutes. Frequency is variable—daily to weekly
Febrile seizures	Tonic-clonic movements that occur in the presence of a fever (greater than 100.4°F or 38°C) and in a child younger than age 6 years. Seizures can range from having no focal features and short duration to including focal features with greater than 30 minute duration
Status epilepticus	Prolonged seizure or repeated seizures without regaining consciousness. Usually refers to generalized grand mal seizures. Can result in hypoxia; hypotension; cardiac arrhythmias; respiratory depression. Constitutes a medical emergency that requires immediate treatment

determined. Grand mal seizures usually are not difficult to identify, but petit mal or psychomotor seizures can be difficult to diagnose.

Complete general physical and neurologic examinations are performed. Particular attention is given to determining any localized neurologic signs, head circumference, neurocutaneous lesions, or other findings that might help to diagnose the underlying brain dysfunction.

Various laboratory tests might be performed depending on the indications. These tests include a complete blood count and fasting glucose, serum calcium, phosphorus, and lead levels. Other tests are indicated if an underlying metabolic disturbance is suspected.

An electroencephalogram (EEG) is done to detect any abnormality in electrical activity and determine the type of seizure and focus, if any. The EEG might or might not show alterations between seizures; therefore, a normal EEG does not rule out a seizure disorder. Conversely, an abnormal EEG is not necessarily diagnostic. The EEG is most helpful in differentiating the characteristic patterns of different seizure types such as petit mal or psychomotor seizures.

Radiographic examinations of the skull frequently are

performed to rule out intracranial calcifications and asymmetric skull development or when trauma is suspected. A CT scan can help to identify any atrophy, tumors, or other anatomic abnormalities associated with seizures. More definitive studies, such as arteriography or radioisotope brain scans, are used when vascular or focal lesions are indicated that cannot be differentiated by CT scan.

A lumbar puncture is not done routinely but is indicated for seizures occurring in infants under 6 months of age, children with fever and seizures, and children suspected of having meningitis (Low and Downey, 1982b).

Treatment Children with recurrent seizures are treated with appropriate anticonvulsant medications. Depending on the type of seizure, one drug is chosen to begin treatment, and the dosage is adjusted until the seizures are controlled or the maximum tolerated dose is reached. If the drug is inadequate in controlling seizures, a second drug might be added slowly.

For some children, a combination of medications is more effective, and a third or even fourth drug might be added. The goals of treatment are to eliminate seizures or reduce their frequency without any side effects of drug therapy seriously affecting the child. Many children respond well to medication, with seizures occurring rarely or not at all. Other children's conditions are more difficult to manage, with seizures persisting and varying in frequency or type. Children with mixed seizure disorders, especially minor motor seizures, tend to be more resistant to treatment.

Medications more frequently prescribed for major motor seizures include diphenylhydantoin (Dilantin) and phenobarbital. Valproic acid (Depakene), ethosuximide (Zarontin), or trimethadione (Tridione) might be used for petit mal seizures. Other agents used for seizure control include carbamazepine (Tegretol), clonazepam (Clonopin), and primidone (Mysoline).

Febrile seizures might be treated with phenobarbital, which can be prescribed prophylactically for 2–4 years. Children who are candidates for phenobarbital therapy include those with a family history of epilepsy, children with neurologic deficits, children with prolonged focal seizures, and infants. Otherwise, fever reduction methods (see Chapter 20) are used to control fever and prevent seizures.

Caution should be exercised when any anticonvulsant drugs are used because of the side effects the child might experience. Drowsiness, irritability, gastrointestinal problems, and blood dyscrasias are among the possible side effects of seizure medications. Diphenylhydantoin might cause gingival hypertrophy. Good oral hygiene, gum massage with an electric toothbrush, and regular dental examinations will help to decrease this problem. Clonazepam can cause excessive upper respiratory secretions. Because of the risk of aspiration, this drug needs to be used with caution for severely disabled children.

All anticonvulsants must be given daily, usually in divided doses, to maintain therapeutic serum levels. Abrupt cessation of medication can lower the seizure threshold and precipitate status epilepticus (see the section on status epilepticus later in the chapter).

Another form of treatment for recurrent seizures is dietary therapy. The *ketogenic diet* is based on inducing ketosis by high fat and low protein and carbohydrate intake. Its use is reserved for young children (2–5 years of age) with minor motor or petit mal seizures refractive to anticonvulsant medication. This special diet is designed to induce a state simulating the ketosis and acidosis of starvation, which reduces seizure activity by an unknown mechanism. Adequate protein (1–1.5/g/kg of body weight), high fat, and low carbohydrate are calculated in a rigidly controlled diet, and vitamin supplements are given.

Surgery is considered if anticonvulsant treatment is unsuccessful and a focus of seizure activity is proven amenable to surgery.

Nursing management Nurses play an important role in both the acute management of seizures and the ongoing care of the child and family. Seizures can elicit fear, misunderstanding, and feelings of helplessness in the child and those around the child, including nurses and other health care professionals who are unfamiliar with seizures. Nursing responsibilities include not only health supervision and teaching with the child and family but also community education to help reduce the stigmas and negative attitudes associated with seizures.

Acute care Nursing management begins with being prepared for the occurrence of seizures in any child who is at risk from alteration in cerebral function (such as head trauma, meningitis or other neurologic disease, brain tumor, or drug ingestion). Seizure precautions include padding side rails to prevent injury and keeping oropharyngeal suctioning equipment, oxygen, and a soft rubber airway at the child's bedside. Additional safety measures involve close supervision during ambulation or mealtimes to protect the child from injury caused by falls or the aspiration of food during a seizure.

During the acute stage of a seizure, nursing care focuses on protecting the child from injury, maintaining an airway, and observing the seizure activity. At the onset of a grand mal seizure, the child becomes rigid and falls. If the child is not in bed, the nurse attempts to break the child's fall and ease the child to the floor. The nurse loosens any tight clothing around the neck and holds the child's head gently

TABLE 31-5 Nursing Observations During a Seizure

Time	Criteria for observation
Preseizure	Activity or status of the child Awake or asleep Febrile Excited
	Aura Behavior changes Complaints of abdominal pain, fear, or unusual sensations
	Antecedent events Flickering or bright lights Loud or buzzing noises Emotional stress
Seizure activity	Time of onset
	Cry
	Fall—forceful or slow drop
	Description of body movements Localized or full-body involvement Position of head and body Tone—rigid or limp Clonic jerking or twitching Sequence and type of movements
	Facial characteristics Color—cyanotic, or flushed Twitching—parts of face involved Eye position and movements Pupil changes Jaw clenching Frothing of secretions
	Respirations Absence of respiratory effort—length, depth, and quality of respirations Adequacy of airway
	Bladder or bowel incontinence
	Length of seizure
Postseizure (postictal phase)	Activity or status of the child Awake or sleeping Oriented Drowsy Confused Changes in motor function—weakness, movement Complaints of headache or pain Assessment of any injuries sustained at the onset of the seizure

to the side with the neck extended to maintain the airway and facilitate the drainage of secretions.

Nothing should ever be forced into the child's mouth to prevent tongue biting. Any injury caused by the teeth clenching shut usually occurs at the onset of the seizure, and trying to insert tongue blades, spoons, or other objects after a seizure has begun can cause more severe damage to the teeth and mouth. If the child's mouth is open, the nurse may place the edge of a soft piece of gauze between the child's teeth to avoid repetitive biting.

The nurse does not attempt to restrain the child's movements; any attempt to do so can result in musculoskeletal injury. Objects that the child might strike should be moved away, and the nurse places a small pillow or other soft object under the child's head to prevent it from banging against the floor. Unless the child is in a dangerous position (such as near a radiator, stove, or stairs), the nurse does not move the child until the seizure subsides.

The nurse allows the seizure to run its course, attending the child constantly to maintain the airway and prevent injury. The nurse also observes the seizure manifestations, times the duration, and monitors for complications of aspiration or status epilepticus. During a prolonged grand mal seizure, the nurse might need to suction excessive secretions from the child. Oxygen administration and airway placement is indicated when respiratory effort is impaired. Parenteral anticonvulsant medication might be necessary to halt prolonged or repetitive seizures.

Following the seizure, the nurse helps the child (carries if necessary) to a private area to rest. The nurse explains simply and calmly that the child has had a seizure, that the child is all right, and that someone will stay with the child. The child often will sleep deeply after a major motor seizure and should not be roused or disturbed unnecessarily. The nurse takes the child's vital signs, which often are altered temporarily during and immediately after a seizure. It is important for the nurse to determine whether the child is febrile because an elevated body temperature can trigger seizures in some children. The nurse identifies other precipitators of seizures by the history and clinical examination. These might include an inadequate serum anticonvulsant level, metabolic alteration, or illness.

The child with recurrent seizures does not require medical attention every time a seizure occurs. Most major motor seizures stop spontaneously, without any need for intervention other than protection and observation. Accurate observation and description of seizure activity are extremely valuable in diagnosis and management. (The observations the nurse makes before, during, and following a seizure are outlined in Table 31-5.) These observations also can be useful in eliciting a history of the child's seizures and should include the time of day, frequency, and whether the child sustained any injury from the seizure.

Chronic care The child with a seizure disorder needs long-term monitoring and care directed toward achieving the best possible control of the seizures and promoting optimal adjustment. The nurse's role in both acute and outpatient settings includes teaching the child and family about anticonvulsant medications, monitoring the child for medication effects and seizure activity, and providing support and counseling for the family.

The nurse manages the child with a newly diagnosed seizure disorder and the family carefully, helping them to cope with the initial crisis period. The child and family often are frightened by the term *epilepsy* and are affected by their concept of the stigmas associated with this condition. They will have many questions about the diagnosis, treatment, prognosis, and handling of the child. The nurse offers information, being careful not to overwhelm the child and parents with lengthy, extensive explanations that they might not be ready to hear. The nurse is alert to cues from the family about what they are able to absorb in the early stages. Often, the nurse needs to repeat material over a period of time as the family goes through the process of adjustment.

Instructing the family about the seizures and how to manage the child during a seizure are initial teaching goals. The specific aspects of management will vary depending on the type of seizure disorder. For major motor seizures, the parent is instructed to protect the child from injury, maintain the child's airway, and seek emergency medical care if the seizure is prolonged or recurs immediately.

A common misconception is that the tongue will be swallowed if something is not placed in the child's mouth. The nurse often needs to instruct the family not to force anything into the child's mouth during a seizure. The nurse explains that the child usually will sleep or be lethargic following the seizure and encourages the family to allow the child to rest during recovery.

The nurse describes other types of seizures as indicated and teaches the family the appropriate safety precautions. Depending on the seizure manifestations and the degree of control achieved with medication, these precautions might include close supervision in situations where a sudden loss of consciousness could produce injury (such as swimming or climbing to heights). Children who fall frequently because of seizures must wear protective helmets or faceguards to prevent head and facial injuries.

Teaching about anticonvulsant medication, the effects, side effects, and importance of cooperation is an essential nursing responsibility. The child and family are taught how to take the medication, what side effects to watch for, and why periodic laboratory monitoring is necessary. If the child's seizures are well controlled, the need for continuing to take the anticonvulsant medication might not be apparent to the child and family. The nurse stresses the important fact that the medication be administered regularly to prevent the seizures from recurring. The nurse works out a convenient schedule of medication administration that best fits in with the child's daily routine. Older children can be taught to assume responsibility for taking their own medication.

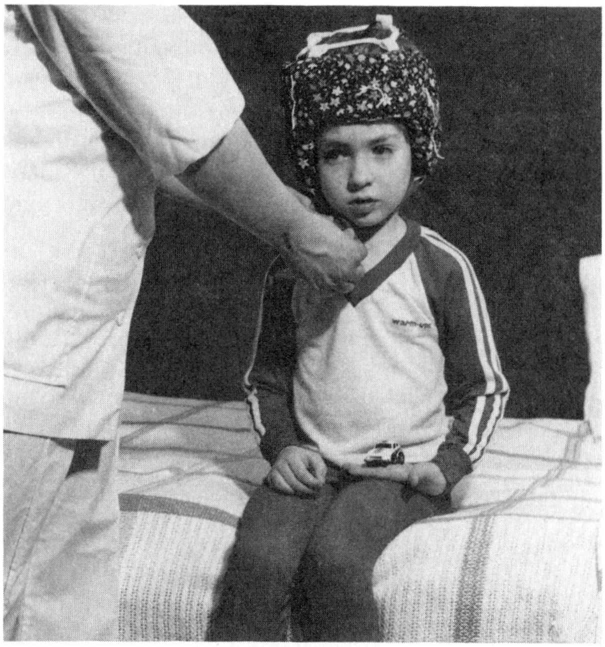

The child who experiences frequent seizures might require a protective helmet to prevent head injury. (From Swearingen PL: The Addison-Wesley Photo-Atlas of Nursing Procedures. *Addison-Wesley, 1984, p. 611, with permission.)*

Families often are concerned about the risks of toxicity, undesirable side effects, and dosage adjustments. The nurse instructs the family to keep a record of the child's seizures and responses to medication because this information is vital to ongoing management. Repeated medication changes are needed to try to control seizures in some children with seizure disorders.

At times, the degree of impairment caused by the seizures must be weighed against the impairments caused by the side effects of anticonvulsant medications, such as drowsiness. Achieving a balance of the best control possible with the fewest side effects can be a lengthy, frustrating process, during which the family requires consistent, responsive support and guidance.

The nurse advises the child and family about the factors that can precipitate seizure activity. A lowered seizure threshold often occurs with fever. The nurse therefore teaches the family fever control measures, which are important for preventing seizures.

The child who has an illness that results in vomiting

might be unable to tolerate anticonvulsant medication, which can result in seizures. The nurse advises the family to consult their physician for procedures to follow when the child has missed doses of medication. The child might be given antiemetic medications or parenteral anticonvulsant medications temporarily.

Increased seizure activity also can accompany other illnesses, alterations in the fluid and electrolyte balance, excessive fatigue, or severe stress. Certain stimuli, such as flickering lights (such as from televisions, strobe lights, or fluorescent lights) or particular sounds (rhythmic mechanical buzzing or sudden, sharp noises), can precipitate seizures in a few children. The child often is more likely to have seizures while drifting off to sleep or awakening, which is associated with changes in the brain's electrical activity during the transition from sleeping to waking states and vice versa.

Seizure activity might increase during puberty, although many children have fewer seizures as they mature. Premenstrual fluid retention can precipitate seizures, and diuretics might be prescribed for girls who encounter this problem. In addition, some medications, such as antihistamines, central nervous system stimulants, and alcohol, can lower the seizure threshold. The nurse urges both the child and family to follow prescribed guidelines in taking other medications and encourages them to always ask if they are unsure about a particular drug's effects. Adolescents must be informed adequately about the potential hazards of drug or alcohol use precipitating seizures or interacting with anticonvulsant medications.

The nurse pays particular attention to the psychosocial adaptation of the child and family to the seizure disorder. The family might feel a natural tendency to overprotect and expect less of the child. They might feel guilty about the child's condition or fear that disciplining the child might provoke a seizure.

The nurse corrects their misconceptions and stresses the importance that the child's developing independence be fostered. Safety and supervision requirements for each child are determined on an individual basis and depend on the severity and type of seizures and any other disabilities present (such as physical handicaps or cognitive or sensory limitations).

The activities of most children with good seizure control do not need to be limited or restricted beyond the minimal precautions for swimming or climbing. The family often is faced with the dilemma of protecting the child adequately while simultaneously fostering growth. The family often can benefit from the sharing offered by support groups composed of other parents of children with epilepsy.

As the family members become more confident about their ability to care for the child, they often are more receptive to interventions geared toward promoting the child's independence, which might involve some risks. For example, allowing the child to travel on the school bus, stay at a friend's house, or ride a bicycle might provoke intense anxiety and fear that the child might have a seizure. The family needs ongoing support and encouragement in their continual struggle to accept and manage appropriately the child with a seizure disorder.

Public attitudes and acceptance regarding seizures are continuing problems for the child and family. Social stigmas associated with seizures are common and reflect a general misunderstanding of epilepsy. As a liaison and advocate, the nurse promotes the child's acceptance in school and the community by correcting misinformation, dispelling myths, and increasing public awareness of the facts about epilepsy. The Epilepsy Foundation of America (4351 Garden City Drive, Landover, MD 20785) is an excellent resource for educational materials, support groups, and special services.

Nurses in community health and school settings can contribute greatly to educating the public about seizures and helping to demystify the disorder. The school nurse is in an ideal position to both monitor the child with a seizure disorder and promote understanding of seizures by teachers and other children. The child who has seizures in school might need a rest period after a major seizure but most often is able to resume class activities and should not be sent home or isolated unnecessarily. Teachers and others dealing with the child must be prepared for the possible occurrence of seizures and instructed in how to manage them.

The reactions of other children to a seizure tend to reflect the responsible adult's response. If adults react in a calm and reassuring manner and provide simple explanations about what has occurred, the child's classmates will not be fearful or overreact. If, on the other hand, those in charge respond with panic and revulsion to the child's seizure, the other children will react accordingly, perpetuating the negative attitude toward the disorder. The school staff should be instructed to protect the child from embarrassment by asking curious onlookers not to stand and stare. Following the seizure, the child should be allowed privacy to rest and change clothes if incontinence occurred.

Many children with seizure disorders attend a regular school program and can participate in a range of normal activities with few restrictions. The needs of some children with poorly controlled seizures or other disabilities (physical, cognitive, or sensory deficits) are best met in a specialized educational program that offers individual therapeutic services.

The child with a seizure disorder, like any child with a disability, will experience additional stresses related to poor self-image, dependency needs, and feeling different. The child's sense of self-control and mastery are particularly vulnerable because the loss of control during seizures can leave the child feeling inferior and insecure. The child often is acutely embarrassed after having a seizure, particularly

STANDARDS OF NURSING CARE *The Child with a Seizure Disorder*

GUIDE FOR NURSING MANAGEMENT

Nursing diagnosis	Intervention	Rationale	Outcome
1. Potential knowledge deficit concerning seizure management (stressors: anxiety, unfamiliarity with procedure or resources, misconceptions)	Teach the child and family about what happens during a seizure, alterations in electrical activity in the brain, and types of seizures. Correct misperceptions about etiology, trigger factors, and mental disturbance.	Knowledge about what happens during a seizure decreases fear.	The family can describe the causes of seizures and correct management of a seizure. Family members accurately report seizure activity and recognize the need for emergency care if status epilepticus occurs.
	Teach the family how to care for the child during a seizure: Break the child's fall when possible. Turn the child's head to the side. Extend the child's neck to open the airway. Remove tight neck clothing. Place a soft pad under the child's head. Move surrounding objects. *Do not* place anything in the child's mouth. Do not restrict the child's movements. Move the child when the seizure is over.	Learning a step-by-step method of handling a seizure can increase the parent's feeling of confidence and decrease anxiety.	
	Instruct the family to keep a record of seizures and to describe and report them to the child's physician. Describe status epilepticus and instruct the family when to call for emergency help if it occurs.	Accurate descriptions of seizures can help pinpoint a diagnosis.	
	Promote epilepsy education in the schools and community.	Epilepsy education can decrease misunderstandings about children with seizures and promote rapid acceptance of the child into the community.	
2. Potential injury (stressors: uncontrolled random movements, misconceptions of seizure management, falls)	In the hospital, maintain seizure precautions—padded side rails, side rails fully raised, oxygen, suction and airway equipment at the bedside; supervise ambulation and mealtimes; take rectal or axillary temperatures.	These measures ensure the child's safety in the hospital.	The child remains free from injury during a seizure. The parents can describe safety precautions.

(Continues)

STANDARDS OF NURSING CARE *The Child with a Seizure Disorder (Continued)*

GUIDE FOR NURSING MANAGEMENT

Nursing diagnosis	Intervention	Rationale	Outcome
	Teach the family about the potential risks of injury from a seizure while climbing or swimming. Help the family to obtain a protective helmet/faceguard for the child who falls frequently. Advise the family about safety measures in the home as appropriate: Padded table edge Carpeted stairs Use of stove Use of sharp utensils Care while bathing or showering	These measures increase the child's safety at home.	
	Prepare adolescents for possible restrictions in obtaining a driver's license.	Knowing what the restrictions will be helps the adolescent deal with them.	
3. Potential knowledge deficit concerning seizure prevention (stressors: fever, medication administration and interaction)	Teach the child and family the importance of giving anticonvulsant medication consistently. Instruct the family to notify the physician if the child is unable to take medication by mouth.	Consistent medication administration can control seizures.	The child's seizure activity is not increased as a result of high fever or inconsistent medication administration.
	Teach the family the methods of fever control.	Some seizures are triggered by fever.	
	Advise the family to check with the child's physician before giving the child any other medication (especially antihistamines).	Other medications might react adversely with the seizure medication.	
	Inform the physician of any increase in seizure frequency or change in the type of seizure.	Changes in the pattern or frequency of seizures might call for a medication change.	
	Teach the family about the adverse effects of medication, the necessity to monitor blood levels, and methods of alleviating side effects (eg, oral hygiene for gum hypertrophy).	Knowledge of adverse side effects can enable the family to identify and report them early or take measures to counteract them.	
4. Potential ineffective individual coping (stressors: anxiety, anger, fear of inability to handle social or school situations)	Use age-appropriate method to encourage the child to express fears, anger, sense of loss of control, and rejection.	Verbal expression of fears allows the child to be more realistic and increases coping.	The child is able to express fears and face them realistically. The child states feelings of confidence and the ability to handle a stressful situation.
	Encourage the child to make choices about care and activities whenever possible.	Encouraging choices gives the child a feeling of control.	

STANDARDS OF NURSING CARE *The Child with a Seizure Disorder (Continued)*

GUIDE FOR NURSING MANAGEMENT

Nursing diagnosis	Intervention	Rationale	Outcome
	Encourage the child's independence as much as possible, taking safety precautions as appropriate.	Independence can increase self-esteem and assist with coping.	
	Provide anticipatory guidance and problem solving to help the child handle seizures at school and reactions from peers.	Role playing gives the child an opportunity to handle potentially stressful situations in a nonstressful environment.	
	Refer the child for individual or peer group counseling.	Peer support can increase coping strategies.	

when it occurs in the presence of peers. Being labeled "weird" or different because of seizures is a social catastrophe for the child. Friends might reject the child at a time during childhood or adolescence when peer group acceptance is vitally important. Both the child and family might try to hide the condition in an attempt to avoid others' reactions.

The adolescent with a seizure disorder faces special stresses from restrictions on obtaining a driver's license, worries about getting and keeping a job, peer pressures to try alcohol and drugs, and anxieties about dating. The adolescent's struggle for independence is a difficult task, and the adolescent might react by denying the condition, stopping the medication, and rebelling against parental restrictions.

The nurse caring for the child with a seizure disorder encourages the child and family to share their fears and express their frustrations. The nurse explores coping strategies the family might use. The nurse helps the family to develop a plan for action if a seizure occurs in different situations, allowing them to solve problems ahead of time. Assessing the child's and family's adaptation and recognizing problems that require referral for more intensive counseling are important nursing functions.

Status Epilepticus

Status epilepticus is a condition in which seizures are prolonged or repeated without the child's regaining consciousness. This condition presents a medical emergency because hypoxia, hypotension, cardiac arrhythmias, and respiratory depression or arrest are potential complications. Failure to adhere to anticonvulsant medication regimens is a frequent cause of status epilepticus in children with a previously diagnosed seizure disorder. Other precipitants include metabolic disturbances (hypoglycemia, hypocalcemia), central nervous system infection, and intracranial trauma or hemorrhage.

Status epilepticus must be treated promptly to prevent life-threatening complications. It requires rapid assessment of respiratory and cardiac functions and readiness in the event of cardiopulmonary arrest. Treatment is directed toward maintaining an airway and promoting effective gas exchange, administering intravenous anticonvulsants, correcting metabolic alterations, and treating the underlying cause of the episode.

An episode of status epilepticus requires critical nursing assessments and care. In addition to the same care associated with seizures, the nurse monitors for signs of cardiopulmonary arrest, signs of metabolic and electrolyte disturbances, and effects of intravenous medications.

Following the cessation of status epilepticus, the nurse monitors the child closely, assessing vital signs and level of consciousness and watching for abnormal neurologic signs such as a recurrence of seizure activity or focal neurologic deficits. The child often will be unconscious for prolonged periods following the seizure activity because of both postictal exhaustion and sedation from medications given.

The Child with Congenital Malformations of the Central Nervous System

Hydrocephalus

Hydrocephalus is a condition with multiple causes that results in an increased amount of CSF within the ventricles of the brain. Increased CSF can be caused by obstructions to normal flow of the CSF system, overproduction of CSF, or inadequate reabsorption of CSF in the subarachnoid villa. Hydrocephalus might be present at birth as a result of embryonic malformation or might occur secondary to injury, infection, or space-occupying lesions.

Hydrocephalus can be classified as *noncommunicating* or *communicating* depending on the mechanism of alteration in CSF. Noncommunicating hydrocephalus results from obstruction of CSF flow from the ventricles of the brain to the subarachnoid space. This obstruction can occur at any point in the ventricular system. Aqueductal stenosis, a narrowing or obstruction of the aqueduct of Sylvius between the third and fourth ventricles is the most frequently seen type of noncommunicating hydrocephalus. Communicating hydrocephalus results when CSF flow is not obstructed through the ventricles but is inadequately circulated or reabsorbed in the subarachnoid space.

Postinfectious, posthemorrhagic hydrocephalus involves meningeal inflammation or subarachnoid hemorrhage and can result in fibrous tissue formation in the subarachnoid space or ventricular obstruction. Bacterial meningitis, toxoplasmosis, and cytomegalic inclusion disease can result in this type of hydrocephalus.

In addition to infection, acquired hydrocephalus of both types can result from cerebral trauma or tumors interfering with CSF circulation at any point in the system.

Clinical manifestations The signs and symptoms of hydrocephalus depend on the age at onset and the degree of increased CSF volume within the brain. From infancy through 2 years of age, enlarging head size, bulging, nonpulsating fontanelles, and downward rotation of the eyes with scleras visible above the iris ("setting sun sign") are characteristic signs of hydrocephalus. Scalp veins might be distended and cranial sutures separated. Poor feeding, vomiting, lethargy, irritability, and developmental delays accompany progressive hydrocephalus. A characteristic high-pitched cry and abnormal muscle tone might be present.

In older children the cranial sutures are closed and head circumference changes are less common. Signs of increased ICP such as vomiting, ataxia, and headache are common. Late signs include alterations in consciousness and papilledema. Cognitive development might be impaired and accompanied by behavioral (hyperactive) and learning disabilities in chronic forms of hydrocephalus.

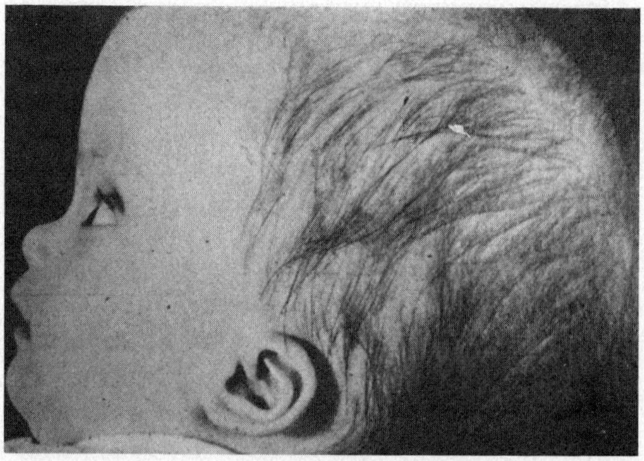

Infant with hydrocephalus. Note enlarged occipital area and lateral view of the sunset eyes.

Diagnostic evaluation Head circumference changes in infancy that increase faster than the normal rate indicate the need for further diagnostic assessment of enlarged head size. Transillumination of the skull with a flashlight and special rubber adapter is performed in a darkened room to determine the presence of asymmetric areas of increased light. Transillumination usually does not reveal asymmetric light areas in hydrocephalus but does with subdural hematomas (bleeding in the subdural space, usually a result of trauma). Serial transilluminations are performed to detect increases in light areas.

CT scanning is performed to determine the size and position of the ventricles and subarachnoid spaces. Dilatation of the ventricles can be determined readily, as well as the presence of tumors or other space-occupying lesions. Cerebrospinal fluid circulation and obstructions to CSF flow or reabsorption can be evaluated by injecting dye into the lumbar subarachnoid space and obtaining CT scans several times to measure the course of the CSF. In most instances the CT scan has replaced pneumoencephalography in the diagnosis of hydrocephalus. Other studies, such as angiography or radioisotope scanning, might be needed in the diagnosis of hydrocephalus.

Treatment Hydrocephalus is treated by surgery either to correct an obstruction to CSF circulation or to implant a shunting device to divert the CSF. When a mass, lesion, or adhesions within the CSF system are identified and surgically accessible, they are treated directly. More commonly, progressive hydrocephalus is managed by ventricular shunting procedures.

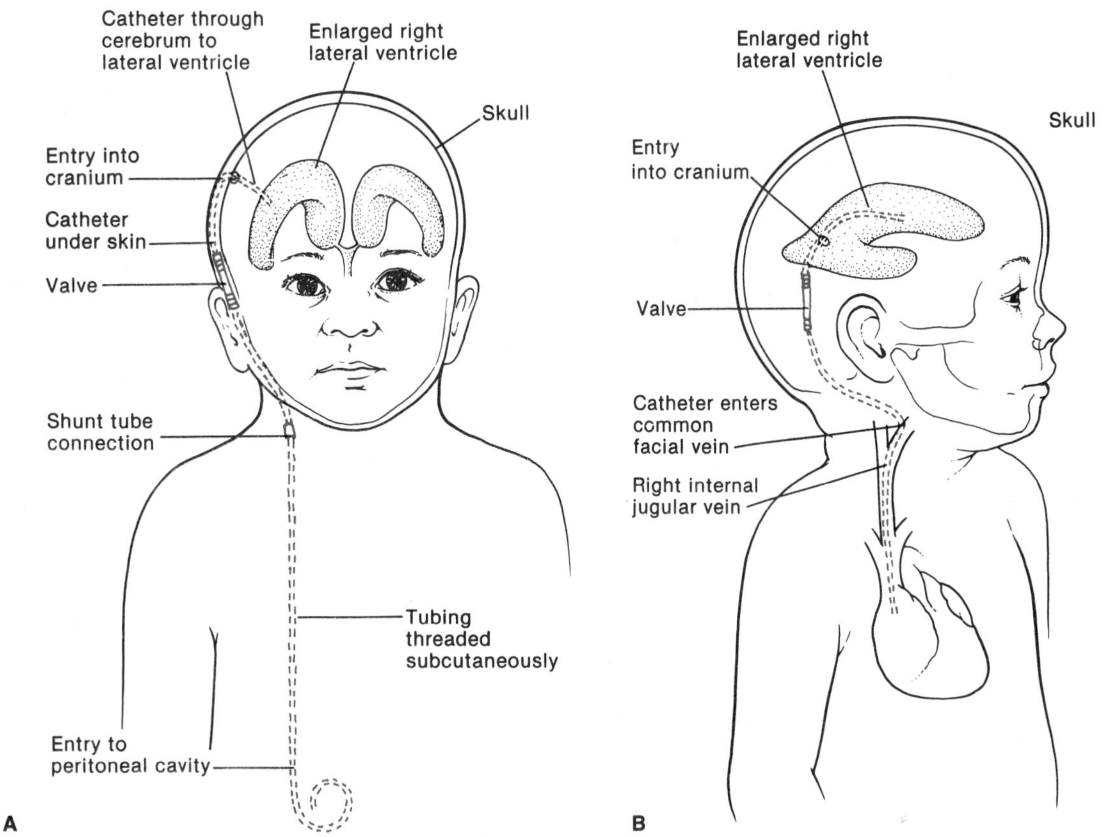

FIGURE 31-2

A. *Ventriculoperitoneal shunt with the distal end of the tubing located in the peritoneum and coiled to allow lengthening as the child grows.* ***B.*** *Ventriculovascular shunt with the distal end of the tubing located in the superior vena cava.*

Both types of hydrocephalus can be treated with bypass shunts, which carry the CSF from the ventricle, divert it extracranially, and drain it into another body compartment. The shunt is made up of a ventricular catheter, one-way valve, and distal catheter. A reservoir might be placed in the ventricular catheter near the valve to give access to the shunt to measure pressure, culture CSF, or instill antibiotics.

Various types of valves are used that permit one-way flow of CSF away from the ventricles. The valves are set to open at different intraventricular pressures depending on the degree of increased CSF pressure. The distal catheter attaches to the valve and is directed to the designated body cavity for drainage.

Although other sites occasionally might be used, most ventricular shunts in children drain either into the peritoneum or the superior vena cava. *Ventriculoperitoneal (VP) shunts* are threaded subcutaneously against the cranium and down the chest to the abdominal wall, where the catheter is inserted to drain the CSF into the peritoneal cavity. The end of the catheter might be coiled to allow the shunt to "grow" with the child without displacing the distal tip (Fig. 31-2A). Ventriculovascular shunts are threaded similarly extracranially but then are routed into the venous system to the superior vena cava. The drained CSF enters the vascular flow to the right atrium (Fig. 31-2B).

Both types of shunts might require periodic revision as the child grows or if a shunt obstruction occurs. Obstruction might be due to tissue particles, venous clotting, or bacterial colonization. Common shunt complications are obstruction, infection, and disconnection of the tubing. With obstruction, sudden or gradual symptoms of increased ICP develop. Infection might be acute in onset or develop gradually over time. An infected shunt is removed, and the child is treated with appropriate antibiotics.

Alternative shunting devices are placed if the child continues to need CSF diversion. One complication of ventriculovascular shunts is bacterial endocarditis and bacteremia, which requires antibiotic treatment and shunt revision. If the shunt becomes disconnected, surgery is performed to reconnect the tubing.

Nursing management Preoperative nursing care for the child with hydrocephalus is similar to that for any preoperative child, with several special considerations. The nurse monitors the child's neurologic status periodically. The nurse pays particular attention to the child with acute-onset hydrocephalus, watching for changes indicative of increasing ICP.

The child might have a markedly enlarged head, the weight of which prevents the child from moving or being held easily. The nurse positions the child carefully and uses sheepskin or cushions to prevent skin breakdown. The child can be held with the child's head on a pillow and support from an armchair (McElroy, 1980).

Postoperatively, the nurse assesses the child frequently for changes in vital signs or neurologic status (see Standards of Nursing Care, The Child Following Neurosurgery). Any preoperative medications, such as anticonvulsants, are continued postoperatively. A follow-up CT scan is done to determine ventricular size.

The child who has had surgery to revise the distal portion of a shunt will have a briefer recovery period than the child who has had an initial shunt placed. In children who demonstrated preoperative lethargy and decreased awareness, marked improvements often occur in the level of consciousness postoperatively.

The family needs a clear explanation of the shunting procedure, support through the operative period, and education in preparation for discharge. The family might be afraid of displacing the shunt by handling the child or might restrict the child's activity level unnecessarily. The nurse helps the family members to palpate the shunt and valve and reassures them that normal activity will not interfere with shunt function. The physician might recommend that activities that place the child at higher risk for head injury (such as contact sports) be avoided. Guidance is geared to the specific child's age and developmental level.

The nurse describes the signs of shunt obstruction and infection to the family. The family members are taught to observe the child for lethargy, headache, vomiting, eye turning, visual disturbances, or pupil changes. A child with a shunt infection might exhibit increased ICP and fever, stiff neck, nausea, vomiting, and seizures. The family is encouraged to contact the child's primary health care provider if shunt problems are suspected.

The family members might or might not be instructed to "pump" the reservoir of the shunt to check for patency. Some physicians demonstrate this maneuver to parents but advise them not to pump the shunt reservoir routinely. It is important for parents to understand the basic mechanics of the shunt, but it generally is unnecessary or contraindicated for them to compress the reservoir or valves.

Children with hydrocephalus might have developmental or focal neurologic deficits that persist after shunting because of cerebral damage or nervous system malformation. The types and severity of impairment depend on the original disorder (such as congenital, tumor, trauma, or infection) and the degree of hydrocephalus present before shunting. Frequent follow-up evaluations are essential to monitor the child's development and plan rehabilitative interventions early.

Myelodysplasia

The term *myelodysplasia* encompasses a group of related central nervous system disorders characterized by malformations of the neural tube that occur during embryonic development. They include syndromes involving abnormalities in the vertebral column, spinal meninges, and spinal cord (that is, spina bifida occulta, meningocele, and myelomeningocele).

Failure of the midline of the neural plate to close as it forms the neural tube during the third and fourth weeks of gestation is believed to be responsible for these overt and occult spinal defects. The severity of these defects ranges from asymptomatic to severely disabling. Other CNS anomalies might be associated with these defects.

The specific cause of myelodysplasia is not known. Combined hereditary and environmental factors are believed to contribute, and the familial incidence is known to be higher than that for the general population. For families with one affected child, the risk of recurrence increases to 1 in 20–50. With two affected children, the risk of recurrence is 1 in 10 (Carmel, 1982). Siblings and other family members also are at greater risk than the general population of having a child with a neural tube defect.

The incidence estimates vary, but spina bifida occulta is known to occur widely in the general population without evidence of neural dysfunction. A small percentage of affected individuals develop some lower extremity involvement, usually with increasing age (Passo, 1980). Meningocele without neural involvement occurs less often than myelomeningocele. The incidence of these defects, referred to collectively as *spina bifida cystica,* varies worldwide, with the highest number of cases found in Great Britain.

Clinical manifestations *Spina bifida occulta* is a defect in closure of the vertebral laminae in which the meninges or neural tissue are not exposed at the skin surface (Fig. 31-3A). The usual site of this condition is the lumbosacral area. Underlying malformation of the spinal cord and nerve roots might or might not be present.

Although most cases of spina bifida occulta go undetected throughout life, external skin abnormalities such as a small nevus or hemangioma, dimple, or hair tuft might be present. A dermal sinus often is associated with the vertebral abnormality, forming a blind tract that does not extend to the dura mater or spinal cord. This tract, referred

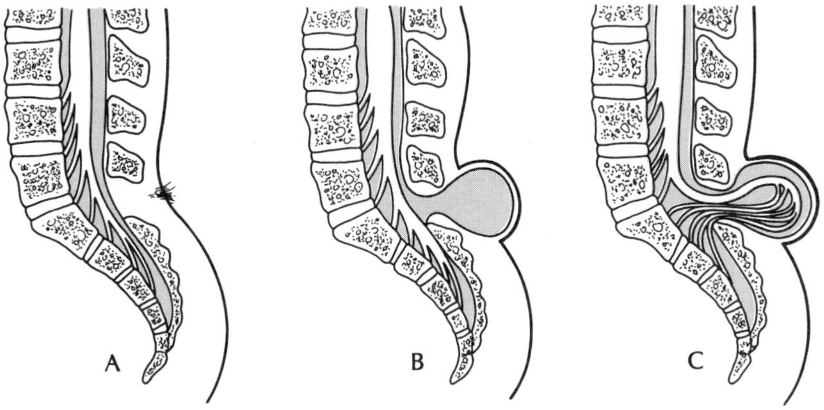

FIGURE 31-3

Midsaggital view of the spinal column showing various degrees of neural defect. ***A.*** *Spina bifida occulta. Note that the vertebral arches have not fused. There is no herniation of the spinal cord.* ***B.*** *Meningocele. The meninges protrude through the spina bifida, forming a saclike cyst that is visible on the infant's back.* ***C.*** *Myelomeningocele. Meninges, elements of the spinal cord and its nerves, and cerebrospinal fluid protrude through the spina bifida. Externally, this defect resembles a meningocele.*

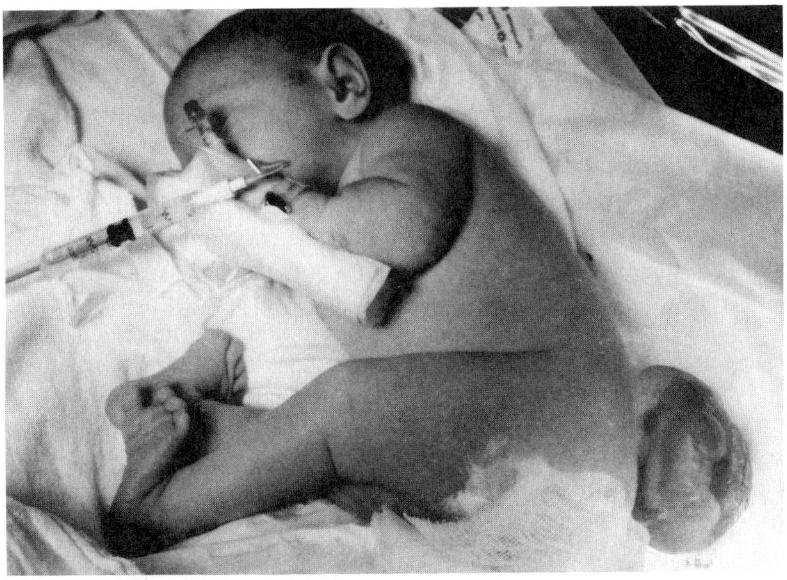

Infant with lumbar myelomeningocele. (Courtesy of Dr. Paul Winchester.)

to as a pilonidal sinus, might become a focus of infection and require surgical closure later in life.

Meningocele is a defect in which the meninges and CSF protrude through the unfused vertebral arches, appearing as a saclike cyst at the defective area (Fig. 31-3B). The spinal cord is not involved. A soft, cystic mass containing meninges and CSF is apparent at birth, usually in the lumbosacral or sacral area. The cyst might be covered with a thick membrane or epithelial tissue and can be completely transilluminated. The spinal nerve roots might be displaced, but their function remains intact. The absence of neurologic involvement is evidenced by normal motor, sensory, reflex, and sphincter function. Hydrocephalus might be associated with the meningocele.

Myelomeningocele is a cystlike protrusion at the area of vertebral defect that resembles a meningocele but includes the distended abnormal portion of the spinal cord as well as the meninges and CSF (Fig. 31-3C). Myelomeningocele occurs at a rate of 1 in every 1000 live births, making it the second most frequent birth defect (Richardson et al., 1985).

When spinal cord segments are involved in the cystic malformation, the most prominent clinical manifestation is flaccid paralysis of the lower extremities. Varying degrees of motor, sensory, reflex, and sphincter dysfunction are present, depending on the location and severity of the spinal abnormality. A large majority of defects occur in the lumbar or lumbosacral area.

In general, lesions at L3 or above result in total paraplegia, sensory loss, and bowel and bladder incontinence. Involvement at lower spinal cord levels is accompanied by partial preservation of muscular, sensory, or sphincter function; the lower the lesion, the less the neurologic deficit.

Almost all children with lumbar or lumbosacral myelomeningocele develop hydrocephalus of varying severity. This abnormality usually is due to associated embryonic malformations of the CSF circulation in the brain, most notably the *Arnold-Chiari malformation* (malformation of the lower brain stem and cerebellum). Functional motor disability is greatest in children with spinal cord lesions at L3 and above. Motor paralysis often results in musculoskeletal deformities, which can compromise the child's mobility further. Partial innervation of muscle groups (flexor and extensor muscles) causes unequal pull at various joints, resulting in dislocation and contractures.

Hip dislocation occurs frequently, which in turn contributes to the development of scoliosis. Contractures of the hips, knees, and ankles result from muscle imbalance and are progressive if not prevented through positioning and surgical correction. Various foot deformities, commonly the equinovarus type, occur with myelomeningocele.

Small muscle bulk and osteoporosis result from the lack of normal innervation and use. Fractures of the lower extremities are a common complication of bony atrophy in these children. Sensory deficits and circulatory alterations predispose the child to pressure decubiti and unnoticed heat or traumatic injuries of the affected areas of the body.

Bowel and bladder dysfunction usually results in incontinence, with sphincter paralysis, chronic retention of urine, and constipation. The child dribbles urine intermittently or continuously without effective bladder evacuation. Incomplete bladder emptying can lead to the serious urologic complications of recurrent infection, ureteral reflux, and renal impairment. Lack of bowel tone often results in the retention of feces. Rectal prolapse might accompany rectal sphincter paralysis and poor bowel tone.

Other neurologic sequelae might accompany myelomeningocele, caused by structural deformities and neuronal damage. Cognitive, perceptual, and learning disabilities of varying severity can be present, most often associated with hydrocephalus.

Treatment Meningocele is treated by surgical closure of the defect at birth. The child is observed carefully for complications of meningitis, hydrocephalus, and spinal cord dysfunction. Close neurologic follow-up is important to monitor the child's head circumference and sensorimotor development.

Management of the child with myelomeningocele is complex, beginning at birth and continuing throughout the child's lifetime. Most neonates with this condition are transferred immediately to tertiary care centers, where surgery is performed to close the myelomeningocele (dura mater, connective tissue, and skin) within 24 hours of birth. This reduces the risk of infection and might prevent further neurologic impairment.

Skin grafting often is necessary to repair the defect. The presence of hemorrhage, infection, or rapidly expanding hydrocephalus contraindicate surgery on the myelomeningocele until these conditions are controlled. The decision not to perform surgery in the early neonatal period also might be related to the severity of the malformation and associated congenital anomalies.

Prophylactic antibiotics are administered before, during, and following surgery. The operative site is protected from contamination and pressure by positioning. The infant is observed for signs of hydrocephalus, which might follow closure of the myelomeningocele. The obstruction to the CSF flow usually existed prior to surgery, but CSF pressure is elevated when the cystic outlet for the fluid is removed. If indicated, a ventricular shunt is created to divert CSF and reduce ICP.

Urologic evaluation is performed early, and treatment is initiated to prevent urinary retention, infection, and renal damage. Periodic urine cultures, intravenous pyelograms, cystometrograms, and measurement of residual urine are done to monitor the child's urologic status. In infants the bladder might be emptied by Credé's method at regular (2- to 4-hour) intervals. *Credé's maneuver* is the exertion of manual pressure over the bladder to promote emptying. Because of the potential for bladder injury from Credé's maneuver, intermittent catheterization (see Chapter 28) might be preferred. Intermittent clean catheterization is used with good results in a large percentage of children. With increasing maturity, the child can be taught to perform this procedure.

Medications can be used to alter abnormal bladder tone and promote complete bladder emptying. A hypotonic bladder might respond to cholinergic agents to increase tone, and a hypertonic bladder can benefit from antispasmodic agents. Acute or chronic urinary tract infections are treated with appropriate antibiotics. The child might receive prophylactic urinary antiseptic medication for its bacteriostatic action.

When these measures fail to prevent secondary urologic complications, surgical diversion of the urinary tract might be necessary. In an ileal loop bladder procedure, the ureters are diverted to an artificial bladder that is formed from a resected ileal segment, which drains urine through an abdominal stoma to an external collecting bag. Other surgical procedures include the placement of artificial sphincter devices.

Bowel dysfunction is managed with dietary measures to alter stool consistency and with adjunctive methods to help the child achieve continence. Bisacodyl or glycerin suppositories; regular, timed toileting; and abdominal straining are often effective in a bowel program. Enemas and disimpaction might be necessary should constipation become severe.

Promoting the child's mobility and preventing musculoskeletal deformity are early and continuing goals of treatment. Orthopedic care involves exercise, braces, casts, and surgical correction to achieve these goals. Equipment such as body jackets and long or short leg braces maintain good anatomic alignment and give the child more functional posture and support.

Ambulation is often possible for young children with myelomeningocele with bracing of the lower extremities and use of a walker or crutches. Older children with higher-level lesions might become more dependent on wheelchairs as functional ambulation becomes more difficult (Carmel, 1982). The child is still encouraged, however, to bear as much weight as possible using assistive devices to prevent osteoporosis and contractures.

Nursing management Nursing care for the child with myelodysplasia might involve acute care during infancy, care during subsequent hospitalizations, and outpatient or community follow-up in the long-term management of complex needs. The lifelong care of children with these conditions and their families is best achieved with coordinated treatment by a multidisciplinary team to promote optimal development and prevent secondary complications.

Immediate care at birth During infancy, the child with myelodysplasia requires intensive care both pre- and postoperatively.

Preoperatively, the meningeal sac is inspected for signs of abrasion, infection, or leakage of CSF. Topical antibiotics and a moist saline dressing to the cele might be prescribed. The infant is positioned on the abdomen with the head turned to the side to protect the sac from irritation, contamination, or rupture. The infant's hips are abducted with a pad to reduce hip dislocation, and the infant's feet are kept in a neutral position with a small blanket roll under the ankles. Sandbags might be used on either side of the infant to prevent rolling. Diapers and clothing are not used, and the infant is kept in an isolette to maintain warmth. The nurse changes the diaper pads beneath the infant frequently to prevent skin excoriation and protect the cele from contamination.

The nurse assesses the infant's sensorimotor function, noting spontaneous movement, response to stimulation, and any changes indicative of neurologic deterioration. The nurse also observes the infant closely for early signs of meningeal infection (elevated or subnormal temperature, irritability, pallor, vomiting, or nuchal rigidity).

Following surgery, the nurse observes the infant's vital and neurologic signs, head circumference, wound (for leakage of CSF or hemorrhage), and elimination. The infant is kept prone, and the operative site is protected from pressure or contamination until the wound is well healed. Behavioral changes such as restlessness, irritability, lethargy, or fever, vomiting, and pallor could indicate complications of meningitis or hydrocephalus and must be detected early.

Family support and teaching begin with the birth of the infant and continue as the infant matures. Within a short period of time, the family must adjust to the birth of an infant with a serious defect, consent to surgical treatment, and learn how to provide the infant's specialized physical care. Parent-infant bonding is encouraged by allowing the parent to participate in as much of the infant's care as possible. The nurse provides careful, repetitive explanations of the multisystem observations and care required as the family prepares to take the infant home. The nurse establishes liaisons and referrals for long-term care. Ongoing guidance, support, and treatment are best provided by the coordinated efforts of a multidisciplinary team that can communicate effectively with the family.

Chronic care The nurse teaches the family to avoid skin breakdown and injury resulting from the child's lack of sensory awareness. The nurse emphasizes the importance of avoiding pressure and temperature extremes and proper positioning and skin care measures. The nurse demonstrates how to perform range-of-motion exercises and apply braces, splints, or casts.

The child's ability to explore the environment and development are enhanced by devices to aid sitting and mobility, which are adapted to the individual child's needs. Low-sitting caster carts and prone scooter boards can be employed at early ages to allow children to move about with upper-extremity control. As the child begins ambulation using assistive devices, specialized programs are undertaken to teach the child transfers, gait, self-help skills, and safety measures.

If the child is at risk for hydrocephalus or has a shunt in place, the symptoms of increased ICP are explained to the family, and they are instructed to contact their neurologist or primary care provider should any concerns arise. As is the case with any child with hydrocephalus, shunt malfunctions can occur, requiring revision or removal of the shunt. Other neurologic sequelae, such as seizures, might require specialized therapy and teaching.

Management of elimination is a major focus of care to prevent serious complications. The nurse teaches the family to carry out the chosen elimination program, explains the rationale for the treatment, and describes the symptoms of urinary tract infection the family should watch for. With increasing maturity, the child can be involved increasingly in the bowel and bladder program. The nurse emphasizes prevention of urinary tract infections by ensuring adequate fluid intake and frequent bladder emptying.

A bowel program is begun when the child is around 2 years of age. The parent is encouraged to develop a regular daily routine of placing the child on the toilet and to use suppositories if needed. Problems with stool consistency are managed by dietary adjustments when possible, and the use of laxatives is avoided.

Incontinence remains a major problem for children with

myelomeningocele, and the psychosocial implications become increasingly negative as these children get older. Bowel continence usually can be achieved with some success if regularity is maintained, but bladder continence can be more difficult. The nurse works with the child and family to adapt the frequency and timing of the child's bladder emptying program and provide measures to prevent wetness, such as protective incontinence pads for girls or external catheter devices for boys.

The Spina Bifida Association of America (343 South Dearborn Street, Chicago, IL 60604) provides resource and educational materials and can refer families to local support groups.

Dietary guidance is important in ensuring adequate nutrition and managing elimination problems and also in preventing obesity, a common problem associated with myelomeningocele.

The child with myelomeningocele might be hospitalized repeatedly for orthopedic, urologic, or neurologic treatment. As much as possible, the child's mobility and elimination routines are maintained. When orthopedic surgery is performed, resulting in immobility and casting, the nurse pays special attention to skin care and observes the child carefully for circulatory or pressure complications that the child does not notice immediately because of sensory deficits. Urinary stasis and infection might occur more rapidly in these children, and the nurse observes the child for bladder distension and signs of urinary tract infection. Constipation is avoided with suppositories and enemas, and usual regimens are maintained when possible. Getting these children mobile as soon as possible aids not only elimination but also helps to prevent further osteoporosis and contracture deformities.

Adolescence is a particularly difficult time for children with myelomeningocele. The combination of altered body image, concerns about sexuality, and independence issues accentuates the typical adolescent turbulence. The child's cognitive and social maturity might lag behind physical development, delaying some of the peer-related adolescent issues. Appropriate sex education and sensitive counseling are begun at an earlier age for teenagers with myelodysplasia to help their adjustment during this period.

The lifelong care of children with myelomeningocele requires an interdisciplinary team approach. The nurse plays a major role in both acute care and long-term management through the coordination of specialized programs, child and family teaching, and psychosocial counseling. Parents with an affected child in the immediate family can be referred for genetic counseling. Spina bifida can be diagnosed by amniocentesis. A less invasive diagnostic method is the serum alpha fetoprotein (AFP) test that can screen the fetus for a neural tube defect during pregnancy.

The Child with an Infection of the Central Nervous System

Acute Bacterial Meningitis

Bacterial meningitis is a significant pediatric health problem, and immediate diagnosis and treatment are necessary to prevent morbidity and mortality. Central nervous system invasion by the causative organism produces inflammation of the meninges, resulting in acute illness. Different organisms are responsible for meningitis, and the prevalence of each organism varies depending on the age of the child.

Haemophilus influenzae type B is the primary causative organism of meningitis in children between 3 months and 5 years of age (Overturf and Wehrle, 1986). *Streptococcus pneumoniae* (a pneumococcus), *Neisseria meningitidis* (a meningococcus), and staphylococci cause the remainder of the cases of bacterial meningitis in children beyond the neonatal period. Neonatal meningitis differs both in the causative organism and clinical course from that of older infants and children. Gram-negative enteric bacilli (*Escherichia coli*), other gram-negative rods, and group B streptococci cause most cases of meningitis in neonates (Overturf and Wehrle, 1986).

Bacteria most often are carried to the meningeal area in the blood from another site in the body. Direct invasion can occur in traumatic injury, neurosurgical procedures, or from adjacent infections such as sinusitis or otitis. Predisposing factors that increase the incidence of meningitis include central nervous system anomalies (myelomeningocele), immune deficiencies, immunosuppression therapy, and sickle cell disease.

The invading organism most often causes an upper respiratory infection, otitis media, or some other infection. Secondary spread to the meninges occurs when bacteria in the venous drainage from the naospharynx, ear, or sinus pass into the meningeal vasculature. Meningeal inflammation evolves rapidly, and purulent exudate is released into the CSF system. The infection spreads through vascular and CSF circulation to adjacent brain tissue and nerve roots. Cerebral edema results from vascular congestion and cortical inflammation, and neuronal damage results if the infection is not treated.

Clinical manifestations Acute bacterial meningitis often is preceded by an upper respiratory or gastrointestinal infection. Fever, headache, vomiting, irritability, photophobia, and nuchal (neck) and spinal rigidity develop and can progress rapidly to decreased level of consciousness and seizures. Irritation of the meninges and spinal roots causes pain and resistance to neck flexion (nuchal rigidity), a positive *Kernig's sign* (resistance to knee extension in the supine position with the hips and knees flexed against the body), and a positive *Brudzinski's sign* (flexion of the knees and hips when the neck is flexed forward rapidly). With severe meningeal irritation, the child might demonstrate opisthotonic posturing (rigid arching of the back with the head extended).

Infants and young children often have less specific signs; irritability, crying, poor feeding, and vomiting are the initial manifestations. The fontanelle becomes full and tense and ICP is increased in a later stage of meningitis. The infant might exhibit a characteristic high-pitched cry.

Meningococcal meningitis, which is more common in older children and adults, can produce a characteristic petechial rash. Occasionally, petechiae also are seen with *H. influenzae* and pneumococcal meningitis. The course of meningococcal meningitis is more rapidly fulminant and progressive than other forms, with a higher mortality rate when accompanied by septicemia, shock, and disseminated intravascular coagulation (DIC) (Rimar and Goschke, 1985).

Increased ICP results from cerebral edema and might be increased further by obstruction to CSF circulation. Thickened meninges and pus in the subarachnoid space at the base of the brain obstruct the CSF, resulting in communicating hydrocephalus. Less commonly, obstruction of a ventricular foramina occurs, producing a noncommunicating hydrocephalus.

Subdural effusion, a collection of fluid in the subdural space, is a complication of meningitis that occurs primarily in infants under 2 years of age and following *H. influenzae* infections. Nonspecific signs of vomiting, irritability, and increasing head circumference together with failure of clinical improvement after 72 hours of antibiotic treatment might indicate subdural effusion.

Other signs of meningitis include cranial nerve involvement, abnormal reflexes and muscle tone, sensorimotor alterations, and seizures (most common with *H. influenzae*) (Conway-Rutkowski, 1982). Metabolic alterations in fluid and electrolytes might occur as a result of dehydration, septic shock, cerebral edema, or inappropriate secretion of ADH.

The incidence of serious residual neurologic deficits has been decreased with early diagnosis and aggressive treatment, but bacterial meningitis continues to result in neurologic sequelae in a significant number of cases. Seizures; vision or hearing loss; cognitive, language, or perceptual deficits; motor dysfunction; and behavioral alterations are possible residual impairments.

Diagnostic evaluation When the signs and symptoms suggest meningitis, the diagnosis must be confirmed by examination and culture of the CSF. A lumbar puncture is performed prior to initiating antibiotic therapy to accurately identify the causative organism. If acute increased ICP is suspected, the lumbar puncture is performed cautiously, with a parenteral line in place and emergency equipment available to anticipate brain stem herniation from the sudden reduction of high ICP. This complication occurs rarely but needs to be considered.

Initial CSF pressure is characteristically high and the CSF is cloudy in the child with meningitis. The white cell count is elevated with predominantly polymorphonuclear leukocytes. The CSF glucose level is decreased, and protein and lactic acid levels are increased (see Essentials of Structure and Function, p. 1060). Gram stain and culture of CSF are performed to identify the causative organism. Nasopharyngeal, blood, and urine cultures also help determine the cause.

Other laboratory tests that are useful include a complete blood count, serum electrolyte levels, blood urea nitrogen, and urinalysis. If other predisposing factors are suspected, additional tests might be performed, such as serologic, immunoglobulin, or radiographic studies. CT scan can be used to determine hydrocephalus, subdural effusion, or abscess formation.

Treatment Acute bacterial meningitis is a pediatric emergency that requires swift diagnosis, antibiotic treatment, and supportive care to reduce the risks of death or permanent disability. The initial antibiotic is broad spectrum, the choice of which is determined by the most likely infecting organism depending on the patient's age, results of CSF Gram's stain, and any known predisposing factors. Once the specific pathogen has been identified and its sensitivities determined, antibiotics are adjusted accordingly.

Antibiotics are administered intravenously in sufficiently high dosages to cross the blood-brain barrier. The dosage is calculated by body surface area or weight, and the drugs are administered by bolus or continual drip. Parenteral antibiotics are continued until the child has been afebrile for 5 days but at least for a total of 10–14 days, depending on the clinical response and repeat culture results. The lumbar puncture often is repeated 24–36 hours after the end of treatment to demonstrate that the CSF is sterile. If clinical improvement is not as good as expected, the CSF is reexamined at any point in the treatment course.

Infants with meningitis caused by gram-negative organisms are treated longer, for 2 weeks after repeat CSF cultures are sterile or for a minimum of 3 weeks.

The patient's fluid and electrolyte balance is managed with parenteral replacement. Initially, fluid intake usually is kept low (two-thirds of maintenance) to decrease cerebral edema. If the child demonstrates signs of inappropriate secretion of ADH, fluid restrictions are critical to prevent overhydration and a resulting increase in cerebral edema. If cerebral edema results in increased ICP, the child is treated accordingly.

Fever is controlled by antipyretics, tepid sponge baths, or a hypothermia mattress, if necessary. If the child becomes febrile after the first 3 or 4 days of treatment, sources of secondary infection must be sought. Seizures are treated promptly with anticonvulsant medication.

The child is monitored continually for the development of complications associated with both the disease process and therapeutic measures. Hypovolemia from septic shock or aggressive fluid restriction, respiratory insufficiency, and renal and metabolic alterations are detected early and treated appropriately. If the bacterial meningitis is associated with other disorders, such as trauma, shunt infection, or other systemic foci of infection, additional treatment is undertaken accordingly.

Nursing management Nursing care of the child with acute bacterial meningitis involves continual assessment of status, maintenance of prescribed medical therapies, and supportive measures. An intensive care setting is indicated for neonates, infants, and severely ill older children. The child is isolated and respiratory precautions are taken for 24 hours after specific antimicrobial therapy is initiated to prevent spread of the meningitic infection.

In the diagnostic and initial treatment period, the nurse assists in accomplishing procedures (lumbar puncture, obtaining blood samples, starting intravenous infusions). Required specimens are obtained and other diagnostic tests performed if indicated (such as CT scan, radiographs). A baseline assessment of the child's neurologic and vital signs is made, and the nurse reassesses these parameters frequently to detect changes and the response to treatment. The lumbar puncture can be extremely stressful to the acutely ill, frightened child. During the procedure, the nurse comforts the child as much as possible and observes the child's respirations carefully for signs of distress.

Bed rest is required, with the head of the bed elevated slightly and the child in a position of comfort. This helps to decrease cerebral edema and allows the child to rest. Safety measures are taken to prevent injury should seizures occur and to maintain the patency of the intravenous infusion. Most children with meningitis are irritable, photophobic, and respond with pain to external stimuli. The nurse ensures that excessive manipulations, noise, bright lights, and stressful stimuli are reduced or eliminated during the acute period.

The child's level of consciousness is the most sensitive indicator of neurologic status. The nurse remains alert to subtle changes in responsiveness, behavior, and activity that indicate alterations in consciousness. The nurse assesses the child's vital signs, including temperature, frequently during the initial period.

Temperature elevation increases cerebral metabolic activity and oxygen demands, increases fluid requirements, and places the child at higher risk for febrile seizures. Fever is reduced by external measures (light coverings, tepid sponge baths, and a hypothermia mattress) and by administering antipyretics. Extra fluids usually are not given in the early acute period because they might contribute to increasing cerebral edema.

The nurse monitors the child's blood pressure and pulse for changes indicative of increased ICP or signs of shock. The nurse assesses the child's respiratory effort, rhythm, and rate frequently. Impaired oxygenation can result in cerebral hypoxia, which increases cerebral edema further.

The child's hydration and electrolyte balance are managed by carefully maintaining the fluid intake at the prescribed amount and composition and accurately measuring output. The nurse measures the specific gravity of urine initially and with each void or once each shift. The child is weighed each day to assist in determining hydration. If the child is alert without vomiting, small amounts of clear liquids by mouth might be allowed. After the acute period, the diet might be advanced as the child's condition improves.

The nurse describes and reports any seizures carefully and administers anticonvulsant medications as prescribed. The nurse observes the child for other complicating conditions such as increasing head circumference, motor or sensory deficits, or other infectious sites. Pneumonia, joint effusions, otitis, or abscess formation can develop secondary to meningitis. The prolonged intravenous therapy that is a necessary part of treatment might result in phlebitis. The nurse monitors infusion sites closely and changes them if appropriate.

Within several days, the child usually begins to improve clinically and gradually tolerates increased activity. The nurse offers quiet games, books, and music to provide entertainment while preventing fatigue. Developmentally appropriate stimuli are provided as the child recovers and to the degree warranted by the child's condition. The child works through the traumatic experiences brought about by the meningitis, particularly repeated intravenous insertions and having blood drawn, by hospital play. A follow-up lumbar puncture most likely will be performed to determine the adequacy of treatment. The nurse helps to prepare the child through age-appropriate explanations, play, and rehearsal.

A continuing nursing concern is maintaining the child's intravenous infusion, which is needed for the administration of antibiotics for 10–14 days or longer. Treatment is continued at least 5 days after signs and symptoms subside, when the child has become increasingly active, and even longer for infants. In younger children the intravenous site must be protected, including the use of restraints when the child is unattended. The nurse makes every effort to see that the parent and staff members spend as much time as possible with the child so that restraints can be removed. For example, a heparin lock device is placed to free older children from the constant infusion between medication doses.

The nurse provides emotional support to the child and parent during the initial stages of the child's disease. Parents might feel guilty that they did not recognize the child's illness earlier. The nurse explains the disease process and reassures them that the child's preceding mild illness would not have alerted them to central nervous system infection. The nurse describes all procedures (such as lumbar puncture, isolation, or treatments) and explains their rationale. First and foremost the parent might be concerned about the child's prognosis and possible neurologic damage. The nurse avoids false reassurances but corrects misconceptions and helps the family to talk about their fears. If neurologic sequelae result, they might not be apparent initially, and the nurse stresses the importance of follow-up appointments to the family.

The nurse is concerned that immediate family members receive prophylactic treatment and encourages them to contact the physician. In most cases therapy with rifampin is effective for preventing meningitis in family members. Vaccination against *Haemophilus influenzae* type B, the organism that causes meningitis in younger children, is available (see Chapter 11).

If residual deficits persist from the recovery period, a specialized rehabilitative treatment might be developed. The nurse evaluates visual, hearing, speech, motor, or other impairments early and makes therapeutic recommendations. (See the section on habilitation and rehabilitation.) If seizures have occurred and the child is to continue receiving anticonvulsant medication, the nurse teaches the parent and child about seizures and how to manage them.

Aseptic (Viral) Meningitis

Aseptic meningitis is a usually benign illness that is most often caused by a virus. Coxsackie viruses, echoviruses, and other enteroviruses or mumps viruses are commonly responsible, although arboviruses, herpes viruses, and nonviral (toxic, postinfectious) agents can cause aseptic meningitis (Overturf and Wehrle, 1986).

Seasonal variations in incidence correlate with viral occurrence, with enteroviruses the most common causative agents during warm weather. The virus is transmitted by enteric means, droplets, or an arthropod vector. Viremia might result, and the organism in turn then invades the meninges. Young adult populations get aseptic meningitis more often than children.

Clinical manifestations Nonspecific prodromal signs of malaise, gastrointestinal disturbance, and flu symptoms might precede the acute onset of fever, headache, and stiffness and pain in the neck and back. Such mild neurologic signs as lethargy, irritability, and transient reflex changes might occur. In rare cases motor impairment or cranial nerve involvement occurs. A reddened, maculopapular rash can appear with echovirus infections (Conway-Rutkowski, 1982). The disease is self-limited, with complete recovery usually occurring within 7–10 days. Older children and adults might experience transient weakness and fatigue that can last for a few weeks to months, but permanent residual deficits are extremely rare.

Because of the similarity in initial manifestations of aseptic meningitis to bacterial meningitis, diagnostic procedures must be performed to rule out other infectious etiologies. Most often, the CSF is clear, with normal to elevated pressure. Cell counts might range from 100 to several thousand cells per cubic millimeter but are generally less than 500 cells/mm^3 (predominantly lymphocytes). The glucose level is normal, and the protein level can be normal or slightly elevated (Conway-Rutkowski, 1982). Bacterial cultures of CSF are negative. Viral cultures might be performed to identify the specific causative agent, but the results do not affect treatment.

A blood count usually reveals a viral profile, with a normal or decreased white blood cell count and lymphocyte predominance. Other cultures (blood, nasopharyngeal secretions, urine, stool) are obtained to detect a concurrent bacterial infection.

Treatment The child with aseptic meningitis is treated symptomatically with antipyretics, analgesics, and bed rest. Until bacterial meningitis is definitely ruled out, the child might be placed in isolation and treated with intravenous antibiotics. Hospitalization usually is brief, and the child is allowed to recover at home.

Nursing management Nursing care includes monitoring the child's neurologic status, vital signs, and hydration. The nurse focuses care on regulating the child's temperature, assuring adequate hydration and nutrition, and providing comfort measures. The nurse instructs the parent about caring for the child at home and advises the family to schedule a follow-up appointment with their primary health care provider.

Other Neurologic Infections of Childhood

Children can acquire infections of the central and peripheral nervous systems as a result of direct organism invasion

TABLE 31-6 Other Neurologic Infections of Childhood

Cause	Clinical manifestation
Encephalitis	
Primary Arboviruses (these spread to humans from insects), mumps, measles, varicella zoster viruses, herpes viruses, and enteroviruses *Secondary* Postinfection complication of viral illness, postvaccination complication, unknown	Headache, vomiting, and fever followed by neurologic signs, including behavior changes, stiff neck, seizures, high-pitched cry, and lethargy. May proceed to coma and death
Rabies	
Viral Transmitted by saliva of infected animals. Enters nervous system at wound and travels along peripheral nerve pathways to CNS. Causes degeneration of neurons with phases of encephalopathy and paralysis	1–3 month incubation (severity of disease and length of incubation related to amount of exposure and proximity of wound to the head) *Phase 1* Numbness and tingling at wound site, fever, malaise, headache *Phase 2* Irritability, excitement, insomnia, photophobia. Laryngeal spasm, particularly in response to sight or sound of liquids (hydrophobia). Inability to handle secretions. Delirium alternating with lucid periods *Phase 3* Paralysis, stupor, and coma lead to death
Postinfectious polyneuritis (Guillain-Barré syndrome)	
Might appear following viral illness and some immunizations. Prevalent age 4–9 years. Possible autoimmune reaction (Menkes, 1980) causing temporary progressive inflammation of peripheral nerves with myelin breakdown	Onset of symptoms within 2 weeks following viral illness. Sudden pain and weakness of feet and legs progress upward in ascending paralysis of trunk and all four extremities. Can result in paralysis of respiratory muscles and respiratory arrest. Cranial nerve paralysis might appear. Impaired autonomic function can lead to cardiac irregularities, urinary retention, and eventually to collapse. CSF shows increased protein, normal cell count, and negative culture. Acute stage of illness might last several weeks followed by gradual return of function. Recovery might take up to 2 years

or secondarily as a response to a previous illness. (Some of these infections and their care are presented in Table 31-6.)

Tetanus

Tetanus is an acute disease caused by the toxin of the bacillus *Clostridium tetani*, which is introduced into the body through open wounds via contaminated soil. The toxin acts on the neurons of the central nervous system, resulting in extreme muscle spasticity and convulsions. The incubation period varies from 5 days to 5 weeks depending on the amount of exposure, the speed with which the bacterium reproduces, and the amount of toxin produced. The fatality rate ranges from 35%–70% depending on the severity of the disease, the age of the patient, and the time lapse between initial exposure and the initiation of treatment.

The symptoms of tetanus primarily are painful muscular contractions of the neck and jaw and of the trunk, leading to spastic rigidity. Reflexes are hyperactive, and the child is irritable and restless. Convulsions can be precipitated by minor motion such as jarring of a bed or a loud noise. Intensive therapy is necessary because tetanus might affect the muscles of respiration, causing asphyxia and death. Thus, the person suspected of having tetanus is always hospitalized and usually requires intensive care nursing.

Tetanus is a preventable disease, and immunization should begin at 2 months of age (see Chapter 11). Because tetanus can result from relatively minor wounds, children

Prognosis	Treatment	Nursing Management
Course lasts days to weeks. Complete recovery possible, but child often left with neurologic deficits	Directed toward life support. Treatment of cerebral edema, antibiotics until bacterial etiology ruled out. Anticonvulsants for seizures. Fever therapy and correction of fluid and electrolyte imbalances	Intensive monitoring of vital and neurologic signs. Assessment and management of child with increased ICP. If child is unconscious, care of comatose child includes preventing hazards of immobility. Support child and family through rehabilitation management
Fatal in Phase 2 from cardiorespiratory arrest or anoxia Fatal in Phase 3	Wound cleansing with iodine or alcohol application. Administration of antirabies vaccine. Human diploid cell vaccine (HDCV) preferred because of greater effectiveness and fewer side effects. HDCV IM in 5–6 doses over 28–90 days. Passive immunization with rabies immune globulin (RIB) or hyperimmune rabies serum provides fast, temporary protection	Prepare child and family for antirabies prophylaxis. Prophylaxis is administered when exposure is known or cannot be reasonably ruled out according to US Center for Disease Control Guidelines. Health teaching to children to avoid occasions which would precipitate animal bites. Promotion of rabies control education in community. Report all suspected cases of rabies to CDC
20% mortality (Gellis and Kagan, 1982). Most children recover completely	Supportive. Directed toward maintaining life functions. Intubation and respiratory assistance might be required. Medications for cardiac alterations. Orthopedic program during recovery	Intensive care nursing with particular attention to respiratory and cardiac status. Prevention of joint contractures and other hazards of immobility. Assist child and family with rehabilitation

who receive any injury in which there is a laceration should receive tetanus prophylaxis according to their immunization status (see Chapter 24). All wounds should be thoroughly cleaned as a preventive measure.

Reye's Syndrome

Reye's syndrome is a relatively recently described syndrome that affects children, primarily from ages 5 to 14 years. The incidence appears to be increasing in the adolescent population and decreasing in children of younger ages. The disease causes encephalopathy and fatty degeneration of the visceral organs, most frequently the liver. If treated in time, the prognosis is relatively good. Most children who survive the acute stage recover completely. The mortality is high for children in coma or who exhibit progressively worsening neurologic signs.

Clinical manifestations The signs of Reye's syndrome follow a relatively mild viral illness by a few days to several weeks. Just as the child appears to be recovering from a "flu," upper respiratory infection, or chickenpox, the child's condition suddenly worsens. The child exhibits rapid behavioral changes such as irritability, confusion, apathy, and hostility. The stages of Reye's syndrome progress rapidly, and the child's neurologic condition deteriorates within 24–48 hours (Table 31-7).

Liver involvement is indicated by elevated aminotrans-

TABLE 31-7 Stages of Reye's Syndrome

Stage	Symptoms
0	Alert, wakeful
I	Lethargic, sleepy, difficult to arouse, vomiting
II	Delirious, combative, semipurposeful motor responses, hyperactive reflexes, responds to painful stimuli
III	Unarousable, decorticate position, comatose
IV	Unarousable, decerebrate position, large fixed pupils, deepened coma
V	Unarousable, flaccid paralysis, loss of deep tendon reflexes, seizures, respiratory arrest

ferases (formerly SGOT and SGPT). The serum bilirubin might be elevated to greater than 4.0 mg/dL (see Chapter 27). Prolonged prothrombin time and high serum ammonia levels support the diagnosis. The child might exhibit associated hypoglycemia, respiratory alkalosis, and metabolic acidosis (see Chapter 21).

Treatment Treatment is supportive and directed toward maintaining life functions, controlling cerebral edema, and reversing metabolic alterations. An IV of 10% or a higher concentration of glucose might be needed to correct hypoglycemia. Anticonvulsants are prescribed for seizures. Clotting or bleeding difficulties are corrected. The child is cared for in an intensive care setting.

Nursing management Intensive care nursing includes assessment and management of the child with altered neurologic signs, altered vital life functions, and increased ICP. The nurse uses a calm approach to the anxious, disoriented child. Care of the comatose child is instituted should the child progress to stage III or beyond. The nurse initiates seizure precautions. During the acute and rehabilitative phases, the nurse provides support to the child and family.

An important nursing function is public education. The occurrence of Reye's syndrome has been linked to the administration of aspirin during the preceding viral infection. The connection between aspirin and Reye's syndrome has been investigated by the United States Public Health Service. The recently released findings of this study establish a positive correlation between children who take aspirin during a viral episode and those that develop Reye's syndrome (Mitchell, Mitchell, & Mandell, 1987).

Because of the publicity regarding the connection between aspirin use and Reye's syndrome, parents of young children with viral illnesses or chickenpox have begun to avoid aspirin. This avoidance has resulted in a decrease in the incidence of Reye's among young children. Aspirin use has not decreased dramatically in adolescents, however, and therefore the incidence of Reye's appears to be increasing among children of that age group.

During well-child visits, the nurse cautions parents against giving aspirin to treat fever in children with influenza, upper respiratory illness, or chickenpox. The nurse explains to parents that should the child appear to be recovering from an illness and suddenly exhibit behavioral changes, irritability, and hostility, Reye's syndrome needs to be considered. The parent is advised to take the child immediately to the closest medical center and tell the medical personnel that Reye's is suspected. The earlier the child can be treated for Reye's the better the prognosis.

The Child with a Traumatic Lesion of the Central Nervous System

Cerebral Palsy

Cerebral palsy is a nonspecific term that refers to impairment of motor function resulting from an insult to the brain (motor cortex, basal ganglia, or cerebellum). The disorder is nonprogressive and can have a variety of causes. Prenatal and perinatal factors account for the largest percentage of cases, including maternal infection, toxemia, irradiation, placental insufficiency, and anemia. Prematurity, low birthweight, anoxia, and perinatal trauma are considered high-risk factors in the etiology of cerebral motor impairment. Postnatal infection, trauma, or cerebral anoxia can result in damage to upper motor control areas.

Regardless of the specific cause, cerebral palsy carries the essential clinical finding of neuromotor impairment as a result of insult to the immature central nervous system. Sensory, language, perceptual, and cognitive impairments occur frequently. The exact incidence of cerebral palsy is difficult to determine, but estimates vary from 1.5 to 5 cases per 1000 live births.

Clinical manifestations Although certain prenatal and perinatal conditions are known to place the infant at higher risk for neuromotor deficits, the diagnosis of cerebral palsy at birth is difficult. Cerebral control of movement develops as the infant matures, and it is during this maturational process that developmental abnormalities and delays are detected (Taft and Barabas, 1982).

The earliest manifestations of cerebral palsy in the neonate who has suffered serious brain injury include poor feeding with weak sucking and swallowing, hypotonia ("floppy infant"), absent or abnormal grasp, Moro or stepping reflexes, and seizures. As the infant develops, muscle tone might change from hypotonic to hypertonic, which is manifested as spasticity and abnormal rigidity of the extremities.

More often, the lack of specific neuromotor data in early infancy delays diagnosis until deviations from normal development can be discerned. Delays in gross motor performance are characteristic, with poor head control and failure to sit, crawl, and attain other motor milestones. The delays might range from subtle weaknesses to more obvious impairments accompanied by abnormal posturing and muscle tone.

The infant with cerebral palsy might show signs of increased muscle tone and spasticity, manifested by spinal and leg extensor thrust when the infant is supine or suddenly lifted under the arms. Arching of the back and head, scissoring of the legs, and stiffness or rigidity when held are early manifestations of spasticity. Hands held in a fisted position after 4–5 months of age also indicates spasticity of the upper extremities.

Early hand preference (before 18 months to 2 years of age), asymmetric crawling, using one arm and leg more, and abnormal posturing or weakness of one side of the body might indicate hemiplegia (paralysis on one side).

Feeding difficulties include poor suck, regurgitation, frequent thrusting of the tongue outward, and swallowing and oromotor incoordination. The infant might exhibit poor lip closure and impaired swallow and gag reflexes, resulting in both trouble with food intake and aspiration of fluids.

As the child develops, other indications of motor dysfunction might become noticeable. Standing on the toes can reflect spasticity of the legs, as can persistent hip adduction and hyperextension of the knees. Crawling using only the upper extremities and dragging the lower extremities might indicate diplegia. Uncoordinated, uncontrolled muscle movements occurring spontaneously or as the child attempts to move to reach for an object reflect underlying motor deficits.

Infantile reflexes persisting beyond the expected ages are a cause to suspect cerebral palsy. A tonic neck reflex or Moro or palmar grasp reflex that remains after 6 months of age indicates neurologic dysfunction. Sustained tonic neck posturing (obligatory) at any age is abnormal. The absence of later developing postural reflexes (neck righting, equilibrium) also suggests impairment of motor mechanisms.

Types of cerebral palsy The primary neuromotor dysfunctions seen in cerebral palsy are divided into three types: spastic, athetoid, and ataxic. The differing degrees of involvement of each of these types as well as the combinations of types result in great variation of clinical manifestations.

Spastic cerebral palsy Up to 65% of all cases of cerebral palsy are manifested by increased muscle tone, increased stretch reflexes, and muscle weakness (Low and Downey, 1982a). Spasticity may be mild or severe, resulting in contractures of affected joints. One side of the body might be affected (hemiparesis), or all four extremities might be involved (quadriparesis).

Hemiparetic cerebral palsy is the most frequent of all the clinical types. The child's extremities are smaller on the affected side, and the arm is usually weaker and more spastic than the leg. The characteristic posturing is flexion at the elbow, wrist, and knee, with equinus extension of the foot. The most severe impairment is fine motor function of the hand. Sensory deficits might accompany the motor dysfunction, as may cortical neglect or unawareness of the paretic side. Affected children almost always become ambulatory and are able to perform most activities with one hand, assisting with the paretic hand and arm.

The child's overall motor function often is more severely impaired with spastic cerebral palsy than with other types. Oromotor involvement causes tongue protrusion, impaired swallowing, and dysarthric (stammering) speech (Low and Downey, 1982a). Oculomotor deficits frequently result in strabismus. The usual motor pattern seen is hip adduction spasticity with scissoring of the legs, plantar flexion of the feet, poor trunk control, and fisted hands. Mass flexion-extension spastic movements of the arms, legs, trunk, or head might be the only voluntary motor control present.

Athetoid cerebral palsy The second most frequent type of neuromotor abnormality is *athetosis,* or abnormal involuntary movements. These movements are writhing, uncontrolled muscular activity that first appears when the child is 18 months of age or older. Facial grimacing, tongue and mouth movements, and rotary or twisting movements of the hands and feet are seen first. Later, the trunk and all extremities show the characteristic involuntary movements of purposeless, "wormlike" writhing, flailing, and distorted positioning.

In purely athetotic forms of cerebral palsy, increased muscle tone and spasticity are not present consistently. Muscle tone fluctuates, as does the intensity of abnormal movements. The movements disappear during sleep and become more intense when the child is anxious or physically stimulated. The movements interfere significantly with voluntary control of motor function. Elements of spasticity and athetosis can be found together in a mixed pattern of cerebral motor deficit.

Ataxic cerebral palsy Ataxic cerebral palsy, which is characterized by cerebellar impairment of balance and coordination, is the least frequent clinical type seen. Children show hypotonia and delay in achieving motor milestones. They have a wide-based, unsteady gait and clumsy, uncoordinated upper extremity function. Most ataxic forms of cerebral palsy improve somewhat as the child matures (Low and Downey, 1982a).

Associated conditions Children with cerebral motor deficits often have other central nervous system impairments. Cognitive deficits occur in many children with cerebral palsy. (Nursing care of the child with a mental deficiency is discussed in Chapter 15.) True assessment of learning and reasoning abilities is difficult when the child's motor and speech impairments make standardized testing inappropriate.

Other conditions that might be associated with cerebral palsy include manifestations of attention deficit disorder (see Chapter 16), visual and hearing impairments, and language or perceptual deficits. Seizures occur in about one-half of children with cerebral palsy and are more often associated with spastic forms (Menkes and Batzdorf, 1980). Children who have poor function of the respiratory musculature or impaired swallow and gag reflexes have difficulty clearing secretions, which might result in respiratory disturbances.

Treatment Because cerebral palsy is caused by permanent damage to the central nervous system, treatment efforts are directed toward improving motor function and preventing further handicap rather than toward curing the disability. Intervention begins early, is long term, and is best managed by interdisciplinary methods that are integrated to meet the child's particular needs. Specialists from neurology, orthopedics, pediatrics, nursing, physical therapy, speech and language pathology, occupational therapy, psychology, education, and other disciplines collaborate as a therapeutic team to foster the child's optimal development and functional potential.

Early intervention is desirable and depends on the early detection of initial signs of cerebral motor dysfunction. Most treatment in the early period involves teaching the family and guiding them in the care of the child. The family is taught specialized techniques for handling the child and methods of stimulation to encourage sensorimotor development. Adapted feeding, positioning, musculoskeletal exercises, and appropriate play activities are among the early intervention strategies employed. The importance of sensorimotor experience in developing cognitive and motor skills is emphasized as parents are guided in providing early therapeutic measures (Low and Downey, 1982a).

Orthopedic management includes the use of braces, casts, and corrective appliances, which help the child to maintain functional position and prevent contracture formation when supplemented by therapeutic stretching exercises and, when possible, functional use.

Orthopedic surgery might be undertaken to improve the child's functional ability and correct deformities that affect movement or self-care. The child with plantar flexion of the feet might be helped by heel cord lengthening. Other common surgical procedures include hamstring release for knee flexion contractures, obturator neurectomy and adductor myotomy for hip flexion or dislocation, and various wrist and foot procedures to release contractures and provide stabilization.

The relative benefits and goals of surgical intervention must be evaluated carefully and communicated clearly to the family to avoid unrealistic expectations of postoperative outcome. Gait, stability, or progressive deformity might be ameliorated, but the underlying motor dysfunction will remain (Low and Downey, 1982a).

The use of cerebellar implants with pacemakers providing electrical stimulation to relax spastic muscles is a newer surgical intervention that has been suggested for some children. The long-term effects of such treatment have not yet been evaluated (Conway-Rutkowski, 1982). Other neurosurgical procedures for specific lesions or deformities are indicated in a limited number of cases.

Medications to reduce spasticity or athetotic movements generally have not proven to have sufficient benefit to outweigh their side effects (Menkes and Batzdorf, 1980). Selected children might be helped by diazepam or dantrolene sodium, with careful monitoring for adverse side effects. The child with seizures is treated with appropriate anticonvulsant therapy. Other associated conditions, such as attention deficits, might respond to adjunctive medication therapy (see Chapter 16).

Physical therapy is an important part of the child's long-term management. The therapist works with the child, family, and other team members to maximize the child's functional motor skills, facilitate mobility, and prevent fixed deformities. The program approaches vary, and the conceptual bases for treatment differ. Active and passive exercise of muscle groups, practice of gross motor activities, and strengthening of equilibrium responses are some of the methods used.

Adaptive equipment enhances mobility and provides postural and skeletal alignment. The occupational therapist facilitates the child's performance of activities of daily living by modifying feeding and dressing methods that help the child achieve independence.

Language and speech disorders are identified early and treated as are any visual or hearing impairment. Programs are developed that use nonverbal communication systems ranging from yes-or-no indicators to multi-item communication boards to electronic devices.

Educational programming is an integral part of the child's management. The educational plan is individualized for each child depending on the child's motor, cognitive, language, perceptual, and associated abilities. Special settings or partial integration or full participation in a regular school program are appropriate for different children with cerebral palsy. Regardless of the type of program, integration of the various therapeutic goals into the child's educational program is essential to optimal learning.

Nursing management The nurse's role with children with cerebral palsy and their families involves long-term management in community, home, school, and hospital settings. The nurse's observations of the child's early development might provide the first clues that motor dysfunction exists. Newborn care and contacts in outpatient and hospital visits offer opportunities for developmental screening and the detection of abnormal signs.

The early recognition of potential neuromotor difficulties depends on a sound knowledge of normal development, application of appropriate screening measures, and follow-up with serial assessments. Indicators such as asymmetric strength and movement of the infant's limbs, legs held in extension, rigidity when held, and difficulty sucking and swallowing alert the nurse to the need for more specialized evaluation.

Delayed achievement of motor milestones might be the first indication of the disability; often, this does not become apparent until the infant is 6 months of age or older. The family might be the first to suspect that the child is not progressing normally and want rapid diagnosis of the condition and prognosis of the child's function. Caution must be used in interpreting isolated areas of deficit and predicting outcomes because the extent of disability in cerebral palsy cannot be determined early in life.

Parental anxiety and feelings of helplessness can be reduced by offering the concrete services of an early intervention team to develop a home program and provide family support. The family becomes more confident about caring for their child when they are guided carefully by the therapeutic team.

Nurses teach parents stimulation activities, motor exercises, and specialized feeding and handling techniques. At the same time, they encourage these activities as adaptations of normal parent-child interaction and play and not as exhausting "treatments." The nurse models, demonstrates, and suggests ways to incorporate recommendations into everyday life.

As they gain mastery in the care of their children, families feel that they are doing something actively to improve their children's disabilities. This might reduce feelings of guilt and frustration but also carries the danger of raising unrealistic expectations for the child's progress. An unfortunate outgrowth of various therapeutic programs is that parents sometimes believe erroneously that if a little therapy is good, a lot of therapy must be better. Nurses can be extremely helpful in assisting parents to view the child's developmental level realistically, recognize their own and the child's fatigue, and achieve a balance between the demands of the child's particular disability and other aspects of life.

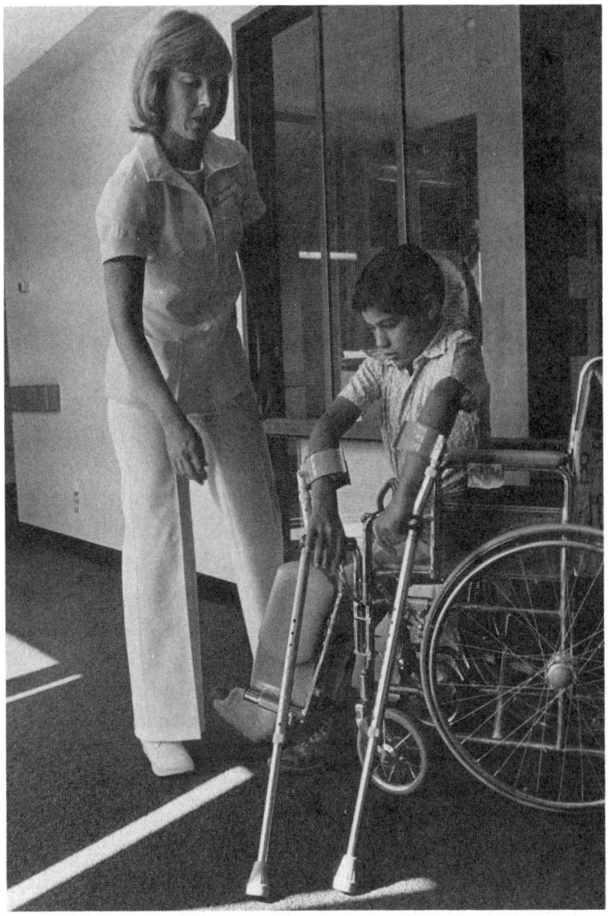

Nursing care for long-term management involves teaching the child to use assistive devices.

Specific tips and training for handling the child with spasticity focus on promoting relaxation and reducing reflexive postures. The child should not be picked up from a flat position but rather brought to a flexed sitting position first and then lifted by the underarms with support under the thighs to maintain the flexed position. This technique avoids the reflexive hyperextension thrust. Positioning the child in a sitting position with the head and neck flexed slightly forward, trunk supported, and hips abducted both decreases extensor tone and provides a functional position for activities. Other measures are directed toward facilitating mobility and promoting independence in activities of daily living (as described in the Nursing Care Guide on habilitation and rehabilitation).

Helping the family to adapt to the special demands of caring for a child with cerebral palsy involves emotional support as well as teaching specialized techniques. Many parents describe their child's early years as a nightmare, with conflicting opinions about the child's disability, improper advice, and exhaustive days of appointments, therapy, and basic care.

Parents must attempt to cope with the new and changing family organization and with their grief about having a child with defects. The nurse helps the family to mobilize supports within the family and refers them to community agencies for counseling, parent groups, and concrete services such as respite child care. Sharing their concerns with other parents of children with similar problems can reduce the isolation and insecurities many parents feel. The nurse helps the family to find more inventive means of play, interaction, and gratification.

Children with cerebral palsy also face adjustment problems in learning to live with their disabilities. This becomes particularly acute as these children approach adolescence. Difficulty with speech and motor movements sets these children apart, often causing peers to misunderstand and shun them. Their understanding and reasoning might be at or above their age level, yet they might be treated like younger children because of their appearance and dependency needs. Especially in unfamiliar situations such as hospitalization, it is important for the nurse to know the child's developmental level, system of communication, and usual routines of activity and care to provide continuity and interact appropriately with the child.

Head Injury

Head injury is one of the leading causes of death and disability in children. Craniocerebral trauma from accidents is the most frequent neurologic condition for which individuals under 19 years of age are hospitalized. Many children with minor head trauma are not hospitalized, so the overall incidence of the problem is even higher.

The causes of head injury vary with age. In the perinatal period, birth trauma due to cephalopelvic disproportion and injury from forceps are the primary causes. During infancy and early childhood, falls from heights, (arms, beds, stairs, and so forth) and child abuse account for many of these injuries. Athletic injuries, skateboard and bicycle accidents, and falls are frequent causes of head trauma in older children and adolescents. In all age groups of children, motor vehicle accidents are a leading cause of serious head trauma.

Craniocerebral trauma might range from mild head injury to severe, life-threatening nervous system insults. Children have more flexible skulls and tissues, which might enable them to withstand head trauma better than adults. Their greater tissue fragility and proportionally higher cerebral blood volume, however, place them at higher risk for brain damage and complicating hemorrhage (Walleck, 1980).

Trauma results from several types of physical forces acting on the skull and its contents. The mechanism may be direct (coup) when the injury is at the site of impact or indirect (contrecoup) when the injury occurs on the side of the brain contralateral to the blow. The contrecoup phenomenon results when the impact drives the brain contents against the opposite side of the skull. Acceleration and deceleration forces acting on the brain cause pressure changes and shearing forces as different parts of the brain are shifted at different rates. Strain or actual damage to neuronal tissue, dura, bone, and blood vessels occurs, producing various types of injuries.

Clinical manifestations Clinical manifestations of head injury depend on the type of injury.

Skull fractures Skull fractures are less common with head trauma in children than in adults because of the greater elasticity of the child's skull in withstanding impact. Skull fractures alone do not signify underlying cerebral injury and can occur with or without accompanying neurologic manifestations.

Depressed skull fractures occur with direct blunt trauma, directing fragmented bone inward against the brain. In infants and young children, the pliable skull might be depressed on impact, without an actual fracture occurring. The symptoms of depressed fractures depend on the area of the brain compressed and whether blood vessels, dura, or cerebral tissue is lacerated. Cerebral scarring can result from depressed skull fractures.

Basilar skull fractures, which occur infrequently in children, involve anterior fossa or temporobasal fracture. The symptoms might include vertigo, orbital ecchymoses (bruising) (Raccoon's sign), CSF or blood drainage from the ears or nose, postauricular ecchymoses (*Battle's sign*), and cranial nerve deficits. Cerebrospinal fluid leakage can predispose the child to meningitis, which is a complication of basilar skull fracture. Diagnosis is confirmed by associated signs because the fracture seldom is visible by radiography. Resolution of symptoms might take days to weeks.

Concussion Concussion is the most common type of closed-head injury other than minor head trauma. *Concussion* is defined as an immediate, transient impairment of neural functions due to trauma. The victim characteristically loses consciousness briefly and has no recall of the events surrounding the injury. The loss of memory for

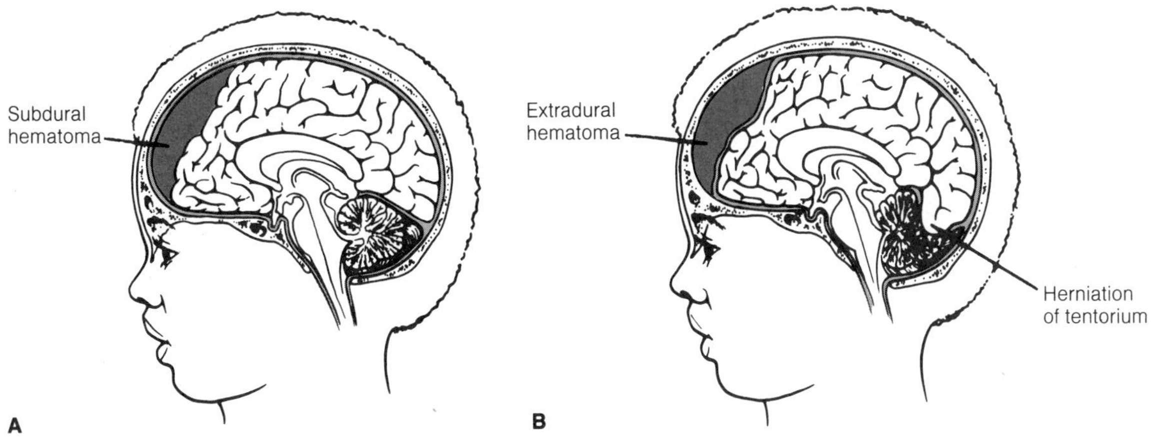

FIGURE 31-4

***A.** Subdural hematoma. **B.** Epidural hematoma with herniation through the tentorium.*

events immediately prior to the injury is termed *retrograde amnesia,* and the loss of memory for events following the injury is called *anterograde amnesia.* After consciousness is regained (several minutes), confusion, lethargy, irritability, pallor, headache, and vomiting might be seen. Symptoms usually resolve within 24–48 hours.

Subtle behavior changes (attentional problems, personality changes) and dull headaches constitute a postconcussion syndrome, which can occur and might persist for up to 6 months to a year following the injury.

Contusion and laceration More severe head injuries can bruise or lacerate brain tissue, causing petechial hemorrhages, edema, and actual tearing of cerebral matter. The clinical manifestations might be the same as those for concussion but are more severe, and focal neurologic deficits are present. Alteration of consciousness is more profound, lasts longer, and may progress rapidly to coma. The focal neurologic deficits seen reflect the contused area of the brain and might be manifested as focal seizures, aphasia, hemiplegia, eye deviations, or other localizing signs.

The frontal and temporal lobes are the most frequent sites of contusions. Recovery from cerebral contusion and laceration is variable, depending on the location and severity of the injury, development of complications, and treatment received.

Subdural hematoma A subdural hematoma is a collection of blood between the dura and the brain, which results from the rupture of subdural veins or, less commonly, arteries. It might occur acutely within 24 hours of the initial injury, manifesting symptoms of severe head injury. More often, subdural hematoma develops gradually, taking weeks or months to become symptomatic. The clot tends to encapsulate, becoming cystlike and filling with fluid. This fluid enlargement and slow bleeding combine to enlarge the hematoma, causing a gradual, insidious onset of symptoms related to compression of an area of the brain and increased ICP (Fig. 31-4A).

Subdural hematoma is quite common in infancy, occurring most often in infants between 2 and 6 months of age. Birth trauma and inflicted injury account for most of the cases. The infant often appears chronically ill, with anemia, vomiting, and developmental delays. Seizures, either focal or generalized, and a bulging fontanelle are indicators of cerebral pathology. In older children headache, increasing lethargy, unsteady gait, and seizures occur. A CT scan and subdural tap can be used, if necessary, to diagnose a subdural hematoma.

Extradural (epidural) hematoma Extradural hematoma is an acute condition that results from bleeding between the skull and dura, most often due to disruption of the middle meningeal artery (Fig. 31-4B). The hemorrhage is usually arterial, with rapid progression compressing the brain and causing the brain to herniate inferiorly through the tentorium. Death results if surgical treatment is not undertaken immediately. A CT scan generally is diagnostic.

The characteristic course is of an initial injury with a temporary recovery (lucid interval) of minutes to several hours, which is followed by progressive deterioration, with headache, seizures, stupor, coma, and focal signs of unequal pupils and contralateral hemiparesis. In children the initial injury might not be apparent, and the symptoms might take longer (up to several days) to appear. The manifestations of extradural hematoma are associated with increased ICP and brain stem involvement as the brain is displaced downward.

Intracranial hematoma Bleeding may occur anywhere within the brain as a result of trauma. Intracerebral hematomas are relatively uncommon in children but are possible; the symptoms are related to the site of involvement. Alterations in consciousness and focal neurologic signs might be seen, depending on the areas of the brain affected and the size of the hematoma.

Complications of head injury

Cerebral edema Contusions, lacerations, and hematomas of the brain are accompanied by cerebral edema, which further jeopardizes the functional integrity of brain tissue by increasing ICP and hypoxia. Focal swelling and vasodilatation with venous stasis decrease cerebral blood flow, resulting in cerebral hypoxia. The hypoxia in turn causes the fluid balance mechanisms to fail, and the resulting accumulation of sodium and water in the cerebral tissues leads to further edema and hence hypoxia. If not treated, the cycle repeats until death occurs.

Increased intracranial pressure Both cerebral edema and the mass effect of accumulations of blood can increase ICP (see p. 1076). Interruption of CSF circulation by trauma also can contribute to increasing ICP.

Posttraumatic sequelae Posttraumatic seizures may occur early (within 24–48 hours of injury) or late (up to 2 years after the injury). Major cerebral contusions or depressed or compound fractures are more likely to result in posttraumatic seizures, whereas more minor trauma less often leads to a seizure disorder (Low and Downey, 1982b).

Seizures may be either generalized or focal. Petit mal seizures are not caused by trauma. The seizure manifestations reflect the cerebral area damaged, with cerebral scarring forming a focus for abnormal electrical discharges.

Anticonvulsant therapy is used to treat posttraumatic seizures and might be employed prophylactically to prevent seizures following severe head trauma. Use of anticonvulsants for prevention of posttraumatic seizures is controversial (Evans and Hansen, 1985).

Focal neurologic deficits following head trauma can include impaired cognitive, language, motor, or sensory function, depending on the area and degree of cerebral injury. Forms of hemiplegia, aphasia, cranial nerve dysfunction, and alterations in memory and cognitive skill can occur. Behavioral changes and emotional disturbances can appear during recovery, which can be either transient or persistent. Anxiety, depression, and phobic reactions have been described following head injury in children.

Treatment The goal of immediate treatment of head injury is life support, controlling cerebral edema and increased ICP. The child's vital signs are obtained, a thorough neurologic examination is performed, a history of the trauma is elicited, and the indicated diagnostic tests are performed (skull and spine radiographs, CT scan, cerebral angiography, and blood analysis—hematocrit, electrolyte levels, and blood gases).

The child with a concussion is observed for changes in neurologic status for 24–48 hours. The child who has experienced a loss of consciousness or demonstrates abnormal neurologic signs usually is admitted to the hospital for close observation. If the child is allowed to go home, the family is instructed to observe for changes in consciousness, persistent vomiting, motor function changes, or severe headache. The child is seen for periodic neurologic evaluations following a concussion to detect any subsequent changes.

For the child who has suffered more severe head trauma, establishing an airway and providing life-support measures might be the first treatment steps. Emergency measures to decrease cerebral edema through glucocorticoids, hyperosmolar agents, and hyperventilation might be required. Vigorous treatment of increased ICP is undertaken. Anticonvulsant medication might be administered for postinjury seizures.

Surgical treatment is undertaken to reduce depressed skull fractures that compress brain tissue. Removal of hematomas and the control of cerebral bleeding also are managed surgically. Subdural hematomas might need to be evacuated repeatedly because they tend to reaccumulate in infants.

Nursing management The child with head trauma can develop complications related to hemorrhage or cerebral edema rapidly, and continuous neurologic assessments are needed to detect any changes in condition early. The nurses' observations are critical in the management of cerebral trauma to determine interventions and prevent complications.

In the immediate postinjury period, the nurse might be involved with emergency care in placing an airway, establishing parenteral lines, obtaining baseline diagnostic assessments (vital signs, neurologic signs, and radiographic and laboratory tests). Because head trauma often is accompanied by other injuries, the nurse examines the child for other signs of injury. The nurse handles the cervical and spinal areas with particular care until injury to these areas is ruled out.

Following initial assessment and treatment, the nurse monitors the child's vital signs and neurologic status frequently. The child is kept at rest, and stimulation is reduced to a minimum. The head of the child's bed is elevated 30° to increase venous return from the brain. The child's head and neck are maintained in correct alignment. If the child is excessively restless, the nurse applies the fewest restraints necessary to prevent self-injury. Fighting restraints can in-

NURSING CARE PLAN *The Comatose Child*

Assessment data: Lucy, a 13-year-old girl, suffered severe closed head injury (cerebral contusion) when she was struck by a car while riding her bicycle. Emergency management included tracheal intubation, assisted ventilation, treatment of cerebral edema, and anticonvulsant prophylaxis. Initial loss of consciousness was characterized by flexion response to pain (decorticate posturing) and no eye opening or verbal responses (Glasgow Coma Score 5). Ten days postinjury, she no longer requires intubation, her vital signs have stabilized, and she has been transferred from the intensive care unit to the pediatric unit. Although still unconscious, she now opens her eyes in response to verbal stimuli and no longer demonstrates decorticate posturing. Lucy is the youngest of four children; her parents feel guilty about the accident because it followed an argument with Lucy about her curfew.

Nursing diagnosis	Intervention	Rationale
1. Sensory-perceptual alteration related to impaired ability to respond to stimuli secondary to depressed level of consciousness	Talk to Lucy while caring for her. Touch her soothingly.	Sensory stimulation promotes the child's potential for increasing orientation and provides comfort.
	Have the parents bring tapes of family conversations, comments from friends, and favorite music to play for Lucy. Refrain from inappropriate discussions within Lucy's hearing.	The comatose child might perceive auditory stimuli despite a lack of response.
	Hang pictures of family and friends within Lucy's field of vision.	Familiar faces can be comforting even though the child might not be able to communicate this.
	Monitor Lucy's neurologic signs and vital signs every 2–4 hours. Include a Glasgow Coma Scale assessment.	The early detection of changes in neurologic status allows for prompt diagnosis and treatment, which improves the prognosis. Accurate observation of neurologic state can identify change in level of consciousness.
Outcome: Lucy begins to respond with gestures or verbalizations to environmental stimuli.		
2. Impaired physical mobility (level IV) related to uncompensated neuromuscular impairment secondary to head trauma	Maintain Lucy's body alignment with pillows and sandbags to support her position.	Functional body alignment helps to prevent stress on the joints and contractures.
	Change Lucy's position (from side to side and semiprone) every 2 hours.	Position changes promote circulation and joint flexibility and help to prevent respiratory congestion and skin pressure sites.
	Perform range-of-motion exercises every 4 hours.	Range-of-motion exercises increase circulation and maintain joint mobility.
	Apply ankle and foot orthoses and hand splints. Remove every 4 hours for range of motion and skin care.	The proper application of orthoses prevents foot drop and wrist drop.
Outcome: Lucy's joints remain mobile and she does not exhibit any signs of joint contractures. She advances from passive to active exercises.		
3. Total self-care deficit (level IV) related to uncompensated neuromuscular impairment secondary to head trauma	Inspect skin condition and provide skin care, giving special attention to bony prominences, every 2 hours.	The child is not able to inform the nurse about any pressure sensation to the skin.
	Insert in-dwelling catheter if Lucy is incontinent, and provide catheter and perineal care at least once a shift as ordered.	An in-dwelling catheter reduces skin excoriation from incontinent urine.

(Continues)

NURSING CARE PLAN *The Comatose Child (Continued)*

Nursing diagnosis	Intervention	Rationale
	Note urinary drainage and take a specimen for culture if urine appears cloudy or has sediment.	Cloudy urine can indicate urinary tract infection.
	Provide gastrostomy feedings as ordered.	Lucy's level of consciousness precludes oral feeding; nutritional needs therefore are met with gastrostomy feedings.
	Provide mouth care at least every 4 hours.	This increases the child's comfort, removes excess secretions, or provides moisture to dry mouth and lips if child is mouth breathing.
	Dress Lucy in nightgowns or other clothing from home.	The child is more comfortable in her own clothes, and seeing familiar items might increase her level of consciousness.
	Encourage Lucy to do more for herself as she is able.	Encouraging self-care helps reduce the child's self-care deficit and increases positive sense of one's own ability.

Outcome: Lucy gradually assists with self-care and achieves greater independence with activities of daily living.

Nursing diagnosis	Intervention	Rationale
4. Potential ineffective family coping (stressors: knowledge deficit, emotional conflict, change in expectations)	Encourage Lucy's parents to express their feelings. Allow them to express their sense of guilt, but reinforce that they did not cause Lucy's accident.	The verbalization of feelings helps parents to begin to adapt to a crisis situation and resolve any grief.
	Empathize with the parents' sense of loss and anxiety about Lucy's potential for recovery.	Empathic listening will comfort parents in their grief and uncertainty.
	Answer the parents' questions sensitively but realistically. Repeat information as needed, and explain all treatments and care.	Accurate information will help to prevent parental misperceptions and unrealistic hopes.
	Encourage the parents to talk to Lucy and touch and comfort her. When the parents indicate their readiness, encourage them to participate in Lucy's care.	Interacting with their child and assisting in care reduces the parents' feeling of helplessness and reaffirms the parent-child relationship.
	Offer referral to support and counseling (pastoral care, social services).	Outside support can provide additional comfort to the parents and increase their coping abilities.

Outcome: The family communicates effectively with each other and with the health care staff. The family utilizes resources appropriately and plans for the future.

crease ICP, and the nurse avoids using them whenever possible.

The nurse obtains information from the family about the child's normal behavior and responses, which is essential in detecting any changes. The parents are encouraged to remain with the child, and the nurse also observes the child's response to them.

Changes in the child's level of consciousness are the most sensitive indicators of changes in ICP. An in-depth nursing assessment is essential. Nursing interventions are directed toward management of increased ICP and any seizures or coma if they develop (see pp. 1076, 1085, and 1078 for discussions of ICP, seizures, and coma).

The nurse reports the amount and nature of any drainage from the ear or nose (that is, clear, bloody) because it might represent an undetected skull fracture. The conscious child who is vomiting receives nothing by mouth and then is given clear liquids in small amounts when they are tolerated, depending on fluid allowance or other conditions present (gastrointestinal or renal impairment). As the child improves, the diet is advanced.

Environmental stimulation in the form of familiar objects, quiet music, positional changes, and interaction is provided as the child recovers. The assessment of possible developmental changes continues past the acute period. Regression or behavioral changes might occur as transient phenomena or as longer-term posttraumatic sequelae.

Family support in both the acute and recovery phases is an important aspect of nursing management. During the acute period, the family needs to be informed at all times about the child's condition and have all treatment measures explained to them. They should be allowed to spend as much time as possible with the child, with the staff readily available to answer questions and help them cope with the trauma. Feelings of guilt and anger about the circumstances of the accident and fears that the child will not recover fully can overwhelm the parent. The nurse uses crisis intervention methods, listening supportively, correcting misconceptions, and exploring other supports available to the family.

As the child recovers and the nurse undertakes discharge preparation, the family is informed about the posttraumatic syndrome effects they might encounter. The family should be aware that behavioral changes, mood alterations, and poor concentration are possible transient sequelae following head injury. More significant posttraumatic sequelae such as seizures or sensorimotor or other impairments require specific parent education regarding medication, management, and rehabilitative care. Follow-up evaluations are mandatory for all children who have had cerebral trauma to determine any new or persisting neurologic signs.

Spinal Cord Injury

Traumatic injury to the spinal cord resulting in paraplegia or quadriplegia occurs more often in older children and adolescents than in young children. The causes of spinal cord injury vary with age. Falls from high places or diving or athletic injuries can produce indirect trauma by sudden hyperflexion, hyperextension, or compression of the spinal cord. The most frequent cause of spinal cord trauma at all ages is motor vehicle accidents.

The mechanism of injury is most often indirect trauma. Fracture or dislocation of vertebrae might accompany the injury but are not always present. Common sites of injury in children are the twelfth thoracic and first lumbar segments and the fifth and sixth cervical segments.

Cord injury often is caused by spinal concussion or contusion. Less often, the spinal cord is actually severed. Early changes indicative of cord contusion include edema, petechial hemorrhage, neuronal changes, and an inflammatory reaction. The damaging effects of compression or overstretching on tissue from the initial insult are compounded by the resulting edema and circulatory impairment. Neuronal tissue disruption and ischemia cause necrotic changes in the spinal cord, partially or completely disrupting function.

Clinical manifestations In spinal concussion a transient loss of cord function follows a traumatic incident. Immediate flaccid paralysis below the injured site occurs, which lasts for minutes to hours. Recovery of function is complete, and pathologic abnormalities of the cord are not seen.

More severe injuries produce permanent neurologic dysfunction of the spinal cord; the manifestations vary depending on the level and degree of damaged neuronal tissue. Complete lesions refer to total loss of functional motor activity and sensation below the level of insult. Incomplete lesions result in varying degrees of functional loss in which partial motor and sensory activities are intact. Partial lesions might have symptoms similar to incomplete lesions with a scattered return of function.

The higher the location of the lesion on the spinal cord, the more extensive the body involvement. For example, in high thoracic and lower cervical lesions, respiratory effort can be impaired by loss of accessory muscle function. At level C4 or above, phrenic nerve function is lost, resulting in diaphragmatic paralysis and respiratory failure.

The spinal cord responds to traumatic insult in characteristic stages (see Table 31-8).

Treatment Emergency care of the child with a spinal cord injury involves maintaining cardiovascular and respiratory function and preventing further damage to the neuronal tissue. Initial care and transport is of utmost importance because moving the injured site increases the risk of permanent damage. If resuscitation is necessary in the child with suspected cervical injury, it is accomplished with the head in a neutral position rather than hyperextended. Hasty actions such as the removal of a young athlete's football helmet can seriously aggravate spinal cord injury, as can any flexion, extension, or rotation of the spine. The child is transported on a firm, flat surface, and stabilizing aids such as a cervical collar, straps, and sandbags are used. Airway maintenance, ventilation, and the treatment of associated injuries are carried out with the child's spine immobilized.

A history of the trauma is helpful in determining the site and mechanism of the injury. Neurologic evaluation of motor, sensory, and reflexive functions gives an initial indication of the impairment and serves as a baseline for later comparisons. Only essential diagnostic measures are performed to avoid manipulating the child unnecessarily. The spine is examined radiographically to identify any fractures and dislocations, and contrast studies are performed to detect compression of the subarachnoid space.

The spine is then stabilized by skeletal traction (cervical tongs, halo apparatus), body jackets, or positioning on a

TABLE 31-8 Stages of Spinal Cord Injury

Spinal shock	
Lasts 2–6 weeks. The shorter the duration the better the prognosis. Best prognosis if there is some return in 48 hr	*Musculoskeletal* immediate flaccid paralysis and sensory and reflex loss below the level of the lesion. Immobility leads to muscle atrophy and negative nitrogen balance. Potential for joint contractures, decubiti, and osteoporosis from immobility *Cardiovascular* reduction in cerebral blood flow and syncope (fainting) from decrease in cardiac output and plasma volume from inactivity. Increased autonomic reflexes (hyperreflexia) might cause hypertension, often related to bladder or bowel distension. Orthostatic hypotension occurs in response to postural changes, causing blood pooling in lower extremities *Genitourinary* bladder atony and distension as a result of reflex loss and urinary retention. Residual urine increases chance of infection and urinary calculi *Gastrointestinal* atony with constipation as a result of bowel reflex loss. Poor nutritional intake *Neuroendocrine* loss of temperature regulation below level of lesion. Excessive sweating above lesion level is sometimes a reflex response to bladder or bowel distension
Gradual return of reflexes	
Continues for months to a year or longer. Outcomes range from purely reflexive activity to partial return of function	Reflex return accompanied by improvement in movement and sensation. There might be progressive spasticity of affected parts. Reflex bladder function produces hypertonicity of the bladder with partial involuntary emptying. Excessive sphincter resistance might result in bladder distension and its associated complications. Bowel function returns. Many of the initial clinical manifestations might remain although improvement in voluntary movement and contraction of spastic muscles reduces the hazards of immobility

horizontal turning frame with sandbags and pads to maintain alignment. Surgical intervention in the acute period usually is avoided except in cases in which debridement of compound injuries is necessary or in which ascending loss of function develops. Fracture reduction and decompressive laminectomy (excision of a lamina) are performed selectively, depending on the type of injury.

Children with high cervical injuries require respirator-assisted ventilation for an indefinite period of time, depending on the degree of diaphragmatic impairment. Decreased or absent respiratory effort combined with atelectasis and pooling of secretions from inactivity necessitate early and thorough respiratory therapy.

The child's fluid and electrolyte balance is monitored closely, and replacement and correction initially are provided parenterally. Initial paralytic ileus is managed with gastric decompression. Following the return of peristalsis, nutrition is provided by oral or nasogastric feeding. Indwelling or intermittent catheterization is employed for bladder drainage. Bowel atony is managed by rectal tubes or enemas.

Throughout the acute and recovery periods, the child is given frequent neurologic assessments to determine the extent of injury and return of reflex and functional neuronal activity.

Nursing management Acute nursing care is directed toward maintaining vital functions and immobilizing the injured area. The long-term nursing management involves working with the child and family to handle the necessary aspects of ongoing care. Musculoskeletal, bladder, bowel, skin, temperature, and respiratory regimens are lifelong concerns. Family adaptations to accommodate the child's physical state are accompanied by major psychosocial changes as the child and family adjust to the new situations they face. The child's self-image changes significantly, as does the family's perception of the child.

Nursing care of children with spinal cord injury in both the acute and rehabilitative phases is an integral part of a multidisciplinary team effort, the goals of which are to maximize postinjury function and prevent secondary complications. If at all possible, care is provided in a regional spinal injury center where specialized management is available.

TABLE 31-9 Selected Degenerative Neurologic Disorders

Disease	Pathophysiology	Clinical manifestations	Management
Infantile cerebromacular degeneration (Tay-Sachs disease)	Abnormal accumulation of lipid material in the cells of central nervous system due to an enzymatic defect (gangliosidosis)	Onset between 3 and 10 months of age; hypotonia; loss of vision; irritability; cherry-red spot on the macula; exaggerated startle response to noise (hyperacusis); seizures; muscle spasticity, macrocephaly, and deterioration of psychomotor functions in later stages; progresses to death by 2 or 3 years of age	Symptomatic and supportive care. Care of the child with vision impairment (see Chapter 32). Gentle handling to decrease reflex spastic responses. Care of the child with seizures. Care of the terminally ill child (see Chapter 17). Referral for genetic counseling
Familial dysautonomia (Riley-Day syndrome)	Autonomic nervous system dysfunction suggestive of neurohormone metabolism defect	Onset within 0–3 months of age; swallowing difficulties; vomiting; lack of adequate tear formation; excessive perspiration; erratic temperature regulation; skin blotching; labile blood pressure; hypotonia; psychomotor retardation; impaired sensation; chronic respiratory failure due to aspiration and pneumonia; variable course; death usually occurs during childhood from pulmonary complications or unknown causes	Symptomatic and supportive care. Adapted feeding techniques. Respiratory care to reduce pulmonary complications. Eyedrops to protect cornea from ulceration. Acute care for persistent vomiting. Protection from injury secondary to impaired pain sensation. Care of the chronically ill child (see Chapter 14)
Infantile muscular atrophy (Werdnig-Hoffman disease)	Progressive degeneration of anterior horn cells of the spinal cord and motor nuclei of the brain stem	Present at birth or within the first months of life; Muscle weakness, hypotonia, and atrophy; typical frog-leg position; progressive loss of motor and cranial nerve function; respiratory and feeding difficulties; variable course; most cases are fatal in early childhood	Symptomatic and supportive care. Adapted feeding techniques. Respiratory care to improve ventilation and decrease congestion. Cognitive and sensory stimulation for the child with severe motor deficits. Parent-child support for a potentially fatal illness (see Chapter 17)
Spinocerebellar ataxia (Friedreich's ataxia)	Progressive degeneration of spinal cord tracts ("demyelinization" and proliferation of interstitial tissue); degenerative changes in the cerebellum, brain stem, and cortex	Onset in late childhood or early adolescence; ataxia, clumsy gait, easy fatigability; skeletal deformities of the feet and spine; slowly progressive loss of balance and motor control, first of the lower and then of the upper extremities; nystagmus, myocarditis; diabetes; variable course and severity	Orthopedic care for skeletal deformities (see Chapter 30). Rehabilitation management. Supportive care for progressive loss of motor function

The Child with a Degenerative Neurologic Disorder

A number of degenerative disorders of the central nervous system occur in childhood. Most of these conditions are hereditary and involve one or more areas of the brain and spinal cord. A specific enzymatic defect can be demonstrated for some children, but in many cases the mechanism of degeneration is obscure. Neurologic manifestations depend on the metabolic or structural changes and the anatomic site affected. Several of the more prevalent types of childhood degenerative disorders are listed in Table 31-9.

Essential Concepts

- The nervous system consists of the brain, which is composed of the cerebrum, cerebellum, and brain stem; the spinal cord; the cerebrospinal fluid system; and the peripheral nervous system, which includes the cranial and spinal nerves and the autonomic nervous system.
- Assessment of the child's cerebral function includes observation of the child's behavior, level of consciousness, orientation, memory, and integrative function.
- Assessment of the child's motor function includes examination of muscle tone, muscle strength, motor control and coordination, and movement and posture.
- For the child with neurologic dysfunction, preparation for diagnostic tests involves helping the child become familiar with the equipment, describing the sensations the child will feel, and explaining the position that the child will need to assume for the test.
- Diagnostic tests and procedures common to neurologic function include electroencephalogram, radiographic studies, lumbar puncture, subdural tap, electromyography, and nerve conduction studies.
- Rehabilitation for children with neurologic disorders involves special exercises; assistive devices such as casts, splints, and braces; and mobilizing aids.
- Nursing management for the child requiring rehabilitation to improve neurologic deficits involves physical care, teaching the use of adaptive equipment, developmental stimulation, and behavior management.
- Nursing goals for the child with increased intracranial pressure are to reduce intracranial volume and treat the underlying disorder.
- Nursing management for the child with increased intracranial pressure involves administering diuretics, reducing fluid intake, preventing an elevated body temperature, monitoring the child's level of consciousness, and elevating the child's head to promote drainage from the brain.
- Nursing management for the comatose child involves serial monitoring of neurologic status, which includes assessment of vital signs, neurologic signs, and level of consciousness.
- Nursing measures for the comatose child are directed toward preventing the secondary effects of immobility and altered sensory perception.
- Nutritional needs for children with neurologic dysfunction may be met through adaptive equipment to compensate for impaired motor control and tube feedings for children whose disabilities prevent their handling food orally.
- Children with neurologic dysfunction often require special interventions to provide stimulation within a structured environment, facilitate learning adaptive skills, enhance socialization with peers, and achieve as much independence as possible.
- Seizures are classified as generalized or partial, are usually self-limiting, are sometimes directly preceded by an aura, and might be followed by varying degrees of headache or fatigue.
- Acute care for the child experiencing a seizure is directed toward protecting the child from injury and maintaining an airway. Following the seizure, nursing interventions include calm explanations to the child, monitoring vital signs and temperature, and documenting seizure activity.
- Chronic care for the child with a seizure disorder is directed toward teaching the child and family to control seizures through anticonvulsant medications and to prevent complications of seizure activity through attention to safety needs and to conditions that lead to the child's seizures.
- Children with neurologic dysfunction might experience problems related to congenital defects, central nervous system infection, trauma, or nerve degeneration. Each of these conditions might result in sensory-perceptual alterations, motor deficits, increased intracranial pressure, or seizures.

References

Carmel PW: Spinal dysraphism. In: *The Child With Disabling Illness,* 2nd ed. Downey JA, Low NL (editors). Raven, 1982.

Conway-Rutkowski BL: *Carini and Owen's Neurological and Neurosurgical Nursing,* 8th ed. Mosby, 1982.

Evans M, Hansen B: *A Clinical Guide to Pediatric Nursing.* Appleton-Century-Crofts, 1985.

Gellis SS, Kagan BM: *Current Pediatric Therapy.* Vol. 10. Saunders, 1982.

King RB, Dudas S: Rehabilitation of the patient with a spinal cord injury. *Nurs Clin North Am* (June) 1980; 15(2):225–243.

Low NL, Downey JA: Cerebral palsy. In: *The Child With Disabling Illness,* 2nd ed. Downey JA, Low NL (editors). Raven, 1982a.

Low NL, Downey JA: Lower motor neuron diseases. In: *The Child With Disabling Illness,* 2nd ed. Downey JA, Low NL (editors). Raven, 1982b.

McElroy DB: Hydrocephalus in children. *Nurs Clin North Am* (March) 1980; 15(1): 23–34.

Menkes JH, Batzdorf U: Postnatal trauma and injuries by physical agents. In: *Textbook of Child Neurology,* 2nd ed. Menkes JH (editor). Lea & Febiger, 1980.

Mitchell P, Mitchell A, Mandell F (editors): Aspirin as a cause of Reye's syndrome—is the question at last resolved? *Child Health Alert* (April) 1987; 1–3.

Myers SJ: The spinal injury patient. In: *The Child With Disabling Illness.* 2nd ed. Downey JA, Low NL (editors). Raven, 1982.

Overturf GD, Wehrle PF: Central nervous system infections. In: *Infectious Diseases of Children and Adults.* Pickering LK, DuPont HL (editors). Addison-Wesley, 1986.

Passo SD: Malformations of the neural tube. *Nurs Clin North Am* (March) 1980; 15: 5–21.

Richardson K et al: Biofeedback therapy for managing bowel incontinence caused by myelomeningocele. *MCN* (Nov/Dec) 1985; 10: 388–392.

Rimar JM, Goschke B: Fulminant meningococcemia in children. *Heart Lung* (July) 1985; 14(4): 385–389.

Taft LT, Barabas G: Infants with delayed motor performance. *Nurs Clin North Am* (Feb) 1982; 29(1): 137–149.

Walleck C: Head trauma in children. *Nurs Clin North Am* (March) 1980; 15(1): 115–127.

Additional Readings

Aadelen SP, Stroebel-Kahn F: Coping with quadriplegia. *Am J Nurs* (Aug) 1981; 81(8): 1471–1478.

Austin JK, McBride AB, Davis HW: Parental attitude and adjustment to childhood epilepsy. *Nurs Res* (March/April) 1984; 33(2): 92–96.

Belkengren RP, Sapala S: Reye's syndrome, clinical guidelines for practitioners in ambulatory care. *Pediatr Nurs* (March/April) 1981; 7(2): 26–28.

Bleck EE, Nagel DA (editors): *Physically Handicapped Children, A Medical Atlas for Teachers.* Grune & Stratton, 1982.

Casey R et al: Minor head trauma in children. *Pediatrics* (Sept) 1986; 77: 497–502.

Challenor YB: Orthoses for children. In: *The Child With Disabling Illness,* 2nd ed. Downey JA, Low NL (editors). Raven, 1982.

Chuang S: Perinatal and neonatal hydrocephalus: Incidence and etiology, part 1. *Perinat-Neonat* (Sept/Oct) 1986; 10(5): 8–14, 19.

Committee on Infectious Diseases of the American Academy of Pediatrics: Aspirin and Reye's syndrome. *Pediatrics* (June) 1982; 69(6): 810–812.

Connolly R, Zewe GE: Update: Head injuries. *J Neurosurg Nurs* (Aug) 1981; 13(4): 195–201.

DeLong R, Glick TH: Encephalopathy of Reye's syndrome: A review of pathogenetic hypotheses. *Pediatrics* (Jan) 1982; 69(1): 53–65.

Demarest CB: Suspected meningitis: Emergency handbook, part 5. *Patient Care* (Oct 15) 1985; 19(17): 123–126, 131, 134.

Frye BA: Brain injury and family education needs. *Rehabil Nurs* (July/Aug) 1982: 27–28.

Haughey CW: What to say . . . and do . . . when your patient asks about CT scans. *Nurs '81* (Dec) 1981; 11(12): 72–77.

Hausman KA: Critical care of the child with increased intracranial pressure. *Nurs Clin North Am* (Dec) 1981; 16(4): 647–656.

Hurwitz ES et al: Public Health Service study on Reye's syndrome and medications: Report of the pilot phase. *N Engl J Med* (Oct 3) 1985; 313(14): 849–857.

Icenogle DA, Kaplan AM: A review of congenital neurologic malformations. *Clin Pediatr* 1981; 20(9): 565–576.

Igoe JB et al: *School Nurses Working With Handicapped Children.* American Nurses' Association Publication No. NP-60, 2M, May, 1980.

Leonidas JC et al: Mild head trauma in children: When is a roentgenogram necessary? *Pediatrics* (Feb) 1982; 69(2): 139–143.

Maker AB: Dealing with head and neck injuries. *RN* (March) 1985; 48(3): 43–46.

Manley LK: Pediatric trauma: Initial assessment and management. *JEN* (Mar/Apr) 1987; 13(2): 77–87.

Marshall JG et al: Hydrocephalus: Ventriculoperitoneal shunting in infants and children. *AORN J* (Dec) 1984; 40(6): 842–846, 853–857.

Martelli ME: Teaching parents about Reye's syndrome. *Am J Nurs* (Feb) 1982; 82(2): 260–263.

Martelli ME: Reye's syndrome: An update. *JEN* (Nov/Dec) 1984; 10(6): 287–293.

Morris LA, Klimburg R: A survey of aspirin use and Reye's syndrome awareness among parents. *Am J Public Health* (Dec) 1986; 76(12): 1422–1423.

Nelson JD: Management problems of bacterial meningitis. *Pediatr Infect Dis* 1985; 4(suppl): 41–45.

Neu HC: CNS infection: First things first. *Hosp Pract* (Nov 30) 1985; 20(11): 69–73, 76, 79–81.

Pallett P, O'Brien MT: *Textbook of Neurological Nursing.* Little, Brown, 1985.

Parrish MA: A comparison of behavioral side effects related to commonly used anticonvulsants. *Pediatr Nurs* 1984; 10(2): 149–152.

Perude P: Urgent priorities in severe trauma: Life-threatening head and spinal injuries. *RN* (June) 1981; 44(6): 36–41, 102.

Rich J: Action STAT: Generalized motor seizure. *Nurs '86* (April) 1986; 16(4): 33.

Spaniolo AM, Van Antwerp J: Case study of a child with meningococcemia. *Pediatr Nurs* 1986; 1(6): 396–403.

Vogt G, Miller M, Esluer M: *Manual of Neurological Care.* Mosby, 1985.

U.S. Department of Health and Human Services: *Morbidity and Mortality Weekly Report* 1985; 33 (3SS): 9SS–10SS.

Chapter 32

Perception and Communication

Implications of Impaired Sensory Function

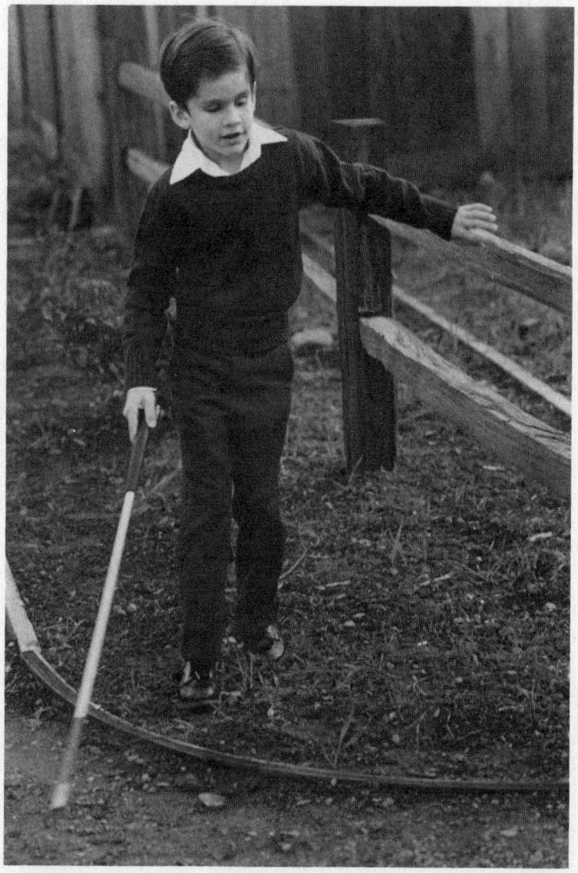

Chapter Contents

Alteration in nutrition: less than body requirements related to altered taste sensation

Developmental Needs

Potential for altered growth and development

Emotional Needs

Potential anxiety

Potential body image disturbance

Health Maintenance Needs

Potential injury

Potential for infection

The Child with a Visual Deficit Related to Structural Alterations of the Eye

Refractive Errors
Strabismus
Cataract
Glaucoma

The Child with Inflammation of the Eye

Conjunctivitis
Orbital Cellulitis
Corneal Ulcers

The Child with Traumatic Injury to the Eye

Corneal Abrasion
Subconjunctival Hemorrhage
Chemical Injury
Hyphema
Penetrating Eye Injuries

The Child with an Auditory Deficit Related to Structural Alterations of the Ear

Hearing Deficits
Structural Anomalies of the External Ear
Structural Anomalies of the Internal Ear

Cross Reference Box

To find these topics, see the following chapters:

Learning disabilities	Chapter 16
Otitis externa	Chapter 18
Retinoblastoma	Chapter 33
Retrolental fibroplasia	Chapter 34

The Child with an Ear Infection or Inflammation

Suppurative Otitis Media (SOM)
Nonsuppurative Otitis Media (NOM)
Mastoiditis

The Child with Ear Trauma

The Child with a Disorder of the Nasal Cavity

The Child with a Language Disorder

Childhood Aphasia
Expressive Language Disorders

Objectives

- Describe how perception and communication are affected by alterations in sensory organs.
- Describe the structure and function of the eye, ear, and oral cavity.
- Delineate the information obtained from the nursing assessment of a child with a sensory dysfunction, including data from the history, physical assessment, and diagnostic studies.
- List the principles of nursing care related to a child with alterations in sensory function, including acute care, nutritional, developmental, emotional, and health maintenance needs.
- Describe the nursing approach in the care of a child with a specific problem affecting the eye, the ear, and the nasal and oral cavities.
- Identify the interruptions in development of the child who is blind, deaf, or speech impaired.

ESSENTIALS OF STRUCTURE AND FUNCTION
The Senses

Glossary—Structures of the Eye

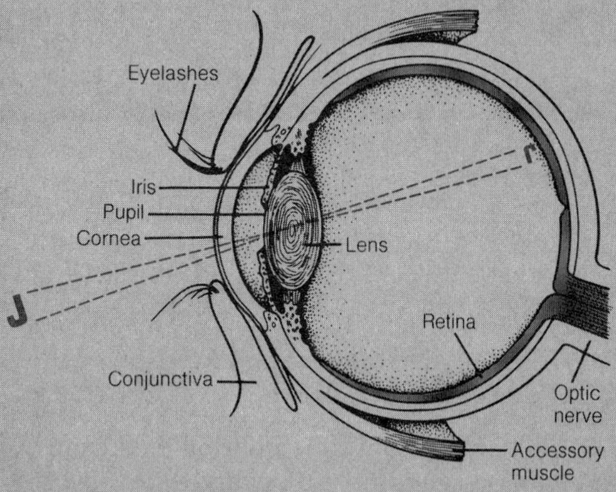

Refraction is the process of focusing light onto the retina. Light passes through the cornea, the aqueous humor, the lens, and the vitreous humor before creating an image on the retina. Retinal images are reversed (left to right) and upside down.

Accessory muscles Muscles that attach the eye to the skull and move the orbs in conjunction to achieve precise vision.

Aqueous humor Clear serous fluid between the lens and the cornea.

Conjunctiva Vascular lining that secretes mucus for lubrication.

Cornea Transparent membrane covering the colored iris and its open center, the pupil. The shutterlike iris controls the passage of light into the eye.

Lacrimal gland Gland that secretes tears to lubricate the eye, located in the upper outer portion of the eye.

Lens Clear convex structure that changes its shape (accommodation) to focus light from various distances onto the retina.

Retina Inner layer of the eye containing rods and cones, which receive the light stimulus and send messages via the optic nerve to the brain.

Sclera White covering of the eye.

Vitreous humor Jellylike fluid that fills the posterior chamber between the lens and retina. Both aqueous and vitreous humors maintain the internal pressure of the eye.

The developing eye is first evident in the twenty-second day of embryonic development. By the eighth gestational week, the eye is fully developed, although some structures will differentiate further. The retina continues to develop, and myelination of the optic nerve fibers is complete at the time of birth. During the first 4 months of life, the foveal retinal receptors differentiate, completing eye development.

The neonate can see and track objects, although visual acuity is limited. Neonates can see objects 8–12 inches from the face with reasonable clarity. Visual accommodation, the ability to alternately focus on close and distant objects, is minimal. Binocular vision (use of both eyes together) develops from about 9 months of age until the child reaches age 6, when 20/20 vision is achieved. During that early childhood period the child is farsighted, but at 6 years of age the child has developed the ability to focus clearly on close objects and is ready to read (see Table 10-4 for visual acuities at various age levels).

Another critical time in visual development is adolescence. At puberty, the adolescent is able to both fixate (seek and hold an image) and focus (define an image). Because the eyeball lengthens during the adolescent growth spurt, however, visual problems related to alterations in eyeball shape can occur.

Glossary—Structures of the Ear

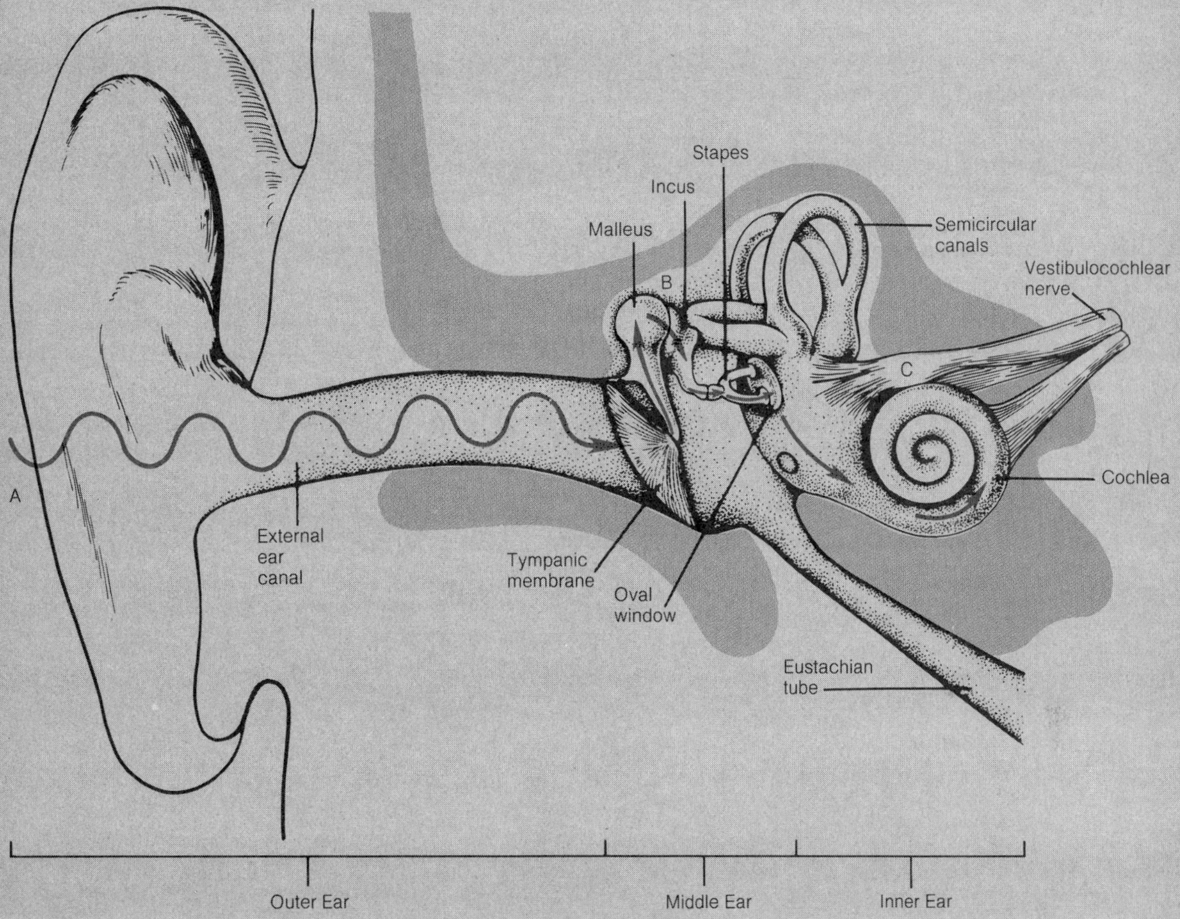

A. Sound waves travel through air into the external ear canal and cause the tympanic membrane to vibrate. B. The tympanic membrane movement causes movement of the ossicles and vibration of the fluid in the inner ear chamber. C. Fluid motion in the inner ear causes cells to generate afferent impulses, which are then transmitted to the brain via the vestibulocochlear nerve.

Cerumen Earwax that prevents the lining tissue of the ear canal from drying and forms a barrier against dirt and insects.

Eustachian tube Passage from the middle ear to the nasopharynx. It equalizes pressure between the middle and outer ear and allows for drainage of excess secretions from the middle ear to the nasopharynx. The eustachian tube in children is shorter than in adults.

Inner ear Portion that contains nerve endings for hearing, located in the cochlea, a fluid-filled snail-shaped chamber. The inner ear also controls balance by way of nerve endings in three semicircular canals, each oriented to a different plane.

Middle ear Portion that contains three small bones (ossicles)—the malleus, the incus, and the stapes—which touch both the tympanum and the inner ear.

(Continues)

ESSENTIALS OF STRUCTURE AND FUNCTION *(Continued)*
The Senses

Outer ear Portion that includes the auricle and external ear canal, which leads into the middle ear.

Tympanum Flexible membrane that separates the outer from the middle ear. It vibrates to conduct sound waves to the ossicles.

The three divisions of the ear (outer, middle, inner) develop separately during embryonic development and gradually join. As the mandible (lower jaw) forms, the ears move to the sides of the head at the level of the eyes. This process is not completed until about the thirty-second week of gestation. The sensitive period for disruption in ear development extends through the middle of the ninth week of gestation.

Auditory discrimination improves during the first 18 months of life. This period is critical, as anything that interferes with proper hearing during this time interferes with adequate speech development.

The Oral Cavity

The oral cavity is a rich source of sensations. Taste buds contain the end-organs for the perceptions of salt, sweet, sour, and bitter (see illustration of tongue areas). The condition of the oral cavity affects not only sensation but also speech and nutrition. The precise articulation of sounds requires the use of all the oral structures and control of air past the vocal cords.

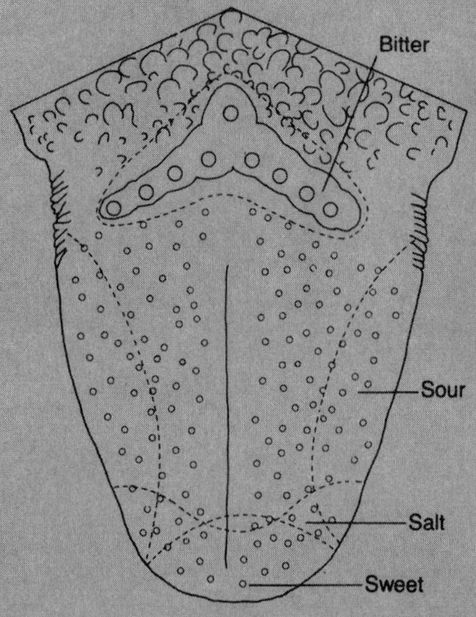

Areas of the tongue that are most sensitive to particular taste sensations. (From Vick R: Contemporary Medical Physiology. *Addison-Wesley, 1984, with permission.)*

Through the perception of events and communication of ideas and feelings, infants and children come to understand the world around them. Any alteration in either perceptive or communicative abilities can have an adverse effect on successful development. Alterations particularly can affect the attachment process of the parent and child.

The senses of vision, hearing, taste, smell, and touch are the vehicles through which children gain perception, whereas language is the major tool of communication. The sensory systems of infants and children are especially sensitive to malfunction, and when malfunction occurs, the potential impact on overall development is great. For this reason, prompt recognition of inadequate or abnormal sensory function is essential.

Nurses often recognize deviations from normal sensory function before others. Nurses caring for newborn infants and practicing in primary care settings such as well-child clinics and schools often identify sensory deficits. Nurses also play an important role in minimizing the long-term effects and maximizing rehabilitative efforts after acute, chronic, or permanent changes in sensory function. In this way the impact of sensory malfunctions on the child's development can be reduced.

Assessment of the Child with Sensory Dysfunction

History

The nursing history related to a child with sensory dysfunction includes all the elements recommended for the initial interview for any child entering a health care facility. For the child with a sensory problem, however, certain aspects of the history deserve special emphasis.

Prenatal history Some alterations in sensory function can be attributed to prenatal factors. The nurse obtains information about several maternal factors when compiling the history.

Maternal infections and the use of drugs or alcohol might affect fetal development by adversely affecting the mother. For example, rubella and other visual infections have the potential to cause hearing, visual, and neurologic deficits in the developing fetus. Even prescription drugs can cause fetal damage, especially if taken during the first trimester of pregnancy. Increasing concern has focused on the possible adverse influences of environmental pollutants such as smog, pesticides, and toxic fumes.

Sensory dysfunctions might be hereditary, for example, those associated with facial clefts, cataracts, strabismus, glaucoma, and nerve deafness. For this reason, the nurse elicits information about the presence or history of any congenital anomaly in the family, including those other than the one affecting the patient. Some congenital anomalies such as cleft lip, cleft palate, and widely spaced eyes (hypertelorism) are related to one another.

Developmental history A careful description of the child's development contributes useful information. The nurse asks at what age the child first began to attend to the parent's voice or sought eye contact and when the child first began to explore the environment through visual scanning, reaching, and creeping. The Revised Denver Developmental Screening Test (Appendix C) can be used to remind the nurse what questions should be asked to obtain a complete developmental history.

The nurse also questions the parent about the specific sensory deficit. For example, if impaired vision is suspected, the nurse asks whether the child squints while watching television, whether the child sits close to the television in order to see or hear better, and when the parent first noticed the child's behavior. The answers to specific questions such as these can yield important information related to the sensory systems of an infant or child.

Other specific areas to explore include reflexive and deliberate responses of the infant or child to stimuli, coordination skills, feeding difficulties, and speech and language patterns. Documentation of these data can be helpful in the assessment of any developmental delay related to the sensory dysfunction and in the identification of areas of development in which remedial or educational efforts should be applied.

Past infections The history includes data about past infections: the site of the infection, course of the illness, treatment and medications used, and age of the child at the time of the illness. These data are useful in understanding the cause of sensory loss or dysfunction. Hearing loss, for example, can be caused by recurrent ear infections in which the eardrum was ruptured. Some antibiotics, such as streptomycin, can cause permanent damage to the auditory nerve. In addition, a history of infections can suggest areas for health teaching to help the parent recognize infections earlier or prevent their occurrence.

Past trauma Data about any trauma include the child's age at the time of the injury and the circumstances surrounding the trauma. The site of the injury, treatment and medications used, and the healing process are important pieces of information. Head trauma might result in speech, hearing, or vision difficulties. Direct trauma to the eye or ear can cause permanent sequelae. A history of frequent accidents and trauma might be related to an undetected loss of visual or auditory acuity or motor dysfunction in the child, parent neglect, or abuse.

Environment Although health histories generally include questions about the home environment, some home environmental factors are especially important in assessing problems of hearing, vision, or speech. The amount of environmental stimulation can influence the child's attentiveness to stimuli. Some busy, disorganized households include adults who continually shout at the children, and the children soon learn what sounds or messages are safely disregarded. This lack of attention might be puzzling to adults, who become concerned about the children's hearing acuity.

On the other hand, if too little stimulation is present, the child might become apathetic and fail to attend or might become fearful and vigilant when in a noisy environment. Children who are not spoken to develop speech more slowly than children whose caregivers talk to them. Children who are spoken to mimic adult speech and receive positive reinforcement from adult responses to their early efforts at language. Children who live in crowded, economically deprived homes might be more vulnerable to ear and

ASSESSMENT GUIDE *The Child with Impaired Sensory Function*

Assessment questions	Supporting data
Has the child experienced a recent upper respiratory infection or allergy?	Rhinorrhea; thick, purulent nasal discharge; pain and edema in the sinus area; fever; anorexia. Itching or watering of the eyes; reddened conjunctiva; possible mucus discharge. Pain or feeling of fullness in the ear (infant might tug or bat the affected ear); decreased hearing; fever; purulent discharge from the ear; bulging red or gray tympanic membrane; alteration in tympanogram
Has the child sustained any trauma to the nose, eye, or ear?	
Nose	Epistaxis; edema; bruising
Eye	Presence of blood in the anterior chamber; loss of visual acuity; headache; feeling of foreign body in the eye; history of exposure to chemicals, heat, or ultraviolet light; flashing lights or dimming vision might indicate retinal detachment
Ear	History of foreign body in the ear; purulent discharge; diminished hearing in affected ear; laceration of external ear; exposure to ototoxic medications
Does the child have any obvious structural or functional abnormality?	
Eye	Blindness; squinting; altered visual acuity; corneal haze and enlarged corneal diameter in infants; tonometry readings of greater than 22 mm Hg; opacity of the lens; nystagmus (involuntary eye movements); strabismus (deviation of the iris); change in color of the iris or in pupil size and reactivity
Ear	Deafness; abnormal results of routine hearing tests; abnormalities of the external ear; delayed or distorted speech; consistently loud speech or inattention to the environment
Speech	Speech dysfunction or dysfluency; vocal changes; delayed speech development; persistent tongue thrust

Additional data: Family history of disorders affecting the senses; presence of a neuromuscular deficit; prenatal maternal infection or exposure to medications; history of meningitis or other severe viral infections

eye infections because of close contact with many other people, poor hygiene, or inadequate nutrition. If these environmental factors are identified and changed early, sensory delay can be corrected and parental concerns removed.

Changes in behavior In addition to general questions, the nurse probes or encourages the parent to provide specific information about changes in the child's behavior that could be related to sensory deficits. Changes in motor skills, decreased attention span, an increase in disruptive behavior, or changes in voice tones or volume might indicate decreased visual or auditory acuity.

Physical complaints A history of specific physical complaints of dizziness, headache, nausea, or vomiting also might serve as a diagnostic aid. It is important to record the onset of the symptom and whether it is continuous or intermittent. The frequency and duration of its occurrence is important to note. In addition, any other condition or syndrome needs to be noted, regardless of whether it is associated with the sensory problem. The plan of care needs to take into account the child's overall physical condition.

Physical Examination

Physical examination of a child with a problem of the special senses includes a review of body systems and assessment of sensory structures. (Visual examination of the retina and tympanic membrane is discussed in Chapter 10.)

Validating Diagnostic Tests

Vision and hearing are assessed with a variety of diagnostic tests. (Table 32-1 summarizes the most frequently used diagnostic tests for assessing eye and ear function.)

Assessment of taste in an older, cooperative child can be accomplished by giving the child a variety of substances that will elicit a response from the taste buds in the appropriate section of the tongue (see Essentials of Structure and Function, p. 1124). Sugar affects taste at the tip; salt is perceived in the forward portion; lemon elicits a sour taste in the middle of the tongue; and quinine's bitterness demonstrates taste bud activity in the back. The child rinses the mouth with water between each taste for a more accurate response (Systems of Life 88, 1982).

Assessment of speech adequacy depends on listening to a child's verbalizations. When the nurse listens to spontaneous speech, the general intelligibility of the child's speech and the correctness of the articulation of specific vowels and consonants can be identified. These data should be noted in detail in the health record so that any changes can be observed. The nurse also documents any speech dysfunction such as lisp, stuttering, and consistent substitution of one letter sound for another.

TABLE 32-1 Diagnostic Tests Related to Altered Sensory Function

Test	Description	Preparation
Visual acuity measurement		
Snellen charts	Consists of the alphabet chart and E chart (see Chapter 10)	See Chapter 10; this test can be used only with children old enough to follow directions
Allen cards	Uses schematic picture cards (see Chapter 10)	See Chapter 10
STYCAR test (Screening Test for Young Children and Retardates)	Consists of a chart with the letters *T, H, V,* and *O* set up in rows of decreasing size letters; also, a set of four cards, each of which is inscribed with one of the four letters. Children are asked to match the designated letter with one of the cards in their hands	Children should be encouraged to stand at the prescribed distance from the chart
Optokinetic drum (for infants)	A drum with alternating black and white stripes is rotated before the infant's eyes to elicit nystagmus (involuntary eye movements). Stripes of decreasing width are presented and visual acuity is the point at which the nystagmus disappears	The infant should be well rested and fed prior to the test to maintain attention and visual fixation on the drum
Other tests for infant visual acuity	Tests involve presenting disks of varied width, alternating black and white stripes against a gray background to the right or left of the infant's visual field. An independent observer judges whether the infant's eyes move in the direction of the disk. Facial outlines in black and white stripes have been used instead of striped disks. Visual acuity is determined by the infant's ability to discriminate the stripes from the gray background	The parents need to be informed that the infant's eyes will be patched one at a time; the infant should be well rested and fed prior to the test; the infant may sit on the parent's lap during the test
DEST (Denver Eye Screening Test)	Uses a combination of Snellen E, Allen cards, and tests used to assess eye and extraocular muscle function (see Chapter 10). Test distance is 15 ft; the 2- to 3-year-old child's acuity is normal if three of seven Allen cards are identified. Older children demonstrate 20/30 vision if the E is correctly positioned in one of three trials. Infants are checked for visual fixation by presentation of a moving toy, checking the pupil light reflex, and the cover test (see Chapter 10)	
Tonometry	Screens for glaucoma. The child's eyes are anesthetized and the child is placed in a recumbent position; after asking the child to fixate, intraocular pressure is measured with the tonometer. Normal intraocular pressure is less than 20 mm Hg	Tonometry can only be done with an older, cooperative child. A thorough explanation of the procedure is necessary to ensure cooperation

(Continues)

TABLE 32-1 Diagnostic Tests Related to Altered Sensory Function *(Continued)*

Test	Description	Preparation
Auditory acuity measurement		
Crib-o-gram	Measures the infant's arousal response to sound. The infant is placed on a motion-sensitive recording device; motor activity is recorded before, during, and after the presentation of sounds. Infant response includes the presence of a Moro reflex or turning in the direction of the sound	None
Evoked brain stem potential test	Electrodes, which record changes in brain stem potential when sounds are introduced, are placed on the infant's head	The parent should be aware that the infant might have to be restrained while the electrodes are in place
Audiometry	Headphones or earphones are placed on the child, and tones of varying frequencies are presented one ear at a time; the child indicates by raising a hand when the tone is heard. Frequencies are tested at various decibel (dB) levels. Mild hearing loss is failure to hear frequencies at 30 dB. Moderate loss is failure at 50–60 dB, while severe loss is failure at over 60 dB	The child must be able to follow directions. The tester needs to check the child's understanding of the directions given
Tuning fork test (Weber)	The tester activates the tuning fork and holds the handle against the midline of the child's head; sound should be equal in both ears. Tests for bone and air conduction	The child needs to know what to listen for and that vibrations might be felt on the head
Tuning fork test (Rinne)	Fork tines are placed near the child's ear canal; tests air conduction of sound	
Tympanometry	An airtight probe is fitted into the external ear canal, and pressure and movement of the tympanum are recorded electronically. A flat tracing on the graph (Fig. 32-2B) indicates excessive middle ear pressure	The child should be told that the probe will not hurt. An explanation of the procedure ensures cooperation
Articulation screening		
DASE (Denver Articulation Screening Examination)	Children age 2½ to 6 years are asked to repeat one- and two-syllable words spoken by the tester. The score is derived from the number of correctly articulated sounds and compared with percentile-ranked scores by age to assess normal language development. The tester makes a judgment regarding overall intelligibility of the child's speech, which also is ranked by age	None. If performance is abnormal, the child should be screened for auditory acuity

Nursing Management for Procedures and Treatments—Preparation for Diagnostic Tests

The nurse prepares each child for diagnostic tests on an individual basis that is suited to each child's abilities and developmental level. If appropriate, the nurse explains the purpose of the test, what the child will experience, and what is expected of the child. Visual and hearing acuity tests have a gamelike quality that enhances the child's willingness to participate. Because the results depend on the accuracy of the child's report, however, the atmosphere should be friendly but businesslike. If otoscopy (visual examination of the internal ear) or ophthalmoscopy (visual examination of the internal eye) or any other intrusive test is to be done, the infant or young child might need to be restrained to prevent injury. The restraint should be only as much as is needed for safety, and the child should be reassured that the holding is for only a short time.

Eyedrops and eardrops might be required in the testing

and treatment of conditions of the eye or ear. (The procedures and precautions for instilling eyedrops and eardrops are described in Chapter 20.) Eardrops might be needed to soften impacted cerumen before an ear examination or to treat an external otitis. To soften impacted cerumen, drops might be needed only once or for several days.

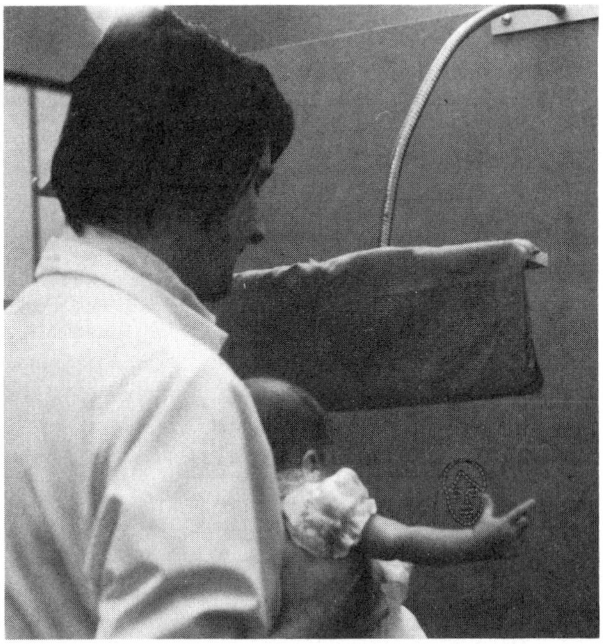

Infant eye examination for visual acuity.

Principles of Nursing Care

Acute Care Needs

Nursing care might begin with case finding in a well-child clinic or in a newborn nursery (eg, the child with a cleft palate). Deviations from normal, such as abnormal appearance, blurred vision, or deficits in hearing require medical intervention and are referred to a physician. The urgency of this referral depends, of course, on the nature of the abnormality.

In general, dysfunction or abnormalities of the sensory organs and systems require prompt attention to prevent or

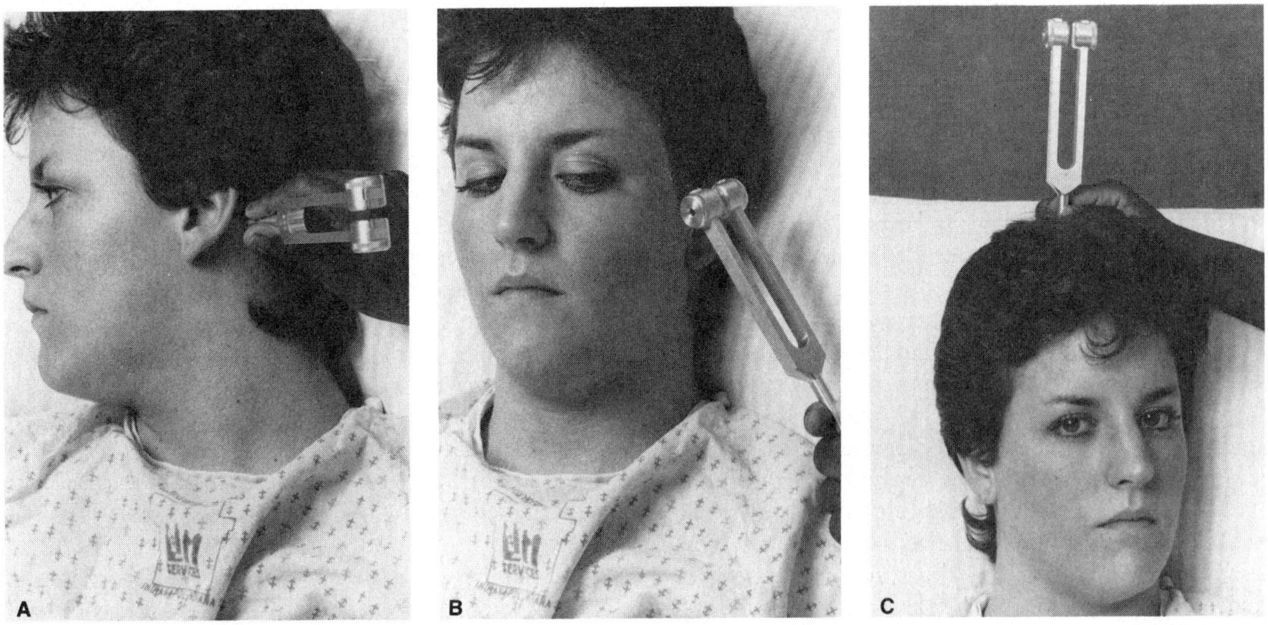

Rinne and Weber tests. ***A.*** *For the Rinne test, the child covers one ear, and the activated tuning fork is placed on the mastoid process of the uncovered ear. The nurse notes the amount of time during which the child heard the sound.* ***B.*** *Prongs of the tuning fork are moved in front of the uncovered ear. Unless the child has conductive hearing loss, the child should be able to hear the sound twice as long in this position.* ***C.*** *In the Weber test, the activated tuning fork is placed on top of the child's head; normally, the child hears the sound equally in both ears. (From Swearingen PL:* The Addison-Wesley Photo-Atlas of Nursing Procedures. *Addison-Wesley, 1984, p. 627.)*

reduce the severity of long-term effects. Nursing care includes explaining to parents why the medical referral will be made and emphasizing the importance of immediate follow-up.

Special nursing measures are required when a child with a chronic or acute sensory deficit is admitted to an ambulatory or inpatient facility for acute health care problems. These special needs and nursing measures depend on the degree of the sensory impairment.

Children with sensory deficits who are hospitalized are cared for best by assigning a primary nurse or, at the least, a limited number of persons responsible for care. The nurse who works most closely with the child continually assesses and records the most effective means of communication. Parents can provide additional help and validate the nurse's observations.

⊛ Sensory-perceptual alteration: input deficit related to visual deficit

Mild visual impairment Nursing care of children with mild visual impairments (eg, visual acuity better than that constituting legal blindness) consists of visual screening and parent education for early detection, referral, and teaching. The nurse encourages children who have corrective lenses to wear them, not because failure to do so will worsen the vision but because corrected vision promotes safety and the enjoyment of optimal visual acuity. The wearing of eyeglasses or eyepatches is not a negotiable issue. Children should be taught the proper care and cleaning of eyeglasses (eg, putting them in the case when not in use, cleaning the lenses with lens paper or soft lint-free cloth).

Parents might have difficulty encouraging children to wear corrective lenses or eyepatches. It is important to discover how the parent feels about the use of these devices. If the parent feels that eyeglasses or eyepatches are stigmatizing or uncomfortable, the child will perceive that attitude and protest or refuse to wear the devices. The parents will be better able to ensure that the devices are used by demonstrating positive attitudes and an expectation that the child will cooperate. Glasses will be more acceptable to the child if the frames are attractive, straight, and fit properly and if the lenses are kept clean and free from scratches. Head straps are useful for small children to keep the glasses from annoying slippage and to prevent breakage. Straps are useful also for older children who participate in athletics. Older children might find glasses more acceptable if they are permitted to choose the style of the frames.

An increasing number of children are wearing contact lenses instead of eyeglasses for the correction of visual impairment. As with eyeglasses, proper care and maintenance of contact lenses is crucial for optimal visual acuity. Cleaning and storage instructions differ depending on the type of lens used. Because contact lenses are so easily lost, children should be discouraged from wearing them in the hospital if they have eyeglasses available. If lenses are brought to the hospital, the nurse makes certain that the case is well labeled and that the contacts are stored in an easily accessible location. Nurses also need to be aware that without the lenses, children, especially those who use contact lenses as cataract replacements, cannot see appropriately and might become disoriented.

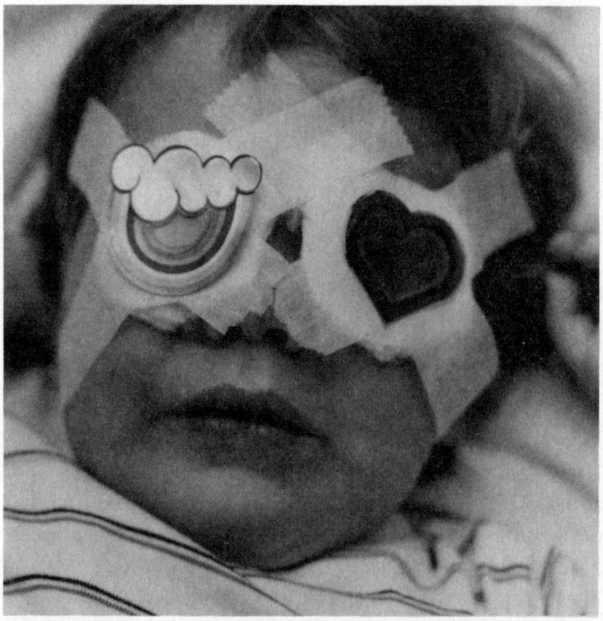

A child with bilateral eyepatches requires careful orientation to the environment.

Families are encouraged to provide regular eye checkups for all children wearing contact lenses. The risk of corneal abrasions is increased in contact lens wearers. Also, children who wear contact lenses for long periods of time can have a decreased supply of oxygen to their corneas. The newer gas-permeable contact lenses seem to alleviate this problem.

Sudden, severe visual impairment Sudden, traumatic dysfunction of the eyes is a terrifying experience for children and their parents. Temporary loss of vision can be due to trauma, infection, or surgery. Frequently, both eyes are patched to reduce the movement of the affected eye. This loss of vision adds to the child's confusion, fear, and discomfort.

Nursing care of the child who is temporarily blind includes providing as quiet an environment as possible. The level of distress can be reduced if the child is not bombarded with the sounds of the emergency room or hospital unit when unable to see what is happening.

The parent's distress can be telegraphed to the child. Prompt attention to the parent's needs and questions can reduce parental anxiety and benefit the child as well. The timely administration of pain medication and treatments such as compresses, ointments, or irrigations reduce the child's pain and discomfort and alleviate anxiety for both the child and parent.

Double patching a child whose sight previously was normal can result in the classic symptoms of sensory deprivation—confusion, withdrawal, nightmares, impaired thought processes and perceptions, and in severe cases hallucination and psychosis (Ashworth, 1979). Nursing interventions directed toward preventing sensory deprivation include the following:

1. Creating an environment that limits sensory overload but does not allow for isolation and sensory deprivation
2. Orienting the child to the environment, being as descriptive as possible to help the child create an internal visual image
3. Helping the child to perceive correctly the events that are occurring
4. Providing reality orientation, particularly to time, by relating time to events with which the child can identify (such as mealtime or *Sesame Street* time)
5. Encouraging self-care
6. Facilitating the use of cognitive thought processes by reading stories, playing music, or playing a tape of family members' voices
7. Providing enough sleep and time free from interruptions
8. Varying the external stimuli to maintain the child's attention such as by wheeling the child to a playroom

Existing, severe visual impairment When a child with existing severe visual impairment is hospitalized, special attention is needed to orient the child to the new setting. The child's degree of difficulty with orientation will depend on the degree of impairment and the recency of onset. Because infants rely on their parents for orientation and a sense of safety, it is especially important that the parent remain with and participate in the care of an infant who is blind. The older child might be able to accept care by a stranger if the nurse has obtained information from the parent about the child's daily routine and usual manner of communication, as well as the child's preferred arrangement of items in the hospital setting.

The nurse needs to know the degree of visual impairment. If the child cannot see at all, more supervision and assistance will be required in the strange environment than would be required for a child who is able to see shapes and forms and light and dark. On the other hand, the child with a partial loss of vision might be more frightened because of misperception of visual images. In either case the nurse describes the setting in detail to the child—the hospital room and unit for the child who has been admitted to the hospital and the examining room and waiting area for the child in an outpatient setting.

The nature of the description will depend on the child's age at the onset of the impairment. Children who are blind from birth will not understand visual references to colors and abstract measurements that are comprehended by children who are recently impaired. The nurse questions the parent about the means used to orient the child who is blind from birth. Methods include describing distances by referring to familiar settings, the number of steps away, or some other personal referent. The task of describing objects, distances, or persons even to recently impaired children requires inventiveness and patience to be sure that the references or comparisons are understood.

In general, orienting the blind child to the strange environment of a hospital ward can be accomplished best by guiding the child around the rooms and corridors of the patient division and encouraging the child to note sounds, odors, and surface textures to aid in establishing a mental picture of the special relationships. Bedside equipment such as the call bell, water glass, and bedside stand should be kept in their usual locations so that the child can learn where to reach for them as needed. The child who is blind, just like any other new patient, needs to learn to operate the call bell and the television conrols and to know where the bathroom is and when and where meals are served.

The need to announce to a blind child any changes in the environment seems self-evident, but it is easy to forget to supply a running commentary on the activities that a sighted child would be able to discern without assistance. It is important to identify oneself and one's purpose before touching the visually impaired child. Noises in the environment need to be identified immediately to prevent worry over their possible meanings, even when the activity is not related to the child's care. For example, the sound of a wheelchair or stretcher being brought into a room for another child might be interpreted by children who are blind as an indication that they are about to be taken somewhere without warning. The feeling of vulnerability in the strange environment might make children who are blind even more vigilant and aware of sounds, odors, and skin sensations.

Hospitalized children who are blind should be encouraged to maintain the same level of independence and self-care that they have achieved at home, within the limitations of the illness and the strange environment. Autonomy and independence are important for any child but will be more difficult to maintain for a blind child. Home routines of hygiene and other self-care activities should be preserved as much as possible, even if the nurse could do things for the child more quickly and effectively. When a child is forced back into dependency because of illness, help should be offered with tact and assurances that the need for assistance is temporary.

Children who have correctable visual impairments might need encouragement or assistance in the use of eyeglasses or contact lenses. It is important to help hospitalized children to keep their lenses clean and in a safe place when not in use.

Documentation of assessment and nursing care always is important, but record keeping is especially important in the care of the child who is visually disabled. The nurse notes mobility limitations and aids, the degree of independence in the activities of daily living, and the child's preferences for care in order to ensure safe and consistent care and to encourage maximum independence.

❀ Potential knowledge deficit concerning eye surgery

The nurse in an acute-care setting offers preoperative preparation to children and families when surgical correction is planned. In addition to the routine preoperative teaching, preparation includes describing the administration of eyedrops to prepare the eyes for surgery and explaining about the possible use of eyepatches immediately after surgery. Parents and older children need to be prepared for the typical bloodshot appearance of the eye after surgery. The nurse also determines whether the parent or child holds the common misconception that the eye is removed from the socket during surgery. The physician should describe the incision and sutures accurately, and the nurse can review and clarify the procedures, as needed.

Preoperative preparation emphasizes descriptions of the sounds, odors, and sensations of touch that the child will experience. It might be useful for the nurse to spend some time in the patient unit, operating room, and recovery room with the eyes closed, attending to sounds and sensations to become better able to prepare children who are blind for these experiences. Blind children benefit from actually handling new equipment or materials that will be used preoperatively and postoperatively, such as syringes, eye patches, dressings, or arm restraints.

Parents need to learn postoperative care. An eyepatch might be recommended for several weeks at naptime and during the night to protect the eye from accidental rubbing and to maintain lubrication during sleep. Antibiotic ointments or eyedrops might be instilled into the eye to prevent infection. Infants and young children will need to be restrained whenever they are not directly supervised by a responsible adult. Elbow restraints are particularly effective.

When eyepatches, eyedrops, ointment, or eyeglasses are prescribed postoperatively, parents might need help in enforcing their use. It is important that parents avoid allowing cooperation to become a power issue. They should make the child understand that wearing the patch, receiving the eye medication, or wearing the corrective lens is expected rather than negotiable. Parents often slip into the use of bribery and rewards if the nurse does not caution against this practice.

❀ Sensory-perceptual alteration: input deficit related to auditory deficit

Emergency or acute situations related to the ear can be encountered in the hospital, school, community, or home. Acute conditions include the presence of foreign bodies and acute external and middle ear infections. Each of these conditions is accompanied by pain of varying degrees and, frequently, nausea, vomiting, and vertigo. Nursing management includes the prompt administration of analgesics, medications for vertigo, antibiotics, and other prescribed medications and treatments. Fear and anxiety, which contribute to vertigo and nausea, are reduced in a quiet, calm environment. Like the child who is visually impaired, the child who is hearing impaired is at greater risk for developing adverse effects of sensory deprivation. The nurse intervenes to prevent this occurrence.

Partial hearing loss (30–80 dB) Problems arise for children with partial hearing losses. Strangers might be unaware of the impairment or of the specific loudness or pitch of sounds that can or cannot be perceived. Children who experience temporary losses of hearing from otitis media might have been scolded for a lack of attention or disobedience before the impairment was discovered. These children might be reluctant to say that they do not hear clearly. The speaker watches closely for facial expressions of confusion, doubt, or strain.

Other signs of hearing loss include disruptive behavior caused by the child's frustration and uncertainty about what is expected, or passivity and social withdrawal caused by the child's lack of normal auditory stimulation and the usual social interaction. On the other hand, children who wear hearing aids might suffer from persons shouting at them, even though their ability to hear normal tones has been restored. Careful history taking and recording of the character of the hearing disability can prevent some of these difficulties. In addition, careful, unobtrusive assessment of the child's ability to hear should be part of the hospital admission process. The nurse might speak the child's name when the child is not watching and note the response or lack of response. The nurse might ask the child to review what has been said to be sure that the child was able to hear and comprehend.

STANDARDS OF NURSING CARE *The Child Undergoing Eye Surgery*

GUIDE FOR NURSING MANAGEMENT

Nursing diagnosis	Intervention	Rationale	Outcome
1. Potential for sensory-perceptual alterations (stressors: eye patches, strange environment, impaired vision)	Preoperatively, familiarize the child with the environment (call light, bed controls, hospital staff), and implement age-appropriate preparation such as puppet play, "dress up" using eyepatches, and audiovisual instruction.	Preparing the child thoroughly relieves anxiety.	The child is alert, oriented, and interested in surroundings. The child can verbally express frustration at limitations without getting overly upset.
	Postoperatively, minimize unfamiliar environmental stimuli that can increase anxiety, such as unfamiliar noises or movements.	The child will feel more relaxed if noises are familiar or if the nurse describes what is happening in the environment.	
	Reorient the child to the environment.	The child might have forgotten where things are because of preoperative anxiety.	
	Provide reality orientation by relating time to events with which the child is familiar (eg mealtimes, time for a favorite television program).	Keeping the child in touch with reality and the passage of time will prevent disorientation and other adverse effects of sensory deficit.	
	Encourage auditory and tactile activities such as story tapes, music, and water play.	Promoting use of the other senses assists with providing reality orientation.	
	Encourage self-care activities.	Performing self-care provides the child with a measure of control.	
	Facilitate the expression of frustration through play activities and therapeutic communication.	Play activities provide an appropriate outlet for frustration while encouraging the use of other senses.	
2. Potential for injury (stressors: developmental level, impaired vision)	Maintain eyepatches or shield placement as ordered.	Eyepatches or shields protect the eye from further trauma.	The child remains free of injury during the postoperative period. The child cooperates with activity and play restrictions, thus demonstrating understanding of what could cause injury.
	Restrain as necessary (remove restraints every 1–2 hours to evaluate skin condition and provide range of motion).	Proper restraining prevents the child from rubbing the eye and causing further trauma.	
	Remove blunt objects or hard toys from the child's reach. Pad the siderails of the crib or bed.	Young children might accidentally hit themselves and reinjure the eye. Padded rails prevent injury.	

(Continues)

STANDARDS OF NURSING CARE *The Child Undergoing Eye Surgery (Continued)*

GUIDE FOR NURSING MANAGEMENT

Nursing diagnosis	Intervention	Rationale	Outcome
	Minimize intraocular pressure by administering analgesics if ordered and limiting coughing.	Analgesics limit agitation from pain and decrease the potential for injury. Coughing and straining increase intraocular pressure.	
3. Potential for infection (stressors: surgical incision, invasive procedure, or mobility restrictions)	Observe, record, and report eye redness, itching, discharge, pain, excessive edema, and change in appearance.	Any of these might be a sign of postoperative infection.	The child does not exhibit signs of infection, as evidenced by an afebrile state, a lack of purulence from the operative site, and a decrease in pain.
	Clean the eye from the inner to the outer canthus if cleaning is ordered; clean the external orbit using aseptic technique.	Aseptic technique reduces the chance for microorganism invasion; washing from the inner canthus out reduces the chances of spreading any infection to the unaffected eye.	
	Observe the child for any hazards of immobility if mobility is restricted to decrease intraocular pressure.	See Chapter 20.	
4. Potential knowledge deficit concerning home care of child following eye surgery (stressors: unfamiliarity with procedures, anxiety)	Teach the parent the proper method for administering eyedrops or ointment.	The proper method of administering drops or ointment will reduce the risk of infection.	The parent can demonstrate proper home management of medications, corrective lenses, patches, and/or prosthesis.
	Encourage the parent to be firm if the child is uncooperative about wearing patches or corrective lenses; role play how the parent can respond.	The wearing of patches or corrective lenses is nonnegotiable for optimal recovery and visual acuity; role playing assists the parent with feeling more secure.	
	Teach care of the prosthesis if appropriate.	Proper care prolongs the life of the prosthesis.	

Profound hearing loss (80–90 dB or greater) When children with profound hearing losses are admitted to the hospital, problems similar to those encountered by children who are blind can arise in dealing with the strange environment. Although children who are deaf can see, they might have difficulty understanding new activities and preparation for surgery or treatments.

The child with a total hearing loss might understand sign language or be able to read lips. If signing is the usual mode of communication, it is important to obtain help from a person skilled in sign language, just as one would enlist the help of a translator to communicate with a client who does not understand English. Pantomime, photographs, and picture books might serve to communicate simple requests, but more complex communications are needed to prepare fully deaf children for surgery or treatments.

To assist with simple sign communication, a chart of common positions for finger spelling is helpful. If a deaf child is able to read lips, it is essential that the nurse makes sure before speaking that the child is paying attention. The nurse touches the child to initiate eye contact before speaking. The nurse stands facing the child at the child's eye level and with the face well lighted. Important communications should be made in a setting with minimal visual distractions.

As with the child who is blind, the nurse can help the child who is profoundly deaf adjust to the hospital routine. Showing the child equipment and demonstrating its use on a doll is helpful. Making a time chart with clock faces and symbols of hospital routine is helpful for the older child's adjustment (Fig. 32-1).

⊛ Impaired verbal communication related to physical barrier secondary to hearing deficit

Additional problems for the hearing impaired child might involve inadequate speech development and the inability to communicate with others, especially strangers, who are not familiar with the signals and sounds with which the child communicates in the home. Children who are deaf from birth have particular trouble with learning speech because they are unable to hear others talk or to hear their own sound productions. The nurse therefore needs to remember that children who are deaf might have difficulty not only perceiving events and interpreting communications but also communicating their needs to others. If a sign translator is not available, the nurse might supply older deaf children with paper and pencil so that they can write down what they want to communicate. Even children who do not read can communicate by drawing or pointing out pictures in a book, so these materials should be readily available.

Children who are deaf attend more carefully to visual cues. Nurses need to be aware that facial and body language might unintentionally communicate information that can be misinterpreted by the deaf child.

Nursing management associated with a hearing aid

Some children who are hospitalized require hearing aids for auditory assistance. Four types of hearing aids are in general use:

1. Behind the ear—the most common type
2. In the ear—the most compact
3. Eyeglass
4. Body—for severe hearing loss (Holder, 1982)

All hearing aids have batteries, on-off switches, volume controls, and molds that fit into the outer ear. Hearing aids

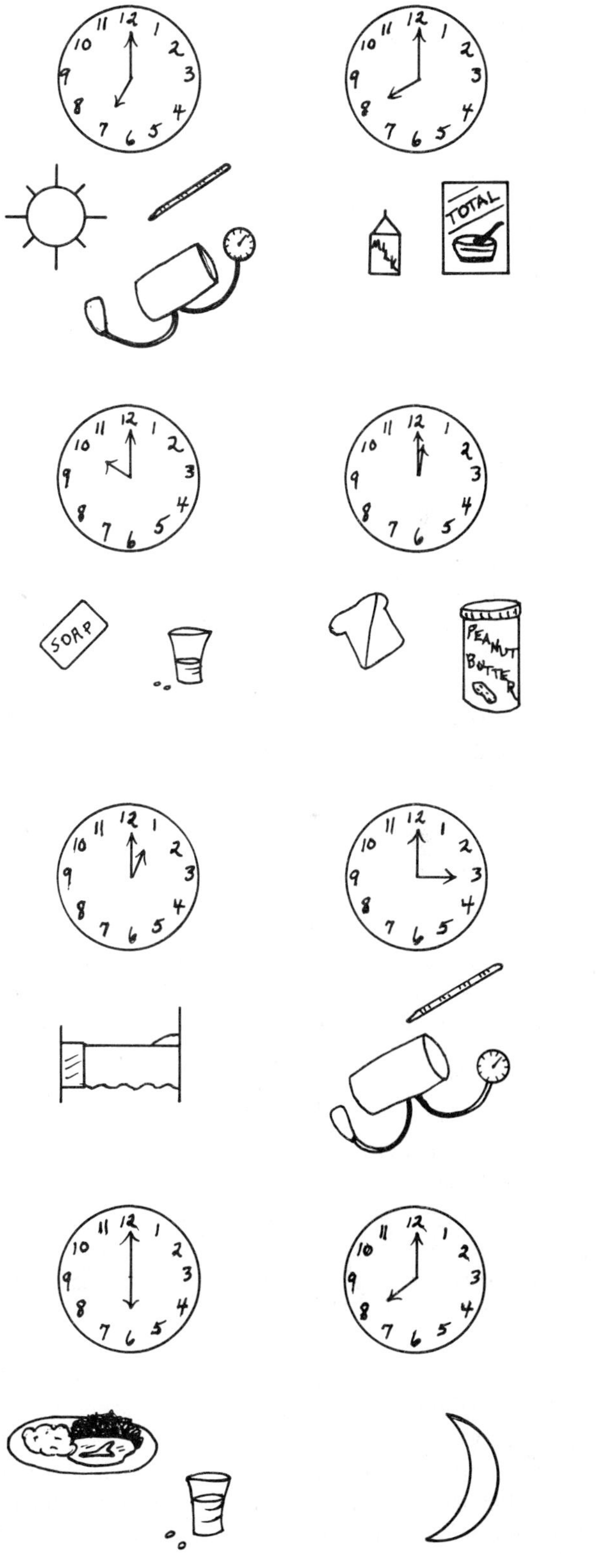

FIGURE 32-1

The nurse can use a chart to indicate hospital routine for the child who is hearing impaired.

function by converting sound waves into electrical impulses through the amplification of the sound signals. With children the volume can be set to maximize effectiveness and the volume control taped to prevent the child from turning the volume off and "tuning out" (Kamenir et al., 1982).

The information the nurse needs to know to care properly for the hearing aid includes the type, make, and serial number (to be recorded on the child's chart); how to insert the hearing aid; how to change the battery; how often the hearing aid is cleaned; and whether the child can clean it (Kamenir et al., 1982). The ear mold and tube are the only portions of the hearing aid that should be cleaned; cleaning in warm water and mild soap is all that is required. It is important to be certain that the mold and tube are completely dry before they are reinserted into the ear.

If the hearing aid does not appear to be working properly, the nurse checks that the switch is on (and not on the "telephone" setting), that the battery is not dead, and that the hearing aid is placed correctly in the ear. If the battery is working, a whistling sound can be heard by covering the mold with a hand prior to insertion. If the hearing aid is inserted incorrectly, a whistling sound can be heard when it is in the ear. The nurse remembers to remove the child's hearing aid prior to any radiographic studies because radiation can adversely affect its function.

⊛ Potential knowledge deficit concerning ear surgery

Orientation to the hospital and preoperative and postoperative preparations are necessary for the child who is deaf just as for the child who is blind. Considering the developmental level of the child and the degree of impairment, the nurse provides concrete descriptions of settings and anticipated events such as preoperative injections, transport by stretcher, and so on. Demonstration and role-play are especially useful for children with total hearing loss and minimal verbal ability.

When surgery is contemplated, preoperative preparation includes the expected postoperative conditions of discomfort, drainage, or temporarily reduced hearing acuity. A frequent minor surgical procedure is incision of the tympanic membrane (*myringotomy*) with the insertion of plastic tubes in the tympanum. This procedure is performed under general anesthesia. Children are admitted to the hospital for day surgery or a brief overnight stay.

An important nursing intervention is to teach the parent and child how to manage the child postoperatively at home. The nurse reminds the parent that drainage lasting several days is expected. If drainage is excessive, the parent can apply petroleum jelly to the auricle and apply a cotton fluff dressing to protect the skin. The parent needs to monitor and report any frank bleeding or purulent drainage (which might signify infection). The parent is given instructions to keep the child's head out of water. Cotton balls dipped in petroleum jelly can be placed in the ear orifice during bathing. Because spontaneous extrusion of the tubes is not unusual, the parent observes regularly for the presence of the tube in the ear canal. The nurse advises the parent to keep the child away from sources of upper respiratory infection to prevent further auditory infection.

Occasionally, when damage to the tympanic membrane has been severe, a *tympanoplasty* might be considered to restore hearing loss. This involves the insertion of a Silastic film to replace the defective tympanic membrane (Bridges, 1982). Postoperatively, the child might have a bulky dressing over the ear and an ear packing. The child should lie on the affected side to facilitate drainage and should avoid sudden movement and be medicated for pain if needed. Sudden nausea, dizziness, or vomiting might indicate disturbance of the cochlea (Bridges, 1982). Home care of the child following tympanoplasty is similar to that of the child following a myringotomy.

Less common ear surgery involves repair of the ossicles. Regardless of the type of ear surgery, nursing interventions are directed toward the prevention of infection, most specifically mastoiditis, which can lead to meningitis.

⊛ Impaired verbal communication related to anatomic defects

Children develop speech impairments from a variety of causes. The impairment might be a temporary failure to pronounce specific words clearly (articulation defect) or a permanent impairment caused by malformations of the palate or difficulty controlling the passage of air over the vocal cords. Whatever the cause or duration of the problem, it is important for the nurse to assess the amount and type of speech the child understands and the extent of the child's ability to use speech to communicate with others. The nurse cannot assume that a child has equal receptive and expressive speech abilities. Children with speech impairments might experience much frustration and embarrassment when they enter a new environment and others have difficulty understanding what they say. Nurses can decrease the child's frustration by attending very carefully to the child's speech, asking the child to communicate using other words if the initial words cannot be understood, and remaining calm, pleasant, and accepting of the communication difficulties. Children with speech impairments communicate most clearly when they are unrushed and feel accepted by the listener.

Many speech problems can be corrected with corrective surgery and speech therapy. Children with cerebral palsy or other neuromuscular problems can be helped to control the expiratory phase of respiration to improve the quality of speech. Children with malformations of the mouth, palate, posterior pharynx, or vocal cords can be helped by cor-

STANDARDS OF NURSING CARE *Postoperative Management of the Child Undergoing Tympanoplasty*

RISKS

Assessed risk	Nursing action
Postoperative bleeding	Place the child in a side-lying position to facilitate drainage. Monitor the amount and color of drainage on the dressing. Report any bright red bleeding that appears to increase. Monitor the child's vital signs. Report any marked decrease in blood pressure and increase in pulse.
Postoperative infection	Change the dressing only when ordered, using aseptic technique. Administer antibiotics as ordered. Monitor the child for any purulent drainage, fever, neck stiffness, or headache that might signal neurologic infection.

GUIDE FOR NURSING MANAGEMENT

Nursing diagnosis	Intervention	Rationale	Outcome
1. Potential anxiety (stressors: unfamiliarity with procedures, the unknown aspects about surgery, or separation)	Review the purpose of the procedure with the child and parent according to level of understanding.	Knowledge reduces the anxiety level.	The child and parent can state the purpose of the operative procedure and how the dressing will appear postoperatively. The child and parent express their anxieties and ask appropriate questions.
	Use puppets to demonstrate the appearance of the dressing. Use puppets or dolls to rehearse the pre- to postoperative sequence.	Puppets provide a visual image for the child and also allow the child to play out anxieties.	
	Encourage the child and parent to ask questions; spend time answering questions and offering reassurance. Support their verbalizations of anxiety.	Knowing that questions are appropriate and answers will be given reduces anxiety.	
2. Potential sensory-perceptual alteration (stressors: occlusive dressing, invasive procedure affecting equilibrium)	Speak to the child in a normal tone of voice; touch the child prior to speaking.	There might be a temporary hearing deficit related to bulky ear dressings. Attracting the child's attention prior to speaking will help the child understand what is being said.	The child responds appropriately to what is said. The child's dizziness is minimal.
	Assist the child with sitting up and getting out of bed; support the child firmly while the child is ambulating. Report any severe dizziness.	Dizziness is a frequently seen after-effect of ear surgery. The nurse needs to ensure the child's safety should any dizziness occur.	
3. Potential knowledge deficit concerning home care of child following tympanoplasty (stressors: unfamiliarity with medication procedure, new procedures, and precautions to practice, restricted activities)	Teach the parent how to administer the antibiotic if one is required; encourage antibiotic compliance.	Occasionally, antibiotic powder might be ordered to dust around the ear.	The parent and child (if old enough) describe any procedures or medications to be administered at home. The parent and child explain the child's limitations and reasons for them.
	Caution the parent against using eardrops unless specifically ordered by the physician.	Ear drops can adversely affect the graft.	

(Continues)

STANDARDS OF NURSING CARE *Postoperative Management of the Child Undergoing Tympanoplasty (Continued)*

GUIDE FOR NURSING MANAGEMENT

Nursing diagnosis	Intervention	Rationale	Outcome
	Instruct the parents to keep the child's head out of water; no swimming is allowed; cotton fluffs dipped in petroleum jelly can be placed in the ear orifice during bathing and hair washing.	Water in the ear will compromise the graft.	
	Teach the parents how to change the dressing if applicable.	Drainage is normal for several days.	
	Tell the parents to notify the physician if the child develops a high fever, neck stiffness, nausea, vomiting, headache, or nuchal rigidity.	Meningitis is a serious complication of ear surgery.	
	Encourage the parents to keep the child away from sources of upper respiratory infection.	Upper respiratory infection might lead to further ear damage.	

rective surgery and speech therapy. Some children with chronic hoarseness might be helped by voice training in which they are taught to project the voice without strain and to avoid voice abuse such as shouting.

Nursing care associated with deafness and blindness The effects of one of these sensory deficits can be devastating to the child and family. Unfortunately, some children have multisensory impairments. For example, children with congenital rubella syndrome might be deaf, develop glaucoma or cataracts, and be delayed in speech development because of sensory deficits or because of associated mental retardation.

Children who are deaf and blind communicate almost entirely through touch, and the use of touch needs to be heavily incorporated in their nursing care. These children require persistent and vigorous habilitation programs if they are to function with any degree of independence. Children who become impaired in several senses through trauma, brain tumor, or some other cause have the advantage of the learning, orientation, and skills gained before the impairment. These achievements can be built on by devising alternative modes of communication with objects, the environment, and other people.

Nutritional Needs

Alteration in nutrition: less than body requirements related to limited ability to feed self secondary to visual deficit

Children who are blind or are temporarily wearing eyepatches have additional nutritional needs during hospitalization. These needs are related to their eating habits and preferences and the adaptations or modifications that are required because of hospitalization. Children who are blind might have difficulty eating without assistance when hospitalized. Even if the family has developed ways to assist the child, these adaptations might not be communicated to the hospital staff.

A visually impaired child should be assisted to wash before meals, oriented to the type of food and the location of the food on the plate or tray, and provided with pleasant mealtime companions. To orient the young child to the type and location of the food, the nurse secures the plate with a suction cup or places it on a towel if the table is slippery. The nurse guides the child's hand to touch each food as the food is named. The nurse tells older children the location of the food on the plate by referring to the position of the numbers on a clock dial. If the child does not comprehend the clock dial, the nurse shows the location of the food by guiding the child's hand over the plate or tray. Cups and glasses are placed in the same position at each meal and should be wide based to reduce accidental spilling. The nurse might need to cut, butter, or season food for the young child, but the child's preferences need to be considered to promote independence.

Alteration in nutrition: less than body requirements related to altered taste sensation

Children with acute infections might have loss of appetite because nasal congestion interferes with taste and fever reduces energy. They require frequent, small meals. These meals need to include the important nutrients of protein, vitamins, and minerals, as well as increased fluid intake, all of which are essential to restore health and promote healing. Children undergoing surgery need to be in the best possible nutritional condition preoperatively. As soon as the postoperative condition permits, a well-balanced diet can be offered that will enhance healing and prevent developmental delays.

Alteration in nutrition: less than body requirements related to altered taste sensation

A child with a hearing impairment caused by chronic ear infections might have a decreased sensitivity to the taste of food because if the chronic infection is related to upper respiratory infections or allergies, the sense of smell is diminished. Smell is an important component of the sensation of taste. Children with chronic ear infections also might have unpleasant tastes in the mouth caused by drainage from the upper air passages. This unpleasant taste also diminishes pleasure in the taste of food.

Because appetite might lag when food is tasteless, color and attractiveness of the food need to be enhanced as much as possible. Seasonings such as catsup and spices can be added to the food if not contraindicated by dietary restrictions.

Developmental Needs

Potential for altered growth and development

Developmental needs are affected whenever a child has a health problem. Children who experience even temporary disruptions in sight or hearing during infancy or early childhood are particularly vulnerable because optimal development is so dependent on sensory input. Early case finding and prompt treatment are the most effective ways of minimizing the impact of temporary sensory dysfunction. However, even when the dysfunction is temporary and brief, nursing management follows the plan of care for children with more prolonged or permanent dysfunction.

Children who are blind or deaf from birth need to participate in sensory stimulation programs from the time of diagnosis. Parents of infants who are blind can help their children gain mobility and pass other developmental milestones in a timely fashion. Focusing on skin stimulation and the use of sound and games to encourage their infants' hand-to-mouth manipulation of objects and environmental exploration is important. Parents are encouraged to speak frequently to their infants so that the infants will begin to recognize their parents by voice and know where their parents are.

Attachment and separation are developmental concepts that describe the close ties between a child and parent and the loosening of the ties as the child gains skills and abilities in self-care. When the child cannot see and obviously needs protection from unseen hazards, it is difficult for both the child and the parent to initiate the separation process. One mechanism used by sighted infants is visual checking back to the parent as the infant gathers the courage to wander farther away. Such checking back is denied the child who is blind. Parents of blind children can offer the sound of their voices to reassure their children. Some children who are blind learn to call out when they need parental reassurance.

Children who are deaf can manage separation only to the degree that they can see their parents. These children are unable to recapture a sense of their parents' presence by hearing their voices or the sounds of their activity. Parents should check on these children frequently and allow the children to keep track of them as they move from location to location. Both children who are blind and children who are deaf have difficulty learning how to predict the behaviors of other people, which would help them gain confidence in their parents or other caregivers.

Congenitally deaf children require early language training. There is still much controversy over whether children who are deaf should be taught to communicate by signs or taught to speak. Deaf children can learn to speak, although their speech is often monotone or difficult to understand.

On the other hand, the child who has learned to communicate by sign language can communicate with others who know the hand signals. Often, the child who is deaf communicates both with spoken and with sign language simultaneously.

Other controversies continue over the comparative value of residential schools, special day schools, or public school education for children who are blind or deaf. For some children, residential school might be necessary, whereas supplemental day school programs might be needed in addition to public school programs for other children. Still other children might be able to be placed exclusively in public schools with the aid of Braille books, sign language readers, or other devices.

Whatever program is carried out and in whatever setting, the aim is to assist children to develop physically, emotionally, cognitively, and socially toward independence and full realization of their potential. To meet these aims, family involvement and support are essential so that the child receives consistent discipline and encouragement in self-care as appropriate to age and physical limitations. (Chapter 14 discusses the effect of chronic conditions on families).

Emotional Needs

⊛ Potential anxiety

Children whose hearing or sight problems are acute in onset are vulnerable to severe and long-lasting emotional upset. Children have difficulty believing or comprehending that the loss of sight or hearing is temporary. Even after function has been restored through treatment or surgery, the child might fear recurrence of the loss.

Young children are unable to understand that illness or disability can happen without being caused by someone. A child who is suddenly deprived of sight or hearing might believe that the disability is a punishment for some real or imagined wrongdoing. The child whose sensory disability occurred as a result of an accident such as a firecracker explosion is even more likely to consider the disability as a punishment.

Nurses can explain to children that accidents are not punishments, but the most useful approach to guilt in a child is to continuously demonstrate a nonjudgmental, accepting manner. The nurse can encourage the family to talk with their child about guilty feelings, reassuring the child of continued love and esteem from family members.

⊛ Potential body image disturbance

Because of the nature of their disabilities, children with sensory deficits such as blindness or deafness (with or without communication problems) are vulnerable to delays in emotional development. Development of a positive body image is hampered by sensory deficits. Children who are blind learn to know their bodies by feel and cutaneous stimulation. They are unable to see admiration or love in the gaze of others. Consequently, they need much physical demonstration of the regard their parents have for them. Gentle touch and lots of hugging by parents assists in the development of a positive body image.

Because blind children frequently are delayed in achieving mobility and autonomy, their concept of body boundaries might be delayed. It is important for parents or other caregivers to be aware of the need to help blind children establish body boundaries and gain a sense of the potential of their bodies and pride in their accomplishments. Parents can assist their children in these tasks by touching them frequently, naming body parts as they are touched, and deliberately making approving and admiring comments to their children.

Children who are deaf are able to see their own bodies and can enjoy the visual stimulation. Children who are deaf can discern love, caring, and admiration in their parents' expressions. Although deaf children have these advantages as compared with blind children, deafness will always be a part of their body images. The degree of disability that deaf children perceive will depend on their ability to develop articulate communication with others and on their parents' acceptance.

Children with sensory deficits are imperiled by the negative reactions of strangers and others to their disabilities. These responses, either directly or indirectly expressed, become part of the child's self-image. Family members and health care providers can prepare the child for these reactions. Adults can explain that some persons do not know how well children who are blind or deaf can manage, and as a result, they become uncomfortable, feel sorry for the children, and make silly, insensitive remarks.

To foster healthy self-images and to counterbalance the negative reactions they receive from others, children need admiration and respect from their families. Families and health care providers can emphasize the child's skills and accomplishments and establish plans for continued independence. Older children need to be encouraged to talk about other people's reactions and their responses to these reactions. Role-play might be helpful in assisting children to develop effective defenses and responses.

Health Maintenance Needs

⊛ Potential injury

Children with problems affecting the sensory organs are at risk for injury. (Teaching associated with accident prevention for the child who has a sensory impairment is discussed in Chapter 12.)

Potential for infection

Eye infections pose a threat to vision. As part of anticipatory guidance, nurses discuss eye hygiene with parents, explaining that the eye is self-cleansing and that eye washes are not needed. The eyelids are cleansed with clear water on a clean washcloth, lightly stroking from the inner corner of the eye to the outer corner. A clean portion of the cloth needs to be used for each eye. If any signs of redness, swelling, or discharge appear, the parent should consult with the nurse or a physician.

Parents need information about ear hygiene. Many parents believe that wax in the external canal should be removed with cotton-tipped applicators, so nurses might need to explain that the wax in the canal is normal and healthy. Only the shell of the ear needs to be cleansed; nothing should be introduced into the canal. If the external canal should become irritated, inflamed, or swollen or if the child does not respond to sounds, the parent should consult the nurse or a physician. Parents should not give eardrops or probe the child's ear without medical advice.

Nurses in primary care settings include information about the prevention of ear infections as part of the anticipatory guidance. The nurse describes the relationshp between the nasopharynx, the eustachian tube, and the middle ear and the ease with which infectious material can move from the throat to the ear of an infant or young child.

Parents need to know how to recognize an upper respiratory infection or an allergic response and be alert to possible signs of *otitis media* (middle ear infection), a frequent complication of upper respiratory illnesses. Some physicians recommend the use of a decongestant with any upper respiratory infection or allergy to prevent eustachian tube blockage, otitis media, and permanent ear damage.

Hearing and vision screening The nurse also advises the parents to have their children's visual acuity and auditory discrimination evaluated during early childhood and prior to entering school. Some conditions such as amblyopia (reduced vision) are somewhat correctable if recognized early enough.

The child who squints, tilts the head persistently, moves close to objects to see them, has excessive tearing or blinking of the eye or eyes that do not move together while watching a moving object needs to be examined earlier. Vision is assessed best while the nurse examines the infant's or child's eyes during a well-child examination.

The child who asks "What?" frequently or who sits very close to the television set in order to hear needs to be evaluated as soon as the behaviors are noticed. The behaviors might be due to fluid in the ears that prevents the child from hearing clearly or might be due to hearing loss from another cause. In either case an early evaluation can possibly prevent further auditory speech dysfunction.

During each well-child visit, the nurse assesses the adequacy of the child's speech production and vocabulary. Parental concerns are elicited as part of the interval history.

The Child with a Visual Deficit Related to Structural Alterations of the Eye

A number of visual acuity problems can arise because of structural anomalies of the eye and accessory muscles.

Refractive Errors

Refractive errors in vision are visual difficulties resulting from alterations in the path of light rays through the structures of the eye. Most refractive errors are caused by an abnormally shaped orb. Elongation or flattening of the orb results most frequently in hyperopia or myopia. *Hyperopia* means far-sighted, or the inability to focus on near objects. *Myopia* means near-sighted, or the inability to focus on distant objects. Children are mildly hyperopic until middle childhood, so findings of hyperopia prior to age 6 years are not cause for concern. More severe hyperopia or myopia is treated with corrective lenses.

Another frequently seen visual deficit is *astigmatism,* asymmetric curvature of the cornea. Although astigmatism can occur in one or both eyes, the condition usually is bilateral. Astigmatism is corrected with glasses or contact lenses to restore visual acuity.

The clinical manifestations of refractive errors usually include complaints by children that they are unable to see clearly, or children are observed squinting, frowning, or holding objects close to their faces or far away. The lenses do not cure or change the condition but do improve visual acuity, and the nurse encourages the proper wear and care of lenses.

Strabismus

Strabismus is a dysfunction of the muscular coordination that affects the relative alignment of the two eyes. It results in double vision (*diplopia*) or the suppression of vision from one eye (*amblyopia,* or "lazy" eye) in response to double vision. Strabismus can be normal in very young infants and will disappear as the infant matures and eye muscles become better developed.

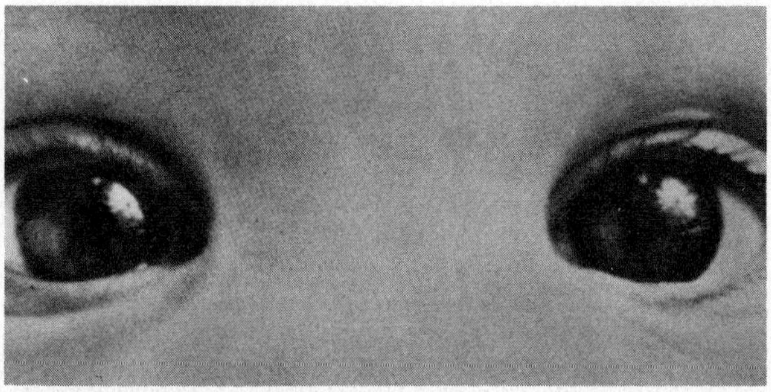

Transient strabismus might be present in the neonate and is caused by poor neuromuscular control. (Courtesy Mead Johnson Laboratories, Evansville, Ind.)

An infant over 4 months of age with strabismus might be referred to an ophthalmologist for evaluation, particularly if there is a close family history of strabismus. Strabismus needs to be recognized and treated in infancy, if possible, because the resulting amblyopia and consequent visual deficit can be irreversible.

The type of strabismus is classified according to the position of the affected eyes. In *esotropia* the eye or eyes turn in toward the nose ("cross-eyes"); in *exotropia* the eyes deviate outward ("wall-eyes"); and in *hypertropia,* strabismus upward rather than sideways, the eyes are at different levels. Estropia is the most common type of strabismus.

Strabismus is diagnosed through observation and the use of the corneal light reflex and the cover test (see Chapter 10). Visual acuity tests might reveal a vision deficit.

Treatment Neuromuscular coordination can be improved through eye muscle exercises, patching, or corrective lenses if refractory errors are present. Eye muscle exercises, known as *orthoptics,* require cooperation from the child and dedication from the parent. The exercises, which are done at least several times each week, consist of the use of a binocular projector or hand-held cards. The child consciously contracts the eye muscles to merge the images projected to each eye.

Corrective lenses are ground so that the "lazy eye" receives an image that is compatible with that received by the unaffected eye. This prevents double vision or amblyopia. Muscle coordination might not be corrected, but vision is restored.

Patching the unaffected eye to force the eye muscles and vision to be used in the affected eye is another method of treatment. Parents might be puzzled at the decision to cover the eye that functions best and will need to have the rationale for the treatment explained to them. If these methods fail to correct the strabismus, surgery might be required.

Binocular vision needs to be restored as soon as possible after the strabismus is recognized. If correction has not been achieved by 6 years of age, the likelihood of restoring vision in the affected eye is remote.

Nursing management Nurses in outpatient settings are alert for the occurrence of strabismus in young children and make appropriate referrals. Emphasizing to the child and family the importance of wearing the corrective lenses or patch is a nursing responsibility. The child might feel embarrassed by having to wear a patch to school, and the nurse is particularly sensitive to this issue. The patient is encouraged to allow the child to express feelings about this issue at home. The parent needs to emphasize the child's positive qualities because excessive teasing from peers can severely undermine the child's confidence.

If surgery is required, nursing management is comparable to care for any child undergoing eye surgery.

Cataract

A cataract is an opacity of the lens of the eye. It can be detected by ophthalmoscope, or the cataract can be seen without the use of a light. Its appearance is like an "oil droplet" visible in the pupillary area. Cataracts are associated with metabolic diseases such as galactosemia, congenital infections such as rubella, eye trauma, and the long-term use of cortisone therapy. Cataracts might be present at birth or develop during childhood. Visual impairment also varies widely from no reduction in sight to complete interference with the passage of light to the retina.

Treatment When sight is impaired, treatment is surgical removal of the lens. Modern surgical procedures have greatly reduced the risk of infection or other postoperative complications. If the remaining eye structures are normal, sight can be restored after surgery through the use of corrective eyeglasses or contact lenses. Intraocular lens implants have been used successfully in adults, but this procedure is seldom done on children, especially those under 1 year of age. The implant results are better if the cataract is caused by trauma rather than congenital. This surgery holds great promise for children because it not only improves visual acuity but also improves cosmetic appearance since thick glasses are no longer required to substitute for the removed lens.

If a cataract is left in place, untreated for a period of time, irreversible occlusional amblyopia might occur. *Occlusional amblyopia* is the term given to the functional blindness that occurs when the brain "blots out" the confusing double or blurred vision from the affected eye. If a cataract is in one eye only, postoperative treatment is difficult. The corrective lens does not provide the same clarity of vision as the unaffected eye. The child tends not to attend to the faulty image from the affected eye, resulting in permanent suppression of vision from that eye. The part-time use of an eyepatch on the unaffected eye might force sufficient use to preserve vision in the affected eye.

Nursing management After surgery and discharge, infants and young children are encouraged to return to their usual daily activities, which helps them to recover more quickly. The distraction these activities provide decreases problems with scratching the eye. The parent is instructed to inspect the eye each time the eye ointment or drops are administered to observe for any signs of infection such as thickened discharge, increased inflammation, and increased complaints of itching or soreness and for any signs of opacities in the eye. Any changes in the eye should be reported to the surgeon immediately.

Glaucoma

Glaucoma is a condition caused by elevated intraocular pressure in the anterior chamber. In infancy glaucoma is characterized by enlarged, hazy corneas. Photophobia, tearing, and poor vision are late signs. Glaucoma can occur in association with systemic disease, trauma, infection, or as an isolated disorder. Tonometry reveals an elevated intraocular pressure.

Treatment The treatment for children is surgery to remove the obstruction to the aqueous humor flow from the anterior chamber. Careful and frequent medical follow-up is important to detect any recurrence of increased pressure due to inflammation or scarring.

Nursing management Preoperative and postoperative care of a child who has had surgery for glaucoma might include the administration of miotic eyedrops to enhance the flow of the aqueous humor and antibiotic ointments. Miotic eyedrops cause the pupils to constrict. The parent needs to know the signs of acute increased intraocular pressure (pain, inflammation of the eye, and nausea and vomiting) and understand that any inflammation, temperature elevation, or other signs of increased intraocular pressure should be reported to the surgeon immediately.

The Child with Inflammation of the Eye

Three major inflammatory eye diseases are conjunctivitis, orbital cellulitis, and corneal ulcer. Each of these problems has the potential to cause permanent damage to the eye; therefore, prompt detection, referral, and treatment are essential.

Conjunctivitis

Conjunctivitis is an inflammation of the conjunctiva, or lining, of the eyelids and covering of the sclera. The inflammation can be caused by mechanical irritation, viral or bacterial organisms, or allergens. The clinical manifestations of conjunctivitis vary depending on the cause but usually include erythema, edema of the lids, itching and tearing, and mucoid or purulent discharge. The treatment consists of antibiotics, such as erythromycin (Ilotycin), in topical ointments or eyedrops.

Children with conjunctivitis usually are cared for at home, so nursing management includes referral for medical care and parent teaching. The nurse informs the parents about the spread of eye disease and the importance of preventing other children from coming in contact with the discharge from the affected child's eye. No one else should use the affected child's washcloth or towel. The affected child should not share a pillow or bed if at all possible while the infection is present.

The parent also needs to be instructed about home treatment of the conjunctivitis. The nurse emphasizes the importance of thorough hand washing before and after cleansing the eyelids and administering the topical medication. The parent cleans the child's eyelids with plain, warm tap water, using a clean cloth or cotton balls and being certain to wipe from the inner canthus outward. After treatment, the cloth needs to be washed thoroughly or the cotton balls discarded. The nurse describes ways to restrain infants and toddlers from rubbing the eye, such as by elbow restraints (see Chapter 20). If such restraint is needed, the nurse emphasizes the importance of removing the restraints frequently and putting the child's arms through full range of motion before replacing the restraints.

Orbital Cellulitis

Orbital cellulitis is a more serious inflammation of the tissues behind the orb, usually caused by ethmoid sinusitis (inflammation of the ethmoid sinus) or by infected skin disruptions or injuries near the eye. The eyelids are swollen, and the orb is displaced anteriorly. Intravenous antibiotics and sinus decongestants are the usual medical treatments to prevent further spread of infection into the cranium.

Nursing management of orbital cellulitis includes administering the intravenous infusion, administering the medications, observing for side effects, and assessing the sinus drainage and appearance of the eye.

Children and parents might be surprised or frightened at the vigorous treatment of what might appear to be a minor problem. The nurse explains that the infected area is very close to the brain and that the vigorous treatment is necessary to prevent brain abscess. The nurse also keeps the family informed of signs of recovery—normal temperature, reduced inflammation, and changes in the white blood cell count. The parents might be concerned that they did not recognize that the child was ill sooner. The nurse reviews the signs of sinusitis and inflammation in the facial area and encourages parents to seek medical consultation if these signs are noted again.

Children often become restless and bored during the long intravenous therapy regimen, especially after the first day or so when they begin to feel well again. Very young children or infants might require restraints to safeguard the intravenous insertion or to prevent them from rubbing the affected eye. These children need the companionship of their parents and other children. Play and other diversionary activities will foster cooperation with the therapy and reduce the boredom of prolonged hospitalization.

Corneal Ulcers

Corneal ulcers can develop as a result of infection. The clinical signs of corneal ulceration are moderate to severe pain, blurred vision, and watery or purulent discharge from the eye. Prompt and vigorous medical treatment is essential to prevent permanent scarring and subsequent loss of visual acuity caused by changes in the refractive surface of the eye. Nursing management includes the administration of topical medications and analgesics. The nurse teaches the parent how to administer eyedrops and ointments and to prevent infections or irritation caused by the child rubbing the eye.

The Child with Traumatic Injury to the Eye

Corneal Abrasion

Corneal abrasion is a direct injury to the cornea caused when an object such as sand is blown into the eye or a projectile such as a tree limb brushes against the cornea. The protective mechanisms of blinking and tearing are usually but not always adequate to remove a small foreign object from the eye. If the object is loose, the nurse can attempt to remove it gently with the corner of a small gauze pad that has been dipped in normal saline. When protective mechanisms fail or a foreign object remains in the eye, an abrasion can occur.

When a child complains of continuing pain in the eye, the nurse suspects a corneal abrasion. The child's eye might tear excessively, and the child might be sensitive to light. Immediate assessment is important. The nurse first examines the conjunctiva and cornea for obvious foreign bodies. If a foreign body is not present or not removable, the nurse refers the child immediately to an ophthalmologist.

Subconjunctival Hemorrhage

Subconjunctival hemorrhage appears as a small red area on the sclera and might be due to increased ocular pressure from something as minor as a cough. Although subconjunctival hemorrhages resolve on their own, they might be associated with other ocular problems and should be evaluated.

Chemical Injury

Chemical burns of the eye are caused by accidental contact with corrosive agents, usually household cleaning products. These products can be acidic, such as bleach, or alkalis, such as lye and commercial drain cleaners. Regardless of the acidity of the substance, the eye should be flushed for at least 20 minutes (as described in Chapter 12). Injuries from alkalis should be flushed for a longer period of time (over 30 minutes) than acids because they penetrate more rapidly and thus are more difficult to remove. The child needs to be transported to the hospital immediately for ophthalmologic evaluation.

Treatment After irrigation, the eye is examined for injury. A mydriatic or cycloplegic drug such as atropine sulfate might be administered to rest the ciliary musculature and relieve pain (Tumulty and Resler, 1984). Severely burned corneas no longer have sensation. An antibiotic ointment is instilled to prevent infection, and the affected eye is patched. The eye is reexamined within 24 hours for injuries that might not have been apparent at the first examination.

Nursing management Nursing management includes emergency eye irrigation or, if the initial inquiry was by telephone, instructing the parent to irrigate the child's eye. Prompt referral to an ophthalmologist is essential. Equally important as first aid is prevention of injury. Parent teaching needs to include the safe storage and use of corrosive liquids or powders (see Chapter 12).

Hyphema

Hyphema, the presence of blood in the anterior chamber of the eye, is caused by a blunt injury. Such an injury occurs with or without orbital fracture and other injuries to the structures of the eye. Hyphema can result from any head injury, such as from a car accident, or from a direct blow to the eye with an object such as a baseball or bat. These injuries are most frequently seen in the active and accident-prone years of early and middle childhood and adolescence.

Hyphema can be observed as a light red color in front of the lower portion of the iris. The presence of blood can be seen by shining a light laterally into the orb. The blood usually is absorbed without further damage, but the bleeding can recur or can cause increased intraocular pressure. For these reasons, it is important to observe a child with hyphema closely for several days.

Treatment Treatment of hyphema includes patching the eye, placing the child on strict bed rest, and instilling ophthalmologic preparations. Medications might be prescribed for pain, and attention is given to associated injuries.

Nursing management Nursing care of the hospitalized child with hyphema includes careful observation for complications and administration of medications. If the child is being cared for at home, the nurse teaches the parents what to watch for and how to administer any medications. Any complaints of diminished vision or sudden flashes of light might indicate retinal detachment (separation of the retina from the choroid) and require prompt notification of an ophthalmologist. Severe, sudden headache associated with nausea and/or vomiting might be a sign of glaucoma with increasing intraocular pressure, another complication of blunt trauma. Acute glaucoma is an ocular emergency and requires immediate attention (Welch, Tyler, & Quinn, 1984).

The nurse emphasizes the importance of observing the child but does so without frightening the parent. If the injury is severe, eyepatches and strict bed rest might be required. The degree to which the child's activity is restricted depends on the severity of the bleeding and other suspected or diagnosed injuries such as a skull fracture. Elevation of the head of the bed to 30° assists in preventing increased intracranial pressure, which might occur from an associated head injury.

The temporary loss of sight and the restricted activity will be difficult for the child, and the nurse and family's ingenuity will be taxed to find ways to help the child cope with the restrictions. Storytelling, records, word games, and other activities that can be enjoyed in bed and without sight are helpful. The most important nursing measure is to reduce the child's anxiety by frequent assurances that the restriction and loss of sight are temporary.

The child with hyphema might become withdrawn or be drowsy. For this reason, frequent neurologic checks are essential in trying to discriminate the effects of hyphema from neurologic problems such as concussion. Hyphema usually resolves in less than 1 week, but complications such as retinal detachment, glaucoma, or displaced lens might develop at a later time.

Penetrating Eye Injuries

Injuries to the eye from darts, arrows, or other thin objects can cause severe ocular damage and possible loss of vision, depending on the severity and extent of the injury. As with blunt trauma, the sequlae of penetrating injuries include detachment of the retina and glaucoma. In addition, cataracts can develop from even minor penetrating injuries (Tumulty and Resler, 1984). Infection is an ever-present danger.

Treatment Treatment of penetrating injuries includes vigorous antibiotic therapy, tetanus prophylaxis, pain relief, sedation, and the administration of antiemetics because vomiting raises intraocular pressure (Tumulty and Resler, 1984). The penetrating object needs to be removed surgically and not at the scene of the accident (see Chapter 12). In severe cases of ocular damage, enucleation (removal of the eye from the socket) might be necessary.

Nursing management (First aid for penetrating eye injuries is discussed in Chapter 12.) Nursing care of the child with a penetrating eye injury is similar to that of a child with hyphema. The nurse observes for any change in eye drainage, level of pain, or presence of extraordinary ocular edema, all signs of an infection. The child and family might experience psychologic problems related to the injury. Anxiety and guilt are common reactions that might be part of the child and family's coping repertoire. If loss of vision is documented, the nurse needs to help the child to adjust to the resulting alteration in body image.

If the child is to be fitted for an artificial eye after enucleation, the nurse needs to ensure that both the child and family understand how to take care of it. The prosthesis can be removed from the eye socket by gently depressing the lower lid and allowing the eye to slide out, or by use of a suction device. After washing the artificial eye in normal saline and cleaning the socket as directed, the prosthesis is replaced. This is done by lifting the upper lid, depressing the lower lid, and sliding the eye into place. The eye is held in place by the restraint of both lids. The prosthesis can be

NURSING CARE PLAN *The Child with Hyphema*

Assessment data: Robert, a 17-year-old high school junior, was admitted to the hospital with a diagnosis of hyphema of the right eye. He suffered a blunt trauma to the eye during football practice and was brought immediately to the hospital when it became apparent that he had sustained an injury. Ophthalmoscopic examination revealed a small area of hemorrhage into the anterior chamber. No other complications were evident at the time other than a right periorbital hematoma. Both eyes were patched, and strict bed rest was ordered. Admission vital signs and laboratory studies were within normal limits, and there was no fracture of the orbital bone. Robert appeared listless and withdrawn.

Nursing diagnosis	Intervention	Rationale
1. Potential anxiety (stressors: unknown outcome of injury, unfamiliar surroundings, inability to see, feelings of helplessness)	Explain to Robert and his family that hyphema usually resolves within several days and that complications are not common.	Giving a realistic time frame relieves the anxiety and concern associated with permanent blindness.
	Explain the nature of the injury, the body's response, and the treatment plan.	Increased knowledge decreases anxiety.
	Spend time with Robert, encourage him to verbalize his concerns relative to his injury and return to school and activities.	Verbalization of concerns helps put them in perspective and any misinformation can be corrected.

Outcome: Robert and his family verbally express any feelings of anxiety. They express relief from anxiety after explanations are given and questions are answered.

Nursing diagnosis	Intervention	Rationale
2. Alteration in comfort: pain related to physical injury to eye secondary to trauma	Administer sedatives or analgesics as ordered.	Analgesics will provide pain relief. Sedatives promote relaxation and a subsequent decrease in pain. The administration of cycloplegic eyedrops, if ordered, will promote paralysis of the ciliary muscle and provide rest for the eye.
	Keep both eyes patched.	Patching prevents movement of the affected eye by reducing movement of the unaffected eye, thus relieving pain by reducing strain. Patching also prevents the child from rubbing the eye.
	Apply ice to the hematoma.	The application of cold reduces the injury-induced edema.
	Provide quiet diversion such as music and conversation.	See Chapter 20 for an explanation of the use of diversionary strategies to reduce pain.
	Explain to Robert the reasons for his pain and encourage him to request pain relief when needed.	Realistic explanations decrease anxiety and correspondingly relieve pain.
	Assist Robert to change position; the bed should be elevated 30°; caution Robert against sudden movements.	Bed elevation of 30° decreases intracranial and intraocular pressure; sudden movements increase pain.

Outcome: Robert expresses his need for pain relief. The pain appears to be diminishing as evidenced by increased relaxation, stable vital signs, and increased interest in his surroundings.

NURSING CARE PLAN *The Child with Hyphema (Continued)*

Nursing diagnosis	Intervention	Rationale
3. Sensory-perceptual alteration: input deficit related to temporary visual deficit secondary to bilateral eyepatches	Organize nursing care to allow Robert periods of uninterrupted rest; develop and post a schedule of activities and nursing care so a similar pattern of events can be followed daily.	Lack of sleep contributes to confusion, increased anxiety, and altered perception of events. Posting a schedule for all staff to follow ensures regular rest.
	Orient Robert to his environment by describing his surroundings as clearly and descriptively as possible; orient Robert frequently to time; can use a digital watch that makes a sound on the hour.	Verbal description provides visual images and allows the child to interact with the surroundings; it also identifies spatial limits that enhance safety.
	Identify self and others as they enter the room.	This provides reality orientation.
	Speak to Robert before touching him.	This will avoid startling the child and will decrease anxiety.
	Explain all care and treatments to Robert. Allow him to feel any equipment before using it; tell him how it might feel.	Knowledge of what is to happen decreases anxiety and provides reality orientation.
	Tell Robert when leaving the room. Make certain that he has a call button secured within reach.	Providing security that the nurse can be reached invites the child to maintain verbal contact when needed.
	Provide stimulation by changing Robert's environment, allowing family and friends to visit or providing distraction.	Changes in the environment maintain attention and enhance the perception of reality.
	Encourage self-care activities such as feeding, bathing, and dressing; assist Robert to be as independent as possible by placing needed articles within reach and describing their location (right, left, up, or down or according to the face of a clock).	Regular participation in care increases the perception of reality and attention to the environment.
	Provide diversion that is age appropriate and is not overstimulating. Read to Robert, provide quiet music, play word memory games. Have phone within easy reach and encourage him to use it.	Diversion using the other senses can prevent sensory deprivation.

Outcome: Robert sleeps well without nightmares. Robert appears to be free of confusion and perceptual distortion. He expresses interest in his surroundings and willingness to participate in his care.

Nursing diagnosis	Intervention	Rationale
4. Potential for injury (stressors: disorientation from eyepatches, fragility of eye while healing, hazards of immobility)	Inform Robert not to blow his nose forcefully. Provide a diet high in bulk and fluids to avoid straining with bowel movement.	Straining of any type can increase intraocular and intracranial pressure.
	Take Robert's vital signs frequently and perform regular neurologic checks.	Increased blood pressure, severe headache, lethargy, pupil alterations, confusion, and vomiting are signs of increased intracranial pressure caused by head injury.
	Encourage Robert to report immediately any signs of decreased vision, particles moving across the visual field, or flashes of light.	These symptoms might indicate retinal detachment, a complication of blunt trauma to the eye. They will be evident when the patches are removed.

(Continues)

NURSING CARE PLAN *The Child with Hyphema (Continued)*

Nursing diagnosis	Intervention	Rationale
	Observe Robert for any signs of severe, sudden headache associated with nausea and vomiting and signs of decreased visual acuity.	Glaucoma can occur secondary to trauma.
	Alert Robert and his family to the possibility of these complications occurring after discharge.	Preparing the family with appropriate information will facilitate the prompt recognition and treatment of complications.
Outcome: Robert and his family describe the symptoms of increased intracranial pressure, retinal detachment, and glaucoma and explain who they will contact should any of these symptoms appear.		
5. Potential for ineffective individual and family coping: compromised (stressors: role changes, interruption in individual routines, lack of knowledge, emotional and situational stress)	Encourage Robert and his family to verbalize feelings of guilt, anger, or fear.	Verbalization of feelings assists with coping.
	Allow Robert to express any feelings he might have relative to missing the rest of the football season.	He might have fears that he might lose popularity or social standing by not participating in the sport; verbalizing fears allows the child to deal with them.
	Suggest alternative activities, which will allow him to continue his social contacts and satisfy his need to participate; involve Robert in decision making.	Decision making increases control and reduces ineffective coping.
Outcome: Robert exerts some control over his activities. He experiences little interruption in his educational or social life as a result of his injury. Robert and his family identify strengths that will promote effective coping.		

cleaned as often as necessary or at the physician's direction. Children can assume care of their own prostheses but must be cautioned against dropping them because this might cause scratches or breakage.

The prevention of eye injuries is infinitely preferable to treating them (see Chapter 12). The nurse includes preventive teaching during well-child visits.

The Child with an Auditory Deficit Related to Structural Alterations of the Ear

Hearing Deficits

Hearing loss in children can be divided into two major categories. *Conductive hearing loss* occurs when the transmission of sound waves between the external ear and the inner ear is interrupted but the inner ear is not affected. For example, conductive hearing loss can be caused by a cerumen-occluded auditory canal, interference with tympanic membrane motility, or ossicle fixation. Many problems that cause conductive hearing loss can be treated successfully medically or surgically (Saxton et al., 1983).

Sensorineural deafness involves alteration of inner ear function in which sound waves are carried successfully to the inner ear but are improperly analyzed there (Saxton et al., 1983). Factors contributing to sensorineural deafness include damage from certain medications, head trauma, infections, or noise pollution (Saxton et al., 1983). Some nerve deafness might be hereditary. Unfortunately, little can be done to treat sensorineural deafness, which forces the child to learn alternate methods of communication.

Hearing loss is determined by whether the child can hear certain sound frequencies (eg, various pitches) at various decibles (dB) by audiometry. The extent of hearing loss can be divided into four major categories. Mild hearing loss occurs when the child fails to hear frequencies at 30 dB. The child with moderate hearing loss cannot hear frequencies at

50–60 dB, while severe hearing loss occurs with failure at over 60 dB. The child is considered to be profoundly deaf with hearing loss at 90 dB.

Structural Anomalies of the External Ear

Structural anomalies of the external ear might not cause hearing problems but can be a source of embarrassment and unhappiness for the child and family. *Lop ear* is the term used to describe large external ears that protrude from the head in a very noticeable fashion. Other malformations include extra skin tabs in the tragus of the ear, absent skin folds on the helix, and a low-set position on the head. Some of these malformations are associated with syndromes of varying seriousness; therefore, the nurse notes any abnormality of the ear and refers the child for medical diagnosis.

Hearing is not affected by these external ear abnormalities, except for those children who have syndromes that include nerve deafness. Arrested development of the external ear sometimes includes failure of the external ear canal to develop, resulting in air conduction deafness. The treatment for malformed external ears is plastic surgery to achieve as normal an appearance as possible. The surgery for malformed ears needs to be completed by 6 years of age and prior to the child's entering school, if possible. Early repair avoids embarrassment for the child from questions by new acquaintances.

Specific postoperative care includes special attention to protecting the operative site by maintaining the integrity of the dressing, observing for circulatory compromise, and discouraging the child from activities that involve roughhousing or have the potential for falls. Parents and children need to be prepared for the appearance of the operative site before the dressing is removed. The sight of swollen, ecchymotic structures will be very disappointing if parents do not understand the normal process of healing. Parents and children often have unrealistic expectations of the final results of plastic surgery. Much can be done to construct the external ear, but exact replication is not possible.

Structural Anomalies of the Internal Ear

Structural anomalies of the internal ear include stenosis (narrowing) or atresia (abnormal closure) of the middle ear and absence or fusion of the ossicles. Some of these anomalies are related to other craniofacial problems.

Surgery to correct internal structural anomalies needs to be done as soon as possible after diagnosis to preserve hearing acuity. Microsurgery can be done to replace or realign the ossicles, open an atretic external canal, and replace tympanic membranes. The postoperative course might include vertigo and pain. Nursing care includes administering drugs for analgesia and the relief of vertigo and providing safety measures for the ambulatory child. Vertigo is a distressing symptom for children. Vertigo can be reduced by encouraging the child to move slowly as the head is moved or the body is raised or turned. The nurse reassures the child that the symptom is temporary.

The Child with an Ear Infection or Inflammation

Ear infections are seen frequently in young children and can cause permanent hearing loss through scarring of the membranes that conduct sound. Temporary hearing loss can occur during the acute phase of the infection or inflammation. The temporary loss of hearing is a result of accumulation of fluid in the middle ear. Fluid accumulation limits the conduction of sound waves by not allowing the same free movement of the ossicles as does the normal air media in the middle ear. Permanent loss of hearing can result from scarring of the tympanic membrane related to repeated infections. Scarring reduces the motility of the membrane and its sensitivity to sound waves.

Infection of the middle ear (otitis media), is caused by microorganisms or allergies. Either of these can cause closure of the eustachian tube. The eustachian tube normally opens and closes regularly to equalize pressure between the middle ear and the outside and to drain secretions produced in the middle ear. Adequate hearing depends on equal pressure because the tympanic membrane vibrates most effectively when pressure is equal on both sides. When the eustachian tube is closed for long periods, fluid accumulates in the middle ear and can create a medium for the growth of infectious organisms. Fluid accumulation also can alter the motility of the tympanic membrane.

Infants and children under 5 years of age are affected by middle ear infection most frequently. The eustachian tube is shorter and straighter than that of the older child or adult, and because of this, it is closer to the nasopharynx. Organisms from the nasopharynx have easier access to the middle ear through the shorter eustachian tube. Additional factors predisposing the child to middle ear infection include (1) obstruction of the eustachian tube from pressure by the relatively large amount of lymphoid tissue in the area (eg, adenoid tissue), (2) immaturity of the young child's immune system, and (3) pooling of liquids or secretions in the nasopharangeal area from the large amount of time an infant or young child spends lying down. Otitis media can be acute or chronic, suppurative or nonsuppurative (with effusion).

Suppurative Otitis Media (SOM)

Suppurative otitis media usually is caused by the *S. pneumoniae* or the *H. influenzae* organisms, although other organisms can be implicated. SOM frequently follows an upper respiratory infection, during which swollen mucosa closes the eustachian tube. Organism growth along with retention of fluid in the middle ear causes classic symptoms in children.

Clinical manifestations The child might experience pain in the affected ear, fever, irritability, dizziness, anorexia, and nausea. In young infants, tugging or pulling at the affected ear along with other symptoms of infection indicates probable middle ear involvement. The fever can be relatively high and often is 40°C (104°F). Cervical lymph node enlargement might occur with SOM.

Diagnostic evaluation Otoscopy reveals an inflamed, red, bulging tympanic membrane with diffusion of the normal light reflex. When air is introduced into the ear canal to test for mobility, the eardrum moves sluggishly or not at all. Audiometry might show decreased auditory acuity, although children who most frequently experience SOM usually are too young to cooperate with audiometric testing. Tympanometry (Fig. 32-2) might reveal a flat pattern indicating relatively little tympanic membrane movement.

Treatment Antibiotics are prescribed to treat SOM. The antibiotic chosen usually is an antibiotic that is effective against both organisms that most frequently cause SOM. Ampicillin, amoxicillin, trimethoprim-sulfamethoxazole (Bactrim, Septra), and cefaclor (Ceclor) are the agents most frequently used. Amoxicillin might be preferred in the treatment of young children since it can be given with meals and is available in chewable tablets. If the child does not respond to treatment after 48 hours, aspiration of the middle ear fluid (tympanocentesis) might be performed to determine more accurately the causative organism. Children who experience repeated attacks of SOM can be placed on prophylactic low doses of trimethoprim-sulfamethoxazole (Bactrim) or sulfisoxazole (Gantrisin). These have been effective in reducing recurrent attacks of SOM.

Nursing management Uncomplicated cases of otitis media usually can be cared for in the home. The nurse encourages the parent to increase the child's fluid intake and

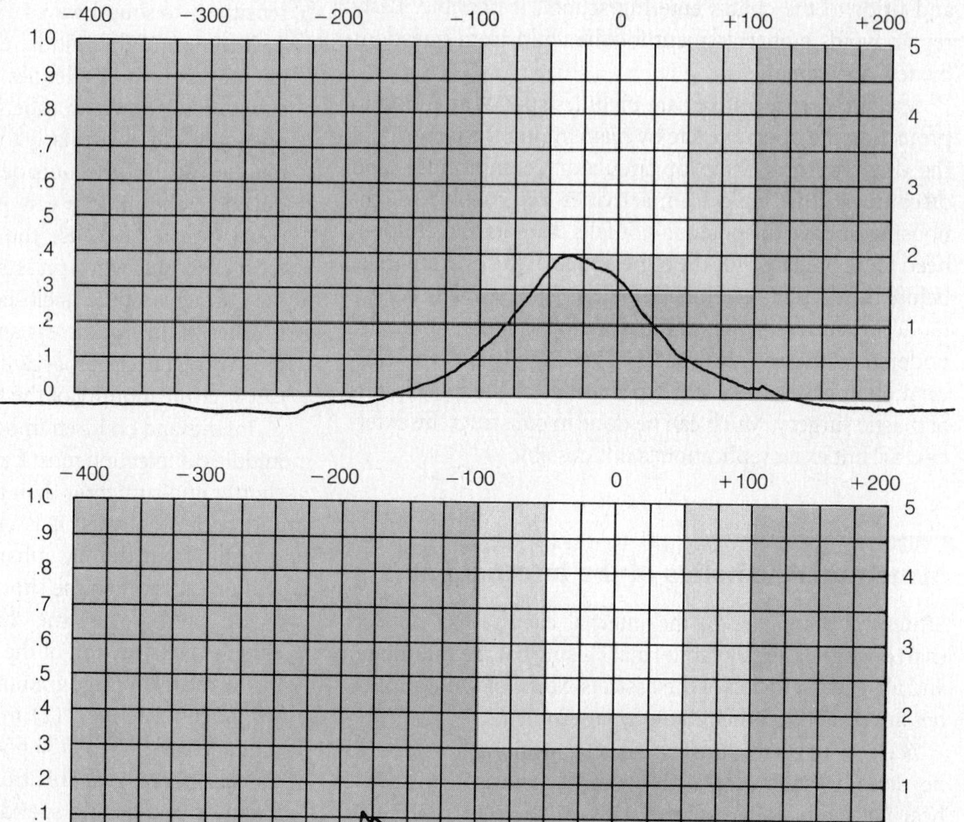

FIGURE 32-2

A. *Normal tympanograph.* ***B.*** *Abnormal tympanograph.*

to relieve discomfort or fever with acetaminophen in appropriate doses. With very young children, it is sometimes necessary to find ingenious methods to encourage fluid intake. The parent needs to provide juices and drinks that the child likes along with ice cream, jello, and frozen drinks or Popsicles.

The parent or caregiver is instructed to bring the child back for evaluation in 48 hours if there is no improvement. In addition, the parent needs to observe the child for a perforated eardrum, evidenced by sudden pain with bloody drainage from the affected ear, followed by relief of pain. Should this occur, the parent needs to notify the physician. The parent is instructed to give the child the antibiotic for the full prescribed period. Because ear infections are sometimes difficult to cure, the nurse emphasizes to the parents the need to recheck the child when the antibiotics are completed, usually 10–14 days after treatment is initiated.

Nonsuppurative Otitis Media (NOM)

Episodes of nonsuppurative otitis media, often called otitis media with effusion, are related to abnormalities in the eustachian tube, congenital abnormalities such as cleft palate that are associated with pooling of secretions in the nasopharynx, upper respiratory infections, enlargement of the adenoids, and previous SOM. Allergy, causing edema of the respiratory passages, has been strongly linked to repeated episodes of NOM (Castiglia, Aquilina, & Kemsley, 1983).

With NOM, closure of the eustachian tube causes fluid retention in the middle ear. The trapped air, which normally equalizes pressure against the tympanic membrane, is absorbed by the circulation. This causes negative air pressure in the middle ear with retraction of the eardrum. The trapped fluid in the middle ear thickens and darkens in color, often referred to as "glue ear." Mild conductive hearing loss can occur from the restricted movement of the tympanic membrane and the small ossicles in the middle ear.

Clinical manifestations The child with NOM does not appear ill, as does the child with SOM. The child might complain about a fullness in the ear, or hearing crackling or popping sounds. The parent might notice that the child's hearing seems reduced. For example, the child might say "What?" quite frequently in conversation or seem to be inattentive when spoken to.

Diagnostic evaluation Otoscopic examination reveals a dull, gray or yellow tympanic membrane. Often, fluid or bubbles can be seen through the membrane. Membrane mobility is markedly decreased with the introduction of air. Audiometric testing might reveal failure at 25–30 dB, indicating mild hearing loss. The tympanograph shows a diminished curve and negative pressure. The Rinne and Weber tests might be positive in children old enough to cooperate (see Table 32-1).

Treatment NOM that follows an episode of SOM or an upper respiratory infection might resolve spontaneously within a few weeks to three months. For this reason, and because decongestants have proved to be ineffective, no treatment is prescribed. The child is observed frequently for resolution of the problem. Attempts are made to correct any underlying problems such as allergy, cleft palate, or enlarged adenoids. Occasionally, bacteria can be found in the fluid of children with NOM. If a subclinical infection is suspected, or if the child has not been treated with antibiotics for a recent SOM, a course of antimicrobial therapy might be indicated.

Any NOM that lasts longer than 3 months is cause for concern. Chronic NOM can cause difficulties with speech development in the young child as a result of chronic diminished hearing. A myringotomy with tube insertion to drain fluid from the middle ear might be considered for any child with chronic otitis media. Any decision for surgery needs to weigh the potential for long-term adverse effects of diminished hearing against the potential hazards of surgery.

Chronic otitis media can result in *cholesteatoma* (pus and debris in the middle ear), mastoiditis (inflammation of the mastoid), brain abscess, and permanent hearing loss. Surgery might be needed to remove debris and promote drainage. Children with severely damaged tympanic membranes from chronic otitis media can recover some hearing with a tympanoplasty.

Nursing management Identification of children with chronic diminished hearing is an important nursing function. The child who exhibits language delays, inattention, or learning disorders needs to be evaluated for hearing impairment.

The nurse supports parents who might feel guilty that they did not recognize the child's problem quickly. The nurse allows the parents to express any feelings of guilt and explains that often the signs go unrecognized by parents because they are so subtle.

If the child is experiencing hearing loss, the nurse teaches the parents to improve their communication techniques with the child. The parent is encouraged to face the child while speaking. The parent might have to speak slightly louder than usual and be closer to the child. The parent might want to have the child verify what has been said. The nurse encourages the parent to communicate the problem to the child's teacher. The child's seat in school might need to be moved closer to the teacher for maximum learning.

If the child is scheduled for surgery, the nurse prepares the child according to age and developmental level (see the Standards of Nursing Care for postoperative management). The nurse teaches the parent how to handle the child at home after surgery and to avoid sources of upper respiratory infection.

Mastoiditis

Mastoiditis is an infection of the mastoid air cells, which are located in the bony cranium just behind the ear. The clinical signs are fever, earache, pain, and tenderness over the mastoid area. Facial paralysis is a serious sign that indicates that the infection has spread to the facial nerve sheath. Radiographs of the area might reveal destruction of the bone. Children usually are hospitalized and treated with intravenous antibiotics. If bone destruction has occurred, surgical incision and drainage are done.

Nursing management of a child with mastoiditis might include detection in an outpatient facility and referral to medical care. Nursing care in the hospital includes the maintenance of intravenous infusions, administration of medications, pain management, and preoperative and postoperative management if surgery is required. The nurse explains the condition to the parent, emphasizing the need for vigorous treatment to prevent complications and the spread of infection. Any signs of meningeal irritation need to be reported immediately (see Chapter 31). During convalescence, the nurse assesses the child's hearing acuity to discover if any permanent damage has occurred to the auditory nerve or internal structures of the ear.

The Child with Ear Trauma

The ear can be injured by a sharp blow to the head, laceration of the external ear, and introduction of foreign objects into the external canal. Laceration of the external ear frequently is caused by animal bites. Ear laceration is treated as any other skin injury, with pressure applied to the bleeding site and suturing if needed to achieve clean and undistorted healing. Tetanus prophylaxis is indicated (see Chapter 24).

Sharp blows to the ear or foreign bodies might rupture the eardrum. The child will complain of severe pain and loss of hearing in the affected ear. Prompt medical attention is needed to prevent infection and promote healing of the eardrum without scarring.

Foreign bodies, such as small beads, pebbles, and earrings might be introduced into the external canal and be undetected for a time. The object might not be noticed until a discharge appears, the external canal becomes irritated, and hearing acuity is decreased. Removal of the foreign body in the external canal requires professional skill and should not be attempted by the parent.

Nursing management includes anticipatory guidance about the potential dangers of allowing toddlers to play with small objects without supervision. Parents might need to be taught not to attempt to clean the ear with cotton swabs; that cerumen serves a function in maintaining ear health.

Sudden exposure to loud noises can rupture the eardrum or damage the auditory nerve (Saunders et al., 1979). Although most of the evidence for damage from loud noises has come from studies of industrial hazards, many researchers believe that similar injuries can occur from stereophonic music turned up to the highest volume. Some loss of hearing acuity might be caused by nerve damage, but the practice of constantly listening to excessively loud sounds also might result in decreased attention to low-volume sounds. Children and parents need to know about the potential dangers of exposure to loud noises.

The Child with a Disorder of the Nasal Cavity

Young children, particularly those in early childhood, are prone to putting small objects in their nares, often without subsequent discovery by the parent. The parent should suspect a foreign body when the child exhibits a malodorous or blood-stained nasal discharge. Medical consultation is advised because the object will need to be removed after diagnosis via a nasal speculum.

Anything that causes nasal obstruction, whether it be a foreign object or swollen nasal membranes from the common cold, will not only interfere with the sense of smell but also with the sense of taste. Nurses need to make parents aware of this to decrease parental concern about anorexia during bouts of upper respiratory infections or during allergy season.

Trauma to the nose is more frequent in children in late childhood or adolescence who participate in athletics. Force from a bat, ball, or other athletic equipment can fracture the nose. If the fracture is not displaced, no treatment is required except to control the resulting epistaxis (nosebleed). Ice packs can be applied for comfort and to reduce edema. Unfortunately, repeated nasal fractures can lead to cosmetic alteration. The child with a deviated septum might require surgery to restore appearance and function.

The Child with a Language Disorder

Language disorders are complex dysfunctions that can adversely affect the child's communicative abilities. Difficulties can be concentrated in any of the following areas of language development.

1. Difficulty formulating ideas, or conceptualizing
2. Difficulty learning the symbols that represent ideas
3. Learning symbols that are not congruent with accepted symbols
4. Inability to use symbols for verbal communication
5. Developmental delay in comparison with peers' language development (Bloom and Lahey, 1978).

Normal language development can be interrupted by any number of physical and emotional factors, including structural or neurologic abnormalities, impaired hearing, impaired cognitive skills, nonstimulating environment, and emotional disease (psychosis).

When managing a child with dysfunctional language development, the nurse needs to be aware of the difference between receptive and expressive language. Children with receptive language problems find it difficult to decode information; that is, they might not understand the verbal symbols of language and/or might have limited ability to comprehend and organize ideas (Goldberg, 1984). Children with expressive disabilities manifest difficulties of speech—poor grammar, alterations in the sound or pattern of speech, or delays caused by environmental deprivation (Goldberg, 1984).

Childhood Aphasia

Childhood aphasia is a disorder of the central nervous system that results in a child's inability to process symbols and abstract ideas. Childhood aphasia also can include an expressive dysfunction in which the child has difficulty translating ideas into speech. Childhood aphasia can be caused by inadequate development in the language realm or by some trauma that impairs language processing capabilities. Occasionally, the trauma has been minor and the parent is unaware of it until the aphasia is diagnosed (Emerick and Hatten, 1979).

Nurses working with hospitalized aphasic children need to be aware that these children do not process information normally and that they have difficulty relating their past experiences to the present. Any explanations of procedures need to be given one piece at a time. A description of even a simple procedure might need to be broken down into component parts and repeated frequently.

Because aphasic children do not express themselves well, it is necessary for the nurse to find out from the parent the child's usual mode of communication. If the child has been in speech therapy, patterns of communication might be established. If at all possible, the parent should remain with the child during hospitalization to reassure and support the child as well as to act as interpreter. The nurse is understanding of the child's difficulties and patient with this often frustrating condition.

Expressive Language Disorders

Speech dysfunctions can be grouped into three distinct categories: (1) voice disorders, (2) articulation disorders, and (3) dysfluency. Voice disorders are variations in pitch that are not considered normal for the child's age and sex. Signs include excessively loud or soft speech, nasal speech, hoarseness, and pitch that is too high or too low. Some voice disorders can be caused by underlying medical problems such as cleft palate or laryngeal nodules. Nurses in outpatient settings can identify voice disorders in children, but more often than not, children with voice disorders are referred for speech therapy by their parents.

Articulation defects Problems with the articulation of sounds not only make communication difficult but might be related to other health problems. Proper articulation requires coordination of breathing, sucking, or swallowing; respiratory muscle strength; the ability to control the muscles of the face and lips; the movement of the tongue; and the ability to control the flow of air to the nasal cavity. A number of neuromuscular diseases can contribute to dysfunctional articulation of sounds, as well as structural deformities of the nose, throat, palate, teeth, and tongue. Some children have problems with articulation because of hearing deficits or because they are imitating another person's improper articulation of sounds. Articulation defects also might be idiopathic (no known cause).

Articulation defects are the most common of the speech disorders. They can take the form of omissions or additions of word syllables, substitutions of incorrect letters for the appropriate ones, or distortions such as lisping. Consonant sounds are affected most frequently. Some children are born with an abnormally attached lingual frenulum ("tongue-tied"). Although this condition can interfere with articulatory speech, it has been found that the frenulum stretches with age. If the child experiences difficulty with developing speech because of severe tongue tie, the frenulum might be clipped after 10 months of age.

Nurses in well-child clinics are in an excellent position to assess children's developing speech patterns and recognize difficulties early. It is important to discover if the misarticulation is related to other health problems that should be identified and treated. If articulation problems persist, the child's speech should be assessed by a speech specialist and appropriate treatment prescribed. It is important to treat speech articulation problems as early as possible, certainly before entry into school.

Dysfluency Stuttering is the major problem disrupting the fluency of speech. Stuttering is a speech problem that is particularly troublesome to parents. It is annoying and often appears to be deliberate. A young child under 3 years of age might stutter but be unaware that this form of speech is a problem. After children are 3 or 4 years old, they begin to realize that their speech is different, and this self-consciousness might make fluency even more problematic.

The major characteristics of stuttering are:

1. Its onset is usually prior to 6 years of age
2. Is is seen more frequently in boys
3. It might be familial and related to high parental expectations
4. It occurs primarily at the beginning of words
5. It can cause adverse psychologic effects such as a decrease in self-esteem

Treatment includes parental guidance. The parent watches for events or situations in which stuttering occurs. When these situations are known, the parent tries to modify or change them to reduce the child's stress. The nurse suggests ways in which the parent can reduce stressful situations for the child. The child should not be scolded for stuttering. The parent should try to be patient and allow the child to complete sentences without interference. The nurse also encourages the parent to identify the child's accomplishments and praise the child as much as possible to build up the child's self-esteem.

Stuttering in the young child can and should be ignored because it is most often a developmental phase of language acquisition. If stuttering continues past the age of 5 years, the child should have professional assistance to help control the stuttering before entering school. The nurse can refer the child and family to a speech specialist.

Essential Concepts

- Through the perception of events and communication of ideas and feelings, infants and children gain an understanding of the world. Any alteration in perception or communication impinges on successful development.
- Nurses play an important role in the recognition and referral of children with sensory deficits as well as in minimizing the long-term effects of such deficits.
- The eye, the ear, and the oral cavity develop early in gestation, and any interference in development results in interference in perception or communication.
- The history of a child with a sensory dysfunction includes data regarding the prenatal environment, familial incidence of sensory deficits, the child's developmental status, incidences of infections or trauma, home environmental factors, changes in the child's behavior, and physical complaints.
- Many diagnostic studies are available to screen children of all ages for sensory deficits. Most of these studies are noninvasive.
- Acute care needs of the child who is visually impaired include prevention of sensory-perceptual alterations related to mild or severe vision impairment. Prevention includes screening and identifying children with mild visual impairments, teaching prescribed exercises and proper use and care of corrective devices, and preventing sensory deprivation in the child who is hospitalized for severe visual impairment.
- Effective preoperative preparation is a nursing challenge with the child who has a sensory deficit.
- Acute care needs of the child who is hearing impaired include prevention of sensory-perceptual alterations, provision of opportunities for adequate communication, and information about the use and proper care of a hearing aid.
- Children with speech deficits experience much frustration and embarrassment when confronted with new situations, and nursing care needs to be directed toward facilitating verbal or nonverbal communication.
- Attention is given to the nutritional needs of the child with a sensory impairment and is directed toward providing proper nutrients for healing as well as providing food that is particularly colorful and attractively served to children with altered taste.
- Special consideration is given to meeting the nutritional needs of children who are blind or whose eyes

are patched; the nurse ensures that the child is able to locate food on the tray and that food is ready to be eaten easily.

- Children with sensory deficits from birth might experience developmental delays and might have had problems with the attachment-separation process.
- Interventions to meet the emotional needs of children with sensory deficits are directed toward reducing anxiety and promoting development of a positive body image.
- Health maintenance needs include prevention of injury and infection because adequate preventive efforts can reduce the incidence of disease and injury.
- Specific structural conditions that can cause visual deficits in a child include refractive errors, strabismus, and glaucoma.
- Frequently seen eye infections include conjunctivitis, orbital cellulitis, and corneal ulceration.
- Eye injury can be the result of abrasion, chemical burns, or blunt or penetrating eye trauma.
- Structural anomalies of the ear might be external, such as abnormal ear placement, or internal, such as the absence or fusion of the ossicles.
- Hearing loss in children can be divided into two major categories—conductive hearing loss and sensorineural hearing loss (nerve deafness).
- Repeated middle ear infections can contribute to conductive hearing loss by damaging the tympanic membrane.
- Foreign bodies in the ear and noise pollution also can contribute to hearing loss.
- Other than inflammation from allergy or virus, difficulties with the nose most often arise from trauma.
- The child with a language disorder might exhibit dysfunction in receptive language, expressive language, or both.
- Speech dysfunction can be identified by nurses in outpatient settings and include disorders of articulation, fluency, or voice.

References

Ashworth P: Sensory deprivation—the acutely ill. *Nurs Times* (Feb 15) 1979; 75:290–294.

Bloom L, Lahey M: *Language Development and Language Disorders.* Wiley, 1978.

Bridges M: Extended cortical mastoidectomy and tympanoplasty for chronic otitis media. *Nurs Times* (Jan 20) 1982; Vol. 78: 101–107.

Castiglia P, Aquilina S, Kemsley M: Focus: Nonsuppurative otitis media. *Pediatr Nurs* (Nov/Dec) 1983; 9(6): 427–431.

Emerick L, Hatten J: *Diagnosis and Evaluation in Speech Pathology.* 2nd ed. Prentice-Hall, 1979.

Goldberg R: Identifying speech and language delays in children. *Pediatr Nurs* (July/Aug) 1984; 10:252–259.

Holder L: Hearing aids: Handle with care. *Nurs '82* (April) 1982; 12:64–67.

Kamenir S et al: Hands-on skills for dealing with hearing aids. *Can Nurse* (Dec) 1982; 78:44–45.

Saunders W et al: *Nursing Care in Eye, Ear, Nose and Throat Disorders.* Mosby, 1979.

Saxton D et al: *Manual of Nursing Practice.* Addison-Wesley, 1983.

Systems of Life 88: Examining the cranial nerves completed. *Nurs Times* (Apr 7–13) 1982; center pages.

Tumulty G, Resler M: Eye trauma. *Am J Nurs* (June) 1984; 84:740–743.

Welch J, Tyler J, Quinn B: Dealing with eye injuries. *RN* (March) 1984; 47:53–54.

Additional Readings

Adams J, Evans G, Roberts J: Diagnosing and treating otitis media with effusion. *Am J Matern-Child Nurs* (May) 1984; 9:22–28.

Bernhardt J: Sensory capabilities of the fetus. *Am J Matern-Child Nurs* (Jan/Feb) 1987; 12(1): 44–46.

Bess F, McConnell F: *Audiology, Education, and the Hearing-Impaired Child.* Mosby, 1981.

Brandes PJ, Ehinger DM: The effects of early middle ear pathology on auditory perception and academic achievement. *J Speech Hearing Dis* (Aug) 1981; 46:301–307.

Brown M, Collar M: Effects of prior preparation on preschoolers' vision and hearing screening. *Am J Matern-Child Nurs* (Sept/Oct), 1982; 7:323–328.

Bullerdieck KM: Minimal hearing loss may not be benign. *Am J Nurs* (July) 1987; 87(7): 904, 906.

Caldarelli D: *Pediatric Otolaryngology.* Medical Examination, 1983.

Cavalier JP: When moments count . . . the two eye emergencies that demand instant intervention. *RN* (Nov) 1981; 44:41–43.

Clarke M: Psychology: A sense of perception. *Nurs Mirror* (June 12) 1980; 150:41–43.

Crawford, J, Morin JD: *The Eye in Childhood.* Grune & Stratton, 1983.

DiChiara E: A sound method for testing children's hearing. *Am J Nurs* (Sept) 1984; 84:1104–1106.

Gerber S: *Audiometry in Infancy.* Grune & Stratton, 1977.

Helveston E: *Pediatric Ophthalmology Practice.* 2nd ed. Mosby, 1984.

Harley R: *Pediatric Ophthalmology.* Vols I and II. 2nd ed. Saunders, 1983.

Liston T, Harbison R: Sulfisoxazole chemoprophylaxis and recurrent otitis media. *West J Med* 1984; 140:47–49.

Ludington-Hoe S: What can newborns really see? *Am J Nurs* (Sept) 1983; 83:1286–1289.

McDermott J: Immittance screening for aural problems in school children. *J School Health* 1982; 52:462–468.

Meadow K: *Deafness and Child Development.* University of California Press, 1980.

Morgan RH: Breaking through the sound barrier . . . your deaf patient. *Nurs '83* (Feb) 1983; 13:112, 114.

Pickering LK, DuPont HL: *Infectious Diseases of Children and Adults.* Addison-Wesley, 1986.

Reichman J, Healey WC: Learning disabilities and conductive hearing loss involving otitis media. *J Learn Disabil* (May) 1983; 16:272–278.

Schwartz RH: A practical approach to the otitis-prone child. *Contemp Pediatr* (Jan) 1987; 4(1):30–42, 47, 50–53.

Shanks S: *Nursing and the Management of Pediatric Communication Disorders.* College-Hill Press, 1983.

Thompson L: Understanding tympanometry. *Pediatr Nurs* (May/June) 1982; 8:193–197.

Tyers A, Westaby S (editors): Wound care #17—wounds of the eye. *Nurs Times* (March 30) 1983; 79:65–68.

Wassenberg C: Common visual disorders in children. *Nurs Clin North Am* (Sept) 1981; 16:469–485.

Wright K: An update on amblyopia and strabismus. *Consultant* 1982; 22:97–99, 103, 106–107.

Chapter 33

Aberrant Cellular Growth

Implications for the Child and Family

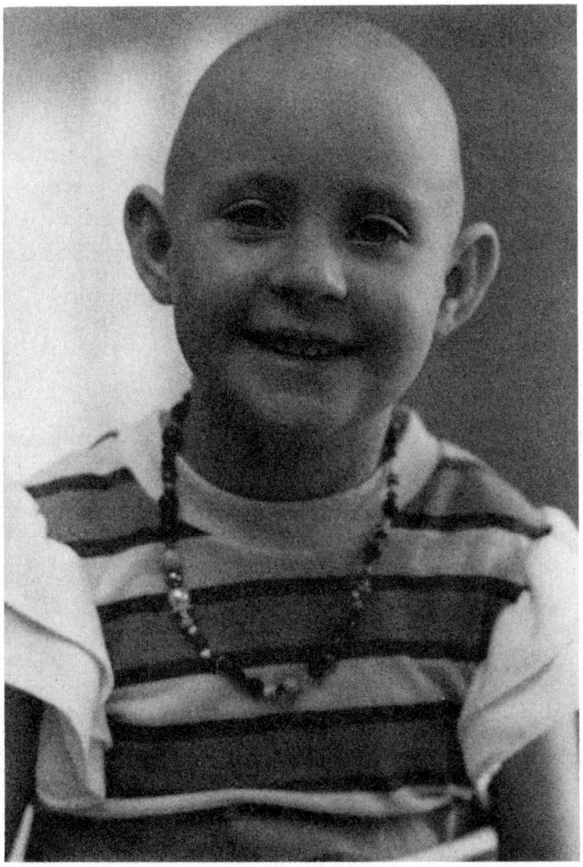

Chapter Contents

(Continues)

Fluid volume deficit related to active loss of body fluid secondary to vomiting and diarrhea
Alteration in oral mucous membrane related to oral cavity radiation or drug induced stomatitis
Alteration in comfort: pain related to chemical injuring agents affecting oral cavity
Impaired tissue integrity related to chemical or radiation irritants resulting in alopecia
Impaired skin integrity related to inflammation and altered pigmentation secondary to radiation therapy
Potential activity intolerance
Potential for infection
Potential for injury
Activity intolerance related to imbalance between oxygen supply and demand
Potential alteration in body temperature
Alteration in comfort: pain related to physical and psychologic injuring agents secondary to the diagnosis of cancer

Nutritional Needs
Potential alteration in nutrition: less than body requirements

Developmental Needs
Potential altered growth and development

Emotional Needs
Potential body image disturbance
Potential ineffective individual coping
Alteration in family processes related to situational crisis secondary to the child's illness and hospitalization

Health Maintenance Needs
Potential knowledge deficit concerning child's home care management

The Child with a Neoplasm

Acute Leukemias
Hodgkin's Disease
NonHodgkin's Lymphoma (Lymphosarcoma)
Brain Tumors
Retinoblastoma
Neuroblastoma
Wilms' Tumor
Rhabdomyosarcoma
Osteosarcoma
Ewing's Sarcoma

Objectives

- Describe tumor characteristics.
- List the types of childhood cancer.
- Describe how childhood cancers differ from adult cancers.
- Describe the assessment criteria related to a child with a neoplasm.
- List the diagnostic tests related to a diagnosis of childhood cancer.
- Describe the main features of medical management of a child with a neoplasm.
- Discuss nursing management related to the side effects of chemotherapy.
- Discuss nursing management related to the side effects of radiation therapy.
- Relate nursing management to the acute-care needs stemming from bone marrow suppression, surgery, and cancer-related pain.
- Discuss the need for optimal nutrition and the nursing strategies to maintain nutritional status.
- Explain the developmental, emotional, and health maintenance needs of children with neoplasms and their families.
- Explain the clinical manifestations, diagnostic evaluation, treatment, and nursing management appropriate for children with various specific neoplasms.

ESSENTIALS OF STRUCTURE AND FUNCTION
Aberrant Cellular Growth

Depending on the system involved, cancer can manifest itself as a growth, or tumor, or can be the result of an extensive multiplication of cells that are not in tumor form, such as in white blood cells. Cancer cells vary in size, rate of growth, and function, depending on the specific cancer involved.

Glossary

Benign tumor Tumor cells that grow at a fairly slow rate and generally within a capsule (encapsulated). The capsule prevents invasion of surrounding tissue and, thus, localizes the tumor. (See table for characteristics of benign vs malignant tumors.)

Cell differentiation A process by which body cells develop specific function. Cancer cells can range from being well differentiated to being nonfunctional, or *anaplastic*.

Doubling time The time it takes for tumor cells to reproduce themselves. The rate of tumor growth depends on its doubling time, the characteristics of the particular cancer, the rate of cell death, and the tumor's nutritional supply.

Embryonal tumors Arise from immature, nonfunctional, fetal tissue. They originate in intrauterine life, manifest themselves in early childhood, and are rarely seen in adults.

Histologic classification A classification system used to identify cells. Tumor cells are classified by cell type and location. Benign tumors generally are classified by adding the tissue type of the tumor to the suffix "oma" (eg, a fibroma is a tumor of fibrous tissue). Malignant tumors add the tissue type and location to the suffix "oma" (eg, osteosarcoma, osteo = bone, sarcoma = connective tissue tumor). There are exceptions, however, to these classifications (eg, lymphoma is malignant lymphoid tissue). Embryonal tumors, those arising from embryonic tissue, have "blast" before the suffix (eg, neuroblastoma is an embryonal neurologic tissue tumor).

Malignant tumor Mass of cells that escapes the control for orderly growth. Malignant cells multiply rapidly and usually are nonfunctional. Unlike benign tumors, malignant cells can invade surrounding tissue or break off and spread throughout the body.

Metastasis The ability of malignant cells to break away and spread to body tissue in other locations. Malignant cells can be carried to other sites through serous fluid in body cavities (serous spread), through the lymph node system (lymphatic spread), or through the veins (venous spread). For metastasis to occur, malignant cells need to implant in the tissues to which they were carried (see illustration).

Tumor An abnormal mass of cells that can be located in body tissue. The suffix "oma" refers to a tumor.

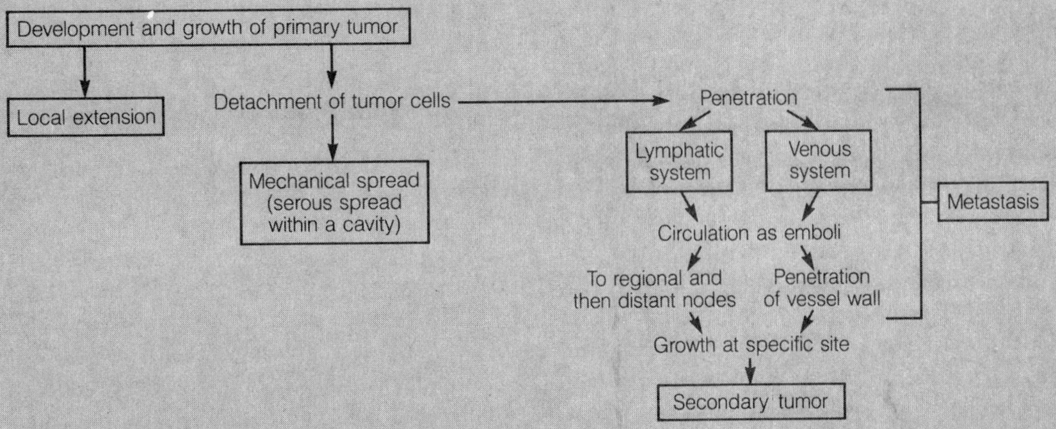

Metastasis of tumor cells.

(Continues)

ESSENTIALS OF STRUCTURE AND FUNCTION *(Continued)*
Aberrant Cellular Growth

Contrast Between Benign and Malignant Tumors

Property	Benign	Malignant
Microscopic features	Cells usually closely resemble tissue of origin	Cells usually do not closely resemble tissue of origin; poorly differentiated
Rate of growth	Grow slowly	Grow according to individual tumor doubling time, which is dependent on tumor and host factors
Mode of growth	Grow by expansion, compressing adjacent tissue, usually encapsulated	Rarely encapsulated, grow by infiltrating adjacent tissue
Tissue destruction	Minimal tissue destruction	May produce necrosis and extensive tissue damage
Surgical resection	Generally do not recur after surgical removal	Often recur after surgical removal because of infiltration into adjacent tissue
Metastasis	Remain localized, do not spread	Frequently spread from site of origin and establish secondary site of growth in distant organs

Aberrant cellular growth refers to pathologic cell proliferation resulting in the development of a neoplasm, or tumor. A neoplasm may be benign, that is, not life threatening, or it may be malignant, that is, life threatening or cancerous.

Cancer in children is relatively rare. In spite of the rarity of childhood cancer, it is the leading cause of death from disease in children between 1 and 14 years of age (Vital Statistics of the United States, 1984). Death from childhood cancer is surpassed only by accidents as the major cause of death in children of this age group. Childhood cancer needs to be viewed as a chronic disease rather than as an inevitably fatal illness. During the past 30 years, tremendous advances have been made in both the diagnosis and successful treatment of childhood cancers, reducing the death rate from childhood cancer from 8.3 per 100,000 in 1950 to 4.4 per 100,000 in 1979 (Vital Statistics of the United States, 1984). Treatment goals are no longer limited to support preparation for death. Instead the emphasis is on total eradication of the disease or significant long-term survival. The overall task for the child and family is to adapt successfully to the chronic disease and live fully in spite of it.

Because a diagnosis of cancer brings an uncertain prognosis, the child and family continually live from day to day with the unknown. The social isolation that can be a consequence of cancer, the extreme discomfort associated with its treatment, and the ongoing fear of death are stressors that can be overwhelming for the child and family. Optimal nursing skill and talent are required to assess and provide effective care for the unique physiologic and psychologic needs that cancer causes. The quality of the nursing care will directly affect the quality of life for the child and family.

Cancer in Children

Cancer in children differs markedly from cancer in adults. Childhood cancer tends to occur in tissues that are reproducing at a rapid rate, such as blood, lymphoid, bone, and nerve. Cancer in adults usually affects epithelial tissue (carcinoma) or connective tissue (sarcoma). Children can have sarcomas, but children rarely experience carcinomas. While adult carcinomas usually occur in response to prolonged exposure to environmental carcinogens (cancer-causing agents), children have not lived long enough to experience prolonged exposure to carcinogens. Embryonal tumors are seen in children but rarely in adults. (Table 33-1 illustrates the suspected causes of childhood cancers.)

Leukemia (cancer of blood-producing tissue) accounts for nearly one-third of all childhood cancers. Tumors of the central nervous system, primarily of the brain, account for the second largest group. The remaining childhood cancers are much less common. Neuroblastoma is an embryonal tumor of the sympathetic nervous system. Wilms' tumor (nephroblastoma) is an embryonal tumor of the kidney. Rhabdomyosarcoma is a tumor of soft tissue, specifically, striated muscle. Other frequently seen childhood cancers include lymphomas (cancer of lymphoid tissue) and bone tumors.

About 45% of all childhood cancers are diagnosed from birth through 4 years of age. This is particularly true of embryonal tumors, because they begin during fetal development and appear very early in childhood. The remaining incidences of childhood cancers are almost evenly divided between the two remaining age groups. Approximately 27% of childhood malignancies occur between the ages of 5 and 10, and 28% occur between the ages of 10 and 14.

Cancer in children often is misdiagnosed initially. Signs and symptoms of malignancy are, for the most part, identical to many acute, easily treatable childhood illnesses. For this reason and because cancer is so rare in children, the true diagnosis might be missed while other, less serious interpretations are applied to the presenting signs and symptoms.

The delay that results is unfortunate. Childhood cancers generally are rapidly growing malignancies. By the time the abnormal cells have multiplied enough to cause significant signs and symptoms, several additional weeks of delay have occurred. Many tumors have already metastasized. The earlier the clinician suspects cancer and the earlier the appropriate assessment is completed, the greater the likelihood of successful treatment.

TABLE 33-1 Factors Suspected of Influencing the Occurrence of Cancer in Children

Factor	Influence
Genetic and familial	Incidence of childhood cancer is increased in children with some chromosome and congenital abnormalities (eg, Down's syndrome, neurofibromatosis). There is an increase in the incidence of leukemia in children whose siblings have leukemia
Immune	Cancer incidence in children is linked to ineffective immune surveillance by T-lymphocytes (see Chapter 25). The occurrence of cancer is higher in children with immune deficiency diseases or in children who have had their immune systems artifically suppressed. Some children experience secondary cancers after radiation or chemotherapy treatment for an initial cancer
Viruses	There is a suspected link between certain viruses and the occurrence of specific types of cancer (eg, Epstein-Barr virus with Burkitt's lymphoma)
Environment	Environmental carcinogens transmitted to a fetus in utero have been linked to the development of certain cancers (eg, diethylstilbesterol [DES] and vaginal cancer)

Assessment of the Child with a Neoplasm

The signs and symptoms of childhood cancer vary with the type and particularly the location of the presenting malignancy. Skill in assessment and a complete understanding of a wide range of diagnostic tools are required when dealing with childhood cancer.

History

Childhood cancer might be identified when the parent brings the child to the physician for examination for a specific complaint, or it might be discovered during a routine physical exam without specific symptoms. Rarely does the parent or child initially suspect the illness might be cancer.

Once cancer is considered to be a possibility, the nurse obtains a systematic history directed toward obtaining data regarding the appropriate etiologic factors (see Table 33-1). A prenatal history of maternal exposure to radiation or specific drugs that have been linked to childhood cancer is noted carefully. A family history is taken to identify hereditary syndromes known to predispose a child to cancer or to identify siblings with malignant disease.

The presenting concern that brings the child in for evaluation varies depending on the location of the malignancy. The parent and child are questioned carefully about the presenting concern. The onset and duration of the symptoms are noted. A detailed description of the nature of the problem is most helpful. Are there patterns to the symptoms? Does anything aggravate or alleviate the symptoms? The nurse determines whether any treatments, either home remedies or physician-prescribed, have been tried, and the nurse asks about the child's response to those treatments. A thorough description of the problem by the family can provide areas of focus for the physical examination.

Physical Examination

A complete evaluation includes both a general health assessment and a detailed examination of the area of concern. A developmental assessment of the child is useful if a developmental delay is apparent. Because many children with cancer experience significant weight loss, a nutritional assessment might be indicated.

The child's general health status is documented, particularly regarding any repeated infections that might indicate altered immune system function. The child is examined for any pallor, bleeding, or bruising. These symptoms along with complaints of fatigue, fever, or slow wound healing indicate changes in the hematopoietic system seen frequently in childhood cancers.

Complaints of pain are important to note, along with descriptions of its location, intensity (eg, sharp, dull), and duration (eg, continuous, intermittent). The child is asked whether certain body positions are more painful than others. For example, the child's leg might hurt more when the child is walking than when the child is at rest.

Lymphadenopathy (enlarged lymph nodes) and splenomegaly (enlarged spleen) can accompany malignant disease. Malignancies affecting lymphoid tissue or white blood cells of the immune system (see Chapter 25) can alter the composition and size of the nodes and spleen. Other less serious conditions than cancer, such as an infection, also involve enlarged spleen and lymph nodes, so cautious investigation is necessary. Systematic evaluation of lymph nodes needs to include observation of all nodes accessible to palpation (see Chapter 10). Size, location, and character of any enlarged lymph node is noted.

Suspicious nodes often are larger than 2.5 cm. They are firm and nontender. These nodes differ from the movable, tender, and hot nodes enlarged because of inflammatory disease. Enlarged nodes located in the supraclavicular or axillary chains are more likely to be involved in malignant disease than cervical or inguinal nodes. Benign, palpable lymph nodes are much more common in children than in adults, making assessment by palpation alone inconclusive and further diagnostic evaluation necessary.

Splenomegaly needs to be carefully documented. Again, an enlarged spleen can be present in conditions other than cancer. In the child under 4 years of age a spleen palpable 1 to 2 cm below the left costal margin can be a normal finding. When the spleen is palpable in the child over 4 years of age, it is usually 2 or 3 times its normal size. A description of its size, consistency, and direction of enlargement (eg, toward the umbilicus) is helpful. Once splenomegaly is documented by plapation, further diagnostic study is warranted.

The nurse notes and describes any noticeable masses. Abdominal masses are evaluated carefully. Palpation of abdominal masses is gently undertaken and kept to a minimum because abdominal pressure caused by palpation can contribute to peritoneal serous spread of tumor cells. A malignant tumor usually feels hard. Movement of the tumor with external pressure or position change is documented. The shape and regularity of the tumor is recorded also, along with its location (eg, left, right, crossing the midline). Any dyspnea or increased respiratory effort can be related to abdominal pressure on the diaphragm and is documented by the nurse.

Alteration in urinary output or in urine appearance is noted. The nurse reports any blood in the urine, urinary retention, or signs of obstruction (see Chapter 28). Central nervous system signs are evaluated during the neurologic examination and the developmental assessment. Head circumference is charted and fontanelle closure evaluated. Ophthalmic and visual examination might reveal eye or vision changes such as optic nerve pressure, nystagmus, double vision, or strabismus. The nurse assesses the child's mental status, altered sensorium, cerebellar signs of ataxia (poor muscle coordination), head tilting, and loss of balance. Any changes in the child's behavior, such as the development of headache, irritability, or learning difficulties, can indicate central nervous system involvement. (Additional assessment data relative to dysfunctions affecting particular body systems can be found in the assessment guides in Chapters 22–32.)

Validating Diagnostic Tests

To delineate the significance of the problem, a number of diagnostic studies are performed. Together with the results of the history and physical examination, the diagnostic studies provide the basis for determining whether or not a biopsy (excision of tissue for microscopic examination) is needed to establish the diagnosis. Diagnostic studies also provide information about the extent of the disease and whether metastasis has occurred. Such information is important in determining the surgical procedure required should a malignancy be confirmed.

Diagnostic studies also provide information about the general health status of the child. Because treatment can affect many organ systems, baseline data of all organ systems is needed prior to beginning treatment.

Laboratory and other diagnostic studies Suspected malignancies of the hematopoietic system require evaluation by performing a complete and differential blood count. The type and number of circulating cells provides valuable data about the functional capabilities of the hematopoietic and immune systems. For example, large numbers of circulating immature white blood cells would diminish the child's ability to fight infection.

Blood chemistries provide important baseline information about other organ systems. Of particular importance are chemistries that evaluate renal and liver function. Serum levels of blood urea nitrogen (BUN) and creatinine (see Chapter 28) can be elevated in renal malignancies. Increases in uric acid reflect increased tissue destruction related to cancer cell breakdown. Elevated serum glutamic pyruvic transaminase (SGPT) and serum glutamic oxaloacetic transaminase (SGOT) can be associated with liver damage (see Chapter 27). An elevated bilirubin indicates increased destruction of red blood cells, or liver dysfunction. Extensive bone involvement often is reflected by increased levels of serum calcium, serum phosphorus, and alkaline phosphatase. (Additional diagnostic studies are presented in Table 33-2.)

Biopsy The diagnosis of a malignancy can be confirmed only by a biopsy. This procedure allows the removal of all or a portion of the abnormal tissue for pathologic examination and the determination of a precise histologic diagnosis.

TABLE 33-2 Studies Used to Evaluate Malignacies

Study	Significance
Intravenous pyelogram (IVP)—visualizes the renal system through use of a contrast medium (see Chapter 28)	Useful for evaluation of abdominal masses. Can differentiate the two most frequently seen abdominal tumors in children—neuroblastoma and nephroblastoma
Angiography—visualizes blood vessels through use of a contrast medium and radiographs	Can evaluate the blood supply to and around a tumor. Useful for differentiating malignancies from benign tumors. Assists with defining an area for surgical resection
Scanning—visualizes tumors or tumor displacement of normal tissue through the use of radionuclides [radioactive materials that concentrate in tumors (direct) or in normal body tissue (indirect)]	Can evaluate tumors of most body tissue. Both false positives and false negatives are associated with direct scanning (scanning of the tumor itself)
CT scan—visualizes characteristics and geography of a tumor in various body structures (see Chapter 31)	Can help determine whether a mass is cystic, solid, or lipid
Lymphangiography—visualizes lymph nodes through use of a contrast material injected into the lymphatic system	Reveals enlarged lymph nodes suspected of disease involvement. Difficult to use in the child because of small lymphatic vessels
Ultrasonography—uses recorded ultrasonic waves to visualize tumor masses	Can precisely establish the size, shape, and location of the kidneys, liver, spleen, and major blood vessels. Is useful for evaluating masses in the pelvis, retroperitoneum, and abdominal cavity
Lumbar puncture—removal of cerebrospinal fluid for cell examination (see Chapter 31)	Identifies malignant cells in the cerebrospinal fluid

Biopsy

Aspiration The use of a needle and syringe and application of suction to collect the specimen

Excisional The removal of the entire lesion including a margin of normal tissue

Exploratory The survey and biopsy of a suspected lesion to determine the exact location and extent of disease

Incisional The biopsy of only a selected portion of the lesion and perhaps some adjacent normal tissue

Needle The insertion of a needle into the lesion and withdrawal of a specimen through its adherence to the lumen of the needle

Most biopsies are performed under general anesthesia. A substantive diagnosis might be determined while the child is still under the anesthesia so that the appropriate surgical intervention can be performed along with the biopsy. Sometimes it is desirable to perform the biopsy only, without planning for subsequent surgery. This approach provides the pathologist with more time to evaluate the tissue samples before determining the diagnosis. The appropriate surgical procedure can then be selected by the surgical team. Thus the biopsy and surgical intervention are separate procedures.

Needle biopsies and biopsies done under local anesthesia are not commonly used in childhood cancer. Biopsy by aspiration of the bone marrow, however, is used to establish the diagnosis or follow the course of malignancies of blood-forming and lymphoid tissue and those solid tumors known to metastasize to the bone. This examination of developing blood cells is performed under local anesthesia and is the definitive means to establish histologically the diagnosis of a hematologic malignancy or bone marrow involvement as a metastatic site (see Chapter 26 for a description of bone marrow aspiration).

TABLE 33-3 TNM Staging Classification

Area of involvement	Staging criteria
Tumor	
T_0	No evidence of primary tumor
T_1, T_2, T_3, T_4	Progressive increase in tumor size and involvement
T_x	Tumor cannot be assessed
Lymph nodes	
N_0	Regional lymph nodes not demonstrably abnormal
N_1, N_2, N_3, N_4	Increasing degrees of demonstrable abnormality of regional lymph nodes
N_x	Regional lymph nodes cannot be assessed clinically
Metastasis	
M_0	No known distant metastasis
M_1	Distant metastasis present, indicate site

SOURCE: Data from American Joint Committee for Cancer Staging and End Results Reporting, 1977.

Medical Management of the Child with a Neoplasm

Staging

The determination of the extent of disease is called *staging*. The results of the physical examination, diagnostic studies including those documenting metastatic sites, and the biopsy are used to evaluate the stage of the disease. Staging is useful to determine the kind of therapy that would be most effective, and to some extent staging indicates prognosis. Although the stage of disease can be changed throughout the course of the illness, the initial staging at diagnosis is most critical.

Staging involves a wide range of criteria and terminology. These vary depending on the specific tumor and the particular treatment facility. Two major classifying systems exist. The first identifies the extent of disease with a Roman numeral system of I through IV. Stage I indicates localized disease without evidence of metastatic spread. Each stage thereafter identifies more extensive disease according to size, structural involvement, and evidence of metastatic disease. Stage IV represents extensive disease with widespread metastatic sites. The child with stage I or II disease generally has a much more favorable prognosis and requires less aggressive therapy than a child with stage III or IV disease.

The second staging system was developed to provide a more precise and universally consistent terminology in cancer treatment. There is often confusion when treatment results are compared among institutions that classify the same tumor and disease status differently. This second staging system, called the TNM system (Tumor size, Node involvement, Metastasis), endeavors to provide a basic language that can be understood by all who treat cancer. Each category is weighted from 0 to 4 depending on extent of disease (Table 33-3).

Approaches to the Treatment Plan

Three approaches to a treatment plan for the child with a malignancy are therapy for (a) curative, (b) adjuvant, or (c) palliative purposes. *Curative therapy* attempts to eradicate the disease completely and is usually the goal for all newly diagnosed childhood cancers.

Adjuvant therapy assists in the eradication of disease. The assumption is that although the child might appear free of disease after an initial surgical procedure, it is highly likely that subclinical micrometastases still exist. The additional therapy directed at micrometastasis is called adjuvant therapy. The third approach is *palliative therapy*. This means that the treatments are not able to cure the child but instead provide the child with a long-term quality survival with a significant degree of symptom control.

The best possible approaches for treating a child with cancer include an optimal combination of available treatment modes—surgery, radiation, and chemotherapy. Radiation and chemotherapy kill malignant cells; surgery removes them. Surgery and radiation offer treatment for localized diseases; chemotherapy treats systemic disease.

The specific treatment plan for the child ideally is chosen by an interdisciplinary health team called a tumor board. At the meeting of the board the physicians present the pertinent histologic, laboratory, and roentgenographic data. Appropriate developmental and psychosocial assessment of the child and family is presented. It is important for nursing personnel to be represented and their input to be presented. The surgeon, radiation oncologist, and medical oncologist discuss treatment possibilities, and the optimal treatment plan is chosen.

The systematic treatment plan, which can include a number of experimental therapies, is referred to as a *protocol*. The protocol outlines the specific treatment, including the surgery, radiation, and chemotherapy, the child will receive. It includes the sequence of treatment and the specific doses that will be administered (Table 33-4). Protocols are based on data obtained from research with combinations of standard and experimental treatments. Should initial treatment prove ineffective during the course of the disease, the tumor board might meet again to review the status of the child and recommend further treatment.

Surgery Surgical resection serves as a primary treatment for solid tumors. It is often the initial treatment the child receives, although radiation or chemotherapy or both can precede surgery. Pretreatment with radiation or chemotherapy can decrease the size of the tumor and facilitates later resection.

There are four categories of surgical intervention

1. *Staging*—the primary purpose is to determine the extent of disease and obtain the biopsy.
2. *Curative*—this surgical treatment requires that the tumor mass be completely removed along with a margin of normal tissue around it.
3. *Palliative*—the procedure does not involve removal of the entire malignancy but allows for increased effectiveness of radiation and chemotherapy by reducing the size of the tumor. Other palliative surgery removes solitary metastatic lesions or removes obstructions caused by tumor growth.
4. *"Second-look"*—the procedure is performed after the initial courses of therapy are completed, and the disease status cannot be determined with less invasive tests.

Radiation Radiation therapy is an important mainstay of cancer treatment. The purpose of radiation therapy is to destroy cancer cells in the localized area receiving treatment. Radiation causes damage to both normal and cancer cells. Rapidly reproducing cells such as those of the skin and bone marrow are most vulnerable to damage. The

TABLE 33-4 Example of a Treatment Protocol

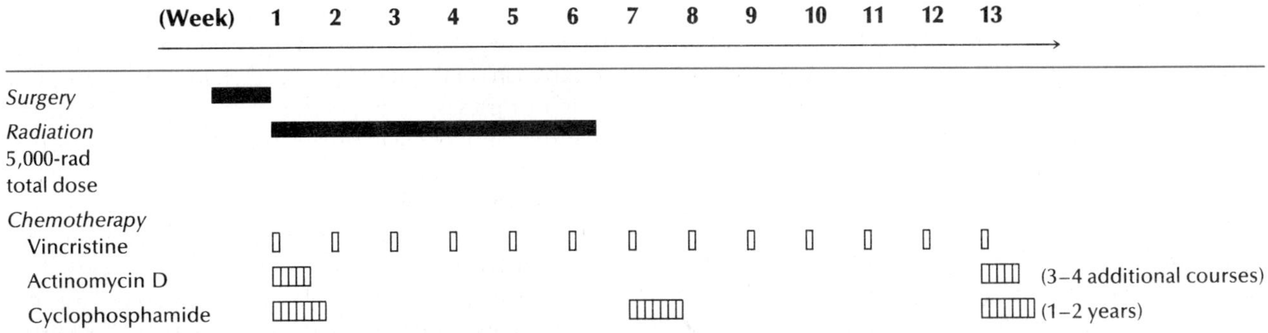
(Week) 1 2 3 4 5 6 7 8 9 10 11 12 13
Surgery
Radiation
5,000-rad
total dose
Chemotherapy
Vincristine
Actinomycin D
Cyclophosphamide
(3–4 additional courses)
(1–2 years)

Vincristine	2 mg/m² intravenously weekly for 12 weeks (maximum dose = 2 mg)
Actinomycin D	0.015 mg/kg/day intravenously for 5 days (maximum dose = 0.5 mg)
Cyclophosphamide	10 mg/kg/day intravenously or orally for 7 days every 6 weeks

NOTE: ▯ = number of doses.

many side effects of radiation are caused by this destruction of rapidly reproducing tissue in the area being radiated.

External radiation is the most common type of therapy for children. External radiation means the electromagnetic energy sources come from a machine outside the child's body. These machines produce either x-rays, which are generated by electrical machines, or gamma rays, which are emitted from radioisotopes.

Megavoltage machines are used frequently in the treatment of childhood cancer. They produce their greatest effect several centimeters into the body, thus having an important skin-sparing function. This allows for higher doses of radiation to be delivered without serious skin damage. Childhood cancers usually are at some distance from the skin, making this feature of the megavoltage machines most appropriate for therapy with children.

Once the radiation has affected a cell, actual cell death might not occur for a period of time. *Lethal damage* is a term that refers to cells that can no longer divide subsequent to radiation. This can occur immediately, or the cell can still divide a few more times before death takes place. *Sublethally damaged cells* are those disrupted by the radiation but able to repair the damage. Ideally, the goal of radiation therapy is to cause as much lethal damage to cancer cells while producing sublethal damage to normal cells. In fact, normal cells might be better able than cancer cells to repair sublethal damage.

To encourage normal cell recovery, radiation treatment is divided into small exposures over a period of weeks until the total dose to be administered, measured in rad, is reached. For example, a child may receive 3000 rad over 6 weeks of 5-day-a-week treatments or 100 rad per treatment. By delivering radiation therapy over time, normal cells can recover from damaging effects, which will reduce toxicity, yet a higher degree of tumor cell death is achieved.

Radiation therapy is not used with all tumors. Although radiation can kill any type of cancer cell, the dose required might be too toxic to surrounding vital tissue. The relationship between tumorcidal doses of radiation and surrounding normal tissue tolerance is referred to as radiosensitivity. Tissues that reproduce most rapidly are the most radiosensitive. Thus lymphoma, leukemia (malignancy of the blood-forming tissue), nephroblastoma, and neuroblastoma are most radiosensitive.

Chemotherapy Chemotherapeutic agents act to kill cancer cells by destroying the cell or preventing the cell from dividing. Unfortunately, these drugs are not tumor-specific, so they destroy normal cells as well as cancer cells. In giving chemotherapy, the goal is to kill as many cancer cells as possible without sustaining severe damage to normal cells.

The drugs used in chemotherapy act on cells by several different mechanisms that can be categorized into two major methods. Drugs can be identified as either cell cycle-specific, killing cells during a specific phase of cell cycle, or cell cycle-nonspecific, killing cells no matter what the phase of the cell cycle (Fig. 33-1).

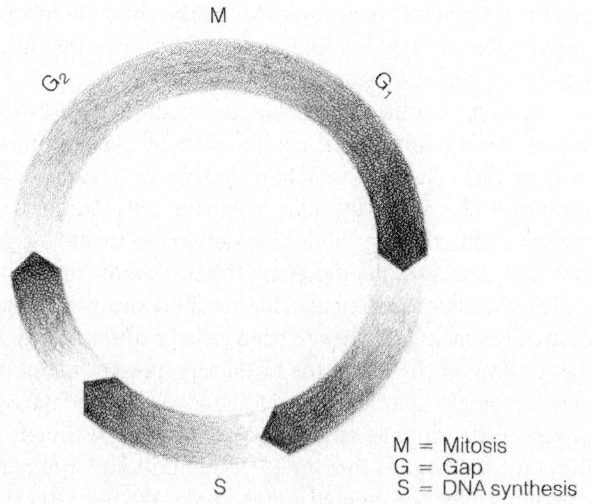

FIGURE 33-1

Phases of the cell cycle. (From Jenkins JB: Human Genetics. *Benjamin/Cummings, 1983, with permission.)*

By combining drugs with different actions rather than administering a single drug, greater tumor kill is accomplished. A combination of drugs can ensure cell death by attacking tumor cells at different phases of their cell cycles. Because of the different activity potentials of cancer cells, no tumor can be completely eradicated with one cycle of drugs. Thus groups of drugs are administered over a protracted time and in a specific sequential fashion to coincide with tumor growth and activity. The hope is that each cycle of drug therapy will continue to reduce the tumor burden.

Different drugs have toxic effects on different normal tissues. This is another reason why chemotherapeutic drugs are given in combination. A child, therefore, might receive a drug that causes moderate bone marrow suppression but limited gastrointestinal toxicity, combined with a drug that has the opposite toxicities—limited bone marrow but moderate gastrointestinal effects. (Some of the chemotherapeutic agents used in the treatment of childhood cancer are presented in Table 33-5.)

All chemotherapeutic agents are handled with care. Because cytotoxic drugs can affect normal cells, local irritation and allergic reactions can occur with some drugs if they are spilled or if the powder is inhaled. Ideally, cancer drugs are prepared under a vertical laminar airflow hood. Masks, eye protection, and polyvinylchloride gloves are recommended for reconstituting drugs in powder form if a laminar airflow

TABLE 33-5 Some Chemotherapeutic Drugs Used in the Treatment of Childhood Cancer

Drug classification	Mode of action	Example
Antimetabolites	Act as falsely similar structures to normal metabolites; mistakenly incorporated into the cell where they interfere with DNA and RNA synthesis; cell cycle specific for S phase	B-Cytosine arabinoside (Cytosar, Ara C), methotrexate, 6-mercaptopurine, 6-thioguanine
Alkylating agents	Act by replacing a hydrogen ion in the DNA chain with an alkyl group; interfere with DNA synthesis and RNA transcription	Cyclophosphamide (Cytoxan), nitrogen mustard, BCNU (carmustine), CCNU (lomustine), methyl-CCNU (semustine), dicarbazine
Antitumor antibiotics	Components inserted with components of the DNA helix	Doxorubicin, daunorubicin, dactinomycin, bleomycin
Plant alkaloids	Stop the formation of the spindle during the metaphase of cell reproduction; cell cycle specific for M phase	Vincristine, vinblastine, VM-26
Hormones	Unclear	Corticosteroids, prednisone
Miscellaneous	Varies with specific drug or action unclear	L-Asparaginase, procarbazine, hydroxyurea, cisplatin
Allopurinol	Not an anticancer drug but given in association with chemotherapy; inhibits the production of uric acid, which is increased as a result of cell death from chemotherapy; interferes with reactions preceding the formation of uric acid; not given with 6-mercaptopurine because it enhances 6MP's potency	

hood is not available (Stolar, Power, & Viele, 1983). Spills are cleaned immediately with disposable cloths and soap and water. Any waste medication or equipment is bagged and disposed of as hazardous waste (Oncology Nursing Society, 1984).

Because chemotherapy doses are calculated close to the toxicity level for the child's height, weight, and body surface area, they must be administered carefully. Doses and the child's identification need to be double-checked before administration. Some chemotherapeutic agents are light sensitive, and intravenous administration sets need to be covered.

Most chemotherapeutic agents cannot cross the blood-brain barrier and become effective against cancer cells in the central nervous system. If cells in the brain and spinal fluid are to be killed, the medication must be given directly into the spinal fluid through a lumbar puncture (ie, intrathecal administration).

Many cancer cells can be present but clinically undetectable. When the initial disease has been controlled so that no cancer cells can be clinically detected, the child with cancer is said to be in *remission*. Remission does not mean that the child is cured, since many undetectable cells are thought to be still present. Thus chemotherapy continues even after remission has been achieved. Because it is difficult to determine the number of remaining cells, for most childhood cancers chemotherapy is generally administered 1–2 years before therapy is terminated. It is important for parents to understand this accurate definition of remission so they understand the importance of continuing drug treatment even when the child seems well and clinically disease-free.

Once the child is in remission, continual evaluation and diagnostic studies are undertaken to identify recurring disease. Although the cancer might be extremely sensitive to the initial drugs, resistance often develops, and *relapse* (recurrence of malignant cells) occurs. The reasons that cells become resistant to the cytotoxic effects of chemotherapy are not well understood. By administering a variety of chemotherapeutic agents, resistance should be minimized. Some chemotherapy protocols therefore involve switching to a new combination of drugs once remission has been obtained.

Bone marrow transplantation Bone marrow transplantation is being used more and more frequently to treat severe dysfunction of the hematopoietic and immune systems. This includes such conditions as malignancies of the bone marrow and lymphatic system (leukemia and lymphoma) as well as the nonmalignant aplastic anemia (see Chapters 25 and 26). Children with cancer respond better to bone marrow transplantation when in remission.

For bone marrow transplantation to be successful, the child's immune system needs to be suppressed totally prior to the procedure. High doses of chemotherapy and total-body radiation cause profound bone marrow failure. This prevents an immune response to reject the marrow transplant.

Bone marrow is removed from a compatible donor in the operating room. Bone chips and fat molecules are filtered out, and the remaining cells are infused intravenously into the child in the child's own room. If the transplantation is successful, the transplanted marrow cells begin to produce functioning blood cells in the patient. The process takes 2–4 weeks, during which the child is subject to severe complications related to hematopoietic and immune suppression.

In addition to rejection of the transplanted bone marrow, bleeding from reduced platelets, and infection from immune suppression, a serious hazard of bone marrow transplantation is graft-versus-host disease (GVHD). Because the donor's bone marrow contains immunocompetent lymphocytes that have the capacity to attack and reject foreign tissue, the donor's bone marrow can actually attack and destroy tissues in the child's body. The donated lymphocytes have the capacity to destroy cells of the skin, liver, and gastrointestinal tract. Severe involvement can cause skin sloughing, serious liver dysfunction, and copious diarrhea and sloughing of the intestinal mucosa. New immunosuppressive drugs, such as cyclosporine, are being successfully used to combat this debilitating and life-threatening complication. They act by selectively inhibiting T-cell (T-lymphocyte) functions. This action prevents donor T cells from recognizing the child's body tissue as foreign (see Chapter 25 for a discussion of T cells).

Although progress has been made in recent years to decrease the many life-threatening complications that occur with bone marrow transplantation, the procedure is not routinely used. Currently, bone marrow transplantation is considered only for those children who have a dismal prognosis because conventional treatment does not offer them long-term survival or who have received conventional therapy and it has failed. For these children with refractory disease, bone marrow transplantation offers them hope where no other hope exists. The technology and intensive care that is required makes the procedure available at only selected cancer specialty centers.

Communicating the diagnosis When the diagnostic tests, investigation of potential metastatic sites, and biopsy have confirmed the presence of a malignancy, the diagnosis and treatment plan are explained to the family. This is the primary responsibility of the physician, but the nurse has an important role at this critical time for the child and family. From the beginning of diagnostic suspicion, the family should know that a serious illness is being investigated.

When the diagnosis has been confirmed, a conference should be called with the family when both sufficient time and a private conference room are available. It is important for the nurse to participate in the conference. The physician gently yet honestly imparts the diagnosis to the family. Realism with hope is the basis of the message. Even if the family was anticipating the diagnosis, it will come with profound shock, sadness, and fear. Family members' initial shock and numbness often interferes with their ability to listen and understand the discussion of prognosis and treatment plan presented by the physician. The nurse can play a key role in later assessing the family members' understanding of the illness and reinforcing the information and treatment plan outlined by the physician.

The nurse assists family members by clarifying understanding and promptly answering innumerable questions they will have in the days ahead. The family is advised to write down any questions for the physician so that all questions will be remembered when the physician is available to answer them.

During the initial conference, plans are made to tell the child and also the child's siblings about the diagnosis and the need for long-term treatment. A parent might wish to tell the child or might wish for assistance from the physician. Whatever the parent's decision, the child and other family members need an honest yet hopeful explanation. The information needs to be age appropriate, with words chosen so that the child can understand. Withholding the diagnosis or minimizing the actual illness serves only to isolate and frighten the child. Children know when they are seriously ill and refusing them the opportunity to confront this and deal with their feelings is a great disservice. Concern does not focus on whether or not to tell the child but on how to tell the child appropriately.

Nursing Management for Procedures and Treatments

For the child with cancer, the nurse develops a specific plan for preparation based on the assessment, an understanding of the developmental norms, and the particular procedure the child is to undergo. Generally it is better to explain the sensations and feelings and their duration rather than give a detailed account of the actual procedure. (General principles for preparing children for procedures are discussed in Chapter 20.)

For example, in preparing a child for a bone marrow aspiration, rather than explaining that a 6-in. diameter of skin will be cleansed, it is more useful for the child to know that when the area is cleansed, it will feel cold. For the younger child, use of dolls for demonstration or rehearsal also might be useful. If the child will be required to lie still for a long period of time, making a game out of practicing lying still in the appropriate position can aid compliance during the actual procedure. For older children or adolescents, a trip to the laboratory to see their blood cells under a microscope or their actual radiographs often intrigues their developing scientific minds and gains their cooperation. When preparing a child for a study that uses contrast medium, the nurse needs to be particularly careful not to use the word "dye." The term "special medication" is preferred.

Because invasive diagnostic tests and treatments are common to the experience of childhood cancer, researchers are investigating additional techniques to reduce the child's distress. Most promising is the use of relaxation technique with visual imagery while the child is undergoing invasive procedures (Dash, 1980). Prior to the beginning of the procedure, the child participates in a relaxation technique. Visual imagery of a pleasant childhood experience then is reinforced while the relaxing child undergoes the invasive procedure.

Principles of Nursing Care

The nursing care of the child with cancer is based on the philosophy that the child should be able to live life fully in spite of life-threatening disease. Every attempt is made to assist the child to continue developmentally appropriate growth and activities. For this reason, whenever possible, treatment for childhood cancer is delivered on an outpatient basis with hospitalization kept to an absolute minimum. Continued socialization and participation in family activities, school, and peer relationships are encouraged and only restricted if absolutely necessary.

The nurse plays a major role in assisting the child and family to adapt to the disease and continue normal development. This includes comprehensive education of the child and family so that they can anticipate and effectively deal with complications of the disease and treatment that might occur while the child is at home. Often health professionals concentrate only on the child's immediate treatment needs and fail to assess fully and provide guidance to families in their day-to-day adjustment at home. Particular encouragement is needed to help the parents to keep from spoiling the child or neglecting other siblings. To provide effective and total nursing care to the child, the nurse integrates a philosophy of quality living in spite of serious illness. The focus is not on the patient as a sick child.

Acute Care Needs

⊛ Knowledge deficit related to anxiety and limited understanding of extent of surgery and postoperative care

Preoperative preparation Preoperative care of the child undergoing a surgical procedure is similar to any major surgical procedure during childhood. The child and family need an honest explanation of the expectations of surgery and the anticipated course of recovery. Preoperative rehearsal, orientation to the intensive care unit if the child will be placed there, and the opportunity to see and manipulate appropriate postoperative equipment are beneficial to the child.

The parent needs to understand clearly the purpose of the surgery, and complete informed consent should be obtained. The parent is encouraged to ask questions and needs to receive honest, complete answers. Parents need to be kept informed during surgical procedures and need to know the anticipated length and where and when children may be seen after surgery is completed. The surgeon should speak to the parent about the outcome of the surgery and the condition of the child as soon as the procedure is finished. The more completely the parent is prepared for the child's surgical procedure and postoperative care, the easier it will be for the child and family to cope with the surgery.

Preoperative physiologic preparation of the child is similar to other pediatric surgical procedures. Depending on the surgeon's routine and the location of the tumor, the actual preparation will vary. Respiratory, cardiovascular, and renal function are evaluated; drug allergies need to be carefully noted. The hematologic status of the child is carefully monitored. Because of the disease process, anemia and bleeding tendencies might be present and must be corrected prior to surgery. Any fluid and electrolyte imbalance should be corrected during the preoperative period.

Postoperative care Specific areas of postoperative concern and need for monitoring depend on the location and extent of the surgical procedure. The nurse carefully evaluates respiratory, cardiovascular, and hematologic functioning along with the fluid and electrolyte balance. Dressings are checked frequently for evidence of bleeding. Oral feedings are resumed as tolerated, beginning with clear liquids. If the surgery has involved the intestines or if a paralytic ileus is suspected, oral feedings are withheld until bowel sounds are present and the child is passing flatus. The nurse

STANDARDS OF NURSING CARE *The Child with Bone Marrow Suppression*

GUIDE FOR NURSING MANAGEMENT

Nursing diagnosis	Intervention	Rationale	Outcome
1. Potential for infection (stressor: compromised immune system)	Place the child with roommate(s) with no infections, and make sure staff and visitors with infections do not enter the room.	Separating the child from sources of infection confers protection from infection.	The child remains free of nosocomial infection. The parent understands and can explain the need for infection prevention measures.
	Monitor vital signs every 4 hours, including respiratory status. Report any signs of upper respiratory infection or other infection immediately.	Signs of infection include elevated or subnormal body temperature, increased pulse, chills, and respiratory difficulties.	
	Follow strict aseptic technique, using laminar airflow if the child is neutropenic.	White blood cells assist the body's immune system function; neutropenia increases the risk of infection.	
	Keep hospitalization to a minimum to prevent nosocomial infections.	Increased contact with the hospital in which invasive treatments are performed can increase the risk of infection.	
	Examine the child regularly for signs of inflammation at all potential sites of infection such as skin breaks (biopsy site, wounds, pierced ears, etc.), oral and rectal mucosa, perineum, or groin. Use axillary or oral method for monitoring temperature, never rectal.	Skin breaks, catheters, and intravenous lines are frequent sources of hospital-acquired infection.	
	Do not give live virus vaccines to the immunosuppressed child; caution parents to avoid exposing the child to chickenpox or measles.	A depressed immune system cannot fight a viral invasion even when given as a vaccine.	
2. Potential injury (stressors: decreased platelets with poor clotting, developmental characteristics)	Institute safety precautions such as padding the bed, using a soft helmet, and other preventive measures (see Chapter 26).	The child who is thrombocytopenic bleeds easily and requires protection from injury.	The younger child is protected from trauma. The older child explains the need for and cooperates with the safety precautions.
	Monitor the child for the appearance of petechiae, ecchymoses, or hematomas. Give meticulous skin care; monitor thrombocyte levels.	The appearance of petechiae or other signs of bleeding can indicate a lowered platelet count and might be indication for transfusion.	
3. Activity intolerance related to imbalance between oxygen supply and demand	Test all body excretions for blood and take vital signs q. 2–4 hours.	Positive blood in stool, urine, or mucus can indicate internal bleeding.	The child identifies activities associated with fatigue and those tolerated. The child helps to plan a daily schedule and expresses decreased fatigue with uninterrupted rest periods.
	Arrange furniture and objects in the home or hospital room to be within easy reach of the child.	The child conserves energy if exertion is kept to a minimum.	

STANDARDS OF NURSING CARE *The Child with Bone Marrow Suppression (Continued)*

GUIDE FOR NURSING MANAGEMENT

Nursing diagnosis	Intervention	Rationale	Outcome
	Determine with the child which self-care activities will require nursing assistance and offer help in those areas.	Although the child might be fatigued, independence with certain activities needs to be encouraged.	
	Plan care so that the child can rest undisturbed for extended periods.	Increased rest without interruption conserves energy.	
	Arrange pillows around the child's head or elevate the head of the bed to allow optimal breathing.	Elevating the head of the bed decreases respiratory effort and thus, fatigue.	
	Note pallor in skin, oral mucosa, conjunctiva, and nail beds. Monitor hemoglobin, hematocrit and reticulocyte count. (See Chapter 26 for care of the child with anemia.)	These are signs of decreased hemoglobin and hematocrit. Decreased hemoglobin and hematocrit indicate anemia.	
4. Potential alteration in nutrition (stressors: traumatized oral mucosa from chemotherapy, pain, anorexia, altered taste)	Continue regular and thorough mouth care. Clean mouth prior to eating.	If the mouth is kept as clean and fresh as possible, the child will be more likely to eat. Mouth care alleviates pain from oral lesions and allows for more comfortable oral intake.	Child assists with mouth care and identifies foods that are preferred. Child's intake is adequate for current status of required nutrients.
	Apply dry tea bags to gingival bleeding points.	Dry tea bags can control local bleeding.	
	Monitor the child's mouth and gums regularly for changes in mucous membrane.	Prompt, continuous assessment can result in prompt treatment.	
	Avoid irritating foods, such as extremely dry, hot, or acidic solids and liquids (citrus juices, carbonated sodas, bread, or hot beverages) if the child does not tolerate them. Offer chilled yogurt, gelatin, and nonirritating liquids such as chocolate milk; give small, frequent feedings with high-protein liquids. Encourage quality foods and avoid empty calories.	Cool liquids and soft solids can be soothing to oral ulcerations while maintaining adequate nutrition.	

observes the child for evidence of infection, particularly if immune function has been altered prior to surgery.

Pain medication is administered frequently. It is often better to give pain medications on a routine, round-the-clock basis for the first few days rather than when needed. It is better for the child to prevent postoperative pain rather than to try to interrupt the pain cycle once it has begun. Children frequently are reluctant to ask for injectable pain medication. The nurse therefore observes the child and administers medication frequently. As soon as the child can tolerate oral medication, any order for injectable medication should be recalculated for oral usage.

Children generally are encouraged to resume their former activity level as soon as possible. By the second postoperative day the child should be allowed to sit upright if this has not already been done. The parents should be encouraged to participate in the child's care. Questions that the parent has about postoperative procedures or treatments should be promptly answered. The nurse also encourages close contact between parent and child. The parent needs to know that the child can still be touched or cuddled in spite of tubings and dressings. The nurse assists the parent to maneuver the tubing and equipment so the parent can hold or be close to the child.

❀ Knowledge deficit related to limited understanding of the procedure and side effects associated with radiation therapy

The child and family need an explanation of and orientation to the radiation equipment and purpose of treatment. Because the child needs to remain absolutely still during the treatment, rehearsal is useful. The child can practice lying still on a table for a few minutes and slowly build to the actual period required for immobility during treatment. Shells, casts, or sandbags can be used to assist the child to remain still. In the very young child, sedation approaching anesthesia might be necessary to ensure cooperation and total immobility.

Children need to be told that they will be left alone during the few minutes of each radiation treatment. Although the child will feel nothing when the radiation is administered, some children feel frightened by the machine and the isolation. The nurse or parent can maintain verbal contact with the child from the control room.

Lead shields designed to protect vulnerable organs in the radiation path from the damaging rays are essential. These lead shields must be individually cut to conform to the actual shape of the child's organ. The child needs to know that the lead shield is necessary and that it might feel heavy.

The delivery of radiation is tailored to the individual child. When surgery has been performed prior to radiation, radiologic markers might have been attached to the site of residual tumor or around the margins of normal tissue. By viewing diagnostic radiographs, the radiation oncologists can determine the specific area requiring radiation. Margins of radiation therapy ("ports") are determined. Multiple lower-dose entry sites spare skin and other tissue, while the tumor itself receives the full dose. Once the final ports are identified, the child's skin is marked with indelible ink to provide an accurate, consistent lineup of the radiation beam for each treatment the child receives. The child and family are told not to remove or alter the skin markings in any way, as these will serve as a guide for direction of the energy beam.

Many myths are associated with therapeutic use of radiation. Allowing the family to identify their fears and clarify misconceptions is essential for cooperation with the treatment.

Side effects of radiation therapy occur as normal tissue in the radiated field is damaged. The severity of side effects is also dose-related. The child and parents need to anticipate potential side effects and need to be taught how to handle them if they occur. Radiation side effects can be immediate, intermediate, or late developing. (Table 33-6 lists potential side effects of radiation therapy and their management.)

The child is closely observed for signs and symptoms of developing toxicities. Nausea and vomiting, if the gastrointestinal tract is included in the field of radiation, are the most immediate side effects. Other toxicities develop after one to several weeks of therapy. A few toxicities, such as cataracts, growth retardation, or learning disabilities might not occur until months to a year after therapy has been completed. Depending on the severity of toxicity, radiation treatments might be stopped for a few days to allow recovery of normal tissue. Nursing management of radiation-induced side effects focuses on symptom control and comfort measures.

❀ Knowledge deficit related to limited understanding of chemotherapy and associated side effects

The child and parents need to know that the side effects of chemotherapy result from damage done to normal cells. Because chemotherapy is not selective for only cancer cells, normal cells also are vulnerable. Chemotherapy is most destructive to rapidly reproducing cells—both normal and malignant. Rapidly reproducing normal tissues in the body include gastrointestinal epithelial cells, developing blood cells in the bone marrow, and mature reproductive cells (in pubescent children). Thus the side effects of chemotherapy often involve these vulnerable tissues.

The degree of toxicity and specific normal tissues affected vary with each drug and with the dose of drug administered. Side effects of chemotherapy can be acute, intermediate, or of late onset. (Table 33-7 presents the side effects of frequently used chemotherapeutic agents.) Not all the agents cause all the side effects. Some medications affect some body systems more than others. Regardless of whether the drugs were administered to the child on an inpatient or outpatient basis, the child usually is at home when symptoms of side effects develop. The parent and child need to know what to expect and how to handle the side effects from the particular drug the child is receiving.

The nurse assumes an important role in assessing, and

TABLE 33-6 Side Effects of Radiation Therapy

Site radiated	Side effect	Nursing management
Brain	*Intermediate:* edema; nausea and vomiting (stimulation of vomiting center in brain stem medulla)	Give steroids as ordered; monitor for headache. Give antiemetic on a round-the-clock schedule; monitor hydration status
	Late: learning disabilities, development of secondary tumors	Follow up assessment of school achievement; refer for psychologic testing
Scalp, ear, mouth	*Intermediate:* alopecia, otitis media, loss of taste, decreased salivation	Assist with wigs, scarfs, and support; observe for signs and symptoms of otitis media; encourage adequate nutrition and dietary changes to increase taste; consider artificial saliva; offer hard candies to stimulate salivation; offer popsicles
Throat	Stomatitis, dysphagia, parotitis	Provide frequent oral hygiene; observe for secondary fungal infection; medicate as needed for pain
Eyes, teeth	*Late:* cataracts, dental caries	Encourage follow-up eye examination; promote regular dental examination and treat with fluoride
Pulmonary area	*Intermediate:* inflammatory pneumonitis *Late:* fibrosis	Observe for signs and symptoms of nonproductive cough, low-grade fever, mild chest pain
Cardiac area	*Intermediate:* pericarditis	Observe for signs and symptoms of chest pain, friction rub; note ECG changes
Gastro-intestinal area	Anorexia, nausea and vomiting	Give small frequent feedings; give antiemetic on a round-the-clock schedule
	Intermediate: diarrhea/cramping, dehydration, weight loss	Give antispasmodics and kaolin pectin as needed; monitor intake and output and replace fluids; monitor weight, encourage high calorie feedings and vitamin supplements
	Rectal irritation, tenesmus (spasm of the anal sphincter)	Provide comfort measures (sitz baths, soothing preparations, heat)
	Late (but uncommon): radiation hepatitis, esophageal stricture, pancreatitis	Observe for signs and symptoms
Kidney	*Intermediate (but uncommon):* acute nephritis	Observe for signs and symptoms: malaise, nocturia, leg edema, proteinuria, microhematuria, weight gain
Bladder	*Intermediate:* dysurea, cystitis	Observe for signs and symptoms: malaise, microhematuria, fever, painful urination; encourage hydration, monitor intake and output
Bone	*Possible late (but uncommon):* secondary cancers (sarcomas), pathologic fractures, growth alterations (growth retardation, asymmetrical growth)	Encourage follow-up medical evaluations after therapy is discontinued
Bone-forming tissue (bone marrow)	*Intermediate:* bone marrow suppression (decreased erythrocytes, decreased leukocytes, decreased platelets)	Observe for signs and symptoms of anemia, infection, bleeding
Skin	*Intermediate:* radiodermatitis (dry desquamation, wet desquamation)	Keep skin clean, dry, and open to the air; avoid creams (unless prescribed); avoid sun exposure and tight clothing
	Late: hyperpigmentation	
Testes or ovaries	*Late:* sterility, testicular hypertrophy *Intermediate:* delay in secondary sexual characteristics *Late:* sterility, early menopause	Encourage adequate counseling so family understands potential effects of treatment; assist with referral for fertility evaluations as needed; explain potential sperm banking for adolescent male
Nonspecific	*Intermediate:* radiation fatigue (malaise, weakness, headache, nausea, anorexia)	Encourage rest and good nutrition; provide symptom management as needed; reassure family that this is a treatment effect *not* a disease effect

TABLE 33-7 Potential Side Effects of Chemotherapy

Side effect	Agent	Nursing action
Integumentary		
Acute: hives (urticaria) and other signs of anaphylactic reaction	Daunorubicin 6-Mercaptopurine Methotrexate	Have epinephrine, diphenhydramine (Benadryl), and hydrocortisone readily available
Photosensitivity	Actinomycin D Bleomycin Daunorubicin Methotrexate	Have child avoid sun exposure for one to two days following medication administration
Intermediate: alopecia	Actinomycin-D Bleomycin Cyclophosphamide Daunorubicin Doxorubicin Nitrogen mustard Vincristine	Allow child and family to express feelings about altered body image Recommend a wig
Gastrointestinal		
Acute: nausea and vomiting	Actinomycin D 5-Azacitidine Carmustine Cisplatin Cyclophosamide Cytosine arbinoside Dacarbazine Daunorubicin Doxorubicin Lomustine Nitrogen mustard Procarbazine Semustine Vinblastine	Administer antiemetics Monitor intake and output and hydration status
Intermediate: ulcers and stomatitis	Bleomycin Cytosine arabinoside Daunorubicin Doxorubicin 6-Mercaptopurine Methotrexate 6-Thioguanine	Provide a systematic schedule of oral hygiene
Cumulative: hepatic dysfunction (uncommon)	Carmustine 6-Mercaptopurine Methotrexate L-Asparaginase	Reassure child and parents that it is reversible approximately 14–28 days after the drug is withheld
Constipation	Vincristine	Institute a bowel regimen of stool softeners and laxatives if necessary
Cardiovascular		
Acute: vein phlebitis with tissue necrosis and sloughing	Actinomycin D Dacarbazine Daunorubicin Doxorubicin Nitrogen mustard Vinblastine Vincristine	Monitor IV and discontinue if infiltrated. Apply cold compresses. Administer antidote or hydrocortisone as ordered. Do not use agents near a joint because of potentially impaired mobility from tissue damage

TABLE 33-7 *(Continued)*

Side effect	Agent	Nursing action
Cardiovascular ***(Continued)***		
Intermediate: bone marrow suppression, anemia, decreased platelet count	Actinomycin D 5-Azacitidine Carmustine Cyclophosphamide Cytosine arabinoside Daunorubicin Doxorubicin Hydroxyurea Lomustine Nitrogen mustard Methotrexate Procarbazine Semustine Vinblastine	Prevent infection and protect from injury causing bruising or bleeding
Cumulative: cardiac toxicity	Cyclophosphamide Daunorubicin Doxorubicin	Monitor for impending cardiac failure (see Chapter 23) Keep accurate cumulative dosage records
Respiratory		
Cumulative: possible pneumonitislike syndrome with rales, cough, dyspnea (uncommon)	Bleomycin Carmustine Cyclophosphamide (uncommon)	Reassure parents that recovery can be expected 1–2 months after drug is discontinued
Genitourinary		
Cumulative: tubular obstruction or necrosis, cystitis	Cisplatin Methotrexate Cyclophosphamide	Encourage increased fluid intake. Monitor intake and output. Administer preventive medications as ordered
Neuroendocrine		
Acute: fever	Bleomycin Cyclophosphamide Cytosine arbinoside Dacarbazine Daunorubicin Doxorubicin 6-Mercaptopurine Methotrexate Procarbazine Vinblastine Vincristine	Administer acetaminophen as ordered and institute cooling measures
Cumulative: peripheral nerve damage manifested by numbness, tingling, and weakness	Vincristine Vinblastine	Discontinue or reduce drug dose as ordered. Assist the child with activities of daily living if needed
Pancreatitis with hyperglycemia	L-Asparaginase	Administer insulin as ordered. Monitor blood sugar and urine for sugar and acetone

teaching the parent to assess, the effects of chemotherapy. Skillful interventions are needed to control the side effects the child is experiencing. The nurse assesses the child daily for new and ongoing problems. Creative intervention strategies are necessary to control side effects effectively. Parents need to be included as much as possible in providing comfort to the child.

❀ Fluid volume deficit related to active loss of body fluid secondary to vomiting and diarrhea

Many cytotoxic drugs cause nausea and vomiting that generally begins 2–6 hours after the drug has been administered. This probably does not represent a direct effect on the gastrointestinal lining but rather stimulation of the vomiting center in the brain. Vomiting due to chemotherapy generally does not last longer than 48 hours. Vomiting and diarrhea can occur as acute and intermediate effects of radiation therapy, as radiation destroys normal cells in the gastrointestinal tract. Occasionally, a child can experience anticipatory vomiting, particularly prior to chemotherapy. Fluid alterations associated with vomiting and diarrhea are particularly critical in infants and young children due to their precarious fluid balance (see Chapter 21).

Effective treatment to prevent nausea and vomiting and the resultant fluid loss has not yet been developed, although control of gastrointestinal symptoms can be achieved. Currently the most effective drugs come from the phenothiazines. Chlorpromazine (Thorazine) or promethazine (Phenergan) are commonly used with the child to control vomiting. Prochlorperazine (Compazine), which is frequently used with adults, has a high risk of undesirable effects in children and should therefore be avoided if possible. Investigational studies are exploring the effectiveness of Δ-9-tetrahydrocannabinol (THC), the active ingredient in marijuana. For research purposes, THC is available in synthetic form, but to date, its usefulness has not been determined. Antihistamines such as Benadryl and hydroxyzine pamoate (Vistaril) also have been used. Antidiarrhea drugs such as diphenoxylate hydrochloride (Lomotil) and atropine sulfate are sometimes useful in the control of radiation-induced diarrhea, but Lomotil is not recommended for children under 2 years of age and is used with caution for children under 5 years of age. Its effects in young children are unpredictable, therefore the danger of toxicity is increased.

Antiemetic drugs should be started prior to the onset of nausea and vomiting. Children's tolerance to chemotherapy varies. The nurse therefore tries to determine a pattern of nausea and vomiting for each child so that the particular antiemetic drugs and schedule of administration optimal for the individual child can be identified. Antiemetic drugs are administered on a regular schedule rather than when needed.

The child's intake and output are closely monitored. Fluid and electrolytes are administered to maintain balance. Oral fluids are offered in small amounts. Fluid in the form of popsicles might be one of the few fluids tolerated. Should the child receive chemotherapy treatment as an outpatient, family members are instructed about recording intake and output, rehydrating the child orally, and bringing the child back to the hospital for intravenous hydration if fluid loss necessitates this. (See Chapter 21 for care of the child with a fluid and electrolyte imbalance.)

❀ Alteration in oral mucous membrane related to oral cavity radiation or drug induced stomatitis

The rapidly reproducing tissue of the gastrointestinal tract can be destroyed by certain cytotoxic agents and radiation. As destroyed cells slough off, inflammation and ulceration occur. Ulcers can develop throughout the entire gastrointestinal tract but are most frequently manifested in the mouth and throat as oral stomatitis. Inflammation and ulcers usually begin 7–10 days after drug administration or about the same time the peripheral blood counts decrease. Stomatitis follows radiation by approximately 2 weeks.

Nursing goals for the child with stomatitis focus on prevention of secondary infection of the oral mucosa. The nurse institutes a systematic schedule of oral hygiene. Researchers have not been able to demonstrate a superior mouth care agent, although solutions such as half-strength hydrogen peroxide and antibiotic solutions frequently are used. It is more important to keep the mouth clean and free of debris and mucus than to use a particular agent. Commercial mouth care preparations containing alcohol are avoided because they tend to dry the mouth, causing increased risk of infection through compromised mucous membranes.

Creativity often is necessary to convince a reluctant child with painful stomatitis to perform mouth care. Soft-sponge applicators rather than stiff toothbrushes might be more comfortable for the child. Use of a tube-feeding bag suspended from a comfortable height and filled with an irrigating solution of a small amount of table salt and baking soda dissolved in water is often a tolerable way for the child to keep the mouth rinsed. Using the bag filled with solution, the child can lean over a sink or bed basin and rinse the mouth while controlling the flow of the solution.

Radiation to the mouth can cause salivary gland dysfunction. Saliva becomes scanty. Thick, ropy mucus might develop. Frequent mouth care and removal of mucus is imperative. Oral-pharyngeal suctioning might be necessary and should be undertaken carefully as the mucosa is extremely fragile. Because radiation of the mouth causes decreased salivation, dental caries are more likely to develop. The child needs to have a complete dental evaluation prior to treatment. Fluoride treatments can reduce the incidence of dental caries.

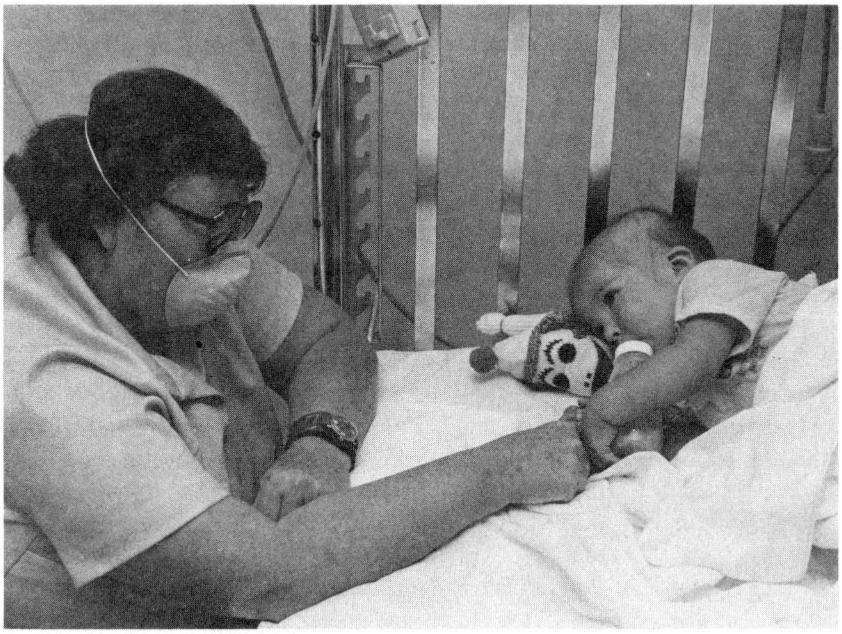

Parents need to maintain closeness to their children even when equipment makes this difficult.

The nurse assesses the child's mouth daily. Tenderness or changes in color or texture in any area of the mouth are recorded. Family members are instructed about the signs and symptoms of stomatitis and appropriate treatment measures so they can encourage mouth care during hospitalization and maintain treatment at home.

The most common infection involves the fungal organism *Candida albicans,* which appears initially as an inflamed patch in the mouth and progresses to white plaques. The organism is treated with the drug nystatin. Liquid suspension of the drug is available and lozenges are available for the older child. Nystatin needs to be held in contact with the oral mucosa for as long as possible for maximum effectiveness.

Alteration in comfort: pain related to chemical injuring agents affecting oral cavity

Local pain control might be necessary to relieve the discomfort of stomatitis, and a variety of solutions and sprays can be ordered by the physician. A combination of diphenhydramine (Benadryl Elixir), Maalox antacid, and lidocaine (viscous Xylocaine), Orabase ointment, or Vince's mouthwash solution are examples. Each will have varying degrees of acceptability to the individual child. Often, simply having the child suck on Popsicles or ice chips provides a sufficient numbing effect.

Impaired tissue integrity related to chemical or radiation irritants resulting in alopecia

Alopecia (hair loss) can be caused by radiation to the skull. Radiation causes destruction of basal cells in the epidermis, resulting in cell death. Alopecia also can occur subsequent to chemotherapy. Hair follicles contain rapidly growing cells and are therefore vulnerable to damage from some chemotherapeutic agents.

Significant hair loss can be a devastating side effect of radiation or chemotherapy even though it is not life threatening. Children need to be prepared for hair loss and need to know that often the hair comes out in large clumps when it is being combed and that the clumps might be found on the bedclothes in the mornings. The child and family need to know also that hair loss usually is not permanent and that regrowth will occur once the drugs producing alopecia are discontinued or approximately 2–3 months after low to moderate doses of radiation therapy are complete. The new hair might look quite different from the original hair. The texture might be finer, and the color can be a lighter or darker shade. Occasionally, when high-dose radiation is indicated, as for some brain tumors, hair will not regrow.

The nurse needs to be sensitive to the impact of hair loss on the child and family. Anger and sadness over hair loss also might be compounded because this might be the first visible sign to the family that the child is seriously ill and needs intensive treatment. This is particularly true if the child appeared healthy at diagnosis.

Wigs or scarves can be used during periods of alopecia. The child needs to select a wig before significant hair loss has resulted. The nurse can direct the family to stores that stock child-size wigs, and the child is encouraged to select the color and style. As the hair begins to fall out, the nurse removes the hair that accumulates on the bedding or clothing of the hospitalized child. Cutting the child's hair shorter also makes hair loss less distracting to the child.

Parents are instructed in managing hair loss for the child at home. Some children adjust rather quickly to the hair loss, but their families might need a longer period of adjustment. These children might prefer not to wear a head covering, and this might in turn become a source of conflict to the parent who wants the child to appear "normal" by wearing a wig or scarf.

Using scalp tourniquets and cooling the scalp with special ice caps during chemotherapy have been used with inconsistent success to decrease blood flow and prevent or retard hair loss. Tourniquets can decrease drug transport to the scalp. Cooling causes vasoconstriction and thus decreases blood flow to the area. The scalp is cooled 20 minutes before the agent is administered. The tourniquet or ice cap remains on the child's head 10–30 minutes after the drug has been injected. These techniques can be used only when the drug is administered intravenously and clears quickly from the blood plasma.

Because the scalp vasoconstriction prevents the cytotoxic drugs from reaching scalp veins, some physicians discourage the use of these techniques because theoretically they allow cancer cells, particularly leukemia and lymphoma cells, to remain in the scalp veins and therefore escape the lethal effects of chemotherapy.

Hair loss also can extend to the entire body. Occasionally the child might lose eyebrows, eyelashes, or even pubic hair. Once the hair has regrown, later disease relapse might necessitate administration of other agents that cause alopecia. Hair loss for the second time usually is much more psychologically traumatic for the child and family.

⊛ Impaired skin integrity related to inflammation and altered pigmentation secondary to radiation therapy

Epidermatitis is an inflammatory skin reaction that is first apparent over a radiated site approximately 2 weeks after therapy has been initiated. Radiation dermatitis is classified by its severity into one of four groups: first-, second-, third-, and fourth-degree epidermatitis. First-degree epidermatitis causes alopecia.

Second-degree reactions are characterized by dry desquamation (peeling). The radiated skin develops erythema, and the child might complain of itching. The skin might peel in a similar manner to a mild sunburn. Once the skin reaction has healed, a permanent increased pigmentation might result.

Third-degree reactions are characterized by wet desquamation. A deep-purple erythema and blisters form. The blisters eventually erupt, resulting in a moist serum exudate. With symptomatic management, healing occurs in about 3 weeks. Again, a permanent hyperpigmentation might remain. A major danger during the wet desquamation reaction is infection. Because of the compromised skin and the presence of the exudate, organisms can flourish. Nurses rarely see a fourth-degree reaction, which is characterized by tissue necrosis and general deep-tissue sloughing. With the use of megavoltage machines, the skin is spared.

Symptomatic treatment of skin reactions varies among radiation oncologists. Generally, keeping the skin dry and exposed to air is recommended. Sometimes the physician will prescribe a lotion or spray containing corticosteroids. The child and parent are instructed not to apply any additional lotions, soaps, deodorants, or ointments since some of these can enhance burning of the skin during radiation therapy. The child is encouraged not to scratch, as even mild scratching can impair the integrity of already-fragile skin. Tight or restrictive clothing and coverings over the radiation field are avoided. Because the skin tissue is very fragile, the area should not be scrubbed, rubbed, or scratched. Using lukewarm water and gently patting the skin dry is recommended when cleansing the area, taking care not to remove radiation ink markers. Sun exposure or application of hot or cold compresses is avoided because it can increase the skin reaction. Radiation usually is avoided for 1–2 weeks after surgery for tumor removal because the child's skin needs to be allowed to heal sufficiently prior to experiencing destructive effects of radiation.

⊛ Potential activity intolerance

A nonspecific side effect of radiation is fatigue. The cause of radiation-induced fatigue is not well understood or studied. Cell destruction due to therapy might stimulate the release of toxic by-products that accumulate in the blood and are slow to be excreted. These toxic by-products could serve as an explanation of radiation fatigue. A second explanation is natural body conservation of energy to direct remaining energy resources to healing normal tissue.

When radiation fatigue is observed in the child undergoing therapy, additional periods of rest need to be planned. The child should not be pushed to keep up a busy activity schedule. Parents need to understand that fatigue is a natural reaction to radiation therapy. Fatigue does not mean that the disease is getting worse, nor does it mean the child is not responding to treatment.

⊛ Potential for infection

Causes of infection Most cytotoxic drugs cause some degree of bone marrow suppression, which decreases the numbers of circulating blood cells. The degree of suppression and specific blood components (erythrocytes, leukocytes, and platelets) affected vary among the different agents and dosage schedules. Generally, peripheral blood counts show signs of suppression 7–10 days after drug administration. The *nadir,* or lowest blood count level, is reached

14 days after the therapy. Recovery and return of blood components to normal levels occur 3–4 weeks after drug administration.

Bone marrow suppression can result from radiation therapy also. The extent of bone marrow suppression is directly related to the dose and extent of bone marrow and lymphoid tissue in the field of radiation. Reduction of circulating platelets and leukocytes is seen initially in the blood count, with a later reduction in circulating erythrocytes. When significant reduction of these blood components results, the child is at risk for developing infection, bruising, bleeding, and anemia.

The child with leukemia or lymphoma is at even greater risk because the disease itself can cause bone marrow dysfunction. The child's hematologic status is carefully monitored. Periods of vulnerability can be predicted through evaluation of laboratory findings and knowledge of the time of greatest risk during the treatment cycle.

Leukopenia (decreased white blood cells) from bone marrow suppression predisposes the child to infection. Many other factors contribute to the risk of infection in the child with cancer. These factors generally are related to compromised body defense. Infections can be bacterial, viral, or fungal in origin.

Disturbance of the first line of defense, the skin, can occur when tissue becomes fragile as a result of chemotherapy and radiation. Stomatitis and fragile erythematous skin, for example, provide easy access to infective agents. Intrusive diagnostic procedures and supportive care measures such as hyperalimentation catheters, lumbar punctures, and venipunctures also encourage infection.

Humoral and cell-mediated immunity can be altered. This leaves the child open to infection as well as to an increase in cancer cells from ineffective surveillance capabilities. Malnutrition, which can be present during times of active treatment, is another factor in susceptibility to infection. Malnutrition contributes to immune defense dysfunction by affecting both humoral and cell-mediated immunity.

Managing infection in the hospital The nurse needs to be knowledgeable about normal blood values (see Table 26-1) and alterations in those values that indicate the child is at risk. Careful systematic assessment of the child on a daily basis during the chemotherapy periods of vulnerability is necessary to determine the presence of complications. Effective nursing management of the child who is experiencing bone marrow suppression requires careful attention to both preventive and supportive measures.

Children are most vulnerable to infection when their absolute granulocyte count falls below 1000 mm. This is referred to as *neutropenia* (see Chapter 25). The nurse observes the neutropenic child closely for signs of infection. Prompt action is required whenever an infection is suspected. If left untreated, a neutropenic child can die of sepsis within 8 hours.

Unfortunately, it is often difficult to document the classic signs and symptoms of infection. Because the child has inadequate numbers of functional white blood cells, pus, inflammation, and therefore pain might not be present. A wound that looks clean and healing might actually be a focal point of infection.

Temperature is monitored every 4 hours as an indicator of infection. Occasionally, it is possible to have an infectious process without a significant temperature elevation. The septic child, for example, might exhibit a subnormal temperature. In spite of exceptions, temperature is one of the better indicators of infection. Nurses on the night shift often find it difficult to imagine waking the sleeping child to record the vital signs, but this procedure should not be skipped for the neutropenic child, as treatment for infection must begin immediately. If no action is taken until morning, the infection might be unresponsive to treatment.

Whenever infection is suspected, and routinely if the temperature is above 39°C (101°F) and the child is neutropenic, the child needs to be evaluated for infection. Cultures of blood, throat, sputum, urine, stool, and any specific lesion or suspicious area are collected for examination. Ideally, all cultures should be obtained before antibiotic therapy is begun. A chest radiograph might be ordered to evaluate subclinical pneumonia.

Strict hand washing technique and care in handling intravenous lines and catheters or other tubings are extremely important and must be consistently practiced. Protective isolation or a laminar airflow environment might be ordered for the hospitalized child, although protective isolation is no longer recommended as effective in preventing infections. Neutropenic children are infected most often by organisms found in their own bodies. During periods of neutropenia, these organisms become pathogenic, so children actually become infected by their own gut flora.

Meticulous rectal care is performed so that the natural microbial flora, particularly *Escherichia coli,* is not introduced into a break in the mucosa. For this reason, rectal temperature, suppositories, and enemas are avoided. Dietary, and other measures if necessary, are initiated to prevent constipation.

The child is monitored for the presence of skin lesions or entry sites from diagnostic or treatment procedures. Band-aids and old blood are promptly removed since they provide excellent media to promote infection. Should lesions, abscesses, or other sources of infection develop, early treatment and continued close observation are required. The nurse also provides comfort measures to decrease pain from the inflammatory process and discomfort from fever should they be present.

Because any infection can be life threatening and the specific causative agent not known or only suspected, broad-spectrum bactericidal coverage with intravenous antibiotics is begun. Although specific drugs vary among institutions and physician preference, broad coverage is most commonly instituted by triple antibiotic therapy of a penicillin derivative, an aminoglycoside, and a cephalosporin. Because of heightened susceptibility, the child might have multiple pathogens responsible for the infection and might have multiple repeated infections of the same organism.

What initially appears to be a localized infection can quickly become a septicemia. The nurse therefore monitors the child for signs of septic shock. Hypotension, confusion and apprehension, shortness of breath, chills, and a subnormal temperature are classic warning signs. Aggressive treatment is required whenever septic shock is suspected. Treatment includes vasopressors, corticosteroids, antibiotics, and granulocyte transfusion. Oxygen administration and even mechanical ventilatory assistance might be necessary to maintain tissue oxygenation. Renal failure is a possible complication. If renal failure is suspected, the rate of fluid administration is altered and drug doses, particularly potassium and aminoglycosides, are lowered to prevent serious toxicity.

If the child does not respond to systemic antibiotics within 48–72 hours, granulocyte transfusions might be done. These transfusions are given on a daily basis until the child shows improvement. Infusion of granulocytes can be associated with hypersensitivity blood reactions. The nurse needs to be alert for signs and symptoms of these reactions, such as chills, rash, hives, blood pressure change, and tachycardia.

Managing infection at home Because the child is more vulnerable to nosocomial (hospital-caused) infections, hospitalization is kept to a minimum. Parents are taught preventive care, how to recognize an infection, and when to seek additional care so they can provide proper supervision of the neutropenic child at home.

Viral infections are common in the immunosuppressed child, particularly the child in remission. Serious viral infections in the child with cancer include chickenpox (varicella), rubella, herpes zoster, and herpes simplex. Although chickenpox and rubella are benign illnesses in normal children, they can be life threatening in the immunosuppressed child with cancer. The child with cancer must carefully avoid exposure to other children with these viruses. When children with rubella and chickenpox are present in the child's school or neighborhood, appropriate steps need to be taken to isolate the child with cancer. If the child has been exposed to chickenpox, zoster immunoglobulin (ZIG) or zoster immune plasma (ZIP) can be given within the first 72 hours after exposure. Gamma globulin can be given for measles exposure. Measles vaccination or any other childhood immunization with live virus vaccine is not given to the immunosuppressed child, as this might cause the disease rather than prevent it.

Pneumocystis carinii is a protozoal infection seen in children with cancer. It appears as a diffuse pneumonia and occurs most frequently in individuals who are immunosuppressed and malnourished. It is also likely to occur during periods of remission. The disease is difficult to diagnose and treat. Previously, deep intramuscular injection of pentamidine isethionate was the drug of choice, but use of oral sulfamethoxazole-trimethoprim (Bactrim or Septra) has proved more effective.

⊛ Potential for injury

Platelets, also known as thrombocytes, play a major role in blood coagulation (see Chapter 26). When the number of available platelets is reduced (thrombocytopenia), the child is at risk for bruising and bleeding. Circulating platelets might be decreased because of the effects of treatment on bone marrow production. They might also be consumed at an increased rate during periods of fever and infection. These complications are much more frequently seen with leukemia, as platelet production is suppressed because of disease activity as well as treatment.

Bruising might be characterized by petechiae or by ecchymoses. Petechiae occur most frequently over pressure points. If the child has been lying in bed, petechiae can be found on the back and sacrum; if the child has been standing, petechiae might appear on the feet and legs. If the child has been crying or coughing, the nurse checks the eyes, head, and chest. Bleeding can vary in amount from mild blood loss to life-threatening hemorrhage.

In addition to platelet suppression, bleeding can be caused by liver involvement, which can decrease circulating coagulants. An enlarged spleen can reduce the number of circulating platelets, resulting in fewer platelets available for clotting. A primary bleed can be due to tumor erosion of vessels.

The child becomes vulnerable to bleeding episodes when the platelet count drops below 50,000/mm^3, and special caution is warranted when the count is below 20,000/mm^3. Platelet transfusions are considered for a count below 20,000/mm^3. Because the platelet concentrate contains some leukocytes and antibodies, immune response can develop after a number of transfusions, destroying many of the newly infused platelets. Once the child has become sensitized, even larger volumes of platelet concentrate do not raise the circulating platelet count significantly, leaving the child vulnerable to hemorrhage. This can be prevented somewhat by using carefully chosen single donor platelets.

Hemorrhage can be spontaneous or a result of trauma. Any number of sites are prone to bleeding. If sufficient blood has been lost, packed red blood cells or whole blood will be administered. Circulatory volume needs to be restored quickly. Fresh-frozen plasma, which contains clotting factors, might reduce bleeding, especially if there is liver dysfunction. The nurse observes the child with a decreased platelet count for warning signs of impending internal hemorrhage. Sudden restlessness and confusion, often called *air hunger;* loss of consciousness; or drop in blood pressure alerts the nurse to possible hemorrhage. Stool, urine, and emesis are guaiac-tested for the presence of blood. Epistaxis is a common occurrence. Nursing care to prevent injury for the child with bone marrow suppression is similar to that for the child with hemophilia. (See Chapter 26 for discussion of nursing care during bleeding episodes.)

⊛ Activity intolerance related to imbalance between oxygen supply and demand

Anemia results from decreased production of red blood cells with corresponding decrease in hemoglobin and hematocrit levels. This can occur from the effects of treatment, although it is less frequently seen than infection and bleeding tendencies. Anemia occurs also from periods of poor nutrition. Additionally, tumor by-products might actually interfere with red blood cell production. At diagnosis and during periods of relapse, the child with leukemia might have significant anemia. This is the result of leukemic cell replacement of normal blood components.

When the hemoglobin value drops below 9 g, the child begins to show such symptoms of hemoglobin deficiency as fatigue, shortness of breath, and dizziness. Children are able to tolerate low hemoglobin levels quite well, however, and symptoms might not be evident until the child becomes profoundly anemic.

The decision to administer packed red blood cells to correct anemia varies among physicians. If the child is asymptomatic and the nadir has passed with recovery expected within a short time, transfusion might not be given. If, however, anemia is profound and complicated by nutritional factors, if recovery is not expected to occur for a number of weeks, or if the child is symptomatic, transfusions will be administered. There is some theoretic evidence that treatment, in particular radiation therapy, is more effective in the presence of well-oxygenated tissue. Thus there might be some effort to keep the child's hemoglobin above 10 g during periods of treatment.

The child with anemia will need to conserve energy to prevent fatigue. Nursing care is organized to provide the maximum amount of rest for the child. Quiet, passive activities and play are recommended. (See Chapter 26 for additional discussion of nursing management of the anemic child and administration of blood components.)

⊛ Potential alteration in body temperature

Fever is associated with the administration of several medications (see Table 33-7). The presence of a fever in the child can be confusing because it can result from a number of causes. Infection always should be investigated since immediate treatment is required, particularly in the immunosuppressed and bone marrow-suppressed child. The fever, however, might actually be caused by the chemotherapy, radiation, immunotherapy, or tumor activity. If the fever is related to one of these causes, comfort measures rather than antibiotics are required. Administration of acetaminophen and sponging or other cooling measures might be useful in reducing fever discomfort.

⊛ Alteration in comfort: pain related to physical and psychologic injuring agents secondary to the diagnosis of cancer

During all phases of treatment, comfort measures should be a high nursing priority. Discomfort can be caused by many factors, including the disease process, fever, nausea, stomatitis, and diagnostic procedures. The child's perception of pain depends on developmental level. For example, the young child might perceive pain and discomfort as punishment.

Therapeutic play programs are an integral part of any childhood cancer program. The child strives to deal with the overwhelming demands of the disease and treatment. A structured play program assists the child to gain psychologic mastery over the perceived threats to stability and sense of self. (Therapeutic play is discussed in Chapter 19.)

Cancer-related pain There are a number of physiologic and psychologic variables in cancer pain. First, pain perception is an individual matter. Perception, meaning, and response to pain vary from child to child. Pain is also a physiologic response. Disease-related causes of pain include tumor infiltration, compression, obstruction, and partial or complete occlusion of pain-sensitive structures. Necrosis, inflammation, and infection as a result of the disease process or side effects of treatment also cause pain. Psychologic aspects related to fear, apprehension, and anxiety can enhance the pain experience.

The initial goal of pain control is to identify the factors causing the pain. Ideally the source of the pain, whether physiologic or psychologic, is removed. For example, if pain is related to infection, antibiotic therapy might remove the source of pain. Bone pain caused by disease infiltration and stretching of the pain-sensitive periosteum often results in excruciating pain. Several low-dose treatments of radiation therapy reduce the pressure on the periosteum and offer dramatic pain relief.

Until therapeutic intervention can remove the source of pain, narcotic treatment and comfort measures are instituted. When pain is caused by disease-related processes, particularly when advanced disease is present, treatment that removes the source of pain might not be possible. If this occurs, pain control by narcotic treatment and comfort measures is the focus of therapy.

Pain is not synonymous with cancer, although this is a frequent misconception of the public. Because the child and family might fear that severe pain is a part of cancer, reeducation is necessary. The child and family are assured that should pain develop, effective pain control techniques are available.

Pain management

Narcotic management When pain is due to a chronic condition, narcotic treatment does not follow the same guidelines as for acute pain management. Because the cause of the pain is not amenable to treatment and will not go away over time, administering drugs on an as-needed basis is inappropriate. Drugs offered on an as-needed basis require the pain to recur before further drugs are given. This regimen simply increases apprehension and anxiety because the child continues to experience pain periodically throughout the day. Thus drugs are administered on a routine (not an as-needed) basis so the pain cycle is halted.

There is no one ideal pain control drug. A narcotic is chosen because of the degree of pain and its effectiveness with the particular child. An appropriate dosage level and schedule needs to be tailored to the individual child. Sometimes very high doses of drugs are given and will not cause the drowsiness or significant respiratory suppression that would be expected in an otherwise-normal child. The exact reason for this is not known but is thought to relate to an alteration in the pain receptors in the brain.

The route of drug administration should also receive consideration. As long as a drug can be absorbed through the gastrointestinal tract, the oral route is used. Because the child is receiving the drug on a routine basis, there is no advantage to intramuscular or intravenous injection. The latter routes offer more rapid absorption than oral administration, but since a constant blood level is maintained when the drug is given routinely, absorption speed is not a factor. Several narcotics such as morphine and methadone are available in liquid form. This allows easier individual measurement of a therapeutic dose for each child. It also might be easier to swallow than pills or capsules. If nausea, vomiting, or swallowing prevent oral administration, rectal suppositories can be considered if the leukocyte count is adequate. When less invasive methods of drug administration are not effective, then intramuscular injection, if the platelet count is adequate, or intravenous injection might be necessary.

The nurse needs to remember that dosage levels change with the route of administration. An adequate dose must be given if pain control is to be achieved, and the nurse assumes a major role in documenting the effectiveness of pain medication. Data are gathered from the child, the parent, and through observation. The nurse carefully records the child's response to medication and any continuing pain patterns. When pain control is inadequate, the nurse provides additional information to the physician so that the drug or dosage can be adjusted.

Nausea and constipation can be problematic side effects of narcotic administration. An antiemetic can be administered to control nausea. Bowel function is carefully monitored. The nursing focus is on preventing rather than treating constipation. Stool softeners or stimulants might be required.

Nonnarcotic interventions In addition to administration and evaluation of pain medication, the nurse uses other intervention strategies to provide comfort and decrease pain perception. Basic comfort measures are a part of nursing care. Bathing and positioning and providing oral hygiene and a clean, uncluttered environment are standard requirements of good nursing care. Encouraging the parent to hold and rock the young child also is therapeutic.

Distraction is another useful intervention. The nurse keeps in mind, however, that distraction is not a substitute for adequate pain medication but instead provides an additional resource.

Interventions that promote relaxation are excellent comfort techniques. A warm bath can effectively reduce muscle tension and encourage relaxation. Children are very suggestible and therefore are good candidates for progressive relaxation techniques combined with guided imagery. Relaxation techniques are easy-to-learn, beneficial resources for every nurse to use.

The child is also an excellent candidate for hypnosis. Recent studies have found hypnosis to be a positive adjuvant to other cancer pain-control measures (Barbora and Gitelson, 1980). Before a nurse uses hypnosis as a method of pain control, however, specific training in hypnotic technique is required.

The nurse also needs to remember that psychologic variables play a significant role in pain perception. If the child feels isolated or anxious and fearful about the disease status or family relationships, administration of narcotics will not totally ease the pain. The nurse carefully assesses the child's emotional response to the illness and family interactions. Supportive counseling or referral to child psychologic services are necessary to deal effectively with the psychologic variables of pain control.

Nutritional Needs

⊛ Potential alteration in nutrition: less than body requirements

The disease process and the effects of treatment contribute to malnutrition in the child with cancer. Because treatment is more effective and potential side effects, such as infection, are less common in the well-nourished child, maintaining optimal nutrition is a high nursing priority.

Cancer cachexia Severe weight loss and wasting of body tissue characterize *cancer cachexia,* the general state of ill health and malnutrition associated with a neoplastic illness. Many factors contribute to cancer cachexia, including an increased metabolic rate due to tumor activity. Side effects of treatment, which cause nausea, vomiting, and stomatitis, reduce the child's desire and ability to eat and drink. Additionally, tumor metabolites in the circulation can directly cause anorexia and alteration in taste perceptions. Once cachexia is evident, it is difficult to halt. Intravenous administration of hyperalimentation (total parenteral nutrition) might be necessary.

Psychologic factors also contribute to cancer cachexia. When the child does not feel well, is frightened by unfamiliar surroundings, or is receiving foods not usually served at home, food and fluid intake can decrease. The parent might become alarmed when the child continues to eat poorly and lose weight. It is important that eating not become a battle between parent and child. The parent needs to understand the importance of good nutrition but at the same time needs to be taught how and when to approach the child about eating so that conflict does not develop. For example, the child might be more comfortable eating while watching a favorite television show, or the parent might determine that the child eats better after a nap. The parent needs to be open to the child's wishes and not be afraid to back off and try another approach if one does not succeed.

By teaching the parent how to make the child's preferences for food more nutritious and assisting the parent to assess the child's needs regarding eating, the nurse promotes participation in the child's care. This allows the parent some control in a situation that, for the most part, is out of the parent's control. In doing this, however, nurses need to be willing to accept the recommendations of parents regarding their children's particular nutritional needs and preferences.

Nutritional assessment The nurse obtains a dietary history and observes the child's current eating pattern. Can decreased eating habits be related to fear of impending treatments, pain, or nausea? Would better timing of pain medication or antiemetics increase eating? What is the social setting during meals? Is the child isolated? Is the general setting conducive to eating or are there unpleasant noises or odors? The nurse also observes the child-parent interaction during meals.

Dietary modifications Taste alterations that might occur include intolerance to some meats and an increased threshold for sweets. If a protein aversion develops, the child will refuse meats such as beef and pork. Other sources of protein are offered, including poultry, fish, cheese, nuts, and protein-rich beans. Children are not forced to continue eating foods they cannot tolerate. Besides finding these foods distasteful, forcing the child to eat intolerable foods can create a generalized aversion to all foods. The child might dislike sweet-tasting foods because these foods no longer taste sweet; additional sweetening can make the food more palatable. Some children simply will not eat any sweet foods because of their altered taste.

Meals are based on the child's individual preference and emphasize maximum calories and nutrients. Calories can be increased by adding butter, cream, mayonnaise, honey, or granola to appropriate foods during cooking. Cheese also can be added to many foods, thus increasing both calories and protein. Milkshakes, puddings, and other nutritional snacks can be offered between meals. Although "junk foods" should not become the mainstay of the child's diet, many of these foods can be made more nutritious. For example, additional cheese and meats (if tolerated) can be added to pizza.

Small, frequent feedings rather than large meals are most acceptable. It might be better to avoid serving liquids with meals since they can quickly make the child feel full. Determining which time of the day is most agreeable to the child helps the child to eat a larger meal. Many children feel better in the morning, and breakfast might be the best time of the day to maximize calories and protein.

For the child with stomatitis, eating might be difficult due to pain and altered taste. The child needs to avoid foods that are too hot, too spicy, and firm textured. Foods that tend to appeal to children with stomatitis include soft, bland food (eg, puddings, ice cream, gelatin).

Developmental Needs

⊛ Potential altered growth and development

The child's life needs to be kept as normal as possible in spite of the illness. Routines are patterned after the child's preillness activities. In keeping the child's life as normal as possible and promoting normal development, both the parents and the health care team can maintain discipline. This can be very difficult for parents who feel guilty placing limits on a sick child. Children need the continued security of appropriate discipline and limits. The nurse thus provides anticipatory guidance, allowing parents to express their reluctance to discipline their children but reinforcing the children's need for continued discipline. (See Chapter 14 for further discussion of the implications of chronic illness for the child.)

Return to school is encouraged. The child's reentry to school is facilitated by the hospital-based or outpatient nurse directly contacting the school or by referral to the school or community health nurse. Teachers need to understand accurately the child's condition and any limitations. They also need reassurance and encouragement to treat the child normally and not single the child out as "special."

One way to help meet the child's developmental needs, especially the need to lead as normal a life as possible, is to continue care of the child at home, particularly when hospitalization and active treatment measures are no longer beneficial. A family who chooses this alternative needs support and education so that the members are comfortable with the child's physiologic care and the family's emotional well-being at home. Hospice programs also provide comprehensive psychosocial and physiologic care in the home setting. (Further discussion of the needs of the dying child and of the role that hospices play can be found in Chapter 17.)

Emotional Needs

⊛ Potential body image disturbance

The child's body image can be altered by the disease and treatment, and this might result in feelings of self-consciousness and withdrawal from peers and activities. Body changes as a result of disease have a particular impact on adolescents, since the usual body changes that occur with puberty can be problematic themselves. The additional stress of hair loss, weight loss, and other consequences of cancer or its treatment can cause overwhelming feelings of inadequacy for an adolescent who is trying to be as much like peers as possible.

Nurses need to offer sensitive support and encouragement to children dealing with problems of body image alterations. The nurse allows the child to verbalize any feelings of anger or resentment. Emphasizing qualities in the child that are not connected with appearance can help. Allowing the child as much control as possible over appearance, such as choosing clothing or a wig, helps the child cope with the altered body image. Children are encouraged to maintain social contacts in spite of changes in appearance. The nursing staff also needs to guard against sheltering the child in the hospital setting, making it so emotionally comfortable for the child that the child resists return to the home and community.

⊛ Potential ineffective individual coping

The general emotional needs of the child relevant to aberrant cellular growth vary, depending on whether the child is hospitalized, is in a state of remission or chronic illness, or is in the terminal stages of the disease. The following stressors, however, can be particularly significant on children with childhood cancer.

- The publicity and fear surrounding cancer in today's society might intensify the anxiety felt by parents and children when the diagnosis is communicated.
- The severity of the side effects of many cancer treatments can exacerbate the child's emotional response to the disease.
- The uncertainty over whether a given treatment will be effective will prolong the fear and anxiety of all concerned.

The child might have difficulty accepting the diagnosis and is likely to go through anticipatory grieving. Denial, fear, anger, hostility, depression, and withdrawal are only a few of the emotions experienced by children with cancer. Adolescents particularly begin to realize that their long-term goals might not be achievable and might mourn their loss. The child with cancer might be avoided by friends who are embarrassed because they don't know what to say or how to act.

The nurse helps the child to cope by allowing the child to express, either verbally or nonverbally, feelings of fear, anger, or depression. Long-term goals might have to be telescoped, with the child focusing on daily achievements instead. The child is assisted to identify personal strengths, such as cooperativeness or humor, and encouraged to use these assets in coping with the disease or its treatments. Role play can be helpful in assisting the child to communicate with peers and to maintain needed peer support.

⊛ Alteration in family processes related to situational crisis secondary to the child's illness and hospitalization

In addition to the stressors placed on the child with cancer, the family unit experiences difficulties for a range of reasons:

1. The treatment for childhood cancer can severely tax the financial resources of the family, creating emotional stress over normal family function.

2. The stress of the child's illness might place a strain on the marital relationship of the parents, driving them apart rather than bringing them closer together. The divorce rate is high because both spouses go through the grief process in different ways and at different times, thus blocking effective communication.
3. A sibling might experience not only the normal emotions of fear, guilt, or resentment but also the fear of contracting the same disease, especially if the sibling and the ill child are twins. Because the major portion of attention is being given to the ill child, siblings might feel unloved.

The nurse can play a major role in helping the family meet its own emotional needs by

1. Promoting open and honest communication among all family members, especially between the parents, to offset any tendency toward individual isolation
2. Referring the family to community resources and parental support groups, such as Candlelighters, to provide financial assistance, needed information, and emotional and social support
3. Providing opportunities for the siblings to express their feelings and to give them as much contact with the ill child as appropriate, while making sure they understand that they cannot "catch" their sibling's disease
4. Being aware of the family's anxieties and thus possibly preventing the members from not hearing or understanding important information (thus the nurse needs to be ready to take more time to prepare the child and family for treatments and procedures, to repeat explanations more frequently, and to answer more questions than usual)
5. Encouraging parents and siblings to participate as much as possible in the care of the ill child and encouraging ill children to participate in their own care

The family who must face advanced disease and the impending death of the child requires tremendous nursing support and assistance. The nurse encourages open expression of feelings and anticipatory mourning. The death of a child is one of the most profound crises a parent can face. Unfortunately, traditional health care services are often terminated at the death of the child. The family must then deal with their bereavement alone. A parental support group, Compassionate Friends, is available for parents who have experienced the death of a child. Follow-up with bereaved families should be encouraged and integrated into health care services. (See Chapter 17 for further discussion of the family who must face the death of a child.)

Health Maintenance Needs

⊛ Potential knowledge deficit concerning child's home care management

The child during remission The nurse assumes a major role assisting the family to understand the child, the disease, the treatment, and the side effects that can occur. Because the child spends the most time at home, parents need to be knowledgeable about and comfortable with the care of their child at home. When the child is hospitalized, the parent is encouraged to participate in the child's care, continuing the important nurturing and caregiving role. The nursing staff develops a systematic educational program for parents that can be adapted to each family's unique situation. Written materials and care directions are given to the family so that the members can refer to them should problems develop at home.

Throughout the course of the illness, parents are confronted with well-meaning friends and relatives and media sources who advocate the use of unproven cancer treatments. Wanting to do everything possible to assure their children's cure, parents might seriously consider alternatives to conventional therapy. Generally, parents choose to investigate unproven treatments (a) during the initial diagnostic period—hoping to find someone who will offer a more favorable diagnosis and treatment or (b) when metastatic disease has been identified—hoping to find someone who can guarantee a cure. Parents need to know that interest in investigating other treatments is normal and that even if they do not actively look for alternatives, friends and relatives or sometimes even unsolicited strangers might contact them. The attitude and sensitivity of the health care professionals is critical in helping parents to feel comfortable in discussing their concerns about current treatments and alternative methods. The nurse encourages parents to bring in information and assists the parents in finding out what is scientifically known about the treatment. Parents need to see the health professional as a supportive ally who might personally discourage the use of unproven treatments but will not condemn and reject the family for investigating other treatments.

The "cured" child A child is considered cured of cancer when free from the disease for longer than 6 years. Discharging a child cured of cancer is a very satisfying experience, although those cured of childhood cancer still must face residual and late effects of the treatment. The child's growth into adulthood and adjustment in society is a matter of keen interest to health professionals. The goal of treating the child with cancer is not only to cure the child but also to make the treatment and long-term consequences of the treatment compatible with a normal lifestyle. Now that many children with cancer can be cured, clinicians are dealing with the new challenges of the cured child.

The child can be left with long-term physical and psychosocial consequences. Physical problems might include (1) permanent physical impairments and dysfunction, (2) reproductive dysfunction, (3) growth and learning disabilities, and (4) mutations causing new cancer. Psychosocial problems might include (1) concerns over body image and sexuality that delay marriage, (2) employment discrimination, and (3) health insurance denial.

To receive satisfaction from curing the child with cancer, consequences after treatment must not be so great as to impair successful social adjustment. Appropriate guidance and advocacy for these individuals needs to be available so they can successfully enter into productive adulthood.

The Child with a Neoplasm

Acute Leukemias

Leukemia is a primary malignancy of the bone marrow and certain white blood cells. Because the white blood cells are immature and nonfunctional, infection is a primary consequence. Leukemia is the most common malignancy of childhood, accounting for 34% of all childhood cancers. There are several types of leukemia, which are divided into two major classifications: (a) acute leukemia and (b) chronic leukemia. The acute leukemias constitute 98% of childhood leukemia. The remaining 2% are chronic myelogenous (granulocytic) leukemias. Acute and chronic leukemia are differentiated by the maturity of the involved cell. Acute leukemia involves immature blast cells, whereas chronic leukemia primarily involves mature cells. (Table 33-8 identifies the different types of acute leukemia along with subclasses that help determine treatment and prognosis.)

Of the subgroups of acute lymphocytic leukemia (ALL), the pre-B cell and null cell leukemias have the best prognosis. Fortunately over 75% of children with ALL have null cell disease. Other prognostic factors have been identified. The child with the most favorable diagnosis is, at diagnosis, between the ages of 2 and 6; has a peripheral white blood cell count below 10,000; has no lymphadenopathy, hepatosplenomegaly, or central nervous system involvement; and has null cell disease. The overall survival rate is 50%; with good prognostic factors the survival rate is closer to 60%–70% (Simone and Rivers, 1984).

There are two other general types of acute leukemia in childhood besides ALL: (a) acute undifferentiated leukemia (AUL), which is the least common type of acute leukemia, and (b) acute nonlymphocytic leukemia (ANLL). Generally, these have a much poorer prognosis than ALL, although progress is being made.

Clinical manifestations The presenting symptoms of leukemia result from the overproduction of immature, leukemic (blast) cells in the bone marrow (Fig. 33-2). The

TABLE 33-8 Types of Acute Leukemia in Childhood

Type	Abbreviation	Primary involved cell line	Percentage of occurrence
Acute lymphocytic leukemia	ALL	Overproduction of immature lymphocytes (lymphoblasts)	80%
Subclass by immunologic marker			
T cell			
B cell			
pre–B cell			
null cell			
Acute undifferentiated leukemia	AUL	Unable to determine	5%
Acute nonlymphocytic leukemia	ANLL	Rapid overproliferation of immature cells coming from one of several cell lines	15%
Subclass by involved cell line			
Acute myelocytic leukemia	AML	Myeloblast	
Acute myelomonocytic leukemia	AMML	Combination myeloblast and monoblast	
Acute monocytic leukemia	AMoL	Monoblast	
Erythyrocytic leukemia		Combination erythroblast and myeloblast	

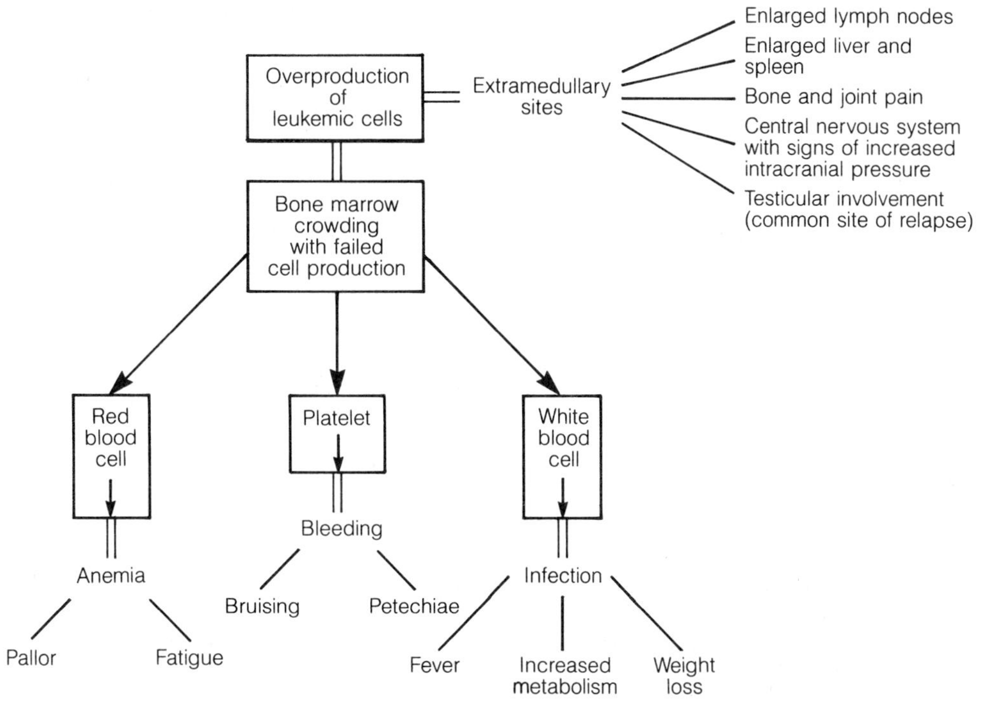

FIGURE 33-2
Effects of leukemia on the body.

increased number of leukemic cells crowds out other normal cell lines. This causes bone marrow failure from decreased production of red blood cells, platelets, and white blood cells, resulting in anemia, bleeding tendencies, and infection. As a direct result of bone marrow failure, over 50% of children have fever, pallor, and bruising/bleeding at diagnosis.

Leukemia cells can migrate from the bone marrow and infiltrate extramedullary (outside the marrow) sites such as lymph nodes, liver, and spleen. Depending on the location and degree of these infiltrations, lymphadenopathy, mediastinal mass, hepatomegaly, and splenomegaly might be present at diagnosis. Leukemia cells also invade bones and the central nervous system, presenting as bone and joint pain, with meningeal symptoms manifested by vomiting, headache, and papilledema. The reproductive organs, particularly the testes, also can be involved.

Diagnostic evaluation History, physical examination, and peripheral blood count showing the presence of blast cells raise the clinical suspicion of leukemia. The total white blood cell count can reach as high as $300{,}000/mm^3$ because of the proliferation (overproduction) of immature cells.

The definitive diagnosis and identification of the actual type of leukemia is, however, determined by bone marrow aspiration. Examination of the bone marrow generally will reveal 80%–90% of the bone marrow replaced with immature blast cells. Normally there are fewer than 5% immature white blood cells in the bone marrow and only rare cells in the peripheral blood. Because the blast cells have replaced normal cell lines, there is also a decrease in developing red blood cells, platelets, and granulocytes. A lumbar puncture is performed to determine whether there are cancer cells in the cerebrospinal fluid.

Treatment

Acute lymphocytic leukemia

Remission induction The initial treatment, called remission induction, is intended to reduce the number of leukemic cells so there is no evidence of leukemia. Currently used is a combination of vincristine and prednisone, with or without a third drug such as L-asparaginase. The child with poor prognostic factors might receive an alternative "high-risk" treatment protocol. Approximately 95% of children with ALL obtain a remission in 2–4 weeks after treatment is instituted (Simone and Rivers, 1984).

Central nervous system prophylaxis Once the child is in remission, prophylactic treatment for central nervous system disease is begun. In the past, standard treatment has included both cranial radiation and intrathecal methotrex-

NURSING CARE PLAN *The Child with Leukemia*

Assessment data: Billy is a 9-year-old boy admitted to the hospital to confirm the diagnosis of acute leukemia. For the past 3 weeks Billy has had an upper respiratory tract infection with fevers that recurred after oral antibiotic treatment. A complete blood count done in the physician's office showed a white blood cell count of 15,000/mm^3, hemoglobin of 11g/dL, and platelet count of 30,000/mm^3. Billy appears pale and lethargic and has both bruises and petechiae on his extremities. Physical assessment reveals a fever of 39°C, absence of lymph node adenopathy or bone pain, and moderate hepatosplenomegaly. Chest radiograph reveals no mediastinal mass, and blood chemistries are within acceptable limits with the exception of the uric acid level, which is moderately elevated. Nose, throat, urine, and blood cultures are obtained, and Billy is started on a combination of three broad-spectrum antibiotics. A bone marrow biopsy and lumbar puncture are performed. Results confirm the diagnosis of acute lymphocytic leukemia with null cell immunologic markers. The bone marrow was hypercellular with 86% blasts. The lumbar puncture showed no evidence of central nervous system disease. Billy is placed in a private room because the pediatric unit has a number of children who harbor chronic infections. Billy is considered to be in the most favorable diagnostic category. He begins his remission induction therapy with vincristine, prednisone, and L-asparginase.

An interview with Billy's parents reveals the following information. Billy is the middle child. He has an older brother, Brian, who is 10, and a younger sister, Kerry, who is 6. Up until the present illness Billy has been a healthy, active child who has developed normally in all areas. The other children also are characterized as completely normal by their parents.

Billy's mother is 33 years old and has been a homemaker since she was married 12 years ago. Recently she has been working part-time as salesperson in an antique shop. Billy's father is 35 years old and operates a gas station. Neither parent has had much experience with health professionals and only see a doctor when an illness "doesn't clear up in a few days." Although they have several good friends, neither has relatives close by. They say that Billy's diagnosis of leukemia confirmed their worst fears and is the most devastating thing that has happened to them.

RISKS

Assessed risk	Nursing action
Hyperuricemia secondary to cell lysis	Monitor serum uric acid level. Encourage fluids. Administer allopurinol, bicarbonate, and intravenous fluids as ordered. Check urine for pH and specific gravity. Observe and report any clinical signs of hyperuricemia, such as pain and inflammation in joints, fever, and chills.
Peirpheral nervous system dysfunction related to chemotherapy (vincristine)	Observe for and report signs of neurotoxicity, such as weakness, numbness, jaw pain, foot drop, or decreased deep tendon reflexes. Teach the family about signs to observe for and encourage them to report symptoms immediately.
Side effects from chemotherapy—infection, bone marrow suppression, stomatitis, alopecia	(See Table 33-7 and Standards of Nursing Care, The Child with Bone Marrow Suppression, p. 1170)

NURSING CARE PLAN *The Child with Leukemia (Continued)*

GUIDE FOR NURSING MANAGEMENT

Nursing diagnosis	Intervention	Rationale
1. Potential for infection (stressors: compromised secondary defenses, introduction of pharmaceutical agents potentially causing immunosuppression)	Obtain cultures as ordered.	Cultures identify current organisms.
	Administer antibiotics as ordered.	Antibiotics control current organisms.
	Monitor temperature every 4 hours and as warranted.	Early identification prevents serious infection.
	Reduce fever if greater than 39°C by promoting cooling of skin and mucous membranes, preventing chilling, and administering acetaminophen as ordered.	Interventions provide comfort and reduce accelerated metabolic need.
	Institute a private room as ordered.	Preventive measures keep the immunosuppressed child from being exposed to others with chronic infection.
	Observe potential sites for further infection development.	Early identification prevents seriously infected sites.
	Achieve and maintain optimal nutrition. (Billy likes milkshakes, apple juice, toasted cheese sandwiches, and pizza.)	Malnutrition negatively affects immune function. (Children are most likely to eat the foods they like.)
	Maintain the integrity of the skin and mucous membranes. Teach Billy and his family the importance of good personal hygiene. Use aseptic technique when performing intrusive procedures. Avoid rectal temperatures, suppositories, or enemas. Teach Billy and his family about infection risk and preventive treatment.	Skin is the first line of defense against microorganisms.

Outcome: Billy's temperature returns to 37°C within 48 hours of admission. Billy does not demonstrate any new evidence of local or systemic infection.

Nursing diagnosis	Intervention	Rationale
2. Potential impairment of skin integrity (stressors: decreased platelets in circulation, chemotherapy and depressed immune response, increased fragility of mucus membranes)	Monitor susceptibility to bleeding. Monitor platelet count, presence of additional bruising and petechiae, guaiac urine, stool, emesis.	Decreased platelet count and bruising and petechiae can indicate bleeding.
	Maintain skin integrity. Hold puncture sites for 5 minutes. Avoid intramuscular injections. Do not take rectal temperatures.	Preserving skin integrity decreases likelihood of capillary damage, skin breakdown, and entry of pathogens.
	Protect mucous membranes. Use a soft bristle or sponge toothbrush to avoid trauma. Lubricate tips. Avoid forceful nose blowing.	Protecting membranes decreases likelihood of capillary damage and mucous membrane breakdown.
	Do not give products that contain aspirin. Teach Billy and his parents about bleeding potential and preventive treatment.	Aspirin destroys platelets.
	Institute safety precautions.	Protecting the child from falls or other trauma decreases risk of bruising or bleeding.

Outcome: Billy's skin and mucous membranes remain intact. Billy's parents understand safety precautions, including avoidance of aspirin.

(Continues)

NURSING CARE PLAN *The Child with Leukemia (Continued)*

Nursing diagnosis	Intervention	Rationale
3. Potential alteration in bowel elimination (stressors: constipation secondary to anticancer medication, decreased mobility, decreased appetite)	Begin administration of stool softener before chemotherapy is started. Force fluids and encourage a high-fiber diet.	Preventive measures combat vincristine-induced constipation.
	Monitor frequency and consistency of bowel movements. Teach Billy and his parents about constipation as a side effect of vincristine and as a preventive treatment.	Early assessment of constipation allows additional intervention.

Outcome: Billy passes soft stool at his usual frequency (once a day). Billy's parents describe preventive measures and relate the occurrence of constipation to the administration of the vincristine.

Nursing diagnosis	Intervention	Rationale
4. Diversionary activity deficit related to monotony of hospital environment secondary to confinement to private room	Elicit information about Billy's normal activity pattern. Determine what activities can be continued while confined in a private room and determine a rest pattern.	Identifying normal activity level, interests, and developmental tasks for Billy allows the plan to be personalized.
	Encourage the family to bring in special toys such as his puzzles, space creatures, and tape player and headset with his favorite tapes. Decorate room with cards, posters, pictures of family and friends.	Billy needs familiar objects and toys to feel comfortable with the environment and to increase his interest in his surroundings.
	Refer Billy to a child-life worker for additional activities.	Billy, although confined, needs a therapeutic and recreational outlet to prevent boredom and withdrawal.

Outcome: Billy demonstrates interest in allowable activities. Billy requests activities appropriately, taking into consideration his limitations. Billy does not appear to be bored (no restlessness, irritability, passiveness).

Nursing diagnosis	Intervention	Rationale
5. Potential for social isolation (stressors: separation from peers, confinement to a private room, fatigue)	Explain to Billy the need for the private room; allow him to express frustration over confinement.	If the medical reason for isolation is clarified, Billy feels less rejected, alienated, or lonely.
	Encourage Billy to keep in touch by phone with his friends.	Billy needs to maintain contact with the normal environment and needs to continue his social development to avoid feeling isolated.
	Arrange for school tutorial service so that Billy may keep on with his schoolwork.	Billy needs to keep up with cognitive development and maintain interest in activities that normally provide social interaction.
	Encourage family visitation and interaction. Assist siblings to deal with feelings of abandonment and rivalry.	Continued contact with the family is necessary during period of crisis.

Outcome: Billy maintains contacts on a regular basis with family and peers within imposed limitations.

Nursing diagnosis	Intervention	Rationale
6. Knowledge deficit concerning the implications of the diagnosis related to incomplete understanding	Prepare Billy and his family for each diagnostic procedure (lab work, radiographs, bone marrow, etc.).	Preparation decreases stress and provides positive coping.

NURSING CARE PLAN *The Child with Leukemia (Continued)*

Nursing diagnosis	Intervention	Rationale
	Determine Billy's and his family's understanding of the diagnosis of leukemia by providing the written materials, encouraging Billy (when out of isolation) and his siblings to visit the lab and see blood and bone marrow slides; encourage the family to keep a list of questions that come to mind.	The emotional response to the diagnosis of a life-threatening illness often clouds understanding of information. Explanations need to be repeated and additional information given gradually.
	Begin a teaching program regarding leukemia, its treatment, side effects, and their control. Topics to be covered are leukemia; chemotherapy and how it works; side effects and what to do about infection, bleeding, anemia, constipation, peripheral neuropathies, moon face, mood changes; and follow-up care. Use procedure and equipment play as part of teaching. Plan follow-up visits for further education after discharge or refer to a visiting nurse for follow-up.	A systematic teaching program provides the foundation for parent and child participation in the treatment of childhood cancer.
Outcome: Billy tolerates procedures and demonstrates effective coping. Family members can individually explain basic information about leukemia. Family members freely ask questions as needed. Family members can correctly describe treatment plan, side effects which might occur, and appropriate management of side effects.		
7. Fear (parents' and child's) related to perceived inability to control event secondary to diagnosis of leukemia	Encourage the family to express fears and feelings. Accept feelings expressed; provide hopeful, realistic support.	Expression of feelings is the basis for identifying effective coping mechanisms.
	Encourage the parents to support each other and keep lines of communication open.	Parents dealing with the crisis of a child's life-threatening illness can discharge feelings of stress and frustration onto each other unless they are sensitive to each other's needs and share feelings.
	Encourage the family to participate in a support group.	Group support with people also experiencing a child's life-threatening disease provides a supportive network and a forum for expressing feelings.
	Refer the family to the American Cancer Society or the Leukemia Society for financial or emotional assistance.	These societies are a good resource for help during a long-term, financially and emotionally draining illness.
Outcome: Family members identify fears, frustrations, guilt and resentments over impact of diagnosis. Parents spend time together. Lines of communication are kept open. Parents have joined a support group and find it helpful.		

ate. Because of the incidence of learning disabilities in the child who has received radiation, some clinicians are omitting it and administering intrathecal methotrexate over an extended period of time (Klopovich and Cohen, 1984).

Maintenance therapy The third phase of treatment, maintenance therapy, is intended to reduce leukemic cells further so that a cure is obtained. A common maintenance protocol includes daily doses of 6-mercaptopurine and weekly doses of methotrexate. Periodic pulses (short-term, intermittent drug doses) of additional drugs such as vincristine and prednisone also might be included. Treatment is continued for 30–36 months.

Reinduction If bone marrow relapse occurs, a second reinduction protocol will be started. The likelihood of cure after bone marrow relapse is poor, but second remissions can be achieved in most children. These remissions usually are shorter than the initial one, however. Bone marrow transplantation might be considered after the child has obtained a second remission since further relapse, eventually leading to death, is common.

If relapse occurs in extramedullary sites, bone marrow relapse generally follows. Testicular leukemia infiltrates occur in approximately 10% of males with ALL. Prophylactic therapy is not given because of the relatively low incidence, because symptomatic treatment does not prevent disease development, and because treatment can result in sterility. When testicular leukemia occurs, radiation to the testes is given (Askin et al., 1981). Aggressive systemic therapy is also begun because of the likelihood of subsequent bone marrow relapse.

Acute nonlymphocytic leukemia Because the prognosis for ANLL is worse than ALL, treatment is more intensive. Remission induction includes protocols such as cytosine arabinoside, vincristine, and daunorubicin. In contrast to the 95% remission response in ALL, only 60%–70% of children with ANLL ever achieve a first remission (Simone and Rivers, 1984). Because long-term survival was not common with ANLL, prophylactic central nervous system treatment was not routinely given. As the length of survival increases, prophylactic central nervous system treatment has become standard practice.

Bone marrow transplantation can be considered for the child with ANLL when the first remission is achieved. If bone marrow transplant is not an option, additional combinations of chemotherapy are administered in phases. The object of the phased chemotherapy is both to reduce the number of leukemic cells and to prevent drug resistance.

Nursing management Nursing management of the child with bone marrow suppression is the basis for caring for the child with leukemia. In addition to bone marrow suppression, hyperuricemia (increased blood uric acid) is a problem in the child with leukemia. Hyperuricemia results from breakdown products during cell death. The leukemia process causes turnover of a large number of cells. Additionally, treatment destroys many cells. The combination of these two processes can cause very high serum uric acid levels. Urinary excretion of uric acid causes the uric acid to precipitate, leading to obstruction and renal failure.

To prevent hyperuricemia, allopurinol, which blocks the formation of uric acid, might be ordered. Liberal hydration and alkalinization of the urine by administration of sodium bicarbonate also reduce the renal toxicity of hyperuricemia.

The nurse assists the child and family to adapt to the disease and treatment requirements. Comprehensive physical care and emotional and social support is based on the individuals needs of each child and family during every phase of the disease process.

Hodgkin's Disease

Lymphomas are broadly separated into two categories: Hodgkin's disease and nonHodgkin's lymphoma (also called lymphosarcoma). Hodgkin's disease is characterized by abnormal cellular production in the lymph nodes. There might be proliferation of lymphocytes, eosinophils, histiocytes, and collagen and fibrous tissue. A classic diagnostic finding of Hodgkin's disease is the presence of a large cell known as the Reed-Sternberg cell. Hodgkin's disease is considered to have one focus of origin with spread to nearby lymph nodes.

Hodgkin's disease is more frequently seen in males than females. It is rare before the age of 5. There is a gradual increased incidence throughout childhood with a marked increase during adolescence. It accounts for 6.5% of childhood cancers.

Clinical manifestations The most common presenting sign of Hodgkin's disease is painless swelling of a lymph node or several nodes generally in the cervical chain. Axillary, inguinal, mediastinal, or retroperitoneal nodes are less frequently the presenting site. Other presenting symptoms include anorexia, lassitude, and malaise. The child might complain of fever, night sweats, weight loss, or organ specific signs of pressure from enlarged lymph nodes (eg, dyspnea, cough, laryngeal paralysis from pressure on the upper respiratory tract).

Staging of the disease helps determine the prognosis (Table 33-9). Staging takes into account the extent of lymph node and extranodal (tissue outside the nodes) involvement. Extranodal involvement can occur in the spleen, liver, mediastinum, lung, central nervous system, and bones. A more favorable prognosis is associated with disease that is located on just one side of the diaphragm and without extranodal involvement. The presence of a group of systemic symptoms—fever, significant weight loss, and night sweats—lends a less favorable prognosis. Prognostic factors also depend on the histologic type: lymphocyte predominant Hodgkin's disease has a good prognosis; nodular sclerosing and mixed cellular Hodgkin's have a guarded prognosis; while lymphocyte depletion Hodkin's has a poor prognosis (Hoffmann, 1983).

Diagnostic evaluation Laboratory studies of serum copper level and erythrocyte sedimentation rate (ESR) are performed at diagnosis and throughout the course of the ill-

TABLE 33-9 Staging for Hodgkin's Disease

Stage	Extent of involvement
I	Disease is limited to a single lymph node, lymph node region, or a single extranodal organ
II	Involves two or more lymph node regions on the same side of the diaphragm (eg, cervical and axillary)
III	Involvement of lymph node regions on both sides of the diaphragm along with involvement of an extranodal organ, usually the spleen
IV	Moderate involvement of one or more extranodal organs or tissues

NOTE: Stages can be further defined by adding: **A,** absence of systemic signs and symptoms; **B,** presence of systemic signs and symptoms (eg, fever, night sweats, 10% weight loss).

ness. Levels are frequently elevated when Hodgkin's disease is present. Therefore, serum copper and ESR are good indicators of disease activity.

Radiographic studies might include a chest radiograph, lymphangiogram (radiographic examination of the lymphatic system), and inferior venacavogram (radiographic visualization of the large abdominal vessels).

Additional tests required include abdominal computed tomographic (CT) scan, liver function tests, bone marrow aspiration, skeletal survey, and liver and spleen scan. Definitive diagnosis is made by biopsy of the enlarged lymph node with documented evidence of the Reed-Sternberg cell. An abdominal laparoscopy or laparotomy might be performed to evaluate intra-abdominal lymph nodes and for purposes of staging. If needed, a liver biopsy and the bone marrow aspiration also are performed at that time. Splenectomy can be useful for staging because the spleen retains a large number of abnormal cells. Pneumococcal vaccine can be given to children who have had splenectomies because of the increased risk of the occurrence of pneumococcal infection in children without spleens.

Treatment Well-established treatment protocols have been developed for Hodgkin's disease. They are based on the clinical stage of disease. For early-stage disease [stages I, II, and IIIA (without systemic symptoms)], radiation therapy can be sufficient to cure the disease. If extensive disease is present (stages III and IV with systemic symptoms) chemotherapy or a combination of chemotherapy and radiation are given. The most commonly used chemotherapeutic protocol for Hodgkin's disease uses nitrogen mustard, vincristine (Oncovin), procarbazine, and prednisone (MOPP). Other drug protocols have been used for the child who has relapsed or not responded to MOPP therapy. The overall prognosis is quite good. The child with early-stage disease has the most favorable prognosis. This is a very treatable tumor. The overall 5-year survival rate can be up to 90%.

Nursing management Nursing care of the child with lymphoma is similar to that of any child with cancer and will be based on the specific treatment and course of disease for the specific child. When the spleen has been removed, the child is at long-term risk of infection. Infections are most frequently bacterial. The risk of infection seems to be particularly high in the younger child and less common in the adolescent. Some physicians might prescribe prophylactic penicillin. The nurse observes the child for signs of infection. Because the child is at home during much of the treatment period, the nurse teaches the parent how to recognize signs of infection and how to protect the child from acquiring one.

From the initial contact with the child and family, the nurse prepares them for impending multiple intrusive procedures. Emotional outlets that include therapeutic play allow the child to master the stress of unpleasant diagnostic and treatment measures. If a laparotomy or splenectomy is planned, nursing management includes preoperative preparation and general postoperative care.

Side effects of radiation and chemotherapy are related to the specific locations, drugs, and doses that the child receives (see Tables 33-6 and 33-7). Helping the child conserve rest and providing adequate nutrition are important nursing measures. Nitrogen mustard can cause severe vomiting with subsequent alterations in nutrition and fluid balance. The nurse administers any ordered antiemetics. Fluid encouragement and a high-calorie and protein diet after vomiting ceases can be given in small frequent meals.

The nurse assists the child to remain active during periods of hospitalization. School tutoring might be necessary so that the child does not get behind in school.

The parents and child are supported and allowed to express feelings of anger and frustration. Referral to community support groups might be necessary.

NonHodgkin's Lymphoma (Lymphosarcoma)

NonHodgkin's lymphoma represents a group of diseases involving malignant cells of lymphoid tissue. Unlike Hodgkin's disease, they are considered to have no single focal origin and therefore are rarely localized. There is no staging classification that is generally agreed on. NonHodgkin's disease represents 6% of childhood cancers. It also is more common in males than females. The disease occurs equally in all ages.

Clinical manifestations The presenting symptoms of nonHodgkin's lymphoma depend on the specific location of the disease. The most frequently seen signs include lymphadenopathy, abdominal involvement, and mediastinal mass. Symptoms associated with abdominal involvement are abdominal pain, vomiting, and diarrhea. Occasionally a palpable mass can be felt.

Abdominal nonHodgkin's lymphoma also is associated with gastrointestinal bleeding and intussusception. Immediate surgical intervention is required for intussusception. If a mediastinal mass is present, the child might complain of dyspnea and cough. Pleural effusions might be present at diagnosis. NonHodgkin's lymphoma that occurs in the mediastinum often infiltrates the bone marrow, transforming the disease into an acute lymphocytic leukemia.

Burkitt's lymphoma is a type of nonHodgkins lymphoma. It is a tumor that generally involves the jaw and can grow to enormous size around the maxilla or eye. Bone marrow involvement does occur. Burkitt's tumor was originally identified in children living in Africa, where it has a high incidence and has been related to the Epstein-Barr virus. The tumor is much less common in the United States.

Diagnostic evaluation Diagnostic studies for nonHodgkin's lymphoma are similar to those performed for Hodgkin's disease with several exceptions. Serum copper and ESR are not useful disease activity indicators; the staging laparotomy is generally not performed because it offers no therapeutic or prognostic value. A lumbar puncture, however, is performed to identify any central nervous system involvement.

Treatment Definitive therapy for nonHodgkin's lymphoma has not been developed. Generally, treatment includes radiation of masses and intensive chemotherapy. Chemotherapy protocols often are similar to those used in the treatment of high-risk leukemia. Remission should occur in 4–6 weeks after therapy has begun.

Prophylactic central nervous system treatment identical to acute lymphocytic leukemia protocols might be used for those at risk for central nervous system involvement. As with other cancers, the child with limited disease has a more favorable prognosis, however the prognosis is generally extremely poor. Once relapse occurs, treatment is only palliative.

Nursing management Because the child with nonHodgkin's lymphoma receives intensive chemotherapy, side effects are common. Drugs such as cytosine arabinoside might be infused over time, requiring periodic hospitalization. The nursing care for the child with nonHodgkin's lymphoma is similar to that for the child with Hodgkin's disease. It also might include care of the dying child (see Chapter 17).

Brain Tumors

Central nervous system tumors constitute the second most frequent childhood cancer, accounting for approximately 19% of all childhood malignancies. Brain tumors are by far the most common central nervous system tumor. Two-thirds of brain tumors are located below the roof of the cerebellum, usually in the cerebellum or brain stem. They also are referred to as *infratentorial,* meaning they are below the tentorium in the posterior third of the brain. The remaining third of brain tumors are located above the cerebellum in the anterior two-thirds of the brain. These tumors are referred to as *supratentorial* (above the tentorium) and generally occupy the cerebrum.

In contrast to those in children, most brain tumors in adults are supratentorial. The actual location of the tumor determines the type and extent of presenting signs and symptoms. It also determines how amenable the tumor is to surgery and therefore ultimately the prognosis. (See Fig. 33-3 for the location of brain tumors in children.)

Most childhood brain tumors arise from glial tissue and are termed *gliomas*. Glial tissue is the structural tissue of the brain. Less commonly, tumors might arise from other tissue such as nerve cells, cranial nerves, the pineal gland, blood vessels, or neuroepithelium. Brain tumors are classified by the tissue involved. The specific location also is noted.

Clinical manifestations It is difficult to determine early signs and symptoms of brain tumors. This is particularly true in the young child, whose skull sutures have not yet closed. Thus tumors might be very large before detection. Children are also less likely to report symptoms of visual change or headache, adding to the delay in making a diagnosis.

The most common initial symptoms often are caused by increased intracranial pressure and include headache and vomiting. Headache is most notable in the morning, gradually improving during the day but returning the next morning.

Vomiting often is not preceded by nausea. The child might be ready to eat immediately after vomiting. Vomiting also occurs more frequently in the morning and can become projectile. With increased cranial pressure, papilledema might be present.

Because most childhood brain tumors involve the cerebellum, coordination and balance are affected. Cerebellar signs include loss of balance, ataxia, wide-based gait, and head tilting. Widening sutures in the infant will be reflected in enlarging head circumference. Visual defects, altered reflexes, motor deficits due to cranial nerve involvement or paralysis, and altered consciousness and personality are additional signs and symptoms. Seizures are only associated with supratentorial tumors. Brain stem tumors might

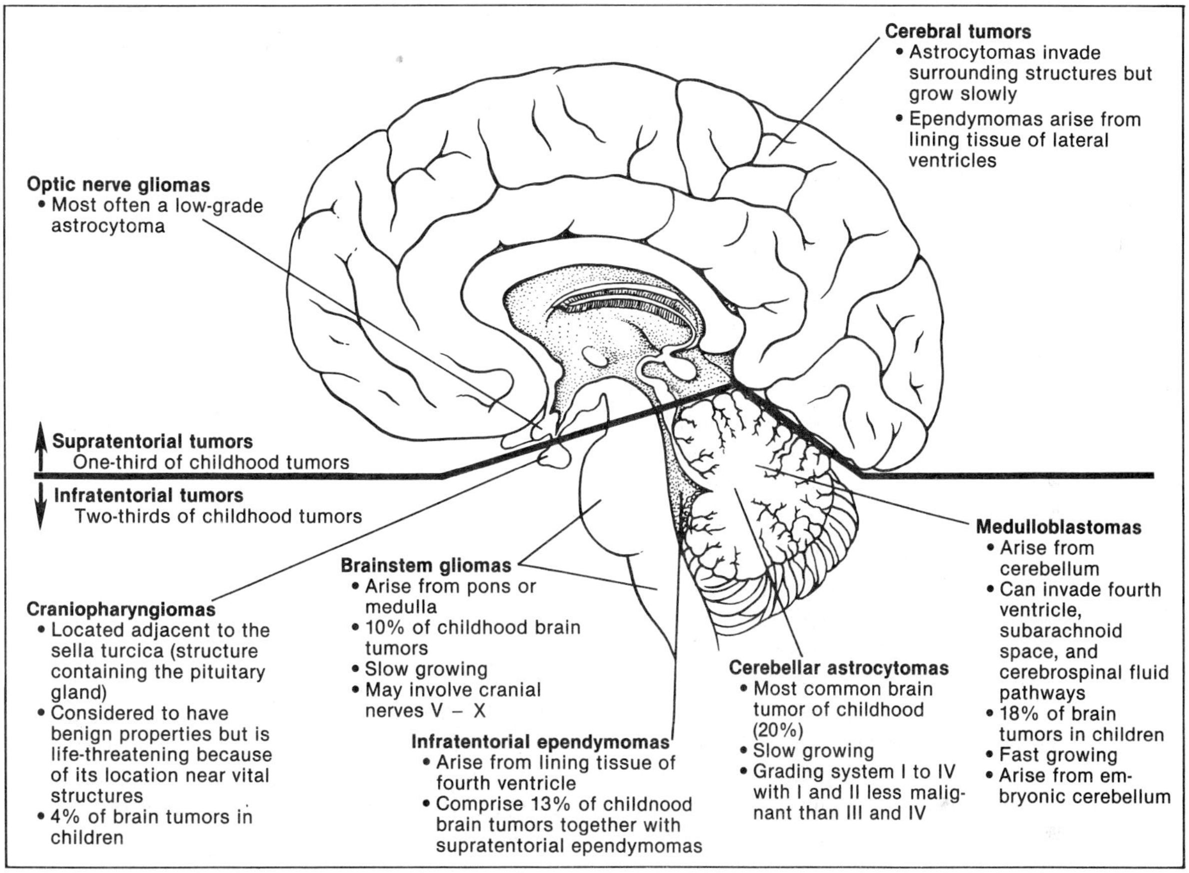

FIGURE 33-3

Types and locations of brain tumors in children.

cause disturbance of the vital sign regulatory mechanisms, resulting in decreased pulse and respirations, increased blood pressure, and difficulty in maintaining normal body temperature.

Diagnostic evaluation When signs and symptoms of a brain tumor are present, complete neurologic, developmental, and ophthalmic examinations are indicated. Radiologic studies can include skull radiograph, radioisotope brain scanning, and CT scan. With the development of the CT scan, invasive procedures such as pneumoencephalogram and cerebral angiography rarely are necessary.

Treatment The initial and most useful treatment is surgical resection. Astrocytomas and medulloblastomas might be entirely resectable. If complete resection is not possible, then partial resection is attempted. Because of their location, some brain stem tumors are not amenable to resection. Biopsy might even carry too much risk.

Postoperative radiation therapy is used with many of the brain tumors and serves as either a primary or palliative treatment. Medulloblastomas, brain stem gliomas, and ependymomas are most commonly treated by radiation therapy. Because medulloblastomas and ependymomas tend to spread to the spinal cord, radiation therapy might include the spine.

Chemotherapy has been used for recurrent brain tumors. Some cancer treatment centers also are studying the effectiveness of chemotherapy as a primary treatment. Drugs include vincristine, lomustine (CCNU), procarbazine, and intrathecal methotrexate. Both single-agent and multiple-drug protocols have been studied. Chemotherapy has not been as effective with brain tumors as with other childhood malignancies because many chemotherapy agents do not adequately cross the blood-brain barrier and tumor cell growth might not be sufficient to be affected by the drugs. Until further studies can establish a beneficial role for chemotherapy in childhood brain tumors, surgery and radiation will remain the primary forms of treatment.

The overall 5-year survival rate for the child with a brain

tumor is only about 20% (Gumbina, 1983). The most favorable prognosis is the child with a low-grade astrocytoma. The 5-year survival rate for these children is 65%.

Nursing management The child undergoing brain surgery requires extensive nursing care (see Chapter 31). On admission, the child and parent might be very apprehensive about the impending diagnostic studies and surgery. Both parents and child should be prepared for each procedure. The nurse assesses the child for developmental and behavioral alterations. Neurologic assessment including vital signs; pupil size, equality, and response to light; level of consciousness; and strength and equality of grip are closely monitored for any changes. Postural changes also are observed and recorded. Head circumference is measured and followed in the infant. Seizure precautions are followed for the child suspected of a supratentorial tumor (see Chapter 31). The quality and pattern of headache is recorded.

The nurse assists in preparing the child for surgery. Because any surgery involving the brain is extremely stressful, the child and parent need much emotional support. Focusing on what the child will experience, rather than the type of surgery, might be helpful. The child should be told if hair is to be cut or shaved. Hair might be cut either prior to surgery or after the child has been anesthetized. The child needs to know that the head will be bandaged when the child wakes up after the surgery. There also can be considerable facial edema.

Both parent and child are prepared for the postoperative appearance of the child. The family needs to know also that the child might experience postoperative headache after awakening. The child who will be transferred to the intensive-care unit needs to be oriented to the unit and equipment preoperatively.

Postoperative care is similar to that for a child undergoing any neurologic surgery (see the Standards of Nursing Care, p. 1080). Postoperative neurologic signs are checked at frequent intervals. Proper positioning and maintenance of a patent airway are important immediate postoperative considerations. Positioning avoids pressure on the operative site. The child can be positioned on either side and the head can be elevated without pillows to facilitate cerebrospinal fluid flow and facial edema drainage. If the child's head is kept in the midline position, venous drainage also will be facilitated. Eye care to prevent corneal ulceration and drying should be instituted. Methylcellulose eye drops are administered frequently. Drainage on the surgical dressing is closely monitored. Profuse drainage, frank bleeding, or clear fluid indicating leaking cerebrospinal fluid require immediate physician attention.

Cerebral edema and increased intracranial pressure are postoperative concerns. The nurse monitors fluid balance carefully. Osmotic diuretics and steroids are administered. Headache might be the result of cerebral edema. Occasionally, anticonvulsants also might be necessary. The nurse monitors the child for postoperative seizures, which can develop from infection or intracranial bleeding.

Once the child has regained consciousness, orientation and grip strength are assessed frequently and any residual surgical motor deficits are determined. When the child has improved and returned to the original admitting nursing unit, safety precautions are observed if ataxia, skeletal weakness, or paresthesia are present.

The nurse prepares the child and parent for any radiation or chemotherapy treatments. The frequency of treatments and the adverse side effects will be draining on the child and family. The nurse offers support and recommends sources for community support groups. Referral for financial or transportation assistance might be necessary. Principles of nursing care for the dying child (see Chapter 17) might be needed.

Retinoblastoma

Retinoblastoma is a rare malignant tumor of the eye. Most of these tumors are diagnosed before the child is 2 years of age. The tumor can result from genetic transmission of a defective gene or spontaneous cell mutation. Most tumors are thought to represent cell mutation rather than hereditary transmission. The disease might be unilateral or, in 29% of cases, bilateral. The child with bilateral disease is considered to have hereditary retinoblastoma.

The tumor might originate in the external retinal layers and extend into the subretinal space, causing retinal detachment, or in the internal nuclear retinal layers and extend to the vitreous cavity. Tumors of the internal retinal layers occupying the vitreous cavity are diagnosed more easily because they are readily visible on ophthalmic examination. The tumor can metastasize through blood vessels serving the tumor or extend to the vascular choroid, resulting in bone marrow, liver, lymph node, or bone involvement. Occasionally, the tumor can involve the optic nerve, gain access to the subarachnoid space, and thereby produce brain and spinal metastases.

Clinical manifestations The most noticeable sign of retinoblastoma is a cat's eye reflex, also called *leukokoria.* This reflex, which makes the child's pupil have a whitish glow, occurs when light is reflected off the tumor. Depending on the location of the tumor, the cat's eye reflex can be seen when the tumor is quite small or not until it is quite large. Strabismus or exophthalmos also are presenting signs. Occasionally, a variety of alterations in the iris can be seen at diagnosis.

Those families who have histories of retinoblastoma

should have their young children evaluated frequently. Diagnostic evaluation includes intraocular echography, CT scan, and ophthalmic examination. Diagnosis is made by a special ophthalmic examination under general anesthesia. Liver and bone scans, lumbar puncture, and bone marrow aspiration are used to determine the presence of metastases.

Staging of the tumor indicates the likelihood of retaining useful vision rather than indicating survival or prognosis. The staging system places the child in one of five groups, ranging from favorable vision preservation (group I) to unfavorable vision preservation (group V). The overall cure rate of retinoblastoma is 85%–90% (Foley, 1982).

Treatment Radiation is the treatment of choice if curative doses can be delivered while preserving vision. Therefore, unilateral tumors of groups I through III might be treated initially with radiation therapy. Because the child must be absolutely still during treatment to avoid damage to the eye lens, short-acting general anesthesia or heavy sedation and positioning the child's head in a half-cast might be necessary.

In more advanced disease, surgical enucleation of the affected eye is the primary treatment. When both eyes are involved, as in bilateral disease, the less affected eye is radiated, and the severely affected eye is enucleated. In bilateral disease, if both eyes are affected equally, treatment depends on the extent of disease. In early disease, both eyes will be radiated, and in advanced disease, enucleation must be considered as a life-saving procedure. If brain or spinal metastases are present, craniospinal radiation might be given. Potential complications of radiation include retinal detachment, vitreous hemorrhage, glaucoma, cataracts, and secondary malignancies.

Chemotherapy is used for recurrent disease or when the tumor has extended into the choroid. Drugs that might be administered include cyclophosphamide, vincristine, doxorubicin, and intrathecal methotrexate. Additional therapies for localized disease such as laser surgery and cryotherapy are being investigated.

Nursing management The enucleation of a child's eye is traumatic for parents. Introducing the parent to a family and child who has experienced the surgery and is doing well with an artificial eye eases fears that the procedure leaves a gross deformity. There is usually some postoperative swelling and bruising of the face. After enucleation no deep crater is left in the socket because a sphere is implanted during surgery so that the eye prosthesis can be applied easily. The child returns to the unit with a small bandage covering the eye.

The eye socket requires little care. The parent needs to view the site and learn appropriate care soon after the surgical procedure. Saline irrigation and application of antibiotic cream might be ordered postoperatively. An eye patch is placed over the socket for a number of days, primarily to keep the child from touching the site and contaminating the area.

The eye prosthesis is designed to match the color and size of the child's other eye. It may be fitted approximately 3 weeks after surgery. The artificial eye need not be removed except for periodic cleaning if a mucus film develops over the prosthesis (see Chapter 32 for care of a prosthesis).

Parents might desire genetic counseling if they are considering additional children. The disease cannot be detected by amniocentesis. Risk percentages are available. For unaffected parents there is a 1%–10% risk that additional children also might develop retinoblastoma. For children who survive retinoblastoma, risk for children they might have varies from 7%–15% for previous unilateral disease in the parent and 50% for previous bilateral disease in the parent (Wong and Dornan, 1982).

Neuroblastoma

Neuroblastoma is a tumor of tissue arising from the embryonal neural crest. Normally, in the developing fetus, embryonal neuroblast cells become mature ganglion tissue of the adrenal medulla and sympathetic ganglia. Why the tissue does not differentiate and instead becomes malignant is not known. In contrast to a few other childhood malignancies, this tumor is not associated with chromosomal abnormalities or any congenital defects.

Neuroblastoma is the second most frequent solid tumor of childhood, yet it only accounts for between 7% and 8% of all childhood malignancies. Because of its embryonal origin and rapid growth, the tumor is almost always diagnosed before the child is 4 years old. Half of the children with neuroblastoma are diagnosed by 2 years of age. The disease can be present at birth.

Clinical manifestations The child with neuroblastoma generally appears quite ill at diagnosis. Because the sympathetic ganglia run along each side of the spinal cord, the tumor can arise in a variety of locations, including the neck, mediastinum, abdomen, and pelvic areas. Tumor involvement of the cervical sympathetic ganglia will present as a mass in the neck. A mediastinal mass can cause airway obstruction, resulting in breathing difficulties.

If the ophthalmic sympathetic nerves are involved, the child's irises can be different colors. Dual eye color is known as *heterochromia*. Because of the proximity of the spinal column, the tumor can extend into the vertebrae and cause spinal compression and paralysis.

By far the most frequent site for neuroblastoma (65%) is the adrenal medulla. Unfortunately, this location has the

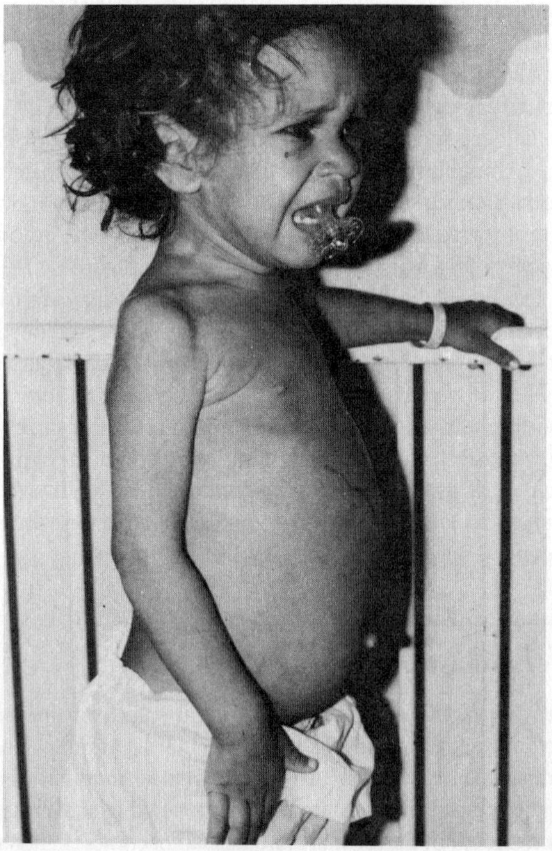

A young child with neuroblastoma. (From Purtilo DT: A Survey of Human Diseases. *Addison-Wesley, 1978, with permission.)*

least favorable diagnosis. The most common presenting sign is a palpable abdominal midline mass. Many times, however, abnormalities due to a metastatic site can be the first indication of neuroblastoma.

More than 60% of children with neuroblastoma have metastatic disease at diagnosis, possibly involving multiple organs. The liver is a common site of metastasis. Metastasis to the long bones and skull is a frequent occurrence. Bone pain or a pathologic fracture might be the presenting symptom. Bone marrow infiltration occurs in over 50% of children and is not necessarily associated with bone involvement. Bone marrow metastasis can result in anemia, bleeding, and infection. Neuroblastoma can also produce profuse diarrhea, which might be caused by tumor metabolites. Skin and soft tissue lesions containing neuroblastoma cells occur infrequently in the infant. General systemic signs and symptoms include weight loss, fatigue, and irritability.

Diagnostic evaluation Because neuroblastoma cells can synthesize and metabolize catecholamines, increased levels of metabolites of catecholamines are found in the urine. HVA and VMA are the metabolites most frequently monitored in the urine; HVA and VMA levels are useful both as diagnostic and clinical course indicators. For urinary catecholamine results to be accurate, the child needs to be on a VMA-restricted diet, which includes foods such as bananas, chocolate, citrus fruits, and vanilla flavoring, for 3 days prior to the specimen collection (see Chapter 29).

Diagnostic studies are used to evaluate the tumor site and extent of metastatic disease. Initial studies will include complete blood count, serum chemistries, 24-hour urine for catecholamine metabolites, chest radiographs, skeletal survey, intravenous pyelogram (IVP), liver and bone scan, and bone marrow aspiration. Definitive diagnosis is made by pathologic confirmation of neuroblastoma by tissue biopsy.

Staging of neuroblastoma is based on a I-to-IV scale. There is also a special IV-S classification for tumors that would otherwise be classified as stage I or II (limited disease) but have additional involvement of liver, skin, or bone marrow without direct bone metastases. Interesting is that stage IV-S disease has an excellent prognosis in spite of significant advanced disease. This is attributed to the frequency of spontaneous regression for the child with this particular stage. Overall, the survival rate for neuroblastoma is poor, but infants below 1 year of age, regardless of the disease stage, have a good prognosis.

Treatment Surgery is the initial treatment to obtain a biopsy and remove as much of the tumor as possible. Stage I and II disease are often completely resectable. During surgery, metallic clips might be placed around the margins of the tumor site to aid in the delineation of radiation therapy ports and to follow treatment response by radiograph. The child with stage IV disease at diagnosis might not be treated surgically since it has not been determined if debulking the primary tumor will extend survival time.

Radiation therapy often is administered after surgery when residual disease remains. Neuroblastoma is considered to be a radiosensitive tumor. Radiation also can be used initially to shrink large tumors near vital structures so that an inoperable tumor becomes amenable to surgery. Additionally, radiation therapy is the primary treatment for spinal cord compression or respiratory distress due to large mediastinal masses.

Chemotherapy is used in the treatment of advanced stage IV disease. Drugs that have shown some effectiveness include cyclophosphamide, vincristine, DTIC, VM-26, cisplatin, and doxorubicin. The use of chemotherapy in stages I through III and stage IV-S is controversial and might not contribute to survival.

Because spontaneous remission is likely, infants with stage IV-S disease might receive no disease treatment and simply be followed and provided symptomatic support.

After an initial waiting period, very small doses of radiation or a short course of small-dose chemotherapy might be given if the disease does not regress in the infant with stage IV-S disease.

Nursing management It is often difficult for the nurse and parent to care for the very ill young child with neuroblastoma, particularly if a poor prognosis is anticipated. The parent is encouraged to participate in the day-to-day care and remain close to the child. The nurse facilitates parent-child contact, including holding and rocking the child. The parent might be particularly uneasy if the infant has stage IV-S disease, especially if the child looks quite ill and yet no therapy is prescribed. The parent needs reassurance about the favorable outcome for the child.

The nurse also is challenged to carry out 24-hour urine collections on the young child. This often necessitates a bit of creativity to collect the entire urine specimen successfully, particularly with the child who is not toilet-trained. Parents also should be taught to collect 24-hour urine samples since once the child is discharged, the parent will be responsible for obtaining these specimens.

Wilms' Tumor

Wilms' tumor, or nephroblastoma according to its historic name, is an embryonal tumor of the kidney. Because it is embryonal, most children are between 1 and 5 years of age at diagnosis. The peak incidence is between 3 and 4 years of age. Approximately 15% of children with Wilms' tumor also have congenital abnormalities such as aniridia (absence of the iris), hemihypertrophy (overgrowth of half of the body), and genitourinary anomalies. The tumor originates from immature renoblast cells located in the kidney parenchyma and extends into the renal cavity and often distorts the renal calices.

Clinical manifestations The most frequent sign of Wilms' tumor is an increase in abdominal girth or a palpable abdominal mass. Unlike the abdominal mass found in neuroblastoma, the mass in Wilms' tumor is on one side of the abdomen only, unless both kidneys are affected. The tumor might be discovered in the course of a routine physical examination, or the parent might note the abdominal enlargement. Often the child appears otherwise healthy and active. The mass usually is smooth, firm, and painless. It is important not to palpate the abdomen if Wilms' tumor is suspected since palpation or manipulation can seed tumor cells throughout the abdomen through rupture of the renal capsule. If pain is evident, it is due to the rapid growth of the tumor.

Diagnostic evaluation Essential diagnostic evaluation includes IVP and inferior cavogram. Additional studies such as angiography and ultrasonography can be useful. Metastasis most commonly occurs to the lung and secondarily to the liver. Therefore, diagnostic radiographs or scans of the lung and liver are appropriate initial studies. Uncommon but possible sites of metastases include the brain, bone, and bone marrow. Tissue biopsy provides the histologic diagnosis.

The most common staging system is based on the recommendation of National Wilms' Tumor Study, classifying the tumor on a group I through group V scale. Groups I and II represent completely resectable disease; Group III represents partial resection but no evidence of metastatic spread; Group IV represents metastatic spread; and Group V represents bilateral kidney disease. Wilms' tumor is one of the most curable solid tumors of childhood. With the latest treatment, the overall survival approaches 90% for localized disease and 50% for advanced disease (Belasco et al., 1984). The specific histology, extent of the disease, and age of the child at diagnosis influence the prognosis for any specific child.

Treatment Initial therapy is begun by laparotomy, definitive biopsy, and total nephrectomy with excision of all tumor. Care is taken not to rupture the tumor or seed the abdominal cavity with tumor cells. If the tumor has spread to regional lymph nodes or involvement of the vena cava is found, a less favorable prognosis is suspected. Metallic clips are placed around any residual tumor that is unresectable so radiation therapy guidelines are evident. The liver is grossly examined for evidence of spread, and lesions are excised if possible. If bilateral kidney involvement is present, the most severely affected kidney will be removed with possible heminephrectomy of the remaining kidney.

Radiation therapy is of value in the treatment of Wilms' tumor since the tumor is considered radiosensitive. Treatments might begin a few days after surgery, particularly to destroy any cells that might have seeded the abdominal cavity during surgery. Radiation therapy generally is not necessary in the young child with stage I disease. The radiation field size and appropriate dose are determined by the stage at diagnosis. Radiation therapy also is beneficial to the lungs if pulmonary metastases are evident.

Chemotherapy is useful postsurgically. Successful drug combinations include vincristine and daunorubicin. Doxorubicin has also been used.

Nursing management Initial nursing goals focus on orienting the child and family to the nursing unit and preparing them for the necessary radiologic studies and surgery. Because diagnosis, surgery, and radiation therapy can occur in rapid succession, the family has little time to adjust to the diagnosis. This can be particularly stressful since the child appears well at diagnosis and may have been quite active before hospitalization.

Preoperatively, the nurse handles the child's abdomen carefully. All medical personnel should refrain from undue abdominal examination, and a sign is placed on the child's bed indicating this.

Postoperative care follows normal guidelines after general abdominal surgery. Fluid intake and output, electrolytes, and vital signs, particularly blood pressure, are monitored. Nasogastric suction is used to preserve gastric decompression. The dressing is checked for drainage, and abdominal girth should be monitored for evidence of distension or internal hemorrhage. The parent is prepared for post-discharge radiation or chemotherapy if necessary.

Rhabdomyosarcoma

Rhabdomyosarcoma is a malignant tumor of striated muscle (*rhabdo* = "striated" and *myo* = "muscle"). It accounts for most soft-tissue tumors in childhood. The peak incidence of rhabdomyosarcoma is 2–6 years of age with a second incidence peak during the adolescent years of 15–19.

Because it originates in striated muscle, there are a number of primary sites for tumor growth. These sites differ according to histologic classification and might include bladder, vagina, uterus, nasopharynx, trunk, and extremities. The most common sites for rhabdomyosarcoma are the head, orbit, and neck, and these account for approximately 40% of tumors. Genitourinary and abdominal sites account for 35%, and trunk or extremity tumors account for 25%.

Clinical manifestations The most common presenting sign is a painless mass or functional impairment of the site. Tumors that involve the orbit present with proptosis (downward displacement of the eyeball). Nasopharyngeal tumors are manifested by nasal discharge, serous otitis media, and nasal-sounding speech. The tumor might actually protrude from the nostrils.

Urinary tract obstruction or palpable mass occur with urinary rhabdomyosarcoma. Vaginal tumors contain grape-like tissues extending out of the vaginal canal. A paratesticular tumor is manifested by a firm, painless mass that is often translucent. Rhabdomyosarcoma of the extremity most frequently involves the lower extremities and presents as a painless mass.

Diagnostic evaluation Diagnostic studies are determined by the site of the tumor and potential metastatic sites. Head and neck tumors require ear, nose, and throat (ENT) evaluation; skull radiographs or tomograms; arteriography; and CT scan. Genitourinary and abdominal tumors require cystoscopy, IVP, upper- and lower-GI series, and abdominal CT scan. The evaluation of extremity tumors includes bone radiograph and other radiographic scans.

Rhabdomyosarcoma is a highly malignant disease that demonstrates both blood and lymph node spread. Metastatic sites include lungs, bone marrow, bone, liver, brain, and lymph nodes. Up to 40% of affected children have metastatic disease at diagnosis. Staging of the disease is based on a standard I-to-IV grading system. Prognosis is based on the primary site, histologic type, stage of the disease at diagnosis, and age of the child. The child with the most favorable diagnosis is between 1 and 7 years of age with sarcoma of the orbit in its earliest stages. The overall survival rate for stage I or II disease is approximately 70%. Two-year survival rates for more advanced stages are poor (about 25%) (Altman and Schwartz, 1983).

Treatment Rhabdomyosarcoma is treated aggressively with combination surgery, radiation, and chemotherapy. Surgery can be curative for localized disease that is amenable to surgical excision. Because radiation therapy and chemotherapy can be effective in controlling disease, mutilating surgeries to the head and neck or pelvic area are not necessary. Amputation for extremity disease might be contraindicated also. Sometimes surgical resection is postponed until radiation therapy and chemotherapy are initially used to shrink or control disease.

Radiation therapy is administered to the tumor site in doses of 5000–6000 rad over a 6-week period. Chemotherapy can be begun concurrently with radiation. The drugs most commonly used are vincristine, cyclophosphamide, and daunorubicin with the occasional addition of doxorubicin.

Nursing management The care of a child or adolescent with rhabdomyosarcoma requires the utmost nursing skill. Because several treatment modes can be used at one time, side effects are potentiated. This is particularly true in the management of head and neck cancers when combined radiation and chemotherapy in addition to the presence of tumor can obstruct a patent airway. The child is also likely to be quite anxious when these combined effects make breathing difficult and affect appearance. The nurse continually monitors the child's progress and symptoms. Supportive nursing care and comfort measures provide the basis of the care plan.

Osteosarcoma

Primary bone tumors account for about 4.5% of childhood cancer. The peak incidence rate occurs during adolescence. The two most common bone tumors are osteosarcoma and Ewing's sarcoma.

Osteosarcoma, which arises from bone-producing mesenchymal cells, is histologically classified by the appearance of large spindle cells in biopsied tissue. The disease occurs most commonly in the end of long bones with almost 50% located near the knee. The two most frequent sites are the distal ends of the femur and the proximal end of the tibia. The tumor is more common in boys than girls and can be related to the adolescent growth spurt.

Some adolescents have reported a recent injury or trauma to the area prior to the tumor appearance, but trauma does not appear to be significantly related to tumor development. Approximately 4% of osteosarcomas can be directly related to previous radiation of the tumor site. The tumor is uncommon before the age of 10 and is most frequently diagnosed between the ages of 10 and 25.

Clinical manifestations The most common presenting symptom is pain and possible swelling of the affected area. Delay in diagnosis is a frequent problem since symptoms often are attributed to athletic activity or injury. Other symptoms can include functional limitation, erythema, and warmth in the affected area.

Diagnostic evaluation Diagnostic evaluation by radiograph can confirm the suspicion of a malignant tumor. Osteosarcoma normally grows from the center of the bone, damaging the cortex and extending into the soft tissue. The lung is the most frequent site of disease spread. Bones might also be secondary sites. Investigation of metastatic sites includes chest radiograph or lung tomograms, bone scan, and skeletal survey. Tissue biopsy confirms the presence of osteosarcoma. Historically the overall survival rate for this tumor has been poor (approximately 20%). With recent therapy advances and better management techniques for lung metastases, the long-term survival rate is about 50% (Gaddy-Cohen, 1982).

Treatment The initial treatment is amputation of the limb above the site of the tumor. Because most lesions appear in the leg, above-the-knee amputation is required for tumors of the tibia. Hip disarticulation is required for tumors of the femur. Some surgeons might avoid total hip disarticulation and instead perform cross-bone amputation around the upper thigh so that the limb prosthesis is easier to fit.

In the adolescent who has passed the growth spurt and nearly attained adult height, limb-sparing bone replacement technique might be indicated rather than amputation. The tumor and often the adjacent joint is removed, followed by artificial implant or bone graft.

For disease in the distal femur, the total femur and knee joint are removed and replaced with a femur implant and total-knee prosthesis. This technique is used at only a few cancer treatment centers and is probably appropriate only for a limited number of children who have attained adult height and have small osteosarcoma lesions around the knee. Although limb-sparing techniques show promise, up to a third of adolescents eventually require traditional amputation. Complications of limb-sparing procedures, such as breakage of the prosthesis, infection, or recurrent disease, necessitate amputation.

Osteosarcoma is a radioresistant tumor. Very high doses of radiation (600–1200 rad) might not sufficiently control tumor growth and instead cause considerable damage to normal tissue and functional loss. For this reason, radiation therapy is used primarily for nonresectable tumors of the rib, skull, or pelvis.

Micrometastasis of osteosarcoma frequently causes metastasis, generally to the lung, within a year after amputation. Because of the likelihood of micrometastasis, chemotherapy has become an important component of treatment. The agents used for micrometastasis or known residual disease include doxorubicin, cisplatin, and high-dose methotrexate followed by leucovorin rescue. Cyclophosphamide, vincristine, bleomycin, doxorubicin, and daunorubicin also have been used in combination.

Prophylactic lung radiation with or without additional chemotherapy also has been attempted because of the likelihood of lung metastases. Whether this substantially contributes to disease-free survival is unclear. For known lung metastases, resection of specific lesions by thoracotomy might contribute to longer survival.

Nursing management The rigorous treatment of osteosarcoma requires skillful psychologic and physiologic nursing intervention. Limb amputation is traumatic and can be particularly damaging to the emerging self-identity of the adolescent. The child is carefully prepared for the impending amputation with full disclosure of the necessary procedure. Immediate reaction to the news of amputation can range from denial to overt refusal and hostility. The parent and child require time and sensitive support to deal with their feelings.

A normal grief reaction generally occurs after surgery as the adolescent adjusts to the loss of the limb. Preoperative or postoperative introduction to another child who has successfully adapted to amputation and has mastered the use of a prosthesis can be very helpful to the child and parent.

Postoperative care of the stump or surgical site depends on the location and extent of surgery. The child might be bothered by phantom limb pain. The nurse monitors the stump for evidence of bleeding or drainage. A Hemovac suction might be used to drain the stump postoperatively for a few days.

The child is mobilized with physical therapy and rehabilitation as soon as possible after surgery. Crutch walking is taught within the first few postoperative days. The nurse encourages proper crutch-walking techniques. The prosthesis can be fitted within 4–6 weeks after surgery. The child requires instruction on the proper care of the stump and application and maintenance of the prosthesis. Nursing goals focus on successful rehabilitation and ambulation with the prosthetic device.

Aggressive chemotherapy requires judicious skill and monitoring of drug infusions. Treatment with high-dose methotrexate necessitates precise infusion of the drug with accurate follow-up administration of the leucovorin rescue so that life-threatening toxicities do not develop.

Encouraging the child to participate in as many activities as possible helps maintain self-esteem. Adjustment to the alteration in body image is difficult but can be made easier by encouraging independence and self-care.

Ewing's Sarcoma

In contrast to osteosarcoma, Ewing's sarcoma occurs in the midshaft of long bones and in flat bones such as the pelvis, scapulae, and ribs. Histologically, this tumor has small, round cells rather than the characteristic large spindle cells of osteosarcoma. The peak incidence is in the second decade of life, and it is rare after age 30.

Clinical manifestations Symptoms of Ewing's sarcoma are similar to osteosarcoma, with pain and swelling over the affected site. Metastasis usually is not evident at diagnosis but occurs later in the disease, with spread to other bones and the lung. Diagnostic workup includes plain radiograph of the bone, bone scan or skeletal survey, and chest radiograph or lung tomograms. Definitive diagnosis is confirmed by tissue biopsy.

The best prognosis is associated with localized disease at diagnosis without subsequent relapse. The 3-year disease-free survival rate for children who present without metastatic disease is 50% (Nesbit et al., 1981). Those with metastatic disease at diagnosis or who develop metastatic disease have a poor prognosis.

Treatment Initial surgery generally is not performed except to obtain a tissue biopsy. Surgical resection or amputation has not significantly contributed to long-term survival, but surgical resection after other primary treatment might be indicated. High-dose radiation therapy and chemotherapy offer the best chance of disease control. Adjuvant chemotherapy has been effective with the use of cyclophosphamide, doxorubicin, and daunorubicin in combination. Other chemotherapy protocols have used carmustine (BCNU), mithramycin, and 5-fluorouracil.

Nursing management The nursing management of the child with Ewing's sarcoma follows the basic guidelines of assisting child and family to adjust to the disease and treatment program. Because the disease rarely necessitates amputation or disfiguring surgery, function and self-image are not altered by a traumatic surgery.

Essential Concepts

- Despite the rarity of childhood cancer, it is the leading cause of death from disease in children between 1 and 14 years of age. Half of all children with cancer are cured, and the remainder experience significant long-term survival.
- Cancer is a cluster of many diseases that share the same pathologic feature of uncontrolled cell growth.
- Compared to benign tumors, malignant tumors have a faster rate of growth, can invade nearby tissue, and can metastasize to other parts of the body.
- Leukemia and cancers of the central nervous system, particularly the brain, account for the largest proportion of childhood cancers.
- Genetic, immunologic, viral, and environmental factors are all being studied for their relationship to the causes of cancer.
- With the steady improvement in the treatment of childhood cancer over the past 10–20 years, the focus of therapy is on the quality of life.
- The presenting symptoms of a child with a neoplasm will vary, depending on the location and size of the tumor.
- A thorough physical examination of a child suspected of having a malignancy includes a general health assessment, a detailed examination of the area of concern, and careful palpation of the suspected tumor location.
- The diagnostic tests for childhood cancer, especially lumbar puncture and biopsy, can be particularly stressful for the child and require a specific nursing plan for preparation.

- The three approaches to the medical treatment plan are curative therapy, adjuvant therapy, and palliative therapy.
- The medical treatment of the child with cancer is directed toward communicating the diagnosis to the child and family and initiating the treatment plan. The appropriate therapeutic regimen then depends on determining the stage of the disease.
- The major focus of nursing care is to assist the child and family to adapt to the life-threatening nature of cancer while facilitating normal development.
- Nursing management is directed toward minimizing complications of surgical procedures and alleviating the physical and emotional stresses of chemotherapy and radiation.
- The side effects of chemotherapy are due to the damage of normal cells and will vary, depending on the dose, combination of drugs used, and the amount of time after drug administration.
- Acute, intermediate, and cumulative side effects of chemotherapy require a daily assessment for new and ongoing problems, leading to creative interventions, strategies, and frequently updated nursing care plans.
- Nursing management during radiation therapy focuses on preparation for the treatment, comfort measures, and control of side effects affecting the mouth, gastrointestinal tract, skin, and blood.
- Bone marrow suppression, a general side effect of chemotherapy and radiation, predisposes the child to anemia, infection, and bleeding and bruising and requires both preventive and supportive nursing measures.
- In providing narcotic management of the child's pain, the choice of drug, dose, and schedule must be tailored to the individual needs of the child. The effectiveness of pain medication also must be thoroughly documented.
- Nonnarcotic pain management strategies, such as distraction, relaxation techniques, and hypnosis, can be effective nursing measures.
- Cancer cachexia and taste alterations that result in aversions to some meats affect the child's nutritional status and necessitate a thorough and ongoing nutritional assessment.
- The nurse helps the family meet its own emotional needs by promoting communication, referring the family to other resources, and encouraging interaction between other family members, especially siblings, and the ill child.
- During remission the nursing staff provides a systematic educational program for the parents and children concerning the illness and helps them deal with information concerning alternatives to conventional therapy.
- For the child cured of cancer, the nurse can provide assistance in dealing with the physiologic concerns of possible sterility, atrophy or uneven physical growth, learning disabilities, and new cancer formation. The nurse also deals with the psychosocial concerns of body image, sexuality, and social adjustment.
- The most common childhood neoplasms, which require comprehensive medical and nursing management, are acute leukemias, lymphomas, brain tumors, retinoblastoma, neuroblastoma, Wilms' tumor, rhabdomyosarcoma, osteosarcoma, and Ewing's sarcoma.

References

Altman A, Schwartz A: *Malignant Diseases of Infancy, Childhood and Adolescence*. Saunders, 1983.

Askin F et al: Occult testicular leukemia: Testicular biopsy at three years of continuous remission of childhood leukemia. *Cancer* 1981; 47:470.

Barbora J, Gitelson J: Cancer pain: Pyschological management using hypnosis. *Cancer J Clin* 1980, 30:130.

Belasco J et al: Wilms' tumor. In: *Clinical Pediatric Oncology*. Sutow W et al. (editors). Mosby, 1984.

Dash J: Hypnosis for symptom amelioration. In: *Psychological Aspects of Childhood Cancer*. Kellerman J (editor). Thomas, 1980.

Foley G: Retinoblastoma. In: *Nursing Care of the Child with Cancer*. Fochtman D, Foley G (editors). Little, Brown, 1982.

Gaddy-Cohen D: Nursing care in childhood cancer update. *Am J Nurs* 1982, 82:416.

Gumbina M: Tumors of the central and peripheral nervous system. In: *Malignant Diseases of Infancy, Childhood and Adolescence*. Altman A, Schwartz A (editors). Saunders, 1983.

Hoffmann AD (editor): *Adolescent Medicine*. Addison–Wesley, 1983.

Klopovich P, Cohen D: An overview of pediatric oncology for the adult oncology nurse. *Oncol Nurs Forum* 1984; 11:56.

Nesbit M et al: Multimodal therapy for the management of primary nonmetastatic Ewing's sarcoma of bone: An intergroup study. *Nat Cancer Inst Monogr* 1981; 56:279.

Oncology Nursing Society: *Cancer Chemotherapy Guidelines and Recommendations for Nursing Education and Practice,* 1984.

Simone J, Rivers G: Management of acute leukemia. In: *Clinical Pediatric Oncology.* 3rd ed. Sutow W, Feinbach D, Vietti T (editors). Mosby, 1984.

Stolar M, Power L, Viele C: Recommendations for handling cytotoxic drugs in hospitals. *Am J Hosp Pharm* (July) 1983; 40: 1163–1171.

Vital Statistics of the United States, 1980, Mortality volume. U.S. Department of Health and Human Services, 1984.

Wong D, Dornan L: Nursing care in childhood cancer—retinoblastoma. *Am J Nurs* (March) 1982; 82:425–431.

Additional Readings

Adams DW, Deveau EJ: *Coping with Childhood Cancer: Where Do We Go from Here?* Reston, 1984.

Altman A, Schwartz A: The soft tissue sarcomas. In: *Malignant Diseases of Infancy, Childhood and Adolescence.* Altman A, Schwartz A (editors). Saunders, 1983.

American Cancer Society: *Cancer Facts and Figures 1984.* American Cancer Society, 1984.

Chekryn J, Deegan M, Reid J: Impact on teachers when a child with cancer returns to school. *Child Health Care* (Winter) 1987; 15(3): 161–165.

Cleaveland MJ: Nursing care in childhood cancer: Brain tumors. *Am J Nurs* 1982; 82:422.

Feinbach D: Natural history of acute leukemia. In: *Clinical Pediatric Oncology.* Sutow W, Feinbach D, and Vietti T (editors). Mosby, 1984.

Fochtman D: *Nursing Care of the Child with Cancer.* Little, Brown, 1983.

Fochtman D, Foley G: *Nursing Care of the Child with Cancer.* Little, Brown, 1982.

Hayes V, Knox JE: Hospital-related stress in parents of children with cancer. *Can Nurs* (Nov), 1983:225–228.

Lipman A, Mooney K: Management of pain. In: *Clinical Pharmacology and Therapeutics in Nursing.* 2nd ed. Weiner M, Pepper G (editors). McGraw-Hill, 1984.

Martinson IM et al: Home care for children dying of cancer. *Research in Nurs and Health* 1986; 9(1): 11–16.

Mulvihill J: Ecogenetic origins of cancer in the young: Environmental and genetic determinants. In: *Cancer in the Young.* Levine A (editor). Masson USA, 1982.

National Study Commission on Cytotoxic Exposure: *Recommendations for Handling Cytotoxic Agents.* August, 1983.

Niehaus CS et al: Oral complications in children cancer therapy. *Cancer Nurs* (Feb) 1987; 10(1): 15–20.

Nurs Clin North Am: The Leukemias: Definition, treatment, and nursing care. *Nurs Clin North Am* (Sept) 1983; 18(3): 523–541.

O'Malley J et al: Psychiatric sequelae of surviving childhood cancer. *Am J Orthopsychiatry* 1979; 49:608.

Schorlemer V: Reflections: A mother's and son's struggle with acute lymphocytic leukemia. *Child Health Care* (Spring) 1984; 12(4): 163–168.

Spinetta J: Behavioral and psychological research in childhood cancer: An overview. *Cancer,* 1982; 50:1921.

Spinetta J, Deasy-Spinetta P: *Living with Childhood Cancer.* Mosby, 1981.

Strong L: Genetics, etiology, and epidemiology of childhood cancer. In: *Clinical Pediatric Oncology.* 3rd ed. Sutow W, Feinbach D, Vietti T (editors). Mosby, 1984.

Sullivan M, Fuller L, Butler J: Hodgkin's disease. In: *Clinical Pediatric Oncology.* 3rd ed. Sutow et al. (editors). Mosby, 1984.

U.S. Department of Health and Human Services. Public Health Service. National Institutes of Health: *Recommendations for the Safe Handling of Parenteral Antineoplastic Drugs.* Publication no. 83-2621, 1983.

Waters J: Coping with a leg amputation. *Am J Nurs,* 1981; 81:1349.

Waaru W et al: *Clinical Pediatric Oncology.* 3rd ed. Sutow et al. (editors). Mosby, 1984.

Weinstein H et al: Chemotherapy for acute myelogenous leukemia in children and adults. VAPA update. *Blood* 1983; 62:315.

Chapter 34

Ongoing Care of the High-Risk Infant

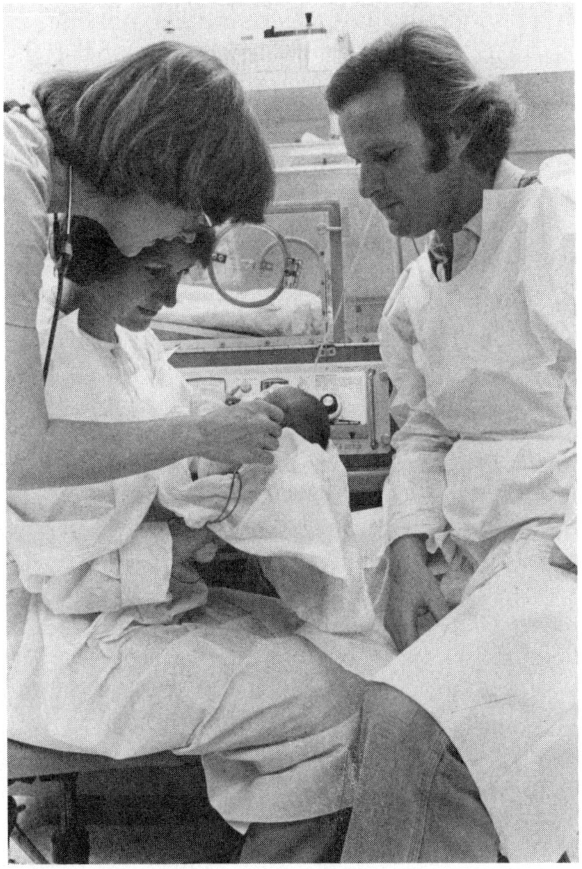

Chapter Contents

(Continues)

Specific Problems of High-Risk Infants

Respiratory Disorders
Necrotizing Enterocolitis (NEC)
Sudden Infant Death Syndrome

Cross Reference Box

To find these topics, see the following chapters:

Child abuse	Chapter 13
Congestive heart failure	Chapter 23
Failure to thrive	Chapter 13
Hyperbilirubinemia	Chapter 26
Neonatal assessment	Chapter 4
Patent ductus arteriosus	Chapter 23

Objectives

- Describe the impact of high-risk infants and neonatal intensive care on the infants' families.
- List risk factors associated with the birth of a high-risk infant.
- Define the terms used to classify high-risk infants.
- Compare the growth and development of premature infants to the growth and development of normal full-term infants.
- List the special problems of high-risk infants.
- Describe the assessment criteria, nursing goals, and nursing management associated with heat regulation and metabolic imbalances.
- Explain the implications of the immaturity of the immunologic, respiratory, gastrointestinal, circulatory, and neurologic systems for the premature infant's physiologic state.
- Describe the assessment criteria, nursing goals, and nursing management associated with specific disorders of the high-risk infant.
- Describe the causes, assessment criteria, nursing goals, and nursing management associated with developmental delays.
- List the causes of alterations in parenting for high-risk infants.
- Describe the assessment criteria, nursing goals, and nursing management associated with both parenting problems and neonatal death.

Although infant mortality has decreased significantly in the past 100 years, early infancy remains a high-risk period. More than one-fifth of all infants require medical treatment after birth, often in neonatal intensive care units (NICU). The decrease in infant mortality has been related directly to the improvement in care for the high-risk infant. The smallest and the youngest infants are surviving in large numbers, with little increase in morbidity (illness).

A high-risk infant is any infant who is at risk for medical, developmental, or psychologic problems persisting into later years. Identification and treatment of these infants can prevent many of these problems. The needs of high-risk infants and their families do not end with hospital discharge. Thus, nurses will come into contact with high-risk infants in many different settings.

Regionalization of care for high-risk infants has helped improve prognoses. Because the equipment required for neonatal intensive care is expensive and NICU personnel—neonatologists, nurses, laboratory technicians, and respiratory therapists—require special training, it is not economically feasible for all hospitals to provide this care. Most intensive care facilities are located in large urban, teaching hospitals that take referrals from the smaller hospitals in a large geographic region. Although this system has its advantages, the major problem is the difficulty parents have in traveling long distances to visit. Some parents are unable to visit at all, a problem that can jeopardize parent-child interactions.

Because society views pregnancy as a happy event that results in a healthy infant, parents are unprepared to deal with an infant who requires medical care. Nurses working with high-risk infants provide not only skilled care to assist infants in their adaptation to extrauterine life but also support and information for the parents.

Impact of High-Risk Infants on Families

Although family structures vary greatly, a family environment of some kind is probably best suited to meet the physical and psychologic needs of infants. High-risk infants spend the first weeks of life in an environment very different from a normal home. The NICU emphasizes medical needs over all others. Most of the infant's interactions are receptive, that is, interaction comes from the professional to the infant. Behavioral cues from the infant, such as crying, visual attention, or smiling, which would normally be recognized by a parent, go unrecognized in the NICU. The infant receives little affectionate handling. Instead, infants are exposed to bright fluorescent lights, loud noises, and stressful procedures.

Even when they are well, high-risk infants do not return to normal home environments. Family members have had to adjust to the stressors involved with the infant's care. Normally, infants establish social relationships with a primary caregiver, but the infant's social development also relies on interactions with other family members—the other parent and siblings—and close friends and relatives. When an infant is admitted to an NICU, these normal relationships are not allowed to develop properly. This can have an adverse effect on family functioning.

Parents

The parents of a high-risk infant usually do not have enough time with the high-risk infant to begin or continue the normal process of attachment (see Chapter 4). Parental visits might be infrequent, so the hospitalized neonate has little opportunity to learn one-to-one interaction. For the parents, the birth of a high-risk infant represents a crisis. Kaplan and Mason (1960) described four tasks that parents of premature infants must accomplish to establish relationships with their infants: (a) preparing for the possible death of the infant, (b) overcoming the guilt caused by the failure to deliver a normal infant, (c) resuming the process of relating to the infant, and (d) developing an understanding of the infant's special needs. These tasks are relevant to parents of any high-risk infant. Parents need to overcome their isolation from their infants and their feelings that these infants belong to the unit personnel (Klaus and Kennell, 1982).

In addition to inadequate opportunities for attachment, parents undergo additional stress with a high-risk infant. The energy required to deal with the family disruption can cause emotional problems. The costs of neonatal intensive care can average as high as $50,000, which places severe financial stress on parents.

Siblings

Siblings can be affected by the birth of a high-risk infant. They are seldom allowed to see the infant prior to discharge because nursery personnel are concerned about infection and about upsetting the siblings. Yet, children's fantasies are usually far worse than the realities of an NICU. If their fears and fantasies are not addressed, siblings might develop behavior problems to attract parental attention.

Young siblings have special fears. The "magical thinking" characteristic of early childhood might cause a child to believe that a new baby's illness is due to the child's desire to eliminate the baby. These children might believe that the parent's emotional upset is due to their own misbehavior.

Characteristics of High-Risk Infants

Risk Factors

Although most of the infants admitted to NICUs are born prematurely, a large number of infants at risk are full-term births. The high-risk infant usually is the result of a high-risk pregnancy. Factors such as maternal chronic disease, blood group incompatibilities, exposure to toxic agents or infection, trauma, multiple births and number of previous pregnancies, age of parents, and socioeconomic factors can increase the risk of infant problems.

Complications during delivery can create problems for the infant. These complications include prolonged or difficult labor or delivery, trauma or asphyxia to the infant during delivery, medication or anesthesia administration, and complications leading to cesarean section. Infants born with certain congenital anomalies are also at risk.

Nurses need to consider psychosocial risk factors because many of these factors are associated with biologic risk. For example, a premature infant might have an unwed adolescent mother, or a woman might develop complications during her pregnancy because she lacked the money to obtain adequate prenatal care. In addition, apparently normal infants with psychosocial risk factors might develop subtle biologic problems at later ages.

Classification of High-Risk Infants

High-risk infants are classified on the basis of gestational age (GA) at birth and body size. These factors can affect mortality and morbidity rates as well as medical treatments.

Gestational age The gestational age of an infant usually is somewhat uncertain because few mothers know the date of conception. Gestational age is calculated from the first day of the mother's last menstrual period. For example, at 40 weeks from the date of the mother's last menstrual period, the infant is considered to have a GA of 40 weeks. Some mothers, however, are vague about the first day of their last menstrual period. Ultrasound examinations can be performed in the second trimester to estimate GA, but because this method is based on head growth, it is not accurate when there is early intrauterine growth retardation.

Because it is necessary to know GA to plan treatment correctly for a high-risk infant, researchers have developed methods of assessing GA by using neurologic and physical criteria. Dubowitz et al. (1970) developed criteria that could estimate GA within 1 to 2 weeks of the actual GA when the assessment is performed within 24 hours after birth. Ballard et al. (1977) developed an abbreviated version of the Dubowitz assessment, and it is this version that is used most frequently in neonatal intensive care units today.

GA is divided into three age divisions: (a) *full-term,* born between 38 and 42 weeks GA (b) *premature* or *preterm,* born prior to 38 weeks, and (c) *postterm,* born after 42 weeks. The term *postmaturity* is used only when a postterm infant exhibits the *postmature syndrome* (alert infant; dry, cracking skin; long arms and legs; thin with malnourished appearance; and meconium staining). The postmature syndrome is a result of prolonged pregnancy and placental insufficiency.

Size Four terms are used to classify infants on the basis of body size: (a) *low birthweight,* less than 2500 g (5.5 lb), (b) *average for gestational age,* birthweights between the 10th and 90th percentiles for gestational age, (c) *small for gestational age (SGA),* weight less than 10th percentile for gestational age, and (d) *large for gestational age (LGA),* weight greater than 90th percentile for gestational age. Most low-birthweight infants are premature. Intrauterine growth retardation is a common cause of SGA infants, while infants of diabetic mothers usually are LGA.

Any estimation of body size needs to take into consideration the child's ethnic background. Average sizes have been determined by looking at a limited cultural sample that excludes some ethnic groups. For example, an Indo-Chinese infant might be below the 10th percentile and still be within the normal range for Indo-Chinese infants.

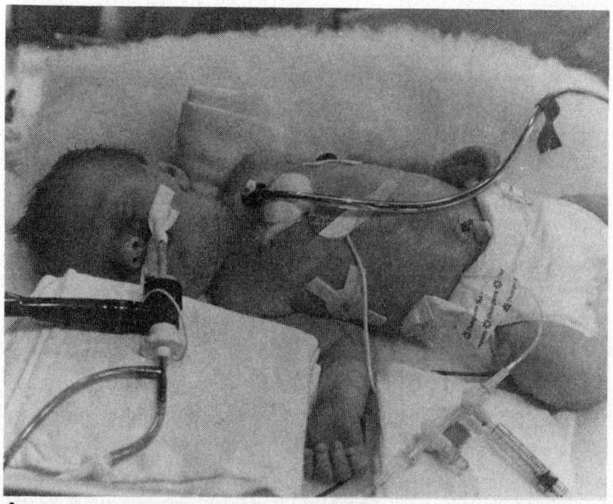

A

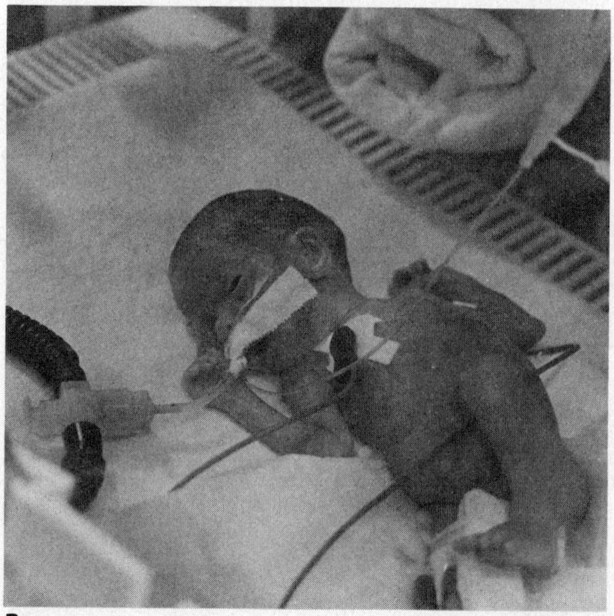

B

Differing appearances of two high-risk infants requiring mechanical ventilation. ***A.*** *A newborn, full-term infant.* ***B.*** *A two-week-old premature infant born at 26 weeks' GA. (Photograph by Christine Acebo.)*

Growth and Development of High-Risk Infants

The capabilities of infants change rapidly during the first year of life. These developmental changes are particularly dramatic during the preterm and early postterm periods, so nurses working with high-risk infants need to know the normal course of growth and development during infancy (see Chapter 4).

In general, high-risk infants without major disabilities show a pattern of growth and development that is similar to that of normal full-term infants. Severe illness or prolonged hospitalization can alter this course. Thus infants born more than 2 months prematurely frequently exhibit delays in development. Specific disabilities also alter an infant's developmental pattern.

Biophysical and cognitive development depend on gestational age. Affective and social development depend on experience as well as age. Therefore, when assessing the development of a premature infant, the infant's age needs to be corrected by subtracting the amount of prematurity from the birth age. A premature infant develops at the same rate as a full-term infant with the same gestational age. Therefore, an infant born 2 months prematurely never "catches up" with a full-term infant born at the same time because the central nervous system of the preterm infant is always 2 months less mature. Clinicians stop correcting for prematurity between 1 and 5 years because the rate of development slows after age 1.

Although age cannot be altered, the social experiences necessary for development can be planned. Therefore, an infant who exhibits developmental delays after prolonged hospitalization or severe illness might experience rapid development once the problem is resolved. These rapid changes often continue until the infant's development is normal.

Biophysical development

Growth When high-risk infants receive adequate nutrition, body weight and length grow at generally the same rate as normal full-term infants of the same biologic age (see Chapter 4). Small premature infants, however, usually experience some malnutrition due to feeding difficulties, and thus they often remain somewhat light for length throughout life (Desmond et al., 1980; Kimble et al., 1982). Infants who are SGA who experienced intrauterine malnutrition may remain below the 10th percentile in both length and weight (Desmond et al., 1980).

The head growth of premature infants and normal full-term infants differs dramatically. This difference is more pronounced for infants at a greater degree of prematurity. Premature infants tend to have large, thin heads. The sides of the head are flatter, and the distance between the temples is narrower than that in full-term infants.

Neuromuscular development The central nervous system develops rapidly during the preterm and neonatal periods. Unless there is neurologic damage, the neuromuscular development of high-risk infants remains very similar to that of healthy infants. The differences most affect the very premature infant, and central nervous system effects can be seen in reflex and sleep-wake behaviors.

The premature infant exhibits weaker and more asymmetric reflexes at term than a full-term infant of comparable gestational age. In addition, improper positioning during hospitalization might cause the infant to develop external rotation of hips, knees, and ankles or increased abduction tone in the shoulders, which will interfere with later efforts to bring the hands to the midline (Desmond et al., 1980).

Sleep-wake states are patterns of behavior that occur together and determine the infant's ability to respond to stimulation. The sleeping and waking states of high-risk infants have a developmental course similar to that of normal full-term infants (see Chapter 4). Certain conditions seen frequently in high-risk infants, such as hyperbilirubinemia, can alter sleep-wake states. Some medications can have the same effect.

The stability of the infant's sleep-wake states is predictive of developmental outcome. Infants who exhibit erratic patterns in the early weeks are more likely to develop later problems (Thoman et al., 1981).

Social development The social skills of young infants include both inborn reflex behaviors (eg, sucking, swallowing, and grasping) and learned behaviors. The reflexes mature at the same rate for both normal and high-risk infants and are fully developed at term. During the preterm period, all reflexes are weak. Therefore, a premature infant might demonstrate difficulties with grasping, sucking, and swallowing. For example, sucking and swallowing are not coordinated enough to permit oral feedings in an infant younger than 32–34 weeks GA. This can cause feeding difficulties with subsequent disturbance in social interaction.

After birth, infants learn social skills. To develop and learn these skills, however, the infant needs to have the opportunity for reciprocal interactions with nurturing adults. Thus, the appearance of social skills such as vocalization, social smiling, laughing, and visual following of parents will be delayed in infants who experience long hospital stays.

In addition, the short periods of alertness in premature infants prevent them from maintaining prolonged visual contact with adults. The nurse who counsels parents can prevent them from interpreting this lack of social responsiveness as rejection or mental retardation.

The extent of delayed social development in premature infants can be reduced if parents and nurses provide an appropriate environment for social growth. For example, evidence now shows that healthy premature infants who receive adequate nurturing begin social smiling early.

General Problems of High-Risk Infants

Immaturity of Heat Regulatory Mechanisms

An infant should maintain a core body temperature of approximately 37°C (98.6°F). When core temperature is significantly lower or higher than 37°C, metabolic rate and oxygen and glucose consumption increase. A lowered core body temperature, or *cold stress,* is often due to exposure to a cold environment. An elevated core temperature is due to exposure to a hot environment, or overheating. Overheating occurs when the core temperature is above 37.5°C (99.6°F) and the infant's high temperature is not related to illness. The increased metabolic rate in both of these conditions leads to acidosis, hypoxia, and hypoglycemia. These problems are worsened by vasoconstriction caused by cold stress, which decreases blood flow to peripheral tissues. Overheating, on the other hand, causes vasodilation, which might lead to shock.

Neonates have limited abilities to regulate their body temperatures. They become overheated in excessively warm environments because they are unable to sweat adequately. In cool environments, infants lose heat more readily than older children because they have less subcutaneous fat to act as insulation, and they have large surface areas for their body volumes. Infants are also unable to shiver effectively in response to cold and must instead rely on increasing activity.

Unlike older children, however, neonates are able to produce heat through *brown fat metabolism.* Brown fat is distributed in several areas on the trunks of infants (Fig. 34-1). When temperature sensors in the skin cause norepinephrine release in response to cold, the norepinephrine stimulates the brown fat to release heat. This mechanism enables healthy full-term infants to maintain their body temperatures in moderately cold environments.

Persistent cold stress, however, can exhaust an infant's brown fat supply. Neurologic damage can interfere with the ability of the skin sensors to stimulate norepinephrine release. In addition, the free fatty acids released by brown fat metabolism interfere with bilirubin binding and might increase the likelihood of kernicterus, or indirect bilirubin in the blood.

Premature infants have even less ability to regulate their body temperatures than do full-term infants. They have higher surface-to-volume ratios than full-term infants and less subcutaneous fat. Consequently, they lose heat more rapidly. Moreover, they have less brown fat and poorer defenses to overheating because their sweating mechanisms are particularly ineffective (Harpin and Rutter, 1982).

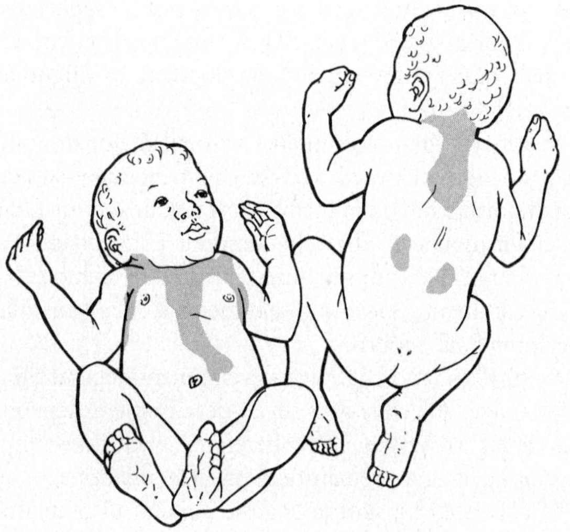

FIGURE 34-1
Distribution of brown fat.

Assessment Principal criteria for assessing heat regulation are physical signs of cold stress such as overheating and body temperatures. The nurse assesses the body temperatures of each hospitalized infant at least every 4 hours. Measurements should determine whether core temperature is between 36.5°C and 37.5°C (97.6°F and 99.6°F) and skin temperature is between 35.8°C and 36.7°C (96.5°F and 98°F). Either rectal or axillary temperature can be used although axillary is preferred for small infants. Skin temperatures can be obtained from skin probes on incubators and radiant warmers or, more crudely, by comparing the temperature of the extremities and abdomen. If the abdomen feels significantly warmer than the legs, cold stress is probably causing vasoconstriction in the legs, which in turn causes peripheral cyanosis.

When the infant is in an incubator, the environmental temperature is also recorded because it affects the nursing diagnosis concerning the infant's temperature regulation. When the incubator temperature and the infant's temperature are both falling, the infant is experiencing cold stress. If the infant's temperature is falling while the incubator's temperature is rising, the infant is experiencing hypothermia, which signals a serious insult such as sepsis.

Infants experiencing early cold stress increase their activity levels and appear restless and irritable. Severe cold stress causes respiratory problems with symptoms of rapid breathing, difficult breathing, pallor, and hypoactivity. The vasodilation of overheating, on the other hand, causes infants to appear flushed. Their skin feels warm, and they might be sweating.

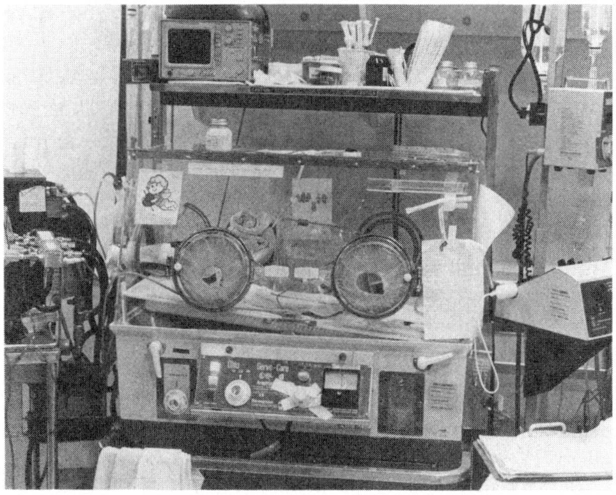

An incubator. (Photograph by Christine Acebo.)

Large fluctuations in core temperature or environmental temperature are also stressful. Graphs of the infant's temperature are analyzed to make certain that the infant is in a neutral thermal environment. In addition, infants who fail to gain weight despite adequate calorie intake might be experiencing mild cold stress.

The nursing diagnosis for an infant experiencing cold stress generally is **ineffective theomoregulation.** The factors related to the nursing diagnosis, however, depend on the specific assessment data gathered for each infant.

Nursing management The goal of nursing care for infants with problems in heat regulation is to maintain the infant in a neutral thermal environment. This requires an environmental temperature at which metabolic rate and oxygen consumption are minimized, and the infant's core body temperature is between 36.5°C and 37.5°C.

Various methods minimize heat loss and provide a neutral thermal environment. Most high-risk infants are initially placed in incubators in which the air is heated to maintain either a constant air temperature or a constant skin temperature. When the portholes are closed, convection and conduction are minimized. Evaporation is reduced by humidifying the air in the incubator. Air is sometimes not humidified, however, to prevent bacterial colonization of the water, which might in turn cause infection. Some radiant heat loss to the walls of the incubator does occur, but these walls are warmer than the walls of the room. For small infants, the radiant heat loss can be further reduced by placing a clear plastic heat shield over the infant.

Infants who require frequent assessment are placed in radiant warmers with a radiant heat supply located above the infant and used to maintain a constant skin temperature. Because the infant in such a warmer is open to the air, convective heat loss to air currents in the NICU and radiant losses to the walls of the room occur, causing the infant's metabolic rate to increase. Thus infants in warmers usually have higher metabolic rates than infants in incubators (LeBlanc, 1982).

Full-term infants and recuperating high-risk infants are placed in open bassinets. Infants in bassinets are exposed to all four types of heat loss, but the nurse minimizes this process by clothing and covering the infant. Covering the head with a hat also reduces heat loss, because the brain is a major heat-producing organ and the head has a proportionately large surface area.

If the infant is showing signs of cold stress or overheating, the environmental temperature should be changed, although temperature changes should not be excessive. The temperature settings on warmers and incubators can be adjusted, and clothing and blankets can be added or removed for infants in bassinets.

Overheating while correcting a low core temperature is also possible. To prevent this, the nurse warms the infant slowly, while monitoring temperature. Metabolic rate returns to normal as soon as skin temperature is normal even though core temperature is still low. Thus, once skin temperature is normal or core temperature begins to rise rapidly, the temperature in the incubator or warmer is returned to that of a neutral thermal environment.

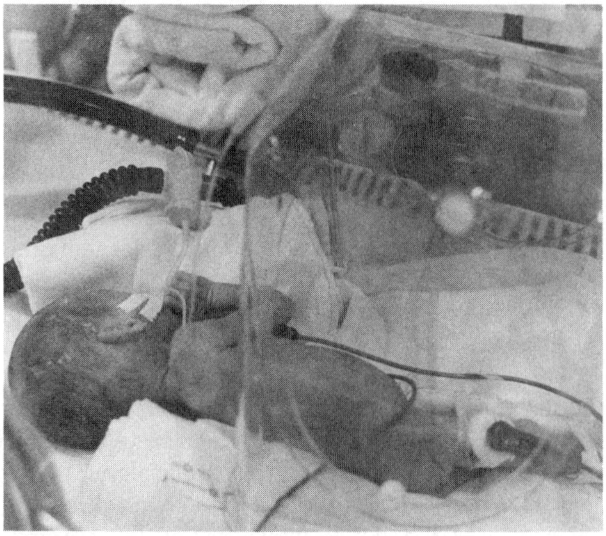

A small, premature infant (weight = 760 g) under a heat shield in an incubator. (Photograph by Christine Acebo.)

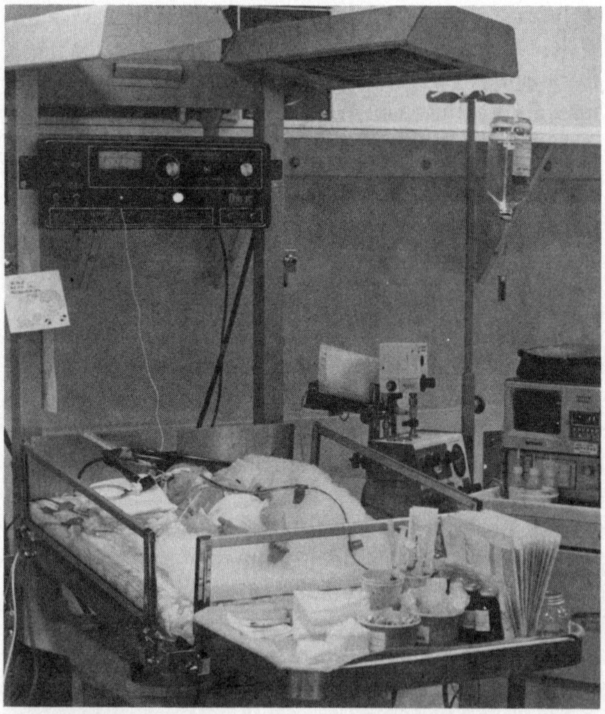

A radiant warmer. (Photograph by Christine Acebo.)

Complications Uncorrected cold stress can lead to hypoxia, acidemia, respiratory failure, and death. A number of infants have been placed on mechanical ventilators because of severe cold stress.

Improper use of incubators and radiant warmers can also cause complications. Incorrect temperature settings can lead to either cold stress or overheating. Using radiant warmers without skin probes might cause burns.

Immaturity of the Immunologic System

Because of the immaturity of their immunologic systems, all infants, especially premature infants and those undergoing invasive procedures, are susceptible to infections. Their leukocytes are less efficient in migrating to the sites of infections and engulfing pathogens than those of older children. All neonates have very few actively acquired antibodies because antibody production depends on exposure to specific infective agents. Therefore, their immunologic systems depend on short-lived maternal antibodies that cross the placenta, especially during the third trimester. Not until 3 months postterm has the infant produced enough antibodies to replace the rapidly declining supply of maternal antibodies. Premature infants are even more vulnerable to infections because they are not in the uterus for the entire third trimester and thus receive fewer antibodies.

Immaturity of the immunologic system also leaves the infant susceptible to infections caused by organisms that are not ordinarily pathogenic in older children. For example, one nursery experienced an outbreak of diarrhea caused by *Staphylococcus epidermidis,* a normally harmless bacterium found on the skin of adults. In addition, infections of infants are more often generalized, involving meningitis, septicemia, or pneumonia.

Assessment The symptoms of infections in infants are seldom specific. Because of the immaturity of their heat regulation mechanisms, infants rarely develop fevers. Instead, hypothermia in an adequately warm environment indicates sepsis (systemic infection). Other symptoms include poor feeding, jitteriness, hyperbilirubinemia, apnea, diarrhea, abdominal distension, respiratory distress, lethargy, cyanosis, irregular or rapid respirations, vomiting, edema, bleeding, pallor, hypotension, jaundice, and rapid heart rate.

Because sepsis can mimic a number of other conditions, the nurse needs to know that an infant has been exposed to an infection. Infants contract illnesses from their mothers during pregnancy or birth and from other patients or staff during the neonatal period. Infection needs to be suspected whenever the mother develops an illness during the perinatal period or the amniotic membranes are ruptured more than 24 hours prior to birth.

The nursing diagnosis in such cases is **potential for infection.** Exposure to bacteria may be secondary to invasive procedures, maternal infection, or other environmental factors. The specific nursing diagnosis thus depends on the assessment of each client.

Nursing management The goals of nursing care are to prevent infection whenever possible and to identify infections in the early stages. Because prevention of infection is always the best intervention, all nurseries need to practice preventive measures that include

1. Good hand washing with an antibiotic soap on entering the nursery and between handling infants
2. Wearing scrub suits or gowns over street clothes when in the nursery
3. Wearing a different gown for directly handling each infant
4. Placing particularly vulnerable infants in incubators
5. Isolating all infants with infections

Another essential aspect of prevention is determining whether an infection is hospital acquired and thus preventable. In most hospitals, an infection control nurse routinely cultures surfaces to determine whether possible infective agents are present. Some nurseries also routinely culture high-risk infants. Also important is determining how well the nursery staff is conducting the infection control measures.

Definitive diagnosis of infections can only be made from bacterial cultures. The sites of serious infection in neonates are the central nervous system, urinary tract, lungs, and circulatory systems, so cultures of spinal fluid, urine, tracheal aspirations, and blood are included in the usual septic workup. Cultures are also repeated often to determine whether the infection is resolving.

A serious infection is treated with antibiotics and determination of antibiotics depends on the culture. Therefore, until results of cultures are available, infants are treated for both gram-positive and gram-negative bacteria and are thus given both a penicillin (ampicillin, oxacillin, or penicillin) and an aminoglycoside (kanamycin or gentamicin). If the pathogen is resistant to these drugs, cephalosporins or chloramphenicol may be given.

Complications Both the infection and the antibiotics used to treat it might cause complications. For example, meningitis, septicemia, and pneumonia can cause death or residual damage.

Prolonged antibiotic use might lead to superinfection from fungus or yeast. Localized superinfections are treatable, but generalized superinfections often cause death because the antifungal drugs are toxic to infants. Prolonged use of the aminoglycosides might lead to deafness due to nerve damage; chloramphenicol might cause aplastic anemia.

Immaturity of the Respiratory System

Because of the immaturity of the lungs and the cerebral respiratory centers, respiratory problems are common in the neonatal period. The lungs are among the last organs to develop in the fetus; the alveoli are not fully developed until 26–28 weeks' GA. Surfactants, chemicals that reduce the surface tension in the alveoli and allow a small amount of air to remain in them after expiration, develop in the second and third trimesters. Synthesis of surfactant begins at 22–24 weeks' GA and is present in fairly adequate amounts by 35 weeks' GA. Thus, an infant born prior to 35 weeks' GA can have insufficient levels of surfactant and resultant respiratory difficulties.

The cerebral controls on breathing are immature in the early months after birth and more so in the premature infant. Brief respiratory pauses of less than 10 seconds are common during this period.

Assessment Assessment of the respiratory system involves taking vital signs, observing physical symptoms, and obtaining blood gases. Vital signs are taken for all hospitalized infants at least every 4 hours. A respiratory rate above 60 breaths per minute (tachypnea) and a cardiac rate above 160 beats per minute (tachycardia) are common signs of respiratory distress. A heart rate less than 100 beats per minute (bradycardia) and apnea might result in hypoxia or respiratory failure.

The physical signs of respiratory distress include cyanosis or pallor, nasal flaring, retractions of the chest wall, and expiratory grunts. Severely ill infants are usually flaccid, hypoactive, and edemic. In addition, respiratory problems alter the breath sounds heard on auscultation. The specific changes depend on the problem.

Blood gases need to be monitored in all infants suspected of having respiratory problems. Normal arterial P_{O_2} in infants ranges from 60–80 mm Hg, which is lower than the level in older children. P_{CO_2} and pH levels are similar to those of older children. The three types of blood gases obtained in infants are: (1) capillary, (b) arterial, and (c) transcutaneous (see Chapter 22).

Vital signs are taken at least every 4 hours and more often if respiratory symptoms are present. The nurse then records descriptions of the infant's color, degree of respiratory distress, and breath sounds at the same time. The assessment data determine the specific nursing diagnosis. Respiratory dysfunction suggests

Ineffective airway clearance
Ineffective breathing pattern
Impaired gas exchange

Nursing management The goal of nursing care for high-risk infants with respiratory problems is to maintain adequate oxygenation by modifying the environment and by treating the underlying problem. The nurse also monitors the infant's status to identify complications of treatment as early as possible.

Supportive interventions to treat respiratory problems include reducing cold stress, metabolic disturbances, and the stress of infections. During the acute phase, however, excessive handling might cause hypoxia, although infants should be repositioned every 2–4 hours to prevent pooling of secretions. Elevating the head slightly tends to increase oxygenation. A diaper roll placed behind the neck helps keep the airway patent, but overextending the neck, which tends to close off the trachea, should be avoided.

In addition, chest physiotherapy and suctioning might eliminate excess secretions. Chest physiotherapy consists of positioning to promote drainage of congested lobes and percussion and vibration to loosen secretions. This treatment can cause hypoxia, so it should be done with caution in severely ill infants (Dingle et al., 1980). The nose and mouth of each infant with respiratory dysfunction are suctioned to remove secretions that might block the upper airway. Endotracheal tubes require suctioning every 1–4 hours (depending on the amount of secretions) to maintain the patency of the tube.

Respiratory support is provided in one of four ways: (a) environmental oxygen, (b) continuous positive airway pressure (CPAP), (c) mechanical ventilation, and (d) continuous negative chest wall pressure. Environmental oxygen is extra oxygen mixed with the air the infant is breathing. Low concentrations of oxygen can be supplied directly to the incubator, but higher concentrations must be administered through an oxygen hood, which is a small, clear plastic box that covers the infant's head. Oxygen is administered to older infants by nasal cannula or oxygen tent. Whenever oxygen is administered, it must be humidified and warmed to prevent cold stress. The nurse monitors its concentration at least once every hour.

Continuous positive airway pressure provides oxygen and continuous pressure on the distending airway to prevent alveolar collapse without overdistending the alveoli. By maintaining positive pressure at the end of expiration, alveolar air is retained, representing the functional residual capacity necessary for continued diffusion of oxygen into the blood and less airway resistance, thereby lessening the work of breathing. The infant breathes unaided. The oxygen is administered by endotracheal tube to the lower airways or by nasal prongs to the upper airways. A head hood or face mask might be used, but these devices restrict accessibility for nursing care. Both oxygen concentration and pressure level are monitored closely. Local irritation might occur to the infant's nares or lips at the site of the delivery system.

Severe respiratory problems must be treated with mechanical ventilators, which provide breaths of oxygen for the infants. Some ventilators are time cycled, whereas others are volume cycled. The ventilator is set to provide a given volume of oxygen with each breath at a given pressure. The settings vary, but the criterion is normalization of arterial oxygen and carbon dioxide. The breathing rate of the ventilator can be varied and is sometimes set fast enough that the machine does all the breathing. At a slow rate (below 20 breaths per minute), the infant is able to breathe between the ventilator breaths. A small positive pressure is usually maintained at the end of a breath so that the alveoli do not collapse. Continuous negative chest wall pressure is rarely used.

Drugs given to treat respiratory problems include sodium bicarbonate to correct acidosis that does not improve after adequate oxygenation, theophylline, and caffeine. The last two are closely related drugs given to treat apnea.

Complications Complications can result either from the initial respiratory problems or from their treatment. Inadequate or ineffective treatment might result in respiratory failure. Respiratory failure occurs when the PCO_2 level is above 60 mm Hg, PO_2 is below 45 mm Hg, and pH is below 7.2. Clinical signs include severe apnea and bradycardia, which, if untreated, will result in death. Infants are usually placed on cardiac and respiratory monitors to detect episodes of bradycardia and apnea.

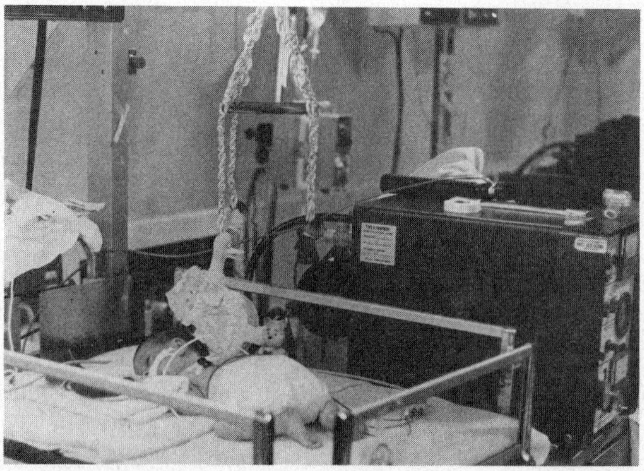

A premature infant at 36 weeks' GA receiving mechanical ventilation. The ventilator is the large box behind the infant. (Photograph by Christine Acebo.)

Significant complications might also result from treatment such as CPAP and mechanical ventilation, which might cause pneumothorax. A pneumothorax occurs when alveoli are ruptured, allowing air to escape into the pleural spaces. The negative pressure between the lungs and the chest wall is thus disrupted, and part of the lung collapses, causing hypoxia. Pneumothorax occurs in 10% of infants receiving CPAP and in 33% of infants receiving mechanical ventilation; only 3% of infants receiving only environmental oxygen develop it (Stavis and Krauss, 1980).

Endotracheal intubation also can cause complications. It provides a route for bacterial infection because repeated suctioning through the endotracheal tube causes irritation of the trachea and bronchial tubes, which predisposes the lungs to infection. Improper placement of the tube, accidental extubation, and plugging of the tube with mucus result in hypoventilation and hypoxia and are major causes of mortality and morbidity among high-risk infants (Stavis and Krauss, 1980).

Umbilical artery catheters also might cause significant complications. Thromboemboli form at the end of a large percentage of umbilical catheters (Stavis and Krauss, 1980). Small emboli break away from the catheters frequently, and occasionally large emboli are formed, resulting in major damage or death. Transient blanching of one or both legs occurs frequently, probably because of arterial spasm or emboli. Bacterial colonization of umbilical catheters is also common and causes serious infections.

The supplemental oxygen used to treat respiratory problems also causes complications. Oxygen toxicity causes retrolental fibroplasia (RLF), an eye condition in some infants that can result in blindness. The etiology of RLF is the high level of oxygen that creates changes in the retinal vasculature, which in turn lead to scarring and retinal detachment. The elevated oxygen levels do not have to be prolonged. RLF might result from brief elevations, as when extra oxygen is given an infant after an apneic attack. The very immature infant is more vulnerable to this problem. Generally, RLF is associated with PO_2 levels above 100 mm Hg, but it sometimes occurs at lower levels, especially in infants with GAs less than 30 weeks.

Immaturity of the Gastrointestinal System

Premature infants are vulnerable to nutritional problems because they have less subcutaneous fat and diminished stores of glycogen, calcium, and iron. Their ability to digest protein, fats, and lactose (milk sugar) is impaired because gastric acidity and the amount of some digestive enzymes are decreased. The stomach capacity of premature infants is very small. The sucking reflex is not fully developed and coordinated with swallowing until 35–36 weeks' GA (Boettcher and Pereira, 1983).

Thus, the nutritional needs of high-risk infants are difficult to meet. Serious illness can impair an infant's ability to suck, and calorie and nutrient needs are increased by the stress of illness. After oral or gastric feedings, high-risk infants tend to regurgitate milk into the lower half of the esophagus, which causes an increased respiratory rate (Fanaroff and Klaus, 1979).

Assessment The nurse assesses the nutritional status of every high-risk infant on a daily basis. The nutrition available to an infant for growth equals the calories consumed minus the calories expended and excreted (Boettcher and Pereira, 1983). Infants receiving and using adequate calories and nutrients show adequate growth. Therefore, repeated measurements of length, weight, and head circumference are used to assess the nutritional status of high-risk infants (see Appendix A).

Every high-risk infant needs to be weighed daily, and length and head circumference should be recorded once a week. All infants lose weight for the first few days after birth and continue to lose weight until feedings are well established. After feedings are well established, premature infants can gain weight at a rate faster than a full-term infant of comparable age (Nelson and Heitman, 1986).

The adequacy of an infant's growth is determined by comparing it with a standard growth chart. When comparing a premature infant to growth charts, it is important that the infant's GA be used for comparison purposes. Adequate growth is probably occurring if head circumference, weight, and length remain at or above the percentiles they reached at birth and all three measurements are at approximately the same percentile.

Assessment also determines how well infants are tolerating feedings. Symptoms of feeding intolerance or gastrointestinal disease include gastric aspirate larger than half the hourly food intake (Boettcher and Pereira, 1983), bile-tinged aspirate or emesis, large emesis, abdominal distension, and occult blood in the stool. Some premature infants have difficulty absorbing sugar and thus excrete it in the stool.

Assessment of feeding tolerance therefore involves estimating the amount of any residual. Before each tube feeding, the contents of the stomach are aspirated and measured. The abdomens of all small premature infants, and all infants with severe illnesses should be measured at least once every 8 hours and their stools checked for occult blood and sugar. (See Chapter 27 for discussion of procedure for tube feedings.)

Generally, the nursing diagnosis for infants with nutritional deficiencies is **alteration in nutrition: less than body requirements.** To provide adequate nutrition, however, it is important to determine not only whether an infant's growth is adequate but also the cause of any inadequacy. The cause of the inadequacy completes the nursing diagnosis and defines the circumstances that result in fewer nutrients than the body's requirements.

Excess expenditure of calories occurs because of cold stress or serious illness, so environmental stresses should be minimized and seriously ill infants should be given additional calories. When an infant is receiving inadequate calories or nutrients for growth, dietary supplementation will improve nutritional status. Some infants excrete excess calories through vomiting or in the stool, and nutrients must therefore be provided by another route until absorption improves. Other infants, because of congenital enzyme deficiencies, are unable to use nutrients even though they are provided with adequate nutrition and can absorb it.

Nursing management The long-term goal of nursing care is to provide an adequate balance of calories and nutrients for brain and body growth and to prevent diseases caused by deficiencies of specific nutrients. High-risk infants receiving adequate nutrition maintain adequate growth in weight, length, and head circumference.

The selection of the type of food and its delivery route is important to providing each infant with adequate nutrition. The route of administration for feeding should progress from parenteral fluids, to continuous tube feedings, to gavage feedings, and finally to oral feedings.

Types of food As long as the mother is not taking medication, infants should be given their mothers' milk, which is easily digested and contains maternal antibodies to protect against infections. In addition, breast-feeding enables the mother of a high-risk infant to play a unique role in the infant's recovery. The breast milk of mothers of preterm infants contains extra protein necessary to meet their increased needs (Pittard, 1981), but breast-fed premature infants still require nutrient supplements, particularly of phosphorus, copper, vitamins B_{12}, D, and E, and folic acid, for ideal growth (Boettcher and Pereira, 1983).

Even so, fewer mothers of high-risk infants breast-feed than mothers of healthy infants, usually because these mothers are separated from their infants during the infants' hospitalization and often have had difficult pregnancies and deliveries. The mothers of these infants must also pump their breasts to provide breast milk. To initiate a milk supply, each breast must be pumped for about 10 minutes every 2–3 hours during the day (Boggs and Rau, 1983). Not every mother is willing or able to make that large a commitment to breast-feeding.

If the infant's mother is unable to breast-feed, the infant may be fed donated breast milk. This provides adequate nutrition but no protection from infection because milk from a breast milk bank must be pasteurized to destroy pathogenic bacteria that might have contaminated it (Lemons, 1981).

Most high-risk infants are instead fed commercial formulas that are universally available and have assured nutrient contents. Special formulas have recently been developed, and these contain the types of proteins, carbohydrates, and fats that are easily digested and meet the nutritional needs of premature infants. Extra vitamins and nutrients are also included in these formulas.

High-risk infants not receiving these special formulas require dietary supplements to meet their nutritional needs, and multivitamins are therefore given with feedings. Premature infants in particular require additional amounts of liposoluble vitamins during the first 2 months of life. Vitamin D supplementation prevents rickets, and vitamin E is given to prevent hemolytic anemia. Medium-chain triglyceride oil (MCT oil) is sometimes given to provide extra calories for infants who have difficulty gaining weight or who are on fluid restrictions.

Feeding methods Feedings can be provided in several ways. Ideally, infants should be allowed to suck from a bottle or breast. For some infants, feedings can be given by the parents and thus promote closeness between parents and infants. Many high-risk infants are unable to suck well enough to receive oral feedings. Instead, they receive tube feedings, usually by gavage, in which a tube is inserted through the nose or mouth and passed into the stomach, and feedings of formula, breast milk, or sugar water are given every 2–4 hours and allowed to drain into the stomach by gravity. The tube is usually inserted just before the feeding and removed when it is completed.

Continuous tube feedings are also given by placing the feeding tube in the stomach, duodenum, or jejunum and pumping feedings through the tube by an infusion pump at a slow, constant rate. Placement of the tube creates certain risks. Locating the tube in the stomach occasionally causes regurgitation. This problem is avoided by intestinal placement, but digestion and absorption are less complete, and intestinal perforation and intussusception might occur, particularly if the tube is placed in the jejunum.

When infants are unable to tolerate gastrointestinal feedings, they must receive fluids and nutrients parenterally. Immediately after birth, parenteral fluids (usually 10% dextrose in water) are given to prevent dehydration and hypoglycemia until a feeding regimen can be established. If infants have difficulty tolerating feedings, they are given parenteral fluids in addition to feedings for several weeks.

Because of extreme prematurity or surgical problems, some infants are unable to tolerate gastrointestinal feedings for long periods and are instead given parenteral nutrition. This is either in the form of intralipids (a high-calorie solution of fats) or hyperalimentation (a concentrated solution of dextrose, proteins, electrolytes, and vitamins). Both intralipids and hyperalimentation with a low sugar content (no more than 10% dextrose) are infused through peripheral veins, but hyperalimentation with higher concentrations of sugar must be infused into the superior vena cava through a cutdown of the internal or external jugular vein. Because of the risk of infection with hyperalimentation, the solution should never be infused through an umbilical catheter.

No matter how they receive their feedings, all infants need opportunities for sucking. In the uterus, fetuses develop this ability by sucking on their fingers, but because infants receiving tube feedings or hyperalimentation may be restrained or otherwise prevented from sucking their fingers, they should be offered pacifiers frequently. Sucking on a pacifier calms an infant and raises the oxygen level (Anderson et al., 1980). Evidence also suggests that sucking aids digestion.

Complications Inadequate nutrition can lead to serious complications. Severe malnutrition can result in inadequate brain growth and permanent mental retardation. Fortunately, however, the brain receives nutrition in preference to other parts of the body so inadequate brain growth occurs only after prolonged nutritional deficiency.

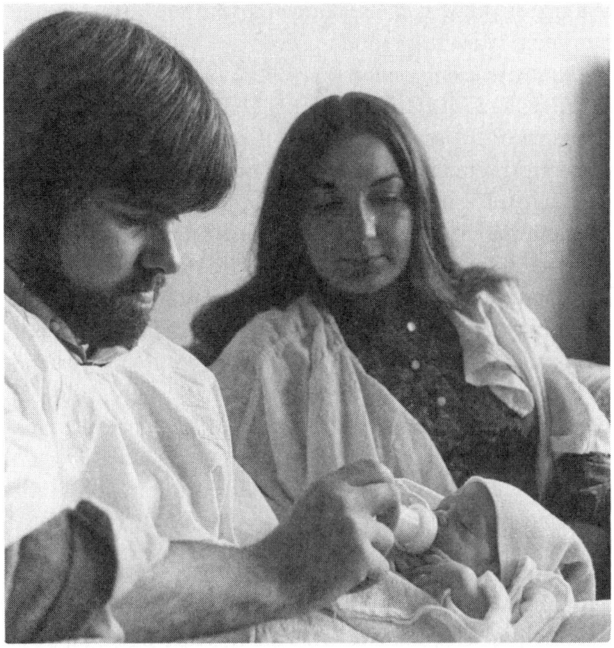

Parents feeding their premature infant shortly before discharge. (Photograph by Christine Acebo.)

The feeding techniques used with high-risk infants might also cause complications. Regurgitation after oral or tube feeding might cause aspiration of formula or breast milk. Positioning the infant on the right side or on the abdomen increases the rate of gastric emptying and thus decreases the risk of aspiration. Perforation of the stomach, esophagus, or intestine occurs, although rarely, during the insertion of tubes for gavage or continuous feedings (Stavis and Krauss, 1980).

Hyperalimentation and intralipids cause other complications. The high glucose content of central hyperalimentation might cause hyperglycemia if the infusion rate is too rapid. Using an infusion pump therefore helps to maintain a constant infusion rate. This high sugar content is also an excellent medium for bacterial growth. Intralipids cause hyperlipidemia (elevated fats in the blood), so serum lipids should be checked daily. Hyperlipidemia can interfere with the binding of bilirubin to albumin and intralipids might rarely cause fat emboli. Symptoms of this condition include dyspnea, cyanosis, and bradycardia or tachycardia. Because of these potential problems, intralipids are not given when the infant has hyperbilirubinemia or lung disease.

Inorganic failure-to-thrive syndrome is another serious consequence of inadequate nutrition. Failure to thrive can occur when inappropriate nurturing and stimulation are accompanied by improper feeding techniques or inadequate calories or nutrients (see Chapter 13).

Immaturity of the Circulatory System

The immaturity of a neonate's circulatory system can lead to significant problems. Occasionally, as a result of hypoxia, the circulatory areas involved in the fetal right-to-left shunt reopen. A patent ductus arteriosus (PDA) is the most common result and occurs primarily in premature infants (see Chapter 23). A PDA should be suspected whenever recovery from respiratory problems is prolonged or the infant's condition deteriorates suddenly (Liebman et al., 1979). PDAs occur in 32% of infants born prior to 36 weeks' GA (Stahler-Miller and Gewitz, 1983).

Congestive heart failure (see Chapter 23) results from the inability of the heart to pump all of the blood returned to it from the peripheral circulation and the lungs. Heart failure occurs as a result of fluid overload, left-to-right shunting from a PDA, or a pulmonary disease. Cardiac problems related to fluid excess are significant because of the relatively small fluid capacity of the infant's circulatory system, less than 100 mL per kilogram. Thus it is relatively easy to cause fluid overload in high-risk infants.

Assessment The circulatory status of high-risk infants is assessed to identify the early stages of PDA and congestive heart failure and to monitor their progression. Vital signs are taken frequently, as tachypnea and tachycardia are common signs of PDA and heart failure. Blood pressure elevations might occur in heart failure, and infants with PDAs usually have wide pulse pressures. Cardiac and apnea monitors should be used, as apnea is often worsened by these conditions, and the drugs used to treat heart failure might also cause arrhythmias and bradycardia. Heart sounds and breath sounds should be auscultated whenever vital signs are taken.

Because metabolic imbalances can mimic the symptoms of cardiac problems, the nurse also monitors electrolyte and glucose levels in all infants suspected of cardiac problems. Moreover, the fluid retention in congestive heart failure and the drugs used to treat it can cause electrolyte imbalances.

The nursing diagnosis for the infant with cardiac dysfunction is **alteration in cardiac output (decreased)**. Furthermore, because these infants are at risk for fluid overload, nursing care is also based on the **potential for alteration in fluid volume**.

Nursing management The goals of nursing care are to prevent fluid overload and to detect circulatory problems as early as possible. While a circulatory problem is being treated, nursing care focuses on maintaining adequate oxygenation of tissues and reducing the workload of the heart. (Specific interventions depend on the underlying cardiac problem and are discussed in Chapter 23.)

Complications The complications of PDA and congestive heart failure are frequently fatal. When cardiac output is very low, tissue perfusion is inadequate, a problem that can lead to cardiogenic shock. Symptoms of shock are similar to those of severe heart failure, with the addition of hypotension (less than 35 mm Hg in a full-term infant).

Pulmonary edema occurs when large amounts of blood pool in the lungs. Fluid enters the interstitial spaces and interferes with the diffusion of oxygen through the alveoli. Symptoms include dyspnea, tachypnea, and pink-tinged mucus. Treatment of both conditions involves treating the underlying cardiac failure, supporting respiration (often mechanical ventilation), restricting fluids, and providing diuretic therapy. Occasionally, rotating tourniquets or leg wraps are used to decrease the volume of blood returning to the heart. Infants with pulmonary edema also require frequent suctioning. Infants receiving digoxin for cardiac dysfunction need to be observed closely since toxicity to digoxin can cause cardiac arrest.

Immaturity of the Neurologic System

The last trimester of pregnancy and the period of early infancy are times of rapid brain growth. The gray and white matter in the brains of neonates is poorly differentiated, and most of the neurons are immature in form and function. The central nervous system of a premature infant is even less developed. Therefore, any insult that occurs during this period can cause extensive brain damage.

On the other hand, the central nervous systems of infants can compensate in order to minimize some types of brain damage. For example, damage to the speech centers in the brain does not affect language acquisition even though damage to these areas in adults causes aphasia.

Additional factors, such as other health problems and the home environment, affect neurologic outcome, so the nature and extent of disabilities are not predictable from the size and location of brain damage. Although, generally, the larger the lesion, the more disabled an infant will be, many individuals are exceptions.

The four main causes of neurologic damage in the neonatal period are hypoxia, birth trauma, hemorrhage, and infection. Episodes of hypoxia caused by birth asphyxia or by cardiac or respiratory abnormalities can damage neural tissues directly or cause brain edema. Tissue compression caused by edema leads to further brain damage. Birth trauma causes brain damage through tissue compression and tearing.

Several different types of hemorrhage can occur. *Intracranial hemorrhage* is caused by both trauma and hypoxia. Subdural hemorrhage occurs in full-term infants because of tearing of dura, falx, or tentorium during birth trauma. Symptoms vary from mild to severe.

Intraventricular hemorrhage (IVH) occurs in premature infants as a result of hypoxia, anoxia, and subsequent hypernatremia or hyperglycemia. IVH is seen to a certain extent in many premature infants with weights below 1500 g (3 1/2 lb). Tissue damage occurs at the site of the hemorrhage. In severe IVH, blood fills the ventricle, causing dilatation, tissue compression, and further brain damage.

Subarachnoid hemorrhage occurs in both full-term and preterm infants as a result of trauma or hypoxia. Infants with small hemorrhages have symptoms of hypotonia and irritability, which resolve within the first week of life. In more severe hemorrhages, the blood in the subarachnoid space causes tissue compression. Meningitis can also cause significant neurologic damage and is more common in the neonatal period than at any other age.

Assessment Physical symptoms, behavioral changes, and laboratory tests are used to assess infants for possible neurologic problems. The diagnosis of neurologic problems has two parts: (a) identifying the cause of the problem—hypoxia, trauma, hemorrhage, metabolic imbalance, or infection—and (b) determining the extent of neurologic disabilities.

Disabilities that can be diagnosed in the neonatal period include alterations in muscle tone, weakness or paralysis of an extremity, abnormal sleep-wake state patterns, and seizure activity. These disabilities might resolve prior to hospital discharge, might continue for several months, or might last throughout the infant's life. Other neurologic disabilities, such as mental retardation and cerebral palsy, might not appear until the infant is older. Nursing care therefore is based on diagnoses of

Potential self-care deficit
Potential impaired physical mobility
Potential for altered growth and development

The specific diagnosis depends on the assessment data gathered for each infant.

Signs and symptoms Abnormalities in vital signs—especially bradycardia and hypotension—might be symptoms of intracranial hemorrhage. Any episode of hypoxia, which might occur during prolonged apnea or bradycardia, can cause brain damage. Because rapid head growth is a sign of hydrocephalus, daily measurements of head circumference are performed on all infants suspected of neurologic problems. The fontanelles of infants also are palpated when vital signs are performed, since bulging or full fontanelles are signs of hydrocephalus. In subdural hemorrhage, only the anterior fontanelle feels full.

A number of behavioral changes signal neurologic problems. Neurologic damage causes weak, asymmetric, or hypoactive reflexes. Muscle tone also is affected frequently and becomes either hypotonic or hypertonic. Because premature infants have less muscle tone than full-term infants, their muscle tone should be compared with that of normal preterm infants rather than the muscle tone of a full-term infant. If muscle tone is weaker on one side, hemiparesis might be present. Optimal performance on muscle tone and reflexes are best obtained when the infant is in an alert state.

Neurologic problems might diminish spontaneous activity, so the nurse assesses the infant's activity level. Because mild abnormalities of tone, reflexes, or activity level are often transient in high-risk infants, all infants with any of these problems should be reassessed.

Neurologic problems can be manifested by alteration in the infant's sleep-wake state. For example, infants with neurologic problems frequently appear irritable or lethargic, with abnormal cries. When awake, infants with neurologic insults might appear unresponsive, although prematurity alone can have a similar effect on the quality of alertness.

Seizures and jitteriness are other signs of neurologic problems, and nurses therefore need to be able to distinguish between them. According to Gale (1981), these phenomena are differentiated by three criteria: (a) jitteriness is not accompanied by abnormal eye movements or gaze abnormalities, (b) episodes of jitteriness can be affected by stimulation, and (c) jittery movements are of equal amplitude and rate, whereas the movements of seizures have fast and slow components. A number of different problems, including neurologic damage, metabolic imbalance, and drugs, also can cause jitteriness or tremulousness in neonates.

Seizures are more ominous symptoms than jitteriness since they can cause neonatal death or disability. Seizures are caused by neurologic damage, by severe metabolic disturbances, and rarely by withdrawal in the narcotics-addicted infant. Neonates do not exhibit the generalized tonic-clonic seizures typical of adults and older children. Instead, *neonatal seizures* involve intermittent periods of hypertonia with deviation of the eyes and jerking of one or more extremities.

Occasionally, the only symptoms of seizures are eye blinking, repetitive mouthing, apnea, and circumoral cyanosis. In infants, the size or location of neurologic damage is not indicated by the symptoms of the seizure as it is in older children (see Chapter 31). During active sleep, small jerks normally accompany rapid eye movements in the neonate, but these jerks should not be confused with seizures.

Diagnostic tests As with older infants and children, the diagnosis of neurologic damage is supported by diagnostic testing. Diagnostic tests include electroencephalogram (EEG), computed tomography (CT), ultrasonography, lumbar puncture, and subdural taps (see Chapter 31).

Nursing management Nursing care focuses on identifying neurologic problems as early as possible and minimizing residual disabilities. Unfortunately, however, neurologic damage cannot be repaired. Therefore, interventions are supportive.

Because hypoxia can damage brain tissue, infants with suspected neurologic problems should be well oxygenated and placed on cardiac and apnea monitors with vital signs monitored closely. Apnea and bradycardia, which always indicate hypoxic episodes, can also be symptoms of seizure activity. Hypertension or hypotension can be signs of intracranial hemorrhage.

Adequate nutrients and calories are needed to promote brain growth. Infants with neurologic damage might require tube feedings because they frequently have weak sucking reflexes. Metabolic imbalances should be avoided because they can cause brain damage. The nurse also monitors body temperature closely because severe neurologic damage can cause temperature instability. Repeated subdural taps may be done to remove blood in cases of severe subdural hemorrhages.

Neonatal seizures are treated with medication, usually phenobarbital. The duration of therapy depends on the causes and severity of the seizures (Horwitz and Amiel-Tison, 1979). Individual requirements vary, so the nurse monitors blood levels to maintain a level of about 20 $\mu g/mL$.

Interventions are clustered during waking periods so that infants have opportunities for rest. Parents also need support so they do not interpret the infant's abnormal state organization as personal rejection.

Other interventions are planned to minimize neurologic handicaps. Abnormalities of movement, such as paralysis, weakness, and abnormal tone, can be minimized by maintaining flexibility and movement through range-of-motion exercises and positioning. Nurses need to continue to hold infants and to provide opportunities for brief interactions, even if the infant appears lethargic and hypotonic. All infants with these problems also should be referred to occupational and physical therapists.

Complications Hydrocephalus is the major complication of intracranial hemorrhage. The bleeding interferes with the circulation of cerebrospinal fluid (CSF) and the CSF accumulates, causing swelling of the head, increased intracranial pressure, and tissue compression. The infant's head circumference increases rapidly, and the fontanelles bulge, although these symptoms might not appear immediately.

In general, the risk of hydrocephalus increases with the severity of the hemorrhage (Ahmann et al., 1980). Early diagnosis and treatment therefore minimize brain damage.

One-third of the cases of hydrocephalus resolve spontaneously (Ahmann et al., 1980), and another third can be managed medically. In the rest, progressive hydrocephalus is managed by shunting (see Chapter 31).

Permanent neurologic disability and mental retardation also may result from any neurologic problem. The degree to which hypoxia causes permanent damage is unclear, but data from animal studies indicate that significant hypoxia must exist for 20 minutes for permanent brain damage to occur (Nelson and Ellenberg, 1981). The longer infants experience birth asphyxia, the more likely they are to develop residual disabilities (Nelson and Ellenberg, 1981). The extent to which brief hypoxic episodes cause permanent disabilities is therefore unknown, but because high-risk infants experience a large number of hypoxic episodes from birth asphyxia, respiratory problems, apnea, malnutrition, anemia, and cardiac problems, hypoxia is probably also a major cause of neurologic problems.

Two frequently seen neurologic problems are epilepsy and cerebral palsy (see Chapter 31). Infants with epilepsy or seizures associated with cerebral palsy might be discharged on anticonvulsants. Parents should be instructed on the importance of giving medications as ordered and on the value of neurologic and developmental follow-up. Some of the infants are able to discontinue medication at later ages, whereas others require treatment throughout their lives. Infants whose seizure disorders begin after discharge should be examined by a neurologist.

The parents of infants with neurologic problems need emotional support. These infants sometimes show behavioral abnormalities such as hyperresponsivity or irritability, which make caring for them unrewarding. When an infant has experienced a serious neurologic insult, such as meningitis or intracranial hemorrhage, most parents are aware of the possibility of permanent brain damage. If health professionals also raise this possibility, parents might interpret the possibility as a certainty, even though predicting whether an individual infant will develop a permanent disability is impossible. Klaus and Kennell (1982) therefore recommend that the possibility of permanent brain damage not be raised and that nurses can instead encourage parents to express their concerns. Nurses then can discuss these concerns realistically and can explain the impossibility of making accurate predictions in the early months.

Parents need support in dealing with this uncertainty. If the infant develops normally, the parent can be reassured that there is no longer any reason to worry. When permanent disabilities occur, parents need assistance in dealing with them. The severely affected infant or child might require institutional care. The nurse then assists in making this decision and provides support to help deal with any guilt this decision causes.

Metabolic Imbalances

High-risk infants cannot maintain metabolic balance as well as healthy full-term infants. The lungs and kidneys of neonates have limited abilities to compensate for excess hydrogen, and so metabolic and respiratory acidosis is common. Many of the enzyme systems necessary to maintain equilibrium are not fully mature in preterm infants. In addition, some infants have congenital abnormalities of enzyme systems affecting metabolic balance (see Chapter 29). (Table 34-1 presents the common metabolic imbalances of high-risk infants.)

A large number of infants of diabetic mothers (IDM) develop hypoglycemia shortly after birth. This problem occurs both in the infants of women with gestational diabetes and those with insulin-dependent diabetes. In the uterus the infant is exposed to excess blood sugar, and the infant's pancreas produces large amounts of insulin to metabolize this sugar. Thus the infant develops large stores of subcutaneous fat and is large for GA.

After birth the infant no longer receives maternal glucose but continues to produce excess insulin for several hours. Hypoglycemia results. When maternal glucose levels are maintained in the normal range for the last 2 months of pregnancy, infants have a lower incidence of hypoglycemia (Jovanic et al., 1981).

Greater survival rates have been attained by monitoring the maternal uterine estriol levels during the third trimester and terminating the pregnancy either by inducing labor or by performing a cesarean section when the estriol level starts to fall. Declining estriol levels indicate placental insufficiency, which places the fetus at risk. Hypoglycemia seldom occurs in the infants whose mothers have diabetes-caused vascular problems because these problems affect the placental vessels and reduce the circulation between mother and infant. The infant of a diabetic mother can experience additional metabolic problems, as well as prematurity, respiratory difficulties, and third-trimester fetal death.

Assessment A variety of different techniques are used in the assessment of metabolic equilibrium. Vital signs and blood pressure are taken at least every 2–4 hours because many metabolic imbalances cause disturbances in vital signs. Cardiac and apnea monitors are needed because metabolic problems cause apnea and bradycardia. Infants are observed closely for the physical symptoms of metabolic disturbances.

Because infants with mild metabolic imbalances usually are asymptomatic and the symptoms that do occur are not specific, laboratory tests are necessary for definitive diag-

TABLE 34-1 Metabolic Imbalances Common During the Neonatal Period

Imbalance	Cause	Symptom	Treatment
Acidosis (excess hydrogen)	Anaerobic metabolism (lactic acid) caused by hypoxia or cold stress	Pallor Tachypnea	Improve oxygenation Place in neutral thermal environment Give sodium bicarbonate or Tham if acidosis persists
Hypoglycemia (deficient blood sugar)	Increased rate of glucose use due to stress (eg, asphyxia, hypothermia, or RDS) Decreased rate of glucose intake Excess insulin (eg, IDM)	Apnea Jitteriness Convulsions Apathy Hypotonia Poor feeding Cyanosis High-pitched cry Temperature instability	Increase glucose intake Reduce energy needs, place in neutral thermal environment Treat sepsis if present, correct acidosis Use steroids
Hyperglycemia (excess blood sugar)	Excess glucose intake	Brain swelling and intraventricular hemorrhage Dehydration	Decrease glucose intake
Hyponatremia (deficient sodium)	Inadequate sodium intake Excess sodium excretion (eg, inappropriate ADH, CAH, or diarrhea) Excess fluid intake or CHF	Apnea Hypotonia Lethargy Convulsions	Increase sodium intake or decrease fluid intake
Hypernatremia (excess sodium)	Excess sodium intake Dehydration	Tremors Lethargy Hypotonia Convulsions	Correct dehydration Decrease sodium intake
Hypocalcemia (deficient calcium)	Deficient calcium intake Stress Treatment of acidosis with bicarbonate Infusion of citrated blood Immaturity of parathyroid gland due to prematurity	Twitching Increased tone Jitteriness Convulsions Prolonged Q-T segment on ECG High-pitched cry Cyanosis Vomiting	Increased calcium intake
Hypokalemia (deficient potassium)	Excess potassium excretion due to diuretics or diarrhea	Low, broad T wave RS-7 deviations Rapid, irregular pulse Malaise	Increase potassium intake
Hyperkalemia (excess potassium)	Infusion of old blood Salt-losing CAH Renal failure	Tent-shaped T wave on ECG	Decrease potassium intake Give kayexalate enemas Administer partial exchange transfusions in life-threatening situations
Hypomagnesemia (deficient magnesium)	Fetal malnutrition IDM Exchange transfusion	Tetany Jitteriness Convulsions S-T depression and T inversion on ECG	Increase magnesium intake
Hypermagnesemia (excess magnesium)	Treatment of mothers with preeclampsia with $MgSO_4$	Cyanosis during feedings Hypotonia Lethargy Poor feeding Rarely—inadequate respiration	Usually none Administer partial exchange transfusions in cases of respiratory depression

noses. The levels of each electrolyte and of glucose in the blood are monitored closely. Urinalysis may also be performed to determine whether there is an excess of electrolytes or glucose being excreted. Blood testing for glucose can be performed right in the nursery using Dextrostix.

Not all cases of gestational diabetes are diagnosed, so all LGA infants should be screened for IDM. Beginning at birth, Dextrostix blood sugar levels should be monitored hourly for 8 hours or until hypoglycemia resolves and then every 4 hours for 24 hours. If the Dextrostix reading is below 45 mg/100 mL, blood sugar levels need to be drawn. Blood sugar levels are frequently elevated immediately after birth in the IDM, so a single elevated reading is not definitive, and blood levels need to be redrawn in about 15–30 minutes. In addition, laboratory tests to check the levels of bilirubin, calcium, magnesium, and potassium, and phosphate are performed because these infants are at risk for imbalances.

Nursing management The goal of nursing care is the early detection and correction of metabolic imbalances, which might require treatment of the underlying problems. (The treatments for common metabolic imbalances of the neonatal period are given in Table 34-1.) In deficiency states, the intake of the metabolite is usually increased, and in situations of excess, intake is decreased. Active attempts to remove excess electrolytes, such as by exchange transfusion, are limited to life-threatening conditions.

After the metabolic disturbance is corrected, the electrolytes and glucose levels continue to be monitored closely whenever the infant is at risk for further metabolic problems. The times of risk for metabolic disturbances include the early postnatal period for all high-risk infants, the periods of serious illnesses for infants with other medical problems, and a period of several months to entire lifetimes for infants with congenital metabolic abnormalities.

Interventions for the IDM include providing a neutral thermal environment, supporting respiration, and monitoring bilirubin levels. Feedings should be started at 2 hours of age with 10% glucose in water and be given every 2 hours until blood glucose level stabilizes. Earlier feedings are sometimes given when early hypoglycemia is present. Infants who cannot tolerate feedings or have blood sugar levels below 30 mg/100 mL are given parenteral infusions of 10% glucose. Because the symptoms of electrolyte imbalance are similar to those of hypoglycemia, the nurse also monitors electrolyte levels.

Complications If untreated, metabolic imbalances can lead to serious complications and death. Acidosis can result in respiratory failure and arrest. Severe respiratory depression in hypermagnesemia might cause respiratory failure. Hyponatremia might cause apnea or shock. Cardiac arrhythmias and cardiac arrest might result from hypocalcemia, hypomagnesemia, or hyperkalemia. Osmotic changes from hyperglycemia increase renal electrolyte and water loss and lead to dehydration.

Brain damage can be caused by metabolic imbalances in any of the following ways: during seizures from hypoglycemia, hypocalcemia, hypomagnesemia, hypernatremia, or hyponatremia; by generalized swelling of the brain from osmotic changes in hyperglycemia causing fluid shifts and increased brain volume and sometimes intraventricular hemorrhage; or by intraventricular hemorrhaging in preterm infants as a result of anoxia and hypernatremia.

⊛ Potential for altered growth and development

Because a variety of risk factors are associated with developmental delay, high-risk infants are more likely to exhibit developmental delays than are normal full-term infants. Risk factors include prematurity, low birth weight, asphyxia, severe illness, and neurologic insult. Generally, the higher the number of risk factors an infant has, the greater the chance the infant will be developmentally delayed. Accuracy of predictions about the extent of developmental delay is not possible in the neonatal period because of four major factors:

1. The neonate's brain development is immature and later brain development can compensate for some insults.
2. Risk factors that actually cause delay cannot yet be identified.
3. Delays appear at different ages, so only long-term follow-up can identify them (see Fig. 34-2).
4. The quality of the home environment can affect the potential for delay.

Ongoing assessment Because delays manifest themselves at different ages, assessment is an ongoing process with the high-risk infant. Assessment includes not only physical growth status but also cognitive skills, social interaction, language, and motor skills, as the child grows. Neurologic assessment (see Chapter 31) is done along with developmental assessment to determine neurologic status.

Tools such as the Brazelton Neonatal Behavior Assessment Scale (see Chapter 4) and the Denver Developmental Screening Test (DDST) (see Appendix C), among others, help the nurse assess developmental delay. Because learning disabilities and hyperactivity are more frequently seen in children who experienced perinatal problems, the nurse assessing an older child who was a high-risk infant questions the parent about school performance and discipline problems (see Chapter 16). The activity level and behavior of these children should be observed during routine follow-up visits.

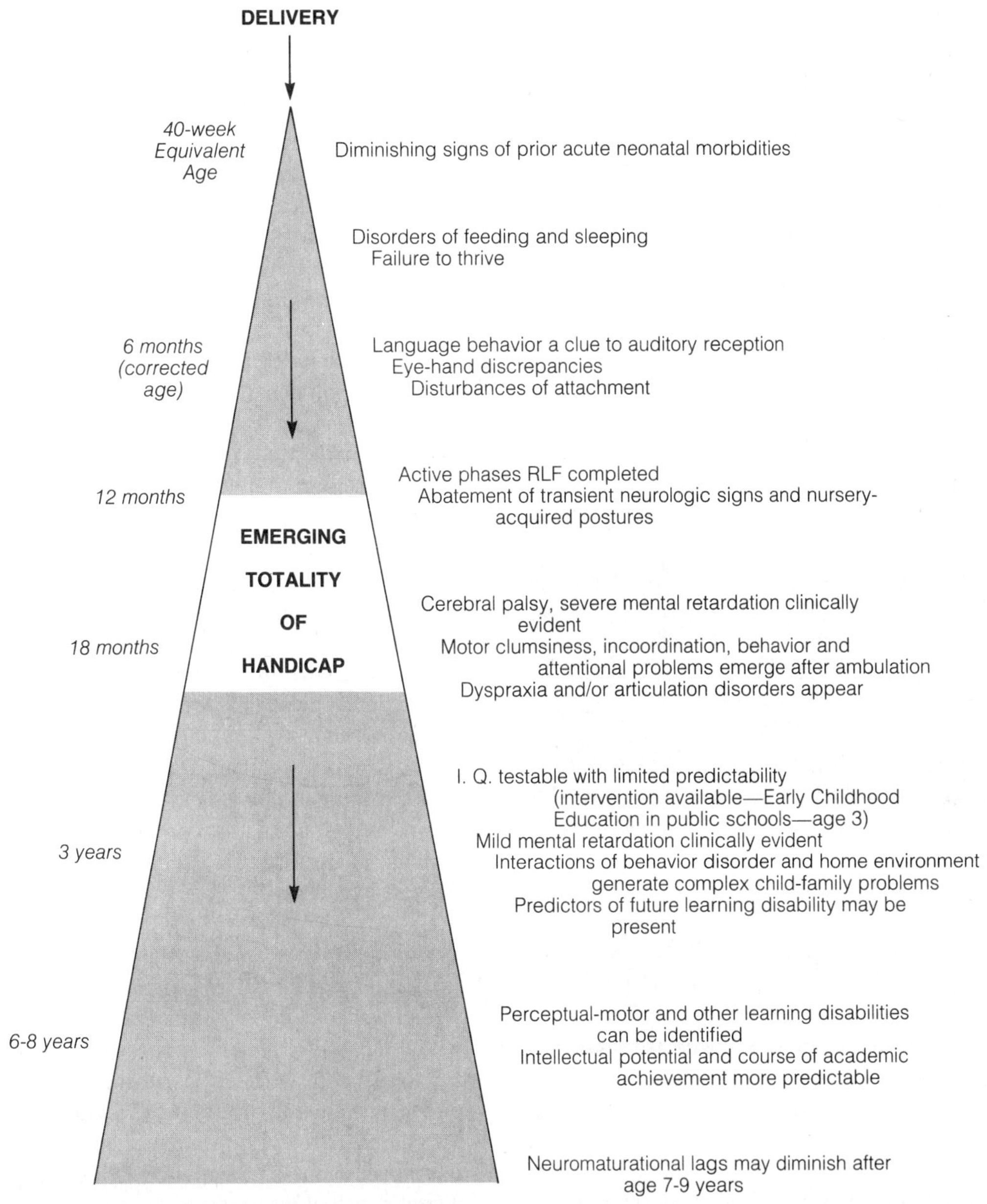
DELIVERY
40-week Equivalent Age
Diminishing signs of prior acute neonatal morbidities
Disorders of feeding and sleeping
Failure to thrive
6 months (corrected age)
Language behavior a clue to auditory reception
Eye-hand discrepancies
Disturbances of attachment
12 months
Active phases RLF completed
Abatement of transient neurologic signs and nursery-acquired postures
EMERGING TOTALITY OF HANDICAP
18 months
Cerebral palsy, severe mental retardation clinically evident
Motor clumsiness, incoordination, behavior and attentional problems emerge after ambulation
Dyspraxia and/or articulation disorders appear
3 years
I. Q. testable with limited predictability (intervention available—Early Childhood Education in public schools—age 3)
Mild mental retardation clinically evident
Interactions of behavior disorder and home environment generate complex child-family problems
Predictors of future learning disability may be present
6-8 years
Perceptual-motor and other learning disabilities can be identified
Intellectual potential and course of academic achievement more predictable
Neuromaturational lags may diminish after age 7-9 years

FIGURE 34-2

Ages at which developmental delays are usually diagnosed in premature and other high-risk infants. (Reproduced with permission from Desmond MM et al: The very low birth weight infant after discharge from intensive care: Anticipatory health care and developmental course. In: Current Problems in Pediatrics. *Gluck L et al (editors). Copyright 1980 by Year Book Medical Publishers, Inc., Chicago.)*

The goals of nursing care are to prevent developmental delays whenever possible, to identify existing delays as early as possible, and to minimize disabilities. Parents need to be informed early about what to look for in infant development. Improving parent awareness of normal development helps parents to identify developmental lags quickly. The nurse explains to the parent exactly what is being observed during any developmental assessment. In this way, the parent can increase observation skills relative to the child's development.

Infant stimulation Many interventions carried out in the NICU can prevent delay in those infants without irreparable neurologic damage. Routine nursing care is modified

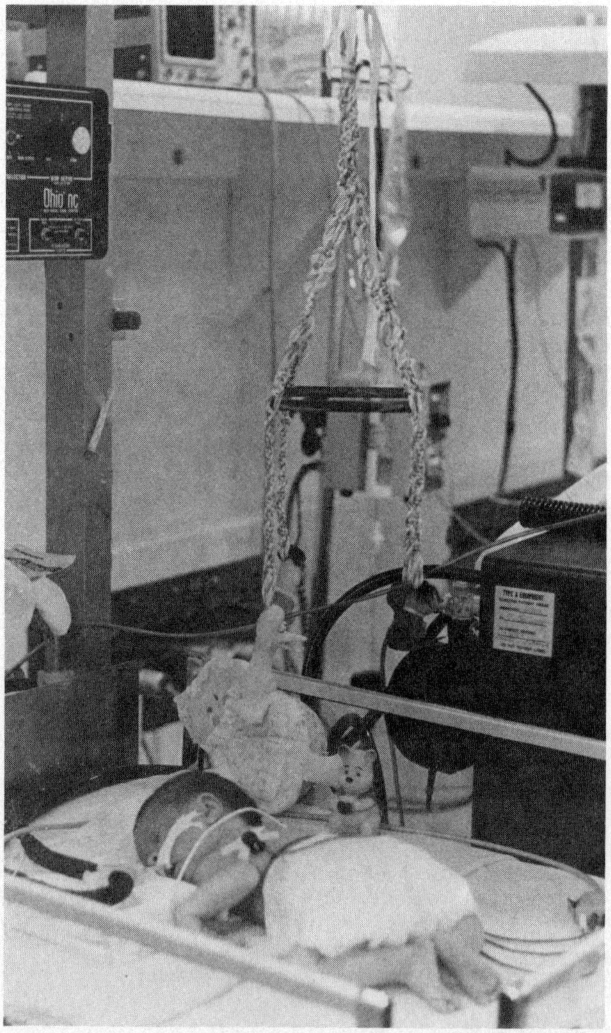

Mobiles and toys hung on a radiant warmer so that a ventilator-dependent infant can see them. (Photograph by Christine Acebo.)

to provide for the infant's developmental needs. During the early stage of illness, the nurse needs to decrease the amount of stimulation that the infant experiences, since even routine nursing care, such as taking vital signs, can be stressful for a sick infant. Infants might actually recover more quickly if they are touched no more frequently than every 4 hours for the first few days of an illness and are instead assessed visually and from monitors. (Suspected deterioration, however, requires interventions that involve touching.)

All infants have a need for rest. Whenever possible, interventions need to be grouped so that infants have periods of undisturbed rest. The lights in the NICU should be dimmed and the sound level decreased several times a day to encourage sleeping.

As the infant's condition improves, the nurse incorporates stimulation lacking in routine NICU care into routine nursing care. Kinesthetic stimulation can be provided by using water beds, by holding and rocking the infant, or by changing the elevation of the infant's head. Affectionate touches and strokes can be given during routine care, and eye-to-eye contact can also be achieved for brief periods. Interesting mobiles, pictures, or toys can be placed where the infant can see them. Responses to infant behaviors, such as picking infants up when they cry, aid the development of the abilities of infants to signal needs, although such stimulation must be individually planned and appropriate to the infant's developmental status.

Parents also are easily included in this type of infant stimulation program and they can assist the nurse to choose stimulation appropriate for the infant. Some types of stimulation—for example, holding the infant during feedings—may be best reserved for the parents.

Overstimulation, a major complication of infant stimulation programs, may be avoided by reducing extraneous stimulation. For instance, one mother of an easily overstimulated premature infant was able to achieve much eye-to-eye contact by placing the infant in an infant seat. Apparently, eye contact while being held was too intense a form of stimulation for this infant (Davis, 1980). Infants attempt to reduce stimulation by gaze aversion or by going into quiet sleep. If excess stimulation continues, oxygen level falls, and the infant might react physiologically by vomiting (Gorski, Hole, & Leonard, 1981).

Multidisciplinary management Most high-risk infants develop normally but have a greater risk of developmental problems than children without perinatal insults. Developmental delays occur despite optimal treatment, but some problems can be avoided. The most common cause of problems is the failure to diagnose a developmental delay and to refer the child to appropriate specialists. Occasionally, pediatricians or nurse practitioners fail to identify a developmental delay because of desire for a positive outcome. Some practitioners also avoid referral in attempts to manage problems on their own.

Multidisciplinary intervention can improve the developmental status of most children. Primary care physicians and nurses seldom have the expertise to plan exercises and games that foster development and coordination of specific muscle groups but should continue to follow these children and provide support for parents.

Alterations in parenting

The birth of a high-risk infant is a crisis for a family, and many psychologic factors can interfere with parenting. These factors include:

1. Premature birth renders the parents unable to prepare for the infant.
2. The appearance of premature infants differs markedly from that of a full-term newborn and parents need to adjust to the characteristics of their infant.
3. The guilt that a parent feels after the birth of a high-risk infant interferes with the ability to form a relationship with that infant.
4. The activities of the NICU interfere with the attachment process between parent and infant.
5. Because of distance or other responsibilities, the parent might not be able to visit the infant, thus preventing the attachment process.
6. Ill high-risk infants are not as responsive as normal full-term infants and are not able to participate in reciprocal interactions early in life.

Because parenting is a process, the relationship between a parent and an infant continues to grow and change. Repeated assessments therefore are necessary to determine both the degree of parental involvement with the infant and the infant's interactional abilities.

Indicators of dysfunctional parenting Because psychologic disturbances can interfere with parental abilities to relate to the infant, parents need to be encouraged to discuss their feelings. Potential parenting problems are indicated by the inability to express guilt or responsibility, apparent lack of anxiety about the infant's condition, and lack of interest in information about the infant. These parents seldom phone for information if they can't be with the infant. Interruptions in usual communication patterns and perceived lack of support can indicate problems. Parents who are still preparing for the possible loss of the infant are not ready to begin a nurturing relationship.

The parent's ability to cope with psychologic problems is related to the parent's developmental stage. For example, adolescents, young adult, and middle-aged parents handle these problems differently. Supportive family and friends can assist parents with psychologic difficulties. Family members and friends involved in the care of the infant also need an opportunity to discuss their feelings, as they too experience emotional difficulties in dealing with a high-risk infant.

Lack of touching behavior is another indicator of problems. The normal touching behaviors of parents with a full-term infant (eg, touching with fingertips, stroking, then encircling and holding) occur within the space of several minutes. Parents of high-risk infants might take several weeks to progress from one to the other. No matter how hesitant parents are to touch their infants at first, they should gradually progress through the various stages of touching and begin to assume some aspects of care.

Nursing goals The general goals to promote parenting remain constant: (1) providing support for parents in resolving their feelings of disappointment, anger, guilt, and responsibility and in progressing through their developmental and psychologic tasks of parenting, (2) helping them to view their infant as an individual with unique characteristics, and (3) promoting positive interactions between parents and infants.

Promoting parent-infant attachment Interventions to promote healthy parenting begin at birth. If desired, the father should be present in the delivery room. In any case, both parents need to have an opportunity to see and touch the infant before transfer to the nursery, and they should be allowed to hold the infant if the infant's condition permits. When the mother has received a general anesthetic and is unable to see the infant immediately after delivery, she should be allowed to see and touch the infant as soon as possible.

Moderately ill infants can sometimes remain with their mothers and be cared for by the recovery room nurse. For example, the blood glucose level and vital signs of a full-term infant of a well-controlled diabetic mother can be monitored by the recovery room nurse, thus reassuring the mother and facilitating bonding.

More seriously ill infants need to be transferred to the nursery, but their parents can still participate in their care. One father bottle-fed his hypoglycemic baby shortly after birth. Later, he was able to reassure his wife that the infant ate well and was not as sick as she had thought.

Some critically ill infants must be transferred to NICUs located in other hospitals. A transport team consisting of a physician and one or more nurses then accompanies the infant, and as this team is usually from the referral hospital, team members can inform the parents about the unit's policies, and consent forms can be signed. Both parents should be allowed to see and touch the infant prior to departure. When the father accompanies the infant, he should be given an opportunity to see the infant as soon as the admission procedures are complete. In addition, the admitting nurse should phone the mother to give her a progress report.

Because infant transport involves medical risks to the infant and separation from the mother, many perinatal centers are accepting transports of high-risk mothers prior to delivery. Thus, medical facilities are readily available to the infant, and the proximity of infant and mother encourages attachment.

Providing support in the NICU A variety of interventions are used in the NICU to provide support. Supportive counseling assists parents in resolving the crisis. Ideally, this support should be provided by the infant's nurse. The nurse develops a plan for parental support and teaching, which includes teaching parents about the infant's capabilities, demonstrating these abilities for parents, and serving as a role model for interactions. The nurse can also promote self-esteem in the parents by emphasizing their essential role in the infant's recovery.

The nurse provides parents with frequent reports about the infant. Even if frequent visits are impossible, parents can begin to relate to their infant if given information about individual activities and developmental accomplishments, such as, "She sleeps best on her right side" or "He looked at your picture today." Incubators can be decorated for special occasions; for example, one group of parents was delighted to find Valentine's Day cards, addressed to them from their infants, on the incubators.

The development of a healthy relationship between parents and high-risk infants may be complicated by several factors. Occasionally, nurses become attached to infants and compete with the parents for the infant's affection. Needless to say, this type of competition prevents nurses from working effectively with families. Nurses develop these attachments as a way of coping with the stresses involved in neonatal intensive care and obtain gratification by feeling parental affection for the infants. (A primary nursing system, in which the nurse immediately develops a commitment to both the infant and the parents, can help avoid the development of this competition, while still providing rewards for the nurse.)

Encouraging parental involvement The nurse also encourages parental involvement in infant care and provides individually planned care for infants and parents as well as goals that can be accomplished together. Schraeder (1980) outlines three stages of parenting behaviors: (a) initial touching and acquaintance, (b) caregiving, and (c) incorporating the infant into the family. Nurses thus assist parents in moving through these stages by demonstrating nurturing behaviors and by encouraging parents to perform activities appropriate to their stage of parenting.

In the acquaintance stage, nurses encourage parents to visit and phone frequently. Most NICUs allow 24-hour visiting for parents, and studies have shown that parents value this opportunity. Parents believe that the infants feel loved when visited (Yu, Jamieson, & Astbury, 1981). Other caregivers also need opportunities to visit; grandparents and siblings, for instance, should see the infant even if only through a viewing window. When the mother is in another hospital, the nurse maintains frequent phone contact and provides photographs or videotapes of the infant.

In the second stage of parenting behavior, parents begin to assume caregiving responsibilities. As the infant's condition permits, they should be encouraged to hold, feed, and change the infant. The nurse also includes parents in decisions about infant care, such as when to feed or bathe the

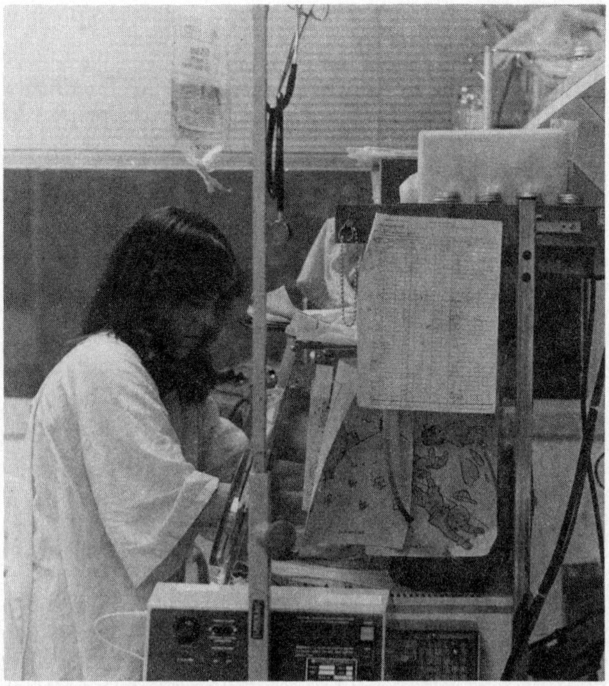

Drawings from siblings have been placed on the incubator of a high-risk infant. (Photograph by Christine Acebo.)

infant. Parents can help the nurse in planning an appropriate infant stimulation program (Schraeder, 1980) and can provide clothes, toys, and photographs of the family to decorate the incubator or warmer. Siblings often feel more involved with the infant when they provide drawings for the baby.

In the final stage, as parents incorporate the infant into the family, they need to assume control over infant care in preparation for discharge and to learn to perform any necessary medical procedures. The nurse plans individual care for the infant, parent, and other caregivers during all three stages.

The period just prior to hospital discharge requires special interventions because the parents are losing the familiar supports of the NICU. Approximately half of the infants are transferred back to the referring hospital prior to discharge, which allows them to complete recovery and to grow in an intermediate care setting, which is closer to their parents' homes. The nurse therefore contacts the other hospital to familiarize the nurses there with the infant's nursing care plan, the degree of parental involvement, and the ongoing plan. The parent is informed about the policies of the new nursery, such as the visiting hours for family and friends and whether rooming-in is possible. After transfer, the nurse can ease the transition by remaining available for phone consultations with the new nursery and the parent.

Preventing family dysfunction Family dysfunction is another complication in the early progress of parenting high-risk infants. Parents are more likely to relinquish high-risk infants to foster care or adoption than they are healthy full-term infants (Klaus and Kennell, 1982).

In addition, the stresses involved with having a high-risk infant can lead to other dysfunctional behaviors. Siblings might develop behavioral problems or parents might fail to communicate with each other except through arguments. Not surprisingly, the divorce and separation rate is higher for parents of high-risk infants than for parents of healthy infants (Klaus and Kennell, 1982). The infant might also become a source of tension between parents and other family members. High-risk infants are more likely to be the victims of child abuse and neglect than are healthy full-term infants (see Chapter 13).

High-risk infants often are unresponsive or irritable in the early weeks. Thus they do not provide many rewards for their parents. As a result, parents might experience mild depression. If parents do not have nursing support available, they might exhibit strange behaviors in an effort to obtain it. One mother of a premature infant refused all help, but a few days after her infant's discharge, she called the NICU and stated that she felt like abusing the infant. Investigation showed that the mother was very good with the infant and that they had many positive interactions. A public health nurse then spent long hours talking with the mother. Although the mother continued to insist that she did not need help, she no longer worried about hurting the infant.

Additional interventions are needed for multiple births. The parents must be helped to view the infants as individuals so that they can develop special feelings for each one (Gromada, 1981; Klaus and Kennell, 1982). A special problem arises when one infant dies and the other lives. The parent must grieve for the one while trying to form a relationship with the other. Because these two activities are mutually exclusive, the parent needs a great deal of support so that both grieving and attachment can occur (Klaus and Kennel, 1982).

Referral for counseling may involve psychologists and psychiatrists who work with parents who have unresolved emotional problems. Social workers assist families with financial difficulties, housing problems, and family problems. Clergy provide assistance with spiritual problems, which is particularly important, as some parents view the birth of a high-risk infant as a punishment from God.

Peer counseling can also help parents in resolving their emotional disturbances. Parents of high-risk infants experience similar anxieties and stresses and thus can provide support for each other. Support can be given by experienced parents of high-risk infants or by support groups made up of new parents and a nurse. Often, support continues after discharge.

⊛ Parental knowledge deficit

Parents of high-risk infants have a special need for education about infant care. Parents usually make their preparations for the infant in the last trimester of pregnancy. At this point, they read child care books and talk with friends and relatives to learn about feeding methods, routine care, and infant development.

During a high-risk pregnancy, however, parents might be afraid to become too involved with the infant, and parents of premature infants have not had this preparation period. Even if the parents did prepare for the infant during pregnancy, their anxiety over the infant's condition might cause them to forget much of what they had learned. In addition, high-risk infants often require medical treatment after discharge, and parents of high-risk infants therefore need education about the infant's special needs along with information about infant care and normal growth and development.

Information about development is especially important for the parents of premature infants. Unless they are taught the importance of age correction, for example, they expect the infant to develop at the same rate as a full-term infant born at the same time. Thus they may come to believe the infant is delayed when the infant is instead developing as expected for the corrected age.

The nurse assesses the parents' level of knowledge about infant care, infant development, and the special needs of their own infant. The parents' and other caregivers' abilities to understand explanations and their readiness to learn also are determined. Information about development is of little value if given to the mother, for instance, when the grandmother will be caring for the baby.

The goals of nursing care are to determine the level of knowledge about infant care of all potential caregivers and to provide any additional information they need to be effective. Anticipatory guidance that includes information about infant needs generally is part of child health nursing (see Chapter 11), but parents of high-risk infants often need special assistance. Parents are unable to make preparations for the infant's care until they believe the baby will survive, so the nurse plans parent teaching after the critical stage of illness has passed.

Anticipatory guidance Specific topics that might need to be covered include infant development up to 3 months of age, feeding methods, bathing, diapering, identifying childhood illnesses, giving medications, taking temperatures, and performing any special medical treatments. The nurse also discusses the importance of affection and appropriate stimulation to an infant. Many parents appreciate being referred to appropriate child care books.

Information about caregiving techniques and medical

treatments is explained and then demonstrated by the nurse. Parents then need opportunities to practice these skills so that prior to discharge they are performing much of the infant's care.

Discharge preparation The rooming-in period is the ideal point to assess parental skills and evaluate the success of parent teaching. Spending a day or two rooming-in with the infant gives the parents a final opportunity to consult with nurses and experience success in providing care to foster their confidence as parents.

If the parents choose not to room-in or if rooming-in is not available for them, this evaluation can be part of routine health care visits. The nurse might need to encourage parents to discuss any questions they have about infant care so that if parents continue to exhibit knowledge deficits, the nurse can use different teaching strategies.

Discharge of the infant is an important step for parents. Suddenly the parent is faced with providing all of the infant's care. Additional interventions thus assist the parent in making the transition from the NICU or community hospital to home. The parent needs competence in performing routine infant care and any special medical treatments that the infant requires. To identify parental concerns about discharge and to plan additional teaching, a predischarge conference is held with the parent, any other caregivers, the nurse, the neonatologist, and other interested staff members. The parent often benefits from rooming-in with the infant for a day or two prior to discharge so that help from experienced professionals is available as the parent begins to provide total infant care (Klaus and Kennell, 1982; Varner, Ossenkop, & Lyon, 1980).

Families are referred to public health nurses so that they can continue to receive support. In addition, the nurse phones the parent within a few days after discharge to learn how the infant is doing. All parents experience a dramatic change in their lives after an infant comes home, but high-risk infants are particularly disruptive. If the infant has been hospitalized for several weeks, the parent has adjusted to life without an infant. The mother has often returned to work to help pay medical bills and with the infant's arrival home must adjust to being a full-time mother.

A recently published study by Brooten et al. (1986) on premature infants discharged early from the hospital yielded interesting data. The study found that premature infants weighing from 2 to 4 pounds experienced a similar course at home as infants of similar weight kept in the hospital. The early release of the premature infant reduced costs by approximately $18,560. Apparently, early discharge of the premature infant not only results in considerable financial savings but also results in a decrease in risk factors for the infant. The project involved healthy low-birthweight infants and required on-call nursing round-the-clock for 18 months. The considerable emotional and developmental savings might make this a viable alternative to hospitalization in the future.

Additional information should be provided as part of nursing follow-up after discharge. Public health nurses and nurses in developmental follow-up clinics need to plan ongoing teaching to inform parents about developmental changes, types of stimulation that infants need at different ages, changes in medical treatments, and care of older infants and children.

Considerations for Home Care of the High-Risk Infant

- Because infants might experience cold stress after discharge, teach parents to recognize symptoms of cold stress: cold hands and feet, peripheral cyanosis, irritability. Minimize heat loss by clothing and covering infant and by preventing exposure to cold surfaces. Also teach parents to recognize signs of overheating.
- Because high-risk infants remain susceptible to infections for at least 3 months postterm, close nursing follow-up is necessary. Instruct parents to avoid crowds and people who are obviously ill. All infants treated with aminoglycosides should have hearing tested.
- If infants are sent home with apnea monitor, assist parents in learning to manage the monitor and to stimulate infant breathing. Support parents in dealing with their anxiety over caregiving responsibility. Refer to support groups of other parents of infants with prolonged apnea, if available.
- High-risk infants continue to have greater-than-normal nutritional needs after hospital discharge. Support mother who chooses to breast-feed infant and counsel on alternative methods of supplementation, such as Lact-Aid system, which requires less sucking ability of the infant.
- To promote maximum development possible in infants with developmental delays, use routine follow-up visits to instruct parents about normal infant development and particular capabilities of their infant. Refer to early intervention programs if available and appropriate. Assist parents to develop realistic expectations for results of intervention.
- Assess for potential parenting problems in follow-up after discharge. Teach parents appropriate behaviors to express feelings of affection for infant while recognizing infant's limited available energy.

Neonatal Death

Despite recent improvement in perinatal care, infant mortality remains a major problem. All nurses working with high-risk infants will thus at some time need to help parents accept the death of a newborn. Parents who have lost an infant experience the same stages of grief as anyone experiencing a major loss (see Chapter 17).

Some factors, however, are unique to a neonatal death. Parental guilt might be prolonged when the parent feels or is partially responsible for the death (for example, a diabetic mother who did not control her blood sugar level). The parent might have to mourn the loss of the hoped-for perfect baby as well as the real one.

Generally, a newborn infant who dies is not recognized as a person. Thus mothers and fathers of first-born infants who die lose their status as parents (Borg and Lasker, 1981). Parents are often comforted with such statements as, "It's for the best," "The baby would have been brain-damaged," or "You can always have another baby," which deny the reality of the parents' grief. Funerals are often not held for infants, especially those who were premature. Therefore, helping the parents to work through their grief is an important nursing role, especially as the degree to which they resolve their grief will influence their relationships with their other children and each other.

Specific Problems of High-Risk Infants

Respiratory Disorders

Several specific respiratory disorders are associated with prematurity and a variety of other risk factors.

Respiratory distress syndrome Respiratory distress syndrome (RDS) is a respiratory problem caused by a deficiency of surfactant in the immature lungs of premature infants. In infants with RDS, alveolar collapse is the cause of inadequate ventilation. RDS occurs primarily in infants with birthweights between 1000 and 1500 g (2 1/4 and 3 1/2 lb) and is a major cause of mortality in the neonatal period. Alveolar collapse results from surfactant deficiency and can lead to the collapse of segments of the lungs (atelectasis).

Symptoms of RDS include expiratory grunting, retractions, nasal flaring, cyanosis, tachypnea, and diminished breath sounds. This syndrome begins within a few hours after birth, progressively worsens for about 2 days, and usually improves within 5 days. Severity of symptoms varies.

RDS is treated with oxygen administration. Some infants require only a small amount of supplemental oxygen to recover. Others die despite mechanical ventilation and intensive nursing care.

Lower airway blockage occurs in transient tachypnea, in meconium aspiration, and in pneumonia. Transient tachypnea is a mild disease that occurs in full-term infants and older preterm infants, particularly those born by cesarean section or depressed by obstetric drugs. Delayed clearing of fluid from the alveoli after birth interferes with gas exchange. Infants with transient tachypnea recover within 48 hours after birth and rarely require more treatment than environmental oxygen. Symptoms are similar to mild RDS.

Meconium aspiration and pneumonia Meconium aspiration and pneumonia may occur in both premature and full-term infants. In meconium aspiration, the infant aspirates meconium-contaminated amniotic fluid, and the foreign material in the lungs then interferes with gas exchange in the alveoli and may cause atelectasis. Pneumonia, an infection of the lungs, occurs as either a congenital infection or a complication of other dysfunctions or procedures. Endotracheal intubation, for example, allows bacteria to enter the lungs, so that when atelectasis is present the collapsed areas provide excellent sites for bacterial growth.

The increased secretions caused by pneumonia also interfere with air exchange. Symptoms of meconium aspiration and pneumonia include cyanosis, mild retractions, tachypnea, and hypoactivity. Breath sounds are diminished over areas of atelectasis, and crepitant rales may be heard in other areas. Both meconium aspiration and pneumonia cause increased pulmonary secretions, but in the early stages of meconium aspiration, the secretions are meconium tinged.

Apnea Apnea (cessation of respiration) is seen in many premature infants. Instead of respiratory pauses, these infants have prolonged apneic episodes that cause hypoxia and bradycardia. The duration of an apneic pause that makes it pathologic is uncertain, but episodes longer than 20 seconds are considered abnormal. Severe apnea can lead to respiratory arrest and death. Because this problem is caused by the immaturity of the central nervous system, it improves as the infant matures. Other conditions that can cause prolonged apnea include sepsis, hypoglycemia, dehydration, hypocalcemia, cardiac abnormalities, and neurologic damage. Apnea caused by these conditions improves only when the underlying problem is treated.

A small percentage of infants with apnea do not improve by term age. Others develop prolonged apnea, which is confirmed by a pneumogram, a 12- to 24-hour recording of an infant's respiratory pattern. These infants often have chronic lung disease, chronic neurologic disabilities, cardiac defects, or siblings who died from sudden infant death syndrome (SIDS). These infants may be treated with theophylline, a bronchodilator, to decrease bronchospasms that may occlude the airway. Infants with prolonged apnea are sent home with apnea monitors to be used during sleep because of the danger that a prolonged apneic episode might lead to respiratory arrest. If breathing ceases for 15 to 20 seconds, the alarm sounds and summons the parent.

Parents need to learn to manage the monitor and to stimulate infant breathing. They need support in dealing with their anxiety about their infants, their knowledge that they are responsible for their infants' survival, and their isolation from other parents (Dimaggio and Sheetz, 1983). Thus these parents often benefit from joining support groups with other parents of infants with prolonged apnea.

Discharge Considerations: The Infant on Apnea Monitoring

- Demonstrate to the parents how to connect the monitor leads and other aspects of the monitor. Remind parents to remove the leads unless they are connected to the infant and to keep the monitor unplugged when not in use (Jackson, 1986). If possible, use a machine similar to what will be used at home.
- Remind parents that the infant needs to be monitored whenever respirations are not being directly observed. Explain that the infant will need direct observation whenever loud noises would obscure the monitor alarm (eg, vacuuming, dishwasher).
- Teach the parents how to assess the infant for apnea (observe color and respirations).
- Teach the parents to attempt to physically stimulate the infant if the infant is apneic (eg, touching the face, sternum, or sole of the foot).
- Demonstrate cardiopulmonary resuscitation to be used if tactile stimulation is not effective.
- Have the parents contact the local emergency personnel and inform them that the child is being monitored. Keep the emergency numbers prominently displayed in the home.
- Recommend electrical inspection of the monitor at frequent intervals.
- Encourage the parents to teach another responsible person resuscitation so that parents can go out together occasionally.
- Encourage the parents to relieve one another to participate in an outside interest.
- Explain that monitoring need not interfere with the infant's development, and encourage the parents to promote normal development as much as possible.
- Refer the family to a community health nurse for follow-up and support and to a monitoring support group.

Bronchopulmonary dysplasia and Wilson-Mikity syndrome Impaired gas exchange is the cause of respiratory problems in *bronchopulmonary dysplasia* (BPD) and *Wilson-Mikity syndrome.* BPD occurs in infants with RDS who have been treated with mechanical ventilation. It is apparently caused by oxygen toxicity and pressure damage in the lungs. Wilson-Mikity syndrome occurs after the first week of life in infants with birthweights less than 1000 g and is not related to oxygen therapy. In both conditions, chronic changes in the lungs, including thickening and necrosis of alveolar walls and bronchiolar linings, impair the diffusion of oxygen from the alveoli to the capillaries. These infants require respiratory support—additional oxygen and often mechanical ventilation—for weeks or months.

Infants who develop chronic lung disease (BPD or Wilson-Mikity syndrome) require long-term hospital treatment and their parents therefore need support in developing positive relationships with their infants. Parents should be encouraged to participate in caregiving and in specific respiratory treatments so that they can learn the needs and capabilities of their infants. A few infants with chronic lung disease require continued respiratory support for months, or even years. These infants should be managed at home, where they can experience normal family stimulation. (These aspects of chronic illness are discussed in Chapter 14.)

For chronically ill infants, oxygen can be administered by nasal catheter or nasal cannula during the day and by an oxygen tent at night. Some of these infants require tracheostomies either with or without a ventilator. Their parents can be taught tracheostomy care, chest physiotherapy, and suctioning.

The physical and psychologic development of infants with chronic lung disease is as important as their respiratory care. Because infancy is marked by development of locomotion and speech, infant jumpers and walkers can enable infants with chronic lung disease to practice their gross motor skills despite the restrictions posed by oxygen equipment. Parents should be encouraged to talk and sing to their infants to stimulate their speech capabilities. Young children with tracheostomies learn to make noises by covering the tracheostomy opening briefly (Kennedy, Johnson, & Sturdevant, 1982).

Necrotizing Enterocolitis (NEC)

A life-threatening complication is necrotizing enterocolitis (NEC), which strikes some high-risk infants, particularly those who are premature. It is characterized by necrosis of the mucosa of the large and small bowel. The necrotic areas are localized at first but spread rapidly and cause bowel perforation or infarction. An episode of hypoxia in the prenatal period predisposes an infant to NEC by causing the blood to be shunted away from the gut. This decrease in tissue perfusion makes the bowel susceptible to infection so infants with immature or compromised immunologic systems are particularly at risk for NEC (Smith, 1981). The carbohydrates of feedings allow the bacteria to proliferate; thus high-calorie formulas (with more than 20–24 calories per ounce) are particularly associated with NEC (Walsh and Kliegman, 1985).

Early symptoms include increases in gastric aspirates, abdominal distension, occult blood in the stool, bile-stained emesis, lethargy, temperature instability, and hypotension. If not treated early, this condition worsens rapidly. Medical treatment is supportive: resting the bowel by discontinuing feedings and providing hyperalimentation, administering antibiotics to treat the infection, ensuring adequate intravenous fluids for hydration, and closely monitoring the infant's vital signs and general condition. If the infant's condition deteriorates, surgery is performed to remove the necrotic bowel. Despite the best treatment, 20%–40% of affected infants die (Walsh and Kliegman, 1985). Early treatment improves the survival rate.

Sudden Infant Death Syndrome

Sudden infant death syndrome (SIDS) is currently the leading cause of postneonatal death in the United States, claiming 7000–10,000 lives each year and accounting for about one-third of all deaths in infants aged 1 week to 1 year (Adams, 1984). A great deal of research, debate, and uncertainty surrounds this phenomenon, which can not only intensify a parent's bewilderment and grief but also cloud the health professional's ability to give care.

Also called "crib death" or "cot death," SIDS refers to the sudden and unexpected death of an infant who has been previously healthy, with the cause of death being still unexplained after a thorough postmortem examination.

The relationship between SIDS and infant apnea has been the focus of much clinical attention and some debate. When an infant is discovered to have stopped breathing for a long period of time (20 seconds or more) but later recovers (frequently in the emergency room), the situation often is termed a case of "aborted" or "near-miss" SIDS. Many hospitals now have home-monitoring programs to allow home care for the infant with apneic spells. Some clinicians, however, feel that the term "near-miss SIDS" is inappropriate and that infant apnea and SIDS are two distinct syndromes, with the latter being confirmed only by an autopsy and therefore unpreventable (Bakke and Dougherty, 1981; Sperhac, 1982). Other authorities feel that the two syndromes are related, with infant apnea being "a symptom as well as a cause" of SIDS, and that home apnea monitoring is in fact a measure to prevent SIDS (Ariagno, 1984). In actuality only 5% of SIDS deaths are related to apnea (McClain, 1985).

Although the incidence of SIDS is increased in siblings, no genetic cause has been found. Current theories propose that SIDS might be the result of a neurologic learning deficit (Greenberg, 1984), or possibly that it might be related to an immature hematopoetic system (Giulian et al., 1987).

Assessment Risk factors associated with SIDS have been identified. SIDS affects primarily boys (61%) aged 2–4 months of age. The incidence is four times higher in low-birthweight infants. Other risk factors are identified as family occurrence of SIDS, mother younger than age 20 years, and a higher incidence in black infants (McClain, 1985).

Nursing management Although studies have drawn attention to the reactions of family members in cases of SIDS and the appropriate nursing interventions (Mandell, McAnulty, and Reece, 1980; Nikolaisen, 1981; Mandell, McAnulty, and Carlson, 1983), these reactions are virtually all identical in kind to those felt by survivors of children who died of other causes—guilt, denial, intellectualization, anger, and so forth. In cases of SIDS, however, the nurse can be instrumental in helping the family deal with the shock caused by the unanticipated nature of the event, the bewilderment resulting from the still unanswered questions concerning the cause, and the parents' own guilt. Parental guilt stems from their assumption that the parents somehow must have been the cause. These feelings can complicate and intensify the grief process.

Another by-product of the lack of a definitive explanation can be a tragic withdrawal of the family's social support because friends, neighbors, grandparents, and even health care providers who are uninformed about SIDS might hold the parents responsible and shun them. The nurse plays an important role in explaining to parents and those around them that SIDS is a specific, identified condition but one that is poorly understood as yet.

With SIDS cases, the nurse's task might be more complex, but it is essentially the same as in other cases of pediatric death. Supporting the family by decreasing feelings of isolation and rejection becomes particularly important. Aiding parents in the detachment process by letting them hold and spend time with the dead infant is another useful intervention. Making sure that the lines of communication among all family members, especially surviving siblings, remain as open as possible is just as important in SIDS as in other cases of childhood death. Parents need to be encouraged to explain the circumstances of the infant's death to the siblings. Families of SIDS infants might be more prone to react to their grief by moving away or breaking up the family, so the nurse should be especially careful to make early intervention after the death of the infant a high priority.

Support either by the community health nurse or by the national SIDS organization can be helpful.

Essential Concepts

- The development of neonatal intensive care has improved the prognosis for high-risk infants and has created a nursing and medical field of specialization.
- Both an infant's social development and the process by which the infant is incorporated into the family are greatly altered by serious illness and the environment of the NICU.
- Risk factors associated with the birth of a high-risk infant are both biologic and psychosocial.
- High-risk infants are classified on the basis of gestational age at birth and body size.
- Developmental assessment for high-risk infants requires correction for prematurity when comparing the assessment data to norms for growth and development.
- Neuromuscular development—including muscle tone, reflexes, and sleep-wake states—is affected by neurologic damage and prematurity.
- To develop and learn social skills, the infant needs to have the opportunity for reciprocal interactions with nurturing adults.
- Inadequate heat regulation in high-risk infants might lead to cold stress, which requires nursing interventions to control environmental temperature and prevent complications.
- Immaturity of the immunologic system in high-risk infants leaves the infants susceptible to infection and thus requires interventions planned to prevent exposure to bacteria.
- Respiratory assessment for high-risk infants involves monitoring vital signs, observing physical symptoms, and taking blood gases.
- Nursing management for respiratory dysfunction in high-risk infants involves supportive interventions to maintain adequate oxygenation and prevent complications.
- Nutritional deficiencies in high-risk infants may be caused by impaired ability to suck, increased calorie requirements due to serious illness, diminished stomach capacity, or impaired digestion.
- Lack of adequate growth is the principal indicator of nutritional deficiency.
- Feedings for high-risk infants may be breast milk, which is preferable, or formula; feedings may be given orally or through gavage, continuous tube feedings, or parenteral fluids.
- Immaturity of an infant's circulatory system may lead to a patent ductus arteriosus, congestive heart failure, or fluid overload.
- Nursing management for circulatory problems is planned to maintain oxygenation, reduce the workload of the heart, and prevent fluid overload and complications.
- Neurologic damage in the neonatal period is usually caused by hypoxia, birth trauma, hemorrhage, or infection.
- Assessment for neurologic dysfunction includes physical symptoms, behavioral changes, and laboratory tests.
- Nursing management for neurologic problems focuses on minimizing disabilities, which may include alterations in muscle tone, weakness or paralysis of an extremity, abnormal sleep-wake state patterns, and seizure activity.
- Maintaining metabolic homeostasis requires early detection and correction of metabolic imbalances.
- Infants of diabetic mothers require assessment for hypoglycemia in the early postnatal period.
- High-risk infants are more likely to exhibit developmental delays than are normal full-term infants.
- Accurate predictions of developmental delays are not possible in the neonatal period, so developmental assessment to identify problems is an ongoing process.
- Nurses can promote positive parenting by assisting parents in resolving their emotional reactions to their infants' status and in helping them to view their infants as individuals capable of positive interactions.
- Parents of high-risk infants have special needs for health teaching to care for their infants.

- Parents should be encouraged to assume as much responsibility as possible for care of their infants before hospital discharge.
- In the event of neonatal death, parents and other family members might need assistance in working through their grief and accepting the infant's death.

References

Adams FE: Six very good reasons why we react differently to various dying patients. *Nurs '84* (June) 1984; 14(6): 41–43.

Ahmann PA et al: Intraventricular hemorrhage in the high-risk pre-term infant: Incidence and outcome. *Ann Neurol* 1980; 7:118–124.

Anderson CC et al: *Nonnutritive Sucking Opportunities: A Safe and Effective Treatment for Premature Infants.* Presented at Int. Conf. on Infant Studies, New Haven, Conn., March 1980.

Ariagno RL: Evaluation and management of infantile apnea. *Pediatr Ann* (March) 1984; 13(3): 210–213.

Bakke K, Dougherty J: Sudden infant death syndrome and infant apnea: Current questions, clinical management, and research directions. *Issues Compr Pediatr Nurs* 1981; 5:77–88.

Ballard JL, Kazmaier K, Driver M: A simplified assessment of gestational age, abstracted. *Pediatr Res* 1977; 11:374.

Boettcher MD, Pereira GR: Nutritional management of the critically ill neonate. In: *Neonatal and Pediatric Critical Care Nursing.* Stahler-Miller K (editor). Churchill Livingstone, 1983.

Boggs KR, Rau PK: Breastfeeding the premature infant. *Am J Nurs* 1983; 83:1436–1444.

Borg S, Lasker J: *When Pregnancy Fails.* Beacon Press, 1981.

Brooten D et al: A randomized trial of early hospital discharge and home follow-up of very-low-birth-weight infants. *N Engl J Med* (October 9, 1986); 315(15): 934–939.

Davis DH: *The Social Competency of Premature Infants Discharged From the Hospital Prior to Forty Weeks Conceptional Age,* Master's degree thesis. University of Connecticut, 1980.

Desmond MM et al: The very low birth weight infant after discharge from intensive care: Anticipatory health care and developmental course. *Curr Probs Pediatr* (Apr) 1980; 10:1–59.

Dimaggio GT, Sheetz AH: The concerns of mothers caring for an infant on an apnea monitor. *Am J Matern-Child Nurs* 1983; 8:294–297.

Dingle RE et al: Continuous transcutaneous O_2 monitoring in the neonate. *Am J Nurs* 1980; 80:890–893.

Dubowitz LMS, Dubowitz V, Goldberg C: Clinical assessment of gestational age in the newborn infant. *J Pediatr* 1970; 77:1–10.

Fanaroff AA, Klauss MH: The gastrointestinal tract—feeding and selected disorders. Pages 113–145 in: *Care of the High Risk Infant.* 2nd ed. Klaus MH, Fanaroff AA (editors). Saunders, 1979.

Gale E: Neonatal seizures. In: *Protocols for Perinatal Nursing Practice.* Perez RH (editor). Mosby, 1981.

Greenberg J: Infant death tied to dopamine excess. *Science News* (Sept 15) 1984; 126(11): 165.

Gromada K: Maternal-infants attachment. The first step toward individualizing twins. *Am J Matern-Child Nurs* 1981; 6:129–134.

Giulian G, Gilbert E, Moss R: Elevated fetal hemoglobin levels in sudden infant death syndrome. *N Eng J Med* (Apr. 30) 1987; 316:1122–1126.

Harpin VA, Rutter N: Sweating in preterm babies. *J Pediatr* 1982; 100:614–618.

Horwitz SJ, Amiel-Tison C: Neurologic problems. Pages 360–381 in: *Care of the High-risk Infant.* 2nd ed. Klaus MH, Fanaroff AA (editors). Saunders, 1979.

Jackson D: Nursing care plan: Home management of children with BPD. *Pediatr Nurs* (Sept/Oct) 1986; 12(5): 342–348.

Jenkins RL, Swatoshtock M: Helping parents bond to their premature infant. *MCN* (Jan/Feb) 1986; 11(1): 32–34.

Jovanic L, Druzin M, Peterson C: Effect of euglycemia on the outcome of pregnancy in insulin-dependent diabetic women as compared with normal control subjects. *Am J Med* 1981; 71:921–927.

Kaplan DM, Mason EA: Maternal reactions to premature birth viewed as an acute emotional disorder. *Am J Orthopsychiatry* 1960; 30:539–552.

Kennedy AH, Johnson WG, Sturdevant EW: An educational program for families of children with tracheostomies. *Am J Matern-Child Nurs* 1982; 7:42–49.

Kimble KJ et al: Growth to age 3 years among very low-birth-weight sequelae-free survivors of modern neonatal intensive care. *J Pediatr* 1982; 100:622–624.

Klaus MH, Kennell JH: *Parent-Infant Bonding.* 2nd ed. Mosby, 1982.

LeBlanc MH: Relative efficacy of an incubator and an open warmer in producing thermoneutrality for the small premature infant. *Pediatrics* 1982; 69:439–445.

Lemons PK: Hospital use of expressed breast milk. *Issues Compr Pediatr Nurs* 1981; 5:195–203.

Mandell F, McAnulty E, Carlson A: Unexpected death of an infant sibling. *Pediatrics* (Nov) 1983; 72(5): 652–657.

Mandell F, McAnulty E, Reece RM: Observations of paternal response to sudden unanticipated infant death. *Pediatrics* (Feb) 1980; 65(2): 221–225.

McClain M: Sudden infant death syndrome: An update. *JEN* (Sept/Oct) 1985; 11(5): 227–233.

Nelson KB, Ellenberg JH: Apgar scores as predictors of chronic neurologic disability. *Pediatrics* 1981; 68:36–43.

Nelson D, Heitman R: Factors influencing weight change in preterm infants. *Pediatr Nurs* (Nov/Dec) 1986; 12(6): 425–428.

Nikolaisen S: The impact of sudden infant death on the family: Nursing intervention. *Top Clin Nurs* (Oct) 1981; 3(3): 45–53.

Pittard WBIII: Special properties of human milk. *Birth Fam J* 1981; 8:229–235.

Schraeder BD: A creative approach to caring for the ventilator-dependent child. *Am J Matern Child Nurs* 1980; 4:165–170.

Smith N: Necrotizing enterocolitis. In: *Protocols for Perinatal Nursing Practice.* Perez RH (editor), Mosby, 1981.

Sperhac AM: Sudden infant death syndrome. *Nurs Pract* (Sept) 1982; 7:38–40, 44.

Stahler-Miller K, Gewitz MH: Current considerations for patent ductus arteriosus in the critically ill newborn. In: *Neonatal and Pediatric Critical Care Nursing.* Stahler-Miller K (editor). Churchill Livingstone, 1983.

Stavis RL, Krauss AN: Complications of neonatal intensive care. *Clin Perinatol* (March) 1980; 7:107–124.

Thoman EB et al: Behavioral state profiles in infancy are predictive of later medical or behavioral dysfunction. *Neuropediatrics* 1981; 12:45–54.

Varner B, Ossenkop D, Lyon J: Prematures too, need rooming-in and care-by-parent programs. *Am J Matern-Child Nurs* 1980; 5:431–432.

Walsh M, Kliegman R: Necrotizing enterocolitis: the spectrum of disease. *Pediatr Basics* 1985; 40:4–7.

Weibley T et al: Gavage tube insertion in the premature infant. *MCN* (Jan/Feb) 1987; 12(1): 24–27.

Yu VYH, Jamieson J, Astbury J: Parents' reactions to unrestricted parental contact with infants in the intensive care nursery. *Med J Aust* 1981; 1:294–296.

Additional Readings

Barnard KE, Blackburn S: Features of the premature infant's animate and inanimate environment in relation to adult activity. In: *Caregiver–Infant Interactions and Stimulation Characteristics of Intensive Care Nurseries.* Gaiter JL (chair). Symposium presented at the biennial meeting of the Society for Research in Child Development, Boston, Mass., April 1981.

Davis DH, Thoman EB: *The Organization of Behavioral States in Premature and Full-term Infants.* Paper presented at the biennial meeting of the Society for Research in Child Development, Detroit, Mich., April 1983.

Dean PG: Monitoring an apneic infant: Impact on the infant's mother. *Matern-Child Nurs J* (Summer) 1986; 15(2): 65–75.

Gorski PA, Hole WT, Leonard CH: Behavioral and physiological observations of infants and their caregivers in an intensive care nursery. In: *Caregiver—Infant Interactions and Stimulation Characteristics of Intensive Care Nurseries.* Gaiter JL (chair). Symposium presented at the biennial meeting of the Society for Research in Child Development, Boston, Mass., April 1981.

Jill A, Perlman JM, Volpe JJ: Relationship of pneumothorax to occurrence of intraventricular hemorrhage in the premature newborn. *Pediatrics* 1982; 69:144–149.

Knobloch H et al: Considerations in evaluating changes in outcome for infants weighing less than 1,501 grams. *Pediatrics* 1982; 69:285–295.

McCarthy M: A home discharge program for ventilator-assisted children. *Pediatr Nurs* (Sept/Oct) 1986; 12(5): 331–335, 380.

Medoff-Cooper B: Temperament in low birth weight infants. *Nurs Res* (May/June) 1986; 35(3): 139–143.

Noga KM: High-risk infants. The need for nursing follow-up. *J Obstet Gynecol Neonatal Nurs* 1982; 11:112–115.

Saigal S et al: Follow-up of infants 501 to 1,500 gm birth weight delivered to residents of a geographically defined region with perinatal intensive care facilities. *J Pediatr* 1982; 100:606–613.

Thoman EB et al: Theophylline affects behavioral state development in premature infants. *Neuropediatrics* 1984. In press.

APPENDIX A
Growth Charts for Infants and Children

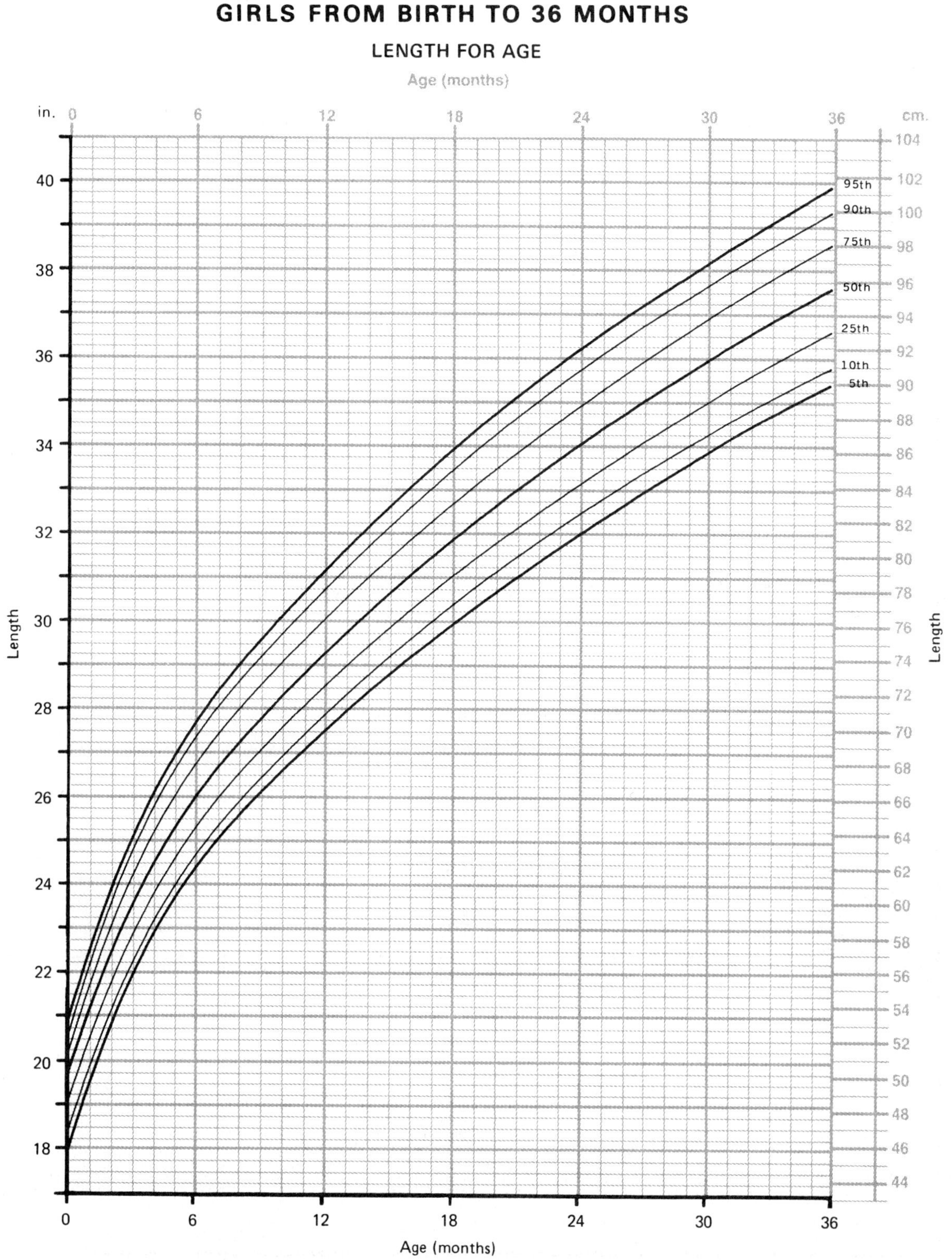

GIRLS FROM BIRTH TO 36 MONTHS

WEIGHT FOR AGE

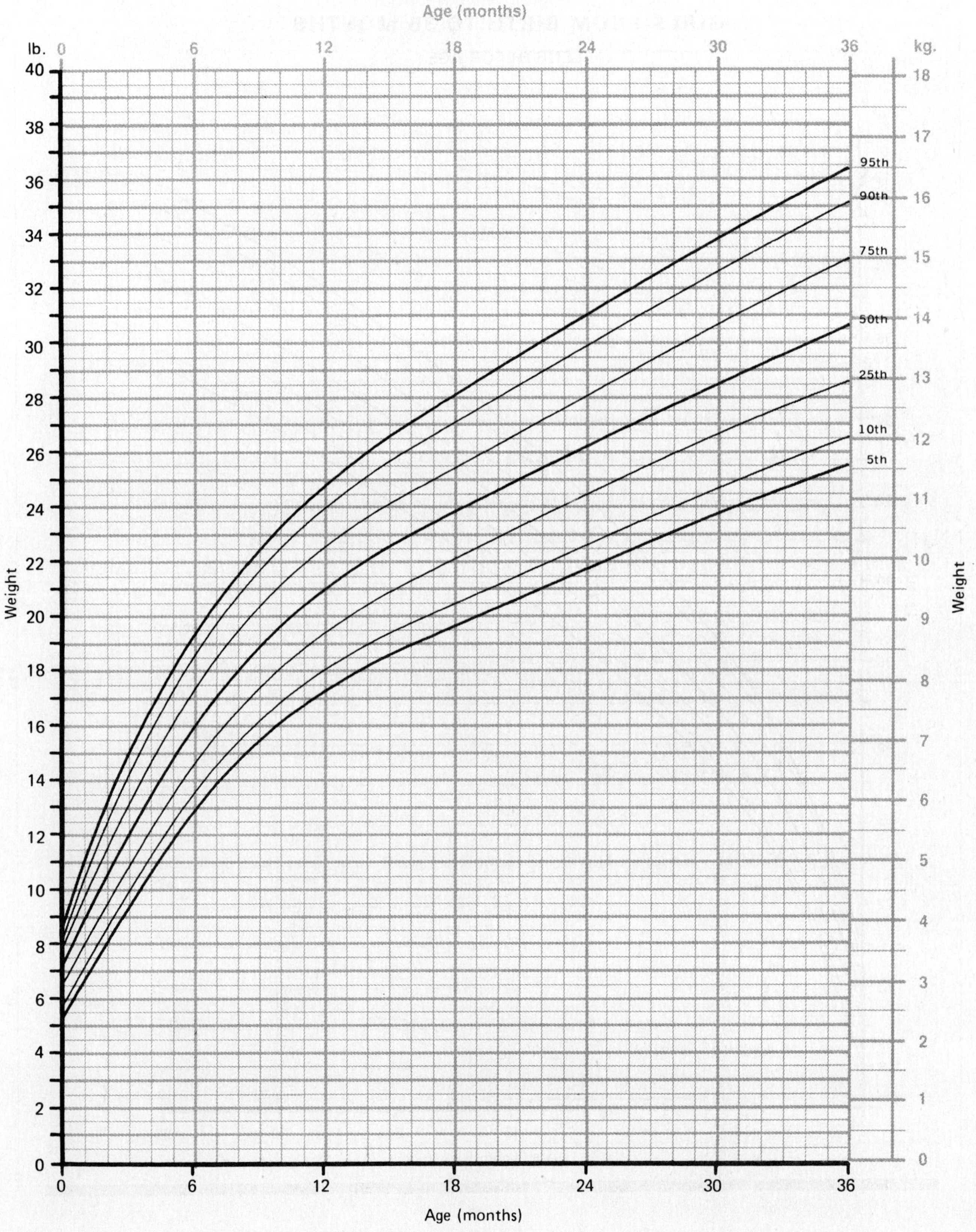

GIRLS FROM BIRTH TO 36 MONTHS

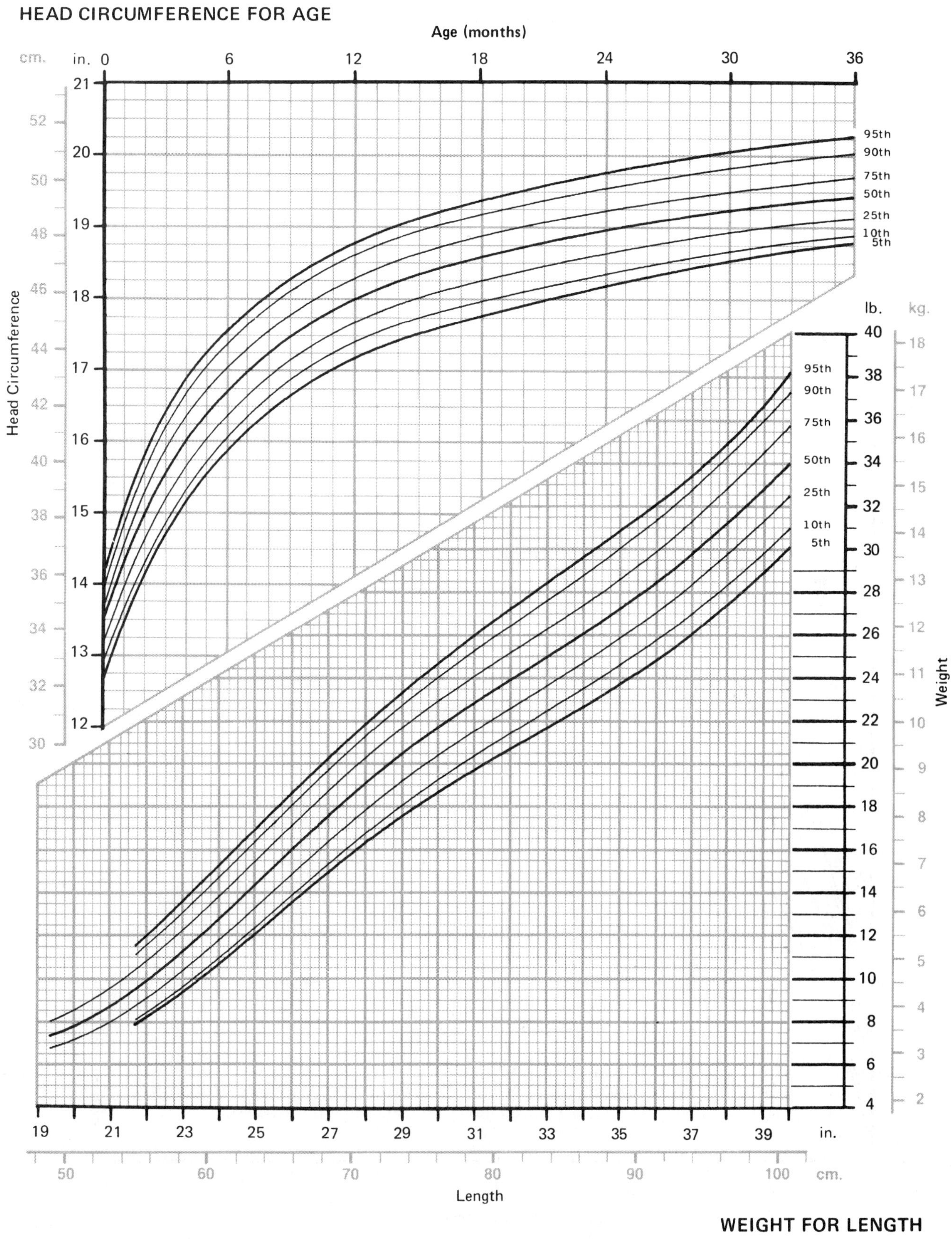

BOYS FROM BIRTH TO 36 MONTHS

LENGTH FOR AGE

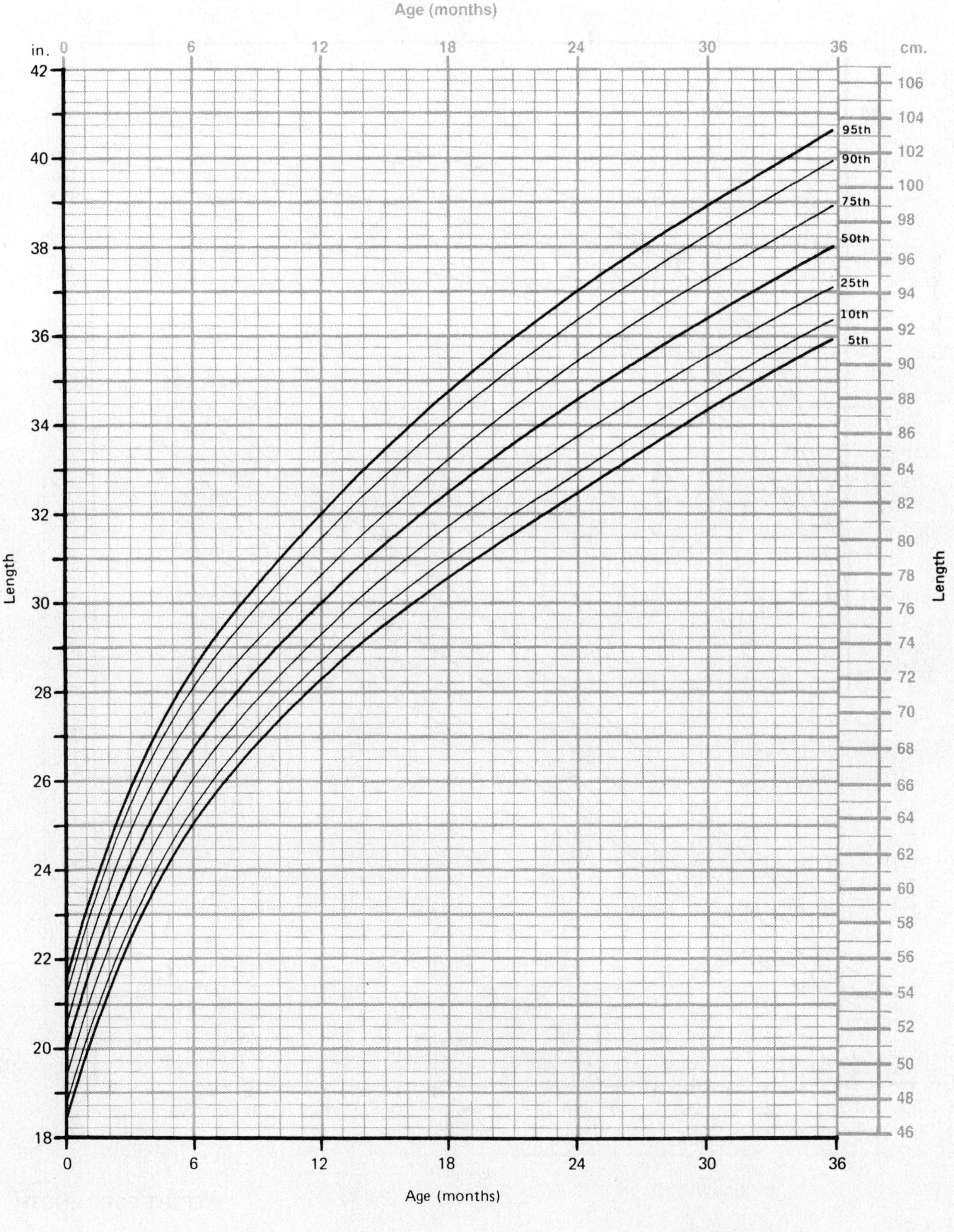

BOYS FROM BIRTH TO 36 MONTHS

WEIGHT FOR AGE

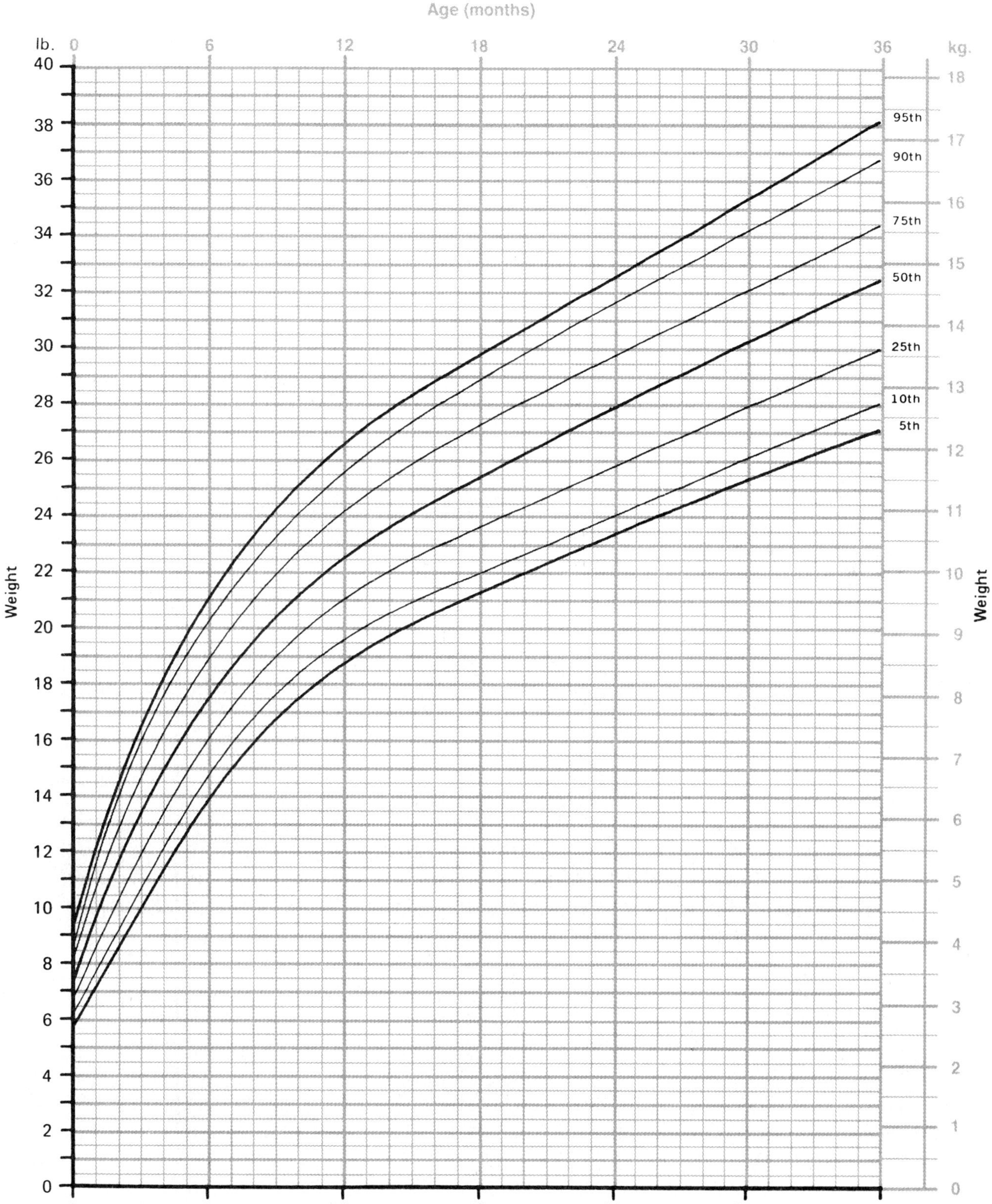

BOYS FROM BIRTH TO 36 MONTHS

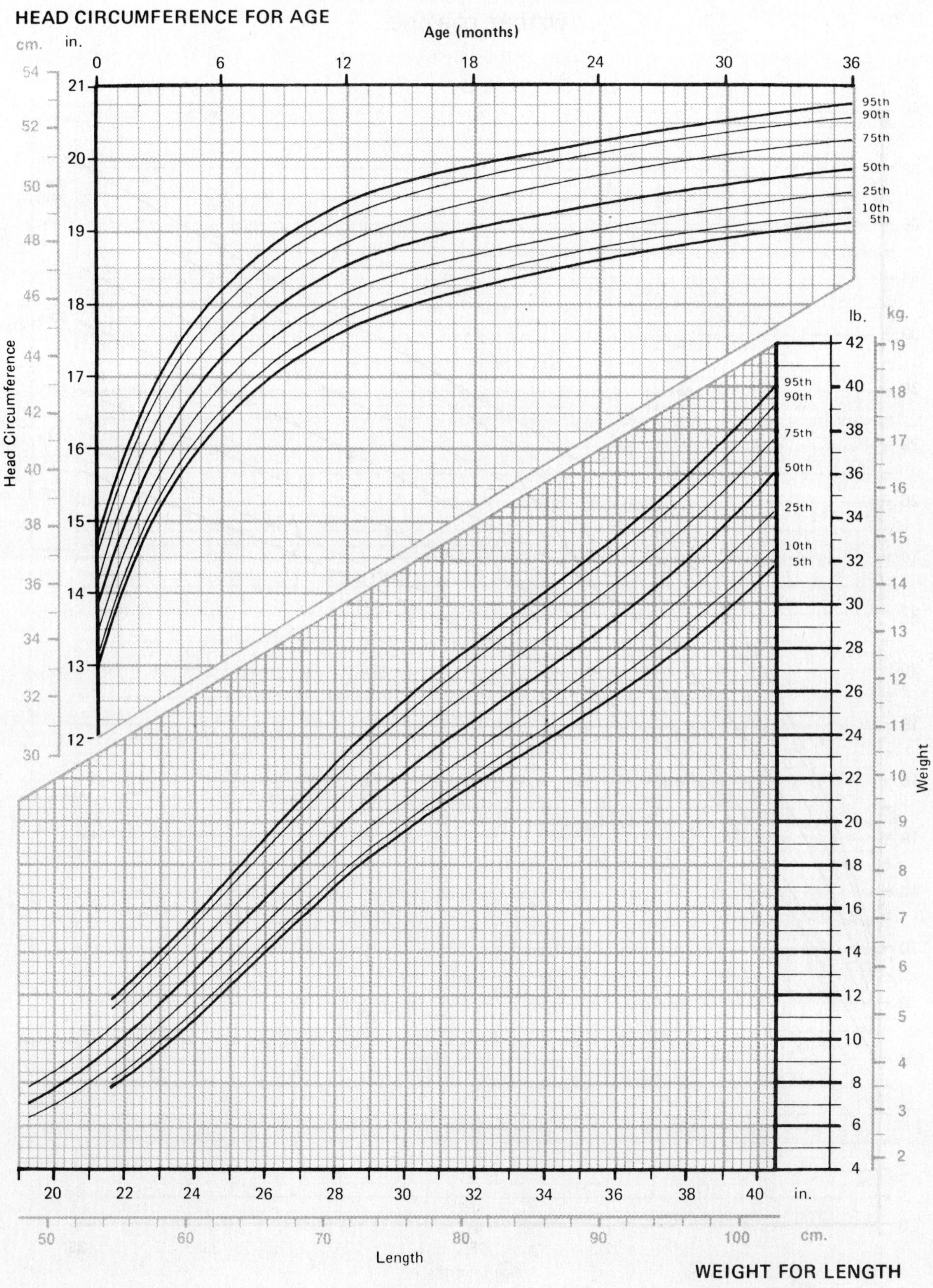

GIRLS FROM 2 TO 18 YEARS

STATURE FOR AGE

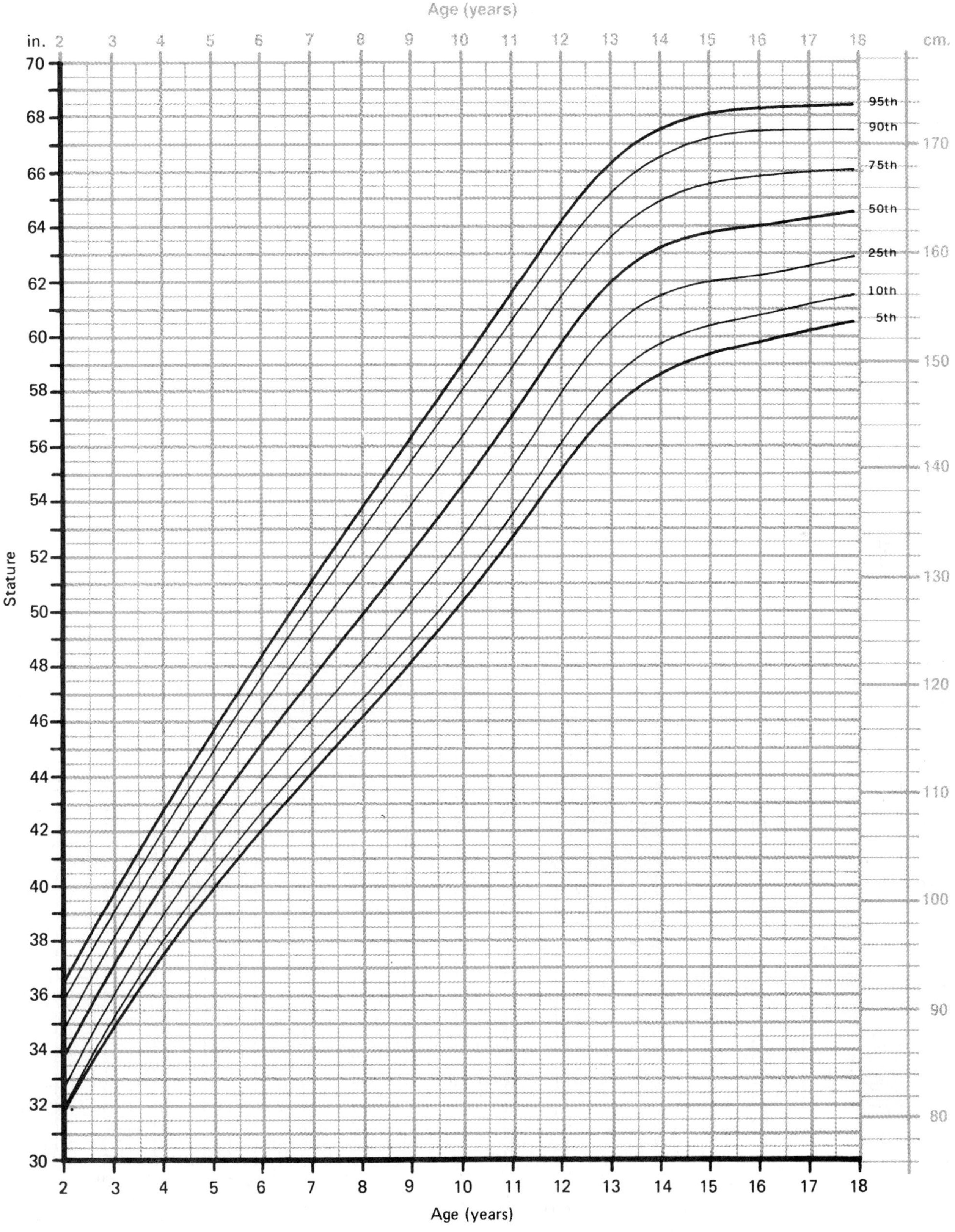

GIRLS FROM 2 TO 18 YEARS

WEIGHT FOR AGE

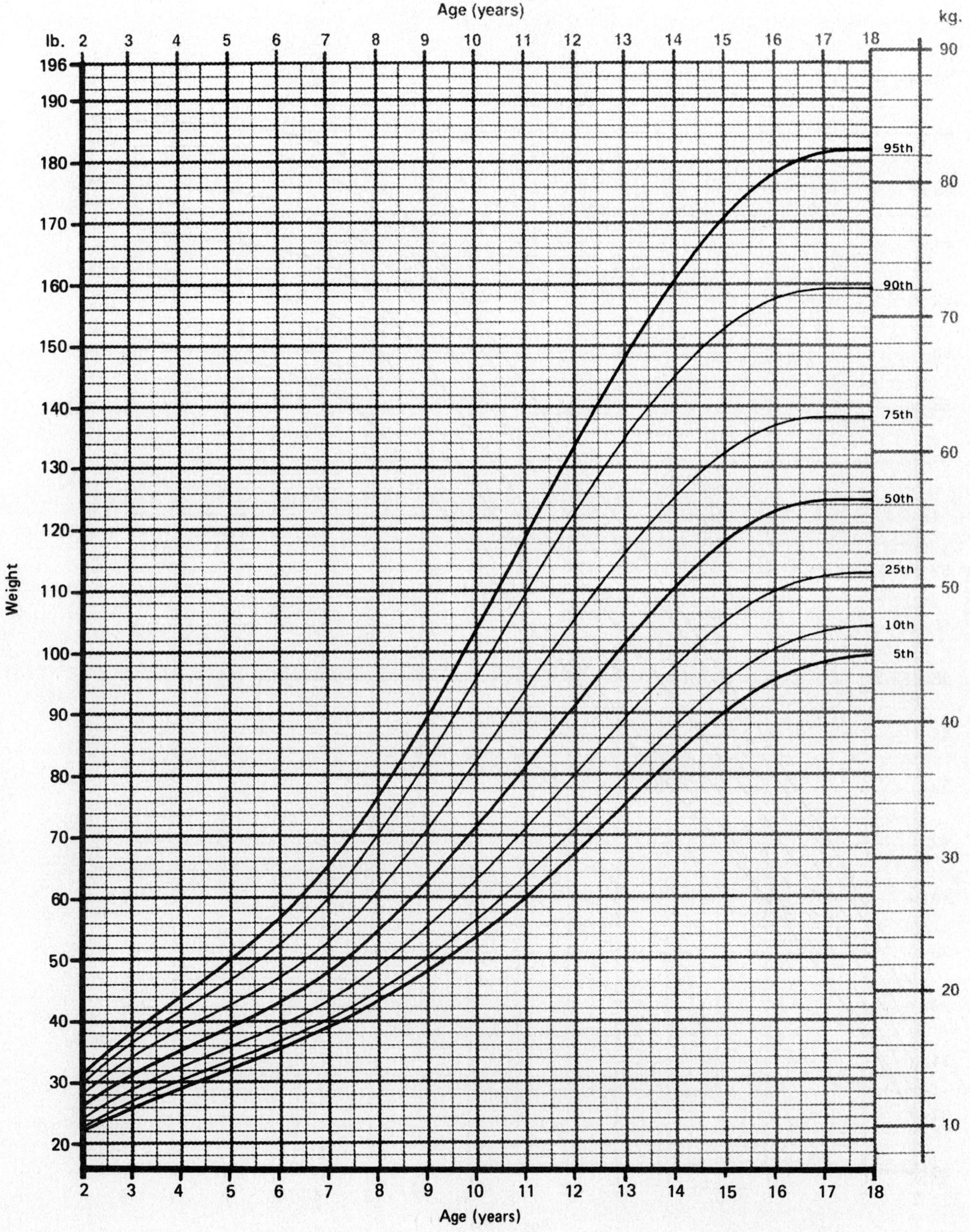

PRE-PUBERTAL GIRLS FROM 2 TO 10 YEARS

WEIGHT FOR STATURE

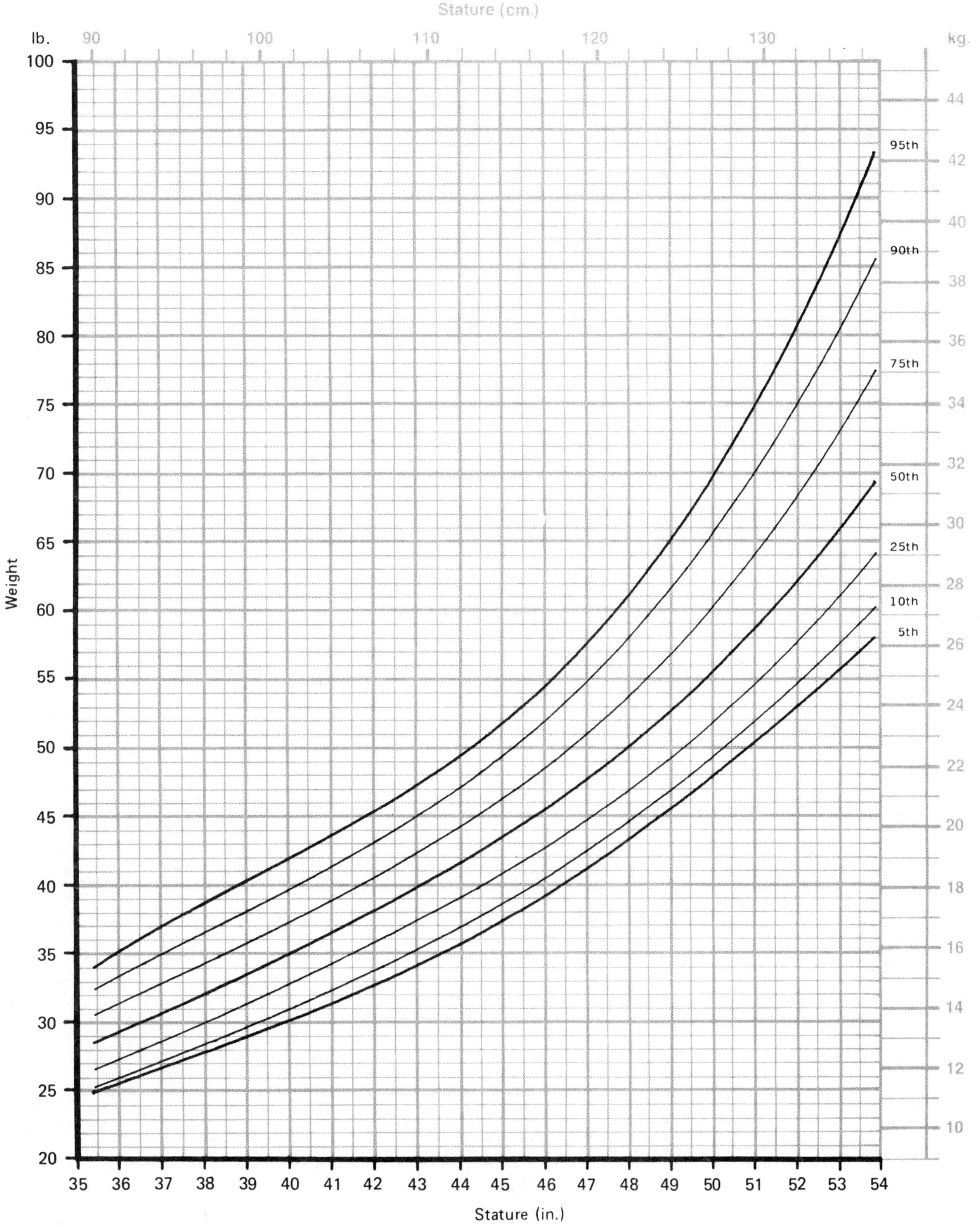

BOYS FROM 2 TO 18 YEARS

STATURE FOR AGE

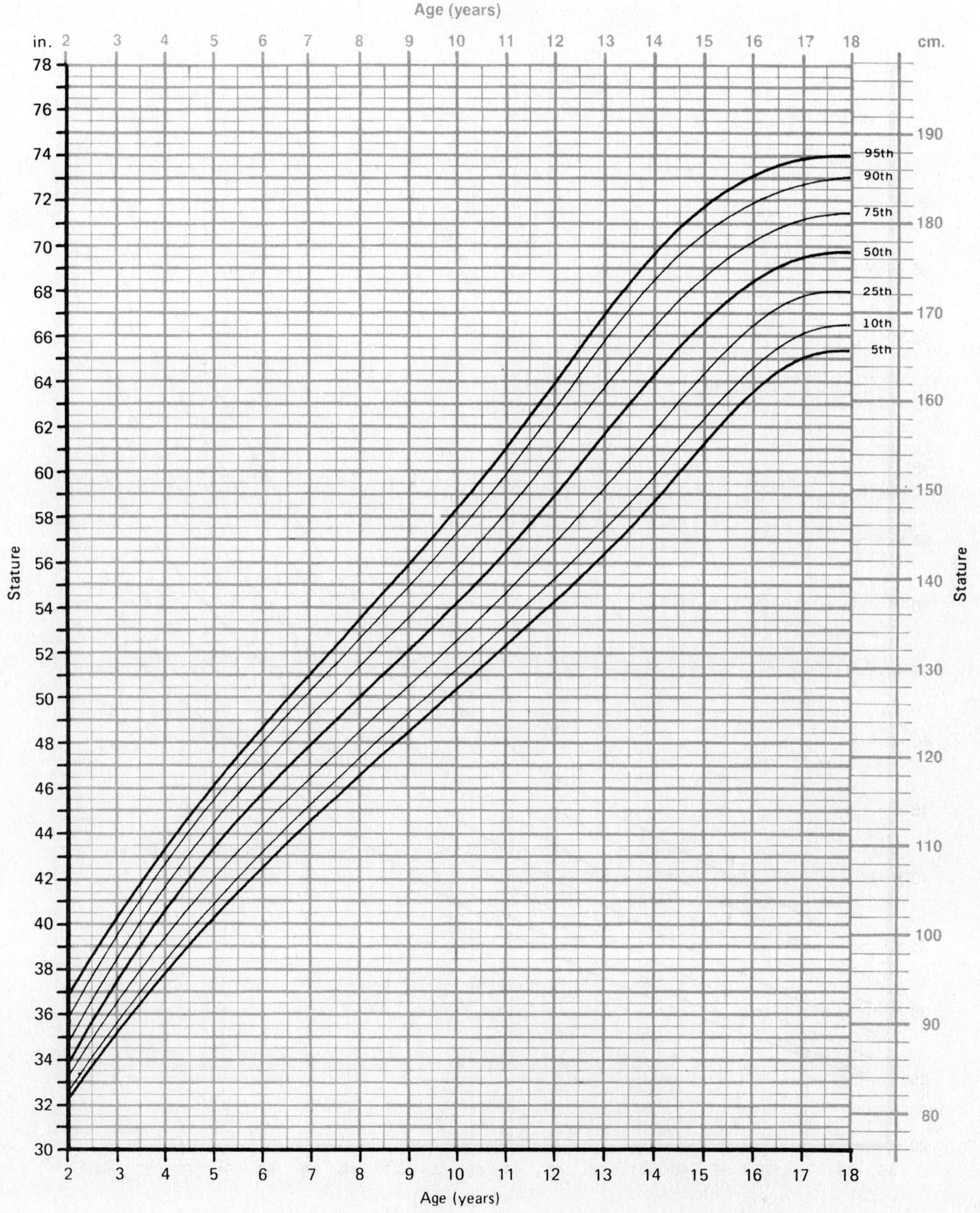

BOYS FROM 2 TO 18 YEARS

WEIGHT FOR AGE

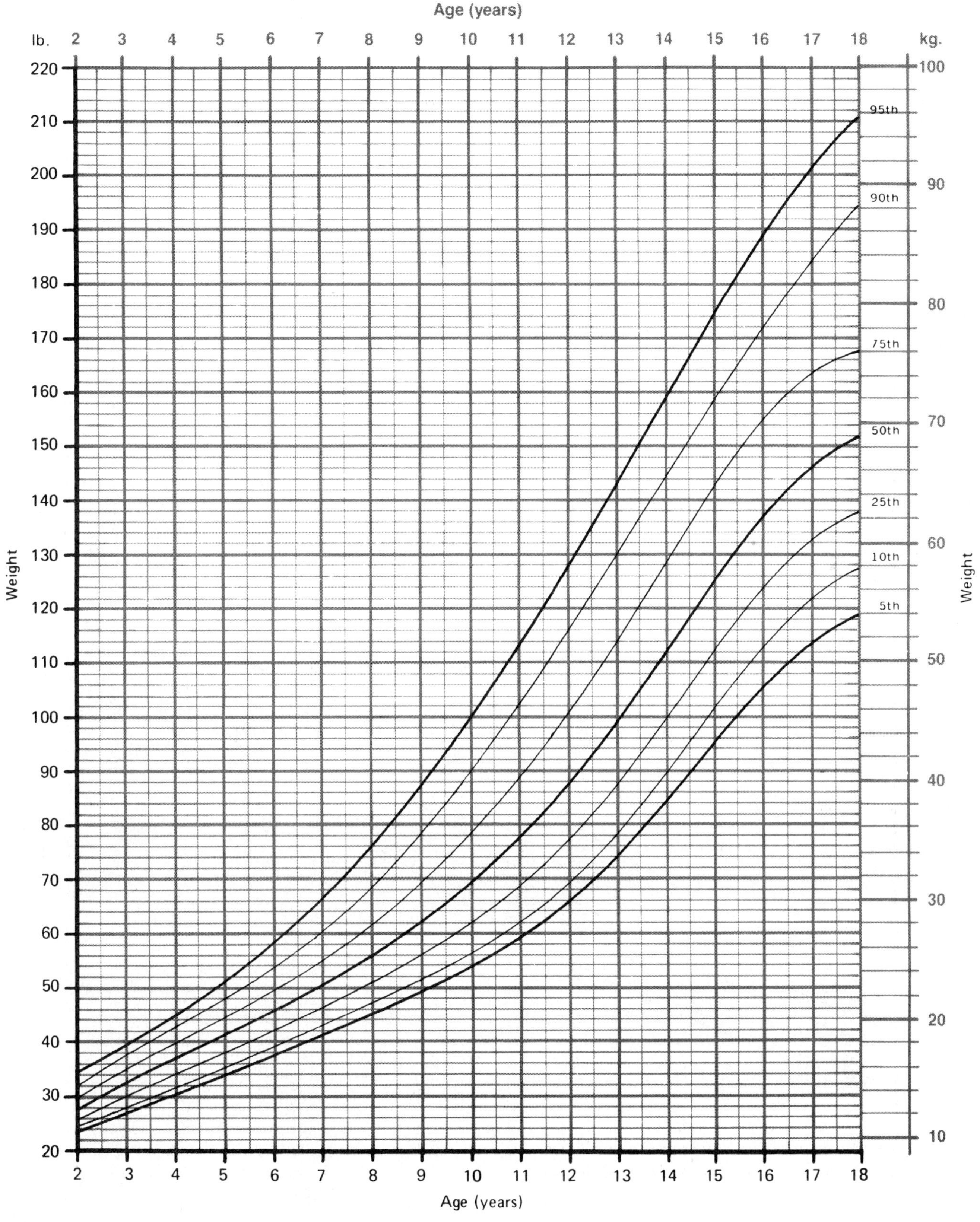

PRE-PUBERTAL BOYS FROM 2 TO 11½ YEARS

WEIGHT FOR STATURE

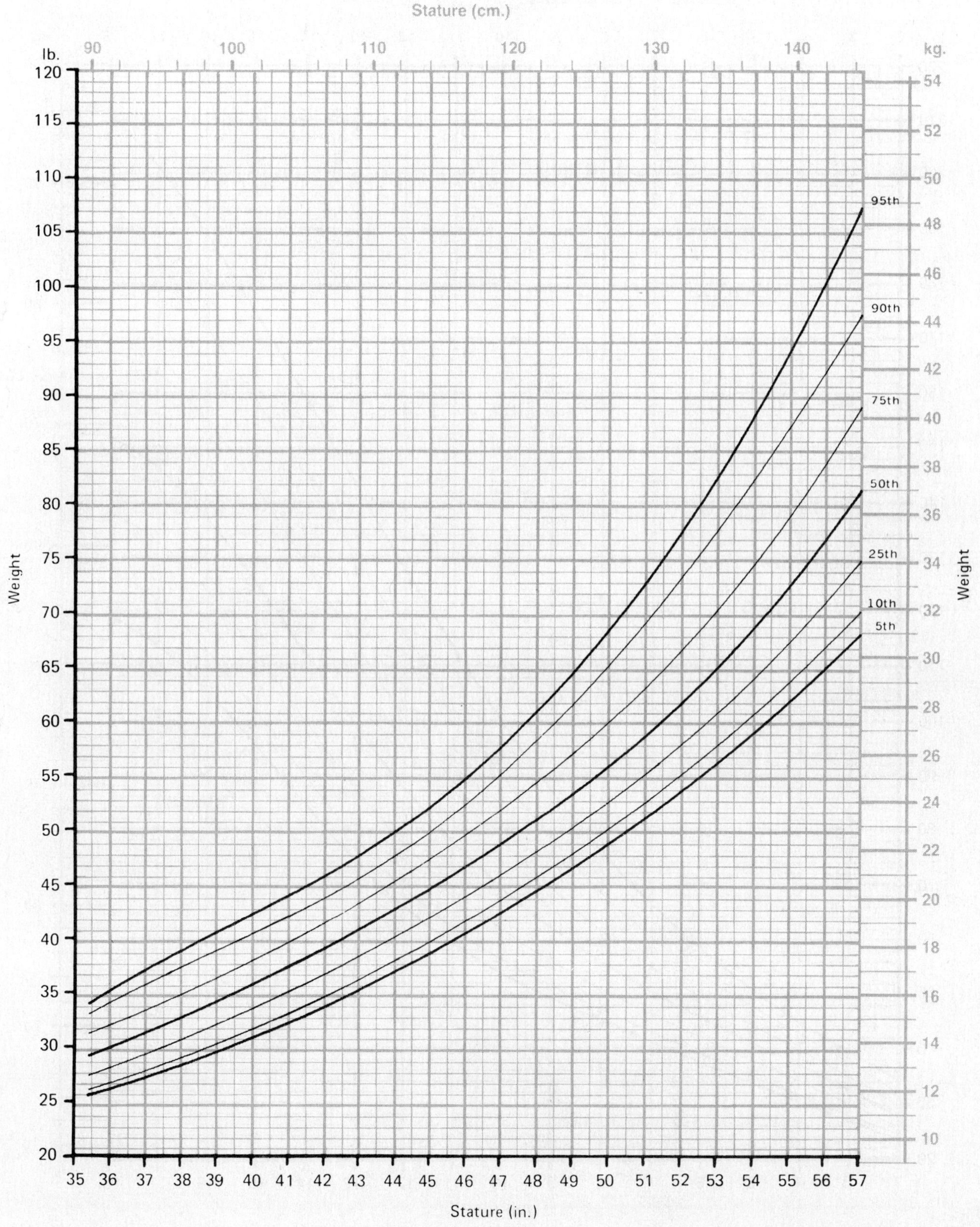

APPENDIX B
Normal Measurements—Variations with Age

Average Heart Rate for Children at Rest

Age	Average rate	2 SD
Birth	140	50
1st mo	130	45
1–6 mo	130	45
6–12 mo	115	40
1–2 yr	110	40
2–4 yr	105	35
6–10 yr	95	30
10–14 yr	85	30
14–18 yr	82	25

SOURCE: Lowrey GH: *Growth and Development of Children.* 7th ed. Year Book, 1978, p. 228.

Variations in Respiration with Age

Age	Rate/min	Tidal air, cc	Vital capacity, L*
Premature	40–90	12	—
Neonate	30–80	19	—
1 yr	20–40	48	—
2 yr	20–30	90	—
3 yr	20–30	125	—
5 yr	20–25	175	1.0
10 yr	17–22	320	2.0
15 yr	15–20	400	3.7
20 yr	15–20	500	3.8

*These represent mean figures from several sources for both sexes. Vital capacity for boys averages about 6% greater than for girls.
SOURCE: Lowrey GH: *Growth and Development of Children.* 7th ed. Year Book, 1978, p. 450.

Normal Blood Pressure for Various Ages (mm Hg)

Infants*		Age	Systolic	2 SD	Diastolic	2 SD
1st day	52	1 day	78	14	42	14
4th day	70	1 mo	86	20	54	18
10th day	80	6 mo	90	26	60	20
2d mo	95	1 yr	96	30	65	25
8th mo	95	2 yr	99	25	65	25
		4 yr	99	20	65	20
		6 yr	100	15	60	10
		8 yr	105	15	60	10
		10 yr	110	17	60	10
		12 yr	115	19	60	10
		14 yr	118	20	60	10
		16 yr	120	16	65	10

*The figures for infants represent averages by the flush method.
NOTE: The figures under 1 year were obtained by the Doppler method. From 1 year on, the figures were obtained by auscultation, using the first change in sound to indicate diastolic pressure.
SOURCE: Lowrey GH: *Growth and Development of Children.* 7th ed. Year Book, 1978, p. 450.

Fluid Maintenance Requirements for Infants and Children

Age	kg weight	Fluid requirement mL/24 hours	Approximate hourly fluid rate	Formula
Newborn (less than 72 h)	3.3	198–330	8–15	60–100 mL/kg body weight
1 wk	3.3	330	15	100 mL/kg (can be increased if no renal or cardiac difficulties)
2 mo	5.0	500	20	
6 mo	8.0	800	35	
12 mo	10.0	1000	40	
3 yr	15.0	1250	50	1000 mL for the first 10 kg plus 50 mL/kg for each kg over 10 kg
5 yr	20.0	1500	60	
8 yr	30.0	1750	70	1500 mL for the first 20 kg plus 25 mL/kg for each kg over 20 kg
12 yr	40.0	1850	80	1750 mL for the first 30 kg plus 10 mL/kg for each kg over 30 kg

SOURCE: Hazinski MF: Nursing care of the critically ill child: A seven point check. *Pediatr Nurs* (Nov/Dec) 1985; 11:453–461.

Clinical Laboratory Values

Test	Normal values*
Arterial blood gases	
Po_2 Partial pressure of oxygen—reflects amount of O_2 diffusing through pulmonary membrane into blood	Sea level: 80%–100% Altitude > 5000 feet: 65%–75%
Pco_2 Partial pressure of carbon dioxide reflects tension exerted by dissolved carbon dioxide in blood	Sea level: 35%–45% Altitude > 5000 feet: 32%–38%
pH Measures the chemical balance in the body	7.35–7.45
Base excess Quantification of total base excess. The sum of the concentration of buffer ions in whole blood	Sea level: −2–+2 Altitude > 5000 feet: −4–+2
Arterial blood gases *(Continued)*	
Blood bicarbonate (HCO_3) Primary buffer union in whole blood, accounts for about half of the total buffer anions	Sea level: 22–26 mEq/L Altitude > 5000 feet: 18–26 mEq/L
Oxygen saturation Measures actual O_2 content of hemoglobin compared to the maximal potential of O_2 carrying capacity	Sea level: 95%
Cerebrospinal fluid values	
Color	Clear
Cell count	Neonate: < 15 leukocytes/mm^3 Child: 0–5 cells/mm^3 (all lymphocytes)
Protein	Neonates: 60–120 mg/dL Child: 15–45 mg/dL
Glucose	One-half to two-thirds serum glucose level
Gram's stain	No organisms

Clinical Laboratory Values *(Continued)*

Test		Normal values*	
Hematology			
Hemoglobin (Hgb)			*(g/dL)*
		Newborn (1–3 da)	14.5–22.5
		Infant (2 mo)	9.0–14.0
		Child (6–12 yr)	11.5–15.5
		Adolescent	
		Male	13.0–16.0
		Female	12.0–16.0
Hematocrit (Hct)			
		Newborn (1–3 da)	44–75
		Infant (2 mo)	28–42
		Child (6–12 yr)	35–45
		Adolescent	
		Male	37–49
		Female	36–46
Red blood cell count (RBC)			*(M/μL)*
		Newborn (1–3 da)	4.0–6.6
		Neonate (1–4 wk)	3.0–6.3
		Infant (1–18 mo)	2.7–5.4
		Child (2–12 yr)	3.9–5.3
		Adolescent	
		Male	4.5–5.3
		Female	4.1–5.1
Mean corpuscular volume (MCV)	Average or mean volume of single RBC; $MCV = \frac{Hct}{RBC}$		*(μm³)*
		Newborn (1–3 da)	95–121
		Infant (0.5–2 yr)	70–86
		Child (6–12 yr)	77–95
		Adolescent	
		Male	78–98
		Female	78–102
Mean corpuscular hemoglobin concentration (MCH)	Average or mean quantity, by weight, of Hgb in a single RBC; $MCH = \frac{Hgb}{RBC}$		*(pg/cell)*
		Newborn (1–3 da)	31–37
		Neonate (1–4 wk)	28–40
		Infant (2–24 mo)	23–35
		Child (2–12 yr)	24–33
		Adolescent	25–35
Mean corpuscular hemoglobin concentration (MCHC)	Average concentration of Hgb in a single RBC; $MCHC = \frac{Hgb}{Hct}$		*(%Hb/cell)*
		Newborn (1–3 da)	29–37
		Neonate (1–2 wk)	28–38
		Infant (1–24 mo)	29–37
		Child/Adolescent	31–37
Reticulocyte count	Percentage of young RBCs that stain positively for basophil reticulin with a supravital stain		*(%)*
		Newborn (1 da)	3.2 ± 1.4
		Neonate (1–4 wk)	0.6 ± 0.3
		Infant (5–12 wk)	0.3–2.2
		Adults	0.5–1.5
White blood cell count (WBC)	Number of WBC in 1 μL (mm³) of blood		*(× 1000 cells/μL)*
		Newborn	9.0–30.0
		Neonate (1 mo)	5.0–19.5
		Infant (1–3 yr)	6.0–17.5
		Child (4–13 yr)	4.5–15.5
		Adult	4.5–11.0
Hematology *(Continued)*			
Differential white count	Percentage of various types of WBC seen on examination of a slide of peripheral blood		
	Neutrophils		*(%)*
		Newborn	32–62
		Infant (1 yr)	23 (%)
		Child (10 yr)	31–61
		Adult	54–75
	Basophils	Newborn	0.5–1.0
		Infant (1 yr)	0.4
		Child (10 yr)	0.5
		Adult	0–1
	Eosinophils	Newborn	2–2.5
		Infant (1 yr)	2.6
		Child (10 yr)	2–2.5
		Adult	1–4
	Lymphocytes	Newborn	26–36
		Infant (1 yr)	61
		Child (10 yr)	28–48
		Adult	25–40
	Monocytes	Newborn	5–6
		Infant (1 yr)	5
		Child (10 yr)	4–4.5
		Adult	2–8
Platelet count	Number of platelets in 1 μL (mm³) of blood	Newborn	84,000–478,000
		Thereafter	150,000–400,000
Bleeding time	Amount of time it takes for bleeding from small superficial wound to stop	Newborn	1–8 min
		Thereafter	1–6 min
Whole blood clotting time	Amount of time it takes for blood to clot in a glass tube	All ages	5–8 min
Prothrombin time (PT)	Amount of time it takes for blood to clot after thromboplastin and calcium chloride are added to blood plasma. Detects deficiencies of Factors V, VII, and X, fibrinogen, and prothrombin	Newborn	< 17 s
		Thereafter	11–15 s

(continues)

Clinical Laboratory Values *(Continued)*

Test	Normal values*	
Hematology *(Continued)*		
Partial prothrombin time (PTT) A clotting test that measures activity of thromboplastin. Detects various factor deficiencies	Newborn Thereafter Nonactivated Activated	< 90 s 60–85 s 25–35 s
Thromboplastin generation time (TGT) Measures the blood's ability to generate thromboplastin. Distinguishes between Factor VIII and IX deficiencies	Newborn Thereafter	8–20 s 8–16 s
Prothrombin consumption time (PCT) Measures thromboplastin generation and prothrombin response	Almost complete consumption is indicated by a clotting time of greater than 20 seconds	
Fibrinogen level Measures fibrinogen levels in the blood	Newborn Thereafter	125–300 mg/dL 200–400 mg/dL
Immunoglobins		
IgG Major (85%) immunoglobin of blood; only one to cross the placenta; possesses antibody activity against some bacteria, toxins, and viruses	Newborn Infant (6 mo) Child (6–12 yr) Adolescent	700–1480 (mg/dL) 300–1000 (mg/dL) 700–1650 (mg/dL) 700–1550 (mg/dL)
IgA Main immunoglobin of body secretions. Accounts for 10%–15% of total, protects mucous membranes in respiratory and gastrointestinal tract. Possesses antibody activity against viruses and some bacteria	Newborn Infant (6 mo–2 yr) Child (6–12 yr) Adolescent	0–2.2 (mg/dL) 14–108 (mg/dL) 29–270 (mg/dL) 81–232 (mg/dL)
IgM Accounts for 5%–10% of immunoglobulin. First antibody to come after antigens enter body. Possesses antibody activity against gram-negative organisms; is a complement activator	Newborn Infant (6 mo–2 yr) Child (6–12 yr) Adolescent	5–30 (mg/dL) 43–239 (mg/dL) 50–260 (mg/dL) 45–240 (mg/dL)

Test	Normal values*	
Immunoglobins *(Continued)*		
IgE Possesses antibody activity for hypersensitivity reactions. Only small amounts present in blood. Might protect against pinworms	Male Female	0–230 (IU/mL) 0–170 (IU/mL)
IgD Only small amount present in blood.	Newborn After newborn	0 (mg/dL) 0–8 (mg/dL)
Serum chemistry		
Alpha 1-antitrypsin (AAT) test. Measures a protein produced by the liver that inhibits protease release by dying cells		130–238 mg/dL
Bilirubin Measures liver function, hemolytic anemias, and newborn hyperbilirubinemia	Total bilirubin Newborn Child Indirect bilirubin Direct bilirubin	mg/dL 1.0–12.0 0.2–0.8 0.2–0.8 0.1–0.4
Ammonia Used as an indicator of hepatic protein metabolism	Values vary widely	40–110 mg/100 ml
Amylase	Children	45–200 dye U/dL
Serum glutamic-oxaloacetic transaminase (SGOT) Presence of the enzyme directly related to number of dying cells and time lapse between injury to the tissue and test	 Newborn (1–3 days) Infant (6 mo–1 yr) Child (1–5 yr) Older child (5 yr–adult)	IU/L 16–74 16–35 6–30 19–28
Serum glutamic-pyruvic transaminase (SGPT) Test of enzyme level found mainly in liver. Evaluates liver function	 Infant Children	IU/L below 54 1–30
Alkaline phosphatase Index of liver and bone disease when matched with other clinical findings	Bodansky units units/dL Children 5–14, adults 1.5–4.5 King-Armstrong units units/dL Children 15–30, adults 4–13 Bessy-Lowery units units/mL Children 3.4–9.0, adults 0.8–2.3	

Clinical Laboratory Values *(Continued)*

Test	Normal values*	
Serum electrolytes		
Potassium	3.5–5.5 mEq/L	
Sodium	130–150 mEq/L	
Calcium	4.5–5.7 mEq/L	
Magnesium	1.2–2.1 mEq/L	
Stool specimens		
pH	7–7.5	
Ova and parasites	0	
Stool culture	No pathologic organisms	
Stool electrolytes		
Fecal fat	(One specimen or 72 hr collection.) On smear, fatty acid globules 1–4 μ in diameter	
Trypsin	2+–4+ in children	
Reducing substances	Negative	
Clinitest of liquid stool	Negative	
Urine studies		
Urinalysis		
Color	Clear, amber	
Turbidity	Clear	
Specific gravity—ratio of density of urine to density of water	1.001–1.040;	
	Usual child	1.003–1.010
	Usual adult	1.015–1.025
pH	4.6–8.0, average 6.0	

Test	Normal values*	
Urine studies *(Continued)*		
Protein	0	
Glucose	0	
Ketones	0	
Cells	Few	
Erythrocytes (RBC)	0	
Leukocytes	Few	
Casts	0	
Crystals	Some	
		(mg/24 hrs)
17-ketosteroids Test of adrenal cortex function	Infant (less than 1 yr)	under 1
	Child (5–8 yr)	under 3
	Child (9–12)	approx. 3
	Adult male	8–25
	Adult female	5–15
		(mg/M/24 hrs)
17-hydroxycorticosteroids Test of adrenal cortex function	Children to 16 yrs	3.1–10.0
Urinary-free cortisol Test of adrenal cortex function	20–100 μg/24 hr	
Urinary calcium	10 mg/dL	
Urinary sodium	40–180 mEq/24 hr	
Urinary vanillymandelic acid (VMA)	*(24-hr specimen mg/g creatinine)*	
	Infant (1–12 mo)	1.40–15.0
	Child (5–10 yr)	0.5–6.0
	Child (10–15 yr)	0.25–3.25

*Normal values may vary with laboratory method used.

APPENDIX C

Denver Developmental Screening Test

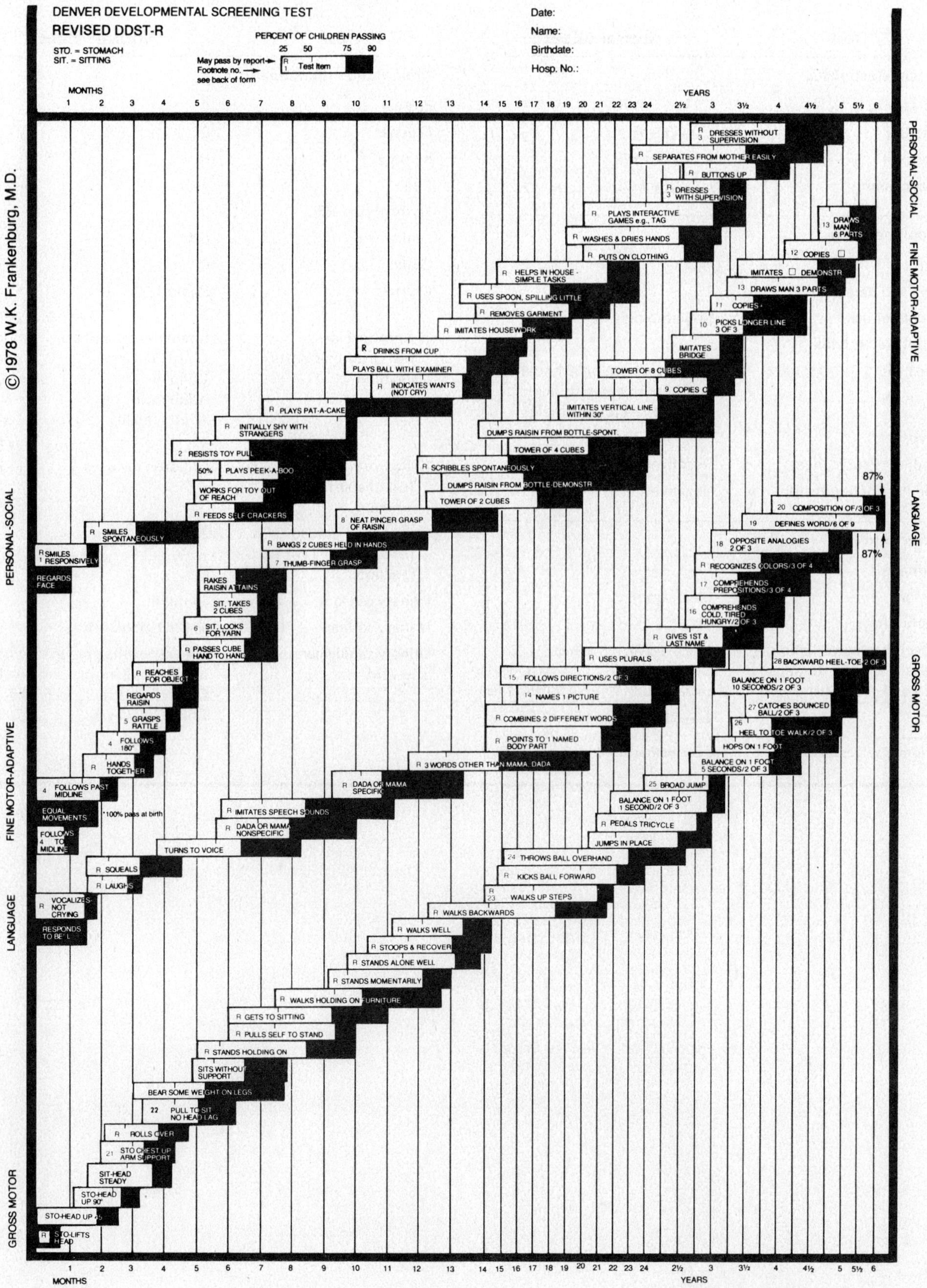

DATE
NAME
DIRECTIONS BIRTHDATE
HOSP. NO.

1. Try to get child to smile by smiling, talking or waving to him. Do not touch him.
2. When child is playing with toy, pull it away from him. Pass if he resists.
3. Child does not have to be able to tie shoes or button in the back.
4. Move yarn slowly in an arc from one side to the other, about 6" above child's face. Pass if eyes follow 90° to midline. (Past midline; 180°)
5. Pass if child grasps rattle when it is touched to the backs or tips of fingers.
6. Pass if child continues to look where yarn disappeared or tries to see where it went. Yarn should be dropped quickly from sight from tester's hand without arm movement.
7. Pass if child picks up raisin with any part of thumb and a finger.
8. Pass if child picks up raisin with the ends of thumb and index finger using an over hand approach.

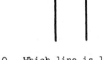

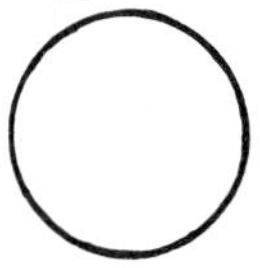
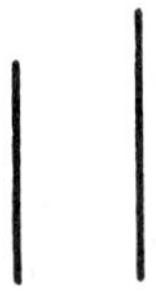
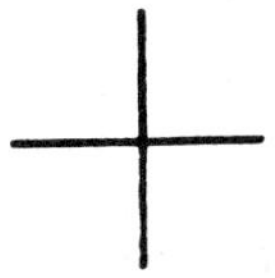

9. Pass any enclosed form. Fail continuous round motions.
10. Which line is longer? (Not bigger.) Turn paper upside down and repeat. (3/3 or 5/6)
11. Pass any crossing lines.
12. Have child copy first. If failed, demonstrate

When giving items 9, 11 and 12, do not name the forms. Do not demonstrate 9 and 11.

13. When scoring, each pair (2 arms, 2 legs, etc.) counts as one part.
14. Point to picture and have child name it. (No credit is given for sounds only.)

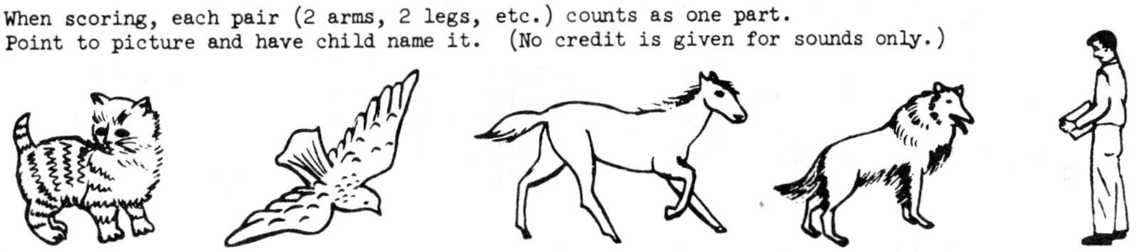

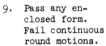

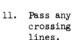

15. Tell child to: Give block to Mommie; put block on table; put block on floor. Pass 2 of 3. (Do not help child by pointing, moving head or eyes.)
16. Ask child: What do you do when you are cold? ..hungry? ..tired? Pass 2 of 3.
17. Tell child to: Put block <u>on</u> table; <u>under</u> table; <u>in front</u> of chair, <u>behind</u> chair. Pass 3 of 4. (Do not help child by pointing, moving head or eyes.)
18. Ask child: If fire is hot, ice is ?; Mother is a woman, Dad is a ?; a horse is big, a mouse is ?. Pass 2 of 3.
19. Ask child: What is a ball? ..lake? ..desk? ..house? ..banana? ..curtain? ..ceiling? ..hedge? ..pavement? Pass if defined in terms of use, shape, what it is made of or general category (such as banana is fruit, not just yellow). Pass 6 of 9.
20. Ask child: What is a spoon made of? ..a shoe made of? ..a door made of? (No other objects may be substituted.) Pass 3 of 3.
21. When placed on stomach, child lifts chest off table with support of forearms and/or hands.
22. When child is on back, grasp his hands and pull him to sitting. Pass if head does not hang back.
23. Child may use wall or rail only, not person. May not crawl.
24. Child must throw ball overhand 3 feet to within arm's reach of tester.
25. Child must perform standing broad jump over width of test sheet. (8-1/2 inches)
26. Tell child to walk forward, → heel within 1 inch of toe. Tester may demonstrate. Child must walk 4 consecutive steps, 2 out of 3 trials.
27. Bounce ball to child who should stand 3 feet away from tester. Child must catch ball with hands, not arms, 2 out of 3 trials.
28. Tell child to walk backward, ← toe within 1 inch of heel. Tester may demonstrate. Child must walk 4 consecutive steps, 2 out of 3 trials.

<u>DATE AND BEHAVIORAL OBSERVATIONS</u> (how child feels at time of test, relation to tester, attention span, verbal behavior, self-confidence, etc,):

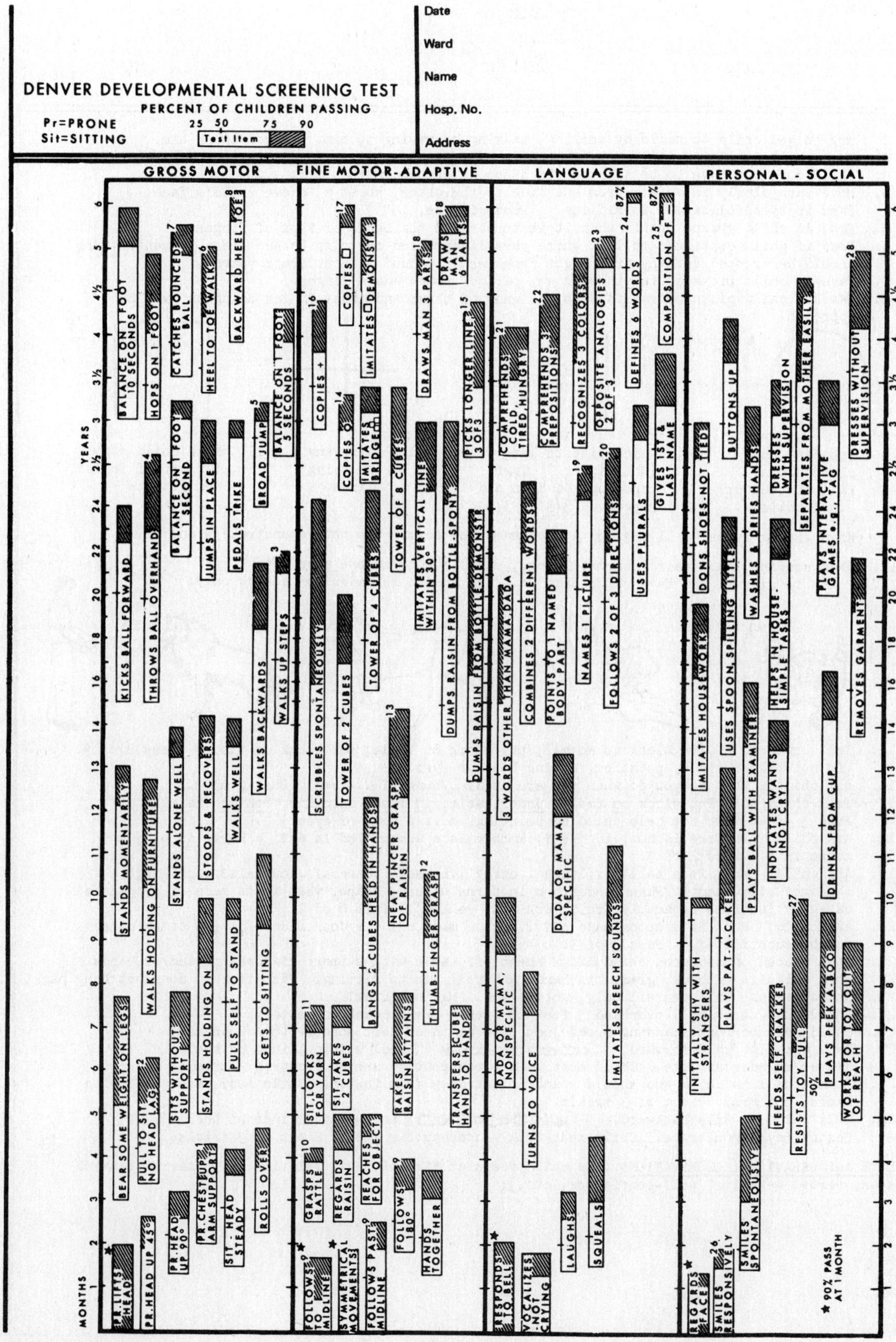

SOURCE: Reprinted with permission of William K. Frankerburg, MD, University of Colorado Medical Center.

APPENDIX D
Resources for Parents

American Foundation of AIDS Research 40 W 57th St New York, NY 10019	AIDS
Asthma and Allergy Foundation of America 1835 K St NW, Suite P-900 Washington, DC 20006	Allergy
Association of Birth Defects in Children 3526 Emerywood Ln Orlando, FL 32806	Birth Defects
March of Dimes Birth Defects Foundation 1275 Mamaroneck Ave White Plains, NY 10605	
American Council of the Blind 1010 Vermont Ave NW, Suite 1100 Washington, DC 20005	Blind
Association of Services for the Blind 919 Walnut Street Philadelphia, PA 19107	
Braille Institute 714 N Vermont Ave Los Angeles, CA 90029	
Cooley's Anemia Foundation 105 E 22nd St, Suite 911 New York, NY 10010	Blood
National Association for Sickle Cell Disease 4221 Wilshire Blvd Los Angeles, CA 90010	
National Hemophilia Foundation 110 Green St, Rm 406 New York, NY 10012	
National Burn Victim Foundation 308 Main St Orange, NJ 07050	Burns
American Cancer Society 90 Park Ave New York, NY 10016	Cancer
Candlelighters Childhood Cancer Foundation 2025 Eye St NW, Suite 1011 Washington, DC 20006	
Leukemia Society of America 733 Third Ave New York, NY 10017	
National Leukemia Association Roosevelt Field, Lower Concourse Garden City, NJ 11530	
United Cerebral Palsy Association 66 E 34th St New York, NY 10016	Cerebral Palsy
National Association for the Craniofacially Handicapped PO Box 11082 Chattanooga, TN 37401	Cleft Lip and Palate
American Association for Deaf Children 814 Thayer Ave Silver Springs, MD 20910	Deaf
Alexander Graham Bell Association for the Deaf 3417 Volta P1 NW Washington, DC 20007	
National Psoriasis Foundation 6443 SW Beaverton Highway, Suite 210 Portland, OR 97221	Dermatology
American Diabetes Association National Service Center PO Box 25757 1660 Duke St Alexandria, VA 22313	Diabetes

Juvenile Diabetes Foundation International
60 Madison Ave
New York, NY 10010

American Anorexia/Bulimia Association — Eating Disorders
133 Cedar Ln
Teaneck, NJ 07666

National Association for Anorexia Nervosa and Associated Disorders
Box 217
Highland Park, IL 60035

National Alliance for the Mentally Ill — Emotional Disorders
1901 N Fort Meyer Dr, Suite 500
Arlington, VA 22209

National Foundation for Ileitis and Colitis — Gastrointestinal Diseases
444 Park Ave S
New York, NY 10016

United Ostomy Association
2001 W Beverly Blvd
Los Angeles, CA 90057

American Heart Association — Heart
7320 Greenville Ave
Dallas, TX 75231

Arthritis Foundation — Immune
1314 Spring St NW
Atlanta, GA 30309

Lupus Foundation of America
11921 A Olive Blvd
St. Louis, MO 63141

National Kidney Foundation — Kidney
2 Park Ave
New York, NY 10016

American Liver Foundation — Liver
998 Pomton Ave
Cedar Grove, NJ 07009

Children's Liver Foundation
7 Highland Pl
Maplewood, NJ 07040

Mental Retardation Association of America — Mental Retardation
211 E 300 South St, Suite 212
Salt Lake City, UT 84111

Muscular Dystrophy Association — Muscular Dystrophy
810 Seventh Ave
New York, NY 10019

National Hydrocephalus Foundation — Neurologic
Rte 1 Box 210 A
River Road
Joliet, IL 60436

National Head Injury Foundation
PO Box 567
Framingham, MA 01701

National Reye's Syndrome Foundation
426 Lewis St
Bryan, OH 43506

Spina Bifida Association of America
3435 Dearborn Ave, Suite 317
Chicago, IL 60604

National Tay-Sachs and Allied Diseases Association
92 Washington Ave
Cedarhurst, NY 11516

Scoliosis Association — Orthopedic
One Penn Plaza
New York, NY 10119

Osteogenesis Imperfecta Foundation
c/o Rosalind James
PO Box 245
Eastport, NY 11941

PKU Parents — PKU
c/o Dale Hillard
8 Myrtle Ln
San Anselmo, CA 94960

American Lung Association — Respiratory
1740 Broadway
New York, NY 10019

Cystic Fibrosis Foundation
6000 Executive Blvd, Suite 309
Rockville, MD 20852

National Sudden Infant Death Syndrome Foundation — SIDS
2 Metro Plaza, Suite 205
8240 Professional Place
Landover, MD 20785

Children's Transplant Association — Transplantation
PO Box 270192
Dallas, TX 75227

APPENDIX E
Admission Assessment—Nursing

A

ADMISSION ASSESSMENT – NURSING

DATE	AGE	SEX
MARITAL STATUS	LANGUAGE SPOKEN AT HOME	

FROM WHOM WAS THIS HISTORY OBTAINED

☐ Patient ☐ Parent(s) ☐ Spouse ☐ Other ______

☐ Legal Guardian/Custody (Name) ______

PREFERRED NAME

ATTENDED CHMC PRE-ADMISSION PROGRAM ☐ Yes ☐ No

REASON FOR ADMISSION

WHERE DO YOU RECEIVE MEDICAL CARE

AGENCIES INVOLVED IN CARE	CONTACT PERSON	TELEPHONE NO.

HT. ______ WT. ______ TEMP. ______ PULSE ______ RESP. ______ B/P ______

RECENT/CURRENT MEDICATIONS ☐ Yes ☐ No (If Yes, give name of medication, frequency taken, who administers medication)

ALLERGIES ☐ Yes ☐ No (Drugs, Food, Environment)

HELPING PATIENT/FAMILY COPE WITH HOSPITALIZATION

PATTERNS OF COPING (Ability to verbalize, comfort measures, identified fears, special needs, words, security objects)

RELIGIOUS OR CULTURAL NEEDS THAT WILL REQUIRE SPECIAL ATTENTION DURING HOSPITALIZATION

EXPRESSED NEED FOR FINANCIAL OR OTHER RESOURCES DURING HOSPITALIZATION

PLANS FOR FAMILY PARTICIPATION IN CARE

03581 5M (Rev. 10/80)

HEALTH CONCERNS/PROBLEMS

REVIEW OF SYSTEMS (Information obtained through interview with patient and/or family)

ASSESSMENT OF PHYSICAL STATUS

Skin ______ Cardiovascular Status ______

Head/Neck ______ Back/Extremities ______

Eyes/Ears/Nose ______ Abdomen ______

Mouth/Teeth ______ Neurological Status ______

Chest/Respiratory Status ______ Genitals/Perineum ______

Psychiatric/Emotional Status ______

Other information important in planning nursing care ______

SIGNATURES OF NURSES COMPLETING FORM

1. ______ Date ______ 2. ______ Date ______

FAMILY STAYING ON DIVISION ☐ Yes ☐ No

FAMILY MEMBERS

	NAME	AGE	GENERAL HEALTH
FATHER (or Spouse)			
MOTHER			
SIBLINGS (or Patient's Children)			

SIGNIFICANT OTHERS

PRIMARY CARETAKER

ISSUES RELEVANT TO CARE IN HOSPITAL

ACTIVITIES OF DAILY LIVING (Performed with or without assistance of another person or device – bathing, brushing teeth, feeding, walking, attending school/work, etc.) Explain:

SCHOOL/WORK

Name of School ____ Grade ____

Special Classes/Learning Needs ____

Type of Work ____

HOBBIES/EXERCISE/SPORTS/PLAY

HEALTH MAINTENANCE

DIET ____

☐ Table Food ☐ Baby Food

Favorite Foods ____

Foods Disliked ____

Special Diet – Cultural/Medical ____

Special Feeding Techniques/Problems ____

Drinks from: ☐ Bottle ☐ Special Nurser ☐ Breast Fed ☐ Cup ☐ Tippy Cup

☐ Special Devices ____

SLEEP

Type of Bed ____ Usual Bedtime ____ Usual Rising Time ____ Nap(s) Time ____ How Long ____

Bedwetter ☐ Yes ☐ No Climber ☐ Yes ☐ No

Special Rituals and Sleeping Habits ____

Problems ____

ELIMINATION (Child's usual toileting routines and patterns – techniques or aids used)

☐ Cloth Diapers ☐ Disposable Diapers ☐ Potty Chair ☐ Toilet Trained (☐ Day ☐ Night)

What terminology is used by child to communicate his/her needs ____

Problems ____

OTHER FACTORS THAT MAY AFFECT HEALTH (Tobacco, Alcohol, Drugs, Sexuality – complete this section only if relevant to care)

GROWTH AND DEVELOPMENT (Note milestones and concerns related to gross motor, fine motor, speech/language development and socialization – record when patient sat, walked, spoke first words)

ROUTINE HEALTH SCREENING (Special needs for infection control)

Recent exposure to communicable diseases ☐ Yes ☐ No

Date ____ Describe ____

Congenital Rubella ☐ Yes ☐ No Hepatitis ☐ Yes ☐ No

Cytomegalic Inclusion Virus ☐ Yes ☐ No Other (e.g., parasites) ☐ Yes (describe) ____ ☐ No

Known Antibiotic Resistance ____

Has had Chicken Pox ☐ Yes ☐ No

IMMUNIZATIONS							TUBERCULIN TESTS	
	INITIAL DATE			BOOSTER DATE				
TYPE	1st	2nd	3rd	1st	2nd	3rd	DATE	RESULTS
DPT								
POLIO								
MMR								

SOURCE: The Children's Hospital Medical Center, Boston, Massachusetts 02115 © 1980.

Index